THERAPY OF
Digestive
Disorders

Dedication

This book is dedicated to all my colleagues and students for providing friendship and purpose, and to my entire family, and especially my children, Jessica, Matthew, and Aliza, for their inspiration, love, understanding, encouragement, unremitting sacrifice, and support, as well as the challenges they continuously provide.

Commissioning Editor: *Karen Bowler*
Project Development Manager: *Shuet-Kei Cheung*
Editorial Assistant: *Katie McCormack*
Project Manager: *Rory MacDonald*
Cover Designer: *Jayne Jones*
Text Designer: *Stewart Larking*
Illustration Manager: *Mick Ruddy*
Illustrator: *Antbits & Tim Loughhead*
Marketing Manager (UK/USA): *Amy Hey & Laura Meiskey*

SECOND EDITION

THERAPY OF
Digestive
Disorders

*GASTRO UNIT
BVH BLACKPOOL*

M. Michael Wolfe MD
Professor of Medicine and Chief,
Section of Gastroenterology
Boston University School of Medicine
Boston, MA, USA

Gary L. Davis MD
Director
Division of Hepatology
Baylor University Medical Center
Dallas, TX, USA

Francis A. Farraye MD MSc
Associate Professor of Medicine and
Clinical Director
Section of Gastroenterology
Boston University School of Medicine
Boston, MA, USA

Ralph A. Giannella MD
Mark Brown Professor of Medicine
Division of Digestive Diseases
University of Cincinnati College of Medicine
Cincinnati, OH, USA

Juan-R. Malagelada MD
Professor Digestive Diseases
Digestive Diseases Department
Hospital Universitari Vall d'Hebron
Barcelona, Spain

Michael L. Steer MD
Professor of Surgery, Chief of General
Surgery
Tufts University School of Medicine
Tufts-New England Medical Center
Boston, MA, USA

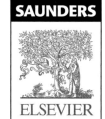

SAUNDERS

ELSEVIER

SAUNDERS
ELSEVIER

An imprint of Elsevier Inc

© 2000, WB Saunders Company.
© 2006, Elsevier Inc. All rights reserved

First edition 2000
Second edition 2006

ISBN 1-4160-0317-7

This book is also available as a package of book and PDA software:
ISBN 1-4160-0318-5

A PDA software version of this book is also available:
ISBN 1-4160-0319-3

British Library Cataloguing in Publication Data
A catalogue record for this book is available from the British Library

Library of Congress Cataloging in Publication Data
A catalog record for this book is available from the Library of Congress

Notice
Medical knowledge is constantly changing. Standard safety precautions must be followed, but as new research and clinical experience broaden our knowledge, changes in treatment and drug therapy may become necessary or appropriate. Readers are advised to check the most current product information provided by the manufacturer of each drug to be administered to verify the recommended dose, the method and duration of administration, and contraindications. It is the responsibility of the practitioner, relying on experience and knowledge of the patient, to determine dosages and the best treatment for each individual patient. Neither the Publisher nor the author assume any liability for any injury and/or damage to persons or property arising from this publication.
The Publisher

Printed in China
Last digit is the print number: 9 8 7 6 5 4 3 2 1

Contents

Contributors

Aijaz Ahmed MD
Gastroenterology Fellow
Hepatology
Stanford University Medical Center
Palo Alto, CA, USA

Vicente Arroyo Perez MD
Professor of Medicine, Director Institute for
Digestive Diseases
Hospital Clinic i Provincial de Barcelona
Universitat de Barcelona
Barcelona, Spain

Bruce R. Bacon MD
James F. King MD Endowed Chair in
Gastroenterology
Director, Division of Gastroenterology and
Hepatology
Saint Louis University School of Medicine
St. Louis, MO, USA

William F. Balistreri MD
Director, Division of Gastroenterology,
Hepatology & Nutrition
Dorothy M.M. Kersten Professor of Pediatrics
Cincinnati Children's Hospital Medical Center
Cincinatti, OH, USA

Carl L. Berg MD
Director of Hepatology
Medical Director, Liver Transplantation
Associate Professor of Medicine
Digestive Health Center of Excellence
University of Virginia Health System
Charlottesville, VA, USA

Adil E. Bharucha MD MBBS
Associate Professor of Medicine
Consultant Division of Gastroenterology &
Hepatology
Mayo Clinic Rochester
Rochester, MN, USA

Cheryl Blank DO
Fellow
Division of Pediatric Gastroenterology
Children's Hospital of Pittsburgh
Pittsburgh, PA, USA

Henry Worth Boyce MD
Professor and Director
Joy McCann Culverhouse Center for Swallowing
Disorder
University of South Florida College of Medicine
Tampa, FL, USA

Lawrence J. Brandt MD
Chief of Gastroenterology
GI Division
Montefiore Medical Center
Bronx, NY, USA

Markus W. Büchler MD
Professor of Surgery
Department of Surgery
University of Heidelberg
Heidelberg, Germany

Theresa A Byrne PhD
Director of Research and Clinical Studies
Nutritional Restart Center
Hopkington, MA, USA

James H. Caldwell MD
Professor, Internal Medicine (Digestive Diseases)
Division of Digestive Disease
The Ohio State University Hospital
Columbus, OH, USA

Michael Camilleri MD MRCP FACP FRCP FACG
Atherton and Winifred W. Bean Professor,
Professor of Medicine
Mayo Clinic College of Medicine
Rochester, MN, USA

Andrés Cárdenas MD MMSc
Instructor in Medicine
Harvard Medical School
Beth Israel Deaconess Medical Center
Boston, MA, USA

Shivakumar Chitturi MD MRCP(UK)
Consultant Hepatologist
Department of Gastroenterology
Apollo Hospitals
Chennai, India

Umesh Choudhry MD
Professor of Gastroenterology
Mease Hospitals
Clearwater, FL, USA

M. T. Clandinin PLQ
Professor of Agriculture, Food & Nutritional
Sciences
University of Alberta
Edmonton, AB, Canada

Ray E. Clouse MD
Professor of Medicine and Psychiatry
Division of Gastroenterology
Washington University
St Louis, MO, USA

Jonathan F. Critchlow MD FACS
Department of Anesthesia & Critical Care
Beth Israel Deaconess Medical Centre
Boston, MA, USA

Srinivasan Dasarathy MD
Assistant Professor of Medicine
Case Western Reserve University
Metro Health Medical Center
Cleveland, OH, USA

Bradley R. Davis MD
Associate Professor of Surgery
Division of Colon and Rectal Surgery
University of Cincinnati
Cincinnati, OH, USA

Gary L. Davis MD
Director
Division of Hepatology
Baylor University Medical Center
Dallas, TX, USA

John Del Valle MD
Professor of Medicine
Department of Internal Medicine
University of Michigan
Ann Arbor, MI, USA

Carlo Di Lorenzo MD
Chief, Division of Pediatric Gastroenterology
Division of Pediatric Gastroenterology
Columbus Children's Hospital
Columbus, OH, USA

Ram Dickman MD
Research Fellow
GI Section
Southern Arizona VA Health Care System
Tucson, AZ, USA

Eric J. Dozois MD
Assistant Professor
Division of Colon and Rectal Surgery
Mayo Clinic College of Medicine
Rochester, MN, USA

Andrew W. DuPont MD
Assistant Professor
Division of Gastroenterology
University of Texas Medical Branch
Galveston, TX, USA

Hashem B. El-Serag MD MPH
Chief, Clinical Epidemiology and Outcomes,
Gastroenterology
Associate Professor of Medicine
Baylor College of Medicine
Houston, TX, USA

Francis A. Farraye MD MSc
Associate Professor of Medicine and Clinical
Director
Section of Gastroenterology
Boston University School of Medicine
Boston, MA, USA

Geoffrey C. Farrell MD FRACP
Department of Gastroenterology & Hepatology
Westmead Hospital
New South Wales, Australia

Ronnie Fass MD FACP FACG
Associate Professor of Medicine
GI Section
Southern Arizona VA Health Care System
Tucson, AZ, USA

David M. Felig MD
Attending Physician
Division of Gastroenterology
Hackensack University Medical Center
Hackensack, NJ, USA

Stephen J. Ferzoco MD
Assistant Professor of Surgery
Department of Surgery
Brigham and Women's Hospital
Boston, MA, USA

Henry S. Fraimow MD
Associate Professor of Medicine
Division of Infectious Diseases
Cooper University Hospital
Camden, NJ, USA

Ronald Fried MD
Consultant for Gastroenterology and Hepatology
Gastroenterology and Hepatology
Merian-Iselin Spital
Basel, Switzerland

Sonia Friedman MD
Instructor of Medicine, Harvard Medical School
Gastroenterology Division
Brigham and Women's Hospital
Boston, MA, USA

Helmut M. Friess MD
Professor of Surgery
Department of Surgery
University of Heidelberg
Heidelberg, Germany

Daniel Gelrud MD
Assistant Professor of Medicine
Department of Gastroenterology
Jacobi Medical Center
Bronx, NY, USA

Ralph A. Giannella MD
Mark Brown Professor of Medicine
Division of Digestive Diseases
University of Cincinnati College of Medicine
Cincinnati, OH, USA

Pere Ginés Gibert MD
Associate Professor of Medicine, Chief of Liver Unit
Hospital Clinic i Provincial de Barcelona
Universitat de Barcelona
Barcelona, Spain

Stuart L.Goldberg MD
Chief, Leukemia Service
Clinical Associate Professor of Medicine
Hackensack University Medical Center
University of Medicine and Dentistry of New Jersey
Hackensack, NJ, USA

Richard C. Golding MD
Senior Attending Physician
Division of Gastroenterology
Hackensack University Medical Center
Hackensack, NJ, USA

Gregory J. Gores MD
Professor of Medicine and Chief
Division of Gastroenterology and Hepatology
Mayo Clinic College of Medicine
Rochester, MN, USA

Annette Grambihler MD
Division of Gastroenterology and Hepatology
Mayo Clinic College of Medicine
Rochester, MN, USA

Norton J. Greenberger MD
Clinical Professor of Medicine, Harvard Medical
School
Senior Physician, Brigham and Women's Hospital,
Division of Gastroenterology
Brigham and Women's Hospital
Boston, MA, USA

David Greenwald MD
Associate Professor of Medicine
Albert Einstein College of Medicine
Associate Director, Division of Gastroenterology
Montefiore Medical Center
Bronx, NY, USA

Francisco Guarner MD PhD
Consultant of Gastroenterology
Digestive System Research Unit
Hospital Universitari Vall d'Hebron
Barcelona, Spain

J. Eileen Hay MBChB FRCP
Professor of Medicine and Consultant
Division of Gastroenterology and Hepatology
Mayo Clinic College of Medicine
Rochester, MN, USA

Ikuo Hirano MD
Associate Professor of Medicine
Gastroenterology Fellowship Training Director
Division of Gastroenterology
Northwestern University School of Medicine
Chicago, IL, USA

Richard Hodin MD
Associate Professor of Surgery
Department of Surgery
Massachusetts General Hospital
Boston, MA, USA

Christopher S. Huang MD
Instructor
Gastro Medicine
Boston University Medical Center
Boston, MA, USA

Richard H. Hunt FRCP FRCPC FACG
Professor of Medicine
Division of Gastroenterology, Department of
Medicine
McMaster University Medical Centre
Hamilton, Ontario, Canada

Brian C. Jacobson MD MD MPH
Associate Director of Endoscopy
Boston University Medical Center
Boston, MA, USA

Maureen M. Jonas MD
Professor and Chairman of Internal Medicine
Division of Gastroenterology
The Children's Hospital
Boston, MA, USA

Emmet B. Keeffe MD
Professor of Medicine, Chief of Hepatology,
Co-Director,
Stanford University Medical Center
Palo Alto, CA, USA

Ciarán P. Kelly MD FRCPI FRCG
Associate Professor of Medicine
Department of Gastroenterology
Beth Israel Deaconess Medical Center
Boston, MA, USA

Robert S. Klein MD
Professor of Medicine, and Epidemiology &
Population Health
Department of Medicine
Division of Infectious Diseases
Montefiore Medical Center
Bronx, NY, USA

Samuel Klein MD
Professor of Medicine & Nutritional Science
Division of Gastroenterology
Washington University School of Medicine
St Louis, MO, USA

Kenneth L. Koch MD
Professor of Medicine, Section Head
Section on Gastroenterology
Wake Forest University School of Medicine
Winston-Salem, NC, USA

Patricia L. Kozuch MD
Instructor of Medicine
Department of Medicine
The University of Chicago
Division of Biological Sciences
Chicago, IL, USA

Edward L. Krawitt MD
Professor of Medicine
Department of Medicine
University of Vermont
Burlington, VT, USA

J. Thomas LaMont MD
Charlotte F. & Irving W. Rabb Professor of
Medicine, Ha
Chief, Division of Gastroenterology
Beth Israel Deaconess Medical Center
Boston, MA, USA

Nicholas F. LaRusso MD
Professor and Chairman of Internal Medicine
Division of Gastroenterology and Hepatology
Mayo Clinic College of Medicine
Rochester, MN, USA

James Y. W. Lau MD
Consultant, Division of Upper
Gastrointestinal Surgery
Department of Surgery
Prince of Wales Hospital
Hong Kong, China

Konstantinos N. Lazaridis MD
Assistant Professor of Medicine
Center for Basic Research in Digestive Diseases
Division of Gastroenterology and Hepatology
Mayo Clinic College of Medicine
Rochester, MN, USA

Mike A. Leonis MD PhD
Research Instructor in Pediatrics, William E.
Cooper Procter Scholar
Division of Gastroenterology, Hepatology and
Nutrition
Department of Pediatrics
Cincinatti, OH, USA

Markus M. Lerch MD
Professor of Medicine and Chair
Department of Gastroenterology, Endocrinology
and Nutrition
Ernst-Moritz-Arndt Universität Greifswald
Greifswald, Germany

Wai K. Leung MD
Associate Professor
Department of Medicine & Therapeutics
The Chinese University of Hong Kong
Shatin
Hong Kong, China

David R. Lichtenstein MD
Associate Professor of Medicine
Director of Endoscopy
Section of Gastroenterology
Boston University School of Medicine
Boston, MA, USA

Gary R Lichtenstein MD
Professor of Medicine, University of Pennsylvania
School
Director, Center for Inflammatory Bowel Diseases
Hospital of the University of Pennsylvania
Gastroenterology Division
Philadelphia, PA, USA

Keith D. Lindor MD
Professor of Medicine and Dean
Mayo Medical School
Division of Gastroenterology and Hepatology
Rochester, MN, USA

Robert M. Lowe MD
Educational Director of Gastroenterology
Assistant Professor of Medicine
Gastroenterology
Boston Medical Center
Boston, MA, USA

Lars Lundell MD PhD
Professor of Surgery
Department of Surgery
Sahlgrens Hospital
Gothenburg, Sweden

Juan-R. Malagelada MD
Professor Digestive Diseases
Digestive Diseases Department
Hospital Universitari Vall d'Hebron
Barcelona, Spain

Paul Martin MD
Professor of Medicine, Associate Director of the
Division
Recanati / Miller Transplantation Institute
The Mount Sinai Hospital
New York, NY, USA

Jeffrey B. Matthews MD
Christian R Holmes Professor and Chairman
Department of Surgery
University of Cincinnati
Cincinnati, OH, USA

Julia Mayerle MD
Lecturer
Department of Gastroenterology, Endocrinology
and Nutrition
Ernst-Moritz-Arndt Universität Greifswald
Greifswald, Germany

Arthur J. McCullough MD
Director of Gastroenterology
Department of Medicine
MetroHealth Medical Center
Cleveland, OH, USA

James E. McGuigan MD
Professor of Medicine
Division of Gastroenterology, Hepatology and
Nutrition
University of Florida College of Medicine
Gainesville, FL, USA

Peter J. Milla MD
Reader in Paediatric Gastroenterology
Gastroenterology Unit
Institute of Child Health
London, UK

Daniel S. Mishkin MD CM
Instructor of Medicine
Section of Gastroenterology
Boston University Medical Center
Boston, MA, USA

Kevin D. Mullen MB FRCPI
Professor of Medicine
Case Western Reserve University
and Consultant of Gastroenterology
GI Division
Metro Health Medical Center
Cleveland, OH, USA

David R. Nelson MD
Associate Professor
Chief, Section of Hepatobiliary Diseases
Director, Adult Liver Transplant Program
Dept of Gastroenterology, Hepatology and
Nutrition
University of Florida
Gainesville, FL, USA

Enders K.W. Ng MD FRCS
Assistant Dean (Clinical), Faculty of Medicine
Professor and Chief, Upper Gastrointestinal Surgery
Department of Surgery
The Chinese University of Hong Kong
Shatin
Hong Kong, China

David P. Nunes MB
Director of Hepatology
Boston University School of Medicine
Boston, MA, USA

Jaime Oviedo MD
Assistant Professor of Medicine
Gastroenterology
Boston Medical Center
Boston, MA, USA

Sareh Parangi MD
Assistant Professor of Surgery
Department of Surgery
Beth Israel-Deaconess Medical Center
Boston, MA, USA

John H. Pemberton MD
Professor of Surgery
Division of Colon and Rectal Surgery
Mayo Clinic
Rochester, MN, USA

David A. Peura MD
Associate Chief of Gastroenterology and
Hepatology
Professor of Medicine
University of Virginia
Charlottesville, VA, USA

Gilda Porta MD
Professor of Pediatrics
University of Sao Paulo
Sao Paulo, Brazil

Charlene M. Prather MD
Associate Professor of Medicine
Saint Louis University School of Medicine
Saint Louis, MO, USA

Sarathchandra I. Reddy MD
Instructor of Medicine, Harvard Medical School
Gastroenterology Division
Brigham and Women's Hospital
Boston, MA, USA

Joachim Richter MD
Assistant Professor of Medicine; Lecturer, Tropical
and In
Tropenmedizinische Ambulanz, Klinik für
Gastroenterologi
Universitätsklinikum Düsseldorf
Düsseldorf, Germany

Malcolm K. Robinson MD
Director, Metabolic Support Services
Brigham and Women's Hospital
Assistant Professor of Surgery
Harvard Medical School
Department of Surgery
Brigham and Women's Hospital
Boston, MA, USA

Juan Rodés MD
Professor of Medicine
Hospital Clinic
University of Barcelona
Barcelona, Spain

Janice G. Rothschild MD, FACS
Assistant Professor of Surgery
Department of Surgery
Tufts-New England Medical Center
Boston, MA, USA

Richard I. Rothstein MD
Professor of Medicine
Assistant Dean Cont. Education
Chief, Section of Gastroenterology
Dartmouth-Hitchcock Medical Center
Lebanon, NH, USA

Deborah C. Rubin MD
Professor of Medicine
Department of Medicine
Director, DDRCC Morphology Core Facility
Washington State University School of Medicine
St Louis, MO, USA

Sherif Saadeh MD
Staff Gastroenterologist & Transplant Hepatologist
Division of Hepatology
Department of Internal Medicine
Baylor University Medical Center
Dallas, TX, USA

Arun J. Sanyal MBBS MD
Charles Caravati Professor of Medicine
Chairman, Division of Gastroenterology and
Hepatology
Medical College of Virginia
Richmond, VA, USA

Miguel Saps MD
Division of Pediatric Gastroenterology
Children's Memorial Hospital of Chicago
Chicago, IL, USA

Lawrence J. Sauberman MD
Assistant Professor of Medicine
Gastroenterology Division
Brigham and Women's Hospital
Boston, MA, USA

Robert E. Schoen MD MPH
Professor of Medicine and Epidemiology
Division of Gastroenterology, Hepatology and
Nutrition
Pittsburgh, PA, USA

Paul C. Schroy III MD MPH
Professor of Medicine
Boston University School of Medicine
Section of Gastroenterology
Boston Medical Center
Boston, MA, USA

Douglas Simon MD FACG
Professor of Clinical Medicine
Department of Medicine
Jacobi Medical Center
Bronx, NY, USA

Adam Slivka MD PhD
Associate Professor of Medicine &
Associate Chief of Gastroenterology, Hepatology
& Nutrition
UPMC Gastroenterology
University of Pittsburgh Medical Center
Pittsburgh, PA, USA

Consuelo Soldevila-Pico MD
Associate Professor of Medicine
Department of Medicine
University of Florida
Gainesville, FL, USA

David I. Soybel MD
Associate Professor of Surgery
Division of General and GI Surgery
Brigham and Women's Hospital
Boston, MA, USA

Stuart Jon Spechler MD
Professor of Medicine
University of Texas Southwestern Medical Center
Chief, Division of Gastroenterology
Dallas VA Medical Center
Dallas, TX, USA

Michael L. Steer MD
Professor of Surgery, Chief of General Surgery
Tufts University School of Medicine
Tufts-New England Medical Center
Boston, MA, USA

**Joseph J.Y. Sung MD PhD FRCP FRCPE
FRACP FACP FHKAM FHKCP**
Professor of Medicine
Chairman Department of Medicine and
Therapeutics
Director, Center for Emerging Infectious Diseases
New Territories
Hong Kong SAR

Christina M. Surawicz MD
Professor of Medicine
Harborview Medical Center
University of Washington
Seattle, WA, USA

Jan Tack MD PhD
Professor of Medicine
Head of Clinic, Department of Gastroenterology
University Hospitals Leuven
Leuven, Belgium

Jayant A. Talwalkar MD MPH
Assistant Professor of Medicine
Mayo Clinic College of Medicine
Rochester, MN, USA

Beth E. Taylor MS RD CNSD FCCM
Nutrition Support Specialist
Department of Food and Nutrition
Barnes-Jewish Hospital Plaza
St Louis, MO, USA

A. B. R. Thomson MD FRCPC
Professor or Medicine
Department of Medicine
University of Alberta
Edmonton, AB, Canada

Tram T. Tran MD
Medical Director, Liver Transplant, Cedar Sinai
Medical
Assistant Professor of Medicine
Geffen UCLA School of Medicine
Los Angeles, CA, USA

Jacques Van Dam MD PhD
Professor and Chief of Clinical Gastroenterology
Division of Gastroenterology and Hepatology
Stanford University Medical Center
Palo Alto, CA, USA

C. Mel Wilcox MD
Division of Gastroenterology and Hepatology
University of Alabama
Birmingham, AL, USA

G. E. Wild MD PLQ
Professor of Medicine
University of Alberta
Edmonton, AB, Canada

Douglas W. Wilmore MD
Professor of Surgery
Harvard Medical School
Department of Surgery
Brigham and Women's Hospital
Boston, MA, USA

Jacqueline L. Wolf MD
Associate Professor of Medicine
Division of Gastroenterology
Beth Israel Deaconess Medical Center
Boston, MA, USA

M. Michael Wolfe MD
Professor of Medicine and Chief,
Section of Gastroenterology
Boston University School of Medicine
Boston, MA, USA

Yuhong Yuan MD MSc PhD
Research Associate
Division of Gastroenterology, Department of
Medicine
McMaster University Medical Centre
Hamilton, Ontario, Canada

Preface to the second edition

During the past three decades, gastroenterologists and other healthcare workers engaged in the management of patients with digestive disorders have been witness to remarkable improvements in the understanding of the biology of these commonly encountered problems. Moreover, advancements in the elucidation of the pathogenesis of various digestive disorders and the exponential increase in therapeutic modalities for the treatment of these diseases have been unsurpassed during this same period of time. The universal availability of fiberoptic, and more recently video and wireless capsule, endoscopy and the widespread employment of minimally invasive surgery, have facilitated the ability of gastroenterologists and gastrointestinal surgeons to investigate and provide therapy for the multitude of persons suffering from the vast array of digestive disorders. This spectacular progress has enabled practitioners to extend the technological advances and improvements in pharmacological treatment to the masses, and in doing so, have diminished morbidity, improved survival, and enhanced the quality of life for the hundreds of millions of individuals afflicted with these diseases.

One prominent example of our remarkable progress during this period of time is the management of gastroesophageal reflux disease (GERD). Beginning in the mid-1970s with the availability of the histamine H2-receptor antagonists and, more recently, the proton pump inhibitors, as well as surgical and endoscopic approaches to the disorder, the treatment of GERD has been revolutionized. A myriad of individuals, who previously received generally inadequate therapy, have benefited significantly by these remarkably effective and safe agents. The significance of gastrointestinal drug development is further evident by the bestowing of two Nobel Prizes in Medicine and Physiology for biomedical research that led to the development of two prominent classes of drugs that affect gastrointestinal function: the histamine H2-receptor antagonists and prostaglandins. Furthermore, the past decade has witnessed the development of a myriad of new classes of medication, including specific immunomodulators and other drugs used for the therapy of inflammatory bowel diseases, antiviral agents for the treatment of viral hepatitides, and neuromodulators for the management of irritable bowel syndrome and other motility disorders of the gastrointestinal tract.

Along with these important advances comes the requisite requirement for practitioners to remain informed, a task generally accomplished by the availability of contemporary textbooks and other literature relevant to their interests and needs. Beginning with its inception and formulation and during the preparation of the second edition of this textbook, *Therapy of Digestive Disorders* was formulated to provide practitioners with an authoritative and evidence-based, yet practical, approach to the optimal management of individuals afflicted with specific digestive disorders. The text of each chapter focuses on diagnosis and treatment, with less emphasis placed on epidemiology and pathogenesis. Nevertheless, all treatment recommendations are based on the biology and pathophysiology of the specific disease entities. In addition to providing updates and expanding the topics included in the first edition, several new chapters and sections and new features have been included in the second edition of this textbook. They include:

(1) A chapter devoted in its entirety to the use of probiotics in the management of gastrointestinal disorders;

(2) A section on the treatment of the ever-increasing problem of nonalcoholic fatty liver disease;

(3) A chapter devoted to the management of gastrointestinal diseases in the elderly;

(4) A chapter that focuses on the management of gastrointestinal diseases in children;

(5) A chapter that considers the special and specific issues encountered during the management of pregnant women with acute and chronic digestive and hepatic disorders;

(6) Owing to the significant recent advances in our understanding of their pathogenesis, as well as marked improvements in the therapy of inflammatory bowel diseases, separate chapters on the management of Crohn's disease and ulcerative colitis;

(7) All chapters now include succinct summaries with specific treatment recommendations;

(8) Annotated references to help guide readers to the review of specific topics;

(9) A PDA version of each chapter for rapid, bedside use.

The full spectrum, from preventive measures to the therapy of complex and advanced disease states, is covered in depth, with the liberal use of tables and treatment algorithms to help guide clinicians. My distinguished colleagues and Section Editors – Doctors Gary L. Davis, Francis A. Farraye, Ralph A. Giannella, Juan-R. Malagelada, and Michael L. Steer – and all the outstanding authors have striven to emphasize, extend, and amplify specific treatment topics and have provided contemporary citations, several of which have been annotated, to further guide the examination of specific topics. In addition to their respective roles as objective authorities, the contributors have interjected their own personal expert opinion regarding the appropriate selection of management, including the proper dosing and administration of specific medication and the judicious employment of procedure-based diagnostic and therapeutic modalities.

The target audience for this textbook includes gastroenterologists, gastrointestinal surgeons, and all practitioners who care for individuals afflicted with digestive disorders. The contributors have used utmost care and discrimination in presenting their materials, and the subject matter has been composed in a concise, yet thorough, format. Accordingly, medical students, internal medicine, family medicine, and surgery residents, and gastroenterology fellows will view this text as an invaluable adjunct to their educational needs, and it should be regarded as germane to the practices of primary care and emergency room physicians, intensivists, hospitalists, pharmacists, and other health care professionals involved in the management of diseases of the alimentary tract and hepatobiliary systems.

Therapy of Digestive Disorders is clearly the product of the enormous effort of its superb contributors, some of the most capable persons in the fields of gastroenterology, hepatology, gastrointestinal surgery, and other medical disciplines, defined in advance by their willingness to respond to the compelling need to share their knowledge and produce quality chapters despite their other endless commitments. These authors were selected primarily for their record of excellence as investigators, clinicians, and educators. All are engaged in clinical or basic investigation and are particularly proficient in the application of basic scientific information to the realm of patient management. The Section Editors and I believe that the second edition of *Therapy of Digestive Disorders* has been built upon the high standards set forth in the initial text, and that the ultimate recipient of its excellence will be the patients with digestive disorders, whose care will optimized by the improved proficiency of their physicians.

M. Michael Wolfe, M.D.

Preface to first edition

The logarithmic increase in medical and technological advances used in the management of individuals with digestive disorders during the past two decades is unparalleled. The universal availability of fiberoptic instruments, and later video, endoscopic, and surgical instruments, has facilitated the ability of gastroenterologists and gastrointestinal surgeons to investigate and provide therapy for the multitude of individuals suffering from the vast array of digestive disorders. These spectacular technological advances have enabled practitioners to extend the use of noninvasive and minimally invasive methods to the masses, thereby producing diminished morbidity, improved survival, and probably most important, enhanced quality of life. Equally important to these remarkable achievements, however, was the development of a myriad of new classes of medication for the treatment of these diseases. Since the mid-1970s, with the introduction of H_2 receptor antagonists, we have experienced a virtual explosion of new drugs that have revolutionized medical therapy for gastrointestinal illnesses. Since 1978, the leading individual drug used throughout the world has been one used to treat digestive disorders. The significance of their importance is further evident by the bestowing of two Nobel Prizes in Medicine and Physiology for biomedical research that led to the development of two prominent classes of drugs that affect gastrointestinal function: H_2 antagonists and prostaglandins.

Beginning with its inception and formulation and during the writing of this companion book, rather than emphasizing specific classes of medication, endoscopic intervention, or surgical procedures, Therapy of Digestive Disorders was developed to provide practitioners with an authoritative and evidence-based, yet practical, approach to the optimal management of individuals with specific digestive disorders. The full spectrum, from preventive measures to the treatment of complex and advanced disease states, is covered in depth, with liberal use of tables and treatment algorithms to help guide the clinician. Rather than merely reiterate the content of Drs. Mark Feldman, Bruce F. Scharschmidt, and Marvin H. Sleisenger's landmark *Sleisenger and Fordtran's Gastrointestinal and Liver Disease*, the authors here have striven to emphasize, extend, and amplify specific treatment topics and have provided up-to-date references to direct further examination of specific topics. Although the contributors have written their chapters as objective authorities, they have also interjected their expert opinions regarding the appropriate selection of therapeutic options, including the proper dosing and administration of specific medications and the judicious employment of diagnostic and procedure-based therapeutic modalities.

The target audience for this text includes all practitioners who care for individuals with digestive disorders. The contributors have used utmost care and discrimination in presenting their materials, and the subject matter is thus appropriate not only for gastroenterologists and gastrointestinal surgeons, but also for medical and surgical residents, primary care and emergency department physicians, intensivists, and other health care professionals specializing in the management of diseases of the alimentary tract and hepatobiliary organs. The superb group of contributors assembled for this book were selected primarily for their record of excellence as investigators, clinicians, and teachers. All are engaged in clinical or basic investigation and are particularly proficient in the application of basic scientifc information to the realm of patient management. This book is clearly the product of the enormous effort of these individual authors, some of the most capable persons in the fields of gastroenterology, hepatology, and gastrointestinal surgery, defined in advance by their willingness to respond to the compelling need to share their knowledge and produce quality chapters despite their other endless commitments.

M. Michael Wolfe

Acknowledgements

I am most pleased to be afforded the opportunity to acknowledge the many teachers and mentors, all of whom have inspired me immeasurably during my training and career as an academic gastroenterologist. It is particularly gratifying for me to have been able to include my medical school advisor, Professor James H. Caldwell, as a contributor to the second edition of *Therapy of Digestive Disorders*. I also acknowledge the invaluable advice and counseling received over the years from the late Professor Walter Rubin, whose recent untimely death was a tragedy to all who revered him. Among the others who played an invaluable and instrumental role are Professors Donald Kaye, Phillip P. Toskes, James E. McGuigan, Gabriel M. Makhlouf, James W. Freston, William Silen, Eugene Braunwald, William W. Chin, and Joseph Loscalzo. I am deeply indebted to the Section Editors — Gary Davis, Frank Farraye, Ralph Giannella, Juan Malagelada, and Mike Steer — for their diligence and efforts in assembling a distinguished, talented, and exceptional group of authors. As a result of their outstanding contributions, we have succeeded in compiling a contemporary textbook that combines a scholarly review of every individual topic with practical guidelines for the management of the wide array of digestive disorders. The ultimate beneficiaries of their efforts will be the hundreds of millions of patients with gastrointestinal diseases, who will receive the most optimal and contemporary care available.

In addition to the Section Editors and authors, the successful completion of the second edition of *Therapy of Digestive Disorders* would not have been possible without the invaluable support of the group of dedicated professionals and assistants. I would like to express my sincere appreciation to Carolyn Dumas, my assistant in the Section of Gastoenterology at Boston University School of Medicine, and to Erin Medley, who provided technical assistance. A special debt of gratitude goes to Linda Neville, Administrator in the Section of Gastroenterology, who helped maintain the excellence of the daily operations of the GI Section when my attention was diverted by the formidable challenges faced during the preparation of a textbook of this magnitude. I thank Joanne Scott, Henrietta Preston, and especially Shuet-Kei Cheung, Project Managers at Elsevier, who approached the formidable task of serving as liaison between the chapter authors, Section Editors, and Elsevier with enthusiasm and zeal, and who made my tasks tolerable by streamlining all the various protocols and processes involved with editing the textbook. In addition to the Project Managers, this project would not have been possible without the support of Sue Hodgson, Publisher at Elsevier, and Karen Bowler, Senior Acquisitions Editor. Finally, a special debt of gratitude goes to Rolla Couchman, Senior Acquisitions Editor at Elsevier, who served as a friend and as an earnest and enthusiastic professional throughout the course of this textbook's inception, planning, organization, and composition.

Finally, I wish to express my personal appreciation to my fellows and colleagues within the Section of Gastroenterology and in the Department of Medicine for their collegiality and friendship. I have been blessed to have the opportunity to work with an unparalleled group of dedicated and accomplished physicians and scientists, who have devoted their careers and lives to research, education, and patient care and for maintaining an environment conducive to creativity and scholarship. I offer my extreme gratitude to my research collaborators and to the devoted members of my laboratory, Mike Boylan, Lisa Jepeal, Diane Song, Carlton Moore, Min Yao, Wei Zhou, Albert Chang, Jon Simon, Tom Liu, and Cherrell Wilson. Their diligent and resolute efforts have consistently produced research of the highest quality that have culminated in publications in most prestigious scientific journals. Lastly, I thank my father, my late mother, sister, brother, wife, and children for their endless patience, encouragement, support, and understanding throughout not only the preparation of this textbook, but during my education and career.

M. Michael Wolfe

Section One

Modes of therapy

CHAPTER ONE

1

Molecular and cellular targets in therapy of acid-related diseases

James E. McGuigan

INTRODUCTION

History

From early recorded antiquity, acid has been thought to be present in the human stomach. Greek scholars more than 2300 years ago remarked on epigastric pain, heartburn, and sour eruptions as potentially caused by problems with the stomach. Celsus, 3 centuries later, concluded that some foods were acidic and recommended that 'if the stomach is infested with an ulcer...acid is to be avoided.' Proof that hydrochloric acid was the acidic material in the stomach awaited the scientific documentation of William Prout in his elegant presentation before the Royal Society in London in 1823 and published the following year entitled 'On the Nature of Acid and Saline Matters Usually Existing in the Stomach of Animals.'[1] Hippocrates was reported to have introduced the term 'pepsis' to describe the process of digestion, far in advance of the much later applications of derivatives of the term to appreciation of the intimate interrelationships of pepsin with gastric acid and to acid-related diseases.

An assortment of clinical symptoms and disorders have been thought to be associated with hydrochloric acid secretion by the stomach. Recognition of acid-related diseases prompted the application of a variety of lifestyle measures, diets, and pharmacological approaches intended to reduce the potentially harmful effects of hydrochloric acid secreted by the stomach. Lifestyle adjustments appeared to offer some adjunctive value for patients with acid-related disorders, but alone provided limited benefits. Various dietary manipulations, although transiently attracting their proponents, proved to be of little value in management of those patients. Major efforts have been directed to the treatment of acid-related diseases by pharmacological agents directed to neutralize secreted gastric acid or, more recently, to inhibit its secretion. Surgical procedures were also developed to reduce gastric acid secretion, principally by gastric resection and/or by interruption of the vagus nerves, recognizing the integral role of the vagus in stimulation of hydrochloric acid secretion by the stomach. Until the latter part of the twentieth century, pharmacologic treatment of acid-related disorders was of limited effectiveness. Antacid preparations of various composition partially neutralized secreted gastric acid, but because of their relatively short residence in the gastric lumen, they proved to be of no prolonged benefit; if sustained effects were sought, frequent repetitive dosing was required. Anticholinergic agents were found to inhibit gastric acid secretion, but for the most part only marginally and with predictable adverse side effects, which prevented their dosing in sufficiently potent quantities.

The treatment of acid-related diseases was revolutionized by the conception, development, and introduction of H_2-receptor antagonists.[2–6] It had long been appreciated that histamine, present in many tissues and organs, including the stomach, was a potent stimulant of gastric acid secretion. However, its role in regulation of acid secretion by the stomach was controversial. Histamine had been used as a provocative stimulant to assess the capacity of the stomach to secrete acid, an effect that could not be inhibited by traditional histamine receptor (histamine 1 receptor) antagonists. This observation predicted and stimulated the search for a separate class of histamine receptors, which if inhibited specifically, would reduce acid secretion by the stomach. The development of structural analogs of histamine that inhibited gastric acid secretion by competitive inhibition of the receptors in the absence of other antihistaminic effects validated the concept and for which Sir James Black was awarded a Nobel Prize in 1988.[2] Cimetidine, the first of this class of agents (H_2-receptor antagonists) which competitively inhibited these histamine$_2$ receptors was introduced in the United States in 1977 for clinical use in reducing gastric acid secretion.[3]

More potent and more prolonged inhibition of gastric acid secretion was achieved subsequently by development of antagonists of the parietal cell hydrogen potassium ATPase (H+, K+-ATPase), which constitutes the parietal cell's final exchange mechanism for hydrogen and potassium ions, resulting in its secretion of hydrochloric acid. Omeprazole was the first clinically available member of this class of inhibitors of H+, K+-ATPase, now commonly referred to as proton pump inhibitors (PPIs).[7,8] Omeprazole was introduced in the United States in 1989.

This chapter will address the neurohumoral regulation of gastric acid secretion and the pharmacologic agents that are used to inhibit gastric acid secretion in the therapy and prevention of acid-related diseases. It will also describe and discuss the molecular and cellular targets of these acid inhibitory agents, as well the behavior of those cells which predispose their susceptibility to these pharmacologic agents and the regulation of acid secretion by these and other factors.

Acid-related diseases

A variety of diseases and disorders are viewed as acid-related diseases. In each of these conditions hydrochloric acid secreted by the stomach is believed to play a crucial pathogenic role. Although similar in this regard, the various acid-related diseases differ in other important aspects. In some instances, acid-related diseases result as a direct consequence of excessive secretion of gastric hydrochloric acid. In other examples, the diseases are caused by diminished mucosal defense mechanisms, rendering the tissues susceptible to injury by secreted gastric acid, usually in patients with normal or often decreased gastric acid secretion. Finally, some acid-related disorders may result from variably, but often modestly, increased gastric acid secretion coupled with some deficiency of mucosal defense.

The Zollinger-Ellison syndrome (gastrinoma) is certainly the prototypic consequence of pure gastric acid hypersecretion (see Ch. 20). Although gastric acid plays a role, ulcers associated with nonsteroidal antiinflammatory drugs appear to develop principally because of deficient mucosal defense, as does stress-related mucosal ulceration (see Ch. 19). Acid-related diseases include gastric ulcer, associated with normal or reduced gastric acid secretion, and duodenal ulcer, usually with normal or modestly increased gastric acid secretion, and are often accompanied by some reduction of mucosal defense (see Chs 18 and 20). Gastroesophageal reflux disease is also an acid-related disease that results from gastric hydrochloric acid refluxing into the esophagus, which is less well equipped to defend itself from gastric acid than the relatively richly defended normal stomach and most proximal duodenum (see Ch. 13). Supra-esophageal reflux disorders also appear to be produced by gastric acid contact with tissues possessing relatively insufficient mucosal defense mechanisms. The role of gastric acid in the pathogenesis of nonulcer dyspepsia is less clearly defined.[9]

Although most patients with acid-related diseases do not have gastric acid hypersecretion, therapy used in prevention and cure of these diseases is directed principally to reduction of hydrochloric secretion by the stomach and the avoidance of its corrosive effects on the gastrointestinal tract.

CELLULAR TARGETS

Parietal cells

The cells responsible for secretion of hydrochloric acid by the stomach are gastric parietal cells.[10,11] These cells are present in glands, often referred to as parietal cell glands or oxyntic glands, which are located principally in the body and fundus of the stomach. Parietal cells are the most frequent cell type found in oxyntic glands. Parietal cells are located singly or in clusters in the mid and slightly deeper portions of the glands. Parietal cells are surface epithelial cells with their mucosal apical surfaces facing the gland lumen. They have a basolateral membrane, which surrounds the remainder of the cell and includes the serosal surface on which the cell is situated. The basolateral membranes of parietal cells contain prominent tight junctions. Parietal cells have several different classes of receptors on their basolateral cell membranes that participate in the regulation of stimulation and inhibition of gastric acid secretion (Fig. 1.1).[11] Parietal cells are somewhat plump and flask shaped, with wide bases and much thinner conical apices abutting the gland lumen, and are primarily secretory, rather than absorptive, cells. In the resting state and in response to stimulation, the extensive canalicular system of the parietal cell is in continuity with the

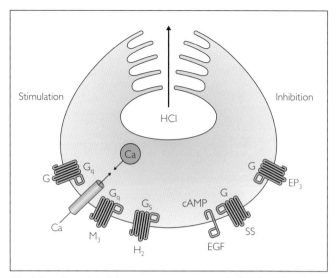

Fig. 1.1 • A model of the receptors present on the basolateral surface of the parietal cell and their intracellular effects. G_q and G_s trimeric G proteins; cAMP, cyclic adenosine monophosphate; G, G protein; M_3, muscarinic receptor; H_2, histamine receptor; EGF, epidermal growth factor; SS, somatostatin; EP_3, subtype of prostaglandin.

gland lumen (Fig. 1.2). The secretory canaliculi are infoldings of the apical membranes of the parietal cells and serve as the channels by which the cells empty their secretory products into the gland lumen. The major secretory products of parietal cells are hydrochloric acid and intrinsic factor, the latter playing an important role in the promotion of active absorption of cyanocobalamin (vitamin B_{12}).

The parietal cell has a prominent nucleus and cytoplasm containing abundant mitochondria. Parietal cells are extremely active metabolically, requiring vigorous mitochondrial synthesis of adenosine triphosphate (ATP), which serves as the source of energy that drives gastric acid secretion. The mitochondria occupy approximately one-third of the cytoplasm of parietal cells. During the resting state, the remainder of parietal cell cytoplasm is filled with an extensive tubulovesicular system, containing numerous membrane-containing tubules.[11,12] Immunolabeling has demonstrated the presence of the H+, K+-ATPase (proton pump) on the tubules of the tubulovesicular system.[12] In the resting (unstimulated) parietal cell, the secretory canaliculi have short and stubby microvilli (see Fig. 1.2). After stimulation, parietal cells expand their intracellular canalicular membranes and exhibit dramatic changes in the appearance of their canalicular membrane microvilli, which become long and slender (Fig. 1.3). When the parietal cell is stimulated (i.e., after eating), the tubules of the tubulovesicles located in the parietal cell cytoplasm fuse with cell membranes of the microvilli projecting on the luminal surface of the secretory canaliculi, inducing an enormous expansion of the canalicular luminal surface area (see Figs 1.2, 1.3). These changes also result in translocation of H+, K+-ATPase from its sequestered position of insertion in the tubular membranes within the parietal cell cytoplasm to the luminal surfaces of its secretory canaliculi. Immunolabeling using high-pressure freezing (HPF) techniques has demonstrated substantial increases in the labeling density of H+, K+-ATPase on the canalicular membranes of parietal cells after stimulation compared with resting parietal cells.[12]

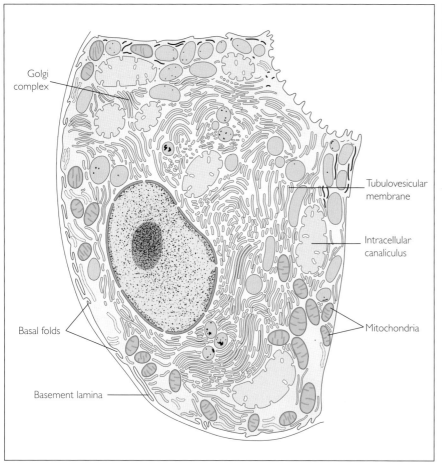

Fig. 1.2 • Electron photomicrograph of parietal cell in the resting (unstimulated) state demonstrating abundant cytoplasmic tubulovesicular membranes to which proton pumps – hydrogen potassium ATPase (H+, K+-ATPase) are inserted.

Golgi complex

Tubulovesicular membrane

Intracellular canaliculus

Mitochondria

Basal folds

Basement lamina

Enterochromaffin-like cells

Enterochromaffin-like (ECL) cells are located close to parietal cells in the oxyntic gland areas in the body and fundus of the stomach, found exclusively in oxyntic glands. In contrast to parietal cells, ECL cells are not luminal epithelial cells. Although ECL cells are located near parietal cells, they are positioned beneath the epithelial cell layer and do not have a cell surface exposed to the gland lumen. ECL cells contain prominent eccentrically located nuclei and have numerous cytoplasmic extensions. The cytoplasm is also packed with conspicuous vacuoles containing the biogenic amine histamine. ECL cells are responsible for synthesis and secretion of histamine, a potent stimulus of gastric acid secretion.[9,13,14] Stimulation of the ECL cell induces the synthesis and activity of parietal cell histidine decarboxylase (HDC), the enzyme responsible for histamine synthesis. Through synthesis and release of histamine, ECL cells play a crucial role in the stimulation of gastric acid secretion. The ECL cell is distinct from mast cells, which are also found in the oxyntic mucosa. Mast cells, like ECL cells, contain histamine but do not participate in the regulatory stimulation of gastric acid secretion.

ECL cells possess receptors in their plasma membranes for gastrin, somatostatin, galanin, and pituitary adenylate cyclase activating polypeptide (PACAP), all of which participate in regulation of histamine release.

REGULATION OF GASTRIC ACID SECRETION

The secretion of hydrochloric acid by the stomach is highly regulated by multiple endocrine, neurocrine, paracrine, enterchromaffin-like cells and autocrine mechanisms responsible for its stimulation and its inhibition.

Endocrine factors

The polypeptide hormone gastrin in the most potent known stimulant of gastric acid secretion. The ingestion of food constitutes the principal physiological stimulus to gastrin release from gastrin-containing G cells located in the gastric antral mucosa, resulting in the stimulation of gastric acid secretion.[15] Gastrin is released into the circulation when the intraluminal pH increases above 3.5–4.0 and in response to protein ingestion and specifically in response to the peptide and amino acid products of protein digestion. Intact protein does not stimulate gastrin release, and ingested fat and carbohydrate inhibit gastrin release. Aromatic amino acid products of protein hydrolysis such as tryosine and phenylalanine are particularly potent in stimulating gastrin release. Gastrin released into the circulation in response to stimulation binds to specific gastrin receptors (CCK-2 receptors) on the membrane surfaces of ECL cells, which are located in intimate proximity to parietal cells. Gastrin binding to ECL cells

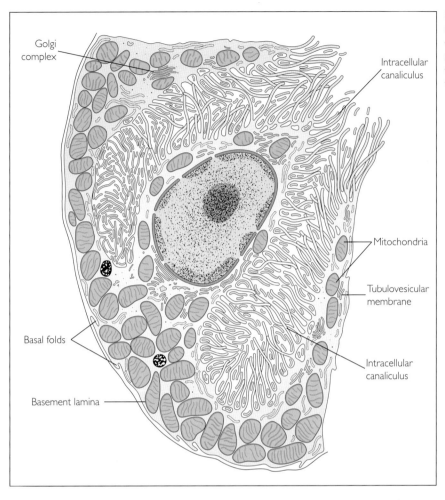

Golgi complex

Intracellular canaliculus

Mitochondria

Tubulovesicular membrane

Intracellular canaliculus

Basal folds

Basement lamina

Fig. 1.3 ● Electron photomicrograph of stimulated parietal cell demonstrating translocation of the tubulovesicular membranes (containing proton pumps) to the intracellular secretory canalicular membranes, facilitating pump exposure to the highly acidic canalicular lumen.

results in increases in intracellular calcium, which induces transcription of histidine decarboxylase, resulting in enhanced synthesis and secretion of histamine. Histamine released from stimulated ECL cells binds to histamine 2 receptors, which are located on the basolateral membranes of parietal cells, resulting in the stimulation of hydrochloric acid secretion. Stimulation of ECL cells, evoking histamine release and histamine-mediated stimulation of parietal cell secretion, is the most important mechanism by which gastrin stimulates hydrochloric acid secretion. The role and importance of direct binding of gastrin to parietal cells are controversial and clearly of less importance than gastrin induction of histamine-stimulated acid secretion by parietal cells.

In addition to its stimulation of release by gastrin, histamine release from ECL cells may also be stimulated by PACAP.[9] This neuropeptide, which is structurally related to vasoactive intestinal peptide (VIP), is localized to enteric nerves distributed throughout the gastrointestinal tract, including the stomach. PACAP administration increases intracellular calcium concentrations and cyclic AMP in ECL cells, resulting in histamine release.

A variety of mechanisms are operative in inhibiting gastrin release and in inhibiting parietal cell secretion of acid.[15] The most important physiologic peptide inhibitor of gastrin release and gastric acid secretion is somatostatin.[16] Somatostatin is a peptide hormone and a neuropeptide widely distributed throughout the body in neurons of the central, peripheral, and enteric

nervous systems and in endocrine cells (D cells). Local release of somatostatin directly inhibits G cells, ECL cells, and parietal cells. In the gastric antrum, somatostatin is present in D cells located in close proximity to gastrin-containing G cells. Antral D cells are classified as open cells since they have a cell surface that is exposed to the contents of the antral gland lumen. In addition to somatostatin-containing D cells in the antrum, somatostatin-containing cells are also located in the body and fundus of the stomach. D cells in the body and fundus of the stomach differ from those in the antrum in that they are closed-type D cells, not having a surface facing the oxyntic gland lumen.

Somatostatin decreases gastric acid secretion by both direct and indirect mechanisms. D cells inhibit gastrin release by a paracrine mechanism in which somatostatin released from cytoplasmic extensions from D cells binds to somatostatin receptors located on the basolateral membrane surfaces of antral G cells. By decreasing gastrin release, somatostatin inhibits gastrin-mediated secretion of hydrochloric acid by parietal cells. Somatostatin, released from cytoplasmic extensions of D cells located close to ECL cells, binds to its receptors on these cells, inhibiting histamine synthesis and release and thereby directly reducing histamine stimulated gastric acid secretion. Finally, somatostatin released from D cells in close proximity to parietal cells binds to somatostatin receptors located on the basolateral membranes of parietal cells, resulting in direct inhibition of parietal cell secretion of hydrochloric acid.[15]

Somatostatin is also the prime mediator of the negative feedback inhibitory control of gastric acid secretion. Acidification of the gastric luminal contents (to pH <3.5) stimulates antral D-cell release of somatostatin, which inhibits gastrin release, resulting in decreased histamine release and inhibition of further acid secretion.[17] In addition to increases in gastric intraluminal pH, the secretion of somatostatin is regulated by several other mechanisms. D cells in the body and fundus of the stomach are stimulated to release somatostatin in direct response to gastrin. Cholecystokinin, VIP, secretin, and gastric inhibitory polypeptide (GIP) also stimulate D cells to release somatostatin.

Neurocrine factors

The regulation of gastric acid secretion involves both stimulatory and inhibitory neurocrine mechanisms. The vagus nerves provide the principal neural stimulation of parietal cells.[18] Acetylcholine released from vagal cholinergic nerve fibers binds to cholinergic muscarinic (M_3) receptors located on the basolateral membranes of parietal cells.[19,20] (There are five different cholinergic muscarinic receptors – M_1 through M_5 receptors – each with different specificity.) Cholinergic stimulation via these receptors increases parietal cell intracellular calcium concentrations by opening plasma membrane calcium channels for calcium entry into parietal cells and by promoting release of calcium from intracellular stores. These increases in cytoplasmic calcium result in the stimulation of gastric acid secretion, and blockade of cholinergic muscarinic receptors decreases gastric acid secretion. There are also inhibitory cholinergic receptors on D cells, by which vagal stimulation promotes gastric acid secretion by the inhibition of somatostatin release.

Gastric acid secretion is also influenced by other neural mechanisms and neuropeptides. Gastrin release is stimulated by the neuropeptide gastrin-releasing peptide (GRP), as well as by PACAP and galanin. PACAP has at least two separate and opposing effects on gastric acid secretion. As stated above, PACAP increases gastric acid secretion by stimulating ECL cells to release histamine. PACAP also binds to VIP receptors on D cells, stimulating somatostatin release and inhibiting gastric acid secretion. PACAP has no effect on gastrin release from antral G cells. Galanin is a 29 amino acid neuropeptide that inhibits gastrin-stimulated gastric acid secretion. Galanin inhibits both gastrin release from antral G cells and histamine release from ECL cells, but does not inhibit cholinergic stimulation of gastric acid secretion.

RECEPTORS INVOLVED IN REGULATION OF GASTRIC ACID SECRETION

H_2 receptors

A variety of receptors participate in acid secretory regulation by inhibition or stimulation of gastric acid secretion. As stated above, histamine plays the dominant role in stimulating gastric acid secretion by its binding to and stimulating H_2 receptors located on the basolateral membranes of parietal cells.[12,14] Parietal cell H_2 receptors are responsible for the greatest portion of the stimulation of the acid secretory response to gastrin.

The H_2 receptor of the parietal cell is a member of the seven transmembrane G protein-coupled receptor superfamily and is imbedded in the basolateral membranes of parietal cells.[21] This receptor possesses seven transmembrane domains with three cytoplasmic loops and three loops located on the external surface of the membrane, as demonstrated in Figure 1.4. The H_2 receptor has an extracellular amino terminal-linked glycosylation site and an extended intracellular carboxy-terminal peptide segment and is comprised of 359 amino acids. H_2 receptors are structurally and functionally distinct from histamine 1 receptors, which account for many allergic-type responses to histamine. Antihistaminic agents that engage H_1 receptors have negligible effects on gastric acid secretion.

The site to which histamine and H_2-receptor antagonists are thought to bind is believed to be located on the external surface of the middle of the extracellular loop located between the fourth and fifth transmembrane segments and to the surface of the transmembrane segments 3 and 5 of the H_2 receptor.[22] Histamine stimulation of parietal cells is mediated principally by intracellular cyclic AMP. Binding of histamine to parietal cell H_2 receptors results in their coupling to a stimulatory G protein (G_s), which activates adenylate cyclase, thereby increasing intracellular cyclic AMP. The increase in intracellular cyclic AMP is also accompanied by increases in intracellular calcium, which exert a limited signal interaction with a G_q trimeric G protein. It has been hypothesized that both cyclic AMP and calcium signals are required because cyclic AMP is necessary for the activation of H+, K+-ATPase, and increases in intracellular calcium appear to be necessary to provide for redistribution of the enzyme in its attachment to the secretory canaliculi.

In addition to their presence on parietal cell membranes, H_2 receptors have been found on membranes of smooth muscle and cardiac myocytes. Cardiac arrhythmias, cardiac arrest, and atrioventricular conduction abnormalities have been reported rarely in patients being treated with H_2-receptor antagonists. Most of those patients were very seriously ill and often they had received the H_2-receptor antagonists by rapid intravenous infusion.[23]

The H_2 receptor in the cell membrane of the parietal cell is the most important receptor involved in stimulation of parietal cell secretion. It is responsible for the stimulation of basal acid output and for gastric acid secretory responses to feeding, principally mediated through gastrin. In addition to H_2 receptors, there are other stimulatory receptors on parietal cells, including the M_3 receptor for acetylcholine and the CCK-2 receptor for gastrin (see Fig. 1.1). However, unlike the parietal cell H_2 receptor, the CCK-2 receptor is believed to promote gastric acid secretion principally through elevations in parietal cell cytoplasmic calcium, with a very minor role played by cyclic AMP.

Gastrin receptors

Binding of gastrin to its receptor on the surrounding cell membranes of ECL cells stimulates histamine synthesis and secretion, resulting in parietal cell activation and gastric acid secretion. Gastrin binding to its receptor induces acid secretion by increases in intracellular calcium by an inositol 1,4,5-triphosphate (IP_3) mechanism. The receptors to which gastrin binds have been classified CCK-2 (also known as CCK-B) because of their relative structural homology to cholecystokinin (CCK) receptors. Gastrin stimulation of acid secretion does require a small increase in cyclic AMP, whereas cholinergic receptor activation of the parietal cell requires only increases in parietal

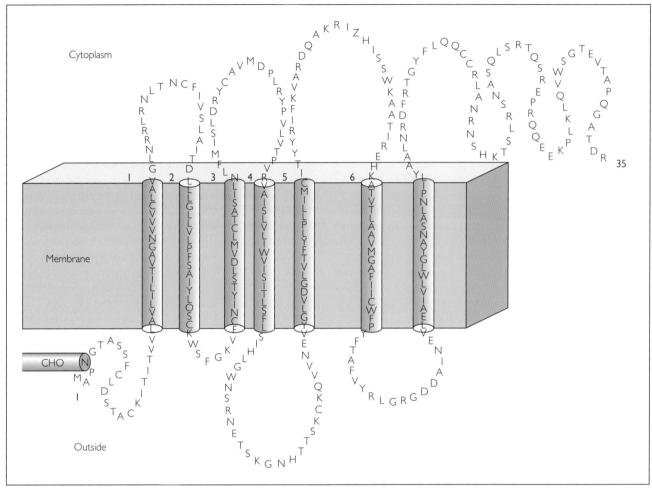

Fig. 1.4 ● The amino acid sequence and membrane arrangement of the H$_2$ receptor with a single external nitrogen glycosylation site (CHO).

cell calcium, without requirements for increased amounts of cyclic AMP.

In addition to gastrin receptors on ECL cells, some CCK-2 receptors may be present on parietal cells, but these receptors, if present, appear to play a minor role in the stimulation of gastric acid secretion. Studies of rat stomachs concluded that CCK-2 receptors were present on ECL cells, but could not be demonstrated on parietal cells.[24]

Somatostatin receptors

Somatostatin receptors are seven transmembrane G protein-coupled receptors located in the plasma membranes of an assortment of cells that participate in the regulation of gastric acid secretion and in many other physiological functions. Five different classes of somatostatin receptors have been identified and are classified as somatostatin receptors one through five (SSR 1, 2, 3, 4, 5). They are structurally distinct receptors, which constitute a defined subgroup of the large seven transmembrane G protein-coupled receptor superfamily. The five distinct somatostatin receptor subtypes range in size from 356 to 391 amino acids and possess a range of 39–57% amino acid sequence identity. One hundred of those amino acid residues are conserved strictly among all five somatostatin receptor amino acid sequences. These receptors, while sharing structural charac-

teristics, possess differences in structure and function that vary according to their interactions with different cell types. All somatostatin receptors involved in various aspects of cellular regulation of gastric acid secretion by parietal cells are members of the somatostatin subtype 2 receptor class (SSR2).

As discussed above, somatostatin plays important roles in the regulation of gastric acid secretion directly on the parietal cell and indirectly by its effects on G cells and ECL cells. Somatostatin-mediated inhibition of ECL cell release of histamine exerts a greater reduction in gastric acid secretion than does its inhibition of gastrin release. In addition to parietal, antral G and corpus and fundic ECL cells, somatostatin 2 receptors are also found in the cell membranes of somatostatin-containing D cells, in which they are believed to serve an autocrine downregulating function, inhibiting further somatostatin release.

Other receptors

As stated above, M$_3$ muscarinic receptors (M$_3$Rs) present on the basolateral membranes of parietal cells provide the mechanism for the stimulation of gastric acid secretion in response to vagal stimulation. Activation of M$_3$Rs, in concert with gastrin/CCK-2 and H$_2$ receptors, stimulates parietal cell secretion of hydrochloric acid principally by increases in intracellular calcium concentrations.[25] Stimulation results from coupling to a G$_q$ trimeric protein, which activates phospholipase C, resulting in the generation of IP$_3$, which in turn releases calcium from intracellular stores accompanied by facilitation of increased calcium entry into parietal cells from the extracellular space.[26] Gastrin stimulation of acid secretion is mediated principally by increases in cytoplasmic calcium concentrations, but does require some participation of cyclic AMP. Cholinergic receptor activation of the parietal cell requires only increases in parietal cell calcium, without requirements for increased cyclic AMP.

Receptors for prostaglandins (EP$_3$ subtype) and epidermal growth factor (EGF) are present on the basolateral membrane of parietal cells. The binding of those receptors by their respective ligands inhibits parietal cell secretion of hydrochloric acid. In addition to H$_2$ receptors, H$_3$ receptors have been found on fundic ECL cells, as well as on enterochromaffin cells in the gastrointestinal tract and in various locations of the central nervous system. Histamine may inhibit somatostatin release by binding to H$_3$ receptors on D cells, consequently increasing gastric acid secretion.

PHARMACOLOGIC INHIBITORS OF GASTRIC ACID SECRETION

Anticholinergic agents

Anticholinergic agents have been used to inhibit secretion of gastric acid in treatment of patients with a variety of acid-related diseases. The participation of vagal stimulation is particularly apparent during the cephalic phase of gastric acid secretion and appears to also play a significant role in regulating nocturnal gastric acid secretion. Anticholinergic agents that have been available for clinical use in the past have not proven beneficial in the management of patients with acid-related diseases due to their association with an assortment of adverse effects, occasionally severe, including dryness of the mouth and eyes, urinary retention, cardiac arrhythmias, and glaucoma. Presently available anticholinergic drugs exhibit specificity insufficient to effect substantial gastric acid inhibition in the absence of significant adverse events. However, pirenzepine and telenzepine, M$_1$-specific receptor antagonists, appear to inhibit gastric acid secretion by a mechanism other than binding to parietal cell cholinergic receptors. Rather, these antagonists appear to bind to an M$_1$ receptor located on the postganglionic neuron of the vagus nerve.[11] Efforts continue to be directed to development of anticholinergic agents with a sufficiently high degree of specificity for the M$_3$ cholinergic receptor to exert effective inhibition of gastric acid secretion with minimal to negligible adverse drug effects.

H$_2$-receptor antagonists

Histamine has been recognized as a powerful stimulant of gastric acid secretion since the early 1900s. Until relatively recently, however, the molecular and cellular mechanisms governing the participation of histamine in the physiological regulation of hydrochloric acid secretion by the parietal cell had not been elucidated. The development of H$_2$-receptor antagonists (H2RAs) accelerated substantially our acquisition of knowledge concerning the biology of histamine and the importance of its role as the major direct stimulant of gastric acid secretion. Histamine is a relatively small organic molecule comprised of an imidazole ring and a single side chain that is positively charged at neutral pH. A series of H2RAs, developed as structural analogs of histamine, have been shown to inhibit effectively gastric acid secretion in response to almost all gastric acid secretory stimuli. These will be discussed below.

Proton pump inhibitors

Stimulated by the success of H2RAs in inhibiting gastric acid secretion and in their application in treatment of acid-related disease, a vigorous search ensued for other pharmacological agents with potent capacities to inhibit gastric acid secretion. This search was rewarded by the identification and development of a series of structurally related benzimidazoles that demonstrated potent and sustained capacities to inhibit parietal cell secretion of hydrochloric acid. These agents act not by competing with histamine but rather by inhibiting the terminal step in acid secretion by binding to and inactivating H+, K+-ATPase. These agents, which inhibit this H+, K+-ATPase, are referred to as proton pump inhibitors (PPIs) and will be discussed below.

H$_2$-RECEPTOR ANTAGONISTS

Biological properties

The four approved and widely used H2RAs are cimetidine (Tagamet®), ranitidine (Zantac®), famotidine (Pepcid®), and nizatidine (Axid®).[3–6] Each of these agents is available by prescription and as over-the-counter (OTC) medications. The H2RAs are competitive inhibitors of histamine-stimulated gastric acid secretion and inhibit gastric acid secretion by competing with histamine for occupancy of H$_2$ receptors located on the basolateral surfaces of parietal cells, blocking the effects of histamine released from ECL cells located in proximity to parietal cells.[2] H2RAs inhibit both basal gastric acid output and gastric acid output stimulated by meals.

H2RAs are efficient and effective in inhibiting gastric acid secretory responses to gastrin, the most potent stimulant of gastric parietal cell acid secretion. The specificity of the gastric acid inhibitory action of H2RAs supports the importance of the intermediate role of histamine in stimulating parietal cell secretion of gastric acid. H2RAs do not inhibit cholinergic stimulation of gastric acid secretion, consistent with an independent role for cholinergic (principally vagal) stimulation of parietal cells.

Although the biological properties of individual H2RAs are remarkably similar, these agents differ based on their relative potency in their abilities to inhibit gastric acid secretion. In clinical application, these differences have been accommodated readily by differences in dosing. Famotidine, the most potent of the H2RAs on a mg per mg basis, is approximately five times as potent as ranitidine and nizatidine, which are about five times as potent as cimetidine.

In addition to inhibiting basal gastric acid output, H2RAs have been shown to be very effective in inhibiting nocturnal gastric acid secretion, with less pronounced inhibitory effects on daytime (postprandial) gastric acid output. The mechanism by which these agents preferentially inhibit nocturnal gastric acid secretion is not known. Cimetidine was initially used at a dose of 300 mg four times daily, but subsequently it was demonstrated to be equally effective when administered as a single dose at night in the treatment of duodenal ulcer (see Ch. 20).

The continued use of H2RAs has been shown to be associated with development of tolerance to H$_2$ receptor blockade, which develops rapidly during therapy.[27] Approximately 50% of potency in reducing gastric acid secretion is lost after one week of treatment with H2RAs. The precise mechanisms accounting for the acquisition of tolerance to the acid secretory inhibitory effects of H2RAs have not been elucidated; however it appears not be due to H$_2$ receptor downregulation nor is it produced by alterations in serum gastrin levels.[27]

Mechanism of action

H2RAs act by inhibiting competitively H$_2$ receptors located on the basolateral membranes of parietal cells. While H$_1$ receptor antagonists have no effect on gastric acid secretion, H2RAs inhibit acid secretion by preventing histamine activation of parietal cell adenylate cyclase and cyclic AMP generation. Famotidine appears to possess a noncompetitive inhibitory mechanism in addition to its competitive inhibition of histamine-stimulated acid secretion.

Structures

Histamine is a relatively compact organic molecule comprised of an imidazole ring and an ethylamine side chain (Fig. 1.5). H2RAs were designed as structural analogs of histamine which were intended to compete specifically with histamine for binding to parietal cell H$_2$ receptors and thereby to inhibit gastric acid secretion.[2]

As discussed above, the four H2RAs were developed and have been used widely in treatment of patients with acid-related diseases.[3–6] Most traditional H$_1$ receptor antagonists were designed by modification of the imidazole ring of histamine without alteration of the ethylamine side chain. While searching for this new form of histamine antagonist, a large number of compounds structurally related to histamine were designed, synthesized, and examined for their safety and effectiveness in inhibiting gastric acid secretion. The cimetidine molecule was designed with retention of the histamine imidazole ring, but with modification of the ethylamine side chain of histamine (see Fig. 1.5). Ranitidine, the second H2RA made available for the treatment of patients with acid-related disorders, was developed differently. Ranitidine was designed by the substitution of a furan ring for the imidazole ring of histamine, as well as a modification of the ethylamine side chain and the addition of another side chain (see Fig. 1.5). Famotidine, the next H2RA, introduced additional modifications by the substitution of a thiazole ring for the imidazole ring of histamine, coupled with two further modified side chains (see Fig. 1.5). Nizatidine, the most recently introduced H2RA, was designed similarly with a thiazole ring substituted for the imidizole ring of histamine, accompanied by more extensive modification of the two side chains (see Fig. 1.5).

Duration of actions

Peak blood levels of H2RAs are achieved within 1–3 hours after oral dosing. Similarly, H2RAs have biological half-lives with respect to gastric acid secretory inhibition of approximately

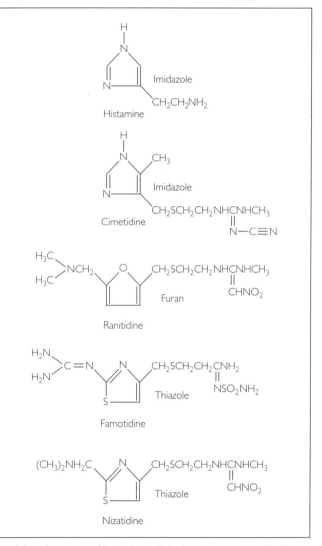

Fig. 1.5 • Structures of histamine and the four currently available H$_2$ receptor antagonists (cimetidine, ranitidine, famotidine, and nizatidine). Demonstration of substitutions of ring structure (imidizole) of histamine by furan and thiazole and extensive R group substitutions and additions in H$_2$ receptor antagonists.

2–3 hours and in this regard are relatively similar to one another. The gastric acid inhibitory effects of cimetidine, rantitidine, and nizatidine decrease substantially after approximately 6–8 hours following their administration; the inhibitory effects of famotidine persist an additional 3–4 hours. When orally ingested, H2RAs are absorbed readily and their absorption is not enhanced, diminished, or otherwise affected by food. However, the concomitant administration of antacids or sucralfate can impair absorption of H2RAs, although the clinical relevance of this effect is minimal.

Metabolism and adverse effects

As a group, H2RAs are safe and effective drugs and possess few serious side effects. There is no individual dominant safety advantage for any one of the H$_2$RAs. These drugs are eliminated by hepatic metabolism and/or by renal excretion. Cimetidine, ranitidine, and famotidine undergo first-pass metabolism by the liver, which reduces their bioavailability by approximately 35–60%. Of orally administered cimetidine, ranitidine and famotidine, 60–80% is cleared by the liver. However, nizatidine, which is eliminated principally by renal excretion, does not undergo first-pass metabolism by the liver, and the bioavailability after oral administration of nizatidine is therefore >90%. After intravenous administration, H2RAs are eliminated principally through renal excretion, and the bioavailability of each of the H2RAs approximates 100%. All H2RAs but nizatidine are available as intravenous formulations in the US. No reductions in the doses of these drugs are required based exclusively on hepatic insufficiency, whereas dose reductions are usually recommended for most patients with clinically significant renal insufficiency.[28]

Cimetidine and ranitidine are metabolized by the hepatic cytochrome P450 mixed function oxidase system. For this reason, these H2RAs may compete with other drugs which are metabolized by the same P450 enzyme system.[29,30] Potential drug interactions include, among others, those with warfarin, lidocaine, quinidine, phenytoin, and theophylline. Some drug interactions have been reported in patients who have been treated with cimetidine, with somewhat fewer interactions having been observed with ranitidine. Because nizatidine and famotidine are metabolized by different enzyme systems, they are not associated with the potential increases in blood levels of those drugs.

In addition to their presence on gastric parietal cells, H_2 receptors have also been identified on suppressor T lymphocytes.[31] Antiandrogenic effects, principally in the forms of impotence and gynecomastia, have been reported in patients receiving very high doses of cimetidine, but not the other H2RAs, most often in treatment of patients with the Zollinger-Ellison syndrome. Central nervous system symptoms have been reported rarely in patients receiving H_2 receptor antagonists.[32] These have been noted most often in seriously ill, mostly elderly patients, commonly in intensive care settings, and it is uncertain whether these very unusual associations actually represent adverse effects from these agents.[32] Bone marrow suppression has been reported as a very uncommon side effect of treatment with H2RAs and is believed to represent an idiosyncratic mechanism. Rarely, drug administration has been associated with some asymptomatic increases in serum liver aminotransferase levels. However, these increased levels return to normal after the drugs are discontinued and do not appear to represent hepatic disease.[33]

H2RAs compete with creatinine for renal tubular excretion, and as a result, their administration has occasionally been associated with small increases in serum creatinine levels.[34] These increases are transient and disappear after discontinuation of therapy. With the exception of famotidine, H2RAs inhibit gastric mucosal alcohol dehydrogenase and may thus increase blood alcohol levels.[35] However, because >90% of alcohol dehydrogenase is hepatic in origin, these increases in blood alcohol concentrations tend to be small and are rarely of clinical significance.

Gastric acid secretory rebound has been reported after discontinuation of chronic H2RA therapy of 1–9 months' duration.[36,37] Acid secretory rebound after the cessation of therapy is usually brief and has been reported to be resolved by 9 days after stopping the drug. Gastric acid rebound may occur as a result of upregulation of parietal cell H_2 receptors due to receptor antagonism.

INHIBITORS OF H+, K+-ATPASE (PPIS)

The proton pump (H+, K+-ATPase)

H+, K+-ATPase is a heterodimeric protein comprised of a much larger α-subunit and a small β-subunit.[38] The much larger α-subunit is the catalytic subunit that contains the ion transport pathway and is directly responsible for the acid secretory activity of the enzyme. The α-catalytic subunit consists of ten transmembrane domains, whereas the smaller β-subunit of the H+, K+-ATPase has only a single transmembrane domain. The ion transport channel is located between transmembrane segments 5 and 6 (and 4 and 8) of the α-subunit. The α-subunit contains the phosphorylation sequence and the ATP binding domain of the enzyme. The β-subunit includes seven N-linked glycosylation sequences that are responsible for the stability of the enzyme and for targeting the enzyme to its positions on the secretory canalicular membrane and the tubulovesicular system.

The parietal cell H+, K+-ATPase transports H+ (technically H_3O+) for secretion in exchange for uptake of K+. This enzyme utilizes a potassium-chloride co-transport system to promote hydrogen potassium exchange.[39] The gastric H+, K+-ATPase (proton pump) has been classified as a P-type ATPase because the enzyme is phosphorylated and dephosphorylated repetitively during its enzymatic cycle. The concentration of H+ in the secretory canaliculi of actively secreting parietal cells, where active proton pumps reside, approximates 160 mmol/L H+, which corresponds to a pH of approximately 0.8. This circumstance contrasts with the resting or unstimulated parietal cell, in which approximately 90–95% of the proton pumps are sequestered in the tubulovesicular membranes located in the cytoplasm of the parietal cells and are thus inaccessible to the intracanalicular acidic environment and to inhibition by PPIs.

PPIs: biological properties and mechanisms of action

The five PPIs currently available for use in inhibiting parietal cell H+, K+-ATPase are omeprazole (Prilosec®), esomeprazole (Nexium®, the S optical isomer of omeprazole), lansoprazole (Prevacid®), pantoprazole (Protonix®) and rabeprazole (Aciphex®) (Fig. 1.6).[40–43] Data suggest a mg per mg equivalency among the different PPIs.[44] Because these drugs are acid labile, they are prepared and used as enteric-coated delayed-release tablets or capsules for oral dosing. Pantoprazole and lansoprazole are also available in intravenous formulations. Recently, an oral liquid suspension preparation of omeprazole with sodium bicarbonate, Zegerid®, has been introduced.[45]

PPIs are administered and absorbed systemically as prodrugs that undergo acid catalyzed chemical arrangement requisite for their activation, and they bind predominantly to actively secreting parietal cells. These agents are all weak bases with a pKa of approximately 4 (5 for rabeprazole), and as a result, PPIs accumulate preferentially in the acidic canalicular spaces of stimulated and secreting parietal cells.[46] Protonation of the pyridine nitrogen atom in the PPI results in accumulation of the PPI in the highly acidic secretory canaliculus.[47] As a result of the low pH (≈0.8), PPIs concentrate in the highly acidic canalicular spaces, achieving concentrations approximately 1000 times greater than those found in plasma. This property ensures PPI accumulation

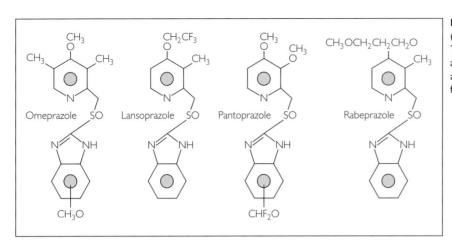

Fig. 1.6 • Structures of proton pump inhibitors. (Esomeprazole is the S-isomer of omeprazole.) They are all ampholytic weak bases and accumulate as prodrugs in the secretory canaliculus of the active parietal cell. They are activated by acid to form the reactive sulfenamide derivative.

exclusively in the very low pH of the canaliculi of the actively secreting parietal cell. The protonated form of the PPI as a weak base is membrane impermeable and thus accumulates in the acidic compartment at a concentration depending on the gradient between the pH and the pKa of the weak base. The pKa of PPIs is sufficiently low to prevent their accumulation in other relatively acidic intracellular compartments, such as lysomes or secretory granules, which have a pH of 4.5–5.

After the PPI prodrugs have been concentrated by the acid gradient-dependent mechanism, they undergo acid catalyzed protonation, converting the prodrugs to the active thiophilic sulfenamide form of the proton pump inhibitor (Fig. 1.7). At a pH <2, PPIs are converted from an inactive prodrug to an active compound in a half-time of activation of less than 1 minute. At a higher pH, the rapidity of activation is slower for all of the PPIs. The rate of acid activation of PPIs in stimulated parietal cells varies among different PPIs, being most rapid for rabeprazole, about the same for omeprazole and lansoprazole, and the slowest for pantoprazole. None of these differences is clinically relevant.

The pH activation curves for the PPIs also differ.[48] The half-maximum rate of activation for pantoprazole is achieved at a pH of 3.0, while for omeprazole and lansoprazole, activation is achieved at a pH of 4.0. The acid catalyzed activated form of the proton pump inhibitor, the thiophilic sulfenamide, which now contains a highly reactive sulfenamide group, is prepared to form disulfide bonds with accessible cysteines on the luminal surface of the proton pump. The sulfenamide form of the activated proton pump inhibitor is a permanent cation and is membrane impermeable in the acid medium of the canaliculus. This property assures that the activated form of the PPI remains in the secretory canalicular lumen and does not diffuse into the parietal cell, and is thereby available for attachment to the sulfhydryl groups of cysteine residues within the enzyme. PPIs, activated and accumulated in high concentration in the acidic space of secreting parietal cells, then bind to selected cysteine residues of H+, K+-ATPase located and accessible on the luminal surface of the α-catalytic subunit of the enzyme (see Fig. 1.7). The different PPIs interact with different cysteine residues located on the α-subunit,[40,49–51] although all bind to cysteine 813. Pantoprazole binds to cysteine 813 and cysteine 822, both of which are located in the ion transport pathway of the α-subunit. These residues are the only cysteines in which disulfide binding by a PPI is associated with inhibition of H+, K+-ATPase.

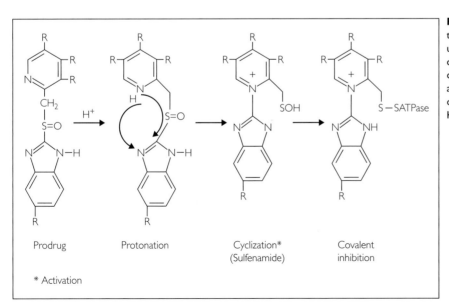

Prodrug   Protonation   Cyclization* (Sulfenamide)   Covalent inhibition

* Activation

Fig. 1.7 • The reaction pathway for inhibition taken by all four proton pump inhibitors in clinical use. They are all concentrated in the secretory canaliculus of the parietal cell, undergo acid-catalyzed conversion to the active sulfenamide, and then form covalent disulfide bonds with cysteines accessible in the luminal domain of the H+, K+-ATPase.

Cysteine 813, which forms disulfide bonds with each of the PPIs, is located at the luminal surface of the sixth transmembrane segment,[40] which positions it directly in the ion transport pathway of the enzyme α-catalytic subunit (Fig. 1.8). Cysteine 813 is nestled in a vestibule, partially enclosed by transmembrane segments 4 and 5 and the exoplasmic loop between transmembrane segments 5 and 6 and transmembrane segment 8, as shown in Figure 1.8. Omeprazole also binds to cysteine 892, which is located in the exoplasmic loop on the luminal surface of transmembrane segments 7 and 8 of the α-catalytic subunit of the enzyme. Cysteine 321, which reacts with both lanzoprazole and rabeprazole, is also located on the luminal surface of the enzyme close to the exoplasmic loop between transmembrane segments 3 and 4. In addition to binding to cysteine 813, rabeprazole also binds to other less selective cysteines of the pump. Pantoprazole is the only one of the PPIs which forms a disulfide bond with cysteine 822, which is located on transmembrane segment 6 deep in the α-subunit, approximately 2.5 α-helical turns from the luminal surface.

PPIs were initially believed to inhibit H+, K+-ATPase activity permanently by their irreversible covalent disulfide bonding to available cysteines on the enzyme.[52] Therefore, acid secretion would be anticipated to be abolished for the life of the enzyme, and consequently, enzyme activity and gastric acid secretion

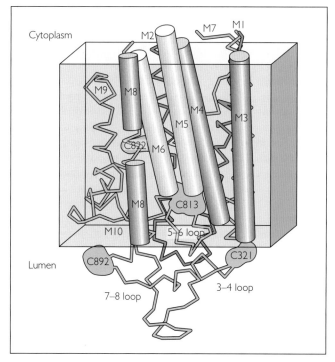

Fig. 1.8 ● The enzyme structure surrounding the PPI-reactive cysteines. A three-dimensional model of the membrane domain of the H+, K+-ATPase showing the positions of cysteine 321, 813, 822, and 892. The structure represented is derived from the E_1 conformation of the sarcoplasmic reticulum ATPase at 2.8-A[10] resolution where the amino acids of the H+, K+-ATPase have been substituted at equivalent positions. The location of the cysteine at position 822 is deeper within the membrane domain compared with the other cysteines and also M8 is split to show the position of this cysteine. The transmembrane helices for M4, 5, 6, and 8 are shown as cylinders overlaying the peptide backbone to illustrate the vestibule surrounding cysteine 813 at the end of the 5–6 exoplasmic loop. (Reprinted from Shin JM, Sachs G, Gastroenterology 2002; 123: 1588–1597. © 2002, with permission from The American Gastroenterological Association.)

would return only when new enzyme was synthesized. More recent studies have refuted this concept and have demonstrated substantial differences between the half-life of the proton pump and the duration of inhibition of H+, K+-ATPase activity or acid secretion by several of the PPIs. The half-life of the α-catalytic subunit of the proton pump protein in rats has been found to be 54 hours.[53] In contrast, the half-time of recovery of gastric acid secretion and H+, K+-ATPase activity in rats following administration of omeprazole was found to be about 15 hours.[54,55] After inhibition of acid secretion by rabeprazole, the return of acid secretion occurred more rapidly than with lansoprazole. The observation that after omeprazole and rabeprazole administration, acid secretion returned in less than the half-life of the enzyme suggested that more than only new protein synthesis may play a role in gastric acid secretory recovery.[40] Differences in the half-lives of inhibition of gastric acid secretion after administration of several of the PPIs have also been detected in humans. The half-life of recovery of acid suppression following lansoprazole was found to be 12.9 hours and for omeprazole the half-life was less than 27.5 hours.[56] Some reports in humans showed more rapid return of acid secretion after rabeprazole than with omeprazole, but in other studies, the rate at which acid secretion returned was similar with omeprazole and rabeprazole.[57–60] With pantoprazole, the half-life of recovery of acid suppression was reported to be approximately 46 hours. The differences in the duration of inhibition by different PPIs may occur as a consequence of variations in the duration of attachment to the H+, K+-ATPase. Pantoprazole is the only PPI that exhibits a half-time return of gastric acid secretion consistent with protein turnover as its sole determinant.

Recovery of gastric acid secretion after PPI inhibition may be due to synthesis of new enzymes and/or to dissociation of the disulfide bonding between the enzyme and the PPI, resulting in reactivation of previously inhibited pumps. Reducing agents such as glutathione and dithiothreitol possess the capacity to disrupt covalent disulfide bonds. Studies have been conducted in rats to determine whether glutathione or dithiothreitol could dissociate PPI disulfide binding to H+, K+-ATPase cysteine residues and thereby accelerate return of enzyme inhibited ATPase activity. Glutathione, a potent naturally occurring reducing agent, arrested acid inhibition produced by omeprazole by dissociating the disulfide bonds between cysteines and the PPI.[40] Complete reactivation of H+, K+-ATPase activity after inhibition with omeprazole was seen with dithiothreitol, and 89% reactivation was demonstrated with glutathione.[40] Similar results were obtained in studies after inhibition with lanzoprazole or rabeprazole. No effect by either reducing agent was observed following inhibition of H+, K+-ATPase activity by pantoprazole.

The differences in duration of inhibition of H+, K+-ATPase activity with different PPIs may occur as a consequence of different rates of enzyme reactivation resulting from differences in accessibility of disulfide binding of cysteines to reducing agents, such as glutathione present in the parietal cell environment. The studies in rats suggest that reversal of H+, K+-ATPase inhibition by omeprazole, esomeprazole, lansoprazole, and rabeprazole, but not pantoprazole, results from both the dissociation of disulfide bonds between the PPIs and cysteine residues and enzyme synthesis. It has been proposed that pantoprazole reversal of acid inhibition may be due exclusively to enzyme synthesis because of pantoprazole binding to cysteine

822, at a location within the ion transport pathway deep within the membrane domain of H+, K+-ATPase, rendering it less accessible to reducing agents. These differences in the reversal of acid inhibition have not been shown to be clinically relevant.

Structures

All PPIs have a common core structure consisting of 2-(pyridine methylsulfinyl) benzimadazole,[61] but vary in their substitutions in the pyridine and benzimidazole moieties (see Fig. 1.6). All except esomeprazole are comprised of S and R optical isomers, while esomeprazole is the S-isomer of omeprazole.[62,63] The R-isomer of omeprazole is metabolized more rapidly by the P450 enzyme CYP 2C19 than the S-isomer, which is metabolized more slowly by CYP 3A4. Esomeprazole was prepared exclusively as the S-isomer to take advantage of its more sustained presence in the circulation in order to enhance its potency in inhibiting gastric acid secretion.

Duration of actions

Peak circulating blood concentrations of orally administered PPIs are reached about 2–5 hours after ingestion. The plasma half-lives of PPIs are relatively short and are slightly less than 2 hours (usually 60–90 minutes). These values for peak circulating blood concentrations and plasma half-lives contrast with the duration of gastric acid secretory inhibition produced by these agents, which are much longer because of the covalent attachment of the protonated PPI derivative to the H+, K+-ATPase enzyme molecule. As stated above, the initial dose of a PPI will inhibit only activated H+,K+-ATPase present in the canalicular membrane.[28] As inactive enzyme is recruited into the secretory canaliculus, acid secretion will resume, albeit at a reduced level. After a second dose, more enzyme will have been recruited and subsequently inhibited, and after a third dose, additional recruitment and further acid inhibition may be expected. Once-daily PPI dosing results in 65–70% steady-state inhibition of maximal acid output after 4–5 days.[28] Based on these pharmacokinetic properties, the occasional use of currently formulated PPIs taken on an 'as needed' basis would not be expected to provide adequate acid inhibition and would be unlikely to produce a consistent or satisfactory clinical response.[28]

The clearance of biologically active PPIs from the circulation is not influenced by renal insufficiency,[64] and the renal secretory products of PPI metabolism are inactive. Although hepatic failure can reduce the rate of hepatic clearance of PPIs, this effect is insufficient to require dose adjustments in patients with liver dysfunction.

Metabolism and adverse effects

PPIs have been documented to be safe and effective in the inhibition of gastric acid secretion for the treatment of patients with acid-related diseases. These drugs are metabolized by the hepatic cytochrome P450 mixed oxidase enzyme system, mostly by CYP 2C19. Serious side effects resulting from PPI administration are rare, the most common being headache, diarrhea, and abdominal pain. These side effects have been found in approximately comparable frequency in those receiving PPIs or placebo. The inhibition of gastric acid secretion can reduce the intestinal absorption of some drugs, such as digoxin or ketoconazole, which are absorbed more efficiently when administration of these drugs is accompanied in the presence of gastric acid. Based on these observations, it has been recommended that serum digoxin levels be monitored in patients being treated with PPIs. Antifungal agents other than ketoconazole are recommended when such therapy is required in patients who are also receiving concomitant PPIs (see Ch. 6). The protracted use of PPIs may reduce absorption of some nutrients. Because of their potency in increasing gastric luminal pH, PPI therapy has been associated with changes in gut flora and/or small intestinal bacterial overgrowth. Moreover, a recent study reported an association between PPI use and community-acquired pneumonia, presumably a result of pathogen colonization of the upper gastrointestinal tract.[65]

Hypergastrinemia may be produced by PPIs in response to the inhibition of gastric acid secretion and secondary increases in intragastric pH.[37] The normal mechanism for inhibition of gastrin release is negative feedback control, whereby acid in the gastric lumen stimulates somatostatin release by paracrine communication with nearby G cells, inhibiting further gastrin release. Elevation of gastric pH by PPIs (or by any agent that increases intragastric pH) interferes with, or abolishes, this feedback control mechanism, permitting continued biosynthesis and release of gastrin. The magnitude of increase in serum gastrin levels by PPIs is usually relatively small. In general, the more potent and the more sustained the inhibition of acid secretion, the greater the likelihood and magnitude of serum gastrin increases. Substantial increases in serum gastrin levels to levels greater than 400 pg per ml have been reported in about 5% of patients receiving prolonged therapy with PPIs.[66] Elevated serum gastrin levels usually return to normal within 2–4 weeks after discontinuance of treatment. H2RAs also possess the capacity to increase serum gastrin levels, but the increases are usually not as great nor do they occur as frequently as those observed with PPIs. Similar to H2RAs, rebound increases in gastric acid secretion may also occur after discontinuation of PPI therapy. Sustained elevations of serum gastrin levels may precipitate ECL cell proliferation and increased histamine release, contributing to increased gastric acid secretion.[37] The clinical consequences of rebound hypersecretion remain undetermined.

In addition to its role in stimulating gastric acid secretion, gastrin is also a trophic hormone and stimulates replication of a variety of cells, including ECL cells. PPIs have been shown to produce ECL cell hyperplasia and carcinoid tumors of ECL cells in rats. The phenomenon of carcinoid tumors in response to PPI-induced hypergastrinemia appears to be unique to rodents. The reasons for such interspecies differences are not entirely evident, but are probably related in part to a lower mucosal ECL cell density and a considerably less-pronounced increase in circulating gastrin in humans compared to rodents in response to antisecretory medications.[28] In some instances, ECL cell hyperplasia may be found in stomachs of patients with hypergastrinemia receiving chronic PPI treatment for acid-related diseases. However, ECL cell carcinoid tumors have not been reported in humans in response to PPIs nor to any other antisecretory drug.[67] Carcinoid tumors of ECL cells have been observed in some patients with the Zollinger-Ellison syndrome, almost always in those with multiple endocrine neoplasia type I (MEN-I), suggesting the contribution of an additional genetic factor(s) in those patients.[68] Carcinoid tumors of ECL cells have also been reported in patients with pernicious anemia and associated chronic atrophic gastritis. In patients with the Zollinger-Ellison syndrome and pernicious anemia, serum gastrin levels are usually substantially greater than those observed in patients with hypergastrinemia produced by PPI therapy. One area of theoretical concern that has not been completely resolved is the possible effect of gastrin and its precursor prohormones on promoting the growth of colonic and other gastrointestinal neoplasms.[28]

SUMMARY

Although most patients with acid-related diseases are not hypersecretors of gastric acid, hydrochloric acid secreted by the stomach plays a crucial role in the pathogenesis of all acid-related diseases. Inhibition of acid secretion by the gastric parietal cell is the basis for current treatment and prevention of acid-related diseases. Multiple endocrine, neurocrine, paracrine, and autocrine factors contribute to the complex regulation of acid secretion by the parietal cell. The most potent physiological stimulus to gastric acid secretion is the release of gastrin in response to products of protein digestion, resulting in gastrin binding to enterochromaffin-like (ECL) cells and in secondary histamine synthesis and release. Histamine binds to H_2 receptors on adjacent parietal cells, stimulating secretion of hydrochloric acid. Histamine, in concert with gastrin, is the major direct physiological stimulus to parietal cell secretion of acid. Somatostatin plays the most important role in the physiological regulatory inhibition of gastric acid secretion. The development of H_2-receptor antagonists and proton pump inhibitors revolutionized the treatment of acid-related diseases. Four H_2-receptor antagonists (cimetidine, ranitidine, famotidine, and nizatidine) have been developed as competitive inhibitors of histamine binding to receptors. The H_2-receptor antagonists are structural analogs of histamine designed with variable substitutions of the imidizole ring of histamine and its single structural side chain. H_2-receptor antagonists are safe and effective and induce rapid inhibition of gastric acid secretion. Continuous treatment with these agents may result in tolerance, which can attenuate acid secretory inhibition by 50%.

Proton pump inhibitors (omeprazole, lanzoprazole, pantoprazole, rabeprazole, and esomeprazole) inhibit parietal cell H+, K+-ATPase, the final step in gastric acid secretion (Fig. 1.9). The proton pump inhibitors are substituted benzimidazoles, which share an identical backbone structure with variable substitutions in their respective side chains. Esomeprazole, the S-isomer of omeprazole, is metabolized more slowly by the P450 enzyme CYP 3A4 than the R-isomer of omeprazole, which is metabolized by CYP 2C19, resulting in slower metabolic disposal of the S-isomer. PPIs are prodrugs with a pKa of 4–5, which are absorbed, secreted, and concentrated in the highly acidic (pH 0.8–2.0) secretory canaliculi of the parietal cells to levels 1000 times greater than the plasma concentration. The prodrug PPIs are concentrated, protonated, and converted to sulfenamide moieties, which form covalent disulfide bonds with available cysteine residues located on the luminal surface of the parietal cell secretory canaliculus.

See Chapters 13, 19, and 20 for dosing of H_2-receptor antagonists and proton pump inhibitors in the treatment of various acid-related disorders.

REFERENCES

1. Prout W. On the nature of the acid and saline matters usually existing in the stomach of animals. Philos Trans 1824; 114:45.

2. Black JW, Duncan WAM, Durant CJ, et al. Definition and antagonism of histamine H_2 receptors. Nature 1972; 236:385–390.

In this publication James Black and colleagues identified and characterized the histamine 2 receptor and demonstrated the ability of a structural analog of histamine to inhibit the activity of this receptor. They showed that burimamide, the first H_2 receptor antagonist evaluated, inhibited pentagastrin stimulated gastric acid secretion. They also noted that this compound, which they referred to as a histamine 2 antagonist, did not inhibit cholinergic secretion. In this article they also quoted F.C. McIntosh who in 1938 proposed that histamine in the gastric mucosa might be the local common mediator for secretion. Black expressed agreement with the position of Charles Code that histamine is involved in the actions of gastrin. Black concluded that the balance of opinion must tip toward the idea that the actions of gastrin are somewhat coupled with those of histamine.

3. Brimblecombe RW, Duncan WAM, Durant CJ, et al. Characterization and development of cimetidine as a histamine H_2 receptor antagonist. Gastroenterology 1978; 74:339–348.

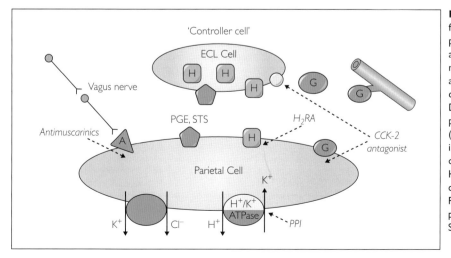

Fig. 1.9 • Schematic representation of the factors influencing gastric acid secretion by the parietal cell, depicting neurocrine (acetylcholine and other neurotransmitters from vagal efferent neurons), paracrine (somatostatin from D cells and histamine from gastric enterochromaffin-like cells), and endocrine (circulating gastrin) factors. Dashed arrows indicate potential sites of pharmacologic inhibition of acid secretion (in italics), either via receptor antagonism or via inhibition of H+,K+-ATPase. A, acetylcholine and other neurotransmitters; H, histamine; H2RA, H_2-receptor antagonist; G, gastrin; CCK-2, cholecystokinin-2 (gastrin) receptor antagonist; PG, prostaglandin; S, somatostatin; PPI, proton pump inhibitor. Adapted from Wolfe MM and Sachs G (reference 28).

4. Grant SM, Lagtry HD, Brogden RN. Ranitidine: An updated review of its pharmacodynamic and pharmacokinetic properties and therapeutic use in peptic ulcer diseases and other allied diseases. Drugs 1989; 37:801–870.

5. Langtry HD, Grant SM, Goa KL. Famotidine: An updated review of its pharmacodynamic and pharmacokinetic properties and therapeutic use in peptic ulcer disease and other allied diseases. Drugs 1989; 38:551–590.

6. Price AH, Brogden RN. Nizatidine: A preliminary review of its pharmacodynamic and pharmacokinetic properties, and its therapeutic use in peptic ulcer disease. Drugs 1988; 36:521–539.

7. Cederberg C, Andersson T, Skanberg I. Omeprazole: Pharmacokinetics and metabolism in man. Scand J Gastroenterol Suppl 1989; 166:33–40.

8. Clissold SP, Campoli-Richards DM. Omeprazole: A preliminary review of its pharmacodynamic and pharmacokinetic properties, and therapeutic potential in peptic ulcer disease and Zollinger-Ellison syndrome. Drugs 1986; 32:15–47.

9. Lindstrom E, Bjorkqvist M, Boketoft A, et al. Neurohormonal regulation of histamine and pancreastatin secretion from isolated rat stomach ECL cells. Regul Pept 1997; 71:73–86.

10. Forte JG, Soll A. Cell biology of hydrochloric acid secretion. In: Forte JG, Schultz SG, Rauner BB, et al., eds. Handbook of physiology, section 6, the gastrointestinal system, vol. 3. Bethesda, MD: American Physiological Society; 1989:207–228.

11. Hersey SJ, Sachs G. Gastric acid secretion. Physiol Rev 1995; 75:155–187.

12. Sawaguchi A, McDonald KL, Forte JG. High-pressure freezing of isolated gastric glands provides new insight into the fine structure and subcellular localization of H+/K+-ATPase in gastric parietal cells. J Histochem Cytochem 2004; 52(1):77–86.

Sawaguchi, McDonald, and Forte utilized immunocytochemical and ultrastructural techniques coupled with high-pressure freezing in the study of the morphology and function of rabbit gastric parietal cells, especially as related to the hydrogen potassium ATPase proton pump. They studied the parietal cell and its subcellular components in the fasting and stimulating state. They found that there was no change in the concentration of ATPase in cytoplasmic tubulovesicles with stimulation compared with the resting state. In contrast, there was at least a fourfold increase in the density of hydrogen potassium ATPase in the intracellular canaliculi of stimulated cells compared with unstimulated parietal cells.

13. Modlin IM, Tang LH. The gastric enterochromaffin-like cell: An enigmatic cellular link. Gastroenterology 1996; 111:783–810.

14. Sachs G, Prinz C. Gastric enterochromaffin-like cells and the regulation of acid secretion. News Physiol Sci 1996; 11:57–62.

15. Feldman M. Gastrin secretion: normal and abnormal. In: Gastrointestinal diseases. Feldman M, Scharschmidt BF, Sleisenger MH, eds. 6th edn. Philadelphia: WB Saunders Company; 1997:587–603.

16. Chew CS. Inhibitory action of somatostatin on isolated gastric glands and parietal cells. Am J Physiol 1983; 245:G221–G229.

17. Walsh JH. Gastrointestinal hormones. In: Johnson LR, ed. Physiology of the gastrointestinal tract. New York: Raven Press; 1994:1–129.

18. Hirschowitz BI, Fong J, Molina E. Effects of pirenzepine and atropine on vagal and cholinergic gastric secretion and gastrin release and on heart rate in the dog. J Pharmacol Exp Ther 1983; 225:263–268.

19. Pfeiffer AH, Rochlitz B, Noelke R, et al. Muscarinic receptors mediating acid secretion in isolated rat gastric parietal cells are of M3 type. Gastroenterology 1990; 98:218–222.

20. Kajimura M, Reuben MA, Sachs G. The muscarinic receptor gene expressed in rabbit parietal cells is the m3 subtype. Gastroenterology 1992; 103:870–875.

21. Gantz I, Schaffer M, Del Valle J, et al. Molecular cloning of a gene encoding the histamine H_2 receptor (erratum). Proc Natl Acad Sci USA 1991; 88:5937.

22. Del Valle J, Gantz I. Novel insights into histamine H_2 receptor biology. Am J Physiol 1997; 273:G987–G996.

23. Hughes DG, Dowling EA, De Meersman RE, et al. Cardiovascular effects of H_2-receptor antagonists. J Clin Pharmacol 1989; 29:472–477.

24. Bakke I, Qvistad G, Sandik AK, Waldum HL. CCK-2 receptors located on the ECL cell but not on the parietal cell. Scan J of Gastroenterol 2001; 36:1128–1133.

25. Petersen OH, Petersen CCH, Kasai H. Calcium and hormone action. Annu Rev Physiol 1994; 56:297–319.

26. Chew CS. Intracellular activation events for parietal cell hydrochloric acid secretion. In: Forte JG, Schultz SG, Rauner BB, et al., eds. Handbook of physiology, section 6. the gastrointestinal system, vol. 3. Bethesda, MD: American Physiological Society; 1989:255–266.

27. Nwokolo CU, Smith JT, Gavey C, et al. Tolerance during 29 days of conventional dosing with cimetidine, nizatidine, famotidine or ranitidine. Aliment Pharmacol Ther 45 (Suppl 1) 1990; 29–45.

28. Wolfe MM, Sachs G. Acid suppression: Optimizing therapy for gastroduodenal ulcer healing, gastroesophageal reflux disease and stress-related erosive syndrome. Gastroenterology 2000; 118:59–531.

Wolfe and Sachs have discussed acid suppression and in particular in regard to optimizing therapy for gastric and duodenal ulcer healing, gastroesophageal reflux disease and stress-related erosive syndrome. In this paper they review some of the fundamental biology that relates to the drugs and their targets as well as to place that in perspective in the various diseases under consideration.

29. Smith SR, Kendall MJ. Ranitidine versus cimetidine: A comparison of their potential to cause clinically important drug interactions. Clin Pharmacokinet 1988; 15:44–56.

30. Hansten PD. Drug interactions with antisecretory agents. Aliment Pharmacol Ther 1991; 5(Suppl 1):121–128.

31. Kumar A. Cimetidine: An immunomodulator, DICP 1990; 24:289–295.

32. Cantu TG, Korek JS. Central nervous system reactions to histamine₂ receptor blockers. Ann Intern Med 1991; 114:1027–1034.

33. Lewis JH. Hepatic effects of drugs used in the treatment of peptic ulcer disease. Am J Gastroenterol 1987; 82:987–1003.

34. Feldman M, Burton ME. Histamine₂-receptor antagonists: Standard therapy for acid-peptic diseases. N Engl J Med 1990; 323:1672–1680; 1749–1755.

35. Miller TA, Robinson M. H_2-receptor antagonists and blood alcohol levels. Gastroenterology 1992; 103:1102–1104.

36. Prewett EJ, Hudson M, Nwokolo CU, et al. Nocturnal intragastric acidity during and after a period of dosing with either ranitidine or omeprazole. Gastroenterology 1991; 100:873–877.

37. Qvigstad G, Waldum H. Rebound hypersecretion after inhibition of gastric acid secretion. Pharmacol Toxicol 2004; 94(5):202–208.

Qvigstad and Waldum in this publication described the observations of rebound hypersecretion after inhibition of gastric acid secretion. They reviewed the phenomenon of acid secretory rebound after periods of treatment with either a histamine 2 receptor antagonist or a proton pump inhibitor. They noted that long-term inhibition of gastric acid output is accompanied by elevated serum gastrin levels which have the capacity to activate ECL cells and cause their proliferation, resulting in increased amounts of histamine mobilized from the cells and made available to stimulate parietal cells. They did note that the clinical consequences of rebound hypersecretion have not been settled.

38. Fellenius E, Berglindh T, Sachs G, et al. Substituted benzimidazoles inhibit gastric acid secretion by blocking (H+ + K+) ATPase. Nature 1981; 290:159–161.

In this publication Fellenius and colleagues identified the capacity of substituted benzimidazoles, which would include all of the modern proton pump inhibitors, to inhibit hydrogen potassium ATPase which they isolated from rabbit and human gastric mucosa. They found this enzyme only on the secretory surface of the parietal cell and noted that it catalyzed exchange of protons and potassium ions. They referred to this enzyme as a proton pump and suggested it may be the terminal or one of the terminal steps in the acid secretory process. They concluded by suggesting such an inhibitory action may be a highly selective clinical means of suppressing the acid secretory process.

39. Sachs G, Shin JM, Briving C, et al. The pharmacology of the gastric acid pump: The H+,K+ ATPase. Annu Rev Pharmacol Toxicol 1995; 35:277–305.

40. Shin JM, Sachs G. Restoration of acid secretion following treatment with proton pump inhibitors. Gastroenterology 2002; 123:1588–1597.

In this publication Shin and Sachs demonstrated the restoration of acid secretion after inhibition of secretion by proton pump inhibitors and the effects of reducing agents, dithiothreitol and glutathione. They demonstrated that these reducing agents have the capacity to cleave disulfide bonds between cysteine and the proton pump inhibitor. These studies in rats showed that they could induce reactivation of ATPase following inhibition by omeprazole or its enantiomers completely with dithiothreitol and 89% with glutathione. Similar data were found for lanzoprazole or rabeprazole. No reaction by either reducing agent was seen following inhibition by pantroprazole. They concluded that recovery of acid secretion after inhibition by all PPIs other than pantroprazole may depend not only on protein turnover but also on reversal of the inhibitory disulfide bond. They suggested that recovery of acid secretion after pantroprazole may depend entirely on new protein synthesis.

41. Sachs G, Carlsson E, Lindberg P, et al. Gastric H,K-ATPase as therapeutic target. Annu Rev Pharmacol Toxicol 1988; 28:269–284.

42. Rabon EC, Reuben MA. The mechanism and structure of the gastric H, K-ATPase. Annu Rev Physiol 1990; 52:321–344.

43. Fujisaki HH, Sahibata K, Oketani M, et al. Inhibitions of acid secretion by E3810 and omeprazole and their reversal by glutathione. Biochem Pharmacol 1991; 42:321–328.

44. Kromer W. Relative efficacies of gastric proton-pump inhibitors on a milligram basis: desired and undesired SH reactions. Impact of chirality. Scand J Gastroenterology 2001; 36(Suppl 234):3–9.

45. [No authors listed]. Omeprazole/antacid-powder suspension-Santarus: Acitrel Rapinex Powder for oral suspension, SAN 05. Drugs RD. 2004; 5(4):234–235.

46. Sachs G. Physiology of the parietal cell and therapeutic implications. Pharmacotherapy 2003; 23:685–735.

47. Shin JM, Cho YM, Sachs G. Chemistry of covalent inhibition of the gastric (H (+), K (+))-ATPase by proton pump inhibitors. J Am Chem Soc 2004; 30:7800–7811.

48. Huber R, Kohl B, Sachs G, et al. The continuing development of proton pump inhibitors with particular reference to pantoprazole. Aliment Pharmacol Ther 1995; 9:363–378.

49. Besancon M, Shin JM, Mercier F, et al. Membrane topology and omeprazole labeling of the gastric HK-adenosine triphosphatase. Biochemistry 1993; 32:2345–2355.

50. Sachs G, Shin JM, Besancon M, et al. The continuing development of gastric acid pump inhibitors. Aliment Pharmacol Ther 1993; 7:4–12.

51. Shin JM, Besancon M, Simon A, et al. The site of action of pantoprazole in the gastric H/K-ATPase. Biochim Biophys Acta 1993; 1148:223–233.

52. Sachs G, Shin JM, Briving C, et al. The pharmacology of the gastric acid pump the H+K+ ATPase. Ann Rev Pharmacol Toxicol 1995; 35:277–305.

53. Munson K, Lambrecht N, Shin JM, et al. Analysis of the membrane domain of the gastric H(+)/K(+)-ATPase. J Exp Biol 2000; 203:161–170.

54. Gedda K, Scott D, Besancon M, et al. Turnover of the gastric H+,K+-adenosine triphosphatase alpha subunit and its effect on inhibition of rat gastric acid secretion. Gastroenterology 1995; 109:1134–1141.

55. Im WB, Blakeman DP, Davis JP. Irreversible inactivation of rat gastric (H+-K+)-ATPase in vivo by omeprazole. Biochem Biophy Res Commun 1985; 126:78–82.

56. Katashima M, Yamamoto K, Tokuma Y, et al. Comparative pharmacokinetic/pharmacodynamic analysis of proton pump inhibitors omeprazole, lansoprazole and pantaoprazole, in humans. J Drug Metab Pharmacokinet 1998; 23:19–26.

57. Dammann HG, Burkhardt F, Wolf N. The effects of oral rabeprazole on endocrine and gastric secretory function in healthy volunteers. Aliment Pharmacol Ther 1999; 13:1195–1203.

58. Prakash A, Faulds D. Rabeprazole. Drugs 1998; 55:261–267.

59. Williams MP, Sercombe J, Hamilton MI, et al. A placebo controlled trial of the effects of 8 days of dosing with rabeprazole versus omeprazole on 24-hr intragastric acidity and plasma gastrin concentration in health young male subjects. Aliment Pharmacol Ther 1998; 12:1079–1089.

60. Ohning GV, Barbuti RC, Kovacs TO, et al. Rabeprazole produced rapid, potent and long-acting inhibition of gastric acid secretion in subjects with *Helicobacter pylori* infection. Aliment Pharmacol Ther 2000; 12:701–708.

61. Lindberg P, Nordberg O, Alminger T, et al. The mechanism of action of the gastric acid secretion inhibitor omeprazole. J Med Chem 1986; 29:1327–1329.

62. Andersson T, Hassan-Alin M, Hasselgren G, et al. Pharmacokinetic studies with esomeprazole, the (S)-isomer of omeprazole. Clin Pharmacokinet 2001; 40:411–426.

63. Andersson T, Rohss K, Bredberg E, et al. Pharmacokinetics and pharmacodynamics of esomeprazole, the S-isomer of omeprazole. Aliment Pharmacol Ther 2001; 15:1563–1569.

64. Andersson T. Pharmacokinetics, metabolism, and interactions of acid pump inhibitors: Focus on omeprazole, lansoprazole, and pantoprazole. Clin Pharmacokinet 1996; 3:9–28.

65. Laheij RJF, Sturkenboom MCJM, Hassingf R-J, et al. Risk of community-acquired pneumonia and use of gastric acid-suppressive drugs. JAMA 2004; 292:1955–1960.

66. Kuipers EJ, Meuwissen SG. The efficacy and safety of long-term omeprazole treatment for gastroesophageal reflux disease. Gastroenterology 2000; 118:795–798.

67. Laine L, Ahnen D, McClain C, et al. Potential gastrointestinal effects of long-term acid suppression with proton pump inhibitors. Aliment Pharmacol Ther 2000; 14:651–658.

68. Maton PN, Lack EE, Collen MJ, et al. The effect of Zollinger-Ellison syndrome and omeprazole therapy on gastric oxyntic endocrine cells. Gastroenterology 1990; 99:943–950.

CHAPTER TWO

2

Pharmacology and therapeutics for motor and sensory disorders of the gut

Michael Camilleri

INTRODUCTION

Gastrointestinal motility and sensation are regulated by a complex balance of inhibitory and excitatory neuronal, humoral, and mechanical factors.[1,2] Disorders of motility can result from a disruption of the balance between these factors and is manifested by a variety of gastrointestinal complaints such as nausea, vomiting, abdominal pain, distention, constipation, and diarrhea. The goal in the management of disorders of motility and sensation is to maintain decreasing symptoms, and maintain adequate nutrition. This can be accomplished by the judicious use of medications, nutritional support, and in some patients behavioral modifications including biofeedback. This chapter reviews the medications available for stimulating coordinated motor function and for reducing symptoms arising in the human gastrointestinal tract in disease.

Prokinetic agents are drugs that stimulate coordinated gastro-intestinal motility. Gastrointestinal motor function is important for the digestion of chyme and aborad movement of residue through the bowel. An element of gastrointestinal motor dysfunction is important in neuromuscular disorders. For example, in one study, about 50% of unselected patients in a diabetic clinic had evidence of gastric emptying disorder (predominantly stasis). However, there is also a component of motor dysfunction in the common clinical syndromes in the spectrum of functional gastrointestinal disorders, such as gastroesophageal reflux, functional dyspepsia, constipation, and irritable bowel syndrome which affects respectively about 30%, 20%, 5%, and 15% of the US population, respectively. All of these conditions are associated with hypersensitivity of the affected viscus.

The anatomical substrate of visceral sensation[3] and the potential approaches for relief of pain is reflected in the neural centers and pathways involved in pain sensation (Fig. 2.1).

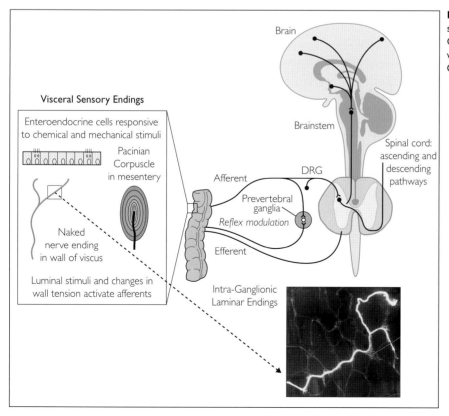

Fig. 2.1 • Anatomical substrate of visceral sensation (Inset: Reprinted from Lynn et al, Gastroenterology 2003; 125:786–794. © 2003, with permission from The American Gastroenterological Association).

Medications may be directed to central processes to reduce the perception of pain or activate centers that are involved in the down-regulation of pain sensation or descending pathways that reduce the ability of the dorsal horn neuron to activate ascending pathways that bring afferent signals to conscious sensation. Antinociception is currently a goal for treatment of many disorders that present features of visceral hypersensitivity. There are few agents that have been recently introduced for treating these disorders of gastrointestinal function.

The common endpoint for many current prokinetics is the M_3 muscarinic receptor on the smooth muscle cells (Fig. 2.2). These receptors are activated by release of acetylcholine from intrinsic cholinergic neurons, which are, in turn, stimulated or inhibited by other neurons. A second common pathway is the activation of cyclic nucleotides in smooth muscle cells which results in contraction or relaxation. Thus, cGMP is activated by extrinsic nitric oxide or by transmitters from other inhibitory neurons (e.g., opiate, somatostatin, VIP). Pharmacological approaches also change intracellular cyclic nucleotide levels, e.g., phosphodiesterase 5 inhibitors, such as sildenafil, increases cGMP levels and results in relaxation of smooth muscle.

This chapter focuses on the compounds that affect motor and sensory functions, and these form the basis for pharmacotherapeutics for several common gastrointestinal disorders. Each section of the chapter includes novel approaches being developed for future application.

LAXATIVES

Mechanism of action

Laxatives may act by changing the bulk of stool, its consistency (osmotic agents), or the frequency of defecation. Laxatives such as psyllium are thought to relieve constipation by increasing the bulk of the stool, therefore physically stimulating the colon, and by decreasing stool hardness. Bulk laxatives also induce irregular unorganized colonic contractions[4,5] and alter small intestinal contractile activity.[6] Ingestion of fiber leads to prolongation of the postprandial disruption of the migratory motor complex, and psyllium has also been shown to induce clustered contractions in the small intestine.

Osmotic laxatives include milk of magnesia, lactulose, and polyethylene glycol-electrolyte solutions. They produce a laxative effect by imposing a nonabsorbable intraluminal osmotic load in the intestine, thereby increasing stool volume and reducing consistency.

Stimulant laxatives such as bisacodyl increase colonic secretion and stimulate reflexes resulting in peristaltic contractile activity. Stimulant laxatives also increase small intestinal secretions and contractile activity. Long-term use of stimulant laxatives such as senna may be associated with habituation and a cathartic colon, that is, an atonic colon without haustrations.

Clinical efficacy

Laxatives play an important role in the patient with chronic constipation or with a decreased ability to initiate defecation. Table 2.1 lists commonly available laxatives, mode of action, and the recommended doses from a recently published review.[7] In patients with anal incontinence of solid stool, the use of a stimulant laxative twice weekly to facilitate emptying of the colon can help decrease the number of episodes of incontinence. In patients with predominantly liquid stool incontinence, fiber may increase stool consistency and decrease incontinence.

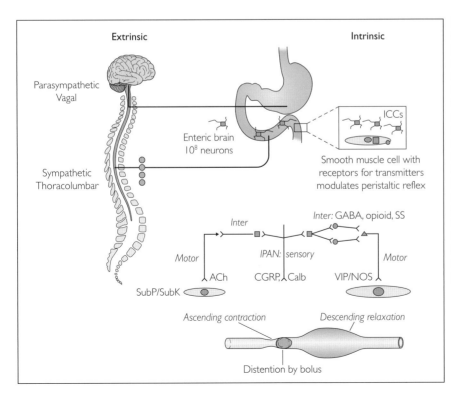

Fig. 2.2 • Control of gastrointestinal motility: extrinsic, enteric, and myogenic. Intrinsic neurons involved in the peristaltic reflex. Note that a distending stimulus within the gut results in ascending excitatory responses through motor neurons that contain predominantly choline acetyltransferase as well as tachykinins such as substance P and substance K. The same distention also results in descending inhibition which relaxes the intestine. This pathway involves several interneurons containing transmitters such as somatostatin, GABA, opiates, and, ultimately, inhibitory motor neurons containing VIP and nitric oxide synthase. SS, somatostatin; GABA, gamma amino butyric acid; VIP, vasoactive intestinal polypeptide; NOS, nitric oxide synthase; Ach, acetylcholine; Sub P, substance P; Sub K, substance K; Calb, calbindin; CGRP, calcitonin gene related peptide; IPAN, intrinsic primary afferant neuron.

Table 2.1 Medications commonly used for constipation
(Adapted from Lembo T, Camilleri M, New England Journal of Medicine 2003; 349:1360–1368. © 2003, with permission from Massachusetts Medical Society)

	Examples and generic name(s)	Dosage	Mode of action; pertinent comments
A) Bulk laxatives	Psyllium, Methylcellulose, Polycarbophil	up to ≈20 g	Natural or synthetic fibers increase colonic residue, stimulating peristalsis; bacterial degradation of *natural* fibers may contribute to bloating and flatus. Allergic reactions such as anaphylaxis and asthma are rare.
B) Osmotic laxatives	Saline Laxatives Magnesium hydroxide Magnesium citrate Sodium phosphate	15–30 mL q.d.-b.i.d 150–300 mL p.rn. 10–25 mL with 12 oz water p.rn.	Draw water into the intestines along osmotic gradient Hypermagnesemia can occur in patients with renal failure and in children. Hyperphosphatemia in patients with renal insufficiency.
	Poorly absorbed sugars Disaccharides e.g. Lactulose Sugar alcohols e.g. Sorbitol, Mannitol Polyethylene Glycols e.g. with electrolyte, or without PEG-3350	15–30 mL q.d-b.i.d. 15–30 mL q.d.-b.i.d. 17–36 g q.d-b.i.d. in 8 oz water p.rn.	Synthetic, resistant to disaccharidases, not absorbed by small intestine. Undergoes bacterial fermentation in the colon to form SCFAs. Gas, bloating common. Poorly absorbed by human intestine; undergo bacterial fermentation. Organic polymers, poorly absorbed and not metabolized by colonic bacteria.
C) Stimulant laxatives	Anthraquinones e.g. Cascara sagrada Senna Ricinoleic acid e.g. Castor oil Diphenylmethanes e.g. Bisacodyl Sodium Picosulfate	325 mg (or 5 mL) qhs 187 mg qd 15–30 mL qhs 5–10 mg qhs 5–15 mg qhs	Stimulate intestinal motility or secretion Converted by colon bacteria to active form May cause pseudo-melanosis coli; No definitive association with colon cancer or myenteric nerve damage Inhibits intestinal water absorption, increases mucosal permeability and stimulates motility by release of neurotransmitters from enteroendocrine cells. Cramping and severe diarrhea are common. Hydrolyzed by endogenous esterases and stimulates secretion and motility of small intestine and colon. Hydrolyzed to its active form by colonic bacterial enzymes; affects only the colon.
D) Stool softener	Docusate sodium	100 mg bid	Ionic detergents soften stool by allowing water to interact more effectively with solid stool; modest fluid secretion.
E) Emollient	Mineral oil	5–15 mL po qhs	Lubrication eases passage of stool. Long-term use may cause malabsorption of fat-soluble vitamins, anal seepage.
F) Rectal preparations	Phophate enema Mineral oil retention enema Tap water/Soap suds enema Glycerin or Bisacodyl suppositories	100 mL prn 500 mL prn 1500 mL prn 10 mg prn	Initiates evacuation by distending the rectum, softening hard stool, and by topically stimulating the colonic muscle to contract. Hyperphosphatemia and other electrolyte abnormalities can occur if the enema is retained.
G) Pro-kinetics	5-HT$_4$ Agonists e.g. Tegaserod, Renzapride (experimental)	6 mg bid 2–4 mg qd	Stimulation of 5-HT$_4$ receptors in the intestines induces peristalsis. Tegaserod, approved for women with constipation predominant IBS.
H) Others	e.g. Colchicine, Misoprostol	0.6 mg tid 600–2400 µg QD	Data for both medications efficacy limited, side effects common, not recommended.

PROSTAGLANDIN ANALOGS

Misoprostol

Mechanism of action

Misoprostol is a synthetic prostaglandin E_1 analog developed for the prevention of gastric ulcer disease in patients taking nonsteroidal antiinflammatory agents. A frequent side effect of misoprostol use is diarrhea. Prostaglandins may cause diarrhea by several mechanisms including an increase in cAMP production in the enterocyte, leading to secretion,[8] and a change in gastrointestinal motility, leading to a decreased transit time.[9] At higher doses (200–800 µg q.i.d.), misoprostol inhibited intestinal motility and significantly decreased orocecal transit time.[9] It has been proposed for treatment of slow transit constipation,[10] and stimulates colonic long-spike burst activity, which typically causes colonic propulsion.

Uses

At doses of 400–800 µg, q.i.d., misoprostol may be an adjunct to conventional treatment of patients with impaired intestinal transit or slow transit constipation. Its beneficial effects appear to decrease within a few months of initiating treatment.

MACROLIDES

Erythromycin and other macrolides

Mechanism of action

Erythromycin induces beneficial prokinetic effects and gastrointestinal side effects through actions on contractile activity.[11] Erythromycin is a macrolide, distinguished by the presence of a lactone ring.[12] Other macrolides include oleandomycin, azithromycin, and clarithromycin.[12,13] The contractile effects of the macrolides appear to correlate with their ability to displace motilin from its receptor (azithromycin >erythromycin >clarithromycin >oleandomycin).

Two major mechanisms for erythromycin's effects on motility have been reported: stimulation of motilin receptors and a cholinergic mechanism. Erythromycin activates L-type calcium channels, increasing intracellular calcium and causing contraction of single muscle cells.[14]

Clinical efficacy

Erythromycin stimulates gastric emptying in normal subjects and in patients with diabetic gastroparesis.[15] Erythromycin (200 mg i.v.) increased the rate of emptying of liquids and solids. In postvagotomy or idiopathic gastroparesis, similar results are obtained with intravenous and oral preparations of the drug. Erythromycin can stimulate intense fundic[16] and antral contractions,[17,18] resulting in the dumping of solids out of the stomach. This may be a disadvantage since nontriturated solids, unprepared for chemical digestion, are delivered to the small bowel.[19] On the other hand, this property is utilized in clinical practice when nondigestible solids (e.g., bezoars, tubes, blood clot) need to be emptied from the stomach.

The long-term efficacy of erythromycin is less clear, as down-regulation of the motilin receptor may reduce its efficacy. However, one study noted sustained effects for a median time of >6 months when dosages were titrated to permit continued use without intolerable side effects.[20] The dose of erythromycin has to be selected carefully according to the indication; there is evidence that doses lower than 2 mg/kg are needed to induce phase III of the MMC,[21] and may be preferable for small bowel dysmotility. The standard dose used to induce clearance of gastric residue is 3 mg/kg i.v. In patients with gastroparesis who develop recurrent bezoars, i.v. erythromycin (3 mg/kg every 8 hr) induces highly propulsive gastric contractions and dumps nondigestible debris out of the stomach.[22] Intravenous erythromycin can also be used to facilitate placement of nasoduodenal tubes.

Erythromycin at low doses (40 mg i.v.) has been shown to increase contractile events in the *small intestine*.[22] Higher doses (350–400 mg i.v.) appear to decrease small intestinal activity. In patients with pseudo-obstruction or ileus, intravenous erythromycin, at doses ranging from 40 to 250 mg, increased duodenal contractions.[23] Short-term oral administration of erythromycin (40 mg t.i.d.) has also been shown to be beneficial in few patients with chronic intestinal pseudo-obstruction and in a patient with intestinal scleroderma.[24] There are anecdotal reports of i.v. erythromycin use in acute colonic pseudo-obstruction.[25] Erythromycin combined with octreotide was effective in inducing motility and reducing symptoms in an open trial of patients with chronic intestinal pseudo-obstruction (neuropathic or myopathic).[26]

New synthetic motilin agonists that are devoid of antibiotic activity constitute a promising addition to the clinical armamentarium in the treatment of disorders of gastric motility. The most clear indication for their use is in the short-term treatment of gastroparesis, though it is also possible that these medications will be indicated for other acute gastrointestinal motility disorders such as acute colonic pseudo-obstruction or postoperative ileus. For longer-term treatment, new agents are being developed that are not likely to induce tolerance and lose efficacy over a few days or weeks. Formal trials are under way.

Serotonergic agents

5-hydroxytryptamine (5-HT, serotonin) mediates several physiological functions throughout the gastrointestinal tract through several different types of receptors (Fig. 2.3).

5-HT$_4$ AGONISTS

Tegaserod

Tegaserod is an aminoguanidine indole derivative of serotonin that acts as a selective agonist at 5-HT$_4$ receptors.[27]

Mechanism of action

Tegaserod activates 5-HT$_4$ receptors located on excitatory cholinergic neurons of the gastrointestinal tract and probably also on intrinsic primary afferent neurons that are important for activation of the peristaltic reflex. It increases gastrointestinal motility in animal models,[28] healthy male volunteers[29] and in patients with constipation-predominant irritable bowel syndrome,[30] and it may reduce visceral sensation in experimental animal models of visceral hyperalgesia[31] and in humans.[32] Tegaserod is absorbed rapidly after oral administration and distributes widely into tissues. No important drug interactions have been identified.[33] No dose adjustment for age or gender is recommended in tegaserod therapy.[34]

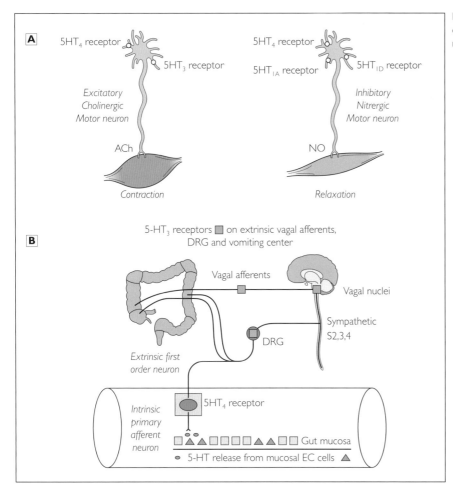

Fig. 2.3 • Summary of the actions of the main currently available serotonergic agents affecting motor (**A**) or sensory (**B**) functions.

Clinical efficacy

Tegaserod, 6 mg, b.i.d., reduces pain and discomfort in the abdominal area, and reduces bloating and constipation. Three studies have appeared in the peer-reviewed literature.[35–37] Improvement of symptoms, particularly constipation, may occur within 1 or 2 weeks of the start of treatment. The efficacy of tegaserod beyond 12 weeks has not been studied extensively.

Adverse effects

The adverse event reported most often in association with tegaserod compared to placebo was diarrhea (9% of patients receiving tegaserod compared to 4% of patients receiving placebo). The discontinuation rate from clinical studies due to diarrhea was 1.6%.[38] Other adverse events such as abdominal pain, flatulence, and headaches appear to be no more frequent with tegaserod than placebo. Safety with long-term use appears good.[39]

Other potential indications

There are several other preliminary reports suggesting the potential use of tegaserod for other conditions, notably chronic constipation, gastroparesis, and functional dyspepsia.

Metoclopramide

Mechanism of action

Metoclopramide antagonizes dopamine at central and peripheral receptor sites. It also activates 5-HT₄ receptors on cholinergic neurons, and it possibly acts directly on smooth muscle.[40,41] Metoclopramide increases lower esophageal sphincter pressure when administered parenterally. Metoclopramide accelerates gastric emptying, relaxes the pyloric sphincter, and increases jejunal peristalsis. Metoclopramide (10 mg, 30 min before meals) increases gastric emptying in diabetic and idiopathic gastroparesis.[40] The symptomatic benefit of metoclopramide in patients with gastroparesis is not always accompanied by a significant acceleration of gastric emptying.[42] Metoclopramide crosses the blood–brain barrier and has direct effects on the vomiting center.

Clinical efficacy

For a decade, cisapride had largely supplanted the use of metoclopramide as an oral prokinetic agent. Side effects occur in approximately 20% of patients given metoclopramide at therapeutic doses.[40] However, with the absence of cisapride and the insufficient studies to date with alternatives such as domperidone and tegaserod, metoclopramide is being used more extensively again. As metoclopramide can be given subcutaneously or parenterally, it has a secondary role (after i.v. erythromycin) during episodes of severe nausea and vomiting when the patient is unable to tolerate oral medications. It can also be administered long-term by the subcutaneous route in patients with gastroparesis.[43]

Adverse effects

Common side effects include anxiety, restlessness, and drowsiness. Extrapyramidal reactions are less common and are usually reversible with diphenhydramine. Tardive dyskinesia is rare,[44] but may be irreversible when it occurs.

NOVEL 5-HT₄ AGONISTS IN DEVELOPMENT

Renzapride

Mechanism of action

Renzapride is a full agonist at 5-hydroxytryptamine 4 (5-HT₄) receptors[45] and is also an antagonist of 5-HT₂ᵦ and 5-HT₃ receptors.[46,47] The 5-HT₄ receptor action mediates increased gut transit rate and perhaps also contributes to the alleviation of symptoms attributed to disordered gastrointestinal motility[46] in constipation-predominant IBS. Activating 5-HT₄ receptors is thought to result in an increase in adenylate cyclase activity that subsequently leads to release of acetylcholine from postsynaptic neurons.[47]

Clinical efficacy

Evidence for renzapride's promise in the treatment of IBS is based on two promising phase IIb trials in constipation-predominant IBS or mixed symptom IBS, which was recently presented in abstract form.[48,49]

A pharmacodynamic study showed that 4 mg renzapride accelerated ascending colon emptying and there was a significant dose-related acceleration of colonic transit in patients with constipation-predominant IBS in whom an evacuation disorder was excluded. The acceleration of transit was associated with an improvement in stool consistency and ease of stool passage during a two-week treatment period.[50]

5-HT₃ AGONISTS

These receptors are located in the motor and sensory apparatus of the rodent gut[51,52] and are the target for antiemetic medications (see section on antagonists below), as well as being antagonized by alosetron and cilansetron in the treatment of IBS. Interestingly, a recent study has shown that an agonist at the 5-HT₃ receptor, MKC 733, slightly delays stomach emptying of liquids and transfer of solids from the proximal stomach, but it significantly accelerates small bowel transit in healthy volunteers.[53] The presumed mechanism of action is activation of cholinergic neurons to stimulate contractions. MKC 733 increased the number of migrating motor complexes recorded in the antrum and duodenum ($p < 0.001$), but had no effect on postprandial motility in healthy volunteers. Effects on colonic transit and trials of clinical efficacy are awaited.

5-HT₃ ANTAGONISTS

Mechanism of action

5-HT₃ receptors are found throughout the enteric nervous system in sensory and motor neurons and in extrinsic sensory neurons, and their activation results in measurable changes in gastrointestinal motility or transit.[54–57]

Granisetron is a 5-HT₃ receptor antagonist which modestly accelerates gastric emptying;[58] this class of compounds (including ondansetron and tropisetron) inhibits chemotherapy-induced

emesis,[59] probably by its effects on visceral afferent function or a direct effect on the vomiting center on the floor of the fourth ventricle.

In healthy volunteers and patients with irritable bowel syndrome, colonic pressure activity increases after a meal. The increase in tone is thought to be mediated by several mechanisms including cholinergic pathways and serotonin through type 3 receptors.[57] Studies in healthy volunteers have shown that *ondansetron* prolongs colonic transit time.[54–56]

Alosetron, the 5-HT₃ receptor antagonist most extensively studied in the gut, exerts effects on several sensorimotor functions. It reduces aggregate symptoms and nausea after a fully satiating meal[60] without altering gastric accommodation[60] or compliance.[61] Alosetron slowed overall and, particularly, ascending colonic transit[62] and increased colonic compliance in diarrhea-predominant IBS, with reduced colonic sensation to volume distention.[63] Alosetron also reduces colonic transit and diarrhea associated with carcinoid syndrome.[64] Recent data from Mayer's group suggest that this class of drug has the ability to change the areas of the brain that respond to visceral pain, and that activation of areas associated with descending modulation may result in reduced sensitivity of the dorsal horn neuron to incoming afferent signals.[65,66]

Clinical efficacy

Although the pharmacology of these compounds is very similar, they are labeled for different indications. The main indications for 5-HT₃ antagonists (e.g., ondansetron) are in the treatment of chemotherapy-induced emesis whereas alosetron is indicated for diarrhea-predominant IBS. 5-HT₃ receptor antagonists such as granisetron and tropisetron have greater in vitro potency, duration of action, and a more linear dose–response relationship when compared to ondansetron. However, clinical trials indicate a similar antiemetic activity and tolerability for all three agents.[67] However, these agents confer no major therapeutic advantage over standard antiemetics after the first couple of days of chemotherapy.

Alosetron is a 5-HT₃ receptor antagonist which has been shown to have potential in clinical practice because of its motor and sensory effects in the gut. Alosetron is approved for the treatment of diarrhea-predominant irritable bowel syndrome. At least six controlled trials have been published with virtually identical efficacy, reviewed in a recent meta-analysis.[68] At a dose of 1 mg daily or 1 mg b.i.d., it is effective in relief of diarrhea, urgency, and pain in IBS. Compared to antidiarrheal agents, it has a favorable efficacy profile, especially since it affords adequate relief of pain and discomfort. Its prescription is restricted to patients with severe IBS.

Adverse effects

About one in four patients receiving alosetron may develop constipation; in trials, this led to cessation of treatment in ≈10% of patients. In practice, this is avoided by spacing out the medication or by using lower doses, e.g., 1 mg per day or every 2 days. Reports of ischemic colitis with use of this medication have led to considerable concern and to its restriction for use in the more severe end of the spectrum of IBS with diarrhea.

Cilansetron

Cilansetron follows on from alosetron with the same presumed mechanism of action, that is, inhibition of cholinergic neurons and of visceral sensory mechanisms (peripherally or centrally). As with alosetron, there is evidence that this 5-HT₃ antagonist is also effective in IBS without constipation, and the benefit-risk ratio will require further appraisal.

5-HT1A AGONIST

Data from studies with buspirone suggest that it may have beneficial effects on rectal sensorimotor function.[69] In a subsequent study, these effects were not observed during colonic distention, and no effect on colonic tone and compliance were observed.[70] Formal studies in IBS are awaited.

REUPTAKE INHIBITORS OF SEROTONIN AND NOREPINEPHRINE

While it has been known for a while that serotonin reuptake inhibitors tend to accelerate small bowel transit,[71] recent data suggest that the combined serotonin and norepinephrine reuptake inhibitors alter colonic tone (preventing the tonic response to feeding), and reduce colonic sensation in response to distention pressures that are in the noxious range, as well as satiation after feeding.[70,72] Other serotonin reuptake inhibitors are being considered for treatment of fibromyalgia and chronic pain syndromes.

μ AND κ OPIOID RECEPTOR MODULATORS

Mechanisms of action

Three types of receptors for opioid peptides have been identified as having effects on human gastrointestinal function: δ, κ, and μ receptors.[73] They all belong to the family of G protein-coupled receptors and reduce intracellular cAMP by inhibiting adenylate cyclase. At the membrane level, they reduce neuronal excitability and neurotransmitter release.[74] Examples of these medications include loperamide (agonist), methyl naltrexone, and alvimopan (antagonists) which are peripherally restricted μ receptor modulators, and fedotozine and asimadoline which are peripherally κ agonists. These agents do not cross the blood–brain barrier. In contrast, other μ agonists such as codeine or morphine and μ antagonists such as naloxone do cross the blood–brain barrier.

The overall effect at the cellular level is thus inhibitory, with reduction in acetylcholine release.

Opioid compounds affect enteric motility, secretion, neurotransmission and inflammation,[75] and nociceptive pathways conducting pain to the central nervous system (reviewed in ref. 76). Clearly, an effective μ opiate such as fentanyl[77] is capable of blunting pain induced by colonic distention, but the central, euphoric, and addictive potential make this an impractical therapy, except in emergencies.

κ agonists such as fedotozine are capable of inhibiting visceral afferents that reflexively inhibit intestinal motility after laparotomy and intestinal handling,[78–80] in contrast the more potent analgesics of the μ opiate variety such as fentanyl and morphine have central effects apart from their peripheral actions.

Clinical efficacy
μ opioids for acute and chronic diarrhea and IBS

Loperamide and diphenoxylate are used worldwide for the treatment of acute and chronic diarrheal states. Stimulation of μ receptors in the myenteric plexus reduces intestinal transit, but this influence seems inferior to the antisecretory effect of that class of compounds.[81] Loperamide appears superior to diphenoxylate in relieving symptoms, in reducing the number of bowel movements, and in improving stool consistency in patients with chronic diarrhea, with less central nervous effects.[82]

In IBS patients who suffer predominantly from diarrhea, treatment with loperamide has proven to be beneficial.[83–85] Loperamide significantly decreased symptoms of diarrhea (mostly reduction in stool frequency and improvement of stool consistency) and urgency in IBS patients compared to controls but did not have a significant effect on the perception of pain.

Alvimopan, a novel μ opioid antagonist

Alvimopan is a selective and competitive antagonist at the μ opioid receptor. The amide hydrolysis product of alvimopan may contribute to the potency and duration of action of alvimopan and the propensity to antagonize the centrally mediated effects of morphine.

Alvimopan has limited (12%) bioavailability with limited absorption and ability to cross the blood–brain-barrier. It reversed oral loperamide effects on GI transit, i.v. morphine, and MS Contin® inhibition of colonic transit ($p<0.01$) without reversing pupillary constriction or analgesia. Alvimopan also prevented nausea following i.v. morphine.

Alvimopan, a selective peripherally acting μ receptor antagonist, can also reduce opioid-induced bowel symptoms without antagonizing centrally mediated opioid effects.[86–88]

Alvimopan relieved symptoms of postoperative ileus, shortened hospitalization, and sped recovery of bowel dysfunction.[86] Alvimopan seems not to interfere with the analgesic effect of concomitant systemic opioids.[87]

Experimental use of novel opioids

Asimadoline, a μ opioid agonist
Mechanism of action

Asimadoline has a high affinity only to μ opioid receptors. In healthy individuals, asimadoline tended to decrease postprandial fullness independent of changes in the gastric volume, increased the capacity for a nutrient drink intake, and decreased fasting colonic tone.[89,90] No serious adverse events were reported with treatment. Adverse events were equally prevalent in the placebo and active treatment groups. Asimadoline reduced colonic sensation in patients with irritable bowel syndrome with minor effects on colonic compliance.[91] There are data to suggest that kappa opiate receptor functions are altered in females, and an effect or interaction with female sex hormones has been postulated.[92,93]

Clinical uses

Clinical trials are awaited.

Fedotozine, a κ opioid agonist

Fedotozine has been proposed as a mediator of visceral hypersensitivity[94] in IBS patients by stimulating κ receptors on peripheral visceral afferent pathways. Fedotozine was slightly superior to placebo in relieving symptoms of abdominal pain and bloating.[95] It also increased thresholds for perception of colonic distention using barostat in IBS patients[94] without affecting colonic compliance. Yet, the clinical efficacy of fedotozine in IBS is unclear.

Naloxone, an opioid antagonist

A study compared *naloxone* versus placebo and showed no significant improvement in the scores for pain, bloating, straining, and urgency in the naloxone group in IBS.[96] However, larger clinical trials are needed to evaluate the usefulness of opioid antagonism in constipation-predominant IBS.

Methylnaltrexone, a nonselective opioid antagonist

Methylnaltrexone is a quaternary ammonium derivative of naltrexone, an opioid antagonist similar to naloxone. It is less lipid soluble than naloxone; thus, it is less likely to cross the blood–brain barrier.[97] It blocks acute morphine-induced delay in orocecal transit time without affecting analgesia,[98] or causing central withdrawal effects. Intravenous methylnaltrexone infusion effectively reversed methadone-induced constipation, increasing stool frequency and decreasing orocecal transit times.[99,100] Orally administered methylnaltrexone showed the same results, attaining very low plasma levels, which suggests that the drug's effect is mainly local in the gut.[101] An enteric-coated form of the compound proved to be even more efficient.[102]

ALPHA-2 ADRENERGIC AGONIST

There is good pharmacodynamic evidence that clonidine reduces colonic pain sensation in response to distention and relaxes colonic compliance and tone.[103–105] A single-center preliminary study of clonidine in IBS with diarrhea suggests that 0.1 mg clonidine b.i.d. may be associated with an improvement in the proportion of patients achieving satisfactory relief of IBS and an improvement in overall bowel function;[106] more definitive studies are required. However, it is clear that excessive somnolence or postural hypotension are dose limiting with clonidine and more gut selectivity would be advantageous with this class of medication.

SOMATOSTATIN ANALOG, OCTREOTIDE

Mechanism of action

Octreotide is a long-acting, cyclized somatostatin analog. In healthy volunteers, octreotide induces a phase III-like wave of motor activity in the duodenum, suggesting a potential role as a prokinetic agent. In a study on 5 healthy subjects and 50 consecutive patients with functional or organic[107] dysmotility, octreotide (50 μg) inhibited antral motility and induced a small intestinal activity front, followed by intestinal quiescence. The activity front was significantly longer and had more rapid propagation than the migratory motor complexes observed in the same individuals. Octreotide also improved abdominal symptoms including nausea, bloating, and abdominal pain in patients with

scleroderma.[108] Symptom improvement may result from decreased visceral perception.[109] Verne et al. used octreotide in combination with erythromycin in an open trial for 6 months.[26] Patients who developed MMC-like activity fronts with octreotide were more prone to derive symptomatic benefit from this treatment.[26] It is unclear which of the two 'prokinetic' agents was responsible for the motor or symptomatic benefit. It is unlikely that symptomatic benefit results from any 'prokinetic' effect, since octreotide retards small bowel transit.[110] In summary, somatostatin analogs are unlikely to be efficacious when used for indications that require prokinetic agents.

In eight healthy volunteers and five patients with diarrhea-predominant irritable bowel syndrome, octreotide (100 μg) increased the threshold to rectal perception, rectal pressure activity, and maximal tolerated volume. Since no effect on rectal compliance was demonstrable, the data suggested inhibition of visceral afferent pathways.[109] Octreotide (50 μg t.i.d) had no significant effect on colonic transit in healthy volunteers with a cleansed colon.[110] However, octreotide reduced the colonic tone increase after a meal in health.

Octreotide (30 or 100 μg) alters gastric accommodation and postprandial sensation.[111]

Clinical efficacy

Octreotide was first used in the treatment of symptoms caused by endocrine tumors such as carcinoid diarrhea and flushing.[112] It is administered as a subcutaneous injection, at typical doses of 50–75 μg t.i.d. Depot preparations are available and have shown some efficacy in short bowel syndrome. Octreotide is unlikely to benefit patients with impaired distal antral motility, and its overall effect in the stomach and small intestine is to delay transit.[110,111] There is a potential role in intestinal scleroderma.[108] In patients with an extrinsic neuropathy, surgical vagotomy with Roux-en-Y gastrojejunostomy, or those with gastric bezoars, octreotide might induce an activity front, but it is unclear whether this actually dumps nondigestible debris out of the stomach. Octreotide is very useful in the treatment of the dumping syndrome, as it retards small intestinal transit and inhibits hormone release[110,113] when administered at modest doses, 25–50 μg s.c., before meals. Somatostatin analogs are best reserved for dumping and accelerated transit.[114] The long-standing depot i.m. preparation retarded small bowel transit in patients with short bowel syndrome.[115] Subcutaneous octreotide is a mainstay for treatment of short bowel syndrome.[116]

CHOLECYSTOKININ MODULATORS

Cholecystokinin (CCK) is a gastrointestinal hormone that is released in response to the ingestion of fat and protein. It plays an important role in the stimulation of pancreatic secretion, gall bladder contraction, regulation of gastrointestinal motility, and induction of satiety.

CCK stimulates discharge of vagal afferent fibers arising from the stomach and intestine, resulting in reflex inhibition of gastric motility, gastric acid secretion, and stimulation of pancreatic enzyme secretion. Thus, endogenous release of CCK (in response to luminal fat or soybean trypsin inhibitor) also alters gastric function through a capsaicin-sensitive pathway, and CCK released from the intestine acts either locally or systemically to stimulate vagal afferent fiber discharge. This alters proximal gastrointestinal function, regulating the entry of food into the duodenum to ensure effective digestion and absorption.[117] CCK is involved in the reflex relaxation of the proximal stomach and effects mediated at least in part by vagal and splanchnic pathways.[117]

CCK receptors in the hypothalamus and CCK-A receptors in the nucleus of the solitary tract are involved in the regulation of food intake.[118–120] Relaxation of the proximal stomach in the postprandial period occurs concurrently with an increase in plasma CCK, and this also coincides with the early phase of intestinal digestion.[121]

CCK-RECEPTOR ANTAGONISTS

Loxiglumide

Mechanism of action

Loxiglumide, a highly specific, competitive CCK-1 antagonist, has been shown to attenuate the effects of CCK on gall-bladder contraction, pancreatic enzyme secretion, and gastric emptying.[122]

Loxiglumide is approximately half as potent as dexloxiglumide but has been shown to produce almost complete and selective blockade of CCK-1 receptors at a dose of 10 mg/kg/h.[123] Dexloxiglumide, the (D-)enantiomer of loxiglumide, is responsible for the pharmacological activity of loxiglumide.[124] Dexloxiglumide is well absorbed and rapidly bioavailable after single oral dose administration in healthy volunteers. Peak plasma concentrations are reached within 1 hour after drug intake; absolute bioavailability is approximately 50% when administered orally as a tablet.

Loxiglumide has been studied as a potential modulator of gastric emptying, accommodation, and colonic motility. Loxiglumide significantly improved constipation in a geriatric population, although its mechanism of action is unclear.[125] Duodenal infusion of 20% lipid resulted in an increase in intragastric volume after placebo which was completely prevented by dexloxiglumide, suggesting that this CCK-1 antagonist has important inhibitory effects on fat-induced, vagally mediated gastric relaxation in the postprandial period.[126]

Clinical efficacy

There is presently no established role for loxiglumide in the clinical management of disorders of gastrointestinal motility. After initial promise, it was decided to discontinue development in the US of dexloxiglumide for constipation-predominant irritable bowel syndrome, based on the outcome of two completed placebo-controlled phase III clinical studies involving over 1400 women and 12 weeks of treatment. Although a numeric trend was observed in favor of dexloxiglumide in both studies, the difference compared to placebo was not statistically significant. On theoretical grounds, one may question whether the choice of the subgroup of IBS patients with predominant constipation was an optimal choice, given the evidence that loxiglumide mimics the effects of atropine on muscle tension of colonic muscle strips and other preliminary data suggesting that dexloxiglumide retards ascending colon emptying.[127]

Potential uses

Given the importance of cholecystokinin in gut physiology in the postprandial period, it is to be expected that this class of compound may eventually find a niche in therapy, such as in gastroparesis, because it accelerates gastric emptying or, in obesity, because it inhibits postprandial accommodation.

CCK AGONIST

Mechanism of action

GI181771X is a 1,5-benzodiazepine that is devoid of classical benzodiazepine properties and is a potent, full CCK-A receptor agonist and a CCK-B receptor antagonist. It reduces food intake in rats; this action is thought to be mediated by activating peripheral CCK-A receptors on vagal afferent fibers and on the pyloric sphincter. Unlike CCK-B, which requires parenteral administration, GI181771 is orally active. The circulating $t_{1/2}$ of GI181771X in healthy humans is ≤4 hours for the solution and suspension formulations and is slightly longer for the tablet formulation. The t_{max} occurs 45 minutes after study drug administration with the solution formulation but is more variable following the tablet.

In a pharmacodynamic study of 61 healthy subjects, GI181771X delayed gastric emptying of solids and increased fasting and postprandial gastric volumes without altering postprandial symptoms. The 1.5 mg oral solution significantly altered these stomach functions relative to placebo. The 5.0 mg form delayed gastric emptying of solids. The increase in fasting gastric volume with this CCK-A agonist suggests the existence of CCK-A receptors that can modulate fasting gastric function.[128]

Clinical uses

The study suggests that further studies are needed to define optimal patients for the medication, such as dyspeptics with reduced gastric accommodation but normal gastric emptying.

SUMMARY

In summary, the main prokinetics used currently in clinical practice are i.v. erythromycin and oral tegaserod. Stimulant laxatives are generally used after bulk and osmotic laxatives prove inadequate in the treatment of constipation. The 5-HT$_3$ antagonist (alosetron) and the 5-HT$_4$ agonist (tegaserod) are approved for the treatment of diarrhea- or constipation-predominant irritable bowel syndrome, respectively. These medications have proven effective repeatedly in well-controlled studies; they impact patients' symptoms in the short- and medium-term (up to 6 months).

Other medications discussed above are either second-line therapies or awaiting confirmatory evidence of clinical efficacy, that is, evidence of symptom relief and facilitation of a return to a state of normal hydration and nutrition in patients with gastrointestinal motility disorders.

REFERENCES

1. Camilleri M. Gastrointestinal motility disorders. In: Scientific American Medicine. Dale DC, ed. New York: Web MD Scientific American Medicine; 2003:788–799.

2. Camilleri M. Enteric nervous system disorders: genetic and molecular insights for the neurogastroenterologist. Neurogastroenterology and Motility 2001; 13:277–295.

3. Camilleri M, Coulie B, Tack JF. Subject review: Visceral hypersensitivity: facts, speculations and challenges. Gut 2001; 48:125–131.

4. Burrows C, Merritt AM. Influence of cellulose on myoelectric activity of proximal canine colon. Am J Physiol 1993; 8:G301–G306.

5. Fioramonti J, Bueno L. Motor activity in the large intestine of the pig related to dietary fibre and retention time. Br J Nutr 1980; 43:155–162.

6. Bueno L, Praddaude F, Fioramonti J, et al. Effect of dietary fiber on gastrointestinal motility and jejunal transit time in dogs. Gastroenterology 1981; 80:701–707.

7. Lembo T, Camilleri M. Chronic constipation. N Engl J Med 2003; 349:1360–1368.

8. Kimberg DV, Field M, Johnson J, et al. Stimulation of intestinal mucosal adenylcyclase by cholera enterotoxin and prostaglandins. J Clin Invest 1971; 50:1218–1230.

9. Soffer EE, Launspach J. Effect of misoprostol on postprandial intestinal motility and orocecal transit time in humans. Dig Dis Sci 1993; 38:851–855.

10. Soffer EE, Metcalf A, Launspach J. Misoprostol is effective treatment for patients with severe chronic constipation. Dig Dis Sci 1994; 39:929–933.

11. Zara GP, Thompson HH, Pilot MA, et al. Effects of erythromycin on gastrointestinal tract motility. J Antimicrob Chemother 1985; 16:175–179.

12. Peeters TL. Erythromycin and other macrolides as prokinetic agents. Gastroenterology 1993; 105:1886–1899.

13. Peeters TL, Depoortere I. Motilin receptor: a model for development of prokinetics. Dig Dis Sci 1994; 39:76S–78S.

14. Corbett CL, Thomas S, Read NW, et al. Electrochemical detector for breath hydrogen determination: measurement of small bowel transit time in normal subjects and patients with the irritable bowel syndrome. Gut 1981; 22:836–840.

15. Janssens J, Peeters T, Vantrappen G, et al. Improvement of gastric emptying in diabetic gastroparesis by erythromycin. N Engl J Med 1990; 322:1028–1031.

Classical paper documenting beneficial effect of macrolides in stimulating gastric emptying.

16. Bruley des Varannes S, Parys V, Ropert A, et al. Erythromycin enhances fasting and postprandial proximal gastric tone in humans. Gastroenterology 1995; 109:32–39.

17. Prather CM, Camilleri M, Thomforde GM, et al. Gastric axial forces in experimentally delayed and accelerated gastric emptying. Am J Physiol 1993; 264:G928–G934.

18. Annese V, Janssens J, Vantrappen G, et al. Erythromycin accelerates gastric emptying by inducing antral contractions and improved gastroduodenal coordination. Gastroenterology 1992; 102:823–828.

19. Lin HC, Sanders SL, Gu YG, et al. Erythromycin accelerates solid emptying at the expense of gastric sieving. Dig Dis Sci 1994; 39:124–128.

20. Richards RD, Davenport K, McCallum RW. The treatment of idiopathic and diabetic gastroparesis with acute intravenous and chronic oral erythromycin. Am J Gastroenterol 1993; 88:203–207.

21. Otterson MF, Sarna SK. Gastrointestinal motor effects of erythromycin. Am J Physiol 1990; 259:G355–G363.

22. Tack J, Janssens J, Vantrappen G, et al. Effect of erythromycin on gastric motility in controls and in diabetic gastroparesis. Gastroenterology 1992; 103:72–79.

23. Chami TN, Schuster MM, Crowell MD, et al. Effects of low dose erythromycin on gastrointestinal motility and symptoms in chronic intestinal pseudo-obstruction. Gastroenterology 1991; 100:A41.

24. Chami TN, Schuster MM, Crowell MD, et al. Pervasive gastrointestinal dysmotility in a patient with scleroderma: response to erythromycin. Gastroenterology 1991; 100:A40.

25. Armstrong DN, Ballantyne GH, Modlin IM. Erythromycin for reflex ileus in Ogilvie's syndrome. Lancet 1991; 337:378.

26. Verne GN, Eaker EY, Hardy E, et al. Effect of octreotide and erythromycin on idiopathic and scleroderma-associated intestinal pseudo-obstruction. Dig Dis Sci 1995; 40:1892–1901.

27. Camilleri M. Review article: tegaserod. Aliment Pharm Ther 2001; 15:277–289.

28. Nguyen A, Camilleri M, Kost LJ, et al. SDZ HTF 919 stimulates canine colonic motility and transit in vivo. J Pharm Exp Ther 1997; 280:1270–1276.

29. Degen L, Matzinger D, Merz M, et al. Tegaserod, a 5-HT4 receptor partial agonist, accelerates gastric emptying and gastrointestinal transit in healthy male subjects. Aliment Pharmacol Ther 2001; 15:1745–1751.

30. Prather CM, Camilleri M, Zinsmeister AR, et al. Tegaserod accelerates orocecal transit in patients with constipation-predominant irritable bowel syndrome. Gastroenterology 2000; 118:463–468.

Pharmacodynamic demonstration of efficacy of 5-HT$_4$-agonist in constipation-predominant irritable bowel syndrome.

31. Schikowski A, Thewissen M, Mathis C, et al. Serotonin type-4 receptors modulate the sensitivity of intramural mechanoreceptive afferents of the cat rectum. Neurogastroenterology and Motility 2002: 14:221–227.

32. Coffin B, Farmachidi JP, Rueegg P, et al. Tegaserod, a 5-HT4 receptor partial agonist, decreases sensitivity to rectal distension in healthy subjects. Aliment Pharmacol Ther 2003; 17:577–585.

33. Appel-Dingemanse S. Clinical pharmacokinetics of tegaserod, a serotonin 5-HT(4) receptor partial agonist with promotile activity. Clin Pharmacokinet 2002; 41:1021–1042.

34. Appel-Dingemanse S, Horowitz A, Campestrini J, et al. The pharmacokinetics of the novel promotile drug, tegaserod, are similar in healthy subjects – male and female, elderly and young. Aliment Pharmacol Ther 2001; 15:937–944.

35. Muller-Lissner SA, Fumagalli I, Bardhan KD, et al. Tegaserod, a 5-HT(4) receptor partial agonist, relieves symptoms in irritable bowel syndrome patients with abdominal pain, bloating and constipation. Aliment Pharmacol Ther 2001; 15:1655–1666

First randomized, controlled trial documenting efficacy of tegaserod in females with constipation-predominant irritable bowel syndrome.

36. Novick J, Miner P, Krause R, et al. A randomized, double-blind, placebo-controlled trial of tegaserod in female patients suffering from irritable bowel syndrome with constipation. Aliment Pharmacol Ther 2002; 16:1877–1888.

37. Kellow J, Lee OY, Chang FY, et al. An Asia-Pacific, double blind, placebo controlled, randomised study to evaluate the efficacy, safety, and tolerability of tegaserod in patients with irritable bowel syndrome. Gut 2003; 52:671–676.

38. Fidelholtz J, Smith W, Rawls J, et al. Safety and tolerability of tegaserod in patients with irritable bowel syndrome and diarrhea symptoms. Am J Gastroenterol 2002; 97:1176–1181.

39. Tougas G, Snape WJ Jr, Otten MH, et al. Long-term safety of tegaserod in patients with constipation-predominant irritable bowel syndrome. Aliment Pharmacol Ther 2002; 16:1701–1708.

40. McCallum RW, Albibi R. Metoclopramide: pharmacology and clinical application. Ann Intern Med 1983; 98:86–92.

41. Cohen S, Morris DW, Schoen HJ, et al. The effect of oral and intravenous metoclopramide on human lower esophageal sphincter pressure. Gastroenterology 1976; 70:484–487.

42. Ricci DA, Saltzman MB, Meyer C, et al. Effect of metoclopramide in diabetic gastroparesis. J Clin Gastroenterol 1985; 7:25–32.

43. McCallum RW, Valenzuela G, Polepalle S, et al. Subcutaneous metoclopramide in the treatment of symptomatic gastroparesis: clinical efficacy and pharmacokinetics. J Pharmacol Exp Ther 1991; 258:136–142.

44. Sewell DD, Jeste DV. Metoclopramide-associated tardive dyskinesia. An analysis of 67 cases. Arch Fam Med 1992; 1:271–278.

45. Dumuis A, Sebben M, Bockaert J. BRL 24924: A potent agonist at a non-classical 5-HT receptor positively coupled with adenylate cyclase in colliculi neurons. Eur J Pharmacol 1989; 162:381–384.

46. Stanniforth DH, Pennick M. Pharmacology of renzapride: a new gastrokinetic benzamide without dopaminergic properties. Eur J Clin Pharmacol 1990; 38:161–216.

47. Dumuis A, Sebben M, Bockaert J. The gastrointestinal prokinetic benzamide derivatives are agonists at the non-classical 5-HT receptor (5-HT$_4$) positively coupled to adenylate cyclase in neurons. Naunyn-Schmiedeberg's Arch Pharmacol 1989; 340:403–410.

48. Meyers, NL, Palmer RMJ, Wray HA, et al. Efficacy and safety of renzapride in patients with constipation-predominant irritable bowel syndrome. Gut 2002; 51:A10.

49. George A, Meyers NL, Palmer RMJ. Efficacy and safety of renzapride in patients with constipation-predominant IBS: a Phase IIb study in the UK primary healthcare setting. Gut 2003; 52:A91.

50. Camilleri M, McKinzie S, J Fox J, et al. Renzapride accelerates colonic transit and improves bowel function in constipation-predominant irritable bowel syndrome (C-IBS). Gastroenterology 2004; 126:A642.

51. Glatzle J, Sternini C, Robin C, et al. Expression of 5-HT3 receptors in the rat gastrointestinal tract. Gastroenterology 2002; 123:217–226.

52. Hillsley K, Grundy D. Sensitivity to 5-hydroxytryptamine in different afferent subpopulations within mesenteric nerves supplying the rat jejunum. J Physiol 1998; 509:717–727.

Basic science demonstration of the importance of 5-HT$_3$ receptors in gut sensation.

53. Coleman NS, Marciani L, Blackshaw E, et al. Effect of a novel 5-HT3 receptor agonist MKC-733 on upper gastrointestinal motility in humans. Aliment Pharmacol Ther 2003; 18:1039–1048.

54. Camilleri M, von der Ohe MR. Drugs effecting serotonin receptors. Bailliere's Clinical Gastroenterology 1994; 8:301–319.

55. Gore S, Gilmore IIT, Haigh CG, et al. Colonic transit in man is slowed by ondansetron (GR 38032F), a selective 5-hydroxytryptamine receptor (type 3) antagonist. Aliment Pharmacol Ther 1990; 4:139–144.

56. Talley NJ, Phillips SF, Haddad A, et al. GR 38032F (Ondansetron), a selective 5-HT$_3$ receptor antagonist, slows colonic transit in healthy man. Dig Dis Sci 1990; 35:477–480.

57. von der Ohe MR, Hanson RB, Camilleri M. Serotonergic mediation of postprandial colonic tonic and phasic responses in humans. Gut 1994; 35:536–541.

58. Akkermans LM, Vos A, Hoekstra A, et al. Effect of ICS 205-930 (a specific 5-HT3 receptor antagonist) on gastric emptying of a solid meal in normal subjects. Gut 1988; 29:1249–1252.

59. Cubeddu LX, Hoffmann IS, Fuenmayor NT, et al. Efficacy of ondansetron (GR38032F) and the role of serotonin in cisplatin-induced nausea and vomiting. N Engl J Med 1990; 322:810–816.

60. Kuo B, Camilleri M, Burton D, et al. Effects of 5-HT$_3$ antagonism on postprandial gastric volume and symptoms in humans. Aliment Pharmacol Ther 2002; 16:225–233.

61. Zerbib F, Bruley des Varannes S, Oriola RC, et al. Alosetron does not affect the visceral perception of gastric distension in healthy subjects. Aliment Pharmacol Ther 1994; 8:403–407.

62. Viramontes BE, Camilleri M, McKinzie S, et al. Gender related differences in slowing colonic transit by a 5-HT$_3$ antagonist in subjects with diarrhea-predominant irritable bowel syndrome. Am J Gastroenterol 2001; 92:2671–2676.

63. Delvaux M, Louvel D, Mamet JP, et al. Effect of alosetron on responses to colonic distension in patients with irritable bowel syndrome. Aliment Pharmacol Ther 1998; 12:849–855.

64. Saslow SB, Scolapio JS, Camilleri M, et al. Medium-term effects of a new 5HT$_3$ antagonist, alosetron, in patients with carcinoid diarrhea. Gut 1998; 42:628–634.

65. Mayer EA, Berman S, Derbyshire SW, et al. The effect of the 5-HT3 receptor antagonist, alosetron, on brain responses to visceral stimulation in irritable bowel syndrome patients. Aliment Pharmacol Ther 2002; 16:1357–1366.

66. Berman SM, Chang L, Suyenobu B, et al. Condition-specific deactivation of brain regions by 5-HT3 receptor antagonist alosetron. Gastroenterology 2002; 123:969–977.

67. Tonato M, Roila F, Del Favero A. Are there differences among the serotonin antagonists? Supportive Care in Cancer 1994; 2:293–296.

68. Cremonini F, Delgado-Aros S, Camilleri M. Efficacy of alosetron in irritable bowel syndrome: a meta-analysis of randomized control trials. Neurogastroenterology and Motility 2003; 15:79–86.

Meta-analysis of six randomized, controlled trials documenting the efficacy of alosetron in the treatment of diarrhea-predominant irritable bowel syndrome.

69. Coulie B, Tack J, Vos R, et al. Influence of the 5-HT1A agonist buspirone on rectal tone and the perception of rectal distension in man. Gastroenterology 1998; 114:G3046.

70. Chial HJ, Camilleri M, Ferber I, et al. Effects of venlafaxine, buspirone and placebo on colonic sensorimotor functions in healthy humans. Clin Gastroenterol Hepatol 2003; 1:211–218.

71. Gorard DA, Libby GW, Farthing MJ. 5-Hydroxytryptamine and human small intestinal motility: effect of inhibiting 5-hydroxytryptamine reuptake. Gut 1994; 35:496–500.

72. Chial HJ, Camilleri M, Burton D, et al. Selective effects of serotonergic psychoactive agents on gastrointestinal functions in health. Am J Physiol 2003; 284:G130–G137.

73. Fickel J, Bagnol D, Watson SJ, et al. Opioid receptor expression in the rat gastrointestinal tract: a quantitative study with comparison to the brain. Molec Brain Res 1997; 46:1–8.

74. Rang HP, Dale MM, Ritter JM. Analgesic drugs. Pharmacology 1999: 579–603.

75. Sternini C. Receptors and transmission in the brain–gut axis: potential for novel therapies. III. Mu-opioid receptors in the enteric nervous system. Am J Physiol 2001; 281:G8–G15.

76. Kurz A, Sessler DI. Opioid-induced bowel dysfunction: pathophysiology and potential new therapies. Drugs 2003; 63:649–671.

77. Lembo T, Naliboff BD, Matin K, et al. Irritable bowel syndrome patients show altered sensitivity to exogenous opioids. Pain 2000; 87:137–147.

78. Bagnol D, Mansour A, Akil H, et al. Cellular localization and distribution of the cloned mu and kappa opioid receptors in rat gastrointestinal tract. Neuroscience 1997; 81:579–591.

79. De Winter BY, Boeckxstaens GE, De Man JG, et al. Effects of mu- and kappa-opioid receptors on postoperative ileus in rats. Eur J Pharmacol 1997; 339:63–67.

80. Salet GAM, Heyligers JMM, Lautenschutz JM, et al. The effects of fedotozine on digestive symptoms following abdominal surgery. Gastroenterology 1995; 108:A682.

81. Awouters F, Megens A, Verlinden M, et al. Loperamide. Survey of studies on mechanism of its antidiarrheal activity. Dig Dis Sci 1993; 38:977–995.

82. Palmer KR, Corbett CL, Holdsworth CD. Double-blind cross-over study comparing loperamide, codeine and diphenoxylate in the treatment of chronic diarrhea. Gastroenterology 1980; 79:1272–1275.

83. Cann PA, Read NW, Holdsworth CD, et al. Role of loperamide and placebo in management of irritable bowel syndrome (IBS). Dig Dis Sci 1984; 29:239–247.

84. Bergman L, Djarv L. A comparative study of loperamide and diphenoxylate in the treatment of chronic diarrhoea caused by intestinal resection. Ann Clin Res 1981; 13:402–405.

85. Akehurst R, Kaltenthaler E. Treatment of irritable bowel syndrome: a review of randomised controlled trials. Gut 2001; 48:272–282.

86. Schmidt WK. Alvimopan* (ADL 8-2698) is a novel peripheral opioid antagonist. Am J Surg 2001; 182:27S–38S.

87. Liu SS, Hodgson PS, Carpenter RL, et al. ADL 8-2698, a trans-3,4-dimethyl-4 (3-hydroxyphenyl) piperidine, prevents gastrointestinal effects of intravenous morphine without affecting analgesia. Clin Pharmacol Ther 2001; 69:66–71.

88. Taguchi A, Sharma N, Saleem RM, et al. Selective postoperative inhibition of gastrointestinal opioid receptors. N Engl J Med 2001; 345:935–940.

    First randomized, controlled trial documentation of a novel pharmacological approach to prevent or treat postoperative ileus.

89. Delgado-Aros S, Chial HJ, Camilleri M, et al. Effects of a kappa opioid agonist, asimadoline, on satiation and gastrointestinal motor and sensory functions in humans. Am J Physiol 2003; 284:G558–G566.

90. Delgado-Aros S, Chial HJ, Cremonini F, et al. Asimadoline decreases satiation and postprandial fullness in humans independently of its effects on gastric volume. Aliment Pharmacol Ther 2003; 18:507–514.

91. Delvaux M, Beck A, Jacob J, et al. Effect of asimadoline, a kappa opioid agonist, on pain induced by colonic distension in patients with irritable bowel syndrome. Aliment Pharm Ther 2004; 15:237–246.

92. van Haaren F, Scott S, Tucker LB. Kappa-opioid receptor-mediated analgesia: hotplate temperature and sex differences. Eur J Pharmacol 2000; 408:153–159.

93. Gear RW, Miaskowski C, Gordon NC, et al. Kappa-opioids produce significantly greater analgesia in women than in men. Nature Med 1996; 2:1248–1250.

94. Delvaux M, Louvel D, Lagier E, et al. The kappa agonist fedotozine relieves hypersensitivity to colonic distention in patients with irritable bowel syndrome. Gastroenterology 1999; 116:38–45.

95. Dapoigny M, Abitbol JL, Fraitag B. Efficacy of peripheral kappa agonist fedotozine versus placebo in treatment of irritable bowel syndrome. A multicenter dose-response study. Dig Dis Sci 1995; 40:2244–2249.

96. Hawkes ND, Rhodes J, Evans BK, et al. Naloxone treatment for irritable bowel syndrome – a randomized controlled trial with an oral formulation. Aliment Pharmacol Ther 2002; 16:1649–1654.

97. Foss JF. A review of the potential role of methylnaltrexone in opioid bowel dysfunction. Am J Surg 2001; 182:19S–26S.

98. Yuan CS, Foss JF, O'Connor M, et al. Methylnaltrexone prevents morphine-induced delay in oral-cecal transit time without affecting analgesia: a double-blind randomized placebo-controlled trial. Clin Pharmacol Ther 1996; 59:469–475.

99. Yuan CS, Foss JF, O'Connor M, et al. Methylnaltrexone for reversal of constipation due to chronic methadone use: a randomized controlled trial. JAMA 2000; 283:367–372.

100. Yuan CS, Foss JF, O'Connor M, et al. Effects of intravenous methylnaltrexone on opioid-induced gut motility and transit time changes in subjects receiving chronic methadone therapy: a pilot study. Pain 1999; 83:631–635.

101. Yuan CS, Foss JF. Oral methylnaltrexone for opioid-induced constipation. JAMA 2000; 284:1383–1384.

102. Yuan CS, Foss JF, O'Connor M, et al. Effects of enteric-coated methylnaltrexone in preventing opioid-induced delay in oral-cecal transit time. Clin Pharmacol Ther 2000; 67:398–404.

103. Bharucha AE, Camilleri M, Zinsmeister AR, et al. Adrenergic modulation of human colonic motor and sensory function. Am J Physiol 1997; 273:G997–G1006.

104. Malcolm A, Camilleri M, Kost L, et al. Towards identifying optimal doses for alpha-2 adrenergic modulation of colonic and rectal motor and sensory function. Aliment Pharmacol Ther 2000; 14:783–793.

105. Viramontes BE, Malcolm A, Camilleri M, et al. Effects of α_2-adrenergic agonist on gastrointestinal transit, colonic motility and sensation in humans. Am J Physiol 2001; 281:G1468–G1476.

106. Camilleri M, Kim D-Y, McKinzie S, et al. A randomized, controlled exploratory study of clonidine in diarrhea-predominant irritable bowel syndrome. Clin Gastroenterol Hepatol 2003; 1:111–121.

107. Haruma K, Wiste JA, Camilleri M. Effect of octreotide on gastrointestinal pressure profiles in health and in functional and organic gastrointestinal disorders. Gut 1993; 35:1064–1069.

108. Soudah HC, Hasler WL, Owyang C. Effect of octreotide on intestinal motility and bacterial overgrowth in scleroderma. N Engl J Med 1991; 325:1461–1467.

109. Hasler WL, Soudah HC, Owyang C. Somatostatin analog inhibits afferent response to rectal distention in diarrhea-predominant irritable bowel patients. J Pharmacol Exp Ther 1994; 268(3):1206–1211.

110. von der Ohe MR, Camilleri M, Thomforde GM, et al. Differential regional effects of octreotide on human gastrointestinal motor function. Gut 1995; 36:743–748.

111. Foxx-Orenstein A, Camilleri M, Stephens D, et al. Effect of somatostatin analog on gastric motor and sensory functions in healthy humans. Gut 2003; 52:1555–1561.

112. Kvols LK, Moertel CG, O'Connell MJ, et al. Treatment of the malignant carcinoid syndrome. N Engl J Med 1986; 315:663–666.

113. Geer RJ, Richards WO, O'Dorisio TM, et al. Efficacy of octreotide acetate in treatment of severe postgastrectomy dumping syndrome. Ann Surg 1990; 212:678–687.

114. Camilleri M, Saslow SB. Somatostatin analogs in the treatment of gastrointestinal motility disorders. Advan Gastroenterol Hepatol Clin Nutr 1996; 1:291–298.

115. Nehra V, Camilleri M, Burton D, et al. An open trial of octreotide long-acting release in the management of short bowel syndrome. Am J Gastroenterol 2001; 96:1494–1498.

116. O'Keefe SJ, Haymond MW, Bennet WM, et al. Long-acting somatostatin analogue therapy and protein metabolism in patients with jejunostomies. Gastroenterology 1994; 107:379–388.

117. Raybould HE, Roberts ME, Dockray GJ. Reflex decreases in intragastric pressure in response to cholecystokinin in rats. Am J Physiol 1987; 253:G165–G170.

118. Glatzle J, Kreis ME, Kawano K, et al. Postprandial neuronal activation in the nucleus of the solitary tract is partly mediated by CCK-A receptors. Am J Physiol 2001; 281:R222–R229.

119. Schick RR, Schusdziarra V, Yaksh TL, et al. Brain regions where cholecystokinin exerts its effect on satiety. Ann NY Acad Sci 1994; 713:242–254.

120. Schick RR, Yaksh TL, Roddy DR, et al. Release of hypothalamic cholecystokinin in cats: effects of nutrient and volume loading. Am J Physiol 1989; 256:R248–R254.

121. Mearadji B, Masclee AA, Onkenhout W, et al. Effect of intraduodenal and intravenous amino acids on proximal gastric motor function in man. Dig Dis Sci 2001; 46:38–45.

122. Walsh JH. Gastrointestinal hormones. In: Johnson LR, ed. Physiology of the gastrointestinal tract. Vol. 1, 3rd edn. New York: Raven; 1994:49–67.

123. Niederau C, Heintges T, Rovati LC, et al. Effects of loxiglumide on gallbladder emptying in man. Gastroenterology 1989; 97:1331–1336.

124. D'Amato M, Rovati LC. Cholecystokinin-A receptor antagonists: therapies for gastrointestinal disorders. Exp Opin Invest Drugs 1997; 6:819–836.

125. Feinle C, Meier O, Otto B, et al. Role of duodenal lipid and cholecystokinin A receptors in the pathophysiology of functional dyspepsia. Gut 2001; 48:347–355.

Pharmacodynamic study demonstrating the role of CCK-1 receptors in functional dyspepsia.

126. Chey WY, Jin HO, Lee MH, et al. Colonic motility abnormality in patients with irritable bowel syndrome exhibiting abdominal pain and diarrhea. Am J Gastroenterol 2001; 96:1499–1506.

127. Cremonini F, Camilleri M, Mc Kinzie S, et al. Effect of CCK-1 antagonist, dexloxiglumide, in female patients with irritable bowel syndrome: a pharmacodynamic and pharmacogenomic study. Am J Gastro 2005; 100:652–663.

128. Castillo EJ, Delgado-Aros S, Camilleri M, et al. Effect of an oral CCK-A agonist, GI181771X, on fasting and postprandial gastric functions in healthy volunteers. Am J Physiol 2004; 287:G363–G369.

Pharmacodynamic study demonstrating the effects of CCK-1 receptors in the control of gastric function, and the first documentation of an effective, orally administered CCK-1 agonist.

CHAPTER THREE

3

Probiotics

Francisco Guarner

GUT FLORA

Host–bacterial relationship in the gut

The term 'microflora' or 'microbiota' refers to the community of living microorganisms assembled in a particular ecological niche of a host individual. The human gut is the natural habitat for a large, diverse, and dynamic population of microorganisms, mainly bacteria, that have adapted to live on the mucosal surfaces or in the lumen.[1] Gut bacteria include native species that colonize permanently the tract, and a variable set of living microorganisms that transit temporarily through the tract. Native bacteria are mainly acquired at birth and during the first year of life, whereas transient bacteria are continuously being ingested from the environment (food, drinks, etc.).

The stomach and duodenum harbor very low numbers of microorganisms adhering to the mucosal surface or in transit, typically less than 10^3 bacteria cells (colony forming units, CFU) per gram of contents, mainly lactobacilli and streptococci. Acid, bile, and pancreatic secretions kill most ingested microbes, and the phasic propulsive motor activity impedes stable colonization of the lumen. There is a progressive increase in numbers of bacteria along the jejunum and ileum, from approximately 10^4 in the jejunum to 10^7 CFU per gram of contents at the ileal end, with predominance of Gram-negative aerobes and some obligate anaerobes. The large intestine is heavily populated by anaerobes with numbers in the region of 10^{12} CFU per gram of luminal contents. In the upper gut, transit is rapid and bacterial density is low, but the impact on immune function is thought to be important by interactions of bacteria with organized lymphoid structures of the small intestinal mucosa. In the colon, however, transit time is slow and microorganisms have the opportunity to proliferate by fermenting available substrates derived from either the diet or endogenous secretions.

The intestinal habitat of an adult individual contains 300–500 different species of bacteria, with 30–40 species comprising up to 99% of the total population. Conventional bacteriological analysis of the fecal flora by isolation of bacteria on selective growth media shows that strict anaerobic bacteria outnumber aerobes by a factor of 100 to 1000. The dominant genera are *Bacteroides*, *Bifidobacterium*, *Eubacterium*, *Clostridium*, *Lactobacillus*, *Fusobacterium*, and various anaerobic Gram-positive cocci. Bacteria present in lower numbers include *Enterococcus* and *Enterobacteriaceae*. Every individual has a particular combination of predominant and subdominant species that is distinct from that found in other individuals. However, over 50% of bacteria cells that are observed by microscopic examination of fecal specimens cannot be grown in culture media. Molecular biology techniques have been developed to characterize nonculturable bacteria, and previously unknown strains are now being identified.[2,3] These techniques show differences in predominant species between proximal and distal colon, and mucosal and fecal communities.[4]

Some of the bacteria in the gut are pathogens or potential pathogens when the integrity of the mucosal barrier is functionally breached. However, the normal interaction between gut bacteria and their host is a symbiotic relationship, defined as mutually beneficial for both partners.[5] The host provides a nutrient-rich habitat and the bacteria can infer important benefits on the host's health.

Primary functions of the microflora

Comparison of animals bred under germ-free conditions with their conventionally raised counterparts (conventional microflora) has revealed a series of anatomic characteristics and physiological functions that are associated with the presence of the microflora.[3,6] Organ weights (heart, lung, and liver), cardiac output, intestinal wall thickness, intestinal motor activity, serum gamma-globulin levels, lymph nodes, among other characteristics, are all reduced or atrophic in germ-free animals, suggesting that gut bacteria have important and specific functions on the host. These functions are ascribed into three categories, i.e. metabolic, protective, and trophic functions.[1]

Metabolic functions consist of the fermentation of nondigestible dietary substrates and endogenous mucus. Gene diversity among the microbial community provides a variety of enzymes and biochemical pathways that are distinct from the host's own constitutive resources. Fermentation of carbohydrates is a major source of energy in the colon for bacterial growth and produces short-chain fatty acids that can be absorbed by the host. This results in salvage of dietary energy, and favors the absorption of ions (Ca, Mg, Fe) in the cecum. Metabolic functions also include the production of vitamins (K, B_{12}, biotin, folic acid, panthotenate) and synthesis of amino acids from ammonia or urea.[4]

Protective functions of gut microflora include the barrier effect that prevents invasion by pathogens. The resident bacteria represent a crucial line of resistance to colonization by exogenous microbes or opportunistic bacteria that are present in the gut, but their growth is restricted. The equilibrium between species of resident bacteria provides stability in the microbial population, but use of antibiotics can disrupt the balance (for instance, overgrowth of toxigenic *Clostridium difficile*). The barrier effect is based on the ability of certain bacteria to secrete antimicrobial substances, bacteriocins, that inhibit the growth of pathogens, and also in the competition for ecological niches.

Trophic functions of the gut microflora include the control of epithelial cell proliferation and differentiation. Epithelial cell turnover is reduced in colonic crypts of germ-free animals as compared with colonized controls. Cell differentiation is highly influenced by the interaction with resident microorganisms as shown by the expression of a variety of genes in germ-free animals mono-associated with specific bacteria strains.[7] Bacteria play also an essential role in the development of a healthy immune system. Animals bred in a germ-free environment show low densities of lymphoid cells in the gut mucosa, specialized follicle structures are small, and circulating immunoglobulin levels are low. Immediately after exposure to microbes, the number of mucosal lymphocytes expands, germinal centers and immunoglobulin producing cells appear rapidly in follicles and in the lamina propria, and there is a significant increase in serum immunoglobulin levels.[6] During life, multiple and diverse interactions between microbes, epithelium, and gut lymphoid tissues are constantly reshaping local and systemic mechanisms of immunity.

PROBIOTICS AND PREBIOTICS

Concept

Symbiosis between microflora and host can be optimized by pharmacological or nutritional intervention with probiotics or prebiotics (Table 3.1). Bacteria known to provide specific health benefits in the host can be used for consumption as a food component or in the form of specific preparations of viable microorganisms. These bacteria are called 'probiotics.' The term was originally proposed in 1954 to designate 'active substances that are essential for a healthy development of life,' as opposed to the antibiotics. In a paper published in Science, Lilly and Stillwell[8] described probiotics as substances secreted by one microorganism that stimulate the growth of another. The term was mainly applied to animal feed supplements specifically designed to improve health. In 1989, Fuller described probiotics as 'live microbial feed supplements which beneficially affect the host animal by improving its intestinal microbial balance.' This definition stressed the importance of viable microbial cells as an essential requirement, and the improvement of the intestinal microbial balance as the mechanism of action. He suggested that the concept was also applicable to human nutrition and medicine.[9] In recent years, the Joint FAO/WHO Expert Consultation defined probiotics as 'live microorganisms which when administered in adequate amounts confer a health benefit on the host.' This definition has been adopted by the International Scientific Association for Probiotics and Prebiotics.[10]

The term prebiotic refers to 'a nondigestible food ingredient that beneficially affects the host by selectively stimulating growth and/or activity of one or a limited number of bacteria in the colon.'[11] A prebiotic should not be hydrolyzed by human intestinal enzymes, it should be selectively fermented by beneficial bacteria, and this selective fermentation should result in a bene-

Table 3.1 Probiotics and prebiotics improve the symbiotic functions of the gut flora

Metabolic effects
  Lactose digestion
  Calcium absorption
  Bowel transit: treatment of constipation
  Hepatic encephalopathy
  Production of intestinal gas: irritable bowel syndrome

Protective effects
  Prevention and treatment of gastrointestinal infections
  Prevention of systemic infections due to bacterial translocation

Trophic effects
  Treatment of inflammatory bowel diseases
  Prevention and treatment of atopic diseases
  Prevention of colorectal cancer

ficial effect on health or well-being of the host. At the present time, all prebiotics described are nondigestible carbohydrates that foster the growth of endogenous lactobacilli or bifidobacteria in the large bowel. Finally, the combination of probiotics and prebiotics is termed 'synbiotic,' and is an exciting new concept to optimize the impact of bacteria on health.

In all human studies published so far, probiotics were administered alive and by oral route or topical preparations (skin, nasal or vaginal applications). Recent experimental work suggests that some dead bacteria or their cellular components (cell wall, DNA motifs, etc.) would have efficacy when given by parenteral route. These preparations, however, would not fulfil the current concept of probiotic as the presence of viable microorganisms is mandatory.[10] Synbiotics and prebiotics must also be administered by oral route.

Metabolic effects

Lactose digestion

The disaccharide lactose, mainly found in milk and dairy products, is hydrolyzed to glucose and galactose by lactase (or beta-galactosidase), that is present in the brush border of epithelial cells in the small intestine. However, a sizable percentage of the adult population develops a deficiency of intestinal lactase after weaning. Prevalence of lactose malabsorption in adult populations is high, and varies from 5% to 15% in Northern European and American countries and 50% to 100% in African, Asian, and South American countries.[12] These subjects may develop gastrointestinal symptoms such as abdominal bloating, pain, flatulence, and diarrhea after ingestion of lactose. They tend to eliminate milk and dairy products from their diet and, consequently, their calcium intake may be compromised.

The bacteria used as starter culture in yogurt (*Streptococcus thermophilus* and *Lactobacillus delbrueckii* subsp. *bulgaricus*) can improve lactose digestion and eliminate symptoms in lactase deficient individuals. The benefit is due to the presence of microbial beta-galactosidase in the bacteria that hydrolyzes lactose during its transit through the small bowel.[13] However, the enzyme is destroyed by gastric secretions if the yogurt is pasteurized or sterilized before consumption (bacterial cell wall protects the enzyme from gastric juice). A large number of human studies in which consumption of live yogurt cultures was compared with consumption of heat-killed bacteria demonstrated better lactose digestion and absorption as well as reduction of gastrointestinal symptoms in subjects that consumed yogurt with live cultures.[14–19] The benefit of yogurt bacteria on lactose absorption was also demonstrated in healthy subjects without lactose maldigestion.[18]

Calcium absorption

Certain prebiotics can improve calcium absorption in adolescents and adults. In controlled human studies, dietary intake of inulin and/or oligofructose at doses of 8–15 g/day increased calcium absorption by 18–54%.[20] Inulin is a polysaccharide composed of glucose and a linear chain of fructose moieties linked by specific beta (2-1) bonds. Oligofructose is an inulin-type oligosaccharide that contains only 2–10 fructose moieties in the linear chain. Both inulin and oligofructose are poorly digested in humans and its recovery from the distal small intestine is equivalent to that of an unabsorbable polyethylenglycol marker. However, they are completely fermented by the microflora of the colon, particularly by bacteria with a specific fructosidase that hydrolyzes the fructose chain. The products of hydrolysis, fructose and glucose, are highly efficient substrates for the growth of saccharolytic bacteria, including lactobacilli and bifidobacteria. Oligofructose and inulin have been shown to increase the number of fecal bifidobacteria in healthy humans, and reduce the concentration of *Bacteroides* and clostridia.[21] As a result of the fermentation of inulin, the production of short-chain fatty acids within the colonic lumen increases, and a slight acidification of colonic contents is observed. At a lower luminal pH, more calcium is soluble and thus is more readily absorbed by epithelial cells in the cecum and proximal colon. Short-chain fatty acids also enhance calcium absorption.

Bowel transit

Inulin and oligofructose have a laxative effect on bowel habit.[21] At daily doses of 10–15 g, they consistently increase stool output. The bulking capacity of these prebiotics is 1.2 or 2.1 g of stool increase per gram of ingested oligofructose or inulin, respectively.[22] The effect is due to increases in bacterial biomass in the colon. In constipated patients, inulin also stimulates bowel movements and increases stool frequency.[23]

Lactulose and other nondigestible carbohydrates with low molecular weight have also been proven effective for alleviation of constipation. These products have an important osmotic effect and increase fecal water content by a mechanism unrelated with a prebiotic effect. However, changes on the microflora may also contribute to the positive effect on bowel transit.[24]

Hepatic encephalopathy

Several randomized controlled trials have shown that lactulose and lactitol are superior to placebo to prevent and treat hepatic encephalopathy in decompensated chronic liver disease and in fulminant liver failure.[24] The effect is very well established and both compounds are commonly used in clinical practice for this indication. The mechanisms of action invoked include acidification of the intracolonic environment by fermentation of the disaccharides, and reduction of the breakdown of nitrogen-containing compounds to ammonia and other potential neurotoxins. In a recent clinical trial with patients with chronic liver disease, minimal hepatic encephalopathy was reversed in 50% of the patients treated with synbiotics (four probiotic strains, and four fermentable fibers, including inulin and resistant starch) for 30 days, a response significantly higher than the 13% observed in the placebo group.[25] In this study, changes in the fecal flora were associated with the beneficial effect.

Production of intestinal gas: irritable bowel syndrome

Fermentations taking place in the colon generate a variable volume of gas. However, some gut bacteria degrade metabolic substrates without producing gas, and some other species may even consume gas, particularly hydrogen. Symptoms of abdominal pain, bloating, and flatulence are commonly seen in patients with irritable bowel syndrome. Hypothetically, administration of appropriate bacteria strains could reduce gas accumulation within the bowel in these patients. In a double-blind clinical trial with 60 patients with irritable bowel syndrome, a *Lactobacillus plantarum* strain or placebo was administered for four weeks. Both probiotic and placebo decreased pain and flatulence in these patients, but scores were significantly lower in the probiotic than in the placebo group.[26] Likewise, another placebo-controlled trial with 25 patients concluded that a probiotic mixture (VSL#3) was useful for the relief of abdominal bloating in patients with diarrhea predominant irritable bowel syndrome. The probiotic had no effect on gastrointestinal or colonic transit.[27] Probiotics need to be evaluated further but they appear to be useful for the control of the symptoms related with the altered handling or perception of intestinal gas in this group of patients.

Protective effects

Gastrointestinal infections

A number of clinical trials have tested the efficacy of probiotics in the prevention of acute diarrheal conditions, including antibiotic-associated diarrhea, nosocomial and community acquired infectious enteritis in children, and traveler's diarrhea. Both the short- and long-term use of antibiotics can produce diarrhea, particularly during regimens with multiple drugs. Coadministration of probiotics to the patients on antibiotic therapy has been shown to reduce the incidence of antibiotic-associated diarrhea in children and in adults. In placebo-controlled studies, diarrhea occurred at a rate of 15–26% in the placebo arms but only in 3–7% of patients receiving a probiotic. Different strains have been tested including *Lactobacillus rhamnosus* strain GG, *Lactobacillus acidophilus*, *Lactobacillus bulgaricus*, and the yeast *Saccharomyces boulardii*. Meta-analysis of controlled trials concluded that probiotics can be used to prevent antibiotic-associated diarrhea (Fig. 3.1).[28,29]

Prophylactic use of probiotics has proven useful for the prevention of acute diarrhea in infants admitted into the hospital ward for a chronic disease condition. Supplementation of an infant formula with *Bifidobacterium bifidum* and *Streptococcus thermophilus* significantly prevented the incidence of diarrhea in hospitalized infants aged 5–24 months[30] (31% in placebo versus 7% in probiotic group). A placebo-controlled, double-blind study in infants (1–36 months old) tested the *Lactobacillus rhamnosus* strain GG, and reported similar findings.[31] Probiotic treatment reduced the risk of nosocomial diarrhea to one-fifth (33% in placebo versus 7% in probiotic group). Prevalence of rotavirus infection was not influenced by probiotic treatment but the risk of symptomatic rotavirus enteritis was markedly reduced (17% in placebo versus 2% in probiotic group). A third published clinical

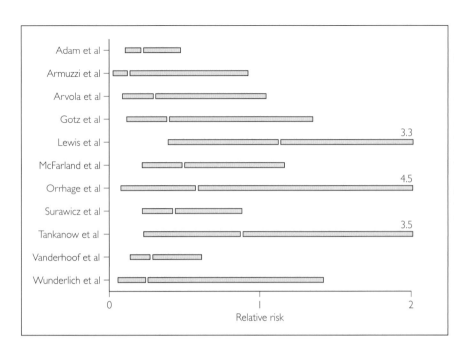

Fig. 3.1 ● Relative risks (and 95% confidence intervals) of diarrhea in subjects on antibiotics and probiotics (*Lactobacillus rhamnosus* GG, *Saccharomyces boulardii*, and others) as normalized by the incidence of diarrhea in control subjects on antibiotics and placebo in 11 controlled clinical trials. Ten out of 11 studies estimated a relative risk lower than 1, and in 5 of these studies the upper limit of the 95% confidence interval was also below 1. Overall, the combined relative risk is significantly reduced, as determined in two published meta-analyses,[28,29] and suggests that probiotic therapy can reduce the risk of antibiotic-associated diarrhea to one-third.

trial on nosocomial diarrhea in infants (1–18 months old)[32] showed no statistically significant benefit associated to *Lactobacillus* GG, but the rate of symptomatic rotavirus enteritis in the placebo arm (20.8%) was higher than in the probiotic arm (13.2%).

Probiotics may also be useful in the prevention of community-acquired diarrhea. The study by Oberhelman and coworkers[33] included 204 infants (6–24 months old) from an indigent peri-urban town that were followed during a 15 month period. Significantly fewer episodes of diarrhea per child per year were observed in children fed with a *Lactobacillus* GG supplemented gelatine than in the placebo control group. In a multicenter, randomized, double-blind trial,[34] conducted over 4 months with 928 healthy children aged 6–24 months, the incidence of acute diarrhea was significantly reduced by supplementation with *Lactobacillus casei* fermented milk (15.9%) as compared with yogurt (22%). The prebiotic oligofructose was tested in a randomized-controlled trial conducted for 12 months with 123 children living in a depressed peri-urban area.[35] Whilst the number of diarrhea episodes per child per year was not affected by the prebiotic, the children on the oligofructose arm showed significantly less severity in these episodes as defined by a lower rate of diarrhea episodes with fever and less frequency of episodes that required medical consultation.

Several studies have investigated the efficacy of probiotics in the prevention of travelers' diarrhea in adults, but methodological deficiencies, such as low compliance with the treatment and problems in the follow-up, limit the validity of their conclusions.[36] In a well-designed study completed by 244 subjects travelling to different parts of the world, oligofructose reduced the incidence of diarrhea episodes that were reported by 20% of the subjects in the placebo group and 11% of the subjects in the prebiotic group.[37] However, the difference was not statistically significant.

Probiotics are useful as treatment of acute infectious diarrhea in children. Different strains, including *Lactobacillus reuteri*, *Lactobacillus* GG, *Lactobacillus casei*, and *Saccharomyces boulardii*, have been tested in controlled clinical trials and were proven useful in reducing the severity and duration of diarrhea. Three meta-

analyses of controlled clinical trials have been published.[38–40] The results of the systematic reviews are consistent and suggest that probiotics are safe and effective. Oral administration of probiotics shortens the duration of acute diarrheal illness in children by approximately one day. As observed by Van Niel and coworkers,[39] there is a direct relationship between the beneficial effect and the dose of probiotic being administered, and a daily intake below 10^{10} CFU is unlikely to have an effect.

Probiotics have been tested as a new strategy for eradication of *Helicobacter pylori* infection of the gastric mucosa in humans. Some strains of lactic acid bacteria are known to inhibit the growth of *Helicobacter pylori* in vitro. However, administration of one of these strains in a specially designed yogurt was not effective for the eradication of *H. pylori* infection.[41] After a 30-day treatment with the probiotic yogurt, only 1 out of 27 subjects showed a negative urea breath test, but eradication was not confirmed by other tests or subsequent follow-up. In other clinical studies, the use of probiotics has been tested as a supplement to the classical triple therapy with antibiotics. The probiotic appears to reduce side effects of the antibiotic therapy and improves compliance, but a higher eradication efficacy has not been demonstrated.[42]

Prevention of systemic infections

Dysfunction of the gut mucosal barrier may result in the passage through the epithelium of a variable quantity of viable micro-organisms that can disseminate throughout the body producing sepsis. Bacterial translocation and its complications have been shown to occur in some pathologic conditions such as postoperative sepsis, severe acute pancreatitis, advanced liver cirrhosis, multisystem organ failure, etc.

Probiotics have been used to prevent sepsis in patients with severe acute pancreatitis. In a randomized double-blind trial, patients were treated with either *Lactobacillus plantarum* or placebo. Infected pancreatic necrosis and abscesses occurred at a significantly lower rate in *L. plantarum* treated patients than in controls.[43] A randomized study involving 95 liver transplant patients compared the incidence of infections among three groups of patients submitted to different prophylaxis procedure: selective bowel decontamination with antibiotics, administration of live *L. plantarum* supplemented with fermentable fiber (synbiotic), and administration of heat-killed *L. plantarum* with the fiber supplement. Postoperative infections were recorded in 15 out of 32 patients (48%) in the antibiotics group, 4 out of 31 (13%) in the live *L. plantarum* group, and 11 out of 32 (34%) in the heat-killed *L. plantarum* group, the difference between antibiotics and live *L. plantarum* groups being significant.[44] In a second study by the same group, patients were randomized to receive a synbiotic preparation (including four probiotic strains, and four fermentable fibers) or a placebo consisting of the four fibers only. Postoperative infection occurred in only one patient in the treatment group (n=33), in contrast to 17 out of 33 in the placebo group.[44] The difference was highly significant. However, another clinical study performed with patients submitted to elective abdominal surgery found no effect of synbiotic treatment (4 bacteria strains plus oligofructose) on prevention of postoperative infections.[45] In this trial, synbiotic treatment after surgery was delayed until patients were able to tolerate oral nutrition. In contrast, the liver transplant studies introduced synbiotic therapy by nasogastric tube immediately after surgery. These data need to be confirmed but suggest that early administration of live probiotics may become an useful and effective therapy to prevent postoperative infections.

Trophic effects

Inflammatory bowel diseases

Clinical and experimental evidence suggests that abnormal activation of the mucosal immune system against the enteric flora is a key event in intestinal inflammatory conditions. In Crohn's disease and ulcerative colitis, patients show an increased mucosal secretion of IgG antibodies against commensal bacteria,[46] whereas the normal physiological response is based on IgA antibodies. Moreover, mucosal T lymphocytes are hyperreactive against antigens of the common flora.[47] Several factors contribute to the pathogenesis of the aberrant immune response towards the autologous flora, including genetic susceptibility, a defect in mucosal barrier function, and a microbial imbalance. There is experimental evidence suggesting that some commensal bacteria are able to down-regulate innate inflammatory responses of the intestinal mucosa.[48] Indeed, certain lactobacilli reduce the release of TNF-α by inflamed mucosa from Crohn's disease patients.[49] Thus, a favorable local microecology could restore the homeostasis of the mucosal immune system and lead to the resolution of the lesions. This hypothesis is currently being investigated by experimental and clinical approaches.

Probiotics and prebiotics have been tested in animal models of bowel inflammation. Selected probiotic strains,[50–52] including a bacterium genetically engineered to secrete the antiinflammatory cytokine IL-10,[53] and the prebiotic inulin[54] were proven effective for prevention and treatment of mucosal inflammation. Both probiotics and prebiotics are also being tested in clinical studies. In ulcerative colitis, two randomized controlled trials investigated the effectiveness of an orally administered enteric-coated preparation of viable *Escherichia coli* strain Nissle 1917 as compared with mesalazine, the standard treatment for maintenance of remission.[55,56] These two studies concluded that this strain has

an equivalent effect to mesalazine in maintaining remission. The same probiotic product was tested for efficacy in maintaining remission in 28 patients with colonic Crohn's disease.[57] This placebo-controlled study showed a lower rate of relapse (33% versus 63%) in the probiotic group than in controls, but the number of patients was low, and no further studies have confirmed this result.

The VSL#3 mixture has been proven highly effective for maintenance of remission of chronic relapsing pouchitis, after induction of remission with antibiotics.[58,59] In the first study,[58] a relapse occurred in only 3 out of 20 patients of the VSL#3 group and in all the 20 patients of the placebo group. Of interest, all patients on remission in the probiotic arm had relapses within 4 months after stopping treatment at conclusion of the trial. In the second study, the probiotic mixture was administered in a once-a-day schedule, and similar efficacy was demonstrated.[59] Treatment with VSL#3 is also effective in the prevention of the onset of pouchitis after ileal pouch-anal anastomosis.[60]

The efficacy of *Lactobacillus* GG in postoperative recurrence of Crohn's disease has been tested in a randomized, double-blind trial. The probiotic showed no effect in the prevention of clinical and endoscopic recurrence as compared with placebo.[61] A second clinical trial confirmed the lack of efficacy of this strain in Crohn's disease patients.[62] The same probiotic strain was ineffective as a primary therapy for induction of a clinical or endoscopic response in patients with chronic pouchitis.[63]

The prebiotic inulin has been tested in patients with an ileal pouch-anal anastomosis and mild chronic pouchitis. Compared with placebo, 3 weeks of dietary supplementation with inulin reduced endoscopic and histological scores.[64] The effect was associated with an increase in fecal butyrate and a decrease in *Bacteroides* counts.

The therapeutical manipulation of the luminal microecology with probiotics and prebiotics is likely to become a new strategic area for the control and prevention of inflammatory bowel diseases. However, with the exception of the studies on pouchitis, results of controlled clinical trials published so far are poor and below the expectations raised. Further research is needed to optimize the use of probiotics or prebiotics for these indications.

Food allergy

Atopic diseases are due to exaggerated or imbalanced immune responses to environmental and harmless antigens (allergens). Prevalence of allergic diseases in Western societies is increasing at an alarming rate whereas it is much lower in the developing world. It has been suggested that this may be the result of inappropriate microbial stimulus during infancy due to improved hygienic conditions. Some epidemiological and experimental studies have indicated that stimulation of the immune system by certain microbes or microbial products may be effective in the prevention and management of allergic diseases.[65]

The effectiveness of probiotic therapy in the prevention of allergic diseases has been clearly demonstrated in randomized controlled trials.[66,67] Likewise, several well-designed studies have provided evidence that specific strains of probiotics can be effective in the management of atopic disorders. Majamaa and Isolauri[68] reported the efficacy of formula supplemented with *Lactobacillus* GG in infants with atopic eczema and cow's milk allergy. Infants receiving the probiotic showed significant improvement in both clinical symptoms and markers of intestinal inflammation (fecal alpha-1-antitrypsin and TNF-α) compared with the placebo group. These findings were confirmed by Rosenfeldt et al.[69] in a crossover study with atopic children (1–13 years of age). Effectiveness in the management of atopic eczema and cow's milk allergy in children is associated with the use of viable but not heat-inactivated probiotics.[70] However, little is known about the efficacy of probiotics in preventing other types of food allergy.

Colon cancer

Experimental studies clearly demonstrate a protective effect of prebiotics such as oligofructose, and probiotics such as some *Lactobacillus* and *Bifidobacteria* strains, or the combination of prebiotics and probiotics, against colon cancer. They can prevent the establishment, growth, and metastasis of transplantable and chemically induced tumors. Several possible mechanisms of protection have been identified.[71] Human intervention trials are needed to corroborate the evidence obtained in experimental studies. Such studies require the validation of intermediate endpoints that can be used as valid biomarkers of colon cancer risk.

Probiotics and prebiotics in evidence-based medicine

Table 3.2 summarizes the grade of recommendations for the use of probiotics in gastroenterology according to the criteria of evidence-based-medicine. Grade A recommendations should be implemented in patient care, and are supported by level 1 evidence (high-quality randomized controlled trials with statistically significant results and few limitations in their design, or by conclusions from systematic reviews of the trials). Grade B recommendations favor a therapeutic option that is supported by level 2 evidence (randomized controlled trials that have some limitations in their study methodology or results showing wide confidence intervals). Grade B recommendations may change in the future, if level 1 evidence from new studies becomes available.

Table 3.2 Probiotics and prebiotics in evidence-based medicine

Grade A recommendation (level 1 evidence)

Treatment of lactose maldigestion (probiotics)
Improvement of the absorption of calcium (prebiotics)
Prevention and treatment of constipation (prebiotics)
Treatment of hepatic encephalopathy (prebiotics)
Treatment of acute infectious diarrhea in children (probiotics)
Prevention of antibiotic associated diarrhea (probiotics)
Prevention of nosocomial and community acquired diarrhea in children (probiotics and prebiotics)
Prevention of pouchitis and maintenance of remission (probiotics)
Prevention and treatment of atopic eczema associated with cow's milk allergy in children (probiotics)

Grade B recommendation (level 2 evidence)

Prevention of travelers' diarrhea (probiotics and prebiotics)
Prevention of sepsis associated with severe acute pancreatitis (synbiotics)
Prevention of post-operative infections (synbiotics)
Maintenance of remission of ulcerative colitis (probiotics)
Treatment of mild pouchitis (prebiotics)

SUMMARY

A large and diverse community of commensal bacteria is harbored in the human gut, in a symbiotic arrangement that influences both physiology and pathology in the host. First, gut microbes conduct a multitude of biochemical reactions and they can be collectively conceived as a 'metabolic organ.' Second, gut bacteria provide an important barrier for defense against invasion by pathogens, and finally, host–bacteria interactions in the gut play a major role in the constitution and reshaping of host's immunity. Microbial ecology in the gut can be modulated by pharmacological and nutritional intervention with probiotics and prebiotics, and a balanced microbial environment would likely help to boost the symbiotic functions of bacteria on host's health. In controlled human studies, probiotics and prebiotics have been used, safely and successfully, for improving certain metabolic functions of the flora (lactose digestion, calcium absorption, stimulation of bowel transit, and prevention of hepatic encephalopathy), for protection against infections (prevention and treatment of acute enteritis, prevention of bacterial translocation), and for modulation of the immune system (prevention and treatment of atopic diseases and chronic pouchitis). Current experimental and clinical research aims at establishing the role and efficacy of probiotics and prebiotics in the prevention and control of inflammatory bowel diseases and colon cancer.

REFERENCES

1. Guarner F, Malagelada JR. Gut flora in health and disease. Lancet 2003; 361:512–519.

   Descriptive review on the impact of gut bacteria on host's health.

2. Suau A, Bonnet R, Sutren M, et al. Direct rDNA community analysis reveals a myriad of novel bacterial lineages within the human gut. Appl Environ Microbiol 1999; 65:4799–4807.

3. Tannock GW. Molecular assessment of intestinal microflora. Am J Clin Nutr 2001; 73(suppl):410S–414S.

4. Zoetendal EG, von Wright A, Vilpponen-Salmela T, et al. Mucosa-associated bacteria in the human gastrointestinal tract are uniformly distributed along the colon and differ from the community recovered from feces. Appl Environ Microbiol 2002; 68:3401–3407.

5. Hooper LV, Midtvedt T, Gordon JI. How host–microbial interactions shape the nutrient environment of the mammalian intestine. Annu Rev Nutr 2002; 22:283–307.

6. Falk PG, Hooper LV, Midtvedt T, et al. Creating and maintaining the gastrointestinal ecosystem: what we know and need to know from gnotobiology. Microbiol Mol Biol Rev 1998; 62:1157–1170.

7. Hooper LV, Wong MH, Thelin A, et al. Molecular analysis of commensal host–microbial relationships in the intestine. Science 2001; 291:881–884.

   This outstanding paper shows how a commensal bacterium can modulate epithelial cell function by stimulating the expression of host genes involved in nutrient absorption, mucosal barrier fortification, angiogenesis, and intestinal maturation.

8. Lilly DM, Stillwell RH. Probiotics: growth-promoting factors produced by microorganisms. Science 1965; 147:747–748.

9. Fuller R. Probiotics in human medicine. Gut 1991; 32:439–442.

10. Reid G, Sanders ME, Gaskins HR, et al. New scientific paradigms for probiotics and prebiotics. J Clin Gastroenterol 2003; 37:105–118.

11. Gibson GR, Roberfroid MB. Dietary modulation of the human colonic microbiota: introducing the concept of prebiotics. J Nutr 1995; 125:1401–1412.

12. de Vrese M, Stegelmann A, Richter B, et al. Probiotics – compensation for lactase insufficiency. Am J Clin Nutr 2001; 73(suppl):421S–429S.

13. Kolars JC, Levitt MD, Aouji M, et al. Yogurt – an autodigesting source of lactose. N Engl J Med 1984; 310:1–3.

14. Savaiano DA, Abou ElAnouar A, Smith DE, et al. Lactose malabsorption from yogurt, pasteurized yogurt, sweet acidophilus milk, and cultured milk in lactase-deficient individuals. Am J Clin Nutr 1984; 40:1219–1223.

15. Dewit O, Pochart P, Desjeux J-F. Breath hydrogen concentration and plasma glucose, insulin and free fatty acid levels after lactose, milk, fresh or heated yogurt ingestion by healthy young adults with or without lactose malabsorption. Nutrition 1988; 4:131–135.

16. Lerebours E, N'Djitoyap Ndam C, Lavoine A, et al. Yogurt and fermented-then-pasteurized milk: effects of short-term and long-term ingestion on lactose absorption and mucosal lactase activity in lactase-deficient subjects. Am J Clin Nutr 1989; 49:823–827.

17. Marteau P, Flourie B, Pochart P, et al. Effect of the microbial lactase (EC 3.2.1.23) activity in yoghurt on the intestinal absorption of lactose: an in vivo study on lactase deficient humans. Br J Nutr 1990; 64:71–79.

18. Rizkalla SW, Luo J, Kabir M, et al. Chronic consumption of fresh but not heated yoghurt improves breath-hydrogen status and short-chain fatty acid profiles: a controlled study in healthy men with or without lactose maldigestion. Am J Clin Nutr 2000; 72:1474–1479.

19. Labayen I, Forga L, González A, et al. Relationship between lactose digestion, gastrointestinal transit time and symptoms in lactose malabsorbers after dairy consumption. Aliment Pharmacol Ther 2001; 15:543–549.

20. Cashman KD. Calcium intake, calcium bioavailability and bone health. Br J Nutr 2002; 87(suppl 2):S169–S177.

21. Gibson GR, Beatty ER, Wang X, et al. Selective stimulation of bifidobacteria in the human colon by oligofructose and inulin. Gastroenterology 1995; 108:975–982.

22. Cherbut C. Inulin and oligofructose in the dietary fibre concept. Br J Nutr 2002; 87(suppl 2):S159–S162.

23. Kleessen B, Sykura B, Zunft HJ, et al. Effects of inulin and lactose on fecal microflora, microbial activity, and bowel habit in elderly constipated persons. Am J Clin Nutr 1997; 65:1397–1402.

24. Clausen MR, Mortensen PB. Lactulose, disaccharides and colonic flora. Clinical consequences. Drugs 1997; 53:930–942.

25. Liu Q, Duan ZP, Ha da K, et al. Synbiotic modulation of gut flora: effect on minimal hepatic encephalopathy in patients with cirrhosis. Hepatology 2004; 39:1441–1449.

26. Nobaek S, Johansson ML, Molin G, et al. Alteration of intestinal microflora is associated with reduction in abdominal bloating and pain in patients with irritable bowel syndrome. Am J Gastroenterol 2000; 95:1231–1238.

27. Kim HJ, Camilleri M, McKinzie S, et al. A randomized controlled trial of a probiotic, VSL#3, on gut transit and symptoms in diarrhoea-predominant irritable bowel syndrome. Aliment Pharmacol Ther 2003; 17:895–904.

28. D'Souza AL, Rajkumar C, Cooke J, et al. Probiotics in prevention of antibiotic associated diarrhoea: meta-analysis. Brit Med J 2002; 324:1361–1366.

29. Cremonini F, Di Caro S, Nista EC, et al. Meta-analysis: the effect of probiotic administration on antibiotic-associated diarrhoea. Aliment Pharmacol Ther 2002; 16:1461–1467.

30. Saavedra JM, Bauman NA, Oung I, et al. Feeding of Bifidobacterium bifidum and Streptococcus thermophilus to infants in hospital for prevention of diarrhoea and shedding of rotavirus. Lancet 1994; 334:1046–1049.

31. Szajewska H, Kotowska M, Mrukowicz JZ, et al. Efficacy of Lactobacillus GG in prevention of nosocomial diarrhea in infants. J Pediatr 2001; 138:361–365.

32. Mastretta E, Longo P, Laccisaglia A, et al. Effect of Lactobacillus GG and breast-feeding in the prevention of rotavirus nosocomial infection. J Pediatr Gastroenterol Nutr 2002; 35:527–531.

33. Oberhelman RA, Gilman RH, Sheen P, et al. A placebo-controlled trial of Lactobacillus GG to prevent diarrhea in undernourished Peruvian children. J Pediatr 1999; 134:15–20.

34. Pedone CA, Arnaud CC, Postaire ER, et al. Multicentric study of the effect of milk fermented by Lactobacillus casei on the incidence of diarrhoea. Int J Clin Pract 2000; 54:568–571.

35. Saavedra JM, Tschernia A. Human studies with probiotics and prebiotics: clinical implications. Br J Nutr 2002; 87(suppl 2): S241–S246.

36. Marteau P, Seksik P, Jian R. Probiotics and intestinal health effects: a clinical perspective. Br J Nutr 2002; 88(suppl 1): S51–S57.

37. Cummings JH, Christie S, Cole TJ. A study of fructo oligosaccharides in the prevention of travellers' diarrhoea. Aliment Pharmacol Ther 2001; 15:1139–1145.

38. Szajewska H, Mrukowicz JZ. Probiotics in the treatment and prevention of acute infectious diarrhea in infants and children: a systematic review of published randomized, double-blind, placebo-controlled trials. J Pediatr Gastroenterol Nutr 2001; 33:S17–S25.

39. Van Niel CW, Feudtner C, Garrison MM, et al. Lactobacillus therapy for acute infectious diarrhea in children: a meta-analysis. Pediatrics 2002; 109: 678–684.

40. Huang JS, Bousvaros A, Lee JW, et al. Efficacy of probiotic use in acute diarrhea in children: a meta-analysis. Dig Dis Sci 2002; 47:2625–2634.

   Systematic review of all clinical trials using probiotics for treatment of acute diarrhea.

41. Wendakoon CN, Thomson AB, Ozimek L. Lack of therapeutic effect of a specially designed yogurt for the eradication of Helicobacter pylori infection. Digestion 2002; 65:16–20.

42. Sheu BS, Wu JJ, Lo CY, et al. Impact of supplement with Lactobacillus- and Bifidobacterium-containing yogurt on triple therapy for Helicobacter pylori eradication. Aliment Pharmacol Ther 2002; 16:1669–1675.

43. Olah A, Belagyi T, Issekutz A, et al. Randomized clinical trial of specific lactobacillus and fibre supplement to early enteral nutrition in patients with acute pancreatitis. Br J Surg 2002; 89:1103–1107.

44. Bengmark S. Use of some pre-, pro- and synbiotics in critically ill patients. Best Pract Res Clin Gastroenterol 2003; 17:833–848.

   Important data from clinical studies using synbiotics in liver transplant patients.

45. Anderson AD, McNaught CE, Jain PK, et al. Randomised clinical trial of synbiotic therapy in elective surgical patients. Gut 2004; 53:241–245.

46. Macpherson A, Khoo UY, Forgacs I, et al. Mucosal antibodies in inflammatory bowel disease are directed against intestinal bacteria. Gut 1996; 38:365–375.

47. Pirzer U, Schönhaar A, Fleischer B, et al. Reactivity of infiltrating T lymphocytes with microbial antigens in Crohn's disease. Lancet 1991; 338:1238–1239.

48. Neish AS, Gewirtz A, Zeng H, et al. Prokaryotic regulation of epithelial responses by inhibition of IκB-a ubiquitination. Science 2000; 289:1560–1563.

Commensal bacteria can down-regulate cytokine responses of intestinal epithelial cells.

49. Borruel N, Carol M, Casellas F, et al. Increased mucosal TNFα production in Crohn's disease can be downregulated ex vivo by probiotic bacteria. Gut 2002; 51:659–664.

50. Madsen KL, Doyle JS, Jewell LD, et al. Lactobacillus species prevents colitis in interleukin 10 gene-deficient mice. Gastroenterology 1999; 116:1107–1114.

51. Schultz M, Veltkamp C, Dieleman LA, et al. Lactobacillus plantarum 299V in the treatment and prevention of spontaneous colitis in interleukin-10-deficient mice. Inflamm Bowel Dis 2002; 8:71–80.

52. McCarthy J, O'Mahony L, O'Callaghan L, et al. Double blind, placebo controlled trial of two probiotic strains in interleukin-10 knockout mice and mechanistic link with cytokine balance. Gut 2003; 52:975–980.

53. Steidler L, Hans W, Schotte L, et al. Treatment of murine colitis by Lactococcus lactis secreting interleukin-10. Science 2000; 289:1352–1355.

54. Videla S, Vilaseca J, Antolín M, et al. Dietary inulin improves distal colitis induced by dextran sodium sulfate in the rat. Am J Gastroenterol 2001; 96:1486–1493.

55. Kruis W, Schutz E, Fric P, et al. Double-blind comparison of an oral Escherichia coli preparation and mesalazine in maintaining remission of ulcerative colitis. Aliment Pharmacol Ther 1997; 11:853–858.

56. Rembacken BJ, Snelling AM, Hawkey PM, et al. Non-pathogenic Escherichia coli versus mesalazine for the treatment of ulcerative colitis: a randomised trial. Lancet 1999; 354:635–639.

57. Malchow HA. Crohn's disease and Escherichia coli. J Clin Gastroenterol 1997; 25:653–658.

58. Gionchetti P, Rizzello F, Venturi A, et al. Oral bacteriotherapy as maintenance treatment in patients with chronic pouchitis: a double-blind, placebo-controlled trial. Gastroenterology 2000; 119:305–309.

Controlled clinical trial showing that probiotics are highly effective in pouchitis.

59. Mimura T, Rizzello F, Helwig U, et al. Once daily high dose probiotic therapy (VSL#3) for maintaining remission in recurrent or refractory pouchitis. Gut 2004; 53:108–114.

60. Gionchetti P, Rizzello F, Helwig U, et al. Prophylaxis of pouchitis onset with probiotic therapy: a double-blind, placebo-controlled trial. Gastroenterology 2003; 124:1202–1209.

61. Prantera C, Scribano ML, Falasco G, et al. Ineffectiveness of probiotics in preventing recurrence after curative resection for Crohn's disease: a randomised controlled trial with Lactobacillus GG. Gut 2002; 51:405–409.

62. Schultz M, Timmer A, Herfarth HH, et al. Lactobacillus GG in inducing and maintaining remission of Crohn's disease. BMC Gastroenterol 2004; 4:5.

63. Kuisma J, Mentula S, Jarvinen H, et al. Effect of Lactobacillus rhamnosus GG on ileal pouch inflammation and microbial flora. Aliment Pharmacol Ther 2003; 17:509–515.

64. Welters CF, Heineman E, Thunnissen FB, et al. Effect of dietary inulin supplementation on inflammation of pouch mucosa in patients with an ileal pouch-anal anastomosis. Dis Colon Rectum 2002; 45:621–627.

65. Matricardi PM, Bjorksten B, Bonini S, et al. Microbial products in allergy prevention and therapy. Allergy 2003; 58:461–471.

66. Lodinova-Zadnikova R, Cukrowska B, Tlaskalova-Hagenova H. Oral administration of probiotic Escherichia coli after birth reduces frequency of allergies and repeated infections later in life (after 10 and 20 years). Int Arch Allergy Immunol 2003; 131:209–211.

67. Kalliomaki M, Salminen S, Poussa T, et al. Probiotic and prevention of atopic disease: 4-year follow-up of a randomised placebo-controlled trial. Lancet 2003; 361:1869–1871.

Follow-up report on the outcome of a well-known clinical trial showing efficacy of probiotic therapy for the prevention of atopic disease in newborns with high risk.

68. Majamaa H, Isolauri E. Probiotics: a novel approach in the management of food allergy. J Allergy Clin Immunol 1997; 99:179–185.

69. Rosenfeldt V, Benfeldt E, Nielsen SD, et al. Effect of probiotic Lactobacillus strains in children with atopic dermatitis. J Allergy Clin Immunol 2003; 111:389–395.

70. Kirjavainen PV, Salminen SJ, Isolauri E. Probiotic bacteria in the management of atopic disease: underscoring the importance of viability. J Pediatr Gastroenterol Nutr 2003; 36:223–227.

71. Rafter J. Lactic acid bacteria and cancer: mechanistic perspective. Brit J Nutr 2002; 88(suppl 1):S89–S94.

CHAPTER FOUR

4

Nutrition support in the patient with gastrointestinal disease

Samuel Klein, Beth E. Taylor and Deborah C. Rubin

Ingestion and absorption of a nutritionally adequate diet is necessary to maintain normal body composition and function. Gastrointestinal (GI) diseases can cause malnutrition by affecting nutrient intake, nutrient absorption, or nutrient requirements. Therefore, it is important for gastroenterologists to understand the principles involved in evaluating and treating malnourished patients.

BASIC NUTRITIONAL CONCEPTS

Energy stores

Endogenous energy stores are continuously oxidized for fuel. Triglycerides present in adipose tissue are the body's major fuel reserve and are critical for survival during periods of starvation (Table 4.1). The high-energy density and hydrophobic nature of triglycerides make it a fivefold better fuel per unit mass than glycogen. Triglycerides liberate 9.3 kcal/g when oxidized, whereas, glycogen produces only 4.1 kcal/g on oxidation. The duration of survival during starvation depends largely on the amount of available body fat and lean tissue mass. Death from starvation is associated with body weight loss of >35% of body weight, protein depletion of >30% of body protein, fat depletion >70% of body fat stores, and body size (body mass index [BMI] of <13 kg/m^2 for men and <11 kg/m^2 for women).

Table 4.1 Endogenous fuel stores in a man weighing 70 kg

Tissue	Fuel source	Mass (g)	Kilocalories
Adipose	Triglyceride	13 000	120 000
Liver	Glycogen	100	400
	Protein	300	1200
	Triglyceride	50	450
Muscle	Protein	6000	24 000
	Glycogen	400	1600
	Triglyceride	250	2250
Blood	Glucose	3	12
	Triglyceride	4	35
	Free fatty acids	0.5	5

Energy metabolism

Energy is continuously required for normal organ function, maintenance of metabolic homeostasis, heat production, and performance of mechanical work. Total daily energy expenditure (TEE) is comprised of resting energy expenditure (REE, normally ≈70% of TEE), thermic effect of feeding (normally ≈10% of TEE), and energy expenditure of physical activity (normally ≈20% of TEE).

Malnutrition and hypocaloric feeding decreases REE to values 15–20% below those expected for actual body size, whereas metabolic stress, such as inflammatory diseases or trauma, often increase energy requirements. Patients with Crohn's disease who do not have an infectious complication have normal metabolic rates,[1] whereas patients with severe burns may have a 40% increase in REE.[2]

Several equations have been generated to estimate resting energy requirements,[3–6] the most commonly used of these is the Harris-Benedict equation.

$$\text{Men:}$$
$$66 + (13.7 \times W) + (5 \times H) - (6.8 \times A)$$
$$\text{Women:}$$
$$655 + (9.6 \times W) + (1.8 \times H) - (4.7 \times A)$$
W, weight in kilograms; H, height in centimeters;
A, age in years.

The equations for normal subjects generate values that are usually within 10% of measured values. However, these equations are much less accurate in persons who are at extremes in weight (either very lean or obese) or who are ill because alterations in body composition and metabolic stress influence energy expenditure. An adjusted body weight (ABW) rather than actual body weight should be used in obese patients with a body mass index (BMI) >30 kg/m^2 to avoid overfeeding.

$$\text{ABW} = \text{ideal body weight} + [(\text{actual body weight} - \text{ideal body weight}) \times (0.25)]$$

Ideal body weight (IBW) can be estimated based on height. For men, 106 lb is allotted for the first 5 ft, then 6 lbs are added for each inch above 5 ft; for women, 100 lb is given for the first 5 ft, with 5 lbs added for each additional inch. Providing total daily energy equal to the Harris-Benedict calculation plus an additional 20% is a reasonable goal for nonobese, non-critically ill patients who have increased metabolic demands. It may be more accurate to utilize the body mass index (BMI) approach to estimate daily total energy for patients who are either very lean or obese.

Recommended Energy Intake in Hospitalized Patients: We have developed a simple method for estimating total daily energy requirements in hospitalized patients based on body mass index (BMI)[7] (Table 4.2). In general, energy given per kilogram body weight is inversely related to BMI. The lower range within each category should be considered in insulin-resistant, critically ill patients, unless they are depleted in body fat, to decrease the risk of hyperglycemia and infection associated with overfeeding.

Protein

Human proteins are composed of 20 different amino acids, some of which (histidine, isoleucine, leucine, lysine, methionine, phenylalanine, threonine, tryptophan, valine, and possibly arginine) are considered essential because the body cannot synthesize their carbon skeletons. Other amino acids (glycine, alanine, serine, cysteine, cystine, tyrosine, glutamine, glutamic acid, asparagine, and aspartic acid) are nonessential because they can be made from endogenous precursors or essential amino acids. Overall, a protein intake of 0.75 g/kg would meet the requirements of 97% of the adult population.

In disease states, nonessential amino acids may become 'conditionally' essential. For example, it has been shown that cysteine is essential in patients with cirrhosis[8] because the transsulfuration pathway is impaired in these patients.

Individual protein requirements are affected by several factors, such as the amount of nonprotein calories provided, overall energy requirements, protein quality, and the patient's nutritional status. Inadequate amounts of any of the essential amino acids result in inefficient utilization. In general, approximately 15–20% of total protein requirements should be in the form of essential amino acids in normal adults. Table 4.3 lists approximate protein requirements during different clinical conditions.[9] Illness, by increasing catabolism and metabolic rate, also increases requirements for protein.

Carbohydrate

Complete digestion of the principal dietary carbohydrates (starch, sucrose, and lactose) generates monosaccharides (glucose, fructose, and galactose). All cells are able to generate energy (adenosine triphosphate) by metabolizing glucose to either three-

Table 4.2 Estimated energy requirements for hospitalized patients based on body mass index

BMI (kg/m²)	Energy requirements (kcal/kg/day)
<15	35–40
15–19	30–35
20–29	20–25
≥30	15–20

These values are recommended for critically ill patients and all obese patients; add 20% of total calories in estimating energy requirements in noncritically ill patients. The lower range within each BMI category should be considered in insulin-resistant or critically ill patients to decrease the risk of hyperglycemia and infection associated with overfeeding.

Table 4.3 Recommended daily protein intake

Clinical condition	Protein requirements (g/kg IBW/day)
Normal	0.75
Metabolic 'stress'	1.0–1.5
Hemodialysis	1.2–1.4
Peritoneal dialysis	1.3–1.5
Continuous dialysis	1.7–2.0

IBW, ideal body weight.
Additional protein requirements are needed to compensate for excess protein loss in specific patient populations, such as patients with burn injuries, open wounds, and protein-losing enteropathy or nephropathy. Lower protein intake may be necessary in patients with chronic renal insufficiency not treated by dialysis and certain patients with liver disease and hepatic encephalopathy.

carbon compounds via glycolysis or to carbon dioxide and water via glycolysis and the tricarboxylic acid cycle.

There is no dietary requirement for carbohydrate because glucose can be synthesized from endogenous amino acids and glycerol. Nevertheless, carbohydrate is an important fuel because of the interactions between carbohydrate and protein metabolism. Carbohydrate intake stimulates insulin secretion (which inhibits muscle protein breakdown),[10] stimulates muscle protein synthesis, and decreases endogenous glucose production from amino acids.[11,12] In addition, certain tissues, such as bone marrow, erythrocytes, leukocytes, renal medulla, eye tissues, and peripheral nerves, cannot metabolize fatty acids and require glucose ($\approx$40 g/day) as a fuel, whereas other tissues, such as the brain, prefer glucose ($\approx$120 g/day) as a fuel. However, once glucose requirements for these tissues are met, the protein-sparing effects of carbohydrate and fat are similar.[13]

Lipids

Lipids consist of triglycerides (fat), sterols, and phospholipids. These compounds serve as sources of energy; precursors for steroid hormone, prostaglandin, thromboxane, and leukotriene synthesis; structural components of cell membranes; and carriers of essential nutrients. Dietary lipids are composed mainly of triglycerides: long-chain triglycerides (LCTs), which contain fatty acids that are >12 carbons in length, or medium-chain triglycerides (MCTs), which are 6 to 12 carbons in length. Medium-chain triglycerides have several advantages over LCTs.[14] The use of MCTs can be beneficial in patients who have disorders of fat digestion (e.g., pancreatic insufficiency, biliary obstruction), fat absorption (e.g., celiac sprue, short bowel syndrome), lipid transport (e.g., intestinal lymphangiectasia, abetalipoproteinemia), or in those who require a reduction in lymphatic flow (e.g., chylous ascites, thoracic duct fistula). MCTs are hydrolyzed more rapidly and more completely in the small intestine than LCTs, do not require bile acids for absorption, and can be absorbed as an intact triglyceride molecule, which is then hydrolyzed in gut epithelium. MCTs are water soluble and are released into the portal vein after absorption and do not require reesterification, chylomicron formation, and lymphatic transport, as do LCTs. In the liver, MCTs can cross the mitochondrial membrane rapidly without carnitine and are readily oxidized.

MCTs also have several disadvantages.[14] They lack linoleic and linolenic acids, so that small amounts of LCTs are still needed to prevent essential fatty acid deficiency. They are also more ketogenic than LCTs and should not be given to patients with diabetes, ketosis, or acidosis. The use of MCTs is also contraindicated in patients with cirrhosis, particularly those with portal-systemic shunts. Finally, MCTs can cause adverse gastrointestinal symptoms such as nausea, vomiting, and diarrhea, which often limit the maximum amount tolerated to ≈500 kcal per day.

Essential Fatty Acids: The use of fat as a fuel requires the hydrolysis of endogenous or exogenous triglycerides and cellular uptake of released fatty acids. Most fatty acids can be synthesized by the liver, but humans lack the desaturase enzyme needed to produce the n-3 (double bond between carbons 3 and 4 counted from the methyl end) and n-6 (double bond between carbons 6 and 7) fatty acid series. Therefore, linoleic acid (C18:2, n-6) should constitute at least 2% and linolenic acid (C18:3, n-6,9, 12) at least 0.5% of the daily caloric intake to prevent the occurrence of essential fatty acid deficiency (EFAD). The plasma pattern of increased triene-tetraene ratio (>0.4) can be used to detect EFAD, even before the presence of clinical manifestations (dermatitis, coarse hair, alopecia, poor wound healing).[15]

Major minerals

Major minerals are inorganic nutrients that are required in large (>100 mg/day) quantities and are important for ionic equilibrium, water balance, and normal cell function. Malnutrition and nutritional repletion can have dramatic effects on major mineral balance. Evaluations of macromineral deficiencies and recommended dietary intake (RDI) for healthy adults are shown in Table 4.4.

Micronutrients

Micronutrients consist of trace elements and vitamins. Both forms of micronutrients are essential because, as constituents of enzyme complexes, they regulate metabolic processes and substrate metabolism.[16] The RDI for trace elements and vitamins (Tables 4.5, 4.6) is set at two standard deviations above the estimated mean so that it covers the needs of 97% of the healthy population. Therefore, the RDI exceeds the micronutrient requirements of most persons. However, patients with disease, particularly those who have decreased GI absorptive function and increased micronutrient GI losses, may have requirements that are considerably higher than the RDI.

Trace elements

Trace minerals are inorganic nutrients that are required in small (<100 mg/day) quantities (see Table 4.5). Fifteen elements have been found to be essential for health in animals: iron, zinc, copper, chromium, selenium, iodine, cobalt, manganese, nickel, molybdenum, fluorine, tin, silicon, vanadium, and arsenic. The recommended daily parenteral intake for manganese may be too high in patients with chronic liver disease or those receiving long-term parenteral nutrition because of excessive manganese deposition in basal ganglia, causing extrapyramidal and Parkinson-like symptoms.[17]

Vitamins

Vitamins are organic compounds that are required in small (<100 mg/day) quantities (see Table 4.6). A negative balance between vitamin intake and vitamin utilization plus losses causes clinical symptoms of vitamin deficiency. The amount of time before the onset of clinical manifestations depends on the cumulative negative vitamin balance and the size of available vitamin stores. In general, water-soluble vitamin body stores are much smaller than fat-soluble vitamin stores, and so the onset of symptoms is more rapid for water-soluble than for fat-soluble vitamin deficiency. Blood test results usually become abnormal before the onset of clinical manifestations and can be used to assess the need for supplementation (see Table 4.6). Plasma levels of vitamins may be affected by disease or injury.[18]

Table 4.4 Major mineral requirements and assessment of deficiency

| Mineral | Recommended daily intake in normal adults | | | | |
	Enteral	Parenteral	Symptoms or signs of deficiency	Test	Laboratory evaluation Comment
Sodium	0.5–5 g	60–150 mmol	Hypovolemia, weakness	Urinary sodium	May not reflect body stores; clinical evaluation is best
Potassium	2–5 g	60–100 mmol	Weakness, paresthesias, arrhythmias	Serum potassium	May not reflect body stores
Magnesium	300–400 mg	5–15 mmol	Weakness, twitching, tetany, arrhythmias, hypocalcemia	Serum magnesium Urinary magnesium	May not represent body stores May not represent body stores
Calcium	800–1200 mg	5–15 mmol	Osteomalacia, tetany, arrhythmias	24 hr urinary calcium Dual energy X-ray absorptiometry	Reflects recent intake Reflects bone calcium content
Phosphorus	800–1200 mg	20–60 mmol	Weakness, fatigue, leukocyte and erythrocyte dysfunction	Plasma phosphorus	May not reflect body stores

Table 4.5 Trace mineral requirements and assessment of deficiency

| Mineral | Recommended daily intake in normal adults | | Symptoms or signs of deficiency | Laboratory evaluation | |
	Enteral	Parenteral		Test	Comment
Chromium	30–200 μg	10–20 μg	Glucose intolerance, peripheral neuropathy, encephalopathy	Serum chromium	Does not reflect body stores
				Glucose tolerance test	Not specific
Copper	2 mg	0.3 mg	Anemia, neutropenia, osteoporosis, diarrhea	Serum copper	Insensitive for body stores
				Plasma ceruloplasmin	Acute phase reactant
Iodine	150 μg	70–140 μg	Hypothyroidism, goiter	Urine iodine	Reflects recent intake
				Thyroid stimulating hormone	Reflects thyroid function
Iron	10–15 mg	1–1.5 mg	Microcytic hypochromic anemia	Serum iron and total iron binding capacity	Poor measure of body stores; high specificity when levels low; poor sensitivity
Manganese	1.5 mg	0.2–0.8 mg*	Hypercholesterolemia, dementia, dermatitis	Serum manganese	Does not reflect body stores
Selenium	55 μg	20–40 μg	Cardiomyopathy (Keshan's disease), muscle weakness	Serum selenium	Insensitive for body stores
				Blood glutathione peroxidase activity	More sensitive for body stores
Zinc	15 mg	2.5–4 mg	Growth retardation, delayed sexual maturation, hypogonadism, alopecia, acro-orificial skin lesion, diarrhea, mental status changes	Plasma zinc	Poor specificity for body stores

* Recent evidence suggests that manganese toxicity, manifested as extrapyramidal and Parkinsonian-like symptoms, can occur in patients with chronic liver disease or those receiving long-term parenteral nutrition. Many clinicians now limit manganese addition to parenteral nutrition solutions to <0.1 mg/d or eliminate it entirely.[17]

STARVATION

During starvation, a complex and carefully integrated series of metabolic alterations decrease metabolic rate, maintain glucose homeostasis, conserve body nitrogen, and increase the use of adipose tissue triglycerides to meet energy needs. Starvation can be divided into four stages: the first 24 hours, 1–14 days of fasting, 14–60 days of fasting, and the final phase. Death commonly occurs when there is a 30% loss of muscle protein.[19] The mechanisms responsible for death from starvation in humans are not well understood. In general, the duration of survival during starvation depends on the amount of available body fuels and lean body mass. In normal-weight men, death occurs after approximately 2 months of starvation, when more than 35% (≈25 kg) of body weight is lost.[20] In contrast, obese persons have undergone therapeutic fasts for more than 1 year without adverse consequences.[21–23] The longest reported fast was that of a 207 kg man who ingested acaloric fluids, vitamins, and minerals for 382 days and lost 61% (126 kg) of his initial weight.[24]

MALNUTRITION

A normal nutritional status represents a healthy balance between nutrient intake and nutrient requirements. Malnutrition repre-

sents a continuum of events caused by nutrient disequilibrium, which alters intermediary metabolism, organ function, and finally body composition. Therefore, in a general sense, malnutrition can be defined as any metabolic, functional, or compositional alteration caused by inadequate nutrient intake. Malnutrition can be caused by specific nutrient deficiencies and a more generalized deficiency in protein and energy.

Specific nutrient deficiencies

A careful history and physical examination, routine blood tests, and selected laboratory tests can be used to diagnose specific macronutrient, major mineral, vitamin, and trace mineral deficiencies (see Tables 4.4–4.6). Replacement of the deficient nutrient usually corrects the biochemical and physical abnormalities but may not cure the underlying cause of the problem. For example, iron therapy corrects iron deficiency anemia but not the factors responsible for the deficiency (e.g., inadequate intake, malabsorption, or iron loss).

Protein-energy malnutrition

The term protein-energy malnutrition (PEM) has been used to describe several nutritional deficiency syndromes, including

Table 4.6 Vitamin requirements and assessment of deficiency

| Vitamin | Recommended daily intake in normal adults | | Symptoms or signs of deficiency | Laboratory evaluation | |
	Enteral	Parenteral		Test	Comment
A (retinol)	5000 IU	3300 IU	Night blindness, Bitot's spots, keratomalacia, follicular hyperkeratosis, xerosis	Serum retinal	Reflects recent intake and body stores
D (ergocalciferol)	400 IU	200 IU	Rickets, osteomalacia, osteoporosis, bone pain, muscle weakness, tetany	Serum 25-hydroxyvitamin D	Reflects body stores
E (alpha tocopherol)	33 IU	33 IU	Hemolysis, retinopathy, neuropathy	Serum tocopherol	Reflects body stores
				Serum tocopherol: total lipid ratio	Ratio is preferred test
K (phylloquinone)	50–100 μg	100 μg	Easy bruising and bleeding, abnormal clotting	Prothrombin time	Not specific for vitamin K
B_1 (thiamine)	1–1.5 mg	3 mg	Beriberi, cardiac failure, Wernicke's encephalopathy, peripheral neuropathy, fatigue, ophthalmoplegia	RBC transketolase activity	Reflects body stores
B_2 (riboflavin)	1.1–1.8 mg	3.6 mg	Cheilosis, sore tongue and mouth, eye irritation, seborrheic dermatitis	RBC glutathione reductase activity	Reflects body stores
B_3 (niacin)	12–20 mg	40 mg	Pellagra (dermatitis, diarrhea, dementia), sore mouth and tongue	Urinary N-methyl-nicotinamide	Reflects recent intake
B_5 (pantothenic acid)	5–10 mg	10 mg	Fatigue, weakness, paresthesias, tenderness of heels and feet	Urinary pantothenic acid	Reflects recent intake
B_6 (pyridoxine)	1–2 mg	4 mg	Seborrheic dermatitis, cheilosis, glossitis, peripheral neuritis, convulsions, hypochromic anemia	Plasma pyridoxal phosphate	Reflects body stores
B_7 (biotin)	100–200 μg	60 mg	Seborrheic dermatitis, alopecia, change in mental status, seizures, myalgia, hyperesthesia	Plasma biotin	
B_9 (folic acid)	400 μg	400 μg	Megaloblastic anemia, glossitis, diarrhea	Serum folic acid	Reflects body stores and recent intake
				RBC folic acid	Reflects body stores
B_{12} (cobalamin)	3 μg	5 μg	Megaloblastic anemia, paresthesias, decreased vibratory or position sense, ataxia, mental status changes, diarrhea	Serum cobalamin	Reflects body stores
				Serum methylmalonic acid	Tests functional block in enzyme
C (Ascorbic acid)	75–90 mg (125 mg in smokers)	100 mg	Scurvy, petechia, purpura, gingival inflammation and bleeding, weakness, depression	Plasma ascorbic acid	Reflects recent intake
				Leukocyte ascorbic acid	Reflects recent stores

kwashiorkor, marasmus, and nutritional dwarfism in children (Table 4.7), and wasting associated with illness or injury in children and adults.[25] The Waterlow classification of malnutrition for children takes into account a child's weight-for-height (wasting) and height-for-age (stunting).[26]

Primary PEM is caused by inadequate nutrient intake, so the functional and structural abnormalities associated with primary PEM are often reversible with nutritional therapy. However, prolonged primary PEM can cause irreversible changes in organ function and growth. Secondary PEM is caused by illness or injuries, which alter appetite, digestion, absorption, or nutrient metabolism. Wasting disorders, such as cancer, acquired immunodeficiency syndrome (AIDS), and rheumatological diseases, are characterized by involuntary loss of body weight and muscle mass in the setting of a chronic illness. These patients often experience wasting because of (1) inadequate nutrient intake caused by anorexia and possibly GI tract dysfunction and (2) metabolic abnormalities caused by alterations in regulatory hormones and cytokines. Alterations in metabolism cause greater loss of muscle tissue than that observed with pure starvation or semistarvation.

Restoration of muscle mass is unlikely with nutrition support unless the underlying inflammatory disease is corrected. Most of the weight that is gained after providing nutrition support is due to increases in fat mass and body water without significant increases in lean tissue. The effect of PEM on tissue mass and function is presented in Table 4.8.

NUTRITIONAL ASSESSMENT TECHNIQUES

The assessment of nutritional status can be divided into techniques that identify specific nutrient deficiencies and those used to assess PEM. The current methods that are used clinically to evaluate PEM in hospitalized adult patients shift nutritional assessment from a diagnostic to a prognostic instrument in an attempt to identify patients who can benefit from nutritional therapy. The best overall approach involves a careful clinical evaluation, which includes a nutritional history and physical examination in conjunction with appropriate laboratory studies to evaluate further the abnormal findings obtained during clinical examination.

Table 4.7 Features of protein-energy malnutrition syndromes in children

	Kwashiorkor	Marasmus	Nutritional dwarfism
Weight for age (% expected)	60–80	<60	<60
Weight for height	Normal or decreased	Markedly decreased	Normal
Edema	Present	Absent	Absent
Mood	Irritable when picked up Apathetic when alone	Alert	Alert
Appetite	Poor	Good	Good

Table 4.8 Effect of protein-energy malnutrition on tissue mass and function

Body composition	Depletion in fat and muscle mass and intravascular volume.
Gastrointestinal tract	Deterioration of the intestinal tract, pancreas and liver; mucosal epithelial cell proliferation rate decreased; intestinal mucosa become atrophic with flattened villi; reduced pancreatic digestive enzyme synthesis; impaired intestinal transport and absorption of free amino acids; protuberant abdomen secondary to hypomotility and gas distention.
Skin	Dry, thin, and wrinkled with atrophy of the basal layers of the epidermis and hyperkeratosis; hyperpigmentation, cracking and stripping of superficial layers leaving epidermis which is friable and easily macerated.
Hair	Thin, sparse, and easily pluckable; eyelashes become long and luxuriant, excessive lanugo hair may be present in children, adults may lose axial and pubic hair.
Heart	Decreased cardiac muscle mass, bradycardia, decreased stroke volume, decreased cardiac output, and low blood pressure.
Lungs	Decreased vital capacity, tidal volume, and minute ventilation.
Kidneys	Decrease in kidney weight, glomerular filtration rate, ability to excrete acid, ability to excrete sodium and to concentrate urine.
Bone marrow	Suppressed red blood cell and white blood cell production.
Immune system	Atrophy of all lymphoid tissues, diminished cell-mediated immunity leading to delayed cutaneous hypersensitivity and anergy, decreased complement and impaired neutrophil function leading to increased risk of infection, decreased gastrointestinal IgA secretion.
Brain	Weight and protein content remains relatively stable preserving brain function at the expense of other organs and tissues.

History

The patient and/or appropriate family members should be interviewed to provide insight into the patient's current nutritional state and future ability to consume adequate amount of nutrients. The nutritional history should evaluate the following issues:

1. *Body weight*: Has the patient had mild (<5%), moderate (5–10%), or severe (>10%) unintentional body weight loss during the last 6 months? In general, a 10% or greater unintentional loss in body weight during the last 6 months is associated with a poor clinical outcome.[27,28] However, the nutritional significance of changes in body weight can be confounded by changes in hydration.

2. *Food intake*. Has there been a change in habitual diet pattern (number, size, and contents of meals)? What is the reason for altered food intake (e.g., appetite, mental status or mood, ability to prepare meals, ability to chew or swallow, GI symptoms)?

3. *Evidence of malabsorption*: Does the patient have symptoms that are consistent with malabsorption?

4. *Evidence of specific nutrient deficiencies*: Are there symptoms of specific nutrient deficiencies, including macrominerals, micronutrients, and water (see Tables 4.4–4.6)?

5. *Functional status*: Has the patient's ability to function and perform normal daily activities changed?

Physical examination

The physical examination corroborates and adds to the findings obtained by history.

1. *Body mass index (BMI)*, which is defined as weight (in kg) divided by height (in m²), can help identify patients at increased risk of an adverse clinical outcome (Table 4.9).[29,30] Patients who are extremely underweight (BMI <16 kg/m²) are at high risk of death and should be considered for admission to the hospital for nutrition support.

2. *Hydration status*: The patient should be evaluated for signs of dehydration (manifested by hypotension, tachycardia, postural changes, mucosal xerosis, decreased axillary sweat, and dry skin), and excess body fluid (manifested by edema or ascites).

3. *Tissue depletion*: A general loss of adipose tissue can be judged by clearly defined bony, muscular, and venous outlines and loose skinfolds. A fold of skin, pinched between the forefinger and thumb, can reveal the adequacy of subcutaneous fat. The presence of hollowness in the cheeks, buttocks, and perianal area suggests body fat loss. An examination of the temporalis, deltoid, and quadriceps muscles should be made to search for muscle wasting.

4. *Specific nutrient deficiencies* (see Tables 4.4–4.6): Rapidly proliferating tissues, such as oral mucosa, hair, skin, and bone marrow, are often more sensitive to nutrient deficiencies than are tissues that turn over more slowly.

Laboratory tests

Serum Albumin: Serum albumin has a half-life of approximately 20 days. During steady-state conditions, approximately 14 g of albumin (22 mg/kg) are produced and degraded daily. Several studies have demonstrated that a low serum albumin concentration is correlated with an increased incidence of medical complications.[31–33] However, illness or injury, not malnutrition, is responsible for hypoalbuminemia in sick patients.[34] Even during chronic malnutrition, plasma albumin concentration is often maintained because of a compensatory decrease in albumin degradation and a transfer of extravascular albumin to the intravascular compartment. Prolonged protein-calorie restriction induced experimentally in human volunteers[23] or observed clinically in patients with anorexia nervosa[35] causes marked reductions in body weight but little change in plasma albumin concentration.

Hospitalized patients may have low levels of plasma albumin for several reasons. Inflammatory disorders cause a decrease in albumin synthesis, an increase in albumin degradation, and an increase in albumin transcapillary losses.[36–38] Specific GI and cardiac diseases increase albumin losses through the gut, whereas some renal diseases can cause considerable albuminuria. Wounds, burns, and peritonitis can cause albumin losses from the injured surface or damaged tissues. During serious illness, vascular permeability increases dramatically and alters albumin exchange between intravascular and extravascular compartments. Albumin losses from plasma to the extravascular space were increased twofold in patients with cancer-related cachexia and threefold in patients with septic shock. Plasma albumin levels do not increase in stressed patients until the inflammatory stress remits. For example, albumin levels failed to increase in patients with cancer after 21 days of intensive nutritional therapy.[39]

Serum Prealbumin: Prealbumin is a transport protein for thyroid hormones and exists in the circulation as a retinol-binding prealbumin complex. The turnover rate of this protein is rapid, with a half-life of 2–3 days. Protein-energy malnutrition reduces the levels of prealbumin, and refeeding restores levels.[40] However, prealbumin levels fall without malnutrition in patients with infections[41] and in response to cytokine[42] and stress hormone infusion.[43] Renal failure increases levels,[44] whereas liver failure may cause a decrease in levels. The influence of disease-related factors on prealbumin concentration makes it unreliable as an index of nutritional status in hospitalized patients.

Overview of nutritional assessment

At present, there is no 'gold standard' for evaluating nutritional status, and the reliability of any nutritional assessment technique as a true measure of nutritional status has never been validated. The best overall approach involves a careful clinical evaluation,

Table 4.9 Classification of nutritional status by body mass index in adults

Body mass index (kg/m²)	Nutritional status
<16.0	Severely malnourished
16.0–16.9	Moderately malnourished
17.0–18.4	Mildly malnourished
18.5–24.9	Normal
25.0–29.9	Overweight
30.0–34.9	Obese (Class I)
35.0–39.9	Obese (Class II)
≥40	Obese (Class III)

which includes a nutritional history and physical examination in conjunction with appropriate laboratory studies to evaluate further the abnormal findings obtained during the clinical exam. The information from this evaluation should help determine the patient's current clinical condition and the anticipated duration of inadequate volitional feeding to identify patients who may require oral, enteral, or parenteral nutrition support.

NUTRITION SUPPORT

It is generally accepted that, whenever possible, enteral rather than parenteral feeding should be used in patients who need nutritional support. In some patients enteral feedings are either contraindicated or cannot be provided in sufficient quantities to meet nutritional requirements. The intestinal tract often cannot be used effectively in patients who have persistent nausea or vomiting, intolerable postprandial abdominal pain or diarrhea, mechanical obstruction, severe ileus, severe malabsorption, or high-output fistulas. These patients can only receive adequate feeding by parenteral nutrition. Some patients have a functional GI tract but are unable to eat enough to meet their nutritional needs because of anorexia associated with medications, illness, or depression. These patients can often be managed with dietary modifications, appropriate liquid formula supplementation, and successful treatment of the primary disease. Another subset of patients has a functional GI tract but cannot eat safely because of impaired consciousness or an inability to swallow. These patients may benefit from tube feedings.

Enteral nutrition

Principles of Enteral Feeding: Enteral nutrition has many advantages compared with parenteral nutrition. First, enteral nutritional therapy is probably associated with fewer serious complications.[45-49] Second, enteral nutrition can supply gut-preferred fuels, glutamine, glutamate, and short-chain fatty acids that are absent from commercially available parenteral formulations. Third, nutrients are needed in the intestinal lumen to maintain the structural and functional integrity of the GI tract.[50] Enteral feeding prevents atrophy of intestinal mucosa and the pancreas,[51-53] maintains mucosal protein and deoxyribonucleic acid concentrations,[54] preserves mucosal[55] and pancreatic[56] digestive enzyme function,[57] and maintains gastrointestinal IgA secretion.[58] Fourth, enteral feeding prevents cholelithiasis by stimulating gallbladder motility.[59]

Feeding regimens

A wide variety of available feeding regimens can be tailored to each patient's clinical condition and particular nutrient requirements. These regimens can be classified into three general categories: whole food diets, defined liquid formulas, and oral rehydration therapy.

Whole Food Diets: Whole food diets include a standard regular diet and modified oral diets. Modified diets are altered in either consistency or nutrient content to meet specific patient requirements (Table 4.10). Diets modified in consistency include clear liquid, full liquid, pureed, and soft diets. Diets with modifications

---

Table 4.10 Characteristics of hospital diets modified in nutrients and consistency

Diet	Characteristics
Modified in nutrients	
Low fiber/residue	Contains mainly eggs, tender meats, milk, white bread or rice, strained juices, cooked vegetables, and cooked or canned fruits. No nuts, seeds, or skins are allowed.
High fiber	Contains total daily fiber intake of more than 20 g/day by increasing the intake of whole grains, raw fruits and vegetables. Additional fluid intake is required to maintain soft stools.
Low fat	Restricts all forms of fat to <50 g/day.
Low sodium	Restricts sodium to <2000 mg/day.
Low protein	Restricts protein to <60 g/day or <0.8 g/kg body weight. A low-protein diet often cannot meet all nutrient needs when protein is limited to ≤40 g/day, so vitamin and mineral supplementation is required.
Modified in consistency	
Clear liquid	Contains clear juices, broth, jello and popsicles.
Full liquid	Contains cream soups, milk, and ice cream. This diet contains lactose and is often high in fat.
Pureed	Contains foods blended to baby food consistency. Often used for patients with dysphagia.
Mechanical soft	Contains ground meat with gravy, soft cooked vegetables, and canned fruit. Often used for patients with poor dentition.
Selected soft	Contains meat, fruit, and vegetables chopped into bite-size pieces. Often used for patients with dysphagia.
Soft	Contains regular textured foods omitting fresh fruits and vegetables.

in nutrients include those with nutrient restrictions, such as low-residue, low-fat, low-sodium, and low-protein diets, and those with increased dietary components, such as a high-fiber diet.

Defined Liquid Formulas: Defined liquid formulas are commercial products with a known or 'defined' nutrient composition. These formulas can be divided into four categories: elemental (monomeric) formulas, semielemental (oligomeric) formulas, intact-protein (polymeric) formulas, and disease-specific formulas (Table 4.11). Table 4.11 provides a comparison of macronutrient composition, caloric content, and osmolality for the different types of formulas, as well as a list of representative products.

Elemental formulas are not palatable and require either tube feeding or mixing with other foods or flavoring for oral ingestion. Absorption of elemental formulas is not clinically superior to that of semielemental or intact-protein formulas in patients with adequate pancreatic digestion function.

The protein present in semielemental formulas consists of hydrolyzed casein, whey, or lactoalbumin, containing different lengths of small peptides and, in some formulas, free amino acids. These formulas also include carbohydrate in the form of simple sugars, glucose polymers, or starch and fat as either LCTs or a combination of LCTs and MCTs. These formulas are purportedly better absorbed and tolerated than are elemental and intact-protein formulas in patients who have impaired intestinal function. The theoretical advantage of semielemental formulas is related to the absorption of dipeptides and tripeptides, which have specific transport mechanisms for their intact uptake and are absorbed more efficiently than are free amino acids or whole protein.[60,61] However, the potential clinical benefits of semielemental formulas compared with intact-protein formula feeding by improving nutrient absorption have not been demonstrated in prospective randomized trials.[61–63]

Intact-protein formulas contain nitrogen in the form of whole proteins, carbohydrate as glucose polymers, and lipid as LCTs or a mixture of LCTs and MCTs (see Table 4.11). These formulas can be used as a dietary supplement to increase nutrient intake, or they can meet complete calorie, protein, essential fatty acid, vitamin, and mineral requirements if given in appropriate quantities. Taste preference in patients being fed orally, individual patient requirements, and tolerance determine which formula should be used in each patient. Intact-protein formulas can be categorized into two main groups: milk-based formulas and lactose-free formulas.

Milk-based formulas usually contain milk as a source of protein and fat, and milk with additional corn syrup solids and sucrose as a source of carbohydrate. These formulas tend to be more palatable than other defined diets and can be taken orally. Although milk-based formulas are not recommended for lactose-intolerant patients, they can be well tolerated when given as a continuous infusion, which diffuses the load of lactose delivered to the intestine over time. Lactose-free formulas, the most commonly used intact-protein formulas for hospitalized patients, usually contain: casein and soy as a source of protein; corn syrup solids, hydrolyzed cornstarch, glucose polymers, and sucrose as a source of carbohydrate; and corn oil, soy oil, and MCT oil as a source of fat. Fiber is not present in most lactose-free formulas, but fiber-enriched products contain 5–15 grams of fiber, as soy polysaccharides, per liter.

Disease-specific formulas have been designed for patients who have specific illnesses, including hepatic insufficiency, renal insuf-

ficiency, pulmonary insufficiency, diabetes, and critical illness. In general, the clinical superiority of the majority of these disease-specific formulas over less expensive, standard intact-protein formulas remains controversial.[64] A double-blind randomized trial compared 1 year of nutritional supplementation with a branched-chain amino acids (BCAA), leucine, isoleucine, and valine, containing formula with two standard formulas, one with an equinitrogenous amount of lactoalbumin (L-ALB) and one with an equicaloric amount of maltodextrins (M-DXT), in 174 patients with advanced cirrhosis.[65] Treatment with BCAA significantly reduced the occurrence of events compared to the L-ALB group, but did not reach significance when compared to the M-DXT group. Events were defined as death (any reason) and deterioration to exclusion criteria. The average hospital admission rate was significantly lower in the BCAA arm than either of the control arms. In addition, BCAA patients who remained in the study demonstrated stable or improved nutritional parameters and liver function tests, as well as health-related quality of life.[65]

Oral Rehydration Therapy: The principle of oral rehydration therapy is to stimulate sodium and water absorption by taking advantage of the sodium-glucose cotransporter present in the brush border of intestinal epithelium. Glucose enhances sodium absorption by an active carrier and water absorption by solvent drag. This carrier process is often preserved during diarrheal illnesses, thereby providing a mechanism for oral sodium and fluid replacement. Oral rehydration therapy has demonstrated profound benefits in treating patients with cholera-induced diarrhea,[66] and has become a lifesaving measure in developing nations where children frequently die from diarrheal illnesses.[67] Oral rehydration therapy may also aid patients with severe GI fluid and mineral losses, such as those with high-output ostomies, short-bowel syndrome, and HIV infection.[68,69] In 2002, the WHO presented a reduced-osmolarity solution with a sodium concentration of 75 mEq/L as opposed to the standard solution with 90 mEq/L. Controversy still exists regarding which is more effective in cholera patients versus acute noncholera patients[70,71] Adult cholera patients lose 120–140 mEq of sodium/liter of stool, and were found to have hyponatremia when supplemented with the lower sodium solution.[72] Similar sodium losses have been found in patients with short bowel syndrome. Therefore, it is particularly important that the sodium concentration of the solution be between 90 and 120 mEq/L to avoid intestinal sodium secretion and negative sodium and water balance in these patients. The characteristics of selected oral rehydration solutions are shown in Table 4.12.

Tube feeding

Feeding through tubes placed in the intestine is useful for providing nutritional support in patients who cannot or will not eat, but who have a functional GI tract. Nasogastric, nasoduodenal, nasojejunal, gastrostomy, jejunostomy, pharyngostomy, and esophagostomy tubes have been used successfully for feeding. The choice of access to the intestinal tract for enteral nutrition is directed by several factors, including clinical prognosis, patency and motility of the gut, risk of aspirating gastric contents, patient preference, and anticipated duration of feeding.

Short-term Tube Feeding: The placement of a soft, small-diameter nasogastric or nasoduodenal tube is the simplest technique for tube feeding in patients who have short-term (<6 weeks) nutritional needs. Most tubes are made of silicone or polyurethane and

Table 4.11 Composition of selected monomeric, oligomeric and polymeric defined enteral formulas

	Calorie content (kcal/ml)	Osmolality (mOsm/kg)	Protein g/L (%kcal)	Carbohydrate g/L (%kcal)	Fat g/L (% kcal)	Representative products
Monomeric formulas	1.0	550–630	21–36 (8–15)	210–230 (82–91)	2–3 (1–3)	FAA Vivonex TEN
Oligomeric formulas	1.0–1.5	300–650	30–94 (13–25)	127–221 (36–82)	5–68 (5–39)	AlitraQ Criticare HN Crucial Diet Optimental Peptamen Peptamen 1.5 Subdue Subdue 1.5 Travasorb HN Travasorb STD Vital HN Vivonex Plus
Polymeric formulas: Blenderized	1.0–1.07	300–450	40–43(12–25)	128–135 (48–53)	37–40 (31–40)	Compleat modified Compleat regular
Milk based	1.0–2.0	510–1130	40–110(12–25)	87–307 (51–64)	10–50 (10–30)	Carnation Instant Breakfast Fortashake Great shakes Mighty shake Scandi shake
Lactose-free: Normal-calorie	1.0–1.2	300–520	34–60 (13–19)	127–169 (50–57)	35–45 (29–37)	Ensure Isocal Isosource Standard Nutren 1.0 Nu Basics Boost Osmolite Resource Standard
Normal-calorie, high-nitrogen	1.0	300–610	45–63(17–25)	113–144(46–54)	26–45(24–37)	Boost HP Ensure HN IsoSource HN VHN NuBasics VHP Osmolite HN Promote Replete Impact
High-calorie, high-nigrogen	1.5–2.0	430–720	53–83 (14–17)	170–250 (39–53)	50–106 (30–45)	Boost Plus Comply Ensure Plus Ensure Plus HN Isosource 1.5 Magnacal Nova Source 2.0 Nubasics Plus/2.0 Nutren 1.5/2.0 Resource Plus Sustacal Plus Two Cal HN Ultracal HN/Plus Impact 1.5

Table 4.11 Composition of selected monomeric, oligomeric and polymeric defined enteral formulas—cont'd

	Calorie content (kcal/ml)	Osmolality (mOsm/kg)	Protein g/L (%kcal)	Carbohydrate g/L (%kcal)	Fat g/L (% kcal)	Representative products
Low-fat/ fat-free	0.7–0.8	480–700	37–41 (20–25)	120–152 (73–80)	0–2 (0–2)	Citrosource Citrotein Enlive Nubasics Jc. Drink Resource Breeze
Fiber-enriched	1.0–1.2	300–520	40–54 (15–18)	127–147 (51–54)	35–42 (30–37)	Boost with fiber Ensure/fiber Fibersource/HN Jevity/Jevity 1.2 Nubasics with fiber Nutren with fiber Probalance Impact with fiber Promote with fiber Replete with fiber Sustacal with fiber Ultracal

may contain weighted tips and insertion stylets to ease placement. Blind bedside placement of these tubes into the small bowel is gaining popularity in the hospital patient population. An experienced professional can achieve first placement success rates of 85–90%, which is similar to fluoroscopy placement success.[73] In addition, the blind bedside technique is less labor intensive and requires less patient manipulation.[74,75]

Long-term Tube Feeding: Gastrostomy tubes may be placed surgically, endoscopically, radiographically, or with fluoroscopy guidance. The most commonly utilized technique is the percutaneous endoscopic gastrostomy (PEG). Potential complications, although uncommon, may include colocutaneous fistula, buried bumper syndrome (characterized by GI bleeding, gastric perforation, and peritonitis) small bowel perforation and leakage into the abdominal cavity causing peritonitis[76–81] The literature suggests feeding can begin 4–6 hours post PEG placement.[82] Conversion of PEGs to percutaneous endoscopic gastrojejunostomies (PEGJs) has been proposed to reduce reflux and aspiration. However, several studies have found that PEGJs are associated with higher rates of tube dysfunction (50–80%) and do not eliminate the risk

Table 4.12 Characteristics of selected oral rehydration solutions

Product	Na mEq/L	K mEq/L	Cl mEq/L	Citrate mEq/L	kcal/L	CHO g/L	mOsm
Equalyte	78	22	68	30 mg	100	30	305
CeraLyte 70	70	20	98	30	165	40	235
CeraLyte 90	90	20	98	30	165	40	260
Pedialyte	45	20	35	30	100	20	300
Rehydralyte	74	19	64	30	100	25	305
Gatorade	20	3	N/A	N/A	210	45	330
WHO	90	20	80	30	80	20	200
Washington University	105	0	100	10	85	20	250

Equalyte also contains fructo-oligosaccharides.
WHO (World Health Organization) formula: Mix ¾-tsp sodium chloride, ½-tsp sodium citrate, ¼-tsp potassium chloride, and 4 tsp glucose (dextrose) in 1 liter (4¼-cups) of distilled water.
Washington University formula: Mix ¾-tsp sodium chloride, ½-tsp sodium citrate, and 3 tbsp + 1 tsp polycose powder in 1 liter (4¼-cups) of distilled water.
Mix formulas with sugar-free flavorings as needed for palatability.

of aspiration.[83–86] A feeding jejunostomy implanted directly into the small bowel provides the most secure means of accessing the small bowel.[87] Surgical jejunostomies placed at the time of laparotomy consist of a subserosa tunnel (Witzell) or needle catheter jejunostomy.[88]

Delivery Systems: The method of nutrient delivery varies with the location of the tube. In patients with a jejunostomy, continuous feeding is preferable because bolus feeding usually creates dumping symptoms. For most patients using gastrostomies, nutritional goals can be achieved with intermittent gravity feedings. Advantages of intermittent gravity feedings include minimal equipment needs and the ability to free patients from the feedings during most of the day. Some patients with a gastrostomy experience nausea and early satiety with gravity feedings and will do better with continuous infusion of the liquid formulas at a slower rate.

Complications: The complications that occur in patients receiving tube feedings can be divided into four categories: mechanical, metabolic, GI, and pulmonary (aspiration).

Mechanical complications: Nasogastric feeding tube misplacement occurs more commonly in unconscious than conscious patients. Intubation of the tracheobronchial tree has been reported in up to 15% of patients;[89] intracranial placement can occur in patients who have had craniofacial surgery or severe head trauma and facial trauma.[90] Erosive tissue damage can lead to nasopharyngeal erosions, pharyngitis, sinusitis, otitis media, pneumothorax, and GI tract perforation.[91–94] Tube occlusion is often caused by inspissated feedings or pulverized medications given through small-diameter (<10 French) tubes. Frequent flushing of the tube with 30–60 ml of water and avoiding administration of pill fragments or 'thick' medications help prevent occlusion. Techniques used to unclog tubes include using a small-volume syringe (10 ml) to flush warm water or pancreatic enzyme preparations through the tube.[95] Commercially made products can be obtained that either dissolve or mechanically remove the obstruction.

Metabolic complications: Disturbances in fluid and electrolytes are common in patients receiving tube feedings. In one study of 100 patients, 30–40% had at least one metabolic complication, with hypokalemia, hyponatremia, hypophosphatemia, and hyperglycemia being the most common.[96]

Gastrointestinal complications: GI side effects of tube feeding include nausea and vomiting, abdominal pain, and diarrhea. Nonocclusive bowel necrosis has been reported in 0.3% of critically ill patients given tube feedings, particularly those patients receiving vasoconstrictive medications to maintain blood pressure.[97] It is likely that the increased intestinal oxygen demands induced by feeding in the presence of compromised GI blood flow is responsible for this adverse event.[97]

Diarrhea occurs in 30–50% of critically ill patients receiving tube feedings and has been shown to correlate most closely with antibiotic use.[98] Antibiotics may cause pseudomembranous colitis (see Chapter 51) or impaired conversion of carbohydrate to SCFAs. Another common source of osmotic diarrhea in tube-fed patients is the surprisingly large dose of the nonabsorbable carbohydrate, sorbitol, given through the tube with common elixirs such as acetaminophen, theophylline, and cimetidine.[99] If diarrhea from tube feeding persists after proper attention to the usual causes, trials of antidiarrheal agents are justified in an effort to maintain adequate delivery of nutrients.

Pulmonary complications: The etiology of pulmonary aspiration can be difficult to ascertain in tube-fed patients because aspiration can occur from refluxed tube feedings or oropharyngeal secretions that are unrelated to feedings. Assessing the color of respiratory secretions after adding several drops of blue food coloring to the feeding formula had been common practice. However, several case reports have documented serious and life-threatening metabolic complications associated with blue food dye administration,[100–102] prompting the FDA to issue a health advisory against its use with enteral feedings in 2003. Prevention of reflux by decreasing gastric acid secretion, keeping the head of the bed elevated during feedings, and avoiding gastric feeding in high-risk patients (e.g., those with gastroparesis, gastric outlet obstruction, or frequent vomiting) is the best management approach.[103,104] Enteric feeding administered past the ligament of Treitz should decrease the risk of aspiration.[105]

Parenteral nutrition

The use of the vascular system to supply nutrient requirements can be an important and even lifesaving therapy. Patients who are unable to consume 'adequate' nutrients for a 'prolonged' period of time by oral or enteral routes require total parenteral nutritional (TPN) therapy to prevent the adverse effects of malnutrition. However, the decision to use TPN can be difficult because the precise definition of these terms is not clear and depends on the patient's amount of body fat and lean tissue mass, the presence of pre-existing medical illnesses, and the level of metabolic stress. In general, parenteral nutrition should be considered if energy intake has been, or is anticipated to be, inadequate (<50% of daily requirements) for more than 14 days and enteral feeding is not feasible. However, the efficacy of this approach has not been tested in clinical trials.

Before initiating intravenous (IV) feeding, an assessment of the patient's nutrient and fluid requirements is needed. As discussed above, the assessment requires a careful medical examination including history, physical examination, and laboratory studies to evaluate for specific nutrient deficiencies and to determine nutritional needs. In particular, a complete blood count and measurement of serum glucose, electrolytes, creatinine, urea nitrogen, magnesium, phosphorus, calcium, triglycerides, and liver biochemistries should be performed before starting nutritional support. Careful monitoring is needed to ensure safety and adequate therapy, and vital signs should be checked daily, as should measurements of body weight, fluid intake, and fluid output. Serum electrolytes, phosphorus, and glucose should be measured every 2 days until stable and then rechecked weekly. If lipid emulsions are being given, serum triglycerides should be evaluated early during the course of TPN to document adequate clearance. In patients who have abnormal glucose homeostasis, finger-stick evaluations for glucose should be performed regularly.

Catheters

The infusion of hyperosmolar (usually >1500 mOsm/L) nutrient solutions requires a large-bore, high-flow vessel to minimize vessel irritation and damage. Percutaneous subclavian vein catheterization with advancement of the catheter tip to the junction of the superior vena cava and right atrium is the most commonly used technique for TPN access. The internal jugular, saphenous, and femoral veins are also used. Although these sites either decrease or eliminate the risk of pneumothorax, they are less desirable because of decreased patient comfort and difficulty in maintaining sterility. Peripherally inserted central catheters (PICCs), which also eliminate the risk of pneumothorax, can be used to provide TPN in patients with adequate antecubital vein access. A retrospective comparison of 135 PICC lines with 135 subclavian lines used for TPN found no significant differences in the total number of catheter-related complications, even though PICC lines remained in place three days longer that subclavian lines.[106] Considerable cost savings can be realized by using PICC lines, if inserted by allied health personnel on the hospital ward.

Nutrient solutions

Parenteral solutions are available to supply all basic nutrient requirements, including fluid, protein, carbohydrate, fat, minerals, trace elements, and vitamins. Typically, these components are given together as an admixture, which reduces handling costs and potential breaks in sterility, or the lipid component is given separately, 'piggy-backed' to the primary nutrient mixture.

Protein: Standard commercially made solutions are composed of crystalline amino acids in concentrations between 2.75% and 15%. These solutions usually contain 40–50% essential and 50–60% nonessential amino acids. The proportion of nitrogen consisting of essential amino acids is more than twice that required by normal adults and increases amino acid biological availability. Most formulas completely lack, or have very little of, the nonessential amino acids glutamine, glutamate, aspartate, asparaginine, tyrosine, and cysteine.

Modified parenteral amino acid solutions have been developed for specific disease states and physiological conditions. Solutions containing higher concentrations of BCAA than standard solutions have been advocated for use in patients who have hepatic encephalopathy (see Chapter 5). These specialized formulas were found to achieve higher amino acid intakes (60–80 g per day) with less risk of encephalopathy than that of standard formulas.[107] Solutions containing large amounts of essential amino acids have been developed for patients who have acute renal failure. Between 67% and 100% of the total amino acids in these formulas are composed of the eight essential amino acids and histidine, which is believed to be essential in patients with renal failure. However, the superiority of administering essential amino acids as the sole source of nitrogen over solutions containing a mixture of essential and nonessential amino acids has not been demonstrated in prospective randomized trials.[108]

Carbohydrate: Carbohydrate is provided in the form of glucose (dextrose), and the amount of infused glucose that is oxidized is directly proportional to the amount administered until a threshold level is reached. Infusing more than 7 mg/kg/minute (≈2800 kcal per day) in stable postoperative patients does not increase glucose oxidation but could have adverse consequences by increasing lipogenesis, carbon dioxide production, and metabolic rate.[109,110] Dextrose is the least expensive and most commonly used IV energy source. Commercially made formulas are available in concentrations ranging 5–70%. Most TPN formulations use 50–70% dextrose, which is diluted to a final concentration of 15–30%. The dextrose in IV solutions is hydrated, so each gram of dextrose monohydrate provides 3.4 kcal.

Fat: Lipid emulsions provide an IV source of fat calories including the essential fatty acids, linoleic and linolenic acids. These emulsions are available as a 10% (1.1 kcal/ml) or 20%

(2.0 kcal/ml) and are ≈6 times more expensive than are equivalent glucose calories. Lipid emulsions contain soybean oil or a combination of soybean and safflower oil triglycerides, egg yolk phospholipids as an emulsifying agent, and glycerin to achieve isotonicity with plasma. The osmolarity of current formulas ranges from 270 to 340 mOsm per liter. Currently available emulsions contain approximately 50–65% of their fatty acids as linoleic acid and approximately 5–10% as linolenic acid. Lipid emulsions should not be given to patients who have triglyceride concentrations of >400 mg/dL. Moreover, patients at risk for hypertriglyceridemia should have serum triglyceride concentrations checked at least once during lipid emulsion infusion to ensure adequate clearance.

The optimal percentage of calories that should be infused as fat is not known. A minimum of ≈5% of total calories as a lipid emulsion is necessary to prevent essential fatty acid deficiency in patients receiving continuous TPN.[111] Administering fat-free TPN can cause biochemical evidence of essential fatty acid deficiency within 2 weeks.[112] A study completed on 11 patients receiving lipid-containing long-term home TPN found the patients to have a suboptimal essential fatty acid status.[113] This observation suggests that the optimal parenteral fat intake for long-term home TPN patients requires further investigation. Most complications associated with IV lipid emulsions occur when lipid calories are provided in excess of 1.0 kcal/kg per hour (0.11 g/kg per hour).[114] Rare complications of IV lipid emulsions include pulmonary dysfunction,[115] hepatic phospholipidosis,[116] impaired immune system function,[117] pancreatitis,[118] decreased platelet aggregation,[119] fat-overload syndrome,[120] hypersensitivity reactions,[121] and delayed gastric emptying.[122]

Complications

The cornerstone in the management of patients receiving TPN is attention to details. Continued adjustment of the nutrient formula is often necessary because of changes in medical therapy or clinical status. The supervision of TPN by an experienced multidisciplinary nutrition support team has been demonstrated to reduce parenteral nutrition-associated complications.[123] The complications associated with the use of parenteral nutrition can be divided into mechanical, vascular, infectious, metabolic, and GI complications.

Mechanical Complications: A misguided approach to central venous catheter insertion can cause pneumothorax, brachial plexus injury, subclavian and carotid artery puncture, hemothorax, thoracic duct injury, and chylothorax.[124] Even when the subclavian vein is cannulated successfully, other mechanical complications can still occur. The catheter may be advanced upward into the internal jugular vein, or the tip can be sheared off completely if it is withdrawn back through an introducing needle.[124]

Vascular Complications: Air embolism can occur during insertion or afterwards if the connection between the catheter and IV tubing is not well secured. The catheter can become occluded because of thrombosis or precipitation of electrolyte salts. Subclavian vein thrombosis occurs commonly (25–50%), but clinically significant manifestations such as upper extremity edema, superior vena cava syndrome, or pulmonary embolism are rare during short-term TPN.[125–127] Fatal microvascular pulmonary emboli, caused by nonvisible calcium and phosphorus precipitate identified in the total nutrient admixtures, have been reported.[128,129] Therefore, strict pharmacy standards regarding physical–chemical compatibility and in-line filters should be used with all parenteral nutrient solutions despite careful inspection of solutions. The smallest pulmonary capillaries are 5 μm in diameter, while the size limit for visually detecting microprecipitates is 50–100 μm.[130]

Metabolic Complications: Most metabolic complications are caused by inappropriate nutrient administration resulting in nutrient excesses or deficiencies or both. Overzealous nutrient administration may provide excess delivery of water and sodium (fluid overload), glucose (hyperglycemia, nonketotic hyperosmolar coma), amino acids (hyperammonemia, azotemia), lipids (hypertriglyceridemia, pancreatitis), and calcium (hypercalcemia, pancreatitis, renal stones).[131] Inadequate nutrient administration can cause glucose, electrolyte, vitamin, trace mineral, and essential fatty acid deficiencies.[132]

Hyperglycemia is a common complication of parenteral nutrition that is associated with leukocyte and complement dysfunction and increases risk of infection when blood glucose is above 200 mg/dL. Therefore, blood glucose should be kept between 100 mg/dL and 200 mg/dL initially and between 100 mg/dL and 150 mg/dL when stable. Blood glucose should be kept below 120 mg/dL in pregnant patients to avoid complications of gestational diabetes and large-for-gestational-age births.

A suggested management scheme for control of hyperglycemia in patients on TPN is included in Table 4.13. In critically ill patients and patients who have undergone coronary artery bypass graft, tighter glucose control of 80–110 mg/dL was found to decrease mortality by approximately 50%.[133,134]

Metabolic bone disease has been observed in patients receiving long-term (>3 months) TPN.[135] The patients with clinical manifestations of bone disease range from those who are asymptomatic but have radiologic evidence of demineralization, to those who have bone pain, and ultimately to those who experience bone fracture.[136] Histological examination has documented osteomalacia, osteopenia, or both. The causes of metabolic bone disease are not known, but several mechanisms have been proposed, including aluminum toxicity, vitamin D toxicity, and negative calcium balance caused by amino acid-induced hypercalciuria.[135,137]

Infectious Complications: Catheter-related sepsis is the most common life-threatening complication in patients receiving TPN. The results from most studies suggest that meticulous catheter insertion and care reduces the prevalence of catheter-related infections to 3% or less.[138] Most prospective trials have demonstrated that multilumen catheters are associated with an increased risk of infection compared with single lumen catheters.[138,139] However, the need for IV access often makes the use of single lumen catheters impractical. Catheter infections can be caused by

---

Table 4.13 Management of hyperglycemia in patients receiving parenteral nutrition

1. If blood glucose is >200 mg/dL or patient has diabetes:
   a. Better control of blood glucose should be obtained before starting CPN
   b. If CPN is started:
      1. limit dextrose to <200 gram/day
      2. add 0.1 unit of insulin for each gram of dextrose in CPN solution (e.g., 15 units for 150 grams)
      3. discontinue other sources of intravenous dextrose
      4. order subcutaneous sliding scale regular insulin with blood glucose monitoring by fingerstick every 4–6 h or sliding scale intravenous regular insulin infusion with blood glucose monitoring by fingerstick every 1–2 h as follows:

Blood glucose (mg/dl)	SQ insulin (unit)	or IV insulin (unit/hr)
150–199	2.0	
200–249	2–3	2.5
250–300	4–6	3.0
301–350	6–8	4.0
351–400	8–12	6.0
>400		8.0

2. If blood glucose remains >200 mg/dl and patient has been receiving:
   a. Subcutaneous insulin: add 50% of sliding scale regular insulin given in last 24 hr to next day's CPN solution; double amount of subcutaneous insulin sliding scale dose for blood glucose values >200 mg/dL
   b. Intravenous insulin: add 50% of IV insulin given in last 24 hr to next day's CPN solution;
   increase sliding scale IV insulin infusion rate by 50% for blood glucose values >200 mg/dL

3. If patient's blood glucose remains >200 mg/dL, consider:
   1. discontinuing CPN until better glucose control can be established
   2. decreasing dextrose content in CPN
   3. initiating insulin drip if not already started

4. Dextrose in CPN may be increased when blood glucose control (100–150 mg/dl) is achieved. Insulin:dextrose ratio in CPN formulation should be maintained while CPN dextrose content is changed

Adapted from McMahon MM, Rizza RA. Mayo Clin Proc 1996; 71:587–594.

entry of organisms at the catheter exit site, contamination at tubing connections, seeding from other sites of infection, and, rarely, contamination of the infusate itself.

Catheter-related sepsis in patients receiving TPN is most commonly caused by *S. epidermidis* and *S. aureus*. In immune-compromised patients (e.g., AIDS, immunosuppressive therapy, absolute neutrophil count <200) and those with long-term (>2 wks) TPN, *Enterococcus*, *Candida* species, E. coli, *Pseudomonas*, *Klebsiella*, *Enterobacter*, *Acinetobacter*, *Proteus*, and *Xanthomonas* should also be considered. Table 4.14 reviews our suggested management approach for suspected catheter-related infection.

The antibiotic lock technique has also been used successfully to treat central catheter infections.[140-143] This technique involves injecting an antibiotic solution (e.g., vancomycin 2 mg/mL) into the central catheter lumen and allowing the antibiotic to reside in the line for at least 12 hours. The catheter can be used to infuse fluids or parenteral nutritional solutions during the remaining 12 hours of the day. The catheter is periodically reinjected for a 14-day course.[141] This approach has the advantage of delivering a higher antibiotic concentration into the catheter, avoiding the side effects of systemic antibiotics, and lower cost.[140] However, this technique is not effective for treating tunnel/skin infections and is probably less efficacious in reservoir-type catheters.[140]

Gastrointestinal Complications: Hepatic abnormalities are the most common GI complications associated with TPN. It is difficult, however, to establish a true causal relationship between the use of TPN and many of the reported liver abnormalities because of the paucity of prospective randomized trials. Many of the hepatic abnormalities in patients receiving TPN might have been caused by clinical factors unrelated to the use of TPN itself. Patients who require TPN often have serious illnesses that are associated with liver disease or have received hepatotoxic therapy, which can cause liver disease.

Several hepatic abnormalities have been observed in adults receiving TPN.[144-146] Although these abnormalities are usually benign and transient, a small subset of patients with more serious and progressive disease has been reported. Most complications occur within 4 weeks of starting TPN, whereas fewer but often more severe complications occur later, usually after 16 weeks of TPN therapy. The hepatic complications include both biochemical (elevated serum aminotransferase and alkaline phosphatase) and histological (steatosis, steatohepatitis, lipidosis and phospho-lipidosis, cholestasis, fibrosis, and cirrhosis) alterations.

The first report of TPN-associated liver disease, published in 1971, was of a premature infant who developed cholestatic jaundice, bile duct proliferation, and cirrhosis after 71 days of TPN therapy.[144] Subsequent studies have shown that cholestasis is the most frequent hepatic complication in TPN-fed infants and correlates directly with decreased gestational age, decreased birth weight, and increased duration of TPN therapy.

The mechanisms involved in the pathogenesis of hepatic complications are not well understood. Many potential contributing factors have been proposed as being responsible for TPN-associated liver disease. These factors include those associated with the patient's clinical condition or therapy, the TPN solution itself (excessive glucose calories, excessive lipid infusion, amino acid degradation products, aluminum toxicity), nutritional deficiencies (essential fatty acid deficiency, choline deficiency,

---

Table 4.14 Management of suspected catheter-related infection

1. Initial evaluation:
   a. Evaluate catheter insertion site and culture any drainage
   b. Obtain blood cultures from peripheral vein and central vein catheter
   c. Consider culture of hub, skin, infusate
   d. Culture catheter tip, if removed
   e. Look for other causes of infection (e.g., urinalysis, chest X-ray, sputum, wounds)

2. Stop TPN for 48–72 hours

3. Indications for central venous catheter removal:
   a. Immediate removal
      1. Purulent discharge or abscess at insertion site
      2. Septic shock without another etiology for the source of infection
   b. Removal of catheters after culture results are obtained
      1. Persistent or recurrent catheter-related bacteremia
      2. *Candida* species or *Pseudomonas* infection
      3. Polymicrobial infection
      4. *S. aureus* infection

4. Antibiotic therapy
   a. Empiric antibiotic therapy administered through central venous catheter until culture results are back:
      1. Vancomycin 1 g q 12 h (adjust dose for creatinine/GFR)
      2. Cefepime 1 g q 12 h (if gram negative infection suspected)
   b. Specific antibiotic therapy administered through central venous catheter once culture results are available
   c. If a catheter is 'irreplaceable,' consider trial of antibiotic therapy with line in place
   d. Duration of antibiotic therapy usually ranges 2–6 wk depending on patient, organism, and whether central line has been left in place

5. Repeat blood cultures in 48 and 72 hours to ensure clearance of bacteremia

6. Fever should resolve within 72–96 h if given appropriate antibiotics; remove catheter if fever persists

carnitine deficiency), and gut factors (intestinal bacteria or endotoxin translocation, bacterial overgrowth, bacterial metabolism of bile acids).

Three types of biliary complications have been associated with the use of prolonged (>4 weeks) of TPN – acalculous cholecystitis,[147] gallbladder sludge,[148,149] and cholelithiasis.[150] Acalculous cholecystitis has been reported to occur in ≈5%,[149] cholelithiasis in ≈30%,[150] and gallbladder sludge in up to 100%[59] of patients receiving prolonged TPN. The pathogenesis of acalculous cholecystitis is unclear, but it occurs in the setting of bile stasis and increased bile lithogenicity. The pathogenesis of gallbladder sludge and stones is related to gallbladder stasis caused by the absence of enteral feeding in TPN-fed patients. The development of gallbladder sludge appears to be a prerequisite for the development of gallstones. Stimulating gallbladder contraction and emptying with either enteral feedings[151] or cholecystokinin injections[152] has been shown to reduce or prevent gallbladder sludge and gallstone formation.

REFEEDING SYNDROME

Because of the structural, functional, and metabolic alterations caused by previously inadequate food intake, injudicious nutritional therapy can have adverse clinical consequences known in part as the *refeeding syndrome*.[153,154] Early evidence of the refeeding syndrome was reported at the end of World War II, when it was found that oral refeeding of chronically semistarved research volunteers and war victims caused cardiac insufficiency and neurologic complications.[155] More recently, refeeding abnormalities and serious complications have been reported after aggressive refeeding in hospitalized cachectic patients.[156,157]

Fluid Overload: Decreased cardiac mass, stroke volume, and end-diastolic volume, bradycardia, and fragmentation of cardiac myofibrils are associated with chronic undernutrition.[158–161] In addition, carbohydrate refeeding increases the concentration of circulating insulin, which enhances sodium and water reabsorption by the renal tubule.[162] These factors place the severely malnourished patient at increased risk for developing fluid retention and congestive heart failure after nutritional therapy containing water, glucose, and sodium.

Mineral Depletion: Of the mineral abnormalities associated with refeeding, phosphate depletion has received the most attention. During starvation, phosphorus requirements are decreased because of the predominant use of fat as a fuel source. Serum phosphate is maintained at normal levels by mobilizing bone stores and increasing renal tubular reabsorption. Refeeding with enteral carbohydrates or glucose-based parenteral formulas stimulates insulin release and intracellular uptake of phosphate.[163] Phosphate is needed for protein synthesis and for the production of phosphorylated intermediates necessary for glucose metabolism.[164] These metabolic processes can cause extracellular phosphorus concentration to fall below 1 mg/dL (severe hypophosphatemia) within hours of initiating nutritional therapy if adequate phosphate is not given. Severe hypophosphatemia, which is associated with impaired diaphragmatic contractility, rhabdomyolysis, erythrocyte dysfunction, hemolysis, myocardial dysfunction, central nervous system dysfunction, and death has occurred in patients receiving enteral or parenteral nutritional repletion.[164–173] Repletion protocols exist so that severe hypophosphatemia can be treated in a prompt and effective manner.[174]

However, it is difficult to determine the contribution of hypophosphatemia per se to the reported clinical complications because of other coexistent medical and nutritional abnormalities.

Potassium and magnesium are the most abundant intracellular cations. Loss of body cell mass in the malnourished patient causes whole body potassium and magnesium depletion. Serum potassium and magnesium concentrations, however, remain normal or near normal during starvation because of their release from tissue and bone stores. The increases in protein synthesis rates, body cell mass, and glycogen stores during refeeding require increased intracellular potassium and magnesium. In addition, hyperinsulinemia during refeeding increases cellular uptake of potassium and can cause a rapid decline in extracellular concentrations.[175]

Glucose Intolerance: The adaptive changes during starvation enhance use of fatty acids and ketone bodies for fuel while glucose is conserved. In addition, the ability of insulin to stimulate glucose uptake and oxidation by peripheral tissues is impaired.[175] Thus, refeeding with high-carbohydrate meals or large amounts of parenteral glucose may not be well tolerated initially and may produce marked elevations in blood glucose, glucosuria, dehydration, and hyperosmolar coma.[176] Furthermore, because of the importance of thiamine in glucose metabolism, carbohydrate refeeding in patients who have thiamine depletion can precipitate Wernicke's encephalopathy.[177]

Gastrointestinal Dysfunction: Starvation and malnutrition cause structural and functional deterioration of the GI tract. The total mass and protein content of the intestinal mucosa and pancreas are markedly reduced. Mucosal epithelial cell proliferation rates, the synthesis of mucosal and pancreatic digestive enzymes, and intestinal transport and absorption of free amino acids are impaired,[178] whereas hydrolysis and absorption of peptides are better maintained.[179] These alterations limit the ability of the GI tract to digest and absorb food. When malnutrition is severe, oral refeeding has been associated with an increased incidence of diarrhea and death.[180] However, most of the adverse consequences of starvation on the GI tract disappear after 1–2 weeks of refeeding.

Cardiac Arrhythmias: Ventricular tachyarrhythmias, which can be fatal, occur during the first week of refeeding.[181] A prolonged QT interval, often documented before death, is a contributing cause of the rhythm disturbances. It is not known whether refeeding per se or the cardiac dysfunction underlying malnutrition precipitated the terminal arrhythmias.

Clinical recommendations

Initial Evaluation: The severity of complications during refeeding cachectic, chronically semistarved patients emphasize the importance of a particularly cautious approach to their nutritional therapy, particularly during the first week of therapy, when the risk of complications is highest. A careful search for cardiovascular and electrolyte abnormalities should be performed before refeeding. In addition, a search for infections (e.g., obtaining a white blood cell count, urine analysis and culture, blood cultures, and chest X-ray) should be considered even in the absence of physical findings, because many patients are not able to mount a normal inflammatory response.

Initial Supportive Care: Judicious resuscitation with fluids and electrolytes may be necessary before beginning feedings to prevent congestive heart failure from excessive fluid. Vitamin supplementation should be given routinely. Because severely malnourished patients are poikilothermic, warm ambient temperature and warming blankets may be necessary to slowly raise core temperature. However, if warming blankets are being used, patients must be carefully monitored to avoid hyperthermia.

Feeding Regimen: Patients can be re-fed orally, by enteral tube feeding, by parenteral nutrition, or through a combination of these methods. Oral or enteral tube feedings are preferred over parenteral feeding because of fewer serious complications and enhanced GI tract recovery. Isotonic feedings should be given in small amounts at frequent intervals to prevent overwhelming the body's limited capacity for nutrient processing and to prevent hypoglycemia, which can occur during brief nonfeeding intervals. Parenteral supplementation or complete parenteral nutrition may be necessary if the intestine cannot tolerate oral/enteral feeding. A combination of many nutrients, particularly nitrogen, phosphorus, potassium, magnesium, and sodium, is needed to restore lean body mass. Inadequate intake of one nutrient may impair retention of others during refeeding.

Although it is impossible to know the precise nutrient requirements of individual patients, some general guidelines are recommended for the first week of refeeding. Fluid intake should be limited to approximately 800 mL/day plus replacement for insensible losses. Adjustments in fluid intake are necessary in patients who have evidence of fluid overload or dehydration. Changes in body weight provide a useful guide for evaluating the efficacy of fluid administration. Weight gain greater than 0.25 kg/day, or 1.5 kg/week, probably represents fluid accumulation. Daily calorie

intake should be approximately 15–20 kcal/kg, containing approximately 100 g of carbohydrate and 1.5 g of protein/kg body weight. Sodium should be restricted to approximately 60 mEq or 1.5 g/day, but liberal amounts of phosphorus, potassium, and magnesium should be given to patients who have normal renal function. All other nutrients should be given in amounts needed to meet the recommended dietary allowance. Daily monitoring of body weight, fluid intake, urine output, and plasma glucose and electrolyte values are critical during early refeeding (first 3–7 days), so that nutritional therapy can be appropriately adjusted when necessary.

MANAGEMENT OF PATIENTS WITH SEVERE MALABSORPTION

Some patients become malnourished because of impaired absorptive capacity of the GI tract. These patients have inadequate functional small bowel length because of intestinal resection or intestinal disease and present the most challenging nutritional management problems for the clinician. The medical management of these patients is often difficult and frustrating but can be simplified by understanding the physiological and clinical principles of treatment (Fig. 4.1).

Clinical considerations

The initial assessment of the patient with chronic malabsorption is meant to provide a logical basis for developing a treatment

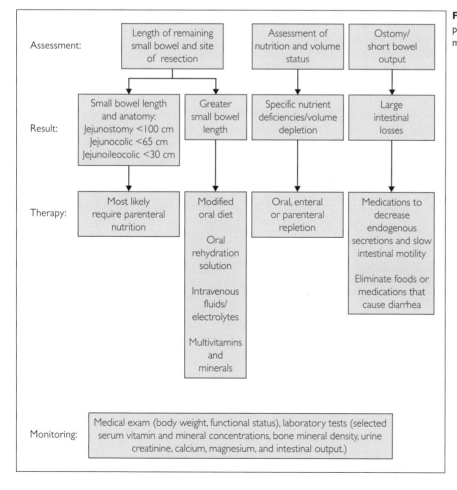

Fig. 4.1 • Algorithm for management of patients with short bowel syndrome and severe malabsorption

strategy to improve the patient's current clinical condition and to prevent future complications. The therapeutic approach depends on the function of the intestinal tract; the presence of macronutrient, micronutrient, electrolyte, and fluid deficits; identification of risk factors for future medical complications; the presence of coexisting diseases that affect the ability to provide nutritional therapy; and an evaluation of factors that affect the patient's daily activities.[182,183]

A careful review of medical records, operative reports, and radiologic studies is needed to evaluate the absorptive capacity of the intestine by determining the length of remaining intestine, the site of intestinal disease or resection, and the presence of diseases that reduce intestinal absorption, such as pancreatic insufficiency or cholestasis. An assessment of fluid losses through diarrhea, ostomy output, and fistula volume should be made to help determine fluid requirements. Knowledge of fluid losses is also useful in calculating intestinal mineral losses by multiplying fluid loss by the estimated electrolyte concentration in intestinal fluid (Table 4.15). In patients who do not respond to treatment as predicted, dynamic studies of intestinal absorptive function by measuring fat, carbohydrate, and nitrogen balance and evaluating ostomy, fecal, or fistula mineral and fluid losses may be helpful in adjusting the treatment program.

The urgency for medical intervention is determined by the severity of hemodynamic and nutritional abnormalities, which requires an evaluation for volume depletion, weight loss, and specific nutrient deficiencies. In addition to standard laboratory tests to evaluate for anemia (iron, folate, or vitamin B_{12} deficiency), prolonged prothrombin time (vitamin K deficiency), and electrolyte abnormalities, more sophisticated measurements to determine vitamin and trace mineral status can be obtained when deficiencies are suspected clinically. Bone mineral densitometry may be useful in many patients to establish a baseline and to screen for unrecognized bone mineral depletion. An accurate dietary history by using food records is useful in evaluating nutrient requirements in nutritionally stable patients and in identifying dietary inadequacies in those with nutrient deficiencies.

Finally, it is also important to consider specific problems that interfere with the patient's quality of life. Maintaining adequate nutritional status with oral feedings at the cost of massive diarrhea and frequent bowel movements may be unacceptable to the patient with an active social or professional life outside the home. In such cases, parenteral supplementation may be necessary to improve lifestyle.

Treatment

The goals of therapy are to control diarrhea, maintain fluid, electrolyte, and nutritional homeostasis, treat and prevent medical complications, and maximize the quality of life. The therapeutic approach depends on the results of the clinical evaluation. Initial therapy often requires subsequent modification using a trial-and-error approach because of individual variability in absorptive function, continued intestinal adaptation, and the development of new medical complications or disease progression. Continued clinical monitoring is critical to adjust medical and nutritional therapy when necessary.

Control of diarrhea

Diarrhea is often caused by a combination of factors, including increased gastrointestinal secretions, decreased intestinal transit time, and osmotic stimulation of water secretion by unabsorbed luminal contents.[182] Therefore, therapy for diarrhea involves limiting endogenous secretions, slowing motility, and improving solute absorption (see Chapter 71)

The stomach normally produces ≈2.5 liters of fluid per day that is absorbed by the small bowel. Gastric secretion and, in some patients, gastric hypersecretion may contribute to diarrhea. The use of H_2-receptor antagonists or proton pump inhibitors may be necessary to reduce gastric secretions (see Chapter 1). The presence of acidic jejunostomy or ileostomy contents after meals is a clear indication for acid-reduction therapy.[184] Large dosages, twice the normal amount used for treatment of peptic ulcer disease or reflux, may be required for adequate control in certain patients because of reduced drug absorption.

The long-acting somatostatin analogue, octreotide acetate (Sandostatin®), can decrease small intestinal secretions. Octreotide has been shown to decrease ostomy or stool volume (by 500–4000 g per day), decrease sodium and chloride output, and prolong small bowel transit in patients with short bowel syndrome.[185–187] However, octreotide therapy does not improve absorption of macronutrients and other minerals. In addition, octreotide is costly, must be given by subcutaneous injections, can decrease appetite, impair fat absorption,[188] increase the risk of gallstones,[189] and decrease the utilization of amino acids for splanchnic protein synthesis.[190] Nevertheless, in patients who have persistent large-volume intestinal output despite standard antidiarrheal therapy, a trial of 100 μg injected subcutaneously three times daily with meals may be useful.

Table 4.15 Electrolyte concentrations in gastrointestinal fluids

	Na (mEq/L)	K (mEq/L)	Cl (mEq/L)	HCO$_3$ (mEq/L)
Stomach	65	10	100	
Bile	150	4	100	35
Pancreas	150	7	80	75
Duodenum	90	15	90	15
Mid-small bowel	140	6	100	20
Terminal ileum	140	8	60	70
Rectum	40	90	15	30

Opiates are the most effective means for slowing intestinal motility and act by delaying gastric emptying, decreasing peristalsis of the small and large intestine, and increasing anal sphincter tone. Loperamide (Imodium®) should be tried first because it is metabolized on first-pass by the liver and does not easily cross the blood–brain barrier, thereby limiting its side effects and potential for drug dependence. If loperamide is not effective, other opiates, such as codeine or deodorized tincture of opium (10–25 drops every 6 hours), should be considered. In addition, the combination of an anticholinergic drug and an opiate may be beneficial. We have found that capsules containing 25 mg powdered opium and 15 mg powdered belladonna are a potent combination. However, these capsules are not commercially available and require a willing pharmacist to formulate them. Diphenoxylate with atropine (Lomotil®) is an effective agent, but is expensive and inconvenient if large doses are needed.

Clonidine, an α_2-adrenergic receptor agonist, may also help to decrease diarrhea. In a small case series, patients with short bowel syndrome successfully reduced intestinal fluid and electrolyte losses utilizing clonidine in conjunction with other antisecretory agents. One of the patients was able to stop home parenteral nutrition (HPN) completely, while the other was able to wean down the amount of HPN by 2 liters per day.[191]

Foods and medications that cause diarrhea should be avoided. Traditionally, it has been recommended to decrease or eliminate lactose-containing foods because of the reduction in intestinal lactase in patients who have had intestinal resection. However, patients with jejunostomies and between 15 cm and 150 cm of jejunum can tolerate 20 g lactose loads as milk or yogurt.[192] Although lactose was better absorbed from yogurt than from milk, there was no difference in clinical symptoms. Foods that have laxative effects, such as caffeine-containing drinks and dietetic products containing osmotically active sweeteners (sorbitol, xylitol, and mannitol), should be avoided. Medications that contain magnesium or sorbitol can also contribute to diarrhea.[193]

Enteral feeding

The ability to use the gut to provide nutritional therapy will depend on intestinal absorptive function, as well as the ability to feed without producing adverse symptoms. Patients with nausea, vomiting, abdominal pain, or severe diarrhea may be unable to tolerate enteral feeding regardless of intestinal absorptive capacity. Specific foods that cause GI complaints should be avoided. However, it is important to evaluate objectively the validity of these complaints to prevent the unnecessary withdrawal of nutritious foods. Patients with gluten-sensitive enteropathy require a strict gluten-free diet.

The goal of feeding is to provide patients with all recommended nutritional requirements. The amount of ingested nutrients needed to reach this goal depends on the normal recommended dietary allowances modified by an estimate of absorptive function

Table 4.16 Guidelines for vitamin and mineral supplementation in patients with severe malabsorption

Supplement (representative product)	Dose	Route
Prenatal multivitamin with minerals*	1 tab q.d.	p.o.
Vitamin D*	50 000 U 2–3 times per week	p.o.
Calcium*	500 mg elemental calcium t.i.d. to q.i.d.	p.o.
Vitamin B$_{12}$†	1 md q.d. / 100–500 µg q 1–2 mo	p.o. / s.c.
Vitamin A†	10 000 to 50 000 U q.d.	p.o.
Vitamin K† (Mephyton; AquaMEPHYTON)	5 mg/d / 5–10 mg/wk	p.o. / s.c.
Vitamin E† (Aquasol E®)	100 U/d	p.o.
Magnesium gluconate† (Magonate®) or magnesium oxide capsules (URO-MAG)	108–169 mg elemental q.i.d.	p.o.
Magnesium sulfate†	290 mg elemental 1–3 times per wk	i.m./i.v.
Zinc gluconate or zinc sulfate†	25 mg elemental zinc q.d. plus 100 mg Elemental zinc/L intestinal output	p.o.
Ferrous sulfate†	60 mg elemental iron t.i.d.	p.o.
Iron dextran†	≤100 mg elemental iron per day based on formula or table	i.v.

po, oral, s.c. subcutaneous, i.m., intramuscular, i.v., intravenous
*Recommended routinely for all patients.
†Recommended for patients with documented nutrient deficiency or malabsorption.

and intestinal losses. This usually requires ingestion of large amounts of fluid, calories, protein, vitamins, and minerals. Even in patients with severe short bowel syndrome, TPN may not be needed when vitamin and mineral supplements and large amounts of calories and protein are provided enterally.[194] Increasing the contact time of food with the intestine may enhance absorption in patients with limited absorptive function. For this reason, total dietary intake should be divided into at least six meals per day. If unsuccessful, defined liquid formulas ingested between meals or administered by continuous tube feedings at night may prevent the need for parenteral nutrition. In general, most patients with severe malabsorption must ingest 40–60 kcal/kg and 1.2–1.5 g of protein/kg per day. Suggested guidelines for vitamin and mineral supplementation are outlined in Table 4.16. The needs of each patient, however, can only be determined by experimentation with different dietary manipulations.

Fat Intake: Fat intake should not be restricted in patients with a jejunostomy or ileostomy despite the presence of steatorrhea. A high-fat, low-carbohydrate diet has been found to be comparable to a low-fat, high-carbohydrate diet with regard to total fluid, energy, nitrogen, sodium, potassium, and divalent ion absorption in patients with short bowel syndrome.[195–197] Furthermore, a high-fat diet facilitates the ingestion of more calories. Limiting fat intake, however, may decrease GI symptoms, colonic water secretion, hyperoxaluria, and divalent cation losses in patients who have steatorrhea and an intact colon.[198,199]

MCTs are theoretically a useful feeding supplement in patients who have impaired fat absorption because they are rapidly hydrolyzed and do not require bile salts and micelle formation for absorption.[200] However, many patients do not find MCT oil palatable. Furthermore, MCT oil can cause nausea, vomiting, and abdominal discomfort. A dosage of 1 tablespoon (15 ml) 3–4 times daily, providing a total of ≈500 kcal, is usually the maximum amount tolerated.

Predigested Formulas: Elemental and semielemental formulas have been recommended for patients with short bowel syndrome. Theoretically, these formulas, which contain nitrogen in the form of free amino acids or small peptides, are absorbed more efficiently over a shorter length of intestine than polymeric formulas or whole food. However, the clinical efficacy of these formulas is not clear.[197,201] Therefore, at present there is not sufficient clinical evidence to justify the routine use of expensive predigested formulas in patients who have short bowel syndrome.

Oral Rehydration Therapy: A subset of patients, usually those with 50–100 cm of jejunum that either ends in a jejunostomy or is anastomosed to the mid-transverse or distal colon, cannot maintain fluid and electrolyte homeostasis but may be able to absorb adequate protein and calories. These patients may benefit from oral rehydration therapy (see Table 4.12). Daily oral administration of 1–2 liters of rehydration solutions has been used successfully to correct fluid and electrolyte abnormalities and allow IV supplementation to be discontinued in patients who have had extensive intestinal resection.[202–205] In some patients, oral rehydration therapy has decreased ostomy output by 4 L/day.[205]

Major Minerals: Major minerals should be supplemented as needed depending on the assessment of body content. Maintaining magnesium homeostasis is often difficult because it is poorly absorbed and because enteral supplementation with magnesium salts may cause diarrhea. Enteric-coated magnesium supplements should not be used because their delayed release reduces contact with the intestine for absorption.[206] Soluble magnesium salts, such as magnesium gluconate, are better tolerated and absorbed than other magnesium complexes and are best given in liquid form (Fleming Inc., St. Louis, MO), added to an oral rehydration solution in doses of 18–27 mmol (432–648 mg of elemental magnesium) per day. This solution should be sipped, not ingested as a bolus, to maximize absorption and avoid diarrhea. Normal serum magnesium levels do not exclude the possibility of magnesium deficiency. The percentage of infused magnesium excreted in urine after magnesium infusion may prove to be a better index of body magnesium stores; excretion of <80% of infused magnesium suggests whole body magnesium depletion.[207]

Supplemental calcium is given routinely because of both reduced intestinal absorption and the limited calcium content of low-lactose diets. Plasma levels of calcium are usually maintained by mobilizing bone stores unless there is concurrent magnesium or vitamin D deficiency. Therefore, urinary calcium excretion, which should be >50 mg per 24 h, is a more reliable index of calcium status. Most patients require 1.5–2 g of elemental calcium daily. Although it has been suggested that calcium citrate is absorbed better than is calcium carbonate,[208] most studies have not demonstrated any differences in calcium bioavailability from calcium ingested as a carbonate, citrate, gluconate, lactate, or sulfate salt.[209,210] However, the amount of calcium present in each calcium salt differs significantly, which will influence the number of tablets needed each day.

Trace Minerals: Data regarding trace mineral requirements in patients with malabsorption disorders are limited. With the exception of zinc and iron, absorption of trace minerals from ingested foods or liquid formulas is often adequate to prevent overt deficiency syndromes. Zinc deficiency is common, and often subclinical, in patients with malabsorption. Large dosages of oral zinc supplements may become necessary because zinc losses are often high and zinc absorption is low. Zinc gluconate is tolerated well and does not cause the gastric distress caused by zinc sulfate. Zinc should not be given with meals, because absorption is reduced by food.[211] Daily zinc supplementation of 25 mg plus an additional 100 mg per liter (or 100 mg per kg) of ostomy or diarrheal output is needed to maintain zinc homeostasis.[212] Thus, many patients will require ≈150 mg of elemental zinc per day. Although zinc ingestion reduces copper absorption and can cause clinically significant copper deficiency,[213] additional copper intake is usually not needed because of the low efficiency of zinc absorption. Treating iron deficiency with oral preparations can be difficult. We recommend a liquid form of ferrous sulfate (300 mg per 5 mL containing 60 mg of elemental iron) mixed in orange juice four times per day. Diluting ferrous sulfate liquid prevents staining of teeth, and the ascorbic acid present in orange juice enhances iron absorption. Some patients, however, will require intermittent administration of parenteral iron.

Vitamins: Patients with malabsorption can usually absorb adequate amounts of most water-soluble vitamins from their diet, but patients with steatorrhea and bile acid depletion have difficulty absorbing fat-soluble vitamins. Vitamin K deficiency is rarely a clinical problem unless patients are receiving antibiotics. However, large doses of vitamins A, D, and E may be required to maintain normal body concentrations. Liquid vitamins present in water-miscible and water-soluble forms are more effective than are standard vitamins in pill form. An assessment of vitamin status should be used to guide therapy.

Parenteral feeding

Parenteral nutrition may be necessary to provide fluids, specific nutrients, or complete nutritional requirements in patients who cannot maintain normal hydration, electrolyte balance, or nutritional status with oral feeding. Some general guidelines are useful in deciding which patients require parenteral therapy. Patients in whom urine output is <1 liter per day are at increased risk for developing renal dysfunction and should receive IV fluids. Adequate levels of certain minerals, such as magnesium, potassium, and zinc, and fat-soluble vitamins are difficult to maintain with oral feedings in patients with severe steatorrhea or large intestinal fluid output and may require parenteral supplementation. Magnesium sulfate can be injected intramuscularly at a dose of 12 mmol (290 mg of elemental magnesium) 1–3 times per week if attempts at oral therapy are unsuccessful. IV infusion of magnesium is preferred, however, because intramuscular injections are painful and can cause sterile abscesses. Monthly intramuscular injections of vitamin B_{12} (200 micrograms per month) are required in patients who have evidence of vitamin B_{12} malabsorption. In patients who have evidence of, or are at high risk for, vitamin K-associated hypoprothrombinemia, 5–10 mg of vitamin K should be given intramuscularly or intravenously each week. In some patients total parenteral nutrition may be lifesaving or needed to limit diarrhea and achieve an acceptable quality of life.

REFERENCES

1. Chan ATH, Fleming CR, O'Fallon WM. et al. Estimated versus measured basal energy requirements in patients with Crohn's disease. Gastroenterology 1986; 91:75.

2. Allard JP, Jeejeebhoy KN, Whitwell J, et al. Factors influencing energy expenditure in patients with burns. J Trauma 1988; 28:199.

3. Harris JA, Benedict FG. Standard basal metabolism constants for physiologists and clinicians. In: A biometric study of basal metabolism in man. Publication 279, The Carnegie Institute of Washington. Philadelphia: JB Lippincott; 1919:223.

4. WHO (World Health Organization). energy and protein requirements. report of a joint FAO/WHO/UNU expert consultation technical report series 724. Geneva: World Health Organization; 1985.

5. Owen OE, Kavle E, Owen RS, et al. A reappraisal of caloric requirements in healthy women. Am J Clin Nutr 1986; 44:1.

6. Ireton-Jones CS, Borman KR, Turner WW. Nutrition considerations in the management of ventilator-dependent patients. NCP 1993; 8:60.

7. Klein S. Nutritional therapy. In: Ahya S, Flood K, Paranjothi S, eds. The Washington manual of medical therapeutics. 30th edn. Philadelphia: Lippincott Williams & Wilkins; 2000:27–42.

8. Rudman D, Kutner M, Ansley J, et al. Hypotyrosinemia, hypocystinemia, and failure to retain nitrogen during total parenteral nutrition of cirrhotic patients. Gastroenterology 1981; 81:1025.

9. Scheinkestel CD, Kar L, Marshall K, et al. Prospective randomized trial to assess caloric and protein needs of critically ill, anuric, ventilated patients requiring continuous renal replacement therapy. Nutrition 2003; 19:909.

10. Fukagawa NK, Minaker KL, Rowe JW, et al. Insulin-mediated reduction on whole body protein breakdown: dose-response effects on leucine metabolism in postabsorptive men. J Clin Invest 1985; 60:648.

11. Biolo G, Fleming RYD, Wolfe RR. Physiologic hyperinsulinemia stimulates protein synthesis and enhances transport of selected amino acids in human skeletal muscle. J Clin Invest 1995; 95:811.

12. DeFronzo RA, Ferrannini E. Regulation of hepatic glucose metabolism in humans. Diabetes Dietab Rev 1987; 3:415.

13. Jeejeebhoy KN, Anderson GH, Nakhooda AF, et al. Metabolic studies in total parenteral nutrition with lipid in man: comparison with glucose. J Clin Invest 1976; 57:125.

14. Bach AC, Babayen VK. Medium-chain triglycerides: an update. Am J Clin Nutr 1982; 36:950.

15. Wene JD, Connor WE, DenBesten L. The development of essential fatty acid deficiency in healthy men fed fat-free diets intravenously and orally. J Clin Invest 1975; 56:127.

16. Cotzias GC. Role and importance of trace substances in environmental health. In: Hemphill DD, ed. Proc First Ann Conf on Trace Subst Environ Health. Columbia, MO: University of Missouri; 1967;1:5.

17. Fitzgerald K, Mikalunas V, Rubin H, et al. Hypermanganesemia in patients receiving total parenteral nutrition. JPEN 1999; 23:333.

18. Long CL, Maull KI, Krishnan RS, et al. Ascorbic acid dynamics in the seriously ill and injured. J Surg Res 2003; 109:144.

19. Hagan SN, Scow RO. Effect of fasting on muscle proteins and fat in young rats of different ages. Am J Physiol 1957; 188:91.

20. Leiter LA, Marliss EB. Survival during fasting may depend on fat as well as protein stores. JAMA 1982; 248:2306.

21. Horowitz JF, Coppack SC, Paramore D, et al. Effect of short-term fasting on lipid kinetics in lean and obese women. Am J Physiol 1999; 276:E278–E284.

22. Horowitz JF, Coppack SW, Klein S. Whole body and adipose tissue glucose metabolism in response to short-term fasting in lean and obese women. Am J Clin Nutr 2001; 73:517–522.

23. Elia M, Stubbs RJ, Henry CJK. Differences in fat, carbohydrate, and protein metabolism between lean and obese subjects undergoing total starvation. Obesity Res 1999; 7:597.

24. Stewart WK, Fleming LW. Features of a successful therapeutic fast of 382 days duration. Postgrad Med J 1973; 49:203.

25. Golden MHN. Severe malnutrition. In: Weatherall DJ, Ledington JGG, Warrell DA, eds. Oxford textbook of medicine. 3rd edn. New York: Oxford University Press; 1996:1278–1296.

26. Waterlow JC. Protein-energy malnutrition. Great Britain: Edward Arnold; 1992.

27. DeWys WD, Begg C, Lavin PT, et al. Prognostic effect of weight loss prior to chemotherapy in cancer patients. Am J Med 1980; 69:491.

28. Stanley KE. Prognostic factors for survival in patients with inoperable lung cancer. J Natl Cancer Inst 1980; 65:25.

29. National Institutes of Health, National Heart, Lung, and Blood Institute. Clinical guidelines on the identification, evaluation, and treatment of overweight and obesity in adults – the evidence report. Obes Res 1988; 6(supplement 2):53S.

30. Madill J, Gutierrez C, Grossman J, et al. Nutritional assessment of the lung transplant patient: body mass index as a predictor of 90-day mortality following transplantation. J Heart Lung Transplant 2001; 20:288.

31. Reinhardt GF, Myscofski JW, Wilkens DB, et al. Incidence and mortality of hypoalbuminemic patients in hospitalized veterans. J Parenteral Enteral Nutr 1980; 4:357.

32. Anderson CF, Wochos DN. The utility of serum albumin values in the nutritional assessment of hospitalized patients. Mayo Clin Proc 1982; 57:181.

33. Apelgren KN, Rombeau JL, Twomey PL, et al. Comparison of nutritional indices and outcome in critically ill patients. Crit Care Med 1982; 10:305.

34. Klein S. The myth of serum albumin as a measure of nutritional status. Gastroenterology 1990; 99:1845.

35. Halmi KA, Struss AL, Owen WP, et al. Plasma and erythrocyte amino acid concentrations in anorexia nervosa. JPEN 1987; 11:458.

36. Cohen S, Hansen JDL. Metabolism of albumin and gamma-globulin in kwashiorkor. Clin Sci 1962; 23:411.

37. Fleck A, Hawker F, Wallace PI, et al. Increase vascular permeability: a major cause of hypoalbuminemia in disease and injury. Lancet 1985; 1:781.

38. Moshage HJ, Janssen JAM, Franssen JH, et al. Study of the molecular mechanism of decreased liver synthesis of albumin in inflammation. J Clin Invest 1987; 79:1635.

39. Gray GE, Meguid MM. Can total parenteral nutrition reverse hypoalbuminemia in oncology patients? Nutrition 1990; 6:225.

40. Prealbumin in Nutritional Care Consensus Group. Measurement of visceral protein status in assessing protein and energy malnutrition: standard of care. Nutrition 1995; 11:169.

41. Hedlund JU, Hansson LO, Ortqvist AB. Hypoalbuminemia in hospitalized patients with community-acquired pneumonia. Arch Intern Med 1995; 155:1438.

42. Nieken J, Mulder NH, Buter J, et al. Recombinant human interleukin-6 induces a rapid and reversible anemia in cancer patients. Blood 1995; 86:900.

43. O'Riordain MG, Ross JA, Fearon KC, et al. Insulin and counterregulatory hormones influence acute-phase protein production in human hepatocytes. Am J Physiol 1995; 269:E323.

44. Cano N, Costanzo-Dufetel J, Calaf R, et al. Pre-albumin retinol-binding protein-retinol complex in hemodialysis patients. Am J Clin Nutr 1988; 47:664.

45. Quigley EM, Marsh MN, Shaffer JL. et al. Hepatobiliary complications of total parenteral nutrition. Gastroenterology 1993; 104:286.

46. Moore FA, Feliciano DV, Andrassy RJ, et al. Early enteral feeding, compared with parenteral, reduces postoperative septic complications. The results of a meta-analysis. Ann Surg 1992; 216:172.

47. Minard G, Kudsk KA. Nutritional support and infection: does the route matter? World J Surg 1998; 22: 213.

48. Kudsk KA, Li J, Renegar KB. Loss of upper respiratory tract immunity with parenteral feeding. Ann Surg 1996; 223:629.

49. Kudsk KA, Croce MA, Fabian TC, et al. Enteral versus parenteral feeding. Effects on septic morbidity after blunt and penetrating abdominal trauma. Ann Surg 1992; 215:503.

50. Macfie J. Enteral versus parenteral nutrition: the significance of bacterial translocation and gut-barrier function. Nutrition 2000; 16:606.

51. Eastwood GL. Small bowel morphology and epithelial proliferation in intravenously alimented rabbits. Surgery 1977; 82:613.

52. Zhao G, Wang C, Wang F, et al. Clinical study on nutrition support in patients with severe acute pancreatitis. World J Gastroenterol 2003; 9:2105.

53. Hughes CA, Prince A, Dowling RH. Speed of change in pancreatic mass and in intestinal bacteriology of parenterally fed rats. Clin Sci 1980; 59:329.

54. Johnson LR, Guthrie PD. Mucosal DNA synthesis: a short term index of the trophic action of gastrin. Gastroenterology 1974; 67:453.

55. Levine GM, Deren JJ, Steiger E, et al. Role of oral intake in maintenance of gut mass and disaccharidase activity. Gastroenterology 1974; 67:975.

56. Johnson LR, Schanbacher LM, Dudrick SJ, et al. Effect of long-term parenteral feeding on pancreatic secretion and serum secretin. Am J Physiol 1977; 233:E524.

57. O'Keefe SJ, Lee RB, Anderson FP, et al. Physiological effects of enteral and parenteral feeding on pancreaticobiliary secretion in humans. Am J Physiol Gastrointest Liver Physiol 2003; 284:G27.

This study of human volunteers examined the effect of oral feeding, duodenal feeding, and parenteral feeding on pancreatic secretion and blood hormone concentrations.

58. Alverdy J, Chi HS, Sheldon GF. The effect of parenteral nutrition on gastrointestinal immunity. The importance of enteral stimulation. Ann Surg 1985; 202:681.

59. Messing B, Bories C, Kunstlinger F, et al. Does total parenteral nutrition induce gallbladder sludge formation and lithiasis? Gastroenterology 1983; 84:1012.

60. Silk DB, Fairclough PD, Clark ML, et al. Uses of a peptide rather than free amino acid nitrogen source in chemically defined elemental diets. JPEN 1980; 4:548.

61. Ksiazyk J, Peina M, Kerkus J, et al. Hydrolyzed versus nonhydrolyzed protein diet in short bowel syndrome in children. J Ped Gastro Nutr 2002; 35:615.

Controlled trial of hydrolyzed versus nonhydrolyzed enteral protein supplementation in short bowel patients showed no differences in nitrogen or energy balance.

62. McIntyre PB, Fitchew M, Lennard-Jones JE. Patients with a high jejunostomy do not need a special diet. Gastroenterology 1986; 91:25.

63. Cosnes J, Evard D, Beaugerie L, et al. Improvement in protein absorption with a small-peptide-based diet in patients with high jejunostomy. Nutrition 1992; 8:406.

64. Russell MK, Charney P. Is there a role for specialized enteral nutrition in the intensive care unit? Nutr Clin Prac 2002; 17:156.

65. Marchesini G, Giampaolo B, Manuela M, et al. Nutritional supplementation with branched-chain amino acids in advanced cirrhosis: a double-blind, randomized trial. Gastroenterology 2003; 124:1792.

Multicenter, randomized study comparing 1 year of nutritional support with branched chain amino acids, lactoalbumin, or maltodextrin in 174 patients with cirrhosis. Primary outcomes including death, deterioration of liver function, and need for hospitalization were improved with branched chain amino acid supplementation.

66. Nalin DR, Cash RA, Rafiqul I, et al. Oral maintenance therapy for cholera in adults. Lancet 1968; 2:370.

67. Hirschhorn N, Cash R, Woodward W, et al. Oral therapy of Apache children with acute infectious diarrhea. Lancet 1972; 1:15.

68. Lennard-Jones JE. Oral rehydration solutions in short bowel syndrome. Clin Ther 1990; 12(Suppl A):129.

69. Winick M. National Task Force on Nutrition in AIDS. Guidelines on nutritional support in AIDS. Nutrition 1989; 5:390.

70. Duggan C, Fontaine O, Pierce NF, et al. Scientific rationale for a change in the composition of oral rehydration solution. JAMA 2004; 291:2628.

This paper and reference 71 discuss the implications of changing the composition and osmolarity of the standard WHO oral rehydration solution, used as therapy for acute diarrhea worldwide.

71. Nalin DR, Hirshhorn N, Greenough W, et al. Clinical concerns about reduced-osmolarity oral rehydration solution. JAMA 2004; 291:2632.

72. Alam NH, Majumder RN, Fuchs GJ, CHOICE Study Group. Efficacy and safety of oral rehydration solution with reduced

osmolarity in adults with cholera: a randomized double-blind clinical trial. Lancet 1999; 354:296.

73. Taylor B, Schallom L. Bedside small bowel feeding tube placement in critically ill patients using a dietitian/nurse team approach. nutrition in clinical practice. Nutr Clin Pract 2001; 16:258.

74. Lenart S, Polissar NL. Comparison of 2 methods for postpyloric placement of enteral feeding tubes. Am J Crit Care 2003; 12:357.

75. Powers J, Chance R, Bortenschlager L, et al. Bedside placement of small-bowel feeding tubes in the intensive care unit. Crit Care Nurse 2003; 23:16.

76. Russell TR, Brotman M, Norris F. Percutaneous gastrostomy: a new simplified and cost-effective technique. Am J Surg 1984; 184:132.

77. Grant JP. Mortality with percutaneous endoscopic gastrostomy. Am J Gastroenterol 2000; 95:3.

78. Stefan MM, Holcomb GW 3rd, Ross AJ 3rd. Cologastric fistula as a complication of percutaneous endoscopic gastrostomy. JPEN J Parenter Enteral Nutr 1989; 13:554.

79. Lattuneddu A, Morgagni P, Benati G, et al. Small bowel perforation after incomplete removal of percutaneous endoscopic gastrostomy catheter. Surg Endosc 2003; 17:2028.

80. Anagnostopoulos GK, Kostopoulos P, Arvanitidis DM. Buried bumper syndrome with a fatal outcome, presenting early as gastrointestinal bleeding after percutaneous endoscopic gastrostomy placement. J Postgrad Med 2003; 49:325.

81. Gencosmanoglu R, Koc D, Tozun N. The buried bumper syndrome: migration of internal bumper of percutaneous endoscopic gastrostomy tube into the abdominal wall. J Gastroenterol 2003; 38:1077.

82. Bell SD, Carmody EA, Yeung EY. Percutaneous gastrostomy and gastrojejunostomy: additional experience in 519 procedures. Radiology 1995; 194:817.

83. Hoffer EK, Cosgrove JM, Levin DQ, et al. Radiologic gastrojejunostomy and percutaneous endoscopic gastrostomy: a prospective, randomized comparison. J Vasc Interv Radiol 1999; 10:413.

84. Simon T, Fink AS. Recent experience with percutaneous endoscopic gastrostomy/jejunostomy (PEG/J) for enteral nutrition. Surg Endosc 2000; 14:436.

85. Wolfsen HC, Kozarek RA, Ball TJ, et al. Tube dysfunction following percutaneous endoscopic gastrostomy and jejunostomy. Gastrointest Endosc 1990; 36:261.

86. DiSario JA, Foutch PG, Sanowski RA. Poor results with percutaneous endoscopic jejunostomy. Gastrointest Endosc 1990; 36:257.

87. McGonigal MD, Lucas CE, Ledgerwood AM. Feeding jejunostomy in patients who are critically ill. Surg Gynecol Obstet 1989; 168:275.

88. Sarr MG, Mayo S. Needle catheter jejunostomy: An unappreciated and misunderstood advance in the care of patients after major abdominal operations. Mayo Clin Proc 1988; 63:565.

89. Bankier AA, Wiesmayr MN, Henk C, et al. Radiographic detection of intrabronchial malpositions of nasogastric tubes and subsequent complications in intensive care unit patients. Intensive Care Med 1997; 23:406.

90. Metheny NA. Case Report: inadvertent intracranial nasogastric tube placement. AJN 2002; 102:25.

91. Caplan ES, Hoyt NJ. Nosocomial sinusitis. JAMA 1982; 247:639.

92. Landis EE Jr, Hoffman HT, Koconis CA. Upper airway obstruction associated with large bore nasogastric tubes. South Med J 1988; 81:1333.

93. Biggart M, McQuillan PJ, Choudhry AK, et al. Dangers of placement of narrow bore nasogastric feeding tubes. Ann R Coll Surg Engl 1987; 69:119.

94. McWey RE, Curry NS, Schabel SI, et al. Complications of nasoenteric feeding tubes. Am J Surg 1988; 155:253.

95. Marcuard SP, Stegall KS. Unclogging feeding tubes with pancreatic enzyme. J Parenter Enteral Nutr 1990; 14:198.

96. Vanlandingham S, Simpson S, Daniel P, et al. Metabolic abnormalities in patients supported with enteral tube feeding. JPEN 1981; 5:322.

97. Marvin RG, McKinley BA, McQuiggan M, et al. Nonocclusive bowel necrosis occurring in critically ill trauma patients receiving enteral nutrition manifests no reliable clinical signs for early detection. Am J Surg 2000; 179:7.

98. Guenter PA, Settle RG, Perlmutter S, et al. Tube feeding-related diarrhea in acutely ill patients. JPEN 1991; 15:277.

99. Edes TE, Walk BE, Austin JL. Diarrhea in tube-fed patients: feeding formula not necessarily the cause. Am J Med 1990; 88:91.

100. Bell R, Fishman S. Eosinophilia from food dye added to enteral feedings. N Engl J Med 1990; 322:1822.

101. Maloney JP. Systemic absorption of food dye in patients with sepsis (Letter). N Engl J Med 2000; 343:1047.

102. Zillich AJ, Kuhn RJ, Petersen TJ. Skin discoloration with blue food coloring. Ann Pharm 2000; 34:868.

103. Kirby DF, DeLegge MH, Fleming CR. American Gastroenterological Association technical review on tube feeding for enteral nutrition. Gastroenterology 1995; 108:1282.

104. Metheny NA, Schallom ME, Edwards SJ. Effect of gastrointestinal motility and feeding tube site on aspiration risk in critically ill patients: a review. Heart Lung 2004; 33:131.

105. Smith HG, Orlando R. Enteral nutrition: should we feed the stomach? Crit Care Med 1999; 27:1652.

106. Alhimyary A, Fernandez C, Picard M. et al. Safety and efficacy of TPN delivered via peripherally-inserted central venous catheters. JPEN 1995; 19:A11;165.

107. Naylor CB, O'Rourke K, Detsky AS, et al. Parenteral nutrition with branched-chain amino acids in hepatic encephalopathy: a meta-analysis. Gastroenterology 1989; 97:1033.

108. Kopple JD. The nutrition management of the patient with acute renal failure. JPEN 1996; 20:3.

109. Wolfe RR, O'Donnell TF Jr, Stone MD, et al. Investigation of factors determining the optimal glucose infusion rate in total parenteral nutrition. Metabolism 1980; 29:892.

110. Covelli HD, Black JW, Olsen MS, et al. Respiratory failure precipitated by high carbohydrate loads. Ann Intern Med 1981; 95:579.

111. Barr LH, Dunn GD, Brennan MF. Essential fatty acid deficiency during total parenteral nutrition. Ann Surg 1981; 193:304.

112. Fleming CR, Smith LM, Hodges RE. Essential fatty acid deficiency in adults receiving total parenteral nutrition. Am J Clin Nutr 1976; 29:976.

113. Ling PR, Ollero M, Khaodhiar L, et al. Disturbances in essential fatty acid metabolism in patients receiving long-term home parenteral nutrition. Dig Dis Sci 2002; 47:1679.

This case series highlights the abnormalities in essential fatty acid status that occur in patients receiving home parenteral nutrition.

114. Miles JM. Intravenous fat emulsions in nutritional support. Curr Opinion Gastroenterol 1991; 7:306.

115. Skeie B, Askanazi J, Rothkopf MM, et al. Intravenous fat emulsions and lung function: a review. Crit Care Med 1988; 16:183.

116. DeGott C, Messing B, Moreau D, et al. Liver phospholipids induced by parenteral nutrition: histologic, histochemical, and ultrasound investigation. Gastroenterology 1988; 95:183.

117. Seidner DL, Mascioli EA, Istfan NW, et al. Effect of long-chain triglyceride emulsions on reticuloendothelial system function in humans. JPEN 1989; 13:614.

118. Lashner BA, Kirsner JB, Hanauer SB. Acute pancreatitis associated with high-concentration lipid emulsion during total parenteral nutrition therapy for Crohn's disease. Gastroenterology 1986; 90:1039.

119. Aviram M, Deckelbaum RJ. Intralipid infusion into humans reduces in vitro platelet aggregation and alters platelet lipid composition. Metabolism 1989; 38:343.

120. Belin RP, Bivins BA, Jona JZ, et al. Fat overload with a 10% soybean oil emulsion. Arch Surg 1976; 111:1391.

121. Hiyama DT, Griggs B, Mittman RJ, et al. Hypersensitivity following lipid emulsion infusion in an adult patient. JPEN 1989; 13:318.

122. Casaubon PR, Dahlstrom KA, Vargas J, et al. Intravenous fat emulsion (intralipid) delays gastric emptying, but does not cause gastroesophageal reflux in healthy volunteers. JPEN 1989; 13:246.

123. Nehme AB. Nutritional support of the hospitalized patient: the team concept. JAMA 1980; 243:1906.

124. Ruesch S, Walder B, Tramer MR. Complications of central venous catheters: internal jugular versus subclavian access – a systematic review. Crit Care Med 2002; 30:454.

    Review of 17 nonrandomized studies that evaluated the complications associated with placement of internal jugular versus subclavian vein catheters. The data suggest that internal jugular vein catheter placement is associated with a greater risk of arterial puncture but lower risk of catheter misplacement than subclavian vein catheter insertion. No conclusions regarding differences in risk of hemothorax, pneumothorax, bloodstream infection, or vessel occlusion could be made because of data heterogeneity.

125. Bozzetti F, Scarpa D, Terno G, et al. Subclavian venous thrombosis due to indwelling catheters: a prospective study on 52 patients. JPEN 1981; 7:560.

126. Brismar B, Hardstedt C, Jacobson S, et al. Reduction of catheter-associated thrombosis in parenteral nutrition of intravenous heparin therapy. Arch Surg 1982; 117:1196.

127. Bern MM, Lokich JJ, Wallach SR, et al. Very low-dose warfarin can prevent thrombosis. A randomized prospective trial. Ann Int Med 1990; 112:423.

128. Hill SE, Heldman LS, Goo EDH, et al. Case report. Fatal microvascular pulmonary emboli from precipitation of a total nutrient admixture solution. JPEN 1996; 20:81.

129. Food and Drug Administration. Safety alert: hazards of precipitation associated with parenteral nutrition. Am J Hosp Pharm 1994; 51:427.

130. Driscoll DF. Total nutrient admixtures: theory and practice. Clin Nutr 1995; 10:114.

131. Daly JM, Long JM. Intravenous hyperalimentation: techniques and potential complications. Surg Clin North Am 1981; 61:583.

132. Rudman D, Williams PJ. Nutrient deficiencies during total parenteral nutrition. Nutr Rev 1985; 43:1.

133. Van den Berghe G, Wouters P, Weekers R, et al. Intensive insulin therapy in critically ill patients. N Eng J Med 2001; 345:1359.

134. Furnary AP, Gao G, Grunkmeier GL, et al. Continuous insulin infusion reduces mortality in patients with diabetes undergoing coronary artery bypass graft. J Thorac Cardiovasc Surgery 2003; 125:1007.

135. Hamilton C, Seidner DL. Metabolic bone disease and parenteral nutrition. Curr Gastro Rep 2004; 6:335.

136. Klein GL, Coburn JW. Parenteral nutrition: effect on bone and mineral homeostasis. Ann Rev Nutr 1991; 11:93.

137. Seidner DL. Parenteral nutrition-associated metabolic bone disease. JPEN 2002; 26:S37.

138. Clark-Christoff N, Watters VA, Sparks W, et al. Use of triple-lumen subclavian catheters for administration of total parenteral nutrition. JPEN 1992; 16:403.

139. Mermel LA. Prevention of intravascular catheter-related infections. Ann Intern Med 2000; 132:391.

140. Johnson DC, Johnson FL, Goldman S. Preliminary results treating persistent central venous catheter infections with the antibiotic lock technique in pediatric patients. The Ped Inf Dis J 1994; 13:930.

141. Messing B. Catheter-sepsis during home parenteral nutrition: use of the antibiotic-lock technique. Nutrition 1998; 14:466.

142. Carratala J, Niubo J, Fernandez-Sevilla A, et al. Randomized, double-blind trial of an antibiotic-lock technique for prevention of Gram-positive central venous catheter-related infection in neutropenic patients with cancer. Antimicrob Agents Chemo 1999; 43:2200.

143. Mermel LA. Prevention of intravascular catheter-related infections. Ann Intern Med 2000; 132:391.

144. Peden VH, Witzleben CL, Skelton MA. Total parenteral nutrition. J Pediatr 1971; 78:180.

145. Chung C, Buchman AL. Postoperative jaundice and total parenteral nutrition-associated hepatic dysfunction. Clin Liver Dis 2002; 6:1067.

    Excellent review of hepatic complications of parenteral nutrition.

146. Klein S. Total parenteral nutrition and the liver. In: Schiff L, Schiff ER, eds. Diseases of the liver. 7th edn. JB Lippincott; Philadelphia: 1993:1505–1516.

147. Barie PS, Eachempati SR. Acute acalculous cholecystitis. Curr Gastroenterol Rep 2003; 5:302.

148. Pazzi P, Gamberini S, Buldrini P, et al. Biliary sludge: the sluggish gallbladder. Dig Liver Dis 2003; 35:S39.

149. Roslyn JJ, Pitt HA, Mann LL, et al. Gallbladder disease in patients on long-term parenteral nutrition. Gastroenterology 1983; 84:148.

150. Pitt HA, King W, Mann L, et al. Increased risk of cholelithiasis with prolonged total parenteral nutrition. Am J Surg 1983; 145:106.

151. Roslyn JJ, DenBesten L, Thompson JE Jr. Effects of periodic emptying of gallbladder on gallbladder function and formation of cholesterol gallstones. Surg Forum 1979; 30:403.

152. Sitzmann JV, Pitt HA, Steinborn PA, et al. Cholecystokinin prevents parenteral nutrition induced biliary sludge in humans. Surg Gynecol Obstet 1990; 170:25,

153. Solomon SM, Kirby DF. The refeeding syndrome: a review. JPEN 1990; 14:90.

154. Apovian CM, McMahon MM, Bistrian BR. Guidelines for refeeding the marasmic patient. Crit Care Med 1990; 18:1030.

155. Burger GCE, Drummond JC, Sandstead HR. Malnutrition and starvation in western Netherlands, September 1944–July 1945, Parts 1 and 2. The Hague General State Printing Office, 1948.

156. Silvis SE, Paragas PD Jr. Parasthesias, weakness, seizures, and hypophosphatemia in patients receiving hyperalimentation. Gastroenterology 1972; 62:513.

157. Weinsier RL, Krumdieck CL. Death resulting from overzealous total parenteral nutrition: The refeeding syndrome revisited. Am J Clin Nutr 1981; 34:393.

158. Keys A, Henschel A, Taylor HL. The size and function of the human heart at rest in semi-starvation and in subsequent rehabilitation. Am J Physiol 1947; 50:153.

159. Garnett ES, Barnard DL, Ford J, et al. Gross fragmentation of cardiac myofibrils after therapeutic starvation for obesity. Lancet 1969; 1:914.

160. Heymsfield SB, Bethel RA, Ansley JD, et al. Cardiac abnormalities in cachectic patients before and during nutritional repletion. Am Heart J 1978; 95:584.

161. Gottdiener JS, Gross HA, Henry WL, et al. Effects of self-induced starvation on cardiac size and function in anorexia nervosa. Circulation 1978; 58:425.

162. DeFronzo RA, Cooke CR, Andres R, et al. The effect of insulin on renal handling of sodium, potassium, calcium, and phosphate in man. J Clin Invest 1975; 55:845.

163. Corredor DG. Sabeh G, Mendelsohn LV, et al. Enhanced postglucose hypophosphatemia during starvation therapy of obesity. Metabolism 1969; 18:754.

164. Rudman D, Millikan WJ, Richardson TJ, et al. Elemental balances during intravenous hyperalimentation of underweight adult subjects. J Clin Invest 1975; 55:94.

165. Silvis SE, Paragas PD Jr. Parasthesias, weakness, seizures, and hypophosphatemia in patients receiving hyperalimentation. Gastroenterology 1972; 62:513.

166. Weinsier RL, Krumdieck CL. Death resulting from overzealous total parenteral nutrition: The refeeding syndrome revisited. Am J Clin Nutr 1981; 34:393.

167. Silvis SE, DiBartolomeo AG, Aaker HM. Hypophosphatemia and neurological changes secondary to oral caloric intake: A variant of hyperalimentation syndrome. Am J Gastroenterol 1980; 73:215.

168. Hayek ME, Eisenberg PG. Severe hypophosphatemia following the institution of enteral feedings. Arch Surg 1989; 124:1325.

169. Subramanian R, Khardori R. Severe hypophosphatemia. Pathophysiologic implications, clinical presentations, and treatment. Medicine 2000; 79:1.

170. Aubier M, Murciano D, Lecocguiec Y, et al. Effect of hypophosphatemia on diaphragmatic contractility in patients with acute respiratory failure. N Engl J Med 1985; 313:420.

171. Singhal PC, Kumar A, Desroches L, et al. Prevalence and predictors of rhabdomyolysis in patients with hypophosphatemia. Am J Med 1992; 92:458.

172. Travis SF, Sugerman HJ, Ruberg RL, et al. Alterations of red-cell glycolytic intermediates and oxygen transport as a consequence of hypophosphatemia in patients receiving intravenous hyperalimentation. N Engl J Med 1971; 285:763.

173. Venditti FJ, Marotta C, Panesai FR, et al. Hypophosphatemia and cardiac arrhythmias. Miner Electrolyte Metab 1987; 13:19.

174. Taylor BE, Huey WY, Buchman TG, et al. Treatment of hypophosphatemia using a protocol based on patient weight and serum phosphorus level in a surgical intensive care unit. Amer Coll Surgeons 2004; 198:198.

175. DeFronzo RA, Soman V, Sherwin RS, et al. Insulin binding to monocytes and insulin action in human obesity, starvation, and refeeding. J Clin Invest 1978; 62:204.

176. Wyrick WJ Jr, Rea WJ, McClelland RN. Rare complications with intravenous hyperosmotic alimentation. JAMA 1970; 211:1697.

177. Mattioli S, Miglioli M, Montagna P, et al. Wernick's encephalopathy during total parenteral nutrition: Observation in one case. JPEN 1988; 12:626.

178. Roediger WEW. Metabolic basis of starvation diarrhea: Implications for treatment. Lancet 1986; 1:1082.

179. Vazquez JA, Morse EL, Adibi SA. Effect of starvation on amino acid and peptide transport and peptide hydrolysis in humans. Am J Physiol 1985; 249:G563.

180. Behar M, Viteri F, Bressani R, et al. Principles of treatment and prevention of severe protein malnutrition in children (kwashiokor). Ann NY Acad Sci 1957; 69:954.

181. Isner JM, Roberts WC, Heymsfield SB, et al. Anorexia nervosa and sudden death. Ann Intern Med 1985; 102:49.

182. Sundaram A, Koutkia P, Apovian CM. Nutritional management of short bowel syndrome in adults. J Clin Gastroenterol 2002; 34:207.

183. Scolapio JS, Fleming CR. Short-bowel syndrome. Gastroenterol Clin North Am 1998; 27:467.

184. Saunders DR, Saunders MD, Sillery JK. Beneficial effects of glucose polymer and an H2-receptor blocker in a patient with a proximal ileostomy. Am J Gastroenterol 1989; 84:192.

185. Cooper JC, Williams NS, King RF, et al. Effects of long-acting somatostatin analogue in patients with severe ileostomy diarrhoea. Br J Surg 1986; 73:128.

186. Ladefoged K, Christensen KC, Hegnhj J, et al. Effect of a long-acting somatostatin analogue SMS 201-995 on jejunostomy effluents in patients with severe short bowel syndrome. Gut 1989; 30:943.

187. O'Keefe SJ, Burnes JU, Peterson ME. Octreotide in the long-term management of HPN patients with massive stomal losses of fluid and electrolytes (Abstract). Gastroenterology 100:A540. 1991;

188. Witt K, Pedersen NT. The long-acting somatostatin analogue SMS 201-995 causes malabsorption. Scand J Gastroenterol 1989; 24:1248.

189. Fisher RS, Rock E, Levin G, et al. Effect of somatostatin on gallbladder emptying. Gastroenterology 1987; 92:885.

190. O'Keefe SJ, Haymond MW, Bennet WM, et al. Long-acting somatostatin analogue therapy and protein metabolism in patients with jejunostomies. Gastroenterology 1994; 107:379.

191. McDoniel K, Taylor B, Huey W, et al. Use of clonidine to decrease intestinal fluid losses in patients with high-output short-bowel syndrome. JPEN 2004; 28:265.

192. Arrigoni E, Marteau P, Briet F, et al. Tolerance and absorption of lactose from milk and yogurt during short-bowel syndrome in humans. Am J Clin Nutr 1994; 60:926.

193. Edes TE, Walk BE, Austin JL. Diarrhea in tube-fed patients: Feeding formula not necessarily the cause. Am J Med 1990; 88:91.

194. Cosnes J, Gendre J-P, Evard D, et al. Compensatory enteral hyperalimentation for management of patients with severe short bowel syndrome. Am J Clin Nutr 1985; 41:1002.

195. Woolf GM, Miller C, Kurian R, et al. Diet for patients with a short bowel: high fat or high carbohydrate? Gastroenterology 1983; 84:823.

196. Woolf GM, Miller C, Kurian R, et al. Nutritional absorption in short bowel syndrome. Evaluation of fluid, caloric, and divalent cation requirements. Dig Dis Sci 1987; 32:8.

197. McIntyre PB, Fitchew M, Lennard-Jones JE. Patients with a high jejunostomy do not need a special diet. Gastroenterology 1986; 91:25.

198. Andersson H, Isaksson B, Sjogren B. Fat-reduced diet in the symptomatic treatment of small bowel disease. Gut 1974; 15:351.

199. Andersson H, Jagenburg R. Fat-reduced diet in the treatment of hyperoxaluria in patients with ileopathy. Gut 1974; 15:360.

200. Greenberger NJ, Skillman TG. Medium-chain triglycerides. N Engl J Med 1969; 280:1045.

201. Cosnes J, Evard D, Beaugerie L, et al. Improvement in protein absorption with a small-peptide-based diet in patients with high jejunostomy. Nutrition 1992; 8:406.

202. Lennard-Jones JE. Oral rehydration solutions in short bowel syndrome. Clin Ther 1990; 12:129.

203. Griffin GE, Hodgson EF, Chadwick VS. Enteral therapy in the management of massive gut resection complicated by chronic fluid and electrolyte depletion. Dig Dis Sci 1991; 27:902.

204. Laustsen J, Fallingborg J. Enteral glucose-polymer-electrolyte solution in the treatment of chronic fluid and electrolyte depletion in short-bowel syndrome. Acta Chir Scand 1983; 149:787.

205. MacMahon RA. The use of the World Health Organization's oral rehydration solution in patients on home parenteral nutrition. JPEN 1984; 8:720.

206. Fine KD, Santa Ana CA, Porter JL, et al. Intestinal absorption of magnesium from food and supplements. J Clin Invest 1991; 88:396.

207. Rude RK, Singer FR. Magnesium deficiency and excess. Annu Rev Med 1981; 32:245.

208. Nicar MJ, Pak CY. Calcium bioavailability from calcium carbonate and calcium citrate. J Clin Endocrinol Metab 1985; 61:391.

209. Patton MB, Sutton TS. Utilization of calcium from lactate, gluconate, sulfate and carbonate salts by young college women. J Nutr 1952; 48:443.

210. Recker RR. Calcium absorption and achlorhydria. N Engl J Med 1985; 313:70.

211. Brewer GJ, Ellis F, Bjork L. Parenteral depot method for zinc administration. Pharmacology 1981; 23:254.

212. Wolman SL, Anderson GH, Marliss EB, et al. Zinc in total parenteral nutrition: requirements and metabolic effects. Gastroenterology 1979; 76:458.

213. Hoffman HN, Phyliky RL, Fleming CR. Zinc-induced copper deficiency. Gastroenterology 1988; 94:508.

CHAPTER FIVE

5

Nutrition and malnutrition in liver disease

Arthur J. McCullough

INTRODUCTION

Protein energy malnutrition (PEM) is common in advanced liver disease with weight loss, nausea, and anorexia occurring in 60%, 55%, and 87% of such patients, respectively.[1] PEM prognosticates clinical outcomes in cirrhosis and nutritional interventions may improve survival, surgical outcome, liver function, and hepatic encephalopathy. These factors have made the recognition and treatment of PEM in chronic liver disease an important factor in the clinical management of these patients.

As the liver is primarily a metabolic organ, it is not surprising that it orchestrates a complex array of physiological and biochemical processes including the regulation of PEM. Therefore, it is not surprising that patients with advanced liver injury commonly have malnutrition in its various forms, including both muscle wasting and obesity. Perhaps more important is the fact that malnutrition may accelerate deterioration of liver function and adversely affect clinical outcome.

The importance of this concept has led to the development of guidelines for the nutritional management of patients with liver disease.[2,3] The rationale for aggressive nutritional therapy in these patients is based on promising clinical information and a number of nutritional axioms relative to chronic liver disease. First, malnutrition is common, but may be difficult to diagnose. Second, these patients have alterations in energy metabolism and nutritional status that mimic starvation. Third, many of the complications associated with chronic liver disease (such as hepatic encephalopathy, ascites, and sepsis) occur pari passu with a negative nitrogen state. Finally, there is the expectation that correction of malnutrition may improve the clinical outcome of these patients.

EPIDEMIOLOGY

Epidemiology evaluates the incidence, prevalence, distribution, and control of a disease or complication of a disease in a specific, selected population. Unfortunately, our knowledge of the epidemiology of malnutrition must be considered wanting in all of these areas.

Definition

Protein energy malnutrition can be defined as the loss of protein stores (both visceral and muscle/somatic) and fat mass. Two forms are described: marasmus (combined protein energy malnutrition) and kwashiorkor (hypoalbuminemic) malnutrition.[4] The former is an insufficient amount of both protein and calories resulting in the loss of muscle and fat mass with relative sparing of visceral proteins, such as albumin and fibrinogen. The latter is predominantly an insufficient amount of protein that results in diminished protein stores that occurs to a greater extent in visceral proteins as compared to muscle proteins.

In addition to these more classical forms of malnutrition, it is also important to realize that overnutrition in the form of obesity is occurring more frequently in patients with liver disease. Obesity – defined as a body mass index (BMI) (weight in kilograms divided by the height in meters squared) =30 – when present in liver disease poses specific and important issues regarding the nutritional management of these patients, as well as a potential etiologic factor for the development of advanced liver disease.[5]

Incidence and prevalence

PEM is uncommon in the precirrhotic stages of liver disease, except in the setting of extrahepatic biliary obstruction or acute liver failure.[6,7] There are no incidence data and the prevalence data are incomplete and in some areas conflicting. However, the prevalence of protein energy malnutrition in cirrhosis has been reported to range between 10% and 100% and may correlate with the severity of disease defined by the Child-Pugh-Turcotte score.[8,9] In one study, PEM was reported to be present in 20% of patients with compensated cirrhosis (Child's A) and in 50–60% of patients with decompensated cirrhosis (Child's C). As shown in Figure 5.1, when albumin and prealbumin are used as markers of malnutrition,[9] there appears to be a clear relation between malnutrition and severity of cirrhosis. The large range in reported prevalence rates may depend on how nutritional assessment is performed. For example, a large study of hospitalized patients with acute alcoholic hepatitis initially reported a 100% prevalence of malnutrition based on at least one abnormal marker of malnutrition. However, the prevalence dropped to approximately 50% when a more complete pattern of marasmus or kwashiorkor was required.[8]

Demographics

Protein energy malnutrition

Although most of the earlier studies have concentrated on patients with alcoholic liver disease, the prevalence of PEM is

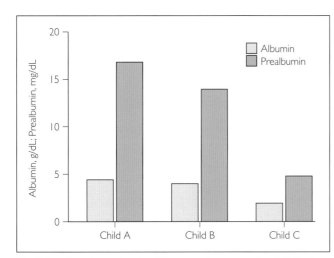

Fig. 5.1 • Prevalence of malnutrition according to severity of cirrhosis.

Table 5.1 Pattern of malnutrition in chronic liver disease

	Muscle wasting	Loss of fat stores	Synthetic function
Alcohol	+++	+	++
Viral	++	++	+
Primary biliary cirrhosis	+++	+++	+
Primary sclerosing cholangitis	++	+	+

+ mild; ++ moderate; +++ severe abnormality, respectively.

high in all forms of cirrhosis.[10] Figure 5.2 shows four studies that have measured nutritional status in both alcoholic and non-alcoholic cirrhosis. These studies show that the prevalence of PEM is high and almost identical in these two different types of cirrhosis. Based on anthropometric measurements of the lowest fifth percentile of a control population, the prevalence of PEM varied between 34% and 62%, and 27% and 67% in these studies for alcoholic and nonalcoholic cirrhosis, respectively. There is also a high prevalence of PEM in patients awaiting liver transplantation with estimates ranging between 18% and 100%.[11] Data from the two most detailed studies of transplant patients are shown in Figure 5.3, which shows that moderate or severe PEM is found in 70–80% of these patients. As listed in Table 5.1, disease-specific patterns of PEM have also been shown in patients with cirrhosis awaiting liver transplantation.[12] Therefore, clinicians need to be aware that PEM is very common in these patients, especially because it has prognostic significance. However, fat mass may be more seriously compromised in alcoholic cirrhosis.[9]

Obesity

The prevalence of obesity is approximately 30% in the adult population of the US and its prevalence is increasing at an alarming rate worldwide.[13] Obesity has also been reported as a

risk factor for the development of cirrhosis in alcoholic, viral, and nonalcoholic fatty liver disease.[5]

Although the prevalence of obesity is unknown in patients with liver disease, obesity has been evaluated in patients awaiting transplantation. Although the definition of obesity differed among the studies, it appears that moderate or severe obesity is present in 6.5–31.5% of patients at the time of transplantation as listed in Table 5.2 (J. Hasse, unpublished data).[14,15] Notably, the prevalence of different degrees of obesity is uniform among the different types of liver disease with the exception of cryptogenic cirrhosis[15] which accounts for an increasing proportion of liver transplants as the severity of obesity increases (Fig. 5.4).

PROGNOSIS

Table 5.3 lists results from a number of studies which suggest a causal relationship between malnutrition and survival in cirrhosis.[11] Malnutrition has prognostic value in patients undergoing liver transplantation and other surgical operations. Similar observations have been made in nonsurgical liver disease patients. Malnutrition predicts impaired immunity and increased susceptibility to infection in patients hospitalized for cirrhosis and ascites. Ascites increases energy expenditure,[16] and the disappearance of ascites following placement of a peritoneovenous shunt improves nutritional status and immunity.[17] Malnutrition has also been

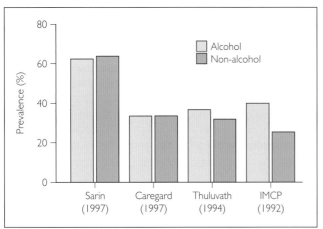

Fig. 5.2 • Prevalence of malnutrition in alcoholic and nonalcoholic cirrhosis from four studies.

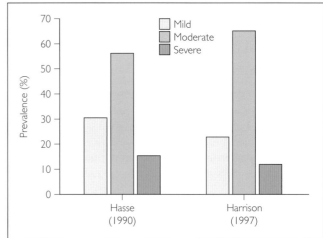

Fig. 5.3 • Prevalence of protein energy malnutrition in patients awaiting liver transplant.

Table 5.2 Prevalence of obesity prior to liver transplantation		
	Moderately obese	**Severely obese**
Keefe (1994)	1.8%	4.7%
Sawyer (1999)	20.4%	11.1%
Hasse (unpublished)		16.5 (Female) 23.2 (Male)

Table 5.3 Influence of protein calorie malnutrition on the clinical outcomes of cirrhosis	
Condition or procedure	**Clinical outcome affected**
Cirrhosis	Survival Immunodeficiency
Cirrhosis with varices	Predicting bleeding Survival
Cirrhotics having abdominal surgery	Survival Post-op complications
Hospitalized patients with ascites/cirrhosis	Survival
Alcoholic hepatitis	Survival Liver function
Liver transplantation	Patient/graft survival
Hepatectomy	Post-op complications

shown to correlate with poor hepatic function and severity of disease in cirrhotic patients. These collective data suggest that the recognition and treatment of malnutrition are important considerations in the management of patients with cirrhosis, especially in those situations listed in Table 5.3.

Protein energy malnutrition

Although it has been difficult to show a direct causal relationship between PEM and survival in patients with chronic liver disease, many studies show the importance of PEM as a prognostic factor in the clinical outcome of patients with cirrhosis, as listed in Table 5.3, which includes liver transplant patients. Most, but not all studies show the importance of nutritional status on graft and/or patient morbidity and mortality.[11] Early data show malnutrition adversely affected survival.[18] Another recent well-performed study of patients awaiting liver transplantation also showed that PEM as well as hypermetabolism predicted decreased survival after transplantation, whereas the Child-Pugh score did not.[19]

Obesity

Recent evidence indicates that obesity associated NASH is also associated with poor prognosis. Cirrhosis develops in 15–25% of NASH patients[20] and up to 40% of these patients may eventually succumb to liver-related death over a 10-year period, a mortality rate similar to cirrhosis associated with hepatitis C.[21,22] NASH is

also now considered the major cause of cryptogenic cirrhosis.[23] NASH-associated cirrhosis can also acutely decompensate, progress to hepatocellular carcinoma (HCC), and recur following transplantation.[24–26] In contrast, steatosis alone is reported to have a more benign clinical course, although progression of fibrosis in cirrhosis has occurred in 3% of these patients with steatosis alone.[20] In addition, obesity leads to steatosis and these lipid-laden hepatocytes then can serve as a reservoir of reactive oxygen species that result from and augment hepatotoxic agents such as alcohol and hepatitis.[27–30]

Although obesity is an important nutritional issue both before and after liver transplant, there is much variability among transplant centers regarding the importance of obesity as a risk factor for patients awaiting liver transplantation. Three studies have shown that graft and patient survival are similar in patients post-transplantation. Nonetheless, many transplant physicians believe that obesity is a significant enough risk factor for liver transplantation to place certain restrictions on transplantation in obese patients. These restrictions are based on the clinical impression that obese patients present significantly increased surgical difficulty and have increased perioperative morbidity compared with nonobese patients. These concerns appear most relevant in obese patients with a BMI of 35 or greater. Table 5.4 shows that obese patients with a BMI greater than 35 compared with patients with a BMI less than 30 required more intraoperative blood transfusions, had an increased number of wound infections, and were more likely to die of multiorgan failure, even though obese and nonobese transplant recipients had similar 3-year survivals.[31]

However, a recent analysis of the United Network of Organ Sharing (UNOS) indicates the degree of obesity influences both primary nonfunction and organ recipient survival. Compared to patients who were mildly obese (BMI 30–35), those with morbid obesity (BMI >40) had more primary graft nonfunction and higher 1-, 2-, and 5-year mortality. This increased mortality was due predominantly to cardiovascular and infectious causes.[31] Therefore, weight loss should be recommended for all overweight patients awaiting a liver transplantation, especially if their BMI is more that 35 kg/m².[14,15,31–33]

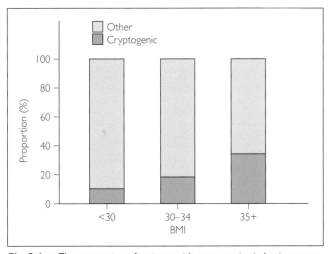

Fig. 5.4 • The proportion of patients with cryptogenic cirrhosis among those undergoing liver transplantation increases with the degree of obesity.

Table 5.4 Complications in obese liver transplant patients

	BMI <30	BMI >35	P value
Operative blood loss (U)	9.1 ± 0.8	16.2 ± 3.5	0.004
Wound infection	4%	20%	0.0001
Graft survival (1 yr)	81%	67%	0.07
Death rate			
Overall (3 yr)	29%	38%	0.30
Pre-discharge	6%	15%	0.10
Multiorgan failure	5%	40%	0.0001

Table 5.5 Factors causing malnutrition in cirrhotic patients

Non-hospitalized patients
Inadequate diet*
    Quantitative
    Iatrogenic
        (protein, fluid/salt restriction)
Malabsorption*
    Pancreatic and bile salt deficiency
    Enteropathy
Anorexia, nausea and vomiting
Alcohol toxicity on energy and protein
Altered protein and energy metabolism
    Amino acid oxidation
    Accelerated fat oxidation and gluconeogenesis
    Increased protein breakdown
    Decreased protein synthesis

Hospitalized patients
Fasting status*
    Diagnostic testing
    Gastrointestinal bleeding
    Altered neurologic status
Purgation and neomycin toxicity
Unpalatable diets*
Stressful complications*

* Indicates factors that can be currently altered or treated.

Finally, the epidemic of obesity is not only causing more end-stage liver disease; it is also decreasing the number of donor organs available for liver transplantation. According to the estimates of 94 transplant surgeons in a recent study,[34] the degree of steatosis ranged 29–40% in approximately half of all retrieved livers, and an additional 14–19% of donor livers showed 40–60% steatosis.[34] The degree of steatosis of donor livers is directly related to primary nonfunction. Potential donor livers containing more than 30–50% fat are usually not accepted. Therefore, obesity has produced an ironic combination of adverse effects for orthotopic liver transplantation, in that obesity and its associated nonalcoholic fatty liver disease has increased the need for donor livers at the same time as decreasing the number of donor livers available.[35]

ETIOLOGY OF MALNUTRITION

There are multiple etiologic factors which accelerate progression of malnutrition in patients with cirrhosis and portosystemic shunting (Table 5.5). Many of these factors can be successfully managed when nutritional status is recognized and treated as a priority.

Nutrient intake

Dietary intake is inadequate in a large percentage of patients with chronic liver disease.[3] Poor intake is prevalent (27–87%) in patients with both alcoholic and nonalcoholic liver disease and has been attributed to anorexia, nausea, early satiety (especially in the presence of ascites), dysgeusia (possibly related to zinc deficiency), and unpalatable sodium- and protein-restricted diets. Inadequate dietary intake is a particular problem in hospitalized patients who typically ingest only 50% of their calculated protein and caloric needs during their first 10 days of hospitalization. This is often iatrogenic and related to diagnostic and therapeutic procedures. The importance of these observations is emphasized by recent work that demonstrated that a regular oral diet can improve PEM in cirrhotic patients.[36]

Absorption and metabolism

Some studies have also demonstrated PEM in cirrhotics despite normal dietary intake. Therefore, other factors (such as those listed in Table 5.5 as 'Altered PEM') must be involved.

Malabsorption

Although malabsorption is not usually considered a major cause of PEM in cirrhosis, moderate steatorrhea (<12 g daily) may occur in as many as 40% of cirrhotic patients with either cholestatic or noncholestatic liver diseases and may exceed 30 g daily in 10% of cirrhotic patients. Malabsorption has been attributed to decreased intestinal bile acids, pancreatic insufficiency, and a diminished capacity for long-chain fatty acid absorption. These abnormalities are more severe in cholestatic liver disease.[6] In patients with extra-hepatic biliary obstruction, the absence of bile acids in the duodenum induces anorexic factors – cholecystokinin and leptin appear to be particularly important. In addition, celiac sprue occurs more frequently in primary biliary cirrhosis, while inflammatory bowel disease and exocrine pancreatic abnormalities are more common in primary sclerosing cholangitis. The use of oral lactulose or neomycin for hepatic encephalopathy may also exacerbate nutrient malabsorption in all forms of liver disease.

Alcohol

Although alcohol is recognized as a direct hepatotoxin, it also has profound effects on PEM as recently reviewed elsewhere.[37] From a practical approach, these adverse effects can be avoided by abstinence from alcohol use.

Protein and energy metabolism

Protein

Underlying pathophysiological factors cause loss of both fat and protein stores. After an overnight fast, cirrhotics have an increased rate of protein breakdown that is not suppressed normally in response to feeding.[38] Additionally, because of alterations in energy metabolism due to glucagon resistance and diminished glycogenolysis, amino acids are oxidized for energy – especially the ketogenic amino acid leucine. This irreversible loss of nitrogen is also associated with an increased rate of gluconeogenesis.[39]

Although increased protein breakdown has usually been considered the major cause of decreased skeletal muscle mass,[38,40] nascent data suggest that diminished protein synthesis may also be involved.[41,42] Factors have been identified that affect skeletal muscle protein synthesis and regeneration of muscle satellite cells. These include myostatin and IGF-1, which are overexpressed and underexpressed in animal models of cirrhosis.[41,43] Therefore, it is likely that diminished IGF-1 and increased myostatin decrease protein synthesis which, when combined with increased protein breakdown, results in rapid skeletal muscle wasting (Fig. 5.5).

Energy

Although highly variable, resting energy expenditure corrected for lean body mass has been shown may be increased in cirrhotics.[44] When measured energy expenditure is compared with predicted energy expenditure, 30%, 20%, and 50% of cirrhotics have high, low, or normal metabolic rates, respectively.[19] Patients with hypermetabolism have increased rates of morbidity and mortality after liver transplantation.[19] A recent study also suggested that alterations in energy metabolism are related to survival in patients with cirrhosis[45] and precede malnutrition in these patients.[46]

Regardless of the rate of energy expenditure, the preferred fuel substrate is clearly altered in cirrhosis.[44] Therefore, a clinician can tailor specific energy requirements for individual patients using simple calculations. Cirrhotics have a decrease in the respiratory quotient, which is the rate of carbon dioxide production divided by the rate of oxygen consumption after an overnight fast. Cirrhotics obtain as much as 75% of their calories from fat after an overnight fast compared with 35% for controls. Individuals without liver disease require 48–72 hours of starvation to obtain the low respiratory quotient levels that cirrhotics obtain after only 12–18 hours. In addition, amino acids are oxidized for energy and converted to glucose via gluconeogenesis in cirrhosis. Therefore, cirrhotics should be considered to have a disease of accelerated starvation with early recruitment of alternative fuels. Consequently, food should not be withheld from cirrhotic patients for any extended period, and frequent enteral feedings need to be encouraged. Cirrhotic patients given an evening snack to supply energy during the sleeping hours have been shown to maintain a greater positive nitrogen balance than those who were given less frequent-interval feedings (Fig. 5.6).

To emphasize this point, Table 5.6 displays the similarities in the metabolic profile in advanced liver disease that resembles a state of stress (such as septicemia) superimposed on that of chronic starvation or prolonged fasting.[47] These similarities between cirrhosis and starvation include decreased glycogen stores and a low respiratory quotient. Features consistent with stress include carbohydrate intolerance, increased lipolysis, negative nitrogen balance, decreased plasma concentrations of branched-chain amino acids, increased energy expenditure, and increased protein breakdown. Recent evidence suggests that leptin may be involved in this process. The protein-bound form of circulating leptin which correlates with energy expenditure is elevated in cirrhotics and may in part be responsible for the abnormal energy expenditure in these patients as described above.[48–50]

DIAGNOSIS

Nutritional assessment

Because PEM has prognostic value and influences clinical decisions regarding nutritional therapy, accurate methods of assessing nutritional status are vital. However, nutritional assessment can be difficult in patients with chronic liver disease. Clinical parameters used to diagnose protein (kwashiorkor or hypoalbuminemic) or combined protein calories (marasmic) forms of malnutrition may be affected by alcohol, liver disease, or renal dysfunction (Table 5.7). Fluid excess related to liver disease may result in an underestimation of malnutrition in chronic liver disease weight-to-height parameters (such as percentage of ideal body weight or body mass index).[51] Liver disease itself may cause alterations in visceral protein synthesis, cellular immunity, and total lymphocyte count independent of PEM which can result in an overestimation of the degree, but not necessarily the prevalence, of PEM. In contrast, markers of muscle mass (creatinine-height index and midarm muscle circumference) and fat mass (triceps skin fold thickness) are less influenced by either alcohol or chronic liver disease.[52–54] When performing a creatinine-height

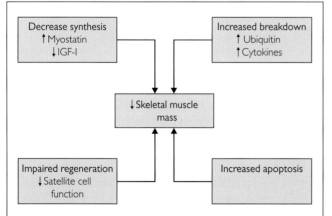

Fig. 5.5 • Factors implicated in loss of skeletal muscle mass in patients with cirrhosis.

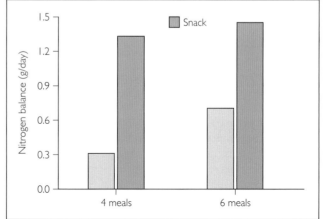

Fig. 5.6 • Effect of frequent feeding and nighttime snacks on nitrogen balance in patients with cirrhosis.

Table 5.6 Comparison of abnormalities in starvation, stress, and cirrhosis

Variable	Starvation	Stress	Cirrhosis
Insulin	NL or ↓	↑	↑
Glucagon	↑	↑	↑
Catecholamines	NL	↑	↑
Cortisol	↑	↑↑	↑
Growth hormone	NL	↑	↑
Energy expenditure	↓	↑	↑
Respiratory quotient	↓	NL or ↓	↓
Nitrogen balance	↓	↓↓	↓
Use of alternative fuels (ketones, fatty acids)	↑	↑	↑
Branched chain amino acids	↑, NL or ↓	↓	↓
Nitric oxide production	NL	↑	↑
Endotoxemia	NL	↑	↑
Body cell mass	↓↓	NL or ↓	↓
Fat stores	↓↓	NL or ↓	↓

Table 5.7 Influence of alcohol, liver disease, and renal dysfunction on nutritional status assessment

	Malnutrition		Factors altered in disease states		
	Protein	Protein/calorie	Alcohol toxicity	Liver disease	Renal function
Visceral proteins	X		X	X	
Lymphocyte count	X		X	X	X
Cellular immunity	X		X	X	X
% Ideal body wt		X		X	X
Anthropometry		X		(?)	(?)
Creatinine height index		X		(?)	X
SGA[a]		X		X	?
BIA[b]		X		X	X
DEXA[c]		X		X	X

[a]SGA, subjective global assessment.
[b]BIA, bioelectrical impedance analysis.
[c]DEXA, dual energy x-ray absorptiometry.

index estimation, creatinine clearance should be measured (not estimated) to confirm the precision of the creatinine-height index.[55]

In addition to these anthropometric and laboratory parameters, bioelectrical impedance analysis (BIA) has been used to estimate total lean body mass rather than just skeletal mass and is logistically convenient and relatively inexpensive. However, this method which correlates with body cell mass (BCM, the metabolically active lean tissue) has a degree of inaccuracy in cirrhotic patients with ascites or edema and even has some imprecision in those without ascites or edema; it may be best used to serially monitor the response to nutritional feeding.[51,56–61] Dual-energy X-ray absorp-

tiometry (DEXA) is a noninvasive method with minimal radiation that provides measurements of total body bone mineral, fat, and fat-free soft tissue mass. However, the accuracy of this method is also influenced by fluid retention, as with BIA.

Subjective global assessment is an evaluation of PEM based predominantly on the following clinical findings: the presence of edema, muscle wasting, subcutaneous fat loss, glossitis, and cheilosis. As a practical method for estimating PEM it compares favorably with standard measures in patients without liver disease.[62] Subjective global assessment in cirrhotic patients appears to be useful when evaluating patients prior to liver transplantation, although not all authors agree.[63] Estimation of handgrip strength may also be important.[64] The combined criteria of handgrip strength of less than 30 kg and midarm muscle circumference (MAMC) of less than 23 cm had a sensitivity of 94% and a negative predictive value of 97% in identifying patients with depleted BCM.[52]

Despite the limitations of these standard methodologies, more sophisticated measurements of BCM provide evidence for PEM in chronic liver disease. The BCM, which comprises the central energy-expending mass of working tissue, has been found to be decreased in both alcoholic and nonalcoholic cirrhosis by three different measurements: (1) total body potassium, (2) intracellular water, and (3) total body protein.[51,65,66]

Therefore, nutritional assessment is useful in all types of cirrhosis, especially when a composite score emphasizing anthropometry; handgrip strength, and creatinine-height index is performed and combined with overall clinical judgment, including subjective global assessment.

CLINICAL FEATURES

Medical history

A complete diet history in addition to a complete medical history should be obtained.[67] The duration, severity, and etiology of liver disease are pertinent to PEM in patients with liver disease (Table 5.8). Other disease processes, such as renal disease and hemochromatosis, should also be evaluated. Factors that may limit nutrient ingestion and absorption, such as anorexia, early satiety, vomiting, taste alteration, and diarrhea should be identified. If possible, dietary recall should estimate macronutrient and micronutrient intake and the consumption of alcoholic beverages. Because cirrhotic patients often self-select a higher proportion of their dietary intake at breakfast, a full day's calorie count is required to obtain an accurate assessment.[68] Weight may be maintained or increased despite the presence of muscle wasting, which makes the weight measurement inaccurate in these patients.

Physical examination

During physical examination, one should look for signs of decompensation, such as mental status changes, asterixis, jaundice, ascites, leg edema, and bruising. Weight should be recorded with specific attention to fluid overload. Signs of specific nutritional deficiency, such as acrodermatitis from zinc deficiency or pellagra from niacin deficiency, should be sought. Patients with cholestatic liver disease and steatorrhea may have skin excoriations related to pruritus, xanthomas due to hyperlipidemia, or dermatitis from essential fatty acid deficiency.

Evaluation of the oral mucosa, skin and hair are particularly important. In the oral mucosa, glossitis (raw tongue), atrophic tongue (slick tongue), and angular stomatitis are common findings and result from deficiencies in the B vitamins, iron, and folate. Less common are gingivitis (vitamin C deficiency) and altered taste/smell (zinc deficiency).

On the skin, petechiae (vitamin C deficiency) and purpura (vitamin A and zinc deficiency) may be present. Hair may demonstrate sparseness (protein, zinc, and biotin deficiencies), follicular hyperkeratosis (vitamins A and C deficiency) or be corkscrewed and coiled (vitamin C deficiency).

NUTRITIONAL REQUIREMENTS

Guidelines have been developed for both nitrogen and energy requirements in patients with cirrhosis.[2,3,69,70]

Nitrogen

In stable cirrhotics, the average protein requirement to maintain positive nitrogen balance is 0.8 g/kg/day, which is similar to that required in the normal population. Because the range of protein requirement is larger in cirrhotics than in controls, compensated cirrhotics should receive at least 1.2 g/kg/day.[71] Although nitrogen balance is achieved at this amount, nitrogen retention continues to improve up to 1.8 g/kg/day.[72] Even stable cirrhotics are protein deficient and this is an important management consideration. Thus, protein restriction should be avoided except for brief periods for management of acute exacerbations of encephalopathy that do not respond to conventional treatment methods. Cirrhotic patients undergoing surgery should receive protein doses between 1.2 and 1.5 g/kg/day (Table 5.9).

Table 5.8 Nutrition assessment in advances in liver disease

History	Physical examination	Laboratory tests
Weight loss >10 of usual weight	Wasting of skeletal muscle mass (temporal muscles)	Visceral proteins albumin, prealbumin and retinol-binding
Loss of appetite	Skin/hairs —Flashing point	
Decrease energy level	Zinc deficiency —Dry rash	Vitamin and mineral levels; assess
Vomiting and/or diarrhea	Purpura and hyperkeratosis —Vitamin A deficiency Oral mucosa —Vitamin B deficiency Peripheral neuropathy —Thiamine deficiency Hyperreflexia —Magnesium deficiency	Micronutrient deficiencies Total lymphocyte count

Table 5.9 Guidelines for nutritional therapy

Liver disease	Protein (g/kg/day)	Energy (Kcal/kg/day)	Energy substrate %CHO	%Fat	Nutritional goal
Hepatitis (acute or chronic[a])	1.0–1.5	30–40	67–80	20–33	Prevent malnutrition Enhance regeneration
Cirrhosis (uncomplicated)	1.0–1.2	30–40	67–80	20–33	Same as above
Cirrhosis (complicated)[b]					
a. Malnutrition	1.2–1.8	40–50	72	28	Restore normal nutritional status
b. Cholestasis	1.0–1.5	30–40	73–80	20–27	Prevent malnutrition
c. Encephalopathy[d]					Treat fat malabsorption[c]
Grade 1 or 2	0.5–1.2	25–40	75	25	Provide nutritional needs without precipitating encephalopathy
Grade 3 or 4	0.5	25–40	75	25	Provide nutritional needs without worsening encephalopathy
Liver transplant					
a. peritransplant	1.2–1.8	30–50	>70	20–30	Restore normal nutritional status
b. post-transplant	1.0	30–35	70–80	≤30	Retain and maintain ideal body weight

a. There are no convincing data indicating any extraordinary vitamin or trace metal requirements in liver disease. A typical substitution solution for parenteral feeding is provided.
   Vitamins: (10 cc/L) – ascorbic acid (20 mg/mL), vitamin A (660 IU/mL), vitamin D (40 IU/mL), thiamine HCL (0.6 mg/mL), riboflavin phosphate (0.72 mg/mL), pyridoxine HCl (0.8 mg/mL) niacinamide (8 mg/mL), d-pantothenic acid (3 mg/mL), vitamin E (2 IU/mL), Biotin (12 μg/mL), folic acid (0.08 mg/5mL), Vitamin B_{12} (1 μq/5mL).
   Trace metals: (1 ml/L) – zinc chloride (10.42 mq/5mL), copper chloride (2.68 mq/5 mL), manganese (1.44 mq/5 mL), chromium chloride (0.012 mq/5 mL).
b. Ascites and sepsis are two complications which are not listed but which should be treated aggressively as part of nutritional therapy (see text).
c. Medium chain triglycerides may be necessary if fat malabsorption is present. Pancreatic enzymes are necessary if pancreatic insufficiency is present; especially in alcoholic cirrhosis and primary sclerosing cholangitis.
d. Branched-chain amino acid (BCAA) formulations may be necessary (see text for formulations). For outpatients, diets high in vegetable protein or casein hydrolysates may be better tolerated than standard dietary protein in the protein intolerant patient with cirrhosis.

Energy

Hypermetabolism may have severe adverse clinical sequelae in cirrhotic patients and therefore it is important to document energy expenditures. Abnormalities in extracellular fluid levels in fat and nonfat body compartments, portosystemic shunting, and variability in energy expenditure between different body requirements all combine to make the prediction of energy requirements quantitatively unreliable in cirrhosis. Therefore, energy expenditure should be measured by indirect calorimetry, if available, especially in hospitalized patients undergoing liver transplantation. If indirect calorimetry is not available, the daily resting energy expenditure for cirrhosis should be assumed to be 25–30 kcal/kg body weight (based on ideal body weight if ascites and/or edema is present) for decisions regarding restorative or maintenance needs. In patients who are severely malnourished, initial calorie provision should be 15–20 kcal/kg to avoid refeeding syndrome,[73] although this concern is less relevant in conditions of insulin resistance, as is the case in cirrhosis.

Energy is proportionally provided by carbohydrates and fat as displayed in Table 5.9. Two points are important. First, insulin resistance is universal in cirrhosis irrespective of the etiology and severity of the disease. Glucose intolerance is not typically an important management issue, except for hypoglycemia, which develops in up to 50% of cirrhotic patients during sepsis. Second, lipid formulations are very useful in cirrhosis because of their low water content and high caloric density. Initial concerns that lipids might precipitate encephalopathy have not been confirmed.[74]

Vitamins

Important points regarding vitamins in patients with liver disease are noted in Table 5.10. Approximately 40% of patients with nonalcoholic liver disease have fat-soluble vitamin deficiencies (vitamin A, D, E, and K), 8–10% have deficiencies in the B complex vitamins (nicotinic acid, thiamine, vitamin B_{12}, riboflavin, and pyridoxine) and 17% have folate deficiency.[75] These abnormalities are related to disordered hepatic function and diminished reserve rather than deficient dietary intake or malabsorption. However, in severe advanced cirrhosis, malabsorption may play a role in both fat-soluble vitamins and the B complex vitamins. These vitamin deficiencies are more prevalent and severe in alcoholic than nonalcoholic liver disease. However, cholestatic liver disease can have severe deficiencies in fat-soluble vitamins.[76–78] This appears particularly important in light of the fact that these vitamin deficiencies are associated with increased risk of hepatocellular carcinoma[79] and lipid peroxidation.[80]

SPECIFIC ALTERATIONS IN LIVER DISEASE

Accelerated starvation

Cirrhosis is a disease of accelerated starvation with early recruitment of alternative fuels.[81] Cirrhotic patients should avoid any extended period of time without feeding. The advantage of a frequent feeding approach has been confirmed by nitrogen balance and indirect calorimetry measurements in cirrhotic patients (Table 5.11) (see Fig. 5.6).[82,83]

Table 5.10 Vitamins in liver disease

Some complications associated with liver disease are manifestations of vitamin deficiencies:
  macrocytic anemia (folate and vitamin B_{12} deficiency)
  neuropathy (pyridoxine, thiamine or vitamin B_{12})
  confusion, ataxia and ocular disturbances (thiamine)
  impaired adaptation to dark (vitamin A)

Pyridoxine phosphate (the major active form of pyridoxine) rather than pyridoxine itself may be required to correct pyridoxine deficiency, especially in alcoholics.

The clinical response to thiamine is usually rapid and effective. However, the neuropathy may be irreversible and abnormalities in red cell transketolase may not improve.

Deficiencies in vitamin B_{12} and folic acid may develop faster in cirrhotic patients due to diminished hepatic storage.

In the presence of active hepatic inflammation, fatty liver or hepatocellular cancer, normal or elevated levels of vitamin B_{12} levels do not exclude a deficiency of this vitamin.

Decreased serum levels of vitamin A do not necessarily reflect vitamin A deficiency. Zinc deficiency may be causing decreased transport out of the liver.

In noncholestatic liver disease, fat-soluble vitamins levels should not be measured or treated in the absence of clinical or laboratory abnormalities which indicate a functional vitamin deficiency. In cholestatic liver diseases, abnormal serum levels of the fat soluble vitamins may be treated even in the absence of clinical symptoms or laboratory abnormalities.

Vitamin supplementation:
  Water-soluble vitamins may be supplied with a multivitamin preparation
  Fat-soluble vitamins should be used in a water-soluble form whenever possible
    Vitamin A, Aquasol 1 capsule daily (50 000 IU)
    Vitamin K, Synkayvite, 1 tablet daily (15 mg)
    Vitamin D treatment should be individualized by monitoring plasma 25-hydroxy vitamin D levels and serum and urinary calcium levels. Vitamin D_2 (ergocalciferol), 1.25 mg (50 000 U), 1 tablet 3–4 times a day, may be adequate.
    Vitamin E (D-α-tocopheryl polyethylene glycol 1000 succinate (TPGS) 23 IU kg^{-1}day). Levels should be checked every 3–4 months.

Hepatic encephalopathy

Advanced acute or chronic liver failure often presents with a constellation of neuropsychiatric abnormalities known as hepatic encephalopathy. These mental status alterations may range from mild behavioral changes to deep coma. Subclinical hepatic encephalopathy is present in up to 70% of patients with cirrhosis and currently does not require any specific nutritional therapy. Overt encephalopathy is almost always associated with some precipitating event such as gastrointestinal bleeding, infection, sepsis, fluid and electrolyte imbalances, constipation, acid–base abnormalities or the use of sedating drugs. In a small minority of cirrhotic patients, hepatic encephalopathy may be precipitated by protein intake (especially animal protein) without any other precipitating factor. These patients are considered protein intolerant. However, it is important to recognize that more than 95% of cirrhotic patients can tolerate diets containing as much as 1.5 g/kg/day of mixed proteins. Therefore, true protein intolerance is rare except for fulminant hepatic failure, or the occasional patient with 'endogenous' chronic encephalopathy or fulminant hepatic failure.[84–87]

Table 5.11 Nutritional considerations for specific clinical situations in patients with liver disease

Clinical presentation	Nutritional management
Accelerated starvation	Frequent feedings with nighttime snack.
Hepatic encephalopathy	Routine or prophylactic protein restriction is discouraged.
Hepatic metabolism of nonessential amino acids	Cysteine and tyrosine may become essential amino acids
Salt restriction	Salt restriction should be balanced against diet palatability
Alcohol toxicity	Abstinence needs to be continually re-enforced
Obesity	Gradual weight loss should be instituted

In those few cirrhotic patients with endogenous protein intolerance, branched-chain amino acid formulations are better tolerated than standard amino acid supplements and can achieve positive nitrogen balance. It should be emphasized, however, that there is no clearly proven benefit of branched-chain amino acids over standard amino acids for the majority of patients with chronic liver disease. Available enteral BCAA preparations are provided in footnotes of Table 5.9. However, the cost of these products may be tenfold higher than standard enteral products. Vegetable protein diets may be beneficial in these patients.[88] However, these diets with increased fiber and decreased caloric and protein density require large volume of dietary intake to meet protein and energy needs. This may not be tolerable in these patients who often have delayed gastric emptying.[89] There are conflicting data regarding the beneficial effects of zinc on hepatic encephalopathy.[90,91]

Non-essential amino acids

Administration of standard or specialized total potential nutrition solutions devoid of the nonessential acids tyrosine and cysteine may not achieve positive nitrogen balance in patients with cirrhosis despite provision of adequate amounts of essential amino acids.[92] This observation suggests that certain intrinsic liver functions, such as the ability to synthesize cysteine from phenylalanine, may be rate-limiting in cirrhosis. Glutamine may also become an essential amino acid in cirrhosis.[45]

Salt restriction

Sodium restriction significantly decreases the palatability of the diet and consequently may diminish food intake. In the hospitalized patient, very low 250–500 mg sodium (0.62–1.3 g salt) diets may be appropriate. In the nonhospitalized patient, every effort should be made to avoid excessive salt restriction. Drastic salt restrictions tend not to be followed well by even motivated patients. Thus, in those patients with fluid overload who otherwise cannot be managed effectively, a no added salt diet (approximately 2.5 g sodium or 6.3 g salt) is generally palatable and should not significantly limit calorie or protein intake.

Alcohol-related alterations

Alcohol has direct deleterious affects on muscle protein status independent from associated liver injury.[37,93] Alcohol is known to inhibit meal-stimulated hepatic protein production which is an important contributor to skeletal muscle and whole body protein synthesis in humans. Alcohol increases intestinal permeability which in turn initiates endotoxin/cytokine-induced muscle proteolysis. In addition, alcohol has a caloric density of seven but produces less efficient energy per gram of nutrient than both carbohydrates and lipids and replaces the amount of other caloric sources.

Obesity

As discussed above, obesity is associated with hepatic steatosis which may not only cause cirrhosis per se, but may also promote fibrosis in patients with alcohol and hepatitis C-associated liver disease. In addition, it is associated with multiorgan failure and decreased survival post-liver transplant.

NUTRITIONAL MANAGEMENT

Goals

Recommendations for nutritional therapy in patients with liver diseases are provided in Table 5.12. Early studies used survival as the primary outcome measure for determining the efficacy of nutritional therapy. Recently, it has been shown that nutritional therapy in cirrhotic patients can improve nutritional status, reduce infection rates, enhance immune function, improve nitrogen balance, and decrease perioperative morbidity. Nutritional therapy is most effective when used for longer periods of time and in certain subgroups such as in those with severe malnutrition, chronic hepatic encephalopathy, and decompensated liver disease. No reliable information is available regarding the cost-effectiveness of nutritional therapy or its effect on the quality of life of cirrhotic patients. Regarding goals specific for liver disease, nutritional therapy needs to correct pre-existing PEM while simultaneously providing sufficient amino acids to encourage hepatic regeneration and normalization of function without precipitating encephalopathy. The clinical emphasis should be placed on supplying the basic requirements of nitrogen and calories.

Specific patient populations

Cirrhosis

Enteral feeding improves liver function, encephalopathy, and perhaps survival in severely malnourished cirrhotics and in patients with decompensated alcoholic liver disease. Nutrient intake is increased by enteral nutrition in all published studies to date and may in part be responsible for those benefits. There have been four published randomized trials that used enteral tube feedings in cirrhosis (with or without alcoholic hepatitis).[86,94–96] Three found enteral tube feedings to be more effective than a conventional diet because food intake was increased.[86,94,96] Two of these trials[86,94] improved liver function and one improved survival.[94] Providing nutritional supplements (1000 cal and 34 g of protein-casein based) for 1 year to patients with complicated alcoholic cirrhosis resulted in higher protein and caloric intake to levels which simply met their required needs.

Alcoholic hepatitis

There have been eight published trials on the use of standard intravenous amino acid formulations as primary therapy for alcoholic hepatitis.[97] The results are conflicting, but six of the eight studies showed improvement in either liver histology or function. One of these studies additionally showed a strong trend toward an improvement in mortality. Two of the studies concluded that supplemental amino acids were of no benefit. In one of these negative studies, the mortality was 3.3% in the 30 patients in whom positive nitrogen balance was achieved, but 58% in those patients who remained in negative nitrogen balance despite nutritional therapy. Therefore, achieving nitrogen balance is an important goal. A recent trial also reported enteral feedings to be equally effective as corticosteroids,[98] but both may be beneficial in different ways. In the initial 10 days of treatment, steroids were more effective (presumably by decreasing the immune and inflammatory injury) while enteral nutrition was more effective after 10 days (presumably by improving gut function and hepatic regeneration).

Table 5.12 Guidelines for the nutritional management of patients with liver disease

Assume protein calorie malnutrition is present in all patients with cirrhosis.

Assume an inadequate dietary intake, particularly in hospitalized patients.

Nutritional assessment is useful in all types of cirrhotic patients.

A composite score (emphasizing anthropometry, hand grip strength, and creatinine-height index) combined with overall clinical judgment should be employed

Determine energy expenditure requirements with indirect calorimetry (if possible) in hospitalized patients or patients listed for liver transplantation. If energy expenditure requirements are estimated from prediction equations, calculate energy need based on weight rather than actual weight if extracellular water (ascites/edema) is present.

The clinician should remember that all the methods for nutritional assessment in cirrhosis are influenced or potentially influenced by the presence of liver disease alone as well as abnormalities associated with liver disease such as renal failure, alcohol ingestion and expansion of the extracellular water compartment.

Treatment of liver disease:

Cirrhotics should never be treated prophylactically with protein restriction to prevent hepatic encephalopathy.

Protein restriction below the required amounts should not be continued for more than 3–4 days.

Neomycin or lactulose may exacerbate malabsorption and this should be considered in the nutritional management plan.

Treat ascites aggressively to decrease energy expenditure.

Diuretic therapy is preferred over large volume paracentesis for the management of ascites in order to minimize protein loss.

Balance the need for sodium restriction with nutritional considerations and diet palatability

Qualitative stool fat should be done intermittently, especially in patients with alcoholic or cholestatic cirrhosis. If malabsorption is present, determine the cause and treat.

Monitor for hypoglycemia and treat aggressively with concentrated glucose solutions recognizing that these may also decrease serum ammonia levels.

Nutritional management:

Nutritional requirements may vary according to the specific type of patient and/or clinical situation (Table 5.9).

Multiple (5–6) small feedings with a carbohydrate-rich evening snack, which consists of approximately 10–15% of caloric needs, should be given. The need for breakfast feeding must also be stressed to the patient.

Complex, rather than simple, carbohydrates should be used for calories. Lipids should supply 20–40% of caloric needs.

Long term nutritional supplements may be necessary to provide recommended protein and caloric supplements.

Severely malnourished or decompensated cirrhotics should be given oral or enteral supplements (Table 5.9).

Patients with severe alcoholic hepatitis should be given supplemental standard protein 1.0 g/kg via an enteral or peripheral parenteral route.

Perioperative nutritional therapy should be given to those cirrhotic patients with significant malnutrition and post-liver transplant patients (Table 5.9).

Standard protein or amino acid mixtures should be supplied to meet the measured estimated nitrogen needs. Branched-chain amino acids should be given only if the required amount of protein results in worsening hepatic encephalopathy.

Enteral feeding is the preferred route of feeding patients with insufficient oral intake. Enteral feeding tubes may be used even if non-bleeding varices are present.

Do not use any nutritional product devoid of cysteine or tyrosine as the only nitrogen source for any prolonged period of time. Be aware of clinically important issues related to vitamins listed in Table 5.10.

Fulminant hepatic failure

Fulminant hepatic failure, defined as the development of hepatic encephalopathy within 8 weeks of the onset of liver disease, is a life-threatening illness associated with a rapid development of protein calorie malnutrition; even when what is calculated to be adequate amounts of calorie and nitrogen are supplied. Up to four times the normal rate of protein breakdown accompanied by decreased hepatic amino acid oxidation leads to the accumulation of potentially toxic levels of certain amino acids (tyrosine, phenylalanine, and methionine). Hypoglycemia occurs commonly and serum glucose levels must be maintained with concentrated glucose infusion (20–40%) to avoid the risks of exacerbating cerebral edema. Lipid emulsions may be particularly useful in this setting.

Administering at least 40–60 g of protein diminishes the rapid depletion of protein stores in patients with stage 1 and 2 encephalopathy. If necessary, the use of branched-chain amino acids may be necessary to achieve this goal in patients with more advanced stages of encephalopathy. However, the efficacy of branched-chain amino acids in this situation remains unproven. If encephalopathy should develop or worsen with protein feeding, the use of specialized formulations of branched-chain amino acids seems indicated.

Obese patients

Serum aminotransferase levels almost always improve with weight loss (with as little as 5–10%) in the obese patient with liver disease, but they are poor predictors of histology. Gradual weight loss (1–2 lb per week) with an overall goal of 10% weight loss over 6 months is recommended as a safe and effective clinical strategy, especially in patients who are more than 30% overweight.[99,100] With success, further weight loss can be attempted, if indicated. Multiple interventions and strategies, including diet modifications, physical activity, behavioral therapy, and pharmacotherapy with Orlistat, or a combination of these treatment modalities is recommended. The particular treatment modality should be individualized, taking into consideration the BMI index and presence of concomitant risk factors and other diseases. Given the lack of clinical trials in this area,[101] these overall recommendations are a useful and safe first step for obese patients with nonalcoholic fatty liver disease (NAFLD). The only prospective study using restrictive bariatric surgery in NAFLD patients was very effective in diminishing hepatic injury.[102]

Liver transplant patients

There is no uniform approach among transplant centers regarding the management of nutrition in transplant patients. There is agreement that malnutrition reflects the severity of chronic liver disease and should generally not be considered as an exclusion for patients receiving liver transplant.[103] Most centers administer postoperative nutrition in a fashion similar to that given other patients after gastrointestinal major surgery. Therefore, the recognition that malnutrition is a significant problem has been gaining momentum.[104–106] In addition, a recent study[107] showed no preoperative nutritional marker was associated with survival or resource utilization. Longer ICU stay and a higher rate of infections were associated with decreased handgrip strength and BCAA levels, respectively. A recent study[108] suggested that enteral nutrition might improve survival in patients awaiting liver transplantation, but it was underpowered. Thus, there are still insufficient data in the pretransplant patient upon which to base any specific recommendations. Consequently, general principles of nutritional management as outlined in Tables 5.9, 5.10, and 5.12 should be followed. In the post-transplant patient, nutritional therapy improves nitrogen balance, decreases viral infection, and shows a trend to shortening ICU stays and lowering hospital costs. Early enteral feeding achieves better nitrogen retention postoperatively. Both nasogastric and jejunostomy tubes have been used successfully in these patients. Available information suggests that enteral and parenteral nutrition are equivalent in their ability to deliver nutrients and improve nutritional status through the tenth postoperative day.

Despite the early benefits of nutritional supplementation, most patients do not appear to achieve normal nutritional status in the long term. Protein breakdown and lipolysis improves after 1 year, but does not normalize. Likewise, total body water and total body fat improve, but there is no change in body cell mass.[109,110] An increasing important nutritional problem, which develops in the first 1–2 years after liver transplant, is obesity which has been reported to occur in 30–70% of patients.[111–113] Therefore, it is important to follow the nutritional status of these patients postoperatively and treat obesity aggressively if it develops. As shown in Figure 5.7, recent data from a four-center study reported that 30% of liver transplant recipients are obese 2 years after liver transplant.[112]

PRINCIPLES AND PRACTICAL IMPLEMENTATION

The nutritional support of patients with liver disease follows the general principles applicable to any other patient. However, there are a number of principles particularly relevant to liver disease patients, with guidelines provided in Tables 5.9, 5.10, and 5.12.

Glucose requirement

Although insulin resistance and hypoglycemia are commonly observed in cirrhosis, hypoglycemia (<50 mg/dL) occurs in up to 50% of cirrhotic patients during episodes of stress. Therefore, serum glucose must be closely monitored in patients with fulminant or decompensated chronic liver disease and supplemented by infusions when necessary.

Route of nutrient administration

The preferred and least invasive route for nutritional supplements is oral, which should be tried first. If attempts of oral supplementation fail, enteral feedings can be administered safely via a small-caliber nasogastric or nasojejunal tube.[94,95,114] The presence of nonbleeding esophageal varices is not a contraindication to the use of enteral feeding tubes in these patients. However, feeding tubes should not be used if there is active esophageal variceal bleeding. The placement of a percutaneous gastrostomy or a jejunostomy tube in cirrhotics with ascites is not recommended due to the possible complications of peritonitis or ascitic fluid leakage. Unfortunately, this limits the potential of long-term enteral feeding in many of these patients.

One study suggests that parenteral feeding may actually be preferred,[115] based on the observation that serum ammonia increases rapidly with enteral but not parenteral feeding in cirrhotic patients with TIPS. However, the risk of catheter-related

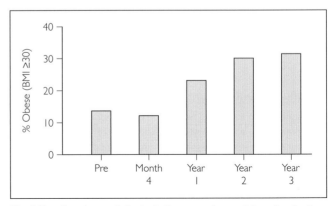

Fig. 5.7 • Prevalence of obesity in liver transplant recipients for the first 3 years post-transplant

sepsis is high in malnourished cirrhotic patients. In addition, parenteral mixtures may be excessive for cirrhotic patients.[116] Parenteral nutrition should be initiated only if nutritional requirements cannot be supplied orally or enterally in situations such as gastrointestinal bleeding, ileus, or after abdominal surgery. Because of its relatively low caloric density, peripheral parenteral nutrition cannot supply total nutritional requirements and is usually not a good choice in cirrhotic patients with sodium and water retention. Peripheral parenteral nutrition may be useful in supplementing enteral or oral feeding, especially for providing amino acids in severe alcoholic hepatitis. Central parenteral nutrition is preferred in most cirrhotic patients despite the risk of central vein catheter replacement in patients with coagulopathy and thrombocytopenia.

The amount of protein recommended for different types of liver disease patients in various situations is provided in Table 5.9. If these amounts of protein cannot be provided without precipitating hepatic encephalopathy, formulations enriched with branched-chain amino acids should be substituted for standard formulations. There are oral or enteral feedings (Nutrihep – 50% BCAA enriched; Hepatic Aid II – 46% BCAA enriched) as well as intravenous formulations (Hepatamine and Hepatasol – both 36% BCAA enriched) available. There are also stress formulations (Freamine HBC and Aminosyn-HBC) that are approximately 45% BCAA enriched. However, these stress formulations have not been evaluated in patients with liver disease.

Dietary supplements

Many patients seek advice regarding the safety and efficacy of vitamins, herbs, or other nutritional supplements. Unfortunately, there is insufficient information in this area to make sound recommendations. General recommendations are provided in Table 5.13.

Obesity

A number of different diets have been suggested, including the American Heart Association healthy heart diet, the Diabetic Diet as recommended by the American Diabetes Association, a low glycemic diet, and diets enriched with omega 3 polyunsaturated fatty acids. However, the effect of these diets in liver is unproven. Diets used to produce weight loss must always be individualized and related to the overall health status of the patient.

In general, patients should follow a well-balanced diet such as the diet recommended by the National Cholesterol Education Program (www.nhlbi.nih.gov/about/ncep). This diet makes specific recommendations regarding total caloric intake, as well as the amount and type of fat and carbohydrate for patients who do not have to lose weight. If the patient has diabetes, specific recommendations have been made by the American Diabetes Association.

Overweight patients (BMI >25 kg/m^2 based on dry weight) should be given a diet with a goal of losing and sustaining an initial weight loss of 10% of body weight. The weight loss should be gradual and should not exceed 2 lb per week. The National Heart, Lung, and Blood Institute (NHLBI) guidelines for weight loss is an excellent model.

SUMMARY

Malnutrition is ubiquitous in all types of cirrhosis. It has prognostic significance and its treatment has been shown to provide beneficial clinical outcomes. Therefore, it is important to identify malnutrition and treat it with increased amounts of conventional feedings while maintaining specialized formulations in only those patients who cannot tolerate standard dietary needs without precipitating encephalopathy.

Specific recommendations for the logistics of managing PEM in patients with liver disease are provided in Tables 5.9, 5.10, 5.12,

Table 5.13 Use of nutritional supplements and medications in nafld

Possibly harmful		Possibly helpful	
Supplements	Medications	Supplements	Medications
St. John's wart	Acetaminophen[4]	Vitamin E[8]	Betaine[11]
Ephedrine containing compounds	Tamoxifen[5]	MVI[9]	Ursodeoxycholic acid[11]
Excessive vitamin A[1]	Amiodarone[5]	SAMe[10,11]	Metformin[11,12]
Glucosamine[2]	Iron[6]	Milk thistle[11]	Statins[11,13]
Others[3]	Estrogen[7]		Thiazolidinediones[11,12]

1. Vitamin A use should not exceed that contained in a daily multivitamin (MVI) which is 5000 IU.
2. Hexosamines cause insulin resistance, so glucosamine should be used with caution.
3. All other herbs should be considered as possible causes of hepatic injury and should be avoided.
4. Acetaminophen should be restricted to less than 2–3 grams daily. Repeated or ongoing use of acetaminophen for longer than 3 days with daily dose above 1.5 grams should be discouraged. Many over the counter (OTC) medications contain acetaminophen. Therefore the amount of acetaminophen in the OTC medications should be carefully sought.
5. This drug may cause hepatic injury that histologically looks similar to NAFLD/NASH. Therefore, the benefit risk of using these drugs in NAFLD/NASH should be carefully considered.
6. Since iron may cause oxidative stress in the liver, iron supplements should only be for treatment of iron-deficiency anemia. Transferrin saturation should not exceed 50%.
7. Estrogens used as oral contraception pills (OCP) or as hormonal replacement therapy (HRT) do not have to be discontinued.
8. Vitamin E should be used at doses less than 400 I.U daily.
9. A daily multivitamin (MVI) with iron content <20 mg should be used.
10. SAMe = S-adenosylmethionine.
11. There are uncontrolled studies that suggest a benefit of this medication in NAFLD, but its use outside of research studies is not encouraged.
12. This agent is approved for use in patients with type II diabetes.
13. The use of the statins as cholesterol lowering agents is not contraindicated (and in fact, may be beneficial) in NAFLD. However, baseline and interval measurements of liver function tests should be performed.

and 5.13. Nutritional therapy should meet and maintain these nutritional requirements. This means that long-term outpatient management is as important to these patients as nutritional supplementation when they are hospitalized for acute illness.

REFERENCES

1. Achord JL. Malnutrition and the role of nutritional support in alcoholic liver disease. Am J Gastroenterol 1987; 82: 1–7.

2. Plauath M, Merli M, Kondrup J, et al. ESPEN guidelines for nutrition in liver disease and transplantation. Clin Nutr 1997; 16:43–45.

   This and the following article provide guidelines for managing nutrition in patients with chronic liver disease.

3. McCullough AJ, Teran JC, Bugianesi E. Guidelines for nutritional therapy in liver disease. In: Klein S, ed. The American Society of Parenteral and Enteral Nutritional Support. Practice manual. Silver Spring, MD: 1998:1–12.

   This and the preceding article provide guidelines for managing nutrition in patients with chronic liver disease.

4. McClave SA, Mitoraj TE, Thielmeier KA. Differentiating subtypes (hypoalbuminemia vs marasmic) of protein calorie malnutrition: Incidence and clinical significance in a University Hospital setting. J Parenter Enter Nutr 1992; 16:337–342.

5. McCullough AJ, Falck-Ytter Y. Body composition and hepatic steatosis as precursors for fibrotic liver disease. Hepatology 1999; 29:1328–1330.

6. Padillo FJ, Andicoberry B, Pera-Madrazo C, et al. Anorexia and malnutrition in patients with obstructive jaundice. Nutrition 2002; 18:987–990.

7. Patton KM, Aranda-Michael J. Nutritional aspects in liver disease and transplantation. Nutr in Clin Prac 2002; 17:332–340.

8. Merli M, Nicotini G, Angeloni S, et al. Malnutrition is a risk factor in cirrhotic patients undergoing surgery. Nutrition 2002; 18:978–986.

9. Roonspisuthipong C, SobhonslidsukA, Nantruj K, et al. Nutritional assessment in various stages of liver cirrhosis. Nutrition 2001; 17:761–765.

10. McCullough AJ, Bugianesi E. Protein-calorie malnutrition and the etiology of cirrhosis. Am J Gastroenterol 1997; 92:734–737.

11. McCullough. Malnutrition in liver disease. Liver Transpl 2000; 6:S85–S96.

12. Dicecio SR, Wieners EJ, Wiesner RAH. Assessment of nutritional status of patients with end-stage liver disease undergoing liver transplantation. Mayo Clin Proc 1989; 69:95–99.

13. Kopelman PG. Obesity as a medical problem. Nature 2000; 404:635–643.

14. Keefe EB, Gettys C, Esquivel CO. Liver transplantation in patients with severe obesity. Transplantation 1994; 57:309–311.

15. Sawyer RG, Pelletier SJ, Pruett TL. Increased early morbidity and morality with acceptable long-term function in severely obese patients undergoing liver transplantation. Clin Transplant 1999; 13:126–130.

16. Dolz C, Ranrich JM, Ibanez J. Ascites increases energy expenditure in liver cirrhosis. Gastroenterology 1991; 100:738–744.

   An important study that demonstrates increased resting energy expenditure in cirrhotic patients with ascites. This may accelerate the appearance of protein energy malnutrition and emphasizes the need to avoid protein restriction in cirrhotic patients.

17. Allard JP, Chau J, Sandokji K, et al. Effects of ascites resolution after successful TIPS on nutrition in cirrhotic patients with refractory ascites. Am J Gastroenterol 2001; 96:2442– 2447.

18. Shaw BW Jr, Wood RP, Gordon RD, et al. Influence of selected patient variables and operative blood loss on six-month survival following liver transplantation. Semin Liver Dis 1985; 5:385–393.

19. Selberg O, Bottcher J, Tusch G, et al. Identification of high and low risk patients before liver transplantation – a prospective cohort study of nutritional and metabolic parameters in 150 patients. Hepatology 1999; 25:652–657.

   Documents the impact of protein-energy malnutrition on survival in patients with chronic liver disease. Patients with increased predicted resting energy expenditure and low body cell mass had significantly increased-year mortality after liver transplantation. These factors predicted survival independently of ascites or Child class.

20. Matteoni CA, Younossi ZM, Gramlich T, et al. Nonalcoholic fatty liver disease: A spectrum of clinical and pathological severity. Gastroenterology 1999; 116:1413–1419.

21. Ratziu V, Bonyhay L, Di Martino V, et al. Survival, liver failure, and hepatoellular carcinoma in obesity-related cryptogenic cirrhosis. Hepatology 2002; 35:1485–1493.

22. Hui JM, Kench JG, Chitturi S, et al. Long term outcomes of cirrhosis in nonalcoholic steatohepatitis compared with hepatitis C. Hepatology 2003; 38:420–427.

23. Caldwell SH, Oelsner DH, Iezzoni JC, et al. Cryptogenic cirrhosis: clinical characterization and risk factors for underlying disease. Hepatology 1999; 32:689–692.

   This study notes that most patients with cryptogenic cirrhosis have features of the metabolic syndrome including obesity and type 2 diabetes. Thus, obesity may be a risk factor for cirrhosis and liver failure. This is an additional nutritional factor to include in the management of patients with liver disease. In addition, obesity may result in progression of other forms of liver disease (see references 27–30).

24. Caldwell SH, Hespenheide EE. Subacute liver failure in obese women. Am J Gastroenterol 2002; 97:2058–2067.

25. Bugianesi E, Leone N, Vanni E, et al. Expanding the natural history of nonalcoholic steatohepatitis: from cryptogenic cirrhosis to hepatocellular carcinoma. Gastroenterology 2002; 123(1):134–140.

26. Younossi ZM, Reddy V, Price LL, et al. Cryptogenic cirrhosis and posttransplantation: nonalcoholic liver disease. Liver Transpl 2001; 7:797–801.

27. McCullough AJ. Obesity and its nurturing effects on hepatitis C. Hepatology 2003; 38:557–559.

28. Naveau S, Giraud V, Borottu F. Excess weight as a risk factor for alcoholic liver disease. Hepatology 1997; 25:108–111.

29. Reeves HL, Burt AD, Woods S, et al. Hepatic stellate cell activation occurring in the absence of hepatitis in alcoholic liver disease and correlates with the severity of steatosis. J Hepatol 1996; 25:677–683.

30. Ortiz V, Berenguer M, Rayon JM, et al. Contribution of obesity to hepatitis C fibrosis progression. Am J Gastroenterol 2002; 97:2408–2414.

31. Nair S, Verma S, Thuluvath PJ. Obesity and its effect on survival in patients undergoing orthotopic liver transplantation in the United States. Hepatology 2002; 35:105–109.

32. Brannfield MY, Chan S, Pregler J, et al. Liver transplantation in obese patients. J Clin Anesth 1996; 8:585–590.

33. Nair S, Cohen DB, Cohen MP, et al. Post-operative morbidity, mortality, cost and long-term survival in severely obese patients undergoing orthotopic liver transplantation. Am J Gastroenterol 2001; 96:842–845.

34. Imber CJ, St. Peter SD, Lopez I, et al. Current practice regarding the use of fatty livers: A transatlantic survey. Liver Transpl 2002; 8:545–549.

35. Burke A, Lucey MR. NAFLD, NASH and orthotopic liver transplantation. In: Farrell GC, George J, Hall Pde la M, et al., eds. Fatty liver disease: NASH and related disorders. London: Blackwell Publishing; 2004:208–217.

36. Campillo B, Bories PPN, Leluan M, et al. Short-term changes in energy metabolism after 1 month of a regular oral diet in severely malnourished cirrhotic patients. Metabolism 1995; 44:765–770

37. Falk-Ytter Y, McCullough AJ. Nutritional effect of alcoholism. Curr Gastroenterol Rep 2000; 2:331–336.

38. McCullough AJ, Mullen KD, Kalhan SC. Defective non-oxidative leucine degradation and endogenous leucine flux in cirrhosis during an amino acid infusion. Hepatology 1998; 28:1357–1364.

39. Bugianesi E, Kalhan SC, Burkett E, et al. Quantification of gluconeogenesis in cirrhosis: response to glucagons. Gastroenterology 1998; 115:1530–1450.

40. Tessari P. Protein metabolism in liver cirrhosis. From albumin to muscle myofibrils. Curr Opin Clin Nutr Metab Care 2003; 6:79–85.

41. Dasarathy S, Dodig M, Muc SM, eet al. Skeletal muscle atrophy is associated with an increased expression of myostatin and impaired satellite cell function in the portacaval anastomosis rat. Am J Physiol Gastrointest Liver Physiol 2004; 287:G1124–G1130.

42. Scharf JG, Schmitz F, Frystyk J, et al. Insulin-like growth factor-1 serum concentrations and patterns of insulin-like growth factor binding proteins in patients with chronic liver disease. J Hepatol 1996; 25:689–699.

43. Picard A, Costa de Oliveira A, Muguerza B, et al. Low doses of insulin-like growth factor-1 improves nitrogen retention and food efficiency in rats with early cirrhosis. J Hepatol 1997; 26:191–202.

44. McCullough AJ, Raguso C. Effect of cirrhosis on energy expenditure. Am J Clin Nutr 1999; 69:1066–1068.

45. Tajika M, Kato M, Muhri H, et al. Prognostic value of energy metabolism in patients with viral liver cirrhosis. Nutrition 2002; 18:224–234.

46. Scolario JS, Bowen J, Stoner G, et al. Substrate oxidation in patients with cirrhosis: Comparison with other nutritional markers. J Parenter Enter Nutr 2000; 24:150–153.

47. Teran JC, Mullen KD, McCullough AJ. Glutamine: a conditionally essential amino acid in cirrhosis. Am J Clin Nutr 1995; 62:897–900.

48. McCullough AJ, Bugianesi E, Marchesini G, et al. Gender-dependent alterations in serum leptin in alcoholic cirrhosis. Gastroenterology 1998; 115:947–953.

49. Cabre E, Gassull MA. Nutritional aspects of liver disease and transplantation. Curr Opin Clin Nutr Metab Care 2001; 4:581–589.

50. Ockenega J, Bischoff SC, Tillman HL. Elevated bound leptin correlates with energy expenditure in cirrhotics. Gastroenterology 2000; 119:1656–1667.

51. McCullough AJ, Mullen KD, Kalhan SC. Measurement of total body extracellular water in cirrhotic patients with and without ascites. Hepatology 1991; 14:1102–1109.

52. Figueiredo FA, Dickson ER, Pasha TM, et al. Utility of standard nutritional parameters in detecting body cell mass depletion in patients with end-stage liver disease. Liver Transpl 2000; 6:575–581.

53. Fiore P, Merli M, Andreoli A. A comparison of skinfold anthropometry and dual-energy X-ray absorptiometry for the evaluation of body fat in cirrhotic patients. Clin Nutr 1999; 18:349–351.

54. Jeong SH, Lee JA, Kim JA, et al. Assessment of body composition using dual-energy X-ray absorptiometry in patients with liver cirrhosis; comparison with anthropometry. Korean J Intern Med 1999; 14:64–71

55. Pirlich M, Selberg O, Boker K. The creatinine approach to estimate skeletal muscle mass in patients with cirrhosis. Hepatology 1996; 24:1422–1427.

56. Pirlich M, Schutz T, Spachos T. Bioelectrical impedance analysis is a useful bedside technique to assess malnutrition in cirrhotic patients with and without ascites. Hepatology 2000; 32:1208–1215.

57. Kyle UG, Genton L, Mentha G. Reliable bioelectrical impedance analysis estimate of fat-free mass in liver, lung and heart transplant patients. J Parenter Enter Nutr 2001; 25:45–51.

58. Schloerb PR, Forster J, Delcore R, et al. Bioelectrical impedance in the clinical evaluation of liver disease. Am J Clin Nutr 1996; 64(Suppl):510–514.

59. Guglielmi FW, Contento F, Laddaga L, et al. Bioelectric impedance analysis experience with male patients with cirrhosis. Hepatology 1991; 13:892–895.

60. Zillikens MC, Van den Berg JWO, Wilson JHP, et al. Whole-body and segmental bioelectrical impedance analysis in patients with cirrhosis of the liver: changes after treatment of ascites. Am J Clin Nutr 1992; 55:621–625.

61. Madden AM, Morgan MY. A comparison of skinfold anthropometry and bioelectrical impedance analysis for measuring percentage body fat in patients with cirrhosis. J Hepatol 1994; 21:878–883.

62. Hasse J, Strong S, Gorman MA, et al. Subjective global assessment alternative nutrition-assessment technique for liver-transplant candidates. Nutrition 1993; 9(4):339–343.

63. Naveau S, Belda E, Borotto E. Comparison of clinical judgment and anthropometric parameters for evaluating nutritional status in patients with alcoholic liver disease. J Hepatol 1995; 23:234–235.

64. Fandersen H, Borre M, Jakobsen J et al. Decreased muscle strength in patients with alcoholic liver cirrhosis in relation to nutritional status, alcohol abstinence, liver function, and neuropathy. Hepatology 1998; 27:1200–1206.

65. Prijamoko D, Strauss BJG, Lambert JR, et al. Early detection of protein depletion in alcoholic cirrhosis: Role of body composition analysis. Gastroenterology 1993; 105:1839–1845.

66. Crawford DHG, Shepherd RW, Halliday JW, et al. Body composition in nonalcoholic cirrhosis: The effect of disease etiology and severity on nutritional compartments. Gastroenterology 1994; 106:1611–1617.

67. Aranda-Michel J. Nutrition in hepatic failure and liver transplantation. Curr Gastroenterol Rep 2001; 3:362–370.

68. Van de Venne WPHGC, Eersterterp KR, vanHook B, et al. Habitual pattern of food intake in patients with liver disease. Clin Nutr 1993; 12:293–297.

69. McCullough AJ, Teran JC, Bugianesi E. Guidelines for nutritional therapy in liver disease. In: Klein ES, ed. The American Society of Parenteral and Enteral Nutritional Support. Practice manual. Silver Spring MD: 1998:1–12.

70. Plauth M. Liver cirrhosis: Rationale and modalities for nutritional support – The European Society of Parenteral and Enteral Nutrition Consensus and beyond. Curr Opin Clin Nutr Metab Care 1999; 2:345–349.

71. Kondrup J, Müller MJ. Energy and protein requirements of patients with chronic liver disease. J Hepatol 1997; 27:239–247.

72. Nielsen K, Kondrup J, Martinsen L, et al. Long-term oral refeeding of patients with cirrhosis of the liver. Br J Nutr 1995; 74:557–567.

73. Solomen SM, Kirby DF. The refeeding syndrome: A review. J Parenter Enter Nutr 1990; 14:90–97.

74. Müller MJ, Rieger A, Willman O, et al. Metabolic responses to lipid infusion in patients with liver cirrhosis. Clin Nutr 1992; 11:193–206.

75. Crawford D. Recent advances in malnutrition and liver disease. What's New in Gastroenterology 1995; 48:1–4.

76. Phillips JR, Angulo P, Peterson T, et al. Fat-soluble vitamin levels in patients with primary biliary cirrhosis. Am J Gastroenterol 2001; 96:2745–2750.

77. Munoz SJ, Neubi JE, Balistreri WF. Vitamin E deficiency in primary biliary cirrhosis gastrointestinal malabsorption frequency and relation to other lipid soluble vitamins. Hepatology 1989; 9:525–531.

78. Sokol RJ. Fat soluble vitamins and their importance in patients with cholestatic liver diseases. Gastroenterol Clin N Amer 1994; 23:673–705.

79. Newsome PN, Beldon I, Moussa Y. Low serum retinol levels are associated with hepatocellular carcinoma in patients with chronic liver disease. Aliment Pharmacol Ther 2000; 14:1295–1301.

80. Moscarella S, Duchins A, Buzzelli G. Lipoperoxidation, trace elements and vitamin E in patients with liver cirrhosis. Eur J Gastroenterol Hepatol 1994; 6:633–636.

81. Mullen K, Denne SC, McCullough AJ, et al. Leucine metabolism in stable cirrhosis. Hepatology 1986; 6:622–630.

82. Chang WK, Chao YC, Tang HS, et al. Effects of carbohydrate supplementation in the late evening on energy expenditure and substrate oxidation in patients with liver cirrhosis. J Parenter Enter Nutr 1997; 21:96–97.

83. Swart GR, Zillikans MC, VonVoure JK. Effect of late evening snack on nitrogen balance in patients with cirrhosis of the liver. Br Med J 1989; 299:1202–1203.

84. Cordoba J, Lopez-Hellin J, Planas M, et al. Normal protein diet for episodic hepatic encephalopathy: results of a randomized study. J Hepatology 2004; 4:38–43.

85. Mullen KD, Dasarathy S. Protein restriction in hepatic encephalopathy: necessary evil or illogical dogma? J Hepatology 2004; 41:147–148.

86. Kearns PJ, Young H, Garcia G, et al. Accelerated improvement of alcoholic liver disease with enteral nutrition. Gastroenterology 1992; 102:200–205.

87. Morgan T, Moritz T, Mendenhall C, et al. Protein consumption and hepatic encephalopathy in alcoholic hepatitis. J Am Coll Nutr 1995; 14:152–158.

88. Uribe M, Marquez MA, Guillermo GR. Treatment of chronic portosystemic encephalopathy with vegetable and protein diets – a controlled cross over comparison. Dig Dis Sci 1982; 27:1109–1115.

89. Galati JS, Holderman KP, Dalrymple GV, et al. Delayed gastric emptying of both liquids and solid components of a meal in chronic liver disease. Am J Gastroenterol 1994; 89:708–712.

90. Reding P, Duchatean J, Bataille C. Oral zinc supplementation improves hepatic encephalopathy. Results of a randomized controlled trial. Lancet 1984; 2:493–494.

91. Riggio O, Ariosto F, Merli M. Short-term oral zinc supplementation does not improve chronic hepatic encephalopathy. Results of a double blind crossover trial. Dig Dis Sci 1991; 36:1204–1208.

92. Chawla R, Wolf DC, Kutner MH, et al. Cysteine may be an essential nutrient in malnourished patients with cirrhosis. Gastroenterology 1989; 97:1514–1520.

93. Halsted CH. Nutrition and alcoholic liver disease. Semin Liv Dis 2004; 24:289–304.

94. Cabré E, González-Huix F, Abad A, et al. Effect of total enteral nutrition on the short-term outcome of severely malnourished cirrhotics: a randomized controlled trial. Gastroenterology 1990; 99:715–720.

95. De Lédinghen V, Beau P, Mannant PR, et al. Early feeding or enteral nutrition in patients with cirrhosis after bleeding from esophageal varices? A randomized controlled study. Dig Dis Sci 1997; 42:536–541.

96. Mendenhall CL, Bongiovanni G, Goldberg SJ, et al. VA cooperative study on alcoholic hepatitis. III: Changes in protein-calorie malnutrition associated with 30 days of hospitalization with and without enteral nutritional therapy. J Parenter Enter Nutr 1985; 9:590–596.

97. Fulton S, McCullough AJ, Treatment of alcoholic hepatitis. Clin Liv Dis 1999; 2:799–819.

98. Cabré E, Rodriguez-Iglesias P, Caballeria J, et al. Short- and long-term outcome of severe alcohol-induced hepatitis treated with steroids or enteral nutrition. A multicenter randomized trial. Hepatology 2000; 32:36–42.

99. Bouneva I, Kirby DF. Management of nonalcoholic fatty liver disease: weight control. Clin Liver Dis 2004; 8:693–713.

100. Agrawal S, Bonkovsky HL. Management of nonalcoholic steatohepatitis. J Clin Gastroenterol 2002; 35:253–261.

101. Wang RT, Koretz RL, Yee HF. Is weight reduction an effective therapy for nonalcoholic fatty liver disease? A systemic review. Am J Med 2003; 115:554–559.

102. Dixon JB, Bhathal PS, Hughes NR, et al. Nonalcoholic fatty liver disease: improvement in liver histological analysis with weight loss. Hepatology 2000; 39:1647–1654.

103. Weimann A, Kuse ER, Bechstein WO, et al. Perioperative and enteral nutrition for patients undergoing orthotopic liver transplantation. Results of a questionnaire from 16 European transplant centers. Transpl Int 1998; 11(Suppl): S289–S296.

104. Pomposelli JJ, Burns DL. Nutrition support in the liver transplant patient. Nutr Clin Prac 2002; 17:341–349.

105. Patton KM, Aranda-Michel J. Nutritional aspects in liver disease and liver transplantation. Nutr Clin Prac 2002; 17:332–340.

106. Campos ACL, Matias JEF, Coelho JCU. Nutritional aspects of liver transplantation. Curr Opin Clin Nutr Metab Care 2002; 5:297–307.

107. Figueiredo F, Dickson ER, Pasha T, et al. Impact of nutritional status on outcomes after liver transplantation. Transplantation 2000; 70:1347–1352.

108. LeCornu KA, McKiernan FJ, Kapadia SA, et al. A prospective randomized study of preoperative nutritional supplementation in patients awaiting elective orthotopic liver transplantation. Transplantation 2000 ; 69:1364–1369.

109. Keogh JB, Tsalamandris C, Sewell RB, et al. Bone loss at the proximal femur and reduced lean mass following liver transplantation: a longitudinal study. Nutrition 1999; 15:661–664.

110. Luzi L, Perseghin G, Regalia E, et al. Metabolic effects of liver transplantation in acirrhotic patients. J Clin Invest 1997; 99:692–720.

111. Reich D, Rothstein K, Manzar Beira C, et al. Common medical disorders after liver transplantation. Semin Gastrointest Dis 1998; 9:110–125.

112. Everhart JE, Lambardero M, Lake JR, et al. Weight changes and obesity after liver transplantation: Incidence and risk factors. Liver Transpl Surg 1998; 4:285–298.

113. Correia MITD, Raego LO, Lima AS. Post-liver transplant obesity and diabetes. Curr Opin Clin Nutr Metab Care 2003; 6:457–460.

114. Keohane PP, Attrill H, Grimble G. Enteral nutrition in malnourished patients with hepatic cirrhosis and acute hepatic encephalopathy. J Parenter Enter Nutr 1983; 7:346–350.

115. Plauth M, Roske AE, Raomaniuk P, et al. Post-feeding hyperammonaemia in patients with transjugular intrahepatic portosystemic shunt and liver cirrhosis: role of small intestinal ammonia and route of nutrient administration. Gut 2000; 46:849–855.

116. Naveau S, Pelletier G, Poynard T. A randomized clinical trial of supplementary parenteral nutrition in jaundiced alcoholic cirrhotic patients. Hepatology 1986; 6:270–274.

Section
2 Two

Special considerations in dosing/ Considerations in special populations

CHAPTER SIX

6

Esophageal infections

Henry S. Fraimow and Robert S. Klein

OVERVIEW OF ESOPHAGEAL INFECTIONS IN THE IMMUNOCOMPROMISED HOST

Introduction

The management of infectious esophagitis has undergone a tremendous evolution since the early 1980s. Esophageal infections are no longer primarily premorbid or autopsy diagnoses. Now clinicians increasingly experienced with these syndromes can rely on improved diagnostic tools to evaluate the growing population of immunocompromised patients at risk for esophageal infections. In addition, the armamentarium of new, less toxic antifungal and antiviral agents available to treat the most common infectious processes continues to expand. Current management strategies must be designed to quickly, effectively, and cost-effectively manage these patients by appropriately integrating these recent advances in diagnosis and treatment.

Epidemiology: populations at risk for esophageal infections

Symptomatic infectious esophagitis is rare in the otherwise healthy population, although both herpes simplex and *Candida* esophagitis can occasionally present in apparently normal hosts.[1-3] Most patients with esophageal infections have one or more underlying alterations in host defense systems, but the type and severity of host defect may differ for specific infectious syndromes. Susceptibility to infection may be secondary to intrinsic or acquired defects in humoral immunity, cell-mediated immunity, or granulocyte number and function. Risk factors also include processes that disrupt host mucosal defenses by direct mechanical irritation or by eliminating the protective barrier of the normal host microbial flora.[4-6]

In general, the risk of esophageal infection increases with the severity of alteration in immune function. The single most important underlying predisposition for severe esophageal infections in the US is infection with HIV. There were over 900 000 HIV-infected individuals in the United States in 2002, including 42 000 newly diagnosed AIDS cases and 380 000 persons living with AIDS.[7] Worldwide, there are estimated to be 38 million HIV-infected individuals.[8] Prior to the recent advances in antiretroviral therapy, one-third of HIV-infected patients would develop esophageal symptoms at some time during their illness.[9-11] The use of highly active antiretroviral therapy has resulted in dramatic decreases in mortality among patients with HIV infection, as well as decreases in the rate of specific opportunistic infectious complications, such as *Candida* esophagitis and cytomegalovirus disease.[12,13] However, there remain large numbers of undiagnosed and inadequately treated individuals with HIV disease at ongoing risk for esophageal infections. Other populations at highest risk for esophageal infections include bone marrow and solid organ transplant patients and patients with neutropenia secondary to cytotoxic therapy.[14,15]

Presentation of esophageal infections

Presenting symptoms of infectious esophagitis most commonly include odynophagia, dysphagia, or retrosternal pain, although these symptoms are not specific for infection. Symptom onset may be either acute or subacute and may be associated with significant weight loss and dehydration secondary to the inability to eat or drink. Other important but less common symptoms may include fever, nausea and vomiting, and hematemesis. Oral pathology, such as oropharyngeal candidiasis, perioral herpes, or oral aphthous ulcer, can occur coincident with esophageal involvement and may provide clues to the diagnosis. Some esophageal infections, especially candidiasis, can also be completely asymptomatic and diagnosed only as incidental findings on endoscopic evaluation.[16-18]

DIAGNOSTIC CONSIDERATIONS FOR SPECIFIC ESOPHAGEAL INFECTIONS

Differential diagnosis and diagnostic methods

A wide variety of pathogens, including viral, fungal, bacterial, mycobacterial, and even protozoal organisms, have been reported to cause infectious esophagitis in healthy and immunocompromised patients. Overall, the vast majority of esophageal infections are caused by *Candida* species, cytomegalovirus, and herpes simplex virus, although the relative importance of each of these varies in different at-risk populations. Idiopathic HIV-associated esophageal ulcers are also an important diagnostic consideration in the HIV-infected population. Less common infections include primarily opportunistic infections, such as bacterial esophagitis and aspergillosis, as well as extremely unusual manifestations of relatively common infections such as *Mycobacterium tuberculosis* and histoplasmosis. The most important as well as less common agents causing infectious esophagitis are listed in Table 6.1. The

Table 6.1 Common and less common causes of esophageal infection

Common	Less common	Uncommon
Candida albicans	Non-*albicans Candida*	Histoplasmosis
Cytomegalovirus	species	Blastomycosis
Herpes simplex	*Mycobacterium*	Zygomyces
virus	*tuberculosis*	Cryptococcus
Idiopathic	Miscellaneous	Epstein-Barr virus
HIV-associated	bacterial species	Papillomavirus
esophageal	Aspergillosis	Cryptosporidiosis
ulcers	Varicella-zoster	Leishmaniasis
	virus	*Pneumocystis carinii*
		Bacillary
		angiomatosis

important clinical features of the most common syndromes discussed below are shown in Table 6.2.

The primary modality for evaluation of esophageal symptoms and diagnosis of esophageal infections in immunosuppressed populations is endoscopy. Endoscopy allows for both direct visualization of the esophageal mucosa and collection of appropriate microbiologic and histologic specimens for establishing specific etiologic diagnosis (see Table 6.2). Endoscopy is also the optimal method for excluding noninfectious diagnoses. Radiographic studies lack sensitivity and specificity, especially in patients with dual infections.[11] Barium studies may still have an occasional role for evaluation in patients too ill to undergo endoscopy or with specific contraindications for endoscopic procedures, such as severe coagulopathy. Radiographic studies may also be helpful for evaluating for motility disturbances and for evaluation and follow-up of specific complications of infection, such as an esophageal fistula. In some populations, such as HIV-infected patients with mild to moderate symptoms, an empiric therapeutic trial of antifungal therapy may also be an appropriate initial diagnostic and therapeutic strategy. Blood cultures, serologic studies, and skin testing may be helpful as adjunctive testing for specific infectious syndromes, but these tests will not eliminate the need for an endoscopic evaluation.

Candida esophagitis

Candida esophagitis remains the single most common cause of esophageal infection in immunosuppressed and debilitated patients, as well as occasionally causing disease in those with minor or no apparent immune deficiencies.[2,4–6] In studies done prior to availability of azole antifungal agents, *Candida* esophagitis was found in 1–8% of unselected patients undergoing upper endoscopy, was diagnosed either antemortem or on autopsy in 5% of patients in cancer hospitals, and was found in up to 20% of severely ill patients with hematologic malignancies on cytotoxic therapy.[2,16,17,19] *Candida* esophagitis remains a common presenting illness in HIV-infected patients and is the AIDS-defining illness in up to 15% of these patients.[9–11] The risk of both oropharyngeal and esophageal candidiasis during HIV infection is related to the level of immune function and stage of

Table 6.2 Characteristics of the most common esophageal infections

Infection	Associated signs and symptoms*	Radiographic findings	Endoscopic findings	Additional diagnostic studies
Candida	Oral thrush	Plaques, cobblestones, ulcerations, 'shaggy esophagus'	Plaques, pseudomembranes, friability	Fungal smears, brush cytology, biopsy with histopathology
Herpes simplex	Oral ulcers, nausea & vomiting, hemorrhage	Linear ulcers, plaques, 'shaggy esophagus' focal ulcerations, normal mucosa	Vesicles, bullae, discrete ulcers, plaques	Viral culture, biopsy with histopathology
Cytomegalovirus	Fever, weight loss, diarrhea		Ulcers on normal mucosa, giant ulcers, diffuse erythema	Biopsy with histopathology
HIV-associated ulcers	Weight loss, oral ulcers	Discrete ulcers in mid or distal esophagus	Single or multiple ulcers on normal mucosa	Biopsy with histopathology (to exclude other pathogens)
Bacteria	Fever, bacteremia	Plaques, ulcers, 'shaggy esophagus'	Single or multiple ulcers on normal mucosa	Biopsy with histopathology, bacterial culture
Tuberculosis	Fever, weight loss, respiratory symptoms	Ulcerations, strictures, masses, sinus tracts	Friable mucosal masses, ulcers, erythema	Biopsy with histopathology, acid fast stains, mycobacterial culture, PPD skin test

* Odynophagia, dysphagia and retrosternal pain seen in all infections.

illness; most cases of *Candida* esophagitis occur with CD4 counts of less than 150 cells/mm[3].[20] *Candida* is a commensal colonizer of the oropharynx and gastrointestinal tract of healthy individuals; disease is related to factors that increase density of *Candida* colonization, such as antimicrobial usage[5] and esophageal stasis, as well as to host defects that predispose to mucosal invasion, such as systemic or inhaled corticosteroids,[21,22] cytotoxic therapy, neutropenia, diabetes mellitus, and HIV infection.[4] Infection is most commonly caused by *Candida albicans*, although other species including the more azole resistant *C. glabrata* and *C. krusei* are occasionally seen.[19,23]

Patients with *Candida* esophagitis present most commonly with complaints of odynophagia with or without associated dysphagia; other symptoms may include retrosternal pain, anorexia, and weight loss. Asymptomatic disease found incidentally at endoscopy or autopsy is reported in up to 40% of cases.[16–18] Oral candidiasis is found in over 80% of untreated patients with esophageal candidiasis,[18,24] but is also commonly seen in patients with other esophageal infections. Fever is rare in the absence of neutropenia or associated disseminated candidiasis, and significant gastrointestinal bleeding is also uncommon. Rarely, patients will present with a severe local complication of *Candida* esophagitis such as esophageal stricture,[25] esophageal necrosis with perforation and fistula formation,[26] or even complete esophageal obstruction.[27] Radiographic features suggestive of early *Candida* infection on double-contrast barium esophagram include plaquelike defects, thickened folds, cobblestoning and mucosal ulcerations. Later findings may include the irregularly contoured 'shaggy esophagus' and long linear ulcers or 'railroad tracks,' found diffusely throughout the esophagus. The sensitivity of barium studies for the diagnosis of *Candida* esophagitis is reported from 65% to as high as 90%,[28,29] but the findings may be difficult to distinguish from those due to viral esophagitis, especially herpes simplex.[30]

The gold standard for diagnosis remains upper GI endoscopy with cytologic or histopathologic studies.[2,4,31] Visual inspection will reveal yellow or white raised plaques or pseudomembranes overlying friable esophageal mucosa, often with associated ulcerations or thickened folds, most commonly in the mid or distal esophagus.[2] With more severe disease, plaques coalesce circumferentially and can impinge on the lumen of the esophagus.[32] A standard grading system for endoscopic findings of *Candida* infection has been proposed.[2] Endoscopic findings are characteristic, but are not pathognomonic, for candidal infection,[10,33,34] and confirmation of the diagnosis requires biopsy, brushings, or fungal smears. Culture results alone may be misleading, as these will not distinguish colonization from invasive disease. Biopsies from involved areas should be stained with routine histopathologic stains as well as silver, periodic acid-Shiff, or Gram stains. Biopsies are more likely to be diagnostic with invasive disease, and specimens from clinically uninvolved areas have a very low diagnostic yield. Brush cytology specimens stained with silver or PAP stains are reported to have a higher yield than biopsy specimens when the techniques have been directly compared, but the two techniques are complementary.[2,32,35] Diagnostic specimens can also be obtained with blind brush cytology of the esophagus without formal endoscopy, although the role of this less invasive and inexpensive procedure has not been completely defined.[36,37] Currently available noninvasive tests such as serologic studies or candidal blood cultures contribute little to the

diagnosis of *Candida* esophagitis in the absence of disseminated disease.

Herpes simplex esophagitis

Herpes simplex (HSV) esophagitis is most commonly described in immunocompromised patients, although numerous cases in otherwise healthy children and adults have been reported.[1,3] Most esophageal disease is caused by HSV type 1, which also causes the majority of oropharyngeal herpes infections. Esophageal involvement occurs either as a severe complication of primary HSV infection, especially in previously healthy individuals, as a local manifestation of reactivation disease, or in the setting of disseminated HSV. Herpes virus that is reactivated in latently infected nerve ganglion cells frequently produces oropharyngeal infection and shedding of virus into the esophagus, but esophageal disease remains rare. Risks for esophageal disease include conditions associated with alterations in cell mediated immunity such as steroid treatment, chemotherapy, radiation, severe burns, and generalized debilitation; granulocytopenia appears to be less important.[34,38] Other risks include direct trauma to the nerve root ganglia and devices, such as nasogastric tubes, that disrupt normal mucosal barriers.[39] In HIV-infected patients, herpes is second only to cytomegalovirus as a viral cause of esophagitis and is the most common viral esophageal infection in solid organ and bone marrow transplants.[10,11,14,15,33]

Patients with herpes esophagitis generally present with odynophagia, dysphagia, and retrosternal pain.[3,38,40] Most esophageal infections occur in the absence of visible oral lesions, although perioral vesicles or ulcers may be an important diagnostic clue.[15,24,40] Non-specific presentations such as nausea and vomiting or unexplained gastrointestinal hemorrhage may occur without other symptoms, and occasional episodes are asymptomatic and diagnosed incidentally.[15,38,40] Fever is uncommon except when esophagitis occurs during primary HSV gingivostomatitis.[3] The most common complication of herpes esophagitis is bleeding, which may be mild or massive and is reported in up to one-third of cases.[38,41] Rare complications include perforation, stricture formation, and tracheoesophageal fistula.[3,42]

Barium studies lack sensitivity for diagnosing early herpetic infection and lack specificity later in the disease.[30,31,34] Studies during early infection may show multiple shallow ulcerations. Later findings include nodular plaques as well as ulcers, most commonly in the distal esophagus, and may mimic findings in candidal infection. The endoscopic appearance of HSV may also frequently be non-specific.[3,15,40,43] Only a few patients will have discrete vesicles in the mid or distal esophagus that are highly diagnostic of HSV. More common findings are superficial ulcers with or without yellowish exudate, seen in up to two-thirds of cases, or plaquelike lesions with erythematous and friable mucosa.[3,38,40,43] Giant ulcers are rarely seen. Diagnosis is confirmed by both histopathology and viral culture. Histopathology is diagnostic in at least 70–80% of cases.[3,38] Biopsy specimens from the ulcer margins are most likely to show the characteristic changes of multinucleated giant cells, cellular 'ballooning' and the presence of eosinophilic intranuclear inclusions.[44] The yield on cytologic brushings may be comparable to that of biopsy, and recovery with both brushings and biopsy can be increased with immunohistochemical stains and hybridization probes specific for

HSV.[38,44] Culture for HSV is considered diagnostic, and in several series had a yield as high as 85–90%.[3,38,40] However, recovery from culture decreases markedly in patients already on appropriate antiviral therapy.

Cytomegalovirus infections

Esophageal infections due to cytomegalovirus (CMV) are generally limited to patients with more severe immunodeficiencies, including advanced HIV disease and transplant recipients, especially bone marrow transplant recipients.[15,46] Evidence of CMV is found in 10–40% of endoscopic biopsies of esophageal lesions in HIV-infected patients and is second to only *Candida* as a cause of esophageal symptoms in this population.[10,33,47] Risk is predominantly in those with CD4 counts of less than 50–100 cells/mm^3.[20] In one study in bone marrow transplant patients, CMV was the most common esophageal infection diagnosed.[15] Like HSV, CMV is a ubiquitous DNA virus that can establish life-long latency after primary infection. Fifty to seventy percent of the adult population has serologic evidence of past CMV infection, with even higher rates in populations also at increased risk for HIV infection. Most CMV disease in AIDS patients is due to reactivation and subsequent hematogenous dissemination of the virus. Disease in transplant patients can occur either from reactivation or from progressive primary infection.

Patients with CMV esophagitis present similarly to those with *Candida* and herpes infections, with odynophagia, dysphagia, and retrosternal pain.[15,33,46] Presentation may be more subacute than that of HSV. As esophageal infection occurs in the setting of systemic viral dissemination, systemic constitutional symptoms of fever and weight loss are common, as are symptoms of involvement of other portions of the GI tract including diarrhea, nausea, and epigastric pain.[4,46] Local complications of CMV infection occur infrequently. Radiographic findings can include superficial mucosal erosions, irregular ulcerations or mucosal thickening, or solitary or a few deep ulcerations in otherwise normal-appearing mucosa.[48] Endoscopy most commonly reveals larger than 1 cm shallow or deep ulcerations, often with heaped-up margins, surrounded by normal-appearing mucosa and occurring predominantly in the mid to distal esophagus; some patients will have diffuse erythema and friability of the entire esophagus.[15,49] The diagnosis of CMV infection often requires multiple deep biopsies from both the ulcer base and edge to find the actively infected fibroblasts predominantly in the submucosal layer that will demonstrate viral inclusions.[50,51] In one recent study of CMV esophageal ulcers in AIDS patients, the diagnosis was established in 80% of confirmed cases with three biopsies, but the others required up to ten biopsy specimens.[50] Immunohistochemical stains may increase the yield of histopathologic specimens.[51,52] A culture positive for CMV without histopathology may lack both sensitivity[52] and specificity for diagnosis of CMV esophageal infection, as shedding of CMV virus occurs in the absence of clinical disease. Brush cytology appears to add little to biopsy for the diagnosis of CMV ulcers.[52]

HIV-associated esophageal ulcers

One infectious syndrome unique to HIV-infected patients is the syndrome of 'idiopathic' or HIV-associated esophageal ulcers. This syndrome was not initially recognized as a discrete clinical entity in HIV-infected patients, but is now reported to be as prevalent as CMV and far more common than HSV as a cause of esophageal ulcers in AIDS patients.[52–54] The pathogenesis of this syndrome remains unknown. Patients with acute HIV infection may have transient, shallow esophageal ulcerations found at endoscopy, but these ulcers appear to represent a different process than the characteristic HIV-associated ulcers found in patients with advanced HIV infection and low CD4 cell counts.[55] HIV viral RNA and other markers of active HIV infection have been found in ulcer biopsy samples, but these same markers may also be found in other biopsy specimens from clinically uninvolved areas.[53,56,57] Patients generally present with subacute onset of severe odynophagia and dysphagia and often with weight loss from inability to eat. Oropharyngeal aphthous ulcerations can occasionally be seen concurrently with esophageal ulcerations.[24] Radiographic studies and endoscopy demonstrate one or multiple moderate to large ulcers in the mid to distal esophagus, surrounded by otherwise normal-appearing esophageal mucosa.[53,58] The diagnosis is made presumptively by the inability to find evidence of other pathogens, especially CMV, in histopathologic specimens from characteristic ulcerated lesions[9,31,52]

Tuberculous esophagitis

Tuberculous esophagitis is uncommon, but is well described in numerous case reports in both immunocompetent and immunocompromised individuals.[59,60] Although the annual incidence of tuberculosis in the United States in 2002 declined to a historically low level, this infection remains a major problem worldwide, and latent tuberculosis infection in immigrants has become a major source of disease in industrialized nations.[61] The esophagus is the gastrointestinal organ least likely to be infected by tuberculosis. Disease may be due to direct extension from contiguous infected mediastinal or cervical lymph nodes or pulmonary foci, via infection of pre-existing esophageal lesions by swallowed mycobacterial organisms, or by hematogenous spread. Active pulmonary disease or visible hilar lymphadenopathy is seen on chest X-ray in only one-third of cases, although PPD reactivity is common among nonimmunocompromised patients with esophageal tuberculosis.[59] HIV infection as well as other immunosuppressive illnesses and therapies increase the risk of reactivation of latent infection and may also increase the frequency of atypical presentations of tuberculosis such as mediastinal lymphadenopathy that could predispose to esophageal involvement. Esophageal tuberculosis can present with typical symptoms of tuberculosis, such as fever, night sweats, and weight loss, or with localized symptoms of retrosternal pain and dysphagia, or even symptoms of esophageal obstruction. Late, potentially catastrophic complications can include fistulization to the bronchus, trachea, or vascular structures.[59,60,62] Radiographic findings are non-specific and may suggest malignancy. Diagnosis is made by findings of typical caseating granulomas on biopsy specimens. Tissue AFB stains are often negative, but cultures are usually positive and are helpful for targeting specific drug therapy in this era of increasing resistance to antituberculous agents.

Bacterial esophagitis

Bacterial esophagitis is uncommon and found primarily in severely immunocompromised, neutropenic patients such as those undergoing bone marrow transplant or aggressive cytotoxic chemotherapy.[63,64] Most cases have been diagnosed at autopsy. Whether bacteria are the primary pathogens or are superinfectors in these settings is not always clear. Patients present with symptoms indistinguishable from other forms of esophageal infection, and endoscopic findings include diffuse esophageal inflammation, pseudomembranes, and even ulcers. Histopathologic findings show evidence of deep bacterial invasion of the mucosal layers without evidence of other pathogens.[63] Many different bacterial organisms have been implicated, although most infections appear to be due to Gram-positive pathogens. Hematogenous spread of infection is common, especially in neutropenic patients.

Other pathogens

A wide variety of other pathogens have been reported to cause esophageal infection in immunocompromised patients, including those with and without HIV infection. Many but not all of these pathogens are listed in Table 6.1. In addition to various *Candida* species, other fungi that have been described include *Aspergillus*,[65] *Cryptococcus*,[66] *Penicillium*,[67] and the zygomycoses, such as mucormycoses.[68] Histoplasmosis and blastomycosis can also infrequently cause esophageal disease in immunosuppressed and immunocompetent patients from endemic areas.[69,70] Other viruses reported to cause symptomatic esophageal infection include varicella-zoster virus,[71] Epstein-Barr virus,[72] human herpes virus-6,[73] enteroviruses, and papovavirus. Lesions due to human papillomavirus have been also described, but these are most often asymptomatic.[74] Other rare causes of esophageal infection in AIDS patients include *Cryptosporidium*,[75] bacillary angiomatosis,[76] *Pneumocystis carinii*,[77] and leishmaniasis.[78] All of these infections are unusual, and would need to be diagnosed specifically by culture or specific histopathologic findings.

TREATMENT OF SPECIFIC ESOPHAGEAL INFECTIONS

Introduction

The treatment of the major causes of infectious esophagitis has been markedly improved in the past two decades by major advances in antifungal and antiviral chemotherapy. Advances in treatment of *Candida* infection include development of potent orally active azole and triazole antifungal agents, as well as the introduction of new classes of parenteral antifungals with significantly less toxicity than amphotericin B, the prior mainstay of parenteral antifungal treatment. There have also been major advances in oral and parenteral options for treatment of herpes viruses and cytomegalovirus. The introduction of new, potent antiretroviral agents and resulting immune reconstitution in HIV-infected individuals has been crucial for improving treatment outcome and preventing recurrences of many HIV-related infections. Factors influencing therapeutic choices from the expanding menu of available agents include severity of illness, presence or absence of associated disseminated disease outside of the esophagus, potential for drug toxicity or drug interactions, and the degree of host immunosuppression. Initial therapy may need to be modified in the face of clinical failure or documented microbiologic resistance to the treatment agent. Although rarely

indicated for routine management of infectious esophagitis, surgery may be required to manage the more severe complications of severe infection, such as fistulization, abscess formation, perforation, and fulminant necrosis.[79] For some immunocompromised patients with sepsis and fulminant necrotizing esophagitis from fungal, viral or bacterial pathogens, emergency esophagectomy may be life saving.[79]

Treatment of *Candida* esophagitis

Introduction

The various options currently available for treating *Candida* esophagitis are listed in Table 6.3. Choices now include topical agents such as nystatin, an expanding array of orally active azole and triazole antifungal agents, and systemic agents that include the various preparations of amphotericin B, as well as novel systemic agents such as caspofungin, the first echinocandin. All

Table 6.3 Treatment of *Candida* esophagitis

Initial therapy

Fluconazole 200 mg p.o. or i.v. daily × 3–4 weeks[a]
or
Itraconazole suspension 200 mg p.o. daily × 3–4 weeks[a]

Alternatives

Ketoconazole 200–400 mg p.o. daily × 3–4 weeks[a]
or
Amphotericin B 0.3 mg/kg i.v. daily × 10–14 days

Mild disease[b]

Nystatin 500 000–1 000 000 units p.o. q.i.d × 3–4 weeks[a]
or
Clotrimazole troches 1 p.o. q.i.d × 3–4 weeks[a]

Severe disease with systemic symptoms or associated neutropenia

Amphotericin B 0.7 mg/kg i.v. daily × 14 days
or
Caspfungin 70 mg i.v. × 1 then 50 mg i.v. daily × 14–21 days[a]

Disease clinically resistant to fluconazole 200 mg q.d.

Fluconazole 400–800 mg p.o. daily × 3–4 weeks[a]
or
Itraconazole oral solution 200–400 mg p.o. daily × 3–4 weeks[a]
or
Voriconazole 200 mg p.o. or i.v. b.i.d × 3–4 weeks[a]
or
Amphotericin B 0.3–0.7 mg/kg i.v. daily × 10–14 days
or
Caspfungin 70 mg × 1 then 50 mg i.v. daily × 14–21 days[a]

Primary prophylaxis[c]

Fluconazole 100 mg p.o. daily

Secondary prophylaxis[c]

Fluconazole 100–200 mg p.o. daily
or
Itraconazole suspension 100–200 mg p.o. daily

[a] Duration typically for 14–21 days after symptomatic improvement.
[b] Not recommended for HIV or moderate to severely immune deficient patients.
[c] See discussion for indication.

recently approved systemic antifungals, as well as those in late clinical development, have been evaluated for treatment of esophageal disease. With the recent emergence of resistance to first-generation oral azole agents, such as fluconazole, demonstration of effectiveness against refractory oropharyngeal and esophageal candidiasis is now a benchmark for the FDA approval of new antifungal agents.

Topical agents

Nystatin, an oral, nonabsorbable polyene antifungal agent, was the agent most commonly employed for the treatment of mild to moderate esophageal candidiasis prior to availability of azole agents and is still widely used for the topical treatment of oropharyngeal candidiasis.[80] Nystatin binds to sterols in the fungal cell membrane, resulting in altered cellular permeability. Other than a bitter taste and gastrointestinal intolerance, there is little significant toxicity associated with nystatin therapy. *Candida* can develop resistance to nystatin in vivo and in vitro.[81] Dosages of nystatin are from 500 000 to 1 000 000 units of oral suspension administered every 4–6 hours. Nystatin's lower efficacy than the newer azole agents and its lack of systemic activity makes it an especially poor option when esophageal disease is associated with deep local invasion or dissemination. Another topical option that has been used for treatment of oropharyngeal candidiasis and mild to moderate esophageal disease, especially in HIV-infected patients, is clotrimazole, a topical azole agent which inhibits fungal sterol synthesis.[82] Unlike newer azole agents such as fluconazole, clotrimazole is poorly absorbed and is rapidly inactivated in the liver, thus providing little systemic activity. Clotrimazole is available as well-tolerated oral troches. The use of oral miconazole has also been reported for the topical therapy of esophageal candidiasis, but experience is limited.[83] Another topical agent used for treatment of refractory or azole resistant oropharyngeal candidiasis in AIDS patients is amphotericin B oral suspension, a nonabsorbable formulation of the parenteral antifungal agent amphotericin B with little or no systemic toxicity.[84] There is little information on the effectiveness of amphotericin B suspension as primary therapy for esophageal candidiasis. A commercially marketed amphotericin B oral suspension is no longer readily available in the US, but some hospital pharmacies have formulated topical preparations using intravenous amphotericin B. In general, although topical agents may be effective in selected patients with mild esophageal candidiasis, most patients, especially immunocompromised patients, will require a systemically active agent for eradication of disease.

Azole agents

Introduction

The treatment of candidal infections has been revolutionized over the past decade by the availability of the new orally active azole and triazole agents. The general mechanism of action of imidazoles and the structurally slightly different triazoles is disruption of ergosterol synthesis in the fungal cell membrane by inhibiting the cytochrome P450-dependent enzyme lanosterol demethylase.[85] Available agents and those in late development differ in potency, oral bioavailability, toxicity profile, and effects on the human cytochrome P450 3A4 enzyme system and resultant potential for drug–drug interactions. There are also differences in the spectrum of activity against various candidal species and modes of resistance, which may have implications for the treatment of drug resistant infections.

Fluconazole

Fluconazole, first introduced in 1988, has become the most widely prescribed azole agent. It is an orally bioavailable, systemically active triazole with good to excellent in vitro activity against most *Candida* species and has approved indications for prophylaxis and treatment of a variety of both mucocutaneous and invasive fungal infections. Fluconazole is available for parenteral or oral administration and has excellent oral bioavailability in healthy individuals, achieving levels after oral administration of >90% of those achieved with parenteral dosing.[85] Fluconazole is a much less potent inducer of the cytochrome P450 system in humans than other azoles, resulting in fewer significant drug–drug interactions than other available agents in this class.[86] Toxicity can include nausea, headache and rash, and elevated liver enzymes; however, clinically significant hepatotoxicity is rare.[85] Unlike ketoconazole, oral absorption is also not affected by decreased gastric acidity.[87] Clinical and endoscopic response rates of *Candida* esophagitis to fluconazole in multiple clinical trails are typically at least 80–90%.[88–90]

With increasing usage of fluconazole in the inpatient and outpatient setting, one predictable consequence has been the emergence of in vitro and in vivo resistance to this and other azole agents.[23,91,92] Fluconazole-resistant candidal infections have been reported most commonly in HIV-infected patients on long-term fluconazole therapy.[23,92,93] Risks for resistance include lower CD4 counts and higher number of prior courses of fluconazole therapy and total prior fluconazole exposure. Primary fluconazole resistance can also occasionally be seen in isolates from patients with no prior azole exposures, including sexual partners of patients with resistant strains.[94] Resistance presents clinically as oropharyngeal or esophageal disease responding only to progressively larger doses of fluconazole of up to 800 mg daily, or disease that is nonresponsive after 14 days of therapy at any dose.[93] One mechanism of clinical resistance is superinfection with species of *Candida* intrinsically more resistant to fluconazole than *C. albicans*, particularly *C. glabrata* or *C. krusei*. In one large study, 9.3% of esophageal isolates from HIV-infected patients were *C. glabrata*.[90] Previously susceptible strains of *C. albicans* can also develop decreased fluconazole susceptibility.[92] Consensus methods for standardized in vitro antifungal susceptibility testing are published. Fluconazole susceptibility testing is now readily available from several reference laboratories, and in vitro results correlate well with clinical outcome of fluconazole therapy and with results of treatment in animal models.[95] Several basic mechanisms of resistance to azoles have been described, including active efflux of the drug and alterations in target pathways. Many isolates intermediately or highly resistant to fluconazole remain moderately susceptible to itraconazole in vitro, and up to two-thirds of cases of fluconazole-resistant candidal esophagitis may respond initially to itraconazole therapy.[96] Voriconazole is also active against many fluconazole-resistant *Candida*,[97] but resistance to voriconazole may emerge when treating fluconazole-resistant strains. Most azole-resistant isolates of *Candida albicans* remain very susceptible to amphotericin B and caspofungin.

Ketoconazole, itraconazole and voriconazole

The first oral azole agent to be approved was the imidazole ketoconazole. Ketoconazole has only modest oral bioavailability and lower overall potency than other azoles. At doses of

200–400 mg daily for 4 weeks, ketoconazole resulted in resolution of symptoms in 70–100% of patients with esophageal candidiasis.[88,98] In a clinical trial directly comparing fluconazole at doses of 100 mg/day to ketoconazole for treatment of esophageal candidiasis, therapeutic efficacy was nearly equivalent, but fluconazole was better tolerated.[88] Ketoconazole has several limiting toxicities, including nausea, vomiting, rash and, most significantly, drug-induced hepatitis, which occurs with a frequency of at least 1 in 10 000.[99] At higher doses, ketoconazole affects human steroid metabolism and can alter testosterone and corticosteroid levels. Ketoconazole is also a potent inhibitor of the hepatic cytochrome P450 3A4 enzyme system, resulting in numerous important drug–drug interactions, including interactions with antiepileptics, antituberculous agents, HIV protease inhibitors, cyclosporine, anticoagulants, sildenafil, certain benzodiazepenes, and certain antihistamines.[86] Effects on cyclosporine and protease inhibitors are particularly important in transplant and HIV-infected patients. Optimal oral absorption requires an acid gastric pH, which can be a major issue in patients on antisecretory agents or those with acquired achlorhydria, such as some AIDS patients.[100] Clinical resistance to ketoconazole was first seen shortly after its introduction.[101]

Another oral triazole in widespread clinical usage is itraconazole. The original capsule formulation of itraconazole has been available since the early 1990s.[102] Like fluconazole, itraconazole has good activity against many candidal species, but has increased activity against some other fungal species, notably *Histoplasma*, *Coccidioides immitis*, and the filamentous fungi including *Aspergillus*.[85] Itraconazole is also generally well tolerated but has a higher incidence of both hepatotoxicity and rash than fluconazole.[85] Itraconazole also has potential for numerous drug interactions through the hepatic cytochrome P450 3A4 system, as well as by effects on protein binding, though interactions are less of an issue than those seen with the structurally similar ketoconazole. The co-administration of itraconazole with terfenadine, astemizole, midazolam, triazolam, and certain statin agents is contraindicated.[102] Other important drug interactions include cyclosporine, digoxin, protease inhibitors, antituberculous drugs, antiepileptics, and oral hypoglycemics. Itraconazole should be taken with food for optimal absorption. Itraconazole capsules have demonstrated effectiveness in the treatment of *Candida* esophagitis.[103] In a large randomized study comparing itraconazole to fluconazole, each at 100 mg twice daily dosing, in over 2000 HIV infected patients with esophageal candidiasis, clinical and endoscopic cure rates were better at two weeks with fluconazole therapy. At the end of one year, however, identically high cure rates of 93% were seen in both groups.[90] A new itraconazole oral solution formulation was approved in 1997 specifically for the treatment of oral and esophageal candidiasis. In this formulation, itraconazole is dissolved in hydroxypropyl B-cyclodextrin, enhancing oral absorption of the drug and resulting in 30% higher plasma drug levels.[104] Itraconazole oral solution also achieves very high salivary levels in HIV infected patients.[104] In a study comparing itraconazole oral solution to fluconazole, both dosed at 100–200 mg daily for 3 to 8 weeks in HIV-infected patients with esophageal candidiasis, no significant differences in the clinically or endoscopically documented response rates were detected, and response rates to both were greater than 90%.[105] Rates of fungal eradication and adverse events in both groups were also similar.[105] A parenteral formulation of itraconazole has also recently been approved for the treatment of systemic candidal infections. Clinical failure of itraconazole has most often been attributed to pharmacokinetic factors, primarily impaired absorption, but true in vitro resistance to itraconazole can also develop.[106] In vitro susceptibility tests correlate with clinical results of itraconazole treatment.[106]

Voriconazole is the newest azole agent to be approved and is available in both oral and parenteral formulations. Voriconazole has similar mechanism of action as the other azoles but has enhanced activity against *Candida* and other fungi, including many fluconazole- and itraconazole-resistant *C. albicans* isolates, as well as the intrinsically more resistant *C. glabrata* and *C. krusei*.[85] In one large study, voriconazole was comparable to fluconazole in treatment of esophageal candidiasis, resulting in cure rates of over 95%, but adverse events, particularly visual disturbances and liver enzyme abnormalities, were more common with voriconazole.[107] Voriconazole has also been used successfully to cure or improve 10 of 12 patients with fluconazole-resistant *Candida* esophagitis[108] and has been used successfully to treat other fluconazole-resistant systemic non-*albicans* candidal infections. Use of voriconazole should be reserved for fluconazole-resistant disease.[109] Other azoles in late stages of development include posaconazole and ravuconazole, both of which appear comparable to fluconazole for treatment of esophageal candidiasis and may also be effective for fluconazole-resistant disease.[97,102]

Amphotericin B formulations

Parenterally administered amphotericin B has an established record as a highly effective, but toxic, treatment for a variety of serious candidal infections. Amphotericin B is a polyene agent with potent activity against fungal cell membranes and is fungicidal in vitro against most *Candida* species, unlike the azole agents.[110] The use of amphotericin is limited by the requirement for intravenous dosing and also by the well-documented toxicity of the drug. Short-term toxicities associated with amphotericin B infusion include fever, chills, headache, nausea, and vomiting, which can be minimized by pretreatment with combinations of antihistamines, meperidine, acetaminophen, non-steroidal agents, and hydrocortisone. More serious adverse effects include a predictable decrease in creatinine clearance that occurs in nearly all patients on this drug, electrolyte abnormalities, and bone marrow toxicity. The appropriate dose of amphotericin B depends on the clinical circumstance. For esophageal disease in the setting of disseminated candidal infection or in febrile neutropenic patients, doses range from 0.5 to 1 mg/kg/day, often given over weeks to months. However, a variety of low-dose short-term regimens, such as 0.3–0.5 mg/kg/day for 10 to 14 days, have been used to treat local esophageal disease refractory to other topical or oral agents.[109,111] Amphotericin is infused over several hours, and vigorous hydration may be beneficial in minimizing deleterious effects on renal function. In an effort to reduce the toxicity and increase the efficacy of amphotericin drug delivery, three new parenteral formulations of amphotericin B have been developed in which the drug is complexed to a lipid or colloid carrier.[110] These preparations appear to provide efficacy at least equivalent to standard amphotericin B with decreased incidence of nephrotoxicity, and are particularly advantageous for the treatment of infections in which high doses of amphotericin are required or in patients at increased risk for renal dysfunction. These products are also significantly more expensive than standard amphotericin B, and the advantages over standard amphotericin B may be less relevant for the lower-dose regimens used in treatment of localized azole-resistant esophageal candidiasis.

Caspofungin and other echinocandins

Echinocandins are a novel class of parenteral agents with broad-spectrum antifungal activity. Their mechanism of action is the inhibition of fungal cell wall beta (1-3) D-glucan synthesis.[112] Caspofungin, the first echinocandin to be approved, has excellent activity against nearly all *Candida* species, as well as activity against *Aspergillus*. In several comparative clinical trials for treatment of esophageal disease, primarily in HIV-infected patients, caspofungin at a dose of 50 or 70 mg/day for 7 to 21 days gave favorable clinical responses in from 67% to more than 90% of patients and was comparable to therapy with fluconazole or intravenous amphotericin B.[112–115] Caspofungin has also been used successfully to treat 71% of AIDS patients with fluconazole-resistant *Candida* esophagitis.[116] Other than the need for parenteral access, the drug is well tolerated. Toxicity includes phlebitis, headache and nausea, and laboratory abnormalities include increased liver enzymes.[112] Resistance to caspofungin can develop clinically and in vitro.[117] Other echinocandins in late clinical development that have been used in open-label studies to treat esophageal candidiasis include micafungin and anidulafungin, both of which appear to have activity comparable to caspofungin.[118]

5-Flucytosine

An older oral agent with in vitro activity against *Candida* is 5-flucytosine (5FC), an antimetabolite similar to the neoplastic agent 5-fluorouracil. Although occasionally effective as a single agent in treatment of *Candida* esophagitis,[119] its use is limited by the emergence of resistance and by toxicity, predominantly rash, diarrhea, and bone marrow suppression. Flucytosine may be useful in combination with either amphotericin B or azoles for refractory disease.[109]

Prevention of *Candida* esophagitis

The development of relatively nontoxic, easily administered agents, such as fluconazole and itraconazole, has stimulated interest in their use for prophylaxis against fungal infections. The relative benefits of prophylaxis in any setting must be measured both by demonstrated effectiveness and by cost, toxicity, and other adverse consequences, including the emergence of resistant strains. Several large studies have shown that oral fluconazole can prevent serious candidal infections in patients undergoing bone marrow and solid organ transplantation and in acute leukemia patients undergoing intensive cytotoxic chemotherapy, and many treatment protocols now incorporate oral azole agents as part of a standard prophylaxis regimen.[120] The risk of superinfection with azole-resistant candidal species such as *C. krusei* may be increased by fluconazole prophylaxis, but the risk of development of acquired fluconazole resistance in susceptible strains appears to be low with the use of prophylaxis in these

settings. Fluconazole prophylaxis has also been studied in other populations at high risk for disseminated candidiasis, such as intensive care unit patients on broad-spectrum antibiotics.[121] Much of the current focus on prophylaxis of mucosal fungal infections is directed at the HIV-infected population. The risk of opportunistic fungal infections increases with falling CD4 cell count, and strategies for primary prophylaxis have thus targeted the highest-risk populations, generally those with less than 200 CD4 cells/mm^3. The major endpoint assessed in initial trials of antifungal prophylaxis has been primary or secondary prevention of cryptococcal infection. The effect of prophylaxis on the development of esophageal candidiasis has also been studied, but this outcome has been considered less important. A delay in initiating treatment for *Candida* esophagitis until symptoms develop is of lesser consequence than a delayed diagnosis of cryptococcal disease. Routine use of fluconazole prophylaxis contributes to cost, increases risk of drug reactions and interactions, and increases potential for emergence of azole resistance in HIV-infected patients.[122] In one study of daily oral fluconazole at a dose of 200 mg/day compared to clotrimazole troches in HIV-infected patients with less than 50 CD4 cells/mm^3, patients on fluconazole prophylaxis showed a significant decrease in visceral fungal infections, including *Candida* esophagitis, but fluconazole prophylaxis was not associated with decreased mortality.[123] Intermittent fluconazole dosing regimens have also been studied as an alternative to daily regimens. Some regimens studied have been 100 mg daily during one of every three weeks and 200–400 mg administered once per week.[124–126] Patients on fluconazole one of every three weeks showed a reduction in cryptococcal disease and invasive candidal infections; however, the effect of this regimen on development of antifungal resistance was not specifically studied.[125] HIV-infected women on a once-weekly fluconazole regimen had a decreased incidence of vaginal and oropharyngeal disease without evidence of development of significant clinical antifungal drug resistance.[124] In a direct comparison of daily versus once a week therapy, 400 mg of fluconazole weekly was less effective than daily therapy in preventing oropharyngeal disease.[126] In the most recently published CDC, NIH and HIV Medicine Association/Infectious Diseases Society of America guidelines for management of opportunistic infections in HIV disease, the routine use of primary antifungal prophylaxis with fluconazole is not recommended.[122] Chronic secondary prophylaxis with either fluconazole at doses of 100–200 mg/day or itraconazole solution at a dose of 200 mg/ day may be appropriate for patients with multiple or severe recurrences of esophageal candidal infections.[122,127] Recent studies in HIV-infected patients comparing continuous fluconazole suppression of mucosal candidal disease to intermittent, symptom-directed treatment of candidiasis have found that patients on suppressive therapy had fewer relapses but may have a higher rate of microbiologic resistance that did not translate into more clinically resistant disease.[128,129]

Treatment of herpes simplex esophagitis

Introduction

Patients with normal immune function may recover from an acute episode of herpes simplex esophagitis without specific therapy, as will some immunocompromised patients.[1,3,45] However, the majority of immunocompromised patients require some form of antiviral therapy.[38,40] Most experience in treatment of herpes esophagitis has involved the use of acyclovir and related drugs, but other agents have also recently become available for the treatment of acyclovir-resistant herpes virus infections.

Acyclovir, famciclovir and valaciclovir

Acyclovir is an orally and parenterally available nucleotide analog that inhibits viral DNA synthesis and is active against a variety of herpes group viruses.[130] The major toxicity of acyclovir is acute renal insufficiency secondary to crystallization of the drug in the urinary tract, which usually is seen only with parenteral dosing and can be prevented with adequate hydration. Other toxicity includes occasional headache, encephalopathy, nausea, and rash[130] Dosing for acute herpes simplex infection is 5–10 mg/kg every 8 hours intravenously or 400 mg 3 to 5 times per day orally, given for 7 to 14 days. In a study of AIDS patients with herpes esophagitis, 70% had complete clinical responses at a mean of 9 days of treatment, with clinical improvement beginning as soon as 24 to 48 hours.[40] Fifteen percent of these patients subsequently relapsed and ultimately required prolonged suppressive therapy. The need for parenteral versus oral therapy for non-central nervous system herpes infections is determined by the severity of disease, underlying immune status, and the ability to take oral medications. Two newer oral agents with activity similar to acyclovir are valaciclovir and famciclovir.[131] Valaciclovir is an L-valyl ester of acyclovir that is well absorbed and subsequently metabolized to acyclovir. It has higher oral bioavailability than the relatively poorly absorbed acyclovir and can be dosed less frequently. Toxicity overall is similar to acyclovir, although there have been rare reports of thrombotic thrombocytopenic purpura-like syndromes in patients on long-term dosing.[132] Famciclovir is an agent similar to acyclovir that also has the advantage of less frequent dosing and may be more active in latently infected cells. Both famciclovir and valaciclovir have demonstrated safety and efficacy in suppressing relapses of HSV infections in HIV-infected individuals.[133,134] Dosing of these agents is shown in Table 6.4.

Treatment of acyclovir-resistant herpes simplex infections

There are numerous reports of acyclovir-resistant herpes simplex infections, especially in immunocompromised patients on intermittent or long-term therapy. In one report, the incidence of acyclovir-resistant herpes simplex infections in patients with late-stage AIDS was as high as 11–17%.[135] Resistance is most commonly due to thymidine kinase deficient viral strains.[136] Acyclovir-resistant mutants may be less hardy, and patients with resistant strains who subsequently relapse may have susceptible strains isolated from later episodes. Some acyclovir-resistant infections have responded to very large doses of parenteral acyclovir, such as 15 mg/kg every 8 hours. Acyclovir-resistant strains are also cross-resistant to famciclovir and valaciclovir, as well as ganciclovir, but are usually susceptible to the systemic antiviral agents foscarnet and cidofovir.[136] Topical antiviral agents have no role in treatment of herpes esophagitis.

Prevention of herpes virus infections

Various strategies for the prevention of herpes simplex infections have been incorporated into treatment protocols for patients undergoing intensive immunosuppressive regimens, such as bone

Table 6.4 Treatment of herpes esophagitis

Initial therapy

Severe disease/unable to tolerate oral Rx
Acyclovir 5–10 mg/kg i.v. q 8 hrs × 7–14 days

Mild to moderate disease
Acyclovir 400 mg p.o. 5 ×/day × 7–14 days
or
Famciclovir 500 mg p.o. tid × 7–14 days
or
Valaciclovir 500 mg p.o. bid × 7–14 days

Acyclovir-resistant disease
Foscarnet 60 mg/kg i.v. q 12 hrs × 2–3 weeks
or
Cidofovir 5 mg/kg i.v. q week × 2 weeks plus probenecid
(2 g p.o. prior to dose and 1 g p.o. 2 and 8 hrs post dose)
or
Acyclovir 12–15 mg/kg i.v. q 8 hrs × 2–3 weeks

Primary or secondary prophylaxis*

Acyclovir 200 mg p.o. t.i.d or 400 mg. p.o. b.i.d
or
Famciclovir 250–500 mg p.o. b.i.d
or
Valaciclovir 500 mg p.o. b.i.d.

* See discussion for indications.

marrow and solid organ transplantation.[137] These regimens most commonly use famciclovir or acyclovir for prophylaxis of HSV and varicella-zoster virus, but regimens that employ ganciclovir for the prevention of CMV disease would also be expected to provide prophylaxis for HSV. The utility of routine primary prophylaxis for HSV infections in HIV-infected patients is less clearly defined. Acute episodes of HSV and other herpes viruses are known to increase HIV viral activation, and some studies prior to availability of potent antiretroviral regimens suggested a survival benefit for HIV-infected patients receiving acyclovir therapy, even in the absence of a demonstrable effect on symptomatic outbreaks of herpes.[138] However, other studies have failed to confirm the benefit of chronic acyclovir in HIV-infected patients, and routine primary prophylaxis for HSV is accordingly not currently endorsed by the CDC guidelines.[122] Patients with frequent or particularly severe recurrences should receive secondary prophylaxis with an effective agent. Oral acyclovir at doses of 200 mg three times daily or 400 mg twice daily, famciclovir at doses of 250 mg or 500 mg twice daily, and valaciclovir at a dose of 500 mg twice daily have all been used for chronic suppressive therapy in HIV-infected patients.[122,133,134]

Treatment of cytomegalovirus infections

Introduction

The high incidence of visceral CMV disease and its morbidity and mortality in AIDS patients and transplant patients has spurred the development of several new CMV active antiviral agents. Strategies for the treatment of gastrointestinal CMV infection in HIV-infected individuals have been in part inferred from experience gained from treatment of the more commonly diagnosed syndrome of CMV retinitis. Significant clinical experience in treating CMV esophagitis in AIDS patients has also been amassed at several centers. The prognosis of CMV infections in AIDS patients is also significantly improved with the use of effective antiretroviral therapy.[54] The options for treatment of CMV esophagitis are shown in Table 6.5.

Initial therapy of CMV esophagitis

For the initial therapy of esophageal CMV infection, both ganciclovir and foscarnet appear to be very effective, and the choice between these agents is generally individualized and based on risk of drug-associated toxicities.[31,46,139,140] Ganciclovir is a nucleoside analog structurally similar to acyclovir but with enhanced activity against CMV. Induction regimens are 5 mg/kg intravenously every 12 hours, with dosage adjustments for

---

Table 6.5 Treatment of cytomegalovirus esophagitis

Initial therapy

Ganciclovir 5 mg/kg i.v. q 12 × 3–4 weeks
or
Valaganciclovir 900 mg p.o. bid x 3–4 weeks
or
Foscarnet 90 mg/kg i.v. q 12 or 60 mg /kg i.v. q 8 hrs × 3–4 weeks

Alternative

Cidofovir 5 mg/kg (plus probenicid) i.v. q week × 2 then q 2 weeks × 3–4 weeks

Relapsing or refractory disease

Switch to alternative agent above
or
Foscarnet 90 mg/kg i.v. q 12 hrs plus ganciclovir 5 mg/kg q 12 hrs × 2–3 weeks
or
Foscarnet 90 mg/kg i.v. q 12 hrs plus valganciclovir 900 mg p.o. b.i.d

Alternative

Cidofovir i.v. (plus probencid) plus either foscarnet or ganciclovir or valganciclovir at initial therapy doses

Primary prophylaxis[a]

Ganciclovir 1–1.5 grams p.o. t.i.d.
or
Valganciclovir 900 mg p.o. daily

Secondary prophylaxis/maintenance[a]

Valganciclovir 900 mg p.o. daily
or
Ganciclovir 5 mg/kg i.v. daily
or
Foscarnet 90 mg/kg i.v. daily
or
Cidofovir 5 mg/kg i.v. (plus probenicid) q 2 weeks
or
Ganciclovir 1–1.5 grams p.o. t.i.d.

Adjuvant therapy in HIV-infected patients

Combination antiretroviral therapy (HAART)

[a] See discussion for indications.

---

renal insufficiency. When indicated, maintenance regimens are 5 mg/kg daily. The primary toxicity of ganciclovir is marrow suppression, particularly neutropenia, which is especially common when ganciclovir is co-administered with zidovudine or cytotoxic chemotherapies.[139] Neutropenia can often be managed with the addition of granulocyte colony stimulating factors. Other less common toxicity includes rash, central nervous system effects, nausea, vomiting, and hepatitis. Oral ganciclovir has poor oral bioavailability and is not recommended for initial therapy, but has been used for maintenance therapy at doses of at least 1000 mg three times per day.[141] Valganciclovir, a new oral prodrug of ganciclovir with higher bioavailability than oral ganciclovir, has recently been approved for maintenance therapy for CMV retinitis, and has also been shown to be effective for induction therapy for CMV retinitis.[142,143] Although no studies specifically demonstrate efficacy of valganciclovir for treatment of CMV esophagitis, this agent is now being used in initial induction therapy for gastrointestinal CMV infections in patients able to tolerate oral therapy. Foscarnet is a parenteral viral DNA inhibitor that is active against CMV and other DNA viruses, including acyclovir-resistant strains of HSV. Response rates to foscarnet as initial therapy for retinal and gastrointestinal CMV disease in HIV-infected patients are similar to that of parenteral ganciclovir.[139,140,144] The initial dose of foscarnet is 90 mg/kg every 12 hours.[139] If required, maintenance therapy is 90–120 mg/kg daily, extrapolating from experience accrued in treatment of CMV retinitis.[139] The primary toxicity seen with foscarnet is nephrotoxicity. Most patients experience some decrease in creatinine clearance, and up to one-third will have a serum creatinine that rises to over 2 mg/dL.[145] Patients should be well hydrated, and infusions should be given over at least 2 hours. Serum creatinine should be monitored at least twice weekly, and foscarnet should be discontinued if there is significant deterioration in renal function. Other toxicity includes electrolyte disturbances, gastrointestinal symptoms, headache, paraesthesias, and rash. Unlike ganciclovir, significant hematologic toxicity is rare. Foscarnet also has modest antiretroviral activity, which may be clinically relevant in the outcome of some AIDS patients with CMV disease.[146] The optimal duration of induction therapy for esophageal disease with either ganciclovir or foscarnet has not been determined, but initial therapy is recommended for a minimum of three weeks.[31,46,139] Approximately 80% of patients have a partial or complete response to 2–3 weeks of therapy with ganciclovir or 3–4 weeks of therapy with foscarnet.[46,139,144] In HIV-infected patients, effective CMV therapy also includes optimization of antiretroviral therapy.[54] CMV ulcers may on rare occasion resolve spontaneously in patients on potent HIV therapy without the use of specific CMV agents.[147]

Salvage therapies

In patients who fail to respond to initial therapy with one agent, the options include changing to the alternate agent or dual therapy with a combination of either parenteral ganciclovir or oral valganciclovir and foscarnet. Dual therapy is superior to switching therapy in the treatment of relapsing CMV retinitis in AIDS patients.[139] Clinical failures may be related to pharmacokinetic issues in drug delivery or to the development of resistant strains of virus. Ganciclovir-resistant strains of CMV have emerged frequently in patients on prophylactic or therapeutic anti-CMV regimens.[148] Ninety percent of resistance is caused by mutations in the CMV UL97 phosphotransferase gene, but mutations in the viral polymerase gene are seen.[148] Foscarnet resistant isolates have also been observed. For patients unable to tolerate either ganciclovir or foscarnet, or failing therapy with these agents, another parenteral drug approved for treatment of CMV infections is cidofovir, a novel nucleotide analog that potently inhibits CMV and herpes virus replication.[149] Cidofovir has the advantage of only once-weekly induction therapy for 2 weeks and then every other week maintenance therapy, simplifying long-term intravenous access requirements.[139] Like foscarnet, the major toxicity of cidofovir is nephrotoxicity, which may be irreversible. Vigorous hydration is essential, and probenecid must be administered before and after infusion to prevent excretion of drug and to achieve adequate systemic drug levels. Cidofovir has been used as monotherapy or in combination with either ganciclovir or foscarnet, although most experience has been in the treatment of retinitis, especially in patients failing or intolerant of other regimens.[139] Resistance to cidofovir develops due to mutations in viral polymerase, and such isolates are also resistant to ganciclovir.[149]

Maintenance therapy for CMV in HIV disease

Unlike experience with retinitis, where lifelong maintenance therapy has been essential to prevent relapse in patients with persistently low CD4 counts, in studies done during the pre-HAART era only 50% of AIDS patients with esophageal disease relapsed after a successful initial course of treatment.[46,139] The risk of relapse of CMV esophageal disease is even lower if CMV therapy is combined with effective antiretroviral therapy.[54] Routine maintenance therapy after an episode of gastrointestinal CMV disease is not recommended in the CPC guidelines.[122] Most experience has been with intravenous ganciclovir at doses of 5 mg/kg daily or foscarnet at doses of 90–120 mg/kg daily.[139] Oral ganciclovir at a total dose of 3–4.5 g/day has been approved and used for maintenance therapy of CMV retinitis, but oral valganciclovir at a dose of 900 mg daily has become the preferred regimen,[122,141,143] and parenteral cidofovir every 2 weeks may represent another alternative.[139] All patients with a subsequent relapse of gastrointestinal disease will require long-term maintenance therapy after acute treatment of their relapse. The role of effective antiretroviral therapy and immune reconstitution on control of CMV disease cannot be underestimated.[147,150] Current guidelines recommend discontinuing chronic maintenance therapy for CMV in asymptomatic patients whose CD4 counts are greater than 100–150 CD4 cells/mm[3] for greater than 6 months, but reinstituting maintenance therapy again if the CD4 count subsequently falls.[122]

Primary prophylaxis for CMV disease

Most CMV disease in immunosuppressed populations is due to reactivation disease. For the minority of immunocompromised patients who are still CMV seronegative, efforts should be made to limit the exposure to CMV-infected body fluids and blood products. Prophylaxis of CMV disease has been extensively studied in clinical trials in solid organ and bone marrow transplant populations. Trials have addressed both therapy for CMV seronegative patients receiving CMV-positive tissues and therapy for the prevention of reactivation disease in patients who are already latently infected. Several regimens have been employed, including acyclovir, valaciclovir, ganciclovir, or oral valganciclovir with or without anti-CMV immune globulin.[151–153] Ganciclovir appears to be more effective than acyclovir, but its use is limited by a high incidence of bone marrow toxicity, particularly in bone marrow transplants.[153] There has been an increase in use of 'preemptive therapy' in targeted patients at highest risk of disease reactivation, rather than routine prophylaxis for all transplant recipients.[151] Quantitative PCR for CMV DNA and the detection of CMV pp65 antigen in serum may help predict patients at higher risk for clinical CMV disease and can also be used to monitor treatment efficacy.[151] The incidence of CMV disease in HIV-infected patients increases with a decrease in the CD4 count, especially below 50 cells/mm[3].[20] Acyclovir prophylaxis showed no effect on the incidence of CMV disease in this population.[138] One trial showed an unexpected increase in mortality in patients receiving oral valaciclovir prophylaxis, and this agent is thus currently not recommended.[132] Oral ganciclovir at a dose of 3 or more grams per day was shown to decrease the incidence of CMV infection in advanced HIV patients; however, no demonstrable effect on overall mortality was detected,[154] and the cost of this intervention is significant. Routine primary prophylaxis for CMV infection is not currently recommended.[122] As in transplant patients, a high quantitative CMV viral load in advanced HIV patients is a marker for higher risk for end-organ CMV disease, and such patients may be candidates for targeted prophylaxis.[155] Effective antiretroviral therapy for HIV can clear CMV viremia in HIV-infected patients without specific anti-CMV therapy.[150]

Therapy of HIV-associated esophageal ulcers

The optimal management of HIV-associated esophageal ulcers not demonstrated to be caused by other infectious pathogens remains a therapeutic challenge (Table 6.6).[31] There are case reports of response of these ulcers to topical steroid preparations, but effective delivery of topical agents to esophageal lesions is problematic. In one report, four patients treated with a slurry of dexamethasone and sulfacrate four times daily had a good clinical response.[156] Most experience thus far has been with the use of systemic corticosteroids, most commonly prednisone.[53,157,158] Prednisone at initial doses of 40 mg/day followed by a slow taper of 10 mg/day per week resulted in clinical and endoscopic responses in 33 of 35 patients.[157] Some patients may require higher doses of up to 60–80 mg of prednisone per day.[158] Symptoms may recur as steroids are tapered, and long-term prednisone therapy may increase the risk for other opportunistic infections, such as CMV infection.[159] Patients with idiopathic HIV-associated ulcers also often have oropharyngeal candidiasis and may benefit from concurrent antifungal therapy, especially while receiving corticosteroids. Patients may also benefit from anti-reflux therapy.[31] A new option for treatment of idiopathic HIV-associated ulcers is thalidomide. Thalidomide, long unavailable in the US due to toxicity concerns, is a potent inhibitor of tumor necrosis factor that is now being re-evaluated for the treatment of a wide variety of infectious, immunologic, and neoplastic conditions. In several clinical trials, thalidomide has been shown to have activity against both oral and esophageal HIV-associated ulcers at doses of 100–400 mg/day for 4 weeks.[160,161] In one randomized, placebo-controlled study of esophageal ulcers treated with 200 mg/day of thalidomide, 8 of 11 patients had complete resolution of ulcers at 4 weeks.[160] In addition to the well-known teratogenic effects of this drug, other toxicities

Table 6.6 Treatment of HIV-associated ulcers

Initial therapy
Prednisone 40 mg/day, taper by 10 mg/day per week or Thalidomide 200 mg p.o./day × 4 weeks

Refractory ulcers
Prednisone 60–80 mg/day, taper by 10 mg/day per week or Thalidomide up to 400 mg p.o./day × 4 weeks

Adjuvant therapy
Fluconazole 200 mg p.o./day Omeprazole 20–40 mg p.o./day (or alternative antireflux agents) Combination antiretroviral therapy (HAART)

limiting the use of thalidomide include sedation, rash, and peripheral neuropathy. Thalidomide at a lower dose of 100 mg three times per week was not effective in preventing recurrent HIV-associated esophageal ulcers,[162] and thalidomide may increase serum HIV RNA levels. Thus, the drug should only be used for the acute therapy of active ulcers. As with other HIV-associated esophageal processes, aggressive treatment of underlying HIV viral infection is important in hastening resolution and preventing relapses of esophageal ulcerations.[54]

Other esophageal infections

Management of other, less common esophageal infections is directed at the specific pathogens involved. Treatment of bacterial esophagitis in the setting of neutropenia includes broad-spectrum antimicrobial therapy directed against Gram-positive and Gram-negative organisms. Culture and susceptibility testing are critical for selecting more specific therapy and for identifying drug-resistant organisms. The initial therapy of tuberculous esophagitis in the era of increased mycobacterial drug resistance includes the initiation of multidrug therapy, usually a four-drug regimen consisting of isoniazid, rifampin, ethambutol, and pyrazinamide.[163] Therapy should be revised based on mycobacterial susceptibility tests. There are no studies that specifically address the optimal duration of therapy for tuberculous esophagitis, but regimens should be similar for those used for other extrapulmonary infections and should include at least 2 active drugs for periods of from 6 to 12 months.[163] In HIV-infected patients, the effects of rifamycins on metabolism of methadone, triazoles, and protease inhibitors must be considered.[164] Atypical mycobacteria such as *Mycobacterium avium* complex only infrequently cause esophageal disease. Treatment for atypical mycobacterial infections generally includes either clarithromycin or azithromycin in combination with one or several other active agents.[165] Options for treatment of opportunistic noncandidal fungal pathogens such as aspergillosis now include itraconazole, voriconazole, and caspofungin, in addition to amphotericin B. The choice of agents depends on the specific pathogen identified. Herpes zoster esophageal infections, like HSV infections, will respond to acyclovir, but higher doses are required than for HSV.

APPROACH TO THE IMMUNOCOMPROMISED PATIENT WITH ESOPHAGEAL SYMPTOMS

HIV-infected patients

As experience has accumulated in the management of HIV-infected patients with esophageal symptoms, strategies have evolved to minimize the need for unnecessary or expensive diagnostic procedures and maximize successful outcomes. Confirming the diagnoses of a specific opportunistic infection, such as *Candida* esophagitis, is no longer necessary for meeting the case definition of AIDS. Therefore, the need for diagnostic studies can be based solely on clinical indications. One algorithm for the work-up of esophageal symptoms in HIV-infected patients is outlined in Figure 6.1. A commonly accepted approach has been to use a trial of antifungal therapy as the initial diagnostic and therapeutic modality for most HIV-infected patients with esophageal symptoms.[9,10,31] *Candida* infection is the most common cause of esophageal symptoms in these patients. Features of the clinical history and the presence or absence of oropharyngeal disease are not sufficiently sensitive or specific for identifying patients who will respond to antifungal therapy. One large randomized trial has compared empiric antifungal therapy using fluconazole to early diagnostic endoscopy followed by specific therapy.[166] In this population, a trial of empiric fluconazole was a safe, effective, and cost-effective strategy, with endoscopy reserved for patients failing to respond after 7–10 days of empiric antifungal therapy. Clinical characteristics of patients who might benefit from earlier endoscopy for esophageal symptoms include those already on antifungal therapy at the onset of symptoms, patients with associated upper gastrointestinal hemorrhage, or those with specific clinical features suggesting a diagnosis other than candidal disease.[166,167] Patients who failed empiric antifungal therapy were most likely to have either CMV esophageal ulcers or idiopathic esophageal ulcerations in 77% of cases.[167,168] Less common diagnoses included HSV, reflux disease, and refractory candidal infection, although up to 20% had entirely normal endoscopic studies. Esophageal motility disorders are also common in HIV infected patients, with or without other infectious diagnoses, and may contribute to esophageal symptoms.[169] As HIV-infected patients are living longer and many have well-controlled disease with higher CD4 counts, the proportion of patients with esophageal symptoms who have noninfectious diagnoses might be predicted to increase. Thus, HIV disease with high CD4 counts should be another indication to proceed directly to endoscopy, similar to the evaluation in otherwise healthy individuals. Endoscopic evaluations should include aggressive collection of samples from abnormal areas for histopathologic and cytologic studies, as noted above. Multiple biopsies should be obtained from ulcerative lesions to optimally distinguish between viral and idiopathic ulcers.[31,52] Barium studies are not generally recommended as the primary investigation due to a lack of sensitivity for diagnoses other than candidal disease and the inability to detect all pathogens in dual infections, which may occur in up to 15% of patients. Barium studies should be reserved for patients too ill to undergo endoscopy or when endoscopy is otherwise contraindicated. Once diagnosed, the treatment of specific infections should follow the recommendations outlined previously.

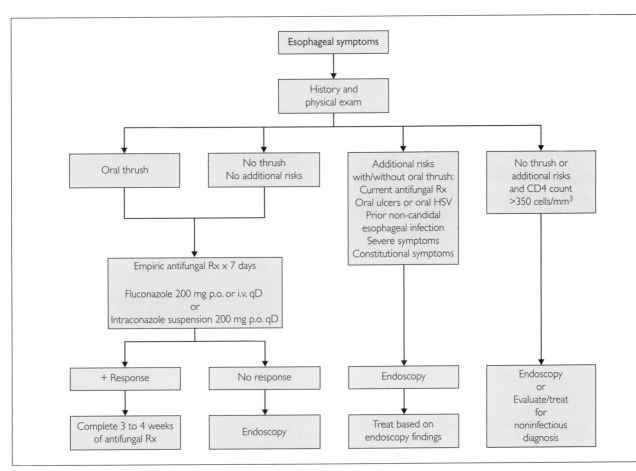

Fig. 6.1 ● Algorithm for initial management of esophageal symptoms in HIV-infected patients

Evaluation of esophageal symptoms in other populations

Strategies for management of esophageal infections in other immunocompromised patients have not been subjected to the same rigorous analysis as have those for patients with HIV disease. In mildly immunocompromised patients, candidal infection or noninfectious diagnoses would be the most likely causes of symptoms. Noninfectious diagnoses to be considered (Table 6.7), depending on the population, include reflux esophagitis, motility disorders, chemotherapy-induced esophageal damage, radiation-induced esophageal necrosis, graft-versus-host disease, and the direct traumatic effects of medications, such as tetracycline and zidovudine.[6,15,170,171] In those patients with mild to moderate symptoms and findings of oropharyngeal candidiasis, empiric

antifungal therapy may be considered, reserving endoscopy for those who fail a trial of fluconazole or itraconazole therapy. For more severely immunocompromised patients, such as bone marrow or solid organ transplant patients or febrile neutropenic patients with no specific contraindication to the procedure, early endoscopy may be the preferred strategy in order to initiate appropriate therapy as expeditiously as possible. As in HIV-infected patients, the role of barium studies would appear to be limited, except in very specific situations.

CONCLUSIONS

Esophageal infections remain a major cause of morbidity in immunosuppressed patients, not only in patients infected with human immunodeficiency virus, but in many other populations as well. There have been major advances in the treatment of the most commonly seen syndromes, including *Candida*, cytomegalovirus, herpes simplex, and idiopathic HIV-associated esophageal ulcerations. Optimal strategies for the prevention and long-term management of these infections are still evolving.

REFERENCES

1. Springer DJ, DaCosta LR, Beck IT. A syndrome of acute self-limiting ulcerative esophagitis in young adults probably due to herpes simplex virus. Dig Dis Sci 1979; 24(7):535–539.

Table 6.7 Common non-infectious causes of esophageal symptoms in immunocompromised patients

Reflux esophagitis
Chemotherapy-induced esophagitis
Radiation esophagitis
Graft-versus-host disease
'Pill'-induced esophagitis
Esophageal tumors
Esophageal motility disorders

2. Kodsi BE, Wickremesinghe PC, Kozinn PJ, et al. *Candida* esophagitis: a prospective study of 27 cases. Gastroenterology 1976; 71(5):715–719.

3. Ramanathan J, Rammouni M, Baran J Jr, et al. Herpes simplex virus esophagitis in the immunocompetent host: an overview. Am J Gastroenterol 2000; 95(9):2171–2176.

4. Baehr PH, McDonald GB. Esophageal infections: risk factors, presentation, diagnosis, and treatment. Gastroenterology 1994; 106(2):509–532.

5. Gundry SR, Borkon AM, McIntosh CL, et al. *Candida* esophagitis following cardiac operation and short-term antibiotic prophylaxis. J Thorac Cardiovasc Surg 1980; 80(5):661–668.

6. Wheeler RR, Peacock JE Jr, Cruz JM, et al. Esophagitis in the immunocompromised host; role of esophagoscopy in diagnosis. Rev Infect Dis 1987; 9(1):88–96.

7. Centers for Disease Control. Cases of HIV infection and AIDS in the United States, 2002. HIV/AIDS Surveillance Report, Vol.14:1–40. October 27, 2003.

8. Joint UN Program on HIV/AIDS. UNAIDS 2004 Report on the Global AIDS Epidemic - Executive Summary, July, 2004. *www.unaids.org/bangkok2004/GAR2004_html/ExecSummary_en/ExecSumm_00_en.htm*

9. Laine L, Bonacini M. Esophageal disease in human immunodeficiency virus infection. Arch Int Med 1994; 154(14):1577–1582.

10. Wilcox CM. Esophageal disease in the acquired immunodeficiency syndrome: etiology, diagnosis and management. Am J Med 1992; 92(4):412–421.

11. Connolly GM, Hawkins D, Harcourt-Webster JN, et al. Oesophageal symptoms, their causes, treatment and prognosis in patients with the acquired immune deficiency syndrome. Gut 1989; 30(8):1033–1039.

12. Kaplan JE, Hanson D, Dworkin MS, et al. Epidemiology of human immunodeficiency virus-associated opportunistic infections in the United States in the era of highly active antiretroviral therapy. Clin Infect Dis 2000; 30(Suppl 1):S5–S14.

13. Palella FJ Jr, Delaney KM, Moorman AC, et al. Declining morbidity and mortality among patients with advanced human immunodeficiency virus infection. HIV Outpatient Study Investigators. N Engl J Med 1998; 338(13):853–860.

14. Alexander JA, Brouillette DE, Chien MC et al. Infectious esophagitis following liver and renal transplantation. Dig Dis Sci 1988; 33(9):1121–1126.

15. McDonald GB, Sharma P, Hackman RC, et al. Esophageal infections in immunosuppressed patients after marrow transplantation. Gastroenterology 1985; 88(5 part 1):1111–1117.

16. Scott BB, Jenkins D. Gastro-oesophageal candidiasis. Gut 1982; 23(2):137–139.

17. Naito Y, Yoshikawa T, Oyamada H, et al. Esophageal candidiasis. Gastroenterol Japan 1988; 23(4):284–290.

18. Porro GB, Parente F, Cernuschi M. The diagnosis of esophageal candidiasis in patients with the acquired immunodeficiency syndrome: Is endoscopy always necessary? Am J Gastroenterol 1989; 84(11):143–146.

19. Jensen KB, Stenderup A, Thomsen JB, et al. Oesophageal moniliasis in malignant neoplastic disease. Acta Medica Scand 1964; 175:455–459.

20. Moore RD, Chaisson RE. Natural history of opportunistic disease in an HIV-infected urban clinical cohort. Ann Intern Med 1996; 124(7):633–642.

21. Simon MR, Houser WL, Smith KA, et al. Esophageal candidiasis as a complication of inhaled corticosteroids. Ann Allergy Asthma Immunol 1997; 79(4):333–338.

22. Wiest PM, Flanigan T, Salata RA, et al. Serious infectious complications of corticosteroid therapy for COPD. Chest 1989; 95(6):1180–1184.

23. Maenza JR, Merz WG, Romagnoli MJ, et al. Infection due to fluconazole-resistant *Candida* in patients with AIDS: prevalence and microbiology. Clin Infect Dis 1997; 24(1):28–34.

24. Wilcox CM, Straub RF, Clark WS. Prospective evaluation of oropharyngeal findings in human immunodeficiency virus-infected patients with esophageal ulceration. Am J Gastroenterol 1995; 90(11):1938–1941.

25. Agha FP. Candidiasis-induced esophageal strictures. Gastrointest Radiol 1984; 9(4):283–286.

26. Obrecht WF Jr, Richter JE, Olympio GA, et al. Tracheoesophageal fistula: a serious complication of infectious esophagitis. Gastroenterology 1984; 87(5):1174–1179.

27. Campero AA, Cambell GD. Complete oesophageal obstruction due to monilia infection. Aust NZ J Surg 1973; 43:244–246.

28. Levine MS, Macones AJ, Laufer I. *Candida* esophagitis: accuracy of radiographic diagnosis. Radiology 1985; 154(3):581–587.

29. Vahey TN, Maglinte DD, Chernish SM. State-of-the-art barium examination in opportunistic esophagitis. Dig Dis Sci 1986; 31(11):1192–1195.

30. Levine MS, Loevner LA, Saul SH, et al. Herpes esophagitis: sensitivity of double-contrast esophagography. Am J Roentgenol 1988; 151(1):57–62.

31. Dieterich DT, Wilcox CM and the Practice Parameters Committee of the American College of Gastroenterology. Diagnosis and treatment of esophageal diseases associated with HIV infection. Am J Gastroenterol 1996; 91(11):2265–2269.

32. Wilcox CM, Schwartz DA. Endoscopic-pathologic correlates of *Candida* esophagitis in acquired immunodeficiency syndrome. Dig Dis Sci 1996; 41(7):1337–1344.

33. Bonacini M, Young T, Laine L. The causes of esophageal symptoms in human immunodeficiency virus infection. A prospective study of 110 patients. Arch Intern Med 1991; 151(8):1567–1572.

34. Agha FP, Lee HH, Nostrant TT. Herpetic esophagitis: a diagnostic challenge in immunocompromised patients. Am J Gastroenterol 1986; 81(4):246–253.

35. Young JA, Elias E. Gastro-oesophageal candidiasis: diagnosis by brush cytology. J Clin Pathol 1985; 38(3):293–296.

36. Bonacini M, Laine L, Gal AA, et al. Prospective evaluation of blind brushing in the esophagus for *Candida* esophagitis in patients with human immunodeficiency virus infection. Am J Gastroenterol 1990; 85(4):385–389.

37. Rosario MT, Raso CL, Comer GM, et al. Transnasal brush cytology for the diagnosis of *Candida* esophagitis in the acquired immunodeficiency syndrome. Gastrointest Endosc 1989; 35(2):102–103.

38. Mc Bane RD, Gross JB Jr. Herpes esophagitis: clinical syndrome, endoscopic appearance, and diagnosis in 23 patients. Gastrointest Endosc 1991; 37(6):600–603.

39. Pazin GJ. Herpes simplex esophagitis after trigeminal nerve surgery. Gastroenterology 1978; 74(4):741–743.

40. Genereau T, Lortholary O, Bouchaud O, et al. Herpes simplex esophagitis in patients with AIDS: report of 34 cases. Clin Infect Dis 1996; 22(6):926–931.

41. Fishbein PG, Tuthill R, Kressel H, et al. Herpes simplex esophagitis: a cause of upper-gastrointestinal bleeding. Dig Dis Sci 1979; 24(7):540–544.

42. Cirillo NW, Lyon DT, Schuller AM. Tracheoesophageal fistula complicating herpes esophagitis in AIDS. Am J Gastroenterol 1993; 88(4):587–589.

43. Byard RW, Champion MC, Orizaga M. Variability in the clinical presentation and endoscopic findings of herpetic esophagitis. Endoscopy 1987; 19(4):153–155.

44. Feiden W, Borchard F, Burrig KF, et al. Herpes oesophagitis. I. Light microscopical and immunohistochemical investigations. Virchows Arch 1984; 404(2):167–176.

45. Lightdale CJ, Wolf DJ, Marcucci RA, et al. Herpetic esophagitis in patients with cancer: ante mortem diagnosis by brush cytology. Cancer 1977; 39(1):223–226.

46. Wilcox CM, Straub RF, Schwartz DA. Cytomegalovirus esophagitis in AIDS: A prospective evaluation of clinical response to ganciclovir therapy, relapse rate and long-term outcome. Am J Med 1995; 98(2):169–176.

47. Gould E, Kory WP, Raskin JB, et al. Esophageal biopsy findings in the acquired immunodeficiency syndrome: Clinical pathologic correlation in 20 patients. South Med J 1988; 81(11):1392–1395.

48. Balthazar EJ, Megibow AJ, Hulnick D, et al. Cytomegalovirus esophagitis in AIDS: radiographic features in 16 patients. Am J Roentgenol 1987; 149(5):919–923.

49. Wilcox CM, Straub RF, Schwartz DA. Prospective endoscopic characterization of cytomegalovirus esophagitis in AIDS. Gastrointest Endosc 1994; 40(4):481–484.

50. Wilcox CM, Straub RF, Schwartz DA. Prospective evaluation of biopsy number for diagnosis of viral esophagitis in patients with HIV infection and esophageal ulcer. Gastrointest Endosc 1996; 44(5):587–593.

51. Theise ND, Rotterdam H, Dieterich D. Cytomegalovirus esophagitis in AIDS: Diagnosis by endoscopic biopsy. Am J Gastroenterol 1991; 86(9):1123–1126.

52. Wilcox CM, Rodgers W, Lazenby A. Prospective comparison of brush cytology, viral culture, and histology for the diagnosis of ulcerative esophagitis in AIDS. Clin Gastroenterol Hepatol. 2004; 2(7):564–567.

   Definitive study comparing diagnostic methodology for the establishing the diagnosis of HIV-associated esophageal ulcers.

53. Kotler DP, Reka S, Orenstein JM, et al. Chronic idiopathic esophageal ulceration in the acquired immunodeficiency syndrome: characterization and treatment with corticosteroids. J Clin Gastroenterol 1992; 15(4):284–290.

54. Bini EJ, Micale PL, Weinshel EH. Natural history of HIV-associated esophageal disease in the era of protease inhibitor therapy. Dig Dis Sci 2000; 45(7):1301–1307.

   A retrospective study demonstrating the dramatic impact of availability of highly active antiretroviral therapy for even a short period of time on the outcome and relapse rate of CMV disease and idiopathic ulcers.

55. Rabeneck L, Popovic M, Gartner S, et al. Acute HIV infection presenting with painful swallowing and esophageal ulcers. JAMA 1990; 263(17):2318–2322.

56. Smith PD, Eisner MS, Monischewitz JF, et al. Esophageal disease in AIDS is associated with pathologic processes rather than mucosal human immunodeficiency virus type 1. J Infect Dis 1993; 167(3):547–550.

57. Bonacini M, Young T, Laine L. Histopathology of human immunodeficiency virus-associated esophageal disease. Am J Gastroenterol 1993; 88(4):549–551.

58. Wilcox CM, Schwartz DA. Endoscopic characterization of idiopathic esophageal ulceration associated with human immunodeficiency virus infection. J Clin Gastroenterol 1993; 16(3):251–256.

59. Damtew B, Frengley D, Wolinsky E, et al. Esophageal tuberculosis: mimicry of gastrointestinal malignancy. Rev Infect Dis 1987; 9(1):140–146.

60. Porter JC, Friedland JS, Freedman AR. Tuberculosis broncho-esophageal fistulae in patients infected with the human immunodeficiency virus: Three case reports and review. Clin Infect Dis 1994; 19(5):954–957.

61. Iademarco MF, Castro KG. Epidemiology of tuberculosis. Semin Respir Infect 2003; 18(4):225–240.

62. Chase RA, Haber MH, Pottage JC Jr, et al. Tuberculous esophagitis with erosion into aortic aneurysm. Arch Pathol Lab Med 1986; 110(10):965–966.

63. Walsh TJ, Belitsos NJ, Hamilton SR. Bacterial esophagitis in immunocompromised patients. Arch Intern Med 1986; 146(7):1345–1348.

64. Ezzell JH Jr, Bremer J, Adamec TA. Bacterial esophagitis: an often forgotten cause of odynophagia. Am J Gastroenterol 1990; 85(3):296–298.

65. Young RC, Bennett JE, Vogel CL, et al. Aspergillosis: the spectrum of disease in 98 patients. Medicine 1970; 49(2):147–173.

66. Jacobs DH, Macher AM, Handler R, et al. Esophageal cryptococcosis in a patient with the hyperimmunoglobulin E-recurrent infection (Job's) syndrome. Gastroenterology 1984; 87(1):201–203.

67. Hoffman M, Bash E, Berger SA, et al. Fatal necrotizing esophagitis due to *Penicillum chrysogenum* in a patient with acquired immunodeficiency syndrome. Eur J Clin Microbiol Infect Dis 1992; 11(12):1158–1160.

68. Lyon DT, Schubert TT, Mantia AG, et al. Phycomycosis of the gastrointestinal tract. Am J Gastroenterol 1979; 72(4):379–394.

69. McKenzie R, Khakoo R. Blastomycosis of the esophagus presenting with gastrointestinal bleeding. Gastroenterology 1985; 88(5 Pt 1):1271–1273.

70. Fosmark CE, Wilcox CM, Darragh TM, et al. Disseminated histoplasmosis in AIDS: an unusual case of esophageal involvement and gastrointestinal bleeding. Gastrointest Endosc 1990; 36(6):604–605.

71. Gill RA, Gebhard RL, Dozeman RL, et al. Shingles esophagitis: endoscopic diagnosis in two patients. Gastrointest Endosc 1984; 30(1):26–27.

72. Kitchen VS, Helbert M, Francis ND, et al. Epstein-Barr virus associated oesophageal ulcers in AIDS. Gut 1990; 31(11):1223–1225.

73. Corbellino M, Lusso P, Gallo RC, et al. Disseminated human herpes virus 6 infection in AIDS. Lancet 1993; 342(8881):1242.

74. Trottier AM, Coutlee F, Leduc R, et al. Human immunodeficiency virus infection is a major risk factor for detection of human papillomavirus DNA in esophageal brushings. Clin Infect Dis 1997; 24(4):565–569.

75. Kazlow PG, Shah K, Benkov KJ, et al. Esophageal cryptosporidiosis in a child with acquired immune deficiency syndrome. Gastroenterology 1986; 91(5):1301–1303.

76. Chang AD, Drachenberg CI, James SP. Bacillary angiomatosis associated with extensive esophageal polyposis: a new mucocutaneous manifestations of AIDS. Am J Gastroenterol 1996; 91(10):2220–2223.

77. Grimes MM, LaPook JD, Bar MH, et al. Disseminated *Pneumocystis carinii* infection in a patient with acquired immunodeficiency syndrome. Hum Pathol 1987; 18(3):307–308.

78. Villanueva JL, Torre-Cisneros J, Jurado R, et al. Leishmania esophagitis in an AIDS patient: An unusual form of visceral leishmaniasis. Am J Gastroenterol 1994; 89(2):273–275.

79. Gaissert HA, Roper CL, Patterson GA, et al. Infectious necrotizing esophagitis: outcome after medical and surgical intervention. Ann Thorac Surg 2003; 75(2):342–347.

Case series that addresses the potential role of surgery for management of severe necrotizing esophageal infection in immunocompromised patients.

80. Quintiliani R, Owens NJ, Guercia RA, et al. Treatment and prevention of oropharyngeal candidiasis. Am J Med 1984; 77(4D):44–48.

81. Martin MV, Dinsdale RCW. Nystatin resistance of Candida albicans isolates from two cases of oral candidiasis. Br J Oral Surg 1982; 20(4):294–298.

82. Ginsburg CH, Braden GL, Tauber AI, et al. Oral clotrimazole in the treatment of esophageal candidiasis. Am J Med 1981; 71(5): 891–895.

83. Deschamps MH, Pape JW, Verdier RI, et al. Treatment of Candida esophagitis in AIDS patients. Am J Gastroenterol 1988; 83(1): 20–21.

84. Nguyen MT, Weiss PJ, LaBarre RC, et al. Orally administered amphotericin B in the treatment of oral candidiasis in HIV-infected patients caused by azole-resistant Candida albicans. AIDS 1996; 10(14):1745–1747.

85. Sheehan DJ, Hitchcock CA, Sibley CM. Current and emerging azole antifungal agents. Clin Microbiol Rev 1999; 12(1):40–79.

86. Baciewicz AM, Baciewicz FA Jr. Ketoconazole and fluconazole drug interactions. Arch Intern Med 1993; 153(17):1970–1976.

87. Blum RA, D'Andrea DT, Florentino BM, et al. Increased gastric pH and the bio-availability of fluconazole and ketoconazole. Ann Intern Med 1991; 114(9):755–757.

88. Laine L, Dretler RH, Conteas CN, et al. Fluconazole compared to ketoconazole for the treatment of Candida esophagitis in AIDS: a randomized trial. Ann Intern Med 1992; 117(8):655–660.

89. De Wit S, Urbain D, Rahir F, et al. Efficacy of oral fluconazole in the treatment of AIDS associated esophageal candidiasis. Eur J Clin Microbiol Infect Dis 1991; 10(6):503–505.

90. Barbaro G, Barbarini G, Calderon W, et al. Fluconazole versus itraconazole for Candida esophagitis in acquired immunodeficiency syndrome. Gastroenterol 1996; 111(5):1169–1177.

91. Parente F, Cernuschi M, Rizzardini G, et al. Opportunistic infections of the esophagus not responding to oral systemic antifungals in patients with AIDS: Their frequency and treatment. Am J Gastroenterol 1991; 86(12):1729–1734.

92. Rex JH, Rinaldi MG, Pfaller MA. Resistance of Candida species to fluconazole. Antimicrob Agents Chemother 1995; 39(1):1–8.

93. Fichtenbaum CJ, Powderly WG. Refractory mucosal candidiasis in patients with human immunodeficiency virus infection. Clin Infect Dis 1998; 26(3):556–565.

94. Goff DA, Koletar SL, Buesching WJ, et al. Isolation of fluconazole resistant Candida albicans from human immunodeficiency virus-negative patients never treated with azoles. Clin Infect Dis 1995; 20(1):77–83.

95. Rex JH, Pfaller MA, Galgiani JN, et al. Development of interpretive breakpoints for antifungal susceptibility testing: conceptual framework and analysis of in vitro-in vivo correlation data for fluconazole, itraconazole and Candida infections. Clin Infect Dis 1997; 24(2):235–247.

96. Eichel M, Just-Nubling G, Helm EB, et al. Itraconazole suspension in the treatment of HIV-infected patients with fluconazole-resistant oropharyngeal candidiasis and esophagitis. Mycoses 1996; 39(Suppl 1):102–106.

97. Pfaller MA, Messer SA, Hollis RJ, et al. In vitro activities of ravuconazole and voriconazole compared with those of four approved systemic antifungal agents against 6,970 clinical isolates of Candida spp. Antimicrob Agents Chemother 2002; 46(6):1723–1727.

98. Fazio RA, Wickremesinghe PC, Arsura EL. Ketoconazole treatment of Candida esophagitis – a prospective study of 12 cases. Am J Gastroenterol 1983; 78(5):261–264.

99. Lewis JH, Zimmerman HJ, Benson GD, et al. Hepatic injury associated with ketoconazole therapy. Gastroenterology 1984; 86(3):503–513.

100. Lake-Bakaar G, Tom W, Lake-Bakaar D, et al. Gastropathy and ketoconazole malabsorption in the acquired immunodeficiency syndrome. Ann Intern Med 1988; 109(6):471–478.

101. Tavitian A, Raufman JP, Rosenthal LE, et al. Ketoconazole-resistant Candida esophagitis in patients with acquired immunodeficiency syndrome. Gastroenterology 1986; 90(2):443–445.

102. Maertens JA. History of the development of azole derivatives. Clin Microbiol Infect 2004; 10(Suppl 1):1–10.

103. Smith PE, Midgley J, Allan M, et al. Itraconazole vs ketoconazole in the treatment of oral and esophageal candidiasis in patients infected with HIV. AIDS 1991; 5(11):1367–1371.

104. De Beule K, Van Gestel J. Pharmacology of itraconazole. Drugs 2001; 61(Suppl 1):27–37.

105. Wilcox CM, Darouiche RO, Laine L, et al. A randomized double-blind comparison of itraconazole oral solution and fluconazole tablets in treatment of esophageal candidiasis. J Infect Dis 1997; 176(1):227–232.

106. Laguna F, Rodriguez-Tudela JL, Martinez-Svarez JV, et al. Patterns of fluconazole susceptibility in isolates from human immunodeficiency virus infected patients with oropharyngeal candidiasis due to Candida albicans. Clin Infect Dis 1997; 24(2):124–130.

107. Ally R, Schurmann D, Kreisel W, et al. A randomized, double-blind, double-dummy, multicenter trial of voriconazole and fluconazole in the treatment of esophageal candidiasis in immunocompromised patients. Clin Infect Dis 2001; 33(9): 1447–1454.

108. Hegener P, Troke PF, Fatkenheuer G, et al. Treatment of fluconazole-resistant candidiasis with voriconazole in patients with AIDS. AIDS 1998; 12(16):2227–2228.

109. Pappas PG, Rex JH, Sobel JD, et al. Infectious Diseases Society of America. Guidelines for treatment of candidiasis. Clin Infect Dis 2004; 38(2):161–189.

Evidence-based guidelines that review treatment of Candida syndromes that discusses alternatives for management of mucosal candidiasis including options for fluconazole-refractory disease.

110. Robinson RF, Nahata MC. A comparative review of conventional and lipid formulations of amphotericin B. J Clin Pharm Ther 1999; 24(4):249–257.

111. Lake DE, Kunzweiler J, Beer M, et al. Fluconazole versus amphotericin B in the treatment of esophageal candidiasis in cancer patients. Chemotherapy 1996; 42(4):308–314.

112. Letscher-Bru V, Herbrecht R. Caspofungin: the first representative of a new antifungal class. J Antimicrob Chemother 2003; 51(3):513–521.

113. Villanueva A, Arathoon EG, Gotuzzo E, et al. A randomized double-blind study of caspofungin versus amphotericin for the treatment of candidal esophagitis. Clin Infect Dis 2001; 33(9):1529–1535.

114. Villanueva A, Gotuzzo E, Arathoon E, et al. A randomized double blind study of caspofungin versus fluconazole for the treatment of esophageal candidiasis. Am J Med 2002; 113(4):294–299.

115. Dinubile MJ, Lupinacci RJ, Berman RS, et al. Response and relapse rates of candidal esophagitis in HIV-infected patients treated with caspofungin. AIDS Res Hum Retroviruses 2002; 18(13): 903–908.

116. Kartsonis N, DiNubile MJ, Bartizal K, et al. Efficacy of caspofungin in the treatment of esophageal candidiasis resistant to fluconazole. J Acq Immune Defic Syndrome Hum Retrovirol 2002; 31(2): 183–187.

117. Hernandez S, Lopez-Ribot JL, Najvar LK, et al. Caspofungin resistance in *Candida albicans*: correlating clinical outcome with laboratory susceptibility testing of three isogenic isolates serially obtained from a patient with progressive *Candida* esophagitis. Antimicrob Agents Chemother 2004; 48(4):1382–1383.

118. Wiederhold NP, Lewis RE. The echinocandin antifungals: an overview of the pharmacology, spectrum and clinical efficacy. Expert Opin Investig Drugs 2003; 12(8):1313–1333.

119. Barbaro G, Barbarini G, Di Lorenzo G. Fluconazole vs. flucytosine in the treatment of esophageal candidiasis in AIDS patients: a double blind, placebo-controlled study. Endoscopy 1995; 27(5): 377–383.

120. Castagnola E, Machetti M, Bucci B, et al. Antifungal prophylaxis with azole derivatives. Clin Microbiol Infect 2004; 10(Suppl 1): 86–95.

121. Sypula WT, Kale-Pradhan PB. Therapeutic dilemma of fluconazole prophylaxis in intensive care. Ann Pharmacother 2002; 36(1): 155–159.

122. Centers for Disease Control and Prevention. Treating opportunistic infections among HIV-infected adults and adolescents: recommendations from the CDC, the National Institutes of Health, and the HIV Medicine Association/Infectious Society of America. MMWR 2004; 53(RR-15):1–112.

Evidence-based guideline that reviews available data and provides recommendations for treatment and primary and secondary prevention of fungal and viral infections in patients with HIV infection.

123. Powderly WG, Finkelstein DM, Feinberg J, et al. A randomized trial comparing fluconazole with clotrimazole troches for the prevention of fungal infections in patients with advanced human immunodeficiency virus infection. N Engl J Med 1995; 332(11):700–705.

124. Schuman P, Capps L, Peng G, et al. Weekly fluconazole for the prevention of mucosal candidiasis in women with HIV infection. Ann Intern Med 1997; 126(9):689–696.

125. Manfredi R, Mastrano A, Coronado OV, et al. Fluconazole as prophylaxis against fungal infection in patients with advanced HIV infection. Arch Intern Med 1997; 157(1):64–69.

126. Havlir DV, Dube MP, McCutchan JA, et al. Prophylaxis with weekly versus daily fluconazole for fungal infections in patients with AIDS. Clin Infect Dis 1998; 27(6):1369–1375.

127. Parente F, Ardizzone S, Cernuschi M, et al. Prevention of symptomatic recurrences of esophageal candidiasis in AIDS patients after the first episode: A prospective open study. Am J Gastroenterol 1994; 89(3):416–420.

128. Pagani JL, Chave JP, Casjka C, et al. Efficacy, tolerability and development of resistance in HIV-positive patients treated with fluconazole for secondary prevention of oropharyngeal candidiasis: a randomized, double-blind, placebo-controlled trial. J Antimicrob Chemother 2002; 50(2):231–240.

129. Revankar SG, Kirkpatrick WR, McAtee RK, et al. A randomized trial of continuous or intermittent therapy with fluconazole for oropharyngeal candidiasis in HIV-infected patients: clinical outcomes and development of fluconazole resistance. Am J Med 1998; 105(1):7–11.

130. Whitley RJ, Gnann JW Jr. Acyclovir: A decade later. N Engl J Med 1992; 327(11):782–789.

131. Naesens L, De Clercq E. Recent developments in herpesvirus therapy. Herpes 2001; 8(1):12–16.

132. Feinberg J, Hurwitz S, Cooper D, et al. A randomized, double-blind trial of valacyclovir prophylaxis for cytomegalovirus disease in patients with advanced human immunodeficiency virus. J Infect Dis 1998; 177(1):48–56.

133. Schacker T, Hui-Lin H, Koelle DM, et al. Famciclovir for the suppression of symptomatic and asymptomatic herpes simplex virus reactivation in HIV-infected persons. Ann Int Med 1998; 128(1):21–28.

134. DeJesus E, Wald A, Warren T, et al, Valacyclovir International HSV Study Group. Valacyclovir for the suppression of recurrent genital herpes in human immunodeficiency virus-infected subjects. J Infect Dis 2003 ;188(7):1009–1016.

135. Erlich KS, Mills J, Chatis P, et al. Acyclovir resistant herpes simplex virus infections in patients with the acquired immunodeficiency syndrome. N Engl J Med 1989; 320(5):293–296.

136. Reusser P. Herpesvirus resistance to antiviral drugs: a review of the mechanisms, clinical importance and therapeutic options. J Hosp Infect 1996; 33(4):235–248.

137. Ljungman P. Prophylaxis against herpesvirus infections in transplant recipients. Drugs 2001; 61(2):187–196.

138. Stein DS, Graham NMH, Park LP, et al. The effect of the interaction of acyclovir with zidovudine on progression to AIDS and survival. Ann Intern Med 1994; 121(2):100–108.

139. Whitley RJ, Jacobson MA, Friedberg DN, et al. Guidelines for the treatment of cytomegalovirus diseases in patients with AIDS in the era of potent antiretroviral therapy: recommendations of an international panel. International AIDS Society–USA. Arch Intern Med 1998; 158(9):957–969.

Evidence-based guideline that reviews available agents and discusses strategies for treatment of CMV disease in HIV infected patients.

140. Nelson MR, Connolly GM, Hawkins DA, et al. Foscarnet in the treatment of cytomegalovirus infections of the esophagus and colon in patients with the acquired immunodeficiency syndrome. Am J Gastroenterol 1991; 86(7):876–881.

141. Drew WL, Ives D, Lalezari JP, et al. Oral ganciclovir maintenance treatment for CMV retinitis in patients with AIDS. N Engl J Med 1995; 333(10):615–620.

142. Martin DF, Sierra-Madero J, Walmsley S, et al. Valganciclovir Study Group. A controlled trial of valganciclovir as induction therapy for cytomegalovirus retinitis. N Engl J Med 2002; 346(15):1119–1126.

143. Reusser P. Oral valganciclovir: a new option for treatment of cytomegalovirus infection and disease in immunocompromised hosts. Expert Opin Investig Drugs 2001; 10(9):1745–1753.

144. Dieterich DT, Poles MA, Lew EA, et al. Treatment of gastrointestinal cytomegalovirus infection with twice daily foscarnet: A pilot study with pharmacokinetics in patients with HIV. Antimicrob Agents Chemother 1997; 41(6):1226–1230.

145. Deray VG, Martinez F, Katlama C, et al. Foscarnet nephrotoxicity: Mechanism, incidence and prevention. Am J Nephrol 1989; 9(4):311–321.

146. SOCA study group. Mortality in patients with AIDS treated with either foscarnet or ganciclovir for CMV retinitis. N Engl J Med 1992; 326(4):213–220.

147. Monkemuller KE, Wilcox CM. Esophageal ulcer caused by cytomegalovirus: resolution during combination antiretroviral therapy for acquired immunodeficiency syndrome. South Med J 2000; 93(8):818–820.

148. Baldanti F, Gerna G. Human cytomegalovirus resistance to antiviral drugs: diagnosis, monitoring and clinical impact. J Antimicrob Chemother 2003; 52(3):324–330.

149. Plosker GL, Noble S. Cidofovir: a review of its use in cytomegalovirus retinitis in patients with AIDS. Drugs 1999; 58(2):325–345.

150. O'Sullivan CE, Drew WL, McMullen DJ, et al. Decrease of cytomegalovirus replication in human immunodeficiency virus infected-patients after treatment with highly active antiretroviral therapy. J Infect Dis 1999; 180(3):847–849.

151. Sia IG, Patel R. New strategies for prevention and therapy of cytomegalovirus infection and disease in solid-organ transplant recipients. Clin Microbiol Rev 2000; 13(1):83–121.

   Excellent review of concepts and general strategies for prevention and therapy of cytomegalovirus disease in transplant patients.

152. Ciancio G, Burke GW, Mattiazzi A, et al. Cytomegalovirus prophylaxis with valganciclovir in kidney, pancreas-kidney, and pancreas transplantation. Clin Transplant 2004; 18(4):402–406.

153. Schmidt GM, Horak DA, Niland JC, et al. A randomized, controlled trial of prophylactic ganciclovir for cytomegalovirus pulmonary infection in recipients of allogenic bone marrow transplants. N Engl J Med 1991; 324(15):1005–1011.

154. Spector SA, McKinley GF, Lalezari JP, et al. Oral ganciclovir for the prevention of cytomegalovirus disease in persons with AIDS. N Engl J Med 1996; 334(23):1492–1497.

155. Erice A, Tierney C, Hirsch M, et al; AIDS Clinical Trials Group Protocol 360 Study Team. Cytomegalovirus (CMV) and human immunodeficiency virus (HIV) burden, CMV end-organ disease, and survival in subjects with advanced HIV infection (AIDS Clinical Trials Group Protocol 360). Clin Infect Dis 2003; 37(4):567–578.

156. Sokol-Anderson ML, Prelutsky DJ, Westblom TU. Giant esophageal aphthous ulcers in AIDS patients: treatment with low dose corticosteroids. AIDS 1991; 5(12):1537–1538.

157. Wilcox CM, Schwartz DA. Comparison of two corticosteroid regimens for the treatment of HIV-associated idiopathic esophageal ulcer. Am J Gastroenterol 1994; 89(12):2163–2169.

158. Wilcox CM, Schwartz DA, Clark WS. Esophageal ulceration in human immunodeficiency virus – causes, response to therapy and long-term outcome. Ann Intern Med 1995; 123(2):143–149.

159. Nelson MR, Erskine D, Hawkins DA, et al. Treatment with corticosteroids: A risk factor for development of clinical cytomegalovirus disease in AIDS. AIDS 1993; 7(3):375–378.

160. Jacobson JM, Spritzler J, Fox L, et al. Thalidomide for the treatment of esophageal aphthous ulcers in patients with human immunodeficiency virus infection. National Institute of Allergy and Infectious Disease AIDS Clinical Trials Group. J Infect Dis 1999; 180(1):61–67.

   Randomized, double-blind study demonstrating the effectiveness of thalidomide for healing of HIV-associated esophageal ulcers.

161. Alexander LN, Wilcox CM. A prospective trial of thalidomide for the treatment of HIV-associated idiopathic esophageal ulcers. AIDS Res Human Retroviruses 1997; 13(4):301–304.

162. Jacobson JM, Greenspan JS, Spritzler J, et al. Thalidomide in low intermittent doses does not prevent recurrence of human immunodeficiency virus-associated aphthous ulcers. J Infect Dis 2001; 183(2):343–346.

163. American Thoracic Society; CDC; Infectious Diseases Society of America. Treatment of tuberculosis. MMWR Recomm Rep 2003; 52(RR-11):1–77.

164. Centers for Disease Control. Updated guidelines for the use of rifabutin or rifampin for the treatment and prevention of tuberculosis among HIV-infected patients taking protease inhibitors or nonnucleoside reverse transcriptase inhibitors. Morb Mortal Wkly Rep 2000; 49(9):185–189.

165. Medical Section of the American Lung Association. Diagnosis and treatment of disease caused by nontuberculous mycobacteria. Am J Respir Crit Care Med 1997; 156(2 Pt 2):S1–S25.

166. Wilcox CM, Alexander LN, Clark WS, et al. Fluconazole compared with endoscopy for human immunodeficiency virus-infected patients with esophageal symptoms. Gastroenterology 1996; 110(6):1803–1809.

   The primary study demonstrating effectiveness of empiric antifungal therapy as an initial diagnostic and therapeutic strategy for HIV-infected patients with esophageal symptoms.

167. Bashir RM, Wilcox CM. Symptom specific use of upper gastrointestinal endoscopy in human immunodeficiency virus-infected patients yields high dividends. J Clin Gastroenterol 1996; 23(4):292–298.

168. Wilcox CM, Straub RF, Alexander LN, et al. Etiology of esophageal disease in human immunodeficiency virus-infected patients who fail antifungal therapy. Am J Med 1996; 101(6):599–604.

169. Zalar AE, Olmos MA, Piskorz EL, et al. Esophageal motility disorders in HIV patients. Dig Dis Sci 2003; 48(5):962–967.

170. Eng J, Sabanathan S. Drug induced esophagitis. Am J Gastroenterol 1991; 86(9):1127–1132.

171. Auguste LJ, Nava H. Postchemotherapy esophagitis: the endoscopic diagnosis and its impact on survival. J Surg Oncol 1986; 33(4):254–258.

CHAPTER SEVEN

7

Enteric infections in immunocompromised hosts

C. Mel Wilcox and Andrew W. DuPont

INTRODUCTION

Significant advancements have been made over the last decade in the management of the immunosuppressed patient including more targeted immunosuppressive therapy, selective use of effective antimicrobial prophylaxis, and the implementation of highly active antiretroviral therapy (HAART) for human immunodeficiency virus (HIV)-infected patients. Nevertheless, gastrointestinal (GI) infections remain important complications in these patients. The GI tract is a natural portal for entry of pathogens into the body and numerous protective mechanisms, most importantly the mucosal immune system, prevent infection. However, with immune compromise, these protective mechanisms are either impaired or lost, thereby predisposing to either local or systemic infection oftentimes by unusual pathogens termed opportunistic infections (OIs). The prototypical syndrome of such an occurrence is the acquired immunodeficiency syndrome (AIDS) where GI infections caused by OIs are almost universal, especially in the late stages of immunodeficiency. For any immunocompromised patient with GI symptoms, the differential diagnosis depends upon the suspected organ(s) of involvement, the type and severity of immune deficiency, and the geographic setting.

This chapter will take a pathogen-based approach to review epidemiology, clinical features, diagnosis, and therapy of luminal GI infections unique to persons immunocompromised by AIDS and those with iatrogenic disease associated with organ transplantation or chemotherapy. Several themes will emerge regarding GI infections in these patients including: (1) the clinical presentation of GI disease is dictated by the infecting pathogen(s), and there is overlap amongst these; (2) the severity and chronicity of infection is dictated by the cause, duration, and type of immunodeficiency; (3) the endoscopic features of GI infection are variable and overlapping, making definitive diagnosis by biopsy essential; and (4) relapse is common despite effective antimicrobial therapy when immunodeficiency persists.

EPIDEMIOLOGY

The prevalence, incidence, and etiology of luminal GI tract infections are influenced by many factors. In the normal host, GI infections generally occur at random following exposure to a pathogen and are self-limited. In any patient, coexisting host factors can attenuate or exacerbate the disease. For immunosuppressed patients, the cause(s), incidence, and severity of infection are linked to the etiology and severity of the immunodeficiency state. For example, patients undergoing solid organ transplantation are at the highest risk of infection early on after transplantation because of profound medication-induced immunodeficiency, and it is during this period that latent infections become manifest and susceptibility to infections is greatest. Over time, as drug-induced immunosuppression is reduced, the incidence of infection falls. The risk may increase, however, if organ rejection occurs as aggressive treatment with medications such as antithymocyte globulin may be required. For human immunodeficiency virus (HIV)-infected patients, the incidence of GI infections rises markedly as immune function deteriorates and the infection risk can be accurately stratified by the absolute CD4 lymphocyte count.[1]

The frequency of GI infections has been evolving in the immunosuppressed patient. Extensive research has defined the time course and spectrum of infections which complicate immune deficiency states.[2] Based on these observations, transplant patients and others with iatrogenic immunosuppression now receive targeted antimicrobial prophylaxis during those periods of greatest vulnerability to these infections. Depending on the risk for infection associated with the specific level of immune impairment, different classes of antimicrobials are utilized at varying time points. More selective immunosuppressive therapies, like cyclosporine, have also played a role in reducing the incidence of infections post transplant.[3] Other preventative strategies for cytomegalovirus (CMV), a frequent OI, in high-risk transplant patients include the use of CMV-seronegative organs and blood products for seronegative recipients and use of leukocyte-depleted platelets for patients following bone marrow transplantation.[4,5] The armamentarium of effective antiviral therapy for HIV continues to expand and the use of HAART for HIV-infected patients has drastically reduced the frequency of GI complications, both infections and neoplasms.[6,7]

OVERVIEW OF GASTROINTESTINAL INFECTIONS IN AIDS

Since the first description of AIDS in 1981, it is estimated that over 12 million people have died from this disease. While the incidence of new infections has fallen markedly in the developed world, new infections are still occurring, and many areas of the world are still plagued by or are at risk for the epidemic. A number of unique abnormalities in AIDS predispose to OIs of the GI tract.

Viral, protozoan, and atypical mycobacterial pathogens are the most numerous of such OIs, and concomitant infection by multiple enteric pathogens is a hallmark of AIDS. Perturbations of the mucosal immune system paralleling those present in peripheral blood[8] are present in the mucosa-associated lymphoid system including reduced numbers of T-helper and T-suppressor cells, altered T-helper/T-suppressor ratios in the lamina propria,[9] and a reduction in both IgA-producing plasma cells and soluble IgA secretion.[10] Interestingly, following HAART, these mucosal immunological abnormalities may be reversed.[11] Also, nonimmune gastrointestinal protective mechanisms are impaired in AIDS. Hypochlorhydria or achlorhydria, of unclear etiology, has been found in 20% of AIDS patients[12,13] and has been correlated with the development of enteric *Mycobacterium avium* complex (MAC) infection and other opportunistic infections.[13] Given these alterations in the native protective mechanisms, it is not surprising that GI infections are so common in these patients.

ENTERIC VIRAL INFECTIONS

Cytomegalovirus and herpes simplex virus (HSV), two highly prevalent species of Herpesviridae, rarely cause enteric infection in the general population; while in contrast, they are among the most common opportunistic pathogens complicating immunodeficiency states especially AIDS.[1,14] A number of other viruses have been found in immunosuppressed patients with GI complaints, most notably diarrhea, but a clear etiologic link remains poorly defined because they are often found in combination with more traditional pathogens.[15] Enteric infection by HIV has also been postulated to cause several GI diseases such as idiopathic esophageal ulcerations and HIV enteropathy, although HIV itself has rarely been identified in the involved tissue.[16,17]

Viral infections

Cytomegalovirus
Epidemiology
Cytomegalovirus (CMV) is one of the most common OIs found across the spectrum of immunosuppressed patients. This frequency relates to the high prevalence of prior exposure to CMV which may be greater than 90% in underdeveloped countries,[18] and the fact that CMV disease generally occurs from recrudescence of latent infection during periods of profound immunosuppression. After transplantation, CMV disease may occur as a result of primary infection, after organ donation by a seropositive donor, or secondary to reactivation of latent infection when the recipient or donor is CMV seropositive.[19] CMV disease is an independent predictor of death in immunocompromised patients with AIDS and contributes significantly to morbidity and mortality.[20] Like all OIs in AIDS, the key determinant of the incidence and perhaps severity of CMV disease is the degree of cell-mediated immunodeficiency.[21] CMV disease is uncommon until the CD4+ cell count falls below 100/mm[3]. In the pre-HAART era, the incidence of gastrointestinal CMV disease in AIDS averaged 30%, with reported rates from 4.4% to 52%.[21,22] Although symptomatic extraintestinal disease is uncommon in most persons with GI CMV disease, occult retinal involvement can be identified in 10% and up to 13% of untreated cases will develop retinopathy over the ensuing 2 weeks.[23] While CMV disease has been documented throughout the entire GI tract, for unclear reasons, the colon and esophagus are the predominant sites of involvement clinically.

Clinical features
Constitutional symptoms are prevalent with active infection and the predominant symptom will be dictated by the site(s) of organ involvement. High-grade fever is uncommon while weight loss is typical regardless of disease location. Esophageal disease is characteristically manifested by odynophagia which is often severe, with large solitary or multiple deep ulcers seen at endoscopy.[24] Gastric involvement presents with epigastric pain which is often constant and associated with nausea, vomiting, and weight loss. Disease of the small intestinal may manifest as abdominal pain, bleeding, or rarely perforation, but significant diarrhea is uncommon. Colonic CMV infection characteristically manifests as a chronic watery diarrhea; abdominal pain is often a prominent feature, and both occult and overt bleeding may occur.[21,25]

Diagnosis
Endoscopic examination with biopsy is required for the diagnosis of CMV enteritis. The endoscopic and histological hallmark of CMV disease is mucosal ulceration. Although variable, deep ulcers are very characteristic for disease in AIDS, whereas in other immunocompromised patients, lesions tend to remain more superficial. An appearance mimicking inflammatory bowel disease, both ulcerative colitis and Crohn's disease, has been described.[25] Unusual findings include a pseudotumor appearance[26] and pseudomembranous colitis.[25] The viral cytopathic effect of CMV is typically located in endothelial and mesenchymal cells in the granulation tissue of the ulcer base. Inclusions are large (cytomegalo) and often have an eosinophilic appearance that may be located either in the nucleus or cytoplasm.[27] Immunohistochemical stains play a valuable role in selected patients to confirm the presence of CMV, and they will often highlight more infected cells than are appreciated by routine hematoxylin and eosin staining.[27,28] For the diagnosis of colonic disease, the yield of sigmoidoscopy ranges from 65% to100% with disease proximal to the left colon found in one-third or more.[29] When rectosigmoid symptoms such as tenesmus or left lower quadrant pain are reported, sigmoidoscopy alone is generally adequate.[30] Random biopsies of normal-appearing mucosa are rarely helpful to exclude CMV, but may identify other infections as a cause of symptoms. Therapy is recommended to all patients, especially those with AIDS, as untreated disease is almost universally progressive and mortality rates are high.[21]

Treatment
A number of effective antiviral agents are available which provide opportunities to individualize therapy (Table 7.1). For all immunosuppressed patients, improving immune function is an integral part of management.

Ganciclovir, a nucleoside analogue of guanosine with structural homology to acyclovir, was the first agent demonstrating efficacy in the treatment of CMV infection in humans. Although CMV does not possess a thymidine kinase, its CMV UL97 gene product is believed to provide the kinase activity needed for initial phosphorylation,[31] and mutation in the *UL97* gene is believed to be one of the primary mechanisms by which resistance to ganciclovir develops.[32] Reversible bone marrow suppression is the

Table 7.1 Treatment of enteric viral infections in immunocompromised hosts

Agent administration	Gastrointestinal indication	Major side effects
Acyclovir (i.v.) 5 mg/kg q8h (7–10 days)	HSV esophagitis/proctitis	Rare, well tolerated
Ganciclovir (i.v.) 5 mg/kg q12h *	CMV disease †	Neutropenia Thrombocytopenia
Ganciclovir (p.o.) 1 g t.i.d.	CMV maintenance/prophylaxis (benefit unproved)	Same as i.v. therapy (less common/less severe)
Foscarnet (i.v.) 60 mg/kg q8h ‡ or 90 mg/kg q12h ‡	CMV disease † Acyclovir-resistant HSV	Electrolyte abnormal Nephrotoxicity
Cidofovir (i.v.) 5 mg/kg every other wk §	CMV disease † Acyclovir-resistant HSV	Nephrotoxicity

i.v., intravenously; q8h, every 8 h; HSV, herpes simplex virus; CMV, cytomegalovirus; p.o., orally; t.i.d., three times daily.
* Ganciclovir should be infused intravenously over a 1 h period at a constant rate. An infusion pump is recommended.
† The lesion should be evaluated endoscopically after 2 wk of therapy. If CMV has been documented and the lesion fails to demonstrate improvement at the interval, a switch to another agent or, if necessary, combination therapy is recommended. A switch is not necessary for partial responders. Such lesions should be re-evaluated after 2 wk of additional therapy.
‡ Foscarnet should be infused intravenously with 750–1000 mL of normal saline.
§ Cidofovir should be infused with 1–2 L of normal saline and administered with probenecid: 2 g 3 h before infusion, 1 g 2 and 8 h after infusion.

most common side effect[33] with leukopenia occurring in 25–68% of patients, usually occurring within the first 2 weeks of treatment. Concomitant use of zidovudine or other bone marrow suppressing agents may exacerbate the bone marrow effects. Ganciclovir-induced neutropenia can be ameliorated by treatment with granulocyte growth factors and thus treatment-related discontinuation is rarely necessary. Since ganciclovir is renally excreted, dose reductions in patients with renal insufficiency are required.[34] The drug must be given intravenously.

Ganciclovir has been extensively studied in immunosuppressed patients for the treatment of CMV infection. In contrast to 17% remission rates for gastrointestinal CMV disease in untreated historical controls,[35] numerous studies have demonstrated responses rates of 56–83% for ganciclovir.[35,36] In contrast to many of the CMV treatment trials in AIDS, transplant trials have generally evaluated responses from disease at all sites rather than the gastrointestinal tract alone. Overall, the use of ganciclovir or foscarnet (see below) has generally been associated with response rates as high as 93–100% in solid organ recipients,[33,35] and treatment of CMV disease has been associated with enhanced allograft and patient survival. Relapse rates range 0–40% over a period of 15–60 weeks.[35] Long-term maintenance therapy is usually not required. Open-label trials of ganciclovir for HIV-infected patients with gastrointestinal CMV disease have demonstrated clinical improvement in ≈75% of patients.[21,35,36] A placebo-controlled trial of ganciclovir for colitis in AIDS found no clinically significant differences between the treatment groups, probably because the treatment period was only for 2 weeks.[23] Although an oral formulation of ganciclovir is available, its very low bioavailability (<10%) makes it an inadequate therapy for the treatment of active infection.[37] A new formulation of ganciclovir, valganciclovir, a prodrug of ganciclovir, has a bioavailability of 60% and when given in therapeutic doses, blood levels equivalent to 5 mg/kg of intravenous ganciclovir are achieved.[38] A controlled trial comparing valganciclovir to intravenous ganciclovir for induction therapy of CMV retinitis in AIDS found no difference in response rates or time to progression.[39] The induction dose of valganciclovir is 900 mg b.i.d. and once daily for maintenance.

While there are no large trials evaluating the efficacy of this agent for active GI disease, its bioavailability suggests a potential role. This drug has become an important option for CMV prophylaxis in the transplant setting (see below).

Foscarnet (phosphonoformate) is an intravenously administered agent whose mechanism of action is inhibition of viral DNA synthesis. Foscarnet inhibits the DNA polymerase of all herpesviruses and also has activity against the reverse transcriptase of retroviruses.[40] The side effects profile and tolerability of foscarnet differs significantly from ganciclovir relegating foscarnet to second-line therapy. Acute tubular necrosis and electrolyte abnormalities, the most common and serious side effects of foscarnet, occur in at least 40% of patients.[41] Electrolyte abnormalities include hypocalcemia (caused by transient chelation of calcium by foscarnet), hypomagnesemia, hypokalemia, and hypophosphatemia or hyperphosphatemia.[42] Less common side effects include anemia, elevated liver enzymes, painful orogenital ulcerations, and particularly with high plasma concentrations (>350 μmol/L), malaise, nausea, vomiting, fatigue, and headache. Vigorous hydration with infusions of isotonic saline, reducing the dosing frequency from every 8 h to every 12 h and avoidance of the concomitant administration of other nephrotoxic agents reduce the risk of renal toxicity.[41] Foscarnet-induced renal impairment is generally reversible in patients with normal baseline renal function.

For patients with major contraindications or failure to respond to ganciclovir, foscarnet is usually effective. Open-label trials of foscarnet have yielded comparable overall efficacy to ganciclovir.[42–45] One randomized study comparing ganciclovir to foscarnet in the therapy of CMV esophagitis found no difference between both agents.[45] Marked endoscopic improvement was observed in 73% of foscarnet-treated and 70% of ganciclovir-treated patients. The symptomatic response was also similar for both treatments: 82% of patients who received foscarnet and 80% of those treated with ganciclovir had a complete or at least a good clinical response.[45] A randomized trial comparing ganciclovir to foscarnet in 48 AIDS patients with gastrointestinal CMV disease also found similar clinical efficacy (73%) regardless of the location of disease (esophagus versus colon) with endoscopic improvement documented in over 80%.[43] Time to progression of disease was similar (13–16 weeks) despite the use of maintenance therapy. Side effects occurred in half the patients in both groups. The recommended dosing schedule is 90 mg/kg i.v. b.i.d. daily for 14–21 days. Salzberger et al.[46] demonstrated in an open-label randomized trial that a frequency reduction of foscarnet from 7 to 5 days a week for 3 weeks was associated with equivalent response and less side effects than using the medication daily for 21 days.

Concomitant administration of ganciclovir and foscarnet show synergistic activity against CMV in vitro.[47] Combination therapy of foscarnet (90 mg/kg b.i.d. daily) and ganciclovir (5 mg/kg b.i.d. daily) may be as effective as primary (induction) therapy and maintenance therapy with a single drug[48] and is also effective for ganciclovir failures.[49] However, the efficacy of available agents coupled with modification of immunosuppressive therapy makes this option rarely necessary today.

Cidofovir is the newest intravenous agent available for treatment of CMV disease. Cidofovir, a nucleotide analogue in monophosphate form, is not dependent on phosphorylation by viral enzymes.[50] Phosphorylation to the active triphosphate metabolite is accomplished by enzymes present in all cells, regardless of whether they are infected by CMV.[51] Thus, cidofovir may be of particular value in the setting of CMV resistance to ganciclovir resulting from mutations in the phosphorylating viral gene product (CMV UL97).[52] Furthermore, cidofovir also demonstrates in vitro and in vivo activity against HSV, Epstein-Barr virus, and varicella-zoster virus.[52]

Published trials of cidofovir have been of relatively small numbers, focused almost exclusively on CMV retinitis in AIDS patients, and have not compared it to other intravenous agents.[53,54] Clinical experience, however, suggests efficacy for the treatment of GI disease. Cidofovir is particularly attractive because of its long half-life which allows intravenous administration on an every other week schedule thereby negating the need for long-term indwelling catheters and associated catheter-related infections. However, cidofovir appears to be more toxic than ganciclovir or foscarnet. The most significant side effect is dose- and schedule-dependent nephrotoxicity, characterized by proximal convoluted tubule degeneration, proteinuria and a rise in serum creatinine.[53] The damage can occasionally be irreversible, particularly with more frequent and higher-dose administration. The addition of concomitant oral probenecid (believed to compete with cidofovir for uptake in the tubules)[51] intravenous saline infusion, extended dosing intervals of 5 mg/kg every other week, preinfusion monitoring of renal function, and limiting its use to those patients without renal insufficiency have all significantly reduced nephrotoxicity.[54] Unfortunately, probenecid use is commonly associated with side effects, with approximately one-third of patients receiving combination therapy experiencing neutropenia ($\approx$15%), gastrointestinal disturbances, headache, hypersensitivity reactions, and fever.[53]

Duration of therapy and follow up

No studies have formally addressed the duration of therapy for isolated gastrointestinal disease. Premature discontinuation of therapy increases the risk of disease recrudescence and potential for development of viral resistance. Symptomatic remission does not necessarily predict endoscopic healing, and most patients require treatment for at least 2–3 weeks, and 4–6 weeks may be necessary for complete healing. Changing to a different anti-CMV agent should be considered whenever minimal or no response is seen during an interval examination. Because of their different mechanisms of action, ganciclovir and foscarnet can be substituted for each other when resistance to one is suspected.[49] Multiple biopsies of any abnormal mucosa should be repeated with each examination to identify previously 'missed' pathogens that might contribute to poor healing. Reduction of immunosuppressive therapy after transplantation, when possible, and improvement of immune function with HAART are cornerstones of management.

Maintenance therapy and prevention of recurrence

Before HAART, maintenance therapy was the standard of care after induction therapy for CMV retinitis in AIDS to prevent the invariably rapid disease recrudescence and progression to irreversible blindness.[55] Recurrence estimates of 22–57% within the first 4 months after completion of therapy have been primarily derived from small uncontrolled trials, many of which failed to separate data on enteric and retinal disease.[43] Most of these studies were performed in the pre-HAART era and do not represent current practices.

As with most OIs in AIDS, improvement in immune function may negate the need for maintenance treatment, and maintenance therapy for CMV disease can be discontinued if HAART increases the CD4 count to >200 cells.[56] Gastrointestinal recurrence is generally less common than retinal recurrence, and responses to retreatment are excellent.[35] While not formally studied for gastrointestinal CMV disease, the available evidence has failed to demonstrate either a reduction in gastrointestinal recurrence rates or a delay in the onset of recurrent disease in patients receiving maintenance therapy.[43] Generally, maintenance doses are half of the induction doses. Indicated at a dose of 1 g three times daily, oral ganciclovir is less effective than either intravenous ganciclovir (5 mg/kg/day) or foscarnet (90–120 mg/kg/day) in preventing reactivation or slowing the progression of retinitis.[57] If maintenance therapy is anticipated, valganciclovir at 900 mg day is a reasonable choice.[58,59]

Primary prophylaxis and preemptive therapy

Oral ganciclovir and valganciclovir have been used for primary prophylaxis in HIV-infected patients when immunodeficiency is severe (CD4 count <100/mm³) and selectively in high-risk transplant patients. Randomized placebo-controlled studies of oral ganciclovir for primary prophylaxis have demonstrated some reduction in the incidence of retinal involvement with no effect on GI involvement.[60] No definite data exist on the effectiveness of primary prophylaxis for decreasing gastrointestinal CMV disease in HIV-infected patients. As noted, secondary prophylaxis with intravenous ganciclovir or foscarnet has not been shown to affect disease progression among HIV-infected patients with gastrointestinal CMV-disease.

Prophylaxis is a common strategy for high-risk patients following transplantation. Prophylactic treatment typically consists of antiviral therapy started at the time of transplantation and continued for at least 100 days post transplantation. This is particularly important for high-risk patients such as those who are donor CMV positive/CMV seronegative recipients. Another strategy employed is termed preemptive, where antiviral treatment is initiated based on the detection of primary or reactivated CMV infection by positive CMV cultures, positive antigenemia assay, or other molecular assays.[61,62] In a study of bone marrow transplant patients, Humar et al.[62] showed that an antigen-based preemptive treatment reduced the incidence of CMV disease at day 400 after transplantation to 1.7% compared to 12.1% when therapy was instituted at the detection of positive cultures on bronchoalveolar lavage fluid obtained at 35 days after transplant. In HIV-infected patients, CMV antigenemia has also been used to predict subsequent CMV disease, thus identifying potential candidates for preemptive therapy.[63] Intravenous ganciclovir is generally considered the drug of choice for very high-risk patients for preemptive therapy whereas prophylactic therapy is typically administered with oral ganciclovir,[64] valganciclovir, or, in older studies, high-dose acyclovir. Currently, valganciclovir is used perioperatively in many patients and is continued until the profound immunosuppression is reversed.

Herpes simplex virus

Epidemiology, clinical features, diagnosis

Herpes simplex virus (HSV) is an uncommon cause of enteritis and, with rare exception, almost all occurrences have been limited to the esophagus and rectum with rare case reports of gastric and/or small bowel disease.[65] Although HSV disease in persons with AIDS may occur as a result of direct extension of primary oropharyngeal or perianal infection, enteric disease is more likely to occur as a result of secondary reactivation of latent viral infection.[66] HSV infection is more likely to be chronic in AIDS patients than in immunocompetent hosts, and CD4+ cell counts are generally less than 50/mm³ in affected individuals.[66]

Symptomatic patients may complain of fever with more specific symptoms localized to the site of disease. Generally, infection is localized to squamous cells and thus the predilection for esophageal and perianal disease. Like CMV, mucosal ulceration is the hallmark of infection and dictates the clinical presentation. Urinary retention and constipation are typical of sacral nerve involvement associated with genital disease.[65] Posterior thigh pain, perineal paresthesias, or impotence may also occur. HSV proctitis is associated with complaints of tenesmus, passage of mucus or blood, and/or purulence. The lesions typically appear in the anorectal areas as small ulcers and perianal disease is usually present in patients with proctitis.

Endoscopic visualization is required to make a definitive diagnosis of HSV esophagogastritis and proctitis. Examination may reveal small, sharply demarcated vesicles (an early finding). Numerous small ulcerations, resembling volcanoes, which may become confluent, are common on upper endoscopy.[67] Biopsy specimens will demonstrate the characteristic findings of multinucleated cells and intranuclear inclusions.[27]

Treatment

For the patient with mild to moderate HSV disease who is able to tolerate pills, oral administration of acyclovir 15–30 mg/kg/day is effective.[68] The drug is usually given in a dose of 400 mg p.o. 5 times a day for 2 weeks. Absorption of oral acyclovir is inconsistent and may be as low as <30%;[65] thus, for patients with more severe disease, a higher dose may be required or intravenous administration is warranted. Intravenous administration, 5 mg/kg (infused for 1 h) every 8 h for 7–10 days,[68] should be given when oral intake is limited or when the patient has not responded to

high-dose oral therapy. Several studies have confirmed the safety and efficacy of foscarnet (40 mg/kg every 12 h) for treatment, as well as supported the utility of this agent as a maintenance therapy by delaying recurrences.[68] Although partial responders may benefit from a prolonged course of therapy, a change to foscarnet may be necessary in these cases. Valaciclovir and famciclovir, two other oral agents, are also highly effective against HSV.[68] Primary prophylaxis is not currently recommended; secondary prophylaxis is usually provided for patients with genital disease or those with frequent relapses of oropharyngeal or esophageal disease. Recurrences may be suppressed with acyclovir (400–600 mg daily). Chronic acyclovir use has been associated with the development of resistance,[69] and foscarnet is the drug of choice in this setting[70] and may be followed by a return to acyclovir sensitivity.[70]

Mycobacterial infections

Mycobacterium avium complex

Epidemiology

Mycobacterium avium and *M. intracellulare* are two atypical mycobacterial species that are ubiquitous in nature,[71] and human infection is largely confined to persons with severe immunosuppression such as those with AIDS. These organisms, referred to collectively as MAC or *M. avium-intracellulare* (MAI) because they are difficult to distinguish, represent one of the most common opportunistic infections in persons with advanced AIDS.[72] MAC infection is 2.5 times as common when CD4+ cell counts are less than 10/mm³ as compared with individuals with CD4+ cell counts of 40–59/mm³ and is rare when CD4+ cell counts are greater than 100/mm³.[72]

Havlik et al.[73] prospectively followed a cohort of AIDS patients with CD4 counts <200 cells/mm³ with blood cultures for MAC every 3 months and found a 23% incidence rate per year. More recent data suggest a fall in disease incidence due to HAART and use of prophylaxis in high-risk patients.[74] MAC lymphadenitis has also been reported as part of the immune reconstitution inflammatory syndrome.[75]

Clinical features and diagnosis

Although MAC infection can manifest with localized symptoms, systemic symptoms dominate the clinical expression of disease.[73] The most common symptoms include fever (87%), night sweats (78%), diarrhea (47%), weight loss greater than 20 lb (38%), abdominal pain (35%), and nausea and vomiting (26%).[73] MAC infiltration of the liver and spleen, which is usually asymptomatic, often causes organomegaly and liver involvement characteristically is associated with elevations of alkaline phosphatase and γ-glutamyl transpeptidase levels that can be striking at 10–20 times the upper limits of normal.

Blood culture using isolator tubes is the most sensitive means of identifying MAC infection. If positive, a presumptive diagnosis may be made and treatment initiated. Once positive, over 97% of subsequent blood cultures remain positive in untreated patients. Liver biopsy appears to be more sensitive than bone marrow biopsy in patients with cholestatic liver tests,[76] and lymph node biopsy may sometimes be necessary. Bone marrow aspirate with AFB staining and culture, especially in patients with evidence of bone marrow dysfunction, may be appropriate prior to liver biopsy as it is safer. MAC appears endoscopically within the small and/or large bowel as yellow plaques or nodules; histology generally shows numerous pathogens which are easily identified by mycobacterial staining. In the patient with diarrhea, stool examination is not generally helpful in making the diagnosis of MAC infection in persons with AIDS and mucosal biopsy with appropriate staining and culture has the highest yield for GI involvement.[77]

Treatment

MAC is much more difficult to treat than *Mycobacterium tuberculosis* because of antibiotic resistance. This resistance is multi-factorial, including its intracellular growth and protective outer polysaccharide wall,[78] the high frequency of genetic diversity within any one infection (multiple strains with heterogeneous patterns of resistance),[79] and the severity of AIDS immuno-suppression in infected patients.[72] Based on in vitro sensitivities, the macrolide antibiotics clarithromycin and azithromycin, rifabutin, ethambutol, clofazimine, ciprofloxacin, and amikacin have all been evaluated for clinical efficacy against MAC (Table 7.2). Of these, clarithromycin[80] and azithromycin[81] have demonstrated the greatest clinical activity against MAC.

Clarithromycin[82] and *azithromycin*[83] effectively reduce MAC bacterial counts in the blood of affected patients with AIDS. Single-drug therapy with either agent, as well as multidrug regimens containing one of these macrolides, has been shown to reduce symptoms and bacteremia colony counts and is far more effective than any regimen of which they are not a component (and with less toxicity). Although clarithromycin (500–2000 mg twice daily) has demonstrated dose-dependent rates of clearance of MAC bacteremia,[80] no difference in MAC-free blood cultures has been seen between high and low doses at 12 weeks.[81] Lower doses have been associated with less gastrointestinal toxicity,[84] a primary cause of discontinuation of therapy, and interrupted drug administration for 7 or more days is a main contributor to the development of resistant organisms.[80] Unfortunately, the use of clarithromycin alone has been associated with recrudescence of MAC infection with clarithromycin-resistant organisms in up to 25% of patients after discontinuation of therapy.[80]

In an attempt to prevent resistance and recurrence, a variety of combination regimens have been studied. *Ethambutol* is well tolerated, has demonstrated clinical efficacy as monotherapy, and has been associated with reduced resistance when used in combination with clarithromycin.[85] The US Public Health Service Task Force on Prophylaxis and Therapy for *Mycobacterium avium* Complex has recommended the use of ethambutol with either clarithromycin or azithromycin in any anti-MAC regimen.[86]

Rifabutin also has demonstrated efficacy as monotherapy for MAC and in combination regimens.[87] The addition of rifabutin to clarithromycin and ethambutol has been associated with a reduced frequency of clarithromycin-resistant relapses. Although a dose–response effect was seen in the rate and frequency of clearance of bacteremia, no difference in median survival was seen with regimens containing rifabutin at doses of 600 or 300 mg/day.[87] Despite its efficacy, therapy with rifabutin has been associated with important side effects, including uveitis and multiple drug interactions, which makes its involvement in combination therapy less clear.[87,88]

A prospective randomized trial compared the outcome of clarithromycin combined with ethambutol and rifabutin, or both, in patients with disseminated MAC.[89] Of the 160 treated patients, after 12 weeks of treatment, no statistical difference was seen in microbiologic response among the three groups, although the clarithromycin plus ethambutol plus rifabutin group had a 51% response as compared to 40% in the clarithromycin plus ethambutol. In all, the triple therapy group had improved survival compared to the other two groups.

Ciprofloxacin (500–750 mg twice daily) and *amikacin* (15 mg/kg) are other agents demonstrating in vitro activity against MAC.[90] However, their contribution to the efficacy of combination regimens has not yet been studied in randomized, controlled fashion. Clofazimine offers reduced benefit over clarithromycin and ethambutol.

As with other OIs, effective antiretroviral therapy, when associated with immune reconstitution, may negate the need for long-term maintenance therapy. In a study of 48 patients who had received a macrolide-containing regimen for MAC and who had responded to HAART and were then followed without long-term MAC therapy, only one patient had disease recurrence.[91]

Mycobacterium tuberculosis

Epidemiology

Gastrointestinal TB is uncommon in immunocompromised hosts from developed countries but its prevalence remains high in Africa and Asia. In a study of 100 hospitalized HIV-infected

---

Table 7.2 Treatment of *Mycobacterium avium* complex in AIDS

Drug	Dosage	Adverse effects and comments
Clarithromycin *	500 mg b.i.d.	GI side effects common, dose limiting in 20%
Ethambutol	15 mg/kg/day	Generally well tolerated
Additional agents for MAC infection		
Rifabutin †	150–300 mg/day	Uveitis
Amikacin	15 mg/kg/day	Nephrotoxicity
Ciprofloxacin	500–750 mg b.i.d.	Well tolerated, least efficacious

AIDS, acquired immunodeficiency syndrome; b.i.d., twice daily; GI, gastrointestinal; MAC, *Mycobacterium avium* complex.
* A minimum of clarithromycin and ethambutol is recommended as initial therapy for MAC. The combination has been associated with less risk of drug resistance and MAC recurrence. Additional agents will frequently be required, however. Although no head-to-head studies exist, azithromycin 500 mg/day, can substitute for clarithromycin.
† Most patients with MAC will be receiving protease inhibitors. When rifabutin is used in such patients, the recommended starting dose is 150 mg/day.

patients from South Africa with CD4 counts <100 cells, the prevalence of disseminated MAC was 10% while 54% for *Mycobacterium tuberculosis*.[92] In most cases, tuberculosis represents recrudescence of prior infection rather than primary infection. While infection may occur at higher CD4 counts than from other opportunistic infections, in many series, however, the CD4 count is often <100 mm³.[93]

Clinical features and diagnosis

The clinical presentation is dependent upon the organ(s) of involvement. Although TB can involve any segment of the gastro-intestinal tract, terminal ileal disease is most common and presents with abdominal pain, diarrhea, and bleeding. Esophageal involvement manifests as chest pain, odynophagia, or due to a symptomatic fistula in the tracheobronchial tree. Bleeding may occur anywhere throughout the gastrointestinal tract when ulceration is present. The diagnosis can be established by appropriate staining of mucosal biopsy specimens, blood cultures, or, in those with pulmonary infection, sputum staining and culture.

Therapy

Multidrug therapy is required for the effective treatment of GI TB. Unlike MAC and other OIs in AIDS, antimicrobial therapy, when taken appropriately and provided there is no drug resistance, results in clinical cure.[94–96] Caution must be exercised when combining TB therapy with HAART as there are many drug interactions. For example, rifampin induces the activity of p-450 CYP3A which reduces serum concentrations of protease inhibitors and non-nucleoside reverse transcriptase inhibitors to subtherapeutic levels.[96]

Enteric protozoan infections in aids

Protozoal infections are among the most common GI infections in patients with AIDS, and less so in other immunocompromised patients. *Giardia lamblia* and *Entamoeba histolytica* are more commonly associated with enteric infection in HIV-seronegative hosts; however, *Giardia* is a frequent intestinal infection in patients with hypogammaglobulinemia.[97] *Cryptosporidium*, Microsporida, and *Isospora* are rarely associated with symptomatic infection outside of persons with AIDS but have rarely been described in outbreaks in normal hosts.[98] Before HAART, these protozoa were responsible for a disproportionate burden of the morbidity and mortality associated with AIDS, but like all OIs, antiretroviral therapy has resulted in a large fall in both prevalence and incidence.

Cryptosporidium, Microsporida, and Isospora
Epidemiology

Cryptosporidium parvum and *Cryptosporidium muris* have been identified in 10–55% of persons with AIDS and chronic diarrhea, the highest prevalence being seen in developing nations.[98,99] Infection can also occur in immunocompetent individuals, where infection generally results in a self-limited diarrhea.[100] Persons at increased risk of exposure to cryptosporidial infection include animal handlers, homosexual men, hospital personnel, children in daycare, and close household contacts of infected individuals.[100] Likewise, Microsporida have been identified in 7–50% of persons with AIDS and unexplained diarrhea.[98,101] Microsporidial infection in persons without AIDS is extremely rare, however, and

infection is limited to two species, *Enterocytozoon bieneusi* and *Septata intestinalis*. In contrast to cryptosporidia and microsporidia, *Isospora belli* has a significantly narrower geographic distribution, endemic primarily to tropical and subtropical regions. Although identified in fewer than 2% of persons with AIDS and diarrhea in the United States, the prevalence of *I. belli* is 8–10 times higher in persons with AIDS from Haiti.[102]

Clinical features

In contrast to the acute, self-limited diarrheal illness observed in the rare immunocompetent individual infected by cryptosporidia, microsporidia, or *Isospora*, infection in persons with AIDS is generally manifested by chronic, watery diarrhea. Affected individuals may experience abdominal cramps, anorexia, nausea, and weight loss. Weight loss is particularly prominent with cryptosporidia, perhaps related to more significant malabsorption. Infection is not generally observed until CD4+ cell counts have dropped below 100/mm³,[98,103] with milder disease observed in those with more preserved immune function. Although diarrhea may be intermittent, it is often severe with reported daily stool frequencies range from 6 to 25 times and stool volumes ranging 1–25 L.[98] Secondary dehydration, malnutrition, and weight loss contribute significantly to the morbidity and mortality of these infections in AIDS. The degree of parasite burden likely explains the variable clinical expression and outcome.[104]

Diagnosis

Stool studies are the mainstay of diagnosis for cryptosporidia, microsporidia, and *Isospora*. The sensitivity of these examinations is frequently low, however, due to erratic fecal shedding, variable protozoan burdens, and differences in operator experience searching for the pathogen in stool specimens. Consequently, diagnosis often requires intestinal biopsies. Although these pathogens may be identified by light microscopy, electron microscopy of small bowel mucosa and special histopathologic stains make identification much easier, particularly for microsporidiosis.[105]

Treatment

Malnutrition, dehydration, and electrolyte abnormalities are common in patients with AIDS and protozoan diarrhea. Nutritional support is essential, with oral intake high in calories and low in fat. Lactose-containing foods should be avoided. Severely affected patients may require short-term parenteral nutrition and volume support. Non-specific antidiarrheal agents, including loperamide or other tincture of opium, are helpful in controlling volume losses and improving quality of life. Although not universally successful in randomized trials, some patients have appeared to respond to subcutaneous administrations of octreotide (100–500 µg three times daily).[106] The higher doses of octreotide may exacerbate diarrhea as a result of inhibition of pancreatic exocrine secretion.

Cryptosporidium: specific therapy

Paromomycin, an aminoglycoside, has been the most extensively studied agent for cryptosporidial diarrhea in patients with AIDS. In vitro cell culture systems have demonstrated cryptosporidial sensitivity to this agent.[107] Prospective placebo-controlled studies have shown short-term response rates from 56% to 92%; however, complete clinical and fecal responses were seen in as few as

20%.[108] The best response rates were seen in patients with the highest CD4+ cell counts (>120–150/mm³).[109] A dose–response effect for paromomycin was suggested by the return of symptoms in patients discontinuing therapy and patients dropping from induction dosing (2 g/day) to maintenance dosing (1 g/day).[108]

One potential therapy is that of passive immunotherapy through ingestion of *hyperimmune bovine colostrum*. Bovine colostrum has been studied because cows are naturally immunized against *C. parvum*, the protozoan being a common bovine pathogen.[110] In contrast to the effect seen with non-amplified bovine colostrum,[110] several small studies have reported positive responses to hyperimmune bovine colostrum in patients with AIDS and cryptosporidial diarrhea.[111]

Other agents under investigation include *letrazuril*,[112] a benzene acetonitrile used in the prevention and treatment of coccidial infections in domestic foul, and nitazoxanide,[113,114] a 5-nitrothiazole compound effective against a broad range of parasites and bacteria, and azithromycin.[115] To date, these studies have demonstrated incomplete responses, particularly with regard to bowel clearance, and symptom responses have been short-lived.

Microsporida: specific therapy

Determinations of therapeutic response to specific agents have been hampered by the lack of prospective, blinded, and controlled studies, the small numbers of patients studied in reported series, erratic protozoan shedding in feces, and the often intermittent nature of associated diarrhea. Although a number of studies have suggested microsporidial sensitivity to *metronidazole* or *albendazole*, reported responses have often been short-lived and little correlation has been observed between symptom response and pathogen clearance.[98,116] The best clinical response rates are with albendazole (400 mg twice daily)[117] with good response in 57% (13/23) and a partial response in 39%; however, all 23 patients demonstrated persistence of microsporidia. It is now clear that albendazole is effective for *Septata* but not for *E. bieunusi*.[98] A study of 19 AIDS patients with albendazole-unresponsive, chronic microsporidial diarrhea demonstrated a complete response to thalidomide (100 mg nightly) in 7 of 19 (37%) and a partial response in 3 of 19 (16%).[118] The mechanism of the potential activity of thalidomide is unclear.

Several studies have demonstrated resolution of OIs in patients receiving only HAART.[119,120] Carr and colleagues[119] demonstrated complete resolution of chronic diarrhea secondary to micro-sporidiosis (five patients), cryptosporidiosis (three patients), or both (one patient) in nine AIDS patients who were treated with combination HIV therapy that included at least one protease inhibitor. A drop in CD4+ cell counts 7 to 13 months later was associated with recurrence of diarrhea in five of nine patients (56%). These results show that immune reconstitution results in remission alone and underscore the importance of preserving the immune system.

Isospora: specific therapy

I. belli is responsive to trimethoprim-sulfamethoxazole (TMP-SMX). A dose of one double-strength (DS) tablet (trimethoprim, 320 mg/sulfamethoxazole, 1600 mg) 4 times daily is given for 10 days, followed by one DS tablet twice daily for 3 weeks.[102] Although most patients will respond to this regimen, relapse occurs in up to 50%. Symptoms are usually responsive to

retreatment, but maintenance therapy is often necessary. As second-line therapy, pyrimethamine (75 mg four times daily) with or without sulfadiazine (4 mg four times daily) is also effective.[121] The widespread use of TMP-SMX for PCP prophylaxis may explain the low rate of *Isospora* infection in developed countries.

Toxoplasma gondii

Epidemiology, clinical features, and diagnosis

T. gondii, an obligate intracellular protozoan parasite, is a common pathogen in the immunocompromised population with approximately 10% of AIDS patients in the US and up to 30% of European AIDS patients estimated to die from toxoplasmosis.[122] Infection occurs by ingestion of tissue cysts in undercooked meat, by ingesting food or water contaminated with oocysts from infected mammals, typically domestic cats, and in the immuno-compromised host, reactivation of latent infection. The most common site of infection is the central nervous system (CNS) followed by the heart and lungs; however, infection may occur in any organ, including the GI tract.[122,123] Reported sites of GI involvement include the stomach, duodenum, and colon with the most prevalent symptoms being abdominal pain, chronic watery diarrhea, nausea, and vomiting.[123] Gastrointestinal involvement usually occurs in patients with concomitant CNS infection. The diagnosis of GI toxoplasmosis is typically made by finding *T. gondii* in host tissue removed by biopsy with microscopic examination revealing cysts filled with bradyzoites and/or crescent-shaped trophozoites. Antibody testing may aid in diagnosis, although the presence of antibodies only establishes that the host has been infected previously, and high titers can remain elevated for several months after infection.[122] Negative *Toxoplasma* titers have also been reported in GI toxoplasmosis.[123]

Treatment

Toxoplasmosis in the immunosuppressed is fatal if not recognized and treated early.[124] Empiric treatment for CNS toxoplasmosis has been applied in cases of gastrointestinal toxoplasmosis; however, the efficacy of this strategy has not been firmly established. Current therapies act mainly against the trophyzoites or proliferative form of disease seen in the acute phase of infection or during reactivation of latent disease in immunocompromised hosts, but do not eradicate the encysted bradyzoites.[125]

The combination of oral pyrimethamine and sulfadiazine is the most effective regimen for treatment of toxoplasmosis in AIDS patients. Leucovorin (folinic acid) 10–25 mg/day should be given to help prevent bone marrow toxicity.[125] In adults, pyrimethamine 200 mg is given as a loading dose on day 1, followed by 75–100 mg/day. Sulfadiazine is given at 1–1.5 gm every 6 hours. These doses are continued for 3–6 weeks at which time pyrimethamine 25–50 mg once a day and sulfadiazine 500–1000 mg every 6 hours are continued indefinitely for maintenance suppressive therapy. Clindamycin 600 mg orally or i.v. every 6 hours in combination with pyrimethamine is an alternative in those who are intolerant of sulfadiazine. Prospective, randomized trials of treatment of toxoplasmic encephalitis showed that pyrimethamine/clindamycin and pyrimethamine/sulfadiazine were equally efficacious during the acute phase of therapy.[126] Trimethoprim-sulfamethoxazole, clarithromycin, azithromycin, dapsone, and atovaquone, in combination with pyrimethamine/folinic acid, have also been used as alternative treatment options.[125] Side effects of pyrimethamine and sulfadiazine are common, requiring frequent monitoring for bone marrow suppression.

Pneumocystis carinii

Epidemiology, clinical features, and diagnosis

P. carinii is a ubiquitous eukaryotic organism that is primarily responsible for pulmonary infection in patients with AIDS and remains one of the most common AIDS-defining illnesses.[1,14] Extrapulmonary disease is rare, and when present, symptoms are generally referable to the site of infection, and pulmonary disease is typically present as well. In many patients with enteric infection, multiple concomitant gastrointestinal sites are involved. Extrapulmonary pneumocystosis is associated with a large tissue burden of organisms and is diagnosed by demonstration of *P. carinii* cysts or trophyzoites in affected tissues.[127]

Treatment

While *P. carinii* has been categorized as a fungal pathogen, it is insensitive to the commonly used antifungal agents.[128] Treatment recommendations for persons with gastrointestinal *P. carinii* infection have been based on clinical experience with pulmonary infection in persons with AIDS.[127] All treatment is given for 21 days and secondary prophylaxis should be continued for life or until CD4 count is greater than 200 for at least three months.[129] TMP-SMX is considered the first-line therapy for *P. carinii*.[130] Oral dosing is 2 double-strength (DS) tablets every 8 hours. When given parenterally, patients with normal renal function are administered 5 mg/kg of trimethoprim plus 25 mg/kg of sulfamethoxazole every 8 hours. Dosing adjustments are necessary in patients with significantly impaired renal function. The most common side effects include neutropenia and anemia (40%), fever (25%), rash (20%); pruritus and rash are significantly more likely in patients with AIDS than in HIV-seronegative persons.[131] As many as 47% of AIDS patients take TMP-SMX. Dapsone (100 mg p.o. q.d.) given with trimethoprim (320 mg p.o. q.d.) is an alternative for patients who cannot take TMP-SMX and appears to be as effective.[132] Clindamycin with primaquine is an alternative for patients unresponsive to TMP-SMX[133] and has been shown to be equally effective. Pentamidine is generally considered second-line therapy,[130] and must be administered parenterally for persons with extrapulmonary pneumocystosis. Less commonly used agents (due either to decreased efficacy or greater toxicity) include atovaquone 750 mg p.o. b.i.d.,[134] trimetrexate plus leucovorin,[135] and eflornithine.[136]

Enteric fungal infections in the immunocompromised

Humans are routinely exposed to multiple fungi present in the environment. With intact host defenses, these organisms rarely cause significant disease except in the case of dimorphic fungi, such as *Histoplasma capsulatum*, which can cause disease even in the normal host. Excluding *Candida* esophagitis (discussed elsewhere), fungal infections of the GI tract are rare, but result in significant morbidity and mortality.

Histoplasma capsulatum

Epidemiology

H. capsulatum, a thermally dimorphic fungus, is endemic in the river valleys of Ohio and Mississippi in the United States and in several other countries, including Guatemala, Mexico, Peru, and Venezuela. Outside of these regions *H. capsulatum* is rarely encountered; however, reactivation of quiescent infection may be seen in those previously exposed while in endemic areas. It is a soil fungus especially seen in soil enriched with bird and bat excrement which accelerates sporulation. Infection is initially confined to the respiratory tract after inhalation of conidia. Infection in the immunocompetent host is typically asymptomatic and spontaneously cleared with approximately 4% developing disseminated disease. In contrast, about 55% of infected immunocompromised patients will develop progressive dissemination.[137] Gastrointestinal involvement, most commonly the colon, is seen in up to 90% of persons with disseminated histoplasmosis.[138]

Clinical features

Enteric involvement is often subclinical, and one-third of cases are not recognized until autopsy. Symptoms depend on the organ(s) involved and systemic symptoms are common.[138,139] The terminal ileum and cecum are the most commonly involved intestinal sites, but mucosal lesions occur anywhere along the GI tract, and multiple sites of involvement are common.[138,139] Up to 25% of patients with microscopically confirmed GI histoplasmosis can have grossly normal GI mucosa. Reported complications include ulceration, hemorrhage (which may be worsened due to coagulopathy and thrombocytopenia), perforation, malabsorption, and small bowel obstruction.[138,139]

Diagnosis

A diagnosis of gastrointestinal histoplasmosis can be made from smears or culture of stool, intestinal biopsy with use of microscopy or culture, or serologic testing. Blood cultures are positive in over 90% of patients with disseminated disease and AIDS but require time and are not specific for gastrointestinal involvement.[140] Serum and urinary *H. capsulatum* antigen levels are useful for diagnosis and may aid in monitoring response to treatment.[141]

Treatment

The mortality of disseminated histoplasmosis without treatment is 80%. Antifungal therapy reduces mortality to <25%.[137,142] For moderate to severe disease in patients with AIDS, therapy consists of a 14-day induction phase with amphotericin B followed by chronic suppressive therapy typically with itraconazole. Amphotericin B, traditionally first-line therapy for patients with AIDS and disseminated histoplasmosis, is associated with an 80–85% response rate when administered at a dose of 0.5–1.0 mg/kg/day for 7–14 days followed by 0.8 mg/kg every other day up to a total dose of 15 mg/kg.[137,143] The traditional form of amphotericin B is associated with significant infusion reactions (rigors, fever, phlebitis) and nephrotoxicity. In a recent randomized, double-blind trial comparing amphotericin B with liposomal amphotericin B for induction therapy of disseminated histoplasmosis in patients with AIDS, the liposomal form of amphotericin B was associated with higher response (88% versus 64%), lower mortality rates (2% versus 13%), fewer infusion-related side effects (25% versus 63%), and less nephrotoxicity (9% versus 37%).[143] In this study, however, there was no difference in mortality after 10 additional weeks of itraconazole in both arms. The recommended dose of liposomal amphotericin B is 3 mg/kg/day i.v. given for 14 days. Amphotericin B may be replaced with itraconazole, 200 mg p.o. b.i.d. (when hospitalization or i.v. therapy is no longer required), to complete a 12-week course of induction therapy. Nevertheless, cost is increased with the liposomal form, and its use is still associated with risk for transfusion reactions and nephrotoxicity. Avoiding dehydration (e.g., hydration before and after infusion with 500 cc normal saline) and the concomitant use of other potentially nephrotoxic agents can reduce the risk of renal toxicity. Itraconazole (300 mg twice daily for 3 days, then 200 mg twice daily for 12 weeks) has also been used effectively as primary therapy for patients with mild disease.[142,144] It is usually given by mouth but can also be given intravenously. Its use by the AIDS Clinical Trial Group was associated with an 85% overall response rate.[144] Neither ketoconazole nor fluconazole is effective as primary treatment of disseminated disease or prevention of relapse in AIDS. Chronic suppressive therapy is necessary to prevent relapse as therapy is not curative for patients with AIDS.[143,145] Itraconazole (200 mg once or twice daily for life) is the treatment of choice for maintenance therapy.[146] Amphotericin B (50–80 mg i.v. twice a week) may be given as an alternative if needed. Itraconazole has been associated with a 5% 2-year relapse rate, similar to that seen with amphotericin. A response to HAART therapy may lessen the need for long-term treatment. Compared to standard amphotericin B, liposomal amphotericin has been shown to have significantly less transfusion-related side effects (rigors, fever, and phlebitis), nephrotoxicity,[143] and fewer breakthrough fungal infections.[147] Itraconazole absorption can be erratic, however, particularly in patients with hypochlorhydria or achlorhydria. Bioavailability of itraconazole is increased when taken with a full meal and should be administered with food. Grapefruit juice should be avoided (or increased dosage of itraconazole might be needed).[86] The concomitant administration of phenytoin, rifampin, and rifabutin should be avoided because these agents result in enhanced hepatic metabolism of itraconazole and significantly reduced drug levels in serum.[86]

Candida albicans

In immunocompromised patients, *C. albicans* is a very rare cause of extraesophageal disease. A large autopsy series of 109 cases of gastrointestinal candidiasis reported *Candida* in the stomach (41%), the small bowel (20%), and the colon (2%) of patients with AIDS.[148] Given the lack of experience with such situations, however, amphotericin B should probably be considered in any patient with AIDS and severe extraesophageal disease secondary to *Candida*. Once symptoms improve, fluconazole, which is very effective, can be instituted.

Aspergillus

Aspergillus species are saprophytic molds found worldwide in the environment, including soil and decaying vegetation. Infection results from direct inoculation or inhalation of aerosolized conidia or spores. Once in the respiratory tract, proliferation of the hyphal form can lead to invasive or disseminated disease by hematogenous spread with visceral organ involvement. Gastrointestinal involvement with *Aspergillus* species is a rare complication of disseminated infection observed primarily in neutropenic patients with clinically apparent pulmonary disease. The most common site of GI aspergillosis is the esophagus, followed by the colon and small intestine.[149,150] Ulceration in the GI tract may result in perforation or infarction.[151] Diagnosis is rarely made antemortem; however, biopsy of the ulceration may demonstrate septate hyphae with dichotomous branching.[151] Prognosis is poor, often due to late diagnosis. Treatment has traditionally been high-dose amphotericin B 1–1.5 mg/kg/day; however, one large randomized trial showed better response and survival in patients with invasive aspergillosis treated with voriconazole.[152] Other treatment options include lipid-based amphotericin B, caspofungin (70 mg i.v. on day 1, then 50 mg i.v. q.d. or 35 mg with hepatic impairment),[153] or itraconazole.[154] Patients who have a good response to amphotericin B may be switched to itraconazole after two weeks.

Intestinal helminthic infection in the immunocompromised

Intestinal helminthic infections such as roundworms, hookworms, tapeworms, and flukes typically cause mild disease, but there are limited data regarding most helminthic infections in the immunocompromised population. However, *Strongyloides stercoralis*, the only helminthic parasite that can complete its life cycle in the human host, has been reported to progress to fulminant fatal disease in patients with compromised immune systems.[155]

Strongyloides stercoralis

Epidemiology, clinical features, and diagnosis

Strongyloides stercoralis, an intestinal nematode (roundworm), generally leads to infection through the transcutaneous route of filariform larvae after exposure to moist, infected soil in tropical and subtropical climates. After penetrating the dermis, the filariform larvae migrate through the venous system to the lungs and tracheobronchial tree and enter the small intestine. In the small intestine the adult female worms lay eggs in the mucosa that hatch into rhabditiform larvae, which are shed in the stool. Filariform larvae lead to an autoinfective cycle either by invading perianally during excretion or directly through the intestinal wall leading to persistent infection with subsequent generations.[155] This autoinfective cycle leads to heavier worm burden which is responsible for serious complications of disease. Chronic infection is typically asymptomatic, but, patients may report episodic vomiting, diarrhea, constipation, and with increased larval burden, intestinal obstruction, ileus, and significant GI bleeding.[155] Immunocompromised individuals are predisposed to develop hyperinfection, an accelerated autoinfection, characterized by development or exacerbation of gastrointestinal and pulmonary symptoms and the presence of increased larvae in stool and/or sputum.[155] This potentially fatal phenomenon has been described in patients with AIDS and patients treated with corticosteroids or immunosuppressive drugs.[156] GI symptoms and manifestations of hyperinfection include abdominal pain or bloating, diarrhea (watery or bloody), constipation, anorexia, weight loss, dysphagia, odynophagia, nausea and vomiting, ileus, small bowel obstruction, frank GI bleeding, and protein-losing enteropathy causing hypoalbuminemia.[156,157] Patients may also have anemia, generalized weakness, fatigue, peripheral eosinophilia, and diffuse myalgias. Endoscopic findings can include mucosal granularity, edema, friability, and frank ulceration involving any portion of the GI tract.[155] Ulceration, when present, is most commonly seen in the small bowel but may occur at any level from the esophagus to the rectum.[155] Hyperinfection may be complicated by spread of gut flora to extraintestinal sites either by invasion through ulcerations or from being carried on or in the larvae themselves. In patients receiving long-term corticosteroids, hyperinfection has yielded mortality rates up to 87%.[158] The diagnosis is established by identification of the organism in stool or in biopsy specimens. In general, however, a single stool examination will fail to detect larvae in up to 70%[158] due to intermittent excretion of larvae; therefore, multiple samples may be required for diagnosis.

Table 7.3 Treatment of protozoan, fungal, and helminthic infections in immunocompromised hosts

Gastrointestinal indication	Agent/administration	Major side effects
Toxoplasma gondii	**Initial treatment (3–6 weeks) *** Pyrimethamine 200 mg p.o. × 1d, then 75–100 mg p.o. q.d.; combined with leukovorin 10–25 mg q.d., and sulfadiazine 1–1.5 gm p.o. q6h	Bone marrow suppression, rash, nephrotoxicity
	Maintenance therapy (indefinitely) Pyrimethamine 25–50 mg p.o. q.d., and sulfadiazine 500–1000 mg p.o. q6h	
Pneumocystis carinii	TMP-SMX 2 DS tabs p.o. q8h, or TMP 5 mg/kg & SMX 25 mg/kg i.v. q8h	Neutropenia, fever, rash, pruritus
	Other † Dapsone 100 mg p.o q.d. with TMP 320 mg p.o. q.d., or Clindamycin p.o./i.v. 300–450 mg q6h with primaquine 15–30 mg i.v. q.d.	Hemolysis, rash, methemoglobinemia, bone marrow toxicity
Histoplasma capsulatum	**Initial treatment (14 days) ‡** Amphotericin B 0.5–1.0 mg/kg/day i.v., or liposomal ampho B 3 mg/kg/day i.v., or	Nephrotoxicity, infusion reactions ¥
	Maintenance therapy (indefinitely) Itraconazole 200 mg b.i.d. then 100 mg q.d. × 7–10 days §	GI disturbances, hepatotoxicity, cardiac toxicity
Candida albicans	Fluconazole 200 mg i.v. or p.o. × 1,	GI disturbances, hepatotoxicity
Aspergillus species	Voriconazole 6 mg/kg i.v. q12h on day 1, then 4 mg/kg i.v. q12 × 7d, then 200 mg p.o. b.i.d.	Generally well tolerated, transient LFT and vision abnormalities
	Other Ampho B 1–1.5 mg/kg/day × 14d, then Itraconazole 200 mg p.o. b.i.d.	Nephrotoxicity, transfusion rxn GI disturbances, hepatotoxicity, cardiac toxicity
Coccidioidomycosis	Amphotericin B 0.6 mg/kg/day; then fluconazole	Nephrotoxicity, transfusion rxn
Cryptococcus	Amphotericin B 0.6 mg/kg/day; then fluconazole	Nephrotoxicity, transfusion rxn
Cryptosporidia	Paromomycin 1 g p.o. b.i.d. Nitazoxanide 0.5–1 gm p.o. b.i.d. Azithromycin 600 mg p.o. q.d	Nausea
Cyclospora	TMP-SMX 2 DS tabs p.o. q8h or ciprofloxacin 500 mg p.o. b.i.d.	Rash, diarrhea
Isopora belli	TMP-SMX 2 DS tabs p.o. q8h or ciprofloxacin or pyramethamine	Rash, diarrhea
Microsporidia	Albendazole 400 mg p.o. b.i.d. /ψ (Encephalitozoon intestinalis) Fumagillin 20 mg p.o. t.i.d. Metronidazole, atovaquone Enterocytozoon bienusi)	Granulocytopenia, pancytopenia Neutropenia Avoid alcohol neuropathy with high dose
Strongyloides stercoralis	Ivermectin 200 μg/kg/day p.o., or Thiabendazole 25 mg/kg p.o. b.i.d., or Albendazole 400 mg p.o. b.i.d. ψ	GI disturbances CNS disturbances, hepatotoxicity, Stevens-Johnson granulocytopenia, pancytopenia

* For sulfadiazine intolerance: clindamycin 600 mg p.o. or i.v. q6h (plus pyrimethamine/leukovorin).
† 3rd-line option for pneumocytosis: pentamidine 4 mg/kg/day i.v. (diluted in 250 mL of 5% dextrose in water given over 1–2 hours).
‡ For mild disease: itraconazole 300 mg p.o. b.i.d. × 3 days.
¥ Fewer side effects with liposomal form.
§ Ampho B or fluconazole 400–800 mg b.i.d. for more severe disease.
ψ Treat until symptom resolution and stools negative for organism for 2 weeks; monitor stools periodically after treatment.

Treatment

The treatment of choice for strongyloidiasis has long been thiabendazole (25 mg/kg p.o. twice a day for 3 days for chronic infection and 7–10 days for hyperinfection). Negative stool studies and symptomatic improvement of chronic strongyloidiasis has been seen in 67–81%.[155] Albendazole (400 mg p.o. b.i.d. for 3 days) has also demonstrated effectiveness with chronic strongyloidiasis with minimal side effects.[159] Currently, ivermectin (200 μg/kg/day p.o. 1–2 days), has become the treatment of choice for strongyloidiasis. Compared with albendazole, ivermectin has a similar side effect profile but with improved effectiveness,[159] has been shown to have better tolerability and a similar stool larvae clearance as compared with thiabendazole,[160] and in disease refractory to thiabendazole.[161] In immunocompromised patients multiple doses are usually required. Because the autoinfective cycle requires at least two weeks, the immunocompromised should be treated until symptom resolution and stools are negative for the organism for 2 weeks.[155] Following therapy, immunocompromised patients should have their stools monitored periodically for *S. stercoralis* while immunosuppressed.

CONCLUSIONS

In summary, the frequency of luminal GI infections, the spectrum of pathogens, severity of infection and organ involvement are dictated by the combination of exposure, predilection (host factors), and organ-specific tropism of the infecting pathogen (Table 7.3). A careful history regarding potential exposure(s), cause, and stage of immunodeficiency, if present, as well as specific epidemiologic factors germane to the clinical presentation will determine the potential causes of infection and thereby direct the appropriate evaluation. A number of antimicrobial agents are available to treat these infections and improvement of immune function also expedites both the short-term response and long-term risk for disease recurrence (Table 7.4).

Table 7.4 Overview of the diagnosis and therapy of enteric infections in the immunocompromised host

1 Immunocompromised patients are susceptible to a wide array of gastrointestinal infections. When immunodeficiency is severe, opportunistic infections are most frequent and usually the cause of the gastrointestinal complaints.

2 The prevalence of specific infections for any gastrointestinal disorder depends upon the severity and duration of immunodeficiency, organ(s) of involvement, and geographic setting.

3 Improvement in immune function plays a key role in the management of all gastrointestinal infections in immunocompromised patients.

4 Immune reconstitution with highly active antiretroviral therapy may not only result in remission of some infections, but discontinuation of long-term maintenance therapy as well.

5 Given the potential efficacy of antimicrobial agents for many of these infections, a thorough evaluation of the immunocompromised patients with gastrointestinal symptoms is warranted.

REFERENCES

1. Bacellar H, Munoz A, Hoover DR, et al., for the Multicenter AIDS Cohort Study. Incidence of clinical AIDS conditions in a cohort of homosexual men with CD4+ cell counts <100/mm³. J Infect Dis 1994; 170(5):1284–1287.

2. Rubin RR. Infections in the liver and renal transplant patient. In: Rubin RH, Young LS, eds. Clinical approach to infection in the compromised host. 2nd edn. New York: Plenum Publishing; 1988:561.

3. Trotter JF, Wallack A, Steinberg T. Low incidence of cytomegalovirus disease in liver transplant recipients receiving sirolimus primary immunosuppression with 3-day corticosteroid taper. Transpl Infect Dis 2003; 5(4):174–180.

4. Boeckh M. Current antiviral strategies for controlling cytomegalovirus in hematopoietic stem cell transplant recipients: prevention and therapy. Transpl Infect Dis 1999; 1(3):165–178.

5. Paya CV. Prevention of cytomegalovirus disease in recipients of solid-organ transplants. Clin Infect Dis 2001; 32(4):596–603.

6. Ives NJ, Gazzard BG, Easterbrook PJ. The changing pattern of AIDS-defining illnesses with the introduction of highly active antiretroviral therapy (HAART) in a London clinic. J Infect 2001; 42(2):134–139.

7. Monkemuller KE, Call SA, Lazenby AJ, et al. Declining prevalence of opportunistic gastrointestinal disease in the era of combination antiretroviral therapy. Am J Gastroenterol 2000; 95(2):457–462.

    This study documents the marked fall in gastrointestinal infections seen in HIV-infected patients in the era of HAART.

8. Lane HC, Masur H, Gelmann EP, et al. Correlation between immunologic function and clinical subpopulations of patients with the acquired immune deficiency syndrome. Am J Med 1985; 78(3):417–422

9. Rodgers VD, Fassett R, Kagnoff MF. Abnormalities in intestinal mucosal T cells in homosexual populations including those with the lymphadenopathy syndrome and acquired immunodeficiency syndrome. Gastroenterology 1986; 90(3):552–558.

10. Kotler DP, Scholes JV, Tierney AR. Intestinal plasma cell alterations in acquired immunodeficiency syndrome. Dig Dis Sci 1987; 32(2):129–138.

11. Miao YM, Hayes PJ, Gotch FM, et al. Elevated mucosal addressin cell adhesion molecule-1 expression in acquired immunodeficiency syndrome is maintained during antiretroviral therapy by intestinal pathogens and coincides with increased duodenal CD4 T cell densities. J Infect Dis 2002; 185(8):1043–1050.

    Improvement of immune function with HAART was associated with corresponding normalization of selected aspects of the mucosal immune system.

12. Wilcox CM, Waites KB, Smith PD. No relationship between gastric pH, small bowel bacterial colonization, and diarrhea in HIV-1 infected patients. Gut 1999; 44(1):101–105.

13. Belitsos PC, Greenson JK, Sisler J, et al. Association of chronic wasting diarrhea with gastric hypoacidity and opportunistic enteric infections in patients with acquired immunodeficiency syndrome (AIDS). J Infect Dis 1992; 166(2):277–284.

14. Jones JL, Hanson DL, Dworkins MS, et al. Surveillance for AIDS-defining opportunistic illnesses, 1992–1997. MMWR CDC Surveill Summ 1999; 48(2):1–22.

15. Thomas PD, Pollok RC, Gazzard BG. Enteric viral infections as a cause of diarrhea in the acquired immunodeficiency syndrome. HIV Med 1999; 1(1):19–24.

16. Zeitz M, Ullrich R, Schneider T, et al. Mucosal immunodeficiency in HIV/SIV infection. Pathobiology 1998; 66(3–4):151–157.

17. Wilcox CM, Zaki SR, Coffield LM, et al. Evaluation of idiopathic esophageal ulceration for human immunodeficiency virus. Mod Pathol 1995; 8(5):568–572.

18. Kothari A, Ramachandran VG, Gupta P, et al. Seroprevalence of cytomegalovirus among voluntary blood donors in Delhi, India. J Health Popul Nutr 2002; 20(4):348–351.

19. Rubin RH. Cytomegalovirus in solid organ transplantation. Transpl Infect Dis 2001; 3(Supple 2):1–5.

20. Gallant JE, Moore RD, Richman DD, et al. Incidence and natural history of cytomegalovirus disease in patients with advanced human immunodeficiency virus disease treated with zidovudine. J Infect Dis 1992; 166(6):1223–1227.

21. Goodgame RW. Gastrointestinal cytomegalovirus disease. Ann Intern Med 1993; 119(9):924–935.

22. Cheung TW, Teich SA. Cytomegalovirus infection in patients with HIV infection. Mt Sinai J Med 1999; 66(2):113–124.

23. Dieterich DT, Kotler DP, Busch DF, et al. Ganciclovir treatment of cytomegalovirus colitis in AIDS: A randomized, double-blind, placebo-controlled multicenter study. J Infect Dis 1993; 167(2):278–282.

24. Wilcox CM, Straub RA, Schwartz DA. Prospective endoscopic characterization of cytomegalovirus esophagitis in patients with AIDS. Gastrointest Endosc 1994; 40(4):481–484.

25. Wilcox CM, Chalasani N, Lazenby A, et al. Cytomegalovirus colitis in acquired immunodeficiency syndrome: a clinical and endoscopic study. Gastrointest Endosc 1998; 48(1):39–43.

26. Rich JD, Crawford JM, Kazanjian SN, et al. Discrete gastrointestinal mass lesions caused by cytomegalovirus in patients with AIDS: Report of three cases and review. Clin Infect Dis 1992; 15(4):609–614.

27. Monkemuller KE, Bussian AH, Lazenby AJ, et al. Special histologic stains are rarely beneficial for the evaluation of HIV-related gastrointestinal infections. Am J Clin Pathol 2000; 114(3):387–394.

28. Beaugerie L, Cywiner-Golenzer C, Monfort L, et al. Definition and diagnosis of cytomegalovirus colitis in patients infected by human immunodeficiency virus. J Acquir Immune Defic Syndr Hum Retrovirol 1997; 14(5):423–429.

29. Bini EJ, Cohen J. Diagnostic yield and cost-effectiveness of endoscopy in chronic human immunodeficiency virus-related diarrhea. Gastrointest Endosc 1998; 48(4):354–361.

30. Wilcox CM, Schwartz DA, Cotsonis GB, et al. Evaluation of chronic unexplained diarrhea in human immunodeficiency virus (HIV) infection: Determination of the best diagnostic approach. Gastroenterology 1996; 110(6):30–37.

31. Littler E, Stuart AD, Chee MS. Human cytomegalovirus UL97 open reading frame encodes a protein that phosphorylates the antiviral nucleoside analogue ganciclovir. Nature 1992; 358(6382):160–162.

32. Limaye AP. Ganciclovir-resistant cytomegalovirus in organ transplant recipients. Clin Infect Dis 2002; 35(7):866–872.

33. Laskin OL, Stahl-Bayliss CM, Kalman CM, et al. Use of ganciclovir to treat serious cytomegalovirus infections in patients with AIDS. J Infect Dis 1987; 155(2):323–327.

34. Laskin L, Cederberg DM, Mills J, Ganciclovir Study Group. Ganciclovir for the treatment and suppression of serious infections caused by cytomegalovirus. Am J Med 1987; 83(2):201–206.

35. Buhles WC, Mastre BJ, Tinker AJ, Syntex Collaborative Ganciclovir Treatment Study Group. Ganciclovir treatment of life- or sight-threatening cytomegalovirus infection: Experience in 314 immunocompromised patients. Rev Infect Dis 1988; 10(Suppl 3):495–504.

36. Wilcox CM, Straub RF, Schwartz DA. Cytomegalovirus esophagitis in AIDS: A prospective evaluation of clinical response to ganciclovir therapy, relapse rate, and long-term outcome. Am J Med 1995; 98(2):169–176.

37. Anderson RD, Griffy KG, Jung D, et al. Ganciclovir absolute bioavailability and steady-state pharmacokinetics after oral administration of two 3000-mg/d dosing regimens in human immunodeficiency virus- and cytomegalovirus-seropositive patients. Clin Ther 1995; 17(3):425–432.

38. Hoffman VF, Skiest DJ. Therapeutic developments in cytomegalovirus retinitis. Expert Opin Investig Drugs 2000; 9(2):207–220.

39. Martin DF, Sierra-Madero J, Walmsley S, et al. A controlled trial of valganciclovir as induction therapy for cytomegalovirus retinitis. N Engl J Med 2002; 346(15):1119–1126.

40. Wagstaff AJ, Bryson HM. Foscarnet. A reappraisal of its antiviral activity, pharmacokinetic properties and therapeutic use in immunocompromised patients with viral infections. Drugs 1994; 48:199–226.

41. Deray GB, Martinez F, Katlama C, et al. Foscarnet nephrotoxicity: Mechanism, incidence and prevention. Am J Nephrol 1989; 9(2):316–321.

42. Palestine AG, Polis MA, De Smet MD, et al. A randomized controlled trial of foscarnet in the treatment of cytomegalovirus retinitis in patients with AIDS. Ann Intern Med 1991; 115(9):665–673.

43. Blanshard C, Benhamou Y, Dohin E, et al. Treatment of AIDS-associated gastrointestinal cytomegalovirus infection with foscarnet and ganciclovir: A randomized comparison. J Infect Dis 1995; 172(3):622–628.

44. Nelson MR, Connolly GM, Hawkins DA, et al. Foscarnet in the treatment of cytomegalovirus infection of the esophagus and colon in patients with the acquired immune deficiency syndrome. Am J Gastroenterol 1991; 86(7):876–881.

45. Parente F, Bianchi Porro G. Treatment of cytomegalovirus esophagitis in patients with acquired immune deficiency syndrome: a randomized controlled study of foscarnet versus ganciclovir. The Italian Cytomegalovirus Study Group. Am J Gastroenterol 1998; 93(3):317–322.

This randomized study shows equivalency of ganciclovir and foscarnet for CMV esophagitis.

46. Salzberger B, Stoehr A, Jablonowski H, et al. Foscarnet 5 versus 7 days a week treatment for severe gastrointestinal CMV disease in HIV-infected patients. Infection 1996; 24(2):121–124.

47. Manischewitz JF, Quinnan GV Jr, Lane HC, et al. Synergistic effect of ganciclovir and foscarnet on cytomegalovirus replication in vitro. Antimicrob Agents Chemother 1990; 34(2):373–375.

48. Cline JJ, Garrett AD. Combination antiviral therapy for cytomegalovirus disease in patients with AIDS. Ann Pharmacother 1997; 31(9):1080–1082.

49. Dieterich DT, Polis MA, Dicker M, et al. Foscarnet treatment of cytomegalovirus gastrointestinal infections in acquired immunodeficiency syndrome patients who have failed ganciclovir induction. Am J Gastroenterol 1993; 88(4):542–548.

50. Sullivan V, Talarico CL, Stanat SC, et al. A protein kinase homologue controls phosphorylation of ganciclovir in human cytomegalovirus-infected cells. Nature 1992; 358(6457):162–164.

51. Lalezari JP, Drew WL, Glutzer E, et al. (S)-1-[3-Hydroxy-2-(phosphonylmethoxy)propyl] cytosine (cidofovir): Results of a phase I/II study of a novel antiviral nucleotide analogue. J Infect Dis 1995; 171(4):788–796.

52. De Clercq E, Sakuma T, Baba M, et al. Antiviral activity of phosphonylmethoxyalkyl derivatives of purine and pyrimidines. Antiviral Res 1987; 8(5-6):261–272.

53. Lalezari JP, Kuppermann BD. Clinical experience with cidofovir in the treatment of cytomegalovirus retinitis. J Acquir Immune Defic Syndr Hum Retrovirol 1997; 14(Suppl 1):27–31.

54. Polis MA, Spooner KM, Baird BF, et al. Anticytomegaloviral activity and safety of cidofovir in patient with human immunodeficiency virus infection and cytomegalovirus viruria. Antimicrob Agents Chemother 1995; 39(4):882–886.

55. Jacobson M, O'Donnell JJ, Brodie HR, et al. Randomized prospective trial of ganciclovir maintenance therapy for cytomegalovirus retinitis. J Med Virol 1988; 25(3):339–349.

56. Jouan M, Saves M, Tubianna R, et al. Discontinuation of maintenance therapy for cytomegalovirus retinitis in HIV-infected patients receiving highly active antiretroviral therapy. AIDS 2001; 15(1):23–31.

57. The Oral Ganciclovir European and Australian Cooperative Study Group. Intravenous versus oral ganciclovir: European/Australian comparative study of efficacy and safety in the prevention of cytomegalovirus retinitis recurrence in patients with AIDS. AIDS 1995; 9(5):471–477.

58. Lalezari J, Lindley J, Walmsley S, et al. A safety study of oral valganciclovir maintenance treatment of cytomegalovirus retinitis. J Acquir Immune Defic Syndr 2002; 30(4):392–400.

59. Somerville KT. Cost advantages of oral drug therapy for managing cytomegalovirus disease. Am J Health Syst Pharm 2003; 60(23 Suppl 8):S9–S12.

60. Spector SA, McKinley GF, Lalezari JP, et al. Oral ganciclovir for the prevention of cytomegalovirus disease in persons with AIDS. N Engl J Med 1996; 334(23):1491–1497.

61. Moretti S, Zikos P, Van Lint MT, et al. Foscarnet vs ganciclovir for cytomegalovirus (CMV) antigenemia after allogeneic hemopoietic stem cell transplantation (HSCT): a randomised study. Bone Marrow Transplant 1998; 22(2):175–180.

62. Humar A, Lipton AJ, Welsh S, et al. A randomized trial comparing cytomegalovirus antigenemia assay vs screening bronchoscopy for the early detection and prevention of disease in allogeneic bone marrow and peripheral blood stem cell transplant recipients. Bone Marrow Transplant 2001; 28(5):485–490.

63. Chevret S, Scieux C, Garrait V, et al. Usefulness of the cytomegalovirus (CMV) antigenemia assay for predicting the occurrence of CMV disease and death in patients with AIDS. Clin Infect Dis 1999; 28(4):758–763.

64. Brosgart CL, Louis TA, Hillman DW, et al. A randomized, placebo-controlled trial of the safety and efficacy of oral ganciclovir for prophylaxis of cytomegalovirus disease in HIV-infected individuals. Terry Beirn Community Programs for Clinical Research on AIDS. AIDS 1998; 12(3):269–277.

65. Kingreen D, Nitsche A, Beyer J, et al. Herpes simplex infection of the jejunum occurring in the early post-transplantation period. Bone Marrow Transplant 1997; 20(11):989–991.

66. Bagdades EK, Pillay D, Squire B, et al. Relationship between herpes simplex virus infections in patients with acquired immunodeficiency syndrome. AIDS 1992; 6(11):1317–1320.

67. Genereau T, Lortholary O, Bouchaud O. Herpes simplex esophagitis in patients with AIDS: Report of 34 cases. The Cooperative Study Group on Herpetic Esophagitis in HIV Infections. Clin Infect Dis 1996; 22(6):926–931.

68. Whitley RJ, Roizman B. Herpes simplex virus infections. Lancet 2001; 357(9267):1513–1518.

69. Erlich KS, Mills J, Chatis P, et al. Acyclovir-resistant herpes simplex virus infections in patients with acquired immunodeficiency syndrome. N Engl J Med 1989; 320(5):293–296.

70. Hardy WD. Foscarnet treatment of acyclovir-resistant herpes simplex virus infection in patients with acquired

immunodeficiency syndrome: Preliminary results of a controlled, randomized, regimen-comparative trial. Am J Med 1992; 92(2A):30S–35S.

71. Yajko DM, Chin DP, Gonzalez PC, et al. Mycobacterium avium complex in water, food, and soil samples collected from the environment of HIV-infected individuals. J Acquir Immune Defic Syndr Hum Retrovirol 1995; 9(2):176–182.

72. Nightingale SB, Byrd LT, Southern PM, et al. Incidence of Mycobacterium-avium-intracellulare complex bacteremia in human immunodeficiency virus-positive patients. J Infect Dis 1992; 165(3):1082–1085.

73. Havlik JA Jr, Horsburgh CR Jr, Metchock BG, et al. Disseminated Mycobacterium avium complex infection: Clinical identification and epidemiologic trends. J Infect Dis 1992; 165(3):577–580.

74. Horsburgh CR, Gettings J, Alexander LN, et al. Disseminated Mycobacterium avium complex disease among patients infected with human immunodeficiency virus, 1985–2000. Clin Infect Dis 2001; 33(11):1938–1943.

75. Hirsch HH, Kaufmann G, Sendi P, et al. Immune reconstitution in HIV-infected patients. Clin Infect Dis 2004; 38(8):1159–1166.

This study reviews the syndrome of immune reconstitution in HIV infected patients.

76. Prego V, Glatt AE, Roy V, et al. Comparative yield of blood culture for fungi and mycobacteria, liver biopsy, and bone marrow biopsy in the diagnosis of fever of undetermined origin in human immunodeficiency virus-infected patients. Arch Intern Med 1990; 150(2):333–336.

77. Gray JR, Rabeneck L. Atypical mycobacterial infection of the gastrointestinal tract in AIDS patients. Am J Gastroenterol 1989; 84(12):1521–1524.

78. Rastogi N, Frehel C, Ryter A, et al. Multiple drug resistance in Mycobacterium avium: Is the wall architecture responsible for the exclusion of antimicrobial agents? Antimicrob Agents Chemother 1981; 20(5):666–677.

79. Von Reyn CF, Jacobs NJ, Arbeit RD, et al. Polyclonal Mycobacterium avium infections in patients with AIDS: Variations in antimicrobial susceptibilities of different strains of M. avium isolated from the same patients. J Clin Microbiol 1995; 33(4):1008–1010.

80. Dautzenberg B, Marc SI, Meyohas MC, et al. Clarithromycin and other antimicrobial agents in the treatment of disseminated Mycobacterium avium infections in patients with acquired immunodeficiency syndrome. Arch Intern Med 1993; 153(3):368–372.

81. Young LS, Wiviott L, Wu M, et al. Azithromycin for treatment of Mycobacterium avium-intracellulare complex infection in patients with AIDS. Lancet 1991; 338(8775):1107–1109.

82. Dautzenberg B, Truffot C, Legris S, et al. Activity of clarithromycin against Mycobacterium avium infection in patients with the acquired immune deficiency syndrome. Am Rev Respir Dis 1991; 144(3 Pt 1):564–569.

83. Ward TT, Rimland D, Kauffman C, et al. Randomized, open-label trial of azithromycin plus ethambutol vs. clarithromycin plus ethambutol as therapy for Mycobacterium avium complex bacteremia in patients with human immunodeficiency virus infection. Veterans Affairs HIV Research Consortium. Clin Infect Dis 1998; 27(5):1278–1285.

84. Chaisson RE, Benson CA, Dube MP, AIDS Clinical Trials Group Protocol 157 Study Team. Clarithromycin therapy for bacteremic Mycobacterium avium complex disease. A randomized, double blind dose ranging study in patients with AIDS. Ann Intern Med 1994; 121(12):905–911.

85. Kemper CA, Havlir D, Haghighat D, et al. The individual microbiologic effect of three antimycobacterial agents,

clofazimine, ethambutol, and rifampin on *Mycobacterium avium* complex bacteremia in patients with AIDS. J Infect Dis 1994; 170(1):157–164.

86. Masur H, Kaplan JE, Holmes KK; U.S. Public Health Service; Infectious Diseases Society of America. Guidelines for preventing opportunistic infections among HIV-infected persons – 2002. Recommendations of the U.S. Public Health Service and the Infectious Diseases Society of America. Ann Intern Med 2002; 137(5 Pt 2):435–478.

Up-to-date source for recommendations regarding prevention of opportunistic infections in HIV-infected patients.

87. Shafran SD, Singer J, Zarowny DP, et al. Determinants of rifabutin-associated uveitis in patients treated with rifabutin, clarithromycin, and ethambutol for *Mycobacterium avium* complex bacteremia: A multivariate analysis. Canadian HIV Trials Network Protocol 010 Study Group. N Engl J Med 1996; 335(6):377–383.

88. Wallace RJ Jr, Brown BA, Griffith DE, et al. Reduced serum levels of clarithromycin in patients treated with multidrug regimens including rifampin or rifabutin for *Mycobacterium avium-M. intracellulare* infection. J Infect Dis 1995; 171(3):747–750.

89. Benson CA, Williams PL, Currier JS, and the AIDS Clinical Trials Group 223 Protocol Team. A prospective, randomized trial examining the efficacy and safety of clarithromycin in combination with ethambutol, rifabutin, or both for the treatment of disseminated *Mycobacterium avium* complex disease in persons with acquired immunodeficiency syndrome. Clin Infect Dis 2003; (9)37: 1234–1243.

This prospective trial shows the efficacy of combination therapy for MAC using a clarithromycin-based regimen.

90. Baron EJ, Young LS. Amikacin, ethambutol, and rifampin for treatment of disseminated *Mycobacterium avium-intracellulare* infections in patients with acquired immune deficiency syndrome. Diagn Microbiol Infect Dis 1986; 5(3):215–220.

91. Aberg JA, Williams PL, Liu T, and the AIDS Clinical Trial Group 393 Study Team. A study of discontinuing maintenance therapy in human immunodeficiency virus-infected subjects with disseminated *Mycobacterium avium* complex: AIDS Clinical Trial Group 393 Study Team. J Infect Dis 2003; 187(7):1046–1052.

This is one of a number of studies now showing that with improvement of immune function with HAART, long-term maintenance therapy for opportunistic infections can be safely discontinued.

92. Pettipher CA, Karstaedt AS, Hopley M. Prevalence and clinical manifestations of disseminated *Mycobacterium avium* complex infection in South Africans with acquired immunodeficiency syndrome. Clin Infect Dis 2001; 33(12):2068–2071.

93. Vajpayee M, Kanswal S, Seth P, et al. Spectrum of opportunistic infections and profile of CD4+ counts among AIDS patients in North India. Infection. 2003; 31(5):336–340.

94. Havlir DV, Barnes PF. Tuberculosis in patients with human immunodeficiency virus infection. N Engl J Med 1999; 340(5):367–373.

95. Hung CC, Chen MY, Hsiao CF, et al. Improved outcomes of HIV-1-infected adults with tuberculosis in the era of highly active antiretroviral therapy. AIDS 2003; 17(18):2615–2622.

96. Justesen US, Andersen AB, Klitgaard NA, et al. Pharmacokinetic interaction between rifampin and the combination of indinavir and low-dose ritonavir in HIV-infected patients. Clin Infect Dis 2004; 38(3):426–429.

97. Washington K, Stenzel TT, Buckley RH, et al. Gastrointestinal pathology in patients with common variable immunodeficiency and X-linked agammaglobulinemia. Am J Surg Pathol 1996; 20(10):1240–1252.

98. Goodgame RW. Understanding intestinal spore-forming protozoa: Cryptosporidia, microsporidia, isospora, and cyclospora. Ann Intern Med 1996; 124(4):429–441.

99. Boagaerts J, Lepage P, Rouvroy D, et al. *Cryptosporidium* species: A frequent cause of diarrhea in central Africa. J Clin Microbiol 1984;20(5):874–876.

100. MacKenzie WR, Hoxie NJ, Proctor ME, et al. A massive outbreak in Milwaukee of cryptosporidiosis infection transmitted through the public water supply. N Engl J Med 1994; 331(3):161–167.

101. Dascomb K, Clark R, Aberg J, et al. Natural history of intestinal microsporidiosis among patients infected with human immunodeficiency virus. J Clin Microbiol 1999; 37(10): 3421–3422.

102. DeHovitz JA, Pape JW, Boncy M, et al. Clinical manifestations and therapy of *Isospora belli* infection in patients with the acquired immunodeficiency syndrome. N Engl J Med 1986; 315(2):87–90.

103. Molina JM, Sarfati C, Beauvais B, et al. Intestinal microsporidiosis in human immunodeficiency virus-infected patients with chronic unexplained diarrhea: Prevalence and clinical and biologic features. J Infect Dis 1993; 167(1):217–221.

104. Goodgame RW, Kimball K, Ou CN, et al. Intestinal function and injury in acquired immunodeficiency syndrome-related cryptosporidiosis. Gastroenterology 1995; 108(4):1075–1082.

105. Schwartz DA, Bryant RT, Weber R, et al. Microsporidiosis in HIV positive patients: Current methods for diagnosis using biopsy, cytologic, ultrastructural, immunological, and tissue culture techniques. Folia Parasitol 1994; 41(2):101–109.

106. Simon DM, Cello JP, Valenzuela J, et al. Multicenter trial of octreotide in patients with refractory acquired immunodeficiency syndrome-associated diarrhea. Gastroenterology 1995; 108(3):1753–1760.

107. Marshall RJ, Flanigan TP. Paromomycin inhibits *Cryptosporidium* infection of a human enterocyte cell line. J Infect Dis 1992; 165(4):772–774.

108. White AC, Chappell CL, Hayat CS, et al. Paromomycin for cryptosporidiosis in AIDS: A prospective, double-blind trial. J Infect Dis 1994; 170(2):419–424.

109. Flanigan TP, Ramratnam B, Graeber C, et al. Prospective trial of paromomycin for cryptosporidiosis in AIDS. Am J Med 1996; 100(3):370–372.

110. Louie E, Borkowsky W, Klesius PH, et al. Treatment of cryptosporidiosis with oral bovine transfer factor. Clin Immunol Immunopathol 1987; 44(3):329–334.

111. Greenberg PD, Cello JP. Treatment of severe diarrhea caused by *Cryptosporidium parvum* with oral bovine immunoglobulin concentrate in patients with AIDS. J Acquir Immune Defic Syndr Hum Retrovirol 1996; 13(4):348–354.

112. Blanshard C, Shanson DC, Gazzard BG. Pilot studies of azithromycin, letrazuril and paromomycin in the treatment of cryptosporidiosis. Int J STD AIDS 1997; 8(2):124–129.

113. Doumbo O, Rossignol JF, Pichard E, et al. Nitazoxanide in the treatment of cryptosporidial diarrhea and other intestinal parasitic infections associated with acquired immunodeficiency syndrome in tropical Africa. Am J Trop Med Hyg 1997; 56(6):637–639.

114. Bailey JM, Erramouspe J. Nitazoxanide treatment for giardiasis and cryptosporidiosis in children. Ann Pharmacother 2004; 38(4):634–640.

115. Kadappu KK, Nagaraja MV, Rao PV, et al. Azithromycin as treatment for cryptosporidiosis in human immunodeficiency virus disease. J Postgrad Med 2002; 48(3):179–181.

116. Eeftinck Schattenkerk JKM, van Gool T, van Ketel RJ, et al. Clinical significance of small-intestinal microsporidiosis in HIV-1-infected individuals. Lancet 1991; 337(8746):895–898.

117. Dieterich DT, Lew EA, Kotler DP, et al. Treatment with albendazole for intestinal disease due to *Entercytozoon bieneusi* in patients with AIDS. J Infect Dis 1994; 169(1):178–183.

118. Sharpstone D, Rowbotton A, Francis N, et al. Thalidomide: A novel therapy of microsporidiosis. Gastroenterology 1997; 112(6): 1823–1829.

119. Carr A, Marriott D, Field A, et al. Treatment of HIV-1-associated microsporidiosis and cryptosporidiosis with combination antiretroviral therapy. Lancet 1998; 351(9098):256–261.

120. Miao YM, Awad-El-Kariem FM, Franzen C, et al. Eradication of cryptosporidia and microsporidia following successful antiretroviral therapy. J Acquir Immune Defic Syndr 2000; 25(2):124–129.

Improvement of immune function alone with antiretroviral therapy can result in remission of opportunistic parasitic diseases of the gut.

121. Pape JW, Verdier RJ, Johnson DW. Treatment and prophylaxis of *Isospora belli* infection in patients with the acquired immunodeficiency syndrome. N Engl J Med 1989; 320(16):1044–1047.

122. Hill D, Dubey JP. *Toxoplasma gondii*: transmission, diagnosis, and prevention. Clin Microbiol Infect 2002; 8(10):634–640.

123. Bonacini M, Kanel G, Alamy M. Duodenal and hepatic toxoplasmosis in a patient with infection: Review of the literature. Am J Gastroenterol 1996; 91(9):1838–1840.

124. Ferreira MS, Borges AS. Some aspects of protozoan infections in the immunocompromised patients. Mem do Inst Oswaldo Cruz 2002; 97(4):443–457.

125. Beaman MH, McCabe RE, Wang SY, et al. *Toxoplasmosis gondii*. In: Mandell HL, Bennett JE, Dolin R, eds. Principles and practice of infectious diseases, 4th edn. New York: Churchill Livingstone; 1995:2455–2475.

126. Katlama C, de Witt S, O'Doherty E, et al. Pyrimethamine-clindamycin vs. pyrimethamine-sulfadiazine as acute and long-term therapy for toxoplasmic encephalitis in patients with AIDS. Clin Infect Dis 1996; 22(2):268.

127. Ng VL, Yajko DM, Hadley WK. Extrapulmonary pneumocystosis. Clin Microbiol Rev 1997; 10(3):401–418.

128. Edman JC, Kovacs JA, Masur H, et al. Ribosomal RNA sequences show *Pneumocystis carinii* to be a member of the fungi. Nature 1988; 334(6182):519–522.

129. Lopez Bernaldo de Quiros JC, Miro JM, Pena JM, et al. A randomized trial of the discontinuation of primary and secondary prophylaxis against *Pneumocystis carinii* pneumonia after highly active antiretroviral therapy in patient with HIV infection. N Eng J Med 2001; 344(3):159–167.

130. Bygbjerg IC, Lund JT, Hording M. Effect of folic and folinic acid on cytopenia occurring during co-trimoxazole treatment of *Pneumocystis carinii* pneumonia. Scand J Infect Dis 1988; 20(6):685–686.

131. Caumes E, Roudier C, Rogeaux O, et al. Effect of corticosteroids on the incidence of adverse cutaneous reactions to trimethoprim during treatment of AIDS-associated *Pneumocystis carinii* pneumonia. Clin Infect Dis 1994; 18(3):319–323.

132. Hughes WT. Use of dapsone in the prevention and treatment of *Pneumocystis carinii* pneumonia: a review. Clin Infect Dis 1998; 27(1):191–204.

133. Toma E, Thorne A, Singer J, et al. Clindamycin with primaquine vs. trimethoprim-sulfamethoxazole therapy for mild and moderately severe *Pneumocystis carinii* pneumonia in patients with AIDS: a multicenter, double blind, randomized trial. Clin In Dis 1998; 27(3):524–530.

134. Hughes W, Leoung GB, Kramer F, et al. Comparison of atovaquone (566C80) with trimethoprim-sulfamethoxazole to treat *Pneumocystis carinii* pneumonia in patients with AIDS. N Engl J Med 1993; 328(21):1521–1527.

135. Sattler FR, Frame P, Davis R, et al. Trimetrexate with leucovorin versus trimethoprim-sulfamethoxazole for moderate to severe episodes of *Pneumocystis carinii* pneumonia in patients with AIDS. J Infect Dis 1994; 170(1):165–172.

136. Smith DE, Davies S, Smithson J, et al. Eflornithine versus co-trimoxazole treatment of *Pneumocystis carinii* pneumonia in AIDS patients. AIDS 1992; 6(12):1489–1493.

137. Wheat LJ, Connolly-Springfield PA, Baker RL, et al. Disseminated histoplasmosis in the acquired immune deficiency syndrome: clinical findings, diagnosis, and treatment, and review of the literature. Medicine 1990; 69(6):361–374.

138. Suh KN, Anekthananon T, Mariuz PR. Gastrointestinal histoplasmosis in patients with AIDS: Case report and review. Clin Infect Dis 2001; 32(3):483–491.

139. Lamps LW, Molina CP, West AB, et al. The pathologic spectrum of gastrointestinal and hepatic histoplasmosis. Am J Clin Pathol 2000; 113(1):64–72.

140. Wheat LJ. Laboratory diagnosis of histoplasmosis: update 2000. Semin Respir Infect 2001; 16(2):131–140.

141. Wheat J. Histoplasmosis. Experience during outbreaks in Indianapolis and review of the literature. Medicine (Baltimore) 1997; 76(5):339–354.

142. Dismukes WE, Bradsher RW Jr, Cloud GC, et al. Itraconazole therapy for blastomycosis and histoplasmosis. NIAID Mycoses Study Group. Am J Med 1992; 93(5):489–497.

143. Johnson PC, Wheat J, Cloud GA, et al. Safety and efficacy of liposomal amphotericin B compared with conventional amphotericin B for induction therapy of histoplasmosis in patients with AIDS. Ann Intern Med 2003; 137(2):105–109.

This trial highlights the difference in side effects of liposomal versus standard amphotericin-B.

144. Wheat J, Hafner R, Korzun AH, et al. Itraconazole treatment of disseminated histoplasmosis in patients with the acquired immunodeficiency syndrome. AIDS Clinical Trial Group. Am J Med 1995; 98(4):336–342.

145. McKinsey DS, Gupta MR, Riddler SA, et al. Long-term amphotericin B therapy for disseminated histoplasmosis in patients with the acquired immunodeficiency syndrome (AIDS). Ann Intern Med 1989; 111(8):655–659.

146. Norris S, Wheat J, McKinsey D, et al. Prevention of relapse of histoplasmosis with fluconazole in patients with the acquired immunodeficiency syndrome. Am J Med 1994; 96(6):504–508.

147. Walsh TJ, Finberg RW, Arndt C, et al. Liposomal amphotericin B for empirical therapy in patients with persistent fever and neutropenia. N Engl J Med 1999; 340(10):764–771.

148. Eras P, Godstein MJ, Sherlock P. *Candida* infection of the gastrointestinal tract. Medicine (Baltimore) 1972; 51(5): 367–379.

149. Denning DW, Stevens DA. Antifungal and surgical treatment of invasive aspergillosis: review of 2,121 published cases. Rev Infect Dis 1990; 12(6):1147–1201.

150. Stevens DA, Kan VL, Judson MA. Practice guidelines for disease caused by *Aspergillus*. Infectious Diseases Society of America. Clin Infect Dis 2000; 30(4):696–709.

151. Young RC, Bennet JE, Vogel CL, et al. Aspergillosis: the spectrum of the disease in 98 patients. Medicine (Baltimore) 1970; 49(2): 147–173.

152. Herbrecht R, Denning DW, Patterson TF, et. al. Voriconazole versus amphotericin B for primary therapy of invasive aspergillosis. New Engl J Med 2002; 347(6):408–415.

153. Keating G, Figgitt D. Caspofungin: a review of its use in oesophageal candidiasis, invasive candidiasis, and invasive aspergillosis. Drugs 2003; 63(20):2235–2263.

154. Denning D, Lee J, Hostetler J, et al. Mycoses study group multicenter trial of oral itraconazole therapy for invasive aspergillosis. Am J Med 1994; 97(2):135–144.

155. Keiser PB, Nutman TB. *Strongyloides stercoralis* in the immunocompromised population. Clin Microbiol Rev 2004; 17(1):208–217.

156. Sarangarajan R, Ranganathan A, Belmonte AH, et al. *Strongyloides stercoralis* infection in AIDS. AIDS Patient Care STDS 1997; 11(6):407–414.

157. Scowden EB, Schaffner W, Stone WJ. Overwhelming strongyloidiasis: an unappreciated opportunistic infection. Medicine (Baltimore) 1978; 57(6):527–544.

158. Siddiqui AA, Berk SL. Diagnosis of *Strongyloides stercoralis* infection. Clin Infect Dis 2001; 33(7):1040–1047.

159. Marti H, Haji HJ, Savioli L, et al. A comparative trial of a single-dose ivermectin versus three days of albendazole for treatment of *Strongyloides stercoralis* and other soil-transmitted helminth infections in children. Am J Trop Med Hyg 1996; 55(5):477–481.

160. Gann PH, Neva FA, Gam AA. A randomized trial of single and two-dose ivermectin versus thiabendazole for treatment of strongyloidiasis. J Infect Dis 1994; 169(5):1076–1079.

161. Torres JR, Isturiz R, Murillo J, et al. Efficacy of ivermectin in the treatment of strongyloidiasis complicating AIDS. Clin Infect Dis 1993; 17(5):900–902.

Biliary infections in the immunocompromised patient

Daniel Gelrud and Douglas Simon

INTRODUCTION

Compared with esophageal and diarrheal diseases, biliary tract diseases are uncommon in patients with the acquired immunodeficiency syndrome (AIDS). Unfortunately, when biliary disorders are present, they cause significant morbidity and mortality and adversely influence the quality of life of affected patients. Prior to the AIDS epidemic, biliary disease caused by opportunistic infections such as CMV or cryptosporidia was unknown. Therefore, the bile ducts of AIDS patients appear to be uniquely susceptible to these types of infections compared to other immunosuppressed patients.[1] Disease of the bile ducts in AIDS patients was first reported by Guarda and colleagues[2] in 1983, and in the same year, Pitlik et al.[3] reported the first case of AIDS-related acalculous cholecystitis. Since that time there have been a several reports that have expanded our understanding of the clinical manifestations, causes, pathophysiology, and management of AIDS-associated biliary disease. Since the mid 1990s coinciding with the widespread use of highly active antiretroviral therapy (HAART) several investigators have noted a steep drop in the incidence of AIDS-associated biliary disease.[4,5]

Disorders of the bile ducts seen in AIDS patients include: (1) non-HIV associated diseases such as gallstone disease, bile duct strictures, etc.; (2) the 'AIDS cholangiopathy syndrome' and; (3) acalculous cholecystitis. The non-HIV associated disorders will not be discussed in this chapter, but it is important to remember gallstone-associated diseases when evaluating HIV-positive patients for biliary symptoms and abnormal liver tests. Gallstones have been reported to be significantly more common in HIV-seropositive individuals than in age-matched seronegative controls and the increase appears to correlate with advanced stage of HIV infection.[6] This chapter will be divided into two sections, acalculous cholecystitis and the AIDS cholangiopathy syndrome. This separation is arbitrary and it is important to realize that in many AIDS patients the two disorders are seen concurrently; this is not surprising since the same opportunistic infections cause each disorder.

ACALCULOUS CHOLECYSTITIS

Introduction

Acalculous cholecystitis appears to be rare in patients infected with HIV, but its actual incidence is unknown. Until 1995 when French and colleagues[7] reported on 136 AIDS patients with gallbladder disease, the pertinent literature consisted of only isolated case reports and small series of patients.[3,8–11]

Pathogenesis

Opportunistic infections associated with acalculous cholecystitis include: cryptosporidia, cytomegalovirus (CMV), microsporidia, *Candida albicans, Isospora belli, Mycobacterium avium intracellulare* (MAC), *Campylobacter, Salmonella entertitis.* and *P. carinii.*[1,12,13] Cryptosporidia and CMV appear to be the most frequent infectious pathogens isolated in such patients.[12] Obstruction of the cystic duct by Kaposi's sarcoma rarely has been reported as a cause of cholecystitis.[14] In 16–53% of patients with acalculous cholecystitis, no infectious pathogen is isolated,[12] but acalculous cholecystitis occurs in the later stages of AIDS when patients are more immunosuppressed and thus more likely to acquire opportunistic infections.[15]

French and colleagues[7] reported on 107 AIDS patients and 29 HIV-seropositive patients without AIDS who underwent cholecystectomy over a 6-year period at a tertiary referral center. Table 8.1

Table 8.1 Findings in 107 AIDS patients undergoing cholecystectomy

Diagnosis	Total (%)
Acalculous cholecystitis (n = 72)	
Microsporidia	7 (10)
CMV	5 (7)
Cryptosporidia	6 (8)
CMV and cryptosporidia	13 (18)
Kaposi's sarcoma	1 (1)
Isospora belli	1 (1)
Pneumocystis carinii	1 (1)
Idiopathic	38 (53)
TOTAL	**72**
Cholecystitis and cholelithiasis (n = 27)	
Microsporidia	1 (4)
CMV	1 (4)
Cryptosporidia	2 (7)
CMV and cryptosporidia	2 (7)
Gallstones only	21 (78)
TOTAL	**27**

summarizes the findings of their report. Most patients had acalculous cholecystitis and an opportunistic infection was identified in half of the cases. Opportunistic infections were more common in patients with acalculous cholecystitis than in AIDS patients with cholecystitis associated with cholelithiasis. Most patients with biliary cryptosporidiosis also had intestinal infection which contrasted with CMV infection of the gallbladder in which there was no evidence of CMV infection elsewhere. Twelve of the 72 patients with acalculous cholecystitis had disseminated MAC infection and 10 of these had no opportunistic infections of the gallbladder. Cacciarelli et al.,[16] in a retrospective study of HIV-seropositive patients undergoing cholecystectomy, found that calculus cholecystitis was more common than acalculous cholecystitis; all subjects with a CD4 count <200/mm³, and therefore AIDS, had acalculous disease. Gathe and colleagues[11] reported that 24 of 30 HIV-seropositive individuals seen with symptomatic gallbladder disease had acalculous cholecystitis. All 30 subjects had CD4 counts <200/mm³, 27 had a previous opportunistic infection, and in 13 patients an etiologic diagnosis was made, most of which were CMV or cryptosporidia.

Clinical presentation

The presentations of acalculous and calculus cholecystitis are similar, with patients complaining of right upper quadrant or epigastric pain and fever. French et al.[7] documented right upper quadrant pain in 90%; nausea in 83%; diarrhea in 59%; and weight loss in 41% of subjects. Serum bilirubin is usually normal; serum alkaline phosphatase is elevated; and the ALT and AST are either normal or minimally elevated. French and colleagues[7] reported a mean serum alkaline phosphatase of 293±394 IU/L in their series and the liver tests were not different for those with or without opportunistic infections. They did note that when the gallbladder exhibited CMV and cryptosporidia infection together, the serum alkaline phosphatase levels (mean = 479±217 IU/L) were higher than when the gallbladder was free of opportunistic infections.

Diagnosis

Right upper quadrant ultrasound examination may reveal a thickened gallbladder wall, gallbladder dilation, dilated and thickened bile ducts, and pericholecystic fluid. Cholangiograms, performed either intraoperatively or during endoscopic retrograde cholangiopancreatography (ERCP), show changes consistent with the 'AIDS cholangiopathy' syndrome[8,10,11,17] in up to 50% of AIDS patients with acalculous cholecystitis, suggesting a common etiology for the two diseases. A HIDA scan showing 'nonvisualization' of the gallbladder is only suggestive of acalculous cholecystitis[18] since calculus and acalculous cholecystitis may not be distinguished by this test. Most patients with cholelithiasis have only abdominal ultrasound as their sole imaging study, whereas patients with acalculous cholecystitis frequently had both ultrasound and HIDA scanning.[7] Nonvisualization of the gallbladder by HIDA scanning is more likely in patients with acalculous cholecystitis and an opportunistic infection than those without such infection, but a normal HIDA scan does not exclude the diagnosis of acalculous cholecystitis. Gathe et al.[11] and French et al.[7] noted that 53% and 74%, respectively, of their patients had a HIDA study suggesting cystic duct

obstruction. French et al.[7] reported that the diagnosis of acalculous cholecystitis was based on decreased gallbladder contractility in response to cholecystokinin injection in 18 of their patients, all of whom had both a normal abdominal ultrasound and HIDA scan.

Management

Surgical removal of the gallbladder is the definitive treatment of acalculous cholecystitis. Mortality in this disorder can be significant if diagnosis is delayed and gangrene and perforation develop. This is especially true with cytomegalovirus infection, since CMV may involve the vascular endothelium resulting in arteritis, thrombosis, and gallbladder ischemia. Patients with AIDS and gallbladder disease typically have end-stage HIV disease with low CD4 counts, coexisting opportunistic infections, and significant malnutrition, all of which contributes to a significant morbidity and mortality. LaRaja et al.[19] reported a 22% postoperative mortality among 904 HIV-seropositive patients undergoing any intra-abdominal surgery. This is in contrast to the 3%, 11%, and 9% mortality reported by Gathe et al.,[11] Cacciarelli et al.,[16] and French et al.[7] in their respective series of AIDS patients undergoing biliary tract surgery. Most deaths in the latter series were due to prolonged hospitalizations resulting from complications of AIDS. In one study[16] laparoscopic cholecystectomy was associated with a lower mortality and postoperative morbidity, compared with open cholecystectomy; laparoscopic removal of the gallbladder has been suggested as the preferred surgical approach. Because of the high prevalence of malnutrition there have been concerns about wound infection and dehiscence in patients with AIDS, but these concerns have not materialized.[20] Surgery should not be withheld solely because of advanced AIDS. Percutaneous ultrasound guided catheter cholecystostomy can be performed in extremely ill or poor surgical risk patients with cholecystitis;[21,22] it is less invasive, requires no general anesthesia, and can serve as definitive therapy or a temporizing procedure until the patient is stable enough to undergo cholecystectomy.

The overall prognosis in AIDS patients with acalculous cholecystitis is poor. However, this is more a function of the severe underlying immunosuppression in these patients rather than their gallbladder disease.

AIDS CHOLANGIOPATHY

Definition

The term 'AIDS cholangiopathy'[23] was first used by John Cello to describe the range of biliary tract disorders that occurs in patients with AIDS. 'AIDS cholangiopathy' is a spectrum of disorders which consist of four distinct entities (Table 8.2): (1) papillary stenosis with dilation of the common bile duct (CBD); (2) sclerosing cholangitis; (3) a combination of papillary stenosis and sclerosing cholangitis; and (4) long extrahepatic stricture formation. Papillary stenosis is defined as a common bile duct >8 mm; delayed emptying of contrast (>30 minutes); a sphincter of Oddi pressure >40 mmHg; and a 2–4 mm tapering of the distal CBD. Sclerosing cholangitis is defined by the presence of focal strictures and dilations of the intra- and/or extrahepatic bile ducts. The combination of papillary stenosis and sclerosing cholangitis is defined by the presence of features of both disorders. Extrahepatic

Table 8.2 Features of the different patterns of aids cholangiopathy

Papillary stenosis	CBD >8 mm
Sclerosing cholangitis	Contrast empties in >30 minutes
Papillary stenosis and sclerosing cholangitis	Sphincter of Oddi pressure > 40 mmHg
Extrahepatic bile duct stricture	2–4 mm tapering of distal CBD
	Focal strictures of dilations of intrahepatic and/or extrahepatic bile ducts
	Features of both
	1–2 cm extrahepatic bile duct stricture
	No prior CBD disease or treatment
	Normal pancreatic duct

bile duct stricture is defined as the presence of a long (1–2 cm), extrahepatic stricture in the absence of common bile duct stones, pancreatic disease, or prior bile duct surgery.

The papillary stenosis with intrahepatic sclerosing cholangitis variant is found in 50–77% of patients with AIDS cholangiopathy (Table 8.3).[12] Sclerosing cholangitis of the intra- and extrahepatic is next most frequent, occurring in 20–40%[12] and papillary stenosis alone with common bile duct dilation is reported in 10–23% of patients. Long extrahepatic stricture is the least common variant of AIDS cholangiopathy, being found in 5% of patients.[12,24] Isolated strictures of the common bile duct usually are due to bile duct neoplasms or pancreatic disease rather than opportunistic infections.[1]

Etiology

If an extensive evaluation, including biopsies of the common bile duct, papilla or duodenum and ova, and parasite examination of bile and duodenal fluid is performed, an infectious etiology will be found in 50–81% of patients with AIDS and cholangiopathy.[1,12,25–27] Infectious cause includes *Cryptosporidium*, CMV, *Microsporidium*, MAC, *Cyclospora*, and *Isospora*.[1,12,26,27] *Cryptosporidium* is the most frequently identified pathogen, being isolated in tissue or secretions in as many as 57% of patients.[1,27] Most cases of cryptosporidiosis occur when the CD4 counts are less than 50/mm³.[28,29] CMV is the second most commonly identified pathogen and multiple pathogens occasionally have been identified (e.g., cryptosporidia and CMV).[1,12] In AIDS patients with only intrahepatic duct abnor-

malities identified by cholangiogram, cryptosporidia, CMV, or both are frequently present.[12] In many patients previously thought to have idiopathic AIDS cholangiopathy, microsporidia are found.[27] Both *Encephalitozoon intestinalis* and *Enterocytozoon bieneusi* have been found in patients with AIDS cholangiopathy.[27,30] The diagnosis of these pathogens can be made by light and electron microscopy of biliary epithelium, liver, bile ducts, gallbladder and duodenal mucosa, as well as ova and parasite examination of biliary and duodenal fluid.[27,30,31] Microsporidia also have been reported in urine and stool from AIDS patients.[30,31] Collectively, these findings indicate the importance of tissue and biliary intestinal fluid analysis in the evaluation of patients with AIDS cholangiopathy.

Both non-Hodgkin's lymphoma (NHL) and Kaposi's sarcoma have been reported[12,13,25,32] to cause the extrahepatic bile duct stricture variant of the AIDS cholangiopathy syndrome;[12] bile duct lymphoma has been reported to cause symptomatic jaundice even with small tumors.[32] Non-HIV-associated causes of biliary disease, including gallbladder or common bile duct stones, postoperative strictures, chronic pancreatitis-associated strictures, and benign ampullary tumors, have been reported in 15% of AIDS patients.[24]

No identifiable cause can be found in 28–50% of patients with AIDS-associated cholangiopathy.[12,27] In these cases a number of possible explanations have been suggested.[12] It is possible that unknown pathogens capable of causing AIDS cholangiopathy have yet to be identified. Conversely, improper sampling, culturing or fixation of tissue or fluid samples may prevent identification of

Table 8.3 Frequency of different cholangiographic patterns

Author (reference)	Cello (17)	Benhamou (29)	Forbes (28)	Ducreux (35)
Number of patients	51	26	19	45
CHOLANGIOGRAPHIC PATTERN (%)				
Papillary stenosis	20	23	15	10
Papillary stenosis and sclerosing	55	77	75	50
Cholangitis	20		10	40
Sclerosing cholangitis extrahepatic stricture	5			

a known infectious pathogen. HIV itself has been proposed as a cause of AIDS cholangiopathy; however, there is no evidence to date suggesting that HIV infects biliary epithelium. Immune-mediated mechanisms associated with specific HLA haplotypes or immune mechanisms stimulated by persistent portal bacteremia also have been proposed as a cause of AIDS-associated cholangiopathy.[12]

The mechanisms by which these pathogens cause the AIDS cholangiopathy syndrome are unclear. Cryptosporidia has been shown to cause biliary epithelial cell death by inducing apoptosis and cytokine production.[33] CMV is known to infect the vascular endothelium and thereby cause thrombosis of vessels, and ischemic damage of the biliary epithelium. Histologically, severe chronic inflammatory infiltrates are seen in the bile duct and these changes may result in the observed cholangiographic abnormalities.[1]

Epidemiology

The incidence and prevalence of AIDS cholangiopathy are not known. Most published studies are descriptive and offer clinical details of patients who present with biliary symptoms or who are found to have biliary disease after evaluation of abnormal liver tests. A study by Chan and Cello[34] suggest that biliary tract disease may be more common in AIDS patients than is appreciated by most physicians. They performed endoscopic retrograde cholangiography in 25 patients undergoing upper tract endoscopy as part of an evaluation of diarrhea and found that 46% of patients had cholangiographic evidence of papillary stenosis or sclerosing cholangitis.[34] AIDS cholangiopathy has been reported more frequently in homosexual men than in AIDS patients with other risk factors.[15] The average age at presentation of patients with AIDS cholangiopathy is 36 years (reflecting the most prevalent age group afflicted with AIDS)[29] and usually have CD4 counts less than 200/mm³, and frequently less than 100/mm³.[12] With the widespread use of HAART, AIDS cholangiopathy is becoming a rare complication of AIDS. Ko et al. reported 94 patients with AIDS cholangiopathy over 2 decades.[5] Only 13 out of 94 received their diagnosis between 1996 and 2003.

Clinical presentation

The clinical presentation of patients with AIDS cholangiopathy is variable; patients with intrahepatic cholangitis without papillary stenosis may be asymptomatic.[1] In asymptomatic individuals, AIDS cholangiopathy may be suspected by the presence of abnormal liver chemistries, but liver tests may be normal.[34] Signs and symptoms of AIDS cholangiopathy generally develop 1 year after the diagnosis of AIDS.[29] Epigastric and/or right upper quadrant pain is the most common symptom and is reported in 73–90% of patients.[12,25,28] Severe abdominal pain is highly suggestive of the presence of the papillary stenosis variant.[1] Fever is present in more than 60% of patients. Other symptoms include vomiting, diarrhea, weight loss, and least frequently, pruritus associated with cholestasis.[25] Diarrhea is a frequent complaint that is not surprising since several of the infections causing cholangiopathy also affect the small and large intestine.[1] Bacterial cholangitis is uncommon in the absence of endoscopic manipulation of the biliary system. Forbes and colleagues

reported that in their series of 20 patients with cholangiographic disease 20% had normal liver tests.[29] Abnormal liver tests frequently are the first clue to the presence of AIDS cholangiopathy, and the serum alkaline phosphatase has been reported to be abnormal in up to 80% of patients, and levels as high as 700–800 IU/L can be seen.[25] Serum transaminase levels are normal or slightly elevated and the serum total bilirubin is rarely abnormal.[12] Jaundice is distinctly uncommon in AIDS patients and its presence should suggest drug-induced liver damage. Most AIDS patients with biliary disease have minimally decreased serum albumin level, hemoglobin, and white blood cell count,[29] most likely due to HIV infection rather than to biliary tract disease.

Diagnosis

Noninvasive

Ultrasound or CT scanning is useful in the evaluation of an AIDS patient with suspected cholangiopathy. In patients with AIDS cholangiopathy proven by cholangiography, abnormalities on ultrasound or CT scan are found in 73–94% of patients.[1,13,25,27] Imaging study abnormalities include dilated intra- and extra-hepatic ducts, thickened bile duct wall, distal tapering of the common bile duct, gallbladder distention, and gallbladder wall thickening.[12] It has been reported that a hyperechoic nodule occasionally is seen on ultrasound which correlated with edema of the ampulla of Vater seen on ERCP and chronic inflammation in ampullary biopsies.[35] Daly and colleagues[36] reported that ultrasound was 98% accurate in predicting a normal common bile duct on ERCP and that it had a 97% and 100% sensitivity and specificity, respectively, for biliary abnormalities.[36] They suggested ERCP was not beneficial in patients with a normal abdominal ultrasound.[36] In contrast, other studies have reported that the biliary system may appear normal on ultrasound or CT scan in 25% of AIDS patients demonstrated to have cholangiographic abnormalities,[29] thus suggesting that a normal ultrasound or CT scan does not exclude biliary disease. Adler et al.[37] have reported that CT has a higher diagnostic yield for dilation of the common bile duct and AIDS-associated neoplasms, whereas ERCP is superior if there is sclerosing cholangitis. Nuclear scintigraphic scanning (i.e., HIDA scan) may suggest biliary obstruction by demonstrating delayed radionucleotide tracer excretion into the bile duct and small intestine.[1] The sensitivity and specificity of a HIDA scan test in AIDS cholangiopathy is 71% and 100%, respectively.[12] Liver biopsy rarely is helpful in the evaluation of AIDS cholangiopathy but if histologic changes of large duct obstruction are seen, the need for extrahepatic biliary duct evaluation is suggested. To our knowledge, there are no studies assessing the efficacy of ERCP or endoscopic ultrasound in the diagnosis of AIDS cholangiopathy, but they may be useful based on their performance in the evaluation of other biliary diseases.

Invasive

The gold standard for the diagnosis of AIDS cholangiopathy is ERCP. The common cholangiographic findings include a dilated common bile duct with strictured and dilated segments of the intrahepatic ducts. Other cholangiographic features include distal common bile duct tapering, 'beaded' mucosal pattern of the common bile duct suggesting submucosal cell infiltration or edema, irregular ductal dilation and sacculations, pruning of the small intrahepatic ducts, and intraductual debris and/or sludge which appears to be due to sloughed mucosa.[29] The right intrahepatic ducts are less commonly involved than the left system.[12] While the cholangiographic features of AIDS cholangiopathy have similarities to those of idiopathic or primary sclerosing cholangitis (PSC), there are differences:[12,29] in PSC the strictures tend to be shorter in length, dilated segments of bile duct are uncommon, intraductular debris is absent and bile ductular beading occurs only occasionally.[12] The common bile duct is irregularly strictured in PSC and frequently involved over its entire length.[24] The cholangiogram findings usually follow one of the four patterns previously presented in this chapter, as described by Cello et al.[23]

In addition to obtaining a cholangiogram, ERCP allows for biopsy of the ampulla of Vater and duodenum, and duodenal and biliary aspirates and bile duct brushings to be obtained. The biliary epithelium can also be biopsied if a papillotomy is performed. Routine histology and special stains can be performed on duodenal, ampullary, and bile duct tissue. Electron microscopy should be performed in patients in whom microsporidia is suspected if other studies are negative.[1] Cytology and ova and parasite examination can be performed on the bile fluid and biliary brushing as well as aspirated biliary and duodenal fluid. Fluid can also be used to culture for viruses and fungi. Biopsies and fluid sampling should be performed routinely during ERCP in AIDS patients with cholangiopathy in order to diagnose cryptosporidia, microsporidia, viruses such as CMV, and (obstructing) tumors including lymphoma.[1,12,32] It has been shown that ERCP has the highest diagnostic yield when multiple small intestinal and papillary biopsies as well as cultures of bile are obtained.[27]

Sphincter of Oddi manometry also can be performed during ERCP and has demonstrated elevated sphincter of Oddi pressures in AIDS patients with the papillary stenosis variant of AIDS cholangiopathy.[38] Auer and colleague[39] reported a number of manometric abnormalities including tachyoddia, a paradoxical response to ceruletid, inability to decrease sphincter pressure or abolition of sphincter waves after ceruletid, and elevated sphincter pressures. Elevated sphincter of Oddi pressures may be due to the chronic inflammation of the ampulla. Auer and colleagues[39] also noted that patients with abnormal sphincter of Oddi manometry had autonomic dysfunction as determined by a series of autonomic neuropathy tests. The elevated pressure may explain the dilated common bile duct in these patients. Sphincter of Oddi manometry may provide a more rational basis for selecting which patients are likely to benefit from sphincterotomy. ERCP also allows for therapeutic implementation (i.e., papillotomy, stent placement, or balloon dilation) in AIDS patients with cholangiopathy.

Therapy

The therapy of AIDS cholangiopathy consists of treating AIDS with HAART and any underlying opportunistic infection or malignancy and performing endoscopic sphincterotomy or stenting in patients with papillary stenosis or a dominant biliary stricture. Medical therapy of the opportunistic infections, associated with AIDS cholangiopathy, has been disappointing[1] but should still be tried for the occasional patient who may respond. The therapy of AIDS cholangiopathy is primarily endoscopic.

Endoscopic retrograde cholangiopancreatography

For AIDS patients with abdominal pain secondary to papillary stenosis, endoscopic sphincterotomy or stenting may provide rapid and lasting symptomatic relief. Cello and coworkers[40,41] reported on their results of 30 patients with papillary stenosis. Long-term relief of pain was obtained in 57%, partial relief in 10%, and 17% of cases had no lasting relief of pain. The mean follow-up of these patients was 7.4 months. Wettestein et al.[42] reported that 79% of their patients had symptomatic response to sphincterotomy compared to 11% of conservatively treated patients. While other investigators have reported similar or better response rates to sphincterotomy in patients with papillary stenosis, others have reported lower response rates (i.e., 32%).[12,43–45] Lyche and colleagues reported that pain relief was not long lasting and that 49% and 16% of their patients required either a repeat diagnostic or therapeutic ERCP, respectively.[43] The reason for these differing results is not clear. Better delineation of baseline characteristics of AIDS patients with papillary stenosis may predict response to sphincterotomy. Sphincter of Oddi manometry has shown elevated pressures in some patients with papillary stenosis and it has been proposed that manometry could potentially predict those most likely to respond.[38] While more studies are required to address these issues, sphincterotomy should be offered to AIDS patients with symptomatic papillary stenosis. The complication rate of sphincterotomy in AIDS patients is not greater than in non-HIV-infected patients.[1] Even in patients with relief of symptoms after sphincterotomy, the serum alkaline phosphatase often continues to rise. This is not surprising since many patients with papillary stenosis also have intrahepatic ductal sclerosing cholangitis. Sphincterotomy has no beneficial effect on pain in HIV-infected patients with sclerosing cholangitis in the absence of papillary stenosis and common bile duct dilation.[1] Dominant extrahepatic bile duct strictures should be stented endoscopically.[12] Stenting also may be appropriate as primary therapy or as a therapeutic trial to determine the potential efficacy of sphincterotomy in patients with papillary stenosis. Lyche et al.[43] treated 33 AIDS patients with papillary stenosis and found no difference in the outcome of the 26 patients who underwent endoscopic sphincterotomy and the seven who underwent stenting. Pain relief was obtained in all, although it frequently recurred and repeat diagnostic or therapeutic procedures were commonly required. The advantage of stenting over sphincterotomy is that the risks of sphincterotomy are avoided in patients with a limited life expectancy. The potential risk of bacterial infection of the indwelling stent has not yet been defined.[1] Biliary balloon dilation is another potential endoscopic approach to papillary stenosis or a dominant common bile duct stricture.[24] However, few studies have addressed the role of balloon dilation in AIDS cholangiopathy or its efficacy or safety compared with sphincterotomy or stenting.

Medical therapy

Medical therapy has included attempts to eradicate any underlying opportunistic infections and the use of symptomatic agents. In two small open-label trials, AIDS patients with symptomatic papillary stenosis who failed to respond to sphincterotomy were treated with ursodeoxycholic acid. Ursodeoxycholic acid did not eliminate but did lessen right upper quadrant pain and improved liver chemistries.[46,47] Therapy with specific agents for cryptosporidia and microsporidia have failed to improve biliary symptoms or cholangiographic abnormalities due to their lack of efficacy.[1] Cryptosporidia and microsporidia can be eliminated or significantly suppressed by the use of HAART.[48–50] While foscarnet and ganciclovir are effective in the therapy of systemic CMV infection, they appear to have no beneficial effect on CMV-associated cholangiopathy. Trimethoprim-sulfamethoxazole has been reported to be curative for *Cyclospora*-associated cholangitis.[1] Multidrug regimens for MAC can be tried for MAC-associated cholangitis in AIDS patients.[12] Chemotherapy has been reported to induce resolution of sclerosing cholangitis secondary to Hodgkin's lymphoma (HD).[51] Therefore, in patients with bile duct involvement secondary to Hodgkin's or non-Hodgkin's lymphoma, Kaposi's sarcoma-specific chemotherapy and/or radiation therapy should be administered in an attempt to alleviate bile duct obstruction.[24]

Other

Finally, when all therapies fail, celiac plexus block and/or neurolysis can be attempted to relieve intractable pain. This can be achieved using CT, MRI, or endoscopic ultrasound guidance.[52] Collazos et al.[53] reported using CT-guided celiac blocks in three patients with AIDS cholangiopathy and pain. All patients had relief of the symptoms. Further studies are needed to assess the efficacy of this technique.

Prognosis

Historically, despite limited data concerning the natural history of AIDS cholangiopathy, there is a consensus that the prognosis is poor. One-year survival rates vary from 14% to 41%[1,12,28] and a median survival of 7.5–10 months have been reported.[1,12] Two-year survival has been reported to be as low as 8%.[29] More recently, Ko et al.[5] reviewed the data on 94 patients with AIDS cholangiopathy who were followed for 2 decades at the San Francisco General Hospital. The median survival after diagnosis of AIDS cholangiopathy was only 9 months. The presence of opportunistic infections of the digestive tract, lung, eye, nervous system, skin, or systemic involvement at the time of the AIDS cholangiopathy diagnosis was associated with poor prognosis. This was especially true for cryptosporidial infection. An alkaline phosphatase level greater than 8 times the upper limit of normal or 1000 IU/L was also a poor prognostic indicator. Interestingly, the CD4 lymphocyte count, the pattern of cholangiopathy, or a previous sphincterotomy did not affect survival. In Ko's study only 13 out of the 94 patients were diagnosed with AIDS cholangiopathy after the universal institution of HAART. Despite the poor prognosis of this disease, 10 out 13 patients on HAART were still alive at the time of publication of this report in 2003 with a mean survival of 55 months. The widespread use of HAART will probably make AIDS cholangiopathy a rare disease, but there will always be patients who cannot take the medications or who have developed resistance to the current regimens.

APPROACH TO BILIARY DISEASE IN AIDS PATIENTS

Since AIDS patients with biliary disease can be asymptomatic and only show abnormal liver tests, the evaluation of biliary disease overlaps with the evaluation of HIV-infected patient with suspected liver disease. Figure 8.1 outlines an approach to AIDS patients with suspected biliary disease. History and physical examination usually will not support any particular diagnosis due to the lack of pathognomonic findings for specific causes of biliary disease. A reasonable first step in evaluating patients with suspected biliary disease is to obtain a CD4 lymphocyte count. If the count is greater than 200/mL, the work-up should be similar to that of an immunocompetent patient. Patients with CD4 lymphocyte counts of less than 200/mL should begin HAART if they are not already on it. Abdominal imaging studies are valuable in the evaluation of AIDS patients with suspected biliary disease. In individuals suspected of having acalculous cholecystitis, an expedited evaluation with either abdominal ultrasound or HIDA scan should be performed. If the diagnosis of acute cholecystitis is made (with or without gallstones) surgery or a percutaneous cholecystostomy should be performed. The relative value of ultrasound compared to CT scan has not been well studied in the evaluation of patients with suspected AIDS cholangiopathy. One strategy recommends use of ultrasound, which is more cost-effective in nonjaundiced[1,23] and CT scans in AIDS patients with marked hepatomegaly, jaundice, suspected mass lesions, or intra-abdominal processes.[1] Liver biopsy may be appropriate if imaging studies suggest hepatic parenchymal disease, a focal or mass intrahepatic lesion, or if the biliary ducts are not dilated.

The pattern of serum liver chemistry abnormalities may be useful in distinguishing hepatic from biliary disease. Significant elevations of the serum transaminases are usually not consistent with biliary disease and suggest a hepatocellular process. Drug-induced liver disease should be high in the differential diagnosis of abnormal liver serum transaminases in any individual with AIDS, since these patients are usually on multiple medications, many of which are hepatotoxic. Disproportionate elevation of the serum alkaline phosphatase is consistent with biliary tract disease but may also be secondary to infiltrative hepatic disease such as TB, MAC, or lymphoma. Thus, an increase in serum alkaline phosphatase could indicate the need for biliary tract evaluation. Jaundice is rare in patients with AIDS and suggests hepatic disease (medications or viral hepatitis) but may also be the result of high-grade bile duct obstruction due to an extrahepatic stricture. ERCP is indicated in patients with ductal abnormalities on imaging studies, especially if they are symptomatic and endoscopic therapy is felt to be necessary.[1,12,15] ERCP also will be useful in the evaluation of those patients with normal imaging studies, RUQ pain and marked elevations in their serum alkaline phosphatase. As discussed previously, when ERCP is performed duodenal, biliary, and ampulla of Vater biopsies as well as biliary and duodenal fluid aspirates should be obtained. Cytological examination of biliary fluid also should be performed. Therapeutic ERCP is primarily reserved for symptomatic AIDS patients with papillary stenosis and a dilated common bile duct. Percutaneous liver biopsy is of little value in the diagnosis of AIDS cholangiopathy.[12]

SUMMARY

While biliary tract disease in HIV seropositive individuals is uncommon, it should always be considered in the differential

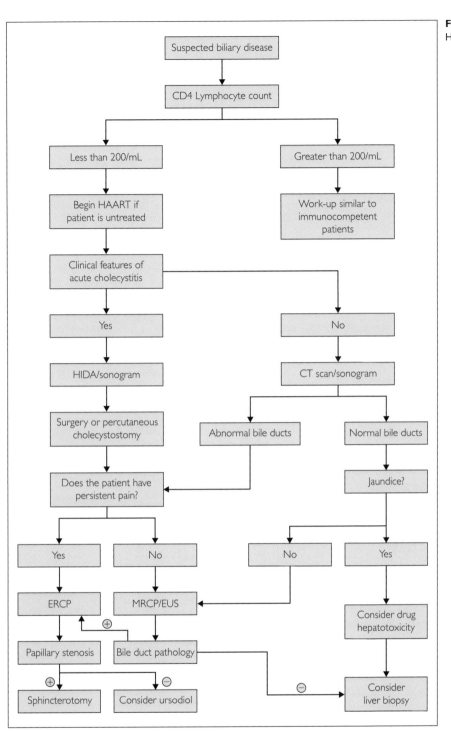

Fig. 8.1 • Approach to biliary disease in HIV-positive patients.

diagnosis of abdominal pain and abnormal liver tests (Table 8.4). Acalculous cholecystitis must be considered in any HIV-seropositive person presenting with biliary colic or an acute abdomen. Failure to consider this diagnosis can lead to gallbladder gangrene, perforation, and resultant death. The pain associated with the papillary stenosis variant of AIDS cholangiopathy does respond in some patients to endoscopic therapy and should be attempted. An attempt to diagnose an opportunistic infection as the etiology of AIDS cholangiopathy should be performed so specific antimicrobial agents can be utilized. Any patient diagnosed with AIDS cholangiopathy also should be treated with aggressive antiretroviral regiments to try to improve survival.

Table 8.4 Summary of approach to biliary infections in the immunocompromised patient

Disorder of the biliary system in AIDS patients include (in order of frequency):

Typical biliary disorders seen in immunocompetent patients such as cholecystitis, choledocholithiasis, etc.

AIDS cholangiopathy syndrome

Acalculous cholecystitis

The first step in the work up of an AIDS patient with suspected biliary disease is to determine the CD4 count

If the CD4 count is above 200 consider conditions of immunocompetent individuals

If the CD4 is below 200 first start HAART if possible

Patients with suspected cholecystitis should have a HIDA or a sonogram performed. If the diagnosis of cholecystitis is made, surgery is the treatment of choice. Cholecystostomy should be reserved for sick or unstable patients

If acute cholecystitis is not likely, start work up with a sonogram or CT scan

Consider a hepatotoxic drug reaction in those patients with normal bile ducts and an elevated bilirubin

There are four patterns of AIDS cholangiopathy:

Papillary stenosis with dilation of the common bile duct

Sclerosing cholangitis

Combination of papillary stenosis and sclerosing cholangitis

Long extrahepatic stricture formation

ERCP with sphincterotomy should be considered for those patients with abdominal pain and papillary stenosis (dilated bile ducts)

The overall prognosis of AIDS cholangiopathy is poor except for those patients who can undergo successful HAART

REFERENCES

1. Wilcox MC. Microbial cholangiopathies in the immunosuppressed patient: Focus on AIDS cholangiopathy. AASLD Syllabus for Postgraduate Course 'Diseases of the bile ducts: Pathogenesis, pathology, and practice' Course Director LaRusso NF. Thorofare, NJ; SLACK Inc.; 1996:67–71.

2. Guarda LA, Stein SA, Cleary KA, et al. Human cryptosporidiosis in the acquired immune deficiency syndrome. Arch Pathol Lab Med 1983; 107:562–566.

   This is the first report of AIDS cholangiopathy.

3. Pitlik SD, Fainstein V, Rios A, et al. Cryptosporidial cholecystitis (Letter). New Engl J Med 1983; 308:967.

4. Enns R. AIDS cholangiopathy: 'an endangered disease' (Editorial) Am J Gastroenterol 2003; 98:2111–2112.

5. Ko WF, Cello JP, Rogers SJ, et al. Prognostic factors for the survival of patients with AIDS cholangiopathy. Am J Gastroenterol 2003; 98:2176–2181.

   In this important study, 94 patients with AIDS cholangiopathy were followed for 2 decades. The presence of other opportunistic infections and an elevated alkaline phosphatase were associated with poor prognosis. More importantly, the authors noted a sharp decrease in the incidence of AIDS cholangiopathy since HAART became widely available.

6. Weber CH, Dancygier H. Increased frequency of gallstones in patients with AIDS. Gastroenterology 1996; 110:A1043.

7. French AL, Beaudet LM, Benator DA, et al. Cholecystectomy in patients with AIDS: Clinical pathologic correlation in 107 cases. Clin Infect Dis 1995; 21:852–858.

8. Margulis SJ, Honiog CL, Soave R, et al. Biliary tract obstruction in the acquired immunodeficiency syndrome. Ann Int Med 1986; 105:2017–2020.

9. Blumberg RS, Kelsey P, Perrone T, et al. Cytomegalovirus- and Cryptosporida-associated acalculous gangrenous cholecystitis. Am J Med l984; 76:1118.

10. Kavin H, Jonas RB, Chowdhury L, et al. Acalculous cholecystitis and cytomegalovirus infection in the acquired immunodeficiency syndrome. Ann Int Med 1986; 106:53–54.

11. Gathe J, Glass H, Ettner E, et al. Gallbladder diseases in AIDS patients: Diagnosis, medical/surgical management. Eighth International AIDS Conference, Berlin, Germany, 1992; Publication 7199:82.

12. Simon DS, Brandt LJ. ERCP in patients with acquired immunodeficiency syndrome: ERCP and its applications. Jacobson I, ed. New York: Raven Press; 1998.

13. Tanowitz HB, Simon D, Weiss LM, et al. Gastrointestinal manifestations of AIDS. Clinic N Amer 1996; 80:1395–1414.

14. Robinson G, Wilson SE, Williams RA. Surgery in patients with the acquired immunodeficiency syndrome. Arch Surg 1987; 122: 170–175.

15. Wilcox M, Rabeneck L, Friedman S. AGA technical review: Malnutrition and cachexia, chronic diarrhea, and hepatobiliary disease in patients with human immunodeficiency virus infection. Gastroenterology 1996; 111:1724–1752.

16. Cacciarelli AG, Marano BJ, Zuretti AR, et al. Gallbladder disease in the HIV population. Gastroenterology 1995; 108:A407.

17. Robinson G, Wilson SE, Willians RA. Surgery in patients with the acquired immunodeficiency syndrome. Arch Surg 1987; 122: 170–175.

18. Cello JP. Gastrointestinal manifestations of HIV infection. Inf Dis Clin N Am 1988; 2:236–245.

19. LaRaja RD, Rothenberg R, Odom JW, et al. The incidence of intra-abdominal surgery in acquired immunodeficiency syndrome: A statistical review of 904 patients. Surgery 1989; 105:175–179.

20. Diettrich NA, Cacioppo JC, Kaplan G, et al. A growing spectrum of surgical diseases in patients with human immunodeficiency syndrome: Experience with 120 major cases. Arch Surg 1991; 126:680–686.

21. Ferrucci JT. Acute cholecystitis: Percutaneous drainage. In: Henderson JM, ed. Hepatobiliary forum: hepato-pancreato-biliary infections. sponsored by AASLD/American Hepato-Pancreato-Biliary Assoc in Chicago: Thorofare, NJ: SLACK Inc; 1996:1–10.

22. Davis CA, Landercasper J, Gundersen LH, et al. Effective use of percutaneous cholecystostomy in high-risk surgical patients: techniques, tube management, and results. Arch Surg 1999; 134(7):727–731.

23. Cello JP. Acquired immunodeficiency syndrome cholangiopathy: Spectrum of disease. Am J Med 1989; 86:539–546.

    This is the first description of the four distinct patterns of AIDS cholangiopathy.

24. Grendell JH, Cello JP. HIV-associated hepatobiliary disease. In: Zakim D, Boyer TD, eds. Hepatology: a textbook of liver disease. Philadelphia: WB Saunders; 1996:1699–1706.

25. Bonacini M. Hepatobiliary complications in patients with human immunodeficiency virus infection. Amer J Med 1992; 92:404–411.

26. Farman J, Brunetti J, Baer JW, et al. AIDS-related cholangiopancreatographic changes. Abdominal Imaging 1994; 19:417–422.

27. Pol S, Romana CA, Richard S, et al. Microsporidia infection in patients with the human immunodeficiency virus and unexplained cholangitis. N Engl J Med 1993; 328:95–99.

28. Bouche H, Housset C, Dumont JL, et al. AIDS-related cholangitis: Diagnostic features and course in 15 patients. J Hepatol 1993; 17:34–39.

29. Forbes A, Blanshard C, Gazzard B. Natural history of AIDS-related sclerosing cholangitis: A study of 20 patients. Gut 1993; 34: 116–121.

30. Wilson R, Harrington R, Stewart B, et al. Human immunodeficiency virus 1 associated necrotizing cholangitis caused by infection with *Septata intestinalis*. Gastroenterology 1995; 108:247–251.

31. Weber R, Deplazes P, Flepp M, et al. Cerebral microsporidiosis due to *Encephalitozoon cuniculi* in a patient with human immunodeficiency virus infection. N Engl J Med 1997; 336:474–478.

32. Herndier BG, Friedman SL. Neoplasms of the gastrointestinal tract and hepatobiliary system in acquired immunodeficiency syndrome. Semin Liver Dis 1992; 12:128–141.

33. Levine SA, Jobin C, Sartor RB, et al. Cryptosporidium cytopathic for human biliary epithelial cells by an apoptotic process associated with cytokine production. Hepatology 1996; 24:246A.

34. Chan MF, Cello JP. Prevalence of AIDS-associated cholangiopathy in asymptomatic patients. Hepatology 1992; 16:127A.

35. DaSilva F, Boudghene F, LeComte I, et al. Sonography in AIDS-related cholangitis: prevalence and causes of an echogenic nodule in the distal end of the common bile duct. Am J Roent 1993; 160:1205–1207.

36. Daly CA, Padley SP. Sonographic predication of a normal or abnormal ERCP in suspected AIDS-related cholangitis. Clin Radiol 1996; 51:618–621.

37. Adler A, Knollmann F, Veltzke W, et al. Value of retrograde cholangiogram (ERC) and computed tomography in hepatobiliary AIDS-related disease. Gastroenterology 1995; 108;A767.

38. Levenson SD, Koch J, Schlueck G, et al. Sphincter of Oddi dysfunction in patients with suspected AIDS cholangiopathy. Gastrointestinal Endoscopy 1994; 40:116A.

39. Auer P, Lubke HJ, Freiling T, et al. Sphincter of Oddi dysfunction in AIDS-related autonomic failure. Gastroenterology 1995; 108:A404.

40. Cello JP. Human immunodeficiency virus-associated biliary tract disease. Sem Liver Dis 1992; 12:213–218.

41. Cello JP, Chan MF. Long term follow-up of endoscopic retrograde cholangiopancreatography sphincterotomy for patients with the acquired immunodeficiency syndrome papillary stenosis. Amer J Med 1995; 99:600–603.

This study reports the long-term effects of sphincterotomy in 30 patients with papillary stenosis. Sixty-seven percent of the patients had complete or partial relieve of their symptoms after sphincterotomy.

42. Wettstein A, Dore G, Murphy C, et al. HIV-related cholangiopathy in Australia. Gastroenterology 1997; 112:A1117.

43. Lyche KD, Savides TJ, Weiner KJ, et al. AIDS cholangiopathy: The role of therapeutic ERCP. Gastrointestinal Endoscopy 1994; 40:117A.

This abstract suggests that stenting may be an alternative to sphincterotomy for patients with papillary stenosis.

44. Benhamou Y, Caumes E, Gerosa Y, et al. AIDS-related cholangiopathy: Critical analysis of a prospective series of 26 patients. Dig Dis Sci 1993; 38:1113–1138.

45. Ducreux M, Buffet C, Lamy P, et al. Diagnosis and prognosis of AIDS-related sclerosing cholangitis. AIDS 1995; 9:875–880.

46. Chan MF, Koch J, Cello JP. Ursodeoxycholic acid (URSO) for symptomatic AIDS-associated cholangiopathy. Gastrointestinal Endoscopy 1994; 40:103A.

47. Castiella A, Iribarren JA, Lopez P, et al. Ursodeoxycholic acid in the treatment of AIDS-associated cholangiopathy. Am J Med 1997; 103:170–171.

This open labeled study suggests that ursodeoxycholic acid may be helpful in patients who failed sphincterotomy for papillary stenosis.

48. Conteas CN, Berlin OG, LaRiviere, et al. Self-limited intestinal microsporidiosis in AIDS patients. Gastroenterology 1997; 112:A952.

49. Carr A, Marriott D, Field A, et al. Treatment of HIV-1-associated microsporidiosis and cryptosporidiosis with combination antiretroviral therapy. Lancet 1998; 351:256–261.

50. Miao YM, Awad-El-Kariem PM, Franzen C, et al. Eradication of cryptosporidia and microsporidia following successful antiretroviral therapy. J AIDS 2000; 25:124–129.

51. Teare JP, Price DA, Foster GR, et al. Reversible AIDS-related sclerosing cholangitis. J Hepatol 1995; 23:209–211.

52. Yusuf TE, Baron TH. AIDS cholangiopathy. Curr Treat Options Gastroenterol. 2004; 7(2):111–117.

53. Collazos J, Mayo J, Martinez E, et al. Celiac plexus block as treatment for refractory pain related to sclerosing cholangitis in AIDS patients. J Clin Gastroenterol 1996; 23:47–49.

Gastrointestinal and hepatobiliary complications of bone marrow transplantation

Stuart L. Goldberg, David M. Felig and Richard C. Golding

Bone marrow and blood stem cell transplantation (BMT) is an integral part of the management of hematologic malignancies, marrow failure syndromes, immunodeficiency states, congenital enzyme defects, and selected solid tumors.

THE PRETRANSPLANT EVALUATION

Before undergoing BMT, candidates undergo extensive evaluation to discover any unrecognized organ dysfunction that may preclude the safe administration of high-dose therapy. The importance of this pretransplant screen has been confirmed by a retrospective multivariate analysis noting abnormalities in serum bilirubin, pulmonary forced expiratory volume, serum creatinine, and overall performance status as independent predictors of toxic mortality during the first 100 days after BMT.[1]

Oropharyngeal evaluation

Poor dentition, tooth abscesses, and normal oral microflora serve as potential sources of septicemia. A thorough pre-BMT dental examination and ultrasonic cleaning (with prophylactic antibiotics for patients with indwelling catheters) are highly recommended.[2]

Esophageal and upper gastrointestinal symptoms

Dysphagia and upper gastrointestinal symptoms may be caused by fungal or viral infections, including *Candida* and herpesvirus. Although empirical therapy with azole antifungal agents or acyclovir may relieve symptoms, endoscopy with biopsy should be considered to exclude other causes. *Helicobacter pylori* infection does not disseminate after BMT and should not delay transplantation. Direct tumor infiltration may result in ulceration and predispose to intestinal bleeding and perforation during chemotherapy. Evaluation for occult tumor in asymptomatic patients is unnecessary given the low frequency of tumor lysis-induced severe bleeding.[3,4]

Diarrhea and lower gastrointestinal symptoms

Transplant candidates may develop diarrhea from enteric infections, prior treatment including radiation-associated enterocolitis, pseudomembranous colitis, medications, or tumor-related malabsorption syndromes. Endoscopic evaluation and stool analysis are essential because infectious causes of diarrhea, including

Entamoeba histolytica and *Strongyloides stercoralis*, may disseminate after BMT. Patients with inflammatory bowel disease have successfully undergone stem cell transplantation and experienced improvement in their bowel disease.[5] Perianal pain is an indication to delay transplantation as neutropenic patients may be unable to form abscesses and have only tenderness or fever. Supralevator and intersphincteric abscesses may not be appreciated by external examination. Surgical debridement and broad-spectrum antibiotics are recommended.[6] Viral causes of perianal pain, including herpesvirus, also require investigation.[7] Granulocyte transfusions, which may assist in abscess formation before surgical drainage, may lead to the development of platelet refractoriness and increased risk of graft rejection.[8]

Liver disease

Abnormalities in liver function have been identified in up to 25% of transplant candidates. Multiple analyses have reported that transplants performed in the setting of prior liver disease result in a higher incidence of complications.[9]

Candidates with prior hepatitis B are at risk for reactivation of virus and liver dysfunction after BMT, which may be fatal in up to 15% without antiviral prophylaxis.[10,11] Allogeneic transplant recipients who require long-term glucocorticoid therapy for graft-versus-host disease (GVHD) are at particular risk. Pre-emptive antiviral therapies with adefovir or lamivudine for 1 year or until all immunosuppressants are discontinued may reduce the rate and severity of post-transplant viral liver disease.[12]

Patients with hepatitis C and elevated AST and ALT, rather than the presence of viremia alone, appear to be at substantially increased risk for early liver toxicity of hepatic veno-occlusive disease. These patients are particularly sensitive to high-dose cyclophosphamide.[13] Oral rather than intravenous busulfan may also increase VOD risk.[14]

Choice of the appropriate stem cell donor may also impact on post-transplant liver disease. Antibodies present in the donor may be transferred to the recipient (adoptive immunity) with subsequent clearance of HBV.[15] If available, donors with naturally acquired HBVsAb would be preferred over nonimmune donors and vaccination of the marrow donor has been proposed.[16]

Hepatitis C RNA positivity has been associated with a high risk of fatal hepatic veno-occlusive disease in some series. Use of interferon and ribavirin therapy if time permits or lower dose non-myeloablative conditioning regimens may be considered. By contrast, HCV infection is not a major cause of late liver dysfunction.[10,17]

Fungal infections are common in transplant candidates, but patients with hepatosplenic candidiasis and prior *Aspergillus* infections have been successful carried through BMT with concurrent antifungal therapy.[18] Magnetic resonance imaging represents the most sensitive non-invasive technique for identifying hepatic fungal infections.[19]

Patients with hepatic fibrosis and/or cirrhosis are at substantially increased risk of fatal toxic liver injury and/or multiorgan failure following high-dose conditioning regimens.[20] Nonmyeloablative transplantation should be considered.

Hepatic VOD is the most frequent early treatment-related liver complication. Potential risk factors include the conditioning regimen, pretransplant elevations in aminotransferase levels, prior infectious hepatitis, liver or fungal disease, treatment of infection soon after BMT, older age, and decreased pretransplant protein C and factor VII levels.[21] Prior exposure to gemtuzumab ozogamicin, a conjugated immunotoxin against CD33 used in acute myeloid leukemia, has been associated with a significantly increased risk (relative risk 19) of VOD.[22]

Donor issues

Hematopoietic stem cell collection from a donor may be accomplished from either multiple aspirations of marrow from the iliac crests or through leukapheresis of the peripheral blood. Donors with autoimmune diseases in whom the use of cytokines needed to mobilize stem cells (such as filgrastim) is not advised, may be better candidates for operative marrow harvests.[23]

Identification of viral hepatitis in a donor presents unique challenges for the gastroenterologist, both in caring for the infected donor and in assessing risks to a potential transplant recipient.

Hepatitis B: HBsAg-positive individuals are infectious but may be used as stem cell donors if the risk of subsequent liver disease is outweighed by the hematologic malignancy requiring transplantation. A review of 24 recipients of HBsAg-positive marrow noted seroconversion in 22%, but only 5.5% became chronic carriers.[24] Risk factors for transmission are high serum levels of HBV DNA.[25] Antiviral therapies result in rapid reduction in HBV DNA levels within weeks potentially reducing transmission risk. Preemptive lamivudine treatment of the recipient of a HBsAg-positive stem cell transplant reduces the rate and severity of subsequent infection.[12] Because less severe liver disease has developed after BMT in previously 'immune' recipients (pretransplant anti-HBs seropositivity), passive prophylaxis of recipients with anti-HBs immunoglobulin or IVIG may also be considered.[24,26] Reverse seroconversion has been reported, so the recipient's prior immune status may not be fully protective in the transplant setting.[27]

Donors who are hepatitis B core antibody positive (anti-HBc) and HBsAg-negative rarely transmit viral infection. Confirmatory HBV DNA studies prior to stem cell donation are recommended.[28] Donors who have antibodies to hepatitis B surface antigen (HBsAb) are not considered infectious.

Hepatitis C: HCV RNA-positive donors transmit infection to their marrow recipients at a rate approaching 100%. By contrast, donors who are anti-HCV seropositive but RNA negative are not infectious. Recipients of hepatitis C-positive stem cells typically develop mild liver disease only after immune reconstitution, and appear to experience minimal morbidity during the first 10 years

following transplantation.[29] Antiviral treatment of the donor may substantially delay the transplant and be toxic for the donor. Since antiviral therapies also may be myelosuppressive and delay marrow engraftment, treatment should be held at least 1–2 weeks prior to stem cell donation.

COMPLICATIONS OF CONDITIONING THERAPY, THE CYTOPENIC PHASE, AND EARLY MARROW RECOVERY (THROUGH DAY 100)

Odynophagia and dysphagia

Oropharyngeal pain and esophageal pain are common early problems after transplantation. Mucosal inflammation and ulceration increase the risk of systemic infection and bleeding and impair adequate nutritional intake.[30]

Mucositis

Oral mucositis (OM), the painful inflammation of tissues of the oropharynx, occurs in upwards of 70–80% of fully ablative transplant recipients.[31] Transplant recipients with severe mucositis are 2–3 times more likely to develop bacteremia, experience more febrile days, and utilize more intravenous antibiotics.[32] Thus, the length of stay and total transplantation costs are significantly increased (US$28000–US$42000).[33] In a survey of BMT patients, 42% of the 38 respondents rated OM as their most significant problem.[34]

Unfortunately, effective preventative or treatment strategies for mucositis are lacking, with empirical symptomatic treatment the mainstay.[35–37] Good oral hygiene with gentle cleaning and saline/sodium bicarbonate rinses is recommended, but oral antibiotic rinses such as chlorhexidine are no longer recommended.[36] Chewing ice chips during chemotherapy administration, an approach to inducing local vasoconstriction and preventing mucositis, has been touted by some centers.[35] As pain develops, topical anesthetics and mucosal coating agents may provide temporary relief. If local measures are inadequate, parenteral narcotic analgesics are indicated.[36] Patient-controlled analgesic devices allow individualized tailoring, resulting in lower total narcotic dosing.[38] In the outpatient setting, transdermal fentanyl may provide an alternative to intravenous therapy. Rarely, in patients with severe inflammation and hemorrhagic tissue breakdown, short courses of steroids or prophylactic intubation may be required to prevent aspiration. Careful serial examinations for other causes of epithelial deterioration, including infection and GVHD, are important. Recognition of α-hemolytic *Streptococcus* as a cause and complication of mucositis supports early antibiotic use.[39]

AES-14 is an oral suspension drug delivery system of L-glutamine, an essential amino acid involved in mucosal healing. A randomized, placebo-controlled trial in 195 BMT patients demonstrated a reduction in the total severity of mucositis by 64% versus placebo in BMT patients (p=0.04) and morphine use was reduced in half (p=0.005).[40] Palifermin (recombinant human keratinocyte growth factor) is a novel cytokine that stimulates epithelial tissue proliferation and differentiation. In a double-blind, placebo-controlled 212-patient study, Palifermin treated patients experienced lower incidence of grades III/IV oral mucositis (63% versus 98%; p=0.001), fewer days of grade III/IV mucositis (mean 3.7 versus 10.4 days; $p<0.001$), and used less narcotic analgesics and nutritional support.[41] Large national trials with novel oral antibiotics (iseganan) and antibiotic/antiinflammatory agents (EN3247) have been disappointing.[42,43]

Infections

Viral causes

Once the most common cause of oral and esophageal complaints (occurring in >80% of patients by the third week), reactivation of latent herpes simplex virus (HSV) is now rare. Seropositive patients, identified during the pretransplant evaluation, should be treated with prophylactic acyclovir therapy through engraftment. Because primary infection with HSV is uncommon, empirical treatment of seronegative transplant recipients is unnecessary. Herpesvirus infections should be considered as a cause of odynophagia/dysphagia in patients not receiving prophylaxis or after a late immunologic insult such as GVHD. Symptoms include nausea, vomiting, and pain. Endoscopy reveals small, 1–2 mm vesicles in the squamous epithelium of the mid to distal portion of the esophagus. These vesicles slough and leave ulcers with reddened, raised borders that may coalesce to form large ulcerations. Because HSV infects only the squamous epithelium in the esophagus, brushings must sample the edges of the ulcer and not the central crater.[3] HSV can be identified by direct microscopy showing multinucleated cells with intranuclear inclusion bodies, by immunohistochemistry, or by viral culture. High-dose intravenous acyclovir or oral valaciclovir is recommended, though ulcer healing may be slow. Although rare in the BMT setting, acyclovir-resistant HSV strains have been identified, but aggressive therapy with the marrow-suppressive drug foscarnet is typically reserved for severe infections.[44]

Varicella-zoster virus (VZV) infection may have similar oropharyngeal-esophageal symptoms as HSV. Primary VZV infection in pediatric BMT patients is uncommon (5% of cases). Reactivation VZV infection is a late occurrence (2–10 months peak, but the risk continues for years).[45] Esophageal symptoms are typically overshadowed by skin and visceral disease. Abdominal pain is a concern. Endoscopic biopsy is diagnostic in cases without easily accessible skin lesions. High-dose intravenous acyclovir and valaciclovir are effective.

Cytomegalovirus (CMV) esophagitis remains a frequent cause of odynophagia and dysphagia occurring 30–100 days after transplantation. CMV esophagitis is typically part of a systemic disease and may foreshadow pneumonia or worsening of GVHD. Because oral cultures are not predictive of esophageal findings, endoscopy is required for an accurate diagnosis. Endoscopic findings are variable and range from normal mucosa to large shallow ulcerations with erythematous borders.[46] Unlike HSV and VZV, CMV does not infect the squamous epithelium but rather involves endothelial cells and fibroblasts of the submucosa. Thus, endoscopic biopsy specimens, under the support of platelet counts above 50 000/mm³, should be taken from the ulcer crater. Rapid diagnosis can frequently be obtained by examination for cytomegalic cells with immunohistochemical stains or by shell-vial centrifugation culture. Ganciclovir suppresses viral replication but has minimal impact on clinical symptoms and the rate of ulcer healing. Unfortunately, a randomized, placebo-controlled trial also failed to show 2 weeks of ganciclovir therapy effective in preventing subsequent life-threatening CMV pneumonia.[47] Prolonged ganciclovir maintenance treatment, high-dose ganci-

clovir, combination ganciclovir with intravenous immune globulin, and foscarnet therapy may be considered.[48,49] Newer therapeutic strategies currently being investigated include long-term suppression of CMV with valganciclovir for the prevention of late CMV infection and disease, adoptive transfer of CMV-specific T cells, and donor/recipient vaccination strategies.[50-53]

Fungal causes

Fungal esophagitis has become rare with widespread prophylactic antifungal use. Fluconazole is effective in decreasing superficial fungal infections and esophageal disease.[54] During the neutropenic-thrombocytopenic phase of BMT, empirical therapy is indicated because endoscopic examination may be difficult. Superficial oral infections should also be treated aggressively to prevent swallowed yeast from causing systemic disease. Endoscopy, performed after marrow recovery, frequently fails to reveal typical fungal exudates, which makes brushing and biopsy for histologic examination important. Antifungal treatment is based on biopsy rather than culture.[55]

Bacterial causes

Bacterial causes of esophagitis are unusual. The most common organisms are anaerobes of the mouth, which cause secondary infection of epithelium injured by acid pepsin reflux.

Peptic esophagitis

BMT patients experience an increased incidence of acid reflux disease. Treatment is similar to non-BMT strategies. Endoscopic diagnosis/confirmation in the absence of fever, or suspicion of infection is typically not required.[56] Stricture formation is uncommon.[57]

Intramural hematoma

Severe retching and emesis after chemotherapy cause an abrupt onset of retrosternal pain radiating to the back, dysphagia, esophageal obstruction, and hematemesis. The diagnosis should be confirmed by noninvasive means, including computed tomography or magnetic resonance imaging. Esophagograms with water-soluble contrast may reveal a double-barrel esophagus or mucosal strip if contrast enters the false lumen.[58] Endoscopy carries a risk of perforation and should be avoided. Management is purely supportive with platelets because hematomas resolve slowly over a 1–3-week period, even with total esophageal occlusion.[59] Surgery is not necessary. Hematomas and perforation may also occur after invasive procedures such as endoscopic biopsy for infection detection. Management is supportive.[60]

Medications

Pill-induced ulceration, which causes direct trauma and local toxicity owing to the delayed transit time of certain drugs (especially doxycycline), is an infrequent cause of odynophagia or dysphagia in these patients. Administration of medications with the patient in a sitting position and liberal intake of fluids are advised.[61]

Acute graft-versus-host disease

Immunologic disparity between the engrafting donor immune system and host tissues may result in GVHD. Lymphocytic infiltrates may invade the squamous epithelium of the oropharynx and esophagus. Esophageal pain is usually accompanied by systemic complaints of nausea, diarrhea, and liver abnormalities.

Anorexia, nausea, and emesis

Patient acceptance of high-dose therapy depends in part on adequate control of nausea.

Conditioning chemotherapy and/or radiotherapy

Nausea and emesis are nearly universal with high-dose therapy and may last for 2 weeks or longer. Protracted anorexia extending for weeks after treatment is also common.[62] Chemotherapy-related symptoms can be subdivided into three components: (1) acute symptoms within 24 h of chemoradiotherapy administration, (2) delayed symptoms, and (3) anticipatory symptoms.

Acute symptoms from high-dose therapy require aggressive management concurrent with initiation of chemoradiotherapy. 5-Hydroxytryptamine type 3 receptor antagonists, including ondansetron, granisetron, and dolasetron, are effective in reducing the severity of symptoms.[63–65] Palonosetron is a new 5-HT$_3$-receptor antagonist with a longer half-life and a higher binding affinity, yielding higher complete response rates.[66] Single, daily bolus dosing of 5-HT$_3$ agents during conditioning appears to be more efficacious than divided schedules.[67] The addition of steroids increases response rates by 10–40%.[68] Although slightly less effective, metoclopramide and phenothiazines have also been used for acute nausea during conditioning therapy.[69] Among patients experiencing breakthrough emesis during the first 24 h, the use of additional doses of 5-HT$_3$ antagonists is generally ineffective and cannot be recommended. In these patients metoclopramide, phenothiazines, benzodiazepines, butyrophenones, and cannabinoids have been used.

Anticipatory nausea occurs in patients with poor emesis control during prior chemotherapy exposure and during the initiation of high-dose treatment and with oral busulfan conditioning. Antianxiolytic medications (lorazepam) can be helpful in these patients. Nonpharmacologic measures, including hypnosis, are useful adjuncts.

Delayed nausea is the most difficult to treat and unfortunately quite common among BMT patients. 5-HT$_3$ antagonists have performed poorly in this situation. Aprepitant is the first agent available in the new drug class of neurokinin-1 receptor antagonists. When added to a standard regimen of a 5-HT$_3$-receptor antagonist and dexamethasone in patients receiving highly emetogenic chemotherapy, it improves the complete response rate of delayed nausea.[66] Other options include prochlorperazine, dexamethasone, and lorazepam. Evaluation for other causes of prolonged nausea, including gastroparesis that responds to promotility drugs, is important in patients failing to improve.[62]

Medications

BMT recipients receive multiple supportive care medications, including antibiotics and narcotics that contribute to nausea. Total parenteral nutrition has been associated with protracted anorexia that can persist for several weeks after administration.[70] The cryoprotectant dimethyl sulfoxide co-administered during stem cell infusion may provoke acute nausea.[71]

Infection

Infectious causes of nausea have become uncommon with the use of prophylactic antiinfectives[72] Central nervous system infections are an unusual cause of nausea, although additional neurologic defects frequently predominate.

Gastric motility disorders

Stem cell recipients with persistent nausea and emesis frequently displayed altered gastric motility.[73,74] CMV, VZV, and GVHD all may cause gastric stasis. Prokinetic agents may be useful.

Acute graft-versus-host disease

The sudden onset of anorexia, dyspepsia, food intolerance, nausea, and vomiting may be the earliest manifestation of acute GVHD in allograft recipients.[75] After day 20, when the acute effects of conditioning treatment have typically resolved, GVHD becomes the most common cause of anorexia.[72] Diagnosis requires endoscopic biopsy of the gastric antrum, which is typically edematous and erythematous. Histologic findings include single-cell epithelial necrosis with associated karyorrhectic debris, dilation of mucosal crypts or glands, and crypt abscesses or obliteration.[76] A classification scheme incorporating upper gastrointestinal symptoms in GVHD has been proposed (Table 9.1). Because upper tract symptoms often precede lower tract disease, early recognition and treatment have been advocated to prevent more serious complications. Initial therapy for most patients consists of high-dose steroids with bowel rest. Oral beclomethasone has also shown promising results.[78] In nonresponsive patients, additional immunosuppressive therapies may be necessary.

A syndrome of lymphocytic gastritis with symptoms and endoscopic findings similar to gastrointestinal GVHD may occur in recipients of autologous transplantation within the first 30–60 days post-transplant. Although self-limited, a short course of prednisone improves symptoms rapidly.[79]

Gastrointestinal bleeding

Occult gastrointestinal bleeding is common after BMT as a result of thrombocytopenia, coagulopathies, and diffuse mucosal injury caused by high-dose therapy and GVHD. Overt bleeding episodes occur only rarely, although mortality rates from severe bleeding approach 40%.[80] Patients with amyloidosis appear particularly susceptible to gastrointestinal bleeding during transplantation.[81]

Conditioning chemotherapy and/or radiotherapy

High-dose therapy results in diffuse mucosal damage. Oral, esophageal, and small intestinal ulcerations are most common, with slow bleeding and rare hemodynamic instability. Endoscopic correction is often ineffective, with cautery techniques leading to increased mucosal damage. Empirical transfusion support to platelet counts >50 000/mm^3 is sufficient. Low-dose steroids and measures to ensure airway protection are infrequently needed. Tumor lysis after conditioning therapy may cause brisk bleeding. Endoscopic and surgical intervention is usually necessary during

Table 9.1 Upper GI GVHD grading classification[77]	
Stage I	Anorexia, nausea, and diarrhea volume greater than 500 mL
Stage II	Food intolerance or vomiting and diarrhea volume greater than 1000 mL
Stage III	Marked decrease in performance status and diarrhea volume greater than 1500 mL
Stage IV	Severe abdominal pain, with or without ileus

these rare events (0.2%).[3] Although emesis and retching may result in direct trauma to the esophagus and stomach with mild bleeding, Mallory-Weiss tears are uncommon.

Acid peptic disease

Pre-existing ulcers may bleed during the severe thrombocytopenic phase of BMT. Peptic esophagitis is a common cause of minimal hematemesis. Transfusion and supportive measures are the mainstay of therapy. Gastric mucosal calcinosis is an unusual cause of ulceration in transplant patients receiving aluminum-containing antacids or sucralfate.[82]

Infection

In the absence of adequate acyclovir prophylaxis, HSV may cause diffuse intestinal necrosis with bleeding. Treatment consists of antiviral therapy and platelet transfusions. CMV ulcers in the esophagus are typically shallow and do not bleed vigorously. However, CMV ulcers in the stomach and intestine are deeper and may cause severe bleeding.[83] Other viruses resulting in minimal ulceration and bleeding include rotavirus and adenovirus.[84]

Candidal infections result in diffuse oozing rather than rapid bleeding. Among patients requiring aggressive immunosuppressive therapy for GVHD or experiencing delayed engraftment, *Aspergillus* infection and mucormycosis can be life threatening. These fungi are angioinvasive and cause arterial occlusion, segmental intestinal infarction, and fatal bleeding.[85] Prophylactic antifungal agents are indicated in high-risk patients. Aggressive antifungal therapy with surgical debridement is required for documented infections.

Neutropenic colitis is uncommon after BMT. Empiric therapy is typically administered. Surgical mortality is high in the BMT setting.[86] *Clostridium difficile* diarrheal disease is associated with minimal bleeding.

Gastric antral vascular ectasia

An unusual cause of bleeding, gastric antral vascular ectasia typically occurs 20–90 days after BMT and is associated with hepatic VOD. Endoscopic biopsy of the gastric antrum reveals capillary dilation, focal capillary thromboses, and fibromuscular hyperplasia.[87] Platelet transfusions and endoscopic laser or argon-plasma photocoagulation are useful in controlling bleeding.

Variceal hemorrhage

Vascular bleeding is an uncommon complication of hepatic VOD and regenerative nodular hyperplasia. Significant hemorrhage requires an urgent reduction in mesenteric blood flow via infusion of octreotide or somatostatin coupled with sclerotherapy or banding.[61,88]

Acute graft-versus-host disease

GVHD, the most common cause of severe bleeding in post-transplant patients, accounts for 60% of episodes and is associated with intestinal infection in half. Sites of immunologic attack may occur anywhere along the gastrointestinal tract, although diffuse mucosal ulceration in the distal portion of the small bowel and cecum is most common. In a patient with concurrent skin changes, diarrhea, and liver abnormalities, the diagnosis is usually obvious. Endoscopic evaluation typically reveals extensive mucosal injury and oozing from multiple sites rather than discrete lesions. Biopsy demonstrates rupture of the capillary basal membrane and extra-

vasated red blood cells. These pericapillary hemorrhages are highly correlated with GVHD severity.[89] Superinfection by fungi or CMV may cause focal bleeding. Treatment of bleeding can be extremely difficult and is aimed at correction of the underlying immunologic disorder, transfusion support with platelets, and identification of secondary causes such as infection. Radionucleotide evaluation may have a role in defining sources of bleeding. Endoscopic corrective measures typically result in ulcer formation and further impair healing. Angiographic embolization of mesenteric blood vessels has been advocated as a temporizing measure.[3]

Abdominal pain

Conditioning chemotherapy and/or radiotherapy

Early crampy abdominal pain in association with emesis and diarrhea is a frequent consequence of high-dose therapy. Control of the accompanying symptoms and reassurance to the patient are sufficient in most cases.

Infection

Because immunosuppressed patients may be unable to mount a typical inflammatory response, serious abdominal infections may occur in the absence of significant pain. Abdominal viral infections such as with HSV and adenovirus are more notable causes of diarrhea and liver disease. VZV is the exception and is occasionally manifested as severe abdominal pain, frequently occurring before classic skin lesions. VZV DNA may be identified in the serum and obviates the need for intestinal biopsy. Skin lesions and rapidly increasing hepatocellular enzymes herald a poor prognosis, and prompt institution of intravenous acyclovir is critical.[90]

Typhlitis is rare.[86] Pain in association with bleeding, diarrhea, and fever are the initial features. *Clostridium septicum* is the most common organism. Rarely, bacterial or fungal liver abscess may result in pain as an initial feature. Patients with *C. difficile*-induced diarrhea may also complain of crampy abdominal pain. *Aspergillus* infection, typically accompanied by pulmonary involvement, may result in intestinal infarction and severe abdominal pain.

Perforation and pneumatosis intestinalis

True abdominal perforation is rare. Infections, including CMV disease and *Aspergillus*, lysis of tumor, and diverticular disease are causative factors. Patients frequently have mild symptoms because of a lack of neutrophil inflammation. Pneumoperitoneum can be identified on plain upright radiographs. Although many BMT recipients will survive initial heroic surgery, the overall mortality in these immunocompromised patients is exceedingly high.[91]

Perforation may be mimicked by pneumatosis intestinalis.[92] The initial features include pain, diarrhea, rectal bleeding, and abdominal distention. Evaluation with plain radiographs reveals gas within the bowel wall, commonly affecting the right colon. Risk factors include prolonged neutropenia and immunosuppression, GVHD, steroids, infection, and prior gastrointestinal instrumentation. Conservative management with bowel rest, and antibiotics in asymptomatic patients, is sufficient. Hemicolectomy should be considered if clinical deterioration occurs.

Pseudo-obstruction and obstruction

A cause of moderate to severe abdominal pain, pseudo-obstruction occurs in patients with gastrointestinal pathology and in patients receiving narcotic analgesics. Common contributors include medications, prior neurotoxic chemotherapy, sepsis, abdominal abscess, pneumonia, pancreatitis, acute GVHD, and electrolyte disturbances.[93] Treatment is directed at the causative underlying factor. Standard conservative management with NPO status and naso-gastric and rectal tube decompression is usually effective. Neostigmine has been used for the treatment of acute colonic pseudo-obstruction.[94] Pseudo-obstructions rarely progress to intestinal perforation. Ogilvie's syndrome induced by VZV denervation, is an infrequent cause of pseudo-obstruction that requires specific antiviral therapy.[95] True obstructions from bezoars are rare.[96]

Hematoma

Intra-abdominal bleeding may cause an acute onset of pain. In the setting of thrombocytopenia, minimal precipitating events such as emesis or falls may result in rectus sheath hematomas and retroperitoneal or intra-abdominal hemorrhage. Computed tomography assists in localization.[97]

Hepatic veno-occlusive disease

The most common cause of abdominal pain in the early (days 10–30) post-transplant setting is hepatic VOD. A consequence of direct toxic effects of the conditioning therapy, three-quarters of patients with VOD have right-upper quadrant pain (tender hepatomegaly). In patients with severe pain in association with ascites, paracentesis may provide temporary symptomatic relief.

Biliary disease

Acute cholecystitis is rare in BMT patients despite the frequent occurrence of biliary sludge.[98] Because ultrasonographic abnormalities are common in the absence of symptoms, clinical examination is most important.

Pancreatic causes

Pancreatitis is uncommon, although pancreatic inflammation is frequent at autopsy. Transplant patients are exposed to multiple precipitating factors for pancreatic disease, including cyclosporine, tacrolimus, steroids, gallstones, and sepsis. GVHD may also contribute to subclinical disease. Large pancreatic pseudocysts (> 6 cm) in this immunocompromised population may require surgical intervention or endoscopic drainage because infected cysts might not be drained adequately with radiographically guided procedures.[99]

Hemorrhagic cystitis

High-dose conditioning regimens may cause hemorrhagic cystitis. Suprapubic pain may be confused with an abdominal source.[100,101]

Acute graft-versus-host disease

Crampy abdominal pain in association with copious diarrhea is the hallmark of lower gastrointestinal GVHD. Progression to severe abdominal pain with or without ileus (clinical stage IV) is ominous. Early empirical therapy, while awaiting biopsy confirmation, with corticosteroids is warranted to decrease mucosal injury.

Diarrhea

Diarrhea is common after high-dose therapy and occurs in nearly half of BMT recipients. Conditioning therapy and infections account for most episodes during the initial phases of BMT,

whereas after marrow engraftment, GVHD becomes the most frequent cause.[102]

Conditioning chemotherapy and/or radiotherapy

Direct mucosal injury by conditioning therapy results in diarrhea in most BMT recipients, starting early in the treatment course and resolving by day 20. When performed, endoscopy reveals diffuse mucosal injury with marked nuclear atypia, epithelial flattening, and crypt cell degeneration. Symptomatic treatment with antidiarrheals and attention to gentle cleansing are important for preventing secondary infections. A randomized trial in severe conditioning-related diarrhea noted loperamide to be superior to octreotide in controlling episodes (86% versus 45%).[103]

Infection

Infectious causes of diarrhea account for approximately 15% of episodes in the BMT setting.[102]

Bacterial and fungal causes

The prevalent use of antibiotics has allowed *C. difficile* infection to emerge as the most common offending organism. Endoscopic evaluation may be unrevealing in as much as pseudomembranes are frequently absent in neutropenic patients. Treatment consists of metronidazole or oral vancomycin, with rifaxin undergoing clinical trials. *C. septicum* is a rare cause of hemorrhagic diarrhea associated with necrotizing enteritis and typhlitis.[86] *Campylobacter*, *Salmonella*, and *Shigella* almost never result in intestinal infections in hospitalized BMT patients.[3] Jejunal vasculitis and necrotizing enteritis are also uncommon but require aggressive surgical intervention. Fungal overgrowth is a rare cause of diarrhea that can be effectively treated by azole antifungals.

Viral causes

Various viruses can contribute to diarrhea, including adenovirus, astrovirus, coxsackievirus, echovirus, and rotavirus. Viral gastroenteritis in BMT patients may cause serious illness or be a marker of significant comorbid conditions. Overall mortality among transplant patients with viral gastroenteritis has been reported to be 55% as compared with 13% in patients without enteric pathogens.[104] Fluid replacement is the mainstay of treatment. Encouraging results with oral immunoglobulin have been described in patients with rotavirus.[105] HSV typically causes esophagitis rather than lower tract disease, but colitis can occur.[106] CMV enteritis is a special problem for the BMT patient. Diffuse CMV ulcerations in the setting of protein-losing diarrheal episodes may both mimic and accompany intestinal GVHD. Endoscopic findings are variable and range from normal mucosa to large shallow ulcerations with erythematous borders.[46] Because CMV infection involves endothelial cells and fibroblasts of the submucosa, endoscopic biopsy specimens should be taken from the ulcer crater, with platelet support above 50 000/mm^3. Rapid diagnosis can frequently be obtained by examination for cytomegalic cells with immunohistochemical stains or by shell-vial centrifugation culture. Endoscopic examination revealing discrete ulcerations favors CMV over GVHD. Weekly screening of the blood for evidence of CMV viremia has not been predictive of enteritis.[107] CMV enteritis may not respond to short-course ganciclovir therapy, although viral replication is suppressed.[47] Ulcer healing is typically slow and recurrence of symptoms is frequent. Prolonged ganciclovir maintenance treatment, high-dose ganciclovir, combination ganciclovir with intravenous immune globulin, and foscarnet therapy may be considered.[49]

Parasitic causes

Pre-BMT screening of individuals from endemic areas is recommended. Rare cases of *Cryptosporidium*, *Giardia*, and *S. stercoralis* infection have been reported.

Medications

The multiple medications used during BMT may contribute to diarrhea. Promotility agents and magnesium supplements are common culprits along with antibiotics and high osmolality nutritional supplements.

Acute graft-versus-host disease

GVHD, the most common cause of significant diarrhea among allogeneic recipients after the second week, accounts for nearly 50% of cases.[102] The onset is typically sudden and explosive. Depending on the degree of immunologic injury, diarrheal volumes can be massive and serve as a basis for the staging system (Table 9.2). The syndrome is characterized as a protein-losing enteropathy with green, watery bowel movements containing strands of tissue debris.[109] Although usually secretory, GVHD may be manifested as an exudative process.[110] The diagnosis is usually suspected by timing and associated symptoms (rash, liver disease), and routine stool cultures are helpful in excluding most infectious causes. Sigmoidoscopy with rectal biopsy is a minimally invasive method to acquire diagnostic tissue.[111] Histologic findings include apoptosis of basal crypt cells, crypt cell dropout, and lymphoid infiltrates. In individuals with symptoms of nausea and emesis, upper endoscopy with gastric antral biopsies results in high diagnostic yields. Exclusion of concurrent CMV enteritis is important in deciding whether to begin antiviral therapy and/or change the level of pharmacologic immunosuppression.[112] Therapy is directed at immune modulation, maintenance of volume and metabolic status, and symptomatic control of diarrhea. It is imperative to start empirical therapy early before severe gastrointestinal ulceration occurs. Corticosteroids are the mainstay of GVHD treatment.[113] Because GVHD diarrhea interferes with the absorption of oral immunosuppressives, standard prophylaxis must be converted to intravenous forms.[114] Treatment of steroid-refractory GVHD has proved difficult and may consist of antithymocyte globulin, mycophenolate mofetil, or investigational trials with monoclonal antibodies including infliximab, denileukin, and daclizumab.[115–120] Gastrointestinal GVHD disease, analogous to the treatment of inflammatory bowel disease, may be particularly sensitive to infliximab.[121] Among patients requiring symptomatic management of diarrhea, high-dose octreotide can be successful if started early in the GVHD course.[122] During the acute syndrome, patients are placed on bowel rest and administered high-protein parenteral nutritional supplementation. Gradual advancement of the diet occurs over weeks.

Intestinal thrombotic microangiopathy

Intestinal thrombotic microangiopathy, causing an ischemic colitis and presenting as severe and refractory diarrhea, is a rare complication of transplantation. Differentiation of this syndrome from GVHD requires colonic biopsy. Intestinal symptoms slowly resolve with reduction of immunosuppressive therapy.[123]

Table 9.2 Lower GI GVHD grading scale[108]

Stage I	More than 500 mL of diarrhea
Stage II	More than 1000 mL of diarrhea
Stage III	More than 1500 mL of diarrhea
Stage IV	More than 2500 mL of diarrhea and severe abdominal pain, with or without ileus

Perianal complications

BMT recipients are at risk for perianal complications as a result of severe neutropenia and immunosuppression, chemotherapy-induced epithelial damage and ulceration, excoriation from diarrhea, GVHD mucosal damage, and trauma from opioid-induced constipation. Emphasis on conservative preventive measures including daily gentle cleansing, sitz baths, warm compresses, and stool softeners is recommended. Neutropenic patients should undergo frequent visual examinations, but instrumentation, suppositories, and digital internal examinations should be avoided. Similar to leukemia patients, infectious causes of pain must be pursued because necrotizing anorectal infections are associated with high mortality rates. Stool cultures are sometimes informative in determining the offending organism. Broad-spectrum antibiotics that include anaerobic coverage, efforts to accelerate marrow recovery with hematopoietic growth factors, and surgery may be necessary.[124]

Nutritional support

Energy needs during the initial 30–50 days have been estimated to be 170% of basal energy expenditure, and protein requirements are approximately twice the recommended daily allowance. During the period of tissue injury caused by conditioning therapy, when endogenous nitrogen levels are high, modest protein support is recommended. Gradually, protein support is increased to allow tissue repair and compensate for GVHD-related diarrheal losses.[125,126] Supplementation of vitamin K is routine to assist in coagulation protein synthesis. The early transition to enteral feeding and the use of elemental diets is under exploration at many centers.[127] Because a severe reduction in brush border enzymes can result in disaccharidase deficiency, low-lactose foods may be advisable. The importance of maintaining hydration in patients receiving potential renally toxic medications, including cyclosporine, must be stressed. Although many myths exist regarding the value of prolonged 'low-bacterial' diets in BMT patients, there is little scientific basis to many restrictions.

Patients with intestinal GVHD present special nutritional problems. Bowel rest is recommended as initial therapy during institution of immunosuppressive treatment. High-protein hyperalimentation and aggressive fluid and electrolyte replacement are necessary to compensate for diarrheal losses. Reinstitution of oral intake should be slow. Initially, isosmotic, low-residue beverages followed by low-lactose, low-fat, low-fiber, and low-acid solids can be taken. Specific GVHD diets have been developed.[61]

Liver disease

Abnormalities in hepatic function are common after high-dose therapy.[128,129] Allogeneic transplant recipients who develop jaundice are at significantly increased risk of nonrelapse mortality before day +200.[130] Liver biopsy may be necessary, especially among allogeneic recipients with viral hepatitis histories.[131]

Hematologic causes

Evaluation for evidence of hemolysis is the first step in the diagnostic work-up of patients with hyperbilirubinemia after BMT. Frequent transfusions and crossing of ABO barriers may result in delayed hemolysis with indirect bilirubinemia. Transfusion support, steroids, gamma globulin, and other hematologic maneuvers are appropriate in these patients.

Hepatic veno-occlusive disease/sinusoidal obstruction syndrome

Hepatic VOD is the most common life-threatening preparative regimen-related toxicity after BMT and the third most common cause of BMT-related death behind sepsis and GVHD.[132] A result of toxic metabolites of high-dose therapy, this clinical syndrome is manifested as a triad of painful hepatomegaly, jaundice, and fluid retention (ascites and peripheral edema), typically within the first 2–3 weeks after BMT.[133-135] Depending on the strictness of definition, patient selection, and conditioning regimens used, VOD has been reported to occur in 1–54% of transplant recipients. Although most cases of VOD resolve spontaneously, VOD may progress to multiorgan failure involving the kidneys, lungs, and heart in 3–67%.[132]

The pathogenesis of VOD is complex and involves direct injury to hepatic venules, sinusoidal epithelium, and hepatocytes; alterations in coagulation proteins; and activation of cytokines. Since damage to the hepatic venules is not essential to the development of clinical symptoms, whereas hepatic sinusoidal injury is critical, McDonald and colleagues have proposed changing the name of this condition to sinusoidal obstruction syndrome.[136] Many putative risk factors have been proposed including most recently polymorphisms of the hepatic urea cycle enzyme carbamoyl-phosphate synthetase and the hemochromatosis allele C282Y.[137]

Liver biopsy specimens reveal subendothelial swelling with narrowing of central veins, dilation and engorgement of sinusoids, closure of sinusoidal fenestrae, and necrosis of hepatocytes in zone 3 of the acinus.[138] Immunohistochemical stains of early VOD lesions have demonstrated deposits of fibrinogen (fibrin), factor VIII, and von Willebrand factor along the interface of the sinusoids and hepatic venules. Hepatic venular occlusion, eccentric luminal narrowing or phlebosclerosis, sinusoidal fibrosis, and hepatocyte necrosis in zone 3 have been associated with severe disease.

Ultrasonic detection of a thickened gallbladder wall has been noted in most patients with VOD but is non-specific. Doppler ultrasound may show an increased mean hepatic artery resistive index or decreased/reversed portal venous flow.[139,140] The role of MRI has yet to be determined.[141]

Obtaining clinically relevant laboratory confirmation of VOD has also proved difficult, although careful studies of the coagulation cascade have revealed several markers. Elevation of the aminopropeptide of type III procollagen, reduction in protein C levels, and elevated plasminogen activator inhibitor type 1 levels correlate with active disease. Elevations of plasminogen activator inhibitor 1 (PAI-1) and interleukin-8 have been proposed as a diagnostic marker for VOD.[142-144] Sudden declines in proteins of the clotting cascade have been advocated as an indication for aggressive VOD management.[145]

Although sepsis, medications, and GVHD can all contribute to early jaundice, the triad of clinical findings in VOD (jaundice, tender hepatomegaly, fluid retention) is so characteristic that invasive liver biopsy is seldom required in this thrombocytopenic population. If the diagnosis is unclear, liver biopsy via a femoral venous approach with the Mansfield biopsy forceps (with a 5% mortality) has been recommended. Transvenous measurement of hepatic venous pressure with balloon-tipped catheters correlates strongly with the histologic diagnosis in VOD when pressure gradients above 10 mmHg are found (approximately 90% predictive value) and can be used for diagnostic confirmation.

Given the frequency and morbidity of VOD, the development of effective preventive measures has been the subject of multiple trials. The central role of the clotting cascade in pathogenesis of the syndrome has focused attention on hemostatic agents. Although several prospective studies have suggested benefit to prophylactic heparin, not all have supported its use.[132,146-150] These contradictory results point to difficulties in VOD research. The wide variations in VOD incidence between trials underscore the importance of patient selection, the effect of differing conditioning regimens, and uniform diagnostic criteria. Infusions of antithrombin III concentrates (a required cofactor of heparin) were also not found to be helpful in a pilot trial.[151] Prophylactic defibrotide infusions, however, have yielded encouraging preliminary results.[152]

Ursodeoxycholic acid protects hepatocytes from damage by toxic bile salts and a randomized trial resulted in a decreased incidence of VOD (14.3% versus 40.6%; $p=0.03$).[153] Minimal effect on VOD was noted in other trials.[154] Prostaglandin E_1 is a vasodilatory molecule that has been suggested to increase blood flow in terminal hepatic venules. Despite initial encouraging reductions in VOD, toxicity has precluded widespread application.[155] Pentoxifylline, an inhibitor of tumor necrosis factor alpha, displayed promising results in phase I/II trials, but it was not substantiated in prospective controlled studies.[294,295] Vitamin E and glutamine are novel approaches under exploration.[296]

Because most cases of VOD resolve spontaneously, the primary goal of treatment is the control of extravascular fluid accumulation without precipitating intravascular volume depletion and renal failure. After the vigorous hydration required with conditioning therapy, maintenance of a euvolemic state through judicious diuretic therapy and intravenous fluid management is necessary. As VOD develops, sodium restriction and potassium-sparing diuretic therapy may be applied. Hypertransfusions, maneuvers to improve intravascular volume, and reduction of renal and hepatic toxic medications are routine. Low-dose dopamine infusions are discouraged. Paracentesis may be necessary for abdominal pain and respiratory comfort. Patients experiencing a combination of weight gain and hyperbilirubinemia early during the BMT course are at greatest risk for fatal VOD. Models have been developed to aid in decision-making.[156]

Case reports have described surgical approaches to severe VOD, including side-to-side portacaval shunts, LeVeen shunts, and orthotopic liver transplantation.[157] Transjugular intrahepatic portosystemic shunting has been attempted as a means of reducing portal hypertension through a minimally invasive procedure.[158] The overall efficacy of these anatomic approaches is unclear.

Thrombolytic therapy was previously used as a heroic measure in patients with severe VOD with approximately 150 cases in the literature and a 30% success rate.[159] A regimen of 20 mg rt-PA over a 4 h period for each of 4 consecutive days (total dose 80 mg) with concurrent heparin, 150 U/kg/day by continuous infusion for 10 days (after a 1000 U bolus), has been recommended. The use of lytic therapy in severely thrombocytopenic post-BMT patients, however, is not without significant risk, including fatal bleeding in up to 10%.

Defibrotide is a novel polydeoxyribonucleotide that has thrombolytic, antithrombotic, antiischemic, and antiinflammatory properties. The drug increases plasminogen activator inhibitor type 1 levels, stimulates thrombomodulin synthesis, increases endogenous t-PA function, and has no systemic anticoagulant activity. Compassionate-use trials in patients at high risk for VOD, including rt-PA failures, have yielded upwards to 60% response rates with minimal drug-related toxicity and no significant bleeding.[160,161]

Minimal effect with infusions of antithrombin III concentrates have been noted among patients with established VOD.[162]

Acute graft-versus-host disease

Liver abnormalities caused by an immunologic attack of donor lymphocytes occur in 70% of patients with GVHD and 20–50% of allogeneic recipients overall.[3] Although most cases of liver GVHD appear after engraftment (after day 21), a hyperacute form occurring early has been reported in recipients of mismatched/unrelated marrow or those receiving inadequate immunosuppression. Liver GVHD is usually accompanied by skin changes (erythematous rash), but occasionally liver involvement is the initial feature. The process is primarily cholestatic, with elevations of serum bilirubin levels forming the basis for staging (Table 9.3). Serum alkaline phosphatase levels can be markedly elevated (10–20-fold increases), but serum aspartate and alanine aminotransferases remain within 5–10 times normal. Hepatic failure with encephalopathy caused solely by GVHD is unusual. Similar to GVHD-related diarrhea, the diagnosis is generally made on clinical grounds and biopsy confirmation is rarely required. Transjugular or laparoscopic biopsy are occasionally performed when the etiology of the jaundice is unclear, such as when coexisting VOD or infections are suspected.[163] Histology reveals cholestasis, scattered acidophil bodies, and portal lymphoid infiltration. Initial therapy typically consists of corticosteroids and continuation of prophylactic cyclosporine or tacrolimus. Liver transplantation for severe GVHD has been reported.[164] Ursodeoxycholic acid reduces cholestasis and may have immunomodulatory effects in GVHD.[165,166] Although unusual, a similar cholestatic syndrome has been reported in autologous transplant recipients.[167]

Medications

The polypharmacy of BMT may contribute to abnormal liver-associated enzymes and jaundice. As permitted, potential offending medications should be withdrawn.

Table 9.3 Liver GVHD classification[108]

Stage I	Bilirubin 2–3 mg/dL
Stage II	Bilirubin 3.1–6 mg/dL
Stage III	Bilirubin 6.1–15 mg/dL
Stage IV	Bilirubin >15 mg/dL

Infections

The prolonged granulocytopenia predisposes to fungal infections during the early course. Viral causes typically have a later onset and become apparent as immune reconstitution occurs.

Bacterial causes

The use of antibiotic prophylaxis during BMT has made hepatic bacterial disease uncommon. Systemic infection with hypotension may result in ischemic liver injury with elevated levels of hepatocellular enzymes. Treatment is directed at stabilization of hemodynamic parameters and antibiotics. Reactivation of mycobacterial disease has been reported. As noted previously, despite a high frequency of gallbladder sludge, acute cholecystis is unusual. Cholangitis lenta, caused by infections outside the liver, is a frequent cause of jaundice.

Fungal causes

Fungal hepatic infections are most commonly identified in patients with prolonged granulocytopenia, those receiving steroid immunosuppression, or those with active GVHD or VOD. Candidal infections are most common, but prophylactic azole antifungal agents have reduced their incidence.[168] BMT recipients may not have the classic symptoms of fungal hepatitis and in the absence of liver tenderness and elevated serum alkaline phosphatase levels, clinical suspicion must be based on persistent unexplained fever. Empirical therapy is indicated because imaging studies may miss early fungal lesions.[3] Late-spiking fevers, anorexia, tender hepatomegaly, and elevated alkaline phosphatase levels after return of marrow function are highly suggestive of hepatosplenic (chronic systemic) candidiasis. Computed tomography, the most reliable non-invasive diagnostic procedure, detects abnormalities in about 90% of late infections. Azole antifungal agents and lipid-complexed amphotericin are the preferred treatments.

Viral hepatitis

Hepatitis B: Post-BMT hepatitis B infection may occur as a result of hepatitis infection of the donor's stem cells, from transfusion support during the transplant, or from reactivation of latent disease. High pretransplant DNA viral load is the most important risk factor for reactivation.[169] During the profound immunosuppression of BMT, asymptomatic viral replication may occur unchecked, leading to fibrosing cholestatic hepatitis. Upon immune reconstitution, attack of virally infected hepatocytes has been reported to cause fulminant hepatic failure. Serial examinations of at-risk recipients after engraftment, especially during withdrawal of BMT immunosuppressive medications, are warranted. The use of pre-emptive lamivudine in HBV-infected allogeneic recipients from the time of transplantation until at least 1 year post-transplant (or until all immunosuppressives are withdrawn, whichever is longer) is recommended.

Hepatitis C: Viral replication occurs asymptomatically during the immunosuppressed early period of BMT. HCV-induced liver abnormalities become clinically apparent upon immune recovery or upon withdrawal of immunosuppressive medications.[170] The vast majority of HCV-positive patients have only mild elevations of transaminases and do not experience significant morbidity during the first 5–10 years post-BMT.[10,17] However, long-term (>10 year) rates of cirrhosis are increased among transplant recipients compared to normal controls infected with HCV. Because immunosuppression and gamma globulin infusions may obscure antibody testing in the transplant recipient, viral RNA detection methods are recommended for evaluation of persistent hepatocellular enzyme abnormalities. Liver biopsy-documented hepatocyte or piecemeal necrosis is an indication for treatment. Despite theoretical concern regarding interferon precipitating marrow aplasia or GVHD, a recent report has indicated that this therapy for HCV is well tolerated.[171]

Hepatitis G: GB virus C is extremely common in BMT recipients (>60% of a British series).[172] The virus appears to be transmitted by blood transfusion. However, no relationship between BMT liver disease and hepatitis G virus infection has been established to date.

Transfusion-transmitted virus: TTV, although common in transplant patients, has not been associated with liver disease.[173]

Adenovirus: The most common viral cause of fulminant hepatitis post-transplant is adenovirus, resulting in rapidly increasing aminotransaminase levels and hepatic coma.[174] Liver biopsy reveals foci of coagulative necrosis surrounded by rims of hepatocytes containing intranuclear inclusions. Viral culture is essential. Management is often difficult, with cidofovir the most active agent for hepatic disease.[175] Rare responses to ribavirin and donor leukocyte infusions have also been reported.[176,177]

Cytomegalovirus: CMV hepatitis is uncommon in the absence of systemic disease. Thus endoscopic biopsy of the colon is the preferred diagnostic procedure. Liver biopsy reveals intranuclear inclusions, microabscesses, and damaged bile duct epithelia.[178] Initial features include moderately elevated aminotransferase and alkaline phosphatase levels. Isolated hepatitis is rarely fatal. Systemic symptoms, including pneumonia, frequently require aggressive management with ganciclovir and gamma globulin infusions. Biliary obstruction by CMV enteritis with involvement of the ampulla of Vater has been reported.[179]

Echovirus: An unusual and fatal cause of severe hepatitis, disseminated echovirus infection has been reported after BMT.[180]

Parvovirus: An uncommon infection during bone marrow transplantation usually causing pancytopenia, hepatitis, and visceral dissemination has been reported.[181]

Herpes simplex virus: HSV may cause an acute illness consisting of fulminant hepatitis with serum aminotransferase enzyme concentrations over 1000 U/L. Liver biopsy and prompt high-dose acyclovir are indicated, although hepatic infection is highly lethal.[182]

Varicella-zoster virus: Acute abdominal pain followed by fever and rapidly rising hepatocellular enzyme levels suggests VZV. High-dose acyclovir is the treatment of choice.[90]

Human herpesvirus-6: HHV-6 infection is a cause of delayed hematologic recovery, encephalitis, pneumonitis, fever, skin rash, and rarely hepatitis. Diagnosis requires PCR assays, with treatment by ganciclovir and growth-factor support.[183]

Human herpesvirus-7: HHV-7 seropositivity is nearly universal in adults. In the transplant setting it may cause a mild febrile illness, with a potential for augmenting CMV disease.[184]

Human herpesvirus-8. HHV-8 may cause a syndrome of fever, rash, and hepatitis. Diagnosis requires PCR assay.[185]

Cholangitis lenta

Sepsis may cause cholestasis with elevated levels of serum bilirubin and alkaline phosphatase. Because infections are common during the first weeks of transplantation, when the patient is also at risk for VOD, culture and fever pattern analysis are important components of the differential diagnosis. Although not recommended, liver biopsy in cholangitis lenta reveals intrahepatic cholestasis, dilation and stasis of bile in cholangioles or ducts of Hering, with minimal hepatocyte necrosis.

Gallbladder disease and extrahepatic biliary obstruction

Despite the high incidence of gallbladder sludge, biliary obstruction is rare. Sludge is noted in over 50% of transplant patients within the first 21 days. Hyperalimentation may contribute to this high incidence. Symptomatic pain management is usually sufficient. Acute acalculous cholecystitis is rare and occurred in only 5 of 770 patients.[186] Unusual causes of biliary obstruction include CMV papillitis, dissecting duodenal hematomas, and inspissated sludge in the distal common bile duct. A neoplastic obstruction caused by chloroma from leukemia has been reported.[187]

LATE COMPLICATIONS OF TRANSPLANTATION (AFTER DAY 100)

Odynophagia and dysphagia

Late oral complications are common after high-dose therapy. Alterations in taste sensation and persistent xerostomia may be noted in patients receiving radiotherapy or in patients in whom chronic GVHD is developing. Dentofacial abnormalities occur in 55% and tooth abnormalities in 62% of pediatric transplant recipients.[188] Candidal and herpesvirus infections may occur in patients receiving prolonged immunosuppression. Yearly dental examinations, fluoride treatments, and staged dental extractions to allow healing and avoid trauma to adjacent teeth are recommended. Observation for secondary buccal mucosal malignancies is important.

Chronic GVHD represents a continuation of the immunologic assault of disparate donor lymphocytes on host tissues. The syndrome has many features of an autoimmune disorder, with autoantibody formation including antinuclear antibodies and anti-smooth muscle antibodies. This syndrome occurs in 30–60% of allogeneic transplant survivors, depending on the degree of HLA match. Oral complications are common and include dryness and pain, especially with acidic foods. Examination of the buccal mucosa reveals lichen planus-like lesions with erythema. Superinfection with *Candida* or oral herpesviruses should be excluded by culture. Symptomatic treatment consists of topical steroid rinses, artificial saliva, and maintenance of good oral hygiene. Recently, a topical cyclosporine preparation in a bioadhesive dressing has begun clinical testing.[189] Esophageal involvement by chronic GVHD is uncommon (<10% of allogeneic survivors) but results in sclerodermatous changes, with dysphagia, insidious weight loss, or retrosternal pain. Esophageal peristalsis is abnormal and esophageal webs can develop.[190] Barium esophagography demonstrates dismotility, webs, rings, and strictures in upper and midportion of the esophagus. Endoscopy should be performed with caution to avoid perforation.[191] Although preventive measures (alternate-day steroids with cyclosporine and antireflux maneuvers) in patients with early chronic GVHD findings are advised, dilatation and nasogastric tube placement may be necessary. Prokinetic agents such as metoclopramide or domperidone may assist in esophageal clearing. Although rare, esophageal carcinomas should be excluded in patients with prolonged dysphagia.[192]

Gastrointestinal bleeding

Late gastrointestinal bleeding after recovery of platelet counts is unusual. Standard evaluation for common causes of bleeding in nonimmunocompromised hosts should be undertaken. New significant bleeding is also a concern for recurrence of malignancy, worsening of chronic GVHD, or Epstein-Barr virus-associated lymphoproliferative disorder.

Diarrhea

In the absence of uncontrolled GVHD, prolonged diarrhea is uncommon. Infectious enteritis with *C. difficile*, *Giardia lamblia*, and *Cryptosporidium* may occur in patients with incomplete immune reconstitution, such as recipients of unrelated volunteer or cord blood grafts.[3] Diarrhea caused by bacterial overgrowth in patients with IgA deficiency secondary to chronic GVHD may respond to antibiotic therapy. Persistent malabsorption and steatorrhea caused by pancreatic insufficiency in patients with chronic GVHD are unusual manifestations.[193] Exocrine enzyme supplementation and treatment of chronic GVHD may be helpful. Pancreatic beta-cell function is not generally affected by BMT.

Abdominal pain

Abdominal pain is also unusual after day 100 but might herald serious infection or intestinal perforation in patients maintained with prolonged immunosuppressives (such as steroids) for the treatment of chronic GVHD. VZV infection typically occurs late. EBV-associated lymphoproliferative disease may also be manifested as abdominal pain. Rare cases of pneumatosis intestinalis have been observed late in patients with chronic GVHD. Late gallstone-related disease is also common. Chronic GVHD may cause late abdominal pain/cramping, nausea/vomiting, weight loss, dysphagia, diarrhea, and early satiety. Endoscopic examination in a series of 22 patients was non-specific for the diagnosis of GI GVHD.[194] Alternate-day corticosteroid therapy remains the cornerstone of treatment. Rare cases of surgical resection, similar to that recommended in localized inflammatory bowel disease, have been reported.[195]

Liver disease

Chronic graft-versus-host disease

Liver involvement in chronic GVHD is common and represents the most frequent cause of late hepatic enzyme elevations in allogeneic recipients.[196,197] Hepatic disease may be the sole manifestation (stage: limited disease) or may be part of a systemic disease (stage: extensive disease) involving the skin, eyes (Schirmer's test, <5 mm wetting), minor salivary glands or oral mucosa, or other organs. Liver involvement is characterized by cholestasis, including alkaline phosphatase elevations 5–15 times normal and aminotransferases 3–5 times normal. Jaundice is variable. Despite the enzyme elevations, patients may appear relatively asymptomatic. Liver biopsy may be necessary to exclude other causes of hepatic disease. Histology typically reveals portal enlargement, small bile duct injury with dropout, marked cholestasis, and variable portal inflammation. Chronic GVHD may also present as an acute hepatitis with markedly elevated aminotransferases.[198] Empirical antiviral therapy for VZV may be required in patients with rapidly deteriorating hepatocellular enzymes while awaiting histologic confirmation by liver biopsy. Variceal hemorrhage requiring sclerotherapy can complicate chronic GVHD. Prolonged alternate-day steroids and cyclosporine/tacrolimus are the most widely used therapies. In patients with limited-stage disease and no evidence of recurrent infections, observation is generally sufficient. Isolated hepatic enzyme elevations may respond to ursodiol therapy, 300–600 mg orally two to three times daily. However, relapses occur after discontinuation of therapy.[199] The role of thalidomide, clofazimine, and other immunosuppressives in hepatic chronic GVHD has yet to be defined.[200,201] Liver transplantation has been attempted in patients progressing to cirrhosis.[202] Rituximab, an antibody directed against CD20 on B cells has entered clinical trials in steroid-refractory disease.[203] Steatorrhea is a rare late complication of chronic GVHD, which may respond to enzyme supplementation.[204]

Medications

Cyclosporine toxicity, and to a lesser extent tacrolimus toxicity, is a common cause of transaminase elevations.[205] Differentiation from GVHD is often difficult and may require liver biopsy. Toxicity from prolonged trimethoprim-sulfamethoxazole (used for *Pneumocystis carinii* pneumonia prophylaxis) is uncommon. The increasing use of herbal and unconventional therapies by transplant survivors also requires careful evaluation of patient practices.

Infections

Hepatic viral infections with CMV, HBV, and HCV after day 100 usually follow a chronic rather than a fulminant course.[206] The immunodeficiency of BMT and use of gamma globulin infusions make early serologic diagnosis difficult. Viral RNA/DNA studies are recommended. Late reactivation of hepatitis B and C are common, especially in patients with GVHD.[207,208] Lamivudine has been successfully used for late hepatitis B infection.[209]

Delayed use of interferon and ribavirin, after resolution of graft-versus-host disease, may be considered for late hepatitis C infection. A recent long-term study of 1078 patients, who underwent an allogeneic transplantation between January 1973 and January 1995, identified 96 patients infected by hepatitis C virus (HCV) during the transplantation period. Fifteen patients developed biopsy-proven cirrhosis, leading to a cumulative incidence of cirrhosis of 11% and 24% at 15 and 20 years, respectively. By multivariate analysis, extrahepatic HCV manifestations and HCV genotype 3 were associated with risk of cirrhosis. The median time to cirrhosis in transplant recipients was 18 years as compared with 40 years in the control population.[210] Delayed use of interferon and ribavirin, after resolution of GVHD, may therefore be appropriate.

Transfusion related hemachromatosis

Iron overload as a result of frequent red cell transfusions is common among transplant recipients.[211] Portal fibrosis, cirrhosis, and hepatocellular carcinoma may be late consequences. Patients with hemosiderosis are also at increased risk of opportunistic infections, and may experience more significant hepatitis C-related disease including fibrosis. Differentiation of iron overload from late chronic graft-versus-host disease involving the liver on clinical grounds may be difficult. Phlebotomy and/or iron chelation therapy should be considered.[212]

Hyperlipidemia

In contrast to the situation in solid organ transplant recipients, hyperlipidemia is a rare occurrence. A case report describes a patient with cholestatic liver disease complicated by high cholesterol levels and end-organ deposits who responded to lovastatin and plasmapheresis.[213]

Epstein-Barr virus-associated lymphoproliferative disease

Immunosuppressed transplant recipients, especially individuals receiving T-cell-depleted allogeneic marrow, are at risk for EBV-associated lymphoproliferative disease. Symptoms include fever, abdominal pain, and lymphadenopathy. Liver involvement is , occurring in up to 50% of cases with sudden hepatosplenomegaly, and elevations of alkaline phosphatase and lactate dehydrogenase.[214] The disease is manifested acutely, 30–500 days after BMT, and may be either monoclonal or polyclonal in origin. Reduction of immunosuppressives, high-dose acyclovir, interferon, and anti-B-cell antibodies have been touted with varying success. In allogeneic recipients, the infusion of donor leukocytes containing cytotoxic T cells presensitized to EBV has emerged as a curative disease even in advanced cases.[215] Antibody therapy directed at CD20 (rituximab) is also effective.[216]

Nodular regenerative hyperplasia

A possible response to altered blood flow, nodular regenerative hyperplasia, is a cause of noncirrhotic portal hypertension, esophageal varices, and ascites months after BMT. Diagnostic liver biopsies reveal nodular regeneration of periportal areas with compression and atrophy of adjacent centrilobular areas. Variable sinusoidal dilatation and congestion without obliterative venulitis are typical. The prognosis is good, with supportive care directed at secondary symptoms because hepatic synthetic activity is preserved.[217]

Idiopathic hyperammonemia

Characterized by the abrupt onset of altered mental status, respiratory alkalosis, and markedly elevated plasma ammonium levels, idiopathic hyperammonemia is a rare cause of encephalopathy occurring late after high-dose therapy. The etiology of this highly fatal syndrome is unknown but may be related to a chemotherapy-induced defect in the urea cycle pathway. Intracranial pressure monitoring, ventilatory support, hemodialysis, avoidance of exogenous nitrogenous sources such as parenteral nutrition, and infusions of sodium benzoate have been tried with variable success.[218] Carnitine infusions have recently been recommended.

Recurrence of tumor and secondary malignancies

Despite the success of high-dose therapy, many patients experience a relapse of their underlying disease. Abnormalities noted on surveillance examinations must always be correlated with the original disease. As the role of BMT expands and patients become long-term survivors, the development of secondary malignancies is emerging as an important health issue.[219] Although hematologic disorders dominate BMT-related secondary malignancies, solid tumors have been reported. A recent review of 19 229 survivors found 80 solid cancers. This figure represents an 8.3% increase over the expected frequency. Buccal mucosa (11-fold increase) and hepatic cancer (7.5-fold increase) were most common. Risk factors for these secondary tumors included younger age at transplantation, total body irradiation, male sex, and chronic GVHD.[220]

SUMMARY

Complications following BMT are common, and the management of patients undergoing transplantation commences prior to the actual procedure. Before undergoing BMT, candidates must

---

Table 9.4 Differential diagnosis of gastrointestinal problems during the 1st 100 days of bone marrow transplantation*

Odynophagia and dysphagia
Mucositis
Infections
Peptic esophagitis
Intramural hematoma
Medications
Acute graft-versus-host disease

Anorexia, nausea, and emesis
Conditioning chemotherapy and/or radiotherapy
Medications
Infection
Gastric motitilty disorders
Acute graft-versus-host disease

Gastrointestinal bleeding
Conditioning chemotherapy and/or radiotherapy
Acid peptic disease
Infection
Gastric antral vascular ectasia
Variceal hemorrhage
Acute graft-versus-host disease

Abdominal pain
Conditioning chemotherapy and/or radiotherapy
Infection
Perforation and pneumatosis intestinalis
Pseudo-obstruction and obstruction
Hematoma
Hepatic veno-occlusive disease
Biliary disease
Pancreatic causes
Hemorrhagic cystitis
Acute graft-versus-host disease

Diarrhea
Conditioning chemotherapy and/or radiotherapy
Infection
Medications
Acute graft-versus-host disease
Intestinal thrombotic microangiopathy
Perianal complications

Liver disease
Hematologic causes
Hepatic veno-occlusive disease/sinusoidal obstruction syndrome
Acute graft-versus-host disease
Medications
Infections
Cholangitis lenta
Gallbladder disease and extrahepatic biliary obstruction

* See text for details

undergo an extensive evaluation to discover any unrecognized organ dysfunction that may preclude the safe administration of high-dose therapy. Moreover, donor candidates should be screened for the presence of viral hepatitis. The critical phases for BMT recipients include the period of conditioning therapy, the cytopenic phase, and the early marrow recovery period (Table 9.4). In addition to opportunistic viral, fungal, bacterial, and parasitic infections, several other complications may develop during these critical periods and warrant a thorough evaluation and therapy. They include mucositis, esophagitis, peptic ulcer, acute and chronic graft-versus-host disease, gastrointestinal motility abnormalities, gastrointestinal hemorrhage due to several different etiologies, visceral perforation, pancreatitis, gallstones and extrahepatic biliary obstruction, cholangitis, hepatic veno-occlusive disease, and other hepatic disorders. Patients who develop abdominal pain, dysphagia, odynophagia, diarrhea, and evidence of bleeding, often associated with fever, should be assessed expeditiously and thoroughly, and supportive care and specific treatment instituted. Finally, adequate nutritional support, including vitamin K and other supplements, are key components of management, keeping in mind that energy needs during the initial 30–50 days after BMT have been estimated to be 170% of basal energy expenditure and protein requirements approximately twice the recommended daily allowance.

REFERENCES

1. Goldberg SL, Klumpp TR, Magdalinski AJ, et al. Value of the pre-transplant evaluation in predicting toxic day 100 mortality among blood stem cell and bone marrow transplant recipients. J Clin Oncol 1998; 16:3750.

2. Raber-Durlacher JE, Abraham-Inpijn L, van Leeuwen EF, et al. The prevention of oral complications in bone marrow transplantation by means of oral hygiene and dental intervention. Neth J Med 1989; 34:98.

3. Strasser SI, McDonald GB. Gastrointestinal and hepatic complications. In: Blume KG, Forman SJ, Appelbaum FR, eds. Thomas' hematopoietic cell transplantation. Malden MA: Blackwell; 2004:796.

    An authoritative review of gastrointestinal complications in the standard BMT reference text.

4. Kaur S, Cooper G, Fakult S, et al. Incidence and outcome of overt gastrointestinal bleeding in patients undergoing bone marrow transplantation. Dig Dis Sci 1996; 41:598.

5. Otero Lopez-Cubero S, Sullivan KM, McDonald GB. Course of Crohn's disease after allogeneic marrow transplantation. Gastroenterology 1998; 114:433.

6. Shaked AA, Shinar E, Freund H. Managing the granulocytopenic patient with acute perianal inflammatory disease. Am J Surg 1986; 152:510.

7. Kalb RE, Grossman ME. Chronic perianal herpes simplex in immunocompromised hosts. Am J Med 1986; 80:486.

8. Klumpp TR, Herman JH, Ennis S, et al. Factors associated with response to platelet transfusion following hematopoietic stem cell transplantation. Bone Marrow Transplant 1996; 17:1035.

9. Chen PM, Liu JH, Fan FS, et al. Liver disease after bone marrow transplantation: The Taiwan experience. Transplantation 1995; 59:1139.

10. Locasciulli A, Testa M, Valsecchi MG, et al. Morbidity and mortality due to liver disease in children undergoing bone marrow transplantation: A 10 year prospective study. Blood 1997; 90:3799.

11. Lau GK, Liang R, Chiu EKW, et al. Hepatic events after bone marrow transplantation in patients with hepatitis B infection: a case controlled study. Bone Marrow Transplant 1999; 19:795.

12. Lau GK, He ML, Fong DY, et al. Preemptive use of lamivudine reduces hepatitis B exacerbation after allogeneic hematopoietic cell transplantation. Hepatology 2002; 36:702.

    In 20 consecutive HBsAg-positive recipients of allogeneic hematopoietic cell transplantation who received lamivudine 100 mg daily (from week −1 through +52), compared to 20 patients not receiving antiviral therapy, only one (5%) developed clinical hepatitis compared to 45% without antiviral therapy. (p<.008).

13. McDonald GB, Slattery JT, Bouvier ME, et al. Cyclophosphamide metabolism, liver toxicity, and mortality following hematopoietic stem cell transplantation. Blood 2003; 101:2043.

14. Lee JH, Lee JH, Choi SJ, et al. Hepatic veno-occlusive disease (VOD) after allogeneic hematopoietic cell transplantation (HCT) in adults conditioned with busulfan (Bu) and cyclophosphamide (Cy) at a single center: A retrospective comparison of oral vs. intravenous Bu (Abstract 6647). Proc Am Soc Clin Oncol 2004; 22:14S.

15. Lau GK, Suri D, Liang R, et al. Resolution of chronic hepatitis B and anti-HBs seroconversion in humans by adoptive transfer of immunity to hepatitis B core antigen. Gastroenterology 2002; 122:614.

16. Brugger SA, Oesterreicher C, Hofmann H, et al. Hepatitis B virus clearance by transplantation of bone marrow from hepatitis B immunised donor. Lancet 1997; 349:996.

17. Ljungman P, Johansson N, Aschan J, et al. Long-term effects of hepatitis C virus infection in allogeneic bone marrow transplant recipients. Blood 1995; 86:1614.

18. Bjerke JW, Myers JD, Bowden RA. Hepatosplenic candidiasis: A contraindication to marrow transplantation? Blood 1994; 84:2811.

19. Anttila VJ, Lamminen AE, Bondestam S, et al. Magnetic resonance imaging is superior to computed tomography and ultrasonography in imaging infectious liver foci in acute leukaemia. Eur J Haematol 1996; 56:82.

20. Lucarelli G, Clift RA, Galimberti M, et al. Marrow transplantation for patients with thalassemia: results in class 3 patients. Blood 1996; 87:2082.

21. Rozman C, Carreras E, Qian C, et al. Risk factors for hepatic veno-occlusive disease following HLA-identical sibling bone marrow transplants for leukemia. Bone Marrow Transplant 1996; 17:75.

22. Goldberg SL, Ellent D, Shtrambrand D, et al. Gemtuzumab ozogamicin (mylotarg) prior to allogeneic hematopoietic stem cell transplantation increases the risk of hepatic veno-occlusive disease. Blood 2002; Abstract 1611.

23. Rowley SD, Goldberg SL, Hsu JW. Practical aspects of stem cell collection. In: Hoffman R, Benz EJ, Shattil SJ, eds. Hematology. 4th edn. Philadelphia: Elsevier Science; 2005:2493.

24. Locasciulli A, Alberti A, Bandini G, et al. Allogeneic bone marrow transplantation from HBsAg+ donors: A multicenter study from the Gruppo Italiana Trapianto di Midollo Osseo (GITMO). Blood 1995; 86:3236.

25. Lau GK, Lie AKW, Kwong YL, et al. A case controlled study on the use of HBsAg-positive donors for allogeneic hematopoietic cell transplantation. Blood 2000; 96:452.

26. Daily J, Werner B, Soiffer R, et al. IGIV: A potential role for hepatitis B prophylaxis in the bone marrow peri-transplant period. Bone Marrow Transplant 1998; 21:739.

27. Goyama S, Kanda Y, Nannya Y, et al. Reverse seroconversion of hepatitis B virus after hematopoietic stem cell transplantation. Leuk Lymphoma 2002; 43:2159.

28. Lau GK, Strsser SI, McDonald GB. Hepatitis virus infections in patients with cancer. In: Wingard JR, Bowdenn RA, eds. Management of infections in oncology patients. London: Martin Dunitz; 2003:321.

29. Strasser SI, Myerson D, Spurgeon CL, et al. Hepatitis C virus infection after bone marrow transplantation: a cohort study with 10-year follow-up. Hepatology 1999; 29:1893.

30. Gralla R, Goldberg SL, Giles FJ. Oral mucositis: Emerging strategies for improving patient care. Oncology Special Edition. March 2003.

31. Sonis ST. The pathobiology of mucositis. Nature Reviews 2004; 4:277.

32. Rapoport AP, Miller Watelet LF, et al. Analysis of factors that correlate with mucositis in recipients of autologous and allogeneic stem-cell transplants. J Clin Oncol 1999; 17:2446.

33. Sonis ST, Olser G, Fuchs H, et al. Oral mucositis and the clinical and economic outcomes of hematopoietic stem cell transplantation. J Clin Oncol 2001; 19:2201.

34. Bellm LA, Epstein JB, Rose-Ped A, et al. Patient reports of complications of bone marrow transplantation. Support Care Cancer 2000; 8:33.

35. Clarkson JE, Worthington HV, Eden OB. Interventions for preventing oral mucositis for patients with cancer receiving treatment. Cochrane Database Syst Rev 3:CD000978, 2003.

36. Rubenstein EB, Peterson DE, Schubert M, et al. Clinical practice guidelines for the prevention and treatment of cancer therapy-induced oral and gastrointestinal mucositis. Cancer 2004; 100(S9):2026.

37. Shubert MM. Oro-pharyngeal mucositis. In: Atkinson KA, ed. Clinical bone marrow and blood stem cell transplantation. 2nd edn. Cambridge: Cambridge University Press; 2000:812.

38. Hill HF, Mackie AM, Coda BA, et al. Patient controlled analgesic administration: A comparison of steady-state morphine infusions with bolus doses. Cancer 1991; 67:873.

39. Ruescher TJ, Sondeifi A, Scrivani SJ, et al. The impact of mucositis on alpha-hemolytic streptococcal infection in patients undergoing autologous bone marrow transplantation for hematologic malignancies. Cancer 1998; 82:2275.

40. Peterson DE, Petit RG. Phase III study: AES-14 in chemotherapy patients at risk for mucositis (Abstract). Proc Am Soc Clin Oncol 2003; 22:2917.

41. Spielberger R, Stiff P, Bensinger W, et al. Palifermin for oral mucositis after intensive therapy for hematologic cancers. N Engl J Med. 2004; 351:2590–8.

42. Giles FJ, Rodriguez R, Weisdorf D, et al. A phase III, randomized, double-blind, placebo-controlled, study of iseganan for the reduction of stomatitis in patients receiving stomatotoxic chemotherapy. Leuk Res 2004; 28:559.

43. Goldberg SL, Pineiro L, Coleman M, et al. Prevention of mucositis by Immunol Oral Rinse: Final results of a randomized vehicle controlled study (Abstract 45). Biol Blood Marrow Transplant 2002; 8:74.

44. Verdonck LF, Cornelissen JJ, Smit J, et al. Successful foscarnet therapy for acyclovir-resistant mucocutaneous infection with herpes simplex virus in a recipient of allogeneic BMT. Bone Marrow Transplant 1993; 11:177.

45. Arvin AM. Varicella zoster virus infections. In; Blume KG, Forman SJ, Appelbaum FR, eds. Thomas' hematopoietic cell transplantation. Malden MA: Blackwell; 2004:732.

46. Goodgame RW. Gastrointestinal cytomegalovirus disease. Ann Intern Med 1993; 119:924.

47. Reed EC, Wolford JL, Kopecky KJ, et al. Ganciclovir for the treatment of cytomegalovirus gastroenteritis in bone marrow transplant patients: A randomized, placebo-controlled trial. Ann Intern Med 1990; 112:505.

48. Nelson MR, Connolly GM, Hawkins DA, et al. Foscarnet in the treatment of cytomegalovirus of the esophagus and colon in patients with the acquired immune deficiency syndrome. Am J Gastroenterol 1991; 86:876.

49. Ljungman P, Cordonnier C, Einsele H, et al. Use of intravenous immunoglobulin in addition to antiviral therapy in the treatment of CMV gastrointestinal disease in allogeneic bone marrow transplant patients. Bone Marrow Transplant 1998; 21:473.

50. Boeckh M, Nichols WG, Papanicolaou G, et al. Cytomegalovirus in hematopoietic stem cell transplant recipients: Current status, known challenges, and future strategies. Biol Blood Marrow Transplant 2003; 9:543.

51. Winston DJ, Yeager AM, Chandrasekar PH, et al. Randomized comparison of oral valacyclovir and intravenous ganciclovir for prevention of cytomegalovirus disease after allogeneic bone marrow transplantation. Clin Infect Dis 2003; 36:749.

52. Ljungman P, de La Camara R, Milpied N, et al. Randomized study of valacyclovir as prophylaxis against cytomegalovirus reactivation in recipients of allogeneic bone marrow transplants. Blood 2002; 99:3050.

53. Reusser P, Einsele H, Lee J, et al. Randomized multicenter trial of foscarnet versus ganciclovir for preemptive therapy of cytomegalovirus infection after allogeneic stem cell transplantation. Blood 2002; 99:1159.

54. Goodman JL, Winston DJ, Greenfield RA, et al. A controlled trial of fluconazole to prevent fungal infections in patients undergoing bone marrow transplantation. N Engl J Med 1992; 326:845.

55. Choi JH, Yoo JH, Chung IJ, et al. Esophageal aspergillosis after bone marrow transplant. Bone Marrow Transplant 1997; 19:293.

56. Vishny ML, Blades EW, Creger RJ, et al. Role of upper endoscopy in evaluation of upper gastrointestinal symptoms in patients undergoing bone marrow transplantation. Cancer Invest 1994; 12:384.

57. Memoli D, Spitzer TR, Cottler-Fox M, et al. Acute esophageal stricture after bone marrow transplantation. Bone Marrow Transplant 1988; 3:513.

58. Ackert JJ, Sherman A, Lustbader IJ, et al. Spontaneous intramural hematoma of the esophagus. Am J Gastroenterol 1989; 84:1325.

59. Wolford JL, McDonald GB. Intramural hematomas of esophagus, stomach and small intestine in marrow transplant patients (Abstract). Gastroenterology 1988; 94:501.

60. Lipson SA, Perr HA, Koerper MA, et al. Intramural duodenal hematoma after endoscopic biopsy in leukemic patients. Gastrointest Endosc 1996; 44:620.

61. Williams DB, Vickers CR. Gastrointestinal complications. In: Atkinson KA, ed. Clinical bone marrow and blood stem cell transplantation. 2nd edn. Cambridge: Cambridge University Press; 2000:903.

62. Hecht JR, Lembo T, Chap L. Prolonged nausea and vomiting after high dose chemotherapy and autologous peripheral blood stem cell transplantation in the treatment of high risk breast carcinoma. Cancer 1997; 79:1698.

63. Hewitt M, Cornish J, Pamphilon D, et al. Effective emetic control during conditioning of children for bone marrow transplantation using ondansetron, a 5-HT3 antagonist. Bone Marrow Transplant 1991; 7:431.

64. Hunter AE, Prentice HG, Pothecary K, et al. Granisetron, a selective 5-HT3 receptor antagonist, for the prevention of radiation induced emesis during total body irradiation. Bone Marrow Transplant 1991; 7:439.

65. Bubalo J, Seelig F, Karbowicz S, et al. Randomized open-label trial of dolasetron for the control of nausea and vomiting associated with high-dose chemotherapy with hematopoietic stem cell transplantation. Biol Blood Marrow Transplant 2001; 7:439.

66. Navari RM. Pathogenesis-based treatment of chemotherapy-induced nausea and vomiting – two new agents. J Support Oncol 2003; 1:89.

67. Beck TM, Hesketh PJ, Madajewicz S, et al. Stratified, randomized, double blind comparison of intravenous ondansetron administered as a multiple-dose regimen versus two single dose regimens in the prevention of cisplatin-induced nausea and vomiting. J Clin Oncol 1992; 10:1969.

68. Matsuoka S, Okamoto S, Watanabe R, et al. Granisetron plus dexamethasone versus granisetron alone in the prevention of vomiting induced by conditioning for stem cell transplantation: a prospective randomized study. Int J Hematol 2003; 77:86.

69. Gilbert CJ, Ohly KV, Rosner G, et al. Randomized, double-blind comparison of a prochlorperazine-based versus a metoclopramide-based anti-emetic regimen in patients undergoing autologous bone marrow transplantation. Cancer 1995; 76:2330.

70. Charuhas PM, Fosberg KL, Bruemmer B, et al. A double-blind randomized trial comparing outpatient parenteral nutrition with intravenous hydration effect on resumption of oral intake after marrow transplantation. J Parenter Enteral Nutr 1997; 21:157.

71. Pavletic ZS, Bishop MR, Tarantolo SR, et al. Infusion toxicity of cryopreserved allogeneic blood stem cells (Abstract). Proc Annu Meet Soc Clin Oncol 1996; 15:5.

72. Wu D, Hockenberry DM, Brentnall TA, et al. Persistent nausea and anorexia after marrow transplantation: a prospective study of 78 patients. Transplantation 1998; 66:1319.

73. Eagle DA, Gian V, Lauwers GY, et al. Gastroparesis following bone marrow transplantation. Bone Marrow Transplant 2001; 28:59.

74. DiBaise JK, Brand RE, Quigley EM, et al. Gastric myoelectrical activity and its relationship to the development of nausea and vomiting after intensive chemotherapy and autologous stem cell transplantation. Am J Gastroenterol 2001; 96:2873.

75. Spencer GD, Hackman RC, McDonald GB, et al. A prospective study of unexplained nausea and vomiting after bone marrow transplantation. Transplantation 1986; 42:602.

In this prospective study of unexplained upper gastrointestinal tract symptoms, 21 of 50 patients (42%) had findings compatible with unsuspected acute GVHD.

76. Ponec RJ, Hackman RC, McDonald GB. Endoscopic and histologic diagnosis of intestinal graft-vs-host disease after marrow transplantation. Gastointestin Endosc 1999; 49:612.

77. Weisdorf DJ, Snover DC, Haake R, et al. Acute upper gastrointestinal graft-versus-host disease: Clinical significance and response to immunosuppressive therapy. Blood 1990; 76:624.

78. McDonald GB, Bouvier M, Hockenberry DM, et al. Oral beclomethasone dipropionate for treatment of intestinal graft-vs-host disease: a randomized, controlled trial. Gastroenterology 1998; 115:28.

79. Tzung S-P, Hackman RC, Hockenbery DM, et al. Lymphocytic gastritis resembling graft-vs-host disease following autologous hematopoietic cell transplantation. Biol Blood Marrow Transplant 1998; 4:43.

80. Schwartz JM, Wolford JL, Thornquist MD, et al. Severe gastrointestinal bleeding after marrow transplantation, 1987–1997: incidence, causes, and outcome. Am J Gastroenterol 2001; 96:385.

81. Kumar S, Dispenzieri A, Lacy MQ, et al. High incidence of gastrointestinal tract bleeding after autologous stem cell transplant for primary systemic amyloidosis. Bone Marrow Transplant 2001; 28:381.

82. Greenson JK, Trinidad SB, Pfeil SA, et al. Gastric mucosal calcinosis. Calcified aluminum phosphate deposits secondary to aluminum-containing antacids or sucralfate therapy in organ transplant patients. Am J Surg Pathol 1993; 17:45.

83. Cohen Y, Paltiel O, Amir G, et al. Unusual cytomegalovirus complications after autologous stem cell transplantation for large B cell lymphoma: massive gastrointestinal hemorrhage followed by a communicating hydrocephalus. Bone Marrow Transplant 2002; 29:715.

84. Willoughby RE, Wee SB, Yolken RH. Non-group A rotavirus infection associated with severe gastroenteritis in a bone marrow transplant patient. Pediatr Infect Dis J 1988; 7:133.

85. Cohen R, Heffner JE. Bowel infarction as the initial manifestation of disseminated aspergillosis. Chest 1992; 101:877.

86. Or R, Mehta J, Nagler A, et al. Neutropenic enterocolitis associated with autologous bone marrow transplantation. Bone Marrow Transplant 1992; 9:383.

87. Tobin RW, Hackman RC, Kimmey MB, et al. Bleeding from gastric antral vascular ectasia in marrow transplant patients. Gastrointest Endosc 1996; 44:223.

88. Ohashi K, Sanaka M, Tanaka Y, et al. Use of octreotide in the management of severe duodenal bleeding after unrelated-donor bone marrow transplantation. Int J Hematol 2003; 78:176.

89. Ertault-Daneshpouy M, Leboeuf C, Lemann M, et al. Pericapillary hemorrhage as criterion of severe human digestive graft-versus-host disease. Blood 2004; 103:4681.

90. David DS, Tegtmeier BR, O'Donnell MR, et al. Visceral varicella-zoster after bone marrow transplantation: Report of a case series and review of the literature. Am J Gastroenterol 1998; 93:810.

91. Shimoda NT, Chauncey TR, Durtschi M, et al. Intestinal perforation in marrow transplant patients: Incidence, risk factors, and clinical features (Abstract). Gastroenterology 1994; 106:27.

92. Lipton J, Patterson B, Mustard R, et al. Pneumatosis intestinalis with free air mimicking intestinal perforation in a bone marrow transplant patient. Bone Marrow Transplant 1994; 149:323.

93. Benya EC, Sivit CJ, Quinones RR. Abdominal complications after bone marrow transplantation in children: Sonographical and CT findings. AJR Am J Roentgenol 1993; 161:1023.

94. Ponec RJ, Saunders MD, Kimmey MB, et al. Neostigmine for the treatment of acute colonic pseudo-obstruction. N Engl J Med 1999; 341:146.

95. Nomdedeu JF, Nomdedeu J, Martino R, et al. Ogilvie's syndrome from disseminated varicella-zoster infection and infarcted celiac ganglia. J Clin Gastroenterol 1995; 20:157.

96. Ben-Yehuda A, Ben-Yehuda-Salz D, Or R, et al. Intestinal obstruction after bone marrow transplantation. Bone Marrow Transplant 1989; 4:137.

97. Koura T, Itoh T, Motimaru J, et al. Rectus hematoma secondary to vomiting: A complication of conditioning regimen for bone marrow transplantation. Intern Med 1995; 34:39.

98. Jacobson AF, Teefey SA, Lee SP, et al. Frequent occurrence of new hepatobiliary abnormalities after bone marrow transplantation: Results of a prospective study using scintigraphy and sonography. Am J Gastroenterol 1993; 88:1044.

99. Shore T, Bow E, Greenberg H, et al. Pancreatitis post-bone marrow transplantation. Bone Marrow Transplant 1996; 17:1181.

100. Akiyama H, Kurosu T, Sakashita C, et al. Adenovirus is a key pathogen in hemorrhagic cystitis after bone marrow transplantation. Clin Infect Dis 2001; 32:1325.

101. Leung AY, Suen CK, Lie AK, et al. Quantification of polyoma BK viruria in hemorrhagic cystitis complicating bone marrow transplantation. Blood 2001; 98:1971.

102. Cox GJ, Matsui SM, Lo RS, et al. Etiology and outcome of diarrhea after marrow transplantation: A prospective study. Gastroenterology 1994; 107:1398.

103. Geller RB, Gilmore CE, Dix SP, et al. Randomized trial of loperamide versus dose escalation of octreotide acetate for chemotherapy-induced diarrhea in bone marrow transplant and leukemia patients. Am J Hematol 1995; 50:167.

104. Yolken RH, Bishop CA, Townsend TR, et al. Infectious gastroenteritis in bone marrow transplant recipients. N Engl J Med 1982; 306:1010.

105. Kanfer EJ, Abramson G, Taylor J, et al. Severe rotavirus associated diarrhoea following bone marrow transplantation: Treatment with oral immunoglobulin. Bone Marrow Transplant 1994; 14:651.

106. Naik HR, Chandrasekar PH. Herpes simplex virus colitis in a bone marrow transplant recipient. Bone Marrow Transplant 1996; 17:285.

107. Mori T, Mori S, Kanda Y, et al. Clinical significance of cytomegalovirus (CMV) antigenemia in the prediction and diagnosis of CMV gastrointestinal disease after allogeneic hematopoietic stem cell transplantation. Bone Marrow Transplant 2004; 33:413.

108. Glucksberg H, Storb R, Fefer A, et al. Clinical manifestations of graft-versus-host disease in human recipients of marrow from HL-A matched sibling donors. Transplantation 1974; 18:295.

109. Weisdorf SA, Salati LM, Longsdorf JA, et al. Graft-versus-host disease of the intestine: A protein-losing enteropathy characterized by fecal alpha-1-antitrypsin. Gastroenterology 1983; 85:1076.

110. Ghilain JM, Martiat P, Fiasse R, et al. Exudative enteropathy caused by an acute graft-vs-host reaction – a propos of a case report. Acta Gastroenterol Belg 1990; 53:488.

111. Epstein RJ, McDonald GB, Sale GE, et al. The diagnostic accuracy of the rectal biopsy in graft-versus-host disease: A prospective study of thirteen patients. Gastroenterology 1980; 78:764.

112. Einsele H, Ehninger G, Hebart H, et al. Incidence of local CMV infection and acute intestinal GVHD in marrow transplant recipients with severe diarrhoea. Bone Marrow Transplant 1994; 14:955.

113. Van Lint MT, Uderzo C, Locasciulli A, et al. Early treatment of acute graft-versus-host disease with high or low dose 6-methylprednisolone: A multi-center randomized trial from the Italian Group for Bone Marrow Transplantation. Blood 1998; 92:2288.

114. Atkinson K, Biggs JC, Britton K, et al. Oral administration of cyclosporine A for recipients of allogeneic bone marrow transplants: Implications of clinical gut dysfunction. Br J Haematol 1984; 56:223.

115. Kienast J, Ippoliti C, Mehra R, et al. Dose intensified antithymocyte globulin in steroid-resistant graft-versus-host disease after allogeneic marrow or blood stem cell transplantation (abstract). Blood 1997; 90(Suppl 1):457.

116. Nash RA, Furlong T, Storb R, et al. Mycophenolate mofetil as salvage treatment for graft-versus-host disease after allogeneic hematopoietic stem cell transplantation: Safety analysis (abstract). Blood 1997; 90(Suppl 1):459.

117. Yamane T, Yamamura R, Aoyama Y, et al. Infliximab for the treatment of severe steroid refractory acute graft-versus-host disease in three patients after allogeneic hematopoietic transplantation. Leuk Lymphoma 2003; 44:2095.

118. Kobbe G, Schneider P, Rohr U, et al. Treatment of severe steroid refractory acute graft-versus-host disease with infliximab, a chimeric human/mouse antiTNFα antibody. Bone Marrow Transplant 2001; 28:47.

119. Ho VT, Zahrieh D, Hochberg E, et al. Safety and efficacy of denileukin diftitox in patients with steroid-refractory acute graft-versus-host disease after allogeneic hematopoietic stem cell transplantation. Blood 2004; 104:1224.

120. Srinivasan R, Chakrabarti S, Walsh T, et al. Improved survival in steroid-refractory acute graft versus host disease after non-myeloablative allogeneic transplantation using a daclizumab-based strategy with comprehensive infection prophylaxis. Br J Haematol 2004; 124:777.

121. Jacobsohn DA, Hallick J, Anders V, et al. Infliximab for steroid-refractory acute GVHD: a case series. Am J Hematol 2003; 74:119.

122. Ippoliti C, Champlin R, Bugazia N, et al. Use of octreotide in the symptomatic management of diarrhea induced by graft-versus-host disease in patients with hematologic malignancies. J Clin Oncol 1997; 15:3350.

123. Nishida T, Hamaguchi M, Hirabayashi N, et al. Intestinal thrombotic microangiopathy after allogeneic bone marrow transplantation: a clinical imitator of acute enteric graft-versus-host disease. Bone Marrow Transplant 2004; 33:1143.

124. Cohen JS, Paz JB, O'Donnell MR, et al. Treatment of perianal infection following bone marrow transplantation. Dis Colon Rectum 1996; 39:981.

125. Raynard B, Nitenberg G, Gory-Delabaere G, et al. Summary of the Standards, Options and Recommendations for nutritional support in patients undergoing bone marrow transplantation. Br J Cancer. 2003; 89(Suppl 1):S101.

126. Weisdorf SA, Lysne J, Wind D, et al. Positive effect of prophylactic total parenteral nutrition on long-term outcome of bone marrow transplantation. Transplantation 1987; 43:833.

127. Malhotra D, DeMeo M, Kruger A, et al. Oral elemental nutrition improves gastrointestinal mucosal integrity in patients undergoing bone marrow transplantation (Abstract). Proc Annu Meet Am Soc Clin Oncol 1996; 15:1406.

128. Arai S, Lee LA, Vogelsang GB. A systematic approach to hepatic complications in hematopoietic stem cell transplantation. J Hematother Stem Cell Res 2002; 11:215.

129. Strasser SI, McDonald GB. Hepatobiliary complications of hematopoietic stem cell transplantation. In: Schiff ER, Sorrell MF, Maddrey WC, eds. Schiff's diseases of the liver. 9th edn. Philadelphia: JB Lippincott; 2003:1636.

130. McDonald GB, Schoch HG, Gooley T. Liver dysfunction and mortality after allogeneic marrow transplantation: analysis of 1419 consecutive patients (Abstract). Hepatology 1999; 30:162a.

   A prospective study noted mortality rates of 19%, 51%, 75%, 83%, and 87% for patients with total serum bilirubin values on day +30 of 1–4, 4–7, 7–10, >10 and >19, respectively.

131. Ma SY, Au WY, Ng IO, et al. Role of liver biopsy in the management of liver dysfunction after hematopoietic stem-cell transplantation in a hepatitis B virus-prevalent patient population. Transplantation 2003; 76:169.

132. Carreras E, Bertz H, Areese W, et al. Incidence and outcome of hepatic veno-occlusive disease after blood or marrow transplantation: A prospective cohort study of the European Group for Blood and Marrow Transplantation. Blood 1998; 92:3599.

133. McDonald GB, Hinds MS, Fisher LB, et al. Veno-occlusive disease of the liver and multiorgan failure after bone marrow transplantation: A cohort study of 355 patients. Ann Intern Med 1993; 118:255.

134. Toh HC, McAfee SL, Sackstein R, et al. Late onset veno-occlusive disease following high-dose chemotherapy and stem cell transplantation. Bone Marrow Transplant 1999; 24:891.

135. Jones RJ, Lee KSK, Beschorner WE, et al. Venocclusive disease of the liver following bone marrow transplantation. Transplantation 1987; 44:778.

136. Strasser SL, McDonald GB. Hepatobiliary complications of hematopoietic stem cell transplantation. In: Schiff ER, Sorrell MF, Maddrey WC, eds. Schiff's diseases of the liver. 9th edn. Philadelphia: JB Lippincott; 2003:1636.

137. Kallianpur AR, Hall LD, Yadav M, et al. Veno-occlusive disease of the liver after hematopoietic cell transplantation: association with the hemochromatosis (HFE) C282Y Allele. Blood 2003; Abstract 677.

138. Shulman HM, Fisher LB, Schoch HG, et al. Venocclusive disease of the liver after marrow transplantation: Histologic correlates of clinical signs and symptoms. Hepatology 1994; 19:1171.

139. Laussau N, Auperin A, Leclere J, et al. Prognostic value of Doppler-ultrasonography in hepatic veno-occlusive disease. Transplantation 2002; 74:60.

140. Lassau N, Leclere J, Auperin A, et al. Hepatic veno-occlusive disease after myeloablative treatment and bone marrow transplantation: Value of gray-scale and Doppler US in 100 patients. Radiology 1997; 204:545.

When findings on Doppler are combined with gray-scale ultrasonography, a positive predictive score of 44% to 89% and a negative predictive score of 91% to 98% have been estimated.

141. Mortele KJ, Van Vierberghe H, Wiesner W, et al. Hepatic veno-occlusive disease: MRI findings. Abdom Imaging 2002; 27:523.

142. Lee JH, Lee KH, Lee JH, et al. Plasminogen activator inhibitor-1 is an independent diagnostic marker as well as severity predictor of hepatic veno-occlusive disease after allogeneic bone marrow transplantation in adults conditioned with busulphan and cyclophosphamide. Br J Haematol 2002; 118:1087.

143. Kaleelrahman M, Eaton JD, Leeming D, et al. Role of plasminogen activator inhibitor-1 (PAI-1) levels in the diagnosis of BMT-associated hepatic veno-occlusive disease and monitoring of subsequent therapy with defibrotide (DF). Hematology 2003; 8:91.

144. Remberger M, Ringden O. Serum levels of cytokines after bone marrow transplantation: increased IL-8 levels during severe veno-occlusive disease of the liver. Eur J Haematol 1997; 59:254.

145. Goldberg SL, Shubert J, Rao AK, et al. Treatment of hepatic veno-occlusive disease with low dose tissue plasminogen activator: Impact on coagulation profile. Bone Marrow Transplant 1996; 18:633.

146. Attal M, Huguet F, Rubie H, et al. Prevention of hepatic veno-occlusive disease after bone marrow transplantation by continuous infusion of low-dose heparin: A prospective, randomized trial. Blood 1992; 79:2834.

Patients were randomized to receive prophylactic heparin, 100 U/kg/day by continuous infusion, or observation from day −8 until day +30 post-BMT. Heparin was found to be highly effective in preventing VOD, which occurred in 11 of 80 patients (13.7%) in the control group versus 2 of 81 (2.5%) in the heparin group (p<0.01).

147. Or R, Nagler A, Shpilberg O, et al. Low molecular weight heparin for the prevention of veno-occlusive disease of the liver in bone marrow transplantation patients. Transplantation 1996; 61:1067.

Sixty-one patients undergoing BMT were randomized to receive subcutaneous enoxaparin (40 mg/day) or placebo beginning before BMT conditioning and continuing until day 40. VOD parameters occurred less frequently in the experimental group, including duration of elevated bilirubin levels (p=0.01) and incidence of hepatomegaly (p=0.04). There was no influence on engraftment or bleeding tendencies.

148. Simon M, Hahn T, Ford LA, et al. Retrospective multivariate analysis of hepatic veno-occlusive disease after blood or marrow transplantation: possible beneficial use of low molecular weight heparin. Bone Marrow Transplant 2001; 27:627.

149. Forrest DL, Thompson K, Dorcas VG, et al. Low molecular weight heparin for the prevention of hepatic veno-occlusive disease (VOD) after hematopoietic stem cell transplantation: a prospective phase II study. Bone Marrow Transplant 2003; 31:1143.

150. Marsa-Vila L, Gorin NC, Laporte JP, et al. Prophylactic heparin does not prevent liver venocclusive disease following autologous bone marrow transplantation. Eur J Haematol 1991; 47:346.

151. Budlinger MD, Bouvier M, Shah A, et al. Results of a phase I trial of antithrombin III as prophylaxis in bone marrow transplant patients at risk for veno-occlusive disease (Abstract). Blood 1996; 88:172.

152. Chalandon Y, Roosnek E, Mermillod B, et al. Prevention of veno-occlusive disease with defibrotide after allogeneic stem cell transplantation. Biol Blood Marrow Transplant 2004; 10:347.

153. Essell JH, Schroeder M, Harman GS, et al. Ursodiol prophylaxis against hepatic complications of allogeneic bone marrow transplantation. A randomized, double blind, placebo controlled trial. Ann Intern Med 1998; 128:975.

154. Ruutu Park SH, Lee MH, Lee H, et al. A randomized trial of heparin plus ursodiol vs. heparin alone to prevent hepatic veno-occlusive disease after hematopoietic stem cell transplantation. Bone Marrow Transplant 2002; 29:137.

155. Schlegel PG, Haber HP, Beck J, et al. Hepatic veno-occlusive disease in pediatric stem cell recipients: Successful treatment with continuous infusion of prostaglandin E$_1$ and low-dose heparin. Ann Hematol 1998; 76:37.

156. Bearman SI, Anderson GL, Mori M, et al. Veno-occlusive disease of the liver: Development of a model for predicting fatal outcome after marrow transplantation. J Clin Oncol 1993; 11:1729.

157. Rapoport AP, Doyle HR, Starzl T, et al. Orthotopic liver transplantation for life-threatening veno-occlusive disease of the liver after allogeneic bone marrow transplant. Bone Marrow Transplant 1991 18:421.

158. Zenz T, Rossle M, Bertz H, et al, Severe veno-occlusive disease after allogeneic bone marrow or peripheral stem cell transplantation: role of trans-jugular intrahepatic portosystemic shunt. Liver 2001; 21:31.

159. Bearman SI, Lee JL, Baron AE, et al. Treatment of hepatic veno-occlusive disease with recombinant human tissue plasminogen activator and heparin in 42 marrow transplant patients. Blood 1997; 89:1501.

160. Chopra R, Eaton JD, Grassi A, et al. Defibrotide for the treatment of hepatic veno-occlusive disease: results of the European compassionate-use study. Br J Haematol 2000; 111:1122.

161. Richardson PG, Murakami C, Wei LJ, et al. Multi-institutional use of defibrotide in 88 patients post stem cell transplant with severe veno-occlusive disease and multi-system organ failure: response without significant toxicity in a high risk population and factors predictive of outcome. Blood 2002; 100:4337.

162. Haire WD, Ruby EI, Stephens LC, et al. A prospective randomized double-blind trial of antithrombin III concentrate in the treatment of multiple-organ dysfunction syndrome during hematopoietic stem cell transplantation. Biol Blood Marrow Transplant 1998; 4:142.

163. Iqbal M, Creger RJ, Fox RM, et al. Laparoscopic liver biopsy to evaluate hepatic dysfunction in patients with hematologic malignancies: A useful tool to effect changes in management. Bone Marrow Transplant 1996; 17:655.

164. Figuera A, Tomas JF, Otero MJ, et al. Orthotopic liver transplantation for acute grade IV hepatic graft-versus-host

disease following bone marrow transplantation (Letter). Am J Hematol 1996; 52:68.

165. Wulffraat NM, Haddad E, Benkerrou M, et al. Hepatic GVHD after HLA-haploidentical bone marrow transplantation in children with severe combined immunodeficiency: the effect of ursodeoxycholic acid. Br J Haematol 1997; 96:776.

166. Ruutu T, Eriksson B, Remes K, et al. Ursodeoxycholic acid for the prevention of hepatic complications in allogeneic stem cell transplantation. Blood 2002; 100:1977.

167. Saunders MD, Shulman HM, Murakami CS, et al. Bile duct apoptosis and cholestasis resembling acute graft-versus-host disease after autologous hematopoietic cell transplantation. Am J Surg Pathol 2000; 24:1004.

168. van Burik JH, Leisenring W, Myerson D, et al. The effect of prophylactic fluconazole on the clinical spectrum of fungal diseases in bone marrow transplant recipients with special attention to hepatic candidiasis: an autopsy study of 355 patients. Medicine 1998; 77:246.

169. Lau GK, Leung YH, Fong DY, et al. High hepatitis B virus (HBV) DNA viral load as the most important risk factor for HBV reactivation in patients positive for surface antigen undergoing autologous hematopoietic stem cell transplantation. Blood 2002; 99:2324.

170. Kanamori H, Fukawa H, Maruta A, et al. Fulminant hepatitis C viral infection after bone marrow transplantation. Am J Med Sci 1992; 303:109.

171. Giardini C, Galimberti M, Lucarelli G, et al. α-Interferon treatment of chronic hepatitis C after bone marrow transplantation for homozygous β-thalassemia. Bone Marrow Transplant 1997; 20:767.

172. Skidmore SJ, Collingham KE, Harrison P, et al. High prevalence of hepatitis G virus in bone marrow transplant recipients and patients treated for acute leukemia. Blood 1997; 89:3853.

173. Kanda Y, Hirari H. TT virus in hematological disorders and bone marrow transplant recipients. Leuk Lymphoma 2001; 40:483.

174. Flomenberg N, Babbit J, Drobyski WR, et al. Increasing incidence of adenovirus disease in bone marrow transplant patients. J Infect Dis 1994; 169:775.

175. Bordigoni P, Carret AS, Venard V, et al. Treatment of adenovirus infections in patients undergoing allogeneic hematopoietic stem cell transplantation. Clin Infect Dis 2001; 32:1290.

176. Liles WC, Cushing H, Holt S, et al. Severe adenoviral nephritis following bone marrow transplantation: Successful treatment with intravenous ribavirin. Bone Marrow Transplant 1994; 12:409.

177. Hromas R, Cornetta K, Srour E, et al. Donor leukocyte infusion as therapy of life-threatening adenoviral infections after T-cell depleted bone marrow transplantation (Letter). Blood 1994; 84:1689.

178. Snover DC, Hutton S, Balfour HH Jr. Cytomegalovirus infection of the liver in transplant recipients. J Clin Gastroenterol 1987; 9:659.

179. Murakami CS, Louie W, Chan GS, et al. Biliary obstruction in hematopoietic cell transplant recipients: an uncommon diagnosis with specific causes. Bone Marrow Transplant 1999; 23:921.

180. Biggs DD, Toorkey BD, Carrigan DR, et al. Disseminated echovirus infection complicating bone marrow transplantation. Am J Med 1990; 88:421.

181. Schleuning M, Jager G, Holler E, et al. Human parvovirus B19-associated disease in bone marrow transplantation. Infection 1999; 27:114.

182. Gruson D, Hilbert G, Le Bail B, et al. Fulminant hepatitis due to herpes simplex virus-type 2 in early phase of bone marrow transplantation. Hematol Cell Ther 1998; 40:41.

183. Ljungman P, Wang FZ, Clark DA, et al. High levels of human herpesvirus 6 DNA are correlated to platelet engraftment and disease in allogeneic stem cell transplant patients. Br J Haematol 2000; 111:774.

184. Clark DA. Human herpesvirus 6 and human herpesvirus 7: emerging pathogens in transplant patients. Int J Hematol 2002; 76(Suppl 2):246.

185. Luppi M, Barozzi P, Schultz TF, et al; Nonmalignant disease associated with human herpesvirus 8 reactivation in patients who have undergone autologous peripheral blood stem cell transplantation. Blood 2000; 96:2355.

186. Jardines LA, O'Donnell MR, Johnson DL, et al. Acalculous cholecystitis in bone marrow transplant patients. Cancer 1993; 71:354.

187. Rotter AJ, O'Donnell MR, Radin DR, et al. Peribiliary chloroma: A rare cause of jaundice after bone marrow transplantation. AJR Am J Roentgenol 1992; 158:1255.

188. Uderzo C, Fraschini D, Balduzzi A, et al. Long-term effects of bone marrow transplantation on dental status in children with leukemia. Bone Marrow Transplant 1997; 20:865.

189. Epstein JB, Truelove EL. Topical cyclosporine in a bioadhesive for treatment of oral lichenoid mucosal reactions: An open label clinical trial. Oral Surg Oral Med Oral Pathol Oral Radiol Endod 1996; 82:532.

190. McDonald GB, Sullivan KM, Schuffler MD, et al. Esophageal abnormalities in chronic graft-versus-host disease in humans. Gastroenterology 1981; 80:914.

191. Schima W, Pokieser P, Forstinger C, et al. Videofluoroscopy of the pharynx and esophagus in chronic graft-versus-host disease. Abdom Imaging 1994; 19:191.

192. Atree SV, Crilley PA, Conroy JF, et al. Cancer of the esophagus following allogeneic bone marrow transplantation for acute leukemia. Am J Clin Oncol 1995; 18:343.

193. Mainghini A, Gertz MA, DiMagno EP. Exocrine pancreatic insufficiency after allogeneic bone marrow transplantation. Int J Pancreatol 1995; 17:243.

194. Akpek G, Chinratanalab W, Lee LA, et al. Gastrointestinal involvement in chronic graft-versus-host disease: a clinicopathologic study. Biol Blood Marrow Transplant 2003; 9:46.

195. Herr AL, Latulippe JF, Carignan S, et al. Is severe intestinal chronic graft-versus-host disease an indication for surgery? A report of two cases. Transplantation 2004; 77:1617.

196. Ma SY, Au WY, Ng IO, et al. Hepatic graft-versus-host disease after hematopoietic stem cell transplantation: clinicopathologic features and prognostic implication. Transplantation 2004; 77:1252.

197. Tomas JF, Pinilla I, Garcia-Buey ML, et al. Long-term liver dysfunction after allogeneic bone marrow transplantation: clinical features and course in 61 patients. Bone Marrow Transplant 2000; 26:649.

198. Maeng H, Lee JH, Cheong JW, et al. Chronic graft-versus-host disease of the liver presenting as an acute hepatitis following nonmyeloablative hematopoietic stem cell transplantation. Int J Hematol 2004; 79:501.

199. Fried RH, Murakami CS, Fisher LD, et al. Ursodeoxycholic acid treatment of refractory chronic graft-versus-host disease of the liver. Ann Intern Med 1992; 116:624.

200. Parker PM, Chao N, Nademanee A, et al. Thalidomide as salvage therapy for chronic graft-versus-host disease. Blood 1995; 86:3604.

201. Lee SJ, Wegner SA, McGarigie CJ, et al. Treatment of chronic graft-versus-host disease with clofazimine. Blood 1997; 89:2298.

202. Rhodes D, Lee WM, Wingard JR, et al. Orthotopic liver transplantation for graft-versus-host disease following bone marrow transplantation. Gastroenterology 1990; 99:533.

203. Canninga-van Dijk MR, Van Der Straaten HM, Fijnheer R, et al. Anti-CD20 monoclonal antibody treatment in six patients with therapy-refractory chronic graft-versus-host disease. Blood 2004; 104:2603.

204. Grigg AP, Angus AP, Hoyt R, et al. The incidence, pathogenesis, and natural history of steatorrhea after bone marrow transplantation. Bone Marrow Transplant 2003; 31:701.

205. Atkinson K, Biggs J, Dodds A, et al. Cyclosporine-associated hepatotoxicity after allogeneic marrow transplantation in man: Differentiation from other causes of post-transplant liver disease. Transplant Proc 1983; 15:2761.

206. Strasser SI, Sullivan KM, Myerson D, et al. Cirrhosis of the liver in long-term marrow transplant survivors. Blood 1999; 93:3259.

207. Locasciulli A, Bruno B, Alessandrino EP, et al. Hepatitis reactivation and liver failure in haemopoietic stem cell transplants for hepatitis B virus (HBV)/hepatitis C virus (HCV) positive recipients: a retrospective study by the Italian group for blood and marrow transplantation. Bone Marrow Transplant 2003; 31:295.

In a study of 90 patients infected with HBV (n=33) or HCV (n=57) receiving allogeneic (n=36) or autologous (n=54) transplant, the risk of death at 2 years was comparable when considering type of infection (3% for HBV, 8% for HCV, p=0.6) or type of HSCT (7% for allogeneic versus 5% for autologous HHSCT, p=0.34).

208. Seth P, Alrajhi AA, Kagevi I, et al. Hepatitis B virus reactivation with clinical flare in allogeneic stem cell transplants with chronic graft-versus-host disease. Bone Marrow Transplant 2002; 30:189.

209. Picardi M, Selleri C, DeRosa G, et al. Lamivudine treatment for chronic replicative hepatitis B virus infection after allogeneic bone marrow transplantation. Bone Marrow Transplant 1998; 21:1267.

210. Peffault de Latour R, Levy V, Asselah T, et al. Long term outcome of hepatitis C infection after bone marrow transplantation. Blood 2004; 103:1618.

211. McKay PJ, Murphy JA, Cameron S, et al. Iron overload and liver dysfunction after allogeneic or autologous bone marrow transplantation. Bone Marrow Transplant 1996; 17:63.

212. Muretto P, Angelucci E, Lucarelli G. Reversibility of cirrhosis in patients cured of thalassemia by bone marrow transplantation. Ann Intern Med 2002; 136:667.

213. Toren A, Nagler A. Solitary pulmonary cholesteroloma, multiple xanthelasma and lipemia retinalis complicating hypercholesterolemia after bone marrow transplantation. Bone Marrow Transplant 1996; 18:457.

214. Markin RS. Manifestations of Epstein-Barr virus associated disorders in the liver. Liver 1994; 14:1.

215. Papadopoulos EB, Ladanyi M, Emanuel D, et al. Infusion of donor lymphocytes to treat Epstein-Barr virus associated lymphoproliferative disorders after allogeneic bone marrow transplantation. N Engl J Med 1994; 330:1185.

216. Faye A, Quartier P, Reguerre Y, et al. Chimaeric anti-CD20 monoclonal antibody (rituximab) in post-transplant B-lymphoproliferative disorder following stem cell transplantation in children. Br J Haematol 2001; 115:112.

217. Snover DC, Weisdorf S, Bloomer J, et al. Nodular regenerative hyperplasia of the liver following bone marrow transplantation. Hepatology 1989; 9:443.

218. Frere P, Canivert JL, Gennigens C, et al. Hyperammonemia after high-dose chemotherapy and stem cell transplantation. Bone Marrow Transplant 2000; 26:343.

219. Bhatia S, Louie AD, Bhatia R, et al. Solid cancers after bone marrow transplantation. J Clin Oncol 2001; 19:464.

220. Curtis RE, Rowlings PA, Deeg HJ, et al. Solid cancers after bone marrow transplantation. N Engl J Med 1997; 336:897.

CHAPTER TEN

10

Pregnancy

Sarathchandra I. Reddy and Jacqueline L. Wolf

In pregnancy women undergo profound changes in anatomy and physiology affecting the gastrointestinal tract and liver. Gastroesophageal reflux disease is common, occurring in over 80% of women, while peptic ulcer disease is reduced. Bowel function is reported by many women to be affected. Conditions of the liver specific to pregnancy may occur and others, such as viral hepatitis, may require specific considerations in pregnancy. Gallbladder sludge is increased and subsequent stone disease is directly related to the total number of pregnancies.

Evaluation and treatment of gastrointestinal disease in pregnancy should take into consideration the health of the mother while attempting to achieve an optimal outcome for the baby. Safety of a drug and any diagnostic procedures have to be assessed. However, in many cases the instinct to delay or withhold treatment out of concern for a healthy pregnancy could potentially produce an adverse outcome.

The safety of drugs used in pregnancy has been assessed through safety in animal studies, trials in pregnant women, and postmarketing studies. There are limited data on the safety of many medications used to treat gastrointestinal disease in pregnancy due to absence of prospective controlled trials in pregnant women. Safety of drugs in animal studies does not necessarily correlate with safety in pregnant women. The safety of several classes of drugs used to treat gastrointestinal and liver disease in pregnancy are defined in Table 10.1. Drugs in categories A and B are considered safe in pregnancy. Drugs in category C are generally safe, and category D drugs should be used only if there is a strong clinical indication.

MONITORING AND DIAGNOSIS OF GASTROINTESTINAL DISEASE DURING PREGNANCY

A number of tests are available for diagnosing and monitoring gastrointestinal disease in pregnancy; however, interpretation of these tests is complicated by their lack of specificity as well as the altered physiologic state of pregnancy. The hematocrit is typically decreased during pregnancy due to increased plasma volume and therefore may not serve as a reliable gauge of gastrointestinal bleeding. Serologic markers such as C-reactive protein and ESR, which can be helpful in assessing inflammatory activity, may also be elevated during pregnancy. Furthermore, in suspected biliary tract disease, serum alkaline phosphatase is difficult to interpret due to the contribution of placental alkaline phosphatase.

Table 10.1 FDA classification of drugs during pregnancy

FDA classification	Definition
Category A	Controlled studies in pregnant women show no fetal risk.
Category B	Animal studies indicate no adverse effect to the fetus, but there are no adequate, clinical studies in pregnant women.
Category C	Animal studies have shown an adverse effect on the fetus, but there are no adequate, clinical studies in humans. Despite potential risks, the drug may be useful in pregnant women.
Category D	There is evidence of risk to the human fetus, but the potential benefits of use in pregnant women may be acceptable, despite potential risks.
Category X	Contraindicated in pregnancy due to fetal abnormalities in animals or humans. The risks involved clearly outweigh any potential benefit from using the drug in pregnant women, regardless of trimester.

Radiologic testing may yield important diagnostic information and potential need for endoscopic or surgical intervention in the pregnant patient; however, radiologic testing is often avoided in pregnant women due to concern about exposure of the fetus to radiation. Ultrasound is safe during pregnancy and is the preferred imaging modality to assess abdominal pain and suspected biliary tract disease during pregnancy. MRI poses no radiation risk to the developing fetus and thus can be used safely during pregnancy; however gadolinium should be avoided during the first trimester.[1,2]

Radiologic studies which expose the developing fetus to ionizing radiation should be utilized with caution, particularly during the first trimester when risk of teratogenicity is greatest. The risk of teratogenicity is greatest if the radiation exposure exceeds 15 rads in the second and third trimesters and 5 rads in the first trimester.[2,3] While abdominal plain films and a CT scan do expose the developing fetus to ionizing radiation, the radiation exposure is relatively small and can be further minimized by obtaining a limited number of images. In contrast, fluoroscopic studies such as endoscopic retrograde cholangiopancreatography (ERCP) entail greater radiation exposure and therefore should only be performed if necessary utilizing techniques to minimize radiation exposure. A single fluoroscopic diagnostic study is considered safe in pregnancy.

Ultimately, endoscopy may be necessary as a diagnostic and treatment modality in the pregnant patient. The safety and efficacy of endoscopy during pregnancy have not been studied extensively. The performance of endoscopy during pregnancy raises concerns regarding risks of inducing premature labor or potential teratogenic risks from medications used during endoscopy. Maternal hypotension and hypoxemia may also pose risks to the fetus if complications arise during endoscopy. Ultimately, the potential diagnostic and therapeutic risks of endoscopy must be weighed against potential harm to the pregnant mother or fetus.

Several studies suggest that both upper and lower endoscopy can be performed safely during pregnancy. In a retrospective study of sigmoidoscopy in 46 pregnant women, Cappell et al. concluded that sigmoidoscopy does not induce premature labor or result in congenital anomalies, low birth weight, or fetal demise.[4] Sigmoidoscopy was particularly beneficial in pregnant women for evaluation of lower gastrointestinal bleeding. Thus, sigmoidoscopy during pregnancy appears to be safe and may be performed in stable patients with important clinical indications such as severe rectal bleeding or the assessment of disease activity in inflammatory bowel disease.

Studies also suggest that colonoscopy may be safely performed in pregnant women.[4] This is technically more difficult, however, due to displacement of the colon by the uterus. During colonoscopy the supine position should be avoided as uterine perfusion can be compromised.[5] While colonoscopy can be performed safely for life-threatening conditions such as bleeding or in cases where colonic surgery is the only alternative, a purely elective colonoscopy should be postponed until the postpartum period.

Upper endoscopy may also be performed safely during pregnancy and may assist in evaluation of bleeding, abdominal pain, and severe nausea and vomiting. A case-controlled study of 83 upper endoscopies performed during pregnancy for various indications found no statistically significant difference in parameters such as maternal complications, premature labor, Apgar scores, low birth weight, infant mortality, or congenital defects.[6] The findings of this study suggested that EGD can be performed safely in pregnant patients with a strong indication for endoscopic evaluation.

The choice and dose of drugs in conscious sedation for gastrointestinal endoscopy should be carefully considered. Many studies of drug effects are either nonexistent or involve very small numbers of patients. Drugs commonly used during endoscopy for sedation and their safety profile during pregnancy are listed in Table 10.2.[5]

NAUSEA AND VOMITING IN PREGNANCY AND HYPEREMESIS GRAVIDARUM

Nausea and vomiting in pregnancy (NVP) are common, occurring in 50–90% of pregnancies.[7] NVP is far more common among patients in the first trimester than in the third trimester, with symptoms usually peaking at 9 weeks' gestation and decreasing significantly by 18 weeks' gestation. A prospective study of 160 pregnant women found that nausea was reported by 74% of women over the course of their pregnancies and usually resolved by 22 weeks' gestation.[8] Nausea and vomiting occur more frequently in women with multiple gestations compared with a single gestation. While it is often a troubling symptom causing significant distress, numerous studies have shown NVP to be associated with a decreased risk of miscarriage, low birth weight, and preterm delivery.[9]

A number of therapies have been investigated in the treatment of nausea and vomiting of pregnancy (see Ch. 70). *Vitamin B₆* (pyridoxine hydrochloride – category A) supplementation may be helpful in certain patients. Small studies suggest that patients with severe nausea and vomiting may benefit from therapy with B₆ at a dose of 10–25 mg orally t.i.d.[10,11]

Doxylamine (category B) is an antihistamine which has also been used with some success in treatment of severe nausea and vomiting. Doxylamine was available in two preparations as doxylamine succinate or in combination with pyridoxine (diclectin, bendectin). Bendectin was withdrawn from the US market due to concern about possible teratogenicity, although a subsequent

Table 10.2 Safety of drugs used in the performance of gastrointestinal endoscopy

Drug	Pregnancy safety category	Recommendation in pregnancy
Meperidine	B	May be used in low dose for endoscopy during pregnancy
Diazepam	D	Use should be restricted during endoscopy during the first trimester due to unproven safety and concern about possible teratogenic effects such as cleft palate and neurologic defects
Midazolam	D	Preferred over diazepam; no association with oral clefts; can be used in low doses and titrated carefully for mild sedation
Fentanyl	C	May be used in low doses in pregnancy; studies of use during labor reveal no neonatal toxicity
Propofol	B	Considered safe during pregnancy; should be administered by anesthesiologist as it may cause respiratory depression

meta-analysis revealed no association between bendectin and birth defects. Diclectin is approved in Canada for nausea and vomiting of pregnancy. A study of 225 patients treated with high-dose diclectin and two meta-analyses revealed no increase in congenital malformations.[12,13]

Antiemetics also offer symptomatic relief in patients with NVP. The safety of the phenothiazines, promethazine (category C) and prochlorperazine (compazine – category C) have not yet been proven although the latter is widely used in pregnancy. Metoclopramide (category B) is widely used for treatment of NVP, and appears to be safe in pregnancy.[14] Finally, odansetron and droperidol are effective antiemetics but there is limited experience using these medications for nausea and vomiting of pregnancy.

In contrast to nausea and vomiting of pregnancy, hyperemesis gravidarum is a serious condition characterized by severe vomiting which may result in dehydration, weight loss, and need for parenteral or enteral nutrition. It occurs most commonly in the first trimester. The condition tends to occur in patients who are overweight, multiparous, and have multiple gestations.[15,16] The true incidence of hyperemesis gravidarum is not known but is estimated between 1 in 100 and 1 in 1000 pregnancies.[17] The condition is likely to recur with subsequent pregnancies. While gastric dysmotility has also been implicated in the pathophysiology, the findings have not been uniform.

Treatment for hyperemesis gravidarum consists of supportive care with rehydration. Patients may also benefit from enteral or parenteral nutrition in severe cases. Correction of dehydration and electrolyte abnormalities such as correction of metabolic alkalosis, and correction of sodium, potassium, and magnesium levels are of crucial importance in the management of hyperemesis gravidarum. Therefore, intravenous hydration and correction of electrolytes are the first treatments for hyperemesis. Thiamine should also be administered intravenously.

Nonpharmacologic treatment includes avoidance of environmental triggers and dietary changes, including a low fat diet. Acupuncture and acupressure are two possible nonpharmacologic interventions which may benefit patients with hyperemesis gravidarum.[18,19]

At present, there are very few evidence-based data to support a particular pharmacologic treatment in hyperemesis gravidarum. Management of hyperemesis involves symptomatic treatments employed for severe nausea and vomiting as well as other agents which have been studied specifically in the context of hyperemesis gravidarum.

Based on its beneficial effects in treatment of nausea, powdered ginger root has been studied in the treatment of hyperemesis gravidarum. In a double-blind, randomized crossover trial, Fischer-Rasmussen et al.[20] studied the effects of ginger root at a dose of 250 mg orally q.i.d. for four days in 30 patients with hyperemesis gravidarum and found significant reductions in severity of nausea as well as decreased number of vomiting episodes. The agent was well tolerated without significant side effects; however, the major limitation of the study was its short treatment period.

Although the mechanism of action is not well understood, corticosteroids (category B) have also been used in women with severe hyperemesis. While uncontrolled trials have shown some benefit, controlled trials have produced varying results.[21] Numerous studies have revealed that use of corticosteroids does not increase the risk of pregnancy complications or congenital anomalies.

Erythromycin (category B) stimulates gastric motility by binding to the motilin receptor. Two case reports have demonstrated improvement in hyperemesis gravidarum when erythromycin was administered orally for 5 days.[21] Large studies do not support an association between erythromycin and congenital malformation.[22]

GASTROESOPHAGEAL REFLUX DISEASE AND PEPTIC ULCER DISEASE IN PREGNANCY

Symptomatic gastroesophageal reflux disease (GERD) is commonly reported in pregnancy with 40–80% of patients experiencing reflux (see Ch. 13). The condition usually begins in the first or second trimester and generally persists throughout pregnancy with significant improvement following delivery.[23] In a large study of over 600 pregnant women, Marrero et al. found that the prevalence of heartburn was associated with gestational age, prior history of heartburn, parity, and inversely related to maternal age. In this same study, the authors reported increasing severity and prevalence of heartburn during pregnancy.[24]

Numerous factors have been implicated in causing GERD during pregnancy. A number of studies have suggested that LES tone is reduced in pregnancy and that the decrease persists during pregnancy but returns to normal after delivery.[25,26] In the setting of lower LES tone, reflux of gastric acid may be facilitated by increased intra-abdominal pressure from the gravid uterus. Abnormal esophageal and gastric motility may also predispose to acid reflux.[25,27] Symptoms of GERD are similar in pregnant and nonpregnant women. Complications of GERD are uncommon in pregnancy.

Peptic ulcer disease (PUD) can present very differently in pregnant patients in comparison to nonpregnant patients. In pregnant patients, the frequency, complication rate, and severity of symptoms are significantly lower than in nonpregnant women. Pregnant women with chronic PUD have been noted to have alleviation of symptoms with onset of pregnancy.[28] Multiple studies also suggest a decreased incidence of PUD in pregnancy.[29] In part this may be due to a lower rate of confirmed diagnosis as standard radiographic and endoscopic assessments are rarely performed during pregnancy. Risk factors for PUD in the pregnant patient are similar to those of the general population.[30]

The diagnosis of GERD and PUD in pregnancy should be based on characteristic symptoms. Barium studies, endoscopy, manometry, and pH studies are unnecessary in the evaluation; however, an upper endoscopy may be warranted to evaluate severe GERD symptoms or to assess for serious complications of GERD and PUD.

There are no published controlled trials of management of GERD and peptic ulcer disease during pregnancy. Most medications utilized in the management of these disorders are considered safe based on case reports and retrospective cohort studies.

Initial treatment of reflux consists of conservative measures such as avoidance of foods and exposures which may provoke reflux symptoms in the individual patient. In particular, the patient should be advised to avoid fatty foods, citric juices, caffeine, chocolate, NSAIDs, alcohol, and smoking. Nocturnal reflux symptoms may be alleviated by elevation of the head of bed by 6 inches at nighttime and decreasing food and fluid intake within 4 hours of bedtime. When symptoms are refractory to these interventions, a trial of medical therapy is appropriate.

Antacids are commonly used and are felt to be safe in pregnancy. Of the antacids which are available, those containing bicarbonate should be avoided as they may precipitate metabolic alkalosis in the mother and fetus. Magnesium- and aluminum-containing antacids are safer although magnesium-containing antacids should be avoided near term as they may act as tocolytics.[31] The safety and efficacy of these antacids was demonstrated by Land et al. who demonstrated that 50% of pregnant women achieved relief of reflux symptoms within two weeks using magnesium- or aluminum-containing antacids without any increase in congenital anomalies.[32]

Sucralfate (category B) is an aluminum-containing sulfated polysaccharide complex which promotes ulcer healing. When orally administered, the agent is safe and poses no risk to the fetus. In an Italian study, a controlled trial of 66 patients with GERD symptoms, sucralfate was found to be a safe and effective therapy and was not teratogenic.[29]

Extensive experience has shown H$_2$ blockers to be safe and effective in pregnancy. In patients with more severe symptoms who have failed antacid therapy, H$_2$ blockers are often effective in controlling symptoms of reflux and promoting ulcer healing. The oldest H$_2$ blocker, cimetidine, has demonstrated safety in several large follow-up and registry studies. A surveillance study of over 200 000 Michigan Medicaid recipients found no increase in congenital anomalies among newborns exposed to H$_2$ blockers in utero, including 460 newborns exposed to cimetidine, 516 newborns exposed to ranitidine, and 33 newborns exposed to famotidine during the first trimester. Similarly, nizatidine has not been shown to cause congenital anomalies. Based on these data, all four drugs in this class are classified as category B drugs during pregnancy.[22]

Proton pump inhibitors (PPIs) are very effective in acid suppression by binding to the acid pump. PPIs have been shown to be effective in the treatment of GERD, esophagitis, and in treatment of peptic ulcer disease. Although generally regarded as safe in pregnancy, there are no extensive clinical data. Studies of omeprazole (category C) in laboratory animals have demonstrated embryolethality; however, large registry studies such as the Swedish Medical Birth Registry did not demonstrate any increase in congenital defects. Registry studies and case reports have demonstrated lansoprazole, rabeprazole, pantoprazole, and esomeprazole to be safe in pregnancy and all these drugs are characterized as category B drugs during pregnancy.[22,33]

Treatment of Helicobacter pylori infection with triple-drug regimens consisting of antibiotics and PPI therapy should be avoided during pregnancy due to potential teratogenicity or other fetal side effects of antibiotics. While ulcer treatment with H$_2$ blockers and PPI therapy can be offered to alleviate symptoms and promote ulcer healing, multidrug therapy for H. pylori infection is best deferred until the postpartum period.[29]

Therefore, there are a number of choices for therapy of GERD and PUD during pregnancy. Based on the safety profiles and clinical experience with these medications, it is reasonable to start with lifestyle modifications and progress to antacid use if symptoms persist. In these patients, magnesium- and aluminum-containing antacids can be administered 1 hour after meals in doses of 15–30 ml, with additional doses administered to patients with severe symptoms. Sucralfate is another therapeutic option for patients with more severe symptoms. If symptoms are refractory, then therapy with H$_2$ blockers can be employed, with ranitidine being the drug of choice based on its improved side effect profile compared with other H$_2$ blockers. In patients who fail H$_2$ blocker therapy, PPI therapy can be instituted with preference given to a category B drug.

PREGNANCY AND BOWEL FUNCTION

Physiologic changes in gastrointestinal function during pregnancy

Small bowel transit time appears to be prolonged in pregnancy. Transit through the small intestine increases in the first trimester throughout the second or possibly third trimester and subsequently falls in the postpartum period.[34,35] Transit times increase as progesterone levels increase from <1 ng/mg to 80 ng/ml but not as levels increase further.

Evaluation of colonic motility or transit in pregnant women has not been done. However, studies in pregnant rats have shown decreased transit times.[36]

Constipation

It is commonly believed that constipation is a frequent complaint in pregnancy. However, many studies have failed to show that a majority of women have constipation. In a 1971 study by Levy[37] of bowel function in 1000 healthy pregnant Israeli women, 55% had no change in bowel frequency, 34% had increased frequency, and 11% had decreased frequency. Other surveys showed an increase in constipation. In Anderson's study of 200 British women interviewed in the third trimester, 38% of women reporting having had constipation sometime during their pregnancy and 18% still had it at the time of the interview.[38] Because of constipation and other ill-defined gastrointestinal complaints, 70% of women reported dietary modification, primarily increasing fiber intake, which likely improved the symptoms of constipation.

Management

The safety of drug therapy of constipation in pregnancy has not been thoroughly evaluated, but most standard therapeutic regiments appear to be safe (see Ch. 71).[22] Dietary[39] modification through increased fiber intake and adequate liquid consumption should be the first line of therapy for constipation in pregnancy. Supplementation of fiber ingested in the diet with psyllium (Metamucil, Konsyl, Effersyllium), methylcellulose (Citrucel), calcium polycarbophil (Fibercon), pectin, and/or flax seed to 25–40 g/day of fiber is safe and often effective. Bloating may occur with some sources of fiber but not others. Therefore, if bloating occurs, changing the source of fiber may be beneficial. Stool softeners used in pregnancy have not been associated with congenital defects.[22] However, their efficacy is questionable. In two large prospective studies, 348 women receiving docusate sodium had no increased risk of fetal malformation. However, there is one report of chronic use of 150–250 mg of docusate sodium throughout pregnancy thought to be the cause of hypomagnesemia in a mother and her newborn infant.[22] Use of hyperosmolar laxatives, polyethylene glycol, nonabsorbable sugars such as lactulose and sorbitol, and glycerin are safe if dietary manipulation fails. A prospective study of 40 pregnant women with constipation treated with 250 ml of PEG-4000 significantly increased evacuation from 1.66 to 3.16 episodes per week and improved pain. Seventy-three percent of women had a resolution of their constipation.[40] The use of nonabsorbable sugars is often limited by induced bloating and cramping. Use of mineral oil should be limited to short periods, because of the possibility of malabsorption of vitamins and nutrients. Ingestion should be limited only to patients without a risk of aspiration and given only with breakfast or lunch. Other laxative use should be limited because of the risk of dependence. The stimulant laxatives, senna and bisacodyl appear to be safe. Senna, and cascara sagrada, anthraquinones, have been used safely in pregnancy and have not been reported to be teratogenic. Oral bisacodyl often produces cramping, limiting its use.

Saline hyperosmotic laxatives, such as phosphosoda and magnesium-containing laxatives, may result in sodium retention in the mother. Laxatives to avoid are castor oil, which may induce uterine contractions in the mother and aloe (casanthranol) which has been associated with congenital abnormalities. Although many women attribute some of their constipation to use of prenatal vitamins that contain iron, the vitamins should be continued if at all possible.

IRRITABLE BOWEL SYNDROME

Epidemiology

Irritable bowel syndrome (IBS) occurs in about 10–20% of the population (see Ch. 48). In industrialized countries female patients predominate: twice as many women as men report symptoms in large studies.

Because IBS is common in women of childbearing age, the effect of the pregnancy on IBS and the safety of IBS drugs in pregnancy are important to understand. No large study has followed women through pregnancy to see what happens to their IBS symptoms. Hence, it is unknown whether or not women require the same or a modified therapeutic regiment during pregnancy. Some interventions are safer than others and therefore it is important to weigh benefit and risk when treating a gravid woman.[22,41]

Constipation in a woman with IBS should be treated as discussed above. Tegaserod (category B) has not produced any ill effects in pregnant animals. However, experience is very limited in pregnant and nursing women and therefore it should only be used when other measures fail to control severe symptoms of constipation-predominant IBS.

Diarrhea does not usually respond to dietary manipulation. One should keep in mind that women, who may be lactose intolerant, often increase their lactose ingestion in pregnancy and consequently develop diarrhea, bloating, and/or abdominal pain. Limitation of lactose intake and providing calcium supplementation may be therapeutic. Loperamide (category B), a peripherally acting opiate receptor agonist, increases intestinal ion and water absorption, decreases intestinal transit by relaxing localized and segmental colonic spasms, and strengthens anal sphincter tone.[42] A surveillance study of Michigan Medicaid recipients reported 108 newborns exposed to loperamide in the first trimester with no increase in major birth defects, although three cardiovascular defects occurred when only one was expected. A subsequent study of 89 women exposed to loperamide in the

first trimester showed no increase in minor or major birth defects of the fetus when compared to control women, although 21 of 105 babies were 200 g lighter than the controls' babies. Loperamide is considered safe in pregnancy and for nursing mothers.[22] Diphenoxylate/atropine sulfate (category C) probably does not cause birth defects.[22] The largest study of 179 newborns exposed to diphenoxylate in the first trimester showed nine major birth defects, when only seven were expected, but this was felt probably to be coincidental. Multiple malformations in an infant exposed at 10 weeks to diphenoxylate was thought to be unrelated to the exposure. Atropine does cross the placenta and could possibly affect the fetal heart rate and decrease fetal breathing. Peptobismol (bismuth subsalicylate) is hydrolyzed in the gastrointestinal tract to inorganic bismuth salts that are poorly absorbed and salicylates that are readily absorbed. Although no reported abnormalities in human fetuses from bismuth has occurred, chronic administration of bismuth tartrate to lambs resulted in poor outcomes. On the other hand, chronic ingestion of salicylates by mothers has resulted in congenital defects, premature closure of the ductus arteriosus in utero, and intra-uterine growth retardation. Therefore, peptobismol should be avoided in pregnancy. Cholestyramine (see Liver Disease below) if used in large doses for prolonged periods of time can potentially cause malabsorption of fat-soluble vitamins.

Antispasmotic medications are frequently given to patients with IBS prior to pregnancy. Their efficacy in pregnancy has not been assessed.[22] Dicyclomine (category B) does not appear to pose a problem to the mother or fetus. In the Michigan Medicaid recipient surveillance study[22] there was no increased occurrence of birth defects in 642 women except perhaps for polydactyly (3 versus 1). Dicyclomine was a component of Bendectin and Debendox that were removed from the market for the concern of teratogenicity, which has not been confirmed. There have been no adverse problems reported in animals. *Hyoscamine* (category C) has not been shown to have adverse effects in women, but has not been well studied. *Tricyclic antidepressants* are common therapies for IBS. *Amitriptyline* and *nortriptyline*[22] are both category D drugs in pregnancy. Nortriptyline is the active metabolite of amitriptyline. Their assignment to this category appears to be due to the report of limb abnormalities in animals and humans. Subsequent analysis of over 500 infants of mothers exposed in the first trimester to amitriptyline and 61 infants of mothers exposed to nortriptyline did not confirm an increase in congenital malformations. Urinary retention in a neonate has been associated with nortriptyline usage in the mother. *Desipramine* (category C), the active metabolite of imipramine, has not been associated with limb abnormalities or other birth defects. However, neonatal withdrawal symptoms have occurred in the newborn of a mother using desipramine throughout pregnancy. In vitro desipramine is a potent inhibitor of sperm motility. Overall, the safety of the tricyclic antidepressants in pregnancy is still questionable[22] and their use should be limited to the severely symptomatic. The selective serotonin reuptake inhibitors (SSRIs) have been used in women with IBS and depression. The main concern with their use is a possible increase in spontaneous abortions (13.8–15.9%) in women exposed to fluoxetine or paroxetine early in pregnancy. Subsequent evaluation of 267 women exposed to fluvoaxamine, paroxetine, or sertraline did not show increased risk of miscarriage.[43] There is no increase in congenital abnormalities in women exposed to sertraline, fluoxetine, fluvoxamine, or paroxetine. Intrauterine exposure of fetuses to tricyclic anti-depressant drugs or fluoxetine does not affect mental, general cognitive, behavioral, or verbal development indices.[44] Lotronex should not be used in pregnant women. Alternative therapies for IBS have not been studied in pregnancy.

INFLAMMATORY BOWEL DISEASE IN PREGNANCY

The two major categories of inflammatory bowel disease (IBD) are Crohn's disease and ulcerative colitis (UC), which are idiopathic inflammatory conditions of the GI tract (see Chs 56 and 57). Symptoms include diarrhea, abdominal pain, bleeding, and weight loss. These disorders are chronic conditions characterized by periods of quiescence and intermittent flares. They are differentiated based on clinical features including history, endoscopic, and radiologic findings. While the etiology of these disorders is unknown, it is likely to be a combination of genetic, environmental, and immunologic factors.

There is a growing literature of the clinical presentation and management of these conditions during pregnancy. Many studies suggest that the presence of active disease increases the risk of pregnancy complications and congenital anomalies in infants born to women with UC and Crohn's disease. In contrast, women with IBD who remain in remission during pregnancy are likely to have an uncomplicated pregnancy without an increased risk of spontaneous abortion, low birth weight, stillbirth, or congenital anomalies.[45–47] Therefore, patients with IBD should be advised to defer pregnancy until their disease is in remission, but the optimal duration of remission prior to conception remains unclear.

Disease activity during pregnancy appears to correlate with disease activity at the time of conception. Pregnancy does not appear to increase the rate of relapse in women with quiescent ulcerative colitis and Crohn's disease. In a large retrospective study, Miller et al. found that in patients with inactive disease, 73% of women with Crohn's disease and 66% of patients with ulcerative colitis did not experience episodes of relapse during pregnancy. In contrast, the presence of active disease resulted in worsened or continued activity in 65% of patients with Crohn's disease and 69% of patients with ulcerative colitis.[48] Thus, active inflammatory bowel disease at the time of conception is likely to remain active and possibly worsen during the course of pregnancy.[47,48] If relapse of IBD occurs during pregnancy, it occurs most commonly during the first trimester for ulcerative colitis and in the first and second trimester and puerperium for Crohn's disease.[49,50]

Medical management of inflammatory bowel disease during pregnancy

Medical management of IBD during pregnancy should be guided by the principle that active disease rather than treatment for disease poses the greatest risk to the pregnancy. Therefore, it is imperative to optimize medical management of inflammatory bowel disease with medications that are safe for the mother and fetus in order to insure a good pregnancy outcome.

There are limited data on the safety of most medications used to treat IBD in pregnancy, as prospective studies in pregnant women are unavailable. However, most medications used for the treatment of IBD in the general population appear to be safe in pregnancy. Symptomatic treatments for IBD patients include antidiarrheals, antispasmodics, and analgesics (see IBS above).

Aminosalicylates including sulfasalazine (category B), mesalamine (category B), and newer 5-ASA agents are the mainstay of treatment for ulcerative colitis and also play an important role in the management of Crohn's disease. Sulfasalazine has been used for treatment of IBD for more than 50 years, and several large studies have demonstrated the safety of sulfasalazine during pregnancy.[51] Patients receiving sulfasalazine should receive folate supplementation to decrease the risk of neural tube defects. Prospective studies have shown that mesalamine and other 5-ASA agents in both oral and topical forms may be used safely in pregnancy.[52,53] In a prospective study of 165 women exposed to mesalamine during pregnancy, there was no significant increase in congenital malformations compared to a control group.[54]

In IBD patients with moderate disease activity, topical and oral corticosteroids (category B) are effective in inducing remission; however these agents have no role in the maintenance of remission. Corticosteroids have not been shown to cause congenital defects in human studies. Use of shorter-acting agents such as prednisone, prednisolone, and methylprednisolone is preferable as these agents are metabolized by placental enzymes, thereby resulting in fetal exposure to only 10% of the maternal dose.[55] While animal studies reveal that high doses of corticosteroids may cause cleft palate, teratogenicity has not been confirmed in human studies.[55] In a large series of pregnant women with IBD treated with steroids, there was no increase in congenital anomalies or in the incidence of prematurity, spontaneous abortion, or still births.[56]

A newer oral corticosteroid agent, budesonide exhibits extensive first-pass hepatic metabolism and may be used for patients with Crohn's disease affecting the ileum or right colon. Because of its topical antiinflammatory activity and low systemic activity, budesonide has fewer steroid side effects compared with other glucocorticoids. However, since controlled studies in pregnant women are unavailable, budesonide is classified as a pregnancy category C drug.[57]

In patients who are steroid dependent, immunomodulatory agents are effective as maintenance therapy for patients with Crohn's disease and ulcerative colitis. Although no large studies exist of the use of immunomodulatory agents such as 6-mercaptopurine (category D), azathioprine (category D), and cyclosporine (category C) for the treatment of IBD during pregnancy, retrospective studies in the IBD literature suggest that they have no increased risk or pose only a minor increase in risk during pregnancy and hence they may be used safely in pregnancy.[58,59] The use of these agents is justified if the patient has active disease refractory to other oral or topical agents.[55,60]

There is significant controversy regarding the teratogenic effect of 6-mercaptopurine (6-MP) taken by fathers at the time of conception. A retrospective study found that the incidence of 6-MP-related complications were increased when fathers used 6-MP within 3 months of conception.[61] This study contradicts the experience in renal transplant patients which suggests that azathioprine and 6-MP use by the father does not increase the risk of congenital anomalies.[62] Many limitations of this study including its retrospective nature, small sample size, lack of a control group, and lack of information about the health of the mothers do not permit a firm conclusion regarding the teratogenic potential of 6-MP or the appropriate duration that the medication should be withheld prior to conception, if at all.

Methotrexate, which has a role in refractory Crohn's disease, is contraindicated in pregnancy due to teratogenic effects including craniofacial and limb defects, central nervous system abnormalities, and myelosuppression.[55] Infliximab is the first biologic agent approved for the treatment of refractory luminal or fistulizing Crohn's disease. Over 100 reports and drug company data suggest that infliximab may be safe in pregnancy, and it is classified as a category B agent.[63]

Limited data are available regarding the safety of antibiotics for treatment of Crohn's disease in pregnancy. While there are no studies assessing the safety of metronidazole (category B) in pregnancy for the treatment of Crohn's disease, a study of over 200 women who received metronidazole for vaginitis during the first trimester revealed no association with spontaneous abortions or congenital abnormalities.[64] However, most clinicians will limit use of metronidazole to the second and third trimesters. Similarly, there are limited data on the safety of fluoroquinolones for treatment of IBD in pregnancy. While there is concern that fluoroquinolones may cause cartilage deformities in the fetus, a few reports suggest that fluoroquinolones when used briefly during pregnancy are not teratogenic.[65] No long-term follow-up is available to determine if arthritis may develop prematurely.

LIVER DISEASE IN PREGNANCY

The liver is affected by the myriad of changes that occur in pregnancy (see Ch. 47). Even in uncomplicated pregnancies, the liver function tests may vary, the gallbladder volume is increased, and the gallbladder motility is decreased. Alkaline phosphatase increases gradually during the first 7 months of pregnancy and then rises rapidly to peak at term. This rise, principally due to placental origin, rarely exceeds two to four times the normal value in the nongravid woman. Serum cholesterol may increase two times the prepregnancy value. In contrast, serum albumin concentration may be decreased to values 10–60% below normal, primarily due to maternal blood volume expansion during pregnancy. In contrast, serum transaminases and bilirubin are generally not altered by pregnancy, and when abnormal the etiology should be identified.

Hepatic disorders in pregnancy may be categorized as those that are present before pregnancy (which may be affected by pregnancy), those that occur exclusively in pregnancy, and those that occur in both pregnancy and the nonpregnant state. Those disorders that may occur independent of pregnancy, such as viral hepatitis and cholelithiasis, present special therapeutic concerns for the mother and fetus when they occur during pregnancy. Those disorders that occur only in the pregnant state include hyperemesis gravidarum, intrahepatic cholestasis of pregnancy, acute fatty liver of pregnancy, preeclampsia/eclampsia, HELLP syndrome (Hemolytic anemia, Elevated Liver function tests and Low Platelets), and hepatic rupture.

Evaluation of the pregnant woman with abnormal liver function tests[66]

History

A careful, detailed history is crucial in determining the cause of abnormal liver function tests during pregnancy and subsequent therapy of the patient. The time of symptom onset in relation to the weeks of pregnancy duration provides an important clue to the etiology of the abnormal tests. For example, severe *nausea and vomiting* are the key features of hyperemesis gravidarum most commonly occurring in the first trimester, but when accompanied by headache and peripheral edema with onset in the second or third trimester may indicate preeclampsia. If nausea and vomiting are accompanied by right upper quadrant abdominal pain with or without hypotension in the third trimester it may indicate acute fatty liver of pregnancy or hepatic rupture. *Pruritus* occurs in normal pregnancy but generally is limited to the abdomen and does not keep the woman awake at night. The pruritus of intrahepatic cholestasis of pregnancy is more severe and is the characteristic symptom. It typically involves the palms of the hands and soles of the feet initially and then disseminates to the rest of the body. Jaundice follows the pruritus in 20% of patients, typically occurring 2–4 weeks after pruritus onset. *Abdominal pain* with associated abnormal liver function tests in pregnancy is a significant symptom. Right upper quadrant and mid-abdominal pain have potential ominous implications, particularly if occurring in late pregnancy and may be indicative of acute fatty liver of pregnancy or hepatic rupture. Colicky pain with or without fever may indicate biliary colic and/or acute cholecystitis. Other symptoms important to elicit are headache, fever, peripheral edema, foamy urine (suggesting possible proteinuria), oliguria, insomnia, change in stools (i.e., acholic or diarrheal), malaise, weight loss or abnormal gain, dizziness, easy bruisability, or neurological symptoms.

Knowledge of the number of fetuses (single versus multiple), past pregnancies elucidating similar symptoms and their time of onset, as well as other complications and similar symptoms between pregnancies or with oral contraceptive medication is helpful in diagnosis. The history should also include symptoms with drug ingestion or injection, previous blood transfusions, alcohol use, skin rashes or sores, a past history of hepatitis or liver function test abnormalities, diabetes mellitus, recent travel history, close contact with others with a similar illness, or pets at home. A family history of preeclampsia, oral contraceptive pill intolerance, pregnancy problems, or cholelithiasis is particularly pertinent.

Laboratory tests

The evaluation of abnormal liver function tests in pregnancy varies only slightly from that in nonpregnancy, with the exception of limiting radiation exposure. Uric acid and bile acid levels may be helpful.

Uric acid elevation usually occurs in acute fatty liver of pregnancy and may occur in preeclampsia. Serum bile acid levels, which may be elevated before the onset of or in conjunction with intrahepatic cholestasis of pregnancy, are helpful in making this diagnosis.

Intrahepatic cholestasis of pregnancy

Intrahepatic cholestasis of pregnancy (IHCP) is a cholestatic disorder that occurs in the second and third trimester of pregnancy.[66,67] It is characterized by pruritus with or without jaundice. The incidence in the United States is unknown, but is reported to be 0.1% in Canada. It is most common in Sweden and Chile with an incidence of 2% and 4%, respectively. There is an increased frequency in those with a past medical or family history of IHCP and in women with a history of intrahepatic cholestasis due to oral contraceptive or estrogen ingestion or with progesterone use in pregnancy. There is a higher incidence of IHCP recently linked to lower plasma levels of selenium in patients with IHCP.[68] There is a clear genetic predisposition for IHCP. Mutations in genes encoding biliary transport proteins may play a role in the pathogenesis of some forms of IHCP.

Maternal and fetal outcomes

The outcome of the mother is excellent with no permanent liver damage, although there may be an increased risk of subsequent gallstones and gallbladder disease. For the fetus there is an increased risk of prematurity, perinatal deaths, fetal distress, and meconium staining of amniotic fluid.[67]

Management

Pruritus improves immediately after delivery, but rarely is preterm delivery the treatment of the disease.[66,67] Management strategies have focused on symptomatic relief for the mother, as well as careful monitoring for signs of fetal distress. General recommendations for alleviation of pruritus have included sleeping in a cool room and applying topical alcohol. Antihistamines and Phenobarbital (category D) are ineffective in relieving pruritus and should not be used.

Cholestyramine,[22,66,67] administered in maximum doses of 8–12 g/day, has had variable success. Cholestyramine acts by binding bile acids in the intestinal lumen and thus decreasing systemic bile acid concentrations. It can produce relief of pruritus within 1–2 weeks and usually works best in cases with moderately increased bile acid levels. However, it does not improve abnormal liver function tests or fetal outcome. Cholestyramine therapy may aggravate malabsorption of fat-soluble nutrients especially when used in high doses.

Ursodeoxycholic acid (UDCA)[66,67,69,70] has been used successfully to treat cholestatic liver disease and many cases of intrahepatic cholestasis of pregnancy.[67] Its proposed mechanisms of action include modification of the bile acid pool by replacement of more hydrophobic and cytotoxic bile salts within hepatocyte membranes, inhibition of intestinal absorption of more hydrophobic bile acids, and modification of immune-mediated liver injury. UDCA up-regulates the bile acid transporter, MRP2, in the placenta in patients with IHCP. In several small case series and in two small randomized, double-blind, placebo-controlled studies, UDCA was found to be effective in reducing pruritus and improving laboratory parameters without adverse maternal or fetal outcomes. In the controlled study[70] of 24 women with IHCP diagnosed before 33 weeks of gestation, who received 1 g/day orally of UDCA or placebo until delivery, no adverse events were noted in the 15 mothers who completed the study or their infants and there were significant improvements in pruritus, serum bilirubin, and transaminases. In patients who received UDCA, deliveries occurred significantly closer to term compared with those in patients who received placebo. Larger and longer-term studies are needed to draw more definite conclusions with regard to the efficacy of UDCA in IHCP and to delineate the long-term effects on mother and fetus.

S-adenosyl-L-methionine therapy showed promise in early studies for symptomatic and laboratory improvement in IHCP.[67] This drug is thought to inactivate estrogen metabolites, increase membrane fluidity, and alter bile acid metabolism. However, in a subsequent double-blind, placebo-controlled trial, no benefit could be demonstrated.[71] In a small study published in 1998,

Nicastri et al.[72] described a benefit of the combination of S-adenosyl-L-methionine therapy (800 mg/day) and UDCA (600 mg/day, a low dose) over placebo or either drug alone with regard to pruritus and serum bilirubin, but not serum SGPT, alkaline phosphatase or bile acids. No side effects were reported in the mother or infant. Given the small size of the study (eight patients in each treatment arm) further studies are needed before definitive conclusions can be reached.

Dexamethasone[67] has also shown promise as a potential therapy for IHCP. Through suppression of fetoplacental estrogen production, which may contribute to IHCP, dexamethasone therapy may lead to amelioration of symptoms. In one small series,[73] 10 women with IHCP received open-label oral dexamethasone at a dose of 12 mg/day for 7 days with subsequent gradual taper over 3 days. After initiation of treatment, pruritus was relieved, serum estrogen and total bile acid levels decreased, and liver function tests improved. No adverse reactions to the steroids were noted. Enthusiasm for dexamethasone has been tempered by a case report of worsening of a patient's status after initiation of dexamethasone.[74] Further clinical studies are needed before dexamethasone can be widely recommended for IHCP.

Other therapies have been reported to be beneficial. Guar gum[75] in a placebo-controlled, double-blind trial of 48 patients decreased pruritus and prevented a rise in the bile acids seen in the placebo group but did not affect the liver function tests. Epomeidol (a terpenoid compound) and peroral activated charcoal[76] have also been reported to improve pruritus but have not been studied in a rigorous manner.

Acute fatty liver of pregnancy

Acute fatty liver of pregnancy (AFLP)[66,77] is a rare and potentially fatal disease that usually occurs after week 35, but can occur as early as 26 weeks and in the immediate postpartum period. It is more common during the first pregnancy and in those women with multiple gestations and with male fetuses. Symptoms include headache, fatigue, malaise, nausea, vomiting, or abdominal discomfort, either localized to the midepigastrium or right upper quadrant or more diffuse. Jaundice, progressive liver failure with encephalopathy, and renal failure may ensue. There is an association between fatty-acid oxidation defects in the fetus and development of AFLP in the mother.[78]

Management

Early delivery is the mainstay of therapy[77] and has improved maternal and fetal survival dramatically compared with conservative therapy and continuation of the pregnancy. Most women experience rapid improvement after delivery. Successful orthotopic liver transplantations in women with AFLP manifesting fulminant hepatic failure despite delivery and intensive supportive care have been reported.

Preeclamsia/eclampsia

Preeclampsia[66,79] is a systemic disorder of the second half of gestation (and occasionally postpartum) and occurs in 5–10% of all pregnancies. The liver is only one of the many target organs which also include the kidney, hematologic system, central nervous system, and placenta. Preeclampsia is characterized by the triad of hypertension, proteinuria, and edema. In mild preeclampsia blood pressure is ≥140/90 mmHg but <160/110 mmHg. In severe preeclampsia blood pressure is ≥160/110 mmHg. Eclampsia includes signs and symptoms of preeclampsia plus convulsions or coma. In severe disease headaches, visual changes, abdominal pain, congestive heart failure, respiratory distress, or oliguria may occur. A variety of etiologies have been proposed. Recently[80] it has been shown the placental soluble fms-like tyrosine kinase 1 (sFlt1) is increased and is associated with decreased circulating levels of free vascular endothelial growth factor (VEGF) and placental growth factor, which leads to endothelial dysfunction[81] in vitro and the classic triad of preeclampsia when injected in rats. Increased perinatal morbidity and mortality for the mother and fetus correlate with preterm delivery, severity of preeclampsia, multiple gestations, and pre-existing maternal medical conditions such as hypertension.

Management

The primary goal in managing preeclampsia/eclampsia is maternal health. The unequivocal therapy for eclampsia and term preeclampsia is delivery.[79] The management of preeclampsia remote from term is more controversial with regard to hospitalization, antihypertensive therapy, and timing of delivery. Close observation is mandatory for those women who are not delivered. However, those women with mild preeclampsia and preterm gestations can often be managed with careful observation. Treatment is the purview of the obstetrician. Hepatic dysfunction and associated liver function test abnormalities generally improve rapidly after delivery.

HELLP syndrome

HELLP[66,82] occurs in the third trimester in 0.1–0.6% of all pregnancies and in 4–12% of women with severe preeclampsia. It is a multisystem disease involving the liver and may be due to abnormal vascular tone, vasospasm, and/or coagulation. Symptoms are non-specific, including epigastric pain, nausea, vomiting, headache, weight gain, and edema. Hypertension may be absent in 15% of patients. Mortality and fetal outcomes do not correlate with the severity of liver involvement. Maternal mortality of 1.0–3.5% or higher are due to DIC, abruptio placenta, and renal, cardiopulmonary or hepatic failure. Infant perinatal mortality is 10–60%.

Prompt recognition and management are critical to the survival of mother and infant. In cases with early signs of maternal and/or fetal distress, delivery is clearly recommended. For other less clear-cut cases, the optimal time of delivery is somewhat controversial. Liver function tests may return to normal soon after delivery without long-term sequelae as long as the patient's course is relatively uncomplicated.

Hepatic rupture

Hepatic rupture[82,83] is rare with most cases occurring in women with pregnancy-induced hypertension including preeclampsia/eclampsia and HELLP. Survival depends on early recognition and prompt therapy. Most experts agree that a ruptured liver capsule mandates emergent surgery and delivery. Surgical options have included direct pressure; evacuation, packing or hemostatic wrapping; application of topical hemostatic agents; oversewing lacerations; hepatic artery ligation, and partial hepatectomy.

Angiographic embolization has been reported but works best when the rupture is limited to only one lobe. Recent literature suggests that liver hematoma without rupture can be managed without immediate surgery if the patient is clinically stable or postpartum. In the setting of an intact liver capsule, if preeclampsia/eclampsia or acute fatty liver of pregnancy is present, early delivery is indicated given the significant maternal and fetal risks. Recombinant factor VIIa has been used in conjunction with other therapy to achieve hemostasis in spontaneous subcapsular liver hemorrhage.[84]

Chronic liver disease

Cirrhosis: Bleeding from esophageal varices[66,85] is more common in women during pregnancy. However, the treatment of the varices is the same and includes sclerotherapy, band ligation, and if necessary transjugular intrahepatic portosystemic shunt placement or portosystemic shunt surgery. The maternal mortality rate is 20% with bleeding varices. The fetal mortality depends on the health and nutrition of the mother. Stillbirths occur in 13% of fetuses and the neonatal mortality rate is about 4.8%.

Wilson's Disease:[66,86] There are potential serious adverse maternal outcomes including death if the copper chelating agents are stopped during pregnancy. Penicillamine is potentially teratogenic in animals and humans, but is considered safe if used in low doses of 0.25–0.5 g/d. Trientene appeared to be safe and effective in a small number of pregnancies, but more data are needed. Because of the teratogenic potential of penicillamine, zinc is recommended as therapy by some authors. The mother's health appears to be protected by all three therapies.

Autoimmune hepatitis:[87,88] Therapy should be continued during pregnancy. However, disease activity may improve in pregnancy, only to flare postpartum. See above for discussion of immunotherapy and steroid therapy during pregnancy.

Viral hepatitis (see Ch. 33)

Hepatitis A[66] occurs in as many as 1/1000 pregnancies in the USA. The course and management is unaffected by pregnancy. Prevention of hepatitis A with immune globulin is safe for the mother and fetus. For infants of mothers infectious at the time of delivery the dose of immune globulin is 0.02 mL/kg i.m.

Hepatitis B[66] occurs acutely in 2/1000 pregnancies and chronically in 5–15/1000 pregnancies in the USA. The transmission to the infant without immunoprophylaxis depends on the presence of HBeAg in the mother and when she was infected. When the mother is HBsAg positive and HBeAg negative the infection rate in the infant is 40%, whereas the infection rate is 90% when the mother is HBsAg positive and HBeAg positive. Ten percent of neonates become HBsAg positive when the mother is infected in the first trimester, while 80–90% of neonates become HBsAg positive when the mother is infected in the third trimester. Combination active (HBV vaccine) and passive (hepatitis B immune globulin) immunotherapy of the newborn is 85–95% effective in preventing transmission from the infected mother to the neonate (Table 10.3).[89]

Interferon-alpha (2A or 2B)[22,57] (category C), used in the treatment of chronic hepatitis, does not cross the placenta. The few cases of use during pregnancy report no toxicity to the fetus. In rhesus monkeys given 20–500 times the human dose there was

Table 10.3 Type and time of treatment of neonates born to mothers with hepatitis B infection

Treatment	Hepatitis B surface antigen in mothers		
	+	Unknown	−
Hepatitis B immune globulin (0.5 ml i.m.)	≤12 h	≤12 h	Not given
Hepatitis B vaccine – first dose	≤12 h	≤12 h	≤1 wk
Subsequent vaccine doses:			
Recombivax HB 5 μg (0.5 ml)	1 mon	1–2 mon	
Engerix-B 10 μg (0.5 ml)	6 mon	6 mon	6–18 mon

Modified from American College of Obstetricians and Gynecologists. Technical Bulletin No. 174; Hepatitis pregnancy. Int J Gynaecol Obstet 1993; 42:189–198.

an increased risk for abortion, which was not seen in treated women. However, because of the antiproliferative activity of this drug, it should be used cautiously during pregnancy and only if necessary. Lamivudine[22,57,90] readily crosses the placenta. It has been well tolerated in pregnancy and has not been associated with any increase in birth defects. It is not clear if perinatal exposure is associated with mitochondrial dysfunction, but if present would be very rare. Lamivudine therapy in pregnancy may decrease the maternal fetal spread of hepatitis B.[90]

Hepatitis C[66] does not adversely affect the pregnancy and the pregnancy does not adversely affect the course of infection. The overall rate of mother-to-infant transmission is generally in the range of 1–5% with higher rates of vertical transmission reported when the maternal viral titers are high or with human immunodeficiency virus coinfection. No effective prevention is available for infants.

Ribovirin[57] (category X) is contraindicated in pregnant women and in male partners of pregnant women and should be discontinued 6 months before conception. It is reported to be teratogenic in low doses in all animals tested. A few healthy births have been reported.

Hepatitis D[66] should be treated by controlling the spread of hepatitis B.

Hepatitis E[91] is more severe in pregnancy with jaundice being 9 times more common in the gravid woman. Disease in the third trimester is more severe than at other times, with a 20% mortality rate, compared with a 0.5–4% mortality rate in nonpregnant patients. There is a 12% risk of abortion and intrauterine death. Vertical transmission occurs. There is no known therapy.

Herpesvirus infections:[92] Disseminated HSV infection during pregnancy is rare, but has been reported usually in late second or third trimester. Pregnancy represents the second largest group of adult patients with HSV hepatitis. Only 50% have skin lesions around the time of presentation. Fever, nausea, vomiting, abdominal pain, leukopenia, thrombocytopenia, coagulopathy, and markedly elevated serum aminotransferase levels are often present. Both types 1 and 2 have been implicated with the latter occurring 63% of the time. Liver biopsy shows extensive necrosis, often hemorrhagic with typical intranuclear viral inclusion particles. Maternal and fetal mortality is close to 40%. Hepatic necrosis, disseminated intravascular coagulation, hypotension, and death can occur rapidly if antiviral therapy is not initiated promptly. Empiric therapy with acyclovir should be initiated for a suspicion

of this entity, especially in a patient with fulminant hepatic failure.

Budd-Chiari syndrome:[66] Twenty percent of cases are associated with pregnancy and oral contraception use. Postpartum onset is rare and is associated with a poor prognosis. The treatment is the same as in a nonpregnant patient. With the acute onset in pregnancy, the maternal mortality rate is as high as 70%.

GALLSTONES AND GALLBLADDER DISEASE[93]

Gallstones are twice as common in women as in men. The increased frequency in women is explained in part by the high rate of gallstone and sludge formation in pregnancy (see Ch. 25). They are the most common cause of acute pancreatitis in pregnancy. Cholecystectomy is the second most common nonobstetric operation, after appendectomy, performed in pregnancy. Prospective studies have shown that biliary sludge develops in up to 31% of women during pregnancy, and new gallstones develop in 2%.[94] The risk is most pronounced during the second and third trimesters and postpartum. In a substantial percentage of affected women, stones and sludge regress or pass in the ensuing year after delivery.

Pregnant women with gallstones have a high frequency of symptoms compared with nonpregnant women with gallstones.[93,94] Up to one-third of affected women have biliary colic during their pregnancies. Although the symptoms are identical in affected pregnant and nonpregnant women, making the correct diagnosis may be difficult because of the expanded differential diagnosis of abdominal pain. Ultrasound is the major tool for the diagnosis of sludge and gallstones during pregnancy, but is limited in its ability to detect common bile duct stones. Oral cholecystography and computed tomography should be avoided because of possible radiation exposure to the fetus. Nuclear medicine scans also should be avoided, although they are probably safe in late pregnancy if required for diagnosis. ERCP with shielding of the fetus and minimal X-ray exposure can be done safely if needed.

Management

Treatment of pregnant women with biliary disease should be undertaken with the understanding that the major risks to the fetus are not from treatment but rather from poor health and complications in the mother. Women with evidence of biliary obstruction, cholangitis, or pancreatitis should undergo immediate endoscopic retrograde cholangiopancreatography, with appropriate fetal shielding. Acute pancreatitis is a particularly dangerous complication in pregnant women, with rates of fetal loss of 10–20%, and maternal mortality of more than 3% in some studies.[93] In women with severe biliary colic, conservative management with intravenous hydration, narcotics, antibiotics, and dietary restriction is the first line of treatment. Nevertheless, 70% of women treated successfully still suffer relapse; the earlier the presentation, the higher this risk.[93] Cholecystectomy is indicated in women with persistent (longer than 4 days) recurrent symptoms, significant nutritional compromise, or weight loss, but is required in less than 0.1% of pregnancies. Surgery is safest during the second trimester. Many older reports suggested increased fetal loss with surgery in the first trimester, although a more recent study questioned the validity of these reports.[95] In the third trimester, cholecystectomy leads to an increased incidence of preterm labor, although it generally can be treated successfully with tocolytic agents.[95] Intraoperative cholangiography can be undertaken after shielding of the fetus. Laparoscopic cholecystectomy is being performed increasingly, although most experience has been in women in the first and second trimesters; there have been case reports of successful laparoscopic cholecystectomy in the early third trimester.[96]

In symptomatic women who deliver without having had a cholecystectomy and who have small (<5 mm) stones, it may be appropriate to consider a trial of ursodeoxycholic acid. There is no justification for a prophylactic cholecystectomy in an asymptomatic woman planning pregnancy. Silent stones should be followed expectantly, as in the general population.

CONCLUSION

In this chapter we have described the presentation of various gastrointestinal diseases in pregnancy and highlighted some features of the natural history, diagnostic modalities, and treatment options for these disorders in pregnant women. Although it may be difficult, it is important to properly assess the potential risks and benefits of treating these disorders with regard to the health of the mother and fetus. The goals of treatment for gastrointestinal disease in pregnancy include patient comfort and avoidance of potential complications which may impact on a healthy pregnancy outcome.

ACKNOWLEDGMENT

We would like to thank Elena A. Voitkov for her expert assistance in preparing this chapter.

REFERENCES

1. Forstner R, Kalbhen CL, Rilly RA, et al. Abdominopelvic MR imaging in the nonobstetric evaluation of pregnant patients. AJR Am J Roentgenol 1996; 166:1139–1144.

2. Wyte CD. Diagnostic modalities in the pregnant patient. Emerg Med Clin N Am 1994; 12:9–43.

3. Toppenberg KS, Hill DA, Miller DP, et al. Safety of radiographic imaging during pregnancy. Am Fam Phys 1999; 59:1813–1820.

4. Cappell MS, Sidholm OA, Colon VJ, et al. A study at ten medical centers of the safety and efficacy of 48 flexible sigmoidoscopies and 8 colonoscopies during pregnancy with follow-up of fetal outcome and with comparison to control groups. Dig Dis Sci 1996; 41:2353–2361.

5. Cappell MS. The fetal safety and clinical efficacy of gastrointestinal endoscopy during pregnancy. Gastroenterol Clin North Am 2003; 32:123–179.

6. Cappell MS, Colon V, Sidhom OA, et al. A study of eight medical centers of the safety and clinical efficacy of esophagogastroduodenoscopy in 83 pregnant females with follow-up of fetal outcome and with comparison to control groups. Am J Gastroenterol 1996; 91:348–354.

7. Koch KL, Frissora CL. Nausea and vomiting during pregnancy. Gastroenterol Clin North Am 2003; 32:201–234.

8. Lacriox R, Eason E, Melzack R, et al. Nausea and vomiting during pregnancy: a prospective study of its frequency, intensity, and patterns of change. Am J Obstet Gynecology 2000; 182:931–937.

9. Weigel RM, Weigel MM. Nausea and vomiting of early pregnancy and pregnancy outcome. A meta-analytical review. Br J Obstet Gynecol 1989; 96:1312–1318.

10. Shahakian V, Rouse D, Sipes S, et al. Vitamin B6 is effective therapy for nausea and vomiting of pregnancy: a randomized, double-blind, placebo-controlled study. Obstet Gynecol 1991; 78:33–36.

11. Niebyl JR, Goodwin TM. Overview of nausea and vomiting in pregnancy with an emphasis on vitamins and ginger. Am J Obstet Gynecol 2002; 186:S258–5.

12. Atanackrovic G, Navioz Y, Moretti ME, et al. The safety of higher than standard dose of doxylamine-pyridoxine (Diclectin) for nausea and vomiting of pregnancy. J Clin Pharmacol 2001; 41:842–845.

13. McKeigue PM, Lamm SH, Linn S, et al. Bendectin and birth defects: A meta-analysis of the epidemiologic studies. Teratology 1994: 20:27–37.

14. Berkovitch M, Elbirt D, Addis A, et al. Fetal effects of metoclopramide therapy for nausea and vomiting of pregnancy. N Engl J Med 2000; 343:445–446.

15. Goodwin TM. Nausea and vomiting of pregnancy: An obstetric syndrome. Am J Obstet Gynecol 2002; 186:S184–189.

16. Klebanoff MA, Koslowe PA, Kaslow R, et al. Epidemiology of vomiting in early pregnancy. Obstet Gynecol 1985; 66:612–616.

17. Tsang IS, Katz VL, Wells SD, et al. Maternal and fetal outcomes in hyperemesis gravidarum. Int J Gynaecol Obstet 1996; 55:231–235.

18. Knight B, Mudge C, Openshaw, et al. Effect of acupuncture on nausea of pregnancy: a randomized controlled trial. Obstet Gynecol 2001; 97:184–188.

19. Roscoe JA, Matteson SE. Acupressure and acustimulation bands for control of nausea: a brief review. Am J Obstet Gynecol 2002; 286:S244–247.

20. Fischer-Rassmussen W, Kjaer SK, Dahl C, et al. Ginger treatment of hyperemesis gravidarum. Eur J Obstet Gynecol Reprod Biol 1990; 38:19–24.

A double blind randomized controlled trial evaluated use of ginger root in 30 patients with hyperemesis gravidarum and found significant reduction in nausea severity and number of vomiting episodes.

21. Koch KL, Frissora CL. Nausea and vomiting during pregnancy. Gastroenterol Clin North Am 2003; 32:201–234.

22. Briggs GG, Freeman RK, Yaffe SY, et al. Drugs in pregnancy and lactation. 5th edn. Philadelphia: Lippincott Williams & Williams; 1998.

23. Richter JE. Gastroesophageal reflux disease during pregnancy. Gastroenterol Clin North Am 2003; 32:235–261.

24. Marrero JM, Goggin PM, De Caestecker JS, et al. Determinants of pregnancy heartburn. British J Obstet Gynaecol 1992; 99:731–734.

This prospective study of 607 pregnant women assessed the prevalence and natural history of GERD symptoms during pregnancy and examined factors associated with the development of GERD symptoms.

25. Nagler R, Spiro HM. Heartburn in late pregnancy: manometric studies of esophageal motor function. J Clin Invest 1961; 40:954–970.

26. Van Thiel DH, Gavaler JS, Joshi SN, et al. Heartburn of pregnancy. Gastroenterology 1977; 72:668–678.

27. Wald A, Van Thiel DH, Hoechstetter BS, et al. Effects of pregnancy on gastrointestinal transit. Dig Dis Sci 1982; 27:1015–1018.

28. Borum ML. Gastrointestinal diseases in women. Medical Clin North Am 1998; 82:21–50.

29. Cappell MS. Gastric and duodenal ulcers during pregnancy. Gastroenterol Clin North Am 2003; 23:263–308.

30. Kurata JH. Epidemiology: peptic ulcer risk factors. Semin Gastrointest Dis 1993; 4:2–12.

31. Broussard CN, Richter JE. Treating gastro-oesophageal reflux disease during pregnancy and lactation: what are the safest therapy options? Drug Safety 1998; 19:325–327.

32. Land GD, Dougall A. Comparative study of Algicon suspension and magnesium trisilicate mixture in the treatment of reflux dyspepia of pregnancy. Br J Clin Pract 1989; 66(Suppl):48–51.

33. Kallen B. Delivery outcome after the use of acid suppressing drugs in early pregnancy with special reference to omeprazole. Br J Obstet Gynaecol 1998; 105:877–881.

This review examines the available data regarding the safety of proton pump inhibitor therapy during pregnancy.

34. Everson GT. Gastrointestinal motility in pregnancy. In: Reily CA, Abell TL, eds. Gastroenterology clinics of North America. Philadelphia: WB Saunders; 1992.

35. Lawson M, Kern F Jr, Everson GT, et al. Gastrointestinal transit time in human pregnancy: prolongation in the second and third trimesters followed by postpartum normalization. Gastroenterology 1985; 89:996–999.

36. Ryan JP, Bhojwani A. Colonic transit in rats: effect of ovariectomy, sex steroid hormones, and pregnancy. Am J Physiol 1986; 251:G46–50.

37. Levy N, Lemberg E, Sharf M, et al. Bowel habit in pregnancy. Digestion 1971; 4:216–222.

38. Anderson AS. Constipation during pregnancy: incidence and methods used in its treatment in a group of Cambridgeshire women. Health Visitor 1984; 12:363–364.

39. Wald A. Constipation, diarrhea and symptomatic hemorrhoids during pregnancy. Gastroenterol Clin North Am 2003; 32:309–322.

An excellent review of the treatment of common problems in pregnancy.

40. Neri I, Blasi I, Castro P, et al. Polyethylene glycol electrolyte solution (Isocolan) for constipation during pregnancy: an observational open-label study. J Midwifery Womens Health 2004; 49:355–358.

41. Hasler WL. The irritable bowel syndrome during pregnancy. Gastroenterol Clin North Am 2003; 32:385–390.

An excellent review of irritable bowel syndrome during pregnancy.

42. Drossman DA. Irritable bowel syndrome, ADHF Part 2: Diagnosis and treatment. Epidemiology and pathophysiology 2000; Monograph.

43. Kulin NA, Pastuszuk A, Sage SR, et al. Pregnancy outcome following maternal use of the new selective serotonin reuptake inhibitors: A prospective controlled multicenter study. JAMA 1998; 279:609–610.

44. Nulman I, Rovet J, Stewart DE, et al. Neurodevelopment of children exposed in utero to antidepressant drugs. N Engl J Med 1997; 336:258–260.

45. Baird DD, Narendranathan M, Sandler RS, et al. Increased risk of preterm birth for women with inflammatory bowel disease. Gastroenterology 1990; 99:987–994.

46. Baiocco PJ, Korelitz BI. The influence of inflammatory bowel disease and its treatment on pregnancy and fetal outcome. J Clin Gastroenterol 1984; 6:211–216.

47. Willoughby CP, Truelove SC. Ulcerative colitis and pregnancy. Gut 1980; 21:469–474.

48. Miller JP. Inflammatory bowel disease in pregnancy: a review. J Roy Soc Med 1986; 79:221–225.

This large retrospective study determined that women with active ulcerative colitis and Crohn's disease at the time of conception are more likely to have worsened or continued activity during pregnancy.

49. Neilsen OH, Andreasson B, Bondesen S, et al. Pregnancy in ulcerative colitis. Scand J Gastroenterol 1983; 18:735–742.

50. Nielsen OH, Andreasson B, Bondesen S, et al. Pregnancy in Crohn's disease. Scand J Gastroenterol 1984; 19:724–732.

51. Kane S. Inflammatory bowel disease in pregnancy. Gastroenterol Clin North Am 2003; 32:323–340.

52. Habal FM, Hui G, Greenberg GR, et al. Oral 5-aminosalicylic acid for inflammatory bowel disease in pregnancy: safety and clinical course. Gastroenterology 1993; 105:1057–1060.

53. Bell CM, Habal FM. Safety of topical 5-aminosalicylic acid in pregnancy. Am J Gastroenterol 1997; 92:2201–2202.

54. Diav-Citrin O, Park YH, Veerasuntharam G, et al. The safety of mesalamine in human pregnancy: a prospective controlled cohort study. Gastroenterology 1998; 114:23–28.

This prospective study of 165 women found that exposure to mesalamine during pregnancy did not increase the risk of congenital malformations.

55. Janssen NM, Genta MS. The effects of immunosuppressive and anti-inflammatory medications on fertility, pregnancy, and lactation. Arch Intern Med 2000; 160:610–619.

56. Mogadam M, Korelitz BI, Ahmed SW, et al. The course of inflammatory bowel disease during pregnancy and postpartum. Am J Gastroenterol 1981; 75:265–269.

57. Micromedex Healthcare Series. Online. Available: http://www.micromedex.com

58. Present D, Meltzer S, Krumholz M, et al. 6-Mercaptopurine in the management of inflammatory bowel disease: short and long-term toxicity. Ann Intern Med 1989; 11:641–649.

59. Alstead EM, Ritchie JK, Lennard-Jones JE, et al. Safety of azathioprine in pregnancy in inflammatory bowel disease. Gastroenterology 1990; 99:443–446.

60. Connell W, Miller A. Treating inflammatory bowel disease during pregnancy: risks and safety of drug therapy. Drug Safety 1999; 21:311–323.

61. Rajapakse RO, Korelitz BI, Zlantanic J, et al. Outcome of pregnancies when fathers are treated with 6-mercaptopurine for inflammatory bowel disease. Am J Gastroenterol 2000; 95:684–688.

62. Kane SV. What's good for the goose should be good for the gander – 6-MP use in fathers with inflammatory bowel disease. Am J Gastroenterol 2000; 95:581–582.

63. Srinivasan R. Infliximab treatment and pregnancy outcome in active Crohn's disease. Am J Gastroenterol 2001; 96:2274–2275.

64. Rosa FW, Baum C, Shaw M, et al. Pregnancy outcomes after first-trimester vaginitis drug therapy. Obstetric Gynecol 1987; 69:751–755.

65. Korelitz BI. Inflammatory bowel disease and pregnancy. Gastroenterol Clin North Am 1998; 27(1):213–224.

66. Wolf JL. Liver disease in pregnancy. Med Clin North Am 1996; 80:1167–1187.

67. Lammert F, Marschall HU, Glantz A, et al. Intrahepatic cholestasis of pregnancy: molecular pathogenesis, diagnosis and management. J Hepatol 2000; 33:1012–1021.

68. Reyes H, Baez ME, Gonzalez MC, et al. Selenium, zinc, and copper plasma levels in intrahepatic cholestasis of pregnancy, in normal pregnancies and in healthy individuals, in Chile. J Hepatol 2000; 32:542–549.

69. Palma J. Effects of ursodeoxycholic acid in patients with intrahepatic cholestasis of pregnancy. Hepatology 1992; 15:1043–1047.

70. Palma J, Reyes H, Ribalta J, et al. Ursodeoxycholic acid in the treatment of cholestasis of pregnancy: A randomized, double-blind study controlled with placebo. J Hepatology 1997; 27:1022–1028.

An important randomized, placebo-controlled trial in women with cholestasis of pregnancy of ursodeoxycholic acid, the current therapy of choice.

71. Ribalta J. S-adenosyl-L-methionine in the treatment of patients with intrahepatic cholestasis of pregnancy: a randomized double-blind, placebo-controlled study with negative results. Hepatology 1991; 13:1084–1089.

72. Nicastri PL. A randomized placebo-controlled trial of ursodeoxycholic acid and S-adenosylmethionine in the treatment of intrahepatic cholestasis of pregnancy. Br J Obstet Gynaecol 1998; 105:1205–1207.

73. Hirvioja ML, Tuomala R, Vuori J, et al. The treatment of intrahepatic cholestasis of pregnancy by dexamethasone. Br J Obstet Gynaecol 1992; 99:109–111.

74. Kretowicz E, McIntyre HD. Intrahepatic cholestasis of pregnancy, worsening after dexamethasone. Aust NZ J Obstet Gynaecol 1996; 34:211–213.

75. Gylling H. Oral guar gum treatment of intrahepatic cholestasis and pruritus in pregnant women: effects on serum cholesterol and other non-cholesterol sterol. Eur J Clin Invest 1998; 28:359–363.

76. Kaaja RJ. Treatment of cholestasis of pregnancy with peroral activated charcoal. Scand J Gastroenterol 1994; 29:178–181.

77. Reyes H. Acute fatty liver of pregnancy: a cryptic disease threatening mother and child. Clin Liver Dis 1999; 3:69–81.

78. Ibdah JA, Yang Zi, Bennett MJ, et al. Liver disease in pregnancy and fetal fatty acid oxidation defects. Molec Genet Metab 2000; 71:182–189.

An excellent review of the association of long-chain 3-hydroxyacyl-CoA dehydrogenase deficiency with acute fatty liver of pregnancy and HELLP syndrome and a discussion of the potential implications for women who develop these problems.

79. Matter F, Sibai B. Preeclampsia: clinical characteristics and pathogenesis. Clin Liver Dis 1999; 3:15–29.

80. Levine RJ, Maynard SE, Qian C, et al. Circulating angiogenic factors and the risk of preeclampsia. N Eng J Med 2004; 350:672–683.

An important study providing evidence for a cause of preeclampsia which has implications for potentially future treatment or prevention of this condition in women.

81. Maynard SE, Min JY, Merchan J, et al. Excess placental soluble fms-like tyrosine kinase 1 (sFlt1) may contribute to endothelial dysfunction, hypertension, and proteinuria in preeclampsia. J Clin Invest 2003; 111:649–658.

82. Barton JR, Sibai BH. HELLP and the liver disease of preeclampsia. Clin Liver Dis 1999; 3:31–48.

83. Coelho T, Braga J, Sequiera M, et al. Hepatic hematomas in pregnancy. Acta Obstet Gynecol Scand 2000; 79:884–886.

84. Merchant SA, Mathew P, Vanderja TJ, et al. Recombinant factor in management of spontaneous subcapsular liver hematoma associated with pregnancy. Obstet Gynecol 2004; 103:1055–1058.

85. Homburg R, Bayer I, Lurie B, et al. Bleeding esophageal varices in pregnancy: a report of two cases. J Reprod Med 1998; 33:784–786.

86. Brewer GJ, Johnson VD, Dick RD, et al. Treatment of Wilson's disease with zinc XVII: treatment during pregnancy. Hepatology 2000; 31:364–370.

87. Heneghan MA, Norris SM, O'Grady JG, et al. Management and outcome of pregnancy in autoimmune hepatitis. Gut 2001; 48:97–102.

88. Buchel E, Steenbergen WV, Nevens F, et al. Improvement of autoimmune hepatitis during pregnancy followed by flare-up after delivery. Am J Gastroenterol 2002; 97:3160–3165.

89. American College of Obstetricians and Gynecologists. Technical Bulletin No. 174: Hepatitis in pregnancy. Int J Gynaecol Obstet 1993; 42:189–198.

90. Su GG, Pan KH, Zhao NF, et al. Efficacy and safety of lamivudine treatment for chronic hepatitis B in pregnancy. World J Gastroenterol 2004; 10:910–912.

91. Aggarwal R, Krawczynski K. Hepatitis E: an overview and recent advances in clinical and laboratory research. J Gastroenterol Hepatol 2000; 15:9–20.

92. Young EJ, Chafizadeh E, Oliveira VL, et al. Disseminated herpesvirus infection during pregnancy. Clin Infect Dis 1996; 22:51–58.

93. Wells RG, Wolf JL. Gastrointestinal disease in pregnancy. In: Brandt LJ, ed. Clinical practice of gastroenterology. Philadelphia: Current Medicine, Inc; 1999; 1586–1597.

94. Maringhini A, Ciambra M, Baccelliere P, et al. Biliary sludge and gallstones in pregnancy: incidence, risk factors, and natural history. Ann Intern Med 1993; 119:116–120.

95. McKellar DP, Anderson CT, Boynton CJ, et al. Cholecystectomy during pregnancy without fetal loss. Surg Gynecol Obstet. 1992; 174:465–468.

96. Eichenberg BJ, Vanderlinden J, Miguel C, et al. Laparoscopic cholecystectomy in third trimester of pregnancy. Am Surg 1996; 62:874–877.

CHAPTER ELEVEN

Treatment of the elderly patient

David Greenwald

INTRODUCTION

The gradual aging of the population is well documented. Physicians treating gastrointestinal diseases are seeing a greater share of 'disease in the elderly,' and need to be familiar with normal physiologic changes associated with aging as well as the presentations and manifestations of gastrointestinal disease in the elderly.

In the year 1900, the percentage of Americans greater than 65 years was only 4%; by 1998 it had climbed to 15%. Estimates are that by 2050, people 65 years and older will represent 21% of the population.[1] As a group, the elderly represent the fastest growing segment of the population. With ever-improving medical care and socioeconomic conditions, the average life expectancy of a United States citizen is now well into the 70s. By 2050, it has been estimated that there will be 18.9 million Americans over the age of 85, termed by some to be the 'oldest old.' Similar changes are occurring worldwide, although longevity may be most pronounced in the United States. Moreover, the number of patients >100 years of age is increasing; some models suggest that by 2050 there will be 900 000 people alive past the century mark.[1]

The rapid growth of the elderly as a segment of the population will have a major impact on future health care costs. Some estimate that Medicare costs in the United States for the oldest old may increase sixfold by the year 2040.[2] Strategies to control healthcare costs will be related to the ability to prevent and/or cure those age-dependent diseases and disorders that produce the greatest needs for long-term care.[2]

This chapter will focus on unique aspects in the treatment of gastrointestinal disease in the elderly. It includes a general approach followed by specific information concerning pharmacotherapy and endoscopy in the elderly. Disease-specific information in the elderly for some of the more common gastrointestinal disorders follows; the sequelae of long-standing gastrointestinal disorders that may afflict patients once they reach older age also are discussed.

APPROACH TO THE TREATMENT OF THE ELDERLY PATIENT

Gastrointestinal complaints are frequent amongst elderly patients, but most gastrointestinal disorders seen in the aged also occur in younger individuals.[3,4] Considerations of differential diagnosis are affected by the age of the subject. Some disorders are less likely to occur or be a significant possibility in an older patient; cystic fibrosis would be an example. In some situations, aging appears to have no influence on disease. For example, liver chemistries and most other laboratory tests are unaffected by age. Finally, some disorders are more likely to occur in older patients; malignancy and diverticulitis are far more prevalent in an older population.

In addition, common gastrointestinal problems that affect all age groups, including swallowing disorders and constipation, may lead to a greater degree of morbidity in an older patient, who may have more difficulty than a younger counterpart in managing these symptoms. What appears to be the same disorder in the aged and the young may have different etiologies, and so mimicry of disease is an important concept when considering gastrointestinal diseases in the elderly. For example, what appears to be inflammatory bowel disease in a younger patient may actually be ischemic colitis or *E. coli O157:H7* infectious diarrhea in an older subject; symptoms of fundal ulcers in the geriatric population may be confused with the presentation of a myocardial infarction.

The same disease may present differently in a younger patient as compared to an elderly subject. For example, a younger patient with celiac disease may have symptoms of steatorrhea, weight loss, and edema, whereas the presenting complaints in the elderly can be subtle. Initial manifestations of celiac disease in the elderly might include metabolic bone disease, osteopenia, fractures, iron deficiency anemia, or even excessive bleeding with anticoagulation, all due to previously unrecognized and 'subclinical' malabsorption. Finally, some disease states have a worse prognosis when they present initially in the elderly. Amongst these are viral hepatitis and peptic ulcer disease.

Hence, an approach to treating gastrointestinal diseases in the elderly must focus on whether a structural or functional change seen in an elderly subject is merely an anatomic or physiologic curiosity, or whether it represents a pathologic change. Understanding that the elderly will have varied presentations of disease, different courses than their younger counterparts, and in some cases an altered prognosis is critical to successfully managing gastrointestinal disease in the elderly. The presence of comorbid illness, increasingly common with advancing age, can make treatment of any new problem more difficult. Lastly, visual and cognitive impairment, as occurs with failing eyesight and progressive dementia in the elderly, may make comprehension of a new illness more difficult, or may lead to treatment difficulties such as inadvertent errors in medication administration.

ALTERATIONS IN DRUG METABOLISM AND POLYPHARMACY IN THE ELDERLY

The elderly are subject to a variety of expected physiologic changes, as well as pathologic changes associated with various disease states, that may affect the way medications are absorbed, metabolized, and excreted. Absorption of orally administered medications may change with aging, particularly if the presence of atrophic gastritis leads to a rise in gastric pH. Other changes may affect absorption, including delayed gastric emptying, a decrease in intestinal blood flow (30–40% decrease from age 20 to 70), changes in intestinal motility, and possibly a decrease in the number of absorptive cells.[5,6]

Changes in body composition with aging, such as a decrease in lean body muscle mass and an increase in body fat, can alter the way that various medications are distributed. In fact, body fat as a proportion of body weight doubles in males and increases significantly in females as they age. Body fluid composition changes as well, with a marked reduction in total body water and extracellular fluid volume over time. Additionally, cardiac output declines with advancing age, generally decreasing 1% per year after age 30. The result of these changes is that the volume of distribution of water-soluble medications is decreased, while that of fat-soluble medication is increased.

Alterations in the hepatic metabolism of medications are well described and adjustments in dose in the elderly are often required.[7] Hepatic blood flow declines by approximately 1% per year in individuals over the age of 30. Aging is associated with a diminution of renal cell mass as well as a decrease in the number and size of nephrons. Age-related decreases in glomerular filtration rate and renal blood flow are expected, and therefore medications that are primarily excreted through the kidneys (e.g., ranitidine, mesalamine) may not be cleared as avidly in the elderly. Clinically, these changes in medication metabolism vary with different agents, and each agent must be considered independently. Overall, most are metabolized more slowly; their effects may last longer, or a smaller dose may be required to achieve the same therapeutic effect. Some drugs such as propranolol, nitrates, and lidocaine have decreased first-pass metabolism, while others such as benzodiazepines and quinidine have decreased phase 1 metabolism (biotransformation of a substance by hepatic enzyme systems to a more polar metabolite). Benzodiazepines are often employed as sedatives in gastrointestinal endoscopy, and partly as a result of the diminished phase 1 metabolism, smaller doses typically are needed when sedating an elderly subject. Indeed, a benzodiazepine dose necessary to adequately sedate a younger patient may result in respiratory depression and cardiovascular compromise in an older patient. By contrast, the metabolism of other medications, such as oxazepam and lorazepam, appears to be unaltered in an older subject. Finally, some medications, such as salicylates, phenytoin, and indomethacin, are bound less well to albumin in older patients; greater doses may be needed to achieve the desired effect. Increased doses, however, also may be associated with an accompanying increased risk of side effects. For example, higher doses of nonsteroidal antiinflammatory medications are associated with a greater risk of gastric erosions, ulceration and bleeding.[8]

For medications commonly used in gastroenterology, including histamine receptor antagonists, proton pump inhibitors, and anti-inflammatory agents used in the treatment of inflammatory bowel disease, overall patterns of safety and effectiveness are similar when these agents are used in older patients as compared to a younger population. In general, dose modifications are not necessary when these agents are used in older subjects. The elderly, however, may have hepatic dysfunction from comorbid disease and, in such circumstances, dose reductions of certain medications, including most proton pump inhibitors, may be necessary.

Polypharmacy is common in the elderly. Elderly patients use more medications than younger patients and the trend of increasing medication use continues past 80 years of age. Studies conducted in a variety of settings have shown that patients over 65 years of age use an average of 2–6 prescribed medications and 1–3.4 nonprescribed medications on a regular basis.[9] There is ample evidence that the elderly often take medications felt on outside analysis to be inappropriate.[10,11] The most common medications used 'inappropriately' are benzodiazepines and NSAIDs, with the most common problems being drug interactions and improper duration of use.[12]

To complicate matters, polypharmacy leads to the presence in the home of multiple medications, and elderly patients with visual and cognitive impairments may take the wrong medicine or an incorrect dose. In addition, the elderly (along with their younger counterparts) often share medication or experiment with medication on the advice of well-intentioned friends, and adverse outcomes may result.

Pharmacological therapies for relief of common gastrointestinal symptoms, e.g., abdominal pain and diarrhea, must be used cautiously in all patients, but particularly in the elderly. Opioids, for example, are used for the treatment of diarrhea, but may be less effective in the elderly because of relatively higher endogenous opioid levels. In addition, use of opioids in the elderly may predispose them to excessive sedation and put them at increased risk for falls and accidents.[13] Anticholinergics often are chosen as antispasmodic medications, but their use may be accompanied by side effects including urinary retention, mental confusion, cardiac arrhythmias, and exacerbation of closed-angle glaucoma. Their use should be avoided in the elderly.[14]

ENDOSCOPY IN THE ELDERLY

Endoscopy plays an important role in the evaluation of gastrointestinal diseases in the elderly. An adequate history may be difficult to obtain and physical examination difficult to interpret, and so endoscopy may yield critical information in establishing an accurate and timely diagnosis. Moreover, endoscopically delivered therapy is playing an ever-increasing role in treatment of gastrointestinal disorders. Some physicians are reluctant to perform endoscopy on the aged for fear of increased complications, but this fear is unfounded.

In fact, gastrointestinal endoscopy is safe and efficacious in the elderly.[15] By some accounts, nearly 30% of all patients undergoing gastrointestinal endoscopy are greater than 70 years of age. Numerous studies have demonstrated that there is no evidence that either upper or lower endoscopy will result in increased complications when performed on patients who are elderly.[16,17] Endoscopy has been shown to be safe in both inpatient and outpatient settings, and also in both routine and emergency situations. When complications occur, they typically are related to problems with the dose of sedating or analgesic medications; clearly the doses of such medications may need to be carefully monitored and adjusted in the elderly.[16]

Indications for upper and lower endoscopy are the same in the elderly as they are in the young. Both only carry increased risk if coexistent cardiorespiratory disease is present. Therefore, the main factor that determines suitability of an elderly person for gastrointestinal endoscopy is the patient's cardiovascular profile.

The cardiorespiratory risk associated with endoscopy clearly decreases when little or no sedation is used. Although some studies have shown the elderly tolerate colonoscopy more readily when analgesia is provided, many older patients can tolerate upper endoscopy without any sedation, particularly with the use of small-caliber endoscopes sometimes passed via the transnasal route.[18]

The main modification to sedation practices in the elderly is the administration of agents at lower doses and slower rates. Benzodiazepines are the agents most commonly employed; they have a short half-life, amnestic properties, and reversal agents are available. In the elderly, initial doses generally are lower, and additional doses added more slowly after the effect of the previous dose has been assessed. The dose of benzodiazepines, and particularly midazolam, required to achieve adequate sedation has been shown to decrease with advancing age.[19]

In addition to the relatively low risk of endoscopy in the elderly is a high yield. Upper endoscopy may produce a diagnostic yield of as high as 77–89%;[16] management often is affected in such patients when a significant abnormality is detected. Colonoscopy has a similarly high yield, and again, changes in therapy based on the results of the endoscopic procedure often ensue.[20] It is important to note that the yield for any given procedure is affected by the indication for which the procedure is being performed. For example, in the elderly, the yield of colonoscopy when performed for evaluation of anemia is likely to be greater as compared to when the same examination is done to evaluate constipation.

The choice of a colon-cleansing agent prior to colonoscopy is an important one in the elderly patient. The 'perfect' bowel preparation combines efficacy and safety with patient tolerance. Polyethylene glycol-based balanced electrolyte solutions are often favored because they are neutral in terms of fluid shifts, and therefore the patient is not subject to fluid overload or dehydration. These considerations are particularly important in patients with known congestive heart failure or renal disease. While phosphate-based preparations allow a patient to drink a smaller quantity of fluid or use a pill-based method, they must be used cautiously in the elderly who may have unsuspected cardiac or renal dysfunction.

Instrument passage may be more difficult in the elderly because of anatomical changes related to senescence. For upper endoscopy, such changes include the presence of cervical osteophyte spurring and esophageal diverticulosis. For colonoscopy, diminished anal tone and ligamentous laxity may make it easy to 'loop' the instrument, increasing the complexity and discomfort of the procedure.

Arterial oxygen desaturation, typically detected by pulse oximetry, is often seen during upper endoscopy.[21] Such desaturation, possibly due to the obstructing presence of the endoscope in the oropharynx, has been felt to be potentially dangerous because significant desaturation might predispose elderly patients to cardiac arrhythmias.[22]

Although studies have confirmed a somewhat increased rate of sustained oxygen desaturation in the elderly as compared with the young, supplemental oxygen administration appears to prevent any endoscopy-induced desaturation both in younger and older patients.[23] Care must be taken to avoid suppressing the hypoxemic ventilatory drive, particularly in elderly patients with established chronic obstructive pulmonary disease.[24] Finally, cardiac dysrhythmias, typically ventricular and supraventricular ectopic beats, found during endoscopy in the elderly do not appear to be associated with the degree of oxygen desaturation occurring during endoscopy; these mild dysrhythmias generally are not associated with adverse hemodynamic events.[25]

TREATMENT OF OROPHAYNGEAL DISORDERS IN THE ELDERLY

Many age-related changes are expected in the oropharynx with aging. Among these are increased periodontal disease and poor dentition, which can make eating and proper nutrition more difficult.[26] Estimates are that 50% of Americans will be edentulous by age 65; the proportion increases to 85% by age 75. The roots of teeth become fragile and susceptible to fracture with advancing age. Gingival recession also contributes to increased rates of periodontal disease. The enamel density in teeth increases, decreasing the tendency towards dental caries, but the dentin layer thickens, leading to a decrease in pain sensitivity.[27] Attention to dental care and proper fitting dentures is critical for the elderly.

Taste perception may be altered in older patients, with a reported diminution in the discrimination of sweet, sour, and salty foods. Olfactory discrimination decreases notably by age 70. Medications being used to treat disease may additionally impact on taste and olfactory perception in an adverse fashion.

Nutritional deficiencies may lead to glossitis; in the elderly, for example, Vitamin B_{12} deficiency may result in a 'bald tongue' and niacin deficiency can lead to a 'magenta tongue.' Some believe that salivary gland secretion diminishes with aging, leading to xerostomia and difficulty swallowing, while others note a decrease in secretory cells in the parenchyma of the salivary glands, but no diminution of stimulated salivation. In any case, nearly half of all elderly complain of a dry mouth.[28] Factors that appear to contribute to this 'dry mouth' include coexistent diseases, side effects of medications, and relatively poor fluid intake.

With a decrease in lean body mass, or sarcopenia, associated with aging, striated muscle function critical to the oropharyngeal phase of swallowing may become impaired. The main physiologic changes in the region of the upper esophageal sphincter (UES) with aging include a decrease in UES resting pressure, a decrease in UES compliance, and an increase in UES resistance.[29,30] Together, these lead to a delay in the normal swallowing mechanism and prolonged oropharyngeal transit. In fact, in one study, only 16% of elderly volunteers had 'normal' deglutition.[29] Zenker's diverticulum, an outpouching of the posterior oropharynx just proximal to the UES, is a consequence of decreased UES compliance. Cricopharyngeal myotomy in indicated in selected patients with demonstrated 'cricopharyngeal achalasia.'

Transfer dysphagia is a common issue in the elderly, and often occurs as a result of neuromuscular disorders affecting the nerves and musculature of the oropharynx.[31] It may be accompanied by nasal speech, dysarthria, and facial weakness. Common causes of transfer dysphagia include cerebrovascular accidents, Parkinson's disease, myasthenia gravis, and thyroid dysfunction.[32] Aspiration is a common clinical disorder resulting from transfer dysphagia. Treatment of the underlying disorder may improve the condition, although in some situations, adjunctive measures such altering food composition or consistency as well as retraining in swallowing techniques may improve the clinical situation.

TREATMENT OF ESOPHAGEAL DISORDERS AND GERD IN THE ELDERLY

Alterations in the physiology of the esophagus with aging are minimal and may be only of mild clinical importance. The only consistently measured manometric abnormality in the esophagus of the elderly is a diminution in the amplitude of peristaltic waves after a swallow; there is no change in lower esophageal pressure as a result of aging.[33] At the same time, there appears to be an increased frequency of synchronous and nonperistaltic contractions in the esophageal body, with resultant symptoms of chest pain in some patients.[34] The esophageal hiatus has increased elasticity with aging, and coupled with a weakening of the surrounding musculature and support structures, an increased frequency of hernias is noted in the elderly.

Gastroesophageal reflux disease (GERD) is a prevalent condition in the elderly, found in an estimated 20–50% of older individuals.[35] GERD appears to be more common in the elderly than in a younger population.[36] Indeed, the elderly have a myriad of potential precipitating factors for symptomatic GERD, including diminished esophageal peristalsis and concomitant poor clearance of refluxate, and a measurable decrease in salivary bicarbonate secretion. In addition, the elderly often take medications that can affect lower esophageal sphincter pressure, such as calcium channel blockers and theophylline.[36]

Elderly patients with GERD tend to have more severe disease with mucosal abnormalities such as erosive esophagitis, ulcers, and Barrett's esophagus than do their younger counterparts with GERD.[37] Such 'pathologic reflux' occurs more frequently in older individuals; the percentage of time in 24 hours that the pH measured in the esophagus is less than four is three times greater (32.5% versus 12.9%) in older as compared to younger patients.[35] Additionally, the severe sequelae of GERD in the elderly are accompanied by a trend towards less severe symptoms of heartburn, possibly due to a decrease in pain sensitivity in the elderly.[38] Studies have shown that patients over 65 with Barrett's esophagus had less severe symptoms of reflux disease as compared to a group of younger patients.[39,40]

Given the fact that mucosal disease may be more severe but with less frequently reported symptoms, an aggressive investigation and treatment of the GERD in the elderly may be necessary.[41] Acid reduction therapy is central to the management of GERD, and should be used assertively in the management of an older individual with GERD.[42] New-onset heartburn in an older patient is an indication for mucosal evaluation with upper endoscopy. Endoscopic examination also is indicated in any patient with 'alarm' symptoms such as dysphagia, anemia, bleeding, or weight loss.

Medication-induced esophageal injury is another important entity seen in an elderly population. On a background of disordered esophageal motility, possibly diminished salivary flow, and altered local anatomy, the elderly often take numerous pills, many of which are quite large.[43] These pills frequently are taken in the supine position and with inadequate fluids. Pill-induced esophagitis, with resultant dysphagia and possible stricture formation, may occur. Common offending agents are listed in Table 11.1.

TREATMENT OF GASTRIC DISORDERS AND PEPTIC ULCER DISEASE IN THE ELDERLY

One of the 'myths' about the aging process has been that gastric acid production decreases with aging. In fact, as long as good health is preserved, gastric acid production, whether basal or stimulated, will remain normal. In the setting of disease, however, acid production may diminish. A decrease in the production of stomach acid is seen in both type A, or autoimmune, atrophic gastritis and the more common type B atrophic gastritis associated with chronic *H. pylori* infection.[44]

If achlorhydria is present, resultant hypergastrinemia is to be expected. Other possible manifestations of diminished gastric acid production seen in the elderly may include esophageal candidiasis, iron and vitamin B_{12} malabsorption, increased rates of certain infections such as *Salmonella* and *Shigella*, and bacterial overgrowth. With aging, mucosal defenses against gastric tissue injury such as prostaglandin synthesis and secretion of bicarbonate appears to decline.[26]

Aging has been associated with alterations in the emptying and motility of the stomach. In particular, as measured by radioactive tagging, liquid emptying may be shown to be impaired, whereas it is less common to see disorders of solid emptying. Clinically, these changes may present with the development of bezoars as well as decreased bioavailability of some medications. Finally, ligamentous laxity may occur and become clinically evident in an elderly patient. With diminished strength of the supporting structures of the stomach, gastric volvulus may occur, both in the organoaxial (about two-thirds of the time) and mesentero-axial (about one-third of the time) directions. Such disturbances may present with symptoms of abdominal pain, vomiting, and weight loss.

Table 11.1 Common causes of medication-induced esophageal injury

Most common

Tetracycline

Alendronate

Potassium chloride

Quinindine

Emepronium (not available in US)

Also

Aspirin

Ascorbic acid

Clindamycin

Nonsteroidal antiinflammatory drugs (NSAIDs)

Theophylline

Helicobacter pylori infection is more prevalent in an older population, and plays a central role in the development of peptic ulcer disease. The prevalence of *H. pylori* in the United States is 50% at age 60, but only 10% at age 20.[45] The prevalence appears to plateau at about age 60, indicating a cohort effect with most people having acquired the infection early in life. Infection with *H. pylori* leads to type B, or bacterial gastritis and subsequent gastric atrophy. Chronic effects of gastric mucosal atrophy include diminished gastric acid production, intestinal metaplasia and, in some patients, gastric carcinoma. *H. pylori* has been associated with the development of MALT lymphoma as well.[45]

Use of nonsteroidal antiinflammatory medications among the elderly is enormous. Estimates are that 10–15% of older Americans use a prescription nonsteroidal daily, and over-the-counter usage may be up to seven times greater.[46] With advancing age, NSAID use leads to an increased risk of developing gastrointestinal symptoms and complications as compared to a younger population. Use of NSAIDs leads to dyspepsia in 40%, erosive changes in 30%, and ulceration in up to 20%, and increased NSAID use corresponds with an increasing risk of gastrointestinal hemorrhage with advancing age.[47]

Peptic ulcer disease is a very common clinical entity, with estimates of over 500 000 newly diagnosed ulcers each year in the United States, and many recurrences.[48] The elderly have more risk factors for developing ulcers than do the young, including a higher prevalence of *H. pylori*, and increased use of NSAIDs. Moreover, in the elderly, peptic ulcer disease is more serious than in younger patients because the elderly have increased complication rates and higher mortality.[48] Other factors that contribute to the overall poorer prognosis of peptic ulcer disease in the elderly include the presence of other comorbid medical conditions, side effects of medication, and dementia.

Typical features of peptic ulcer disease, including epigastric and abdominal pain, which often occur after eating and may lead to nighttime awakening with relief by antacids, may be absent or variable in the elderly.[49] Atypical or absent symptoms may lead to a delay in diagnosis and treatment, and possibly, a poorer prognosis. For example, in one study, pain was absent in 53% of patients over age 60 with an endoscopically proven ulcer; other data suggest elderly patients are four times as likely as younger patients to have no pain in the presence of endoscopically proven peptic ulcer disease.[50]

Physical examination findings in the elderly with peptic ulcer disease may be less obvious given comorbid disease. The ulcers themselves tend to be large and proximally located; the so-called 'geriatric ulcer' is located high up in the proximal stomach in the gastric cardia. Mimicry is an important issue leading to diagnostic confusion in the elderly; symptoms from a gastric ulcer may be confused with chest pain from cardiac disease.[3,51]

Unfortunately, serious complications of peptic ulcer disease, such as bleeding and perforation, may be the presenting symptoms in the elderly, since the more 'typical' pain may be absent. As many as 65% of people older than 80 years with an upper gastrointestinal bleed related to peptic ulcer disease have no antecedent pain.[52] Indeed, significant complications associated with peptic ulcer disease increase with advancing age; the complication rate of 31% found in those aged 60–64 is contrasted with a complication rate of 76% in those 75–79 years. Mortality from gastrointestinal bleeding and perforation complicating peptic

ulcer disease ranges from approximately 25% to 50%, and is substantially greater than in younger individuals.[53]

TREATMENT OF COLORECTAL DISORDERS IN THE ELDERLY

Colorectal disorders in the elderly are frequent, and may be divided into those related to vascular degeneration, including vascular ectasias and colon ischemia, diverticula formation, including diverticulitis and hemorrhage, and motility changes. Inflammatory bowel disease in the elderly may manifest somewhat differently than in younger subjects.

Vascular ectasias, which are found in the right colon and cecum, occur due to age-related degeneration of previously normal colonic blood vessels. Most people found to have ectasias are over the age of 50, and two-thirds are over the age of 70; ectasias are equally prevalent in men and women.[54] Ectasias are likely caused by repeated episodes of partial low-grade obstruction of submucosal veins, leading to dilation and tortuosity of the submucosal venules and the arteriolar-capillary units that supply them, ultimately resulting in a communication between artery and vein.[54,55]

Ectasias may present as acute and significant hemorrhage or as iron-deficiency anemia and occult blood in the stool; different presentations may occur in the same patient over time. When massive bleeding occurs from colonic ectasias, it generally stops spontaneously.[56] Diagnosis typically is established by colonoscopy or angiography. A characteristic early finding on angiography is a 'late-emptying vein,' since low-grade obstruction of intramural veins leads to difficulty in emptying; later changes that can be demonstrated include a vascular tuft and an early filling vein.[57] It is unusual to see contrast material extravasate into the lumen of the bowel because acute bleeding from ectasias is most commonly episodic.

Treatment of ectasias is limited to those patients in whom detected lesions are causing clinical signs of bleeding (anemia, occult blood in the stool, overt hemorrhage, etc.). Ectasias found incidentally during colonoscopy done for another indication should not be treated. When therapy is indicated, thermal modalities including contact coagulation and argon plasma coagulator therapy is typically employed.[58] Diverticular disease is more common with advancing age, but despite the significant prevalence of diverticular disease in the elderly, at least 80–85% of such patients are asymptomatic. Of those who come to clinical attention, most have painful diverticular disease; only a minority has diverticulitis or diverticular hemorrhage.[59]

The diagnosis of diverticular disease in the elderly usually is made by colonoscopy, whereas diverticulitis often is detected by radiographic testing with CT scan in the appropriate clinical setting. Suspected diverticular hemorrhage may be approached by a combination of colonoscopy, angiography, and bleeding scan.

Diverticular hemorrhage usually is brisk, since the source of the bleeding is arterial, but similar to vascular ectasias, most bleeding stops spontaneously. Although most diverticula are in the left colon, most angiographically proven episodes of diverticular bleeding emanates from lesions in the right colon.[60]

Management of diverticular disease in the elderly has long included fiber therapy, but data supporting the efficacy of this intervention are scarce. Treatment for diverticulitis varies with the severity of the clinical illness. In the elderly, uncomplicated diverticulitis is usually managed with antibiotics and oral hydration alone; more complicated disease may dictate intravenous hydration and possible surgery. Many elderly will require hospitalization for complicated diverticular disease, particularly if such patients have significant comorbid disease. While most elderly patients with complicated diverticular disease will respond to 'conservative' therapy, 15–30% of such aged patients ultimately will require surgery.

Diverticular hemorrhage may be managed in a variety of ways, including endoscopic, angiographic, and surgical. While there are few data directly comparing these approaches, the majority of older patients can be managed without surgery. In a study examining diverticular hemorrhage in the elderly, older patients with significant bleeding, defined as requiring an average of 2.8 units of blood, were successfully treated without surgery. Only 18% required surgical resection; the 30-day mortality was 9%.[61]

Ischemic bowel disease is caused by acute or chronic insufficiency of blood flow to all or part of the gastrointestinal tract, and includes acute and chronic mesenteric ischemia and colonic ischemia. Colonic ischemia is the most common manifestation of ischemic injury to the gastrointestinal tract, and the majority of patients with colon ischemia are older than age 60. Acute mesenteric ischemia typically is seen in older patients with other comorbid conditions seen in elderly patients, including congestive heart failure, myocardial infarction, and hypotension.[62]

Diagnosis of colonic ischemia includes typical symptoms of sudden onset of crampy left lower quadrant pain, often followed by bloody diarrhea. Blood loss is usually minimal; hemodynamically significant bleeding should prompt an investigation for another cause. While any part of the colon may be affected, the splenic flexure, descending colon, and sigmoid are the most common sites of injury.[62]

Thumbprinting is the major radiological finding in colonic ischemia; the changes seen on abdominal X-ray are caused by submucosal and mucosal hemorrhage and edema. Colonoscopy may be performed in patients with suspected colonic ischemia, but care should be taken not to overdistend the colon because increasing intraluminal pressure beyond 30 mmHg diminishes intestinal blood flow, especially to the mucosa. At pressures greater than 30 mmHg, which can occur routinely with air insufflation during colonoscopy, there is shunting of blood from the mucosa to the serosa, with a resultant reduction in the arteriovenous oxygen difference; these changes increase the risk of further ischemic damage. Colonoscopy is preferable to

barium studies because it permits mucosal inspection and allows for biopsies.

Therapy for colonic ischemia in the elderly is generally supportive; most cases resolve spontaneously. Management typically includes stabilization of the patient, optimization of cardiac function, and bowel rest. Antibiotics are often administered; systemic glucocorticoids have not been shown to be of benefit. Only 5% of patients experience recurrent episodes. In rare instances, the acute episode may have other outcomes such as severe ischemia leading to infarction and gangrene, and surgery is required.[63]

Acute mesenteric ischemia is much less common, and may be caused by a superior mesenteric artery embolus or thrombus, by nonocclusive mesenteric ischemia, or by mesenteric venous thrombosis. Elderly patients with acute mesenteric ischemia typically complain of severe pain, which can be either localized or diffuse; in fact, it is the combination of severe abdominal pain and a relative lack of substantial physical findings that is the important diagnostic clue in this disorder.[62] Diagnosis is established by angiography, and testing must be initiated promptly if mortality is to be avoided. Waiting for development of peritonitis or for radiologic signs such as thumbprinting or ileus to occur may have catastrophic consequences, as these findings indicate bowel that is no longer viable.

In the elderly, differentiating between colonic ischemia and acute mesenteric ischemia is critical. Features that distinguish these two entities are shown in Table 11.2.

Management of acute mesenteric ischemia involves an aggressive combination of angiography to define the lesion followed by intra-arterial infusion of papaverine to disrupt splanchnic vasoconstriction.[64] Early diagnosis of acute mesenteric ischemia, combined with an aggressive approach to treatment, has improved outcome in the elderly, with survival improved from 20% to 55%.

The inflammatory bowel diseases, including ulcerative colitis and Crohn's disease, once felt to be disorders of the young, are now being noted with increased frequency in the elderly. Up to 32% of new diagnoses of ulcerative colitis are made in elderly patients.[65,66] The presenting symptoms of ulcerative colitis in older persons are similar to those in a younger group, except that diarrhea and weight loss are more common, and abdominal pain and rectal bleeding are less frequent.[67] In general, the elderly with new-onset ulcerative colitis have predominantly distal disease, and it is usually less extensive than in younger patients. Proctitis

Table 11.2 Distinguishing acute mesenteric ischemia and colonic ischemia

Acute mesenteric ischemia	Colonic ischemia
Most patients >50 years old	Most patients >60 years old
Acute precipitating cause is typical	Acute precipitating cause is unusual (myocardial infarction, congestive heart failure, hypotension, arrhythmias)
Predisposing lesion unusual	Some patients have predisposing lesion such as colon cancer, stricture
Patients appear seriously ill	Patients appear mildly ill or well
Severe pain	Mild pain
Rectal bleeding and diarrhea rare	Bloody diarrhea typical

alone is more common in older patients with inflammatory bowel disease.[68] Making an accurate diagnosis of ulcerative colitis in the elderly may be more difficult because other conditions such as infectious colitis, diverticulitis, and ischemia may have similar presentations. A list of conditions that mimic ulcerative colitis in the elderly is given in Table 11.3.

In the elderly, the initial episode of ulcerative colitis is more often protracted, and is more likely to prompt hospitalization with a longer length of stay. While medical therapy is generally as effective as in younger patients, the initial episode in the elderly is more likely to require surgery. Still, the prognosis for elderly patients with ulcerative colitis generally is favorable; outcomes are similar in younger and older populations.[69]

Crohn's disease in the elderly presents in a similar fashion as it does in younger populations, with diarrhea and abdominal pain being typical. About one-quarter of patients with newly diagnosed Crohn's disease are elderly; when Crohn's disease presents later in life, a female preponderance of almost 2:1 has been noted.[70]

Atypical manifestations of Crohn's disease such as weight loss (24%), rectal bleeding, fever (10%) and constipation may be found in Crohn's disease in the elderly.[71] As in ulcerative colitis, the distribution of the disease tends towards the more distal when it is found in the elderly; Crohn's disease limited to the colon

Table 11.3 Conditions that may mimic IBD in the elderly

Infection
Clostridium difficile
Salmonella
Shigella
Campylobacter
E. coli O157:H7
Entamoeba histolytica
Balantidum coli
Schistosomiasis
Ischemic colitis
Diverticulitis
Neoplasia
Medication induced colitis
Antibiotics
Allopurinol
Estrogens
Gold
Laxatives
NSAIDs
Microscopic colitis
Systemic disease
Vasculitis
Amyloidosis
Radiation colitis
Diversion colitis

occurs more commonly in the elderly. The correct diagnosis is often delayed; common misdiagnoses include irritable bowel syndrome, infectious colitis, diverticulitis, and neoplasia. In one study, the time between symptom onset and correct diagnosis was 6.4 years in the elderly and 2.4 years in younger people.[71]

The response to medical therapy in older patients with Crohn's disease is much as it is in younger patients; greater than 80% of elderly patients with Crohn's disease can be managed with medical therapy. Once remission has been achieved, relapses occur less often in the elderly. As in the treatment of ulcerative colitis, surgery is needed more frequently during the initial presentation of Crohn's disease in an older patient and may be done earlier during that individual episode than in a younger patient. While younger patients with Crohn's disease often have substantial disease-related mortality due to their inflammatory bowel disease, death in elderly patients with Crohn's disease is most commonly not related to their Crohn's disease. Elderly patients with Crohn's disease have mortality rates that are similar to those of age- and sex-matched controls without Crohn's disease.

The elderly with inflammatory bowel disease have special issues with medical therapy. As in all drug treatment in the elderly, altered drug metabolism, frequent adverse drug reactions, and polypharmacy make the use of all medications more difficult. In particular, corticosteroid use should be minimized, to avoid complications including hypokalemia, hypotension, mental status changes, diabetes, glaucoma, infection, and myopathy.[72] Aminosalicylates and immunosuppressives may be associated with fewer side effects than corticosteroids, and are generally well tolerated by the elderly.[14,73] Topical therapies for distal disease, such as enemas, foams, and suppositories, may represent the ideal treatment in a given clinical situation, but elderly patients may have difficulty administering or retaining enemas because of arthralgias, decreased flexibility, diminished rectal capacity, and decreased anal sphincter pressure.

CONSEQUENCES OF LONG-STANDING GASTROINTESTINAL DISORDERS IN THE ELDERLY

Some common gastrointestinal disorders, when found in the elderly, may have different outcomes. For example, intestinal infections such as viral enteritis can lead to profound dehydration and electrolyte imbalances, ultimately causing more significant morbidity in the elderly than in younger individuals. Some infections are more serious when they occur in older individuals; *E. coli* O157:H7 has increased morbidity and mortality when it develops in those at the extreme ages of life, including the older ages.

Some common gastrointestinal disorders have important long-term sequelae that may manifest themselves in an older population. An individual may have Barrett's esophagus for many years; in the elderly it may manifest as esophageal adenocarcinoma. Patients who have a gastrectomy early in life are more likely to develop Vitamin B_{12} and iron deficiency, along with their manifestations, later in life; gastric carcinoma is more common in patients who have had partial gastrectomies in the distant past. Long-standing celiac disease may be complicated later in life by the development of a myriad of malignancies, including esophageal and gastric adenocarcinomas and intestinal lymphoma. Finally, those with long-standing inflammatory bowel disease are at increased risk with advancing age for the development of colonic carcinoma.

SUMMARY: AUTHOR'S RECOMMENDATIONS

- Most gastrointestinal disorders seen in the aged also occur in younger individuals; considerations of differential diagnosis are affected by the age of the subject.
- Mimicry of disease is an important concept when considering gastrointestinal diseases in the elderly.
- Polypharmacy is common in the elderly; alterations in drug metabolism and medication interactions need to be considered when prescribing medications in the elderly.
- Endoscopy is safe and efficacious when performed in the elderly. Endoscopic procedures should not be withheld for fear of increased complications.
- GERD in the elderly may present with more severe mucosal disease, including esophagitis and Barrett's esophagus, and less severe symptoms than in the young.
- Peptic ulcer disease in the elderly is common. The presentation may be subtle and atypical, which may lead to a delay in the appropriate diagnosis, in turn causing increased morbidity and a worse prognosis.
- Vascular ectasias are often seen in the elderly and may manifest as an acute or chronic source of bleeding. Asymptomatic lesions detected at colonoscopy should not be treated.
- Differentiation between colon ischemia and acute mesenteric ischemia is critical since diagnostic testing and therapeutic considerations are different.
- The elderly with inflammatory bowel disease tend to have more distal disease and a more protracted initial episode, but outcomes are similar to younger patients.

REFERENCES

1. Hazzard WR. Demographic peristalsis. Implications of the age wave for gastroenterologists. Gastroenterol Clin North Am 2001; 30:297–311.

2. Schneider EL, Guralnik JM. The aging of America. Impact on health care costs. JAMA 1990; 263(17):2335–2340.

3. Brandt LJ. Gastrointestinal disorders of the elderly. In: Brandt LJ, ed. Gastrointestinal disorders of the elderly. New York: Raven Press; 1984:620.

4. Holt PR. General perspectives on the aged gut. Clin Geriatr Med. 1991; May;7(2):185–189.

5. Guay DR, Artz MB, Hanlon JT, et al. The pharmacology of aging. In: Tallis RC, Fillit HM, eds. Brocklehurst's textbook of geriatric medicine and gerontology, 6th edn. Philadelphia: Churchill Livingstone; 2003:155–161.

   An outstanding review of the age-related changes in medication absorption, distribution, metabolism and excretion.

6. Iber FL, Murphy PA, Connor ES. Age-related changes in the gastrointestinal system. Effects on drug therapy. Drugs Aging 1994; 5(1):34–48.

7. Woodhouse K, Wynne HA. Age-related changes in hepatic function. Drugs Aging 1992; 2:243–255.

8. Hanlon JT, Shimp LA, Semla TP. Recent advances in geriatrics: drug-related problems in the elderly Ann Pharmacother 2000; 34(3):360–365.

9. Stewart RB, Cooper JW. Polypharmacy in the aged. Practical solutions. Drugs Aging 1994; 4(6):449–461.

10. Chutka DS, Takahashi PY, Hoel RW. Inappropriate medications for elderly patients. Mayo Clin Proc 2004; 79(1):122–139.

11. Curtis LH, Ostbye T, Sendersky V, et al. Inappropriate prescribing for elderly Americans in a large outpatient population. Arch Intern Med 2004; 164(15):1621–1625.

    This study outlines the relatively high degree of medication use among the elderly in the outpatient setting that can be deemed inappropriate.

12. Hanlon JT, Schmader KE, Boult C, et al. Use of inappropriate prescription drugs by older people. J Am Geriatr Soc 2002; 50(1):26–34.

13. Holt PR. Gastrointestinal disease in the elderly. Curr Opin Clin Nutr Metab Care 2003; 1:41–8.

14. Akerkar GA, Peppercorn MA. Inflammatory bowel disease in the elderly: practical treatment guidelines. Drugs Aging 1997; 10: 199–208.

15. Greenwald DA, Brandt LJ. Endoscopy in the elderly patient. In: Zenilman ME, ed. Problems in general surgery: gastrointestinal surgery in the elderly. Hagerstown, MD: Lippincott-Raven: 1996: 13;32–43.

    Comprehensive review of issues related to safety, yield, hypoxemia, and diagnostic and therapeutic applications of endoscopy in the elderly patient. This chapter includes a section on IBD.

16. Cooper BT, Neumann CS. Upper gastrointestinal endoscopy in patients aged 80 years or more. Age Aging 1986; 15:343–349.

17. Cobden I. Colonoscopy in the elderly patient. Geriatr Med Today 1988; 7:30.

18. Chatrenet P, Friocourt P, Ramain JP, et al. Colonoscopy in the elderly: a study of 200 cases. Eur J Med. 1993; 2(7):411–413.

19. Scholer SG, Schafer DF, Potter JF. The effect of age on the relative potency of midazolam and diazepam for sedation in upper gastrointestinal endoscopy. J Clin Gastroenterol. 1990; 12(2): 145–147.

20. Ure T, Dehghan K, Vernava AM 3rd, et al. Colonoscopy in the elderly. Low risk, high yield. Surg Endosc 1995; 9(5):505–508.

21. Lieberman DA, Wuerker CK, Katon RM. Cardiopulmonary risk of esophagogastroduodenoscopy. Role of endoscope diameter and systemic sedation. Gastroenterology 1985; 88(2):468–472.

22. Lavies NG, Creasy T, Harris K, et al. Arterial oxygen saturation during upper gastrointestinal endoscopy: influence of sedation and operator experience. Am J Gastroenterol 1988; 83(6):618–622.

23. Kinoshita Y, Nishiyama K, Kitajima N, et al. Age-related effects of gastroduodenoscopy on arterial oxygen saturation. Jpn J Geriatr 1992; 29:185–189.

24. Freeman ML, Hennessy JT, Cass OW, et al. Carbon dioxide retention and oxygen desaturation during gastrointestinal endoscopy. Gastroenterology 1993; 105(2):331–339.

25. Solomon SA, Isaac T, Banerjee AK. Oxygen desaturation during endoscopy in the elderly. J R Coll Phys Lond 1993; 27:16–18.

26. Jensen GL, McGee M, Binkley J. Nutrition in the elderly. Gastroenterol Clin North Am 2001; 30:313–334.

27. Shay K, Ship JA. The importance of oral health in the older patient. J Am Geriatr Soc 1995; 43(12):1414–1422.

28. Lovat LB. Age-related changes in gut physiology and nutritional status. Gut 1996; 38(3):306–309.

29. Kern M, Bardan E, Arndorfer R, et al. Comparison of upper esophageal sphincter opening in healthy asymptomatic young and elderly volunteers. Ann Otol Rhinol Laryngol 1999; 108(10):982–989.

30. Shaker R, Ren J, Bardan E, et al. Pharyngoglottal closure reflex: characterization in healthy young, elderly and dysphagic patients with predeglutitive aspiration. Gerontology 2003; 49(1):12–20.

31. Mendez L, Friedman LS, Castell DO. Swallowing disorders in the elderly. Clin Geriatr Med 1991; 7(2):215–230.

32. Ramsey DJ, Smithard DG, Kalra L. Early assessments of dysphagia and aspiration risk in acute stroke patients. Stroke 2003; 34(5): 1252–1257.

33. Schindler JS, Kelly JH. Swallowing disorders in the elderly. Laryngoscope 2002; 112(4):589–602.

34. Achem AC, Achem SR, Stark ME, et al. Failure of esophageal peristalsis in older patients: Association with esophageal acid exposure. Am J Gastroenterol 2003; 98:35–59.

This study finds that reflux in older patients is complicated by disordered esophageal motility, and this in turn may lead to decreased acid clearance, rendering elderly patients more susceptible to GERD complications.

35. Zhu H, Pace F, Sangaletti O, et al. Features of symptomatic gastroesophageal reflux in elderly patients. Scand J Gastroenterol 1993; 28:235–238.

36. Collen MJ, Abdulian JD, Chen YK. Gastroesophageal reflux disease in the elderly: More severe disease that requires aggressive therapy. Am J Gastroenterol 1995; 90:1053–1057.

37. Linder JD, Wilcox CM. Acid peptic disease in the elderly. Gastroenterol Clin North Am 2001; 30:363–376.

38. Lasch H, Castell DO, Castell JA. Evidence for diminished visceral pain with aging: Studies using graded intraesophageal balloon distension. Am J Physiol 1997; 272:G1–G3.

39. Triadafilopoulos G, Sharma R. Features of symptomatic gastroesophageal reflux disease in elderly patients. Am J Gastroenterol 1997; 92(11):2007–2011.

40. Johnson DA, Fennerty MB. Heartburn severity underestimates erosive esophagitis severity in elderly patients with gastroesophageal reflux disease. Gastroenterology 2004; 126(3):660–664.

41. Katz PO. Gastroesophageal reflux disease. J Am Geriatr Soc 1998; 46(12):1558–1565.

This article reviews the presentation, pathophysiology, diagnosis, and treatment of GERD as it relates to the older patient.

42. Freston JW, Triadafilopoulos G. Review article: approaches to the long-term management of adults with GERD-proton pump inhibitor therapy, laparoscopic fundoplication or endoscopic therapy? Aliment Pharmacol Ther 2004; (Suppl 1):35–42.

43. Kikendall JW. Pill esophagitis. J Clin Gastroenterol 1999; 28(4): 298–305.

44. Krasinski SD, Russell RM, Samloff IM, et al. Fundic atrophic gastritis in an elderly population. Effect on hemoglobin and several serum nutritional indicators. J Am Geriatr Soc 1986; 34(11):800–806.

45. Shiotani A, Nurgalieva ZZ, Yamaoka Y, et al. *Helicobacter pylori.* Med Clin North Am 2000; 84(5):1125–1136.

46. Laine L. Approaches to nonsteroidal anti-inflammatory drug use in the high-risk patient. Gastroenterology 2001; 120(3): 594–606.

47. Llewellyn JG, Pritchard MH. Influence of age and disease state in nonsteroidal anti-inflammatory drug associated gastric bleeding. J Rheumatol 1988; 15:691–694.

48. McCarthy DM. Acid peptic disease in the elderly. Clin Geriatr Med 1991; 7:231–254.

49. Hilton D, Iman N, Burke GJ, et al. Absence of abdominal pain in older persons with endoscopic ulcers: a prospective study. Am J Gastroenterol 2001; 96(2):380–384.

50. Clinch D, Banerjee AK, Ostick G. Absence of abdominal pain in elderly patients with peptic ulcer. Age Ageing 1984; 13(2):120–123.

51. Holt PR. Gastrointestinal diseases in the elderly. Curr Opin Clin Nutr Metab Care 2003; 6(1):41–48.

52. Wilcox CM, Clark WS. Features associated with painless peptic ulcer bleeding. Am J Gastroenterol 1997; 92:1289–1292.

53. Booker JA, Johnston M, Booker CI, et al. Prognostic factors for continued or rebleeding and death from gastrointestinal haemorrhage in the elderly. Age Ageing 1987; 16(4):208–214.

54. Boley SJ, Sammartano R, Adams A, et al. On the nature and etiology of vascular ectasias of the colon. Degenerative lesions of aging. Gastroenterology 1977; 72(4 Pt 1):650–660.

Important article describing the mechanism underlying the development of vascular ectasias of the colon.

55. Reinus JF, Brandt LJ. Vascular ectasias and diverticulosis. Common causes of lower intestinal bleeding. Gastroenterol Clin North Am 1994; 23(1):1–20.

56. Farrell JJ, Friedman LS. Gastrointestinal bleeding in the elderly. Gastroenterol Clin North Am 2001; 30:377–407.

57. Boley SJ, Sprayregen S, Sammartano RJ, et al. The pathophysiologic basis for the angiographic signs of vascular ectasias of the colon. Radiology 1977; 125(3):615–621.

58. Bounds BC, Friedman LS. Lower gastrointestinal bleeding. Gastroenterol Clin North Am 2003; 32(4):1107–1125.

59. Farrell RJ, Farrell JJ, Morrin MM. Diverticular disease in the elderly. Gastroenterol Clin North Am 2001; 30(2):475–496.

60. West AB, Losada M. The pathology of diverticulosis coli. J Clin Gastroenterol 2004; 38(5 Suppl):S11–S16.

61. Bokhari M, Vernava AM, Ure T, et al. Diverticular hemorrhage in the elderly – is it well tolerated? Dis Colon Rectum 1996; 39(2): 191–195.

62. Greenwald DA, Brandt LJ, Reinus JF. Ischemic bowel disease in the elderly. Gastroenterol Clin North Am 2001; 30(2):445–473

63. Medina C, Vilaseca J, Videla S, et al. Outcome of patients with ischemic colitis: review of fifty-three cases. Dis Colon Rectum 2004; 47(2):180–184.

64. Brandt LJ, Boley SJ. AGA technical review on intestinal ischemia. American Gastrointestinal Association. Gastroenterology 2000; 118(5):954–968.

This review features several excellent algorithms for the management of the various forms of intestinal ischemia.

65. Tokayer AZ, Brandt LJ. Idiopathic inflammatory bowel diseases of the elderly. In: Kirsner JB, ed. Inflammatory bowel diseases. 5th edn. Philadelphia: Saunders; 2000:335–341.

66. Robertson DJ, Grimm IS. Inflammatory bowel disease in the elderly. Gastroenterol Clin North Am 2001; 30:409–426.

67. Zimmerman J, Gavish D, Rachmilewitz D. Early and late onset ulcerative colitis: distinct clinical features. J Clin Gastroenterol 1985; 7:492–498.

68. Softly A, Myren J, Clamp SE, et al. Inflammatory bowel disease in the elderly patient. Scand J Gastroenterol Suppl 1988; 144:27–30.

69. Lindner AE. Inflammatory bowel disease in the elderly. Clin Geriatr Med 1999; 3:487–497.

70. Polito JM 2nd, Childs B, Mellits ED, et al. Crohn's disease: influence of age at diagnosis on site and clinical type of disease. Gastroenterology 1996; 111(3):580–586.

Data are presented that highlights possibly different phenotypes between those who manifest Crohn's disease at a younger as compared to an older age.

71. Walker MA, Pennington CR, Pringle R. Crohn's disease in the elderly. Br Med J 1985; 291:1725–1726.

72. Akerkar GA, Peppercorn MA, Hamel MB, et al. Corticosteroid-associated complications in elderly Crohn's disease patients. Am J Gastroenterol 1997; 92:461–464.

73. Pardi DS, Loftus EV, Camilleri M. Treatment of inflammatory bowel disease in the elderly: an update. Drugs Aging 2002; 19:355–363.

CHAPTER TWELVE

12

Children

Carlo Di Lorenzo, Cheryl Blank and Miguel Saps

INTRODUCTION

Children have been considered *therapeutic orphans*, a term which describes individuals not routinely included in drug trials. As a consequence, only a small fraction of drugs used in children have pediatric clinical trial data. Package information accompanying sale of drugs routinely include a disclaimer that safety and effectiveness of the medication has not been established in children. It has been reported that during a randomly chosen 5-week period in a Dutch hospital, children admitted to the pediatric ward or the intensive care unit received unlicensed or off-label drugs in 90% of patient-days.[1] In another neonatal intensive care unit in Israel, 93% neonates received at least one off-label medication during their hospital stay.[2] Neonates and toddlers have immature organ systems, considerable patient-to-patient variability in ability to metabolize drugs, and an increased likelihood of clinically important variations in pharmacokinetic and pharmacodynamic responses.[3] In response to these concerns, the United States Food and Drug Administration has recently introduced legislature that offers an incentive to manufacturers of drugs to be used in pediatrics by increasing the duration of the marketing exclusivity.[4] This chapter deals with the treatment of some of the most common conditions encountered in pediatric gastroenterology. We elected to discuss conditions which either have treatments that differ substantially from the adults, such as gastroesophageal reflux and constipation, or conditions that seem to be more prevalent in children, such as cyclic vomiting and eosinophilic esophagitis. We have specifically chosen to highlight the differences in clinical presentation and treatment between children and adults. When available, information obtained from pediatric studies is emphasized. Most of the drug doses are reported on a per kilogram (kg) basis.

GASTROESOPHAGEAL REFLUX

It has been reported that up to 100% of infants, 2% of children (age 3 to 9 years), and 15% of adolescents (age 10–17 years) experience signs and symptoms of reflux on a regular basis.[5,6] The prevalence of gastroesophageal reflux disease (GERD) in children with neurological injuries or development delay is even higher, ranging between 25% and 75%.[5] It has been reported that US$750 million was spent on children hospitalized with GERD in the year 2000.[6]

Signs and symptoms of GERD vary according to different age groups in children. Infants commonly manifest GERD with regurgitation, vomiting, poor weight gain, back arching, and irritability. Older children are more likely to complain of epigastric abdominal pain or substernal chest pain, heartburn, regurgitation, or dysphagia, similar to symptoms seen in adults. Other signs and symptoms that have been associated with GERD in children include reactive airway disease, apnea and bradycardia, chronic cough, and failure to thrive. Observational data show that adults with reflux often recall having similar symptoms in childhood.[7] Adults with GERD are also more likely to have taken antireflux mediations as children and their symptoms as adults were more severe if they had exhibited symptoms of GERD by 11 years of age.

Treatment

Treatment for GERD includes lifestyle modification, pharmacological therapy, and surgical options (see Ch. 13).

Lifestyle modifications differ by age groups, while pharmacological and surgical options are similar. Because symptoms related to GERD in infants usually resolve within 1 year of life, it is reasonable in this age group to begin with conservative management. It has been suggested that a trial of a hypoallergenic formula should be given to infants with suspected GERD because it may be arduous to differentiate GERD from cow or soy protein intolerance.[8] Thickening the formula with rice or oatmeal cereal at a ratio of one tablespoon of cereal to one ounce of formula has been shown to decrease the number of vomiting episodes but does not alter reflux index scores or the amount of reflux as measured by nuclear scintigraphy.[9] Two randomized, controlled trials have been conducted evaluating the effect of infant positioning on GERD. One study evaluated children placed in an infant seat at an angle of 60 degrees[10] and found that infants in the seat had significantly more episodes of reflux when compared to those in the prone position, suggesting that the seat exacerbated reflux. Another study evaluated reflux in infants in the prone position or the prone position plus elevation of the head of the bed at a 30° angle.[11] It was found that there was no difference between the two positions in regards to different parameters of GERD. Prone position for sleeping is beneficial for infants with GERD because prone positioning not only decreases reflux, but also accelerates gastric emptying and decreases the incidence of aspiration.[8,12,13] In 1992, the American Academy of Pediatrics began its 'Back to Sleep' campaign which promotes putting infants to sleep in the supine position to prevent sudden infant death syndrome (SIDS). Because of the wide success of this program in preventing SIDS, prone positioning for sleeping is *no longer* recommended except in cases of very severe infantile GERD. Lifestyle changes in older children are similar to the recommendations in adults although limited data exist in the pediatric population. Weight loss in overweight children, avoidance of foods such as chocolate, spicy foods, and caffeine which are known to cause symptoms of GERD and alcohol avoidance are recommended.[8] Avoiding tobacco smoke exposure in both infants and child not only decreases the risk for reflux, but also decreases the risk for apnea, SIDS, asthma and pneumonia.

Pharmacological treatment

Acid suppressants and prokinetic agents are the mainstay of pharmacotherapy in the treatment of GERD. Antacids (magnesium hydroxide, aluminum hydroxide) are readily available and are known to buffer acid in the stomach, resulting in decreased esophageal exposure to acid.[8] Although there is evidence that high doses of antacid medications are as effective as cimetidine in the treatment of esophagitis in children,[12] such medications are not widely used because significant absorption of aluminum in infants may lead to microcytic anemia, osteopenia, and neurotoxicity.[12]

Histamine-2 (H_2) receptor antagonists (Table 12.1) are the most commonly prescribed medications for the treatment of GERD in infants and children.[14] A recent multicenter, randomized, single-dose, double-blind, placebo-controlled, parallel-design trial evaluated the effects of a single dose (75 mg) of ranitidine. It was found that the pharmacokinetic and pharmacodynamic properties of ranitidine in children and adults were similar. There was an increase in gastric pH within 30 minutes of receiving ranitidine and the effect lasted for up to 5 hours. This study suggested that ranitidine can be given every 6–9 hours to effectively treat childhood GERD. A multicenter, randomized, double-blind, placebo-controlled

withdrawal trial investigating the use of famotidine in infants less than 12 months of age[14] found that both 0.5 mg/kg and 1 mg/kg of famotidine given every 12 hours were effective at reducing symptoms of GERD such as regurgitation frequency and volume as well as crying. The efficacy of cimetidine for treatment of children with GERD has also been well studied. One study measured gastric acid suppression of different doses of cimetidine (5, 7.5, 10, and 15 mg/kg).[15] This study showed that the duration of response was maintained for a significantly longer period of time in the groups receiving both 10 and 15 mg/kg. Nizatidine was studied in infants, children, and adults who were given intravenous, liquid, or capsule formulations of the drug. It was concluded that the biodisposition of nizatidine in children and adults is similar; however, response after a comparable weight-based dose is equal and potentially greater in children.[16]

Proton pump inhibitors (PPIs) are quickly becoming the drug of choice to treat children with GERD although few controlled studies are available in the pediatric literature. PPIs are available in oral and intravenous preparations. Traditionally, these drugs were prepared as capsules containing enteric-coated granules, which were challenging for young children to swallow. Placing the granules in an acid medium such as apple sauce and fruit juices allows the granules to stay intact in the stomach.[17] The granules can also be made into a liquid form by dissolving the granules in 8.4% sodium bicarbonate solution which can be given via a gastrostomy tube.[17] Lansoprazole is now available in an oral suspension form as well as a rapidly dissolving tablet. Both of these preparations are extremely palatable and easy to administer to children. Efforts are under way to package other PPIs in more children-friendly formulations.

Studies of omeprazole and lansoprazole have shown these drugs to be more efficacious in improving esophagitis when compared with histamine-2 receptor antagonists.[5,8] There have also been multiple case reports of children with GERD refractory to H_2-receptor antagonists who improved with PPIs.[8] The International Pediatric Omeprazole study set out to determine the efficacy of this drug and its ideal dose to treat children ages 1–16 years old with erosive esophagitis.[18] The researchers determined the 'healing dose' of omeprazole by demonstrating an esophageal pH less than 4 for less than 6% of a 24-hour intraesophageal pH study. Doses ranged from 0.7 mg/kg to 3.5 mg/kg with a maximum of 80 mg. After 3 months of treatment, this study reported that in 95% of the patients erosive esophagitis had healed. A recent study used oral pantoprazole in children with GERD at a dose of 0.5–1 mg/kg/day[18,19] and found that after 28 days 80% of the patients had complete resolution of at least one of the clinical symptoms and 47% had an improved endoscopy. The widespread awareness of the superior effectiveness of PPIs over H_2-receptor antagonists has led to an increase in use of PPIs in children between the ages of 12 and 17 years old.[5] The FDA has recognized the safety and effectiveness of lansoprazole in pediatric patients ages 1–11 years of age and omeprazole in children 2–16 years of age.

There are several prokinetic agents that have been used to improve motility and decrease symptoms of GERD. Multiple studies with cisapride have been conducted in infants and children with GERD. These studies have shown decreased esophageal acid exposure and improvement in symptoms of GERD.[8,20] Cisapride is no longer available in the United States except on a limited-access basis secondary to its adverse cardiac effects. Metoclopramide has been shown to decrease the frequency of GERD episodes and decrease the volume of refluxate in some studies[20] although other reports

Table 12.1

Type of medication	Recommended dose
Histamine-2 receptor antagonists	
Cimetidine	40 mg/kg/day divided t.i.d. (max 150 mg b.i.d.)
Ranitidine	5–10 mg/kg/day divided t.i.d. (max 300 mg b.i.d.)
Famotidine	1 mg/kg/day divided b.i.d. (max 20 mg b.i.d.)
Proton pump inhibitors	
Omeprazole	1 mg/kg/day q.d. or b.i.d. (max 20 mg b.i.d.)
Lansoprazole	15 mg q.d. (body weight ≤30 kg) or 30 mg q.d. (>30 kg)
Pantoprazole	No pediatric recommendations (adult dose 40 mg q.d.)
Prokinetics	
Cisapride	0.8 mg/kg/day divided q.i.d. (max 20 mg q.d.) *
Metoclopramide	0.1–0.8 mg/kg/day divided q.i.d. (max 15 mg b.i.d.)
Erythromycin	9 mg/kg/day divided t.i.d.

* No longer approved by FDA.

have not confirmed its efficacy.[8] Side effects of metoclopramide including drowsiness, restlessness, fatigue, dystonic reactions, extrapyramidal movement disorders, and tardive dyskinesia limit its use in children. Erythromycin accelerates gastric emptying in individuals with gastroparesis but does not seem to have a beneficial effect on the esophagus and has a limited role in the treatment of pediatric GERD. Baclofen, a GABA type B receptor agonist, has been shown to decrease the frequency of transient relaxation of the lower esophageal sphincter (LES). One study on neurologically impaired children found a decreased frequency of emesis and a reduction of reflux episodes after 1 week of oral or nasogastric tube baclofen treatment at dose of 0.7 mg/kg/day given in three divided doses.[21] Further studies need to be done before recommending the routine use of this medication to treat pediatric GERD.

Surgery

Even with adequate acid suppression, infants and children may continue to have symptoms of nonacid reflux such as aspiration, asthma exacerbation, pneumonia, and failure to thrive. Such children often require a surgical antireflux procedure. There are many descriptive studies and case series regarding surgical fundoplications in children. Relief of symptoms has been reported as occurring in 57–92% of patients. Complications of the surgery include gagging, retching, breakdown of the wrap, small bowel obstruction, gas bloat syndrome, infection, and esophageal obstruction if the wrap is 'too tight.'[22] A comparison between long-term medical management and a fundoplication has not been done in children.

CYCLIC VOMITING SYNDROME

Cyclic vomiting syndrome (CVS) is characterized by recurrent, stereotypical, and explosive bouts of severe nausea and vomiting lasting for hours or days alternating with intervals of normal health between episodes. Due to the recurrent nature and severity of the events, this condition results in an average of 20 school absences per year imposing an important economic and social burden to the family and the child.[23]

Clinical presentation

CVS is characterized by four distinctive phases: prodrome, episode, recovery, and symptom-free interval. The *prodrome* phase signals that an episode of nausea and vomiting is imminent. This phase may last from minutes to several hours or not be present and the patient may just wake up vomiting without any warning (Li BUK, Kagalwalla A. Unpublished data. 2002). The symptoms are non-specific, including nausea, pallor, anorexia, and lethargy. Frequently the patients can identify a condition or event that triggers an episode. The *episode* phase is self-limited and stereotypical within individuals, lasting the same length of time and having a similar clinical presentation and severity. These episodes are frequently associated with headache, photophobia, abdominal pain, anorexia, drowsiness, fever, pallor, lethargy, and excessive salivation.[24] Patients may become thirsty but the ingestion of water usually leads to more vomiting. The episodes usually last anywhere from 1 to 4 days (mean duration of 20 hours),[25] though they can last for up to 10 days. The *recovery* phase begins when the nausea and vomiting stop and the patient is able to tolerate liquids and food. This phase is characterized by a quick return of appetite, energy, and healthy appearance. A *symptom-free* interval phase lasting weeks to months in which the patient remains completely or almost totally asymptomatic follows this phase.

The etiology of CVS is unknown. A number of factors may play a role in the pathogenesis of cyclic vomiting syndrome, including mitochondrial DNA mutations, ion channelopathies, autonomic dysfunction, and excessive hypothalamic-pituitary-adrenal axis activation. Some clinical features of CVS overlap with those of migraines and abdominal migraines, suggesting a common pathogenesis.

Diagnosis

The diagnosis is clinical and based on the presence of typical symptoms and the exclusion of other disorders causing nausea and vomiting. There are no laboratory diagnostic markers to identify this condition. The lack of awareness of, and the existence of, more common conditions presenting with vomiting contribute to a significant delay at diagnosis in children and adults (2, 7, and 8 years, respectively).[26] Pediatric studies have shown that an upper gastrointestinal series with small-bowel follow-through (UGI-SBFT) to exclude any underlying conditions and initiation of an empiric 2 months' trial of prophylactic antimigraine therapy is the most cost-effective approach in children with recurrent episodic vomiting.[27]

Treatment

There is no known cure for CVS. Due to the unknown pathophysiology and lack of controlled trials, diverse therapeutic approaches are often utilized based on personal experience, open-label trials, and case reports. Management should be aimed at preventing or aborting episodes before they occur, ameliorating or interrupting symptoms if they are already present, and preventing future episodes. The choice between daily prophylactic medication and early administration of drugs to abort the episode depends on the intensity and frequency of the episodes. If prodromic symptoms occur, antiemetics, benzodiazepines, prokinetic agents, or cyclooxigenase inhibitors may abort the episode. If these medications fail, the prodromal phase evolves into the vomiting phase. Once a vomiting episode begins, treatment is supportive. Severe nausea and vomiting may require hospitalization and use of intravenous fluids to prevent dehydration. Oral feedings should be discontinued to minimize vomiting, although some patients prefer to consume large volumes of liquids during the episode. The patient should be assessed for metabolic disturbances such as acidosis, hypoglycemia, or electrolyte abnormalities. When present, these abnormalities require prompt correction with higher than maintenance infusion rates and hyperglycemic solutions. During the episode, medications should be given parenterally as the patient will not be able to tolerate oral medications. Commonly used agents include lorazepam, ondansetron, granisetron, ketorolac, diphenhydramine, promethazine, and chlorpromazine often used in combination with anxiolytics such as lorazepam.[28,29]

Avoidance of triggers

Occasionally, the avoidance of certain precipitating factors in combination with prophylactic medications may prevent the appearance of episodes. When stress or excitement is known to trigger episodes, relaxation techniques and anxiolytics may avert the onset of vomiting. Patients are recommended to avoid stressful situations, and have long periods of rest and sleep. Dietary products such as chocolate and cheese, sinusitis, and allergies have also been associated with CVS episodes.

Prophylactic medication

Subjects with frequent or long-lasting episodes need to be treated during the symptom-free intervals in an effort to prevent or ease future episodes. Because of the similarities between migraines and CVS, medications used to treat migraines are commonly used for CVS. They include beta-blockers (propranolol) and tricyclic antidepressants (amitriptyline, nortriptyline), 5-HT$_2$ antagonists (cyproheptadine), GABA inhibitors (phenobarbital), antiepileptic drugs (valproic acid, carbamazepine), and motilin agonists (erythromycin). These agents were amenable to ameliorate symptoms in about 70% of cases in one experience.[28] Another pediatric retrospective study[30] showed 93% and 83% response, respectively, using amitriptyline or cyproheptadine. Regardless of the drug to be used, each treatment should be given time to prove its effectiveness, and a 1–2 months trial may be necessary. Propranolol (10–20 mg p.o. b.i.d. – t.i.d.) is a nonselective beta-blocker with a half-life of 4–6 hours. Initially used as an antimigraine medication, propranolol has also proved to be effective for the prevention of recurrent vomiting.[31] No absolute correlation has been demonstrated between the dose and its clinical efficacy in migraine studies.[30] Beta-blockers can cause drowsiness, lethargy, fatigue, depression, nightmares, hallucinations and memory disturbances, decrease exercise tolerance, and have been associated with orthostatic hypotension and bradycardia. They are contraindicated in patients with asthma, congestive heart failure, and insulin-dependent diabetes. Other medications of the same class such as atenolol have occasionally been used in patients with CVS. Amitriptyline (1–2 mg/kg p.o., q.h.s.) is a tertiary tricyclic antidepressant which increases synaptic noradrenaline and serotonin. The mechanism responsible for its prophylactic effect is uncertain. Similarly to its use in the therapy of headaches and other forms of chronic pain, in CVS amitriptyline is used in lower doses than used for depression. Its anticholinergic properties are responsible for most side effects including sedation, dry mouth, constipation, urinary retention, dizziness, tachycardia, palpitations, and blurred vision. Most worrisome is that this drug can rarely result in life-threatening arrhythmias. The American Heart Association recommends obtaining an EKG before its use. Cyproheptadine (0.3 mg/kg/day divided t.i.d.) is an antihistaminic with antiserotonin and calcium channel-blocking activity that has been frequently used in the prevention of vomiting. Side effects are mostly limited to sedation secondary to its antimuscarinic effects and increased appetite.[30] Erythromycin (3–5 mg/kg/dose repeated q 6–12 hours) is a macrolide with prokinetic effects through its motilin agonist properties. Side effects include diarrhea, abdominal pain, and nausea.[32]

Anticonvulsant medications have been proved to be effective in the prevention of migraines in double-blind, placebo-controlled studies. Much like many other medications used for migraine prophylaxis they are empirically used to prevent the recurrence of vomiting episodes. Valproic acid (500–1000 mg slow-release tablets at nighttime) increases GABA levels by inhibiting its degradation and it enhances the postsynaptic response to GABA. The drug also interacts with the central 5-HT system reducing the firing rate of serotoninergic neurons.[33] The mechanism of action in the prevention of cyclic vomiting is unknown. The use of valproate can occasionally result in idiosyncratic and unpredictable hepatitis and pancreatitis, but self-limited nausea, vomiting, and gastrointestinal distress are the most common side effects. It causes little effect on cognitive functions and rarely causes sedation.

Phenobarbital (2–3 mg/kg/day q.d.), is a barbiturate with antiepileptic and antimigraine action. This drug has also been used in the prevention of vomiting although side effects and the availability of newer drugs have decreased its use. Phenobarbital should not be used in combination with valproic acid due to the potential interaction resulting in severe sedation and coma. L-carnitine is another agent that has been proposed to decrease the frequency of episodes. A pediatric study has shown an increase in the interval between episodes from 1.7 months to 1.1 years using oral L-carnitine (50 mg/kg/day) in six patients in which an evaluation for metabolic disorders did not document any abnormality.[34] The authors suggest that carnitine may bind to a noxious compound as a carnitine ester.

Suggested approach

It is our preference to use prophylactic medications when episodes occur at least 3 times per year or are severe in nature. Although there are no specific guidelines, there is a general consensus among specialists to use drugs with a lower risk of side effects in younger patients. Thus, we usually recommend using cyproheptadine or propranolol in patients younger than 6 years of age while we reserve amitriptyline for older children and more severe cases. Our approach is to titrate the dose over several weeks depending on the evolution of symptoms.

Abortive medication

Sometimes, during the prodrome phase, it is possible to prevent the occurrence of the episode. Exclusive abortive therapy has been recommended in case of infrequent episodes or in patients that break through the prophylactic therapy.[28] Multiple parenteral drugs can be used for this purpose.

Ondansetron (i.v. 0.3–0.4 mg/kg q.i.d.) is a selective 5-HT$_3$-receptor antagonist. Serotonin plays an important role in nausea and vomiting. Serotonin may activate the vomiting center by the stimulation of vagal afferent neurons or by direct activation of the chemoreceptor trigger zone. The use of 5-HT$_3$ antagonists in conjunction with lorazepam increases its efficacy. Ondansetron seems to have a low potential for clinically significant drug interactions. All the 5-HT$_3$ inhibitors have the potential to induce QT prolongation. Sumatriptan, a widely used antimigraine medication, was the first selective 5-HT$_{1B/1D}$ receptor agonist to be developed. The nasal form 20 mg (in patients >40 kg) is the most widely used in pediatric patients with cyclic vomiting. The oral formulation has poor palatability and is not suitable to be used in a patient with vomiting. Sumatriptan delays gastric emptying by activation of 5-HT$_{1P}$ receptors causing relaxation of the fundus through a nitrergic pathway. Sumatriptan has a 46% efficacy rate in aborting vomiting episodes in pediatric patients[28] when used in its intranasal or subcutaneous form. Sumatriptan has the potential for drug interactions with MAO inhibitors. There are no pharmacokinetic studies in children. In adult studies the most frequently reported adverse events were somnolence, nausea, dizziness, fatigue, chest burning, and paresthesias. The utilization of its nasal form reduces greatly the sensation of burning in chest and neck frequently manifested with the subcutaneous form. The use of parenteral ketorolac (0.5–1 mg/kg every 6–8 hours) has also been proposed by some authors as an effective agent in limiting severity and aborting an event of CVS.[35]

Suggested approach

Ondansetron should be considered as soon as the child begins to experience the prodromes of the syndrome, before the onset of vomiting. Patients with a history of repeated and severe events could benefit from early intranasal administration of sumatriptan at the onset of symptoms.

Supportive therapy

Supportive care includes a quiet and dark environment, intravenous fluids, sedatives, antiemetics, antinausea medication, antacids, and analgesics.

Lorazepam (i.v. 0.05–0.1 mg/kg q.i.d.) is a benzodiazepine of rapid onset of action used to abort seizures and severe vomiting episodes not responding to intravenous 5-HT$_3$ antagonist. This drug is particularly useful for its multiple effects as an anxiolytic, sedative, and antiemetic medication. It has been used in an open-label trial[36] at high doses (0.3–0.4 mg/kg/dose) resulting in symptom improvement. In addition, medications to decrease the stomach's acidity (H$_2$-receptor antagonists, proton pump inhibitors) should be initiated promptly during the vomiting episode in order to limit the erosive effect, prevent enamel damage, and reduce pain.

Suggested approach

Early administration of intravenous fluids is critical in the treatment of severe episodes. Lorazepam should be given as soon as the patient begins to vomit.

EOSINOPHILIC ESOPHAGITIS

Eosinophilic esophagitis (EE) is a disorder characterized by isolated eosinophilic infiltration of the esophagus (see Ch. 53).[37] Signs and symptoms of EE are often mistaken as those seen in GERD. They include vomiting, dysphagia, food refusal, heartburn, chest pain, and abdominal pain.[37–39] Unlike GERD, in EE these symptoms do not improve in response to adequate acid suppression.[37,39] Solid foods impactions and esophageal strictures can also be presenting symptoms of EE.[40,41] EE is a male-predominant disorder[37,38,42,43] and occurs in all ages. Increased immunoglobulin (Ig) E levels and peripheral eosinophilia have been reported in up to 60% of patients.[37] Frequently, there is a history of atopy in the patient or family members such as seasonal allergies, asthma, and eczema, as well as food allergies.[37,40,42] The frequent association of EE with atopy suggests that EE is associated with an allergen, either food or inhaled, although the evidence for this is incomplete.[44]

Diagnosis

A definitive diagnosis of EE is made when esophageal biopsies demonstrate greater than 20 eosinophils per high-power field.[37,38] The classic appearance of EE on upper endoscopy includes linear furrowing of the esophagus, esophageal ring formation (trachealization), and granularity.[37,38]

Therapy

The treatment of EE has been based on diet modification and corticosteroids. Elemental diets have been shown to improve clinical symptoms and significantly reduce the number of mucosal eosinophils.[37,45,46] Once children are allowed an unrestricted diet, the majority of the symptoms reoccur.[45] It can be assumed that a strict elemental diet removes the offensive agent that is causing the EE, allowing the esophagus to heal. If a specific food allergy is detected, that food should be removed from the diet. Despite its efficacy, the use of elemental formulas is often not practical. Such formulas are often poorly tolerated in terms of palatability, making long-term compliance a challenge.

Both systemic and topical corticosteroids have been used to treat EE. Corticosteroids inhibit circulating eosinophils and decrease the number of activated inflammatory cells, therefore allowing the esophagus to heal.[39] They have been demonstrated to induce both clinical and histological remission but symptoms often redevelop once steroid therapy is tapered or removed.[43] Oral methylprednisolone (1.5 mg/kg/day divided b.i.d.) was given to 20 children with clinical symptoms and biopsy proven EE for 4 weeks.[47] The average time for improvement of clinical symptoms was 8 days. All of the participants had significant improvement of clinical symptoms, histology, peripheral eosinophils, as well as quantitative IgE at the end of 4 weeks of treatment. A swallowed metered dose of fluticasone (2–4 years old, 44 µg/puff; 5–10 years old, 110 µg/puff; 11 years and older, 220 µg/puff), a trifluorinated steroid preparation, was given to a total of 13 patients with EE for a total of 8 weeks.[39] Two puffs of fluticasone were swallowed twice a day. Patients were instructed not to inhale the medication and a spacing device was not used. All patients experienced clinical improvement and had a decreased number of esophageal eosinophils on repeat endoscopy. Swallowed fluticasone is easily administered and well tolerated by children. Systemic side effects are limited because the medication is rapidly metabolized in the liver by the first-pass effect.[39] Oral and esophageal *Candida* infections have been reported as side effects but have been easily treated.[38,39] Currently there are no specific guidelines to direct duration of treatment of EE with corticosteroids. There are also no recommendations in regards to food and environmental allergen testing.

In an uncontrolled trial, clinical improvement was noted in 8 patients with EE after treatment with montelukast, a leukotriene receptor antagonist that inhibits the cysteinyl leukotriene CysLT$_1$ receptor.[48] Further studies are warranted regarding the use of this medication for EE.

FUNCTIONAL ABDOMINAL PAIN

Chronic abdominal pain is one of the most common pediatric gastrointestinal conditions, accounting for[49] 2–4% all of pediatric office visits (see Ch. 69).[50] Most children with functional abdominal pain (FAP) have symptoms that fulfill the criteria for irritable bowel syndrome (IBS) in adults.[51] Symptoms consistent with IBS occur in 14% of all high school students and 6% of all middle school students.[52] Female patients with a history of FAP may be at increased risk of IBS during adolescence and young adulthood.[53]

Therapy

There is no uniformly successful treatment for FAP. The main goal of the therapy is to reestablish a normal daily life. The physician should educate the patient and the family about the benign nature of the condition by emphasizing the reassuring aspects of the history, physical examination, and laboratory tests. Comparisons with other common entities such as headaches or muscle cramps may help to conceptualize the nature of the condition. The family should be discouraged from reinforcing the symptoms by allowing the child to miss school. Perceived triggering factors and possible psychosocial stressors at home or school should be addressed. The lack of objective diagnostic criteria, unclear pathogenesis,[54] and almost no scientific evidence for any therapeutic intervention pose a challenge to the practitioner who has to make recommendations based on anecdotal experience.

Tricyclic antidepressants

Adult studies have shown a beneficial effect of tricyclic antidepressants (TCA) in the treatment of chronic abdominal pain, but no study has evaluated the efficacy of these drugs in children with FAP. Thus, the type of TCA and the doses used derive from anecdotal reports, personal experiences, and inferences from adult studies. Tricyclic antidepressants in children are generally used at a dose of 0.2–0.4 mg/kg/day (5–50 mg/day), lower than the doses needed to treat clinical depression. The beneficial effect of the TCA starts 3–7 days after the beginning of the treatment,[55] and relief of pain has been documented in the absence of any antidepressant response.[56] When planning to use antidepressants it is fundamental to allocate enough time to discuss in depth with the family why the medication is being proposed in order to address possible misconceptions and warn about side effects. The family should be informed that antidepressants are used to treat various chronic painful conditions in patients without depression. Due to their antimuscarinic and antihistaminic effects this group of drugs is especially effective in patients with diarrhea and difficulty sleeping. Possible side effects and toxicity should be discussed with the family. The American Heart Association recommends obtaining an EKG prior to the use of antidepressants in order to minimize the risk of cardiac arrhythmia.

Selective serotonin re-uptake inhibitors

Much like in the case of TCAs there are no pediatric studies that appropriately demonstrate the efficacy of this group of medications for FAP. The effects of TCA and selective serotonin re-uptake inhibitors (SSRIs) in the GI tract are different, with the TCA slowing intestinal transit and SSRI increasing motility in the small intestine.[57,58] Thus, a patient in whom the main symptom is constipation may benefit from SSRIs, whereas a patient with diarrhea may benefit from an antidepressant with anticholinergic properties. There have been conflicting reports relating to the risk of suicidal episodes among patients receiving SSRIs for treatment of depression. Some authors support the concept of an increased risk of suicidal episodes in depressed adolescents using SSRIs, others attribute the increasing incidence to an inadequate methodological approach.[59–62] While the controversy on the benefit ratio of the use of SSRIs is yet to be solved, it is important to clarify that the controversy seems to be limited to this group of drugs and so far has not involved patients receiving TCAs.

Serotonin modulators

A number of selective 5-HT$_3$-receptor antagonists have been developed. Treatment with alosetron has led to significant relief of abdominal pain and discomfort in adult women with diarrhea-predominant IBS, but this medication has not been approved by the FDA for use in children. Currently, the only available 5-HT$_4$-receptor agonist is tegaserod. Cisapride, a less selective 5-HT$_4$-receptor

agonist is no longer commercially available in the US due to its potentially serious adverse events. Tegaserod stimulates the peristaltic reflex, increases intestinal and colonic transit, increases gas evacuation and may reduce visceral sensitivity. Its most common side effect is diarrhea. Adverse events, particularly loose stools, are compatible with an exaggerated pharmacological response to tegaserod and are most common during the first 2 days of therapy.[63]

Laxatives

Patients with IBS or FAP and constipation may find relief by combining fiber with a laxative. It is our preference to use polyethylene glycol solution without electrolytes (PEG 3350 at 0.5–0.8 g/kg/day), but other laxatives may be used according to the practitioner's preference.

Anticholinergic and antidiarrheal medications

Antispasmodics are widely used in pediatrics in the treatment of abdominal pain. Although anecdotal experience seems to indicate that some patients find relief by using antispasmodics, there is little evidence suggesting efficacy of this group of medications in the treatment of FAP in children or adults. Hyoscyamine and dicyclomine are the most commonly prescribed drugs in this class in the United States, acting by decreasing tone and motility of the gut through antimuscarinic properties. The recommended dose for dicyclomine is 10–40 mg by mouth q.i.d. in adult patients, although is often used at lower doses. In children, the recommended dose for hyoscyamine is 0.125–0.25 mg by mouth or sublingual q.i.d. High doses may exhibit atropine-like side effects such as visual disturbances, urinary retention, constipation, and dry mouth. These agents are best used on a sporadic basis, whenever the symptoms are present, much like analgesics are used for headaches.

Peppermint oil

Peppermint oil (mentha piperita), an over-the-counter preparation, is one of the few products that have proved to be effective in double-blind, placebo-controlled studies in the relief of chronic abdominal pain and IBS.[64,65] This drug is a spasmolytic agent that relaxes gastrointestinal smooth muscle relieving pain.

Antidiarrheal preparations

Some patients with diarrhea seem to benefit from antidiarrheal preparations that inhibit the peristalsis and prolong the transit time (loperamide 0.08–0.24 mg/kg/day maximum 2 mg per dose divided once or twice a day). Diphenoxylate/atropine preparation (0.1–0.4 mg/kg/day p.o. divided 4 times daily) is not approved for use in children less than 2 years of age.

CONSTIPATION

Childhood constipation is a prototypical example of a condition in which a team effort is required to achieve success (see Ch. 71). Physician, nurses, teachers, family, and the patient should work together in order to obtain best results.[66] Education of the family and the patient, including a comprehensive but simple explanation of the pathogenesis of constipation, is a major component of the therapy. As parents may have misconceptions on the nature and consequences of constipation, demystification constitutes the initial step of the intervention. Parents should be instructed in what is considered a normal stool pattern at different ages and reassured that there is no serious disease underlying the symptom. In addition, parents should be able to recognize the clinical features of stool withholding and differentiate them from an attempt to defecate.

Overflow fecal soiling (the involuntary passage in the underwear of stools leaking around a rectal fecal mass) constitutes a particular problem as parents may interpret it as a purposeful and defiant act. A comprehensive explanation is usually effective to reverse the connotations associated with soiling. Parents should be encouraged to maintain a positive and supportive attitude and should be informed that the therapy is a long process in which setbacks should be expected but long-term results are almost always satisfactory. Parents should always be advised not to interrupt the therapy in case of improvement or apparent success as that may result in a recurrence of the problem. A thorough discussion of possible side effects and the availability of the medical staff for changes in doses or medication are essential to the success of the therapy. However, a careful balance is required in order not to allow stools and defecation pattern to become the center of the child's life and family functioning.

Key to successful treatment is maintaining the rectum devoid of stools. The chronic presence of large amount of stools in the rectum causes the rectum to enlarge, decreasing the sensitivity to distention, a factor often associated with worse outcome.[67] In order to achieve complete and successful evacuations, the North American Society for Pediatric Gastroenterology and Nutrition (NASPGHAN), in its position paper on guidelines for the management of constipation, recommends a number of options. The actual choice of medication is not as important as an adequate dosage of any of them and the will and ability of the child and parents to comply with the treatment plan. Laxatives can be divided into several types: dietary fiber and bulking agents, osmotic and saline laxatives, lubricating agents, and laxatives that stimulate colonic motility (Table 12.2). A common myth about laxatives is that they cause physical dependence, 'lazy' bowels, or irreversibly damage the colon. There is no credible scientific evidence supporting any of these misconceptions. Tolerance, another frequently quoted side effect, may be easily solved by increasing the dose. Addressing these issues in the consultation may contribute to improve adherence to treatment.

Fiber

Constipated children as a group have lower fiber intake than those with normal bowel movements.[68] Unfortunately, achieving a significant increase in the fiber content of the diet is a difficult task. A double-blind, randomized, placebo-controlled crossover study has found fiber (glucomannan) to be beneficial in the treatment of constipation in children.[69] Bulk-forming laxatives such as cellulose and methylcellulose are not commonly used in pediatrics. This group of agents is not digested, absorbs liquid in the intestines and swells to form a softer and larger stool that stimulates the bowel. Bulk-forming laxatives take several days to exert their effect and are not suitable for acute relief.

Osmotic laxatives

Osmotic laxatives include saccharated osmotics (lactulose), PEG-based osmotic laxatives, and saline osmotics (e.g., magnesium or sodium salts). There is evidence for the efficacy and safety of some medications of this group for the therapy of functional consti-

Table 12.2

Mineral oil	Maintenance: 1–5 mL/kg/d divided 1–2 doses. Disimpaction: 25 mL/yr of age up to 240 mL/day
Lactulose	1–3 mL/kg/d divided 1–2 doses
Sorbitol	1–3 mL/kg/d divided 1–2 doses
Milk of magnesia	1–3 mL/kg/d divided 1–2 doses
Magnesium citrate	<6 years 1–3 mL/kg/d, 6–12 years: 100–150 mL/day, >12 years: 150–300 mL/day divided 1–2 doses
Polyethylene glycol 3350	0.7–1.4 g/kg/d divided 1–2 doses
Polyethylene glycol-electrolyte solution: lavage	Disimpaction: 25 mL/kg/hr (up to 1000 mL) PO/NG tube until clear or 20 mL/kg/hr 4 hrs/day
Phosphate enemas	≥6 mL/kg up to 135 mL. Contraindicated <2 years of age
Senna	5 mL or 1 tablet with breakfast, maximum 15 mL or 3 tablets with breakfast
Bisacodyl	5 mg/day for children under 5 years; 10 mg/day for children over 5 years. ≥2 years of age: 0.5–1 suppository (10 mg suppository) or 1–3 tablets per dose (5 mg tablets)

pation in children (magnesium hydroxide, lactulose and sorbitol, PEG).[70] Lactulose is a stool softener that is not systemically absorbed and requires colonic flora for metabolism and primary activation. Lactulose can be taken 'as is' or diluted with milk, juice, and water, or taken into a food. In children, lactulose is effective and generally well tolerated.[71] However, it may be associated with flatulence, bloating, and abdominal cramping. Polyethylene glycol acts by hydrating bowel contents, leading to decreased stool consistency, lubricating and softening the stools, and increasing fecal bulk. Polyethylene glycol is not metabolized and remains virtually unchanged and not absorbed through the whole gastrointestinal tract. There are different formulations of polyethylene glycol (PEG 3350 and PEG 4000), with and without the addition of electrolytes. PEG 3350 is an odorless osmotic laxative used to treat constipation in children. It is indicated for the treatment of occasional constipation, but has also been successfully used for the treatment of fecal impaction in children.[72] A capful of the powder (17 g) is dissolved in 240 mL of any beverage making it particularly easy to use for children. Studies in adults and children have reported long-term efficacy of PEG in the long-term therapy of chronic constipation. A study of 43 constipated children with and without encopresis receiving an average dose of 0.7 g/kg/day (range, 0.3–1.8 g/kg/day) demonstrated significant improvement in stool frequency, consistency, and symptoms and signs of constipation after more than 3 months of therapy.[73] PEG 3350 was found to be more palatable and better accepted by children than lactulose.[74]

Phosphate salts also are frequently used osmotic laxatives. As phosphate can be absorbed by the small intestine, a large dose must be ingested orally to produce a laxative effect, resulting in problems with compliance with treatment. Phosphate and sodium absorption can potentially result in hypernatremia and hyperphosphatemia, leading to compensatory hypocalcemia. Because the colon is less permeable to phosphate, phosphate salts can be used in an enema to clear the colon. Phosphate enemas and other medications of this type such as magnesium salt laxatives can cause serious metabolic disturbances in babies and young children.[75] Milk of magnesia (1–4 mL/kg/daily) is an osmotic laxative with the additional effect of stimulating the secretion of cholecystokinin that in turn increases the secretions and motility of the gut. Overdose can lead to hypermagnesemia, hyperphosphatemia, and secondary hypocalcemia. This medication should not be used in patients with renal insufficiency. Infants are also more susceptible to magnesium poisoning. Magnesium citrate is a similar medication with comparable side effects and contraindications. There have been adult reports of transient severe muscle weakness and paralytic ileus, respiratory and cardiac dysfunction caused by neuromuscular blockade as a result of magnesium imbalance due to this medication.[76] Sodium docusate is a stool softener with detergent properties that allows water to mix with hard stools thereby softening stools. There is some evidence of its efficacy on the maintenance treatment of constipation in children.[77] It is available for pediatric use only in oral form (capsules, drops, or syrup). In order to mask the taste, its liquid or syrup form may be mixed with milk, juice, or infant formula.

Lubricants

Mineral oil (liquid petrolatum, liquid paraffin) and certain digestible plant oils, such as olive oil, soften fecal contents by coating them and thus preventing colonic absorption of fecal water. Mineral oil (2 6 mL/kg/daily) is a transparent, colorless, tasteless, odorless (when cold), and oily liquid that is insoluble in water. It is a mixture of complex hydrocarbons derived from crude petroleum. Although the conversion of mineral oil into hydroxy fatty acids may result in an osmotic effect, mineral oil action is primarily as a stool lubricant. Lubricants are frequently used in pediatrics due to the low cost, ease of titration, and good tolerability when compared with osmotic or stimulant laxatives that are more commonly associated with abdominal cramps, flatulence, or electrolyte disturbances. There is good evidence of the efficacy of mineral oil in the therapy of children with constipation and encopresis with and without fecal impaction.[78–80] Oral mineral oil is contraindicated in patients younger than 1 year old, debilitated or neurologically impaired, and when there is swallowing difficulty or any other case with risk of aspiration with resultant lipid pneumonitis. Although previously thought to cause fat-soluble vitamin malabsorption, a controlled study of patients on chronic therapy with mineral oil revealed that patients had similar prothrombin time, serum retinol, and alpha-tocopherol concentrations to the control group.[81] =

Stimulant laxatives

Senna-containing compounds and bisacodyl act by increasing intestinal motility and secretions of the intestine by local irritation of the mucosa or by a more selective action on the nerve plexus of the intestinal smooth muscle. In patients with very dilated or less active colons the exclusive use of osmotic laxatives may not suffice to produce appropriate stool evacuation. In these cases, osmotic laxatives may soften the stools but in the presence of abnormal propulsion making the stools more liquid may result in increasing overflow soiling. Stimulant laxatives have a fast onset of action. In some children the timing of the onset of the laxative-provoked defecation is very predictable but in others it is not and may lead to embarrassing episodes of incontinence. Due to its need for activation by colonic bacteria, senna has a longer mode of action (often 24 hours from ingestion), so it can be helpful in cases where the evening dose is likely to provoke a stool during school time on the next day. Senna is available in the United States as tablets, granules, oral solution, and syrup, while bisacodyl is available for oral use or in enema form. Glycerine is a safe laxative frequently used as suppository in infants. There is some evidence of its efficacy to treat fecal impaction in infants.[70]

Fecal impaction

In the presence of a fecal impaction, disimpaction is necessary before initiation of maintenance therapy. Disimpaction can be achieved by the oral route, the rectal route, or a combination of both routes. The oral approach is preferred when possible as it is the least invasive, but adherence to therapy may constitute a problem. In a prospective double-blind, randomized study with PEG 3350, the success of disimpaction was significantly greater for patients who received PEG 3350 1 or 1.5 g/kg/day for 3 days.

Behavioral modification

Although compliance may be an issue, behavioral modification based on regular toilet habits with unhurried time on the toilet after meals has proved to be as useful as the use of medications for the treatment of constipation.[82] Toileting after meals takes advantage of the gastrocolonic reflex. A program consisting of counseling and education, twice-daily toileting, and laxatives resulted in no episodes of encopresis in 51% of children after 1 year.[83] Children and caregivers should be encouraged to keep diaries of stool frequency. Every successful evacuation of stool into the toilet can be rewarded with a sticker on a calendar that is later exchanged for a preestablished prize. An additional advantage of the chart is to provide the health care provider with the opportunity to assess the progress of therapy. Patients with motivational or behavioral problems interfering with successful treatment should be referred to a mental healthcare provider.

Biofeedback is a simple and morbidity-free technique that has been used for many years for the treatment of constipation in children. Biofeedback can be used to train patients to relax and coordinate relaxation of pelvic floor and sphincter with abdominal maneuvers to enhance evacuation. Despite its wide use a review of the literature does not indicate clear evidence of its advantage in the management of encopresis and constipation in children.[84,85]

Extreme cases of functional constipation unresponsive to medical management may require temporary diversion to allow the colon to restore its normal size,[86] and may benefit from a variety of other surgical interventions including segmental resection, subtotal colectomy with ileo-rectal anastomosis, and the placement of an appendicostomy or a cecostomy for administration of antegrade enemas.[87]

Suggested approach

When present, we prefer to eliminate the fecal impaction by using oral administration of high-dose PEG 3350. We suggest use of PEG 3350 or lactulose for long-term maintenance treatment.

When a stimulant laxative is needed, senna provides the best safety and efficacy. The maintenance treatment should last until the child has 3 months with normal bowel frequency and painless stooling without episodes of fecal incontinence.

INFLAMMATORY BOWEL DISEASE

The pediatric gastroenterologist dealing with the management of inflammatory bowel disease (IBD) has a number of issues to confront specific to the pediatric patient (see Chs 56 and 57). Children, more often than adults, present with growth failure or delayed pubertal development as their sole presenting sign of IBD.[88] One study found that 31–58% of children with IBD presented with weight loss and 3–13% of children presented with height less than the third percentile.[89] Pubertal development and longitudinal growth delay should be considered a measurement tool of inflammation along with clinical signs and symptoms.[90] One of the goals of medical therapy of pediatric IBD includes optimizing growth and development. Because IBD is a chronic illness, children with this diagnosis will use medications for the rest of their lives. The long-term effects of these medications must be considered prior to committing a patient to any therapy, and such effects are unknown for some of the most recently developed drugs.[90] Noncompliance is an issue for every physician, but is especially relevant for physicians treating children and adolescents, whose rebellious attitude often manifests itself with the refusal of following prescribed treatments.

The therapeutic options used to manage IBD in children are similar to those available for adult patients. The most striking difference in treatment options in children is the use of nutritional therapy. Nutritional therapy has been used to induce remission in children with Crohn's disease, especially when the small bowel is predominantly involved. Enteral nutrition, in the form of an elemental, semi-elemental, or polymeric formula, has been shown to induce remission and promote mucosal healing in children with active IBD.[90,91] It is thought that these formulas reduce inflammation by altering the proinflammatory cytokine cascade. Enteral nutrition has also been demonstrated to decrease intestinal motility, reduce antigenic load, decrease stool output, and promote weight gain, all contributing to the general well-being of children with IBD.[90] Several studies have demonstrated that the remission rate for children with Crohn's disease being treated with enteral nutrition only (elemental, semi-elemental, or polymeric formulas) compared favorably to those being treated with corticosteroids. It has also been shown that children with newly diagnosed Crohn's disease respond better to nutritional therapy than children with recurrent flares.[90] One study found no difference in inducing remission with the use of either an elemental formula or a polymeric formula,[91] and indicated that patients taking a polymeric formula gained more weight than children on an elemental diet. In most children, formulas are given via a nasogastric tube. Rarely, a gastrostomy tube is necessary. Children are often taught to pass the nasogastric tube on their own and receive the formula as continuous feeds overnight.

Immunomodulators are commonly used in the treatment of IBD in both adults and children. A hallmark multicenter, prospective, double-blind, placebo-controlled study in children demonstrated that 6-mercaptopurine (6-MP) decreased the need for corticosteroids in children with newly diagnosed moderate to severe Crohn's disease.[92] This was the first study to evaluate the effectiveness of 6-MP as part of the initial treatment of patients with Crohn's disease.

Despite the lack of randomized clinical trials in children, 62% of pediatric gastroenterologists surveyed by the North American Society of Pediatric Gastroenterology and Nutrition report using infliximab in patients with Crohn's disease refractive to conventional therapy.[90] A recent prospective, open-label study examined the efficacy and tolerance of infliximab in children with severe refractory Crohn's disease. The authors reported improvement of clinical symptoms in all patients receiving infliximab, with complete remission occurring in 90% of patients.[93] All perianal fistulas resolved and inflammatory markers significantly improved after receiving three infusions of infliximab (5 mg/kg on days 0, 15, and 45). Similarly to adult studies, the authors reported that 90% of patients relapsed within 1 year despite maintenance therapy with immunomodulators. A recent report of a 1.5% increased annual incidence of lymphoma in patients receiving infliximab[94] has caused both pediatric and adult gastroenterologists to reassess the long-term usefulness of this medication. Future studies in pediatric patients with refractory Crohn's disease should address the role of infliximab as a maintenance medication. The chronicity of this disease and increased risk of lymphoma may prove to limit the use of this medication in pediatrics.

OTHER CONDITIONS

Congenital gastrointestinal diseases, such as intestinal atresias and stenoses, anorectal malformations, and meconium plugs usually present at birth with obstructive symptoms. There are also other gastrointestinal conditions which are much more common in infants and children than in adults, such as necrotizing enterocolitis, hypertrophic pyloric stenosis, Meckel's diverticulum, intestinal intussusception, or mid-gut volvulus. Treatment of such entities is surgical in most cases and has not been discussed in this chapter.

SUMMARY

There is a dire need for further studies of newly introduced and already existing drugs in children. The desire to protect children and prescribing physicians from unsafe drug use has led in the past to much guesswork when administering medications to children. We hope that governments and regulatory agencies will recognize the special pediatric needs, allowing the medical community to use medications based on well-accrued scientific evidence rather than continuing the practice of performing uncontrolled experiments whenever prescribing drugs for children.

REFERENCES

1. Jong GW, Vulto AG, de Hoog M, et al. A survey of the use of off-label and unlicensed drugs in a Dutch children's hospital. Pediatrics 2001; 108:1089–1093.

2. Barr J, Brenner-Zada G, Heiman E, et al. Unlicensed and off-label medication use in a neonatal intensive care unit: a prospective study. Am J Perinatol 2002; 19:67–72.

   A provocative study uncovering the dire need for more studies of commonly used drugs in pediatrics.

3. Cote CJ, Alexander J. Drug development for children: the past, the present, hope for the future. Paediatr Anaesth 2003; 13:279–283.

4. Best Pharmaceuticals for Children Act. Public Law 107-1-9, 107th Congress, 115 Stat 1408 (2002 Jan 4). 2004.

5. Gold BD, Freston JW. Gastroesophageal reflux in children: pathogenesis, prevalence, diagnosis, and role of proton pump inhibitors in treatment. Pediatr Drugs 2002; 4(10):673–685.

6. Gold BD. Outcomes of pediatric gastroesophageal reflux disease: in the first year of life, in childhood, and in adults . . . oh, and should we really leave *Helicobacter pylori* alone? J Pediatr Gastroenterol Nutr Treatment Pediatr Gastroesophageal Reflux Disease: Current Knowledge and Future Research 2003; 37(Supplement 1):S33–S39.

7. Waring JP, Feiler MJ, Hunter JG, et al. Childhood gastroesophageal reflux symptoms in adult patients. J Pediatr Gastroenterol Nutr 2002; 35(3):334–338.

8. Rudolph CD, Mazur LJ, Liptak GS, et al. Guidelines for evaluation and treatment of gastroesophageal reflux in infants and children: recommendations of the North American Society for Pediatric Gastroenterology and Nutrition. J Pediatr Gastroenterol Nutr 2001; 32(Suppl):31.

A practical, evidence-based review of the evaluation and treatment of GERD directed to the primary care physician.

9. Orenstein SR, Magill H, Brooks P. Thickening of infant feedings for therapy of gastroesophageal reflux. J Pediatr 1987; 110:181–186.

10. Orenstein SR, Whitington P, Orenstein DM. The infant seat as treatment for gastroesophageal reflux. N Engl J Med 1983; 309:760–763.

11. Orenstein SR. Prone positioning in infant gastroesophageal reflux: is elevation of the head worth the trouble? J Pediatr 1990; 119(pt 1):184–187.

12. Gremse DA. Gastroesophageal reflux: life-threatening disease or laundry problem? Clin Pediatr 2002; 41(6):369–372.

13. Orenstein SR. Gastroesophageal reflux. Pediatr Rev 1999; 20(1):24–28.

14. Orenstein SR, Shalaby TM, Devandry SN, et al. Famotidine for infant gastro-oesophageal reflux: a multi-centre, randomized, placebo-controlled, withdrawal trial. Aliment Pharmacol Ther 2003; 17(9):1097–1107.

15. Lambert J, Mobassaleh M, Grand R. Efficacy of cimetidine for gastric acid suppression in pediatric patients. J Pediatr 1992; 120(3):474–478.

16. Abdel-Rahman SM, Johnson FK, Connor JD, et al. Developmental pharmacokinetics and pharmacodynamics of nizatidine. J Pediatr Gastroenterol Nutr 2004; 38:442–451.

17. Gibbons TE, Gold BD. The use of proton pump inhibitors in children: a comprehensive review. Pediatr Drugs 2003; 5(1):25–40.

18. Hassall E, Israel D, Shepherd R, et al. Omeprazole for treatment of chronic erosive esophagitis in children: a multicenter study of efficacy, safety, tolerability and dose requirements. International Pediatric Omeprazole Study Group. J Pediatr 2000; 137(6):800–807.

19. Madrazo-de la Garza A, Dibildox M, Vargas A, et al. Efficacy and safety of oral pantoprazole 20 mg given once daily for reflux esophagitis in children. J Pediatr Gastroenterol Nutr 2003; 36(2):261–265.

20. Maier I, Wu GY. Prokinetic therapy for gastroenterological diseases. Chinese J Dig Dis 2003; 4(4):151–159.

21. Kawai M, Kawahara H, Hirayama S, et al. Effect of baclofen on emesis and 24-hour esophageal pH in neurologically impaired children with gastroesophageal reflux disease. J Pediatr Gastroenterol Nutr 2004; 38:317–323.

22. Di Lorenzo C, Orenstein S. Fundoplication: friend or foe? J Pediatr Gastroenterol Nutr 2002; 34(2):117–124.

23. Fleisher DR, Matar M. The cyclic vomiting syndrome: a report of 71 cases and literature review. J Pediatr Gastroenterol Nutr 1993; 17(4):361–369.

24. Li BU. Cyclic vomiting: the pattern and syndrome paradigm. J Pediatr Gastroenterol Nutr 1995; 21(Suppl):10.

25. Abu-Arafeh I, Russell G. Cyclic vomiting syndrome in children: a population-based study. J Pediatr Gastroenterol Nutr 1995; 21:454–458.

26. Prakash C, Clouse RE. Cyclic vomiting syndrome in adults: clinical features and response to tricyclic antidepressants. Am J Gastroenterol 1999; 94(10):2855–2860.

27. Olson ADM, Li BUK. The diagnostic evaluation of children with cyclic vomiting: A cost-effectiveness assessment. J Pediatr 2002; 141(5):724–728.

One of the first systematic studies of the societal impact of cyclic vomiting in children.

28. Li BU, Misiewicz L. Cyclic vomiting syndrome: a brain-gut disorder. Gastroenterol Clin North Am 2003; 32(3):997–1019.

29. Stein MT, Katz RM, Jellinek MS, et al. Cyclic vomiting. J Devel Behav Pediatr 2001; 22(2:Suppl):42.

30. Andersen JM, Sugerman KS, Lockhart JR, et al. Effective prophylactic therapy for cyclic vomiting syndrome in children using amitriptyline or cyproheptadine. Pediatrics 1997; 100(6):977–981.

31. Ludvigsson JF. Propanolol in treatment of migraine in children. Lancet 1973; 2:799.

32. Vanderhoof JA, Young R, Kaufman SS, et al. Treatment of cyclic vomiting in childhood with erythromycin. J Pediatr Gastroenterol Nutr 1995; 21(Suppl):2.

33. Moskowitz MA. Neurogenic versus vascular mechanisms of sumatriptan and ergot alkaloids in migraine. Trends Pharmacol Sci 1992; 13(8):307–311.

34. Van Calcar SC, Harding CO, Wolff JA. L-carnitine administration reduces number of episodes in cyclic vomiting syndrome. Clin Pediatr 2002; 41(3):171–174.

35. Pasricha PJ, Schuster MM, Saudek CD, et al. Cyclic vomiting: association with multiple homeostatic abnormalities and response to ketorolac. Am J Gastroenterol 1996; 91(10):2228–2232.

36. Fleisher DR. The cyclic vomiting syndrome described. J Pediatr Gastroenterol Nutr 1995; 21(Suppl):5.

37. Liacouras CA. Eosinophilic esophagitis in children and adults. J Pediatr Gastroenterol Nutr Treatment Pediatr Gastroesophageal Reflux Dis: Current Knowledge and Future Research 2003; 37(Suppl 1):S23–S28.

38. Khan SM, Orenstein SR, Di Lorenzo C, et al. Eosinophilic esophagitis: strictures, impactions, dysphagia. Dig Dis Sci 2003; 48(1):22–29.

39. Teitelbaum JE, Fox VL, Twarog FJ, G et al. Eosinophilic esophagitis in children: immunopathological analysis and response to fluticasone propionate. Gastroenterology 2002; 122(5):1216–1225.

This study points out that eosinophilic esophagitis is characterized by immunologically active esophageal mucosa and that fluticasone propionate significantly reduces mucosal inflammation.

40. Munitiz V, Martinez de Haro LF, Ortiz A, et al. Primary eosinophilic esophagitis. Dis Esophagus 2003; 16(2):165–168.

41. Straumann A, Spichtin HP, Grize L, et al. Natural history of primary eosinophilic esophagitis: a follow-up of 30 adult patients for up to 11.5 years. Gastroenterology 2003; 125(6):1660–1669.

42. Cheung KM, Oliver MR, Cameron DJS, et al. Esophageal eosinophilia in children with dysphagia. J Pediatr Gastroenterol Nutr 2003; 37(4):498–503.

43. Khan S, Orenstein SR. Eosinophilic gastroenteritis: epidemiology, diagnosis and management. Paediatr Drugs 2002; 4(9):563–570.

44. Mishra A, Hogan SP, Brandt EB, et al. An etiological role for aeroallergens and eosinophils in experimental esophagitis. J Clin Invest 2001; 107(1):83–90.

45. Kelly KJ, Lazenby AJ, Rowe PC, et al. Eosinophilic esophagitis attributed to gastroesophageal reflux: improvement with an amino acid-based formula. Gastroenterology 1995; 109(5):1503–1512.

46. Markowitz JE, Spergel JM, Ruchelli E, et al. Elemental diet is an effective treatment for eosinophilic esophagitis in children and adolescents. Am J Gastroenterol 2003; 98(4):777–782.

47. Liacouras CA, Wenner WJ, Brown K, et al. Primary eosinophilic esophagitis in children: successful treatment with oral corticosteroids. J Pediatr Gastroenterol Nutr 1998; 26(4):380–385.

48. Attwood SE, Lewis CJ, Bronder CS, et al. Eosinophilic oesophagitis: a novel treatment using montelukast. Gut 2003; 52(2):181–185.

49. Alfven G. The covariation of common psychosomatic symptoms among children from socioeconomically differing residential areas: an epidemiologic study. Acta Paediatrica 1993; 82:484–487.

50. Starfield B, Hoekelman RA, McCormick M, et al. Who provides health care to children and adolescents in the United States? Pediatrics 1984; 74, 991–997.

51. Hyams JS, Treem WR, Justinich CJ, et al. Characterization of symptoms in children with recurrent abdominal pain: resemblance to irritable bowel syndrome. J Pediatr Gastroenterol Nutr 1995; 20(2):209–214.

52. Hyams JS, Burke G, Davis PM, et al. Abdominal pain and irritable bowel syndrome in adolescents: a community-based study. J Pediatr 1996; 129(2):220–226.

A very important epidemiologic study uncovering a very high prevalence of IBS in middle and high school children.

53. Walker LS, Guite JW, Duke M, et al. Recurrent abdominal pain: a potential precursor of irritable bowel syndrome in adolescents and young adults. J Pediatr 1998; 132(6):1010–1015.

54. Sperling MS, McQuaid KR. Rational medical therapy of functional GI disorders. In: KW Olden, ed. Handbook of functional gastrointestinal disorders. New York: Marcel Dekker; 1996:269-328.

55. Fishbain D. Evidence-based data on pain relief with antidepressants. Ann Med 2000; 32(5):305–316.

56. Couch JR, Hassanein RS. Migraine and depression: effect of amitriptyline prophylaxis. Trans Am Neurol Assoc 1976; 101:234–237.

57. Gorard DA, Libby GW, Farthing MJ. Ambulatory small intestinal motility in 'diarrhoea' predominant irritable bowel syndrome. Gut 1994; 35(2):203–210.

58. Gorard DA, Libby GW, Farthing MJ. Effect of a tricyclic antidepressant on small intestinal motility in health and diarrhea-predominant irritable bowel syndrome. Dig Dis Sci 1995; 40(1):86–95.

59. Teicher MH, Glod C, Cole JO. Emergence of intense suicidal preoccupation during fluoxetine treatment. Am J Psychiatry 1990; 147:207–210.

60. Healy D, Langmaak C, Savage M. Suicide in the course of the treatment of depression. J Psychopharmacol 1999; 13:94–99.

61. Khan A, Khan S, Kolts R, et al. Suicide rates in clinical trials of SSRIs, other antidepressants, and placebo: analysis of FDA reports. Am J Psychiatry 2003; 160:790–792.

62. Grunebaum MF, Ellis SP, Li S, et al. Antidepressants and suicide risk in the United States, 1985–1999. J Clin Psychiatry 2004; 65:1456–1462.

63. Wagstaff AJ, Frampton JE, Croom KF. Tegaserod: a review of its use in the management of irritable bowel syndrome with constipation in women. Drugs 2003; 63(11):1101–1120.

64. Kline RM, Kline JJ, Di Palma J, et al. Enteric-coated, pH-dependent peppermint oil capsules for the treatment of irritable bowel syndrome in children. J Pediatr 2001; 138(1):125–128.

One of the very rare double-blind, randomized, controlled study of any therapeutic intervention in children.

65. Pittler MH, Ernst E. Peppermint oil for irritable bowel syndrome: a critical review and meta-analysis. Am J Gastroenterol 1998; 93(7):1131–1135.

66. Youssef NN, Di Lorenzo C. Childhood constipation: evaluation and treatment. J Clin Gastroenterol 2001; 33(3):199–205.

67. Loening-Baucke V. Clinical approach to fecal soiling in children. Clin Pediatr 2000; 39(10):603–607.

68. Vitolo MR, Aguirre AN, Fagundes-Neto U, et al. [Estimated dietary fiber intake in children according to different food composition reference tables]. [Portuguese]. Archivos Latinoamericanos de Nutricion 1998; 48(2):141–145.

69. Loening-Baucke V, Miele E, Staiano A. Fiber (glucomannan) is beneficial in the treatment of childhood constipation. Pediatrics 2004; 113(3:Pt 1):64.

70. Baker SS, Liptak GS, Colletti RB, et al. Constipation in infants and children: evaluation and treatment. A medical position statement of the North American Society for Pediatric Gastroenterology and Nutrition. J Pediatr Gastroenterol Nutr 1999; 29(5):612–626.

An evidence-based review of evaluation and treatment of constipation directed to the primary care physician.

71. Perkin JM. Constipation in childhood: a controlled comparison between lactulose and standardized senna. Curr Med Res Opin 1977; 4(8):540–543.

72. Youssef NN, Peters JM, Henderson W, et al. Dose response of PEG 3350 for the treatment of childhood fecal impaction. J Pediatr 2002; 141(3):410–414.

Four doses of PEG 3350 were compared in this study aimed at assessing efficacy in the treatment of fecal impaction.

73. Pashankar DS, Bishop WP, Loening-Baucke V. Long-term efficacy of polyethylene glycol 3350 for the treatment of chronic constipation in children with and without encopresis. Clin Pediatr 2003; 42(9):815–819.

74. Gremse DA, Hixon J, Crutchfield A. Comparison of polyethylene glycol 3350 and lactulose for treatment of chronic constipation in children. Clin Pediatr 2002; 41(4):225–229.

75. Gattuso JM, Kamm MA. Adverse effects of drugs used in the management of constipation and diarrhoea. Drug Safety 1994; 10(1):47–65.

76. Swift TR. Weakness from magnesium-containing cathartics: electrophysiologic studies. Muscle & Nerve 1979; 2(4):295–298.

77. Liebman WM. Disorders of defecation in children: evaluation and management. Postgrad Med 1979; 66(2):105–108.

78. Nolan T, Debelle G, Oberklaid F, et al. Randomised trial of laxatives in treatment of childhood encopresis. Lancet 1991; 338(8766):523–527.

79. Sondheimer JM, Gervaise EP. Lubricant versus laxative in the treatment of chronic functional constipation of children: a comparative study. J Pediatr Gastroenterol Nutr 1982; 1(2):223–226.

80. Tolia V, Lin CH, Elitsur Y. A prospective randomized study with mineral oil and oral lavage solution for treatment of faecal impaction in children. Aliment Pharmacol Ther 1993; 7(5):523–529.

81. Clark JH, Russell GJ, Fitzgerald JF, et al. Serum beta-carotene, retinol, and alpha-tocopherol levels during mineral oil therapy for constipation. Am J Dis Child 1987; 141(11):1210–1212.

82. Nolan T, Oberklaid F. New concepts in the management of encopresis. Pediatr Rev 1993; 14(11):447–451.

83. Levine MD, Bakow H. Children with encopresis: a study of treatment outcome. Pediatrics 1976; 58(6):845–852.

84. Brazzelli M, Griffiths P. Behavioural and cognitive interventions with or without other treatments for defecation disorders in children. Cochrane Database of Systematic Reviews 2001;(4):CD002240.

85. Heymen S, Jones KR, Scarlett Y, et al. Biofeedback treatment of constipation: a critical review. Dis Colon Rect 2003; 46(9):1208–1217.

86. Youssef NN, Barksdale JE, Griffiths JM, et al. Management of intractable constipation with antegrade enemas in neurologically intact children. J Pediatr Gastroenterol Nutr 2002; 34(4):402–405.

87. Pensabene L, Youssef NN, Di Lorenzo C. Success of antegrade enemas in children with functional constipation. Pediatria Medica e Chirurgica 2003; 25(2):126–130.

88. Ballinger AB, Savage MO, Sanderson IR. Delayed puberty associated with inflammatory bowel disease. Pediatr Res 2003; 53(2):205–210.

89. Sawczenko A, Sandhu BK. Presenting features of inflammatory bowel disease in Great Britain and Ireland. Arch Dis Child 2003; 88(11):995–1000.

90. Escher JC, Taminiau JA, Nieuwenhuis EE, et al. Treatment of inflammatory bowel disease in childhood: best available evidence. Inflam Bowel Dis 2003; 9(1):34–58.

91. Ludvigsson JF, Krantz M, Bodin L, et al. Elemental versus polymeric enteral nutrition in paediatric Crohn's disease: a multicentre randomized controlled trial. Acta Paediatrica 2004; 93(3):327–335.

92. Markowitz J, Grancher K, Kohn N, et al. A multicenter trial of 6-mercaptopurine and prednisone in children with newly diagnosed Crohn's disease. Gastroenterology 2000; 119(4):895–902.

   A very important study which has had a substantial impact on how pediatric gastroenterologists care for children with Crohn's disease.

93. Cezard JP, Nouaili N, Talbotec C, et al. A prospective study of the efficacy and tolerance of a chimeric antibody to tumor necrosis factors (remicade) in severe pediatric Crohn disease. J Pediatr Gastroenterol Nutr 2003; 36:632–636.

94. Ljung T, Karlen P, Schmidt D, et al. Infliximab in inflammatory bowel disease: clinical outcome in a population based cohort from Stockholm County. Gut 2004; 53(6):849–853.

Section

3 Three

Management of esophageal disorders

CHAPTER THIRTEEN

13

Gastroesophageal reflux disease

Robert M. Lowe, Lars Lundell, Richard I. Rothstein, and M. Michael Wolfe

INTRODUCTION

Gastroesophageal reflux disease (GERD) is one of the most common gastrointestinal disorders, affecting more than 60 million Americans.[1] Although the majority of persons experience symptoms of GERD infrequently, approximately 14% of Americans report GERD episodes at least once per week, and up to 7% describe daily symptoms of heartburn or regurgitation. In addition, the extraesophageal manifestations of GERD, including asthma, chronic cough, and laryngitis, are being recognized with increasing frequency. The management of GERD has evolved over the past 3 decades to the point at which the use of proton pump inhibitors permits highly effective treatment of even the most severe disease. Effective surgical therapy is available, and the utility of several new endoscopic therapies is being evaluated; the mainstay of GERD treatment, however, remains the use of antisecretory drugs, which have a proven record of effectiveness and safety.

PATHOGENESIS OF GASTROESOPHAGEAL REFLUX DISEASE

Gastroesophageal reflux disease results from exposure of the esophageal mucosa to gastric contents, particularly acid and pepsin. Bile acids and other substances also play a role in mucosal injury, albeit to a lesser extent.[2] Factors that play a role in promoting esophageal acid exposure include the anatomic structure and function of the lower esophageal sphincter (LES), esophageal clearance mechanisms that act to limit contact time with noxious substances, and protective factors intrinsic to the esophageal mucosa.

The LES is a 3–4 cm long region of smooth muscle located at the esophagogastric junction that provides a zone of high pressure separating the esophageal and gastric compartments. The diaphragmatic crura surround the LES and assist in the maintenance of a tonically closed sphincter. Although a low resting LES pressure may precipitate gastroesophageal reflux, it is the primary cause of GERD in only a minority of patients and, when present, is associated with more severe reflux disease and erosive esophagitis.[3]

The contribution of hiatal hernia to GERD is well known, although reflux may occur in its absence. The hiatal hernia eliminates the contribution of the crural diaphragm to LES function and thereby promotes gastroesophageal reflux, especially when intragastric pressure is increased due to gastric distention or straining of the abdominal musculature. The severity of reflux disease in patients with hiatal hernia has been positively correlated with the size of the hernia sac.[4]

While a hypotensive LES or hiatal hernia may be important contributors to gastroesophageal reflux disease, the most common cause of gastroesophageal reflux is an excessive exposure of the esophagus to acid and pepsin during transient lower esophageal sphincter relaxation (TLESR). These periods of relaxation last for approximately 10–30 seconds, and occur in response to gastric distention and vagal stimulation. This physiologic process may serve to vent gas from the stomach, and each TLESR is not necessarily associated with gastroesophageal reflux. Patients with GERD, however, have a larger fraction of TLESRs associated with reflux than normal controls and, as a consequence, a significantly longer duration of esophageal acid exposure.[5] The contribution of TLESRs to GERD is greatest for patients with nonerosive or mild erosive disease. Patients with more severe grades of esophagitis often have other factors, such as hiatal hernia or decreased LES pressure, as major causes of prolonged acid exposure.[6]

Once acid and pepsin reflux into the esophagus, clearance mechanisms are activated in an attempt to limit exposure of the esophageal mucosa to gastric secretions. The presence of gastric juice in the lower esophagus stimulates muscular contractions (secondary peristalsis) that rapidly propel the bolus back into the stomach. Bicarbonate present in saliva and in the secretions of esophageal glands serves to neutralize residual esophageal acid. Thus, patients with impaired esophageal motility or decreased salivary secretion have a predisposition to GERD as a result of impaired esophageal acid clearance.

MEDICAL THERAPY OF GASTROESOPHAGEAL REFLUX DISEASE

Gastroesophageal reflux disease, as described above, is principally a motility disorder, and the majority of patients with GERD do not secrete excessive quantities of gastric acid. Nevertheless, the treatment of GERD is generally not directed at the underlying pathophysiology, but rather is aimed at rendering the refluxate less noxious (i.e., less acidic) to the esophageal mucosa, tilting the balance between offensive and defensive forces toward the side of mucosal protection. An effective therapy for GERD should accomplish three goals; symptom control is the primary focus of treatment, and the expectation of complete symptom relief is not unreasonable. Additionally, an effective therapy should heal esophageal mucosal breaks (erosive esophagitis). It should be noted that the severity of symptoms does not correlate with the presence or severity of erosive disease.[7] Lastly, effective therapy of GERD should prevent the esophageal complications of chronic reflux, including esophageal ulceration, stricture, and intestinal metaplasia.

Lifestyle modifications

The treatment of GERD begins with educating patients regarding the factors that contribute to gastroesophageal reflux and the nonpharmacologic measures that may reduce symptom frequency (Table 13.1). Supine reflux, a common cause of nocturnal symptoms, can be reduced by elevating the head of the patient's bed by 6 inches. The use of multiple pillows is not effective, but rather elevation is accomplished by the placement of solid blocks under the bedposts. Alternatively, the use of a firm wedge that elevates both the head and thorax may provide benefit. Sleeping with the left side down may also improve the anatomic barrier to supine reflux. Patients should be advised not to lay supine for at least 2–3 hours after a meal, to allow for gastric emptying, and to reduce the quantity of gastric secretions available for reflux into the esophagus. A recent study of patients with nocturnal GERD symptoms reported that these practices provide 'completely satisfactory' relief of nighttime symptoms in approximately 50% of patients who used them.[1] Dietary modification may be helpful in ameliorating GERD symptoms, and many patients can easily identify foods that exacerbate their symptoms. While no specific diet is recommended for GERD patients, they need to be made aware of the most common provocative factors, including fatty foods, citrus fruits, tomato-

based foods, coffee (including decaffeinated brands), chocolate, and alcohol. Patients can then evaluate their own diet and eliminate the agents that precipitate symptoms. Smoking is also positively associated with GERD symptoms, and smoking cessation should be encouraged both to control reflux and for a number of other health benefits. A careful review of the patient's medications is essential, as many common antihypertensives, bronchodilators, and psychotropic agents promote gastroesophageal reflux, including calcium-channel blockers, oral beta-2 agonists, and antidepressants with anticholinergic properties.

Despite the large number of potential lifestyle modifications available, pharmacological therapy is typically required to control symptoms, and although these measures should be discussed with patients, the use of medication should not be delayed except in cases of very mild and infrequent heartburn.

Antacids

Antacids are a class of medications that directly neutralize gastric acid. They are among the earliest medications used for gastrointestinal disorders, with ground coral powder (calcium carbonate) employed as a remedy for dyspepsia among the ancient Greeks. Currently available antacid preparations include magnesium or aluminum hydroxides and calcium carbonate. Powdered sodium bicarbonate is also available, but it is less frequently used. These agents all provide rapid, but short-lived, relief of heartburn (30–60 min) and as a result require frequent dosing. There are few well-designed studies evaluating the use of antacids in treating GERD, and they have generated conflicting results. A number of trials have shown no significant difference between antacids and placebo in the control of heartburn,[8] while others demonstrate a clear benefit of antacid therapy in symptom relief.[9,10] No trials, however, have demonstrated antacids to be effective in healing esophagitis. Currently, antacid therapy is useful in the management of uncomplicated GERD in patients with infrequent symptoms.

Alginic acid has been used in combination with antacids. This agent creates a viscous layer atop the gastric acid pool and may decrease acid reflux by physically preventing acid from entering the esophagus, as well as by delivering coadministered antacids to the esophagus. Small studies have demonstrated that antacid/alginic acid combinations are superior to placebo for the relief of GERD symptoms,[11] but this therapy should also be reserved for the treatment of mild and infrequent heartburn.

Although antacids are a very safe class of drug, adverse effects may be associated with their use, including diarrhea (with magnesium-containing formulations) or constipation (with aluminum-based formulations).

Prokinetic agents

Agents that modify esophageal and gastric motility are conceptually attractive for the treatment of GERD, which, as described above, is primarily a motility disorder. Currently available prokinetic agents, however, have demonstrated only modest efficacy in a number of small trials, and the side-effect profile of several of these agents renders them less useful in the therapy of GERD.

Cisapride, a 5-HT$_4$ receptor agonist which also promotes the release of acetylcholine from the myenteric plexus, was more

---

Table 13.1 Lifestyle modifications for patients with GERD

Positional modifications

Elevation of the head of the bed

Sleeping left side down

Avoidance of lying supine for 2–3 hours after a meal

Dietary modifications

Avoidance of:
Foods that precipitate symptoms

High-fat foods

Citrus fruits

Tomato-based foods

Coffee (including decaffeinated brands)

Chocolate

Alcohol

Others

Smoking cessation

Weight loss

Examination of prescribed medication list and avoidance of classes of drug known to cause reflux (calcium channel blockers, anticholinergic medications, oral beta-2 agonists)

effective than placebo in controlling postprandial heartburn[12] and compared favorably with histamine-2 receptor antagonist (H2RA) therapy in small randomized trials.[13] Compared with proton pump inhibitor (PPI) therapy, however, cisapride was significantly less effective in controlling heartburn.[14] Cisapride is no longer widely available, as it was associated with over 300 cases of cardiac arrhythmia and 80 patient deaths.[15] Cisapride can still be obtained on a limited basis for patients who cannot tolerate alternative therapies.

Metoclopramide, a dopamine antagonist, has also been evaluated in the treatment of GERD. Most of the clinical studies of metoclopramide suffer from small sample sizes and a lack of placebo controls. The few well-designed studies demonstrate an improvement in symptom control with metoclopramide 10 mg p.o. q.i.d. compared with placebo.[16] Compared with H2RA therapy, however, metoclopramide is less effective in both symptom control and healing of esophagitis.[17] The unfavorable side-effect profile of metoclopramide remains the principal justification against its widespread use. Metoclopramide crosses the blood–brain barrier and induces a number of CNS side effects, including drowsiness, agitation, and motor symptoms. These side effects occur in up to 30% of patients and often necessitate discontinuation of therapy. More serious side effects, including depression, dystonia, and tardive dyskinesia, are less common.[15]

Domperidone is a dopamine antagonist available outside the United States. It does not cross the blood–brain barrier and thus has a better safety profile than metoclopramide, with no significant CNS side effects and only a small incidence of gynecomastia and galactorrhea. The clinical effectiveness of domperidone in the therapy of GERD has not been well established, with small studies providing inconsistent results with regard to the control of heartburn and mucosal healing.[18] Small trials comparing ranitidine to domperidone found similar efficacy in symptom control and the resolution of esophagitis, but demonstrated no benefit of combination therapy with domperidone and an H2RA.[19]

H₂-receptor antagonists

H₂-receptor antagonists (H2RAs) inhibit acid secretion by binding to the histamine-2 receptor on the basolateral membrane of the parietal cell (see Fig. 1.9). Secreted by the gastric enterochromaffin-like cell, histamine is the principal stimulus for acid secretion, and the inhibition of this paracrine effect significantly decreases gastric acid production. The initial clinical studies evaluating H2RAs in the treatment of GERD demonstrated little benefit. The disappointing results may have been due, however, to the fact that the dose of H2RA required to effectively treat duodenal ulcer is generally insufficient to treat GERD. Later studies using appropriate H2RA dosing have consistently demonstrated a clinical effect greater than placebo, both in the control of reflux symptoms and the healing of esophageal erosions. The available H2RAs (cimetidine, ranitidine, famotidine, and nizatidine) appear to be equally effective in treating GERD. Pooled results from clinical trials have demonstrated a 50–75% rate of symptom control and mucosal healing.[20] The effectiveness of H2RA therapy is inversely correlated with the severity of erosive disease, with response rates of nearly 80% in grade I–II esophagitis, but response rates of only 30–50% in grade III–IV disease.[21–23]

H2RAs are particularly effective at inhibiting nocturnal acid secretion; thus, dosing of H2RAs at bedtime or after the evening meal provides effective nighttime relief, especially in patients with mild erosive esophagitis. Patients with more severe mucosal inflammation may require twice-daily dosing.[24] Moreover, owing to their rapid onset of action, H2RAs, particularly when coadministered with antacids, are very effective in treating episodic heartburn.

H2RAs are associated with a low rate of adverse effects (<4%). Concern had been expressed regarding drug interactions due to the effects of cimetidine (and to a lesser extent ranitidine) on the cytochrome P450 system. Altered drug levels have been reported, but these have not proven clinically relevant. The newer H2RAs, nizatidine and famotidine, have not been associated with significant drug interactions. Intravenous ranitidine, used in the hospital setting, may be associated with altered mental status, especially in elderly patients.[2]

Tachyphylaxis, or the development of tolerance to H2RAs, has been demonstrated in several studies, and may occur after as little as 2 weeks of therapy.[25] This phenomenon may be responsible for the decreased efficacy of H2RAs in the control of GERD.

Proton pump inhibitors

Proton pump inhibitors (PPIs) are the most effective class of agents employed in the treatment of GERD. They act on the final common pathway of acid secretion, the H+/K+ ATPase enzyme located on the apical membrane of the gastric parietal cell (see Fig. 1.9). All PPIs are prodrugs, with a pKa of 4–5, which are absorbed from the small bowel, transported via the blood stream to the gastric mucosa, and ultimately are transported to the parietal cell secretory canaliculus. Owing to their pKa, at the neutral pH of blood and of the parietal intracellular milieu, PPIs are inactive. After transport into the secretory canaliculus of the *stimulated* parietal cell, however, with an ambient pH of approximately 0.8–1.0, PPIs become protonated and thereby activated. The resulting thiophilic sulfenamide then forms a covalent disulfide bond with the H+/K+ ATPase, which inactivates the proton pump and produces a profound and durable decrease in acid secretion. It must be emphasized that PPIs only bind to *activated* proton pumps; thus, the appropriate time to administer a PPI is *before* a meal to ensure that drug is circulating during the period of parietal cell activation. Maximal pump activation occurs with the initial meal of the day after an overnight fast, making breakfast the optimal time to administer a PPI. If twice-daily dosing is required, the second dose should be given before the evening meal, rather than at bedtime.

The effectiveness of PPIs in the treatment of GERD has been demonstrated in numerous studies, the majority of which compared PPI therapy to H2RAs. Two large studies comprising 476 patients compared lansoprazole 30 mg per day with ranitidine 150 mg twice daily in patients with erosive esophagitis. Healing rates at 8 weeks were >90% in the lansoprazole groups, compared with 53–69% in the ranitidine groups.[26,27] A comparison of standard dose lansoprazole and high-dose ranitidine (300 mg p.o. b.i.d.) demonstrated similar results, with 8-week healing rates of 91% and 66%, respectively.[28] A large meta-analysis of 43 randomized controlled trials comparing PPIs to H2RA or placebo demonstrated aggregate healing rates of 84% for PPIs versus 52% for H2RA (Fig. 13.1).[29] Thus, standard-dose PPI therapy appears to heal erosive disease in 85–95% of patients with reflux esophagitis.

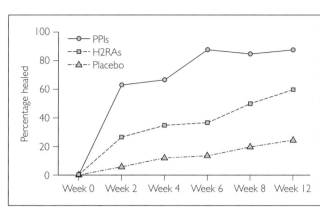

Fig. 13.1 • A comparison of PPI, H2RA, and placebo in the healing of erosive esophagitis, demonstrating the superiority of PPI therapy. (Reprinted from Chiba N et al, Gastroenterology 1997; 112: 1798–810. © 1997, with permission from The American Gastroenterological Association.)

The available PPI formulations have demonstrated similar efficacy in head-to-head trials. A meta-analysis of randomized controlled trials using PPIs to treat erosive esophagitis found no significant difference among omeprazole, lansoprazole, pantoprazole, and rabeprazole in control of heartburn symptoms and in rates of mucosal healing.[30] The most recent addition to the PPI class of drugs is esomeprazole. This drug is composed of the S-enantiomer of omeprazole, which is a racemic mixture of the active S-enantiomer and rapidly metabolized R-enantiomer. A large randomized controlled trial (n=2425) compared esomeprazole to omeprazole in patients with erosive esophagitis.[31] Esomeprazole was associated with significantly greater rates of healing and control of symptoms than omeprazole (93.7% versus 84.2%). This result is to be expected, given that esomeprazole contains only the active enantiomer found in omeprazole. In comparison with other PPIs, however, esomeprazole does not demonstrate clear superiority. A large study (n=5241) compared esomeprazole 40 mg p.o. q.d. to lansoprazole 30 mg p.o. q.d. in the treatment of erosive esophagitis. Healing rates with esomeprazole were 92.6% compared with 88.8% in the lansoprazole group.[32] Although this difference was statistically significant, the absolute rates were very similar, underscoring the comparable clinical effectiveness of most PPI formulations.

Patients who fail to respond to daily-dose PPI therapy should be questioned regarding the timing of therapy and should be encouraged to take the PPI before the first meal of the day. A second dose of PPI, to be taken before dinner, may then be added. A recent study by Barrison et al.[33] reported that approximately 70% of primary care physicians prescribed PPIs before bedtime or without instruction, suggesting that inadequate acid suppression with PPI therapy may occur as a result of suboptimal administration. Patients who remain refractory to PPI therapy should undergo EGD and pH monitoring *on therapy* to determine whether appropriate acid suppression has been achieved and whether the patient's symptoms are indeed due to gastroesophageal reflux. Although the PPIs are equally effective as a class of drug, some patients may experience idiosyncratic responses to different PPIs, and changing to another formulation may be indicated if a true failure of acid suppression is documented on pH monitoring.

Refractory GERD

The term 'refractory GERD' is used to describe patients who continue to have symptoms of gastroesophageal reflux despite maximal pharmacological therapy, which is defined as twice-daily PPI administration. Many patients with 'refractory' symptoms are noncompliant with medications, while others take PPIs inappropriately (at bedtime or several hours before their first meal of the day). The consistent use of PPIs before breakfast and, if needed, before dinner, often improves the response in so-called 'refractory' GERD. There are, however, patients who fail to maximally suppress gastric acid despite appropriate PPI therapy, a situation that can be diagnosed using ambulatory pH monitoring. Such patients may respond to an alternate PPI formulation as a result of patient-specific responses to different PPIs. Patients who are truly refractory to twice-daily PPIs should be evaluated for an acid hypersecretory state (i.e., Zollinger-Ellison syndrome) with a fasting serum gastrin level performed after a two-week period off PPI therapy. In patients with gastrinoma, adequate acid secretion can often be achieved with the use of higher doses of PPI (equivalent to 60–80 mg of omeprazole b.i.d.).

A subset of patients with 'refractory GERD' may demonstrate adequate acid suppression on ambulatory pH monitoring. One explanation for continued symptoms despite acid suppression is the possibility of 'functional heartburn,' essentially a subset of nonulcer dyspepsia manifesting as symptoms of GERD. Alternatively, patients with persistent GERD symptoms may have a 'hypersensitive esophagus,' a situation in which a less acidic refluxate still induces classic symptoms of reflux. Current pH monitoring protocols define acid reflux as an esophageal pH <4; a pH of 5 or 6, however, remains acidic, and may be the cause of symptoms, without causing injury, in a subset of patients with GERD. In such patients, higher doses of PPI may further decrease gastric acidity and relieve symptoms.[34]

Another possible cause of persistent GERD symptoms in the face of effective acid suppression is *bile acid reflux*, in which duodenal contents mix with gastric secretions and comprise a portion of the refluxate that reaches the esophageal mucosa. Bile acids are thought to be the toxic moiety in duodenal secretions; in the presence of acid, these components of bile are protonated and therefore acidic in themselves, adding to the damaging effects of acid and pepsin.[35] In the presence of acid suppression, bile acids exist as neutral bile *salts*, which are less likely to incite esophageal mucosal injury. While bile acid reflux clearly plays a role in patients who have undergone gastric surgery for prior malignant disease or peptic ulcer (i.e., subtotal gastrectomy with Billroth I or II anastamosis), the contribution of bile acid reflux to GERD remains an active area of research. A recent study by Tack and colleagues examined patients with GERD symptoms refractory to daily PPI therapy. Standard pH monitoring was performed to measure esophageal acid exposure, and duodenogastroesophageal reflux was determined using a spectrophotometric method (Bilitec) that identifies bilirubin in the refluxate by measuring its characteristic light absorption spectrum. Sixty-five patients were examined, and 38% exhibited only bile acid reflux, with no pathologic acid exposure.[36] Although these patients were not treated with maximal PPI therapy, the results of this trial suggest that bile acid reflux may indeed play a role in symptomatic GERD. The treatment of bile acid reflux is at present limited; aluminum hydroxide antacids and liquid sucralfate are capable of binding bile acids and may offer some relief. Ursodeoxycholic acid is an orally available bile acid that is effective in the treatment of gallstone disease and primary biliary cirrhosis. Entering the bile salt pool, it displaces more toxic bile acids and may decrease the noxious effects of duodenal reflux on the esophageal mucosa. While the pharmacology is conceptually attractive, no clinical studies to date have demonstrated the efficacy of ursodiol in this scenario.

Maintenance therapy

Gastroesophageal reflux disease is a chronic disorder, with frequent relapses occurring after discontinuation of antisecretory therapy. Chiba and colleagues performed a meta-analysis of clinical trials using PPIs and H2RAs in the treatment of erosive esophagitis; approximately 80% of patients experienced recurrence of heartburn within 1 year after the discontinuation of therapy.[37] The highest recurrence rates were seen in patients with grade III–IV esophagitis.[38] Maintenance therapy for GERD has been shown to be safe and effective, with long-term omeprazole therapy maintaining remission for up to 11 years in one long-term study, although a number of patients required transient PPI dose increases for periods of symptomatic relapse.[39] Vigneri et al. performed a study comparing the effectiveness of ranitidine, cisapride, omeprazole, ranitidine+cisapride, and omeprazole+cisapride in maintaining remission in patients with erosive esophagitis. All patients (n=175) underwent initial therapy with omeprazole for 4–8 weeks, with healing documented by endoscopy. Patients were then randomized to one of the five therapy groups. The results of this trial are presented in Figure 13.2. After 12 months, omeprazole maintained remission in 80% of patients, compared with 49% in the ranitidine group and 54% in the cisapride group. The combination of omeprazole and cisapride yielded the highest rate of remission (89%), which was not significantly different from omeprazole alone.[40] It is thus clear that PPIs provide the most effective therapy for the maintenance of remission in patients with erosive GERD.

'Step therapy' in the treatment of GERD

The approach to treatment of patients with GERD has evolved with the addition of new medical therapies, and the concept of 'step therapy' includes two approaches to treatment. 'Step-up' therapy begins with lifestyle modifications and treatment with over-the-counter antacids and/or low-dose H2RAs, proceeds to prescription-strength H2RAs, and finally to PPI therapy if symptoms are not fully controlled. In contrast, 'step-down' approaches initiate therapy with PPIs to afford the greatest chance of success. Once relief has been achieved, patients are changed to H2RA therapy to determine whether relief of symptoms can be maintained with less potent acid inhibition. These approaches have been evaluated in a small number of trials. Howden and colleagues randomized 593 patients with GERD to one of four treatment arms. Patients received either continuous ranitidine therapy (150 mg p.o. b.i.d.), continuous lansoprazole therapy (30 mg p.o. q.d.), or one of two 'step regimens.' These regimens consisted of either ranitidine twice a day for 8 weeks followed by a 'step-up' to lansoprazole daily for 12 weeks, or lansoprazole daily for 8 weeks followed by a 'step-down' to ranitidine twice daily for 12 weeks. At the end of 20 weeks, the greatest degree of symptom control (measured as 'heartburn-free days') was demonstrated in the continuous lansoprazole group.[41]

In contrast, a study of 'step-down' therapy by Inadomi and colleagues reported very different results. A total of 73 patients with GERD symptoms who responded to initial PPI therapy had their PPI dose decreased and then discontinued over a 4-week period. Those who experienced a return of symptoms were treated with twice-daily H2RA therapy with or without promotility agents. At the end of one year, 58% of the cohort were no longer taking PPIs. Only 15% of patients were off medication entirely, while 35% required H2RA therapy and 7% were on prokinetic agents.[42] Younger patients and those with heartburn as a primary symptom were more likely to fail step-down therapy and require continuous PPI treatment.

Despite conflicting results from studies of step therapy, the step-up approach has gained popularity in an era of managed care

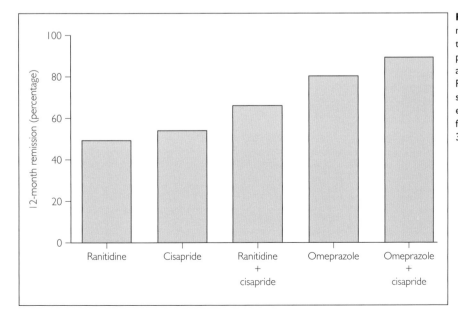

Fig. 13.2 • A comparison of five regimens for maintenance of remission in GERD. Omeprazole therapy was superior to both H2RA and prokinetic therapy. While the combination of PPI and prokinetic therapy was slightly better than PPI alone, this difference was not statistically significant. (From Vigneri S, Termini R, Leandro G, et al. A comparison of five maintenance therapies for reflux esophagitis. N Engl J Med 1995; 333(17):1106–1110.)

cost controls. This strategy is not unreasonable, as many patients with nonerosive GERD or mild erosive esophagitis will be controlled with H2RA therapy. Patients with more severe disease may experience a delay in achieving symptom relief, which needs to be balanced against the total cost savings of any 'step therapy' regimen.[24]

A staged approach to the treatment of GERD

It must be emphasized that nearly all studies evaluating various approaches to treating GERD have included subjects with either documented mucosal abnormalities (erosive esophagitis) or severe and frequent episodes of heartburn. The majority of individuals with GERD, however, do not have erosive disease and experience symptoms infrequently (<2–3 episodes per week). Endoscopy is typically reserved for patients with longstanding symptoms (>5 years duration) to exclude the possibility of Barrett's metaplasia; alarm symptoms such as weight loss, dysphagia, or signs of gastrointestinal bleeding; or onset of symptoms at an age greater than 45 years. Thus, many patients are treated on the basis of symptoms, rather than on endoscopic findings. Moreover, the presence of esophageal mucosal breaks cannot be accurately predicted from a patient's symptom complex or from their response to therapy.[7] Many patients would prefer an 'on-demand' approach to therapy over a daily medical regimen, and such a strategy can be effective in patients with less severe symptomatic disease.

Nocturnal GERD symptoms are common, affecting a majority of patients with frequent reflux symptoms. The importance of nighttime GERD has been underestimated, but a recent Gallup study demonstrated significant morbidity related to nocturnal acid reflux. In a sample of 1000 Americans who reported GERD symptoms at least once per week, 79% reported nighttime symptoms of heartburn or regurgitation, and 63% noted that GERD symptoms interfered with their quality of sleep. Moreover, 40% reported that their daily activities were negatively affected by their nighttime reflux symptoms (Fig. 13.3).[1] Of this group, 71% of patients reported trying OTC medications for their nighttime symptoms, but only 29% found this approach 'completely satisfactory.' Only 41% of patients in this cohort reported using prescription medication for their nocturnal

GERD, and while 49% found this regimen to give complete relief, a full 51% remained dissatisfied with the symptom control afforded by prescription medication. Fifteen percent of patients reported the use of concurrent prescription and OTC medications, although the effectiveness of this regimen was not reported in this study. It is clear that nighttime symptoms of GERD are common and may be difficult to treat with current medical therapy. Of concern is the possibility that nocturnal acid reflux may be associated with a greater incidence of erosive esophagitis and complications of GERD.[43] Lagergren and colleagues, in a retrospective case-control study, demonstrated that symptomatic GERD was a risk factor for adenocarcinoma of the esophagus. Patients with recurrent symptomatic reflux had a relative risk of 7.7, but patients with nocturnal symptoms had an even greater relative risk (approximately 11).[44] Thus, nighttime GERD symptoms have important implications both with regard to patient quality of life and in the clinical sequelae of GERD.

Nocturnal acid breakthrough

The concept of nocturnal acid breakthrough (NAB) was first described by Peghini et al. in a study of GERD patients taking PPIs twice daily. Twenty-four-hour pH monitoring revealed that 73% of study patients had an esophageal pH below 4 for at least 60 minutes during the nighttime hours,[45] a finding confirmed by subsequent studies. The same authors also demonstrated that a single dose of an H_2-receptor antagonist taken at night prevented acid breakthrough in a small cohort of normal volunteers.[46] This approach is based on sound pharmacologic principles, as H_2-receptor antagonists are particularly effective at controlling nocturnal acid secretion, while PPIs are more effective in blocking meal-stimulated acid secretion. Further studies of nocturnal acid breakthrough, however, have reported conflicting results. Fackler and colleagues in a prospective study of 40 subjects found that the addition of an H_2-receptor antagonist to twice daily proton pump inhibitor therapy was effective only during the first 24 hours after initiation of the H2RA. At 7 and 28 days, however, pH monitoring demonstrated no difference in acid control between the two groups.[47] In contrast, Xue et al. conducted a retrospective review of 105 patients on twice-daily

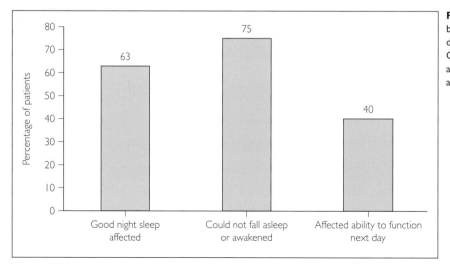

Fig. 13.3 • Results of a Gallup poll sponsored by the American Gastroenterological Association, demonstrating that patients with nocturnal GERD symptoms at least once per week have a significantly decreased quality of sleep, which affects daytime functioning.

PPI therapy alone (60 patients) or b.i.d. PPI therapy along with an H2RA at bedtime (45 patients). The median percentage duration of gastric pH >4 was 96% in the group taking an H2RA compared with 51% in the group taking PPIs only. Mean esophageal acid exposure time was also significantly decreased in the combination therapy group.[48] It should be noted that the pH studies were performed at least 4 weeks after initiation of H2RA therapy in a subset of patients. A recent prospective study[49] compared four antisecretory regimens in a group of 22 subjects (13 with symptomatic GERD and 9 normal volunteers). Patients had baseline pH monitoring and then had repeat pH studies after each of four regimens, including twice-daily PPI therapy (before breakfast and dinner), b.i.d. PPI therapy plus an H2RA given at bedtime, PPI therapy given *three* times daily, and PPI therapy given before breakfast and at bedtime. This study revealed several interesting findings. The dosing of proton pump inhibitors at bedtime, rather than with the evening meal, produced the least suppression of NAB (9%) compared with pretreatment pH studies. PPIs dosed b.i.d. *with meals* suppressed NAB in 18% of patients, and b.i.d. PPI therapy plus a nighttime dose of H2RA suppressed NAB in 41% of patients. This difference was not statistically significant, but the number of subjects in the study was small. It should be noted, however, that NAB persisted in 59–91% of patients using these various regimens, suggesting that none of these options is very effective at controlling nocturnal acid secretion. Despite these conflicting results, it appears that nighttime H2RA therapy *may* be effective in patients with nocturnal GERD symptoms who are taking b.i.d. proton pump inhibitors. Larger prospective studies are needed to confirm or refute this concept, but it remains a reasonable choice for clinicians dealing with seemingly refractory nocturnal GERD.

Caution must be exercised when recommending an H2RA to patients on PPIs since the *concomitant* administration may *decrease* the acid inhibitory properties of PPIs.[24,33] Because H2RAs suppress parietal cell activation, the conversion of the inactive PPI prodrug to the active thiophilic sulfenamide may be retarded. Patients should accordingly be instructed *not* to take both agents simultaneously, but rather to take them several hours apart.

Intermittent therapy with proton pump inhibitors

PPI therapy for GERD is usually continuous, with either daily or twice-daily dosing. Such dosing has been conclusively demonstrated to both control symptoms and heal erosive esophagitis in several studies. Moreover, as stated above, relapse rates after discontinuation of therapy were approximately 75%, confirming the need for long-term maintenance therapy, which has been proven effective in controlling symptoms and erosive disease over a 5–10-year period.[50] Recent studies, however, have examined the possibility of intermittent therapy with PPIs, also known as 'on-demand' therapy, in patients with nonerosive reflux disease or mild reflux esophagitis. Early studies of 'weekend PPI therapy' given 3 days per week were disappointing, with symptom relief at 1 year significantly lower with weekend therapy compared with daily dosing (32% versus 89%).[51] Other studies, using alternate-day dosing regimens, unfortunately published only in abstract form, were more promising.

Lind and colleagues conducted a large randomized controlled trial of on-demand therapy in 424 patients with nonerosive GERD. Patients with typical heartburn symptoms and no endo-scopic evidence of erosive disease were treated for 4–8 weeks; those in whom heartburn resolved were randomized to receive omeprazole 20 mg, omeprazole 10 mg, or placebo.[52] These medications were to be taken 'on-demand,' meaning that if heartburn recurred, patients would take the study drug *daily* until symptoms resolved, and then discontinue therapy. The primary endpoint was discontinuation of the study protocol due to poorly controlled heartburn. After 6 months of follow-up, 83% of patients remained on the 'on-demand' omeprazole 20 mg. In the 10 mg omeprazole group, 69% remained on therapy, while only 56% in the placebo group remained on therapy. The authors concluded that because >50% of patients required no active maintenance therapy, the remainder could be effectively treated 'on demand' with a resultant decrease in total drug costs. It must be emphasized that this approach assessed the effect of PPI therapy given for days to weeks and not therapy 'as needed.' The use of PPIs on an 'as needed' basis (i.e., a single dose when symptoms occur) has not proven effective.[24]

Talley et al. conducted a similar study of 342 patients with nonerosive GERD, using on-demand esomeprazole. After 6 months, only 14% of patients discontinued the study medication due to inadequate symptom control, compared with 51% receiving placebo. The frequency of dosing during relapses in the 'on-demand' esomeprazole group were as follows: 52% took the drug for 1–3 consecutive days, 22% for 4–6 days, and 11% for 7–13 days.[53] These two trials demonstrate that on-demand PPI therapy is tolerated by patients who experience heartburn after initial GERD therapy. Although this approach is less costly in terms of medication expenditures, it remains to be determined whether patients outside the realm of clinical trials will prefer interrupted relief of symptoms to complete relief afforded by daily maintenance therapy.

A recent review by Bardhan summarized the data from several randomized controlled trials and uncontrolled studies.[54] He recommends on-demand or intermittent PPI therapy for younger patients with nonerosive or mild erosive GERD that responds rapidly to initial PPI therapy. Patients who do not meet these criteria should be treated with daily maintenance PPI therapy. It must be emphasized, however, that 'on-demand' therapy as defined in these trials is not in keeping with patients' conception of 'as needed' therapy. The goal of having rapid-onset relief and long-lasting symptom control with a PPI taken once or twice in a single day is not realistic given the pharmacokinetic profile of PPIs. At least 4–5 days of continued PPI therapy are required to maximally inhibit gastric acid secretion and provide the benefit of continuous PPI therapy.[24] Thus, it is unlikely that a patient using PPIs 'as needed' will have adequate symptom relief unless the PPI is taken for several days at a time.

The future of pharmacological therapy for GERD

Antisecretory therapy currently represents the most effective pharmacological means of controlling GERD symptoms; however, even PPI therapy has limitations, as detailed above. Current research is focused both on improving antisecretory medications and on modifying gastrointestinal motility. New proton pump inhibitors are in development, including a competitive inhibitor that reversibly binds near the K+ binding site of the H+/K+ ATPase.[55] Superiority of these so-called 'acid pump inhibitors' over existing PPIs has yet to be determined. More interesting, however, is the ongoing development of prokinetic agents that aim to reverse the abnormal motility underlying the pathogenesis of GERD. Baclofen, a $GABA_B$ receptor antagonist, has been shown to reduce the frequency of TLESRs in both healthy volunteers and GERD patients.[56–58] Randomized, controlled trials of baclofen therapy have yet to be performed, and are necessary before $GABA_B$ receptor antagonists can be added to the armamentarium for the treatment of GERD.

The role of serotonin in gastrointestinal motility has been the subject of considerable research, and tegaserod, a selective 5-HT_4 receptor agonist, has been demonstrated to be effective in irritable bowel syndrome. As serotonin stimulates peristaltic contractions and increased gastric motility, the use of serotonin agonists has the potential to ameliorate GERD symptoms by promoting gastric emptying and enhancing esophageal acid clearance. Early studies demonstrated a decrease in reflux episodes in patients treated with tegaserod,[59] and larger controlled studies with this agent and newer 5-HT_4 agonists are in progress.

Other approaches to the treatment of GERD include inhibition of gastrin-mediated acid secretion with CCK antagonists, inhibition of histamine-mediated acid secretion via histamine-3 receptor blockade, and enhancement of esophageal mucosal protection with agents such as PGE_2, EGF, and TGF alpha. These remain in early phases of development and are not available for use at present.

EXTRAESOPHAGEAL MANIFESTATIONS OF GERD

Manifestations of acid reflux outside the esophagus have been recognized with increasing frequency (Table 13.2). As these extra-esophageal symptoms may occur without concomitant heart-burn or regurgitation, the clinician must maintain a high index of suspicion when patients present with any of these symptoms. The association between GERD and pulmonary symptoms is well established. El-Serag and colleagues evaluated a cohort of over 100 000 service veterans with erosive GERD and demonstrated a significantly increased risk of asthma, COPD, and pulmonary fibrosis.[60] Conversely, patients with asthma have a higher inci-

Table 13.2 Extraesophageal manifestations of GERD
Pulmonary
Asthma
Chronic cough
Otolaryngeal
Hoarseness/laryngitis
Globus sensation
Chronic sore throat
Excessive throat clearing
Dental
Caries
Erosion of enamel
Other
Noncardiac chest pain

dence of GERD symptoms than the general population, with up to 80% of asthma patients reporting significant heartburn.[61,62] The contribution of reflux to adult-onset asthma in patients *without* GERD symptoms has been recently evaluated; Harding et al. performed 24-hour pH monitoring of patients with nocturnal asthma but no GERD symptoms. Abnormal esophageal acidity was documented in 62% of this cohort.[63]

Empiric PPI therapy for presumed GERD-induced asthma has been evaluated in a number of small trials, with conflicting results. Kiljander and colleagues performed a randomized, controlled trial in 52 patients with asthma and abnormal 24-hour pH studies. Treatment with omeprazole 40 mg twice daily for 8 weeks was associated with a significant improvement in nocturnal asthma symptoms; similar results were reported in an additional uncontrolled trial.[64,65] Two other randomized, controlled trials, however, comprising 50 patients reported no improvement in symptoms after PPI therapy.[66,67] Despite these conflicting studies, an empiric 12-week trial of PPI therapy, typically with dosing before both breakfast and dinner, represents a reasonable approach if GERD-induced asthma is suspected. Patients most likely to respond to such a trial include those with adult-onset asthma, nocturnal asthma, or concurrent GERD symptoms.

The contribution of GERD to otolaryngeal symptoms, including hoarseness, globus sensation, and excessive throat clearing, is an area of active research. Koufman et al. studied 225 patients presenting to an otolaryngology service with suspected GERD-induced symptoms. Abnormal esophageal acid exposure was demonstrated in 62%, and pharyngeal reflux was documented in 30%.[68] 'Typical' GERD symptoms were present in only 43% of study patients. This study reported one of the highest rates of GERD-induced otolaryngeal disease; the results of other trials suggest that approximately one-third of otolaryngeal symptoms result from unsuspected GERD. It is clear that physicians must have a high index of suspicion for GERD in patients with hoarseness, chronic cough, or globus sensation, even in the absence of classic reflux symptoms.[69,70] The use of empiric PPI therapy in this patient population has been evaluated in a number of small trials. El-Serag et al. performed a randomized controlled trial comparing lansoprazole 30 mg twice daily versus placebo in 22 patients with reflux laryngitis and reported a 50% response in the treatment group, compared with 10% in the placebo group.[71] A similar trial by Noordzij and colleagues using omeprazole 40 mg twice daily for 8 weeks demonstrated a significant reduction in hoarseness and throat clearing.[72] Thus, in a patient with suspected GERD-induced otolaryngeal symptoms, a trial of proton pump inhibitor b.i.d. for 8–12 weeks is reasonable. Recently, however, the diagnostic accuracy of such empiric therapy has been called into question,[73] and it is recommended that patients who fail to respond to empiric therapy undergo 24-hour pH monitoring to confirm or rule out a diagnosis of GERD.

Noncardiac chest pain (NCCP), discussed in detail in Chapter 68, is defined as angina-type chest pain (substernal pressure or heaviness) in the absence of demonstrable cardiac disease. It is a common condition, with a prevalence of 23% reported in one study based in the northern United States.[74] The syndrome has multiple etiologies, including musculoskeletal pain and psychiatric illness, but esophageal disorders are the most prevalent inciting factor. Of the esophageal causes of NCCP, GERD is the most common, accounting for 25–60% of cases in a number of studies.[75,76] Given the absence of typical reflux symptoms in a subset of patients with NCCP, the diagnosis of GERD is established with 24-hour pH monitoring, which is abnormal in up to 60% of patients.[77,78] Although the association of NCCP with GERD does not necessarily imply causation, several studies of PPI therapy in NCCP demonstrate improvement in symptoms with adequate acid suppression.[77,79] These observations have led to the use of empiric PPI therapy as a diagnostic test for reflux-induced NCCP. PPI therapy is administered twice daily (before breakfast and dinner) for 8–12 weeks, and patients whose symptoms resolve are considered to have GERD as a cause of their chest pain. Patients who fail to respond to a therapeutic trial require 24-hour pH monitoring, as the 'PPI test' has a sensitivity of approximately 80%.[80]

ENDOSCOPIC THERAPY FOR GASTROESOPHAGEAL REFLUX

Endoscopic therapies for GERD have recently provided an alternative to medical or surgical treatments. These interventions can provide long-term benefit for GERD sufferers. Moreover, they may be considered a 'bridge' therapy because patients who undergo endoscopic treatments can still elect to be treated with chronic medications or surgical intervention if the endoscopic therapy does not provide full symptom relief or if symptoms later recur. These endoscopic or endoscopy-assisted treatments include sewing/plication techniques, radiofrequency thermal therapy, and injection/implantable biopolymer therapies (Table 13.3). Some of these treatments are reversible, and many are repeatable. They are designed for the outpatient arena, utilizing conscious sedation and rapid recovery. It must be emphasized that these novel endoscopic antireflux treatments continue to evolve, and most initial reports have addressed symptom relief in short-term follow-up studies of patients with mild GERD. Unfortunately, few peer-reviewed original reports have been published for each of these new techniques, and as discussed below, only one published sham-controlled trial has been conducted. While other data have been presented in abstract form, few studies have incorporated the large numbers of subjects and intention-to-treat analysis required to provide valid demonstration of effect. Long-term outcome studies and sham-controlled trials are currently underway for many of these devices and techniques and will presumably provide much needed peer-reviewed evidence for their use.

Table 13.3 Endoscopic treatments for GERD
Plication/sewing – submucosal
Bard EndoCinch
Wilson-Cook Endoscopic Suturing Device
Plication/sewing – full-thickness
NDO Plicator
Syntheon Anti-Reflux Device
Radiofrequency thermal treatment
Curon Stretta
Injection/implantable
Plexiglas (pmma) microspheres
Boston Scientific Enteryx
Medtronic Gatekeeper

Sewing/plication devices – submucosal

The first endoscopic sewing/plication instrument was designed more than 15 years ago, and techniques to apply this instrument were developed over subsequent years.[81–86] This early work evolved into the currently FDA-approved Bard EndoCinch™ system (Bard Endoscopic Technologies, Billerica, MA), and more than 5000 clinical procedures have now been performed worldwide utilizing this device. This system requires the mounting of a specialized sewing capsule to the distal end of a videoendoscope, which is passed to the cardia via an oroesophageal overtube. The procedure is done in the outpatient setting under conscious sedation and takes about 30–60 minutes to perform, depending on the number of plications created (10–15 minutes per plication). Typically, two to four plications (pleats) are formed just beneath the squamocolumnar junction, with the goal of remodeling the gastric cardia. Various configurations of the multiple pleats have been proposed: circumferential, longitudinal, and helical; none has yet been determined to yield superior results.

The initial US multicenter EndoCinch™ gastric plication trial included 64 patients from 8 sites and reported significant improvement in GERD symptom scores and regurgitation in short-term follow-up.[87] To be included, subjects were required to have three or more episodes per week of heartburn when off antisecretory medications, dependency on continued use of antisecretory drugs for symptom control, and documented acid reflux, as determined by ambulatory pH monitoring. Exclusion criteria included dysphagia, significant erosive esophagitis (more than Savary-Miller grade II), body mass index greater than 40 kg/m^2, GERD refractory to antisecretory therapy, and a hiatal hernia over 2 cm in length. No increase in LES pressure was demonstrated, and only a mild improvement in distal esophageal acid exposure was noted (with normalization in a minority of patients). Whereas 25% of subjects had erosive esophagitis initially, 19% had esophagitis six months following treatment. No differences were detected in outcomes following linear versus circumferential placement of the plications. Short-term efficacy has also been reported by many other investigators, with an overall improvement of GERD symptoms scores in the 70–80% range, and 20–65% of patients remaining off PPIs 6–12 months after the procedure.[88] Normalization of 24-hour pH has occurred in 30–40% of treated subjects in selected studies. Longer-term follow-up (26 month) of the pivotal trial cohort has demonstrated that approximately 25% of subjects were off all antisecretory medications, while another 25% were on minimal doses of medications to control symptoms. The EndoCinch™ treatment appears safe, with no significant serious early or long term complications. This therapy may be valuable in the management of the nonerosive GERD patient. A sham-controlled, randomized, blinded single institution EndoCinch™ study has recently been completed and at three months, the EndoCinch™ procedure significantly decreased heartburn frequency score, acid exposure, and daily antisecretory medication use compared to sham controls.[89] However, no significant improvement in heartburn symptom severity or regurgitation scores, the ability to discontinue all antisecretory medications, or in quality of life (QOL) parameters were found. This study underscores the significant sham-response rate and the need for randomized, controlled trials of sufficient size to determine the true effectiveness of these novel endoscopic therapies for GERD.

Another submucosal stitching instrument, the Wilson-Cook Endoscopic Suturing Device (Wilson-Cook Medical, Winston-Salem, NC), was recently approved by the FDA. The flexible sewing (Sew-Right™) and knot-tying (Ti Knot™) devices are passed via an accessory channel mounted to a flexible videoendoscope and no oroesophageal overtube is required. The Sew-Right™ device has a diameter of 5.2 mm and uses a dual-needle system with a continuous loop of suture. Similar to the technique for EndoCinch™, the Ti Knot™ device can cut and crimp together the suture ends in a fastener. As for the EndoCinch™ technique, each plication takes 10–15 minutes to perform. No consensus has been formulated regarding the number and location of these pleats for optimal effect. Both preclincial and clinical experience with this device is quite limited, and no treatment outcome data are yet available for the Wilson-Cook device.

Sewing/plication devices – full-thickness

The NDO Plicator™ (NDO Surgical, Mansfield, MA) is an instrument designed to create a full-thickness serosa-to-serosa apposition of the proximal cardia. It has recently been evaluated in a US multicenter trial[90] and received FDA approval for marketing as a form of antireflux therapy. In the pivotal open-label trial, the earliest version of the NDO device was placed via an esophageal overtube and a 5.9 mm videogastroscope was inserted through the core of the instrument to provide direct visualization of the cardia while the plication was being created. The most recent version of the instrument can be passed without an overtube and still accepts a small pediatric videogastroscope for viewing the operative field. After identifying a target area for plication in the proximal stomach, a corkscrew-shaped tissue-grasping catheter is embedded into the cardia. The two instrument arms are opened while the proximal stomach is pulled between them, and as they close together a pre-tied monofilament suture implant is deployed to fix the tissue in apposition. The instrument arms are opened to release the plicated tissue, and subsequently closed to allow removal of the NDO instrument.

The preclinical and initial pilot study data reported this technique to be a successful antireflux therapy.[91] Six months after performance of the procedure, 63% of patients reported improvement of their symptom score, with 83% of patients off their usual PPI medications.[90] However, normalization of pH occurred in only 31% of the participants at the short-term follow-up, similar to that seen for the other endoscopic therapies. Although 70% of patients remained off PPIs in a recent follow-up assessment at 12 months, no sham-controlled study has yet been completed. Moreover, in the pilot NDO trial, only one plication was placed, and further study comparing single with multiple plications would be valuable. Procedure time for one NDO plication (mean of 17 minutes) is shorter than that to complete the typical Bard EndoCinch™ or Wilson-Cook Endoscopic Suturing Device procedure (assuming at least two plications placed per session with those instruments). Some significant safety issues (including perforation) emerged with the initial NDO device, which must be addressed by the design modifications of the most recent instrument version.

The Syntheon Anti-Reflux Device™ (Syntheon/ID, Miami, FL) is another full-thickness plicator and is now undergoing study in an open-label multicenter clinical trial. The Syntheon instrument is passed over a guidewire, and a standard gastroscope is passed alongside the device rather than through it (as described above for the NDO). The Syntheon plicator places a titanium metal implant to appose the serosal surfaces. Once in place in the proximal stomach, and under direct visualization from the retroflexed gastroscope, the Syntheon instrument arms are opened, allowing for proximal stomach tissue to be pulled between them with a special tissue grasper deployed through the biopsy channel of the observing endoscope. The arms are subsequently closed to apply the metal fastener and then reopened to release it. Closed again, the instrument is then removed from the stomach behind the gastroscope as it is withdrawn. The time to perform the technique is comparable to that for the NDO plicator and, similarly, only one plication is performed. This initial trial is nearing completion and outcome results and safety details are awaited. Whether transmural plication will ultimately prove to be more effective and durable than submucosal stitching (or other endoscopic treatments for GERD) remains to be seen.

Radiofrequency thermal therapy

A system has been developed and is currently FDA approved to deliver radiofrequency (RF) thermal energy to the gastroesophageal junction for the treatment of GERD (Stretta System™, Curon Medical, Sunnyvale, CA). The system employs a special 20 French diameter balloon catheter that contains 4 radially distributed 25 gauge, 5.5 mm length nickel-titanium needles with dual thermocouple temperature sensors to maintain consistent energy delivery to the LES muscular layer. Ports in the catheter provide intraprocedural cold-water irrigation in order to reduce mucosal heating and prevent surface tissue injury. A computerized control module controls and delivers the RF energy to the needle electrodes. The catheter is advanced into the esophagus over a guidewire placed during a standard upper endoscopy performed with usual conscious sedation in an outpatient setting. The Stretta procedure involves deploying thermal RF treatment in four antegrade rings that straddle the gastroesophageal junction from 1 cm above to just beneath the squamocolumnar junction, and two retrograde 'pull-back' rings in the cardia. The procedure takes ≈45 minutes to complete.

Preclinical and early human studies provided evidence of the feasibility of this system for GERD therapy, highlighting some mechanical and neurological effects of RF thermal treatment. Using a porcine model and incorporating the use of botulinum toxin to relax the lower esophageal sphincter pre-treatment, RF energy delivery to the gastroesophageal junction demonstrated significant augmentation of lower esophageal sphincter pressure and gastric yield pressure.[92] Two human trials reinforced the findings from an earlier animal trial and showed significant reductions in transient lower esophageal sphincter relaxations (TLESRs) following the RF treatment.[93–95]

In the uncontrolled initial Stretta multicenter trials, the 6-month and 1-year results showed significant improvement in all GERD-specific parameters including heartburn scores, GERD health-related quality of life scales, and distal acid exposure time post-treatment.[96,97] At the longer-term follow-up, PPI use fell from 88.1% to 30%, while 40% were off all antireflux medications at 12 months. Lower esophageal sphincter pressure did not increase, and the percentage of patients with esophagitis before or after treatment was not significantly different. No major complications were seen in these initial reports, and a subsequent study has reported no adverse effects on vagal nerve function or gastric emptying. This device has been released commercially, and over 4000 procedures have now been performed. Although there has been no systematic collection of outcomes data from the majority of these cases, a registry of 558 patients who were treated with Stretta at 33 institutions with a mean follow-up of 8 months showed significant GERD symptom control, with 51% no longer using antisecretory medication, and high patient satisfaction.[98] Unfortunately, there have been several perforations and two deaths now associated with the Stretta procedure, although these occurred early after marketing release. No additional serious complications have been reported, and the provision of adequate training to address the learning curve of this, and any new, treatment will help to avoid further device-related problems. Similar to the other endoscopic antireflux treatments, Stretta has been performed primarily in patients with mild GERD without hiatal hernia or with a hernia smaller than 2 cm in length.

A recent sham-controlled study of 64 GERD patients reported the Stretta treatment to be superior to sham for control of heartburn symptoms and improvement in quality of life at 6 months after the intervention.[99] Interestingly, while there were more treated than sham subjects without heartburn symptoms at 6 months (61% versus 30%), no differences in reduction of daily medication use was evident between the groups. Moreover, no differences in esophageal acid exposure times were detected between the 2 groups at 6 months. This finding emphasizes the utility of endoscopic GERD treatment for the patient with nonerosive GERD (the majority of individuals), with no demonstrated consistent ability of these minimally invasive procedures to effectively heal erosive esophagitis.

Injection/implantation therapies

For the past 20 years, implantation therapy for the treatment of GERD has been examined intermittently, with the hope of finding and using the ideal implant material meeting the so-called 'Lehman criteria.' The characteristics of these criteria include: low viscosity, biologically inert, low side effect profile, nonbiodegradable, high persistence at implantation site, low cost, capable of resisting mechanical strain, sterile, favorable elasticity, favorable plasticity, no adverse effect on adjacent musculature, and no required refrigeration.[100] In a small clinical trial reported in 1988, 10 GERD patients who were being managed with H_2-receptor antagonists, antacids, and prokinetics, and were still symptomatic, were treated with submucosal collagen injections.[101] Treated patients were found to experience a 50–75% reduction in their reflux symptoms and medication requirements, with improvement in their distal esophageal acid exposure. At 12-month follow-up, the patients had recrudescence of their symptoms and the implants were observed to be partially or fully degraded.

In search of a more 'ideal' implant, other groups have investigated a variety of injectable or implantable biopolymers and treatments. These inert biocompatible substances include Plexiglas (pmma) spheres in bovine collagen, ethylene vinyl alcohol (Enteryx™, Boston Scientific, Natick, MA) and an expandable hydrogel prosthesis (Gatekeeper™, Medtronic, Minneapolis, MN), all of which may be easily placed in an outpatient setting under conscious sedation.

A pilot clinical trial using submucosal injection of polymethylmethacrylate (Plexiglas, pmma) microspheres in 3.5% bovine gelatin solution has been reported.[102] Ten patients who were on PPIs to control reflux-related symptoms and who had abnormal esophageal acid exposure times were recruited to the study. Treatment sessions took 10–30 minutes, with a mean volume of about 32 mL implanted. Patients were followed up at 6 and 14.5 months after therapy. Results showed significant improvement in GERD symptom scores and distal acid exposure times following the intervention compared to baseline values, although no patients normalized their 24-hour total time of pH <4. Seven of ten subjects were completely off antireflux medications at short-term follow-up. Two patients experienced transient chest pain at the time of the implantation, and no serious complications developed post-treatment. Clusters of pmma microspheres were identified by endoscopic ultrasonography 6 months post-implantation and were seen to be scattered circumferentially in the submucosa and occasionally in the muscular layer. No further clinical study has been reported using this agent since this pilot project.

The Enteryx™ agent is an 8% ethylene vinyl alcohol (EVA) copolymer in a solution of dimethylsulfoxide (DMSO) containing micronized tantalum powder for radiographic visualization. When the implanted mixture is exposed to tissue fluids, the DMSO dissipates and the EVA becomes a spongy mass. Enteryx™ is injected into the lower esophageal sphincter area at the squamocolumnar junction, using a 4 mm, 23-gauge needle introduced through the gastroscope. Patients undergo conscious sedation, and X-ray fluoroscopy is required to visualize the intramural placement of the implant. The Enteryx™ is injected slowly under continuous observation, and 6–8 mL are typically delivered in multiple circumferential blebs. The procedure takes approximately 30 minutes to perform.

In a porcine model, injection of EVA resulted in augmentation of the gastric yield pressure.[103] In that study, the intentional injection of EVA implant into multiple extraesophageal tissues did not result in discernable harm. A pilot study was reported on 15 subjects with GERD, who demonstrated augmentation of LES pressure and improvement in heartburn score post-treatment.[104]

The results of the pivotal international multicenter Enteryx™ study were recently published and showed PPI use to be eliminated in 74% of treated subjects at 6 months and in 70% of these subjects at 12 months.[105,106] pH scores significantly improved, with 38.8% normalization at 12 months in studied subjects, and LES length was augmented by 1 cm following therapy. No effect on the incidence or severity of esophagitis after treatment was detected. At 2-year follow-up, 64% of patients remain off PPIs.[107] Although there was significant chest pain post-procedure, no serious adverse events were reported from this cohort of treated patients. A postmarketing long-term assessment study and a multicenter, randomized, sham-controlled Enteryx™ trial are currently underway.

The Gatekeeper™ device uses an overtube-style instrument through which is passed a standard or pediatric-sized videogastroscope that is used to monitor the treatment field and to provide suction within the overtube. This suction will draw mucosal tissue into multiple shallow holes in the distal part of the Gatekeeper™ instrument to stabilize it in place as the hydrogel prostheses are introduced submucosally. With the subject receiving conscious sedation, a typical upper endoscopic examination is carried out, noting the landmarks and the distance to the squamocolumnar junction. After placing a guidewire into the distal stomach, the endoscope is removed and the Gatekeeper™ tube is advanced over the wire to straddle the squamocolumnar junction. The flexible gastroscope is then introduced through the appropriate channel of the Gatekeeper™ instrument and advanced to its distal end. Suction is applied within the endoscope to draw the adjacent mucosa into the device. Using a flexible sclerotherapy-type needle, saline is injected submucosally to create a pocket into which the hydrogel implant will be placed after the pocket is pierced by a sharp trocar. The implant is directed into submucosal position by a pushrod. The polyacrylonitrile-based hydrogel implants are small and resemble pieces of 'pencil lead' when introduced, but swell to their full size within a day when hydrated. Typically, 4–6 implants are placed in a radial fashion into the submucosa at a treatment session, each implantation taking about 5 minutes to perform. One advantage of this implantation technique is its easy reversibility if needed, accomplished by using a needle knife to incise over the edge of an implant, which can then be gently suctioned out from its submucosal pocket by employing a variceal banding 'cup' attached to the distal endoscope.

While the Gatekeeper™ technique requires specific training to place the hydrogel implants in the correct manner, data from an animal trial using farm pigs demonstrated that 98% of delivery attempts were successful.[108] Eighty-eight percent of the hydrogel implants were present for up to 6 months, and 18 of 19 prostheses were retained at three years in long-term follow-up. The implants were easily removable in less than 5 minutes.

A pilot study initiated at the Academic Medical Center of the University of Amsterdam in the Netherlands in which 10 GERD patients underwent the Gatekeeper™ procedure showed that the implants were successfully placed in 97% of attempts.[109] The procedures, which were accomplished in 22 minutes or less, improved the median reflux symptom scores at 1- and 6-months follow-up. Four of nine patients were off their antisecretory medication, while three reduced their PPI dosage by at least 50% at the short-term follow-up. In a follow-up European multicenter trial, 30 additional patients underwent the Gatekeeper™ procedure. The introduction of the implant was successful in 94% of attempts, with a mean procedural time of 23 minutes. At 1 month post-implantation, 110 of 128 prostheses were still in position, while at 6 months, 47 of 62 were in correct position. Two serious adverse events occurred in this cohort: one patient suffered a pharyngeal perforation which resolved following conservative management and was thought related to the older design of the now-modified overtube instrument, and severe postprandial nausea occurred in another subject that resolved after endoscopic removal of the prostheses.

An international, multicenter, randomized, sham-controlled Gatekeeper™ trial has recently commenced and will be a pivotal trial for efficacy and safety outcomes using this technique.

The future of endoscopic GERD therapy

It is early in the evolution of endoscopic treatment of gastro-esophageal reflux disease. The utility of these new endoscopic techniques as successful GERD treatments will be determined from longer-term follow-up, additional sham-controlled studies, and from the careful scientific study of the effect of the endoscopic treatments on GERD pathophysiologic parameters. To date, most studies have enrolled patients with mild GERD, and the role of these treatments in controlling extraesophageal reflux symptoms is not known. They neither appear effective in healing erosive esophagitis nor do they consistently normalize the distal acid exposure, which will certainly limit their use in the patient with erosive esophagitis or Barrett's metaplasia. Whether this failure to control acid reflux is due to suboptimal techniques or devices must be determined. The optimal number, location, and depth of treatments, whether suturing, applying heat, or implanting materials, is not known, and may differ from that chosen by consensus in the pivotal trials. All of the data from the initial studies were from procedures performed during the investigators' learning curve, and it will be important to determine outcomes after additional experience has been accrued.

The majority of GERD patients have nonerosive disease, and these endoscopic treatments may serve well for that cohort of reflux sufferers. Ultimately, cost-effective analyses and post-marketing documentation of complications will better define the role of these new endoscopic therapies in the management of GERD patients. Although much remains to be learned, from the initial studies it appears that these treatments can improve the symptoms of selected individuals with GERD.

ANTIREFLUX SURGERY FOR THE MANAGEMENT OF GERD

Although generally very effective, pharmacological therapy of GERD is not without its drawbacks, including tachyphylaxis with H2RAs and acid rebound after cessation of antisecretory therapy.[110] In addition, severe reflux disease often requires twice-daily doses of PPIs for extended periods of time. Another issue of concern is the potential effect of nonacid components of the refluxate on the occurrence of intestinal metaplasia and the subsequent risk of developing adenocarcinoma of the esophagus. The rising incidence of adenocarcinoma within the esophagus and gastric cardia has been shown recently to be strongly associated with chronic reflux, particularly in obese subjects.[44,111]

Uncomplicated reflux disease

In the past, antireflux surgery was recommended in cases where medical treatment could not prevent the disease from having a significant negative impact on patient quality of life. Although still valid, the effectiveness of modern PPI therapy is such that only a small minority of patients fail to get substantial or complete relief of their symptoms. Nevertheless, even when effective, many patients experience rapid and consistent relapse of symptoms and esophagitis upon cessation of therapy.[39,112] Continuing symptoms of reflux with only a partial response to high-dose PPI therapy may be considered an indication for antireflux surgery,[113] but more studies will be required to assess the postoperative risk profile in this subset of patients.

Peptic stricture

The treatment of peptic strictures has been greatly improved by the introduction of PPIs.[114] In the past, surgery was the only effective treatment for strictures and when the stricture was tight and fibrotic, an esophageal resection was often required.

Resection is still indicated in extremely dense and undilatable fibrotic strictures associated with shortening of the esophagus, but the majority of strictures can be treated with endoscopic dilation and PPI therapy. However, dilatable strictures in young, fit patients may still constitute an indication for fundoplication and dilatation.

Tracheopulmonary complications

Tracheopulmonary complications due to reflux have been considered indications for antireflux surgery, although the scientific evidence for its benefit has yet to be established.[66,115,116] In clinical practice, it may be difficult to precisely select patients with concomitant reflux and tracheopulmonary symptoms in whom a beneficial effect of antireflux surgery could be predicted. It thus may be worthwhile to evaluate the effect of high-level acid suppression on symptoms to better select those individuals who might benefit from an operation.

Barrett´s esophagus

Whether the presence of Barrett's metaplasia is an indication for antireflux surgery has not been determined. Evidence suggest that continued reflux may enhance the process of neoplastic changes in the esophageal mucosa, and the results of randomized clinical trials suggest that antireflux surgery may have advantages over medical therapy in this setting.[117-119] However, it must be stressed that a fully comprehensive comparison between antireflux surgery and modern PPI therapy has as yet not been conducted. It can presently be concluded that the aim of antireflux surgery in patients with Barrett's metaplasia should be to control reflux rather than primarily to prevent progression and/or induce regression of the columnar lined segment.

Open versus laparoscopic antireflux surgery

During recent years, the rapid development of minimal access surgical techniques have emerged that have been made available by the development of new technological advances applicable to the operating room. A laparoscopic approach to antireflux surgery has gained rapid acceptance as the preferred surgical treatment since the introduction of laparoscopic Nissen fundoplication in 1991.[120] Nonrandomized comparisons have shown that laparoscopic antireflux surgery reduces hospital treatment costs and early surgical morbidity,[121,122] similar to other operations, such as inguinal herniorrhaphy, appendectomy, and cholecystectomy. However, these advantages, reported in uncontrolled studies, have not been supported by data from prospective randomized clinical trials.[123,124] Although laparoscopic antireflux surgery generally requires a longer operating time than does an equivalent open surgical procedure, the difference diminishes with increasing experience. The incidence of postoperative complications has likewise been reduced by at least 50%, and the length of postoperative stay has generally been reported to be shortened by a few days. Patients have also been shown to return to full physical function earlier following laparoscopic antireflux operations.[125-128] Short- and medium-term efficacy in controlling reflux differs little between the two different surgical approaches.[121] Two randomized clinical trials, using advanced clinical research methodology, comparing open and laparoscopic Nissen fundoplication have

recently been performed and reported.[123,124] Neither of these studies was able to demonstrate any clinically significant advantage with the laparoscopic approach. In fact, the largest study, performed in the Netherlands, had to be prematurely abandoned due to a large number of severe obstructive complaints in the laparoscopic group, requiring re-operation in a substantial proportion of patients.

Hiatal hernia repair was traditionally not a major issue during the era of open fundoplication, but it appears that this issue has become more important when performing a laparoscopic operation. The incidence of early paraesophageal herniations in patients undergoing laparoscopic operations (10%) seems to be greater than previously reported.[129-131] Circumstantial evidence exists from the old surgical literature, covering the open surgical approach, to suggest that hiatal hernia repair should generally be included when performing laparoscopic fundoplication.

Cost-effectiveness of antireflux surgery

To obtain a comprehensive picture of the merits of antireflux surgery, the cost-effectiveness of therapy must be taken into account, with a comprehensive cost analysis incorporating both direct and indirect costs. It is obvious that the total cost for medical and surgical treatment of GERD will not only vary from one country to another, but also from one time period to another.[132,133] Within the framework of a recent randomized clinical trial comparing medical and surgical antireflux therapy,[134] surgical treatment appeared to be associated with a substantial initial investment, followed by comparatively low annual costs. Furthermore, surgical treatment purportedly becomes relatively less expensive in comparison with medical therapy with the passage of time. Irrespective of the methodology used, the specific time span that must be applied to compare different therapeutic alternatives and treatment options is unclear. For example, with the introduction of laparoscopic antireflux surgery, it is obvious that the cost estimates should be adjusted. Many studies have suggested that laparoscopic antireflux surgery is less costly than open surgery based on the fact that the numbers of the days in hospital and on work absence are reduced.[135,136] A recent prospective controlled clinical trial[137] reported that, by applying the laparoscopic operative technique, the total management cost during the first postoperative year was reduced by 40%. However, in other countries when similar or even more advanced clinical research methodology has been applied, it has been difficult to demonstrate any cost benefit afforded by the laparoscopic antireflux surgical approach.

Antireflux surgery appears to be most cost-effective when performed in specialized centers with documented experience and efficacy, as reflected in the therapeutic outcome. The break-even point, compared to conventional dosing of PPIs purchased at the current retail prices, has generally been reported to occur after 5 years on therapy, after which a surgical approach may be more cost-effective in patients with a history of chronic GERD. However, such calculations assume long-term durability of laparoscopic fundoplication, an assumption that must first be corroborated by carefully performed clinical studies. Finally, the anticipated widespread availability of generic PPIs, as well as over-the-counter preparations, will add to the complexity of determining cost-effectiveness. Thus, at present, the decision to continue medical treatment or proceed with a surgical approach will

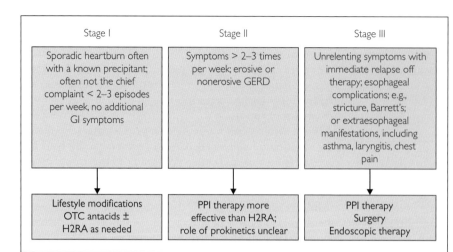

Stage I	Stage II	Stage III
Sporadic heartburn often with a known precipitant; often not the chief complaint < 2–3 episodes per week, no additional GI symptoms	Symptoms > 2–3 times per week; erosive or nonerosive GERD	Unrelenting symptoms with immediate relapse off therapy; esophageal complications; e.g., stricture, Barrett's; or extraesophageal manifestations, including asthma, laryngitis, chest pain
Lifestyle modifications OTC antacids ± H2RA as needed	PPI therapy more effective than H2RA; role of prokinetics unclear	PPI therapy Surgery Endoscopic therapy

Fig. 13.4 • A suggested approach to the use of antisecretory therapy in the treatment of GERD, based on symptoms at presentation.

require careful case-by-case discussions between patients and their physicians.

SUMMARY

A suggested approach to patients with GERD symptoms is outlined in Figure 13.4. In this schema, GERD is divided into discrete stages based on the frequency and severity of symptoms, as well as the presence of complications of GERD or extraesophageal manifestations of GERD. Stage I GERD is defined as intermittent heartburn (fewer than 2–3 episodes per week) with no complicating factors; this level of disease may be treated with lifestyle modifications, over-the-counter antacids, nonprescription H2RAs, or both as needed. Stage II disease is characterized by more frequent symptoms (more than three times per week). Although full-dose H2RA therapy may be used initially, PPI therapy is more effective in providing symptomatic relief and healing of esophagitis, if present. The role of prokinetic drugs as sole agents to treat GERD is presently undefined. Stage III GERD is defined as daily symptoms that remit as soon as symptomatic therapy is discontinued. Patients with complications of GERD, such as strictures or Barrett's esophagus, should be considered Stage III, as should patients with extraesophageal manifestations of GERD, such as asthma, laryngitis, or chest pain. These patients usually require PPI therapy either once or twice daily to relieve symptoms and prevent complications. This schema is widely applicable in clinical practice as it is based on presenting symptoms rather than the finding of endoscopic esophagitis, and it promotes tailored therapy rather than an inflexible regimen of PPIs. Patients with stage III GERD may also be considered candidates for surgical therapy, as well as for the various endoscopic approaches to treatment.

REFERENCES

1. Shaker R, Castell DO, Schoenfeld PS, et al. Nighttime heartburn is an under-appreciated clinical problem that impacts sleep and daytime function: the results of a Gallup survey conducted on behalf of the American Gastroenterological Association. Am J Gastroenterol 2003; 98(7):1487–1493.

   This is the first paper to examine the impact of nocturnal GERD symptoms. In a nationwide poll conducted in 2000, 79% of 1000 respondents reported nocturnal heartburn symptoms, 75% of which reported decreased quality of sleep, which commonly affected daytime performance. Interestingly, 41% of subjects reported using prescription medication, but only 49% of this cohort reported them to be extremely effective.

2. Katz PO. Optimizing medical therapy for gastroesophageal reflux disease: state of the art. Rev Gastroenterol Disord 2003; 3(2):59–69.

3. Kahrilas PJ. GERD pathogenesis, pathophysiology, and clinical manifestations. Cleve Clin J Med 2003; 70(Suppl 5):S4–S19.

4. Jones MP Sloan SS, Rabine JC. Hiatal hernia size is the dominant determinant of esophagitis presence and severity in gastroesophageal reflux disease. Am J Gastroenterol 2001; 96:1711–1717.

5. Mittal RK, McCallum RW. Characteristics and frequency of transient relaxations of the lower esophageal sphincter in patients with reflux esophagitis. Gastroenterology 1988; 95(3):593–599.

6. van Herwaarden MA, Samsom M, Smout AJ. Excess gastroesophageal reflux in patients with hiatus hernia is caused by mechanisms other than transient LES relaxations. Gastroenterology 2000; 119(6):1439–1446.

7. Pace F, Santalucia F, Bianchi Porro G. Natural history of gastro-oesophageal reflux disease without oesophagitis. Gut 1991; 32(8):845–848.

8. Graham DY, Patterson DJ. Double-blind comparison of liquid antacid and placebo in the treatment of symptomatic reflux esophagitis. Dig Dis Sci 1983; 28(6):559–563.

9. Weberg R, Berstad A. Symptomatic effect of a low-dose antacid regimen in reflux oesophagitis. Scand J Gastroenterol 1989; 24(4):401–406.

10. Farup PG, Weberg R, Berstad A, et al. Low-dose antacids versus 400 mg cimetidine twice daily for reflux oesophagitis. A comparative, placebo-controlled, multicentre study. Scand J Gastroenterol 1990; 25(3):315–320.

11. Tytgat GN, Nio CY. The medical therapy of reflux oesophagitis. Baillieres Clin Gastroenterol 1987; 1(4):791–807.

12. Castell D, Silvers D, Littlejohn T, et al. Cisapride 20 mg b.i.d. for preventing symptoms of GERD induced by a provocative meal. The CIS-USA-89 Study Group. Aliment Pharmacol Ther 1999; 13(6):787–794.

13. Arvanitakis C, Nikopoulos A, Theoharidis A, et al. Cisapride and ranitidine in the treatment of gastro-oesophageal reflux disease – a comparative randomized double-blind trial. Aliment Pharmacol Ther 1993; 7(6):635–641.

14. Galmiche JP, Barthelemy P, Hamelin B. Treating the symptoms of gastro-oesophageal reflux disease: a double-blind comparison of omeprazole and cisapride. Aliment Pharmacol Ther 1997; 11(4):765–773.

15. Maton PN. Profile and assessment of GERD pharmacotherapy. Cleve Clin J Med 2003; 70(Suppl 5):S51–S70.

16. McCallum RW, Fink SM, Winnan GR, et al. Metoclopramide in gastroesophageal reflux disease: rationale for its use and results of a double-blind trial. Am J Gastroenterol 1984; 79(3):165–172.

17. Guslandi M, Testoni PA, Passaretti S, et al. Ranitidine vs metoclopramide in the medical treatment of reflux esophagitis. Hepatogastroenterology 1983; 30(3):96–98.

18. Ramirez B, Richter JE. Review article: promotility drugs in the treatment of gastro-oesophageal reflux disease. Aliment Pharmacol Ther 1993; 7(1):5–20.

19. Masci E, Testoni PA, Passaretti S, et al. Comparison of ranitidine, domperidone maleate and ranitidine + domperidone maleate in the short-term treatment of reflux oesophagitis. Drugs Exp Clin Res 1985; 11(10):687–692.

20. Sontag SJ. The medical management of reflux esophagitis. Role of antacids and acid inhibition. Gastroenterol Clin North Am 1990; 19(3):683–712.

21. Sabesin SM, Berlin RG, Humphries TJ, et al. Famotidine relieves symptoms of gastroesophageal reflux disease and heals erosions and ulcerations. Results of a multicenter, placebo-controlled, dose-ranging study. USA Merck Gastroesophageal Reflux Disease Study Group. Arch Intern Med 1991; 151(12):2394–2400.

22. Tytgat GN, Nicolai JJ, Reman FC. Efficacy of different doses of cimetidine in the treatment of reflux esophagitis. A review of three large, double-blind, controlled trials. Gastroenterology 1990; 99(3):629–634.

23. Cloud ML, Offen WW, Robinson M. Nizatidine versus placebo in gastroesophageal reflux disease: a 12-week, multicenter, randomized, double-blind study. Am J Gastroenterol 1991; 86(12):1735–1742.

24. Wolfe MM, Sachs G. Acid suppression: optimizing therapy for gastroduodenal ulcer healing, gastroesophageal reflux disease, and stress-related erosive syndrome. Gastroenterology 2000; 118(2 Suppl 1):S9–S31.

This comprehensive review of acid suppression therapy provides a detailed outline of the pathophysiology of acid secretion and the role of acid in the pathogenesis of peptic ulcer, GERD, and stress erosive gastritis. The authors review the mechanisms of pharmacologic acid inhibition and summarize the clinical trial data regarding the use of acid suppressive therapies in the management of acid-peptic diseases.

25. Colin-Jones DG. The role and limitations of H2-receptor antagonists in the treatment of gastro-oesophageal reflux disease. Aliment Pharmacol Ther 1995; 9(Suppl 1):9–14.

26. Bardhan KD, Hawkey CJ, Long RG, et al. Lansoprazole versus ranitidine for the treatment of reflux oesophagitis. UK Lansoprazole Clinical Research Group. Aliment Pharmacol Ther 1995; 9(2):145–151.

27. Robinson M, Sahba B, Avner D, et al. A comparison of lansoprazole and ranitidine in the treatment of erosive oesophagitis. Multicentre Investigational Group. Aliment Pharmacol Ther 1995; 9(1):25–31.

28. Jansen JB, Van Oene JC. Standard-dose lansoprazole is more effective than high-dose ranitidine in achieving endoscopic healing and symptom relief in patients with moderately severe reflux oesophagitis. The Dutch Lansoprazole Study Group. Aliment Pharmacol Ther 1999; 13(12):1611–1620.

29. Chiba N. Proton pump inhibitors in acute healing and maintenance of erosive or worse esophagitis: a systematic overview. Can J Gastroenterol 1997; 11(Suppl B):66B–73B.

30. Caro JJ, Salas M, Ward A. Healing and relapse rates in gastroesophageal reflux disease treated with the newer proton-pump inhibitors lansoprazole, rabeprazole, and pantoprazole compared with omeprazole, ranitidine, and placebo: evidence from randomized clinical trials. Clin Ther 2001; 23(7):998–1017.

31. Richter JE, Kahrilas PJ, Johanson J, et al. Efficacy and safety of esomeprazole compared with omeprazole in GERD patients with erosive esophagitis: a randomized controlled trial. Am J Gastroenterol 2001; 96(3):656–665.

32. Castell DO, Kahrilas PJ, Richter JE, et al. Esomeprazole (40 mg) compared with lansoprazole (30 mg) in the treatment of erosive esophagitis. Am J Gastroenterol 2002; 97(3):575–583.

33. Barrison AF, Jarboe LA, Weinberg BM, et al. Patterns of proton pump inhibitor use in clinical practice. Am J Med 2001; 111(6): 469–473.

34. Watson RG, Tham TC, Johnston BT, et al. Double blind cross-over placebo controlled study of omeprazole in the treatment of patients with reflux symptoms and physiological levels of acid reflux – the 'sensitive oesophagus.' Gut 1997; 40(5):587–590.

35. Katz PO. Review article: the role of non-acid reflux in gastro-oesophageal reflux disease. Aliment Pharmacol Ther 2000; 14(12):1539–1551.

36. Tack J, Koek G, Demedts I, et al. Gastroesophageal reflux disease poorly responsive to single-dose proton pump inhibitors in patients without Barrett's esophagus: acid reflux, bile reflux, or both? Am J Gastroenterol 2004; 99(6):981–988.

37. Chiba N, De Gara CJ, Wilkinson JM, et al. Speed of healing and symptom relief in grade II to IV gastroesophageal reflux disease: a meta-analysis. Gastroenterology 1997; 112(6):1798–1810.

This meta-analysis of 43 randomized controlled trials examined the effectiveness of medical therapy in the healing of erosive esophagitis. PPI therapy was most effective, with a mean healing rate of 84%, compared with H2RA therapy (52%), sucralfate (39%), and placebo (28%). In addition, PPI therapy had a faster rate of healing and relief of heartburn symptoms than H2RA or other therapies.

38. Hetzel DJ, Dent J, Reed WD, et al. Healing and relapse of severe peptic esophagitis after treatment with omeprazole. Gastroenterology 1988; 95(4):903–912.

39. Klinkenberg-Knol EC, Festen HP, Jansen JB, et al. Long-term treatment with omeprazole for refractory reflux esophagitis: efficacy and safety. Ann Intern Med 1994; 121(3):161–167.

40. Vigneri S, Termini R, Leandro G, et al. A comparison of five maintenance therapies for reflux esophagitis. N Engl J Med 1995; 333(17):1106–1110.

This randomized prospective trial compared the effectiveness of various maintenance therapies in patients with erosive esophagitis and confirmed the superiority of PPI in the maintenance of remission.

41. Howden CW, Henning JM, Huang B, et al. Management of heartburn in a large, randomized, community-based study: comparison of four therapeutic strategies. Am J Gastroenterol 2001; 96(6):1704–1710.

42. Inadomi JM, Jamal R, Murata GH, et al. Step-down management of gastroesophageal reflux disease. Gastroenterology 2001; 121(5):1095–1100.

43. Orr WC, Allen ML, Robinson M. The pattern of nocturnal and diurnal esophageal acid exposure in the pathogenesis of erosive mucosal damage. Am J Gastroenterol 1994; 89(4):509–512.

44. Lagergren J, Bergstrom R, Lindgren A, et al. Symptomatic gastroesophageal reflux as a risk factor for esophageal adenocarcinoma. N Engl J Med 1999; 340(11):825–831.

This Swedish study confirmed the relationship between GERD and the development of adenocarcinoma of the esophagus and gastric cardia. The odds ratio for the development of esophageal adenocarcinoma was 7.7 in patients with symptomatic reflux compared to those without reflux, with an odds ratio of 2.0 for adenocarcinoma of the cardia. The risk increased with increasing duration and severity of symptoms.

45. Peghini PL, Katz PO, Bracy NA, et al. Nocturnal recovery of gastric acid secretion with twice-daily dosing of proton pump inhibitors. Am J Gastroenterol 1998; 93(5):763–767.

46. Peghini PL, Katz PO, Castell DO. Ranitidine controls nocturnal gastric acid breakthrough on omeprazole: a controlled study in normal subjects. Gastroenterology 1998; 115(6):1335–1339.

47. Fackler WK, Ours TM, Vaezi MF, eet al. Long-term effect of H2RA therapy on nocturnal gastric acid breakthrough. Gastroenterology 2002; 122(3):625–632.

48. Xue S, Katz PO, Banerjee P, et al. Bedtime H2 blockers improve nocturnal gastric acid control in GERD patients on proton pump inhibitors. Aliment Pharmacol Ther 2001; 15(9):1351–1356.

49. Ours TM, Fackler WK, Richter JE, et al. Nocturnal acid breakthrough: clinical significance and correlation with esophageal acid exposure. Am J Gastroenterol 2003; 98(3):545–550.

50. Klinkenberg-Knol EC, Nelis F, Dent J, et al. Long-term omeprazole treatment in resistant gastroesophageal reflux disease: efficacy, safety, and influence on gastric mucosa. Gastroenterology 2000; 118(4):661–669.

This study demonstrated the safety and efficacy of long-term PPI therapy in the maintenance of remission in patients with severe reflux esophagitis. With a mean of 6.5 years of follow-up, PPI therapy was effective in controlling reflux symptoms and maintaining mucosal healing without evidence of significant adverse events.

51. Dent J, Yeomans ND, Mackinnon M, et al. Omeprazole v ranitidine for prevention of relapse in reflux oesophagitis. A controlled double blind trial of their efficacy and safety. Gut 1994; 35(5):590–598.

52. Lind T, Havelund T, Lundell L, et al. On demand therapy with omeprazole for the long-term management of patients with heartburn without oesophagitis – a placebo-controlled randomized trial. Aliment Pharmacol Ther 1999; 13(7):907–914.

53. Talley NJ, Lauritsen K, Tunturi-Hihnala H, et al. Esomeprazole 20 mg maintains symptom control in endoscopy-negative gastro-oesophageal reflux disease: a controlled trial of 'on-demand' therapy for 6 months. Aliment Pharmacol Ther 2001; 15(3): 347–354.

54. Bardhan KD. Intermittent and on-demand use of proton pump inhibitors in the management of symptomatic gastroesophageal reflux disease. Am J Gastroenterol 2003; 98(3 Suppl):S40–S48.

55. Vakil N. Review article: new pharmacological agents for the treatment of gastro-oesophageal reflux disease. Aliment Pharmacol Ther 2004; 19(10):1041–1049.

56. Vela MF, Tutuian R, Katz PO, et al. Baclofen decreases acid and non-acid post-prandial gastro-oesophageal reflux measured by combined multichannel intraluminal impedance and pH. Aliment Pharmacol Ther 2003; 17(2):243—251.

57. van Herwaarden MA, Samsom M, Rydholm H, et al. The effect of baclofen on gastro-oesophageal reflux, lower oesophageal sphincter function and reflux symptoms in patients with reflux disease. Aliment Pharmacol Ther 2002; 16(9):1655–1662.

58. Koek GH, Sifrim D, Lerut T, et al. Effect of the GABA(B) agonist baclofen in patients with symptoms and duodeno-gastro-oesophageal reflux refractory to proton pump inhibitors. Gut 2003; 52(10):1397–1402.

59. Kahrilas PJ, Quigley EM, Castell DO, et al. The effects of tegaserod (HTF 919) on oesophageal acid exposure in gastro-oesophageal reflux disease. Aliment Pharmacol Ther 2000; 14(11):1503–1509.

60. el-Serag HB, Sonnenberg A. Comorbid occurrence of laryngeal or pulmonary disease with esophagitis in United States military veterans. Gastroenterology 1997; 113(3):755–760.

61. Field SK, Underwood M, Brant R, et al. Prevalence of gastroesophageal reflux symptoms in asthma. Chest 1996; 109(2):316–322.

62. Sontag SJ, O'Connell S, Khandelwal S, et al. Most asthmatics have gastroesophageal reflux with or without bronchodilator therapy. Gastroenterology 1990; 99(3):613–620.

63. Harding SM, Guzzo MR, Richter JE. The prevalence of gastroesophageal reflux in asthma patients without reflux symptoms. Am J Respir Crit Care Med 2000; 162(1):34–39.

64. Kiljander TO, Salomaa ER, Hietanen EK, et al. Gastroesophageal reflux in asthmatics: A double-blind, placebo-controlled crossover study with omeprazole. Chest 1999; 116(5):1257–1264.

65. Harding SM, Richter JE, Guzzo MR, et al. Asthma and gastroesophageal reflux: acid suppressive therapy improves asthma outcome. Am J Med 1996; 100(4):395–405.

This study examined the role of acid suppression in patients with asthma and symptomatic GERD. Thirty patients with documented asthma and GERD were treated with omeprazole, with dose titration to achieve adequate acid suppression on pH monitoring. After 3 months of therapy, patients reported significant improvement, supporting a contributory role of proximal acid reflux in symptomatic asthma.

66. Ford GA, Oliver PS, Prior JS, et al. Omeprazole in the treatment of asthmatics with nocturnal symptoms and gastro-oesophageal reflux: a placebo-controlled cross-over study. Postgrad Med J 1994; 70(823):350–354.

67. Boeree MJ, Peters FT, Postma DS, et al. No effects of high-dose omeprazole in patients with severe airway hyperresponsiveness and (a)symptomatic gastro-oesophageal reflux. Eur Respir J 1998; 11(5):1070–1074.

68. Koufman JA. The otolaryngologic manifestations of gastroesophageal reflux disease (GERD): a clinical investigation of 225 patients using ambulatory 24-hour pH monitoring and an experimental investigation of the role of acid and pepsin in the development of laryngeal injury. Laryngoscope 1991; 101(4 Pt 2 Suppl 53):1–78.

69. Batch AJ. Globus pharyngeus: (Part II), Discussion. J Laryngol Otol 1988; 102(3):227–230.

70. Irwin RS, Corrao WM, Pratter MR. Chronic persistent cough in the adult: the spectrum and frequency of causes and successful outcome of specific therapy. Am Rev Respir Dis 1981; 123(4 Pt 1):413–417.

71. El-Serag HB, Lee P, Buchner A, et al. Lansoprazole treatment of patients with chronic idiopathic laryngitis: a placebo-controlled trial. Am J Gastroenterol 2001; 96(4):979–983.

This was the first randomized placebo-controlled trial of acid suppression in patients with 'idiopathic' chronic laryngitis. Despite small sample size, a significant number of patients treated with twice-daily PPI therapy for 3 months experienced a complete resolution of symptoms, supporting the hypothesis that a subset of chronic laryngitis is a result of GERD and is amenable to therapy with acid suppression.

72. Noordzij JP, Khidr A, Evans BA, et al. Evaluation of omeprazole in the treatment of reflux laryngitis: a prospective, placebo-controlled, randomized, double-blind study. Laryngoscope 2001; 111(12):2147–2151.

73. Numans ME, Lau J, de Wit NJ, et al. Short-term treatment with proton-pump inhibitors as a test for gastroesophageal reflux disease: a meta-analysis of diagnostic test characteristics. Ann Intern Med 2004; 140(7):518–527.

74. Locke GR 3rd, Talley NJ, Fett SL, et al. Prevalence and clinical spectrum of gastroesophageal reflux: a population-based study in Olmsted County, Minnesota. Gastroenterology 1997; 112(5): 1448–1456.

75. Richter JE, Bradley LA, Castell DO. Esophageal chest pain: current controversies in pathogenesis, diagnosis, and therapy. Ann Intern Med 1989; 110(1):66–78.

76. Azpiroz F, Dapoigny M, Pace F, et al. Nongastrointestinal disorders in the irritable bowel syndrome. Digestion 2000; 62(1):66–72.

77. Fass R, Fennerty MB, Ofman JJ, et al. The clinical and economic value of a short course of omeprazole in patients with noncardiac chest pain. Gastroenterology 1998; 115(1):42–49.

This study examined the clinical reliability and cost-effectiveness of a brief empiric trial of PPI therapy as a diagnostic maneuver in patients with noncardiac chest pain. In twenty-three patients with documented GERD on pH monitoring, a 7-day course of omeprazole twice daily had a sensitivity of 78% and specificity of 86% for the diagnosis of GERD. A concurrent economic analysis demonstrated cost savings when the 'omeprazole test' was utilized in the diagnostic work-up of noncardiac chest pain.

78. Hewson EG, Sinclair JW, Dalton CB, et al. Twenty-four-hour esophageal pH monitoring: the most useful test for evaluating noncardiac chest pain. Am J Med 1991; 90(5):576–583.

79. Achem SR, Kolts BE, MacMath T, et al. Effects of omeprazole versus placebo in treatment of noncardiac chest pain and gastroesophageal reflux. Dig Dis Sci 1997; 42(10):2138–2145.

80. Fass R. Empirical trials in treatment of gastroesophageal reflux disease. Dig Dis 2000; 18(1):20–26.

81. Swain CP, Mills TN. An endoscopic sewing machine. Gastrointest Endosc 1986; 32:36–37.

82. Swain CP. Endoscopic sewing and stapling machines. Endoscopy 1997; 29:205–210.

83. Swain CP, Brown G, Mills TN. An endoscopic stapling device: development of a new flexible endoscopically controlled device for placing multiple transmural staples in gastrointestinal tissue. Gastrointest Endosc 1989; 35:338–339.

84. Gong F, Swain CP, Kadirkamanathan SS, et al. Cutting thread at flexible endoscopy. Gastrointest Endosc 1996; 44:667–674.

85. Kadirkamanathan SS, Evans DF, Gong F, et al. Antireflux operations at flexible endoscopy using endoluminal stitching techniques: an experimental study. Gastrointest Endosc 1996; 44:133–143.

86. Swain P, Park P, Mills T. Bard EndoCinch: the device, the technique, and pre-clinical studies. Gastrointest Endoscopy Clin N Am 2003; 13:75–88.

87. Filipi C, Lehman G, Rothstein RI, et al. Transoral endoscopic suturing for gastroesophageal reflux disease: a multicenter trial. Gastrointest Endosc 2001; 53:416–422.

88. Rothstein RI, Filipi CJ. Endoscopic suturing for gastroesophageal reflux disease: clinical outcomes with the Bard EndoCinch. Gastrointest Endoscopy Clin N Am 2003; 13:89–101.

89. Rothstein RI, Hynes M, Grove M, et al. Endocopic gastric plication (EndoCinch) for GERD: a randomized, sham-controlled, blinded, single-center study [Abstract]. Gastrointest Endosc 2004; 59:AB679.

90. Pleskow D, Rothstein R, Kozarek R, et al. Endoscopic full-thickness plication for GERD: a multicenter study. Gastrointest Endosc 2004; 59:163–171.

91. Chuttani R. Endoscopic full-thickness plication: the device, technique, pre-clinical and early clinical experience. Gastrointest Endoscopy Clin N Am 2003; 13:109–116.

92. Utley DS, Kim MS, Vierra MA, et al. Augmentation of lower esophageal sphincter pressure and gastric yield pressure after radiofrequency energy delivery to the gastroesophageal junction: a porcine model. Gastrointest Endosc 2000; 52:81–86.

93. DiBaise JK, Brand RE, Quigley EMM. Endoluminal delivery of radiofrequency energy to the gastroesophageal junction in uncomplicated GERD: efficacy and potential mechanism of action. Am J Gastroenterol 2002; 97:833–842.

94. Tam WCE, Schoeman MN, Zhang Q, et al. Delivery of radiofrequency energy (RFe) to the lower esophageal sphincter (LES) and gastric cardia inhibits transient LES relaxations and gastroesophageal reflux in patients with reflux disease. Gut 2003; 52:479–485.

95. Kim MS, Holloway R, Dent J, et al. Radiofrequency energy (RFe) delivery to the gastric cardia inhibits triggering of transient lower esophageal sphincter relaxations in dogs. Gastrointest Endosc 2003; 57:17–22.

96. Triadafilopoulos G, DiBiase JK, Nostrant TT, et al. Radiofrequency energy delivery to the gastro-esophageal junction for the treatment of GERD. Gastrointest Endosc 2001; 53:407–415.

97. Triadafilopoulos G, DiBaise JK, Nostrant TT, et al. The Stretta procedure for the treatment of GERD: 6 and 12 month follow-up of the U.S. open label trial. Gastrointest Endosc 2002; 55:149–156.

98. Wolfsen HC, Richards WO. The Stretta procedure for the treatment of GERD: a registry of 558 patients. J Laparoendosc Adv Surg Tech 2002; 12:395–402.

99. Corley DA, Katz P, Wo J, et al. Radiofrequency energy to the gastroesophageal junction for treatment of GERD (the Stretta procedure): a randomized, sham-controlled, multicenter clinical trial. Gastroenterology 2003; 125:668–676.

This randomized, sham-controlled trial evaluated the effectiveness of endoscopic radiofrequency therapy (STRETTA) for GERD. At 6 months of follow-up, patients in the active treatment arm had significantly improved heartburn symptoms and quality of life scores compared with sham controls. Medication use and acid exposure time, however, were not significantly different. This early trial suggests a role of endoscopic radiofrequency ablation for the control of GERD symptoms.

100. Lehman GA. The history and future of implantation therapy for gastroesophageal reflux disease. Gastrointest Endoscopy Clin N Am 2003; 13:157–165.

101. O'Connor MD, Lehman GA. Endoscopic placement of collagen at the lower esophageal sphincter to inhibit gastroesophageal reflux – a pilot study of 10 medically intractable patients. Gastrointest Endosc 1988; 34:106–112.

102. Feretis C, Benakis P, Dimopoulos C, et al. Endoscopic implantation of Plexiglas (PMMA) microspheres for the treatment of GERD. Gastrointest Endosc 2001; 53:423–426.

103. Mason R, Hughes M, Lehman G, et al. Endoscopic augmentation of the cardia with a biocompatible injectable polymer (Enteryx) in a porcine model. Surg Endosc 2002; 16:386–391.

104. Deviere J, Pastorelli A, Hubert L, et al. Endoscopic implantation of a biopolymer in the lower esophageal sphincter for gastroesophageal reflux: a pilot study. Gastrointest Endosc 2002; 55:335–341.

105. Johnson DA, Ganz R, Aisenberg J, et al. Endoscopic, deep mural implantation of Enteryx for the treatment of GERD: 6-month follow-up of a multicenter trial. Am J Gastroenterol 2003; 98:250–258.

106. Johnson DA, Ganz R, Aisenberg J, et al. Endoscopic implantation of Enteryx for the treatment of GERD: 12-month results of a prospective multicenter trial. Am J Gastroenterol 2003; 98:1921–1930.

107. Cohen L, Johnson DA, Ganz R, et al. Enteryx solution, a minimally invasive injectable treatment for GERD: analysis of extended follow-up through 24 months [Abstract]. Am J Gastroenterol 2003; 98:A71.

108. Easter DW, Yurek M, Johnson G. Long-term retention of endoscopically placed hydrogel prostheses at the lower esophageal sphincter in pigs. Surg Endosc 2004; 18:448–451.

109. Fockens P. Gatekeeper reflux repair system: technique, pre-clinical and clinical experience. Gastrointest Endoscopy Clin N Am 2003; 13:179–189.

110. Scarpignato C, Galmiche JP. The role of H_2 receptor antagonist in the area of proton pump inhibitors. In: Lundell L, ed. Guidelines for management for symptomatic gastroesophageal reflux disease. London: Science Press Ltd; 1988:55–66.

111. Pera AM, Cameron AJ, Trastec VF. Increasing incidence in adenocarcinoma of the oesophagus and esophagogastric junction. Gastroenterology 1993; 104:510–513.

112. Bardhan KD. The role of the proton pump inhibitors in the treatment of gastro-esophageal reflux disease. Aliment Pharmacol Therapeut 1995; 9(suppl 1):15–25.

113. Lundell L, Dalenbäck J, Hattlebakk J, et al. Nordic GORD Study Group. Outcome of open antireflux surgery as assessment in a Nordic multicenter, prospective clinical trial. Eur J Surg 1998; 164:751–757.

114. Marks RD, Richter JE, Rizzo J, et al. Omeprazole versus H_2-receptor antagonists in treating patients with peptic stricture and oesophagitis. Gastroenterology 1994; 106:907–915.

115. DeMeester TR, Bonavina L, Lascone C, et al. Chronic respiratory symptoms and occult gastro-esophageal reflux: a prospective clinical trial and results of surgical therapy. Ann Surg 1990; 211:337–345.

116. Ruth M, Bake B, Sandberg N, et al. Pulmonary function in gastro-esophageal reflux disease. Effects of reflux controlled by fundoplication disease of the oesophagus. Dis Oesophagus 1994; 7:268–275.

117. Ortiz A, Martinez LF, Parrilla P, et al. Conservative treatment vs antireflux surgery in Barrett's oesophagus: long-term results of a prospective study. Br J Surg 1996; 83:274–278.

118. Csendes A, Braghetto I, Burdiles P, et al. Long-term results of classic antireflux surgery in 152 patients with Barrett's oesophagus: clinical radiologic, endoscopic, manometric and acid reflux test analysis before and late after operation. Surgery 1998; 123:645–657.

119. Parrilla P, Martinez LF, DeHaro LF, et al. Long-term results of randomised prospective study comparing medical and surgical treatment of Barrett's oesophagus. Ann Surg 2003; 237:291–298.

120. Dallemagne B, Weerts JM, Jehaes C, et al. Laparoscopic Nissen fundoplication: preliminary report. Surg Laparosc Endosc 1991; 1:138–143.

121. Peridikis G, Hinder RA, Lund RJ, et al. Laparoscopic Nissen fundoplication: where do we stand? Surg Laparosc Endosc 1997; 7:17–21.

122. Watson DI, Jamieson GG. Antireflux surgery in laparoscopic era. Br J Surg 1998; 85:1173–1184.

123. Bais JE, Bantelsman JF, Bonjer HJ, et al. Laparoscopic or conventional Nissen fundoplication for gastro-esophageal reflux disease: randomised clinical trial. The Netherlands Antireflux Surgery Study Group. Lancet 2000; 355:170–174.

124. Nilsson G, Larsson S, Johnsson F. Randomised clinical trial of laparoscopic versus open fundoplication: blind evaluation of recovery and discharge period. Br J Surg 2000; 87:873–878.

125. Frantzides CT, Carlson MA. Laparoscopic versus conventional fundoplication. J Laparoendosc Surg 1995: 5:137–143.

126. Richards KF, Fisher KS, Flores JH, et al. Laparoscopic Nissen fundoplication: cost, morbidity and outcome compared with open surgery. Surg Laparosc Endosc 1996; 6:140–143.

127. Rattner DW, Brooks DC. Patient satisfaction following laparoscopic and open antireflux surgery. Arch Surg 1995; 130:289–294.

128. Champault G, Volter F, Rizk N, et al. Gastro-esophageal reflux: conventional surgical treatment versus laparoscopy. A prospective study of 61 cases. Surg Laparosc Endosc 1996; 6:434–440.

129. Seeling MH, Hinder RA, Klinger PJ, et al. Paresophageal herniation as a complication following laparoscopic antireflux surgery. J Gastrointest Surg 1999; 3:95–99.

130. Edye MB, Canin-Endres J, Gattorno F, et al. Durability of laparoscopic repair of paraoesophageal hernia. Ann Surg 1998; 228:528–535.

131. Watson DI, Jamieson GG, Devitt PG, et al. Paraoesophageal hiatus hernia: an important complication of laparoscopic Nissen fundoplication. Br J Surg 1995; 82:521–523.

132. van der Boom G, Go PMMUH, Hameeteman W, et al. Cost effectiveness of medical versus surgical treatment in patients with severe or refractory gastro-esophageal reflux disease in the Netherlands. Scand J Gastroenterol 1996; 31:1–9.

133. Heudebert G, Marks R, Wilcox C, et al. Choice of long-term strategy in the management of patients with severe esophagitis: a cost utility analysis. Gastroenterology 1996; 112:1078 1086.

134. Myrvold HE, Lundell L, Liedman B, et al. The cost of omeprazole versus open antireflux surgery in the long-term management of reflux esophagitis. Gut 2000; 49:488–494.

135. Incarbone R, Peters JH, Heimbucher J, et al. A contemporaneous comparison of hospital charges for laparoscopic and open Nissen fundoplication. Surg Endosc 1995; 9:151–155.

136. Laycock WS, Oddsdottir M, Franco A, et al. Laparoscopic Nissen fundoplication is less expensive than open Belsey Mark IV. Surg Endosc 1995; 9:426–429.

137. Blomqvist AMK, Lönroth H, Dalenbäck J, et al. Laparoscopic or open fundoplication? A complete cost analysis. Surg Endosc 1998; 12:1209–1212.

Barrett's esophagus

Stuart Jon Spechler

INTRODUCTION

History

Barrett's esophagus is the condition in which an intestinal-type epithelium (called specialized intestinal metaplasia) that is predisposed to malignancy replaces esophageal squamous epithelium that has been damaged by gastroesophageal reflux disease (GERD).[1] GERD and Barrett's esophagus are the major risk factors for esophageal adenocarcinoma, a tumor whose frequency has increased more than fourfold in frequency over the past several decades.[2,3] The condition is named for Norman Rupert Barrett, an Australian surgeon practicing in England, who drew attention to the 'short esophagus' in a treatise that he published in 1950.[4] The eponym 'Barrett's esophagus' has been retained despite the fact that Norman Barrett was not the first to describe the esophagus lined by columnar epithelium, and that his speculations regarding the nature and pathogenesis of the condition were incorrect.[5]

Early controversies about Barrett's esophagus focused on whether the condition was congenital or acquired, and on whether the esophageal columnar epithelium was gastric or intestinal in type.[5] Today, it is widely accepted that the condition is acquired as a consequence of chronic GERD, and that the demonstration of intestinal metaplasia in the esophagus is required for the diagnosis. For decades, Barrett's esophagus generally was not recognized unless the distal esophagus was lined by at least 3 cm of columnar epithelium. Since the demonstration by Spechler et al. in 1994 that short segments of intestinal metaplasia are found frequently in the distal esophagus, Barrett's esophagus has been categorized as 'long-segment' when columnar epithelium lines more than 3 cm of the distal esophagus, and as 'short-segment' when there is less than 3 cm of columnar lining.[6]

Epidemiology

Barrett's esophagus has been described in young children, but the condition usually is discovered in middle-aged and older adults.[7,8] The average age at the time of diagnosis is approximately 55 years, and white men predominate in most series. For unknown reasons, Barrett's esophagus is uncommon in blacks and Asians. In most cases, Barrett's esophagus is discovered during endoscopic examinations performed for the evaluation of chronic GERD symptoms such as heartburn, regurgitation, and dysphagia. Long-segment Barrett's esophagus can be found in 3–5% of such patients, whereas 10–15% have short-segment Barrett's esophagus.[1]

The prevalence of Barrett's esophagus in the general population is not known, but a recent study has shed some light on this issue. Among 961 patients scheduled for elective colonoscopy who agreed to have an upper gastrointestinal endoscopy performed for research purposes, Barrett's esophagus (predominantly short-segment) was found in 6.8%.[9] Among the 556 patients who had no heartburn, Barrett's esophagus was found in 5.6%, whereas 8.3% of 384 patients who complained of heartburn had Barrett's esophagus. The difference in the frequency of short-segment Barrett's esophagus between the patients with and without heartburn was not significant.

PATHOGENESIS

Barrett's esophagus develops through the process of metaplasia in which one adult cell type replaces another.[10] This metaplasia is judged to be a sequela of chronic esophageal inflammation caused by GERD, and a number of physiological abnormalities that predispose to severe GERD have been described in patients with long-segment Barrett's esophagus. For example, some patients exhibit gastric acid hypersecretion and duodenogastric reflux.[11–13] In these patients, the refluxed gastric juice contains high concentrations of caustic acid and bile that can be exceptionally damaging to the esophagus. Manometric studies have revealed extreme hypotension of the lower esophageal sphincter (an important barrier to gastroesophageal reflux), and patients with this abnormality are exceptionally predisposed to reflux.[14] Some have poor esophageal contractility, an abnormality that may delay the clearance of noxious material from the esophagus.[15] Diminished esophageal pain sensitivity has been demonstrated, and so the reflux of caustic material may not cause heartburn.[16] Decreased salivary secretion of epidermal growth factor, a peptide that enhances the healing of peptic ulceration, has been reported in some patients.[17] This abnormality might delay healing of the reflux-damaged esophagus. Individual patients may exhibit none or all of these abnormalities, and their frequency in Barrett's esophagus is disputed. For example, Hirschowitz did not find gastric acid hypersecretion in his patients with Barrett's esophagus.[18]

The frequency with which physiological abnormalities that predispose to GERD affect patients with short-segment Barrett's esophagus is not clear. Many patients with short-segment disease have no GERD symptoms and no endoscopic signs of esophagitis.[19] Some studies suggest that the length of metaplastic mucosa in Barrett's esophagus is related to the duration of esophageal acid exposure.[20] Thus, patients with long-segment disease may have protracted esophageal acid exposure, whereas patients with short-segment Barrett's esophagus may have esophageal acid exposure values that are normal or only minimally increased.

Recent studies have shown that the gastroesophageal junction (GEJ) region is an especially hostile place. After meals, there is a pocket of acid at the GEJ that escapes the buffering effects of ingested food.[21] This postprandial acid pocket has a mean length of 2 cm, beginning in the most proximal stomach and extending more than 1 cm above the squamocolumnar junction into the distal esophagus. Another recent study has shown that the very distal esophagus (5 mm above the squamocolumnar junction) of healthy volunteers is exposed to acid for more than 10% of the day.[22] Potential consequences of such persistent acid exposure at the GEJ include not only acid-peptic injury, but also exposure to high concentrations of nitric oxide (NO) generated from dietary nitrate (NO_3^-) in green, leafy vegetables. Most ingested nitrate is absorbed by the small intestine and excreted unchanged in the urine, but approximately 25% is concentrated by the salivary glands and secreted into the mouth where bacteria on the tongue reduce the recycled nitrate to nitrite (NO_2^-). When swallowed nitrite encounters acidic gastric juice, the nitrite is converted rapidly to nitric oxide (NO). After nitrate ingestion, high levels of NO have been demonstrated at the GEJ.[23] NO in these concentrations can be genotoxic and, potentially, carcinogenic. Thus, the GEJ is exposed repeatedly to acid, pepsin, NO, and other noxious agents in gastric juice. Chronic exposure to these agents may induce the injury and inflammation that results in the intestinal metaplasia of short-segment Barrett's esophagus.[24]

DIAGNOSIS

Requisite diagnostic factors for Barrett's esophagus

Endoscopic examination is required to diagnose Barrett's esophagus. Two diagnostic criteria must be fulfilled:[25] (1) the endoscopist must document that columnar epithelium lines the distal esophagus, and (2) histological examination of biopsy specimens of the esophageal columnar epithelium must reveal specialized intestinal metaplasia. To document that columnar epithelium lines the esophagus, the endoscopist must identify both the squamo-columnar and gastroesophageal junctions (Fig. 14.1). Columnar epithelium has a reddish color and coarse texture on endoscopic examination, whereas squamous epithelium has a pale, glossy appearance. The juxtaposition of these epithelia at the squamo-columnar junction forms a visible line called the Z-line. The gastroesophageal junction, in contrast, is the imaginary line at which the esophagus ends and the stomach begins anatomically. The gastroesophageal junction can be recognized endoscopically as the level of the most proximal extent of the gastric folds.[26] When the squamocolumnar and gastroesophageal junctions coincide (Fig. 14.2), the entire esophagus is lined by squamous epithelium. When the squamocolumnar junction is located proximal to the gastroesophageal junction (see Fig. 14.1), there is a columnar-lined segment of esophagus. If biopsy specimens from that segment show specialized intestinal metaplasia, then the patient has Barrett's esophagus. Such a patient has long-

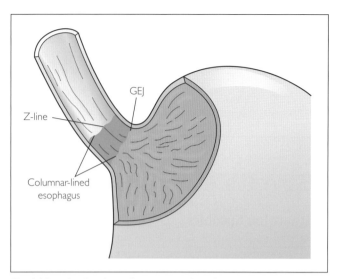

Fig. 14.1 ● Landmarks at the gastroesophageal junction region. The squamocolumnar junction (SCJ or Z-line) is the visible line formed by the juxtaposition of squamous and columnar epithelia. The gastroesophageal junction (GEJ) is the imaginary line at which the esophagus ends and the stomach begins. The GEJ corresponds to the most proximal extent of the gastric folds. When the SCJ is located proximal to the GEJ, there is a columnar-lined segment of esophagus. (Reprinted from Spechler SJ, Gastroenterology 1999; 117:218–228. © 1999, with permission from The American Gastroenterological Association.)

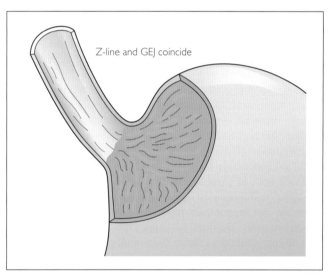

Fig. 14.2 ● The SCJ and GEJ coincide. In this situation, there is no apparent columnar-lined esophagus (i.e., the entire esophagus is lined by squamous epithelium). (Reprinted from Spechler SJ, Gastroenterology 1999; 117:218–228. © 1999, with permission from The American Gastroenterological Association.)

segment Barrett's esophagus if the distance between the Z-line and the GEJ is 3 cm or more, and short-segment Barrett's esophagus if that distance is less than 3 cm.

Controversies regarding the normal squamocolumnar junction

Both the histological type and the precise anatomical location of the columnar epithelium at the normal Z-line are disputed.

Traditional teaching holds that the normal Z-line is a junction between squamous epithelium and cardiac epithelium, a glandular, columnar mucosa comprised almost exclusively of mucus-secreting cells.[27] It has been alleged that cardiac epithelium can line up to 2 cm of the most distal esophagus, and may extend several centimeters below the GEJ to line the gastric cardia.[27,28] However, the evidence on which these claims are based is dubious. Endoscopically, the gastric folds that delimit the stomach are dynamic structures whose proximal extent may vary with respiration and gagging, and with the degree of gastric distention. Surgical and autopsy specimens of the esophagus and stomach can be manipulated mechanically so that the landmarks used to identify the GEJ (e.g., the proximal extent of gastric folds, the angle of His) vary considerably in location. Without a fixed and precise marker for the GEJ, it is difficult to establish whether the Z-line normally is located precisely at or slightly proximal to the junction of esophagus and stomach. Thus, it is not clear whether it is normal to have a short segment of columnar-lined esophagus.

Pathologists disagree on the fundamental, histological characteristics of cardiac epithelium. Some feel that the presence of any parietal cells in the glands precludes a histological diagnosis of cardiac epithelium, and recommend the terms 'oxyntocardiac mucosa' or 'transitional mucosa' to describe a cardiac-type epithelium that has occasional parietal cells.[29] Others contend that cardiac epithelium can have occasional parietal cells provided that other architectural features of the glands are typical of cardiac mucosa.[30] Furthermore, authorities dispute whether cardiac epithelium is even a normal structure. Chandrasoma and colleagues have proposed that the normal Z-line is a junction between squamous and oxyntic epithelia, and that cardiac epithelium is a metaplastic mucosa acquired as a consequence of chronic inflammation in the distal esophagus caused by GERD.[29,31]

A recent study of 40 patients who had subtotal esophagectomy with intrathoracic esophagogastrostomy, an operation frequently complicated by severe reflux esophagitis in the esophageal remnant, supports the notion that cardiac epithelium is metaplastic.[32] Endoscopic examinations performed at a median of 36 months postoperatively showed that 19 of the 40 patients had developed columnar metaplasia in the esophageal remnant (10 cardiac epithelium, 9 intestinal metaplasia). Seven patients who had serial endoscopic examinations showed progression from cardiac epithelium on the initial postoperative endoscopy to specialized intestinal metaplasia on subsequent studies. The median time to the development of cardiac epithelium was 14 months, whereas specialized intestinal metaplasia was found at a median of 27 months postoperatively. These findings suggest that cardiac epithelium is metaplastic, and the precursor of the specialized intestinal metaplasia of Barrett's esophagus.

Finally, it appears that cardiac epithelium occupies a considerably shorter segment of the GEJ than suggested by traditional texts. Cardiac epithelium, if present at all, rarely extends more than a few millimeters below the Z-line.[33–35] One group reported that cardiac mucosa always was located on the gastric side of the GEJ,[33] but it is unlikely that the gross landmarks that this group used to identify the GEJ have the precision necessary to localize a structure whose extent is measured in millimeters. In summary, it remains unclear whether the tiny band of cardiac mucosa at the GEJ is a normal structure, and whether it normally lines the esophagus, the gastric cardia, or both.

Intestinal metaplasia at the gastroesophageal junction

Intestinal metaplasia can develop in the stomach, the esophagus, or both. On routine histological examination, intestinal metaplasia in the stomach cannot be distinguished from intestinal metaplasia in the esophagus. Since the GEJ cannot be identified with great precision, it can be difficult to determine whether short segments of intestinal metaplasia found in the GEJ region are lining the esophagus (short-segment Barrett's esophagus) or the proximal stomach (intestinal metaplasia of the gastric cardia).[10] The term 'intestinal metaplasia at the GEJ' has been used to describe the condition in which intestinal metaplasia is found at a Z-line that appears to coincide precisely with the GEJ. Rather than constituting an independent condition, however, intestinal metaplasia at the GEJ almost certainly represents either short-segment Barrett's esophagus or intestinal metaplasia of the cardia.

Intestinal metaplasia in the stomach often results from the chronic gastritis caused by *H. pylori* infection,[36] whereas chronic reflux esophagitis causes intestinal metaplasia in the esophagus. For some patients, therefore, intestinal metaplasia at the GEJ is due to *H. pylori* gastritis, whereas, for others, the condition results from GERD that causes intestinal metaplasia in segments of esophagus so short that they cannot be distinguished from the serrations of a normal Z-line. Some studies even suggest that *H. pylori* infection protects against Barrett's esophagus and other complications of GERD, perhaps by causing a diffuse gastritis that decreases gastric acid secretion.[37] *H. pylori* gastritis is not rare in patients with Barrett's esophagus, however, and testing for *H. pylori* is not a reliable way to distinguish short-segment Barrett's esophagus from intestinal metaplasia of the gastric cardia.[38]

For patients with intestinal metaplasia at the GEJ, it may be important to distinguish short-segment Barrett's esophagus from intestinal metaplasia of the gastric cardia because the former condition appears to have a substantially higher risk of malignancy. For example, Sharma et al. found dysplasia (the precursor of malignancy) in 20 of 177 patients (11.3%) with short-segment Barrett's esophagus, but in only 1 of 76 patients (1.3%) with intestinal metaplasia in the gastric cardia.[39] Authorities recommend endoscopic cancer surveillance routinely for patients with Barrett's esophagus, but not for patients with intestinal metaplasia in the stomach.[40,41] Therefore, the distinction between these two conditions has important implications for patient management. A number of histochemical and immunological biomarkers have been proposed to differentiate intestinal metaplasia of the cardia from short-segment Barrett's esophagus including cytokeratin staining patterns,[42–45] immunoreactivity for mAb Das-1 (a monoclonal antibody raised against colonic epithelial cells),[46] and mucosal expression of colonic-type sulfomucins.[44] However, a recent review has concluded that the utility of biomarkers in distinguishing short-segment Barrett's esophagus from intestinal metaplasia of the gastric cardia has not been established, and clinical decisions should not be based on the presence of these biomarkers.[47]

Dysplasia in Barrett's esophagus

Dysplasia is the histological expression of DNA damage that favors cell growth and neoplasia.[48] The histological features of dysplasia include nuclear changes such as enlargement, pleomorphism, hyperchromatism, stratification, atypical mitoses, and architectural abnormalities such as crowding of tubules and villiform surfaces.[49] These histological abnormalities suggest that the tissue has sustained DNA damage resulting in clonal proliferations of cells with abnormal differentiation and a predisposition to malignancy. Dysplasia is categorized as low-grade or high-grade depending on the degree of histological abnormalities, with more pronounced abnormalities reflecting more severe genetic damage and greater potential for carcinogenesis.

Histological changes similar to those of low-grade dysplasia can be seen in non-neoplastic tissue that is regenerating in response to injury, and it can be difficult for pathologists to distinguish low-grade dysplasia in Barrett's esophagus from reactive changes caused by reflux esophagitis. Interobserver agreement among experienced pathologists for the diagnosis of low-grade dysplasia may be less than 50%, whereas interobserver agreement for distinguishing high-grade dysplasia from lesser lesions is approximately 85%.[50–52] Furthermore, there can be substantial interobserver disagreement when distinguishing high-grade dysplasia from intramucosal carcinoma, a lesion which has potential for lymphatic dissemination.[53]

Dysplasia in Barrett's esophagus often is flat, inconspicuous, and patchy both in extent and severity.[54,55] Endoscopists rely on random biopsy sampling techniques to identify dysplasia and, consequently, dysplastic areas easily can be missed because of biopsy sampling error. For patients found to have dysplasia, furthermore, foci of higher-grade lesions (including invasive cancer) can be missed. In series of patients who had esophagectomies because endoscopic examination revealed high-grade dysplasia in Barrett's esophagus with no apparent tumor mass, invasive cancer (missed because of biopsy sampling error) has been found in 30–40% of the resected esophagi.[56] Extensive biopsy sampling of the Barrett esophagus can reduce biopsy sampling error, but cannot eliminate the problem entirely.[57,58]

A number of molecular markers for cancer risk and endoscopic techniques for recognizing early esophageal neoplasia have been proposed as alternatives to random biopsy sampling to seek dysplasia in Barrett's esophagus.[59,60] Promising molecular markers include abnormalities in p53 and cyclin D1 expression, and abnormal cellular DNA content demonstrable by flow cytometry, all of which have been associated with carcinogenesis in Barrett's esophagus.[61–63] Techniques to identify neoplastic areas for biopsy sampling during endoscopy include mucosal staining with vital dyes (chromoendoscopy), endosonography, optical coherence tomography, and spectroscopy using reflectance, absorption, light-scattering, fluorescence, and Raman detection methods.[64–68] Although preliminary study results are promising, none of these tests and techniques has yet been shown to provide sufficient clinical information to justify its routine application for surveillance purposes.

Natural history of dysplasia

Much circumstantial evidence suggests that cancers in Barrett's esophagus evolve through a sequence of genetic alterations that are heralded by histological changes of progressive severity. Few studies document the natural history of dysplasia, however, and the rate with which low-grade dysplasia progresses to high-grade dysplasia and cancer is not clear. Furthermore, the fact that low-grade dysplasia in Barrett's esophagus is not diagnosed reliably is a major problem that confounds the interpretation of all studies on this condition. Diagnostic difficulties may underlie the large disparities among published series regarding the prevalence and incidence of low-grade dysplasia in Barrett's esophagus. In one large series, low-grade dysplasia was described in approximately 70% of patients.[69] However, a recent study that reviewed the pathology archives of three large university hospitals using strict diagnostic criteria for dysplasia identified low-grade dysplasia in only 37 (4.7%) of 790 cases of Barrett's esophagus.[70] For comparison, high-grade dysplasia was found in 20 (2.5%) of those 790 cases.

One study of 48 patients with low-grade dysplasia found that 5 (10%) progressed to high-grade dysplasia (4 patients) or adenocarcinoma (1 patient) during a mean follow-up of 41 months.[71] Another group described a 12% cumulative incidence of adenocarcinoma at 5 years for 43 patients with low-grade dysplasia on baseline endoscopy.[63] Skacel et al. followed 25 patients with low-grade dysplasia for a mean duration of 26 months, during which 7 (28%) progressed to high-grade dysplasia (5 patients) or adenocarcinoma (2 patients).[51] In this series, agreement among pathologists in the diagnosis of low-grade dysplasia was associated with neoplastic progression. Seven of the 17 patients (41%) in whom at least 2 of the 3 study pathologists agreed on the diagnosis of low-grade dysplasia exhibited progression, whereas progression was seen in 4 of the 5 patients (80%) for whom there was unanimous agreement among the study pathologists.

Reported estimates on the rate at which high-grade dysplasia in Barrett's esophagus progresses to cancer vary considerably. One report described 8 patients with high-grade dysplasia in Barrett's esophagus, 5 (63%) of whom were found to have adenocarcinomas on repeat endoscopic examinations performed within one year.[71] Reid et al. reported a 59% 5-year cumulative cancer incidence among their 76 patients with high-grade dysplasia in Barrett's esophagus.[63] In Buttar's series of 100 consecutive patients with high-grade dysplasia found by surveillance endoscopy, cancers were detected in 32% during a follow-up period of up to 8 years.[72] In contrast, Schnell reported that only 12 (16%) of his 75 patients with high-grade dysplasia in Barrett's esophagus developed adenocarcinoma during a mean follow-up period of 7.3 years.[69] The reasons underlying the large disparities in the results of these studies are not clear. Buttar found that the extent of high-grade dysplasia in Barrett's esophagus correlated with the risk for adenocarcinoma,[72] but other investigators have not confirmed this observation.[73,74]

Screening and surveillance for Barrett's esophagus

To decrease mortality from esophageal adenocarcinoma, it has been proposed that patients with GERD symptoms should be screened endoscopically for Barrett's esophagus, and that patients found to have Barrett's esophagus should have regular endoscopic surveillance for dysplasia. The rationale for this proposal includes the following assumptions: (1) screening will reliably identify those individuals at highest risk for developing esophageal adenocarcinoma, (2) without intervention, patients with Barrett's esophagus will have decreased survival because of deaths from esophageal adenocarcinoma, (3) surveillance will reliably detect dysplasia in Barrett's esophagus, and (4) treatment of the dysplasia found by surveillance will prolong survival and improve quality of life by preventing death and morbidity from esophageal cancer. All of these assumptions are unproved and questionable.

First, it is not clear that screening patients with GERD symptoms reliably identifies those individuals at high risk for esophageal adenocarcinoma. Indeed, available studies suggest that 40% of patients with esophageal adenocarcinoma have no history of GERD symptoms.[3] Therefore, screening programs that target only patients with heartburn can have only limited impact on cancer mortality rates, and there is little evidence that these programs have prevented deaths from esophageal adenocarcinomas. In published series of patients found to have these tumors, fewer than 5% were known to have had Barrett's esophagus before they sought medical attention for symptoms of esophageal cancer.[75]

A number of studies have suggested that Barrett's esophagus does not affect survival.[76–79] In these series, survival for patients with Barrett's esophagus did not appear to differ significantly from that for control subjects in the general population. However, those studies comprised predominantly older patients who often succumbed to common comorbid illnesses such as coronary artery disease rather than to esophageal adenocarcinoma. Proponents of surveillance argue that the results of those studies may not be applicable to younger, healthier patients with Barrett's esophagus.

Observational studies have documented that endoscopic surveillance can detect curable neoplasms in Barrett's esophagus, and that asymptomatic cancers discovered during surveillance are less advanced than those found in patients who present with cancer symptoms such as dysphagia and weight loss.[80–83] Those studies are highly susceptible to a number of biases, however, and it is not appropriate to conclude that surveillance is beneficial based solely on the observation that patients with asymptomatic neoplasms survive longer than patients who have symptoms due to esophageal cancer.[84] No study has established the reliability of surveillance in detecting curable dysplasia, and a number of reports have documented the development of incurable malignancies in some patients despite adherence to endoscopic surveillance programs[80,81] Furthermore, hazardous invasive therapies for dysplasia, such as esophagectomy, ultimately might do more harm than good.

Some computer models have suggested that endoscopic screening and surveillance for Barrett's esophagus can be beneficial provided that certain baseline assumptions are valid.[85–88] It is important to appreciate that these models do not provide a single definitive answer, but rather a range of possible outcomes that vary with changes in the baseline assumptions. One group used a decision tree to explore the utility of one-time endoscopic screening for high-grade dysplasia in 60 year-old patients with GERD symptoms. The model estimated that screening might cost US$24 700 per life-year saved, provided that a number of baseline conditions were favorable (e.g., relatively high prevalence of dysplasia in the group screened, low cost for endoscopy, good health-related quality of life after esophagectomy).[86] Another group used a Markov model to construct a computer cohort simulation of 10 000 middle-aged patients with Barrett's esophagus, and assumed that esophagectomy would be performed for those whose surveillance endoscopies showed high-grade dysplasia. For an annual cancer incidence rate of 0.4%, this analysis suggested that endoscopic surveillance performed every 5 years was the preferred strategy, costing US$98 000 per quality-adjusted life year gained.[85] Another, more recent cost-utility analysis contra-

dicted the findings of the latter model, concluding that whereas screening for Barrett's esophagus might be cost-effective, surveillance is not.[88] None of these computer models can be considered definitive, however, because all incorporate numerous layers of soft data and questionable assumptions.

In a recent editorial, Spechler summarized the dilemma regarding screening and surveillance for Barrett's esophagus as follows:[89] (1) endoscopy is expensive; (2) there is no proof that endoscopic screening of patients with GERD for Barrett's esophagus has any impact on survival; (3) no 'proof' in the form of a randomized controlled trial is likely to become available in the near future; (4) available observational studies, which are subject to numerous forms of bias, suggest that screening and surveillance are beneficial; (5) available computer models, which are based on some soft data and questionable assumptions, suggest that screening can be beneficial, and (6) although endoscopic screening clearly can be associated with risks (i.e., complications resulting both from endoscopy and from the invasive procedures used to treat conditions found by endoscopy), no study has shown an overall survival disadvantage for patients in screening and surveillance programs. In this murky situation, where the indirect evidence available suggests that screening and surveillance are beneficial and the major objection is cost, it seems better to err by performing unnecessary endoscopy rather than by missing curable esophageal neoplasms.

TREATMENT OF BARRETT'S ESOPHAGUS

Treatment of GERD in Barrett's esophagus

The primary goals of antireflux therapy, irrespective of the presence of Barrett's esophagus, are elimination of the symptoms and signs of reflux esophagitis, and prevention of GERD complications such as peptic esophageal stricture. The general principles of antireflux therapy are discussed elsewhere in this book, and this section is devoted only to those features that pertain specifically to the treatment of GERD in Barrett's esophagus.

Authorities debate whether proton pump inhibitors (PPIs) or histamine H_2-receptor antagonists (H2RAs) should be used as initial therapy for patients with GERD of mild to moderate severity.[90] Reliable healing of severe GERD generally requires treatment with PPIs, however, and there is a consensus that PPIs should be initial therapy for patients with severe GERD.[89,91] Whereas long-segment Barrett's esophagus is associated with severe reflux esophagitis, PPIs usually are prescribed as first-line therapy for GERD in such patients.[92] Patients with short-segment Barrett's esophagus often have mild GERD, however, and H2RA therapy might be sufficient to control their symptoms and signs of reflux disease. Some patients with Barrett's esophagus have no signs or symptoms of active GERD, and it is not clear that any antireflux therapy is warranted in these cases.[93]

Conventional-dose antisecretory therapy reduces, but does not abolish gastric acid secretion in most patients with Barrett's esophagus. The effect of antisecretory therapy on GERD symptoms in these patients does not accurately reflect the level of acid suppression achieved. Esophageal pH monitoring studies frequently reveal pathological levels of acid reflux in patients with Barrett's esophagus rendered asymptomatic by PPIs administered in conventional dosages.[94] Approximately 80% of patients with Barrett's esophagus treated with a PPI twice daily experience the phenomenon of nocturnal gastric acid breakthrough (defined as a fall in gastric pH below 4 for more than 1 hour at night) which is often associated with episodes of acid reflux.[95]

It is sometimes possible to achieve almost complete achlorhydria by administering PPIs in high dosages, or by adding a bedtime dose of an H2RA to a regimen of high-dose PPI therapy.[96] Authorities now debate the advisability of prescribing such aggressive antireflux therapy, designed to eliminate rather than merely reduce acid reflux, for all patients with Barrett's esophagus, irrespective of the severity of their underlying GERD. Proponents of this aggressive approach contend that gastroesophageal reflux is the major factor promoting carcinogenesis in specialized intestinal metaplasia, and that elimination of acid reflux by pharmacological or surgical means should prevent cancer. Opponents argue that the role of acid reflux in promoting carcinogenesis in Barrett's esophagus is not clear, and available data on this issue are too weak to support the routine prescription of aggressive antireflux therapy (with its considerable expense and inconvenience) in all cases.

There is only indirect evidence to support the notions that GERD promotes malignancy in established Barrett's esophagus, and that GERD treatment might prevent cancer. For example, biopsy specimens of specialized intestinal metaplasia maintained in organ culture have been shown to exhibit hyperproliferation and increased expression of cyclooxygenase-2 (a mediator of proliferation) when exposed to acid for 1 hour.[97,98] Brief esophageal acid exposure also has been shown to activate the mitogen-activated protein kinase (MAPK) pathways that can increase proliferation and decrease apoptosis in Barrett's esophagus.[99] These observations suggest, by inference, that acid reflux in patients with Barrett's esophagus might stimulate hyperproliferation, suppress apoptosis, and promote carcinogenesis in their specialized intestinal metaplasia.

One group of investigators took biopsy specimens from 39 patients with Barrett's esophagus at baseline and after 6 months of therapy with PPIs given only in doses sufficient to eliminate GERD symptoms.[100] The expression of PCNA (a proliferation marker) decreased and the expression of villin (a differentiation marker) increased significantly in biopsy specimens from the 24 patients in whom PPIs normalized esophageal acid exposure, but not in the 15 with persistently abnormal acid reflux during PPI therapy. Another group found no significant change in the proliferative activity of Barrett's esophagus (as assessed by in vitro labeling with 5-bromo-2-deoxyuridine) in 22 patients treated with a PPI for 2 years, whereas proliferative activity increased significantly in 23 patients treated for the same time with an H2RA.[101]

Extrapolation of the results of these studies to the practice of prescribing aggressive antireflux therapy for patients with Barrett's esophagus requires assumptions that may not be warranted. The acute effects of acid exposure on tissue maintained in organ culture ex vivo may not reflect the chronic effects of GERD on Barrett's esophagus in vivo. Even if the ex vivo observations are valid, it is unclear to what extent acid exposure must be reduced in order to be beneficial to patients with Barrett's esophagus. It is often difficult to achieve achlorhydria even with PPIs administered in high dosages and in combination with H2RAs,[102] and the ex vivo experiments suggest that a treatment that reduces acid reflux to brief episodes conceivably could stimulate cellular proliferation and promote carcinogenesis. The aforementioned clinical studies suggest that reduction of esophageal

acid exposure can be beneficial,[100,101] but this conclusion is based on the dubious assumption that effects on MAPK pathways, PCNA, and villin expression, and on 5-bromo-2-deoxyuridine labeling reflect important changes in cancer risk.

Another line of evidence suggesting that aggressive antireflux therapy might prevent carcinogenesis in Barrett's esophagus is the observation that such therapy can cause partial regression of the specialized intestinal metaplasia.[103] During chronic PPI therapy, most patients develop islands of squamous epithelium (evidence of partial regression) within their metaplastic columnar lining.[104] It is not clear that this partial regression is beneficial, however. Biopsy specimens of the squamous islands show underlying intestinal metaplasia in approximately 40% of cases, suggesting that the islands may result from an overgrowth of squamous epithelium rather than a regression of the metaplastic mucosa.[105] Furthermore, biopsy specimens from the squamous islands frequently exhibit abnormalities in Ki-67 staining (a proliferation marker) and p53 expression that might favor carcinogenesis.[106] These observations suggest that the partial regression of metaplasia induced by antireflux therapy might not decrease the cancer risk in Barrett's esophagus.

Surgeons have proposed that fundoplication might be more effective than antisecretory therapy for preventing cancer in Barrett's esophagus.[107] This proposal is based on weak evidence, however. For example, two small, uncontrolled studies found fewer cases of dysplasia and cancer among patients with Barrett's esophagus who had antireflux surgery than among those who had received medical treatment.[108,109] Some have even proposed that antisecretory therapy might predispose to malignancy,[110,111] and that the increasing use of antisecretory medications might underlie the rising frequency of esophageal adenocarcinoma in Western countries.[112] However, the limited studies that have addressed this issue directly have not found a significant association between esophageal adenocarcinoma and the use of antisecretory agents per se.[113,114]

A recent report describing the long-term outcome of a randomized trial of medical and surgical therapies for 247 veteran patients with complicated GERD (including 108 with Barrett's esophagus) does not support the contention that fundoplication prevents esophageal cancer better than antisecretory therapy.[115] During 10 to 13 years of follow-up, 4 of 165 patients (2.4%) in the medical group and 1 of 82 (1.2%) in the surgical group developed an esophageal adenocarcinoma. The difference between the treatment groups in the incidence of this tumor was not statistically significant but, with such a low observed rate of cancer development, the study did not have sufficient statistical power to detect small differences in the incidence of esophageal cancer. However, any potential cancer-preventive benefit of surgery was offset by an unexplained, but significant, decrease in survival for the surgical patients due to excess deaths from heart disease. Another recent report describing the results of a large, Swedish, population-based cohort study also refutes the contention that antireflux surgery prevents esophageal adenocarcinoma.[116] In this study, patients with GERD were followed for up to 32 years. The relative risk for developing esophageal adenocarcinoma (compared to the general population) among 35 274 men who received medical antireflux therapy was 6.3 (95% CI 4.5–8.7), whereas the relative risk for 6406 men treated with fundoplication was 14.1 (95% CI 8.0–22.8). These studies suggest that antireflux surgery should not be advised with the expectation that the procedure will prolong life by preventing esophageal cancer.

Treatment of dysplasia in Barrett's esophagus

General considerations

Patients treated for epithelial malignancies traditionally are deemed cured if there is no evidence of recurrence at 5 years, because it is assumed that any cancer cells that survived the treatment would have proliferated and become clinically manifest within that time period.[116] As discussed above, studies on the natural history of dysplasia in Barrett's esophagus suggest that, with antireflux therapy alone, fewer than 60% of patients with high-grade dysplasia will develop a demonstrable cancer within 5 years. In theory, if a treatment for dysplasia leaves even one dysplastic cell behind, that cell can proliferate and eventually become malignant. Even established esophageal cancers can take years to become manifest clinically.[117] Consequently, it may not be appropriate to conclude that the cancer risk has been eliminated for a patient who has survived 5 years after treatment of dysplasia in Barrett's esophagus. Five years might be considered the absolute minimum for a meaningful follow-up of this condition, and many more years would be required before one could reasonably consider that the risk of dysplasia-associated cancer has been eradicated. Unfortunately, the follow-up duration in most studies on treatments for dysplasia in Barrett's esophagus is considerably less than 5 years.

For patients with verified high-grade dysplasia in Barrett's esophagus, there are generally four proposed management options: (1) esophagectomy, (2) endoscopic therapies that ablate the neoplastic tissue, (3) endoscopic mucosal resection, and (3) intensive endoscopic surveillance in which invasive therapies are withheld until biopsy specimens reveal adenocarcinoma. All four choices are associated with substantial risks and unclear benefits.

Esophagectomy

Esophagectomy is the only therapy for high-grade dysplasia that clearly removes all of the neoplastic epithelium. Unfortunately, this definitive therapy also has the highest rates of procedure-related mortality and long-term morbidity. Studies on esophagectomy for high-grade dysplasia in Barrett's esophagus typically have involved small numbers of patients from a single institution, and generally have focused on the observation that many patients have foci of adenocarcinoma discovered in the resected esophagus. Such reports are of limited value for estimating the morbidity and mortality of esophagectomy for dysplasia. Much larger series are available on the results of esophagectomy for esophageal cancer, but it may not be appropriate to extrapolate the results of surgery performed on patients with esophageal cancer, who often have substantial comorbidities, to otherwise healthy patients with precancerous lesions. Nevertheless, there are some important lessons to be learned from the larger series.

One lesson is that the mortality rates for esophagectomy among institutions vary inversely with the frequency with which the operation is performed. In one study of 340 esophagectomies performed at 25 different hospitals, the mortality rate was 3.0% for patients who had the operation at institutions that did 5 or more esophagectomies per year, compared to 12.2% for patients treated at institutions where the operation was performed less frequently.[118] In a study of data from the Dutch National Medical Registry, the mortality rates for esophagectomy were 12.1%, 7.5%, and 4.9% at centers performing 1–10, 11–20, and >50 esophagectomies per year, respectively.[119]

Esophagectomy can have substantial short- and long-term morbidity. The average hospital stay for open esophagectomy is approximately 2 weeks, and 30–50% of patients develop at least one serious postoperative complication such as pneumonia, arrhythmia, myocardial infarction, heart failure, wound infection, and anastomotic leak.[118–121] Available data on minimally invasive techniques for esophagectomy are promising but limited, and it is not yet clear that these approaches are preferable to the open procedure.[122,123]

Although esophagectomy frequently is associated with long-term problems such as dysphagia, weight loss, gastroesophageal reflux, and dumping, limited data suggest that the impact of these symptoms on quality of life is surprisingly small. One group performed a utility assessment of patients who had esophagectomies at least 1 year earlier, and found that they rated their median quality of life at 0.97 on a scale of 0 to 1 (where 0=death and 1=perfect health).[85] In another study of 53 patients who had esophagectomies for high-grade dysplasia in Barrett's esophagus and who completed the MOS SF-36 Health Status Questionnaire, there appeared to be few important differences between the patients and a normal control population.[124]

Specialized intestinal metaplasia develops frequently in the esophageal remnant in patients who have had esophagectomy with esophagogastrostomy, presumably as the result of the reflux esophagitis that often accompanies this procedure.[125–127] Conceivably, those patients might be at risk for developing esophageal dysplasia and adenocarcinoma in the future. No such occurrence has been reported to date, however.

Endoscopic ablative therapies

Endoscopic ablative therapies (e.g., KTP, argon, Nd:YAG laser; multipolar electrocoagulation; argon plasma coagulation; photodynamic therapy) use thermal or photochemical energy to ablate the abnormal epithelium in Barrett's esophagus.[128,129] After the epithelium is ablated, patients are given potent antireflux therapy so that the injured mucosa heals with the growth of new squamous epithelium. The relative merits of the various endoscopic ablative therapies are disputed, and there appears to be a trade-off between the completeness of mucosal ablation and the frequency of complications. Simply stated, the deeper the mucosal injury inflicted, the more complete the ablation, and the greater the rate of complications like esophageal perforation and stricture.

One major concern regarding endoscopic ablative therapies for dysplasia is that the procedures will not eradicate all of the dysplastic cells. Endoscopic ablation commonly leaves visible foci of metaplastic mucosa behind.[128,129] Partially-ablated metaplastic mucosa can heal with an overlying layer of squamous epithelium that hides the 'buried' metaplastic tissue from the endoscopist. There are reports of adenocarcinoma developing from buried metaplastic tissue.[130] Furthermore, partially ablated metaplastic epithelium can develop new abnormalities in the expression of proliferation markers and p53, raising the possibility that incomplete ablation of Barrett's esophagus might even increase the risk of carcinogenesis.[131]

The conclusions that can be drawn from reports on ablative therapies for dysplasia in Barrett's esophagus are limited because most studies are not randomized or controlled, involve relatively few patients, and have a short duration of follow-up. Photo-dynamic therapy (PDT) is the most extensively studied of the ablative techniques. For PDT, patients are given a systemic dose of a light-activated chemical (usually a porphyrin or porphyrin precursor) that is taken up by the esophageal cells. The esophagus is then irradiated using a low-power laser that activates the chemical, which transfers the energy acquired from laser light to oxygen. This results in the formation of singlet oxygen, a toxic molecule that destroys the abnormal cells and their vasculature.

Overholt et al. recently published the results of PDT using porfimer sodium for 103 patients with early cancer or dysplasia in Barrett's esophagus who were followed for an average of 51 months (range 2–122 months).[132] For 9 patients with early-stage cancers, the malignancy appeared to be eliminated in 4 cases (44%). Follow-up endoscopy showed no dysplastic epithelium in 62 of 80 patients (78%) who had PDT for high-grade dysplasia, and in 13 of 14 patients (93%) who had the procedure for low-grade dysplasia. Although this report did not discuss procedure-related complications, a similar study from the same group showed that most patients experienced chest pain and dysphagia, most developed small pleural effusions, and several developed transient atrial fibrillation during the week after treatment.[133] Patients who did not adequately shield themselves from sun exposure in the weeks following the porfimer injection experienced skin injury, and 34% of patients developed esophageal strictures that required one or more sessions of dilation therapy.

The results of a large, multicenter, randomized trial of PDT using porfimer sodium for ablation of high-grade dysplasia in Barrett's esophagus recently has been presented in abstract form.[134] Two-hundred and eight patients with high-grade dysplasia were randomized to receive either PDT with omeprazole 20 mg b.i.d., or omeprazole 20 mg b.i.d. alone (without PDT). Patients were followed for 2 to 4.5 years with endoscopic surveillance performed every 3 months. No dysplasia was seen on follow-up in 77% of the patients treated with PDT, and in 39% of the patients who received omeprazole alone (p<0.0001). Thirteen percent of the PDT patients developed cancer, compared to 28% of those treated with omeprazole alone (p=0.006). There was no procedure-related mortality, but esophageal strictures developed in 37% of those who received PDT. These results show that PDT clearly is superior to omeprazole alone for eradicating dysplasia and preventing cancer in Barrett's esophagus. Nevertheless, it is disconcerting that 13% of the patients who received PDT developed cancer during less than 5 years of follow-up.

The reports discussed above document the feasibility of ablating neoplastic epithelium with PDT, but they do not establish the benefit of the technique. PDT is an expensive treatment that entails substantial risk and inconvenience. Without histological examination of the resected esophagus or duration of follow-up well beyond 5 years, it is not possible to verify claims that dysplasia and cancer are indeed 'eliminated' by PDT. Residual foci of metaplasia remain in most patients after PDT, and some of these foci may be buried under a superficial layer of squamous epithelium where they are invisible to the endoscopist. No study yet has established that PDT decreases the long-term risk for cancer development in Barrett's esophagus.

Endoscopic mucosal resection

In endoscopic mucosal resection (EMR), a diathermy snare or endoscopic knife is used to remove a large segment of esophageal mucosa down to the submucosa.[135,136] Endoscopic ultrasonography usually is performed first to estimate the depth of the neoplastic lesion. If there is no ultrasonographic evidence of extension into the submucosa, which is a contraindication to EMR, the endoscopist elevates the mucosal target by injecting saline into the submucosa. For the snare EMR methods, the saline-elevated mucosa is removed either by a strip biopsy technique using the snare alone or by a 'suck and cut' technique in which the mucosa first is suctioned into a cap that fits over the tip of the endoscope, and the snare is tightened around the suctioned area. In the endoscopic knife techniques, a large segment of mucosa is dissected and removed en bloc. Unlike the endoscopic ablative techniques, EMR provides large tissue specimens that can be examined by the pathologist to determine the character and extent of the lesion, and the adequacy of resection.

Although there is theoretical potential for lymphatic dissemination of neoplastic cells that enter the esophageal lamina propria, limited data from surgical series suggest that fewer than 5% of patients with intramucosal adenocarcinoma in Barrett's esophagus have lymph node metastases.[137,138] In contrast, for esophageal squamous cell carcinomas with a similar early T stage, lymphatic spread appears to be more common.[139] It has been proposed that the reflux esophagitis that often accompanies Barrett's esophagus may occlude mucosal lymphatic channels and thereby prevent lymphatic spread of early esophageal adenocarcinomas.[138] Once the tumor cells breach the muscularis mucosae to enter the submucosa, however, the frequency of lymph node metastases exceeds 20%, even for patients without bulky tumors.[137,138]

EMR cannot be considered definitive therapy for neoplasms that extend into the submucosa. Consequently, accurate staging of the neoplasia is critical for patients treated with this procedure. Unfortunately, one recent study on EMR for dysplasia in Barrett's esophagus has shown that the accuracy of endoscopic biopsy and high-frequency endosonography for assessing the depth of neoplasia is limited.[140] Among 15 patients for whom staging by these techniques showed intramucosal adenocarcinoma, EMR specimens showed submucosal invasion in 6 (40%). Among 27 patients for whom pre-EMR staging showed what appeared to be only high-grade dysplasia confined to the mucosa, none had submucosal cancer in the EMR specimens, but 5 (19%) had intramucosal adenocarcinoma.

Preliminary studies have established the feasibility of EMR, either alone or in combination with an ablative therapy like PDT, for treating high-grade dysplasia in Barrett's esophagus.[141–146] Considering the depth and size of the mucosal resection, reported series have documented surprisingly few serious complications (bleeding, perforation, stricture) and, as yet, no procedure-related mortality. The mean duration of follow-up reported (10–36 months) are woefully inadequate for meaningful conclusions regarding the efficacy of EMR in decreasing the risk of cancer development. Furthermore, a recent report has raised serious questions regarding the adequacy of cap-assisted EMR as a treatment for high-grade dysplasia.[147] Histological examination of EMR specimens from 88 patients with high-grade dysplasia revealed dysplasia at the margins of the specimens in 72 cases (82%). This suggests that cap-assisted EMR leaves neoplastic cells behind in the large majority of cases. An alternative approach is circumferential EMR, in which the endoscopist attempts to remove all of the metaplastic epithelium, not just a localized segment as in the cap-assisted technique. Preliminary results for circumferential EMR are promising, but as yet too limited to make meaningful conclusions regarding the safety and efficacy of the technique.[148]

Intensive endoscopic surveillance

Some authorities recommend a program of expectant management with intensive endoscopic surveillance (i.e., endoscopic examinations every 3–6 months) for patients with high-grade dysplasia in Barrett's esophagus. These authorities withhold invasive treatments such as esophagectomy until biopsy specimens reveal adenocarcinoma.[69,149] Although this practice has been endorsed as a management option by the American College of Gastroenterology,[40] few published data directly support the safety and efficacy of intensive surveillance for high-grade dysplasia.

Schnell described 12 patients who developed adenocarcinomas during intensive endoscopic surveillance for high-grade dysplasia in Barrett's esophagus.[69] The cancers were deemed potentially curable at the time of detection in all 11 patients who were compliant with the surveillance program, but one patient who was lost to follow-up returned 10 years later with an unresectable tumor. In Reid's series of 32 patients with high-grade dysplasia who developed adenocarcinoma during intensive endoscopic surveillance, only one patient (3%) had incurable disease (metas-tases) when the cancer was first detected on surveillance endoscopy.[150] Weston performed intensive endoscopic surveillance in 15 patients with high-grade dysplasia for a mean duration of 36.8 months, during which four developed adenocarcinoma.[74] One of those four had metastatic disease, and the authors concluded that an observational approach to the management of high-grade dysplasia should be discouraged.

MANAGEMENT RECOMMENDATIONS

Clinicians should appreciate that no management strategy for patients with Barrett's esophagus has been verified by studies demonstrating that the strategy prolongs life. An algorithm for management is proposed in Figure 14.3. This algorithm incorporates most of the patient management policy that has been endorsed by the Practice Parameters Committee of the American College of Gastroenterology.[40] Key features of this policy include the following:

- Patients with chronic GERD symptoms are those most likely to have Barrett's esophagus and should undergo upper endoscopy.
- Patients found to have Barrett's esophagus should have regular surveillance endoscopy to obtain esophageal biopsy specimens. GERD should be treated prior to surveillance to minimize confusion caused by inflammation in the interpretation of dysplasia.

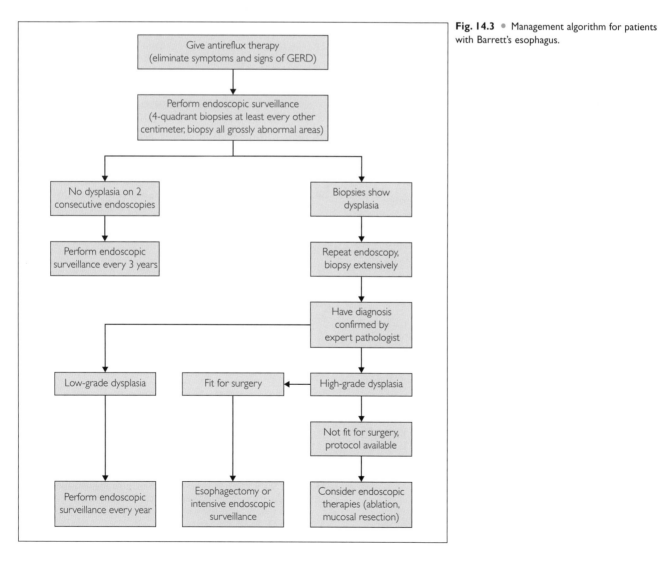

Fig. 14.3 • Management algorithm for patients with Barrett's esophagus.

- For patients who have had two consecutive endoscopies that show no dysplasia, surveillance endoscopy is recommended at an interval of every 3 years.
- If dysplasia is noted, the finding should be verified by consultation with another expert pathologist.
- For patients with verified low-grade dysplasia after extensive biopsy sampling, yearly surveillance endoscopy is recommended.
- For patients with verified high-grade dysplasia, the risks of intervention (e.g., esophagectomy) must be weighed against those of intensive endoscopic surveillance (e.g., every 3 months) in which intervention is withheld until surveillance biopsy specimens show adenocarcinoma. (Note: The ACG guidelines recommend different management strategies for focal and multifocal high-grade dysplasia, but this recommendation is based primarily on data from a single institution and have been disputed by others. It is not clear that this is a useful clinical distinction, and the author presently does not recommend that clinical decisions should be based on an assessment of the focality of dysplasia.) The author feels that esophagectomy is the preferred management strategy for young patients with high-grade dysplasia.

Although not specifically recommended in the practice guidelines, clinicians can consider the use of experimental ablative therapies such as photodynamic therapy and endoscopic mucosal resection for their patients with high-grade dysplasia in Barrett's esophagus, *provided the therapy is administered as part of an established, approved research protocol*. The use of ablative therapies outside of research protocols cannot be condoned at this time.

REFERENCES

1. Spechler SJ. Barrett's esophagus. N Engl J Med 2002; 346: 836–842.
2. Brown LM, Devesa SS. Epidemiologic trends in esophageal and gastric cancer in the United States. Surg Oncol Clin N Am 2002; 11:235–256.
3. Lagergren J, Bergstrom R, Lindgren A, et al. Symptomatic gastroesophageal reflux as a risk factor for esophageal adenocarcinoma. N Engl J Med 1999; 340:825–831.
4. Barrett NR. Chronic peptic ulcer of the oesophagus and 'oesophagitis'. Br J Surg 1950; 38:175–182.
5. Spechler SJ, Goyal RK. The columnar lined esophagus, intestinal metaplasia, and Norman Barrett. Gastroenterology 1996; 110:614–621.
6. Sharma P, Morales TG, Sampliner RE. Short segment Barrett's esophagus. The need for standardization of the definition and of endoscopic criteria. Am J Gastroenterol 1998; 93:1033–1036.
7. Cameron AJ. Epidemiology of columnar-lined esophagus and adenocarcinoma. Gastroenterol Clin N Am 1997; 26:487–494.
8. Hassall E. Barrett's esophagus: new definitions and approaches in children. J Pediatr Gastroenterol Nutr 1993; 16:345–364.
9. Rex DK, Cummings OW, Shaw M, et al. Screening for Barrett's esophagus in colonoscopy patients with and without heartburn. Gastroenterology 2003; 125:1670–1677.
10. Spechler SJ. Intestinal metaplasia at the gastroesophageal junction. Gastroenterology 2004; 126:567–575.
11. Collen MJ, Lewis JH, Benjamin SB. Gastric acid hypersecretion in refractory gastroesophageal reflux disease. Gastroenterology 1990; 98:654–661.
12. Mulholland MW, Reid BJ, Levine DS, et al. Elevated gastric acid secretion in patients with Barrett's metaplastic epithelium. Dig Dis Sci 1989; 34:1329–1335.
13. Gillen P, Keeling P, Byrne PJ, et al. Implication of duodenogastric reflux in the pathogenesis of Barrett's oesophagus. Br J Surg 1988; 75:540–543.
14. Iascone C, DeMeester TR, Little AG, et al. Barrett's esophagus. Functional assessment, proposed pathogenesis, and surgical therapy. Arch Surg 1983; 118:543–549.
15. Zaninotto G, DeMeester TR, Bremner CG, et al. Esophageal function in patients with reflux-induced strictures and its relevance to surgical treatment. Ann Thorac Surg 1989; 47:362–370.
16. Johnson DA, Winters C, Spurling TJ, et al. Esophageal acid sensitivity in Barrett's esophagus. J Clin Gastroenterol 1987; 9:23–27.
17. Gray MR, Donnelly RJ, Kingsnorth AN. Role of salivary epidermal growth factor in the pathogenesis of Barrett's columnar lined oesophagus. Br J Surg 1991; 78:1461–1466.
18. Hirschowitz BI. Gastric acid and pepsin secretion in patients with Barrett's esophagus and appropriate controls. Dig Dis Sci 1996; 41:1384–1391.
19. Spechler SJ. The columnar lined oesophagus: a riddle wrapped in a mystery inside an enigma. Gut 1997; 41:710–711.
20. Oberg S, DeMeester TR, Peters JH, et al. The extent of Barrett's esophagus depends on the status of the lower esophageal sphincter and degree of esophageal acid exposure. J Thorac Cardiovasc Surg 1999; 117:572–580.
21. Fletcher J, Wirz A, Young J, et al. Unbuffered highly acidic gastric juice exists at the gastroesophageal junction after a meal. Gastroenterology 2001; 121:775–783.
22. Fletcher J, Wirz A, Henry E, et al. Studies of acid exposure immediately above the gastro-oesophageal junction: evidence of short segment reflux. Gut 2004; 53:168–173.
23. Iijima K, Henry E, Moriya A, et al. Dietary nitrate generates potentially mutagenic concentrations of nitric oxide at the gastroesophageal junction. Gastroenterology 2002; 122:1248–1257.
24. Spechler SJ. Are we underestimating acid reflux? Gut 2004; 53:162–163.
25. Spechler SJ. The role of gastric carditis in metaplasia and neoplasia at the gastroesophageal junction. Gastroenterology 1999; 117:218–228.
26. McClave SA, Boyce HW Jr, Gottfried MR. Early diagnosis of columnar-lined esophagus: a new endoscopic criterion. Gastrointest Endosc 1987; 33:413–416.
27. Fawcett DW. The esophagus and stomach. In: Fawcett DW, ed. Bloom and Fawcett. A textbook of histology. 11th edn. Philadelphia: WB Saunders; 1986:619–640.
28. Hayward J. The lower end of the oesophagus. Thorax 1961; 16:36–41.
29. Chandrasoma P. Pathophysiology of Barrett's esophagus. Semin Thorac Cardiovasc Surg 1997; 9:270–278.
30. Goldblum JR, Vicari JJ, Falk GW, et al. Inflammation and intestinal metaplasia of the gastric cardia: the role of gastroesophageal reflux and *H. pylori* infection. Gastroenterology 1998; 114:633–639.
31. Oberg S, Peters JH, DeMeester TR, et al. Inflammation and specialized intestinal metaplasia of cardiac mucosa is a manifestation of gastroesophageal reflux disease. Ann Surg 1997; 226:522–532.

32. Dresner SM, Griffin SM, Wayman J, et al. Human model of duodenogastro-oesophageal reflux in the development of Barrett's metaplasia. Br J Surg 2003; 90:1120–1128.

33. Kilgore SP, Ormsby AH, Gramlich TL, et al. The gastric cardia: fact or fiction? Am J Gastroenterol 2000; 95:921–924.

34. Sarbia M, Donner A, Gabbert HE. Histopathology of the gastroesophageal junction. A study on 36 operation specimens. Am J Surg Pathol 2002; 26:1207–1212.

35. Chandrasoma PT, Der R, Ma Y, et al. Histology of the gastroesophageal junction. An autopsy study. Am J Surg Pathol 2000; 24:402–409.

36. Correa P. Helicobacter pylori and gastric carcinogenesis. Am J Surg Pathol 1995; 19(Suppl 1):S37–S43.

37. Vicari JJ, Peek RM, Falk GW, et al. The seroprevalence of cagA-positive Helicobacter pylori strains in the spectrum of gastroesophageal reflux disease. Gastroenterology 1998; 115:50–57.

38. Couvelard A, Cauvin JM, Goldfain D, et al. and members of the Groupe d'Etude de l'Oesophage de Barrett. Cytokeratin immunoreactivity of intestinal metaplasia at normal oesophagogastric junction indicates its aetiology. Gut 2001; 49:761–766.

39. Sharma P, Weston AP, Morales,T, et al. Relative risk of dysplasia for patients with intestinal metaplasia in the distal oesophagus and in the gastric cardia. Gut 2000; 46:9–13.

40. Sampliner RE and The Practice Parameters Committee of the American College of Gastroenterology. Updated guidelines for the diagnosis, surveillance, and therapy of Barrett's esophagus. Am J Gastroenterol 2002; 97:1888–1895.

41. Fennerty MB. Gastric intestinal metaplasia on routine endoscopic biopsy. Gastroenterology 2003; 125:586–590.

42. Ormsby AH, Goldblum JR, Rice TW, et al. Cytokeratin subsets can reliably distinguish Barrett's esophagus from intestinal metaplasia of the stomach. Hum Pathol 1999; 30:288–294.

43. Jovanovic I, Tzardi M, Mouzas IA, et al. Changing pattern of cytokeratin 7 and 20 expression from normal epithelium to intestinal metaplasia of the gastric mucosa and gastroesophageal junction. Histol Histopathol 2002; 17:445–454.

44. Glickman JN, Wang H, Das KM, et al. Phenotype of Barrett's esophagus and intestinal metaplasia of the distal esophagus and gastroesophageal junction. An immunohistochemical study of cytokeratins 7 and 20, Das-1 and 45 MI. Am J Surg Pathol 2001; 25:87–94.

45. El-Zimaity HMT, Graham DY. Cytokeratin subsets for distinguishing Barrett's esophagus from intestinal metaplasia in the cardia using endoscopic biopsy specimens. Am J Gastroenterol 2001; 96:1378–1382.

46. Das KM, Prasad I, Garla S, et al. Detection of a shared colon epithelial epitope on Barrett epithelium by a novel monoclonal antibody. Ann Intern Med 1994; 120:753–756.

47. Morales CP, Spechler SJ. Intestinal metaplasia at the gastroesophageal junction: Barrett's, bacteria, and biomarkers. Am J Gastroenterol 2003; 98:759–762.

48. Spechler SJ. Dysplasia in Barrett's esophagus: limitations of current management strategies. Am J Gastroenterol 2005; 100:927–935.

49. Goldblum JR. Barrett's esophagus and Barrett's-related dysplasia. Mod Pathol 2003; 16:316–324.

50. Reid BJ, Haggitt RC, Rubin CE. Observer variation in the diagnosis of dysplasia in Barrett's esophagus. Hum Pathol 1988; 19:166–178.

51. Skacel M, Petras RE, Gramlich TL, et al. The diagnosis of low-grade dysplasia in Barrett's esophagus and its implications for disease progression. Am J Gastroenterol 2000; 95:3383–3387.

52. Montgomery E, Bronner MP, Goldblum JR, et al. Reproducibility of the diagnosis of dysplasia in Barrett esophagus: a reaffirmation. Hum Pathol 2001; 32:368–378.

53. Ormsby AH, Petras RE, Henricks WH, et al. Observer variation in the diagnosis of superficial oesophageal adenocarcinoma. Gut 2002; 51:671–676.

54. Reid BJ, Weinstein WM, Lewin KJ, et al. Endoscopic biopsy can detect high-grade dysplasia or early adenocarcinoma in Barrett's esophagus without grossly recognizable neoplastic lesions. Gastroenterology 1988; 94:81–90.

55. Cameron AJ, Carpenter HA. Barrett's esophagus, high-grade dysplasia, and early adenocarcinoma: a pathological study. Am J Gastroenterol 1997; 92:586–591.

56. Collard JM. High-grade dysplasia in Barrett's esophagus. The case for esophagectomy. Chest Surg Clin North Am 2002; 12:77–92.

57. Levine DS, Haggitt RC, Blount PL, et al. An endoscopic biopsy protocol can differentiate high-grade dysplasia from early adenocarcinoma in Barrett's esophagus. Gastroenterology 1993; 105:40–50.

58. Falk GW, Rice TW, Goldblum JR, et al. Jumbo biopsy forceps protocol still misses unsuspected cancer in Barrett's esophagus with high-grade dysplasia. Gastrointest Endosc 1999; 49:170–176.

59. Reid BJ, Blount PL, Rabinovitch PS. Biomarkers in Barrett's esophagus. Gastrointest Endosc Clin N Am 2003; 13:369–397.

60. Guindi M, Riddell RH. Dysplasia in Barrett's esophagus. Chest Surg Clin N Am 2002; 12:59–68.

61. Skacel M, Petras RE, Rybicki LA, et al. p53 expression in low-grade dysplasia in Barrett's esophagus: correlation with interobserver agreement and disease progression. Am J Gastroenterol 2002; 97:2508–2513.

62. Bani-Hani K, Martin IG, Hardie LJ, et al. Prospective study of cyclin D1 overexpression in Barrett's esophagus: association with increased risk of adenocarcinoma. J Natl Cancer Inst 2000; 92:1316–1321.

63. Reid BJ, Levine DS, Longton G, et al. Predictors of progression to cancer in Barrett's esophagus: baseline histology and flow cytometry identify low- and high-risk patient subsets. Am J Gastroenterol 2000; 95:1669–1676.

64. Canto MIF, Setrakian S, Willis J, et al. Methylene blue-directed biopsies improve detection of intestinal metaplasia and dysplasia in Barrett's esophagus. Gastrointest Endosc 2000; 51:560–568.

65. Scotiniotis IA, Kochman ML, Lewis JD, et al. Accuracy of EUS in the evaluation of Barrett's esophagus and high-grade dysplasia or intramucosal carcinoma. Gastrointest Endosc 2001; 54:689–696.

66. Kobayashi K, Izatt JA, Kulkarni MD, et al. High-resolution cross-sectional imaging of the gastrointestinal tract using optical coherence tomography: preliminary results. Gastrointest Endosc 1998; 47:515–523.

67. Georgakoudi I, Jacobson BC, Van Dam J, et al. Fluorescence, reflectance, and light-scattering spectroscopy for evaluating dysplasia in patients with Barrett's esophagus. Gastroenterology 2001; 120:1620–1629.

68. Kendall C, Stone N, Shepherd N, et al. Raman spectroscopy, a potential tool for the objective identification and classification of neoplasia in Barrett's oesophagus. J Pathol 2003; 200:602–609.

69. Schnell TG, Sontag SJ, Chejfec G, et al. Long-term nonsurgical management of Barrett's esophagus with high-grade dysplasia. Gastroenterology 2001; 120:1607–1619.

70. Lao CD, Simmons M, Syngal S, et al. Dysplasia in Barrett esophagus: implications for chemoprevention. Cancer 2004; 100:1622–1627.

71. Hameeteman W, Tytgat GNJ, Houthoff HJ, et al. Barrett's esophagus: development of dysplasia and adenocarcinoma. Gastroenterology 1989; 96:1249–1256.

72. Buttar NS, Wang KK, Sebo TJ, et al. Extent of high-grade dysplasia in Barrett's esophagus correlates with risk of adenocarcinoma. Gastroenterology 2001; 120:1630–1639.

73. Dar MS, Goldblum JR, Rice TW, et al. Can extent of high-grade dysplasia in Barrett's oesophagus predict the presence of adenocarcinoma at oesophagectomy? Gut 2003; 52:486–489.

74. Weston AP, Sharma Prateek S, Topalovski M, et al. Long-term follow-up of Barrett's high-grade dysplasia. Am J Gastroenterol 2000; 95:1888–1893.

75. Dulai GS, Guha S, Kahn KL, et al. Preoperative prevalence of Barrett's esophagus in esophageal adenocarcinoma: a systematic review. Gastroenterology 2002; 122:26–33.

76. Cameron AJ, Ott BJ, Payne WS. The incidence of adenocarcinoma in columnar-lined (Barrett's) esophagus. N Engl J Med 1985; 313:857–859.

77. Van der Veen AH, Dees J, Blankensteijn JD, et al. Adenocarcinoma in Barrett's oesophagus: an overrated risk. Gut 1989; 30:14–18.

78. Eckardt VF, Kanzler G, Bernhard G. Life expectancy and cancer risk in patients with Barrett's esophagus: a prospective controlled investigation. Am J Med 2001; 111:33–37.

79. Anderson LA, Murray LJ, Murphy SJ, et al. Mortality in Barrett's oesophagus: results from a population based study. Gut 2003; 52:1081–1084.

80. Streitz JM Jr, Andrews CW Jr, Ellis FH Jr. Endoscopic surveillance of Barrett's esophagus. Does it help? J Thorac Cardiovasc Surg 1993; 105:383–388.

81. Peters JH, Clark GWB, Ireland AP, et al. Outcome of adenocarcinoma arising in Barrett's esophagus in endoscopically surveyed and nonsurveyed patients. J Thorac Cardiovasc Surg 1994; 108:813–822.

82. Corley DA, Levin TR, Habel LA, et al. Surveillance and survival in Barrett's adenocarcinomas: a population-based study. Gastroenterology 2002; 122:633–640.

83. Fountoulakis A, Zafirellis KD, Dolan K, et al. Effect of surveillance of Barrett's oesophagus on the clinical outcome of oesophageal cancer. Br J Surg 2004; 91:997–1003.

84. Shaheen NJ, Provenzale D, Sandler RS. Upper endoscopy as a screening and surveillance tool in esophageal adenocarcinoma: a review of the evidence. Am J Gastroenterol 2002; 97:1319–1327.

85. Provenzale D, Schmitt C, Wong JB. Barrett's esophagus: a new look at surveillance based on emerging estimates of cancer risk. Am J Gastroenterol 1999; 94:2043–2053.

86. Soni A, Sampliner RE, Sonnenberg A. Screening for high-grade dysplasia in gastroesophageal reflux disease: is it cost-effective? Am J Gastroenterol 2000; 95:2086–2093.

87. Sonnenberg A, Soni A, Sampliner RE. Medical decision analysis of endoscopic surveillance of Barrett's oesophagus to prevent oesophageal adenocarcinoma. Aliment Pharmacol Ther 2002; 16(1):41–50.

88. Inadomi JM, Sampliner R, Lagergren J, et al. Screening and surveillance for Barrett esophagus in high-risk groups: a cost-utility analysis. Ann Intern Med 2003; 138:176–186.

89. Spechler SJ. To screen or not to screen: scoping out the issues. Am J Gastroenterol 2004; 99:2295–2296.

90. DeVault KR, Castell DO, and The Practice Parameters Committee of the American College of Gastroenterology. Updated guidelines for the diagnosis and treatment of gastroesophageal reflux disease. Am J Gastroenterol 1999; 94:1434–1442.

91. Klinkenberg-Knol EC, Nelis F, Dent J, et al. and Long-Term Study Group. Long-term omeprazole treatment in resistant gastroesophageal reflux disease: efficacy, safety, and influence on gastric mucosa. Gastroenterology 2000; 118:661–669.

92. Ter RB, Castell DO. Gastroesophageal reflux disease in patients with columnar-lined esophagus. Gastroenterol Clin North Am 1997; 26:549–563.

93. Cameron AJ. Management of Barrett's esophagus. May Clin Proc 1998; 73:457–461.

94. Ouatu-Lascar R, Triadafilopoulos G. Complete elimination of reflux symptoms does not guarantee normalization of intraesophageal acid reflux in patients with Barrett's esophagus. Am J Gastroenterol 1998; 93:711–716.

95. Katz PO, Anderson C, Khoury R, et al. Gastro-oesophageal reflux associated with nocturnal gastric acid breakthrough on proton pump inhibitors. Aliment Pharmacol Ther 1998; 12:1231–1234.

96. Peghini PL, Katz PO, Castell DO. Ranitidine controls nocturnal gastric acid breakthrough on omeprazole: a controlled study in normal subjects. Gastroenterology 1998; 115:1335–1339.

97. Fitzgerald RC, Omary MB, Triadafilopoulos G. Dynamic effects of acid on Barrett's esophagus. An ex vivo proliferation and differentiation model. J Clin Invest 1996; 98:2120–2128.

98. Shirvani VN, Ouatu-Lascar R, Kaur BS, et al. Cyclooxygenase 2 expression in Barrett's esophagus and adenocarcinoma: ex vivo induction by bile salts and acid exposure. Gastroenterology 2000; 118:487–496.

99. Souza RF, Shewmake K, Terada LS, et al. Acid exposure activates the mitogen-activated protein kinase pathways in Barrett's esophagus. Gastroenterology 2002; 122:299–307.

100. Ouatu-Lascar R, Fitzgerald RC, Triadafilopoulos G. Differentiation and proliferation in Barrett's esophagus and the effects of acid suppression. Gastroenterology 1999; 117:327–335.

101. Peters FT, Ganesh S, Kuipers EJ, et al. Effect of elimination of acid reflux on epithelial cell proliferative activity of Barrett esophagus. Scand J Gastroenterol 2000; 35:1238–1244.

102. Fackler WK, Ours TM, Vaezi MF, et al. Long-term effect of H2RA therapy on nocturnal gastric acid breakthrough. Gastroenterology 2002; 122:625–632.

103. Peters FTM, Ganesh S, Kuipers EJ, et al. Endoscopic regression of Barrett' oesophagus during omeprazole treatment: a randomised double blind study. Gut 1999; 45:489–494.

104. Srinivasan R, Katz PO, Ramakrishnan A, et al. Maximal acid reflux control for Barrett's oesophagus: feasible and effective. Aliment Pharmacol Ther 2001; 15:519–524.

105. Sharma P, Morales TG, Bhattacharyya A, et al. Squamous islands in Barrett's esophagus: what lies underneath? Am J Gastroenterol 1998; 93:332–335.

106. Garewal H, Ramsey L, Sharma P, et al. Biomarker studies in reversed Barrett's esophagus. Am J Gastroenterol 1999; 94:2829–2833.

107. DeMeester SR, DeMeester TR. Columnar mucosa and intestinal metaplasia of the esophagus. Fifty years of controversy. Ann Surg 2000; 231:303–321.

108. McCallum RW, Polepalle S, Davenport K, et al. Role of anti-reflux surgery against dysplasia in Barrett's esophagus. Gastroenterology 1991; 100:A121.

109. Katz D, Rothstein R, Schned A, et al. The development of dysplasia and adenocarcinoma during endoscopic surveillance of Barrett's esophagus. Am J Gastroenterol 1998; 93:536–541.

110. Theisen J, Nehra D, Citron D, et al. Suppression of gastric acid secretion in patients with gastroesophageal reflux disease results in gastric bacterial overgrowth and deconjugation of bile acids. J Gastrointest Surg 2000; 4:50–54.

111. Kauer WKH, Peters JH, DeMeester TR, et al. Mixed reflux of gastric and duodenal juices is more harmful to the esophagus than gastric juice alone. The need for surgical therapy re-emphasized. Ann Surg 1995; 222:525–533.

112. Wetscher GJ, Hinder RA, Smyrk T, et al. Gastric acid blockade with omeprazole promotes gastric carcinogenesis induced by duodenogastric reflux. Dig Dis Sci 1999; 44:1132–1135.

113. Chow WH, Findkle WD, McLaughlin JK, et al The relation of gastroesophageal reflux disease and its treatment to adenocarcinomas of the esophagus and gastric cardia. JAMA 1995; 274:474–477.

114. Garrow DC, Vaughan TL, Sweeney C, et al. Gastroesophageal reflux disease, use of H2 receptor antagonists, and risk of esophageal and gastric cancer. Cancer Causes Control 2000; 11:231–238.

115. Spechler SJ, Lee E, Ahnen D, et al. Long-term outcome of medical and surgical treatments for gastroesophageal reflux disease. Follow-up of a randomized controlled trial. JAMA 2001; 285:2331–2338.

116. Ye W, Chow WH, Lagergren J, et al. Risk of adenocarcinoma of the esophagus and gastric cardia in patients with gastroesophageal reflux diseases and after antireflux surgery. Gastroenterology 2001; 121:1286–1293.

117. Guanrei Y, Songliang Q, Guizen F. Natural history of early esophageal squamous carcinoma and early adenocarcinoma of the gastric cardia in the People's Republic of China. Endoscopy 1988; 20:95–98.

118. Swisher SG, DeFord L, Merriman KW, et al. Effects of operative volume on morbidity, mortality, and hospital use after esophagectomy for cancer. J Thorac Cardiovasc Surg 2000; 119:1126–1134.

119. Van Lanschot JJB, Hulscher JBF, Buskens CJ, et al. Hospital volume and hospital mortality for esophagectomy. Cancer 2001; 91:1574–1578.

120. Karl RC, Schreiber R, Boulware D, et al. Factors affecting morbidity, mortality, and survival in patients undergoing Ivor-Lewis esophagogastrectomy. Ann Surg 2000; 231:635–643.

121. Young MM, Deschamps C, Trastek VF, et al. Esophageal reconstruction for benign disease: early morbidity, mortality, and functional results. Ann Thorac Surg 2000; 70:1651–1655.

122. Nguyen NT, Schauer P, Luketich JD. Minimally invasive esophagectomy for Barrett's esophagus with high-grade dysplasia. Surgery 2000; 127:284–290.

123. Luketich JD, Alvelo-Rivera M, Buenaventura PO, et al. Minimally invasive esophagectomy: outcomes in 222 patients. Ann Surg 2003; 238:486–494.

124. Headrick JR, Nichols FC III, Miller DL, et al. High-grade esophageal dysplasia: long-term survival and quality of life after esophagectomy. Ann Thorac Surg 2002; 73:1697–1703.

125. Oberg S, Johansson J, Wenner J, et al. Metaplastic columnar mucosa in the cervical esophagus after esophagectomy. Ann Surg 2002; 235:338–345.

126. Franchimont D, Covas A, Brasseur C, et al. Newly developed Barrett's esophagus after subtotal esophagectomy. Endoscopy 2003; 35:850–853.

127. O'Riordan JM, Tucker ON, Byrne PJ, et al. Factors influencing the development of Barrett's epithelium in the esophageal remnant postesophagectomy. Am J Gastroenterol 2004; 99:205–211.

128. Van den Boogert J, van Hillegersberg R, Siersema PD, et al. Endoscopic ablation therapy for Barrett's esophagus with high-grade dysplasia: a review. Am J Gastroenterol 1999; 94:1153–1160.

129. Sampliner RE. Endoscopic ablative therapy for Barrett's esophagus. Gastrointest Endosc 2004; 59:66–69.

130. Van Laethem JL, Peny MO, Salmon I, et al. Intramucosal adenocarcinoma arising under squamous re-epithelialisation of Barrett's oesophagus. Gut 2000; 46:574–577.

131. Garewal HS, Ramsey L, Sampliner RE, et al. Post-ablation biomarker abnormalities in Barrett's esophagus (BE): Are we increasing the cancer risk? Gastroenterology 2001; 120:A79.

132. Overholt BF, Panjehpour M, Halberg DL. Photodynamic therapy for Barrett's esophagus with dysplasia and/or early stage carcinoma: long-term results. Gastrointest Endosc 2003; 58:183–188.

133. Overholt BF, Panjehpour M, Haydek JM. Photodynamic therapy for Barrett's esophagus: follow-up in 100 patients. Gastrointest Endosc 1999; 49:1–7.

134. Overholt BF, Lightdale CJ, Wang K, et al. International, multicenter, partially blinded, randomised study of the efficacy of photodynamic therapy (PDT) using porfimer sodium (POR) for the ablation of high-grade dysplasia (HGD) in Barrett's esophagus (BE): results of 24-month follow-up. Gastroenterology 2003; 124:A20.

135. Soetikno RM, Gotoda T, Nakanishi Y, et al. Endoscopic mucosal resection. Gastrointest Endosc 2003; 57:567–579.

136. Pech O, May A, Gossner L, et al. Management of pre-malignant and malignant lesions by endoscopic resection. Best Pract Res Clin Gastroenterol 2004; 18:61–76.

137. Rice TW, Zuccaro G, Adelstein DJ, et al. Esophageal carcinoma: depth of tumor invasion is predictive of regional lymph node status. Ann Thorac Surg 1998; 65:787–792.

138. Feith M, Stein HJ, Siewert JR. Pattern of lymphatic spread of Barrett's cancer. World J Surg 2003; 27:1052–1057.

139. Siewert JR, Stein HJ. Lymph-node dissection in squamous cell esophageal cancer – who benefits? Langenbeck's Arch Surg 1999; 384:141–148.

140. Lightdale CJ, Larghi A, Rotterdum H, et al. Endoscopic ultrasonography (EUS) and endoscopic mucosal resection (EMR) for staging and treatment of high-grade dysplasia (HGD) and early adenocarcinoma (EAC) in Barrett's esophagus. Gastrointest Endosc 2004; 59:AB90.

141. Nijhawan PK, Wang KK. Endoscopic mucosal resection for lesions with endoscopic features suggestive of malignancy and high-grade dysplasia within Barrett's esophagus. Gastrointest Endosc 2000; 52:328–332.

142. Ell C, May A, Gossner L, et al. Endoscopic mucosal resection of early cancer and high-grade dysplasia in Barrett's esophagus. Gastroenterology 2000; 118:670–677.

143. Buttar NS, Wang KK, Lutzke LS, et al. Combined endoscopic mucosal resection and photodynamic therapy for esophageal neoplasia within Barrett's esophagus. Gastrointest Endosc 2001; 54:682–688.

144. May A, Gossner L, Pech O, et al. Local endoscopic therapy for intraepithelial high-grade neoplasia and early adenocarcinoma in Barrett's oesophagus: acute-phase and intermediate results of a new treatment approach. Eur J Gastroenterol Hepatol 2002; 14:1085–1091.

145. May A, Gossner L, Pech O, et al. Intraepithelial high-grade neoplasia and early adenocarcinoma in short-segment Barrett's esophagus (SSBE): curative treatment using local endoscopic treatment techniques. Endoscopy 2002; 34:604–610.

146. Pacifico RJ, Wang KK, Wongkeesong LM, et al. Combined endoscopic mucosal resection and photodynamic therapy versus esophagectomy for management of early adenocarcinoma in Barrett's esophagus. Clin Gastroenterol Hepatol 2003; 1:252–257.

147. Lewis J, Lutzke L, Smyrk T, et al. The limitations of mucosal resection in Barrett's esophagus. Gastrointest Endosc 2004; 59:AB101.

148. Seewald S, Groth S, Brand B, et al. Circumferential EMR – future endoscopic management of HGIN and IMC in Barrett's esophagus? Preliminary results of an ongoing study. Gastrointest Endosc 2004; 59:AB101.

149. Levine DS, Haggitt RC, Blount PL, et al. An endoscopic biopsy protocol can differentiate high-grade dysplasia from early adenocarcinoma in Barrett's esophagus. Gastroenterology 1993; 105:40–50.

150. Reid BJ, Blount PL, Feng Z, et al. Optimizing endoscopic biopsy detection of early cancers in Barrett's high-grade dysplasia. Am J Gastroenterol 2000; 95:3089–3096.

CHAPTER FIFTEEN

15

Management of achalasia

Ikuo Hirano

INTRODUCTION

Achalasia is an uncommon but important disease that is the best understood and most readily treatable esophageal motility disorder. It serves as a prototype for disorders of the enteric nervous system with degeneration of the myenteric neurons that innervate the lower esophageal sphincter (LES) and esophageal body. The clinical manifestations, as well as treatment of achalasia, center upon the integrity of the LES. This chapter focuses on therapeutic strategies in the management of achalasia.

CLINICAL FEATURES

Two regional studies conducted in the United States have estimated the incidence of achalasia at 0.6 cases per 100 000 per year, with a prevalence of approximately 10 cases per 100 000. Other features of note are an equal frequency among males and females and an increased incidence with age, particularly after age 70.[1]

Dysphagia and regurgitation are the most commonly reported symptoms in patients with achalasia. While regurgitation is most common during the postprandial period, it can also occur independently of meals due to the prolonged stasis of retained food and saliva in a dilated esophagus. Nocturnal regurgitation of esophageal contents is common and can lead to nighttime cough and aspiration. With progressive disease over prolonged periods, weight loss can occur. Interestingly, during the course of the disease, occasional patients deny symptoms of dysphagia in spite of radiographic and manometric confirmation of the diagnosis of achalasia.[2] The absence of dysphagia may be due to lifestyle adaptations to chronic partial obstruction, acquired accommodation of retained food in a dilated esophagus, or impairment of visceral sensation.[3]

Chest pain is a recognized phenomenon in achalasia and has been reported in 17–63% of patients. The mechanism for chest pain is unclear, although proposed etiologies include secondary or tertiary esophageal contractions, esophageal distention by retained food, gastroesophageal reflux and esophageal irritation by retained medications, food and bacterial or fungal overgrowth. Inflammation within the esophageal myenteric plexus could also be a causative factor. More than one mechanism for pain is likely operative in an individual patient. Pain occurring with food impactions may be secondary to esophageal distention, whereas paroxysmal pain episodes may be neuropathic in origin. A prospective study found no association between the occurrence of chest pain and either manometric or radiographic abnormalities.[4] Patients with chest pain were younger and had a shorter duration of symptoms compared to patients without pain. In this same study, treatment of achalasia had little impact on the reporting of chest pain, in spite of adequate relief of dysphagia. In contrast, a recent surgical series reported adequate relief of chest pain following Heller myotomy.[5] Importantly, chest pain is not a feature in every patient with achalasia. In fact, many patients appear unaware of either esophageal distention or the prolonged retention of food in their esophagus. Recent studies using barostat stimulation of the esophagus have demonstrated that some patients with achalasia have diminished mechanical and chemosensitivity of the esophagus.[3] It is possible that differences in intrinsic and sensory neural degeneration, as well as varied mechanisms for inciting visceral pain, may explain the heterogeneity of visceral sensitivity in the achalasia population.

Heartburn is another notable symptom in achalasics. Patients with untreated achalasia are thought to be 'immune' to gastroesophageal reflux due to impaired LES relaxation. Spechler et al., however, found that a surprising 30% of achalasia patients reported symptoms of what they termed 'heartburn.'[6] In approximately one-third of these patients, the heartburn disappeared coincident with the onset of dysphagia, consistent with the protective nature of achalasia against reflux. However, the remaining two-thirds reported persistent heartburn symptoms at the time of presentation with achalasia. Poor esophageal clearance of even small amounts of refluxed acid and acidic byproducts of bacterial metabolism of retained food are two possible mechanisms for heartburn symptoms. In other cases, the symptom of heartburn may have nothing to do with acidification of the esophageal lumen and instead may represent functional chest pain. Abnormal amounts of acid reflux have been detected in as high as 20% of untreated achalasics by 24-hour ambulatory pH monitoring, suggesting that the first two mechanisms may be significant.[7] Additionally, there are reports, albeit rare, of transient LES relaxations occurring in patients with achalasia.[8–10] Gastroesophageal reflux is, of course, a recognized sequela of successful treatment of achalasia.

The majority of patients with achalasia report difficulty belching. The belch reflex requires not only relaxation of the lower, but also the upper, esophageal sphincter. Massey et al. found that some achalasia patients failed to relax their upper sphincter in response to distention of the esophagus and were thereby unable to belch.[11] This mechanism along with the failure of LES relaxation are important factors responsible for episodes of upper airway obstruction secondary to a massively dilated esophagus that has been reported in achalasia.

DIAGNOSTIC EVALUATION

Upper endoscopy is one of the first tests performed to evaluate patients with dysphagia or suspected achalasia. Findings include esophageal dilatation with retained saliva or food and annular constriction of the gastroesophageal junction. In idiopathic achalasia, the basal LES pressure should not significantly impede intubation of the stomach. Significant difficulty passing an endoscope through the gastroesophageal junction should instead raise the index of suspicion for pseudoachalasia due to neoplastic infiltration of the distal esophagus or gastric cardia. In spite of these recognized endoscopic features, upper endoscopies were reported as normal in 44% of a series of newly diagnosed patients with achalasia.[12] A barium esophagram can be highly suggestive of the diagnosis of achalasia, particularly when there is the combination of esophageal dilatation with retained food and barium and a smooth, tapered constriction of the gastroesophageal junction. However, in the same series mentioned above, the diagnosis of achalasia was suggested in only 64% of barium examinations. The test with the highest sensitivity in the diagnosis of achalasia is esophageal manometry, with defining features that include

aperistalsis of the distal esophagus and incomplete or absent LES relaxation (Fig. 15.1A, C). Additional supportive features include a hypertensive lower esophageal sphincter and low amplitude esophageal body contractions. To exclude the diagnosis of achalasia, esophageal manometry should be performed in patients with dysphagia whose etiology is not evident by endoscopic or radiographic examination. High-resolution esophageal manometry combined with contour plot topographic analyses are recent enhancements to conventional manometry that may improve the diagnostic accuracy of esophageal manometry (Fig. 15.1B, D).

While manometry is regarded as the gold standard for making the diagnosis of achalasia, heterogeneity does exist in the manometric presentation. The most commonly recognized variant of achalasia is known as 'vigorous achalasia,' variably defined by the presence of normal to high-amplitude esophageal body contractions in the presence of a nonrelaxing LES. Such contractions are generally simultaneous and can be difficult to distinguish from common cavity phenomena. While vigorous achalasia may represent an early stage of achalasia, studies have failed to demonstrate differences in terms of clinical presentation in such patients, although botulinum toxin has been reported to be more effective in patients with vigorous achalasia. Additional manometric variants of achalasia include rare individuals with intact peristalsis through the majority of the esophageal body and with preservation of either deglutitive or transient LES relaxation.[10] The significance in defining these variants of achalasia lies in the

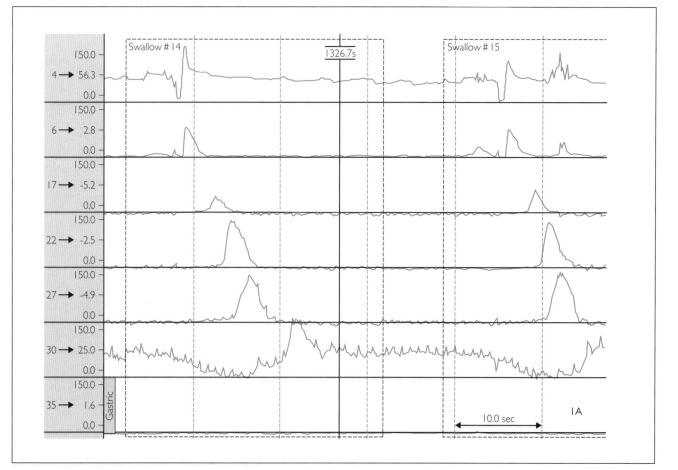

Fig. 15.1 • Esophageal manometric findings in achalasia and contour plot topographic analysis of esophageal motility in achalasia. **(A)** Illustration of a normal esophageal motility recording characterized by peristaltic esophageal body contractions and complete relaxation of the LES.

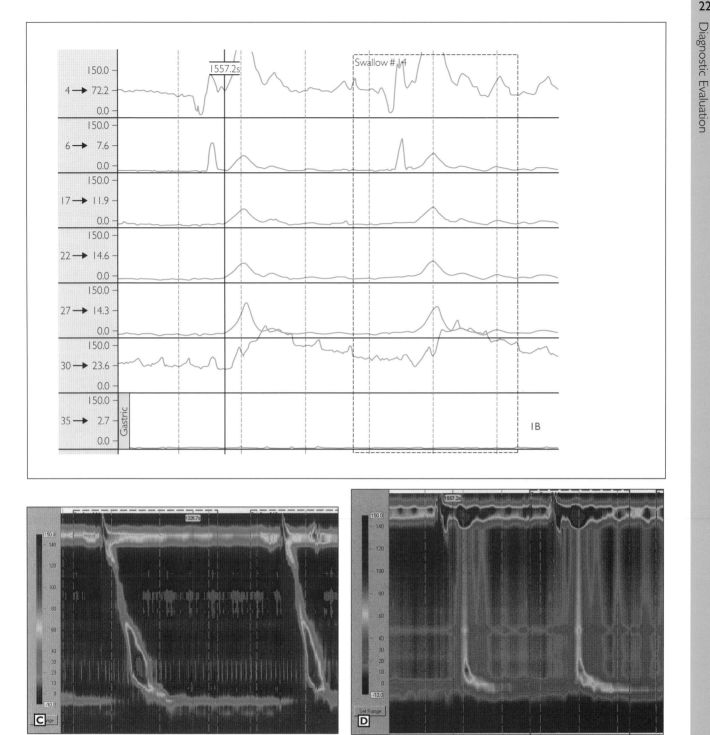

Fig. 15.1 • Cont'd **(B)** Illustration of the findings in classic achalasia, with low-amplitude simultaneous esophageal body contractions and failed relaxation of the lower esophageal sphincter.

Topographic analysis is a method of axial data interpolation derived from computerized plotting of data from multiple, closely spaced, solid state recording transducers. The interpolated pressure information is plotted as a two dimensional contour plot in which pressure amplitude is coded by color. **(C)** Illustration of normal esophageal study with propagation of the peristaltic wave and relaxation of the LES. The upper esophageal sphincter is also depicted at the top of the panel demonstrating a higher basal pressure and shorter relaxation phase. **(D)** Illustration of a study from a patient with achalasia with complete esophageal aperistalsis and incomplete relaxation of the hypertensive lower esophageal sphincter. An esophagogastric pressure gradient is evident in the distal esophagus.

recognition that these sometimes confusing manometric findings are still consistent with achalasia when combined with additional clinical data supportive of the diagnosis.

Secondary forms of achalasia are important considerations during the diagnostic evaluation. The most concerning secondary etiology is cancer, which can present as achalasia by one of three mechanisms. The first, and most common, occurs through direct mechanical obstruction of the gastroesophageal junction. This clinical entity is referred to as pseudoachalasia, and has been described with a number of cancers, most commonly distal esophageal and proximal gastric adenocarcinomas (Table 15.1). Cancer can also infiltrate the submucosa and muscularis of the lower esophageal sphincter and disrupt the myenteric neurons,

resulting in achalasia without an endoscopically visible mucosal abnormality. Finally, tumors remote from the esophagus can cause achalasia through a paraneoplastic syndrome with circulating autoantibodies that are directed at the myenteric neurons. This syndrome is a rare, but important, complication of small cell lung cancer.

Additional secondary causes of achalasia are numerous (see Table 15.1). Of these, the most important to recognize are Chagas' disease and postfundoplication achalasia. Chagas' disease is a parasitic infection caused by *Trypanosoma cruzi* that is endemic to regions of Central and South America and Mexico. While any portion of the gastrointestinal tract can be involved, the esophagus is most commonly affected, and manifests as secondary achalasia in 7–10% of chronically infected individuals.[13] Postfundoplication achalasia is typically caused by constriction of the gastroesophageal junction by the fundoplication or diaphragmatic crura closure. The importance of this complication is in differentiating it from the inadvertent fundoplication in a patient with achalasia whose symptoms were mistaken for 'refractory GERD.' A preceding history of dysphagia and preoperative manometry can generally differentiate postfundoplication achalasia from primary achalasia.

PATHOGENESIS

Histopathologic studies in achalasia have demonstrated chronic inflammatory infiltration of the myenteric plexus with marked paucity and often complete absence of ganglion cells. Such descriptions led to a working model of achalasia in which both the excitatory, cholinergic neurons and inhibitory, nitric oxide/vasoactive intestinal peptide neurons are absent (Fig. 15.2). However, a number of physiologic studies have uncovered an intact cholinergic innervation to the esophagus in some patients with achalasia, leading to a second model for achalasia that incorporates the selective loss of inhibitory neurons.[14] This latter model provides the rationale for the use of botulinum toxin, a potent anticholinergic agent.

The etiology of primary achalasia remains unknown. Several hypotheses have been proposed to account for the loss of ganglia from the esophageal myenteric plexus. A number of studies have implicated viral agents in the pathogenesis. A preliminary report noted a statistically significant increase in antibody titers against measles virus in patients with achalasia compared with controls.[15] While this study has not been substantiated, another study using DNA hybridization techniques found evidence of varicella-zoster virus in three of nine myotomy specimens from patients with achalasia.[16] The predilection of the herpes viruses for squamous epithelium as opposed to columnar epithelium could explain why achalasia targets the esophagus while sparing the remainder of the gastrointestinal tract. More recent studies using polymerase chain reaction techniques, however, failed to detect the presence of measles, herpes, or human papillomaviruses in myotomy specimens of 13 patients with achalasia.[17,18] These negative studies do not exclude the possibility of either alternative viral agents or remote viral infection with subsequent disappearance of the inciting viral pathogen from the host tissue.

Lymphocytic inflammatory infiltration of the affected regions of the esophagus in achalasia led to speculation of an autoimmune etiology. Immunohistochemical staining characterized the infiltrative cells as T-cells positive for CD3 and CD8.[19] An association between achalasia and class II histocompatibility

Table 15.1 Secondary forms of achalasia

Achalasia
Postfundoplication
Allgrove's syndrome (AAA syndrome)
Hereditary cerebellar ataxia
Familial achalasia
Sjögren's syndrome
Sarcoidosis
Postvagotomy
Autoimmune polyglandular syndrome type II
Achalasia with generalized motility disorder
Chagas' disease (*Trypanosoma cruzi*)
MEN IIb (Sipple's syndrome)
Neurofibromatosis (von Recklinghausen's disease)
Paraneoplastic syndrome (Anti-Hu antibody)
Parkinson's disease
Amyloidosis
Fabry's disease
Hereditary cerebellar ataxia
Achalasia with associated Hirschsprung's disease
Hereditary hollow visceral myopathy
Achalasia secondary to cancer (pseudoachalasia)
Squamous cell carcinoma of the esophagus
Adenocarcinoma of the esophagus
Gastric adenocarcinoma
Lung carcinoma
Leiomyoma
Lymphoma
Breast adenocarcinoma
Hepatocellular carcinoma
Reticulum cell sarcoma
Lymphangioma
Metastatic renal cell carcinoma
Mesothelioma
Metastatic prostate carcinoma
Pancreatic adenocarcinoma

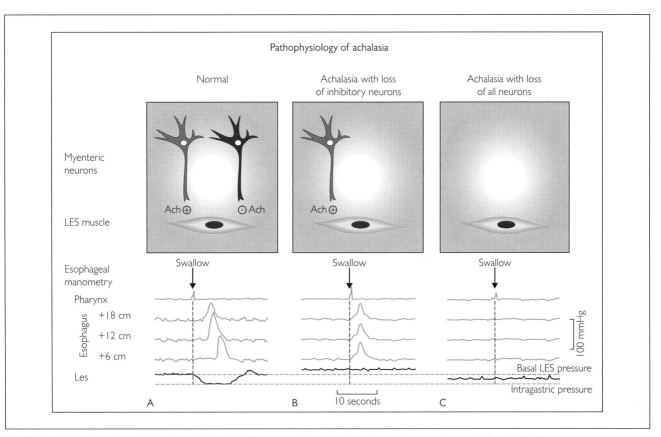

Fig. 15.2 • Pathophysiology of idiopathic achalasia. **(A)** Depiction of the normal condition where excitatory, cholinergic (Ach) motor neurons innervate the smooth muscle cells of the lower esophageal sphincter and contribute to the genesis of basal pressure of the LES (LESP). Inhibitory nitric oxide (NO) motor neurons also act on the LES to produce the relaxation that accompanies a swallow. **(B)** Illustration of the case of achalasia resulting from the loss of inhibitory neurons. In this situation, the absence of nitric oxide motor neurons results in an elevation in the basal LESP and absence of swallow-induced relaxation of the LES. Esophageal aperistalsis is defined by simultaneous esophageal body contractions. **(C)** Depiction of achalasia with complete loss of myenteric neurons. Here the basal LESP is low due to the absent excitatory neurons and swallow-induced relaxation is absent due to the lack of inhibitory neurons. Esophageal aperistalsis is defined by the absence of esophageal body contractions.

antigen has been described. Class II antigen expression on myenteric neurons could be targeted as foreign antigens.[20] Two studies supporting an autoimmune etiology for achalasia demonstrated the presence of serum antibodies against myenteric neurons in achalasia patients.[21,22] The patients' antibodies bound to neurons in enteric plexi from sections of both the esophagus and intestine of rodents. However, because the defect in primary achalasia is specific for the esophagus, the significance of a circulating antibody that targets not only esophageal, but also intestinal, myenteric neurons is unclear. Furthermore, antibodies were also demonstrated in patients with gastroesophageal reflux disease. Thus the circulating antibody detected may be a secondary rather than causative phenomena in the pathogenesis.

Neurodegeneration is a third proposed etiology for primary achalasia. Loss of neurons within the dorsal motor nucleus and degenerative changes of the vagal nerve fibers have been noted.[23] Such findings led investigators to speculate that the site of primary involvement in achalasia was in the dorsal motor nucleus and vagus nerve and that the myenteric abnormalities were secondary. The majority of pathologic studies, however, have found that the predominant abnormalities exist within the myenteric plexus. Furthermore, primary defects in vagal innervation would be expected to lead to prominent autonomic nervous system abnor-

malities outside the esophagus, including gastric emptying disorders, which are uncommon in achalasia. Conversely, clinically significant abnormalities in esophageal function are uncommon in patients who have had surgical vagotomy. Therefore, it is likely that the neurodegenerative changes in achalasia are secondary to viral or autoimmune-mediated destruction of the enteric ganglia.

THERAPY

All forms of therapy for achalasia seek to reduce the LES pressure to allow for improved esophageal clearance by gravity since the esophageal peristaltic pump is characteristically impaired. Treatment options include medical therapy, endoscopic botulinum toxin injection, endoscopic pneumatic dilation, and surgical myotomy (Table 15.2).[24,25] The response given for each therapy represents the pooled response of the referenced studies that enrolled more than 10 patients weighted by sample size. Table 15.2 includes data collected from controlled and uncontrolled studies as well as retrospective studies. Furthermore, the definition of response, follow-up intervals, and disease severity are not standardized among studies, and thus the values given only represent estimates.

Table 15.2 Pooled estimate of response rate of achalasia treatments across referenced studies

Therapy	Total n	Weighted mean response ($\hat{p}$) ± SE %†	Weighted mean follow-up	Weighted mean perforation
Botulinum toxin (27, 38, 40–43, 46, 93–97)	638	78 ± 33	1 mon	NA
	412	58 ± 36	6 mon	
	225	49 ± 23	12 mon	
Pneumatic dilation (Rigiflex) (27, 48, 59, 98–107)	374	85 ± 30	20 mon	2.6
Heller myotomy Thoracotomy (80, 108–119)	1221	84 ± 20%	5 y	NA
Laparotomy (78, 79, 110, 112, 119–125)	732	85 ± 18%	7.6 y	NA
Laparoscopy (68, 70, 122, 126–134)	365	91 ± 13%	1.4 y	NA

$$\dagger \hat{p} = \frac{n_1 p_1 + n_2 p_2 + n_x p_x}{n_1 + n_2 + n_x} \quad SE(\hat{p}) = \sqrt{\frac{p_1(1 - p_1)}{n_1} + \frac{p_2(1 - p_2)}{n_2} + \frac{p_x(1 - p_x)}{n_3}}$$

In calculating the weighted mean response for each treatment modality ($\hat{p}$), included studies were characterized by the number of subjects included (n) and the response rate for those subjects (p). Both controlled and uncontrolled studies reporting more than 10 patients are included. (Modified and updated from reference 24.)

Definition of response

A discussion of the therapy of achalasia should begin with an examination of the goals of therapy. Certainly, symptom relief, particularly relief of dysphagia, is accepted as the primary desired outcome. However, several recent studies have suggested that objective measurement of improvement and sustained response should be considered as additional parameters defining success. Radiographic follow-up studies using barium emptying as an objective measure of the esophageal function have reported that nearly one-third of the patients who reported near-complete symptom improvement following pneumatic dilation had less than 50% improvement in barium emptying.[26] Multiple prospective studies using botulinum toxin demonstrated significant symptom relief but less impressive improvement in objective esophageal function.[27,28] These studies highlight limitations on the use of symptoms alone as the only measure of success of achalasia treatment. The poor correlation between symptoms and objective parameters may be partly due to impaired visceral sensitivity in patients with achalasia.[3]

The concern with using only a symptom profile to define success, while ignoring objective measures of esophageal function, is that inadequate esophageal emptying may lead to not only symptom relapse but also long-term complications, such as progressive esophageal dilatation and an increased risk of esophageal neoplasm. Objective measures of esophageal function include measurements of LES pressure and esophageal emptying by barium radiographs or nuclear scintigraphy. Although an LES pressure of less than 10 mmHg has been shown to be a significant predictor of long-term response to pneumatic dilation,[29] poor patient tolerance for repeated motility studies limits the use of this test. In light of this limitation, semi-quantitative assessment of esophageal emptying using a timed barium swallow has been recommended.[26,30,31] The technique involves the ingestion of a fixed aliquot of barium with serial radiographs obtained at 1, 2, and 5 minutes following ingestion, with comparisons made in the height of the barium column (Fig. 15.3).

Given that symptoms are presently the primary determinant indicating the potential need for additional therapy for patients treated for achalasia, the definition of severity and type of symptom becomes relevant. Most studies use improvement of dysphagia, regurgitation, and chest pain as the primary outcome variables for successful therapeutic response. In most studies, these three symptoms are given equal weight in an overall symptom score, but such weighting has not been well validated. Some studies use grading schemes that rely on symptom frequency, whereas others rely on a patient's perception of symptom severity using terms of 'excellent, good, tolerable, and bad.' The latter terms are, of course, subjective and may be influenced by factors such as patient or physician interpretation and severity of symptom at presentation. The same degree of objective improvement might be interpreted differently in a patient with very mild, intermittent dysphagia compared to one with severe, daily problems. It is worth mentioning that many patients with achalasia continue to experience varying degrees of dysphagia despite an adequate response in objective parameters of esophageal function, such as LES pressure or barium clearance. This disparity may be due to the fact that esophageal body peristaltic function generally does not recover following therapy directed at reducing LES pressure, as the underlying neuropathic process targets not only the LES, but the entire esophagus. Thus, patients are counseled prior to treatment that even successful therapy will improve but not make their swallowing function 'normal.'

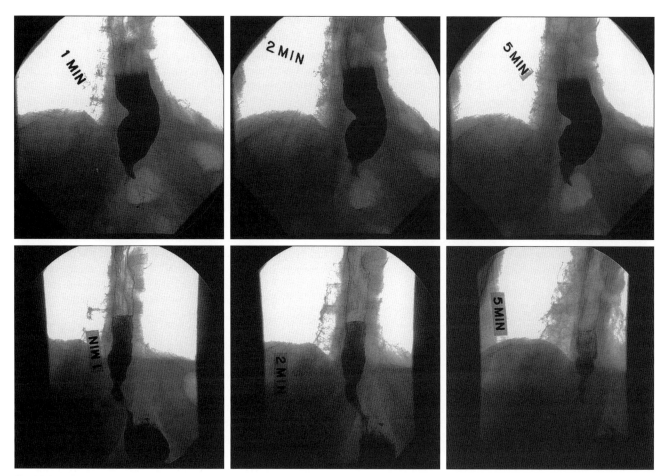

Fig. 15.3 • Timed barium swallow. Following the ingestion of a fixed volume of barium, sequential radiographs are taken at 1, 2, and 5 minutes. The top three panels demonstrate lack of emptying with a fixed column of barium persisting at 5 minutes. The bottom three panels demonstrate the same patient after therapy was performed with pneumatic dilation. An improvement in emptying and degree of esophageal dilatation is shown.

Medical therapy

Medical therapy of achalasia consists of the use of orally administered agents that cause smooth muscle relaxation and thereby improve LES patency. The primary agents in clinical use are nitrates and L-type calcium channel antagonists. Small, randomized controlled trials using sublingual nifedipine and isosorbide dinitrate have demonstrated a significant reduction in LES pressure and symptom relief. However, the long-term effectiveness of medical therapy has generally been limited by both side effects as well as efficacy that is less than the more invasive therapies.

The use of nitrates as therapeutic for achalasia was reported as long ago as 1940, over one-half a century before the mechanism of nitrates as donors of nitric oxide was discovered. Since the inhibitory, nitric oxide-producing myenteric neurons characteristically are destroyed in achalasia, the therapeutic use of an NO donor has good rationale. Unfortunately, systemic vasodilatory effects of nitrates limit their tolerability by patients. Calcium channel antagonists have a better side effect profile compared to nitrates. Two prospective studies, one of which was a placebo-controlled trial, demonstrated the manometric and symptomatic benefit of nifedipine in doses of 10–30 mg sublingually.[32,33] A small, crossover study comparing nifedipine with verapamil failed to show improvement with either therapy, although the agents

were administered orally instead of by the sublingual (SL) route. A prospective study compared the efficacy of isosorbide dinitrate 5 mg SL with nifedipine 20 mg orally three times daily in 15 patients with achalasia.[34] Significantly more patients responded both in terms of symptoms and radionuclide emptying with isosorbide dinitrate compared with nifedipine, although the route of administration was different. Nifedipine (10–20 mg SL) has been compared with pneumatic dilation using Rider-Moeller dilators in a prospective study of 30 patients with achalasia. After a mean follow-up period of 21 months, both treatments led to a significant reduction in LES pressure and a good to excellent symptom response in 75% of the patients.[35] However, in a long-term follow-up report from the same investigators studying a cohort of achalasia patients selected by an initial response to nifedipine, only one-third of patients remained on medical therapy after a mean follow-up period of 2.8 years.[36]

A recent study by Bortolotti et al. demonstrated a significant decrease in LES pressure following the administration of sildenafil (Viagra®).[37] Sildenafil is an inhibitor of phosphodiesterase type 5 that breaks down cyclic GMP, the second messenger stimulated by nitric oxide. The efficacy of sildenafil in achalasia demonstrates the integrity of the nitric oxide second messenger system in the smooth muscle of the LES in achalasia. Side effects and cost are important limitations to the use of sildenafil in the therapy of achalasia. Furthermore, nitrates that also activate the cyclic GMP pathway are available and can be administered by the sublingual pathway.

Overall, medical therapy does have demonstrated efficacy in achalasia, but is limited by a less than optimal response, need for frequent administration, and side effect profile. Given the degree of reduction in LES pressure achieved and short half-life of available agents, medical therapy would be expected to be less effective in the prevention complications of salivary regurgitation, nocturnal aspiration, and megaesophagus compared with pneumatic dilation or Heller myotomy. Medical therapy thus has a limited role in the management of achalasia and is generally restricted to patients awaiting more definitive therapy or patients who are not candidates for more invasive therapies and have not responded to treatment with botulinum toxin. When used, the sublingual route is preferable, given the unreliable delivery via oral administration. Doses should usually be given 10–30 minutes prior to meals, with nitrates having a shorter interval to onset of action compared with nifedipine.

Endoscopic therapy

Botulinum toxin

Botulinum toxin was first used in the treatment of neurologic and ophthalmologic disorders affecting skeletal muscle in the 1970s. It is a protein synthesized by *Clostridium botulinum* that acts at the nerve terminals of the neuromuscular junction by cleaving SNAP-25, a cytoplasmic protein involved in the exocytosis of acetylcholine-containing presynaptic vesicles, thus leading to muscular paralysis. Selective loss of inhibitory neural function in achalasia with preservation of excitatory, cholinergic innervation has been demonstrated in achalasia (see Fig. 15.2). The intact cholinergic neurons constitute a therapeutic target for botulinum toxin. Pasricha et al. introduced the use of botulinum toxin for achalasia in 1995 in a randomized, placebo-controlled trial in 21 patients,[28] demonstrating symptom improvement in 82% after botulinum toxin injection compared with 10% in those received placebo. Significant reductions in LES pressure and improved esophageal radionuclide retention were also demonstrated. This trial was followed by a prospective, long-term follow-up study of 31 patients that reported a response in two-thirds of patients at a mean follow-up of 2.4 years.[38]

Response rates and predictors of success

Botulinum toxin has emerged as a novel therapy that is both easy and safe to administer. To date, there have been over 15 prospective studies involving over 450 patients from around the world that have examined the efficacy of botulinum toxin. Response rates at 1 month following administration average 78% (range 63–90%). The clinical response decreases to 58% (range 25–78%) at 6 months and to 49% (range 15–64%) at 12 months (see Table 15.2). It should be noted that the 12-month data was strongly influenced by a single, multicenter study of 118 patients by Annese et al. that reported the highest response rate of 64%.[46] The transient efficacy of botulinum toxin and the wide range of reported response rates are apparent. With repeated injections, the response rates reported in limited studies are similar or lower to that achieved with the initial injection. This observation implies that with repeated injections, the absolute number of patient responders decreases. The diminishing effect may be due to the development of protective antibodies against the botulinum toxin

molecule that have been demonstrated in approximately 5% of patients treated with botulinum toxin for skeletal muscle disorders.[39] Use of a different serotype of botulinum toxin may be a way of prolonging response rates, although this approach remains to be proven.

The variable response rates to botulinum toxin may be in part due to patient selection as well as definition of response. Predictors of response to botulinum toxin include age >50 years and the presence of vigorous achalasia defined by the presence of esophageal contractile waves with amplitudes in excess of 40 mmHg. In the study by Pasricha et al., the response rate was 82% for patients >50 years and 43% in younger patients.[38] Duration of illness, baseline radiographic features, initial symptom severity, and gender have not been shown to be predictive of response. The clinical definition of response is another important variable between studies. Most studies utilized a scoring system incorporating the symptoms of dysphagia, chest pain, and regurgitation. Response was variably defined in some studies by an absolute point score and in others as achievement of a percent improvement in the symptom score.

Limitations

Most studies have emphasized the clinical efficacy of botulinum toxin therapy for relief of symptoms. Objective measures of response to therapy such as a reduction of lower esophageal sphincter pressure and improvement in esophageal emptying by barium swallow or radionuclide emptying scans, have demonstrated statistically significant, but clinically modest, results. While an approximate 40% reduction in basal LES pressure has been reported, the residual LES pressure post botulinum toxin has averaged approximately 20 mmHg. This residual pressure is clinically relevant as post-treatment LES pressure has been shown to be an important predictor of response to therapy and the need for future therapy. Similarly, studies incorporating measures of esophageal emptying by means of barium radiography or nuclear scintigraphy have demonstrated statistically significant, but modest, improvements in esophageal transit. The apparent disproportionate symptom and objective functional improvement has led to the speculation that botulinum toxin may also be affecting afferent neural function, resulting in impairment of visceral sensation. Highlighting this point is the study by Vaezi et al., a randomized study comparing botulinum toxin with pneumatic dilation. At 1 month post therapy, the response rates were similar. At 1 year, however, 70% of patients treated with pneumatic dilation and only 32% of patients treated with botulinum toxin were in symptomatic remission.[27] Four other randomized studies comparing botulinum toxin to pneumatic dilation have also demonstrated significantly greater symptom and objective esophageal functional improvement with pneumatic dilation.[40-43] Although the Vaezi study did not allow for repeated injections of botulinum toxin, the lower response rate was seen at nearly all intermediate time points beyond 2 months. Of greater concern was the observation that objective parameters of esophageal function, including LES pressure and esophageal emptying by barium swallow, did not significantly improve after botulinum toxin, while substantial reductions were seen after pneumatic dilation. While many patients treated with botulinum toxin showed a decrement in LES pressure following treatment, one-third of the patients were noted to have a paradoxical increase in LES pressure. These results conflict with the majority of other published series that have reported a consistent and statistically significant decrease in LES pressure among treated patients, although two abstracts also reported a lack of improvement following botulinum toxin.

Indications

Given these limitations to the efficacy and durability of response, botulinum toxin is generally reserved for use for patients who are not candidates for more invasive treatments with pneumatic dilation or Heller myotomy. Such patients might include elderly patients with comorbidities and patients awaiting more definitive therapy. Given the concerns of modest objective esophageal functional improvement in spite of symptom improvement, some assessment of esophageal emptying following botulinum toxin is reasonable. Recent reports have also raised concerns about adverse effects of botulinum toxin therapy on subsequent esophagomyotomy. These reports have noted technical difficulty with the surgical procedure, with a risk of intraoperative esophageal perforation perhaps secondary to obliteration of tissue planes from an inflammatory reaction created by the biologic agent.[44,45] However, other studies have not confirmed this observation, and previous botulinum toxin therapy does not appear to affect the overall outcome of surgery should it be indicated.

Dosing and technique of administration

The optimal dose of botulinum toxin therapy was examined by Annese and colleagues.[46] In this multicenter study from Italy, 118 patients were randomized to treatment with 50, 100, and 200 units of botulinum toxin. Responders to the 100 unit dose were administered a second 100 units after 30 days. At a mean follow-up of 12 months, relapse was seen in 19% treated with the double injections of 100 units compared with 47% and 43% for the 50 and 200 unit doses, respectively. The effect of intermittent versus scheduled dosing of botulinum toxin on clinical efficacy has not been studied. Other potential variations on technique of administration of botulinum toxin include retrograde injection into the gastric aspect of the LES under retroflexed positioning of the endoscope and EUS guidance of the injections. Neither of these techniques has been shown to have increased efficacy over the standard botulinum toxin administration method. A suggested protocol for use of botulinum toxin is given in Table 15.3.

Side effects

Botulinum toxin injection for achalasia has been extremely safe. Concerns about potential muscular paralysis have not been realized in the gastrointestinal or neurological applications as the doses used are 20 to 30 times less than the per kilogram lethal dose reported in primates. Transient chest pain is usually mild and has been reported in approximately 20% of patients. Significant heartburn is reported in approximately 5–10% of patients. Isolated case reports of potential adverse events have included heart block, urinary retention, and pneumothorax.

Pneumatic dilation

Dilation system

Dilation of the esophagus is the oldest form of therapy for achalasia with the earliest use credited to the use of a whale bone by Willis in 1674. Since that time, a number of different techniques have been employed, all with the purpose of mechanically disrupting the LES. Bougienage using dilators with diameters of

---

Table 15.3 Botulinum toxin (Botx) injection technique for achalasia

1. Botx is stored at or below −5°C until ready for use.

2. Botx is contraindicated in patients with an allergy to eggs.

3. Reconstitute Botx 100 IU with 5 mL of preservative-free normal saline immediately prior to use (yields 20 IU per mL). Care is taken to avoid excess agitation and frothing of Botx during the process.

4. Five-millimeter sclerotherapy catheter/needle is primed with Botx. A preservative-free normal saline flush is used to expel the final 1–2 mL of Botx from the catheter.

5. Standard upper endoscopy is performed with aspiration of any retained esophageal contents and close inspection of the gastroesophageal junction and cardia.

6. Injection is performed into the proximal aspect of the constriction or 'rosette' at the gastroesophageal junction. This typically is located 1–2 cm proximal to the squamocolumnar junction. The needle is angled at approximately 45° to penetrate the muscularis propria and avoid a submucosal injection. Four quadrant injections are performed for a total of 80 to 100 IU.

7. Standard postendoscopy recovery with follow up at 4 weeks with consideration for objective assessment of esophageal emptying.

---

less than 60 French had been advocated in the past but have since been supplanted by use of pneumatic or mechanical dilators with diameters exceeding 90 French (see Table 15.2). A more recent retrospective study compared symptom response following 56-French mercury bougienage with pneumatic dilation and reported responses of 50% and 83%, respectively.[47] While the smaller diameter bougienage is clearly inferior to pneumatic dilation, it is a safer procedure and might be considered in patients at high risk for more invasive therapies, either as an alternative or perhaps in combination with botulinum toxin.

Currently, the Rigiflex™ pneumatic dilator (Boston Scientific Corp, Boston, MA) is the most widely used and readily available dilating system for achalasia (Fig. 15.4). The polyethylene balloon is noncompliant and is available in three sizes designed to inflate to fixed diameters of 3, 3.5, or 4 cm. This system offers a safety advantage over earlier compliant, latex balloons that delivered variable diameters depending upon inflation pressure.

Dilation technique and predictors of success

Kadakia and Wong reported the results of 47 patients treated with the Rigiflex™ system using a stepwise approach, in which dilation was started with a 3 cm balloon with progression to a 3.5 cm and 4 cm balloon for patients not responding to prior dilator size.[48,49] In this series, 62% of patients responded to a 3 cm balloon, with 45% of the nonresponders achieving success with a 3.5 cm balloon. Six patients went on to receive a 4 cm dilation, with 67% responding, yielding an overall response to dilation of 93% over a mean follow-up period of 47 months (range 3–72 months).

Over 20 retrospective and prospective studies have been reported on the effectiveness of pneumatic dilation for achalasia using the Rigiflex™ balloon dilator. The overall response rates,

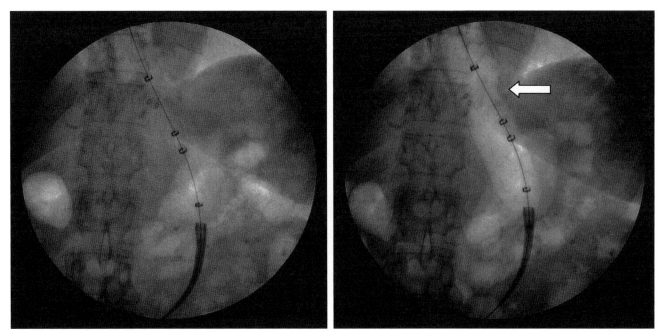

Fig. 15.4 ● Pneumatic dilation for achalasia using Rigiflex balloon dilator. The left panel shows an uninflated balloon being positioned across the gastroesophageal junction. The four radio opaque rings are centered upon the junction that is visualized endoscopically and generally situated at the level of the diaphragm. The right panel depicts the balloon being inflated, with evidence of a constriction or waist created at the midpoint of the balloon (arrow) due to the LES.

defined by good to excellent relief of symptoms, averages 85% (range 70–92%) with mean follow-up period of 20 months (see Table 15.2). As discussed below, a marked decrement in the response rate has been noted in several, recent, long-term follow-up studies of pneumatic dilation using balloon dilators that are no longer available. It is therefore reasonable to expect that the response rate in Table 15.2 will decrease with long-term follow-up studies using the Rigiflex™ system.

A protocol for pneumatic dilation is listed in Table 15.4.[49] While the use of the Rigiflex™ dilators with an approach that incorporates stepwise increments in balloon diameter has been accepted, a number of methodological issues have not been standardized. The use of conscious sedation, pressure to which the balloon is inflated, duration of balloon inflation, and number of inflations per session are variables that could affect patient outcomes and complications. The use of conscious sedation could theoretically decrease the efficacy of pneumatic dilation through relaxation of the lower esophageal sphincter. Arguing against this possibility is the uncontrolled observation that the response rates in studies using conscious sedation are similar to those not employing sedation.[29,48] The importance of specific dilation parameters have been addressed in a small number of prospective studies. Khan and Castell randomized 81 patients to either 60- or 6-second dilation with a 3 cm Rigiflex™ dilator and found similar symptom improvement in both groups at 6 month follow-up.[50] Kim and colleagues reported a study of 14 patients randomized to different balloon sizes, one or two inflations per session, and differing inflation times.[51] The problem with these studies is that the small sample sizes limit their statistical power to detect significant differences. Nevertheless, the limited prospective and retrospective studies have not shown that inflation times, inflation duration, or number of inflations significantly affect outcomes.

Studies examining clinical and technical factors have identified age, balloon diameter, post-dilation lower esophageal sphincter pressure, clearance of barium on esophagram, and prior dilation as predictors of success following pneumatic dilation. Similar to the botulinum toxin experience, several studies have reported that older patients respond better than younger patients. Eckardt found a 2-year remission rate of 29% in patients under 40 compared with 67% for those over 40.[29] In this same study, a Browne-McHardy pneumatic dilator was used, and balloon diameter of less than 3.6 cm was associated with a 31% response compared with 68% for diameter greater than 3.6 cm. Post-dilation LES pressure of <10 mmHg was associated with a 100% 2-year remission rate compared with 71% for pressures between 10 and 20 mmHg and 23% for pressures over 20 mmHg. Vaezi and Richter reported that 30% of patients treated with pneumatic dilation had excellent relief of symptoms in spite of poor emptying of barium at 1 month post dilation.[31] This subgroup of patients had a 90% failure rate at one year as defined by the return of symptoms and need for retreatment. Of note, esophageal clearance of barium immediately after pneumatic dilation has not been shown to be predictive of outcome, likely due to confounding factors of transient muscular spasm or edema.[52] Prior pneumatic dilation portends a lower response rate. In a retrospective study by Parkman et al., over a 5-year time period, subsequent treatment was required in 40% after initial dilation, 65% following a second dilation and 75% following a third dilation.[53] However, the overall remission rates are higher in the population of patients undergoing repeated dilations compared to those having single dilations.[54]

Long-term outcomes

Long-term follow-up studies of the effectiveness of pneumatic dilation have reported a substantially lower response rate of

Table 15.4 Pneumatic dilation protocol

1. The patient is consented with specific documentation of discussion of risk of esophageal perforation. On-site availability of thoracic surgeon is confirmed prior to the procedure date.

2. The patient is maintained on liquid diet for 24 hours and kept fasting for 8 hours prior to endoscopy. A longer period of liquid diet may be necessary for patients with megaesophagus.

3. The Rigiflex™ balloon and inflation device are checked prior to use.

4. The patient is positioned in the supine position. Standard upper endoscopy is performed with aspiration of retained esophageal contents and careful attention to the gastroesophageal junction and cardia for possible secondary achalasia.

5. The fluoroscopic position of the constricted gastroesophageal junction is noted by positioning the tip of the endoscope at the GEJ and checking the fluoroscopic image.

6. A Savary™ guidewire is placed into the gastric antrum and the endoscope is withdrawn.

7. The Rigiflex™ dilator is advanced over the guidewire and positioned such that the inner radiopaque markers straddle the previously determined fluoroscopic position of the gastroesophageal junction (usually at the level of the diaphragm).

8. The Rigiflex™ balloon is inflated with fluoroscopic monitoring of the positioning and obliteration of a waist on the balloon that corresponds with the LES. Maximum distention is held at 7–12 psi for 30–60 seconds. Care is taken to maintain traction on the dilation catheter as there is a tendency for the balloon to be drawn into the stomach during inflation. A shorter, second inflation is sometimes performed to confirm obliteration of the LES (absence of waist on the balloon) although the utility of this is unproven.

9. The patient is repositioned on the left side to minimize aspiration risk and the deflated Rigiflex balloon and guidewire are removed simultaneously.

10. Observation in the recovery room is continued for 4 hours.

11. A Gastrograffin® followed by thin barium swallow is performed after 1 hour to look for perforation. Poor emptying on the immediate postdilation study does not translate to a failed procedure.

12. The patient is advised to remain on a liquid diet and to advance diet as tolerated after 24 hours

13. Proton pump inhibitor therapy is strongly considered even in the absence of reflux symptoms.

14. Follow-up is scheduled in 4 weeks with objective reassessment of esophageal emptying by timed barium swallow. If no clinical improvement is evident, repeat dilation with larger-diameter balloon or laparoscopic Heller myotomy are discussed.

30–40%, approximately one-half that reported in the short-term studies. Two long-term studies with mean follow-up periods of 5–6 years did report success rates for pneumatic dilation of over 85%.[53,55] However, both studies were retrospective and defined success as the need for no additional therapy beyond pneumatic dilation. When incorporating a symptom score as well as avoidance of surgery as defining success, Torbey and West reported success rates of pneumatic dilation of 26%, with mean follow-up of 7 years and 50% with mean follow-up of 12 years, respectively.[56,57] In both studies, many patients who were symptomatic did not seek medical attention for retreatment. In the study by Torbey and West, 124 patients were included, and repeated dilations were performed with a median of four dilations per patient over the study period. Thirty-five percent were classified as having a poor response defined as dysphagia more than once a week, lasting longer than 2–3 minutes or accompanied by regurgitation or weight loss. A more optimistic report by Chan et al. followed up on 32 patients reporting cumulative success rates of pneumatic dilation of 74% and 62% at 5 and 19 years, respectively.[58] While the above studies were based on questionnaires mailed to previously treated achalasia patients, Eckardt et al. recently reported the long-term results of a prospective study of pneumatic dilation.[54] Fifty-four patients were followed for a median of 13.8 years, with remission defined by a clinical symptom assessment. Clinical remission was present in 40% of patients at 5 years following a single pneumatic dilation. In the subset of patients in remission at 5 years, 85% remained in remission at 10 years. In patients undergoing repeated dilations, the remission rate was 35% at 5 years. As in the short-term studies, age and post-dilation LES pressure were strong predictors of successful outcome. Patients 40 and younger had a 5-year remission rate of only 16% compared to 58% for those older than 40. Patients with post-dilation pressures less than 10 mmHg had a 75% remission rate at 10 years. These long-term follow-up studies emphasize important limitations of pneumatic dilation as primary therapy for achalasia. The effectiveness of pneumatic dilation appears to diminish over time, and even with repeated dilations, the majority of achalasia patients have clinical relapses. This observation has led to the recommendation that patients treated with pneumatic dilation as primary therapy be followed more vigilantly, perhaps with objective testing of esophageal function. Poor responders might be identified earlier through such an approach and undergo treatment with surgical esophagomyotomy. This approach presumes, of course, that surgical therapy is more effective than pneumatic dilation and offers a more durable response. Although unproven by prospective studies, this conclusion is supported by available uncontrolled studies.

Complications

Complications of pneumatic dilation exist, the most significant of which is esophageal perforation. Published series using the Rigiflex™ dilator and including more than 10 patients have reported perforation rates of 0–8 % with a mean rate of 2.6 % (see Table 15.2). The graded approach to pneumatic dilation starting with the smaller diameter dilators has been associated with a lower perforation risk.[48] However, it should be noted that perforations, albeit rare, have been reported with the 3 cm Rigiflex™ dilator.[58,59] Risk factors for perforation have historically included epiphrenic diverticula, hiatal hernia, inflation pressures exceeding 10 psi, the presence of esophagitis at the time of dilation, presence of vigorous achalasia, and prior esophagomyotomy. Retrospective studies of large numbers of patients treated with pneumatic dilation that included patients with these conditions have not substantiated these concerns.[59,60] Furthermore, inflation pressure is no longer a concern using the noncompliant, Rigiflex™ dilators. Death from pneumatic dilation is very uncommon and not observed in most series. One report examining complications in 504 patients treated with pneumatic dilation reported two deaths, both in patients over 90 years of age, with one developing sepsis and one having a perforation.[60] Delayed recognition of the complication was noted in both cases.

Schwartz and Traube reported the outcomes of seven perforations requiring emergent surgery with esophagomyotomy compared to five patients who had undergone elective esophagomyotomy.[61] No differences in length of hospitalization or long-term outcomes were observed. Assuming an equivalent outcome in these two groups, there would be little downside to recommending that pneumatic dilation be first-line therapy for achalasia. However, the advent of laparoscopic Heller myotomy has substantially challenged this paradigm in favor of surgery since the less invasive laparoscopic option is not an option for perforation from pneumatic dilation. Additional reported complications following pneumatic dilation include transient chest pain, gastrointestinal bleeding, esophageal hematoma formation (usually asymptomatic), and symptomatic esophageal mucosal tears. The latter is usually managed conservatively with inpatient observation and intravenous antibiotics.[62]

Gastroesophageal reflux can complicate pneumatic dilation. Prospective studies using pH monitoring have detected significant acid reflux in 25–35% of patients following dilation.[63,64] Most of the patients with significant gastroesophageal reflux did not report heartburn. Achalasia patients may have impaired visceral sensitivity and have less sensitivity to Bernstein testing.[3] Acid reflux may have important sequelae, including esophagitis, Barrett's esophagus, and peptic stricture formation in patients with treated achalasia. Empiric proton pump inhibitor therapy, therefore, should be considered even in the absence of heartburn.

Surgical therapy

Surgical technique

Surgical treatment of achalasia has undergone substantial changes over the past century. Heller described the original myotomy in 1913 with both an anterior and posterior incision of the muscularis propria of the gastroesophageal junction approached through a laparotomy. Over the next several decades, the surgical approach was modified to include only a single anterior myotomy via thoracotomy. Minimally invasive surgical techniques were first reported by Cuschieri et al. in 1991 and Pellegrini et al. in 1992 using laparoscopic and thoracoscopic approaches, respectively.[65,66] The laparoscopic technique is now the preferred method due to better accessibility of the intra-abdominal portion of the LES and avoidance of the need for a postoperative chest tube.[67] The use of minimally invasive technology has been a significant advance, allowing patients shorter hospital stays of 2–3 days and less recovery time. Success rates reported in large series approximate 90%, with mean follow-up approaching 2 years (see Table 15.2). Perioperative complications of perforation, hemorrhage, or pneumothorax are uncommon and readily managed intraoperatively.

Intraoperative endoscopy and manometry

Intraoperative endoscopy and manometry have been utilized as a method to reduce the potential for incomplete myotomy. Endoscopy allows for visual inspection of patency of the gastroesophageal junction following myotomy.[68–71] The transillumina-tion may also improve the visualization of residual muscle fibers along the myotomy. As mentioned above, post-treatment LES pressure is an important predictor of the success of achalasia therapy. The use of intraoperative manometry was first reported by Del Ginio and Hill as a means of assessing the completeness of myotomy.[72,73] Several studies have reported the manometric detection of a residual high-pressure zone after apparently complete surgical myotomy that led to extension of the myotomy.[74–76] Our experience at Northwestern University has demonstrated a learning curve in terms of the benefits of intraoperative manometry.[74] A residual high-pressure zone requiring myotomy extension was detected in 25% of the first 40 cases, compared with less than 5% after 100 cases. These results point to the potential utility of intraoperative manometry in determining the completeness of surgical myotomy in the early surgical experience with the procedure or perhaps in low-volume surgical centers. Whether manometry adds value to intraoperative endoscopy alone in determining adequacy of the myotomy has not been studied.

Gastroesophageal reflux and surgical anti-reflux procedure

An area of ongoing controversy in the surgical management of achalasia has been the need or lack thereof of an accompanying antireflux procedure. Reflux is not an infrequent complication of both endoscopic and surgical therapies that seek to obliterate LES pressure in the setting of an aperistaltic esophagus. In one of the larger surgical series, reflux was documented by pH testing in 17% of patients following laparoscopic myotomy, with most of these subjects not reporting heartburn.[68] Successful treatment of achalasia effectively transforms the manometric picture from achalasia to one of a 'scleroderma' esophagus, with the concomitant risks of regurgitation and acid reflux disease. Complications of Barrett's esophagus and peptic stricture have been documented in several reported series following Heller myotomy. Reflux and its complications are of particular concern in achalasia patients, who appear to have diminished visceral sensation and may not complain of typical heartburn symptoms.[3] Surgical approaches to the problem have included creation of a loose Nissen, partial posterior Toupet, or partial anterior Dor fundoplication. While the Nissen fundoplication is generally avoided, controversy exists over the superiority of the Toupet and Dor procedure. The Toupet is created by attaching the fundoplication to either edge of the myotomy, whereas the Dor is positioned to directly cover the myotomy site. Angulation of the gastroesophageal junction and the potential for inciting fibrosis of the myotomy site are issues that may reduce the efficacy of the procedure for relieving dysphagia while attempting to prevent gastroesophageal reflux.

Dysphagia post-Heller myotomy

Dysphagia following Heller myotomy can be subclassified into dysphagia that persists following myotomy and dysphagia that redevelops in a delayed manner, months or even years following surgery. Early postoperative dysphagia can be caused by incomplete myotomy, periesophageal scarring, underlying esophageal dysmotility, massive esophageal distention with sigmoid deformity, or mechanical obstruction by the fundoplication, paraesophageal hernia, or crural diaphragmatic hiatus repair. It is important that patients recognize that some degree of dysphagia is anticipated even after successful myotomy given the esophageal aperistalsis that characterizes the disease as it is uncommon for esophageal peristalsis to recover following therapy directed at the LES. Late postoperative dysphagia is most commonly caused by either the development of a recurrent high-pressure zone at the LES or peptic stricture complicating acid reflux. Less commonly, an obstructed fundoplication or the development of esophageal cancer can manifest. The recurrent high-pressure zone may be due to the development of scarring of the myotomy site that leads to connection of the cut edges of the muscularis propria, thus reestablishing the circular integrity of the LES. In cases of post-operative dysphagia due to either an incomplete myotomy or recurrent high-pressure zone, pneumatic dilation can be employed as an alternative to a second operation. Concerns over risks of perforation after a myotomy with only a thin epithelial layer separating the esophageal lumen from the mediastinum exist. However, published series have reported success with pneumatic dilation, commonly requiring a 3.5 cm rather than 3.0 cm balloon.[59,77]

Long-term outcomes

The reported remission rates after Heller myotomy for achalasia reflect a gradual deterioration over time. Csendes et al. reported a 95% success rate at a median follow-up of 62 months following myotomy via an open abdominal approach.[78] Malthaner et al. reported a 95% success rate at 1 year, 77% at 5 years, 68% at 10 years, and 67% at 20 years.[79] Similarly, Ellis reported an 86% remission rate at 15 years and 67% at 20 years.[80] Thus, the effectiveness of even what is considered the most definitive therapy for achalasia appears to wane with time. While the long-term results are not as discouraging as those recently reported for pneumatic dilation, they do highlight potential limitations of surgery and the importance of clinical follow-up. Whether the effectiveness of pneumatic dilation that is performed for recurrent dysphagia following Heller myotomy approximates that of pneumatic dilation performed as primary therapy has not been reported.

Comparison of pneumatic dilation and Heller myotomy

Studies comparing pneumatic dilation and Heller myotomy are limited. Several retrospective studies have reported superior success rates for surgery compared with pneumatic dilation. The potential for selection bias and the varied methods used for pneumatic dilation limit the conclusions that can be drawn from such studies. Two prospective studies have been reported. The first was reported by Csendes et al., who randomized 81 patients to pneumatic dilation with a Mosher bag or Heller myotomy with Dor fundoplasty via laparotomy.[78] The study was conducted at the University of Chile, and 14% of the patients had Chagas' disease. The Mosher bag had a maximum diameter of 4 cm with 2 inflations of 10–20 seconds at 5.4 psi. Atropine was used as a premedication and could have affected the response to balloon dilation through inhibition of LES basal tone. Nevertheless, at long-term follow-up of a median of 62 months, excellent results were achieved in 95% of the surgical group, compared with only 65% of the dilation group, of whom some had undergone a second dilation to maintain their response. The dilations were performed by the same surgeon who performed the myotomy, and blinding was thus not possible. In spite of the criticisms raised regarding the technique of pneumatic dilation employed, the 65% response at 5-year follow-up is similar to the rate reported in other studies of pneumatic dilation. A second prospective study

by Felix et al. from Brazil is the only other prospective comparison of the two techniques.[81] This study randomized 40 patients with Chagas' disease to balloon dilation or laparotomy with Heller myotomy and Toupet fundoplication and found similar efficacy at 3-year follow-up. The balloon dilation technique utilized an aggressive approach that incorporated a rubber balloon with maximum diameter of 4 cm with 3 distentions of 5 minutes each with inflation pressures of 5.4 psi. To date, there are no controlled data comparing the currently used techniques of laparoscopic Heller myotomy with pneumatic dilation using Rigiflex™ dilators. It should be mentioned that laparoscopic treatment has been compared to botulinum toxin injection, with the former being the superior approach,[82,83] which is not surprising since botulinum toxin is less effective than pneumatic dilation.

Studies comparing the cost-effectiveness of pneumatic dilation and Heller myotomy have favored dilation.[53,84] These studies have used a short-term time horizon, generally under 5 years, to define success. However, experience in the minimally invasive surgical approach has resulted in decreases in the length of hospitalization as well as associated costs of surgery. Moreover, several recent publications have reported a less than 40% long-term remission rate with pneumatic dilation, even with repeated dilations. In one series, the median number of dilations over a mean 12-year follow-up period was 4, with 1 patient having received 14 dilations.[57] Such emerging data would likely shift the cost analysis in favor of laparoscopic Heller myotomy, especially in younger patients who would likely require multiple dilations during the course of their lifetime.

Refractory achalasia

In patients with achalasia that is refractory to therapy with Heller myotomy, options are limited. Esophagectomy is considered in patients with marked dilation (exceeding 6 cm in diameter) and sigmoid deformity. Many such patients continue to have symptoms and radiographic evidence of poor esophageal emptying in spite of an adequate myotomy, with patency of the gastro-esophageal junction demonstrable both endoscopically and manometrically. It should be noted that the presence of megaesophagus with sigmoid deformity, but with competency of the lower esophageal sphincter, may respond to Heller myotomy.[85] Esophagectomy is usually performed with a gastric pull-up or Ivor Lewis esophagogastrectomy, but some cases may require colonic interposition. Success rates from larger centers approximate 90%, but significant morbidity and a 2–8% mortality have been reported.[86–88]

Other treatments for refractory achalasia that have been reported include endoscopic esophageal stent and gastrostomy tube placement. Stenting should generally be avoided as there exists a high stent migration rate, likely secondary to the presence of a proximal esophageal dilation above a short, smooth constriction of the gastroesophageal junction.[89] Other potential complications of stent placement, such as bleeding and perforation, need to be considered as well given the benign nature of the underlying disease state. Gastrostomy placement might be considered in patients with a very high risk for either pneumatic dilation or surgery and short survival due to other comorbidities. While providing nutrition and access for medications, gastrostomy tube placement would not reduce the symptoms and complications of salivary accumulation and regurgitation.

DISEASE COMPLICATIONS

The primary complications of achalasia are related to the functional obstruction rendered by the nonrelaxing LES. These include progressive malnutrition and aspiration. Aspiration can be a substantial cause of morbidity, with patients at risk for postprandial and nocturnal coughing and aspiration. Uncommon, but important, secondary complications of achalasia include the formation of epiphrenic diverticula and esophageal cancer. Epiphrenic diverticula presumably form as a result of increased intraluminal pressures and are most commonly detected in the distal esophagus immediately proximal to the LES. Esophageal cancer is also seen with an increased frequency in patients with idiopathic achalasia. Most commonly, the cancers that develop are squamous cell carcinomas, although adenocarcinomas are also reported. A large cohort study from Sweden found a 16-fold increased risk of esophageal cancer during years 1 through 24 after initial diagnosis. Cancers detected in the first year after the diagnosis of achalasia were excluded to eliminate pre-existing cancers that may have presented as secondary or pseudo-achalasia.[90] The overall prevalence of esophageal cancer in achalasia is approximately 3%, with an incidence of approximately 197 per 100 000 per year.[91] The incidence of cancer does significantly increase after 15 years of symptoms referable to achalasia. However, based on the overall low incidence of esophageal cancer, routine endoscopic screening of patients with achalasia is not generally recommended.[92] Nevertheless, some experts still advocate consideration of a surveillance program in patients with long-standing achalasia who would be candidates for esophageal resection were a cancer to be detected.[91] While it is possible that successful treatment of achalasia may reduce the risk of cancer, this possibility has not been proven and several cases have been reported of squamous cell carcinoma arising following therapy with pneumatic dilation or surgical myotomy.

CONCLUSIONS

Despite being considered a single disorder, achalasia demonstrates significant diversity in terms of both clinical manifestations and response to therapy. Variability in the stage at presentation and underlying enteric neural degeneration are likely explanations for this heterogeneity. Current management options include medical, endoscopic, and surgical therapy. Botulinum toxin, while targeting intact cholinergic function in patients with achalasia, has both limited efficacy and durability of response and is reserved for patients at high risk for invasive procedures. Pneumatic dilation and laparoscopic Heller myotomy are both accepted primary therapies for achalasia. However, recent long-term follow-up studies have reported a substantial decrement in effectiveness of pneumatic dilation over time. Whether closer clinical follow-up and more aggressive dilation protocols will improve the long-term success rates remains to be seen. Recent advances in minimally invasive surgery from large-volume centers with excellent response rates and low morbidity have led to laparoscopic myotomy being considered first-line therapy at many institutions, particularly for younger patients. Ongoing investigations into the etiology of the enteric neurodegeneration that characterizes achalasia will lead to more targeted therapeutics.

The management of achalasia is summarized in Table 15.5.

Table 15.5 Management of achalasia: general guidelines

1. The diagnosis of achalasia should be suspected in patients with esophageal dysphagia that is not explained by a mechanical obstruction. Manometry is the most sensitive test and manometric variants of achalasia should be recognized. Secondary achalasia, particularly that associated with cancer, should be excluded in the appropriate clinical setting.

2. Medical therapy consists of sublingual (SL) administration of nitrates or calcium channel antagonists. Agents studied include isosorbide dinitrate 5 mg SL three times per day and nifedipine 10–20 mg SL three times per day prior to meals. Medications are generally used as a temporizing measure while awaiting more definitive therapy.

3. Endoscopic injection of botulinum toxin provides symptomatic relief of dysphagia in about 60% of patients at 6 months. Predictors of response include age >50 and presence of vigorous achalasia. Objective measures of esophageal function do not improve to the same degree as seen with pneumatic dilation. Moreover, the response to botulinum toxin wanes with time and repeated injections have been associated with a decrease in the number of patient responders. Therefore, botulinum toxin is recommended for patients who are poor candidates for more invasive therapies due to medical comorbidities.

4. Pneumatic dilation using the Rigiflex™ balloon is an accepted first line-therapy for achalasia, with reported response rates of 85% at 1–2 years and perforation rates averaging 2.6%. Predictors of response include larger balloon diameter and age >40. A graded approach is recommended that starts with a 3 cm balloon, with incremental balloon diameters reserved for nonresponders. Long-term follow-up studies suggest that the effectiveness of pneumatic dilation diminishes over time, with an approximate 40% remission rate at 5 years even with repeated dilations.

5. Based on limited, mostly uncontrolled observations, laparoscopic Heller myotomy is the most effective therapy for achalasia with response rates of 90% reported from centers with large patient experiences. Improvements in surgical approach have resulted in shortened hospital stays approximating 1 day. Furthermore, the benefits of the minimally invasive surgical approach are not available to patients who have perforations resulting from pneumatic dilation, as these require a traditional thoracotomy. Laparoscopic Heller myotomy is a recommended primary therapy at centers having surgical experience with the procedure, especially for younger patients. Complications of gastroesophageal reflux occur and can be treated with proton pump inhibitor therapy.

REFERENCES

1. Mayberry JF. Epidemiology and demographics of achalasia. Gastrointest Endosc Clin N Am 2001; 11(2):235–248.

2. Salzberg BA, et al. Achalasia: a disease of varied and subtle symptoms that do not correlate with radiographic findings. Am J Gastroenterol 2002; 97(10):2577–2584.

3. Brackbill S, Shi G, Hirano I. Diminished mechanosensitivity and chemosensitivity in patients with achalasia. Am J Physiol – Gastrointest Liver Physiol 2003; 285(6):G1198–G1203.

4. Eckardt VF, Stauf B, Bernhard G. Chest pain in achalasia: patient characteristics and clinical course. Gastroenterology 1999; 116(6):1300–1304.

5. Perretta S, et al. Achalasia and chest pain: effect of laparoscopic Heller myotomy. J Gastrointest Surg 2003; 7(5):595–598.

6. Spechler SJ, et al. Heartburn in patients with achalasia. Gut 1995; 37(3):305–308.

7. Shoenut JP, et al. Reflux in untreated achalasia patients. J Clin Gastroenterol 1995; 20(1):6–11.

8. van Herwaarden MA, Samsom M, Smout AJ. Prolonged manometric recordings of oesophagus and lower oesophageal sphincter in achalasia patients. Gut 2001; 49(6):813–821.

9. Holloway, RH, Wyman JB, Dent J. Failure of transient lower oesophageal sphincter relaxation in response to gastric distension in patients with achalasia: evidence for neural mediation of transient lower oesophageal sphincter relaxations. Gut 1989; 30(6):762–767.

10. Hirano I, et al. Manometric heterogeneity in patients with idiopathic achalasia. Gastroenterology 2001; 120(4):789–798.

   Four manometric variants of achalasia are described including patients with (1) vigorous achalasia, (2) integrity of proximal esophageal peristaltic function (short segment achalasia), (3) apparent intact deglutitive LES inhibition, and (4) intact transient LES relaxation. Histopathology was obtained to support the diagnosis of achalasia in the variants.

11. Massey BT, et al. Alteration of the upper esophageal sphincter belch reflex in patients with achalasia. Gastroenterology 1992; 103(5):1574–1579.

12. Howard PJ, et al. Five year prospective study of the incidence, clinical features, and diagnosis of achalasia in Edinburgh. Gut 1992; 33(8):1011–1015.

13. de Oliveira RB, et al. Gastrointestinal manifestations of Chagas' disease. Am J Gastroenterol 1998; 93(6):884–889.

14. Hirano I, Kahrilas P. Achalasia. In: Spiller R, Grundy D, eds. Pathophysiology of the enteric nervous system. New York: Blackwell; 2004:105–125.

15. Jones DB, et al. Preliminary report of an association between measles virus and achalasia. J Clin Pathol 1983; 36(6):655–657.

16. Robertson CS, Martin BA, Atkinson M. Varicella-zoster virus DNA in the oesophageal myenteric plexus in achalasia. Gut 1993; 34(3):299–302.

17. Birgisson S, et al. Achalasia is not associated with measles or known herpes and human papilloma viruses. Dig Dis Sci 1997; 42(2):300–306.

18. Niwamoto H. et al. Are human herpes viruses or measles virus associated with esophageal achalasia? Digest Dis Sci 1995; 40(4):859–864.

19. Clark SB, et al. The nature of the myenteric infiltrate in achalasia: an immunohistochemical analysis. Am J Surg Pathol 2000; 24(8):1153–1158.

20. Wong RK, et al. Significant DQw1 association in achalasia. Dig Dis Sci 1989; 34(3):349–352.

21. Storch WB, et al. Autoantibodies to Auerbach's plexus in achalasia. Cell Molec Biol 1995; 41(8):1033–1038.

22. Moses PL, et al. Antineuronal antibodies in idiopathic achalasia and gastro-oesophageal reflux disease. Gut 2003; 52(5):629–636.

23. Cassella RR, et al. Achalasia of the esophagus: Pathologic and etiologic considerations. Ann Surg 1964; 160(3):474–485.

24. Spiess AE, Kahrilas PJ. Treating achalasia: from whalebone to laparoscope. JAMA 1998; 280(7):638–642.

25. Spechler SJ. American Gastroenterological Association medical position statement on treatment of patients with dysphagia caused by benign disorders of the distal esophagus. Gastroenterology 1999; 117(1):229–233.

26. Vaezi MF, Baker ME, Richter JE. Assessment of esophageal emptying post-pneumatic dilation: use of the timed barium esophagram. Am J Gastroenterol 1999; 94(7):1802–1807.

27. Vaezi MF, et al. Botulinum toxin versus pneumatic dilatation in the treatment of achalasia: a randomised trial. Gut 1999; 44(2):231–239.

   One of five prospective studies that compare the efficacy of pneumatic dilation with botulinum toxin. Although only a single injection of botulinum toxin was allowed, the 12-month response rates with botulinum toxin of 32% were substantially lower than that the 70% seen with pneumatic dilation. Moreover, objective measures of LES pressure and esophageal emptying by barium swallow did not improve after botulinum toxin.

28. Pasricha PJ, et al. Intrasphincteric botulinum toxin for the treatment of achalasia. N Engl J Med 1995; 332(12):774–778. First double-blind study on the use of botulinum toxin in achalasia.

29. Eckardt VF, Aignherr C, Bernhard G. Predictors of outcome in patients with achalasia treated by pneumatic dilation. Gastroenterology 1992; 103(6):1732–1738.

30. de Oliveira JM, et al. Timed barium swallow: a simple technique for evaluating esophageal emptying in patients with achalasia. Am J Roentgenol 1997; 169(2):473–479.

31. Vaezi MF. Timed barium oesophagram: better predictor of long-term success after pneumatic dilation in achalasia than symptom assessment. Gut 2002; 50(6):765–770.

32. Bortolotti M, Labo G. Clinical and manometric effects of nifedipine in patients with esophageal achalasia. Gastroenterology 1981; 80(1):39–44.

33. Traube M, et al. The role of nifedipine therapy in achalasia: results of a randomized, double-blind, placebo-controlled study. Am J Gastroenterol 1989 84(10):1259–1262.

34. Gelfond M, et al. Effect of nitrates on LOS pressure in achalasia: a potential therapeutic aid. Gut 1981; 22(4):312–318.

35. Coccia G, et al. Prospective clinical and manometric study comparing pneumatic dilatation and sublingual nifedipine in the treatment of oesophageal achalasia [see comments]. Gut 1991; 32(6):604–606.

36. Bortolotti M. Medical therapy of achalasia: A benefit reserved for few. Digestion 1999; 60(1):11–16.

37. Bortolotti M, et al. Effects of sildenafil on esophageal motility of patients with idiopathic achalasia. Gastroenterology 2000; 118(2):253–257.

38. Pasricha PJ, et al. Botulinum toxin for achalasia: long-term outcome and predictors of response. Gastroenterology 1996; 110(5):1410–1415.

39. Brin MF. Botulinum toxin: chemistry, pharmacology, toxicity, and immunology. Muscle Nerve Suppl 1997; 6:S208–S220.

40. Allescher H.D, et al. Treatment of achalasia: botulinum toxin injection vs. pneumatic balloon dilation. A prospective study with long-term follow-up. Endoscopy 2001; 33(12):1007–1017.

41. Mikaeli J, et al. Randomized controlled trial comparing botulinum toxin injection to pneumatic dilation for the treatment of achalasia. Aliment Pharmacol Therapeut 2001; 15:1389–1396.

42. Annese V, et al. Controlled trial of botulinum toxin injection versus placebo and pneumatic dilation in achalasia. Gastroenterology 1996; 111(6):1418–1424.

43. Muehldorfer SM, et al. Esophageal achalasia: intrasphincteric injection of botulinum toxin A versus balloon dilation. Endoscopy 1999; 31(7):517–521.

44. Horgan S, et al. Does botulinum toxin injection make esophagomyotomy a more difficult operation? Surg Endosc 1999; 13(6):576–579.

45. Patti MG, et al. Effects of previous treatment on results of laparoscopic Heller myotomy for achalasia. Dig Dis Sci 1999; 44(11):2270–2276.

46. Annese V, et al. A multicentre randomised study of intrasphincteric botulinum toxin in patients with oesophageal achalasia. GISMAD Achalasia Study Group. Gut 2000; 46(5):597–600.

47. McJunkin B. Assessment of dilation methods in achalasia: large diameter mercury bougienage followed by pneumatic dilation as needed [see comment]. Gastrointest Endosc 1991; 37(1):18–21.

48. Kadakia SC, Wong RK. Graded pneumatic dilation using Rigiflex achalasia dilators in patients with primary esophageal achalasia. Am J Gastroenterol 1993; 88(1):34–38.

    Describes a protocol for pneumatic dilation starting with a 3 cm balloon with progression to 3.5 and 4 cm for nonresponders. This stepwise approach minimizes risk of esophageal perforation. The procedure is detailed in reference 49.

49. Wong RK. Pneumatic dilation for achalasia. Am J Gastroenterol 2004; 99(4):578–580.

50. Khan A.A, et al. Pneumatic balloon dilation in achalasia: a prospective comparison of balloon distention time. Am J Gastroenterol 1998; 93(7):1064–1067.

51. Kim CH, et al. Achalasia: prospective evaluation of relationship between lower esophageal sphincter pressure, esophageal transit, and esophageal diameter and symptoms in response to pneumatic dilation. Mayo Clin Proc 1993; 68(11):1067–1073.

52. Wong RC, Maydonovitch C. Utility of parameters measured during pneumatic dilation as predictors of successful dilation. Am J Gastroenterol 1996; 91(6):1126–1129.

53. Parkman HP, et al. Pneumatic dilatation or esophagomyotomy treatment for idiopathic achalasia: clinical outcomes and cost analysis. Dig Dis Sci 1993; 38(1):75–85.

54. Eckardt VF, Gockel I, Bernhard G. Pneumatic dilation for achalasia: late results of a prospective follow up investigation. Gut 2004; 53(5):629–633.

    An important prospective study that reports on the long-term response to pneumatic dilation. A 5-year remission rate of 40% and 10-year remission rate of 36% were observed, with repeated dilations providing minimal incremental benefit. Dilations were performed using Browne-McHardy dilation rather than Rigiflex dilation but this is unlikely to change the overall conclusion.

55. Katz PO, Gilbert J, Castell DO. Pneumatic dilatation is effective long-term treatment for achalasia. Dig Dis Sci 1998; 43(9): 1973–1977.

56. Torbey CF, et al. Long-term outcome of achalasia treatment: the need for closer follow-up. J Clin Gastroenterol 1999; 28(2):125–130.

57. West RL, et al. Long term results of pneumatic dilation in achalasia followed for more than 5 years. Am J Gastroenterol 2002; 97(6):1346–1351.

    Similar to Eckhardt's study, this report from Australia finds a surprisingly poor long-term response to pneumatic dilation with a 50% success rate at mean follow-up of 12 years.

58. Chan KC, et al. Short-term and long-term results of endoscopic balloon dilation for achalasia: 12 years' experience. Endoscopy 2004; 36:690–694.

59. Vela M, et al. Complexities of managing achalasia at a tertiary referral center: use of pneumatic dilatation, Heller myotomy, and botulinum toxin injection. Am J Gastroenterol 2004; 99(6):1029–1036.

60. Metman EH, et al. Risk factors for immediate complications after progressive pneumatic dilation for achalasia. Am J Gastroenterol 1999; 94(5):1179–1185.

61. Schwartz HM, Cahow CE, Traube M. Outcome after perforation sustained during pneumatic dilatation for achalasia. Dig Dis Sci 1993; 38(8):1409–1413.

62. Molina EG, et al. Conservative management of esophageal nontransmural tears after pneumatic dilation for achalasia. Am J Gastroenterol 1996; 91(1):15–18.

63. Shoenut JP, Duerksen D, Yaffe CS. A prospective assessment of gastroesophageal reflux before and after treatment of achalasia patients: pneumatic dilation versus transthoracic limited myotomy. Am J Gastroenterol 1997; 92(7):1109–1112.

64. Burke CA, Achkar E, Falk GW. Effect of pneumatic dilation on gastroesophageal reflux in achalasia. Dig Dis Sci 1997; 42(5):998–1002.

65. Shimi S, Nathanson LK, Cuschieri A. Laparoscopic cardiomyotomy for achalasia. J Roy Coll Surg Edinb 1991; 36(3):152–154.

66. Pellegrini C, et al. Thoracoscopic esophagomyotomy. Initial experience with a new approach for the treatment of achalasia. Ann Surg 1992; 216(3):291–296; discussion 296–299.

67. Ali A, Pellegrini CA. Laparoscopic myotomy: technique and efficacy in treating achalasia. Gastrointest Endosc Clin N Am 2001; 11(2):347–358.

68. Patti MG, et al. Minimally invasive surgery for achalasia: an 8-year experience with 168 patients. Ann Surg 1999; 230(4):587–593; discussion 593–594.

    One of the largest surgical experiences with laparoscopic Heller myotomy that reports a 90% success rate. Gastroesophageal reflux was detected in 60% of patients after thoracoscopic myotomy compared with 17% after laparoscopic myotomy.

69. Sharp KW, et al. 100 consecutive minimally invasive Heller myotomies: lessons learned. Ann Surg 2002; 235(5):631–638; discussion 638–639.

70. Raiser F, et al. Heller myotomy via minimal-access surgery. An evaluation of antireflux procedures. Arch Surg 1996; 131(6):593–597; discussion 597–598.

71. Tatum RP. et al. Operative manometry and endoscopy during laparoscopic Heller myotomy. An initial experience. Surg Endosc 1999; 13(10):1015–1020.

72. Hill LD, Asplund CM, Roberts PN. Intraoperative manometry: adjunct to surgery for esophageal motility disorders. Am J Surg 1984; 147(1):171–174.

73. Del Genio A, et al. Intraoperative esophageal manometry in the surgical treatment of achalasia. Revista Espanola de Enfermedades Digestivas 1991; 79(1):3–7.

74. Chapman JR, et al. Achalasia treatment: improved outcome of laparoscopic myotomy with operative manometry. Arch Surg 2004; 139(5):508–513.

    Recent report of experience with 136 laparoscopic Heller myotomies. The mean operating time was 2.3 hours with a median postoperative hospital stay of 1 day. Intraoperative manometry was used and influenced the extent of myotomy, particularly early in the surgical experience.

75. Del Genio A, et al. Intraoperative esophageal manometry: our experience. Dis Esophagus 1997; 10(4):253–261.

76. Clemente G, et al. Intraoperative esophageal manometry in surgical treatment of achalasia: a reappraisal. Hepato-Gastroenterol 1996; 43(12): 1532–1536.

77. Zaninotto G, et al. Etiology, diagnosis, and treatment of failures after laparoscopic Heller myotomy for achalasia. Ann Surg 2002; 235(2):186–192.

78. Csendes A, et al. Late results of a prospective randomised study comparing forceful dilatation and oesophagomyotomy in patients with achalasia [see comments]. Gut 1989; 30(3):299–304.

79. Malthaner RA, et al. Long-term results in surgically managed esophageal achalasia. Ann Thoracic Surg 1994; 58(5):1343–1346; discussion 1346–1347.

80. Ellis FH Jr, et al. Ten to 20-year clinical results after short esophagomyotomy without an antireflux procedure (modified Heller operation) for esophageal achalasia. Eur J Cardio-Thoracic Surg 1992; 6(2):86–89; discussion 90.

81. Felix VN, et al. Achalasia: a prospective study comparing the results of dilatation and myotomy. Hepato-Gastroenterol 1998; 45(19):97–108.

82. Andrews CN, Anvari M, Dobranowski J. Laparoscopic Heller's myotomy or botulinum toxin injection for management of esophageal achalasia. Patient choice and treatment outcomes. Surg Endosc 1999; 13(8):742–746.

83. Zaninotto G, et al. Randomized controlled trial of botulinum toxin versus laparoscopic Heller myotomy for esophageal achalasia. Ann Surg 2004; 239(3):364–370.

84. Imperiale TF, et al. A cost-minimization analysis of alternative treatment strategies for achalasia. Gastrointest Endosc Clin N Am 2001; 11(2):409–424.

85. Patti MG, et al. Laparoscopic Heller myotomy relieves dysphagia in achalasia when the esophagus is dilated. Surg Endosc 1999; 13(9):843–847.

86. Patti MG, et al. Esophagectomy for achalasia: patient selection and clinical experience. Surg Endosc 2001; 15(7):687–690.

87. Miller DL, et al. Esophageal resection for recurrent achalasia. Ann Thorac Surg 1995; 60:922–926.

88. Devaney EJ, et al. Esophagectomy for achalasia: patient selection and clinical experience. Ann Thorac Surg 2001; 72:854–858.

89. De Palma GD, et al. Self-expanding metal stents for endoscopic treatment of esophageal achalasia unresponsive to conventional treatments. Long-term results in eight patients. Endoscopy 2001; 33(12):1027–1030.

90. Sandler RS, et al. The risk of esophageal cancer in patients with achalasia. A population-based study. JAMA 1995; 274(17): 1359–1362.

91. Dunaway PM, Wong RK. Risk and surveillance intervals for squamous cell carcinoma in achalasia. Gastrointest Endosc Clin N Am, 2001; 11(2):425–434.

92. [No authors listed]. The role of endoscopy in the surveillance of premalignant conditions of the upper gastrointestinal tract. Gastrointest Endosc 1998; 48(6):663–668.

93. Cuilliere C, et al. Achalasia: outcome of patients treated with intrasphincteric injection of botulinum toxin. Gut 1997; 41(1):87–92.

94. Fishman VM, et al. Symptomatic improvement in achalasia after botulinum toxin injection of the lower esophageal sphincter. Am J Gastroenterol 1996; 91(9):1724–1730.

95. Kolbasnik J, et al. Long-term efficacy of botulinum toxin in classical achalasia: a prospective study. Am J Gastroenterol 1999; 94(12):3434–3439.

96. Gordon JM, Eaker EY. Prospective study of esophageal botulinum toxin injection in high-risk achalasia patients. Am J Gastroenterol 1997; 92:1812–1816.

97. Neubrand M. Long-term results and prognostic factors in the treatment of achalasia with botulinum toxin [see comment]. Endoscopy 2002; 34(7):519–523.

98. Barkin JS, et al. Forceful balloon dilation: an outpatient procedure for achalasia. Gastrointest Endosc 1990; 36(2):123–126.

99. Stark GA, et al. Prospective randomized comparison of Brown-McHardy and microvasive balloon dilators in treatment of achalasia. Am J Gastroenterol 1990; 85(10):1322–1326.

100. Makela J, Kiviniemi H, Laitinen S. Heller's cardiomyotomy compared with pneumatic dilatation for treatment of oesophageal achalasia. Eur J of Surg 1991; 157(6–7):411–414.

101. Kim CH, et al. Achalasia: prospective evaluation of relationship between lower esophageal sphincter pressure, esophageal transit, and esophageal diameter and symptoms in response to pneumatic dilation. Mayo Clin Proc 1993; 68(11):1067–1073.

102. Abid S, et al. Treatment of achalasia: the best of both worlds. Am J Gastroenterol 1994; 89(7):979–985.

103. Lambroza A, Schuman RW. Pneumatic dilation for achalasia without fluoroscopic guidance: safety and efficacy. Am J Gastroenterol 1995; 90(8):1226–1229.

104. Bhatnagar MS, et al. Achalasia cardia dilatation using polyethylene balloon (Rigiflex) dilators. Ind J Gastroenterol 1996; 15(2):49–51.

105. Muehldorfer SM, Hahn EG, Ell C. High- and low-compliance balloon dilators in patients with achalasia: a randomized prospective comparative trial. Gastrointest Endosc 1996; 44(4):398–403.

106. Gideon RM, Castell DO, Yarze J. Prospective randomized comparison of pneumatic dilatation technique in patients with idiopathic achalasia. Dig Dis Sci 1999; 44(9):1853–1857.

107. Kadakia SC, Wong RK. Pneumatic balloon dilation for esophageal achalasia. Gastrointest Endosc Clin N Am 2001; 11(2):325–346.

108. Ferguson MK, Reeder LB, Olak J. Results of myotomy and partial fundoplication after pneumatic dilation for achalasia. World J Surg 1996; 62(2):327–330.

109. Duranceau A, LaFontaine ER, Vallieres B. Effects of total fundoplication on function of the esophagus after myotomy for achalasia. Am J Surg 1982; 143(1):22–28.

110. Donahue PE, et al. Esophagocardiomyotomy – floppy Nissen fundoplication effectively treats achalasia without causing esophageal obstruction. Surgery 1994; 116(4):719–724; discussion 724–725.

111. Sariyannis C, Mullard KS. Oesophagomyotomy for achalasia of the cardia. Thorax 1975; 30(5):539–542.

112. Stipa S, et al. Heller-Belsey and Heller-Nissen operations for achalasia of the esophagus. Surg Gynecol Obstet 1990; 170(3):212–216.

113. Castrini G, Pappalardo G, Mobarhan S. New approach to esophagocardiomyotomy: report of forty cases. J Thoracic Cardiovasc Surg 1982; 84(4):575–578.

114. Okike N, et al. Esophagomyotomy versus forceful dilation for achalasia of the esophagus: results in 899 patients. Ann Thorac Surg 1979; 28(2):119–125.

115. Pai GP, et al. Two decades of experience with modified Heller's myotomy for achalasia. Ann Thoracic Surg 1984; 38(3):201–206.

116. Ellis FH Jr. Oesophagomyotomy for achalasia: a 22-year experience. Br J Surg 1993; 80(7):882–885.

117. Jara FM, et al. Long-term results of esophagomyotomy for achalasia of esophagus. Arch Surg 1979; 114(8):935–936.

118. Menzies-Gow N, Gummer JW, Edwards DA. Results of Heller's operation for achalasia of the cardia. Br J Surg 1978; 65(7):483–485.

119. Mattioli S, et al. Surgery for esophageal achalasia. long-term results with three different techniques. Hepato-Gastroenterol 1996; 43(9):492–500.

120. Di Simone MP, et al. Onset timing of delayed complications and criteria of follow-up after operation for esophageal achalasia. Ann Thoracic Surg 1996; 61(4):1106–1110; discussion 1110–1111.

121. Gallone L, Peri G, Galliera M. Proximal gastric vagotomy and anterior fundoplication as complementary procedures to Heller's operation for achalasia. Surg Gynecol Obstet 1982; 155(3):337–341.

122. Rosati R, et al. Laparoscopic approach to esophageal achalasia. Am J Surg 1995; 169(4):424–427.

123. Picciocchi A, et al. Surgical treatment of achalasia: a retrospective comparative study. Surg Today 1993; 23(10):855–859.

124. Murray GF, et al. Selective application of fundoplication in achalasia. Ann Thoracic Surg 1984; 37(3):185–188.

125. Cosentini E, et al. Achalasia. Results of myotomy and antireflux operation after failed dilatations. Arch Surg 1997; 132(2):143–147.

126. Hunter JG, et al. Laparoscopic Heller myotomy and fundoplication for achalasia. Ann Surg 1997; 225(6):655–664; discussion 664–665.

127. Pandolfo N, et al. Manometric assessment of Heller-Dor operation for esophageal achalasia. Hepato-Gastroenterol 1996; 43(7): 160–166.

128. Robertson GS, Johnstone JM. Laparoscopic Heller's cardiomyotomy without an antireflux procedure. Surg Endosc 1995; 9(7):781–785.

129. Mitchell PC, et al. Laparoscopic cardiomyotomy with a Dor patch for achalasia. Can J Surg 1995; 38(5):445–448.

130. Morino M, et al. Laparoscopic Heller cardiomyotomy with intraoperative manometry in the management of oesophageal achalasia. Int Surg 1995; 80(4):332–335.

131. Rosati R, et al. Evaluating results of laparoscopic surgery for esophageal achalasia. Surg Endosc 1998; 12(3):270–273.

132. Yamamura MS, et al. Laparoscopic Heller myotomy and anterior fundoplication for achalasia results in a high degree of patient satisfaction. Arch Surg 2000; 135(8):902–906.

133. Stewart KC, et al. Thoracoscopic versus laparoscopic modified Heller myotomy for achalasia: efficacy and safety in 87 patients. J Am Coll Surg 1999; 189(2):164–169; discussion 169–170.

134. Dempsey DT, et al. Comparison of outcomes following open and laparoscopic esophagomyotomy for achalasia. Surg Endosc 1999; 13(8):747–750.

CHAPTER SIXTEEN

16

Treatment of esophageal disorders caused by medications, caustic ingestion, foreign bodies and trauma

Umesh Choudhry and Henry Worth Boyce

ESOPHAGEAL INJURY CAUSED BY MEDICATIONS

Introduction

Esophageal injury due to 'pills' was first reported by Pemberton in 1970.[1] Since then, nearly 100 drugs have been reported to incite injury to the esophageal mucosa (Table 16.1).[2-4] Drugs that have been most reported to cause esophageal injury include potassium chloride (especially the slow release, wax matrix form), tetracycline, doxycycline, quinidine gluconate, ferrous sulfate, nonsteroidal antiinflammatory drugs (NSAIDs) and more recently, alendronate, zidovudine, rifampin and lansoprazole.[5,6] Emepronium, a common cause of drug-induced esophageal damage (DIED) in parts of Europe, is not available in the United States.

Esophageal injury caused by medications can be classified into two categories. The first type of injury is an acute, superficial injury of a short duration. Spontaneous healing after discontinuation of the offending agent is the rule. The second type of injury is characterized by deep, intramural inflammation and ulceration, which heals by stricture formation. The late sequelae of this latter type of injury are difficult to treat and place considerable limitations on the patient's lifestyle.

Pathogenesis

The pathogenesis of DIED is best understood by examining the properties of the drug formulation, the shape and form in which the drug is swallowed, the habitus and characteristics of the patient who ingests the medication, and the functional status/anatomy of the esophagus. The most critical factor in the development of DIED is the contact time of the injurious drug with the esophageal mucosa.

Agent factors

The drug delivery vehicle, whether pill or capsule, is important because the latter can adhere to the esophageal wall and dissolve slowly, thereby increasing the contact time of the drug with the mucosa. The hygroscopic property of gelatin capsules and their sticky surface allows them to adhere to the mucosa. Thus, doxycycline tablets were found to be less ulcerogenic than the capsule form of the same medication.[7] Large tablets, especially those larger than 13 mm in size are more likely to get lodged at a site of 'physiological narrowing' in the esophagus, such as at the aortic arch level.[8,9] Oval-shaped, film-coated tablets traverse the esophagus easier than round, uncoated tablets.[9]

The chemical nature of the drug is another important factor. Some medications such as doxycycline, ferrous sulfate, ascorbic acid, or aspirin cause esophageal damage due to their acidic nature.[7,10-12] Aspirin may also increase the permeability of the mucosal barrier, allowing H^+ ions into the cells.[13] Although other medications, such as quinidine gluconate and potassium chloride, have a neutral pH, they incite damage by the hyperosmolar solution produced by dissolution of the drug.[14] Direct thermal injury may be produced by dissolving of the agent/medication, as occurred in the case of Clinitest (copper sulfate) tablets. These tablets, now off the market, were used for detecting urine glucose in diabetics and were ingested accidentally or deliberately.[15]

Host factors

DIED is more common in the elderly, debilitated population because they take more medications and are typically in a recumbent position for longer periods of time. These patients also secrete a reduced amount of saliva. In healthy adults, more than one ounce (30 cc) of water is required to swallow and reliably pass a 13 mm tablet promptly into the stomach.[16] Therefore, when medications are ingested without or with an insufficient amount of liquid, the chance they will persist in the esophagus is increased.[17-19] Even when the esophageal lumen is normal, elderly patients or those confined to a bed are at a higher risk for medications adhering to their esophageal mucosa, due to protracted recumbency.[9,18] In addition, poor memory or visual impairment may interfere with their ability to read and comprehend the instructions on the package.

Esophageal factors

In addition to the natural propensity for medicines to traverse the sites of anatomical narrowing in the esophagus (cervical esophagus, aortic arch level, and lower esophageal sphincter), underlying esophageal pathology, such as abnormal esophageal motility, a pre-existing stricture, or cardiomegaly (left atrial esophageal compression), may compound the risk of injury due to medications. Hiatal hernias, a very common condition in Western populations, have been shown to reduce the transit of ingested pills.[20] Similarly, a Schatzki ring less than 13 mm in diameter may contribute to the delayed transit of tablets.[11]

Table 16.1 Various drugs causing esophageal disease

Class of drug	Agents
Major offenders	
Potassium chloride (delayed release)	Slow K & other KCl formulations
Antiarrythmics	Quinidine gluconate, quinidine sulfate
Antiosteoclastic	Alendronate
Diuretic	Furosemide
Antibiotics	Doxycycline, other tetracyclines, penicillin, clindamycin
Antiinflammatory drugs	Aspirin, indomethacin, piroxicam ibuprofen
Other offenders	
Antiviral agents	Zidovudine
Vitamins	Ascorbic acid, multivitamins
Iron preparations	Ferrous sulfate/succinate
Miscellaneous	Mexiletine, captopril, theophylline, warfarin,
Agents not available in the United States	Emepronium bromide, pinaverium

Prevention of drug-induced esophageal damage

Esophageal injury due to medications is entirely preventable. The lack of knowledge of physicians, pharmacists, and patients is the biggest hurdle in preventing this injury. Dissemination of information regarding the injurious potential of various medications is therefore essential. Pharmaceutical companies have the primary responsibility of informing and educating the medical community, using unambiguous language, about the injurious potential of drugs. Package inserts of such medications should contain explicit instructions regarding their use. All physicians and nursing personnel should similarly educate patients, hospital/nursing, home personnel, and caregivers at all levels. Although potassium chloride (Slow-K) was identified as being injurious to the esophagus over 30 years ago, many internists and cardiologists remain unaware of this potential problem with potassium chloride.[1] Patients should be warned prior to initiation of therapy with these high-risk agents. Periodically during therapy, a careful history for odynophagia, retrosternal pain, and dysphagia should be obtained. Special attention should be given to patients who are taking multiple medications. Medications that reduce salivary secretions or esophageal peristalsis (e.g., antihistamines, anticholinergics) are likely to increase the contact time of injurious medications with esophageal mucosa, thereby worsening the damage. *All patients should be advised to take medications in an upright posture, take at least 2–3 oz water with each tablet, and to remain upright for at least 15 minutes after ingestion.*[21] When medications are prescribed to be taken at bedtime, patients should be informed that 'at bedtime' does not mean at the time of recumbency, but rather 15 minutes or longer before assuming a recumbent position. Liquid preparations should be used for bedridden patients and patients with pre-existing esophageal lesions such as strictures, diverticula, and achalasia.[2,7] Prevention and treatment strategies are summarized in Table 16.2.

Diagnosis and treatment of drug-induced esophageal damage in the acute phase

As previously outlined, an accurate history leads to an early diagnosis in most cases. Patients with DIED present most often with a burning retrosternal pain (60–70%).[4] Odynophagia is the second most common symptom (50–74%); however, dysphagia is relatively infrequent and usually is reported when there is a significant luminal compromise during the later stages of injury.[22] Pain, odynophagia, and dysphagia can develop within hours to 10 days after the initiation of the medication. The first and foremost step in this phase of injury is to identify the offending agent and discontinue its use. If a pill is found adherent to the mucosa or impacted in the esophageal lumen on a barium swallow, early endoscopy may be required for its removal. Symptomatic treatment using antacids, topical xylocaine gel or a combination and oral analgesics are useful in alleviating pain. These combinations may be named variously in different hospitals as 'GI cocktail,' 'Kessler's solution' or 'magic mouthwash.' They are usually short acting and must be administered frequently. Sucralfate, H$_2$-blockers, and proton pump inhibitors have also been used to promote the healing of acid reflux-related ulceration/erosion of the esophagus, although their efficacy in treatment of DIED has not been established.[2,3,23] No further diagnostic evaluation for acute symptoms is recommended in younger patients without immune deficiency states.[3,8]

If symptoms persist or worsen despite the above measures, the patient should undergo an esophagogastroduodenoscopy (EGD). A double-contrast barium esophagogram may be helpful as an initial study, but EGD has the advantage of revealing more mucosal detail. It also provides a more accurate assessment of the degree of injury and gives an opportunity for biopsy. Impacted tablets/capsules, if encountered, can also be removed at the time of the procedure. In 99% of cases, mucosal abnormalities are found on EGD and commonly include a single, shallow, discrete ulcer with exudate at the level of the aortic arch or circumferential mucosal ulceration or nodularity of the mid esophagus with an adherent clot.[4,24]

Table 16.2 DIED: prevention and treatment strategies

Prevention

Physician/pharmacist education

Patient education: upright posture and 100 cc water

Modification of pill size/shape

Substitution of pills by elixir or orally dissolving formulations

Avoid concurrent use of offending agents

Treatment during acute phase

Cessation of offending agent

Symptomatic treatment: topical and oral analgesics, antacids, sucralfate

Treatment after stricture formation

Esophageal dilation

Intralesional triamcinolone injection: questionable benefit

Surgery: almost never required

The mucosa above and below this lesion is generally normal,[7,25] although on occasion, a distal esophageal ulceration maybe be found, especially in the presence of a pre-existing reflux-related injury.[26,27] Pill remnants or pigmentation of the mucosa may also be seen. On histological examination, the pigmentation has been shown to be due to impregnated crystals of the offending medication, viz., ferrous sulfate or doxycycline.[28] Most cases of DIED improve with cessation of the offending medication plus symptomatic therapy in the acute phase and do not require any further treatment.[29] Pre-existing lesions, when identified, should be managed appropriately for complete resolution of symptoms.

Management of delayed sequelae of drug-induced esophageal damage

When medications cause a deep ulceration of the esophageal wall, the healing phase is prolonged and slow. Persistent symptoms often indicate complications such as stricture formation, bleeding, or perforation.[19] The medications usually implicated in this type of injury include a delayed-release wax-matrix form of potassium chloride (Slow-K), quinidine gluconate (Quinaglute), and indomethacin. A recent addition to this list is the daily dosing version of bisphosphonate: alendronate (Fosamax 10 mg).[27,29,30] When patients present with continued symptoms and a history of ingestion of one of the above mentioned 'serious offenders,' it is important to proceed with an early endoscopy due to the serious transmural injury caused by these agents.[31,32] If active ulceration is identified by barium study or EGD, acid suppression in the form of H_2-blockers or proton pump inhibitors is indicated in patients with gastroesophageal reflux. Esophageal dilation is postponed until inflammation/ulceration is completely healed. Esophageal dilation in the presence of ulceration is often ineffective and may be associated with complications.[33] Once inflammation is resolved and stricture formation is confirmed, the stricture should be dilated early and frequently, to prevent contraction of the cicatrix.[19,26] Unfortunately, patients may be seen by gastroenterologists months to years after the initiation of these medications because some drugs such as potassium chloride and quinidine gluconate may not cause odynophagia or retrosternal pain. In other cases, repeated complaints of dysphagia are often ignored until a tight, fibrotic stricture develops, at which point esophageal dilation becomes very difficult. These patients require multiple sessions of esophageal dilation performed at 1–2 week intervals, usually over several months.[26] Almost all patients show gratifying results and have nearly complete resolution of symptoms after adequate esophageal luminal patency has been restored. Since multiple sessions of esophageal dilation are anticipated, the pathophysiology of the condition and treatment plan should be discussed in detail with the patient. The patient may be given appointments for several sessions of dilation in advance to assure proper treatment intervals. The median number of dilation sessions required over 6–12 months to achieve adequate lumen patency for severe quinidine gluconate-related strictures at our center is 14. Dilation over a wire guide is the preferred method for these strictures.

Several investigators have described the use of intralesional injections of triamcinolone in 'refractory' strictures.[34–39] A MEDLINE review of the use of intralesional steroids revealed several case reports, primarily in patients with corrosive strictures, one retrospective study, and one randomized prospective study (in abstract form) of patients with reflux strictures.[34–39] All report a decrease in the frequency of dilation after intralesional steroids. However, none of these reports defined 'stricture' relative to the degree of active inflammation present, and only one patient had a DIED-related stricture. Intralesional injection of steroids is simple and safe, with no serious reported adverse effects. However, it is useful only for strictures less than 1 cm in length. A 23–26-gauge endoscopic needle (sclerotherapy needle) is used to inject 40 mg/mL strength triamcinolone or a larger volume of diluted strength. Four quadrant injections of 0.5 mL each are made at the time of each dilation. The benefit shown with the use of intralesional steroids has likely been due to their antiinflammatory property. However, satisfactory results can be achieved with conventional dilation performed with a proper technique. There is currently no proof that steroid injections relieve obstructions in chronic fibrotic strictures not associated with active inflammation. We ascribe the therapeutic success to the elimination of inflammation, discontinuation of the offending agent, and wire-guided dilation under fluoroscopy. The use of intralesional steroids is not recommended as a standard therapy in patients with DIED.

Role of surgery/stents

Surgery has no proven role in the treatment of DIED, except when perforation or uncontrollable bleeding occurs. All strictures can be successfully managed by wire-guided dilation. The use of self-expanding metal or nonmetallic stents for benign esophageal strictures has been evaluated over the past few years. The experience to date suggests that this approach leads to significant complications and should be avoided in patients with significant life expectancy and who have other treatment alternatives.[40,41]

ESOPHAGEAL INJURY CAUSED BY CANCER CHEMOTHERAPY

Introduction

Cancer chemotherapy alone or in conjunction with radiation therapy often results in esophageal damage. The damage is often diffuse and similar to mucosal injury that occurs elsewhere in the body.[42,43] Patients typically present with severe odynophagia and dysphagia. Intense nausea and vomiting are caused by the chemotherapeutic agents and reduce the ability of the patient to ingest oral liquids. On endoscopy, diffuse erythema with exudation is seen throughout the esophagus. Bleeding may occur and may be potentiated by thrombocytopenia or coagulopathy secondary to bone marrow suppression. Immunosuppression may also result in opportunistic esophageal infections due to *Candida*, herpes simplex virus, or cytomegalovirus.

Symptomatic treatment

Amelioration of retrosternal pain and odynophagia is the first goal of treatment, followed by treatment to promote healing. Topical analgesics are often useful for the mucositis that nearly always accompanies esophagitis. Viscous xylocaine can provide some measure of relief, albeit short-lived, from pain and odynophagia. Due to its short duration of action, xylocaine jelly alone or in combination with antacids needs to be given at frequent intervals (every 1–2 hours, up to a maximum of 8 doses of 15 mL in

24 hours). Oral/parenteral pain medications may be required, in addition to topical analgesics. When used, it is best to prescribe these medications as alcohol-free suspensions since alcohol typically exacerbates pain and odynophagia. Combinations of acetaminophen and codeine or hydromorphone are useful in this situation. Cryotherapy using ice chips in the mouth has been used to prevent oral mucositis in patients receiving chemotherapy.[44] Similarly, sucralfate has been studied in prevention and treatment of chemotherapy-induced stomatitis.[45] It is uncertain if sucralfate has any proven effect in the treatment of chemotherapy-associated esophagitis. Because acid suppression therapy using H_2-blockers or proton pump inhibitors is traditionally used for reflux esophagitis or peptic ulcer disease, these medications are often used in patients with esophagitis due to chemotherapy despite lack of any substantial evidence indicating a benefit.[46] Supportive measures such as adequate nutrition and hydration by the parenteral route or a thin nasogastric tube for enteral feeding are important. It is preferable to pass the nasogastric tube under fluoroscopic guidance. Acid suppression by either an H_2-blocker or a proton pump inhibitor should be given during nasogastric intubation.

ESOPHAGEAL INJURY CAUSED BY LYE/CAUSTIC SUBSTANCE INGESTION

Introduction

Lye-based liquid household cleaners have been commercially available in the United States since 1967. Accidental and intentional ingestion of these substances has resulted in serious morbidity during the past three decades. It is estimated that caustic ingestion and foreign body aspiration are the third most common causes of pediatric death in this country.[47] Nearly 26 000 episodes of caustic substance ingestion occur in the United States every year. Nearly 17 000 of these involve children, 50% of whom are under the 4 years of age. Adults and adolescents account for 20% cases, the majority of which are suicidal gestures. The agents most often reported to be involved in these cases are shown in Table 16.3.

Table 16.3 Common household corrosives

Brand name/product	Chemical name
Red Devil Drain Opener	Sodium hydroxide (96–100%)
Crystalline Drano	Sodium hydroxide (50%)
Clinitest tablets	Sodium hydroxide (50%)
Liquid Drano	Sodium hydroxide (2–10%)
Mr. Clean liquid	Sodium carbonate
Top Job liquid	Sodium carbonate/ammonia
Liquid clorox	Sodium hypochlorite (5.25%)
Lysol deodorizing cleaner	Ammonium chloride (2.7%)
Swish toilet bowl cleaner	Ammonium chloride (1.25%)
Dish water detergents	A combination of sodium hypochlorite, bicarbonate, phosphate, silicate (pH: 12.5)
Battery fluid	Sulphuric acid

Signs and symptoms of caustic injury

Several large series of caustic ingestion esophageal injuries have been reported.[48–50] The signs and symptoms reported include nausea, vomiting, dysphagia, refusal to drink, drooling, and stridor. None of these signs and symptoms appears to accurately predict the degree of injury. Crain and colleagues reported that the presence of two or more of the serious signs/symptoms, namely vomiting, drooling, or stridor, indicated a 50% chance of esophageal injury.[50,51]

Pathogenesis

Vancura and colleagues, using a cat model, demonstrated that alkali at a pH of 12.5 produces esophageal ulceration.[52] Liquid lye, frequently available in the form of drain cleaner, produces its injury by liquefaction necrosis and is thus able to quickly spread into the esophageal and gastric mucosa, thereby producing widespread penetrating injuries. Bacterial infection regularly occurs and potentiates the injury. Acidic caustic substances (except hydrofluoric acid), in contrast, result in coagulation necrosis and form a thick eschar, which may protect the mucosal layers from damage. By 10 days after caustic injury, granulation tissue begins to replace the necrotic tissue, and fibroblast proliferation and scar formation begin by the third week after injury.

Caustic ingestion may cause serious systemic effects by causing airway edema and obstruction, resulting in hypoxia and hypercapnia. Metabolic disturbances can occur and require immediate attention. Infection usually complicates the clinical scenario in cases of esophageal perforation.

Prevention of corrosive injury

In most instances, injury due to corrosive substances is preventable. Educating the public regarding proper storage of these agents away from the reach of infants and children and possibly from suicidal adolescents is required as a continuous effort. Educating prospective parents during prenatal classes when their attention level is heightened may be another strategy. Efforts from industry are needed to minimize the corrosive component of household cleaning solutions. Proper labeling and addition of colors to these agents can prevent their being mistaken for water. In addition to household cleaners, corrosive alkali is present in cylindrical and button batteries. There is thus a need for manufacturing leak-proof battery casings, as merely sucking on a battery by a child has been reported to result in esophageal burns.[53] Some countries such as Norway have taken a lead in this matter and have banned the sale of alkaline corrosives as household cleaners. Ironically, acid injuries now account for a majority of cases in Finland.[54]

Phases of corrosive injury

Three phases of corrosive injury have been described.[55] A thorough understanding of these phases is important in planning a therapeutic strategy.

Acute phase

The first 72 hours after the ingestion of the corrosive substance constitute the acute phase. It is characterized by the initiation of an inflammatory response and vessel thrombosis. Invasion of the esophageal wall by bacteria and polymorphonuclear leukocytes takes place during this phase.

Subacute phase

This phase spans from 3 days to 3 weeks post corrosive ingestion. An intense inflammatory response and further vascular thrombosis occurs during this phase, resulting in sloughing of the superficial layers of mucosa and ulceration. Granulation tissue formation, fibroblast infiltration, and collagen deposition also occur and may be accompanied by significant hemorrhage. The risk of esophageal perforation is increased, especially with blind instrumentation such as nasogastric intubation during this phase.

Chronic phase

Beginning at about 3 weeks post ingestion, the chronic or late phase of corrosive injury is marked by scar retraction, continued fibrosis, mucosal re-epithelialization and possible tracheoesophageal fistula formation. Stricture formation occurs in up to 30% of patients with corrosive esophageal injury, typically in patients with second and third degree injury.[56] These patients have been estimated to have a greater than 1000-fold increase in the incidence of squamous cell carcinoma of the esophagus 15–20 years after corrosive ingestion,[57,58] and periodic surveillance should thus be considered in this group after 15 years. The use of Lugol iodine chromoendoscopy will delineate foci of dysplasia or cancer and can enhance early diagnosis.

Treatment in the acute phase

Patients who can give a reliable history of accidental ingestion, are asymptomatic, have no evidence of oropharyngeal burns, or have only a questionable history of corrosive ingestion may be observed in the emergency room or during an overnight hospital stay. In contrast, patients who show signs of acute injury, may have ingested large amounts of corrosive substances or are suicidal should be admitted to the intensive care unit for observation, further diagnostic tests, and treatment. In either situation, early endoscopy will provide an accurate assessment of the degree of injury.

Airway protection

Emergency tracheostomy or endotracheal intubation is indicated in patients with stridor, hoarseness, or inability to speak. It should be borne in mind that the onset of respiratory symptoms may be delayed up to 24 hours. PA and lateral chest X-rays should be obtained initially and repeated, based on the patient's condition, since aspiration pneumonia is a risk in these patients.

Supportive treatment

Appropriate management of hypotension and shock may be required in the form of intravenous fluids or pressor agents. Surgical consultation should be obtained early in cases of severe esophageal injury as emergency surgery is indicated if evidence of esophageal, gastric, or other visceral perforation is present. Signs of esophageal perforation include pneumomediastinum, subcutaneous emphysema, crepitus, dyspnea, and severe chest or abdominal pain. Care should be taken to avoid the use of emetic agents as they may precipitate additional esophageal and oropharyngeal injury and lead to perforation. The use of neutralizing agents is contraindicated as neutralization reactions lead to heat production and may further aggravate the injury.[59]

Most patients need to be kept NPO in view of the possibility of endoscopy or surgery. Patients who are able to swallow their saliva, do not have any respiratory symptoms, or in whom urgent endoscopy is not contemplated may be allowed ice chips or sips of water.

Endoscopic evaluation and management

As stated above, signs and symptoms do not generally predict the severity of damage. Since treatment options depend greatly on the assessment of injury (Table 16.4), endoscopic examination should be carried out as early as possible. This strategy also minimizes the risk of perforation. Endoscopy should be done 24–48 hours post ingestion or sooner if respiratory and hemodynamic parameters are stable. More than 50% of patients with a history of caustic ingestion are found to have no evidence of esophageal injury on an early endoscopy.[49,50,60,61] The extent of the endoscopic examination has also been debated. In the past, when endoscopes were rigid, a limited examination within the first 24 hours was favored to avoid perforations.[62,63] Endoscopists terminated the exam at the level of the first burn site. With the availability of small-caliber flexible video endoscopes, endoscopy under direct vision is considered safe during any phase of the illness in the absence of obvious evidence of perforation.[64] Some authors recommend gently guiding the instrument through areas of superficial injury and continuing examination until areas of possible full-thickness necrosis are encountered, an approach that allows complete evaluation of the upper gastrointestinal tract and has been reported to be safe.[65–67] If severe full-thickness necrosis is encountered, the examination is terminated and intensive care observation continued for signs of esophageal or gastric perforation. Endoscopic management strategy is summarized in Table 16.5.

Nasogastric tube placement

There have been reports in which acute corrosive injury was managed conservatively by the insertion of a nasogastric tube.[68] Although no controlled data are available regarding this approach, the nasogastric tube appears to act as a stent and prevents complete occlusion of the lumen and assures access for dilation guidewire

---

Table 16.4 Endoscopic grades of corrosive injury

1st degree	Erythema, edema, erosions (bleeding)
2nd degree	Intense erythema, blebs, and deep erosions with exudate
3rd degree	Epithelial loss, ulceration, necrosis, exudate and eschar

---

Table 16.5 Endoscopic management of corrosive injury

General anesthesia usually not required

Early endoscopy post stabilization

Complete, diligent examination of the esophagus and stomach

Repeat EGD after 2 weeks

Initiate dilation before 3 weeks if evidence of stricture

Savary dilation over guide wire under fluoroscopy is optimal technique for initial therapy

placement. If a nasogastric tube is used, it should be connected to low intermittent suction to avoid gastric distention. Measures to prevent acid reflux such as elevation of the head of the bed and acid suppression should also be employed during intubation. Some authors favor this approach if severe esophageal damage has been ruled out by endoscopy. In our opinion, when nasogastric intubation is considered appropriate, the concomitant use of an intravenous proton pump inhibitor is indicated. It is safer to place the nasogastric or nasoduodenal tube under fluoroscopic guidance or over a wire placed through the endoscope after evaluation has been completed. If the nasogastric tube tip is modified prior to placement by removing the blind end tip and smoothing the cut edges, guidewire insertion at the time of dilation can be done through the tube with safe post-dilation replacement of the nasogastric tube over the guidewire.

Use of corticosteroids, antibiotics, and early dilation

Since 1950, the use of systemic corticosteroids has been advocated in the acute and subacute phases of injury. Spain and colleagues reported a reduction in the degree of inflammation in an animal model.[69] However, Anderson and colleagues, in a prospective study, refuted this claim and reported no improvement in the steroid-treated group.[60] This debate may have been rekindled by a recent study by Bautista et al., who showed dexamethasone to be superior to prednisone in preventing strictures and reducing burn severity at 3 weeks. The dexamethasone-treated group also needed fewer dilations.[70] Barring this study, the prevailing belief at the present time is that steroids do not play a role in the treatment of corrosive injury.[71,72] The positive effect of dexamethasone in children may also be related to the fact that children, unlike suicidal adults, are brought to the hospital very early during the postingestion period.

Antibiotics alone have not been shown to be of any benefit in the treatment of corrosive injury. Their use has been limited to the prevention of septic complications in patients on intravenous corticosteroids.[73] Broad-spectrum antibiotic therapy is indicated in patients with signs of esophageal or gastric perforation.

Esophageal dilation carried out in the subacute phase may be associated with an increased risk of perforation.[74,75] In contrast to traditional thinking, esophageal dilation using proper technique and fluoroscopic control may be safe even during the subacute phase. Early dilation and the prevention of stricture formation forms the basis of the modified Salzer technique described by Palmer.[67,76] Using fluoroscopic guidance and proper technique, the patient receives a nasogastric tube within a few hours of the corrosive ingestion. Wire-guided esophageal dilation is then initiated on the third day after an endoscopic examination, with the dilator size chosen based on the age of the patient. Adult patients may be started with a 12 or 13 mm dilator (5–6 mm for a child); the dilation may be gradually progressed by 1–2 mm to reach a 15 mm diameter by the end of the first month. The dilation is discontinued if fresh blood is seen on the dilator. Dilations are carried out at least two or three times per week for several weeks in order to prevent stricture formation. Dilations predictably meet more resistance by the fourth week. The diameter of the lumen and frequency of dilation sessions should be determined by the resistance experienced on passage of each dilator. A progressively less frequent dilation schedule should be set for the next several months to years, using either wire-guided dilation or Maloney bougie dilation under fluoroscopic control to maintain lumen diameter between 15 and 18 mm. Periodic radiographic and endoscopic evaluations

should be continued as indicated for dysphagia and surveillance for the remainder of the patient's life.

Total parenteral nutrition

Maintenance of nutrition is of utmost importance in seriously ill patients. Feeding through the nasogastric tube may not be possible in patients with severe (grade 3) injury or in patients with impending perforation. These patients should receive early total parenteral nutrition (TPN) to avoid malnutrition, while allowing the gastrointestinal tract to rest and heal. DiConstanzo and colleagues reported that TPN protects the damaged mucosa.[77] TPN may also be required during the perioperative period in patients who require surgery.

Surgery

Esophagectomy should be performed when evidence of perforation related to the acute-phase injury is present. When endoscopic examination reveals extensive gastric necrosis, most authors recommend esophagectomy with gastrectomy and anastomosis, as either a one- or two-stage operation. Surgery is performed with the presumption that esophageal perforation is imminent in this situation. Zargar and colleagues proposed a modified classification system for corrosive injury and further subdivided second and third degree injury into grades 2a, 2b, 3a, and 3b. Patients with grade 1 (erythema and edema) and grade 2a injury (friability, hemorrhages, erosions, and superficial ulceration) did not develop any complications. Grade 2b (deep discrete or circumferential ulcers) or deeper injury was associated with complications. Patients with small and scattered areas of necrosis could be managed conservatively in the acute phase. Only 25% of these patients required surgery at a later stage. They recommend emergent esophagectomy only for patients with extensive necrosis (stage 3b).[64] Laparotomy may be needed for an evaluation of the depth of injury in some patients with extensive second or third degree injury. It also provides the option for the placement of a feeding gastrostomy tube and a continuous #4 silk suture, which may be utilized for retrograde dilation should it become necessary at a later date.

Treatment during chronic phase

In patients with severe esophageal injury, strictures typically develop within 3 to 4 weeks. Earlier frequent dilation serves to minimize this risk.[76] A barium esophagogram should be obtained at this time to assess the degree of stricture formation, the site of strictures, and contour of esophageal lumen. A solid bolus challenge may be required for accurate assessment if no stricture is apparent with liquid barium. A detailed regimen of wire-guided esophageal dilation needs to be planned as outlined above in the section on DIED. The dilation strategy should, however, take into account that the transmural fibrosis seen in this condition makes the esophageal wall prone to tearing and perforation. These patients may have pseudodiverticulum formation and require a much more careful approach. It is prudent to begin with a dilator size just below the estimated lumen diameter (by barium esophagogram) and advance only one or two millimeters in dilator diameter in the beginning. The rate of dilator size progression is determined by the resistance encountered, as well as operator experience. Some authors have shown a decrease in the need for repeated dilation when intralesional injections of triamcinolone were used in both pediatric and adult population.[38,39] The mechanism by which intralesional steroids benefit in this condition is not clearly understood. Often patients not properly treated by adequate dilation early in the chronic phase, or who are later neglected during follow-up, will require a series of careful dilation sessions to achieve and sustain adequate esophageal patency. Collagen synthesis inhibitors may have a role in this condition; such agents, however, are currently under investigation and no data presently support their use.[78]

Detection and treatment of late complications

As discussed above, patients with a history of corrosive injury to their esophagus have been estimated to have a 1000 times higher incidence of squamous cell carcinoma.[57,58] It may thus be reasonable to perform periodic surveillance endoscopies with Lugol staining chromoendoscopy in these patients starting 15 years after injury. However, no studies are available to prove or disprove the usefulness, cost-effectiveness or the proper interval of endoscopic surveillance.

TREATMENT ISSUES SPECIFIC TO MINIATURE (BUTTON) BATTERY INGESTION

Introduction

The ingestion of 'button' batteries follows the old axiom that 'toddlers put in their mouth what they get their hands on.' 'Button' battery ingestion represents a relatively new phenomenon. These miniaturized alkaline batteries have rapidly replaced the older cylindrical cells (Fig. 16.1). With electronic toys and quartz watches replacing their mechanical counterparts, these batteries are present in every modern household. They contain a highly concentrated solution of potassium or sodium hydroxide and potentially toxic compounds of mercury and zinc, lithium and cadmium. Over a 10-year period (1982–1992), 2320 cases of button battery ingestion were reported to the National Button Battery Ingestion Hotline at Georgetown University Hospital's National Poison Center (202-625-3333).[79–81]

Pathogenesis

The major mechanism of injury to the esophagus is the leakage of the caustic alkaline solution from the button battery. Esophageal mucosal damage may occur within 1 hour of ingestion, and the degree of damage correlates directly to the duration of contact with the mucosa.[82] The risk of impaction of a disc battery in the esophagus depends on its size, being more likely with batteries larger than 20 mm in diameter. Fortunately, 97% of the ingested

batteries are less than 15 mm in diameter, with 62.5% being 11.6 mm in diameter (range 7–23 mm).[79–81,83] Disc batteries should be considered as a foreign body with severe corrosive properties or a corrosive chemical delivered as a small pellet. Contrary to early belief, Litovitz did not find the severity of injury to be dependent on the electrical status of the battery in a study of 1718 cases in which the battery status and outcome were both known. Instead, they found that lithium batteries with their larger size and higher voltage (3 volts) were associated with more severe damage.

Prevention

Precautions required to prevent ingestion of button batteries are similar to those needed for any foreign body ingestion. However, due to their potential for causing rapid damage, it is extremely important to keep these batteries out of reach of children. Sixty-six percent of battery ingestions occur in children younger than 6 years of age.[79–81] Children who use a hearing aid require closer supervision because nearly one-half of the reported ingestions involve these batteries. Education of audiologists, parents, and children may help reduce these events. Design improvements and industry involvement can likely eliminate this threat. It may be prudent for the manufacturers to use smaller batteries, which are less likely to get impacted in the esophagus. Further miniaturization and the development of batteries that do not contain corrosive materials may eliminate this damage in the coming decades. The development of one such battery was reported in the lay press by researchers at Johns Hopkins University.

Management

Foreign body identification

Prompt identification and location of the battery is the most important first step in this condition. Once a possible case is brought to the notice of a physician, posteroanterior and lateral chest radiographs should be promptly obtained. A 'double-density' opacity is usually produced by a disc battery.[84] The edges of a battery are more rounded than that those of a coin. An abdominal radiograph is also indicated initially to search for other foreign objects that may have been ingested.

Removal

If the battery is lodged in the esophagus, a prompt endoscopic extraction is mandatory. No neutralizing agents have been found to be useful to prevent or decrease esophageal damage while the patient is in transit to a medical center.[85] Emetic agents are generally ineffective and should not be used. Although Foley catheter balloon-assisted removal of foreign bodies is considered safe in patients with a disease-free esophagus, this method is not

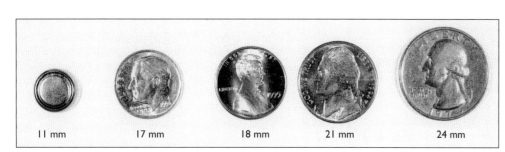

| 11 mm | 17 mm | 18 mm | 21 mm | 24 mm |

Fig. 16.1 ● A photograph of an 11 mm disc battery and common coins, showing the rounded edges of the battery that make its retrieval using forceps difficult. The caustic material leaks out from the gap between front and back covers. The coins have elevated edges, which enable them to be grasped with alligator/rat-tooth forceps.

recommended for disc batteries due to a lack of control.[86–88] The use of a magnetic probe for the removal of button batteries has been reported in European countries.[89] A protocol for the management of ingested button batteries is presented in Table 16.6. Most reviews do not recommend any intervention for batteries that have arrived in the stomach or more distally at the time of diagnosis.[88–90] However, more recent experience tends to suggest that polyethyline glycol solution preparations may be used safely to flush the battery more quickly.[91]

Endoscopic intervention

Oral removal by endoscopy is the treatment of choice for button batteries lodged in the esophagus. General anesthesia or monitored anesthesia care with protection of the airway may be required in infants and children, while adolescents and adults may be able to undergo endoscopy using intravenous sedation. A bronchoscopy prior to endoscopy should be performed if more than 4 hours have elapsed since the ingestion of battery to identify a fistula that may form as a result of full-thickness injury to the anterior esophageal and posterior tracheal walls.

Endoscopic removal of disc batteries from the esophagus is challenging. General principles employed in the removal of disc batteries are similar to those followed for any other foreign body retrieval with the exception of need for removal as early as possible (Table 16.7). Because of their rounded edges, these batteries are difficult to grasp securely with foreign-body forceps or snares. If the exact size and type of the battery is identified, the choice of instrument can be made by prior rehearsal. Common US coins and a disc battery are shown in Figure 16.1. Forceps with magnetic properties may be more useful in these situations, but are not currently available. An overtube may be used to protect the airway or to prevent dropping the battery as it traverses the cricopharyngeal sphincter. A Dormier basket as used for gallstone retrieval

Table 16.6 Management protocol for esophageal button battery

History: establish accurate size and time of ingestion

Initial X-ray (posterior-anterior and lateral chest X-ray plus abdominal X-ray)

Esophageal battery: emergent endoscopic retrieval

Identify the chemical system: mercury levels only when battery disintegrated

For help call (202) 625-3333 in the United States or contact your physician immediately

Table 16.7 Indications for emergent removal of ingested foreign body

Respiratory distress

Foreign body at the cricopharyngeus level

Inability to swallow secretions

Evidence of perforation

Button battery ingestion

Sharp object ingestion

or the Roth Retrieval Net used to retrieve colon polyps may be helpful. Only 33% of attempted removals have been reported as successful.[81] If retrieval is not possible, the battery can be gently pushed into the stomach and removal attempted from the stomach. However, this maneuver should only be done if the lumen beyond the battery is clearly visible, adequately patent, and free of any pathology. If retrieval is not possible even from the stomach, the battery should be left in the stomach and a follow-up radiograph obtained at 48 hours to follow the passage of the battery. Although Willis and Ho reported the perforation of a Meckel's diverticulum by an ingested disc battery, no further intervention is generally required if the battery has passed beyond the pylorus by 48 hours and if no symptoms are reported.[90]

Role of surgery

Early surgery may be indicated if a perforation, full-thickness injury, or fistula formation is detected by endoscopy and/or bronchoscopy. The management is then the same as that of perforation due to any foreign body.

Post-retrieval measures

If a battery has been removed uneventfully without full-thickness damage evident on endoscopy, no further intervention may be required. In patients where progression to full-thickness burn or fistula formation may be likely, a barium swallow using thin barium may be performed during the next 24–48 hours. This study may be repeated in the next several days to delineate stricture formation. Treatment with proton pump inhibitors or sucralfate may be useful if mucosal erosion is seen. The use of laxatives or prokinetics to promote the passage of a gastrointestinal button battery is not recommended since most batteries are excreted within 72 hours.[88]

ESOPHAGEAL FOREIGN BODIES (NONFOOD)

Foreign body ingestion results in approximately 1500 deaths annually in the United States. A large majority of foreign body ingestions occur in children, edentulous elderly, prisoners, and psychiatric patients. In a recent series of 414 adult patients with ingested foreign bodies, 38% were nonfood-related objects. Seventy-five percent of these objects were found in the esophagus (36% cervical, 19.8% mid-esophagus, and 19.1% distal esophagus).[92] Nonfood foreign bodies are ingested primarily by children.[93] These include coins, components of toys, crayons, and small household items such as pens, paper clips, and safety pins. College students have a propensity for accidental ingestion of coins as a consequence of a flip and oral catch game often played under the influence of alcohol. Prisoners, on the other hand, have been reported to indulge in recurrent (3–10%), deliberate ingestion of many types of foreign bodies for secondary gain.[95,96] Nearly 75% of all documented ingested foreign bodies are lodged in the esophagus at the time of diagnosis.[97]

Pathogenesis

Children ingest foreign bodies while playing with them, while the elderly who ingest foreign bodies most often have their palatal sensation reduced or eliminated by a denture plate. One such example is the aluminum foil wrapping on medications with the medication enclosed, which has resulted in esophageal perforation. Although uncommon in children, adults who have esophageal foreign bodies impacted in the esophagus have underlying lesions of the esophagus in up to 88% of cases.[95]

Diagnosis

A history of definite ingestion by the patient/witness or in its absence other associated signs of dysphagia, odynophagia, sialorrhea, chest discomfort, or constitutional, signs of perforation may all point to the diagnosis of foreign body ingestion. Radiography is of paramount importance as most ingested foreign bodies are radiopaque. Since 1982, at the insistence of pediatricians and radiologists, all North American coins have been minted with radiopaque metals.[98] It is important to obtain two axis (AP and lateral) views to estimate the exact location, size, and shape of the object. However, plain films have false-negative rates up to 47% in the detection of foreign bodies.[99] When the suspicion is strong, but plain radiography fails to identify a foreign body, barium contrast radiography is often useful. However, barium should be avoided in patients suspected to have total esophageal obstruction. Also, barium may be retained in enough quantity with incomplete obstruction to hinder endoscopic examination. Radiographic diagnosis assists the endoscopist in planning the procedure and selecting the timing and equipment for retrieval.[94,97] It may also rule out or confirm a suspicion of perforation. CT scanning of the neck and chest with soft tissue and bone windows provide better contrast and are more useful in foreign body detection.[100] Flexible video endoscopy has the advantage of combining diagnostic and therapeutic capabilities. Extreme care should be exercised by the endoscopist during the procedure. It is critical that the passage of the endoscope and accessories be done under constant direct vision and never blindly into or beyond a foreign body.

Prevention

Prevention of foreign body ingestion is far more cost-effective than their extraction. Coins and small objects that can be swallowed should be kept out of the reach of infants and small children. A similar strategy for close supervision should be adopted for the mentally retarded and elderly patients.

Removal of esophageal foreign bodies

Nonendoscopic management

In a retrospective study of esophageal foreign bodies, Crysdale and colleagues[101] reported that 7.8% passed spontaneously within 24 hours, while another 2.5% passed with the use of pharmacological agents. In contrast, Tibbling and Stenquist reported a spontaneous passage rate of 21% within 24 hours,[102] which further increased to 29% if endoscopy was delayed beyond 24 hours. Spontaneous passage is almost universal once the foreign body has reached beyond the lower esophageal sphincter.

Nonendoscopic approaches can be divided into two categories: those that promote the passage of the object distally and those aimed at extraction of the object. Distal passage is promoted primarily by pharmacological means using agents that relax the lower esophageal sphincter. The use of a carbonated drink has been reported to be 100% successful in a small number of patients. This approach may represent a simple strategy, but its safety and efficacy needs to be further tested by a larger study.[103] Other effervescent agents that release large quantities of CO_2 upon ingestion have also been used, with success rates of 75%.[104] However, because effervescent agents in the setting of complete obstruction have resulted in perforation, their use can not be recommended. Their use may be safe prior to endoscopy in patients with nontoxic, blunt/round, small-caliber foreign bodies in the absence of pre-existing esophageal pathology.

A technique usually reported by radiologists and not favored by most gastroenterologists involves the use of a Foley catheter for the removal of esophageal foreign bodies. This technique has been widely reported in emergency medicine and in the pediatric literature and employs the passage of a Foley catheter under fluoroscopic guidance, followed by inflation of its balloon distal to the ingested object.[105–107] The catheter is then withdrawn, thus removing the foreign body. This technique has been shown to be safe in the pediatric population, where pre-existing esophageal pathology is generally not encountered. The technique has an obvious cost advantage because it obviates the need for an endoscopy and minimizes the period of observation in a hospital or emergency room. The primary risk of this strategy is the lack of control when the object passes the hypopharynx. This risk may be overcome either by the use of endotracheal intubation or placing the patient in a Trendelenburg position. In a survey of pediatric radiologists, Campbell and colleagues reported 2500 successful foreign body removals, with only one complication.[108] The use of this method is limited to blunt objects within 12 hours of ingestion.[105]

Gastroenterologists prefer endoscopy over the Foley balloon catheter, perhaps due to their experience with endoscopy and lack of experience with Foley catheter technique.[94,109] Because esophageal disease is so common in patients with esophageal foreign bodies, an endoscopy should be performed in all cases. The blind passage of an esophageal bougie to push the foreign body into the stomach has been described, but should not be done because of the high risk for perforation and the ready availability of safer alternatives.[110] Thompson and colleagues recently described another nonendoscopic technique for the removal of gastric and esophageal metallic foreign bodies, using a magnetic orogastric tube.[111,112] Although their reported success rate was >90%, lack of control is once again an issue. The technique, however, has the potential of being useful as an adjunct to endoscopy and overtube placement.

Endoscopic removal

Rigid esophagoscopy was most widely used for foreign body removal prior to the 1960s and 1970s. However, the availability of flexible fiberoptic endoscopes, and more recently video endoscopy, has brought about a revolution in this field. The diameter of the endoscopes has become progressively smaller, thereby making flexible endoscopy favored for the removal of foreign bodies. Gastroenterologists today are primarily trained in, and prefer to use, flexible video endoscopes, a preference that is widely supported.[93–95,97,113] In his report of 242 foreign body removals, Webb used a flexible endoscope in 211 (87%) cases.[93] Similarly, in a 15-year review of foreign body management, Weiss and colleagues employed flexible endoscopy in 111 of the 132 cases where endoscopic removal was carried out, with a success rate of 90%. In addition, flexible endoscopy has the advantage of being safer, with a reported perforation rate less than one-half that of rigid esophagoscopy (0.9%

versus 2%).[95,110] Rigid endoscopy retains a role for the removal of foreign bodies impacted in the hypopharynx and cricopharyngeus (upper esophageal sphincter) and in those not removable by a flexible endoscope.

Preparation for endoscopy

Indications for emergent foreign body retrieval are summarized in Table 16.7. While performing endoscopy for removal of foreign bodies, one must ascertain that the patient is completely cooperative or adequately sedated and properly monitored, with ample assistance and equipment available to the endoscopist. If intravenous conscious sedation does not achieve this objective, monitored anesthesia care (MAC) using short-acting intravenous agents, such as propofol, is preferred. MAC is especially useful when endotracheal intubation is required for airway protection. Availability of the surgical team, if needed, should be ascertained before beginning any foreign body removal, especially when dealing with sharp object or button battery ingestion or when the object was ingested more than 24 hours previously.

Equipment selection

Most experts in this field practice and recommend a proper selection of equipment and planning (i.e., a 'dry run'), using accessories to practice grasping a similar foreign body prior to the actual procedure.[94,97] This process provides the endoscopist and the endoscopy assistant a feel for both the eventualities that might occur during the retrieval and the suitability of the accessory equipment to be used.

Accessories

Various accessories have enhanced the ability of the endoscopist in successful retrieval of ingested foreign bodies safely (Table 16.8). These include: overtube, alligator forceps, rat-tooth forceps, (both manufactured by Olympus America Inc., Lake Success, NY), Roth retrieval net, (US Endoscopy Group, Inc., Mentor, Ohio), polypectomy

snare, Dormier basket, tripod, hooded sheath, and the Stiegman-Goff adaptor for variceal band ligation (Figs 16.2–16.4). Of these, the plastic overtube is a versatile, multipurpose accessory that should be stocked in every endoscopy unit (Fig. 16.2). It also allows multiple passages of the endoscope with lesser patient discomfort. When back-loaded on an endoscope and advanced after the endoscope tip is beyond the cricopharyngeus, it can be advanced over the scope to provide airway protection. However, injury can occur due to trapping of the mucosa between either an endoscope or a Maloney dilator used as an obturator to introduce the overtube.[114] Introduction of the overtube should be performed gently and carefully regardless of the obturator (endoscope or rubber bougie) used. A 44 French size Maloney dilator is used as the obturator for

Table 16.8

Esophageal foreign body	Suitable extraction accessories
Coin	Roth net, alligator forceps, rat-tooth forceps, snare, basket, TTS balloon, magnetic probe (if available)
Button battery	Roth retrieval net, Dormier basket, magnetic probe
Thumb tacks	Alligator forceps, rat-tooth forceps
Sharp objects (pins, needles, toothpicks, blades, open safety pins, fish bone)	Overtube, hooded sheath, snare, alligator forceps
Marbles, seeds, eraser	Baskets, snare, polyp retriever
Food bolus (meat)	Overtube Stiegman-Goff adaptor, Dormier basket

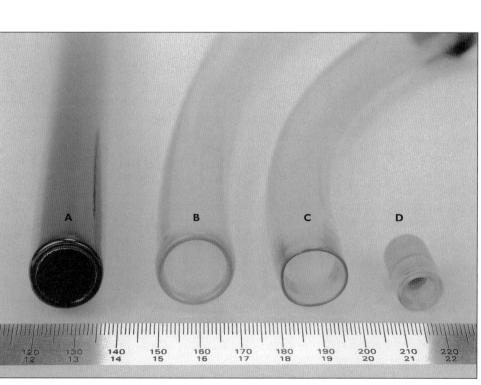

Fig. 16.2 • Overtubes. (**A**) Conventional, black, straight overtube with sharp inner edge; (**B and C**) Newer variety, curved, clear plastic (20 cm long) overtubes. Note their round (B) and tapered (C) distal ends. (**D**) Friction tip (Stiegmann-Goff) adaptor for variceal ligation and meat bolus extraction.

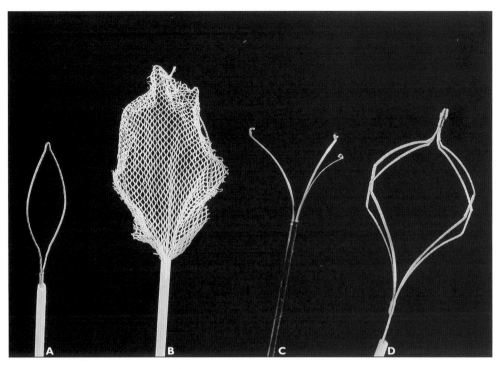

Fig. 16.3 • Photograph showing: (**A**) Snare, (**B**) Roth Retrieval Net, (**C**) polyp retriever, and (**D**) Dormier basket.

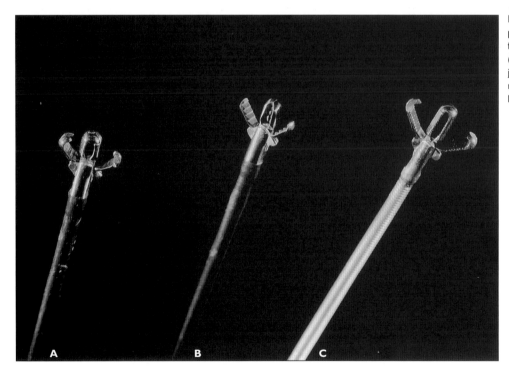

Fig. 16.4 • A dual exposure photograph showing: (**A**) rat-tooth forceps, (**B**) alligator forceps, and (**C**) alligator forceps with rat-tooth jaws. These accessories are useful in removal of a variety of foreign bodies.

passing one standard model of overtube in patients without esophageal foreign bodies; however, this blind overtube passage should not be used for fear of push injury when an esophageal foreign body is suspected. Sharp objects, such as pins, needles, blades and wires, can be withdrawn into the tube, thus protecting the esophageal mucosa from damage. Coins, the most common foreign bodies ingested by children, are best removed using an alligator or a rat-tooth forceps or a Dormier basket (Figs 16.3, 16.4). These forceps have sharp jaws that appose well to grasp an object

with rough and vertical edges. Button batteries, on the other hand, have rounded edges that are difficult to grasp with forceps. In an in vivo comparison of various accessories, Faigel and colleagues demonstrated that button batteries could be removed only by using either a basket or a Roth Retrieval Net (Fig. 16.3), whereas the snare was the best instrument for removing toothpicks and thumb tacks.[115] A through-the-scope (TTS) balloon may at times be used to remove a foreign body under direct visualization via a two-channel operating endoscope, or as a means of opening the lumen distal to a foreign body in the grasp of a snare or forceps.

Body packer syndrome (cocaine-loaded foreign body)

The popularity of cocaine as a recreational drug within the United States has resulted in increased smuggling of this drug across international borders. Its abundant availability in South American countries and the enormous cost difference between these countries and United States has resulted in people devising ingenious ways to smuggle the drug. 'Body packing' or ingesting cocaine-filled latex condoms is one such ingenious method used to conceal the illicit material. Each pack generally contains up to 5 grams of cocaine. Once the 'packer' arrives at his destination, the ingested pack is retrieved after it is passed in feces.

The clinical significance of this crime strikes home when the scheme does not proceed as planned. Complications of this ingestion usually arise when the packages rupture or are not passed in the feces within 24–48 hours. Esophageal impaction with these packages is rare, but may occur as with any ingested foreign bodies. Johnson and Landreneau reported a case of esophageal obstruction and perforation due to ingested marijuana packs by a prisoner in Missouri.[116] The cocaine/drug packs are unique in that endoscopic removal should not be attempted because it may lead to perforation of the pack and release of a fatal dose of the drug. Whenever detected, these packs are best managed surgically. The general condition of the patient merits intensive observation and supportive care if some or all of the packs have traversed the esophagus.

TREATMENT OF FOOD BOLUS IMPACTION

Introduction

A food bolus represents a specific type of foreign body, and most studies deal with the accidentally swallowed, unchewed or unprepared food bolus as a part of ingested foreign bodies. We deal with the specific aspects of management of food bolus separately due to the unique characteristics of this foreign body. Impacted food bolus is the most common type of foreign body encountered in adults. In a large majority of cases, a food bolus impacts in the esophagus due to an underlying disorder. The impacted food is usually a piece of meat that is swallowed without careful chewing. Hence, the commonly used terms include 'meat impaction' or 'steakhouse syndrome.'

Pathogenesis

A distal esophageal ring or a stricture is usually present that prevents the passage of the bolus into the stomach. Patients frequently present several hours after dining at a restaurant or having a big holiday meal. Meat boluses impacted for over 12 hours or those that contain slivers of bone create a higher risk for esophageal perforation during attempts at removal.

Diagnosis/treatment

As discussed in the section on foreign bodies above, diagnosis is often apparent from the history. Most patients receive glucagon,

nitroglycerine, or similar medications in the emergency room before a gastroenterologist is consulted. The statistics presented above for success of these agents in foreign bodies are applicable to the impacted food bolus. Recent experience with glucagon has not been very gratifying. Although esophageal perforation was reported with the use of papain as early as 1968,[117] the use of meat tenderizers (a very reduced concentration of papain) was common in emergency rooms long after that.[118] The use of this agent should no longer be considered a standard treatment. Papain, the active ingredient in meat tenderizer, has no effect on normal mucosa, but contact with inflamed mucosa may incite a marked increase in inflammation,[117] and mural digestion may occur if the tissue is ischemic. Because of its chemical nature and contact with saliva, a food bolus impacted in the esophagus undergoes progressive degradation with passage of time. This feature is of importance in planning its extraction. If the patient can handle salivary secretions, emergent endoscopy is not necessary. Observation and sedation may allow spontaneous passage of the food bolus.[93] If urgent endoscopy is performed, a meat bolus ingested recently can potentially be extracted in one piece using a snare or a basket. However, if more than 12 hours have elapsed since the consumption of the meal, the meat may have become very soft and fragmented. Under such circumstances, multiple passages of the endoscope may be required, necessitating the use of an overtube.[94] The standard forceps and snare accessories often are inadequate for removing such impactions. Saeed and colleagues in 1990 reported the use of the Stiegman-Goff band ligator tip as an accessory for meat bolus extraction (see Fig. 16.2D).[119] This technique produces a suction cup at the tip of the endoscope, thus facilitating removal of a soft food bolus. Despite disintegration with the usual instrumentation, the bolus can be suctioned and anchored into this cup during the passage across the cricopharyngeus. Homemade endoscope tip adaptors fashioned from plastic tubing were, however, in use even prior to this report. The newer variety transparent variceal band ligator adaptors are even more suitable for this task as they do not occlude the endoscopist's field of vision. Other aspects of meat bolus extraction are generally identical to those of ingested foreign bodies.

Any bolus that completely occludes the lumen and prevents visual inspection of the lumen beyond the bolus should not be blindly pushed ahead with the endoscope or any accessory instrument because of an increased risk of perforation.

Treatment of the underlying disorders

An underlying esophageal structural abnormality is present in up to 80% of adults with foreign body impaction in the esophagus. An appropriate therapy of the underlying lesion may thus prevent future recurrences. The lesion most often encountered is a reflux-induced esophageal stricture. Mosca et al. found associated pathology in 83 (30.7%) of their patients (stricture, 50; hiatal hernia, 11; achalasia, 11; and Schatzki ring, varices, diverticula, and cancer, 11).[92] If the ingested object or food bolus is present for more than 12 hours and the esophageal mucosa shows signs of ischemia/inflammation, esophageal dilation should be deferred for at least 1–2 weeks after foreign body removal. A malignant lesion should be appropriately managed. Patients with psychiatric disorders should receive prompt help via psychiatric consultation and should be appropriately treated because of the risk of repeated ingestion or other suicide attempts.

TRAUMATIC INJURY TO THE ESOPHAGUS

Introduction

Traumatic injury to the esophagus can be classified into two groups based on etiological mechanisms. The first and far more frequent is the extrinsic group, which includes instrumentation, such as endoscopy, dilation, surgery, foreign bodies, and thermal ablation of lesions. Recognition of complication risk and efforts at prevention are the key elements in avoiding perforation.[120] The second and less common group is due to intrinsic causes, which includes Mallory-Weiss tear, Boerhaave's syndrome, and malignant strictures.

Pathogenesis

Various etiological factors involved in trauma to the esophagus are summarized in Table 16.9. Instruments such as endoscopes, bougies, hydrostatic or pneumatic balloon dilators, guidewires, tips of hydrostatic (TTS) dilators, and other accessories all may cause disruption of the wall of the esophagus due to a shearing or radial force or a direct puncture. Owing to its unique anatomic characteristic of lacking the serosal layer, the esophagus is especially susceptible to these forces. Trauma during or after surgery, on the other hand, may be either direct laceration or disruption of vascular supply at the time of surgery resulting in an ischemic injury, which finally results in perforation. Modalities such as thermal lasers, multipolar coagulation and heater probe, or photodynamic laser therapy (PDT) may traumatize the esophagus by direct burn

or deep desiccation, which eventually results in necrosis of the tissue and perforation. Barotrauma or forceful distention may take place due to excessive insufflation of air during various procedures, especially in the setting of complete obstruction.

Prevention

Esophageal injury due to instrumentation may increase as newer procedures, instruments, and techniques are adopted for achieving hemostasis and performing esophageal dilation, as well as with the advent of endoscopic antireflux procedures. In our view, adequate emphasis on prevention of iatrogenic injury is likely the most important part of management. The following section deals with issues important for the prevention of iatrogenic esophageal injury.

Barium esophagogram

'Cost containment' issues have also resulted in the endoscopist often not having the luxury of, or making the effort to, obtain a barium esophagogram study prior to endoscopic intervention for stenotic lesions. Identification of pre-existing lesions prior to endoscopy by barium swallow is, however, useful. The value of a barium esophagogram being available prior to endoscopy in stenotic lesions of the esophagus cannot be overemphasized. A detailed history may help in selecting the cases where a barium study must be obtained before endoscopy is attempted. A barium esophagogram helps to identify the site, length, and contour of the stricture. It also alerts the endoscopist to the possibility of more than one stenotic lesion with different characteristics being present in one patient. A barium study will identify necrotic cavities in an esophageal carcinoma prior to endoscopy, dilation, or stent placement that otherwise might be interpreted as a perforation when done following the procedure.

Issues relating to fluoroscopy, wire guidance and TTS balloons

Several developments in the evolution of endoscopy have resulted in esophageal dilation being done routinely without the use of fluoroscopy. These include time constraints, commercial promotion to employ newer TTS balloons for esophageal dilation, the demonstrated safety of esophageal dilation in simple, distal, peptic strictures without the use of fluoroscopy, and the advent of office- or outpatient center-based endoscopy. All have led to the general belief that fluoroscopy may be superfluous for most esophageal strictures. However, fluoroscopy helps in completing a safe, effective dilation of esophageal stricture and is of utmost value when the endoscopist is not familiar with the severity of the lesion. We prefer that patients be in a supine position for this procedure, especially when using fluoroscopy, which helps in the correct anatomical identification of landmarks and helps in following the course of the dilator accurately. Availability of excellent C-arms with digital image quality has brought fluoroscopy out of hospital radiology departments and into modern endoscopy units, thereby making it easily accessible.

Esophageal dilation under wire guidance has made esophageal dilation safer and, in the authors' view, should be the method of choice for most dilation procedures. The wire placement should either be endoscope assisted or under fluoroscopic guidance or both. Advancement of the Savary wire or a thinner, floppy wire under fluoroscopy may prevent inadvertent injury when a patient has

---

Table 16.9 Esophageal trauma: etiology
Extraluminal etiologies
Penetrating wounds
Blunt trauma
Operative injury
Through-the-wall suture
Disruption of blood supply
Laparoscope/other instruments
Intraluminal etiologies
Intrinsic
Mallory-Weiss tear
Boerhaave syndrome
Esophageal malignancy
Ulceration
Extrinsic
Foreign bodies/nonendoscopic instrumentation
Bone/pin ingestion, endotracheal, nasogastric, orogastric tube placement
Endoscopic instrumentation
Dilation, guidewire/endoprosthesis placement, balloon tip
Pneumatic dilation, sclerotherapy, laser or electrocoagulation, overtubes

luminal abnormalities, such as a Zenker diverticulum, cricopharyngeal bar, epiphrenic diverticulum or large hiatal hernia. The Savary wire, although flexible at its tip, has been reported to cause perforation of the gastric or duodenal wall when not fixed diligently in position during advancement of the dilator. Injury occurs when the flexible tip is completely flexed or the wire bent acutely, and force is exerted either at the junction of the flexible tip and stiff steel wire or against the point of the bent wire. Due to its thickness and relative rigidity, the tip may also traverse severely inflamed, friable tissue planes if not observed carefully during endoscopy or under fluoroscopy.

Esophageal TTS hydrostatic balloons have gained increased popularity in recent times for the dilation of esophageal strictures. Although far more expensive than bougie-type dilators, aggressive marketing and relative ease of use form the basis of their increased usage. These balloons, however, have a long, semi-firm tapered tip, which is often several centimeters away from the view of the endoscope (Fig. 16.5). The tip is prone to causing injury to the mucosa in the presence of inflammation, friability, or carcinoma, especially when the endoscope is being repositioned or with respiratory excursion. This possibility is even more important with longer balloons or when a stenotic lesion does not allow the passage of the endoscope to direct safe passage of the balloon dilator tip. The tip should be carefully observed at the time of advancement and at every point when the balloon or the endoscope is advanced. Development of an even more flexible tip may address this problem. Regardless, the endoscopist and the assistant need to diligently fix the endoscope at the mouth and the balloon catheter at the insertion port of the endoscope, which should prevent inadvertent movement of the balloon dilator or its tip during inflation. Another concern is the use of these hydrostatic balloons to dilate strictures due to causes likely associated with deep transmural injury and fibrosis, such as those related to radiation and caustic injury. In our opinion, wire-guided dilation or Maloney dilators under fluoroscopic control are safest in these patients.

Issues relating to thermal or other ablative modalities

Adhering to safe levels of power settings while performing thermo-ablation procedures and becoming familiar with new equipment prior to use may prevent accidental deep burns. Testing the power settings in vitro on comparable animal tissue or in vivo in the stomach (which has a thicker wall) immediately before use may prevent deeper esophageal burns or perforation. Using lower power settings when the tissue is inflamed or treating raised lesions and avoiding excavated lesions may also be helpful. The depth of ablation achieved with equipment made by different manufacturers may differ even with similar settings. Early experience with the radio-frequency technique for treatment of gastroesophageal reflux (STRETTA™) has reportedly resulted in perforation, although added experience has improved its safety profile. The Endo Cinch™ device technique has recently been reported to have caused a perforation of the distal esophagus that was managed laparoscopically.[121] It is obvious that these techniques are best used by adequately trained operators who perform these procedures regularly.

Issues relating to overtubes and foreign-body removal

During endoscopy, intubation and advancement of the endoscope should be done under direct visualization. While attempting foreign body retrieval, the overtube should not be passed until the foreign body and esophageal mucosa have been examined. The use of an overtube should be avoided if possible, but not at the cost of compromising the airway. However, overtubes are important in the protection of the airway and should be used when indicated. Mucosal injuries related to passage of overtubes can be minimized by placing the overtube in warm water prior to insertion and passing the overtube over a proper diameter bougie.[122,123] The largest bougie that can be comfortably moved in and out of the overtube should be used. The use of the newer variety 60F/20 cm length tube with a filed, blunt, rounded leading edge may further reduce this trauma.[124] Inadequate sedation and inability of the assistant to hold the overtube in place are two factors that may precipitate accidental,

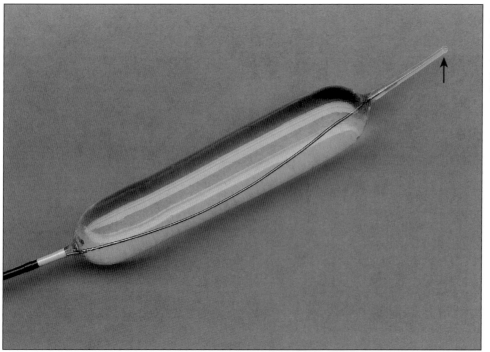

Fig. 16.5 • Photograph showing tip of a TTS balloon. The tip (arrow) can traverse through inflamed, necrotic, or even normal tissue, with sufficient force, during blind placement and cause perforation if caution is not exercised.

uncontrolled, and repetitive repositioning or advancement of the overtube, thereby increasing the chances of mucosal injury. The older, larger, longer, and stiffer overtube (see Fig. 16.2A) should be considered obsolete and removed from the endoscopy units.

As described above, while removing foreign bodies, the sharper end should always be trailing (Fig. 16.6) in order to avoid accidental puncture of the mucosa. Removal of a PEG tube mushroom should be done by the external traction method whenever possible. Cutting of the internal bumper and snare-assisted retrieval should only be done when one-step external traction removal is not possible. If not retrieved carefully, these bumpers can result in esophageal perforation.

Management of perforation of the esophagus

Causes of esophageal perforation have been listed along with causes of esophageal trauma in Table 16.9. Whatever the cause, esophageal trauma and perforation constitute an emergency and require rapid diagnosis and treatment. The signs and symptoms usually depend on the cause, location, and extent of perforation (Fig. 16.7). Patients usually present with tachycardia, chest pain, shortness of breath, and vomiting, and may have subcutaneous or mediastinal emphysema. Efficient management of esophageal perforation begins with an accurate history in high-risk cases. The classic scenario is of a patient presenting after consuming a large meal that includes alcohol, followed by vomiting and/or severe bouts of coughing, chest pain, and dysphagia. Subtle presentations may include a history of consumption of carbonated drinks/beer with forceful retching, blunt trauma to the chest during a fist fight or accident, swallowing a sharp bone or object, or severe coughing episodes. Symptoms of pleuritic chest pain with radiation to shoulder, neck or jaw, or epigastric pain in a patient with the above-mentioned history should alert physicians to the possibility of esophageal perforation. This possibility is especially important for the physicians evaluating patients during the night or in walk-in clinics, where several hours may elapse before the patient is likely to be seen by another physician. Early detection and evaluation of suspicious symptoms with chest radiographs and barium esophagogram can be invaluable in improving the eventual outcome.

Radiographic studies may show subcutaneous emphysema (Fig. 16.8), mediastinal widening, pneumothorax, pleural effusion, or an air–fluid level in the mediastinum. Typically, a water-soluble contrast (Gastrograffin®, meglumine diatrizoate) swallow should be performed if esophageal perforation is suspected. This study should be the first radiographic procedure done for the evaluation of a suspected perforation after a PA and lateral chest X-ray. If negative, a barium esophagogram using a limited volume of thin barium is more likely to reveal small perforations and should be done. If perforation is still suspected, a CT scan will prove most sensitive for revealing barium outside the esophageal lumen. Once esophageal perforation is suspected, regardless of whether initial studies are negative, a thoracic surgeon with significant experience in performing esophageal surgery should be contacted promptly. Preferably, the surgeon should be alerted to the possibility of esophageal perforation and be available on call even before a relatively high-risk procedure, such as pneumatic balloon dilation for achalasia, is actually performed. The patient with suspected esophageal perforation is best managed in the hospital under close observation with surgical consultation until perforation is excluded.

Nontransmural tears of the esophagus can be successfully managed conservatively and patients discharged within 3 to 4 days.[125] Occasionally, limited/nontransmural tears may extend after delayed weakening of the wall by infection or by high intrathoracic pressures generated by gagging, vomiting, or coughing. Thus, the diagnosis should be reviewed and diagnostic studies repeated if the clinical condition of the patient does not improve rapidly.

Esophageal perforation occurring after endoscopy or dilation is considered by some authors to represent a different entity. Although surgery forms the mainstay of therapy, several studies have reported successful management of these patients by conservative

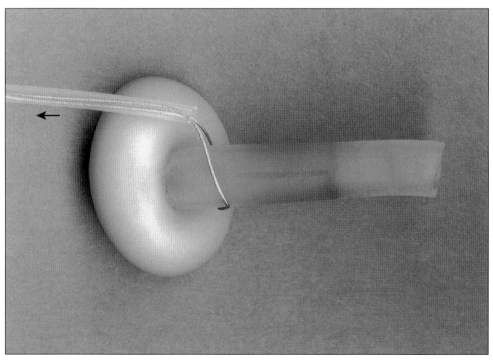

Fig. 16.6 ● Photograph showing the cut internal bumper of a gastrostomy tube. The relatively sharp tube end can cause mucosal injury. Retrieval direction (arrow) should be with the sharp end trailing.

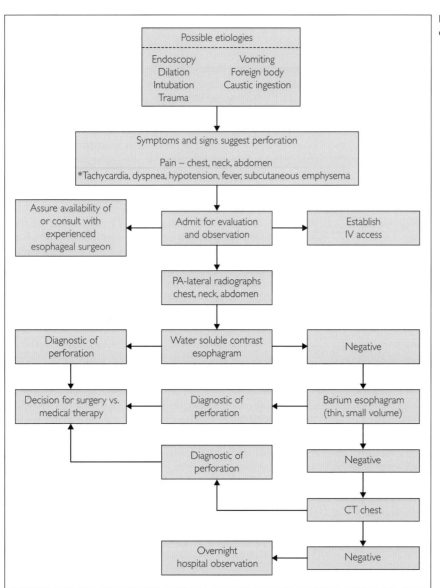

Fig. 16.7 • Algorithm for management of esophageal perforation.

treatment, using intravenous fluids and antibiotics.[126–131] Mortality is generally low compared to noniatrogenic patient groups, although morbidity is higher in patients with delayed (>24 hours) identification of perforation.[132] If the patient is not a surgical candidate and has a limited life span, as in patients with esophageal cancer, immediate placement of a plastic or coated metal expandable endoprosthesis is an option, with 60–90% chances of survival.[133,134] Despite these reports, it must be emphasized that such patients require close observation, preferably in the intensive care unit, aggressive supportive care, broad-spectrum antibiotic therapy and an alternative source of nutrition. Surgery should be considered if clinical improvement does not continue. There has been one case report where perforation following pneumatic balloon dilation for achalasia was treated endoscopically using a metallic clip.[135] In the future, laparoscopic surgery may also play a larger role in the management of small, clean, iatrogenic perforations that are detected early.[120]

Perforation due to noniatrogenic trauma is best managed by early surgical repair.[136] Historically, patients undergoing early surgery

have had a better outcome. Mortality rates as high as 56% with delayed recognition of esophageal perforation are reported.[137,138] More recent reports, although maintaining the trend of poor prognosis for patients with delayed detection, show a comparatively better outcome in both groups.[139] Most patients are able to avoid esophagectomy.

Some of these studies also support conservative management for noniatrogenic perforations. The studies that have evaluated a conservative approach for this group of patients report success in patients with hypopharyngeal perforations.[139] Others who have evaluated this form of treatment with thoracic esophageal perforations have selected larger perforations for surgical treatment.[133] There is also a chance of reporting bias where failures of conservative approach may not be reported. In addition, as emphasized by Pasricha et al., it is quite difficult to predict that a small perforation selected for conservative management will not progress to cause extensive mediastinitis.[138] Thus, early surgery should still be considered the treatment of choice for most patients, with conservative treatment reserved for selected cases (Table 16.10).

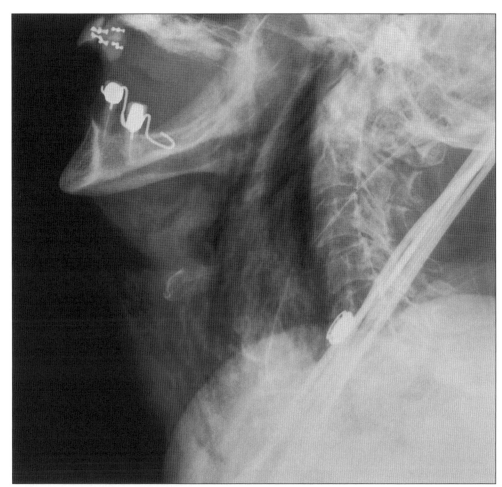

Fig. 16.8 • A radiograph of the neck showing diffuse subcutaneous emphysema. The patient had a microperforation following esophageal dilation for Zenker diverticulum and prominent cricopharyngeal bar.

Table 16.10 Selection guidelines for nonoperative management of esophageal perforation

Minimal pain

Absence of shock

Mild to moderate fever or leukocytosis

No clinical evidence of sepsis

A confined cavity that drains well into the esophagus

Delayed diagnosis >24 hours, no progression or patient improving

Adapted from Pasricha et al.[119]

SUMMARY

Nearly 100 drugs have been reported to cause injury to the esophageal mucosa. Such injury may be an acute, superficial injury that heals rapidly or deep, intramural ulceration, which heals by stricture formation. Esophageal injury caused by medications is entirely preventable. A periodic, careful history for odynophagia, retrosternal pain, and dysphagia should be obtained. Concomitant therapy with anticholinergics should be avoided, and liquid preparations should be used for bed-confined patients or those with esophageal strictures, diverticula, or dysmotility. Early barium swallow or endoscopy is indicated, and symptomatic treatment using antacids, topical xylocaine gel, or both are useful. Drug-induced deep esophageal ulcers are slow to heal and acid suppression is indicated. Tight, fibrotic strictures may require diligent, multiple fluoroscopic and wire-guided dilations, while intralesional corticosteroid injections and surgery have no proven role. Esophageal damage caused by chemotherapy and chemoradiation therapy is often diffuse and involves long segments. Pain control followed by healing is the goal of therapy; viscous lidocaine, systemic analgesics, sucralfate, and PPIs appear to provide benefit.

Lye-based liquid household cleaners along with foreign body aspiration are the third most common cause of pediatric death in the United States. Industry-wide voluntary and legislative efforts are needed for effective prevention. These patients typically present with nausea, vomiting, dysphagia, refusal to drink, drooling, and stridor. In the first 72 hours after ingestion, airway protection is the primary goal. Management in the intensive care unit with intravenous fluids, pressors, and antibiotics is useful. Early surgical consultation is needed when viscous perforation is suspected. In the absence of perforation, early endoscopy with a small, flexible endoscope is safe and necessary for assessment of severity. Acute corrosive injury may be managed conservatively with broad-spectrum antibiotics, thin-caliber nasogastric suction tube placement, and intensive care management with arguable success. Esophageal dilation carried out in the subacute phase (3 days to 3 weeks) is risky but may be successful. Frequent, painfully diligent sessions over several months may be needed.

Due to their potential for causing rapid damage, button batteries must be kept out of the reach of children. Prompt identification and location of the battery by radiography is the most important first step. If the battery is lodged in the esophagus, a prompt endoscopic extraction is mandatory, using a basket or a net device as the method of choice. Airway protection by endotracheal intubation and the use of an overtube are critical. Neutralizing agents and emetic agents are generally ineffective. Early surgery may be indicated if a perforation, full-thickness injury, or fistula formation is detected by endoscopy. Similarly, other foreign bodies or food bolus require emergent removal in the presence of respiratory distress, location of the foreign body at the cricopharyngeus level, inability to swallow secretions, sharp object ingestion, or evidence of perforation.

With increasing availability of diagnostic and therapeutic endoscopy, iatrogenic trauma to the esophagus has become more common. Endoscopic ablation of esophageal lesions by thermo-ablative techniques, photodynamic therapy, and radiofrequency devices has added a new dimension to the iatrogenic esophageal injury. Nevertheless, management principles remain the same, with prompt identification of the injury being the key. Although the use of conservative management is being reported, surgical repair remains the mainstay of management when perforation is strongly suspected.

REFERENCES

1. Pemberton J. Esophageal obstruction and ulceration caused by oral potassium therapy. Br Heart J 1970; 32(2):267.

2. Eng J, Sabanathan S. Drug-induced esophagitis. Am J Gastroenterol 1991; 86(9):1127.

3. Minocha A, Greenbaum DS. Pill-esophagitis caused by nonsteroidal anti-inflammatory drugs. Am J Gastroenterol 1991; 86(8):1086.

4. Kikendall JW. Pill-esophagitis. J Clin Gastroenterol 1999; 28(4):298.

   This is an excellent literature review of the clinical manifestations, risks, complications, management and prevention of pill-related esophageal injury.

5. Smith SJ, LeeAJ. Pill-induced esophagitis caused by oral rifampin. Ann Pharmacother 1999; 33(1):27.

6. Maekawa T, Ohji G. Pill-induced esophagitis caused by lansoprazole. J Gastroenterol 2001; 36(11):790.

7. Carlborg B, Densert O. Esophageal lesions caused by orally administered drugs. An experimental study in cat. Eur Surg Res 1980; 12(4):270.

8. Bott S, Prakash C, McCallum RW. Medication-induced esophageal injury: survey of the literature. Am J Gastroenterol 1987; 82(8):78.

9. Perkins A, Wilson C. The use of scintigraphy to demonstrate the rapid esophageal transit of the oval film-coated placebo risedronate tablet compared to a round uncoated placebo tablet when administered with minimal volumes of water. Int J Pharm 2001; 222 (2):295.

10. Whitney B, Croxon R. Dysphagia caused by cardiac enlargement. Clin Radiol 1972; 23(2):147.

11. Semble EL, Wu WC, Castell DO. Nonsteroidal anti-inflammatory drugs and esophageal injury. Semin Arthritis Rheum 1989; 19(2):99.

12. Schreiber JB, Covington JA. Aspirin-induced esophageal hemorrhage. JAMA 1988; 259(11):1647.

13. Lanas A, Hirschowitz BI. Significant role of aspirin use in patients with esophagitis. J Clin Gastroenterol 1991; 13(6):622.

14. Boley SJ, Allen AC, Schultz L, et al. Potassium-induced lesions of the small bowel. JAMA 1965; 193:997.

15. Burrington JD. Clinitest burns of the esophagus. Ann Thorac Surg 1975; 20(4):400.

16. Gallo SH, McClave SA, Laszlo JK, et al. Standardization of clinical criteria required for use of the 12.5 millimeter barium tablet in evaluating esophageal lumen patency. Gastrointest Endosc 1996; 44(2):181

17. Applegate GR, Malmud LS, Rock E, et al. 'It's a hard pill to swallow' or 'Don't take it lying down' (Abstract). Gastroenterology 1980; 78:1132.

18. Evans KT, Roberts GM. Where do all the tablets go? Lancet 1976; 2(7997):1237.

19. Bonavina L, DeMeester TR, McChesney L. Drug-induced esophagal strictures. Ann Surg 1987; 206(2):173.

20. Smith VM. Association of aspirin ingestion with symptomatic esophageal hiatus hernia. Southern Med J 1978; 71(suppl 1):45.

21. Doman DB, Ginsberg AL. The hazard of drug-induced esophagitis. Hosp Pract 1981; 16(6):17.

22. Wong RKH, Kikendall JW, Dachman AH. Quinaglute-induced esophagitis mimicking an esophageal mass. Ann Intern Med 1986; 105(1):62.

23. Reddy AN, Budhiraja M. Sucralfate therapy for lye-induced esophagitis. Am J Gastroenterol 1988; 83(1):71.

24. Ribeiro A, DeVault KR, Wolfe JT, et al. Aledronate-associated esophagitis: endoscopic and pathologic features. Gastrointest Endosc 1998; 47(6):525.

25. Walta DC, Giddens JD, Johnson LF, et al. Localized proximal esophagitis secondary to ascorbic acid ingestion and esophageal motor disorder. Gastroenterology 1976; 70(5 pt. 1):766.

26. Boyce HW. Drug-induced esophageal and gastric damage. In: Tytgat GNJ, Van Bankenstein M, eds. Current topics in gastroenterology and hepatology. Stuttgart, New York: Georg Thieme; 1990:170.

27. Colina RE, Smith M, Kidendall JW, et al. A new probable increasing cause of esophageal ulceration: alendronate. Am J Gastroenterol 1997; 92(4):704.

28. O'Meara TF. A new endoscopic finding of tetracycline-induced esophageal ulcers. Gastrointest Endosc 1980; 26(3):106.

29. Boyce HW. Editorial: Drug-induced esophagitis damage: diseases of medical progress. Gastrointest Endosc 1998; 47(6):547.

30. deGroen PC, Lubbe DF, Hirsch LJ, et al. Esophagitis associated with the use of alendronate. N Engl J Med 1996; 335(14):1016.

31. Graham D. What the gastroenterologist should know about the safety profiles of bisphosphonates. Dig Dis Sci 2002; 47(8) 1665.

32. Mason SJ, O'Meara TF. Drug-induced esophagitis. J Clin Gastroenterol 1981; 3(2):115.

33. Boyce HW. Definitions, diagnoses and documentation (Editorial). Gastrointest Endosc 1995; 41(3):264.

34. Zein NN, Greseth JN, Perrault J. Endoscopic intralesional steroid injections in the management of refractory esophageal strictures. Gastrointest Endosc 1995; 41(6):596.

35. Kirsch M, Blue M, Desai RK, et al. Intralesional steroid injections for peptic esophageal strictures. Gastrointest Endosc 1991; 37:(2)180.

36. Rupp T, Earle D, Hawes R, et al. Randomized trial of savary dilation with and without intralesional steroids for benign gastroesophageal reflux strictures (Abstract). Gastrointest Endosc 1994; 40:P78.

37. Kochhar R, Ray JD, Sriram PV et al. Intralesional steroids augment the effects of endoscopic dilation in corrosive esophageal strictures. Gastrointest Endosc 1999; 49:509.

38. Lee M, Kubik CM, Polhamus CD, et al. Preliminary experience with endoscopic intralesional steroid injection therapy for refractory upper gastrointestinal strictures. Gastrointest Endosc 1995; 41:(6)598.

39. Kochhar R, Makharia GK. Usefulness of intralesional triamcinolone in treatment of benign esophageal strictures. Gastrointest Endosc 2002; 56(6):829.

40. Fiorini A, Fleischer D, et al. Self-expanding metal coil stents in the treatment of benign esophageal strictures refractory to conventional therapy: a case series. Gastrointest Endosc 2000; 52(2):259.

41. Wadhwa RP, Kozarek RA, France RE, et al. Use of self expanding metallic stents in benign GI diseases. Gastrointest Endosc 2003; 58(2):207.

42. Volkes EE, Haraf DJ, Drinkard LC, et al. A phase I trial of concomitant chemotherapy with cisplatin dose intensification and granulocyte-colony stimulating factor support for advanced malignancies of the chest. Cancer Chemother Pharmacol 1995; 35:304.

43. Hirota S, Tsujino K, Hishikawa Y, et al. Endoscopic findings of radiation esophagitis in concurrent chemoradiotherapy for intrathoracic malignancies. Radiother Oncol 2001; 58(3):273.

44. Loprinzi CL, Foote RL, Michalak J. Alleviation of cytotoxic therapy induced normal tissue damage. Semin Oncol 1995; 22(2):95.

45. Taal BG, Vales Olmos RA, Boot H. Assessment of sucralfate coating by sequential scintigraphic imaging in radiation-induced esophageal lesions. Gastrointest Endosc 1995; 41(2):109.

46. Steer CB, Harper PG. Gastro-oesophageal complications in patients receiving cancer therapy: the role of proton pump inhibitors. Eur J Gastroenterol Hepatol 2002; 14(Suppl 1):S17.

47. Espinola TE, Amedee RG. Caustic ingestion and esophageal injury. J La State Med Soc 1993; 145(4):121.

48. Sellars S, Spence J. Chemical burns of the oesophagus. Laryngol Otol 1987; 101:1211.

49. Gaudreault P, Parent M, McGuigan MA, et al. Predictability of esophageal injury from signs and symptoms: a study of caustic ingestion in 378 children. Pediatrics 1983; 71(5):767.

50. Crain EF, Gershel JC, Mezey AP. Caustic ingestions. Symptoms as predictors of esophageal injury. Am J Dis Child 1984; 138:863.

51. Schaffer SB, Hebert AF. Caustic ingestion. J La State Med Soc 2000; 152(12):590.

52. Vancura EM, Clinton JE, Ruiz E, et al. Toxicity of alkaline solutions. Ann Emerg Med 1980; 9(3):118.

53. Untersweg U. Oesophageal burns caused by licking a 1.5 volt battery. Acta Pediatrica 1996; 85(11):1382.

54. Nuutinen M, Uhari M, Karvali T, et al. Consequences of caustic ingestions in children. Acta Pediatrica 1994; 83(11):1200.

55. Arif A, Karetzky MS. Complications of caustic ingestion. N Engl J Med 1991; 88(3):201.

56. Zargar SA, Kochhar R, Nagi B, et al. Ingestion of strong corrosive alkalis: spectrum of injury to upper gastrointestinal tract and natural history. Am J Gastroenterol 1992; 87(3):337.

57. Isolauri J, Markkula H. Lye ingestion and carcinoma of the esophagus. Acta Chir Scand 1992; 155(4–5):269.

58. Hopkins RA, Postlethwait RW. Caustic burns and carcinoma of the esophagus. Ann Surg 1981; 194(2):146.

59. Penner GE. Acid ingestion: toxicology and treatment. Ann Emerg Med 1980; 9(7):374.

60. Gorman AM, Khin-Maung-Gyi MT, Klein-Schwartz W, et al. Initial symptoms as predictors of esophageal injury in alkaline corrosive ingestions. Am J Emergency Med 1992; 10:189.

61. Anderson KD, Rouse TM, Randolph JG. A controlled trial of corticosteroids in children with corrosive injury of the esophagus. N Engl J Med 1990; 323(10):637.

62. Cardona JC, Daly F. Current management of corrosive esophagitis. Ann Otol Rhinol Laryngol 1971; 80(4):521.

63. Hollinger PH. Management of esophageal lesions caused by chemical burns. Ann Otol Rhin Laryngol 1968; 77:819.

64. Zargar SA, Kochhar R, Mehta S, et al. The role of fiberoptic endoscopy in the management of corrosive ingestion and modified endoscopic classification of burns. Gastrointest Endosc 1991; 37(2):165.

65. Ramasamy K, Gumaste VV. Corrosive ingestion in adults (Review). J Clin Gastroenterol 2003; 37(2):119.

This review summarizes current knowledge and practices for managing acute and chronic complications of caustic esophageal injury.

66. Meredith JW, Kon ND, Thompson JN. Management of injuries from liquid lye ingestion. J Trauma 1988; 28(8):1173.

67. Boyce HW, Palmer ED. Techniques of clinical gastroenterology. Springfield, IL: Charles C. Thomas; 1975; 237–251.

This chapter reviews the classic concepts for managing complications of caustic esophageal injury and the Salzer technique for early dilation.

68. Wijburg FA, Beukers MM, Heymans HS, et al. Nasogastric intubation as sole treatment of caustic esophageal lesions. Ann Otol Rhinol Laryngol 1985; 94:337.

69. Spain DM, Molomut N, Haber A. The effect of cortisone on the formation of granulation tissue in mice (Abstract). Am J Pathol 1950; 26:710.

70. Bautista A, Varela R, Villanueva A, et al. Effects of prednisone and dexamethasone in children with alkali burns of the oesophagus. Eur J Ped Surg 1996; 6(4):198.

71. Howell JM, Dalsey WC, Hartsell FW, et al. Steroids for the treatment of corrosive esophageal injury: a statistical analysis of past studies. Am J Emerg Med 1992; 10(5):421.

72. Berkovitz RNP, Bos CE, Wijburg FA, et al. Caustic injury of the esophagus. Sixteen year experience and introduction of a new model esophageal stent. J Laryngol Otol 1996; 110:1041.

73. Ferguson MK, Migliore M, Staszak VM, et al. Early evaluation and therapy for caustic esophageal injury. Am J Surg 1989; 157:116.

74. Kirsh MM, Peterson A, Brown JW, et al. Treatment of caustic injuries of the esophagus: a ten year experience. Ann Surg 1978; 188(5):67.

75. Kikendall JW. Caustic ingestion injuries. Gastroenterol Clin North Am 1991; 20(4):847.

76. Palmer ED. Esophagitis due to corrosive agents. In: The esophagus and its diseases. New York: Paul B. Hoeber; 1952:299.

77. DiCostanzo J, Noirclerc M, Jouglard J, et al. New therapeutic approach to corrosive burns of the upper gastrointestinal tract. Gut 1980; 21(5):370.

78. Ozelik MF, Pekmezci S, Saribeyoglu K, et al. The effect of halofuginone, a specific inhibitor of collagen type 1 synthesis, in the prevention of esophageal strictures related to caustic injury. Am J Surg 2004;187(2):257.

79. Cowan SA, Jacobsen P. Ingestion of button batteries. Epidemiology, clinical signs and therapeutic recommendations. Ugeskr Laeger 2002; 164(9):1204.

80. Litovitz T, Schmitz BF. Ingestion of cylindrical and button batteries: an analysis of 2,382 cases. Pediatrics 1992; 89(4 pt 2):747.

This report covers an experience with 2383 cases of button battery ingestion reported to a national registry. The chemical pathogenesis, complications, and a management protocol are presented.

81. Yoshikawa T, Asai S, Takekawa Y, et al. Experimental investigation of battery-induced esophageal burn injury in rabbits. Crit Care Med 1997; 25(12):2039.

82. Maves MD, Carithers JS, Birck HG. Esophageal burns secondary to disc battery ingestion. Ann Otol Rhinol Laryngol 1984; 93(4 pt.1):364.

83. Lyons MF, Tsuchida AM. Foreign bodies of the gastrointestinal tract. Med Clin N Am 1993; 77(5):1101.

84. Maves MD, Lloyd TV, Carithers JS. Radiographic identification of ingested disc batteries. Pediatr Radiol 1985; 16(2):154.

85. Tanaka J, Yamashita M, Yamashita M, et al. Effects of tap water on esophageal burns in dogs from button lithium batteries. Vet Hum Toxicol 1999; 41(5)279.

86. Harned RK, Strain JD, Hay TC, et al. Esophageal foreign bodies: safety and efficacy of Foley catheter extraction of coins. Am J Roentgenology 1997; 168:443.

87. Sigalet D, Lees G. Tracheoesophageal injury secondary to disc battery ingestion. J Ped Surg 1988; 23(11):996.

88. Studley JGN, Linehan IP, Ogilvie AL, et al. Swallowed button batteries: is there a consensus on management? Gut 1990; 31(8):867.

89. McDermott VG, Taylor T, Wyatt JP, et al. Orogastric magnet removal of ingested disc batteries. J Pediatr Surg 1995; 30(1):29.

90. Willis GA, Ho WC. Perforation of Meckel's diverticulum by an alkaline hearing aid battery. Can Med Assoc J 1982; 126(5):497.

91. Namasivayam S. Button battery ingestion: a solution to a management dilemma. Pediatr Surg Int 1999; 15(5–6):383.

92. Mosca S, Manes G, Martino R, et al. Endoscopic management of foreign bodies in the upper gastrointestinal tract: report of series of 414 adult patients. Endoscopy 2001; 33:692.

93. Webb WA. Management of foreign bodies of the upper gastrointestinal tract: update. Gastrointest Endosc 1995; 41(1):39.

Management of 242 foreign bodies of the upper gastrointestinal tract (181 in the esophagus), without morbidity or mortality, is reviewed.

94. Weiss KL, Brady PG, LaFontaine P. Management of ingested foreign objects and food bolus impactions [Abstract]. Gastrointest Endosc 1996; 43:361.

95. Rosenow EC. Foreign bodies of the esophagus. In: Payne WS, Olsen AM, eds. The esophagus. Philadelphia: Lea & Febiger; 1974:159.

96. Webb WA, Mc Daniel L, Jones L. Foreign bodies of the upper gastrointestinal tract: current management. South Med J 1984; 77:1083.

97. Quinn PG, Connors PJ. The role of upper gastrointestinal endoscopy in foreign body removal. Gastrointest Endosc Clin N Am 1994; 4(3):571.

98. Neilson IR. Ingestion of coins and batteries. Peds in Review 1995; 16(1):35.

99. Herranz-Gonzalez J, Martinez-Vidal J, et al. Esophageal foreign bodies in adults. Otolaryngol Head Neck Surg 1991; 105(5):649.

100. Braverman I, Gomori JM, Polv O, et al. The role of CT imaging in the evaluation of cervical esophageal foreign bodies. J Otolaryngol 1993; 22(4):311.

101. Crysdale WS, Sendi KS, Yoo J. Esophageal foreign bodies in children: 15 year review of 484 cases. Ann Otol Rhinol Laryngol 1991; 100(4 pt. 1):320.

102. Tibbling L, Stenquist M. Foreign bodies in the esophagus: a study of causative factors. Dysphagia 1991; 6(4):224.

103. Rice BT, Spiegel PK, Dombrowski PJ. Acute esophageal food impaction treated by gas forming agents. Radiology 1983; 146(2):299.

104. Kaszar-Seibert DJ, Korn WT, Bindman DJ, et al. Treatment of acute food impaction with a combination of glucagon, effervescent agent and water. Am J Roentgenol 1990; 154(3):533.

105. Kirks DR. Fluoroscopic catheter removal of blunt esophageal foreign bodies. Pediatr Radiol 1992; 22(1):64.

106. Campbell JB, Quattromani FL, Foley LC. Foley catheter removal of blunt esophageal foreign bodies. Experience with 100 consecutive children. Pediatr Radiol 1983; 13(3):116.

107. Ginaldi S. Removal of esophageal foreign bodies using a Foley catheter in adults. Am J Emerg Med 1985; 3(1):64.

108. Campbell JB, Condon VR. Catheter removal of blunt esophageal foreign bodies in children. Survey of the Society for Pediatric Radiology. Pediatr Radiol 1989; 19(6–7):361.

A nonoperative, low-risk technique is reported successful in 98 of 100 children with blunt esophageal foreign bodies.

109. Berggreen PJ, Harrison ME, Sanowski RA, et al. Techniques and complications of esophageal foreign body extraction in children and adults. Gastrointest Endosc 1993; 39(5):626.

110. Shaffer RD, Klug T. A comparative study of techniques for esophageal foreign body removal with special emphasis on meat bolus obstruction. Wisconsin Med J 1981; 80(11):33.

111. Thompson N, Lowe-Pansford F, Mant AK, et al. Button battery ingestion: a review. Adverse Drug React Toxicol Rev 1990; 93:157.

112. Paulson EK, Jaffe RB. Metallic foreign bodies in the stomach: fluoroscopic removal with a magnetic orogastric tube. Radiology 1990; 174(1):191.

113. Brady PG. Esophageal foreign bodies. Gastroenterol Clin North Am 1991; 20(4):691.

114. Sanowski RA, Harrison ME, Young MF, et al. Foreign body extraction in the gastrointestinal tract. In: Sivak MV Jr, ed. Gastroenterologic endoscopy. Philadelphia: WB Saunders; 2000:801–812.

An excellent review of endoscopic techniques for removal of esophagal and gastric foreign bodies.

115. Faigel DO, Stotland BR, Kochman ML, et al. Device choice and experience level in endoscopic foreign object retrieval: an in vivo study (Abstract). Gastrointest Endosc 1996; 43:334.

116. Johnson JA, Landreneau RJ. Esophageal obstruction and mediastinitis: a hard pill to swallow for drug smugglers. Am Surgeon 1991; 57(11):723

117. Holsinger JW, Fuson RL, Sealy WC. Esophageal perforation following meat impaction and papain ingestion. JAMA 1968; 204:188.

118. Goldner F, Danley D. Enzymatic digestion of esophageal meat impaction. A study of Adolph's Meat Tenderizer. Dig Dis Sci 1985; 30(5):456.

119. Saeed ZA, Michaletz PA, Feiner SD, et al. A new endoscopic method for managing food impaction in the esophagus. Endoscopy 1990; 22:226.

120. Tulman AB, Boyce HW. Complications of esophageal dilation and guidelines for their prevention. Gastrointest Endosc 1981; 27:229.

121. Tuebergen D, Rijcken E, Senninger N. Esophageal perforation as a complication of Endo Cinch endolumenal gastroplication. Endoscopy 2004; 36(7):663.

122. Baehr PH, McDonald GB. Esophageal disorders caused by infection, systemic illness, medications, radiation, and trauma. In: Feldman M, Scharschmidt B, eds. Sleisenger and Fordtran's gastrointestinal and liver disease. 6th edn. Chapter 334. Philadelphia: WB Saunders; 1997:519.

123. Berkelhammer C, Madhav G, Lyons S, et al. Pinch injury during overtube placement in upper endoscopy. Gastrointest Endosc 1993; 39(2):186.

124. Dennert B, Ramirez FC, Sanowski RA. A prospective evaluation of the endoscopic spectrum of overtube-related esophageal mucosal injury. Gastrointest Endosc 1997; 45(2):134.

125. Molina EG. Conservative management of esophageal nontransmural tears after pneumatic dilation for achalasia. Am J Gastroenterol 1996; 91(1):15.

126. Lo AY, Surik B, Ghazi A. Nonoperative management of esophageal perforation secondary to balloon dilation. Surg Endosc 1993; 7(6):529.

127. Dolgin SR, Wykoff TW, Kumar NR, et al. Conservative medical management of traumatic pharyngoesophageal perforations. Ann Otol Rhinol Laryngol 1992; 101(3):209.

128. Sawyer R, Phillips C, Vakil N. Short- and long-term outcome of esophageal perforation. Gastrointest Endosc 1995; 41(2):130.

This is an important report on the long-term outcome in patients who suffer endoscopically related esophageal perforation. A low mortality is related to early diagnosis and therapy.

129. El-Newihi HM, Mihas AA. Esophageal perforation as a complication of endoscopic overtube insertion (Letter). Am J Gastroenterol 1994; 89(6):953.

130. Shaffer HA., Valenzuela G, Mittal RK. Esophageal perforation: a reassessment of the criteria for choosing medical or surgical therapy. Arch Intern Med 1992; 152(4):757.

131. Reeder LB, DeFilippi VJ, Ferguson MK. Current results of therapy for esophageal perforation. Am J Surg 1995; 169(6):615.

132. Port JL, Kent MS, Bacchetta M, et al. Thoracic esophageal perforations: A decade of experience. Ann Thorac Surg 2003; 75:1071.

133. Wesdorp IC. Treatment of instrumental esophageal perforation. Gut 1984; 25(4):398.

134. Hine KR, Atkinson M. The diagnosis and management of perforations of esophagus and pharynx sustained during intubation of neoplastic esophageal strictures. Dig Dis Sci 1986; 31(6):571.

135. Wewalka FW, Clodi PH, Haidinger D. Endoscopic clipping of esophageal perforation after pneumatic dilation for achalasia. Endoscopy 1995; 27(8):608.

136. Weiman DS. Non-iatrogenic esophageal trauma. Ann Thorac Surg 1995; 59(4):845.

137. Moghissi K, Pender D. Instrumental perforations of the esophagus and their management. Thorax 1988; 43(8):642.

138. Pasricha P, Fleischer D, Kalloo A. Endoscopic perforations of the upper digestive tract: A review of their pathogenesis, prevention and management. Gastroenterology 1994; 106(3):787.

A state-of-the-art review of all aspects of instrumental perforations of the esophagus and upper gastrointestinal tract. Important reading for all who perform endoscopy.

139. Stanley RB, Armstrong WB, Fetterman BL, et al. Management of external penetrating injuries into the hypopharyngeal-cervical funnel. J Trauma 1997; 42:675.

CHAPTER SEVENTEEN

17

Approach to the patient with esophageal cancer

Brian C. Jacobson and Jacques Van Dam

INTRODUCTION

Esophageal cancer (EC) is the eighth most frequent cancer worldwide, but ranks sixth in cancer mortality with more than 90% of cases resulting in death.[1] Of the estimated 14 000 new cases of esophageal cancer in the United States each year,[2] the vast majority are either squamous cell carcinoma (SCC) or adenocarcinoma (ADC), with occasional cases of endocrine tumors, carcinoid tumors, choriocarcinomas, small cell carcinoma, and metastatic cancers.[3] The incidence of SCC has been declining gradually over the past few decades while that of ADC has been increasing steadily in both the United States and Europe.[4,5] Men have a greater lifetime risk for developing EC, and incidence rises steadily with age.[6] Black men in the United States have a nearly fivefold increased risk of SCC compared to non-Hispanic white men, while non-Hispanic white men have a fourfold increased risk for AC compared to black men.[7] Squamous cell carcinoma has been strongly linked to chronic heavy alcohol and tobacco exposure[6,8,9] while the majority of cases of AC are associated with Barrett's esophagus and gastroesophageal reflux disease.[10,11] Other risk factors for SCC include poverty;[8,12] frequent consumption of salt-pickled or smoke-cured foods, sun-dried foods, and moldy foods;[9] diets deficient in fruits and vegetables;[9] regular consumption of extremely hot beverages;[13-15] a history of esophageal stricture following caustic ingestion;[16] achalasia;[17] type A tylosis (diffuse palmoplantar keratoderma);[18,19] prior radiation therapy to the chest;[20] and a current or prior history of SCC of the upper aerodigestive tract.[21,22] Increased body mass index, tobacco, and alcohol use appear to be independent risk factors for ADC[8,23-26]

DIAGNOSIS

History, physical examination, and laboratory testing

The majority of EC are diagnosed only after symptoms arise, with only a small percentage found in the setting of surveillance programs, such as for Barrett's esophagus (see below).[27] Patients with EC typically present with dysphagia when eating solid food. Unfortunately, this symptom, as well as a report of weight loss, is often indicative of advanced disease. Other symptoms may suggest invasion of surrounding structures, such as hoarseness from involvement of the recurrent laryngeal nerve, or cough and

pneumonia from a tracheoesophageal fistula. The physical examination is usually normal, but may reveal evidence of rapid weight loss and malnutrition, supraclavicular or axillary lymph node involvement, pleural effusion, and hepatomegaly. There are no laboratory tests specific for EC, although iron deficiency may be present if the tumor has resulted in chronic blood loss. Typically, there are no tumor markers used to diagnose EC, monitor therapy, or survey for early recurrence.

Barium esophagogram

An esophagogram or 'barium swallow' performed to evaluate dysphagia may be the initial diagnostic study demonstrating EC. The esophagogram will define the location of the tumor, the degree and length of stenotic regions, and the presence of fistulae. Tumors may appear as a space-occupying lesion or an irregular stricture. Early lesions may appear as nodular regions or small ulcers.[28]

Endoscopy

Esophagogastroduodenoscopy (EGD) remains the primary method for visualizing esophageal masses and for directing biopsies. Typically, EC will appear as a fungating mass or a stricture with nodularity and friable mucosa (Fig. 17.1). Occasionally, a high-grade malignant stricture will prevent passage of a standard endoscope. When available, an ultrathin endoscope with an insertion tube diameter of 5.3–6 mm may traverse the stricture and allow complete examination of the esophagus and stomach.[29,30]

In order to highlight pathology otherwise difficult to visualize by standard endoscopy, vital staining, or chromoendoscopy, can be used. This entails the application of a dye to the gastrointestinal mucosa, and the two most commonly used stains in the esophagus are iodine and methylene blue. Iodide solutions such as Lugol's iodine stain the glycogen-rich prickle cell layer of the esophageal squamous epithelium. Dysplastic epithelium lacks the glycogen-rich granules present in this epithelial layer and therefore fails to stain.[31] Iodine chromoendoscopy may detect early squamous cell carcinomas of the esophagus that might otherwise be undetected with standard endoscopy.[32-35] Iodine chromoendoscopy may also be helpful in defining the extent of an esophageal SCC.[32,36] During iodine chromoendoscopy patients may experience heartburn, tingling in the chest, or nausea and the technique should be avoided in patients with an allergy to iodine.[37]

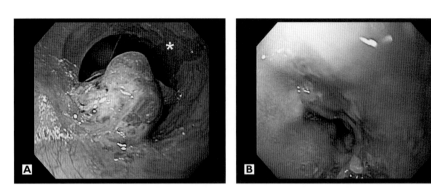

Fig. 17.1 • **(A)** Fungating esophageal adenocarcinoma. A fungating adenocarcinoma can be seen arising from the wall of the esophagus. Barrett's esophagus is demonstrated as well (asterisk). **(B)** This squamous cell carcinoma presented as a tight malignant stricture in the mid-esophagus.

Topically applied methylene blue stains mucin within goblet cells and is therefore useful in highlighting Barrett's epithelium amid normal squamous cell-lined esophageal epithelium.[38–40] As Barrett's epithelium becomes dysplastic, there is a loss of goblet cells and a decreased uptake of dye, which results in highlighting poorly stained dysplastic regions amid more strongly staining nondysplastic mucosa. While methylene blue chromoendoscopy may be useful during Barrett's esophagus surveillance, it has no established role in the diagnosis of adenocarcinoma.

Tissue acquisition

Any lesion suspected of containing cancer should be sampled during diagnostic endoscopy. Standard biopsies are 66–96% sensitive for detecting cancers of the esophagus or gastroesophageal junction.[41–44] While a single biopsy may be adequate, studies have demonstrated that multiple biopsies increase the sensitivity for detecting cancer of the esophagus, with maximum yields resulting from 7 to 10 biopsies.[45,46] Larger-size 'jumbo' biopsy forceps may provide larger specimens, but this method does not necessarily improve the diagnostic yield.[47,48] Brush cytology may also be employed, and is 83–100% sensitive for the diagnosis of esophageal cancer.[42–44] Combining biopsy and brush cytology may improve the diagnostic yield.[42–44] Brushing for cytology is especially important in sampling tight malignant strictures as biopsy forceps may fail to obtain adequate specimens.[49] In cases with a high clinical suspicion for esophageal cancer in which biopsy and brush cytology fail to demonstrate malignancy, endoscopic ultrasound with or without fine needle aspiration may provide a definitive diagnosis.[50]

Screening and surveillance

Survival in the setting of EC is inversely correlated with the stage at diagnosis.[6] Both SCC and ADC develop through a dysplasia–carcinoma sequence, suggesting that high-grade dysplasia or early EC might be detected through a program of screening or surveillance, thereby improving clinical outcomes. The infrequency of EC makes population-based screening inappropriate, but certain high-risk conditions will help identify patients who may benefit from screening/surveillance. Current guidelines recommend screening endoscopy to identify Barrett's esophagus among patients with chronic gastroesophageal reflux disease, and for surveillance endoscopy among those with documented Barrett's esophagus.[51,52] Likewise, patients with a history of esophageal stricture after caustic ingestion and those with type A tylosis should

be enrolled in a surveillance endoscopy program.[16] Prospective studies of screening endoscopy have detected high-grade dysplasia or esophageal SCC among 5% of patients with a history of head and neck cancer[21,22,53–57] and among 4% of patients with a history of chronic, excessive alcohol and tobacco use.[35,58–60] It is not clear whether screening or surveillance among these high-risk populations provides a survival benefit[61,62] or is cost-effective.[63,64]

STAGING

The best prognostic indicator for patients with EC is the extent, or stage, of disease at the time of diagnosis. Five-year survival is 50–80% for stage I EC, 10–40% for stage II EC, 10–15% for stage III EC, and <5 years for stage IV disease.[6] Accurate staging is therefore important for prognostication, therapeutic decision-making, and potentially for reducing the costs of care.[65–67] Both ADC and SCC are staged according to the TNM classification system established by the American Joint Committee on Cancer (AJCC) and the International Union Against Cancer (UICC) (Table 17.1).[68,69] Computed tomography and endoscopic ultrasound are used in staging EC, with an emerging role for positron emission tomography. Bronchoscopy may be useful when a tracheo-esophageal fistula is suspected.

Computed tomography

At the time of diagnosis, a computed tomographic (CT) scan with intravenous contrast enhancement of the chest, abdomen, and pelvis should be obtained to exclude metastatic disease. Spiral CT scans with thin (5 mm) collimation is optimal.[70] CT is not accurate for T staging, but may demonstrate findings suggestive of mediastinal invasion and may detect involvement of the aorta, tracheobronchial tree, and crura.[70] Lymph node staging by CT is also inaccurate, as enlarged nodes in the mediastinum may be reactive. Magnetic resonance imaging (MRI) does not appear to provide added benefit to CT findings and is thus not commonly used in staging.

Endoscopic ultrasound

Endoscopic ultrasound should be performed in all patients with EC after CT has excluded metastatic disease, as it is the most accurate method available for both T and N staging (Fig. 17.2).[71] The accuracy of T stage as determined using a standard echoendoscope is greater for T3 and T4 tumors (>90%) than for T1 and T2 tumors (65%).[72] However, the use of high-frequency

Table 17.1 TNM staging of esophageal cancer

TNM Stage	Definition
T1m	Tumor confined to the mucosa, including the lamina propria
T1sm	Tumor invades the submucosa
T2	Tumor invades into, but not through, the muscularis propria
T3	Tumor extends through the muscularis propria into the adventitia
T4	Tumor invades adjacent structures
N0	No lymph node involvement
N1	Regional nodes involved
M0	No metastatic disease
M1a	Malignant celiac lymph nodes (in distal esophageal cancer) or cervical lymph nodes (in proximal esophageal cancer)
M1b	Distant metastases

Overall Stage	
I	T1 N0 M0
IIa	T2 or T3, N0
IIb	T1, T2, or T3, N1
III	T3 N1 or T4 N0 or T4 N1
IVa	M1a
IVb	M1b

Adapted from references 68 and 69.

(15–30 MHz) ultrasound catheter probes for staging T1 and T2 tumors improves the accuracy to 83–92%.[73–75] Therefore, the T stage of superficial esophageal tumors should be determined using a high-frequency catheter probe whenever possible.

When examining lymph nodes by EUS, particular findings may predict malignant nodal involvement, including a hypoechoic echotexture, a sharply demarcated border, a rounded contour, and a size greater than 1 cm.[76,77] While these individual findings are predictive, sensitivity exceeds 80% only when all four are present, although this occurs in the minority of cases.[76,78,79] Fine needle aspiration (FNA) of nodes improves the accuracy of EUS for determining N stage and should be performed regularly as part of the staging EUS.[79,80] One study demonstrated that three FNA passes were needed to ensure 100% sensitivity.[81] A general caveat is to avoid traversal of the primary tumor by the FNA needle, which can result in a false-positive nodal aspirate.

EUS for esophageal cancer staging should include an assessment of celiac axis lymph nodes as the spread of malignancy to these nodes is considered evidence of advanced disease and may impact management. However, a stricture that restricts passage of an echoendoscope is present in 29% of cases,[82] and indicates a lesion with advanced T stage.[83] Failure to traverse a malignant stricture results in significantly decreased accuracy for both T and N staging.[83,84] When available, catheter ultrasound probes may be used to traverse the stricture and attempt complete T and N staging;[74,85] however lower frequency probes (i.e., 12 MHz) should be used.[86] A 7.5 MHz nonoptical, 7 mm, wire-guided esophagoprobe has also been used to complete staging in the setting of malignant strictures.[82,87] Dilation of the stricture may permit passage of a standard echoendoscope. Savary-Gilliard and balloon dilators have been used with perforation rates ranging from 0% to 24%,[83,88–90] but may not permit passage of the echoendoscope in all cases.[84,88,89] Residual inflammation and fibrosis after chemotherapy and radiation therapy makes EUS too inaccurate to be recommended as a tool for post-therapy restaging.[91–95]

Positron emission tomography

Positron emission tomography (PET) with fluoro-deoxy-glucose (FDG) adds little to the T staging of tumors, but may be accurate

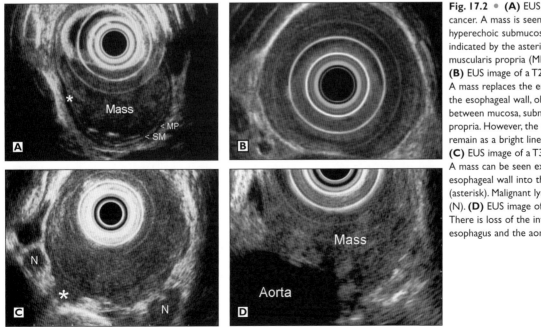

Fig. 17.2 • **(A)** EUS image of a T1 esophageal cancer. A mass is seen extending into the hyperechoic submucosa (SM) at the region indicated by the asterisk. The hypoechoic muscularis propria (MP) is not involved. **(B)** EUS image of a T2 esophageal cancer. A mass replaces the entire circumference of the esophageal wall, obliterating distinctions between mucosa, submucosa, and muscularis propria. However, the confines of the adventitia remain as a bright line surrounding the cancer. **(C)** EUS image of a T3 esophageal cancer. A mass can be seen extending through the esophageal wall into the surrounding adventitia (asterisk). Malignant lymph nodes are also seen (N). **(D)** EUS image of a T4 esophageal cancer. There is loss of the interface between the esophagus and the aorta indicating invasion.

in detecting malignant adenopathy and may be superior to conventional imaging for detecting occult metastases.[96] PET scanning may also prove useful in monitoring response to therapy, but its role in this setting remains preliminary.

Detecting cancer recurrence

Any patient presenting with signs or symptoms of local recurrence after resection of esophageal cancer should undergo endoscopy as part of their evaluation. In this setting, standard endoscopy can yield a diagnosis of recurrent disease in 40% of patients.[97] However, recurrence is often extramucosal and therefore missed with standard endoscopy. EUS has been shown to detect cancer with a positive predictive value of 75–100%.[97,98] While surveillance EUS after cancer resection may detect recurrent cancer, it remains unproven whether this practice has any impact on survival.[98]

THERAPY

Treatment for EC is stage-specific and, in some cases, institution-specific. Different modalities of treatment have been used, including surgery, radiotherapy (RT), chemotherapy, chemoradiotherapy (CRT), and endoscopic therapy. Cancer confined to the esophagus (T1/T2, N0) is generally treated with a primary resection. Cancer with extension through the esophageal wall (T3) or with regional lymph node involvement is usually treated with CRT and subsequent resection when possible. Metastatic disease is treated with palliative measures.

Surgery

Surgery remains the gold standard of treatment for esophageal cancers. The rationale for surgical resection is the potential removal of all neoplastic tissue, including any and all involved lymph nodes. Because EC tends to spread along submucosal planes, limited longitudinal resections are not as effective as more extensive resections. The proximal extent of resection should extend at least 10 cm above macroscopically visible tumor, and the distal margin should be at least 5 cm below the tumor.[70] Radial margins are dictated by the location, with tumors at the esophagogastric junction often requiring resection of portions of the diaphragm. One of two different procedures are typically performed.[99] The transhiatal operation is done completely through the abdominal cavity without complete lymph node resection.[100] The other operation involves an incision into both the chest and abdomen (transthoracic esophagecetomy with extended en-bloc lymphadenectomy) with better exposure, resulting in a more traditional 'cancer operation.' In this latter procedure, an esophagogastric anastomosis is created within the chest (the Ivor-Lewis technique) or within the neck (the three-field technique). The transthoracic esophagectomy is associated with greater morbidity (but not mortality), and does not conclusively prolong 5-year survival.[101] Curative resections (no microscopic disease present at surgical margins) are possible in 54–69% of cases.[6] Even with improved surgical technique and perioperative management, complication rates range 20–40% and operative mortality ranges 3–10%.[102–104] Major complications commonly seen include infection, anastamotic leaks, and cardiopulmonary complications.

Whether surgery alone is sufficient for curative management of EC remains controversial. Obviously, a resection with positive margins or failure to remove involved lymph nodes is not sufficient. However, there may be a role for adjuvant or neoadjuvant therapy, especially in cases where a curative resection is not obtained (see below). For patients with tumors in the cervical esophagus, surgery is often deferred because of the likelihood of early spread to lymph nodes in the neck. However, in some institutions resection is attempted and includes an extensive neck dissection.

The proper selection of patients for surgery should include accurate staging including CT and EUS to exclude patients with T4 or M1 disease. However, selection must also include a thorough preoperative assessment to limit perioperative mortality. This selection process usually includes a detailed medical history and physical examination and often involves consultation with cardiologists, pulmonologists, and anesthesiologists.

Radiation therapy

No trials have randomized patients to radiation therapy (RT) alone versus surgery alone. Uncontrolled series of cases have been published in which patients with high operative risks received RT as their only therapy for SCC. A review of these series found no survival advantage of RT over surgery, but 5-year survival was only 6%.[105] In addition, while primary RT avoids operative morbidity, it may still be associated with local complications such as stricture formation and tracheoesophageal fistulae.

Studies have also examined whether preoperative RT provides benefit compared with surgery alone. A meta-analysis combined five randomized trials of preoperative RT versus surgery and included 1147 patients with a median follow-up of 9 years.[106] This analysis found no significant survival advantage for RT in this setting. Currently, RT is more commonly used in combination with chemotherapy, either before surgery or for nonoperative candidates. In addition, patients with positive resection margins may receive postoperative RT. Radiation therapy has also been used as palliation for malignant dysphagia in nonoperative candidates, but may take several weeks before symptomatic improvement is realized.

Chemotherapy and chemoradiotherapy

Chemotherapy alone is not generally used for curative intent. In patients with localized disease, combination chemoradiotherapy (CRT) using RT and cisplatin/fluorouracil-based regimens may lead to long-term survival in 14–26% of patients.[107,108] A rigorous review of the literature found that CRT provides an absolute reduction in cancer mortality of 7% compared with RT alone, at least within the first 2 years of treatment.[109] CRT is associated with significantly more toxicity than RT alone, and the possibility of toxicity should be considered in any treatment decision-making process. In the setting of proximal esophageal SCC, surgery is often difficult, and CRT has been shown to offer complete pathological response rates in excess of 20%.[70] In this setting, CRT may be a reasonable option in lieu of surgery.

In a long-term follow-up study of CRT without a surgical arm, persistent or local/regional recurrence failures accounted for the majority of deaths, suggesting that the addition of surgery might improve overall survival.[107] However, it remains unclear whether the addition of CRT prior to or following a curative resection is beneficial. Several prospective randomized trials have attempted to address this issue, and conflicting results have been reported.[102,103,110-116] These studies varied with regard to patient selection criteria (including tumor histology and cancer stage), chemotherapeutic regimens used, the inclusion of radiation therapy, and the type of surgery performed. These differences in protocol make interpretation of findings difficult. In general, the use of chemotherapy without RT in the neoadjuvant setting is unlikely to provide a sizeable survival advantage compared to surgery alone.[102,103] In the majority of studies assessing CRT as neoadjuvant therapy, there appeared to be no advantage of CRT over surgery alone.[110,111,114-116] However, a small, but influential, study restricted to patients with adenocarcinoma found a significantly improved 3-year survival advantage of neoadjuvant CRT over surgery alone.[113] Therefore, in an attempt to offer the best survival advantage, most centers currently offer neoadjuvant CRT for EC, although the data supporting this practice are limited. Chemotherapy and radiotherapy regimens used in this setting continue to evolve, and therefore new findings supporting or refuting this practice are anticipated.

Administering CRT in the postoperative setting is hampered by the long delay during recovery following esophagectomy, which may explain the paucity of randomized trials evaluating the role of adjuvant (i.e., postsurgical) chemotherapy. However, two such studies have been conducted, one employing cisplatin and vindesine and the other employing cisplatin and 5-fluorouracil (5-FU), both versus surgery alone for SCC.[117,118] Neither study was able to demonstrate a survival advantage for adjuvant CRT, although disease-free survival among those with node-positive disease was demonstrated in the latter study.[117]

Chemotherapy is often offered alone as palliation for metastatic disease.[119] In this setting, both SCC and ADC are responsive to fluorouracil, taxane, or irinotecan regimens with or without the addition of cisplatin.[6] Unfortunately, responses tend to be partial and short-lived, and adverse effects may limit the dosing of combination regimens.

ROLE OF ENDOSCOPY IN TREATMENT

Effective endoscopic methods are utilized for the treatment of early EC and for the palliation of advanced EC. Definitive treatment of early lesions is limited to those with superficial T1 lesions; i.e., tumors confined to the mucosa. In the United States, endoscopic resection or destruction of early cancer is generally reserved for poor operative candidates or those patients who refuse surgery. However, as more data are collected, endoscopic procedures may emerge as reasonable therapeutic options for more patients. As for palliation, endoscopic techniques are currently the primary means for managing malignant dysphagia and tracheoesophageal fistulae.[71]

Endoscopic mucosal resection

Endoscopic mucosal resection (EMR) removes a region of mucosa, superficial submucosa, and occasionally deep submucosa. Four principal techniques are presently used for EMR of early cancer: (1) the inject and cut; (2) the inject, lift, and cut; (3) cap-assisted EMR (EMRC); and (4) EMR with ligation (EMRL).[120] These methods typically involve the injection of saline into the submucosa below the lesion to provide a cushion of fluid between the mucosa and the muscularis propria, which serves two purposes: (1) the cushion protects the muscularis propria from thermal injury as a relatively large region of mucosa is removed, and (2) lesions that fail to lift on a cushion of saline are more likely to involve the deeper submucosal layer (termed the 'non-lifting sign'[121]), and therefore may not be appropriate for EMR. Once saline has been injected into the submucosa, the lesion is removed by snare excision alone (inject and cut), by being lifted through an open snare using a double-channel endoscope and a grasping forceps prior to snare excision (the inject, lift, and cut), by being aspirated into a variceal banding cap prior to application of a snare (EMRC), or by applying a variceal band ligator to the lesion prior to snare excision (EMRL). After EMR, a second immediate EMR of adjacent residual tumor is possible, and the addition of chromoendoscopy helps determine whether a second EMR is required by delineating tumor margins.

The selection of patients for EMR requires EUS to confirm that the tumor is confined to the mucosa and to exclude the presence of suspicious lymph nodes. Lymph node involvement is rare (<3%) when cancer is confined to the mucosa, but submucosal invasion carries a 14–21% risk of lymph node involvement.[6] Therefore, tumors extending into the submucosa are not generally removed endoscopically. EMR is typically reserved for well- to moderately differentiated tumors 2 cm or less in diameter.[71] Among patients with early (T1m N0) ADC and SCC, EMR has been reported to be successful in removing the entire cancer in 97% or more of cases, with tumor recurrence or metachronous lesions arising in 14–17% of patients.[122-124] This high rate of recurrence and metachronous lesions mandates post-EMR endoscopic surveillance. Complications specific to EMR of EC include bleeding in 2–14% and perforation in <1%.[123,125-127]

Photodynamic therapy

Photodynamic therapy (PDT) requires a light-sensitizing drug, porfimer sodium, which is injected intravenously and concentrates within tumor tissue. An endoscopically guided, low-power laser diffuser exposes the tumor to red light. The light then initiates a photochemical reaction in the sensitized tissue producing cytotoxic singlet oxygen, with resultant tumor necrosis.[71] Red light is used because it achieves the deepest tissue penetration.[128] Photodynamic therapy is technically easy to perform and, due to selective tumor tissue destruction, it can be used to treat cancers that nearly obstruct the esophageal lumen. PDT has also been used prior to or after chemotherapy and radiation. It has been used to limit tumor growth from obstructing the ends of previously placed esophageal stents.[129-131] In addition to this palliative role, there have been cases reported wherein PDT was used successfully as primary treatment for early-stage EC.[132] This indication, however, remains experimental.

The major limiting factors for PDT are the long half-life of porfimer sodium and the expense required for the multiple treatment sessions needed to achieve palliation. Porfimer sodium is retained in the skin for up to 6 weeks after infusion, and patients must avoid sun exposure or risk the likelihood of sustaining severe sunburn. Other complications of PDT include substernal chest pain, odynophagia, fever, pleural effusion, and the development of tracheoesophageal fistulae.[71]

Electrocautery

Thermal debulking by electrocautery is performed for the palliation of short, exophytic, obstructive tumors. Monopolar and bipolar electrocautery[133] and argon plasma coagulation[134] have been shown to be effective in improving malignant dysphagia. Although inexpensive to use, monopolar and bipolar electro-cautery have been limited by inadequate control of the treatment delivery.[133] Argon plasma coagulation is a noncontact method of thermal ablation that uses ionized argon gas to conduct electrical current. Unfortunately, the ablation is fairly superficial, destroy-ing tissue to a depth of approximately 2 mm, making it difficult to obtain a durable response when treating bulky obstructing tumors.[134]

Laser

The high-power Nd:YAG laser can provide deep tissue penetration and palliation for bulky esophageal tumors. The laser is capable of coagulating and vaporizing malignant tissue under endoscopic guidance. Unfortunately, the laser is expensive and technically demanding.[135]

Chemical debulking

The typical agent used in this setting is absolute alcohol because it is inexpensive and easily injected through a standard sclerotherapy needle. Alcohol injected directly into a tumor will result in tissue necrosis and potential relief from malignant dysphagia. Dosing has not been standardized and it may be difficult to limit tissue destruction to the tumor. Relief tends to be of short duration, requiring multiple sessions.[136] In one comparison study, alcohol was as effective as Nd:YAG laser therapy for relief of dysphagia.[137] Treatment may be associated with chest pain.

Bougienage

Malignant strictures may be dilated with either through-the-scope (TTS) balloons or wire-guided polyvinyl bougies with or without fluoroscopic guidance. This type of therapy provides relief of very brief duration and is currently relied upon only for proximal malignant strictures that are not amenable to stenting (see below). Bougienage is much more successful in the relief of radiation-induced strictures for patients who received radiation as part of nonoperative therapy of EC.

Esophageal prostheses

The placement of an expandable metal stent for the purpose of maintaining a patent lumen and to relieve malignant dysphagia has become a major form of endoscopic palliative therapy.[138] One randomized comparative study demonstrated the superiority of stenting over laser therapy for lasting relief of dysphagia.[139] Previously, plastic stents were used in this setting, but were asso-ciated with a 6–8% risk of acute complications during insertion, including esophageal perforation.[140] Expandable metal stents are inserted in a preloaded constrained position using endoscopic and fluoroscopic control. The constrained mechanism minimizes or eliminates the need for stricture dilation. Once placed across the tumor, the constraining device is released, thereby deploying the stent.[71] The rate of successful deployment exceeds 90% among experienced operators.[141]

Although more expensive than plastic stents, the use of metal stents is associated with significantly lower rates of early complications.[140] The incidence of late complications, however, may be as high as 20–40% and include chest pain, migration, hemorrhage, and fistulization.[142] Patients with a history of mediastinal radiation and chemotherapy for their EC may be at greater risk of serious complications.[143]

The most proximal and distal esophagus represents problematic areas for stent deployment. Stents placed proximally may lead to a foreign body sensation or airway compromise.[144] Stents placed at the esophagogastric junction may lead to intractable gastro-esophageal reflux and are prone to migration, ulceration, and food impaction. A recent variant of one stent has a windsock-like valve on the distal end that may reduce severe reflux symptoms.[145] Patients with stents crossing the gastroesophageal junction require chronic acid suppression therapy with a proton pump inhibitor and must maintain an upright or semi-upright position (including the elevation of the head of their bed) to avoid severe esophagitis and aspiration. Furthermore, patients must be instructed to avoid dense and fibrous foods and to limit their diet to liquids and soft mechanical foods as much as possible to avoid stent occlusion.

Tracheoesophageal fistulization is a serious complication of esophageal cancer that can lead to aspiration, recurrent pneu-monia, and respiratory distress. The use of a covered esophageal stent is the treatment of choice in these patients, with closure of the fistula successful in 70–100% of patients.[146]

FUTURE DIRECTIONS

There are several areas of active investigation within the realm of EC. Ongoing trials are addressing the role of neoadjuvant chemotherapy and radiation therapy, as well as less invasive surgical techniques, such as laparoscopic esophagectomy.[147] EMR for cancer confined to the mucosa is also likely to emerge as a more widely available option. However, research into new imag-ing methods such as spectroscopy and optical coherence tomo-graphy is also advancing and may soon offer the possibility for the identification of cancer before macroscopic changes are visible. This option is particularly important for patients undergoing surveillance of Barrett's esophagus and perhaps those at high risk for SCC, such as those with prior upper aerodigestive tract squamous cell carcinoma.

Spectroscopy

Spectroscopy is the study of interactions between light and matter. Several forms of spectroscopy exist and represent the analysis of various fates of photons of light. When a photon strikes the surface of the gastrointestinal lumen, it can be absorbed or reflected by the tissue. Some of the light undergoes scattering within the tissue prior to being reflected. The degree of scattering depends upon the density and size of space-occupying structures such as nuclei, connective tissue fibers, and mito-chondria in the epithelium being illuminated. Scattering occurs when photons of light bounce off and pass through these structures. The information obtained when studying the bulk scattering components of reflected light represents information about the presence of large objects such as collagen within the lamina propria or submucosa. This bulk scattering information combined with the observed absorbance of specific wavelengths is the basis for *reflectance spectroscopy* and provides insight into the structural and biochemical composition of a particular tissue. For instance, reflectance spectroscopy can distinguish dysplastic from nondysplastic Barrett's epithelium.[148] An analysis of minute scattering events represents measures of nuclear crowding and size and can be done after subtracting bulk scattering followed by mathematical modeling.[149] This analysis forms the basis of *light-scattering spectroscopy*, a technique that has also been applied in the setting of Barrett's esophagus.[148,150]

Finally, some photons of light excite tissue fluorophores, biochemical structures that emit longer wavelengths of light when excited by specific incident wavelengths of light, forming the basis of *fluorescence spectroscopy*. Dysplastic epithelium fluoresces with a different intensity than nondysplastic epithelium, thereby providing a method for distinguishing these two entities. Fluorophores that have proven particularly useful for distinguishing dysplastic and nondysplastic epithelium include collagen and nicotinamide adenine dinucleotide (NADH).[151,152] This form of spectroscopy has also been used to distinguish dysplastic from nondysplastic Barrett's mucosa[148,153] and esophageal carcinoma from normal esophagus.[154]

Optical coherence tomography

Optical coherence tomography (OCT) is similar in imaging to ultrasound, except waves of infrared light are focused into the tissue as opposed to waves of sound. A principle known as interferometry is used to measure the time delay between when light leaves the imaging source and returns from a target tissue. This method is accomplished by having a beam of incident light split into two, with one half of the beam traveling to the tissue, while the other half travels to a moving reference mirror. The light reflecting back from both the tissue and the mirror is then analyzed. When light reflecting from within the tissue returns to a detector at the same time as light from the mirror, interference is generated. This interference represents the presence of a reflective structure within the tissue and, by knowing the mirror position, the depth of this structure within the tissue can be determined and mapped. An optical beam scanning the tissue surface creates a two-dimensional image of the tissue architecture with a resolution of approximately 10 μm.

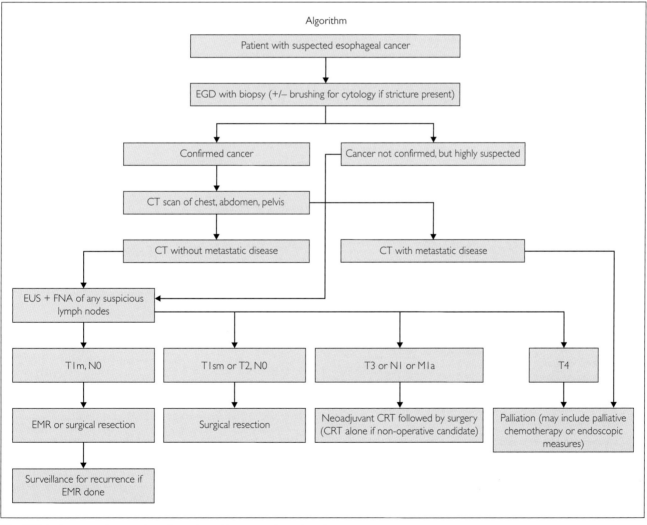

Fig. 17.3 ● A suggested approach to the patient with suspected esophageal cancer.

OCT imaging can distinguish the various layers of the gastro-intestinal tract in a manner similar to that seen with high-frequency endosonography. Systems with 10 μm resolution can delineate surface epithelium, lamina propria, muscularis mucosa, submucosa, and muscularis propria. OCT images are currently detailed enough to accurately detect metaplastic lesions, such as Barrett's esophagus.[155,156] Unfortunately, the resolution of this modality will need to improve further before dysplasia can be diagnosed with certainty, although newer systems may soon provide resolution in the order of 1 μm.[157] Finally, spectroscopic information regarding backscattered light may be incorporated into OCT imaging to combine the diagnostic capabilities of these two powerful imaging techniques.[157]

SUMMARY AND AUTHOR'S RECOMMENDATIONS

Patients with esophageal cancer typically present with dysphagia, and often at an advanced stage (Fig. 17.3). EGD with biopsy is the standard method for making a definitive diagnosis and is followed by CT scanning as the initial staging test to determine the presence or absence of metastatic disease. Because it is the most accurate method for determining T and N stages, EUS with FNA should then be performed. Intramucosal carcinoma may be treated with EMR or surgery. Cancer limited to the esophageal wall is often resected without further therapy, while cancer extending beyond the muscularis propria or involving regional lymph nodes is typically treated with neoadjuvant CRT followed by surgical resection if possible. The data supporting neoadjuvant CRT are limited, but this technique remains the most common approach. CRT is a good alternative for patients with no surgical options, and chemotherapy alone may provide some benefit for patients with metastatic disease. In patients requiring palliation of malignant dysphagia or tracheoesophageal fistulae, endoscopically placed esophageal prostheses appear to offer the most reliable results.

REFERENCES

1. Pisani P, Parkin DM, Bray F, et al. Estimates of the worldwide mortality from 25 cancers in 1990. Int J Cancer 1999; 83:18–29.

2. Jemal A, Tiwari RC, Murray T, et al. Cancer statistics, 2004. CA Cancer J Clin 2004; 54:8–29.

3. Glickman JN, Odze RD. Epithelial neoplasms of the esophagus. In: Odze RD, Goldblum J, Crawford JM, eds. Surgical pathology of the GI tract, liver, biliary tract, and pancreas. Philadelphia: Saunders; 2004.

4. Botterweck AA, Schouten LJ, Volovics A, et al. Trends in incidence of adenocarcinoma of the oesophagus and gastric cardia in ten European countries. Int J Epidemiol 2000; 29:645–654.

5. Devesa S, Blot WJ, Fraumeni JF. Changing patterns in the incidence of esophageal and gastric carcinoma in the United States. Cancer 1998; 83:2049–2053.

6. Enzinger P, Mayer R. Esophageal cancer. N Engl J Med 2003; 349:2241–2252.

An excellent review of esophageal cancer that provides details about various trials supporting and refuting the role of neoadjuvant therapy.

7. Kubo A, Corley DA. Marked multi-ethnic variation of esophageal and gastric cardia carcinomas within the United States. Am J Gastroenterol 2004; 99:582–588.

8. Gammon MD, Schoenberg JB, Ahsan H, et al. Tobacco, alcohol, and socioeconomic status and adenocarcinomas of the esophagus and gastric cardia. J Natl Can Inst 1997; 89:1277–1284.

9. Ribeiro U, Posner MC, Safatle-Ribeiro AV, et al. Risk factors for squamous cell carcinoma of the esophagus. Br J Surg 1996; 83:1174–1185.

10. Lagergren J, Bergstrom R, Lindgren A, et al. Symptomatic gastroesophageal reflux as a risk factor for esophageal adenocarcinoma. N Engl J Med 1999; 340:825–831.

11. Shaheen N, Ransohoff D. Gastroesophageal reflux, Barrett esophagus, and esophageal cancer. JAMA 2002; 287:1972–1981.

12. Brown LM, Hoover RN, Silverman DT, et al. Excess incidence of squamous cell esophageal cancer among US black men: role of social class and other risk factors. Am J Epidemiol 2001; 153:114–122.

13. Munoz N, Victora CG, Crespi M, et al. Hot mate drinking and precancerous lesions of the esophagus: an endoscopic survey in southern Brazil. Int J Cancer 1987; 39:708–709.

14. Castelletto R, Castellsague X, Munoz N, et al. Alcohol, tobacco, diet, mate drinking, and esophageal cancer in Argentina. Cancer Epidemiol Biomarkers Prev 1994; 3:557–564.

15. Castellsague X, Munoz N, De Stefani E, et al. Influence of mate drinking, hot beverages and diet on esophageal cancer risk in South America. Int J Cancer 2000; 88:658–664.

16. American Society for Gastrointestinal Endoscopy Standards of Practice Committee. The role of endoscopy in the surveillance of premalignant conditions of the upper gastrointestinal tract. Gastrointest Endosc 1998; 48:663–668.

17. Sandler RS, Nyren O, Ekbom A, et al. The risk of esophageal cancer in patients with achalasia: a population-based study. JAMA 1995; 274:1359–1362.

18. Maillefer RH, Greydanus MP. To B or not to B: is tylosis B truly benign? Am J Gastroenterol 1999; 94:829–834.

19. Clarke CA, Howel-Evans W, McConnell B, et al. Carcinoma of oesophagus in association with tylosis [Letter]. Br Med J 1959; 2:1100.

20. Ahsan H, Neugut AI. Radiation therapy for breast cancer and increased risk for esophageal carcinoma. Ann Intern Med 1998; 128:114–117.

21. Muto M, Hironaka S, Nakane M, et al. Association of multiple Lugol-voiding lesions with synchronous and metachronous esophageal squamous cell carcinoma in patients with head and neck cancer. Gastrointest Endosc 2002; 56:517–521.

A well-done study that demonstrates the utility of Lugol's iodine staining and the yield of screening for esophageal SCC among patients with other squamous cell carcinomas of the upper aerodigestive tract.

22. Scherubl H, von Lampe B, Faiss S, et al. Screening for oesophageal neoplasia in patients with head and neck cancer. Br J Cancer 2002; 86:239–243.

23. Lagergren J, Bergstrom R, Nyren O. Association between body mass and adenocarcinoma of the esophagus and gastric cardia. Ann Intern Med 1999; 130:883–890.

24. Brown LM, Silverman DT, Pottern LM, et al. Adenocarcinomas of the esophagus and esophagogastric junction in white men in the United States: alcohol, tobacco, and socioeconomic factors. Cancer Causes Control 1994; 5:333–340.

25. Kabat GC, Ng SK, Wynder EL. Tobacco, alcohol intake, and diet in relation to adenocarcinoma of the esophagus and gastric cardia. Cancer Causes Control 1993; 4:123–132.

26. Vaughan TL, Davis S, Kristal AR, et al. Obesity, alcohol, and tobacco as risk factors for cancers of the esophagus and gastric

cardia: adenocarcinoma versus squamous cell carcinoma. Cancer Epidemiol Biomarkers Prev 1995; 4:85–92.

27. Corey K, Levin TR, Habel LA, et al. Surveillance and survival in Barrett's adenocarcinomas: a population-based study. Gastroenterology 2002; 122:633–640.

28. Eisenberg RL. Gastrointestinal radiology: a pattern approach. Philadelphia: Lippincott-Raven; 1996.

29. American Society for Gastrointestinal Endoscopy Standards of Practice Committee. Ultrathin endoscopes esophagogastroduodenoscopy. Gastrointest Endosc 2000; 51:786–789.

30. Mulcahy H, Fairclough P. Ultrathin endoscopy in the assessment and treatment of upper and lower gastrointestinal tract strictures. Gastrointest Endosc 1998; 48:618–620.

31. Inoue H, Rey J, Lightdale C. Lugol chromoendoscopy for esophageal squamous cell cancer. Endoscopy 2001; 33:75–79.

32. Misumi A, Harada K, Murakami A, et al. Role of Lugol dye endoscopy in diagnosis of early esophageal cancer. Endoscopy 1990; 22:12–16.

33. Shimizu Y, Tukagoshi H, Fujita M, et al. Endoscopic screening for early esophageal cancer by iodine staining in patients with other current or prior primary cancers. Gastrointest Endosc 2001; 53:1–5.

34. Sugimachi K, Kitamura K, Baba K, et al. Endoscopic diagnosis of early carcinoma of the esophagus using Lugol's solution. Gastrointest Endosc 1992; 38:657–661.

35. Fagundes RB, de Barros SG, Putten AC, et al. Occult dysplasia is disclosed by Lugol chromoendoscopy in alcoholics at high risk for squamous cell carcinoma of the esophagus. Endoscopy 1999; 31:281–285.

36. Kuwano H, Kitamura K, Baba K, et al. Determination of the resection line in early esophageal cancer using intraoperative endoscopic examination with Lugol staining. J Surg Oncol 1992; 59:149–152.

37. Stevens PD, Lightdale CJ, Green PH, et al. Combined magnification endoscopy with chromoendoscopy for the evaluation of Barrett's esophagus. Gastrointest Endosc 1994; 40:747–749.

38. Wo JM, Ray MB, Mayfield-Stokes S, et al. Comparison of methylene blue-directed biopsies and conventional biopsies in the detection of intestinal metaplasia and dysplasia in Barrett's esophagus: a preliminary study. Gastrointest Endosc 2001; 54:294–301.

39. Sharma P, Topalovski M, Mayo MS, et al. Methylene blue chromoendoscopy for detection of short-segment Barrett's esophagus. Gastrointest Endosc 2001; 54:289–293.

40. Canto MI, Setrakian S, Willis JE, et al. Methylene blue staining of dysplastic and nondysplastic Barrett's esophagus: an in vivo and ex vivo study. Endoscopy 2001; 33:391–400.

41. Graham DY, Schwartz JT, Cain GD, et al. Prospective evaluation of biopsy number in the diagnosis of esophageal and gastric carcinoma. Gastroenterology 1982; 82:228–231.

42. Winawer S, Sherlock P, Belladonna J, et al. Endoscopic brush cytology in esophageal cancer. JAMA 1975; 232:1358.

43. Zargar S, Khuroo M, Jan G, et al. Prospective comparison of the value of brushings before and after biopsy in the endoscopic diagnosis of gastroesophageal malignancy. Acta Cytol 1991; 35:549–552.

44. Young J, Hughes H, Lee F. Evaluation of endoscopic brush and biopsy touch smear cytology and biopsy histology in the diagnosis of carcinoma of the lower oesophagus and cardia. J Clin Pathol 1980; 33:811–814.

45. Graham D, Schwartz J, Cain G, et al. Prospective evaluation of biopsy number in the diagnosis of esophageal and gastric carcinoma. Gastroenterology 1982; 82:228–231.

46. Dekker W, Tytgat G. Diagnostic accuracy of fiberendoscopy in the detection of upper intestinal malignancy. A follow-up analysis. Gastroenterology 1977; 73:710–714.

47. Dandalides S, Carey W, Petras R, et al. Endoscopic small bowel mucosal biopsy: a controlled trial evaluating forceps size and biopsy location in the diagnosis of normal and abnormal architecture. Gastrointest Endosc 1989; 35:197–200.

48. Falk G, Rice T, Goldblum J, et al. Jumbo biopsy forceps protocol still misses unsuspected cancer in Barrett's esophagus with high-grade dysplasia. Gastrointest Endosc 1999; 49:170–176.

49. Kobayashi S, Kasugai T. Brushing cytology for the diagnosis of gastric cancer involving the cardia or the lower esophagus. Acta Cytol 1978; 22:155–157.

50. Faigel D, Deveney C, Phillips D, et al. Biopsy-negative malignant esophageal stricture: diagnosis by endoscopic ultrasound. Am J Gastroenterol 1998; 93:2257–2260.

51. Sampliner RE. Updated guidelines for the diagnosis, surveillance, and therapy of Barrett's esophagus. Am J Gastroenterol 2002; 97:1888–1895.

52. American Society for Gastrointestinal Endoscopy. The role of endoscopy in the surveillance of premalignant conditions of the upper gastrointestinal tract. Gastrointest Endosc 1998; 48:663–668.

53. Atabek U, Mohit-Tabatabai M, Rush BF, et al. Impact of esophageal screening in patients with head and neck cancer. Am Surgeon 1990; 56:289–292.

54. Ina H, Shibuya H, Ohashi I, et al. The frequency of a concomitant early esophageal cancer in male patients with oral and oropharyngeal cancer: Screening results using Lugol dye endoscopy. Cancer 1994; 73:2038–2041.

55. Petit T, Georges C, Jung G-M, et al. Systematic esophageal endoscopy screening in patients previously treated for head and neck squamous-cell carcinoma. Ann Oncol 2001; 12:643–646.

56. Shiozaki H, Tahara H, Kobayashi K, et al. Endoscopic screening of early esophageal cancer with the Lugol dye method in patients with head and neck cancers. Cancer 1990; 66:2068–2071.

57. Tincani AJ, Brandalise N, Altemani A, et al. Diagnosis of superficial esophageal cancer and dysplasia using endoscopic screening with a 2% Lugol dye solution in patients with head and neck cancer. Head Neck 2000; 22:170–174.

58. Yokoyama A, Muramatsu T, Ohmori T, et al. Multiple primary esophageal and concurrent upper aerodigestive tract cancer and the aldehyde dehydrogenase-2 genotype of Japanese alcoholics. Cancer 1996; 77:1986–1990.

59. Meyer V, Burtin P, Bour B, et al. Endoscopic detection of early esophageal cancer in a high-risk population: does Lugol staining improve videoendoscopy? Gastrointest Endosc 1997; 45:480–484.

60. Ban S, Toyonaga A, Harada H, et al. Iodine staining for early endoscopic detection of esophageal cancer in alcoholics. Endoscopy 1998; 30:253–257.

61. Eckardt VF, Kanzler G, Bernhard G. Life expectancy and cancer risk in patients with Barrett's esophagus: a prospective controlled investigation. Am J Med 2001; 111:33–37.

62. MacDonald CE, Wicks AC, Playford RJ. Final results from 10 year cohort of patients undergoing surveillance for Barrett's esophagus: observational study. Br Med J 2000; 321:1252–1255.

63. Inadomi JM, Sampliner R, Lagergren J, et al. Screening and surveillance for Barrett esophagus in high-risk groups: a cost-utility analysis. Ann Intern Med 2003; 138:176–186.

64. Soni A, Sampliner RE, Sonnenberg A. Screening for high-grade dysplasia in gastroesophageal reflux disease: is it cost-effective? Am J Gastroenterol 2000; 95:2086–2093.

65. Hiele M, Leyn PD, Schurmans P, et al. Relation between endoscopic ultrasound findings and outcome of patients with tumors of the esophagus or esophagogastric junction. Gastrointest Endosc 1997; 45:381–386.

66. Mallery S, VanDam J. EUS in the evaluation of esophageal carcinoma. Gastrointest Endosc 2000; 52(suppl):S6–S11.

67. Shumaker D, de Garmo P, Faigel D. Potential impact of preoperative EUS on esophageal cancer management and cost. Gastrointest Endosc 2002; 56:391–396.

68. American Joint Committee on Cancer. AJCC Cancer Staging Manual, 6th edn. New York: Springer-Verlag; 2002.

69. Sobin L, Wittekind C. TNM classification of malignant tumours, 6th edn. UICC. New York: John Wiley and Sons; 2002.

70. Allum WH, Griffin SM, Watson A, et al. Guidelines for the management of oesophageal and gastric cancer. Gut 2002; 50(suppl V):v1–v23.

71. Jacobson BC, Hirota WK, Baron TH, et al. The role of endoscopy in the assessment and treatment of esophageal cancer. Gastrointest Endosc 2003; 57:817–822.

72. Rosch T, Classen M. Staging esophageal cancer: the Munich experience. In: Van Dam J, Sivak M, eds. Gastrointestinal endosonography. Philadelphia: WB Saunders; 1999.

73. Hasegawa N, Niwa Y, Arisawa T, et al. Preoperative staging of superficial esophageal carcinoma: a comparison of an ultrasound probe and standard endoscopic ultrasonography. Gastrointest Endosc 1996; 44:388–393.

74. Menzel J, Hoepffner N, Nottberg H, et al. Preoperative staging of esophageal carcinoma: miniprobe sonography versus conventional endoscopic ultrasound in a prospective histopathologically verified study. Gastrointest Endosc 1999; 31:291–297.

75. Murata Y, Suzuki S, Ohata M, et al. Small ultrasonic probes for determination of the depth of superficial esophageal cancer. Gastrointest Endosc 1996; 44:23–28.

76. Catalano M, Sivak M, Rice T, et al. Endosonographic features predictive of lymph node metastasis. Gastrointest Endosc 1994; 40:442–446.

77. Faigel D. EUS in patients with benign and malignant lymphadenopathy. Gastrointest Endosc 2001; 53:593–598.

78. Bhutani M, Hawes R, Hoffman B. A comparison of the accuracy of echo features during endoscopic ultrasound (EUS) and EUS-guided fine-needle aspiration for the diagnosis of malignant lymph node invasion. Gastrointest Endosc 1997; 45:474–479.

79. Chen VK, Eloubeidi MA. Endoscopic ultrasound-guided fine needle aspiration is superior to lymph node echofeatures: a prospective evaluation of mediastinal and peri-intestinal lymphadenopathy. Am J Gastroenterol 2004; 99:628–633.

This study, like reference 78, demonstrates clearly that endosonographic features alone are not reliable enough for providing nodal staging. Results of fine needle aspiration can improve accuracy and should be obtained whenever possible.

80. Vazquez-Sequeiros E, Wiersema M, Clain JE, et al. Impact of lymph node staging on therapy of esophageal carcinoma. Gastroenterology 2003; 125:1626–1635.

81. Wallace M, Kennedy T, Durkalski V, et al. Randomized controlled trial of EUS-guided fine needle aspiration techniques for the detection of malignant lymphadenopathy. Gastrointest Endosc 2001; 54:441–447.

82. Mallery S, Van Dam J. Increased rate of complete EUS staging of patients with esophageal cancer using the non-optical, wire-guided echoendoscope. Gastrointest Endosc 1999; 50:53–57.

83. Van Dam J, Rice T, Catalano M, et al. High-grade malignant stricture is predictive of esophageal tumor stage. Risks of endosonographic evaluation. Cancer 1993; 71:2910–2917.

84. Catalano M, Vandam J, Sivak M. Malignant esophageal strictures: staging accuracy of endoscopic ultrasonography. Gastrointest Endosc 1995; 41:535–539.

85. Fockens P, van Dulleman H, Tytgat G. Endosonography of stenotic esophageal carcinomas: preliminary experience with an ultra-thin, balloon-fitted ultrasound probe in four patients. Gastrointest Endosc 1994; 40:226–228.

86. Chak A, Canto M, Stevens P, et al. Clinical applications of a new through-the-scope ultrasound probe: prospective comparison with an ultrasound endoscope. Gastrointest Endosc 1997; 45:291–295.

87. Binmoeller K, Seifert H, Seitz U, et al. Ultrasonic esophagoprobe for TNM staging of highly stenosing esophageal carcinoma. Gastrointest Endosc 1995; 41:547–552.

88. Kallimanis G, Gupta P, al-Kawas F, et al. Endoscopic ultrasound for staging esophageal cancer, with or without dilation, is clinically important and safe. Gastrointest Endosc 1995; 41:540–546.

89. Wallace M, Hawes R, Sahai A, et al. Dilation of malignant esophageal stenosis to allow EUS guided fine-needle aspiration: safety and effect on patient management. Gastrointest Endosc 2000; 51:309–313.

90. Pfau P, Ginsberg G, Lew R, et al. Esophageal dilation for endosonographic evaluation of malignant esophageal strictures is safe and effective. Am J Gastroenterol 2000; 95:2813–2815.

91. Giovannini M, Seitz J, Thomas P, et al. Endoscopic ultrasonography for the assessment of the response to combined radiation therapy and chemotherapy in patients with esophageal cancer. Endoscopy 1997; 29:4–9.

92. Laterza E, de Manzoni G, Guglielmi A, et al. Endoscopic ultrasonography in the staging of esophageal carcinoma after preoperative radiotherapy and chemotherapy. Ann Thorac Surg 1999; 67:1466–1469.

93. Isenberg G, Chak A, Canto M, et al. Endoscopic ultrasound in re-staging of esophageal cancer after neoadjuvant chemoradiation. Gastrointest Endosc 1998; 48:158–163.

94. Zuccaro G, Rice T, Goldblum J, et al. Endoscopic ultrasound cannot determine suitability for esophagectomy after aggressive chemoradiotherapy for esophageal cancer. Am J Gastroenterol 1999; 94:906–912.

95. Hordijk M, Kok T, Wilson J, et al. Assessment of response of esophageal carcinoma to induction chemotherapy. Endoscopy 1993; 25:592–596.

96. Annovazzi A, Peeters M, Maenhout A, et al. 18-Fluorodeoxyglucose positron emission tomography in nonendocrine neoplastic disorders of the gastrointestinal tract. Gastroenterology 2003; 125:1235–1245.

97. Catalano M, Sivak M, Rice T, et al. Postoperative screening for anastamotic recurrence of esophageal carcinoma by endoscopic ultrasonography. Gastrointest Endosc 1995; 42:540–544.

98. Fockens P, Manshanden C, van Lanschot J, et al. Prospective study on the value of endosonographic follow-up after surgery for esophageal carcinoma. Gastrointest Endosc 1997; 46:487–491.

99. Krasna M. Surgical staging and surgical treatment in esophageal cancer. Semin Oncol 1999; 26(Suppl 15):9–11.

100. Orringer M, Marshall B, Iannettoni M. Transhiatal esophagectomy: clinical experience and refinements. Ann Surg 1999; 230:392–403.

101. Hulscher JBF, van Sandick JW, de Boer AGEM, et al. Extended transthoracic resection compared with limited transhiatal resection for adenocarcinoma of the esophagus. N Engl J Med 2002; 347:1662–1669.

102. Kelsen DP, Ginsberg R, Pajak TF, et al. Chemotherapy followed by surgery compared with surgery alone for localized esophageal cancer. N Engl J Med 1998; 339:1979–1984.

103. Medical Research Council Oesophageal Cancer Working Party. Surgical resection with or without preoperative chemotherapy in oesophageal cancer: a randomised controlled trial. Lancet 2002; 359:1727–1733.

104. Bosset J-F, Mercier M, Triboulet J-P, et al. Surgical resection with and without chemotherapy in oesophageal cancer. Lancet 2002; 360:1173–1174.

105. Earlam R, Cunha-Melo JR. Oesophogeal squamous cell carcinomas: II. A critical view of radiotherapy. Br J Surg 1980; 67:457–461.

106. Arnott SJ, Duncan W, Gignoux M, et al. Preoperative radiotherapy in esophageal carcinoma: a meta-analysis using individual patient data (Oesophageal Cancer Collaborative Group). Int J Radiat Oncol Biol Phys 1998; 41:579–583.

107. Cooper JS, Guo MD, Herskovic A, et al. Chemoradiotherapy of locally advanced esophageal cancer: long-term follow-up of a prospective randomized trial (RTOG 85-01). JAMA 1999; 281(17):1623–1627.

108. Herskovic A, Martz K, al-Sarraf M, et al. Combined chemotherapy and radiotherapy compared with radiotherapy alone in patients with cancer of the esophagus. N Engl J Med 1992; 326:1593–1598.

109. Rebecca WO, Richard MA. Combined chemotherapy and radiotherapy (without surgery) compared with radiotherapy alone in localized carcinoma of the esophagus. Cochrane Database Syst Rev 2003:CD002092.

110. Apinop C, Puttisak P, Preecha N. A prospective study of combined therapy in esophageal cancer. Hepatogastroenterology 1994; 41:391–393.

111. Nygaard K, Hagen S, Hansen HS, et al. Pre-operative radiotherapy prolongs survival in operable esophageal carcinoma: a randomized, multicenter study of pre-operative radiotherapy and chemotherapy. The second Scandinavian trial in esophageal cancer. World J Surg 1992; 16:1104–1109; discussion 1110.

112. Swanson SJ, Batirel HF, Bueno R, et al. Transthoracic esophagectomy with radical mediastinal and abdominal lymph node dissection and cervical esophagogastrostomy for esophageal carcinoma. Ann Thorac Surg 2001; 72:1918–1924; discussion 1924–1925.

113. Walsh TN, Noonan N, Hollywood D, et al. A comparison of multimodal therapy and surgery for esophageal adenocarcinoma. N Engl J Med 1996; 335:462–467.

One of the only randomized trials that provides evidence supporting the role of neoadjuvant chemoradiotherapy prior to esophagectomy for cancer. The findings in this study are relied upon heavily in justifying the current trend in management of esophageal cancer.

114. Le Prise E, Etienne PL, Meunier B, et al. A randomized study of chemotherapy, radiation therapy, and surgery versus surgery for localized squamous cell carcinoma of the esophagus. Cancer 1994; 73:1779–1784.

115. Bossett J, Gignoux M, Triboulet J, et al. Chemoradiotherapy followed by surgery compared with surgery alone in squamous-cell cancer of the esophagus. N Engl J Med 1997; 337:161–167.

116. Urba SG, Orringer MB, Turrisi A, et al. Randomized trial of preoperative chemoradiation versus surgery alone in patients with locoregional esophageal carcinoma. J Clin Oncol 2001; 19:305–313.

117. Ando N, Iizuka T, Ide H, et al. Surgery plus chemotherapy compared with surgery alone for localized squamous cell carcinoma of the thoracic esophagus: a Japan Clinical Oncology Group Study – JCOG9204. J Clin Oncol 2003; 21:4592–4596.

118. Ando N, Iizuka T, Kakegawa T, et al. A randomized trial of surgery with and without chemotherapy for localized squamous carcinoma of the thoracic esophagus: the Japan Clinical Oncology Group Study. J Thorac Cardiovasc Surg 1997; 114:205–209.

119. Enzinger P, Ilson D, Kelsen D. Chemotherapy in esophageal cancer. Semin Oncol 1999; 26(Suppl 15):12–20.

120. Soetikno RM, Gotoda T, Nakanishi Y, et al. Endoscopic mucosal resection. Gastrointest Endosc 2003; 57:567–579.

An excellent review of the techniques and indications for endoscopic mucosal resection. This reference contains figures that demonstrate methods clearly and also provides information about the proper handling of specimens for optimal histologic interpretation.

121. Uno Y, Munakata A. The non-lifting sign of invasive colon cancer. Gastrointest Endosc 1994; 40:485–489.

122. Shimizu Y, Tukagoshi H, Fujita M, et al. Metachronous squamous cell carcinoma of the esophagus arising after endoscopic mucosal resection. Gastrointest Endosc 2001; 54:190–194.

123. Pech O, Gossner L, May A, et al. Endoscopic resection of superficial esophageal squamous-cell carcinomas: Western experience. Am J Gastroenterol 2004; 99:1226–1232.

124. Ell C, May A, Gossner L, et al. Endoscopic mucosal resection of early cancer and high-grade dysplasia in Barrett's esophagus. Gastroenterology 2000; 118:670–677.

This case series provides good evidence for the utility and safety of EMR for superficial esophageal cancer in selected patients.

125. Nijhawan P, Wang K. Endoscopic mucosal resection for lesions with endoscopic features suggestive of malignancy and high-grade dysplasia within Barrett's esophagus. Gastrointest Endosc 2000; 52:328–332.

126. May A, Gossner L, Behrens A, et al. A prospective randomized trial of two different endoscopic resection techniques for early stage cancer of the esophagus. Gastrointest Endosc 2003; 58:167–175.

127. Shimizu Y, Tsukagoshi H, Fujita M, et al. Long-term outcome after endoscopic mucosal resection in patients with esophageal squamous cell carcinoma invading the muscularis mucosae or deeper. Gastrointest Endosc 2002; 56:387–390.

128. Heier S, Rothman K, Heier L, et al. Photodynamic therapy for obstructing esophageal cancer: light dosimetry and randomized comparison with Nd:YAG laser therapy. Gastroenterology 1995; 109:63–72.

129. Raijman I, Lalor E, Marcon N. Photodynamic therapy for tumor ingrowth through an expandable esophageal stent. Gastrointest Endosc 1995; 41:73–74.

130. Lightdale C, Heier S, Marcon N, et al. Photodynamic therapy with porfimer sodium versus thermal ablation therapy with Nd:YAG laser for palliation of esophageal cancer: a multicenter randomized trial. Gastrointest Endosc 1995; 42:507–512.

131. McCaughan J, Ellison E, Guy J, et al. Photodynamic therapy for esophageal malignancy: a prospective, twelve-year study. Ann Thorac Surg 1996; 62:1005–1009.

132. Overholt BF, Panjehpour M, Halberg DL. Photodynamic therapy for Barrett's esophagus with dysplasia and/or early stage carcinoma: long-term results. Gastrointest Endosc 2003; 58:183–188.

133. Johnston J, Fleischer D, Petrini J, et al. Palliative bipolar electrocoagulation therapy of obstruction of esophagal cancer. Gastrointest Endosc 1987; 33:349–353.

134. Heindorff H, Wojdemann M, Bisgaard T, et al. Endoscopic palliation of inoperable cancer of the esophagus or cardia by argon plasma electrocoagulation. Scand J Gastroenterol 1998; 33:21–23.

135. Lightdale C, Zimbalist E, Winawer S. Outpatient management of esophageal cancer with endoscopic Nd:YAG laser. Am J Gastroenterol 1987; 82:46–50.

136. Payne-James J, Spiller R, Misiewicz J, et al. Use of ethanol-induced tumor necrosis to palliate dysphagia in patients with esophagogastric cancer. Gastrointest Endosc 1990; 36:43–46.

137. Carazzone A, Bonavina L, Segalin A, et al. Endoscopic palliation of oesophageal cancer: results of a prospective comparison of Nd:YAG laser and ethanol injection. Eur J Surg 1999; 165:351–356.

138. Baron T. Expandable metal stents for the treatment of cancerous obstruction of the gastrointestinal tract. N Engl J Med 2001; 344:1681–1687.

139. Adam A, Ellul J, Watkinson A, et al. Palliation of inoperable esophageal carcinoma: a prospective randomized trial of laser therapy and stent placement. Radiology 1997; 202:344–348.

140. Knyrim K, Wagner H, Bethge N, et al. A controlled trial of an expansile stent for palliation of esophageal obstruction due to inoperable cancer. N Engl J Med 1993; 329:302–307.

This controlled trial provides evidence of the superiority of self-expandable metal stents over plastic stents for palliation of malignant dysphagia.

141. Siersema P, Schrauwen S, Blankenstein M, et al. Self-expanding metal stents for complicated and recurrent esophagogastric cancer. Gastrointest Endosc 2001; 54:579–586.

142. Ramirez F, Dennert B, Zierer S, et al. Esophageal self-expandable metallic stents – indications, practice, techniques, and complications: results of a national survey. Gastrointest Endosc 1997; 45:360–364.

143. Kinsman K, DeGregorio B, Katon R, et al. Prior radiation and chemotherapy increase the risk of life-threatening complications after insertion of metallic stent for esophagogastric malignancy. Gastrointest Endosc 1996; 43:196–203.

144. Bethge N, Sommer A, Vakil N. A prospective trial of self-expanding metal stents in the palliation of malignant esophageal strictures near the upper esophageal sphincter. Gastrointest Endosc 1997; 45:300–303.

145. Dua K, Kozarek R, Kim J, et al. Self-expanding metal esophageal stent with anti-reflux mechanism. Gastrointest Endosc 2001; 53:603–613.

146. Raijman I, Siddique I, Ajani J, et al. Palliation of malignant dysphagia and fistulae with coated expanded metal stents: experience with 101 patients. Gastrointest Endosc 1998; 48:172–179.

147. Luketich JD, Alvelo-Rivera M, Beunaventura PO, et al. Minimally invasive esophagectomy: outcomes in 222 patients. Ann Surg 2003; 238:486–494.

An exciting glimpse into the potential future of esophagectomy: minimally invasive means of resecting cancer and harvesting lymph nodes.

148. Georgakoudi I, Jacobson BC, Van Dam J, et al. Fluorescence, reflectance, and light-scattering spectroscopy for evaluating dysplasia in patients with Barrett's esophagus. Gastroenterology 2001; 120:1620–1629.

This study demonstrates the accuracy of various forms of spectroscopy for the detection of dysplastic Barrett's epithelium, including the improved accuracy with the combination of the various methods.

149. Backman V, Wallace M, Perelman L, et al. Detection of preinvasive cancer cells: early warning changes in precancerous epithelial cells can now be spotted in situ. Nature 2000; 406:35–36.

150. Wallace M, Perelman L, Backman V, et al. Endoscopic detection of dysplasia in patients with Barrett's esophagus using light-scattering spectroscopy. Gastroenterology 2000; 119:677–682.

151. Georgakoudi I, Jacobson B, Muller M, et al. NAD(P)H and collagen as in vivo quantitative fluorescent biomarkers of epithelial precancerous changes. Cancer Res 2002; 62:682–687.

152. Römer T, Fitzmaurice M, Cothren R, et al. Laser-induced fluorescence microscopy of normal colon and dysplasia in colonic adenomas: implications for spectroscopic diagnosis. Am J Gastroenterol 1995; 90:81–87.

153. Panjehpour M, Overholt B, Vo-Dinh T, et al. Endoscopic fluorescence detection of high-grade dysplasia in Barrett's esophagus. Gastroenterology 1996; 111:93–101.

154. Panjehpour M, Overholt B, Schmidhammer J, et al. Spectroscopic diagnosis of esophageal cancer: new classification model, improved measurement system. Gastrointest Endosc 1995; 41:577–581.

155. Poneros J, Brand S, Bouma B, et al. Diagnosis of specialized intestinal metaplasia by optical coherence tomography. Gastroenterology 2001; 120:7–12.

156. Jäckle S, Gladkova N, Feldchtein F, et al. In vivo endoscopic optical coherence tomography of esophagitis, Barrett's esophagus, and adenocarcinoma of the esophagus. Endoscopy 2000; 32:750–755.

157. Li X, Boppart S, Van Dam J, et al. Optical coherence tomography: advanced technology for the endoscopic imaging of Barrett's esophagus. Endoscopy 2000; 32:921–930.

Section
4 Four

Management of gastroduodenal disorders

CHAPTER EIGHTEEN

18

Treatment of *Helicobacter pylori* infection

David A. Peura

INTRODUCTION

History

Peptic ulcer and gastric cancer are largely infectious diseases. While this statement is now universally accepted, only 25 years ago, before the rediscovery of *Helicobacter pylori* by Marshall and Warren,[1] such a statement would have been considered preposterous – after all, excessive or deficient acid production causes ulcers or stomach cancer, and no bacteria can survive in the hostile gastric environment. Such was the prevailing belief; research and treatment of upper gastrointestinal conditions accordingly focused on the mechanisms and control of acid secretion. It was in this acid-centered atmosphere of the early 1980s that Marshall and Warren's observations initially provoked skepticism and even ridicule. Although *H. pylori*-like organisms had also been reported by a number of others over the last century, this information was simply ignored, lost, or forgotten. The eventual acceptance that *H. pylori* is a pathogen capable of causing significant morbidity and mortality related to associated gastrointestinal diseases refocused interest on the epidemiology and transmission of infection, bacterial and host factors that determine clinical outcome of infection, and most clinically important, how best to diagnose and treat infection to cure and prevent disease.

Despite two decades of refocused investigation, controversy still remains surrounding whom to test for *H. pylori* and which of the many recommended therapies is the 'treatment of choice.' While ulcer recurrence is reduced (but not totally eliminated) and the risk for subsequently developing gastric cancer diminished after curing infection, dyspeptic symptoms, what actually bother patients and challenge physicians, are often unaffected by treatment. Furthermore, the number of proposed treatment regimens continues to increase, and those that are most effective remain complex. The result is confusion surrounding how to treat, frustration with treatment outcome, and in some cases, inappropriate treatment decisions. To deal with these problems, this chapter addresses *H. pylori* management issues, such as who should be tested for infection and which test to use, which regimen and duration of treatment is best, and what, if any, post-treatment follow-up testing is appropriate to confirm bacterial cure.

Epidemiology

An estimated one-half of the world's population is infected with *H. pylori*, possibly making it the most common worldwide bacterial pathogen.[2] Most infection is acquired early in childhood – usually by age five[3,4] – and persists life-long as an asymptomatic infestation in the majority of those infected. Adult infection, and for that matter re-infection after successful eradication, are unusual even in locations where *H. pylori* prevalence remains high.[5,6] Acquisition is most likely through oral–oral or fecal–oral routes, but the precise mechanism of transmission has yet to be determined. Isolation of genetically identical strains of *H. pylori* from multiple family members,[7] as well as custodial patients in the same institution, suggests spread among individuals sharing the same living environment.[8]

Infection appears to be more frequent in developing countries where socioeconomic conditions are not ideal and exposure to suboptimal sanitation and crowded living conditions are common.[5] Before the 1950s, an era when the United States was socioeconomically less developed, *H. pylori* was quite common as indicated by the >50% prevalence of infection in those older than 60 years of age. Succeeding generations of Americans have progressively lower prevalence of *H. pylori*, which reflects socio-economic progress and more favorable microbiological childhood surroundings.[9] In contrast to the past, today children living in the United States and most similarly developed countries have <5% likelihood of acquiring infection. Yet differences in prevalence among racial and ethnic groups within the United States remain. Hispanics and African-Americans continue to have a higher prevalence of *H. pylori* than age-matched Caucasians, possibly related to socioeconomic differences (Fig. 18.1).[10]

PATHOGENESIS

The eventual clinical outcome of *H. pylori* infection represents a complex interaction between the host and the bacterium, which can be influenced by the environment (smoking or antioxidants, salt, and nitrates in the diet, etc.) and modulated by a number of as yet unknown factors. Organisms reside within or beneath the gastric mucous layer and do not directly invade gastroduodenal tissue, but rather indirectly produce damage by adhering to the gastric epithelium, liberating enzymes and toxins, and inciting a

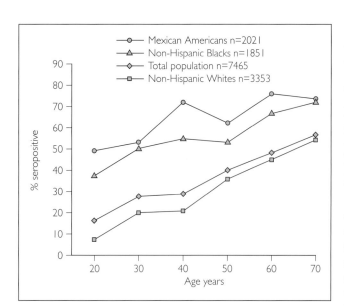

Fig. 18.1 • Seroprevalence of *H. pylori* among US adults. (From Everhart. J Infect Dis 2000; 181:1359.)

chronic immune-related inflammatory reaction. The release of interleukin-8 and other mediators of inflammation from the gastric epithelium activate a cascade of cytokines that, in turn, affect other cells and processes, ultimately weakening mucosal defensive mechanisms and disrupting normal gastric acid secretory physiology (dysregulation of somatostatin [D-cell], gastrin [G-cell], and acid secretion [parietal cell] interaction) (Fig. 18.2).[2] In most individuals the resulting chronic inflammation does not progress and they remain asymptomatic. However, during the lifetime of some individuals, the combination of mucosal injury and acid hypersecretion incites ulcer disease (<20%), gastric inflammation that progresses to atrophy, intestinal metaplasia, and eventually cancer (<1%), or with continuous immune stimulation of gastric lymphoid tissue, gastric MALT lymphoma (<0.001%) (Fig. 18.3).[2]

Differences among strains of *H. pylori* appear to correlate with virulence and tissue injury.[11] For example, *cagA* is a bacterial gene whose protein product, CagA, by itself is not cytotoxic, but is antigenic, enabling serologic strain specific identification. Other bacterial genes, such as *vacA* and *cagE*, which produce more toxic protein products, are co-transcribed with and linked to *cagA*. Strain differences do appear to be clinically important since at least 85% of duodenal ulcer patients harbor CagA strains, compared to 30–60% of infected individuals with no ulcer history.[12] In addition, infection with CagA bacteria is more likely to lead to gastric atrophy and cancer.[13]

Recent reports suggest that host genetics are important in determining clinical outcome of infection. The intensity and distribution (antral predominant or more generalized) of inflammation and the acid secretory profile (hypersecretion or hyposecretion) that results from *H. pylori* infection correlate with specific genetic polymorphisms of IL-1β and other inflammatory cytokines.[14] For example, a study comparing gastric cancer patients with controls suggests that two specific polymorphisms (IL-1β-31T and IL-1RN*2) are associated with low acid secretion and gastric atrophy and possibly an increased risk for gastric cancer.[15] These alleles appear to promote more intense inflammation and directly inhibit acid secretion to a greater degree. Conversely, other cytokine polymorphic profiles may lead to localized antral inflammation, acid hypersecretion, and increased susceptibility to ulcer disease.

Reserving treatment for individuals infected with a more 'virulent' strain of bacteria or those with an unfavorable genetic profile is intellectually attractive, but impractical and unreasonable. Despite contrary views that *H. pylori* infection may in some situations actually be beneficial, the overwhelming evidence supports its role as a pathogen irrespective of strain or host genetics. Testing for infection, as will be discussed, should be selective, while treatment, once infection is detected, should be universal. Pending conclusive evidence to the contrary, the dictum 'the only good *H. pylori* is dead *H. pylori*' remains applicable.

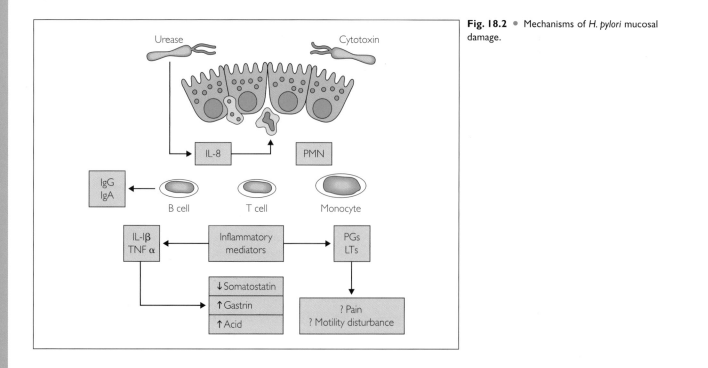

Fig. 18.2 • Mechanisms of *H. pylori* mucosal damage.

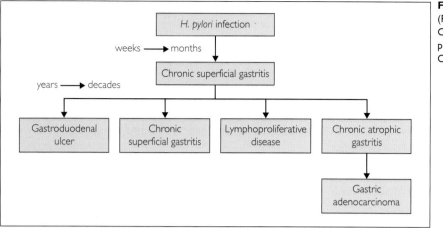

Fig. 18.3 • Natural history of *H. pylori* infection. (Reprinted from Blaser and Parsonnet, Journal of Clinical Investigation 1994; 94:4–8. © 1994, with permission from The American Society for Clinical Investigation.)

Disease associations and effects of treatment

The evidence linking *H. pylori* infection to peptic ulcer disease, gastric cancer, and gastric lymphoma is irrefutable.[2] Less convincing is its association with functional dyspepsia[16,17] and its possible beneficial role in gastroesophageal reflux disease (GERD).[18] Even less compelling is its presumed relationship to nongastrointestinal conditions, such as urticaria, rosacea, coronary artery disease, and short stature.[19]

Worldwide, the majority of peptic ulcers are still caused by *H. pylori* infection. However, as the prevalence of infection decreases, so will the proportion of infectious ulcers.[20] In fact, in some regions, <50% of ulcers are now due to *H. pylori*. Curing infection prevents most, but not all, recurrent ulcers and complications; approximately 20% of ulcers recur despite adequate antibiotic treatment, possibly due to nonsteroidal antiinflammatory drugs (NSAIDs).[21] *H. pylori* and NSAID use are independent risk factors that contribute synergistically to promote ulcers, and thus both deserve attention to avoid subsequent clinical problems.[22] Eradication of *H. pylori* may reduce the likelihood of ulcers and complications in NSAID-naïve patients beginning antiinflammatory drug treatment (Fig. 18.4).[23] The risk of subsequent ulcer complications can also be reduced if infection is cured in high-risk patients taking aspirin.[24] However, *H. pylori* treatment alone is insufficient to prevent recurrent ulcer complications in patients taking traditional NSAIDs.[24] Even patients prescribed presumably safer COX-2-selective NSAIDs are at greater risk of developing ulcers if they are infected with *H. pylori*.[25]

The incidence of gastric cancer is decreasing in developed countries, but it remains one of the leading causes of death worldwide. A number of epidemiological studies link gastric cancer to *H. pylori* infection, and the World Health Organization classifies *H. pylori* as a group I, definite carcinogen.[26] Whether eradication of infection can prevent subsequent cancer remains controversial. Persistent mucosal immune stimulation by *H. pylori* infection can trigger gastric mucosa-associated lymphoid tissue (MALT) lymphoma. Bacterial eradication leads to complete remission in approximately 80% of low-grade stage E1 (limited to mucosa and submucosa) tumors,[27] but monoclonal B cells can persist long after cure of infection and apparent complete histologic and endoscopic remission, which raises questions about the need for continued surveillance endoscopy and gastric biopsy.

Dyspepsia is a common clinical problem in the United States and other Western countries, and the effects of *H. pylori* eradication therapy on dyspeptic symptoms are discussed in Chapter 69. Most epidemiological studies have shown that GERD is less common in those infected with *H. pylori*. However, whether *H. pylori* actually protects against uncomplicated and complicated GERD and whether cure of infection worsens reflux symptoms remain conjectural. A recent study suggests that *H. pylori* eradication does not induce new GERD symptoms, aggravate existing reflux symptoms, or confound ongoing GERD treatment with PPIs.[28] Conversely, there is also little evidence to suggest that *H. pylori* treatment improves reflux symptoms. Therefore, in most situations, the cure of infection will have little impact on GERD, and the presence of reflux symptoms should not deter *H. pylori* treatment in appropriate patients.

Evidence linking nongastrointestinal conditions and *H. pylori* infection is weak, anecdotal at best.[19] Nevertheless, on occasion, 'refractory' iron deficiency, thrombocytopenia, and chronic urticaria improve after bacterial eradication. However, until better evidence justifies dealing with *H. pylori* in the setting of

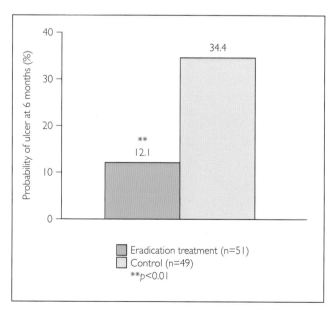

Fig. 18.4 • Effect of *H. pylori* eradication on ulcer risk in NSAID naïve patients medication. (Reprinted from Chan, The Lancet 2002; 359:9, with permission from Elsevier Ltd.)

nongastrointestinal conditions, clinicians should treat infection only in situations with a proven disease association.

Diagnosis of *H. pylori* infection

Tests available to diagnose *H. pylori* infection include both invasive techniques requiring endoscopy and biopsy and noninvasive techniques (urea breath test, stool antigen, and serology).[29] Invasive endoscopic techniques, and in particular histologic evaluation, are very sensitive and specific, but sampling error, improper orientation and handling of specimens, experience of the histopathologist, and concurrent PPI therapy affect their accuracy. While culture to diagnose *H. pylori* is very specific, it is tedious and choice of therapy rarely depends on sensitivity results.

Serology, the most commonly used noninvasive diagnostic test for *H. pylori*, has a positive predictive value too low to guide treatment decisions in areas where prevalence of infection is low (Fig. 18.5).[30] Because serology cannot reliably distinguish past from ongoing infection, positive test results should be confirmed by another method prior to prescribing antibiotics. Moreover, serology has limited value when confirming bacterial eradication after treatment.

The *H. pylori* stool antigen test and urea breath test, unlike serology, are accurate before and after treatment.[31–33] Their accuracy assumes no antibiotic use for four weeks or PPI use for one week prior to testing to avoid false-negative results.[34,35]

Recommendations[36–38] concerning whom to test for *H. pylori* vary considerably, in part because of regional differences in both the prevalence of infection and distinct clinical disease manifestations. Nevertheless, current or past uncomplicated or complicated ulcer disease, MALT-lymphoma, and resected gastric cancer are conditions for which all agree that *H. pylori* testing is appropriate. Most also agree that testing of asymptomatic individuals and routine screening of general populations are not recommended.

Different recommendations concerning dyspepsia stem from inconsistent and unpredictable symptom relief following bacterial eradication. Reports that *H. pylori* treatment benefits patients with uninvestigated or functional dyspepsia originate largely from regions with a high background prevalence of *H. pylori* and ulcer disease whereas reports showing no benefit come from areas with a lower prevalence of infection and ulcers.[16,17] These issues are discussed in detail in Chapter 69.

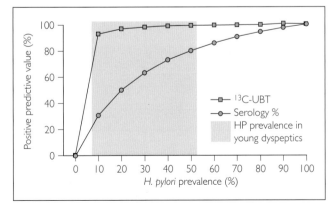

Fig. 18.5 • Positive predictive value of serology and urea breath test versus *H. pylori* prevalence. (Reprinted from Chiba, The Canadian Journal of Gastroenterology 1999; 13:681–683. © 1999, with permission from Pulsus Group Inc.)

Following treatment of *H. pylori*, it is appropriate to confirm successful eradication. The urea breath test and the stool antigen test are the methods of choice to confirm bacterial cure, although testing should be delayed until 4–6 weeks after completion of treatment to avoid possible false-negative results. Post-treatment endoscopic testing is only appropriate when endoscopy is clinically indicated to follow-up a gastric or complicated ulcer or to obtain tissue for culture when antibiotic resistance is suspected and sensitivity testing will direct subsequent treatment. Serology is not useful for follow-up since most patients continue to have detectable antibodies for months and even years after elimination of infection.

TREATMENT OF *H. PYLORI* INFECTION

Selection of *H. pylori* therapy should consider efficacy, cost, side effects, ease of administration and impact of primary or secondary antibiotic resistance. Unfortunately, no single or '*H. pylori* specific' antibiotics can cure infection. Furthermore, although many different treatments have been proposed to treat infection, no one therapeutic regimen has emerged as ideal. Available treatment choices tend to be complicated and include combinations of various antibiotics dosed several times daily for 7–14 days, usually along with acid suppressive medications. Minor side effects of therapy are frequent, patient compliance can be a problem, and bacterial resistance to the most commonly used antibiotics is more prevalent than previously appreciated. Attempts to simplify regimens or shorten treatment duration generally reduce effectiveness. Also, treatment success appears to vary among countries and even within regions of countries.[39] Despite these concerns, available regimens consistently cure *H. pylori* in over 80% of individuals during an initial course of treatment.

Bismuth: For centuries practitioners have used heavy metals, particularly bismuth salts, to treat a variety of conditions, including dyspepsia and ulcer disease.[40] Long before the discovery of *H. pylori*, investigators observed that bismuth compounds could heal ulcers and reduce their recurrence, effects now attributed to the antimicrobial properties of bismuth. Because the absorption of bismuth is limited, its antibacterial mechanism likely involves local direct interaction with *H. pylori* organisms, possibly interfering with bacterial enzymes or mucosal adherence.[41] By directly entering bacteria, bismuth may bind to intracellular structures or facilitate cellular penetration and activity of antibiotics. This synergistic effect of bismuth and antibiotics is useful clinically, especially since bacterial resistance to bismuth does not appear to develop. Colloidal bismuth subcitrate (De-nol™), bismuth subsalicylate (Pepto-Bismol™), and ranitidine bismuth citrate (RBC) have all been used in combination with various antibiotics to cure *H. pylori* infection. Colloidal bismuth, not currently available in the United States, is insoluble in water and forms a colloidal solution after ingestion. Bismuth subsalicylate, which is available by itself in the US or packaged in combination with tetracycline and metronidazole (Helidac™), is soluble in water and gastric juice. RBC, no longer marketed in the US, combines the antimicrobial action of bismuth citrate with the antisecretory effect of ranitidine. While it was available, RBC was particularly useful since it was effective in combination with many different antibiotics and could be dosed twice daily. Bismuth toxicity, especially encephalopathy, does not appear to be an issue with the poorly absorbed, low-dose preparations used to treat *H. pylori*.[42]

Imidazoles: Metronidazole and tinidazole are active against *H. pylori*, presumably by damaging bacterial DNA and disrupting its cell cycle.[43] Both are well absorbed and readily transported from serum to gastric juice.[44] Metronidazole is the most commonly prescribed imidizole, but because of frequent bacterial resistance, it should be reserved as second-line treatment, always given with other effective antibiotics, and administered in sufficient doses (500 mg) to 'overcome' resistance.[43] Imidazoles can cause a metallic taste, dyspepsia, and less commonly peripheral neuropathy, seizures, and a disulfuram-like reaction if taken with alcohol.

Macrolides: Although erythromycin, clarithromycin, azithromycin, and dirithromycin all have in vitro antimicrobial activity against *H. pylori*, clarithromycin is the most effective and the most commonly used macrolide. In fact, clarithromycin is the single most effective antibiotic for *H. pylori,* curing up to 40% of infections when used alone.[45] It works by binding to bacterial ribosomes thereby inhibiting protein synthesis. The anti-*Helicobacter* activity of clarithromycin is significantly reduced in an acid environment – 16-fold lower at pH 5.5 versus pH 7.2[46] – which likely explains why clarithromycin is more effective when administered with PPIs. In addition, the co-administration of PPIs with clarithromycin significantly enhances the concentration of the antibiotic in gastric mucus, another possible explanation for the observed synergy between clarithromycin and PPIs.[47] Although generally well tolerated, it can cause dysgeusia and dyspepsia.

Amoxicillin: With one of the most active in vitro antimicrobial profiles against *H. pylori*, amoxicillin has both topical and systemic bactericidal effects.[48,49] Bacterial resistance to amoxicillin is uncommon. Even though it is quite acid stable and less affected by gastric acidity than clarithromycin, amoxicillin is significantly more effective when co-administered with PPIs. Amoxicillin can cause rash, diarrhea, and allergic reactions in those individuals with penicillin sensitivity.

Miscellaneous Antibiotics:[50] Tetracycline is an acid-stable antibiotic commonly used in bismuth-based regimens. It can cause dyspepsia, photosensitivity, and oral and vaginal candidiasis. Tetracycline should not be used in infants or young children since it can effect bone growth and discolor teeth. The poorly absorbed nitrofuran, furazolidone, is commonly used in less-developed countries because of is low cost. It is available in the US, but only through compounding pharmacies and can be substituted for metronidazole in patients intolerant or resistant to the medication. Side effects of furazolidone include nausea, headache and discoloration of the urine. As with metronidazole, disulfuram-like reactions can occur if taken with alcohol. Rifabutin, an antimycobacterial drug, is an expensive substitute for clarithromycin and should be reserved to 'rescue' patients who fail initial macrolide treatment and bismuth-based re-treatment. Side effects include marrow suppression, dyspepsia, and discolored urine. Levofloxacin is another expensive substitute for clarithromycin reserved for rescue regimens. It can cause typical quinilone side effects that include seizures, photosensitivity, dyspepsia, and restlessness.

Proton-Pump Inhibitors (PPIs): The PPIs possess direct in vitro antimicrobial activity against *H. pylori*, which unlikely plays a major role in eradication of infection.[51,52] Rather, by raising pH and lowering intragastric volume, PPIs act in synergy with antibiotics to increase their gastric luminal concentration, enhance their absorption and mucus penetration, and reduce their degradation. PPIs also play a key role in *H. pylori* management by healing associated ulcers and relieving dyspeptic symptoms.

Multi-drug treatment regimens for *Helicobacter pylori*: dual therapies

The earliest successful treatments for *H. pylori* employed bismuth and single antibiotics. Marshall and colleagues, in the first double-blind trial evaluating the effects of *H. pylori* treatment on duodenal ulcer recurrence, cured infection in 70% on those treated with colloidal bismuth subcitrate (CBS) and tinidazole compared to 27% of those treated with CBS and placebo for 1–10 days.[53] The combination of bismuth and metronidazole taken for 2–4 weeks eliminates infection in 70% of those treated, but metronidazole resistance significantly affects the effectiveness of this combination.[54] The combination of ampicillin and bismuth subsalicylate (BSS) was shown to be effective in clearing *H. pylori* infection in children,[55] while other antibiotics, such as nitrofurantoin combined with bismuth, were less successful.[56] The small numbers of patients studied and the failure to adequately distinguish between suppression and true cure of infection were limitations of these early trials.

Because PPIs heal ulcers and augment the anti-*H. pylori* effects of certain antimicrobials, combining a PPI with an antibiotic was a reasonable treatment approach to investigate.[57] The combination of omeprazole 20 or 40 mg twice daily along with amoxicillin 1.5–3.0 g in divided doses daily (OA) showed initial promise as primary *H. pylori* treatment. Studies from Germany suggested that this simple, well-tolerated regimen taken for 10–14 days could cure >80% of infections.[58,59] These remarkable cure rates could not be consistently reproduced in other centers; in fact, eradication rates with OA in the United States are typically <70%.[60,61] The combination of lansoprazole and amoxicillin has also been studied and shown to have similar efficacy as OA.[62] Based on clinical trial results showing 61% to 70% eradication, the FDA approved dual therapy with lansoprazole 30 mg and amoxicillin 1 g each dosed three times per day for 2 weeks as treatment for *H. pylori* in patients with duodenal ulcer disease. Several factors appear to influence treatment success with the PPI–amoxicillin combination. Poor compliance, short treatment duration, smoking, and pretreatment with PPIs negatively impact treatment success.[63] Older age, more severe gastric inflammation, gastric ulcer disease, higher and more frequent doses of PPI and amoxicillin, and Asian ethnicity (presumably due to slower metabolism of PPIs related to CYP2C19 polymorphisms) all appear to favorably impact efficacy.[63,64] Compliance and tolerance with this simple regimen are good but the inconstant efficacy of dual PPI–amoxicillin treatment preclude its routine first-line clinical use.

Dual treatment with omeprazole 40 mg daily and clarithromycin 500 mg t.i.d. for 2 weeks was actually the first regimen approved by the FDA for treatment of *H. pylori* in patients with duodenal ulcer disease. Although this dual regimen cured >70% of infections during initial clinical trials,[65] subsequent studies showed less consistent bacterial eradication, often <60%. Primary macrolide resistance of *H. pylori* organisms markedly reduced treatment success, and secondary resistance often developed when initial treatment with this regimen failed.[66]

Based on clinical trial results showing >80% cure rates, dual treatment consisting of ranitidine bismuth citrate (RBC) 400 mg twice daily for 4 week and clarithromycin 500 mg three times daily for 2 weeks received FDA approval for *H. pylori* treatment in duodenal ulcer patients.[67] Although worldwide efficacy of this combination was >80% and it was well tolerated, the 4-week duration of therapy and emergence of more popular PPI-based triple-drug regimens relegated RBC to second-line treatment status. Dual treatments combining other individual antibiotics including amoxicillin, metronidazole, and tetracycline with RBC were less effective in curing infection. As discussed below, combinations of two antibiotics and RBC consistently eradicate >85% of *H. pylori* infections, especially when one of the antibiotics is clarithromycin.[68]

Because more effective triple drug treatments are available, dual drug regimens, even those approved by the FDA for *H. pylori* treatment, are no longer recommended, except for the PPI–amoxicillin combination in the rare patient who cannot tolerate metronidazole and clarithromycin.

Multi-drug treatment regimens for *Helicobacter pylori*: triple therapies[68]

Bismuth based triple therapies: Early studies confirmed that bismuth-based regimens with two antibiotics were more effective than dual therapies. Bismuth (either CBS or BSS) combined with metronidazole 250 mg or 500 mg and tetracycline 500 mg (BMT) all generally given four times daily for 2 weeks emerged as the first 'gold standard' *H. pylori* treatment, eliminating >80% of infections.[69] The higher 500 mg dose of metronidazole appears to be more effective since it can 'overcome' imidizole resistance. Twice-daily antisecretory medication, either an H2RA or PPI (termed quadruple therapy), is commonly added, especially if the patient being treated has active ulcer disease. Some feel that the addition of an antisecretory medication, especially a PPI, to BMT improves eradication[70] and ulcer healing, while others believe that the three-drug regimen is sufficient.[71]

Nevertheless, quadruple therapy is commonly used as primary therapy outside the US and as a re-treatment regimen throughout the world.[68,72] The substitution of doxycycline or amoxicillin for tetracycline reduces efficacy,[73] but the regimen remains effective when metronidazole is replaced by either clarithromycin or furazolidone, but not amoxicillin.[74,75] The FDA has approved the BMT regimen of bismuth subsalicylate 525 mg (two 262 mg tablets), metronidazole 250 mg, and tetracycline 500 mg all dosed four times daily with a daily antisecretory medication for two weeks as *H. pylori* treatment in patients with duodenal ulcer disease.

Side effects of BMT are considerable, typically those associated with the individual component medications, as previously described. However, the major drawback is the complexity of this regimen, often 26 pills per day, which adversely affects compliance and treatment effectiveness. Convenient daily-dose blister packaging (Helidac™) of the FDA-approved BMT regimen is an attempt to improve compliance. Treatment for 1 week is generally better tolerated and successful, although cure rates are more consistent with 2-week therapy. Therapy of less than 1 week's duration appears to be inadequate.

RBC 400 mg combined with amoxicillin 1 g and clarithromycin 500 mg (RAC) each given twice daily can cure infection in 92% of patients treated for 2 weeks.[76] RMC (ranitidine bismuth citrate 400 mg, metronidazole 500 mg and clarithromycin 500 mg twice daily), RMT (ranitidine bismuth citrate 400 mg, metronida-

zole 500 mg, and tetracycline 500 mg twice daily), and RAT (ranitidine bismuth citrate 400 mg, amoxicillin 1 g, and tetracycline 500 mg twice daily) are other combinations able to eradicate *H. pylori* in >80% of individuals treated.[77,78] These RBC-based triple therapies compare favorably to other three-drug therapies and are consistently the most effective regimens for primary or rescue treatment, especially when given for 10–14 days.[68] Treatment courses of 1 week are also effective, but offer less consistent eradication.[79] For initial or re-treatment of *H. pylori*, RBC is a very valuable medication since it is effective in combination with so many different antibiotics. While no longer marketed in the US, it is still available in Canada and Europe.

PPI-based Triple Therapies:[68] These regimens are generally regarded as the primary treatments of choice for *H. pylori*, largely based on favorable worldwide experience, tolerability, and aggressive pharmaceutical marketing. Investigators initially combined omeprazole (O) 20 mg with clarithromycin 500 mg or 250 mg (C) and either metronidazole (M) 500 mg (MOC) or amoxicillin (A) 1 g (OAC), each given twice daily for 14 days. The PPI is an essential component of this regimen, significantly augmenting the efficacy of the two antibiotics alone (Fig. 18.6).[80] Early experience in the US with MOC confirmed that the treatment was well tolerated and effective, eradicating infection in 88% of treated adults.[81] It was superior to PPI dual therapy, was as effective but better tolerated than BMT, and was effective in children.[82] Shorter 7–10 day courses of PPI-MC, including those that use a lower 250 mg dose of clarithromycin (to reduce cost) remain effective, but optimistic results with these abbreviated regimens generally emanate from centers outside the US. Recommendations in the US for this combination advise 2-week treatment and full-dose 500 mg clarithromycin (cost of 500 mg and 250 mg doses are similar in US). While there is more experience with omeprazole in combination with metronidazole and clarithromycin, other PPIs are similarly effective.[83] Side effects with a PPI-CM regimen are generally those associated with the individual components previously described, but are usually mild, less common than with BMT, and rarely require discontinuing treatment. *H. pylori* metronidazole resistance can significantly negatively impact treatment with PPI CM[80] (see Fig. 18.6), but clarithromycin resistance

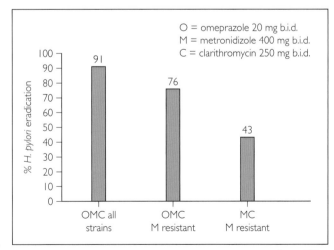

Fig. 18.6 • Effect of a PPI and metronidazole resistance on efficacy PPI triple therapy (OMC). (Reprinted from Lind, Gastroenterology 1999; 116:248. © 1999, with permission from The American Gastroenterological Association.)

renders this combination clinically ineffective. Treatment failure also can lead to emerging resistance to both antibiotics, which can complicate subsequent therapy. Because imidizole resistance among *H. pylori* even in the US is quite common and macrolide resistance so clinically relevant, it is best to avoid co-administration of metronidazole and clarithromycin except in patients who are penicillin sensitive.

The combination of a PPI, amoxicillin, and clarithromycin (PPI-AC) is the most popular and widely recommended treatment for *H. pylori* worldwide. A 7–14 day course of PPI-AC cures infection in approximately 85% of individuals, especially when using the higher 500 mg dose of clarithromycin.[66,84-87] This level of treatment effectiveness is significantly superior to dual treatments and generally better than other PPI or bismuth-based triple therapies. While macrolide resistance does negatively impact treatment success with PPI-AC,[66] imidizole resistance and rarely encountered penicillin resistance do not significantly influence treatment. When azithromycin is used in place of clarithromycin, success of treatment is less consistent. A higher dose of clarithromycin (500 mg) and longer treatment (10–14 days) seem to increase cure rate. However, outside the US, to reduce cost and improve compliance, 7-day treatment with 250 mg clarithromycin is common and generally successful. Shorter course PPI-AC treatment is less often used in the US, but based on comparative studies, the FDA recently approved a 1-week *H. pylori* treatment in patients with ulcer disease (rabeprazole 20 mg, amoxicillin 1g, and clarithromycin 500 mg all twice daily). Other FDA-approved combinations and durations of treatment of *H. pylori* infection in the setting of ulcer disease include amoxicillin (1 g twice daily), clarithromycin (500 mg twice daily) along with lansoprazole (30 mg twice daily for 10 or 14 days), omeprazole (20 mg twice daily for 10 days), or esomeprazole (40 mg once daily for 10 days). Extensive international experience with pantoprazole, amoxicillin, and clarithromycin supports the efficacy of this combination as well, although this specific regimen is not currently approved by the FDA. Lansoprazole-AC is marketed as Prevpac™, a compliance packaging containing each day's component medication in 14 individual blister packs. Side effects with a PPI-AC regimen are generally those associated with the individual components previously described, usually mild, less common than with PPI-CM or BMT, and rarely require discontinuing treatment.

Because the clarithromycin component of PPI-based treatments is expensive, other antibiotics have been substituted to decrease cost. Omeprazole 20 mg, amoxicillin 1 g, and metronidazole 500 mg each dosed twice daily for two weeks (OAM) is one such less expensive regimen that is particularly popular in the United Kingdom. The efficacy of PPI-AM ranges between 70% and 90%, but can be considerably less when treating metronidazole-resistant organisms.[88] A shorter duration of therapy (1 week) results in less consistent cure of infection. Despite its lower cost, PPI-AM is not recommended for primary *H. pylori* treatment because imidizole resistance significantly affects treatment success and because more effective regimens are available.

Ultra-short course and other treatments

A basic principle of treating *H. pylori* is to prescribe one of the available effective regimens for sufficient duration to cure infection. Yet, enthusiastic investigators continue to conduct studies involving multidrug, abbreviated (<7 day) treatment regimens, presumably to improve patient compliance and reduce cost.[89,90] Initial investigator enthusiasm for short-course treatment needs to be tempered since most trials are done in single centers, treat small numbers of patients, and yield inferior results or superior results that cannot be reproduced. Furthermore, treatment failure associated with inadequate therapy can promote antibiotic resistance that will complicate subsequent management. Nevertheless, several recent studies suggest that multidrug short-course regimens are effective in curing *H. pylori* infection. However, until further experience confirms the efficacy of abbreviated treatments, PPI triple therapy for at least 7 days should remain the first-line treatment of choice.

One novel approach to treatment involves pretreating the patient for several days with PPIs and mucolytic agents, followed by balloon occlusion of the pylorus and subsequent nasogastric or endoscopic instillation of antibiotics.[91,92] Continuous bathing of the gastric mucosa with a solution of sodium bicarbonate, bismuth, amoxicillin, and metronidazole for 1–2 hours eliminated infection in >90% of patients in one study and >70% in another. Although this topical treatment is appealing because of its brief duration, it is invasive, expensive when endoscopy is involved, and unlikely to be acceptable to most patients.

Many individuals are attracted to nutraceuticals and homeopathic remedies, which some maintain can cure *H. pylori* infection. None of these natural substances has been rigorously scientifically evaluated and experience with them is anecdotal at best. Currently, they have no place as the sole management of *H. pylori* infection.

Antibiotic resistance and its effect on treatment

H. pylori imidizole resistance is an important clinical problem since it significantly decreases the efficacy of metronidazole-containing treatments.[72,93] PPI-CM, BMT, and especially PPI-AM are less effective in treating metronidazole-resistant strains of bacteria. Prior exposure to metronidazole can lead to resistance, and women, Hispanics, and individuals living in, or emigrating from, less developed areas of the world are more likely to harbor imidizole-resistant bacteria.[94] The prevalence of metronidazole resistance varies considerably. In some parts of the world, the prevalence is >70%, often approaching 100%, while in the US resistance ranges from 25% to 50%.[94-96] The mechanism of metronidazole resistance appears due to a point mutation(s) that prevents the reduction of the drug to its active metabolite.[43] Metronidazole-resistant strains do not remove oxygen from the site of metronidazole reduction, thereby preventing antibiotic activation. Increasing the dose of metronidazole or giving the drug with bismuth can eradicate some resistant strains, suggesting that imidizole 'resistance' is not an absolute phenomenon. However, because of the widespread emergence of metronidazole-resistant strains, an effective nonmetronidazole-containing regimen such as PPI-AC should be the primary treatment of choice.

Macrolide resistance is considerably less prevalent than imidizole resistance, ranging from 5% to 10% in most surveys, and it appears to affect all antibiotics in the drug class (erythromycin, clarithromycin, azithromycin, etc.).[94-96] Its mechanism has been better characterized and involves point mutations within the conserved loop of the 23S strand of ribosomal RNA. Polymerase chain reaction (PCR) methods that detect these point mutations can identify macrolide resistant strains of *H. pylori* in gastric juice and biopsies, but such methods are not clinically available at this time.[97] Unlike resistance to metronidazole, which can be 'overcome' in some instances by administering a higher dose of medication, macrolide resistance is permanent and negatively impacts treatment, even when the dose of antibiotic is increased. In fact, primary macrolide resistance is likely a major cause of treatment failure with clarithromycin-containing three-drug regimens.[66,93] Following initial treatment failure with dual- or triple-drug clarithromycin-containing regimens, secondary macrolide resistance commonly develops. To minimize emergence of secondary resistance, macrolides should not be used alone or in dual therapies. Moreover, it is best to avoid using clarithromycin and metronidazole together since treatment failure would likely result in dual antibiotic resistance, a situation which would complicate subsequent treatment.

To date, *H. pylori* resistance to amoxicillin and tetracycline has not been a clinical problem. In fact, resistance to these antibiotics is so uncommon that most laboratories do not routinely perform sensitivity testing. Quinilone resistance is more common and may increase as quinilones are used more frequently in re-treatment or rescue regimens. A recent analysis evaluated *H. pylori* resistance rates to the commonly used antibiotics (Fig. 18.7) and patient demographic characteristics associated with antibiotic resistance.[94]

Recurrence and re-treatment of *H. pylori* infection

If successfully treated, adults rarely become reinfected with *H. pylori*. Even in regions of the world where the prevalence of infection is high, recurrence is generally <1%, although higher rates of reacquisition have been reported.[98,99] Whether antibodies that develop in response to primary infection confer subsequent immunity or whether adult behavior is less likely to lead to fecal or oral re-exposure to bacteria is not known. Repeat infection, however, appears to be as high as 60% in young children, possibly related to hygiene or behavior that promotes exposure to a variety of infectious agents.[3] In adults, persistent or 'recurrent' infection generally is due to initial treatment failure. In fact, a number of studies using very specific methods to characterize bacterial strains confirm treatment failure, rather than reinfection as the source of persistent *H. pylori*.[99]

Primary care physicians and patients often assume that if symptoms persist or recur despite *H. pylori* treatment, the infection is persistent or has recurred. However, in most circum-stances, functional dyspepsia recurs in the absence of reinfection. Therefore, before initiating any additional antibiotic treatment, the persistence of infection should be confirmed, which is most effectively done by a urea breath or stool antigen test.

The optimal management of persistent *H. pylori* is controversial, but generally involves using antibiotics different from those administered during initial treatment.[100,101] This principle is particularly important with macrolides since emerging resistance to this class of antibiotics is quite common after failed eradication. A simple dual regimen of a PPI and amoxicillin is occasionally effective as re-treatment and it is useful since resistance to penicillins is rare. One such regimen, LA (lansoprazole 30 mg and amoxicillin 1 g each 3 times daily), is approved by the FDA as initial treatment for *H. pylori* infection in patients with ulcer disease. Another option is PPI, metronidazole 500 mg, and amoxicillin 1 g, each given twice daily for 2 weeks.[101] This regimen is appropriate only if initial treatment did not include an imidizole. Different antibiotics combined with ranitidine bismuth citrate are also options for re-treatment outside the US.[101] A popular bismuth-based re-treatment regimen is quadruple therapy, consisting of bismuth, metronidazole 500 mg, and tetracycline 500 mg 4 times daily along with a PPI twice daily for 2 weeks.[101] While relatively inexpensive and effective, clearing persistent infection in >60% of cases, quadruple therapy is cumbersome to take, and its success is influenced by imidizole resistance, although the higher 500 mg dose of metronidazole appears to overwhelm resistant bacteria. The metronidazole dose contained in Helidac™ is only 250 mg so when using this packaged combination, additional medication must be prescribed to ensure sufficient metronidazole, especially during re-treatment. In areas of the world where it is available, furazolidone 100 mg can be substituted for metronidazole in quadruple therapy as another means to counteract antibiotic resistance.[102] Other simpler, but more expensive re-treatment regimens are being used especially outside the US, but experience with these newer regimens is limited. One promising regimen includes PPI, amoxicillin 1 g, and levafloxacin 250 mg b.i.d. for 10–14 days.[103] Optimistic reports suggest >80% success in curing persistent *H. pylori*. Another suggested re-treatment regimen consists of a PPI, rifabutin 150 mg, and amoxicillin 1 g twice daily for 10–14 days. This 'rescue' therapy reportedly eliminates infection in >80% of patients failing one or two courses of more traditional treatments.[104]

FUTURE TREATMENTS FOR *H. PYLORI*

Host immune responses to *H. pylori* not only cause tissue injury, but are also central to any vaccination strategy. Since the organism can survive the immune response to natural infection, the development of an effective vaccine faces significant challenges. However, preliminary studies suggest that immunization with crude bacterial extracts and recombinant subunits of the bacterial enzymes urease and catalase can protect animals from *H. pylori* exposure.[105,106] Efforts are also underway to develop a therapeutic vaccine intended to augment the natural immune response to infection.[107,108] A therapeutic vaccine could promote spontaneous clearance of infection and/or improve the efficacy of antibiotic regimens. An effective therapeutic vaccine could also obviate the widespread use of antibiotics and reduce the emergence of antibiotic-resistant organisms. While preliminary results of human testing of a urease antigen and inactivated whole-cell

	n tested	Rate	95% CI
Clarithromycin	3571	10.1%	9.1–11.1
Metronidazole	2883	36.9%	35.1–38.7
Amoxicillin	3486	1.4%	1.0–1.8

Fig. 18.7 ● *H. pylori* antibiotic resistance rates in the United States (1993–1999). (Reprinted from Meyer JM et al, Annals of Internal Medicine 2002; 136:13–24. © 2002, with permission from American College of Physicians.)

vaccines using heat-labile enterotoxin of *E. coli* as an adjuvant have been reported,[109,110] it is unlikely that an effective, safe vaccine will be available for clinical use in the near future.

Now that the *H. pylori* genome has been sequenced, scientists can identify 'pylori-specific' metabolic mechanisms to target with therapeutic pharmaceuticals. Such a strategy offers the opportunity to eradicate *H. pylori*, while sparing other endogenous organisms. A number of possible candidates for specific targeting are being investigated.[111]

Recommendations regarding management of *H. pylori*

Working parties from the US,[37] Europe,[36,112] and the Asian Pacific region[38] have each developed guidelines intended to assist physicians within their respective localities to appropriately manage *H. pylori* infection. Specific management recommendations are based on factors such as community prevalence and seriousness of *H. pylori*-related disease and the likelihood of altering its clinical course with treatment.

United States guidelines for management of **H. pylori** infection[37]

The most recent US guidelines propose testing for *H. pylori* infection only if subsequent treatment is planned. Appropriate indications for testing and treatment include patients with present or past uncomplicated or complicated gastric or duodenal ulcer, those with gastric MALT lymphoma, or following resection of early gastric cancer. A decision to test a patient with functional or uninvestigated dyspepsia should be made on a case-by-case basis. The guidelines specifically emphasize the lack of data sufficient to recommend routine testing of asymptomatic individuals or those receiving chronic PPI therapy (the latter is a suggestion of the European working group). Diagnostic tests should be tailored to the clinical situation. When endoscopy is not clinically necessary, either serology or a urea breath test is a suitable test. If endoscopy is indicated for patient care, then it is appropriate to obtain a biopsy for diagnosis, but routine culture is not recommended. A PPI or RBC, clarithromycin and amoxicillin or metronidazole or PPI, bismuth, metronidazole and tetracycline given for 2 weeks are recommended therapies. Confirming the cure of infection is suggested for those with complicated ulcer disease, MALT lymphoma, or recurrent symptoms.

These guidelines were established in 1997, and while they remain generally applicable, several modifications and additions may be appropriate. For example, serology is now known to be less accurate when the prevalence of *H. pylori* infection is low, a situation common to many regions of the US.[30] Therefore, if serology is used to screen for *H. pylori* infection, a positive serology test result should be confirmed by a more accurate breath or stool test before initiating treatment.[113] With the widespread availability of these accurate noninvasive tests, it is now also appropriate to document cure of infection in everyone at least 4 weeks following treatment.[114] Initial treatment should be for 10–14 days with a PPI, clarithromycin, and amoxicillin unless the patient is allergic or intolerant of one of the medications. Bismuth-based treatments are now considered second-line therapy. The indications for testing remain well founded, but should be expanded to include other situations. Given the recent information about *H. pylori* and genetic susceptibility to gastric cancer, it is not unreasonable to test individuals, even those with no symptoms, who have first-degree relatives with gastric adenocarcinoma or those of Japanese descent.[115] Recent data question the benefit of *H. pylori* testing in patients with dyspepsia, especially in regions where the prevalence of infection and serious infection-associated diseases are low.[116]

International management of **H. pylori** infection consensus and disagreement

Similarities between the European[36,112] and US guidelines[37] include the treatment of individuals with active or past ulcer disease, MALT lymphoma, or early gastric cancer. Differences include recommended testing of patients with evidence of severe endoscopic or atrophic gastritis and those prescribed long-term PPIs for gastroesophageal reflux disease. Further variations, although not strongly evidence based, include testing young otherwise healthy patients with uninvestigated dyspepsia, persons with functional dyspepsia, those with a family history of gastric cancer, or individuals initiating NSAID therapy.

The development of Asian Pacific recommendations poses a challenge since they need to be applicable in localities with diverse rates of *H. pylori* infection and associated diseases.[38] In harmony with other regional guidelines, testing those with active or past ulcer disease, MALT lymphoma, and early gastric cancer is suggested. The Asian Pacific working group asserts that asymptomatic individuals, those receiving NSAIDs or those solely with a family history of gastric cancer do not need to be routinely tested for *H. pylori*. They also suggest that young healthy individuals with dyspeptic complaints can be initially tested noninvasively for *H. pylori*, but should symptoms not improve, such individuals should have prompt endoscopy because of the high prevalence of gastric cancer in Asian countries.

Diagnosis and treatment recommendations from both Europe and Asian Pacific region support endoscopic diagnosis of *H. pylori*, since ulcer and gastric cancer, which are more prevalent than in the US, need to be excluded. When noninvasive testing is used, a breath test is preferred to serology. As in the US, the treatment regimen of choice in Europe and the Asian Pacific region is a PPI with amoxicillin, and clarithromycin; however, a 7-day course of treatment has been deemed sufficient.

PERSONAL RECOMMENDATIONS FOR *H. PYLORI* MANAGEMENT

Testing for *H. pylori* is appropriate in any patient with an active or past history of duodenal ulcer irrespective of NSAID use (Fig. 18.8). Those with MALT lymphoma, or early gastric cancer, both rare conditions in the US, are also candidates for testing. Although not supported by evidence, individuals at higher risk for gastric cancer, such as those of Japanese descent or with a first-degree relative with gastric cancer, should be tested. *H. pylori* in those with uninvestigated or functional dyspepsia, especially if symptoms are unresponsive to empiric acid suppressive treatments, should be approached on a case-by-case basis, but in practice testing for infection is inevitable. Routine testing of patients with GERD, asymptomatic users of aspirin or NSAIDs, or other asymptomatic individuals is not warranted.

Non-invasive testing for *H. pylori* is the most cost-effective approach. Preferred tests are a urea breath or stool test, but if serology is used, a positive result should be confirmed by another

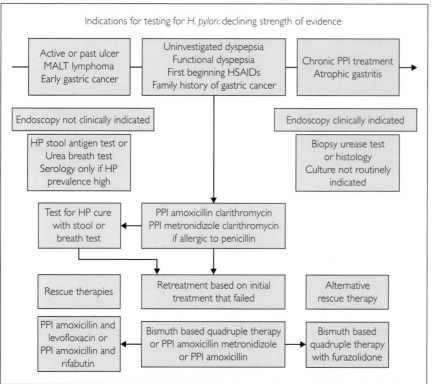

Indications for testing for *H. pylori*: declining strength of evidence

Fig. 18.8 • Current recommendations for *H. pylori* management.

method before starting treatment. Endoscopic testing (i.e., urease test or histology) is appropriate when a procedure is indicated for clinical reasons, but bacterial culture is rarely necessary. All patients should be retested at least 4–6 weeks after treatment to confirm cure.

The treatment of choice is a PPI with amoxicillin and clarithromycin each twice daily for 10–14 days. Metronidazole should be substituted for amoxicillin only if the patient is allergic to penicillin. If initial treatment fails, re-treatment with 14 days of bismuth-based quadruple therapy with high-dose metronidazole (500 mg) is the next best option. 'Rescue therapy' is reserved for third or fourth treatment courses. Experience is limited with rescue regimens, but the author favors the PPI, amoxicillin, levofloxacin combination in the rare patient who fails courses of more conventional therapies.

SUMMARY

Infection with *Helicobacter pylori* is common worldwide, but in many countries such as the United States its incidence is declining. Accompanying this decline is a reduction in associated clinical conditions such as ulcer disease and gastric cancer. Several general principles underlie the management of *H. pylori*. Test and treat only those most likely to benefit. Use a diagnostic test that is accurate, cost-effective, and provides necessary clinical information. Choose an effective, simple, well-tolerated treatment regimen that is less likely influenced by the presence of antibiotic-resistant organisms. Treatment duration and drug dosage should be sufficient to guarantee maximal efficacy since the 'true costs' of managing *H. pylori* are related to the consequences of failed eradication rather than to direct expense of medication (Table 18.1). Given

Table 18.1 FDA-approved regimens for treatment of *H. pylori* in patients with ulcer disease

Regimen	Comment
PPI amoxicillin 1 g clarithromycin 500 mg twice daily for 7–14 days	Treatment regimen of choice
PPI clarithromycin 500 mg twice daily for 14 days	Not recommended
PPI amoxicillin 1 g three times daily for 14 days	Not first-line, but may be useful as re-treatment
Bismuth 2 tabs metronidazole 250 mg tetracycline 500 mg four times daily for 14 days with acid suppressing medication	Not first-line – appropriate for re-treatment but if used need 500 mg metronidazole
RBC twice and clarithromycin 500 mg three times daily for 14 days	RBC not available in the US

the global demographic, socioeconomic, and clinical diversity of patient populations infected with *H. pylori*, application of these principles varies somewhat worldwide and even regionally within countries. During the past two decades, research has centered on the epidemiology, pathogenesis, and management of *H. pylori* and related clinical conditions. Future investigations will ideally lead to a simple cure or optimally to the prevention of infection entirely.

REFERENCES

1. Marshall B, Warren J. Unidentified curved bacilli in the stomach of patients with gastritis and peptic ulceration. Lancet 1984; 1(8390):1311–1315.

2. Suerbaum S, Michetti P. *Helicobacter pylori* infection. N Engl J Med 2002; 347:1175–1186.

   This is an excellent comprehensive review covering all important aspects of *H. pylori*.

3. Rowland M, Kumar D, Daly L, et al. Low rates of *Helicobacter pylori* reinfection in children. Gastroenterology 1999; 117:336–341.

4. Neale KR, Logan RP. The epidemiology and transmission of *Helicobacter pylori* infection in children. Aliment Pharmacol Ther 1995; 9(Suppl 2):77–84.

5. Frenck RW Jr, Clemens J. *Helicobacter* in the developing world. Microbes Infect 2003; 5:705–713.

6. Parsonnet J. The incidence of *Helicobacter pylori* infection. Aliment Pharmacol Ther 1995; 9(Suppl 2):45–51.

7. Kivi M, Tindberg Y, Sorberg M, et al. Concordance of *Helicobacter pylori* strains within families. J Clin Microbiol 2003; 41:5604–5608.

8. Megraud F. Transmission of *Helicobacter pylori*: faecal–oral versus oral–oral route. Aliment Pharmacol Ther 1995; 9(Suppl 2):85–91.

9. Rothenbacher D, Brenner H. Burden of *Helicobacter pylori* and *H. pylori*-related diseases in developed countries: recent developments and future implications. Microbes Infect 2003; 5:693–703.

10. Everhart JE, Kruszon-Moran D, Perez-Perez GI, et al. Seroprevalence and ethnic differences in *Helicobacter pylori* infection among adults in the United States. J Infect Dis 2000; 181:1359–1363.

11. Blaser MJ. Role of vacA and the cagA locus of *Helicobacter pylori* in human disease. Aliment Pharmacol Ther 1996; 10(Suppl 1):73–77.

12. Weel JF, Van Der Hulst RW, Gerrits Y, et al. The interrelationship between cytotoxin-associated gene A, vacuolating cytotoxin, and *Helicobacter pylori*-related diseases. J Infect Dis 1996; 173:1171–1175.

13. Huang JQ, Zheng GF, Sumanac K, et al. Meta-analysis of the relationship between cagA seropositivity and gastric cancer. Gastroenterology 2003; 125:1636–1644.

14. El-Omar EM. The importance of interleukin 1beta in *Helicobacter pylori* associated disease. Gut 2001; 48:743–747.

   The role host response to *H. pylori* infection plays in disease outcome is discussed.

15. El-Omar EM, Carrington M, Chow WH, et al. Interleukin-1 polymorphisms associated with increased risk of gastric cancer. Nature 2000; 404:398–402.

16. Laine L, Schoenfeld P, Fennerty MB. Therapy for *Helicobacter pylori* in patients with nonulcer dyspepsia. A meta-analysis of randomized, controlled trials. Ann Intern Med 2001; 134:361–369.

17. Moayyedi P, Soo S, Deeks J, et al. Eradication of *Helicobacter pylori* for non-ulcer dyspepsia. Cochrane Database Syst Rev 2000: CD002096.

   A systematic review of the effect of *H. pylori* eradication on symptoms in patients with functional dyspepsia suggests a modest benefit of treatment.

18. Vakil NB. Review article: gastro-oesophageal reflux disease and *Helicobacter pylori* infection. Aliment Pharmacol Ther 2002; 16(Suppl 1):47–51.

19. Leontiadis GI, Sharma VK, Howden CW. Non-gastrointestinal tract associations of *Helicobacter pylori* infection. Arch Intern Med 1999; 159:925–940.

20. Ciociola AA, Mcsorley DJ, Turner K, et al. *Helicobacter pylori* infection rates in duodenal ulcer patients in the United States may be lower than previously estimated. Am J Gastroenterol 1999; 94:1834–1840.

21. Laine L, Hopkins RJ, Girardi LS. Has the impact of *Helicobacter pylori* therapy on ulcer recurrence in the United States been overstated? A meta-analysis of rigorously designed trials. Am J Gastroenterol 1998; 93:1409–1415.

22. Huang JQ, Sridhar S, Hunt RH. Role of *Helicobacter pylori* infection and non-steroidal anti-inflammatory drugs in peptic-ulcer disease: a meta-analysis. Lancet 2002; 359:14–22.

   This meta-analysis supports an independent additive role of *H. pylori* and NSAIDs in pathogenesis of ulcers and ulcer complications.

23. Chan F, To K, Wu J, et al. Eradication of *Helicobacter pylori* and risk of peptic ulcers in patients starting long-term treatment with non-steroidal anti-inflammatory drugs: a randomised trial. Lancet 2002; 359:9–13.

24. Chan F, Chung S, Suen B, et al. Preventing recurrent upper gastrointestinal bleeding in patients with *Helicobacter pylori* infection who are taking low-dose aspirin or naproxen. N Engl J Med 2001; 344:967–973.

25. Goldstein J, Correa P, Zhao W, et al. Reduced incidence of gastroduodenal ulcers with celecoxib, a novel cyclooxygenase-2 inhibitor, compared to naproxen in patients with arthritis. Am J Gastroenterol 2001; 96:1019–1027.

26. [No authors listed]. Infection with *Helicobacter pylori*. IARC Monogr Eval Carcinog Risks Hum 1994; 61:177–240.

27. Fischbach W, Goebeler-Kolve ME, Dragosics B, et al. Long term outcome of patients with gastric marginal zone B cell lymphoma of mucosa associated lymphoid tissue (MALT) following exclusive *Helicobacter pylori* eradication therapy: experience from a large prospective series. Gut 2004; 53:34–7.

28. Laine L, Dhir V. *Helicobacter pylori* eradication does not worsen quality of life related to reflux symptoms: a prospective trial. Aliment Pharmacol Ther 2002; 16:1143–1148.

29. Rautelin H, Lehours P, Megraud F. Diagnosis of *Helicobacter pylori* infection. Helicobacter 2003; 8:13–20.

30. Chiba N, Veldhuyzen van Zanten SJ. ^{13}C-Urea breath tests are the noninvasive method of choice for *Helicobacter pylori* detection. Can J Gastroenterol 1999; 13:681–683.

31. Peura DA, Pambianco DJ, Dye KR, et al. Microdose ^{14}C-urea breath test offers diagnosis of *Helicobacter pylori* in 10 minutes. Am J Gastroenterol 1996; 91:233–238.

32. Vaira D, Malfertheiner P, Megraud F, et al. Diagnosis of *Helicobacter pylori* infection by HpSA test. European *Helicobacter pylori* HpSA Study Group. Lancet 1999; 354:1732.

33. Vaira D, Vakil N, Menegatti M, et al. The stool antigen test for detection of *Helicobacter pylori* after eradication therapy. Ann Intern Med 2002; 136:280–287.

34. Laine L, Estrada R, Trujillo M, et al. Effect of proton-pump inhibitor therapy on diagnostic testing for *Helicobacter pylori*. Ann Intern Med 1998; 129:547–550.

35. Manes G, Balzano A, Iaquinto G, et al. Accuracy of the stool antigen test in the diagnosis of *Helicobacter pylori* infection before treatment and in patients on omeprazole therapy. Aliment Pharmacol Ther 2001; 15:73–79.

36. Malfertheiner P, Megraud F, O'Morain C, et al. Current concepts in the management of *Helicobacter pylori* infection: The Maastricht 2-2000 Consensus Report. Aliment Pharmacol Ther 2002; 16:167–180.

These European guidelines for the management of *H. pylori* were developed by a multinational working group.

37. Howden CW, Hunt RH. Guidelines for the management of *Helicobacter pylori* infection. Ad Hoc Committee on Practice Parameters of the American College of Gastroenterology. Am J Gastroenterol 1998; 93:2330–2338.

US guidelines for the management of *H. pylori* are a bit old but generally remain applicable.

38. Lam SK, Talley NJ. Report of the 1997 Asia Pacific Consensus Conference on the management of *Helicobacter pylori* infection. J Gastroenterol Hepatol 1998; 13:1–12.

39. Fischbach LA, Goodman KJ, Feldman M, et al. Sources of variation of *Helicobacter pylori* treatment success in adults worldwide: a meta-analysis. Int J Epidemiol 2002; 31:128–139.

40. Lambert JR. Pharmacology of bismuth-containing compounds. Rev Infect Dis 1991; 13 Suppl 8:S691–S695.

41. Lambert JR, Midolo P. The actions of bismuth in the treatment of *Helicobacter pylori* infection. Aliment Pharmacol Ther 1997; 11(Suppl 1):27–33.

42. Tillman LA, Dixon JS, Wood JR. Review article: safety of bismuth in the treatment of gastrointestinal diseases. Aliment Pharmacol Ther 1996; 10(4):459–467.

43. Van der Wouden EJ, Thijs JC, Kusters JG, et al. Mechanism and clinical significance of metronidazole resistance in *Helicobacter pylori*. Scand J Gastroenterol Suppl 2001; 36:10–14.

44. Lambert JR. Pharmacology of the gastric mucosa: a rational approach to *Helicobacter* polytherapy. Gastroenterology 1996; 111:521–523.

45. Graham DY, Opekun AR, Klein PD. Clarithromycin for the eradication of *Helicobacter pylori*. J Clin Gastroenterol 1993; 16:292–294.

46. Malanoski GJ, Eliopoulos GM, Ferraro MJ, et al. Effect of pH variation on the susceptibility of *Helicobacter pylori* to three macrolide antimicrobial agents and temafloxacin. Eur J Clin Microbiol Infect Dis 1993; 12:131–133.

47. Gustavson LE, Kaiser JF, Edmonds AL, et al. Effect of omeprazole on concentrations of clarithromycin in plasma and gastric tissue at steady state. Antimicrob Agents Chemother 1995; 39:2078–2083.

48. Megraud F, Trimoulet P, Lamouliatte H, et al. Bactericidal effect of amoxicillin on *Helicobacter pylori* in an in vitro model using epithelial cells. Antimicrob Agents Chemother 1991; 35:869–872.

49. Berry V, Woodnutt G. Bactericidal and morphological effects of amoxicillin on *Helicobacter pylori*. Antimicrob Agents Chemother 1995; 39:1859–1861.

50. McNulty CA, Dent JC. Susceptibility of clinical isolates of *Campylobacter pylori* to twenty-one antimicrobial agents. Eur J Clin Microbiol Infect Dis 1988; 7:566–569.

51. Belli WA . Partial characterization and effect of omeprazole on ATPase activity in *Helicobacter pylori* by using permeabilized cells. Antimicrob Agents Chemother 1995; 39:1717–1720.

52. Nagata K, Iwahi T, Shimoyama T, et al. Potent inhibitory action of the gastric proton pump inhibitor lansoprazole against urease activity of *Helicobacter pylori*: unique action selective for *H. pylori* cells. Antimicrob Agents Chemother 1993; 37:769–774.

53. Marshall BJ, Goodwin CS, Warren JR, et al. Prospective double-blind trial of duodenal ulcer relapse after eradication of *Campylobacter pylori*. Lancet 1988; 2:1437–1442.

54. Weil J, Bell G, Powell K, et al. *Helicobacter pylori* infection treated with a tripotassium dicitrato bismuthate and metronidazole combination. Aliment Pharmacol Ther 1990; 4:651–657.

55. Drumm B, Sherman P, Chiasson D, et al. Treatment of *Campylobacter pylori*-associated antral gastritis in children with bismuth subsalicylate and ampicillin. J Pediatr 1988; 113:908–912.

56. Graham DY, Klein PD, Evans DG, et al. Simple noninvasive method to test efficacy of drugs in the eradication of *Helicobacter pylori* infection: the example of combined bismuth subsalicylate and nitrofurantoin. Am J Gastroenterol 1991; 86:1158–1162.

57. Pommerien W, Idstrom JP, Wrangstadh M, et al. Pharmacokinetic and pharmacodynamic interactions between omeprazole and amoxycillin in *Helicobacter pylori*-positive healthy subjects. Aliment Pharmacol Therapeut 1996; 10:295–301.

58. Bayerdorffer E, Miehlke S, Mannes G, et al. Double-blind trial of omeprazole and amoxicillin to cure *Helicobacter pylori* infection in patients with duodenal ulcers. Gastroenterology 1995; 108:1412–1417.

59. Labenz J, Gyenes E, Ruhl G, et al. Amoxicillin plus omeprazole versus triple therapy for eradication of *Helicobacter pylori* in duodenal ulcer disease: a prospective, randomized, and controlled study. Gut 1993; 34:1167–1170.

60. Al-Assi MT, Cole RA, Karttunen TJ, ET AL. Treatment of *Helicobacter pylori* infection with omeprazole-amoxicillin combination therapy versus ranitidine/sodium bicarbonate-amoxicillin. Am J Gastroenterol 1995; 90:1411–1414.

61. Laine L, Stein C, Neil G. Limited efficacy of omeprazole-based dual and triple therapy for *Helicobacter pylori*: a randomized trial employing 'optimal' dosing. Am J Gastroenterol 1995; 90:1407–14010.

62. Harford W, Lanza F, Arora A, et al. Double-blind, multicenter evaluation of lansoprazole and amoxicillin dual therapy for the cure of *Helicobacter pylori* infection. Helicobacter 1996; 1:243–250.

63. Labenz J, Leverkus F, Borsch G. Omeprazole plus amoxicillin for cure of *Helicobacter pylori* infection. Factors influencing the treatment success. Scand J Gastroenterol 1994; 29:1070–1075.

64. Tanigawara Y, Aoyama N, Kita T, et al. CYP2C19 genotype-related efficacy of omeprazole for the treatment of infection caused by *Helicobacter pylori*. Clin Pharmacol Ther 1999; 66:528–534.

65. Logan RP, Gummett PA, Schaufelberger HD, et al. Eradication of *Helicobacter pylori* with clarithromycin and omeprazole. Gut 1994; 35:323–326.

66. Laine L, Fennerty M, Osato M, et al. Esomeprazole-based *Helicobacter pylori* eradication therapy and the effect of antibiotic resistance: results of three US multicenter, double-blind trials. Am J Gastroenterol 2000; 95:3393–3398.

67. Peterson WL, Ciociola AA, Sykes DL, et al. Ranitidine bismuth citrate plus clarithromycin is effective for healing duodenal ulcers, eradicating *H. pylori* and reducing ulcer recurrence. RBC *H. pylori* Study Group. Aliment Pharmacol Ther 1996; 10:251–261.

68. Laheij RJ, Rossum LG, Jansen JB, et al. Evaluation of treatment regimens to cure *Helicobacter pylori* infection – a meta-analysis. Aliment Pharmacol Ther 1999; 13:857–864.

69. Graham DY, Lew GM, Evans DG, et al. Effect of triple therapy (antibiotics plus bismuth) on duodenal ulcer healing. A randomized controlled trial. Ann Intern Med 1991; 115:266–269.

70. De Boer W, Driessen W, Jansz A, et al. Effect of acid suppression on efficacy of treatment for *Helicobacter pylori* infection. Lancet 1995; 345:817–820.

71. Hosking SW, Ling TK, Chung SC, et al. Duodenal ulcer healing by eradication of *Helicobacter pylori* without anti-acid treatment: randomised controlled trial. Lancet 1994; 343:508–510.

72. Houben MH, Van De Beek D, Hensen EF, et al. A systematic review of *Helicobacter pylori* eradication therapy – the impact of antimicrobial resistance on eradication rates. Aliment Pharmacol Ther 1999; 13:1047–1055.

 The authors offer a comprehensive review of *H. pylori* treatment regimens and the impact of antibiotic resistance.

73. Borody TJ, George LL, Brandl S, et al. *Helicobacter pylori* eradication with doxycycline-metronidazole-bismuth subcitrate triple therapy. Scand J Gastroenterol 1992; 27:281–284.

74. Al-Assi MT, Ramirez FC, Lew GM, et al. Clarithromycin, tetracycline, and bismuth: a new non-metronidazole therapy for *Helicobacter pylori* infection. Am J Gastroenterol 1994; 89:1203–1205.

75. Segura AM, Gutierrez O, Otero W, et al. Furazolidone, amoxycillin, bismuth triple therapy for *Helicobacter pylori* infection. Aliment Pharmacol Ther 1997; 11:529–532.

76. Laine L, Estrada R, Trujillo M, et al. Randomized comparison of ranitidine bismuth citrate-based triple therapies for *Helicobacter pylori*. Am J Gastroenterol 1997; 92:2213–2215.

77. Savarino V, Mansi C, Mele MR, et al. A new 1-week therapy for *Helicobacter pylori* eradication: ranitidine bismuth citrate plus two antibiotics. Aliment Pharmacol Ther 1997; 11:699–703.

78. Wyeth JW, Pounder RE, Duggan AE, et al. The safety and efficacy of ranitidine bismuth citrate in combination with antibiotics for the eradication of *Helicobacter pylori*. Aliment Pharmacol Ther 1996; 10:623–630.

79. Gisbert JP, Gonzalez L, Calvet X, et al. *Helicobacter pylori* eradication: proton pump inhibitor vs. ranitidine bismuth citrate plus two antibiotics for 1 week – a meta-analysis of efficacy. Aliment Pharmacol Ther 2000; 14:1141–1150.

80. Lind T, Megraud F, Unge P, et al. The MACH2 study: role of omeprazole in eradication of *Helicobacter pylori* with 1-week triple therapies. Gastroenterology 1999; 116:248–253.

81. Yousfi MM, El-Zimaity HM, Al-Assi MT, et al. Metronidazole, omeprazole and clarithromycin: an effective combination therapy for *Helicobacter pylori* infection. Aliment Pharmacol Ther 1995; 9:209–212.

82. Dohil R, Israel Dm, Hassall E. Effective 2-wk therapy for *Helicobacter pylori* disease in children. Am J Gastroenterol 1997; 92:244–247.

83. Harris AW, Pryce DI, Gabe SM, et al. Lansoprazole, clarithromycin and metronidazole for seven days in *Helicobacter pylori* infection. Aliment Pharmacol Ther 1996; 10:1005–1008.

84. Laine L, Suchower L, Frantz J, et al. Twice-daily, 10-day triple therapy with omeprazole, amoxicillin, and clarithromycin for *Helicobacter pylori* eradication in duodenal ulcer disease: results of three multicenter, double-blind, United States trials. Am J Gastroenterol 1998; 93:2106–2112.

85. Fennerty MB, Kovacs TO, Krause R, et al. A comparison of 10 and 14 days of lansoprazole triple therapy for eradication of *Helicobacter pylori*. Arch Intern Med 1998; 158:1651–1656.

86. Catalano F, Branciforte G, Catanzaro R, et al. Comparative treatment of *Helicobacter pylori*-positive duodenal ulcer using pantoprazole at low and high doses versus omeprazole in triple therapy. Helicobacter 1999; 4:178–184.

87. Miwa H, Ohkura R, Murai T, et al. Impact of rabeprazole, a new proton pump inhibitor, in triple therapy for *Helicobacter pylori* infection – comparison with omeprazole and lansoprazole. Aliment Pharmacol Ther 1999; 13:741–746.

88. Adamek RJ, Suerbaum S, Pfaffenbach B, et al. Primary and acquired *Helicobacter pylori* resistance to clarithromycin, metronidazole, and amoxicillin – influence on treatment outcome. Am J Gastroenterol 1998; 93:386–389.

89. Treiber G, Wittig J, Ammon S, et al. Clinical outcome and influencing factors of a new short-term quadruple therapy for *Helicobacter pylori* eradication: a randomized controlled trial (MACLOR study). Arch Intern Med 2002; 162:153–160.

90. Lara LF, Cisneros G, Gurney M, et al. One-day quadruple therapy compared with 7-day triple therapy for *Helicobacter pylori* infection. Arch Intern Med 2003; 163:2079–2084.

91. Kimura K, Ido K, Saifuku K, et al. A 1-h topical therapy for the treatment of *Helicobacter pylori* infection. Am J Gastroenterol 1995; 90:60–63.

92. Kihira K, Satoh K, Saifuku K, et al. Endoscopic topical therapy for the treatment of *Helicobacter pylori* infection. J Gastroenterol 1996; 31(Suppl 9):66–68.

93. Dore MP, Leandro G, Realdi G, et al. Effect of pretreatment antibiotic resistance to metronidazole and clarithromycin on outcome of *Helicobacter pylori* therapy: a meta-analytical approach. Dig Dis Sci 2000; 45:68–76.

94. Meyer JM, Silliman NP, Wang W, et al. Risk factors for *Helicobacter pylori* resistance in the United States: the surveillance of *H. pylori* antimicrobial resistance partnership (SHARP) study, 1993–1999. Ann Intern Med 2002; 136:13–24.

95. Osato MS, Reddy R, Reddy SG, et al. Pattern of primary resistance of *Helicobacter pylori* to metronidazole or clarithromycin in the United States. Arch Intern Med 2001; 161:1217–1220.

96. Duck W. Antimicrobial resistance incidence and risk factors among *Helicobacter pylori*-infected persons, United States. Emerg Infect Dis 2004; 10:1088–1094.

 Presented in this paper are the latest prevalence statistics relating to *H. pylori* antibiotic resistance.

97. Oleastro M, Menard A, Santos A, et al. Real-time PCR assay for rapid and accurate detection of point mutations conferring resistance to clarithromycin in *Helicobacter pylori*. J Clin Microbiol 2003; 41:397–402.

98. Abu-Mahfouz MZ, Prasad VM, Santogade P, et al. *Helicobacter pylori* recurrence after successful eradication: 5-year follow-up in the United States. Am J Gastroenterol 1997; 92:2025–2028.

99. Xia HX, Talley NJ, Keane CT, et al. Recurrence of *Helicobacter pylori* infection after successful eradication: nature and possible causes. Dig Dis Sci 1997; 42:1821–1834.

100. Kearney DJ. Retreatment of *Helicobacter pylori* infection after initial treatment failure. Am J Gastroenterol 2001; 96:1335–1339.

101. Hojo M, Miwa H, Nagahara A, et al. Pooled analysis on the efficacy of the second-line treatment regimens for *Helicobacter pylori* infection. Scand J Gastroenterol 2001; 36:690–700.

102. Fakheri H, Malekzadeh R, Merat S, et al. Clarithromycin vs. furazolidone in quadruple therapy regimens for the treatment of *Helicobacter pylori* in a population with a high metronidazole resistance rate. Aliment Pharmacol Ther 2001; 15:411–416.

103. Zullo A, Hassan C, De Francesco V, et al. A third-line levofloxacin-based rescue therapy for *Helicobacter pylori* eradication. Dig Liver Dis 2003; 35:232–236.

104. Perri F, Festa V, Clemente R, et al. Randomized study of two 'rescue' therapies for *Helicobacter pylori*-infected patients after failure of standard triple therapies. Am J Gastroenterol 2001; 96:58–62.

105. Chen M, Lee A, Hazell S, et al. Immunisation against gastric infection with *Helicobacter* species: first step in the prophylaxis of gastric cancer? Zentralbl Bakteriol 1993; 280:155–165.

106. Marchetti M, Arico B, Burroni D, et al. Development of a mouse model of *Helicobacter pylori* infection that mimics human disease. Science 1995; 267:1655–1658.

107. Ikewaki J, Nishizono A, Goto T, et al. Therapeutic oral vaccination induces mucosal immune response sufficient to eliminate long-term *Helicobacter pylori* infection. Microbiol Immunol 2000; 44:29–39.

108. Ghiara P, Rossi M, Marchetti M, et al. Therapeutic intragastric vaccination against *Helicobacter pylori* in mice eradicates an otherwise chronic infection and confers protection against reinfection. Infect Immun 1997; 65:4996–5002.

109. Michetti P, Kreiss C, Kotloff KL, et al. Oral immunization with urease and *Escherichia coli* heat-labile enterotoxin is safe and immunogenic in *Helicobacter pylori*-infected adults. Gastroenterology 1999; 116:804–812.

110. Kotloff KL, Sztein MB, Wasserman SS, et al. Safety and immunogenicity of oral inactivated whole-cell *Helicobacter pylori* vaccine with adjuvant among volunteers with or without subclinical infection. Infect Immun 2001; 69:3581–3590.

111. Chalker AF, Minehart HW, Hughes NJ, et al. Systematic identification of selective essential genes in *Helicobacter pylori* by genome prioritization and allelic replacement mutagenesis. J. Bacteriol 2001; 183:1259–1268.

112. Malfertheiner P, Megraud F, O'Morain C, et al. Current European concepts in the management of *Helicobacter pylori* infection – the Maastricht Consensus Report. The European *Helicobacter Pylori* Study Group (EHPSG). Eur J Gastroenterol Hepatol 1997; 9:1–2.

113. Chey WD, Fendrick AM. Noninvasive *Helicobacter pylori* testing for the 'test-and-treat' strategy: a decision analysis to assess the effect of past infection on test choice. Arch Intern Med 2001; 161:2129–2132.

114. Fendrick AM, Chey WD, Margaret N, et al. Symptom status and the desire for *Helicobacter pylori* confirmatory testing after eradication therapy in patients with peptic ulcer disease. Am J Med 1999;1 07:133–136.

115. Parsonnet J, Harris RA, Hack HM, et al. Modelling cost-effectiveness of *Helicobacter pylori* screening to prevent gastric cancer: a mandate for clinical trials. Lancet 1996; 348:150–154.

116. Ladabaum U, Chey WD, Scheiman JM, et al. Reappraisal of non-invasive management strategies for uninvestigated dyspepsia: a cost-minimization analysis. Aliment Pharmacol Ther 2002; 16:1491–1501.

CHAPTER NINETEEN

19

Therapy and prevention of NSAID-related gastrointestinal disorders

Jaime Oviedo and M. Michael Wolfe

INTRODUCTION

History

More than a century has passed since Felix Hoffman, at the suggestion of Hermann Dreser, the chief pharmacologist at Bayer Corporation, synthesized acetylsalicylic acid as the first non-steroidal antiinflammatory drug (NSAID).[1,2] The compound was named 'aspirin,'[3] and it later proved to be a convenient method for the delivery of salicylic acid to treat rheumatic diseases, pain, and fever.[2] The first reports providing endoscopic evidence that aspirin carried the potential to induce gastric mucosal damage in humans date to 1938.[4] Since that time, numerous reports have corroborated these findings,[5–9] and the subsequent introduction of many potent agents with even greater toxicity, such as indomethacin, phenylbutazone, and piroxicam, led to an increase in the occurrence of NSAID-induced gastroduodenal injury and provided the motivation for the development of effective NSAIDs with a more favorable safety profile.

Starting in the early 1970s, numerous new NSAIDs were developed that were purportedly free of gastrointestinal (GI) toxicity. However, because few, if any, of these agents are entirely innocuous, newer compounds were developed to improve the safety profile of NSAIDs while maintaining their antiinflammatory and analgesic properties.

NSAIDS and gastrointestinal toxicity: epidemiology and scope of the problem

NSAIDs are one of the most commonly used medications world-wide. In the United States alone, more than 70 million NSAID prescriptions and 30 billion over-the-counter preparations are sold every year.[10] Although NSAIDs are generally well tolerated, adverse GI events occur in a small, but significant, percentage of patients, resulting in substantial morbidity and mortality. Adverse effects from NSAIDs range from dyspepsia to serious GI complications that may lead to hospitalization and considerable use of resources. The prevalence of dyspepsia while taking NSAIDs may be as high as 50% in some series,[11,12] depending on variations in the terminology used to report GI symptoms. In a recent meta-analysis using a strict definition based on epigastric pain-related symptoms, NSAIDs increased the risk of dyspepsia by 36%.[13] Nearly 15% of patients with rheumatoid arthritis (RA) will choose to discontinue NSAID therapy as a result of dyspepsia and other GI symptoms.[13]

The risk of serious GI complications in patients with RA and osteoarthritis (OA) taking NSAIDs has been estimated at 13 and 7.3 per 1000 patients per year, respectively.[14] The risk of NSAID-induced ulceration and complications is dose-related and increases with age, the concomitant use of corticosteroids or anticoagulants, higher doses of NSAIDs, including the use of more than one NSAID, and a history of prior ulcer disease or serious systemic disorders.[10,15–17] The mortality rate attributed to NSAID-related GI toxicity is 0.22% per year, with an annual relative risk of 4.21, compared with the risk for persons not using NSAIDs.[17] NSAIDs are used regularly by at least 13 million people with arthritides in the US, with a world market for NSAIDs rapidly growing from US$6 billion per year in the mid-1990s,[1] to US$10 billion in 2000.[18] The annual direct costs of managing NSAID-related GI complications exceeds US$2 billion.[19]

PATHOGENESIS OF NSAID-INDUCED GI TOXICITY

More than 90% of gastroduodenal ulcers are associated with the use of NSAIDs or with chronic infection with the bacterium *Helicobacter pylori (H. pylori)*. NSAID-related gastrointestinal damage is, however, not limited to the stomach and duodenum, as these agents are capable of causing injury throughout the length of the GI tract.[20,21] Although NSAID-induced esophageal injury has been reported infrequently, some reports have described pill esophagitis and ulceration associated with the ingestion of these acidic compounds.[22–24] An association between aspirin and NSAID use (including over-the-counter NSAIDs and low-dose aspirin) and esophageal strictures, specially in older individuals, has also been reported.[25] Finally, NSAIDs have been shown to produce a so-called enterocolopathy, which is characterized by a protein- and blood-losing enteropathy, colonic injury resembling inflammatory bowel disease, and the development of small intestinal ulcers, diaphragms, and strictures (Table 19.1).[26–28] This chapter will focus on injury to the upper GI tract.

Damage to the gastroduodenal mucosa occurs as a result of both the topical and systemic effects of NSAIDs.[10] Mucosal injury is initiated topically by the acidic properties of aspirin and many other NSAIDs. In addition, topical mucosal injury may occur as a result of indirect mechanisms mediated through the biliary excretion and subsequent duodenogastric reflux of active NSAID metabolites.[29]

Although topical injury caused by NSAIDs contributes to the development of gastroduodenal mucosal injury, the systemic effects

Table 19.1 Adverse effects of aspirin and NSAIDs on the gastrointestinal tract

Esophagus
Pill esophagitis/ulceration
Esophageal strictures

Stomach and duodenum
Gastroduodenal ulcers

Small bowel
Protein/blood-losing enteropathy
Ulcerations
Diaphragm
Strictures

Colon
Colitis
Colonic perforation
Colonic ulcers/bleeding
Diaphragm-like strictures
? Inflammatory bowel disease (onset and reactivation)
? Development of collagenous colitis

prostaglandins and leukotrienes is catalyzed by the cyclooxygenase (COX) pathway and the 5-lipoxygenase (LOX) pathway, respectively (Fig. 19.1).[1,19,29] Two related but unique isoforms of COX, designated COX-1 and COX-2, have been demonstrated in mammalian cells.[33,34] Despite their structural similarities, each is encoded by distinct genes that differ with regard to their distribution and expression in tissues; the COX-1 gene is primarily expressed constitutively, while the COX-2 gene is inducible.[10]

COX-1 appears to function as a 'housekeeping' enzyme in most tissues, including the gastric mucosa, the kidneys, and platelets, whereas the expression of COX-2 can be induced by inflammatory stimuli and mitogens in many different types of tissue, including macrophages and synovial cells.[35] It has thus been suggested that the antiinflammatory properties of NSAIDs are mediated through the inhibition of COX-2, whereas adverse effects, such as gastroduodenal ulceration, occur as a result of effects on the constitutively expressed COX-1 (Fig. 19.2).[33,35] The discovery of the two COX isoforms led to the development of COX-2-specific inhibitors, drugs that maintain their antiinflammatory properties while preserving the biosynthesis of protective prostaglandins. Standard NSAIDs differ in their relative inhibitory potency against COX-1 and COX-2, ranging from high selectivity ratios favoring COX-1 inhibition to nearly equivalent suppression of both isoforms (Fig. 19.3). The important role of COX-1 in protecting the gastroduodenal mucosa is supported by studies showing that the greatest degree of damage to the gastroduodenal mucosa is generally caused by NSAIDs that preferentially inhibit COX-1, such as naproxen, piroxicam, sulindac, and indomethacin.[36]

RISK FACTORS FOR NSAID-RELATED UPPER GI CLINICAL EVENTS

Because dyspeptic symptoms are not a reliable warning sign for the development of serious NSAID-related mucosal injury, it is crucial to identify patients who are at increased risk of developing serious GI events associated with NSAID therapy.[10] Several factors have been reported to significantly increase the risk of developing NSAID-associated GI events (Table 19.3). Important clinical

of these agents appear to play the dominant role.[1] For example, gastroduodenal ulcers occur with equal frequency using enteric-coated NSAID preparations and cutaneous gels, and following rectal and parenteral administration of these agents.[26–30] These systemic effects are largely the result of the inhibition of endogenous prostaglandin (PG) synthesis, although decreased production of other factors such as nitric oxide (NO), trefoil peptides, and calcitonin gene-related peptide may also be involved. While the entire process by which a reduction in mucosal PG synthesis generates mucosal injury has not been fully elucidated, PGs play a major role by stimulating several local components of the normal defensive properties inherent to the gastroduodenal mucosa (Table 19.2).[23,31] PGs also inhibit acid secretion by reducing the generation of cyclic AMP by the gastric parietal cell.[32]

Prostaglandins are derived from arachidonic acid, which originates from cell membrane phospholipids through the action of phospholipase A2. The metabolism of arachidonic acid to

Table 19.2 Mucosal protective properties inherent to the gastroduodenal mucosa

Pre-epithelial
Enhancement of mucus secretion
Increase in bicarbonate ion secretion

Epithelial
Increase in mucosal blood flow
Enhancement of intercellular tight junctions
Decrease in transmembrane H$^+$ ion permeation

Subepithelial
Increase in rate of cell restitution, i.e., epithelial cell renewal

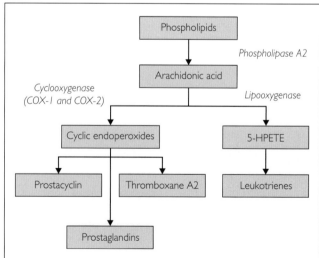

Fig. 19.1 • Biosynthesis of prostaglandins and leukotrienes via the cyclooxygenase and lipoxygenase pathways, respectively. The immediate precursor, arachidonic acid, is derived from membrane phospholipids.

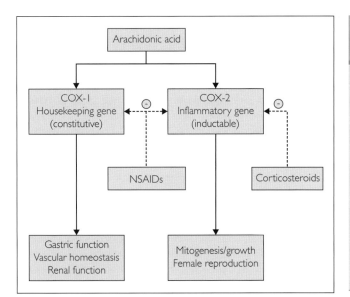

Fig. 19.2 • Depiction of the two cyclooxygenase (COX) isoenzymes that catalyze the synthesis of tissue prostaglandins from arachidonic acid. COX-1 is expressed constitutively and maintains normal homeostasis, including gastric mucosal defense. In contrast, COX-2, the inflammatory gene, is inducible. Although both pathways can be variably inhibited by different nonsteroidal antiinflammatory drugs (NSAIDs), only the COX-2 gene contains a corticosteroid-responsive repressor element in its promoter.

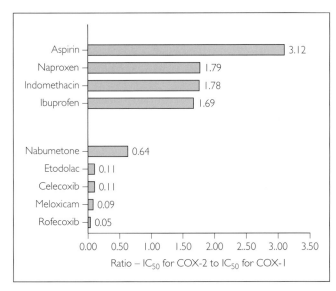

Fig. 19.3 • Selectivity of COX-2 inhibitors. Comparison of in vivo concentration (IC_{50}) ratios (COX-2: COX-1) of selective and nonselective NSAIDs. A lower ratio indicates increased selectivity for COX-2. (Adapted from Feldman M, McMahon AT. Do cyclooxygenase-2 inhibitors provide benefits similar to those of traditional NSAIDs, with less gastrointestinal toxicity? Ann Intern Med 2000; 132:134–143; with permission.)

factors that are validated in multiple studies include increasing age, history of ulcer or GI complications, concomitant anticoagulation therapy, concomitant corticosteroid use, and high-dose NSAID use.[10,37]

Advanced age has consistently been found to represent one of the primary risk factors for GI events.[10,37] The likelihood of serious events appears to increase in linear fashion, with no significant increase in ulcer bleeding reported among patients aged 35–49

Table 19.3 Risk factors for development of NSAID-associated mucosal injury
Proven
Age (older than 60 years)
History of ulcer or GI complications
Concomitant anticoagulation therapy
Concomitant corticosteroid use
High dose of NSAID or use of more than one NSAID
Serious systemic disorder
Duration and severity of arthritis
Possible
Concomitant infection with *Helicobacter pylori*
Cigarette smoking
Ethanol abuse

and a 2.9-fold increase in patients aged 50–64 years.[38] Furthermore, mortality due to upper GI hemorrhage, the most common ulcer complication associated with NSAID use, increases logarithmically with age.[39] While advanced age represents a definite risk, gender-related differences probably do not,[15] and previous suggestions to the contrary likely reflect an increased use of NSAIDs by women.[23,40]

A prior history of gastroduodenal ulcer or GI events may be the most important risk factor for future events.[23,37] A meta-analysis of 10 case-control studies reported an OR of 4.8 (95% CI, 4.1–5.6) for patients with a prior history of a GI event.[41] In addition, a history of ulcer or ulcer complications increases the risk of future GI events in all patients, regardless of their NSAID use.[37] Concomitant use of oral anticoagulants has been reported to increase the risk of hospitalization for bleeding ulcers in NSAID users >65 years old 12.7 times (95% CI, 6.3–25), while the risk in NSAID users not receiving anticoagulants was 4.0 (95% CI, 3.4–4.8).[42,43] Although corticosteroid use alone does not appear to increase the risk of ulcer or ulcer complications,[44] the concomitant use of a corticosteroid and NSAIDs increases the risk of GI events by 10-fold.[16] A meta-analysis of three studies reported an OR for upper GI bleeding of 1.8 (95% CI, 1.2–2.8) for steroid use compared with no steroid use in NSAID users.[15]

Several studies have documented that the risk of upper GI complications increases proportionally to the NSAID dose employed.[45–47] The magnitude of the relative risk varies among the different studies, but increases consistently in a linear fashion. While several epidemiological studies have suggested that the risk of GI complications is highest in the first month of NSAID use,[37,48] and that adaptation occurs with time,[41] other studies indicate that the risk of NSAID-associated GI hemorrhage remains constant or increases steadily over an extended period of observation.[49,50] Therefore, elderly patients who might require high-dose NSAID therapy for a short period or those who might use them intermittently appear to be at highest risk.

Other less well-validated risk factors for the occurrence of NSAID-related upper GI injury include: systemic comorbidities, disability and severity of RA, *H. pylori* infection, type of NSAID use, and presence of dyspepsia. Although supporting data are limited, the presence of concurrent illnesses, such as heart disease, appears to increase the risk of developing NSAID-associated GI events. Furthermore, the presence of comorbidities in patients who develop complications such as GI bleeding will significantly increase the risk of death due to the complication.[51] A multivariate analysis of the MUCOSA trial suggested a modest increase of GI events in NSAID users with heart disease (OR 1.8; 95% CI, 1.1–3.2),[17] but apparently not with other comorbid conditions.[37,52] In a different report, both heart failure and diabetes were found to increase the likelihood of ulcer bleeding in NSAID users.[53] However, a recent multivariate analysis of the Vioxx Gastrointestinal Outcomes Research (VIGOR) study found no evidence of an increased risk of NSAID-related GI complications in patients with heart disease.[43] Although not consistently identified as predictors of GI events, severity of disability and duration of RA has been found to represent significant risk factors in several multivariate analyses.[43,45,52]

Helicobacter pylori

Helicobacter pylori and NSAIDs are both recognized risk factors for the development of ulcer disease, but whether a synergistic relationship between the presence of this organism and NSAID use plays a role in the development of ulcers or ulcer complications is controversial. Most,[54–57] but not all,[58,59] studies have found these two risk factors to be independent. For example, Chan et al.[59] treated *H. pylori*-infected patients with naproxen with or without *H. pylori* eradication therapy for 8 weeks. The study found that individuals treated for *H. pylori* before they began taking naproxen had significantly fewer ulcers (7%) than patients who were given naproxen only (26%). Although the authors concluded that the eradication of *H. pylori* reduces the occurrence of NSAID-induced ulcers, antimicrobial therapy used in this study included the use of a bismuth compound, which possesses ulcer-healing properties independent of its effects on the bacterium.[60]

Other case-control studies have been performed to assess the interaction of *H. pylori* and NSAID use in ulcer bleeding. Although Aalykke et al. reported a borderline significant increase in *H. pylori* infection among NSAID users with ulcer bleeding (OR, 1.8; 95% CI, 1.0–3.2),[61] other studies do not show a significant increase in bleeding with *H. pylori* infection,[62–65] and some studies suggest a possible protective effect of *H. pylori* in ulcer bleeding, especially gastric ulcer bleeding.[62,64,65]

In conclusion, most studies do not support the contention that *H. pylori* infection increases the risk of ulcer formation in individuals receiving NSAIDs. Because both NSAID use and *H. pylori* infection are independent risk factors for ulcer disease, they should be removed when possible in individual patients.[37]

Risk with individual NSAIDs

While all NSAIDs currently in use possess the capacity to induce GI mucosal injury, the relative risk varies among the various preparations. These differences may be due to several factors, including variations in relative potency for inhibiting prostaglandin synthesis, duration of action, systemic absorption, drug solubility in gastric juices, and pH-dependent partition in the gastroduodenal mucosa.[23] Several studies have reported the greatest risk of complications with piroxicam[15,27,46] and ketorolac,[66] and relatively low risk with the use of ibuprofen. Griffin et al.[47] reported relative risks for ulcer formation with several NSAIDs ranging from a low of 2.3 for ibuprofen to a high of 8.7 for meclofenamate. A meta-analysis by Gabriel et al.[15] and a case control study by Henry et al.[27] found the greatest risk of complications with piroxicam, with progressively lower risk ratios for indomethacin, aspirin, naproxen, and ibuprofen. A study by Garcia-Rodriguez and Jick[46] also found piroxicam to carry the greatest relative risk for developing hemorrhage or perforation. In their study, however, the NSAID with the least likelihood of precipitating an ulcer complication, ibuprofen, still carried a relative risk of 2.9 (Table 19.4).[46] Of those nonselective NSAIDs commonly used, ibuprofen appears to carry the lowest risk of developing gastroduodenal ulcers,[67] and low-dose ibuprofen preparations available without prescription in the US are associated with a relative risk of ulcer complications that approaches placebo rates.

Other potential, but unproven, risk factors for NSAID-induced ulcers include smoking and alcohol use. Smoking is an established risk factor in gastroduodenal ulceration and is associated with delayed ulcer healing, but whether smoking (or ethanol) increases this risk in NSAID users is unknown. Nevertheless, owing to other health benefits, cigarette smoking and excessive consumption of ethanol should be discouraged in individuals taking NSAIDs.

Dyspepsia

Although at least 20% of patients who are receiving long-term therapy with aspirin or NSAIDs for arthritis or coronary prophylaxis experience dyspepsia during the course of treatment, dyspeptic symptoms do not predict the presence of gastroduodenal mucosal injury.[10,11,23,68,69] As many as 50% of patients with NSAID-related dyspepsia may have a normal-appearing gastroduodenal mucosa on endoscopy,[10] and conversely, nearly 60% of individuals hospitalized for NSAID-related GI hemorrhage,[70] and up to 70% of patients with arthritis and NSAID-related ulcers report no preceding symptoms.[11]

High doses of any NSAID, as well as any dose of indomethacin, meclofenamate, or piroxicam, increase the risk of dyspepsia by about 3-fold.[71] Whether COX-2 selective inhibitors decrease the prevalence of dyspepsia has not been determined. A recent study by

Table 19.4 Relative risks of upper gastrointestinal tract events in users of individual NSAIDs compared with nonusers

Drug	Relative risk (95% CI)
Ibuprofen	1.9 (1.6–2.2)
Aspirin	1.6 (1.3–2.5)
Diclofenac	3.3 (2.8–3.9)
Sulindac	3.6 (2.8–4.7)
Naproxen	4.0 (3.5–4.6)
Indomethacin	4.6 (3.8–5.5)
Ketoprofen	4.6 (3.3–6.4)
Piroxicam	6.3 (5.5–7.2)
Ketorolac	24.7 (9.6–63.5)

Data from Garcia Rodriguez[66]; Henry[197]; Hernandez-Diaz[198].

Lisse et al.,[72] which did not include a control group, suggested that the use of rofecoxib was associated with a lower rate of NSAID discontinuation and the concomitant use of additional medication.

However, because dyspepsia is quite common, even in patients not taking NSAIDs, a comparison with a control group not taking NSAIDs is necessary to determine the increase in risk. Despite claims to the contrary,[45,48,52,73] dyspepsia is not generally considered a useful predictor for GI events because most complications occur without antecedent symptoms.[29]

TREATMENT

Treatment of NSAID-related dyspepsia

H₂-receptor antagonists

Dyspeptic symptoms are commonly reported by patients taking NSAIDs and include heartburn, abdominal pain, nausea, abdominal distention, and anorexia. In a prospective, double-blind European study,[74] 127 symptomatic individuals using NSAIDs without significant endoscopic abnormalities were randomized to treatment with either cimetidine 400 mg twice daily or placebo. Ninety-five percent of the patients had upper abdominal pain, 60% percent had nausea, and 75% had heartburn. While only 49% of those receiving placebo reported resolution of their symptoms, 72% of those receiving cimetidine reported complete symptomatic remission. In a second study, van Groenendael et al.[75] investigated the efficacy of ranitidine 150 mg twice daily in treating NSAID-related dyspeptic symptoms in patients with RA and osteoarthritis (OA). Among those without endoscopic evidence of any mucosal damage, only 6% and 26% of patients treated with placebo and ranitidine, respectively, had complete disappearance of their dyspeptic symptoms.

In another study, Taha et al.[76] compared placebo with two different doses of famotidine in the prevention of gastroduodenal ulcers in RA and OA patients receiving NSAIDs. As a secondary goal of the study, the effects of famotidine on dyspeptic symptoms were evaluated. At baseline, approximately 30% of patients reported abdominal pain, and at the end of the 24-week study nearly the same percentage of patients (29%) receiving placebo reported abdominal pain. In those randomly assigned to receive famotidine, pain was reported in 19% of those taking famotidine 20 mg twice daily and in 17% taking 40 mg twice daily, reductions of 36.6% and 43.3%, respectively.[76] Taking into account differences in methodology, these studies appear to provide evidence for the beneficial effects of H₂-receptor antagonists (H₂RAs), and it would thus seem reasonable to recommend the use of low doses of H₂RAs for symptomatic relief of dyspeptic symptoms associated with the use of NSAIDs. Although the initial regimen of an H₂RA should generally be low dose (e.g., cimetidine 400 mg, ranitidine or nizatidine 150 mg, or famotidine 20 mg, all twice daily), dosing should be flexible and must be optimized to meet the individual needs of each specific patient.

Proton pump inhibitors

In a study by Ekstrom,[77] patients with no or mild dyspepsia, and with a need for continuous NSAID treatment, were randomized to receive either 20 mg omeprazole once daily or placebo. Gastroduodenal ulcers, erosions, and dyspeptic symptoms were evaluated after 1 and 3 months. The development of moderate to severe dyspepsia requiring active treatment, either alone or in combination with ulcers or erosions, occurred in 15.3% (15 of 85) of patients treated with omeprazole and 35.6% of those who received placebo.

A double-blind trial comparing omeprazole 20 mg once daily and ranitidine 150 mg twice daily in NSAID users demonstrated that omeprazole was significantly more effective than ranitidine in decreasing the incidence of dyspepsia. Over a 4-week period, the proportion of patients with moderate to severe upper GI symptoms decreased from 52% to 6% in those receiving omeprazole, compared to a reduction from 50% to 12% in those taking ranitidine ($p<0.05$).[78]

More recently, two double-blind, placebo-controlled trials, with a total of over 1000 NSAID users, evaluated the use of esomeprazole 20 mg and 40 mg once daily for the control of upper GI symptoms.[67,79,80] Both doses of esomeprazole were significantly more effective than placebo in relieving upper GI symptoms as demonstrated by the change on a 7-point symptom scale. The median time to relief of symptoms was 7–10 fewer days with esomeprazole than with placebo. Esomeprazole was also superior to placebo in maintaining quality of life following the initial improvement of symptoms.[81] The role of antisecretory therapy for treatment of upper GI symptoms in patients receiving low-dose aspirin is less clear. In a recent double-blind trial, when compared with placebo, PPI therapy significantly reduced heartburn, but not other aspirin-associated symptoms.[82]

Treatment of NSAID-related gastroduodenal ulcer complications

When gastroduodenal injury occurs in the setting of chronic NSAID, therapy is usually directed to achieve three goals: management of ulcer complications, such as bleeding, obstruction or perforation, healing of the acute NSAID-induced gastroduodenal ulcer, and prophylaxis of ulcer recurrence. GI hemorrhage is the most common ulcer complication, and as stated previously, the majority of individuals hospitalized for NSAID-related GI hemorrhage reported no antecedent symptoms.[70] In contrast, up to 25% of individuals who develop hemorrhage without prior NSAID use report a history of dyspeptic symptoms preceding the bleeding episode. The reasons for this difference are unknown, but may be related in part to the analgesic properties of NSAIDs. Nevertheless, 'silent' hemorrhage may contribute to increased mortality by several mechanisms, including the precipitation of cardiac and cerebrovascular ischemic events, and the inadvertent progression to severe hemodynamic instability. Regardless of its etiology, the control of hemorrhage is the cornerstone of therapy and is generally achieved by endoscopic hemostatic therapy in conjunction with intensive acid suppression. Treatment of upper GI hemorrhage is discussed in detail in Chapter 21.

Treatment of acute NSAID-related gastroduodenal ulcers

The optimal treatment for patient with NSAID-induced gastroduodenal ulcers is the discontinuation of any potentially causative or aggravating factors. When possible, NSAID therapy should be suspended and replaced with less toxic agents. However, if NSAID use must be continued, the ability to heal ulcers varies among different antisecretory and other agents. The treatment of acute gastroduodenal ulcers is discussed in detail in Chapter 20.

Mucosal protective agents

Sucralfate

Sucralfate, a basic aluminum salt of sucrose octasulfate, is effective in the treatment and prophylaxis of duodenal ulcers (DU) and appears to be as effective as H₂ receptor antagonists (H₂RA) in the healing of gastric ulcers (GU).[83] Similarly, sucralfate heals DUs as effectively as H2RAs whether or not NSAIDs are continued.[83] However, this agent has no proven benefit in the treatment of NSAID-associated GUs.[83]

Prostaglandins

Prostaglandins (PGs) exert their therapeutic effects both by enhancing mucosal defensive properties inherent to the gastroduodenal mucosa and by inhibiting acid secretion.[10] While the protective effect is observed with all doses of PGs, acid secretion is affected only with higher doses, and only antisecretory doses have proven clinical benefit. Although PGs are effective in preventing gastroduodenal mucosal injury associated with the use of NSAIDs, their role in the treatment of NSAID-associated ulcers is less well studied. Roth et al.[84] compared the effects of placebo and misoprostol 200 μg four times daily in RA patients with gastroduodenal mucosal injury associated with high-dose aspirin. Injury ranged from subepithelial hemorrhage to frank ulceration. After 8 weeks of therapy, misoprostol healed 86% of duodenal mucosal injury and 70% of gastric mucosal injury, compared with placebo healing rates of 53% and 25%, respectively. Unfortunately, because clinically irrelevant mucosal lesions were included in the analysis and since complete ulcer healing was not the end point examined in this study, the results are difficult to interpret.

More recently, in the OMNIUM Study, Hawkey et al.[85] compared the ability of misoprostol (200 μg four times daily) and omeprazole (20 mg or 40 mg daily) to heal gastroduodenal ulcers in patients continuing NSAID therapy. After 8 weeks of therapy, omeprazole at both doses healed 89% of the duodenal ulcers, compared to 77% in those receiving misoprostol. Gastric ulcer healing was detected in 80%, 87%, and 73% of those receiving omeprazole 40 mg, omeprazole 20 mg, and misoprostol, respectively.[85] Because misoprostol is clearly less effective than omeprazole and is associated with a significantly greater incidence of adverse effects, the use of prostaglandins cannot be recommended for the treatment of active gastroduodenal ulcers associated with the continued use of NSAIDs.

Antisecretory medication

H₂-receptor antagonists

Although H₂-receptor antagonists (H₂RAs) are quite effective in the healing of gastroduodenal ulcers when NSAIDs are stopped, the healing rates are significantly lower when NSAIDs are continued. Several open, uncontrolled, nonrandomized studies,[86,87] as well as prospective, randomized studies,[88–90] have found that conventional doses of H₂RAs administered for 6 to 12 weeks will heal approximately 75% (50–88%) of GUs and approximately 87% (67–100%) of DUs despite continued NSAID use.

When NSAIDs are continued, healing appears to be delayed and is largely dependent on the initial ulcer diameter. In a randomized study of 190 patients with endoscopically confirmed gastroduodenal ulcers, patients were assigned to continue or discontinue NSAID therapy. All patients were treated with ranitidine 150 mg b.i.d. After 8 weeks, healing of GUs was observed in only 63% of those taking NSAIDs, compared with 95% of those who had stopped them. For DUs, the corresponding 8-week healing rates were 84% in the group continuing NSAIDs and 100% in those who had discontinued them. Extending therapy for an additional 4 weeks improved healing rates to 79% and 92% in those with GUs and DUs, respectively, despite continued NSAID use.[91]

A second study assessed the relevance of the initial gastric ulcer diameter on ulcer healing associated with the use of H₂RAs. An 8-week course of cimetidine combined with unrestricted antacid use demonstrated healing of 90% of small GUs (<5 mm in diameter) notwithstanding the continued use of NSAIDs, whereas only 25% of ulcers >5 mm in diameter healed during the same time period.[90] Extending therapy for an additional 6–26 months resulted in healing of 86% of large ulcers despite continued NSAID use.

Therefore, it appears that although the healing of large gastric ulcers is delayed when NSAID use is continued, healing may be achieved provided H₂RA therapy is continued for an extended period of time. However, with the advent of more potent antisecretory agents such as PPIs, the use of H₂RAs in the healing of NSAID-related ulcers is no longer recommended as first-line therapy.

Proton pump inhibitors

Although the topical effects of NSAIDs are an important factor for the development of gastroduodenal mucosal damage, gastric acid certainly plays an integral role in the pathogenesis of ulcers. Thus, Schwarz's dictum,[92] 'No acid, no ulcer,' initially thought to apply to ulcers associated with infection with H. pylori and with gastric acid hypersecretion, also holds true for ulcers due to NSAIDs. Several studies have demonstrated that healing of DUs is proportional to the suppression of both nocturnal and 24-hour acid secretion.[93,94] A multicenter trial by Walan et al.[95] compared the efficacy of omeprazole (20 mg or 40 mg daily) and ranitidine (150 mg twice daily) in the treatment of patients with GUs, and included a group of 68 patients who continued to take NSAIDs while receiving antisecretory therapy. In this latter group of individuals, GU healing rates at 4 weeks were 81% in the group receiving 40 mg of omeprazole, 61% in the group treated with 20 mg of omeprazole, and 32% in the group receiving ranitidine. The corresponding healing rates after 8 weeks were 95%, 82%, and 53%, respectively, indicating considerable improvement with more potent suppression of gastric acid secretion. Furthermore, patients treated with omeprazole had healing rates similar to ranitidine-treated patients who had discontinued using their NSAIDs.[95] These studies suggest that while GU healing by H₂RAs appears to be impeded by continued NSAID use, proton pump inhibitors (PPIs) possess the capacity to heal GUs at an accelerated rate whether or not NSAIDs are continued.

As stated earlier, Hawkey et al.[85] also found omeprazole to be superior to misoprostol in healing gastroduodenal ulcers in patients who continued to take NSAIDs. After 8 weeks of therapy, GU healing was detected in 80% and 87% of those receiving 40 mg and 20 mg of omeprazole, respectively. DU healing was documented in 89% for both doses of omeprazole. More recently, Agrawal et al.[96] compared the efficacy of lansoprazole (15 mg and 30 mg daily) and ranitidine (150 mg twice daily) in the healing of GUs at least 0.5 cm in diameter in patients continuing NSAID therapy. After 8 weeks, ulcers were healed in 61% of the individuals taking ranitidine, while healing rates were 69% and 73% in those treated with lansoprazole 15 mg and 30 mg, respectively. In the ASTRONAUT study[78] evaluating a group of 541 patients, omeprazole was found to be superior to ranitidine in the treatment of NSAID-related gastroduodenal ulcers. Ulcer healing rates at 8 weeks were 79%, 80%, and 63% in those receiving 40 mg omeprazole, 20 mg omeprazole, and 150 mg ranitidine twice daily, respectively.

Finally, a recent pooled analysis of two studies including 846 patients with confirmed gastric ulcers receiving nonselective COX-2 selective NSAIDs, demonstrated that the PPI esomeprazole at doses of 20 mg and 40 mg daily is more effective than ranitidine in healing GUs associated with the continuous use of NSAIDs. The healing rates at 8 weeks of treatment were 88.6%, 86.6% and 75.3%, for esomeprazole 40 mg, esomeprazole 20 mg daily, and ranitidine 150 mg twice daily, respectively ($p < 0.002$).[97]

These observations demonstrate that PPIs are an effective form of therapy for ulcer healing in patients with NSAID-associated ulcers who continue NSAID treatment. Because their accelerated rates of healing and superior safety profile, PPIs are preferred over both H_2RAs and misoprostol in the treatment of NSAID-associated gastroduodenal ulcers.

Prophylaxis of NSAID-related gastroduodenal ulcers

General principles

Because of the significant rate of serious complications associated to NSAID use and the inability of dyspeptic symptoms to reliably predict the presence of gastroduodenal mucosal injury, the primary prevention of GI toxicity has become the principal goal in the care of patients on chronic NSAID therapy. The ideal strategy to prevent NSAID-related gastrointestinal injury is to minimize the use of these drugs and substitute them with less injurious agents, such as acetaminophen. However, in reality, and because of their superior ability to provide symptomatic relief from the pain associated with inflammatory processes, NSAID use is commonly preferred. Furthermore, aspirin continues to be used widely in the prevention and treatment of ischemic heart disease, peripheral vascular disease, and cerebrovascular disease, as well as more recently in the prevention of colorectal cancer.

Although the effects of aspirin and NSAIDs in inciting gastroduodenal mucosal injury are usually dose-dependent, aspirin doses as low as 30 mg, significantly less than the 81 mg present in 'baby' formulations, inhibit gastric prostaglandin output,[98] and carry the potential to cause injury. The widespread availability of these agents to consumers who may use them without medical supervision will certainly increase the likelihood of their use and the frequency of significant associated GI events.

Significant controversy exists regarding the clinical relevance of endoscopic mucosal damage associated with the use of NSAIDs. In general, acute injury consisting of intramucosal hemorrhage and erosions is commonly observed during short periods of NSAID administration and correlates poorly with the subsequent development of gastroduodenal ulceration and ulcer complications during prolonged use.[10] This spectrum of mucosal changes is known as 'NSAID gastropathy' and, in variable degrees of severity, can be documented with the use of virtually all NSAIDs even at over-the counter doses.[99]

Although the presence of erosions does not correlate well with the development of ulcers, ulcer formation is clearly related to secondary complications, such as hemorrhage and perforation.[17]

Early studies evaluating gastroduodenal mucosal damage and the use of protective agents to prevent mucosal injury produced by NSAIDs often employed endoscopy scores that included superficial lesions such as intramucosal hemorrhages.[100] Because these lesions are generally regarded as clinically irrelevant, most of the subsequent endoscopic studies have only documented the presence or absence of gastroduodenal ulcers.[101] Two strategies have been used to prevent NSAID-related ulcers: the use of concomitant medications such as mucosal protective agents, prostaglandins and antisecretory agents, and the development of safer antiinflammatory agents, such as COX-2 selective inhibitors and nitric oxide (NO)-releasing NSAIDs.

The use of concomitant medication to prevent NSAID-related ulcers

Sucralfate

Despite weak antacid properties, the protective effect of sucralfate is not mediated by acid suppression or neutralization, but by its protective effect on the gastric mucosa, which is mediated by several mechanisms (Table 19.5).[76,102,103]

Sucralfate has been shown to reduce, but not eliminate, gastroduodenal mucosal injury associated with the use of NSAIDs.[104] Caldwell et al.[105] randomized osteoarthritis patients treated with NSAIDs to receive either sucralfate 1 g four times daily or placebo. The endoscopic score and the reported dyspeptic symptoms were significantly better in the group receiving sucralfate than in the placebo group. Sucralfate was therefore portrayed as an effective form of concomitant therapy in patients receiving NSAIDs.[105]

In a study by Agrawal et al.[106] comparing the efficacy and frequency of adverse events of sucralfate and misoprostol in the prevention of GUs in osteoarthritis patients receiving NSAID therapy, 253 individuals receiving NSAIDs were randomized to receive either sucralfate 1 g four times daily or misoprostol 200 μg four times daily. Endoscopy was performed at 4-week intervals for a total of 3 months. The development of a GU at least 3 mm in diameter was regarded as a prophylaxis failure. While only 1.6% of patients receiving misoprostol developed an ulcer, 16.2% of those treated with sucralfate were found to have a GU during the 3-month period of observation. This frequency of ulcer development in the sucralfate-treated group in this study was similar to the incidence found in the placebo arm of other studies. In contrast, in a study by Miglioli et al.[107] evaluating sucralfate gel in the short-term prevention of gastroduodenal lesions in 107 patients with arthritis treated with NSAIDs, subjects were randomized to receive diclofenac 200 mg daily or naproxen 1 g daily plus either sucralfate gel 1 g twice daily (n = 53) or identical placebo (n = 54) for 14 days. All patients had a normal endoscopy at the beginning of the study. At 14 days, the reported frequency of heartburn and epigastric pain, the incidence of erosions, and the mean endoscopic score for both stomach and duodenum were significantly

Table 19.5 Therapeutic effects of sucralfate
Formation of a mucosal protective barrier
Stimulation of gastric mucosal blood flow
Prostaglandin-mediated increase in mucus and bicarbonate secretion
Stimulation of growth factors implicated in ulcer healing

lower in the sucralfate gel group compared with placebo group. The overall difference in the occurrence of gastroduodenal ulcers was also statistically significant (8% in sucralfate-treated patients versus 28% in patients receiving placebo, $p<0.05$).

In summary, although sucralfate may reduce the incidence of symptoms and endoscopic lesions, other agents appear superior and require once-daily use; therefore, the use of this agent cannot be recommended as first-line therapy for the prevention of NSAID-induced ulcers.

H₂-receptor antagonists

Early studies that evaluated the ability of H₂RAs to prevent NSAID-related gastroduodenal ulcers lacked uniformity with regard to experimental design. Specifically, endoscopy score, rather than ulcer development was often used as an end point, follow-up was short, and healthy volunteers, rather than individuals with arthritis, were used as study subjects. Two large placebo-controlled, prospective trials investigated the protective effect of ranitidine in arthritis patients receiving concomitant NSAID therapy.[108,109] An 8-week course of treatment with ranitidine 150 mg b.i.d. proved to be effective in preventing DU formation, with rates of 0% and 1.5% in the two studies, compared to 8% in placebo-treated patients in both.[108,109] In contrast to its beneficial effects in the duodenum, ranitidine was ineffective in preventing GUs in both studies.

In another study, Taha et al.[76] compared placebo with two different doses of famotidine (20 mg and 40 mg twice daily) in the prevention of gastroduodenal ulcers in RA and OA patients receiving NSAIDs for 24 weeks. Endoscopy was performed at baseline and after 4, 12, and 24 weeks of therapy. The cumulative incidence of GUs was 20%, 13%, and 8% in those receiving placebo, famotidine 20 mg and 40 mg twice daily, respectively, and the cumulative incidence of DUs in the three groups was 13%, 4%, and 2%, respectively.[76] As stated previously, the incidence of abdominal pain decreased by approximately 40% in the two groups receiving famotidine.

In comparative studies, misoprostol has been shown to be more effective than ranitidine for the prevention of NSAID-induced gastric ulcers. In a multicenter, 8-week, double-blind study, patients were randomized to receive ranitidine 150 mg twice daily or misoprostol 200 μg four times daily. Follow-up endoscopy was performed after 4 and 8 weeks of treatment. GUs were found in only 1/180 (0.56%) patient on misoprostol and in 11/194 (5.67%) patients on ranitidine, a difference that was statistically significant ($p<0.01$). DU rates were similar for the ranitidine (2/185 or 1.08%) and misoprostol (2/181 or 1.10%) groups.[110] While both agents appear to effectively prevent NSAID-induced duodenal ulcers, misoprostol appears to be statistically superior to H₂RAs in preventing gastric ulcers associated with the use of NSAIDs, particularly when the latter are used in low doses (e.g., famotidine 20 mg or ranitidine 150 mg twice daily).[110,111] Even at higher doses, such as those used by Taha et al.,[76] H₂RAs appear to be less effective than misoprostol in preventing NSAID-related gastric ulcers.

Finally, a prospective observational cohort study by Singh et al.[12] found that asymptomatic RA patients taking H₂RAs had a significantly *higher* risk for GI complications compared to those not taking these drugs. Therefore, although effective in reducing dyspeptic symptoms associated with the use of NSAIDs, the routine use of H₂RAs in the prophylaxis of NSAID-associated gastroduodenal ulcers cannot be recommended.

Proton pump inhibitors

Several studies have clearly demonstrated that PPIs reduce the incidence of NSAID-associated ulcers. Scheiman et al.[112] randomized 20 healthy volunteers to a double-blind, placebo-controlled crossover study to determine whether omeprazole 40 mg daily could prevent gastroduodenal mucosal injury due to the use of 2 weeks of aspirin 650 mg four times daily. Fifty percent of patients developed duodenal mucosal injury while on placebo, including 15% who developed frank ulceration. Omeprazole completely protected the duodenal mucosa from aspirin-induced injury. Seventy percent of patients developed gastric mucosal injury while on placebo, including 25% with gastric ulcers. Omeprazole reduced the severity of gastric mucosal injury by 45%, and only one subject developed an aspirin-associated ulcer while on omeprazole.[112] In a study by Cullen,[113] omeprazole 20 mg once daily was better than placebo in the prophylaxis of gastroduodenal ulcers in patients using NSAIDs. Four percent of patients on omeprazole developed ulcers, compared to 16% in the placebo group. A reduction in the incidence of both GUs (4% versus 11%) and DUs (0% versus 7%) was reported.

In addition to examining ulcer healing, the ASTRONAUT study[78] compared omeprazole and ranitidine in the prevention of gastroduodenal ulcers in 432 patients (425 available for evaluation) arthritic patients in whom ulcers had healed and NSAID therapy was continued for 6 months. Patients were randomized to receive omeprazole 20 mg daily or ranitidine 150 mg twice daily. At the end of 6 months, 16.3% and 4.2% of those given ranitidine developed GUs and DUs, respectively, while only 5.2% developed a GU and 0.5% a DU in the omeprazole group.

In the OMNIUM study,[85] the ability of omeprazole and misoprostol in preventing ulcer recurrence was compared in patients with arthritis on continuous NSAID therapy. In this double-blind, placebo-controlled trial, 732 patients in whom ulcers had healed were randomized to receive placebo, 20 mg of omeprazole once daily or 200 μg of misoprostol twice daily as maintenance therapy. After 6 months, DUs were detected in 12% and 10% of those treated with placebo and misoprostol, respectively, while only 3% of those treated with omeprazole developed a DU. GU relapse occurred in 32%, 10%, and 13% of the individuals receiving placebo, misoprostol, and omeprazole, respectively. Recently, Agrawal et al.[114] confirmed that PPI therapy is more effective than ranitidine in the healing of GUs in patients who continue taking NSAIDs. Their study showed that lansoprazole 15 mg and 30 mg once daily, healed 69% and 73% of GUs, respectively, compared to 53% healed with ranitidine 150 mg twice daily. These studies suggest that PPIs are superior to H₂-receptor antagonists in preventing NSAID-induced gastroduodenal mucosal injury and in maintaining patients in remission during continued NSAID use.

Misoprostol

As stated above, the mucosal protective effects of PGs are seen at all doses, while higher doses also inhibit acid secretion by preventing the generation of intracellular cyclic AMP in gastric parietal cells.[32] Paradoxically, doses of misoprostol that inhibit the generation of cyclic AMP in parietal cells *stimulate* its synthesis in the small intestine.[115] As a result, enterocytes secrete more and absorb less fluid and electrolytes, and intestinal smooth muscle contraction is enhanced, all of which precipitate diarrhea, the principal adverse effect of PGs. Numerous studies have shown that misoprostol, a synthetic E1 prostaglandin analogue, is effective in preventing NSAID-induced gastroduodenal ulcers, but only when administered at doses sufficient to inhibit acid secretion and consequently produce diarrhea.

Five multicenter, prospective, randomized, blinded trials have evaluated the ability of misoprostol to prevent gastroduodenal ulceration in patients taking NSAIDs.[85,101,106,116,117] In their landmark study Graham et al.[101] examined patients with OA and associated abdominal pain who were taking ibuprofen, piroxicam, or naproxen. Of the 420 patients enrolled, 139 patients were randomly assigned to receive misoprostol 200 μg four times daily, 143 to misoprostol 100 μg four times daily, and 138 patients to placebo during continued NSAID use. All enrolled patients underwent endoscopy at baseline and at 1, 2 and 3 months after initiating therapy. The cumulative 3-month prevalence of GUs was 1.4% for high-dose misoprostol, 5.6% for low-dose misoprostol, and 21.7% for placebo.[101] These numbers are likely exaggerated as approximately 40% of the ulcers were 2–4 mm in diameter, lesions more likely to be erosions and less likely to precipitate complications. Nevertheless, if only lesions greater than 5 mm in diameter are considered, the results of the study remain proportionally similar, with a corresponding cumulative 3-month GU prevalence of 0.7%, 4.2%, and 12.3%, respectively.[101] This important study led to FDA approval of misoprostol at a dose of 200 μg four times daily for the prevention of NSAID-induced gastric ulcers.

In a direct comparison with sucralfate 1 g four times daily, misoprostol 200 μg four times daily was superior in the prevention of gastric ulceration. At 3 months, GUs occurred in only 2 of 122 (1.6%) of those subjects taking misoprostol, compared to 21 of 131 (16%) of individuals taking sucralfate.[106] When ulcer diameter was restricted to those of greater than 0.5 cm diameter, the ulcer rates were 0.8% and 9.2%, for misoprostol and sucralfate, respectively.[106]

With regard to the prevention of NSAID-associated DUs, neither of the above studies included patient samples sufficiently large to draw meaningful conclusions. Because a retrospective analysis suggested that DU prophylaxis could be achieved using misoprostol, Graham et al. evaluated the ability of this agent to prevent NSAID-induced duodenal ulcers. In a third study,[116] a group of 638 patients with chronic arthritis were randomized to receive either misoprostol 200 μg four times daily or placebo while continuing NSAID treatment. Unlike the previous two studies, symptoms were not required for patient entry. During 3 months of therapy, the capacity of misoprostol to prevent NSAID-induced GUs was confirmed. Furthermore, misoprostol significantly reduced the incidence of DUs from 4.6% in those taking placebo to 0.6% in those taking misoprostol.[116]

In all studies, misoprostol therapy did not interfere with the antiinflammatory effects of the NSAID, and dose adjustments were not required for patients with renal insufficiency. However, despite the efficacy of misoprostol in preventing gastroduodenal ulcers, a beneficial effect in improving dyspeptic symptoms attributable to NSAIDs has not been proven. During the initial study by Graham et al.,[106] 70% of misoprostol patients reported no dyspeptic symptoms after 3 months of treatment. However, 57% of placebo patients were similarly pain-free, a difference not statistically significant. Furthermore, diarrhea developed in 13% of placebo-treated patients, 25% of patients taking the 100 μg dose of misoprostol, and 39% of those taking the 200 μg dose of misoprostol.[106]

Because the incidence of diarrhea associated with misoprostol use is dose-dependent, Raskin et al.[117] conducted a randomized, double-blind, placebo-controlled trial to evaluate the prophylactic efficacy, tolerability, and safety of three different doses of misoprostol (200 μg two, three, and four times daily). The study included 1197 arthritic patients receiving NSAIDs for 12 weeks. Endoscopy was performed at baseline and after 4, 8, and 12 weeks of therapy. In the placebo group, the incidence of gastric and duodenal ulcers at least 3 mm in diameter was 15.7% and 7.5%, respectively. The cumulative incidence of GUs was reduced in all three groups of patients receiving misoprostol: twice daily, 8.1%; three times daily, 3.9%; and four times daily, 4.0%. The GU rate was significantly greater in patients receiving misoprostol twice daily compared with those receiving the drug three times per day. Likewise, misoprostol reduced the incidence of DUs: Twice daily, 2.6%; three times daily, 3.3%; and four times daily, 1.4%.[117] Diarrhea occurred in 10% of patients who received placebo and in 22%, 29%, and 26% of the patients receiving misoprostol 200 μg two, three, and four times a day, respectively.[117] While dyspepsia was similar in all groups, abdominal pain was *more* common in patients receiving misoprostol. Finally, the incidence of withdrawal for adverse events was significantly higher in the group receiving misoprostol four times daily (20%) than in the groups receiving the drug two or three times daily (12% each).[117]

In a subsequent study, Raskin et al. demonstrated clear superiority of misoprostol 200 μg four times daily over ranitidine 150 mg twice daily in reducing the incidence of GUs in matching groups of 269 arthritic patients taking NSAIDs for 2 months. Only one patient in the misoprostol group (0.56%), compared with 11 in the ranitidine group (5.67%) developed ulcers. In the patients treated with misoprostol, however, abdominal pain, flatulence, and diarrhea were all more common, causing early withdrawal from the study in 13% of the patients, compared to a 6.7% withdrawal rate in the ranitidine group.[110,118]

In a continuation of their study comparing ulcer healing with omeprazole and misoprostol, Hawkey et al.[119] assessed the ability of these agents to prevent gastroduodenal ulcers in patients receiving NSAIDs in a randomized, double-blind placebo-controlled fashion. Patients received placebo, misoprostol 200 μg twice daily, or omeprazole 20 mg daily. After 6 months of observation, during which time upper endoscopy was performed at 1, 3, and 6 months, DUs were detected in 12% and 10% of those treated with placebo and misoprostol, respectively, while only 3% of those treated with omeprazole developed a DU. GU relapse occurred in 32%, 10%, and 13% of the individuals receiving placebo, misoprostol, and omeprazole, respectively.[119] Thus, in addition to being better tolerated than misoprostol, PPIs appear to be at least as effective as misoprostol in preventing NSAID-associated gastroduodenal ulcers.

Because NSAID-associated ulcers and serious complications often develop in the absence of warning symptoms, and endoscopic injury not always correlate with poor clinical outcomes, complications represent a more reliable indicator to truly assess the adverse effects of NSAID therapy. In the MUCOSA trial, a large, randomized, double-blind, placebo-controlled study, Silverstein and colleagues demonstrated that misoprostol 200 μg four times daily reduced the incidence of serious upper GI complications, such as perforation, gastric outlet obstruction, or bleeding, in elderly patients with arthritis who were receiving NSAIDs. Odds ratio was calculated at 0.598 (95% CI, 0.364–0.982; $p=0.049$) for patients receiving misoprostol (25 of 4404 patients) compared with those receiving placebo (42 of 4439 patients), a reduction of 40% in the incidence of ulcer complications. Once again, the withdrawal rate due to side effects, mainly diarrhea and abdominal pain, was significantly higher in the misoprostol group than in the placebo group (42.0% versus 36.4%, $p<0.001$).[17] This study provided conclusive evidence for the benefit of misoprostol in the prophylaxis of NSAID-associated gastroduodenal ulcer complications and confirmed that a decrease in the incidence of endoscopic ulcers may be associated with a reduction in the rate of complications.

Recent studies comparing misoprostol with PPIs in the prophylaxis of NSAID-induced gastroduodenal injury have confirmed that although effective, the high incidence of adverse effects with misoprostol make the use of this agent impractical. A study by Graham et al.[120] compared misoprostol 200 µg four times daily with lansoprazole 15 mg and 30 mg daily in *H. pylori*-negative chronic NSAID users who had a GU. Misoprostol was shown to be superior to lansoprazole for prevention of gastroduodenal ulcers. For example, at 12 weeks, 93% of patients in the misoprostol group and 80–82% of patients in the two lansoprazole groups showed no evidence of recurrent ulcers. The ulcer rates were 15, 43, and 47 per 100 patient years for misoprostol, lansoprazole 15 mg and lansoprazole 30 mg, respectively. However, because of the higher withdrawal rate in the misoprostol group, there was no practical advantage of misoprostol over lansoprazole.[121]

Another randomized, double-blind study compared the efficacy and tolerability of pantoprazole 20 mg once daily with misoprostol 200 µg twice daily, for 6 months in 515 rheumatic patients who required long-term therapy with NSAIDs. Estimated remission rates at 3 and 6 months were 93% and 89%, respectively for pantoprazole, and 79% and 70% for misoprostol. Pantoprazole was superior to misoprostol ($p=0.005$) with regard to endoscopic injury (occurrence of a peptic ulcer, significant gastroduodenal erosions or reflux esophagitis) after 6 months. Patients withdrawing from the study early due to adverse events related to the study drug accounted for 13/257 (5%) in the pantoprazole and 33/258 (13%) in the misoprostol treatment groups. At the end of the analysis, pantoprazole was found to be superior to misoprostol ($p<0.001$) in the prevention of ulcers, erosions, reflux esophagitis, severe gastrointestinal symptoms, and adverse events leading to study withdrawal.[122]

In summary, the results of all these studies indicate that misoprostol is effective in preventing gastroduodenal ulcers and ulcer complications in chronic NSAID users. However, the high incidence of adverse effects makes the use of this agent impractical. In addition to diarrhea and abdominal pain, another significant side effect of misoprostol is increased uterine contractility that can lead to spontaneous abortion, and it is therefore contraindicated in women of childbearing age who are sexually active. Although lower doses of misoprostol are better tolerated, which is likely to improve patient compliance, the drug still needs to be taken at least three times per day to provide adequate prophylaxis for the development of NSAID-associated GUs. The concomitant use of a PPI and an NSAID appears to be more effective and safe for the prophylaxis of gastroduodenal injury, and will be discussed in detail later in the chapter.

The use of safer NSAIDS with diminished GI toxicity

Several modifications in the formulation of NSAIDs have been introduced in an attempt to reduce their toxicity. Because of their insufficient buffering capacity, conventional over-the-counter buffered aspirin products appear to offer little protection against the risk of mucosal injury. Similarly, enteric-coated preparations result in delayed, but not decreased, salicylate absorption, and lead to a similar degree of gastric mucosal PG inhibition.[123] Another alternative is the use of nonacetylated salicylate as an antiinflammatory agent. For example, salsalate neither inhibits endogenous PG synthesis nor precipitates gastroduodenal mucosal damage.[124] Salsalate, a nonacetylated salicylate that is insoluble at the usual acidic gastric pH, inhibits gastric mucosal PG synthesis minimally and as a result, topical gastroduodenal mucosal injury observed with this agent is generally less than that seen with enteric-coated aspirin, despite equivalent serum salicylate concentrations.[124,125] Attempts to avoid topical mucosal injury by the parenteral administration of an NSAID such as ketorolac or the rectal administration of NSAIDs such as indomethacin have also failed to reduce the development of ulcers and their complications.[26,27] Finally, the development of prodrugs to avoid direct gastroduodenal mucosal injury has provided no relevant clinical benefit. For example, sulindac is a prodrug that undergoes hepatic metabolism to its active moiety, sulindac sulfide, which is then excreted into the biliary tree. The active metabolite not only refluxes back into the stomach to produce indirect topical toxicity, but it also inhibits COX-1 and thus confers no significant protective advantage over other nonselective NSAIDs.[126]

Some NSAIDs are also relatively selective (preferential) for COX-2 at low doses. Nabumetone, etodolac, and meloxicam appear to be more effective inhibitors of COX-2 than COX-1 with an IC_{50} ratio of 10–20 to 1.[127–129] Nabumetone, another prodrug, has been reported to be less toxic due to several factors.[130] Its nonacidic structure avoids mucosal trapping and consequently direct topical mucosal injury, and it is metabolized in the liver to its active moiety, 6-methoxy-2 napthyl acetic acid. However, in contrast to sulindac, it is not excreted into the biliary tree, but rather undergoes renal excretion. At low doses, nabumetone preferentially inhibits COX-2, with little effect on COX-1,[131] which, along with the absence of topical (direct and indirect) toxicity, appears to account for its somewhat improved safety profile. Etodolac also preferentially inhibits COX-2; however, in contrast to nabumetone, it is not a prodrug, but rather is ingested in a metabolically active form.[130] Etodolac, which has some COX-2 selectivity, causes significantly less mucosal injury than traditional NSAIDs (naproxen, ibuprofen, indomethacin), apparently because of a lack of significant effect on mucosal PG production.[132] A recent historical cohort analysis found that etodolac reduced the incidence of upper GI events by 61% compared to naproxen, an effect that was negated by the concomitant administration of aspirin.[133]

In a large 6-week, placebo-controlled endoscopic trial, nabumetone (1500 mg daily) was associated with significantly fewer gastric or duodenal ulcers than naproxen (500 mg twice daily; 11% versus 37%) but significantly more than placebo (11% versus 5%).[134] Although no large-scale studies are available to document that the reduction in mucosal injury translates into a decrease in clinical events, post hoc analyses suggest that nabumetone, and perhaps etodolac, induce fewer significant GI complications.[135,136]

Meloxicam is also a COX-2 preferential agent (at doses =15 mg daily), with efficacy similar to other NSAIDs.[129] In two large 4-week double-blind trials comparing lower-dose meloxicam (7.5 mg daily) with diclofenac (100 mg daily), or with piroxicam (20 mg daily), in 9323 patients with OA, adverse GI events were reported in

5 patients taking meloxicam and 7 taking diclofenac.[137] The piroxicam study of 8656 patients with osteoarthritis reported clinical upper GI events in 7 patients taking meloxicam and 16 patients taking piroxicam.[137] Although these differences were not significant, a meta-analysis of 12 randomized trials suggested a reduction in reported clinical GI events with meloxicam.[129] Low doses of meloxicam were generally used during these trials, which may have contributed to the lower incidence of adverse GI events in this group of patients.

Postmarketing surveillance[138–141] and short-term endoscopic studies[142–145] have reported a lower incidence of gastroduodenal mucosal injury associated with the use of both nabumetone and etodolac. In a study involving 37 arthritic patients, significantly less gastroduodenal ulceration was observed endoscopically with nabumetone 1 g daily when compared to naproxen 500 mg daily.[142] Among those treated with nabumetone, only one patient developed an ulcer and one an erosion after 12 weeks of treatment, while in naproxen treated individuals, five developed an ulcer and five developed erosions during the trial period.[142]

Similarly, Roth et al.[144] reported no significant difference in the incidence of gastroduodenal ulcers in patients treated for 3 months with either nabumetone 1 g daily alone or a combination of ibuprofen 2.4 g daily plus misoprostol 200 μg q.i.d. (1.7% and 0% cumulative incidence, respectively). In the same prospective study, 15.1% of patients treated with ibuprofen alone were found to have endoscopically-verified ulcers at least 5 mm in diameter.[144] In a US postmarketing survey of 1912 arthritic patients treated with nabumetone,[138] ulcers were identified in only 13 (0.7%) and no complications were reported. Likewise, an analysis of 10 800 arthritic patients treated with nabumetone in the United Kingdom reported only 11 (0.1%) serious complications, seven of which were GI hemorrhage.[139] A review of treatment with etodolac from 3702 patients participating in double-blind studies and 8334 patients in open-label clinical trials found a 0.3% incidence of gastroduodenal ulcer formation, with no reports of bleeding or perforation.[140]

In another study, Singh et al.[136] reviewed the serious GI toxicity of 18 NSAIDs during 9570 courses of therapy, corresponding to 19 258 patient years, in consecutively diagnosed rheumatoid arthritis patients from eight American Rheumatism Association Medical Information System (ARAMIS) centers in North America. Serious toxicity was defined as GI hemorrhage and other clinically significant events requiring hospitalization. No events were reported with the use of either nabumetone or etodolac during 221 and 88 patient years of therapy, respectively.[136] These data thus corroborate other studies and are consistent with the hypothesis that the preferential inhibition of COX-2 may improve the safety profile of NSAIDs.[146] Meloxicam was also found to be associated with a lower incidence of ulcer complications in a large global safety analysis of data from clinical studies.[147]

COX-2 selective inhibitors

Based on their markedly diminished capacity to produce gastroduodenal mucosal injury,[146,148–151] highly selective COX-2 inhibitors were developed and marketed as a result of increasing concern over the adverse effects of NSAIDs on the gastrointestinal tract (Table 19.6).

In 1971, Vane[152] and Smith and Willis[153] independently described the inhibition of the cyclooxygenase (COX) enzyme by aspirin, resulting in a reduction in prostaglandin synthesis. This observation led to the hypothesis that both the toxicity and efficacy of NSAIDs are mediated through the inhibition of PG synthesis.[154] The existence of the inducible isoform of COX (COX-2) was first suspected in 1990, when Needleman and his group reported that bacterial lipopolysaccharide (LPS) increased the synthesis of prostaglandins in human monocytes in vitro and in mouse peritoneal macrophages in vivo.[155] This increase was inhibited by dexamethasone and was associated with de novo synthesis of a new COX protein. One year later, Herschman and Simmons independently reported the isolation of an inducible COX identified as a distinct isoform of cyclooxygenase (COX-2) encoded by a different gene from COX-1.[156,157]

As discussed earlier, the two isoforms of the COX enzyme are responsible for prostaglandin biosynthesis (see Figs 19.1, 19.2): the constitutive isoform, COX-1, performs housekeeping functions including gastroprotection, while the inducible form, COX-2, is involved in the inflammatory response. This observation suggested that differential inhibition of these isoforms could account for the

Table 19.6 COX-2 selective inhibitors

Compound	Present status	Approved use
1st generation		
Celecoxib (Celebrex®)	Approved 1998. "black box" warning February 2005	RA, OA, pain
Rofecoxib (Vioxx®)	Approved 1999. Withdrawn September 2004.	RA, OA, pain
2nd generation		
Valdecoxib (Bextra®)	Approved 2001. Withdrawn February 2005	RA, OA, dysmenorrhea
Lumiracoxib	Awaiting approval	
Parecoxib	Awaiting approval	Parenteral route
Etoricoxib	In development	
COX-189	In development	

RA, rheumatoid arthritis; OA, osteoarthritis

variable toxicity of NSAIDs.[157] Although all the effects of NSAIDs cannot be attributed to their inhibition of COX, it is generally accepted that inhibition of COX-2 contributes to an NSAIDs efficacy, whereas inhibition of COX-1 contributes to its GI toxicity.

The landmark discovery of the two COX isoforms and the perceived distinction between their biological roles sparked a concerted effort by the pharmaceutical industry to design safer NSAIDs. The culmination of this process was the development of two COX-2-specific inhibitors, celecoxib and rofecoxib, drugs that maintain their antiinflammatory properties while preserving the biosynthesis of protective PGs. As mentioned above, standard NSAIDs differ in their relative inhibitory potency against COX-1 and COX-2, ranging from high selectivity ratios favoring COX-1 inhibition to nearly equivalent suppression of both isoforms (see Fig. 19.3). The important role of COX-1 in protecting the gastroduodenal mucosa is supported by studies showing that the greatest degree of damage to the gastroduodenal mucosa is generally caused by NSAIDs that preferentially inhibit COX-1, such as naproxen, piroxicam, sulindac, and indomethacin.

In February 1999, celecoxib, the first 'highly selective' COX-2 inhibitor, became available in the US, followed 6 months later by rofecoxib. Selective COX-2 inhibitors received approval from the US Food and Drug Administration (FDA) for use in RA (celecoxib) and OA (celecoxib and rofecoxib). These drugs have at least a 200- to 300-fold selectivity for inhibition of COX-2 relative to COX-1.[158] COX-2 selective inhibitors maintain their antiinflammatory properties while preserving the biosynthesis of protective COX-1-derived prostaglandins. Although some differences in selectivity do exist within the class,[159] these agents appear to be as effective as nonselective NSAIDs in suppressing inflammation and providing analgesia, while reducing the incidence of endoscopic ulcers to levels similar to those seen with placebo.[160,161]

Two large trials have addressed the efficacy of coxibs and the associated risk of gastrointestinal complications, the Celecoxib Long-Term Arthritis Safety Study (CLASS) trial,[162] and the Vioxx Gastrointestinal Outcomes Research (VIGOR) trial (Table 19.7).[50] The CLASS study,[162] a 6-month randomized, double-blind, controlled trial, compared the GI toxicity of celecoxib with traditional NSAIDs in individuals with OA and RA. The study included 7968 patients who were randomly assigned to receive 400 mg of celecoxib twice daily (two and four times the maximum FDA-approved dosages for RA and OA, respectively); ibuprofen, 800 mg three times daily; or diclofenac, 75 mg twice daily. Baseline characteristics of the treatment groups were similar in terms of risk factors for ulcer complications, including age, primary rheumatologic disorder, prior history of GI bleeding or ulcer, *H. pylori* infection, tobacco or alcohol use, and concurrent use of aspirin, corticosteroids, or anticoagulants. The predetermined primary outcome to be assessed was the occurrence of ulcer complications termed POBs (perforation, gastric outlet obstruction, and bleeding). The annualized 6-month incidence of POBs plus symptomatic ulcers in patients taking celecoxib was 2.08% compared to 3.54% for those receiving ibuprofen or diclofenac ($p=0.02$). The annualized incidence rates of ulcer complications alone for celecoxib and nonselective NSAIDs were 0.76% and 1.45%, respectively ($p=0.09$), a trend favoring celecoxib that did not achieve statistical significance (Fig. 19.4).

The increased ulcer complication rate for celecoxib can be partially attributed to the use of a supratherapeutic dosage of celecoxib and possibly the inclusion of patients taking low-dose (<325 mg/d) aspirin for cardiovascular prophylaxis. Twenty-one percent of the patients enrolled in this trial were receiving low-dose aspirin, twice the rate reported in other celecoxib clinical trials.[163] Even this small dose of aspirin has been shown to increase the risk of upper GI hemorrhage in several studies,[98,164] and may have offset some of the protective effect of COX-2 selectivity for celecoxib in this trial. Within the celecoxib group, the relative risk (RR) of an ulcer complication was 4.5 when low-dosage aspirin was taken ($p=0.01$). Moreover, for patients taking aspirin, the annualized incidence rates of ulcer complications alone for celecoxib and nonselective NSAIDs were 2.01% and 2.12% ($p=0.92$), respectively; for complications combined with symptomatic ulcers, the rates were 4.7% and 6.0% ($p=0.49$), respectively. Therefore, a small ulcer risk reduction for celecoxib among

Table 19.7 Comparison of VIGOR and CLASS study designs

	VIGOR (n=8076)	CLASS (n=7982)
Drug	Rofecoxib 50 mg/day (2 times maximum dose)	Celecoxib 400 mg/day (2 times maximum dose)
Patients	Rheumatoid arthritis	Osteoarthritis 72% Rheumatoid arthritis 28%
Comparator	Naproxen 500 mg b.i.d.	Diclofenac 75 mg t.i.d. Ibuprofen 800 mg t.i.d.
Low-dose aspirin	No	Yes (21%)
Duration	Median 9 months Maximum 13 months	Median 9 months Maximum 13 months
Analysis	Intent to treat	Excluded events 0–2 days and >6 months
1E endpoint	Clinically significant UGI events	Complicated ulcers
2E endpoint	Complicated UGI events	Clinically significant ulcers

VIGOR, Vioxx Gastrointestinal Outcomes Research
CLASS, Celecoxib Long-Term Arthritis Safety Study
b.i.d., twice daily; t.i.d., three times daily

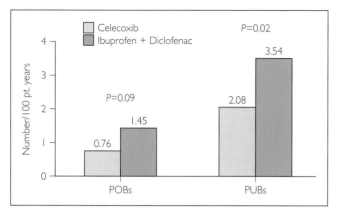

Fig. 19.4 • Six-month annualized data from the CLASS study comparing the incidence rates of GI events per 100 patient (PT)-years. POBs denote ulcer complications (perforation, obstruction and bleeding), whereas PUBs comprise ulcer complications and symptomatic ulcers. (Data from Silverstein F et al. JAMA 2000; 284:1247–1255; with permission.)

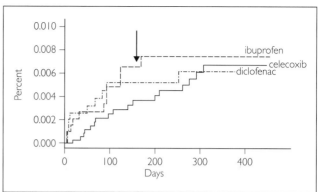

Fig. 19.6 • Kaplan-Meier estimator for incidence of clinically significant GI events associated with CLASS study. Arrow indicates point in time where incidence of GI events was measured and annualized. The annualization of 6-month data may have led to an underestimation of the true prevalence of significant GI events. (Data from FDA Arthritis Advisory Board, February 2001.)

patients taking low-dose aspirin may exist that cannot be conclusively discerned by the study due to the small number of patients taking aspirin (type II error). Conversely, for patients not taking aspirin the annualized incidence of POBs was significantly lower with celecoxib than with ibuprofen and diclofenac: 0.44% versus 1.27% (p=0.04). The annualized incidence of ulcer complications combined with symptomatic ulcers in patients not taking aspirin was also significantly lower with celecoxib than with the comparator drugs: 1.40% versus 2.91% (p=0.02) (Fig. 19.5). Because a placebo group was not included in this study, it is not possible to calculate accurately an ulcer complication risk attributable to celecoxib. Furthermore, because 6-month data were annualized, investigators may have underestimated the incidence of clinically significant upper GI events with prolonged use of celecoxib, as illustrated in a Kaplan-Meier plot (Fig. 19.6).

Although the difference in the primary outcome measure did not reach statistical significance, the results of the CLASS study suggest that celecoxib and possibly other COX-2-selective NSAIDs effectively reduce the risk of symptomatic ulcers and ulcer complications, at least among individuals who do not take aspirin.[165]

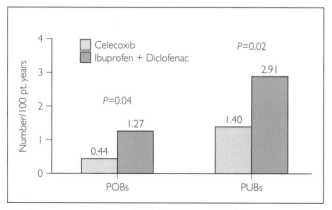

Fig. 19.5 • Six-month annualized data comparing incidence rates of GI events for subjects not taking aspirin and participating in the CLASS study. POBs denote ulcer complications (perforation, obstruction and bleeding), while PUBs comprise ulcer complications and symptomatic ulcers. (Data from Silverstein F et al. JAMA 2000; 284:1247–1255; with permission.)

The VIGOR trial was conducted to compare the incidence of clinically important GI events in patients on rofecoxib with those on the traditional NSAID naproxen. Previous endoscopic studies demonstrated that rofecoxib is associated with a reduced incidence of gastroduodenal ulcers when compared to traditional NSAIDs.[166,167] A total of 8076 patients with RA were randomized to receive rofecoxib (50 mg once daily) or naproxen (500 mg twice daily) for a planned minimum follow-up of 6 months. The median duration of treatment was 9 months. The primary end point was confirmed clinical upper GI events (gastroduodenal perforation or obstruction, upper GI bleeding, and symptomatic gastroduodenal ulcers, i.e., 'PUBs'). The incidence of confirmed GI events per 100 patient-years was lower in the rofecoxib group than in the naproxen group (2.1 and 4.5 per 100 patient-years, respectively [RR 0.46; 95% CI 0.3–0.6; p<0.001]) (Fig. 19.7). The respective rates of complicated confirmed events (perforation, obstruction, and severe upper GI bleeding) i.e., POBs (secondary outcome), were 0.6 per 100 patient-years and 1.4 per 100 patient-years (RR 0.43; 95% CI, 0.2–0.8; p=0.005) (Fig. 19.8). This significant difference was apparent within 6 weeks of starting treatment. The data indicated that only 41 patients would need to be treated with rofecoxib rather than naproxen to avert one clinical upper GI event during a one-year period. A subgroup analysis confirmed that the lower risk of GI adverse events with rofecoxib was maintained in patients with significant risk factors, including age >65, steroid use, prior history of upper GI perforations or obstructions, symptomatic ulcers and bleeds, and *H. pylori* infection. In addition, the risk of bleeding from anywhere in the upper or lower GI tract was also significantly lower in the rofecoxib group than the naproxen group (1.1% versus 3.0%, p<0.001). A subsequent analysis of this cohort,[73] with stratification of risk factors based on individual clinical characteristics, showed that elderly patients (>75 years of age) and individuals with prior upper GI events or severe RA disability, appeared to derive an even greater benefit from protective strategies such as the use of selective COX-2 inhibitors. Only 10–12 of these high-risk individuals would need to be treated with rofecoxib in place of naproxen to avert a clinical GI event.[73]

Discontinuation of therapy due to upper GI symptoms, common with traditional NSAIDs, was significantly lower with rofecoxib

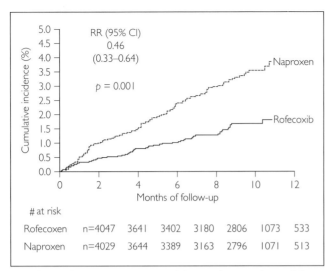

Fig. 19.7 • Kaplan-Meier estimator of the cumulative incidence of the primary end point of confirmed upper GI events among all randomized patients in the VIGOR study. (Bombardier C, et al. N Engl J Med 2000; 343:1520–1528, with permission.)

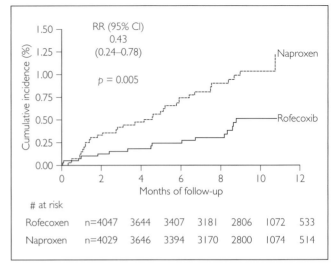

Fig. 19.8 • Kaplan-Meier estimator of the cumulative incidence of the secondary end point of confirmed complicated upper GI events among all randomized patients in the VIGOR study. (Bombardier C, et al. N Engl J Med 2000; 343:1520–1528, with permission.)

than with naproxen (3.5% versus 4.9%). The investigators concluded that in patients with RA, treatment with rofecoxib was associated with significantly fewer clinically important upper GI events than treatment with naproxen, a nonselective COX inhibitor. In summary, VIGOR is the first study to demonstrate a 63% risk reduction in the occurrence of major upper GI bleeds (RR=0.37, p=0.004) and a 54% reduction in lower GI bleeds (RR=0.46, p=0.032) (Table 19.8). The evidence from this trial also demonstrates that the decreased incidence of ulcers is associated with improved clinical outcomes and increased safety.[165]

Since the clinical introduction of celecoxib and rofecoxib, new 'second-generation' COX-2 inhibitors have been developed and evaluated by the FDA. In 2001, valdecoxib received approval in the US for use in patients with OA and RA at a recommended dose of 10 mg once daily. Second-generation COX-2 inhibitors are approximately four times more selective than their predecessors.[168] Although a greater degree of COX-2 selectivity might theoretically confer an enhanced clinical benefit, the majority of clinical trials data do not suggest an improvement in efficacy or safety profiles when compared with 'first-generation' agents. In clinical studies lasting 3 to 6 months, valdecoxib 10 mg once daily was as effective as traditional NSAIDs for the treatment of OA,[169] and doses of 10–40 mg daily were significantly less likely to cause

endoscopically documented gastroduodenal ulcers than traditional NSAIDs. To date, no studies examining the effects of this agent on ulcer complications have been performed. In a recent study, Goldstein et al.[170] randomized 186 healthy elderly subjects to receive naproxen 500 mg twice daily, valdecoxib 40 mg twice daily (4 times the FDA-approved dose), or placebo, and evaluated the short-term effect on the upper GI mucosa. At 7 days, 18% of those receiving naproxen (11/60) had significantly more gastroduodenal ulcers than those receiving placebo (2/61, 3%; p<0.01) or valdecoxib (0/60, 0%; p<0.001).

Lumiracoxib, another coxib in development, has a distinct pharmacology and allegedly increased affinity for inflamed tissues and synovial fluid. In a small study in healthy volunteers, lumiracoxib was found to produce as potent inhibition of COX-2 as the comparator naproxen, with little or no endoscopically detected gastroduodenal injury.[171] A recent large trial involving 18 325 individuals age 50 years or older showed that lumiracoxib reduced the incidence of ulcer complications by 3- to 4-fold compared to ibuprofen and naproxen, a benefit that was attenuated by the concomitant administration of aspirin.[172]

Although all available coxibs are associated with a reduced incidence of gastrointestinal injury compared with traditional NSAIDs, reduced incidence does not equal absolute absence of

Table 19.8 Incidence of gastrointestinal endpoints in the VIGOR study (rates per 100 patient years)

Outcome	Rofecoxib (n= 4047)	Naproxen (n= 4029)	Relative risk (95% CI)	Relative risk p value reduction
Clinical UGI events	2.1	4.5	0.46 (0.33–0.64)	54% p<0.001
Complicated UGI events	0.6	1.4	0.43 (0.24–0.78)	57% p=0.005
Any GI bleeding	1.2	3.0	0.38 (0.25–0.57)	62% p<0.001

Data from Bombardier C, Laine L, Reicin A, Shapiro D, Burgos-Vargas, Davis B, et al. Comparison of upper gastrointestinal toxicity of rofecoxib and naproxen in patients with rheumatoid arthritis. VIGOR study group. N Engl J Med 2000; 343:1520–1530.

risk. Careful monitoring of high-risk patients receiving long-term therapy with these agents is still necessary, and, while no studies have provided unequivocal evidence of proven benefit, the co-administration of antisecretory agents should also be considered in high-risk patients.

In September 2004, the data safety monitoring board overseeing a long-term trial evaluating the use of rofecoxib in patients at risk of developing recurrent colon polyps recommended that the study be terminated because of the recognition of an increased risk of serious thrombotic events, including myocardial infarctions and cerebrovascular accidents, some of which resulted in death, among patients taking rofecoxib compared to patients receiving placebo. In response to these findings, Merck & Co., the manufacturer of Vioxx®, announced the voluntary withdrawal of their rofecoxib product from the market. In April 2005, the FDA withdrew valdecoxib from the US market because of both serious cardiovascular adverse events and serious skin rashes associated with its use. Although celecoxib remains available, as discussed below, an FDA advisory panel that met in February 2005 concluded that the prothrombotic properties and increased risk of thromboembolic events are inherent to *all* drugs within this class.

PPI-NSAID cotherapy

Previous studies,[95,114] have demonstrated the ability of PPIs to heal gastric ulcers at an accelerated rate in the setting of continued NSAIDs use. In a recent 6-month, prospective, randomized, double-blind trial, Chan et al.[173] compared celecoxib with the combination of diclofenac plus omeprazole in the prevention of recurrent ulcer bleeding in patients with arthritis. Patients receiving NSAIDs who developed ulcer bleeding, with negative tests for *H. pylori* or successful eradication were randomized after their ulcers were healed, to receive either 200 mg of celecoxib twice daily plus daily placebo or 75 mg of diclofenac twice daily plus 20 mg of omeprazole daily for 6 months. The end point was recurrent ulcer bleeding. In the group receiving celecoxib (n=144), recurrent ulcer bleeding occurred in 7 patients, compared to 9 patients in the group receiving diclofenac plus omeprazole (n=143). The probability of recurrent bleeding during the 6-month period was 4.9% (95% CI= 3.1–6.7) for patients who received celecoxib and 6.4 % (95% CI= 4.3–8.4) for patients who received diclofenac plus omeprazole (difference =1.5 percentage points; 95% CI for the difference = 6.8–3.8) (Fig. 19.9).

It was concluded that PPIs are effective in maintaining patients in remission during continued NSAID use, and that the combination of omeprazole plus diclofenac may be as effective as treatment with celecoxib, with respect to the prevention of recurrent bleeding. It must be stressed, however, that the number of subjects in this trial was quite small, thus masking a possible beneficial effect of celecoxib. Moreover, as demonstrated in the CLASS trial,[162] diclofenac may be associated with a lower rate of ulcer complications when compared to other nonselective NSAIDs, such as naproxen. Nevertheless, because gastric mucosal injury is largely dependent upon the presence of gastric acid, the use of PPIs appears to offer a rational approach to the prevention of gastroduodenal ulcers associated with NSAID use. Based on two endoscopic studies demonstrating significant reductions in the rate of gastric ulceration, the FDA recently approved the use of esomeprazole for the primary prevention of NSAID-associated

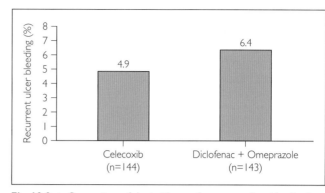

Fig. 19.9 • Comparison of the incidence of recurrent ulcer bleeding in patients using a nonselective NSAID (diclofenac) with omeprazole versus those using celecoxib. (Data from Chan FKL, et al. N Engl J Med 2002; 347:2104–2110.)

ulcers. Although studies demonstrating a reduction in ulcer complications would be valuable, the added benefit of the significant improvement in dyspeptic symptoms afforded by PPIs makes their use an attractive alternative to the use of selective COX-2 inhibitors in patients with arthritis and others requiring NSAID treatment.

Coxibs and cardiovascular disease

As a result of their preferential inhibition of endothelial prostacyclin synthesis without corresponding inhibition of platelet thromboxane, it has been postulated that the use of COX-2-selective inhibitors may be associated with an increased risk for thromboembolic cardiovascular events.[174] Nevertheless, in the CLASS study, the overall incidence of cardiovascular events, and specifically cerebrovascular accidents and myocardial infarction (MI), was comparable in the two treatment groups. The inclusion of patients receiving aspirin for cardiovascular prophylaxis may have provided a protective effect against the prothrombotic effects of COX-2 inhibitors.

In contrast, in the VIGOR study, more patients on rofecoxib experienced an MI and other serious cardiovascular problems than those receiving naproxen. The incidence of MI was lower among patients in the naproxen group than among those in the rofecoxib group (0.1% versus 0.4%; RR, 0.2; 95% CI, 0.1–0.7), while the overall mortality rate was similar in the two groups. Cardiovascular deaths and ischemic cerebrovascular events were also similar in both groups (0.2%). However, the absolute rate of MI among patients treated with rofecoxib was low (0.4%), consistent with rates detected with rofecoxib, placebo, and nonselective NSAIDs in a combined analysis of nine controlled osteoarthritis studies,[165] and comparable to the rate of MI with celecoxib in the CLASS study.[162] When the rates of MI with celecoxib and rofecoxib are recalculated and compared as annualized percentage rates, the results are similar, 0.80% with celecoxib and 0.74% with rofecoxib.[175]

Other than the use of aspirin, pharmacologic differences among the nonselective NSAIDs used as controls may have also contributed to the differences in the incidence of cardiovascular events in the two studies. Diclofenac and ibuprofen, which were used in the CLASS study, have significantly less antiplatelet effects than naproxen, which was used in the VIGOR trial.[50] While naproxen inhibits approximately 90% of thromboxane activity, both diclofenac and ibuprofen inhibit thromboxane by only 45–50%, a level insufficient to attenuate platelet aggregation.

Low-dose aspirin (<325 mg daily) irreversibly inhibits platelet COX-1 activity by acetylating the serine 529 residue, resulting in >95% attenuation of thromboxane A_2 (TXA_2)-mediated platelet aggregation throughout the 24-hour dosing interval.[176] In addition, once COX-1 has been acetylated by aspirin, the substrate cannot gain access to the catalytic site of the enzyme for the lifetime (5 days) of the platelet. Thus, following aspirin withdrawal, the restoration of TXA_2 biosynthesis occurs linearly as a function of platelet turnover.[176] Similar to aspirin, when used in doses of 500 mg twice daily, naproxen produces approximately 90% inhibition of platelet TXA_2 production throughout the dosing interval. The inhibition of TXA_2 by naproxen is, however, less consistent, and unlikely to be greater than that of low-dose aspirin.[177] As mentioned earlier, other NSAIDs do not appear to possess sustained and clinically relevant antiplatelet effects. Therefore, the concomitant use of low-dose aspirin should be strongly considered in patients with a history of coronary artery disease, stroke, TIA, or peripheral vascular disease, even in patients who are using nonselective NSAIDs for arthritis or other inflammatory conditions.

A recent study[178] of a large patient database examined the relation between MIs and ongoing NSAID use. The investigators identified 4425 patients hospitalized for MI during a 5-year period and compared their use of prescribed oral NSAIDs with that of controls. After controlling for different potential confounders, no relationship was observed between NSAID use in the prior 6 months and MI (OR, 1.00; 95% CI, 0.92–1.08; $p=0.92$). However, naproxen use was found to be significantly less common among cases of MI compared with controls, and was associated with a 16–20% reduction in the risk of MI (OR, 0.84; 95% CI, 0.72–0.98; $p=0.03$). While ibuprofen use had no significant association with MI (OR, 1.02; 95% CI, 0.88–1.18), etodolac, a COX-2 preferential inhibitor, appeared to be associated with an increased risk of MI (OR, 1.28; 95% CI, 1.00–1.64; $p=0.05$). Selective COX-2 inhibitors (celecoxib and rofecoxib) were not in use at the time of this study. In general, patients using agents that were nonselective with respect to COX-1:COX-2 ratio had a somewhat lower risk of MI, whereas those taking NSAIDs with preferential COX-2 inhibition appeared to have a small increased risk of MI. Most of the cardiovascular benefit of nonselective NSAIDs appeared to be primarily limited to naproxen.

In another case-control study involving 16 937 patients with RA,[179] the incidence of MI was lower in those taking naproxen (RR, 0.57; 95% CI, 0.31–1.06; $p=0.07$). The incidence of all thromboembolic events was also significantly lower in those taking naproxen compared with those not taking NSAIDs (RR, 0.61; 95% CI, 0.39–0.94; $p=0.03$). A similar study[180] compared the use of naproxen and other NSAIDs in 14 163 patients 65 years or older with acute MI with an equal number of controls. Seven-and-one-half percent of the cases were concurrent users of NSAIDs, and 1.8% were concurrent users of naproxen. In the control group, 5.1% were concurrent users of NSAIDs, and 1.5% were concurrent users of naproxen. Concurrent exposure to NSAIDs or naproxen was defined by prescriptions that covered or overlapped with the date of acute MI (index date). The RR of MI was significantly lower in those taking naproxen than in those taking other NSAIDs (RR, 0.79; 95% CI, 0.63–0.99).

Despite the possible beneficial effects of naproxen, a review of the cardiovascular event rates of four randomized trials, including CLASS, VIGOR, and two smaller trials with approximately 1000 patients each, did suggest a potential increase in the cardiovascular event rates with both rofecoxib and celecoxib.[175] As stated previously, based on an interim analysis, the data safety monitoring board overseeing the APPROVe trial designed to evaluate the use of rofecoxib in patients at risk of developing recurrent colon polyps recommended that the study be terminated because of the recognition of an increased risk of serious thrombotic events among patients taking rofecoxib. In this study of over 3000 individuals, the relative risk of developing a confirmed thrombotic event in patients receiving rofecoxib was 1.92 when compared to placebo.[181] Interestingly, the increased relative risk became apparent only after 18 months of treatment, with event rates similar in the two groups during the first 18 months (Fig. 19.10). It is important to note that 20% of individuals in each group took low-dose aspirin (≤325 mg daily).[181] A similar study of 2035 patients with a history of colorectal neoplasia compared two doses of celecoxib (200 mg twice daily and 400 mg twice daily) with placebo in their ability to prevent recurrent colorectal adenomas.[182] In this study, the hazard ratio for death due to MI, cerebrovascular accident, or heart failure was 2.3 and 3.4 in patients receiving the lower and higher dose of celcoxib, respectively (Fig. 19.11). Similar endpoints were observed for other composite endpoints, and like APPROVe, the data safety monitoring board overseeing this trial recommended early discontinuation of the study.

A third recent trial assessed the use of valdelcoxib and its intravenous prodrug paracoxib in treating postoperative pain in patients undergoing coronary artery bypass grafting.[183] 1671 patients were assigned to receive one of three regimens for ten days: placebo for ten days; placebo for three days, followed by valdecoxib through day ten; or paracoxib for at least three days, followed valdecoxib through day ten. All patients also received 81–325 mg of aspirin orally throughout the course of the study period. Cardiovascular events, including MI, cardiac arrest, stroke, and pulmonary

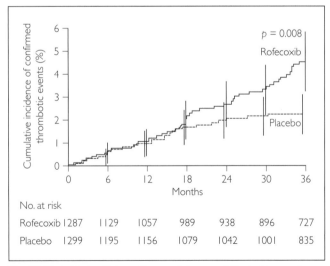

Fig. 19.10 • Kaplan-Meier estimates of the cumulative incidence of confirmed serious thrombotic events. Vertical lines indicate 95% confidence intervals. (Data from Bresalier RS, et al. N Engl J Med 2005; 352:1092–1102, with permission.)

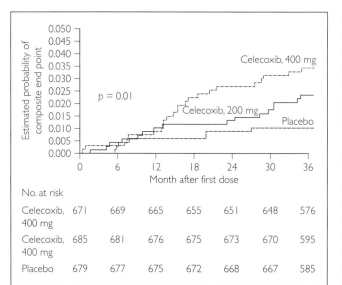

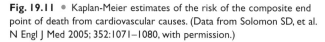

No. at risk							
Celecoxib, 400 mg	671	669	665	655	651	648	576
Celecoxib, 400 mg	685	681	676	675	673	670	595
Placebo	679	677	675	672	668	667	585

Fig. 19.11 • Kaplan-Meier estimates of the risk of the composite end point of death from cardiovascular causes. (Data from Solomon SD, et al. N Engl J Med 2005; 352:1071–1080, with permission.)

embolism, were four times more frequent among patients given paracoxib and valdecoxib than among those given placebo.

The results of these studies clearly indicate that the selective inhibition of COX-2, without the concomitant attenuation of COX-1 enzyme activity, is associated with an increased risk of thrombotic events. This adverse profile is probably due, at least in part, to the unopposed inhibition of prostacyclin without any effect on thromboxane A_2, resulting in a net balance favoring thrombogenesis. As stated above, Merck & Co. voluntarily withdrew rofecoxib from the market in September 2004. However, an FDA advisory panel that met in February 2005 recommended that it be reinstated because of its significant benefit to arthritis patients and others requiring potent analgesia, as well as the panel's conclusion that the observed thrombogenic properties attributed to this agent constitute a class effect. Whether or not rofecoxib is reinstated, the labels of all COX-selective inhibitors, and possibly nonselective NSAIDs, will now include information advising practitioners to exercise caution when prescribing these drugs, in particular to those individuals with a history of heart disease. Despite the valuable information obtained from these trials, additional important clinical questions remain. For example, does the simultaneous administration of aspirin offset the gastro-protective effect of COX-2 inhibitors? A recent endoscopic study by Laine et al.[184] compared the incidence of ulcers in osteoarthritis patients receiving placebo, low-dose aspirin (81 mg daily), ibuprofen (800 mg three times daily), and rofecoxib 25 mg plus 81 mg aspirin. The 12-week cumulative incidence of endoscopic ulcers was 5.8% and 7.3% in the placebo and aspirin group, respectively. The authors also found no difference in the 12-week cumulative ulcer incidence when they compared the groups taking ibuprofen (17.1%) and rofecoxib plus aspirin (16.1%). Unfortunately, the study did not assess the combination of aspirin and ibuprofen, nor did it include a group of patients taking rofecoxib alone. Nevertheless, the study does suggest that the addition of even low doses of aspirin may obviate the gastro-intestinal benefit conferred by selective COX-2 inhibition. Large controlled trials specifically designed to evaluate this specific

issue, as well as the cardiovascular risks of all NSAIDs, will be required to answer these questions. Until these studies are performed, caution should be exercised when prescribing not only COX-2 selective inhibitors, but also nonselective NSAIDs, to patients at risk for cardiovascular morbidity. Most importantly, clinicians must be aware that neither COX-2 selective agents nor nonselective NSAIDs constitute acceptable substitutes for aspirin as prophylaxis for MI and other thromboembolic disorders.

Nitric oxide releasing NSAIDs

Originally described as endothelium-derived relaxing factor, nitric oxide (NO) is a product of the normal endothelial cell that plays a significant role in the regulation of vascular tone. Nitric oxide plays a critical role in maintaining the integrity of the gastro-duodenal mucosa, exerting many of the same effects as endogenous prostaglandins.[185] It has even been suggested that NO and PGs act synergistically to mediate mucosal protective effects, including the maintenance of gastric mucosal blood flow and the prevention of neutrophil adherence to the vascular endothelium. Moreover, Salvemini et al.[186] have demonstrated that NO stimulates COX enzymes. In the GI tract, NO production takes place in the epithelial cells of the mucosa, with minimal NO production in the endothelium.[187] NO donors increase gastric mucus secretion both in vivo[188] and in vitro.[189] NO also contributes to the modulation of mucosal integrity, tissue repair,[190] and maintenance of the microvasculature and mucosal blood flow.[187]

Formulations of NO-linked NSAIDs, in which NO is released to compensate for the suppression of mucosal prostaglandins have been developed. Under these conditions, the desired effects of NSAIDs, including the inhibition of both cyclooxygenase isoenzymes are maintained, while toxicity is minimized. NO-containing compounds appear to possess antiinflammatory and antipyretic properties that are similar to those of the parent compounds with a diminished incidence of gastrointestinal injury. Whether this reduced potential to cause gastroduodenal mucosal lesions will translate into a significant reduction of NSAID-related GI complications and improved clinical outcomes remains to be established. A formulation combining rofecoxib with NO is presently under development. Although not evaluated to date, the antiplatelet effects of NO might in theory provide benefit to those individuals who might be susceptible to the possible thrombotic properties attributed to selective COX-2 inhibition.

The mechanisms by which NO-releasing NSAIDs (NO-NSAIDs) suppress PG synthesis without causing gastric damage are not fully understood. One possibility is that the vasodilator properties of NO prevent the reduction in gastric mucosal blood flow seen following the administration of traditional NSAIDs.[191] Other hypotheses that may explain the effect of NO on the prevention of NSAID-induced gastroduodenal injury include a possible NO-mediated inhibition of neutrophil adherence, increased mucus secretion, and scavenging of oxygen-derived free radicals (Fig. 19.12).[192]

In a study of twenty healthy volunteers,[193] the use of NO-releasing flurbiprofen was associated with fewer gastric erosions than the parent drug, while maintaining its inhibitory effect on gastric mucosal prostaglandin synthesis and serum thromboxane levels. No changes were seen in cardiovascular parameters, and no adverse effects were recorded. Recently, in a randomized, parallel group, blind-observer study of 40 healthy volunteers, two

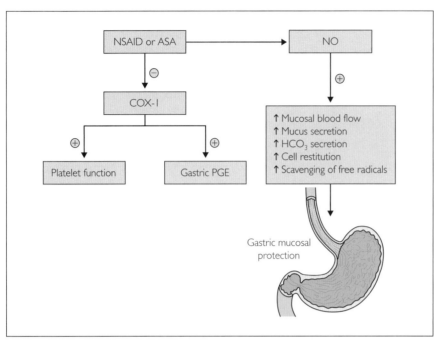

Fig. 19.12 • Postulated mechanism by which nitric oxide releasing nonsteroidal antiinflammatory drugs (NO-NSAIDs) maintain the ability to protect the gastroduodenal mucosa while suppressing the level of endogenous mucosal prostaglandins. NO appears to stimulate some of the inherent defensive properties in the mucosa that are affected by cyclooxygenase-1 (COX-1) isoenzyme inhibition. ASA, acetylsalicylic acid; PGE, prostaglandin E. (Adapted from Wallace J: Nonsteroidal anti-inflammatory drugs and gastroenteropathy: The second hundred years. Gastroenterology 1997;112:1000–1016.)

doses (400 mg and 800 mg twice daily) of the NO-releasing aspirin derivative NCX-4016 were compared with two doses of aspirin (200 mg and 400 mg twice daily) and placebo. Gastric mucosal injury was assessed and scored by endoscopy. At the end of treatment, the two aspirin groups showed a median score of 7.5 and 11.3, while the NCX-4016 groups showed a median endoscopy score of 0.7 and 1.0 ($p<0.001$), confirming the hypothesis that NCX-4016 does not induce macroscopic changes in the gastroduodenal mucosa. Both aspirin and NCX-4016 were effective in reducing platelet aggregation as measured by excretion of urinary thromboxane metabolites. No serious adverse events or significant alteration of cardiovascular parameters were reported.[194]

In summary, NO-NSAIDs inhibit COX-1, COX-2 and prostaglandin synthesis as effectively as the parent NSAID and appear to have comparable antiinflammatory and antipyretic activity, and possibly greater analgesic effects than the parent compound, with a reduced incidence of gastroduodenal mucosal injury. Further large-scale prospective studies need to be performed before these agents can be routinely used in patients with arthritis and other inflammatory conditions, as well as for prophylaxis against thromboembolic events.

FUTURE DIRECTIONS

Lipoxygenase/cyclooxygenase inhibitors

Growing evidence suggests that in addition to COX other mediators are involved in the development of inflammation. Leukotrienes (LTs), which are synthesized by 5-lipoxygenase (5-LOX) in the arachidonic acid pathway, play a major role in the inflammatory process. As a result, dual 5-LOX/COX inhibitors are being developed as potential agents to treat inflammatory conditions. LTs are potent gastrotoxic and proinflammatory mediators, which by virtue of their ability to produce vasoconstriction and reduce mucosal blood flow, promote the breakdown of the mucosal barrier. Because PGs and LTs have complementary effects, it has been postulated that a therapy that inhibits 5-LOX, COX-1, and COX-2 could provide analgesic and antiinflammatory effects with the advantage of improved GI, renal, and systemic tolerability. Based on these principles, the LOX/COX inhibitor licofelone has been developed for the treatment of pain and inflammation in osteoarthritis. Preclinical trials of licofelone have demonstrated an excellent safety profile, as well as good analgesic and antiinflammatory properties.[195,196]

Table 19.9 Recommendations for prevention and treatment of NSAID-related mucosal injury	
Dyspepsia	Empirical H₂RA or PPI
Active gastroduodenal ulcer	
NSAID discontinued	H₂RA or PPI
NSAID continued	PPI
Prophylactic therapy	Use NSAID with low relative risk for injury with concomitant PPI in AM; or concomitant misoprostol, at least 200 μg t.i.d.
	COX-2 selective inhibitor; consider adding PPI in high-risk individuals

H₂RA, H₂-receptor antagonist; PPI, proton pump inhibitor

In a recent, controlled, parallel-group trial evaluating the GI tolerability of licofelone, healthy volunteers were randomized to receive either licofelone 200 mg, 400 mg twice daily, naproxen 500 mg twice daily or placebo all for 4 weeks. At the end of the study, endoscopic ulcers had developed in 20% of the subjects on the naproxen group, compared with 0% of those receiving licofelone at both doses and placebo. Further studies will be required to confirm this potential GI safety advantage of LOX/COX inhibitors over traditional NSAIDs before their use can be adopted in clinical practice.[196]

SUMMARY

The present approach to patients on NSAIDs is summarized in Table 19.9. In general, symptoms associated with the use of NSAIDs are common and can generally be treated empirically with an H_2RA or a PPI. If a gastroduodenal ulcer develops, the most prudent approach would be to discontinue the NSAID and substitute therapy with acetaminophen. If the NSAID must be continued, PPIs appear to heal ulcers at the same rate whether or not NSAID therapy is continued. After the ulcer is healed and it is determined that the NSAID must be continued, prophylaxis is best accomplished either by the concomitant administration of a PPI or the use of a COX-2 selective inhibitor. Many unresolved issues remain regarding the risk of adverse cardiovascular and other thrombotic events associated with the use of the latter option. Thus, along with the added benefit of significant symptomatic improvement afforded by PPIs, their use appears to represent an attractive alternative to selective COX-2 inhibitors in patients with arthritis and others requiring NSAID treatment.

REFERENCES

1. Wallace JL. Nonsteroidal anti-inflammatory drugs and gastroenteropathy: the second hundred years. Gastroenterology 1997; 112(3):1000–1016.

   Excellent review of the development, clinical use, and pathogenesis of NSAID-related gastrointestinal injury. Includes a discussion on preventive measures and some insight into future approaches, which are now widely used to reduce adverse effects on the GI tract.

2. Vane JR, Flower RJ, Botting RM. History of aspirin and its mechanism of action. Stroke 1990; 21(12 Suppl):IV12–23.

3. Dreser H. Pharmacologisches uber aspirin (acetylsalicyl-saure). Pflugers Arch 1899; 76:306–318.

4. Douthwaite AH, Lintott GAM. Gastroscopic observation of effect of aspirin and certain other substances in the stomach. Lancet 1938; 2:1222–1225.

5. Gillies M, Skyring A. Gastric ulcer, duodenal ulcer and gastric carcinoma: a case-control study of certain social and environmental factors. Med J Aust 1968; 2(25):1132–1136.

6. Sun DC, Roth SH, Mitchell CS, et al. Upper gastrointestinal disease in rheumatoid arthritis. Am J Dig Dis 1974; 19(5):405–410.

7. Levy M. Aspirin use in patients with major upper gastrointestinal bleeding and peptic-ulcer disease. A report from the Boston Collaborative Drug Surveillance Program, Boston University Medical Center. N Engl J Med 1974; 290(21):1158–1162.

8. Silvoso GR, Ivey KJ, Butt JH, et al. Incidence of gastric lesions in patients with rheumatic disease on chronic aspirin therapy. Ann Intern Med 1979; 91(4):517–520.

9. [No authors listed.] A randomized, controlled trial of aspirin in persons recovered from myocardial infarction. JAMA 1980; 243(7):661–669.

10. Wolfe MM, Lichtenstein DR, Singh G. Gastrointestinal toxicity of nonsteroidal antiinflammatory drugs. N Engl J Med 1999; 340(24):1888–1899.

    Outstanding clinically oriented review of the gastrointestinal toxicity of NSAIDs. The article provides an overview of the significance and impact of NSAID-related gastrointestinal complications given the widespread use of these agents both as prescription and over-the-counter. Includes informative sections on risk factors, pathogenesis of GI complications, and clinical spectrum of injury, as well as practical recommendations for management.

11. Larkai EN, Smith JL, Lidsky MD, et al. Gastroduodenal mucosa and dyspeptic symptoms in arthritic patients during chronic nonsteroidal anti-inflammatory drug use. Am J Gastroenterol 1987; 82(11):1153–1158.

12. Singh G, Ramey DR, Morfeld D, et al. Gastrointestinal tract complications of nonsteroidal anti-inflammatory drug treatment in rheumatoid arthritis. A prospective observational cohort study. Arch Intern Med 1996; 156(14):1530–1536.

13. Straus WL, Ofman JJ, MacLean C, et al. Do NSAIDs cause dyspepsia? A meta-analysis evaluating alternative dyspepsia definitions. Am J Gastroenterol 2002; 97(8):1951–1958.

14. Singh G, Triadafilopoulos G. Epidemiology of NSAID induced gastrointestinal complications. J Rheumatol 1999; 26(Suppl 56):18–24.

15. Gabriel SE, Jaakkimainen L, Bombardier C. Risk for serious gastrointestinal complications related to use of nonsteroidal anti-inflammatory drugs. A meta-analysis. Ann Intern Med 1991; 115(10):787–796.

16. Piper JM, Ray WA, Daugherty JR, et al. Corticosteroid use and peptic ulcer disease: role of nonsteroidal anti-inflammatory drugs. Ann Intern Med 1991; 114(9):735–740.

17. Silverstein FE, Graham DY, Senior JR, et al. Misoprostol reduces serious gastrointestinal complications in patients with rheumatoid arthritis receiving nonsteroidal anti-inflammatory drugs. A randomized, double-blind, placebo-controlled trial. Ann Intern Med 1995; 123(4):241–249.

    Known as the MUCOSA trial, this landmark study demonstrated a meaningful reduction of NSAID-related GI complications by concomitant use of a prostaglandin analogue.

18. Potential of the COX-2 inhibitor market. 2000. (Accessed Feb, 2002, at www.ims-global.com.)

19. Singh G, Ramey DR, Khraishi M, et al. NSAID-related effects on the GI tract: an ever widening spectrum. Arthritis Rheum 1997; 40(Suppl):S93.

20. Hirschowitz BI, Lanas A. Atypical and aggressive upper gastrointestinal ulceration associated with aspirin abuse. J Clin Gastroenterol 2002; 34(5):523–528.

21. Bjorkman D. Nonsteroidal anti-inflammatory drug-associated toxicity of the liver, lower gastrointestinal tract, and esophagus. Am J Med 1998; 105(5A):17S–21S.

22. Kahn LH, Chen M, Eaton R. Over-the-counter naproxen sodium and esophageal injury. Ann Intern Med 1997; 126(12):1006.

23. Lichtenstein DR, Syngal S, Wolfe MM. Nonsteroidal antiinflammatory drugs and the gastrointestinal tract. The double-edged sword. Arthritis Rheum 1995; 38(1):5–18.

24. Minocha A, Greenbaum DS. Pill-esophagitis caused by nonsteroidal antiinflammatory drugs. Am J Gastroenterol 1991; 86(8):1086–1089.

25. Kim SL, Hunter JG, Wo JM, et al. NSAIDs, aspirin, and esophageal strictures: are over-the-counter medications harmful to the esophagus? J Clin Gastroenterol 1999; 29(1):32–34.

26. Estes LL, Fuhs DW, Heaton AH, et al. Gastric ulcer perforation associated with the use of injectable ketorolac. Ann Pharmacother 1993; 27(1):42–43.

27. Henry D, Dobson A, Turner C. Variability in the risk of major gastrointestinal complications from nonaspirin nonsteroidal anti-inflammatory drugs. Gastroenterology 1993; 105(4): 1078–1088.

28. Zimmerman J, Siguencia J, Tsvang E. Upper gastrointestinal hemorrhage associated with cutaneous application of diclofenac gel. Am J Gastroenterol 1995; 90(11):2032–2034.

29. Wolfe MM, Sachs G. Acid suppression: optimizing therapy for gastroduodenal ulcer healing, gastroesophageal reflux disease, and stress-related erosive syndrome. Gastroenterology 2000; 118(2 Suppl 1):S9–S31.

This article provides an in-depth review of the current knowledge of acid-suppression therapy, as well as practical suggestions for management of the most relevant acid-related disorders.

30. Kelly JP, Kaufman DW, Jurgelon JM, et al. Risk of aspirin-associated major upper-gastrointestinal bleeding with enteric-coated or buffered product. Lancet 1996; 348(9039):1413–1416.

31. Soll AH, Weinstein WM, Kurata J, et al. Nonsteroidal anti-inflammatory drugs and peptic ulcer disease. Ann Intern Med 1991; 114(4):307–319.

32. Wolfe MM, Soll AH. The physiology of gastric acid secretion. N Engl J Med 1988; 319:1707–1715.

33. Crofford LJ. COX-1 and COX-2 tissue expression: implications and predictions. J Rheumatol 1997; 24(Suppl 49):15–19.

34. Masferrer JL, Seibert K, Zweifel B, et al. Endogenous glucocorticoids regulate an inducible cyclooxygenase enzyme. Proc Natl Acad Sci USA 1992; 89(9):3917–3921.

35. Needleman P, Isakson PC. The discovery and function of COX-2. J Rheumatol 1997; 24(Suppl 49):6–8.

36. Beejay U, Wolfe MM. Cyclooxygenase 2 selective inhibitors: panacea or flash in the pan? Gastroenterology 1999; 117(4):1002–1005.

37. Laine L. Approaches to nonsteroidal anti-inflammatory drug use in the high-risk patient. Gastroenterology 2001; 120(3):594–606.

Complete review of the most prominent risk factors for NSAID-related gastrointestinal injury and management strategies for at-risk patients requiring NSAID therapy.

38. Lanza LL, Walker AM, Bortnichak EA, et al. Peptic ulcer and gastrointestinal hemorrhage associated with nonsteroidal anti-inflammatory drug use in patients younger than 65 years. A large health maintenance organization cohort study. Arch Intern Med 1995; 155(13):1371–1377.

39. Lichtenstein DR, Berman MD, Wolfe MM. Approach to the patient with upper gastrointestinal hemorrhage. In: Taylor MB et al, ed. Gastrointestinal emergencies. Baltimore: Williams and Wilkins; 1997:99–129.

40. Aalykke C, Lauritsen K. Epidemiology of NSAID-related gastroduodenal mucosal injury. Best Pract Res Clin Gastroenterol 2001; 15(5):705–722.

41. Gabriel SE, Jaakkimainen L, Bombardier C. Risk for serious gastrointestinal complications related to use of nonsteroidal anti-inflammatory drugs. A meta-analysis. Ann Intern Med 1991; 115(10):787–796.

42. Shorr RI, Ray WA, Daugherty JR, et al. Concurrent use of nonsteroidal anti-inflammatory drugs and oral anticoagulants places elderly persons at high risk for hemorrhagic peptic ulcer disease. Arch Intern Med 1993; 153(14):1665–1670.

43. Laine L. The gastrointestinal effects of nonselective NSAIDs and COX-2-selective inhibitors. Semin Arthritis Rheum 2002; 32(3 Suppl 1):25–32.

44. Conn HO, Blitzer BL. Nonassociation of adrenocorticosteroid therapy and peptic ulcer. N Engl J Med 1976; 294(9):473–479.

45. Singh G, Rosen Ramey D. NSAID induced gastrointestinal complications: the ARAMIS perspective – 1997. Arthritis, Rheumatism, and Aging Medical Information System. J Rheumatol Suppl 1998; 51:8–16.

46. Garcia Rodriguez LA, Jick H. Risk of upper gastrointestinal bleeding and perforation associated with individual non-steroidal anti-inflammatory drugs. Lancet 1994; 343(8900):769–772.

47. Griffin MR, Piper JM, Daugherty JR, et al. Nonsteroidal anti-inflammatory drug use and increased risk for peptic ulcer disease in elderly persons. Ann Intern Med 1991; 114(4):257–263.

48. Hansen JM, Hallas J, Lauritsen JM, et al. Non-steroidal anti-inflammatory drugs and ulcer complications: a risk factor analysis for clinical decision-making. Scand J Gastroenterol 1996; 31(2):126–130.

49. Bjorkman DJ. Nonsteroidal anti-inflammatory drug-induced gastrointestinal injury. Am J Med 1996; 101(1A):25S–32S.

50. Bombardier C, Laine L, Reicin A, et al. Comparison of upper gastrointestinal toxicity of rofecoxib and naproxen in patients with rheumatoid arthritis. VIGOR Study Group. N Engl J Med 2000; 343(21):1520–1530.

Landmark outcomes study demonstrating unequivocal clinical benefit (reduced incidence of gastroduodenal ulcers) associated with the use of the COX-2 selective inhibitor rofecoxib.

51. Rockall TA, Logan RF, Devlin HB, et al. Risk assessment after acute upper gastrointestinal haemorrhage. Gut 1996; 38(3):316–321.

52. Simon LS, Hatoum HT, Bittman RM, et al. Risk factors for serious nonsteroidal-induced gastrointestinal complications: regression analysis of the MUCOSA trial. Fam Med 1996; 28(3):204–210.

53. Weil J, Langman MJ, Wainwright P, et al. Peptic ulcer bleeding: accessory risk factors and interactions with non-steroidal anti-inflammatory drugs. Gut 2000; 46(1):27–31.

54. Goggin PM, Collins DA, Jazrawi RP, et al. Prevalence of Helicobacter pylori infection and its effect on symptoms and non-steroidal anti-inflammatory drug induced gastrointestinal damage in patients with rheumatoid arthritis. Gut 1993; 34(12):1677–1680.

55. Kim JG, Graham DY. Helicobacter pylori infection and development of gastric or duodenal ulcer in arthritic patients receiving chronic NSAID therapy. The Misoprostol Study Group. Am J Gastroenterol 1994; 89(2):203–207.

56. Thillainayagam AV, Tabaqchali S, Warrington SJ, et al. Interrelationships between Helicobacter pylori infection, nonsteroidal antiinflammatory drugs and gastroduodenal disease. A prospective study in healthy volunteers. Dig Dis Sci 1994; 39(5):1085–1089.

57. Laine L, Cominelli F, Sloane R, et al. Interaction of NSAIDs and Helicobacter pylori on gastrointestinal injury and prostaglandin production: a controlled double-blind trial. Aliment Pharmacol Ther 1995; 9(2):127–135.

58. Bianchi Porro G, Parente F, Imbesi V, et al. Role of Helicobacter pylori in ulcer healing and recurrence of gastric and duodenal ulcers in long-term NSAID users. Response to omeprazole dual therapy. Gut 1996; 39(1):22–26.

59. Chan FK, Sung JJ, Chung SC, et al. Randomised trial of eradication of Helicobacter pylori before non-steroidal anti-inflammatory drug therapy to prevent peptic ulcers. Lancet 1997; 350(9083):975–979.

60. Barkin J. The relation between Helicobacter pylori and nonsteroidal anti-inflammatory drugs. Am J Med 1998; 105(5A):22S–27S.

61. Aalykke C, Lauritsen JM, Hallas J, et al. *Helicobacter pylori* and risk of ulcer bleeding among users of nonsteroidal anti-inflammatory drugs: a case-control study. Gastroenterology 1999; 116(6): 1305–1309.

62. Pilotto A, Leandro G, Di Mario F, et al. Role of *Helicobacter pylori* infection on upper gastrointestinal bleeding in the elderly: a case-control study. Dig Dis Sci 1997; 42(3):586–591.

63. Cullen DJ, Hawkey GM, Greenwood DC, et al. Peptic ulcer bleeding in the elderly: relative roles of *Helicobacter pylori* and non-steroidal anti-inflammatory drugs. Gut 1997; 41(4):459–462.

64. Wu CY, Poon SK, Chen GH, et al. Interaction between *Helicobacter pylori* and non-steroidal anti-inflammatory drugs in peptic ulcer bleeding. Scand J Gastroenterol 1999; 34(3):234–237.

65. Santolaria S, Lanas A, Benito R, et al. *Helicobacter pylori* infection is a protective factor for bleeding gastric ulcers but not for bleeding duodenal ulcers in NSAID users. Aliment Pharmacol Ther 1999; 13(11):1511–1518.

66. Garcia Rodriguez LA, Cattaruzzi C, Troncon MG, et al. Risk of hospitalization for upper gastrointestinal tract bleeding associated with ketorolac, other nonsteroidal anti-inflammatory drugs, calcium antagonists, and other antihypertensive drugs. Arch Intern Med 1998; 158(1):33–39.

67. Yeomans ND, Hawkey C, Jones R, et al. Esomeprazole provides effective control of NSAID-associated upper GI symptoms in patients continuing to take NSAIDs. Gastroenterology 2003; 124(4 Suppl 1. Abstract 796):A-107.

68. Brun J, Jones R. Nonsteroidal anti-inflammatory drug-associated dyspepsia: the scale of the problem. Am J Med 2001; 110(1A): 12S–13S.

69. Pounder R. Silent peptic ulceration: deadly silence or golden silence? Gastroenterology 1989; 96(2 Pt 2 Suppl):626–631.

70. Armstrong CP, Blower AL. Non-steroidal anti-inflammatory drugs and life threatening complications of peptic ulceration. Gut 1987; 28(5):527–532.

71. Ofman JJ, Maclean CH, Straus WL, et al. Meta-analysis of dyspepsia and nonsteroidal antiinflammatory drugs. Arthritis Rheum 2003; 49(4):508–518.

72. Lisse JR, Perlman M, Johansson G, et al. Gastrointestinal tolerability and effectiveness of rofecoxib versus naproxen in the treatment of osteoarthritis: a randomized, controlled trial. Ann Intern Med 2003; 139(7):539–546.

73. Laine L, Bombardier C, Hawkey CJ, et al. Stratifying the risk of NSAID-related upper gastrointestinal clinical events: results of a double-blind outcomes study in patients with rheumatoid arthritis. Gastroenterology 2002; 123(4):1006–1012.

74. Bijlsma JW. Treatment of NSAID-induced gastrointestinal lesions with cimetidine: an international multicentre collaborative study. Aliment Pharmacol Ther 1988; 2 Suppl 1:85–95.

75. Van Groenendael JH, Markusse HM, Dijkmans BA, et al. The effect of ranitidine on NSAID related dyspeptic symptoms with and without peptic ulcer disease of patients with rheumatoid arthritis and osteoarthritis. Clin Rheumatol 1996; 15(5):450–456.

76. Taha AS, Hudson N, Hawkey CJ, et al. Famotidine for the prevention of gastric and duodenal ulcers caused by nonsteroidal antiinflammatory drugs. N Engl J Med 1996; 334(22):1435–1439.

77. Ekstrom P, Carling L, Wetterhus S, et al. Prevention of peptic ulcer and dyspeptic symptoms with omeprazole in patients receiving continuous non-steroidal anti-inflammatory drug therapy. A Nordic multicentre study. Scand J Gastroenterol 1996; 31(8):753–758.

78. Yeomans ND, Tulassay Z, Juhasz L, et al. A comparison of omeprazole with ranitidine for ulcers associated with nonsteroidal antiinflammatory drugs. Acid Suppression Trial: Ranitidine versus Omeprazole for NSAID-associated Ulcer Treatment (ASTRONAUT) Study Group. N Engl J Med 1998; 338(11):719–726.

Known as the ASTRONAUT study, this trial demonstrated the superiority of proton pump inhibitors over H$_2$-receptor antagonists to prevent and heal gastroduodenal ulcers in patients receiving NSAIDs.

79. Hawkey C, Yeomans ND, Scheiman J, et al. Maintained symptom control with esopmeprazole following initial treatment of upper GI symptoms of patients on NSAIDs including COX-2-selective NSAIDs. Gastroenterology 2004; 126(4 suppl 2):A-609.

80. Hawkey C, Yeomans ND, Jones R, et al. Esomeprazole improves quality of life in patients with upper GI symptoms associated with long-term NSAID therapy. Gastroenterology 2003; 124(Suppl 1, Abstract 795)(4):A-107.

81. Talley NJ, Hawkey C, Yeomans ND, et al. Maintenance of improvement in quality of life dimensions and symptom control following initial treatment of upper GI symptoms with esomeprazole versus placebo in patients on long term NSAID therapy. Gastroenterology 2004; 126(4 Suppl 2):A-603.

82. Laheij RJ, Van Rossum LG, Jansen JB, et al. Proton-pump inhibitor therapy for acetylsalicylic acid associated upper gastrointestinal symptoms: a randomized placebo-controlled trial. Aliment Pharmacol Ther 2003; 18(1):109–115.

83. McCarthy DM. Sucralfate. N Engl J Med 1991; 325(14):1017–1025.

84. Roth S, Agrawal N, Mahowald M, et al. Misoprostol heals gastroduodenal injury in patients with rheumatoid arthritis receiving aspirin. Arch Intern Med 1989; 149(4):775–779.

85. Hawkey CJ, Karrasch JA, Szczepanski L, et al. Omeprazole compared with misoprostol for ulcers associated with nonsteroidal antiinflammatory drugs. Omeprazole versus Misoprostol for NSAID-induced Ulcer Management (OMNIUM) Study Group. N Engl J Med 1998; 338(11):727–734.

Known as the OMNIUM study, this important trial demonstrated that in patients receiving NSAIDs, omeprazole was more effective and better tolerated than misoprostol in the prevention of ulcer relapse.

86. Croker JR, Cotton PB, Boyle AC, et al. Cimetidine for peptic ulcer in patients with arthritis. Ann Rheum Dis 1980; 39(3):275–278.

87. O'Laughlin JC, Silvoso GR, Ivey KJ. Healing of aspirin-associated peptic ulcer disease despite continued salicylate ingestion. Arch Intern Med 1981; 141(6):781–783.

88. Davies J, Collins AJ, Dixon SA. The influence of cimetidine on peptic ulcer in patients with arthritis taking anti-inflammatory drugs. Br J Rheumatol 1986; 25(1):54–58.

89. Manniche C, Malchow-Moller A, Andersen JR, et al. Randomised study of the influence of non-steroidal anti-inflammatory drugs on the treatment of peptic ulcer in patients with rheumatic disease. Gut 1987; 28(2):226–229.

90. O'Laughlin JC, Silvoso GK, Ivey KJ. Resistance to medical therapy of gastric ulcers in rheumatic disease patients taking aspirin. A double-blind study with cimetidine and follow-up. Dig Dis Sci 1982; 27(11):976–980.

91. Lancaster-Smith MJ, Jaderberg ME, Jackson DA. Ranitidine in the treatment of non-steroidal anti-inflammatory drug associated gastric and duodenal ulcers. Gut 1991; 32(3):252–255.

92. Schwarz K. Uber penetrierende magen-und jejunalgeschwure. Beitr Klin Chirurgie 1910; 24:2–17.

93. Jones DB, Howden CW, Burget DW, et al. Acid suppression in duodenal ulcer: a meta-analysis to define optimal dosing with antisecretory drugs. Gut 1987; 28(9):1120–1127.

94. Burget DW, Chiverton SG, Hunt RH. Is there an optimal degree of acid suppression for healing of duodenal ulcers? A model of the

relationship between ulcer healing and acid suppression. Gastroenterology 1990; 99(2):345–351.

95. Walan A, Bader JP, Classen M, et al. Effect of omeprazole and ranitidine on ulcer healing and relapse rates in patients with benign gastric ulcer. N Engl J Med 1989; 320(2):69–75.

96. Agrawal NM, Campbell DR, Safdi MA, et al. Superiority of lansoprazole vs ranitidine in healing nonsteroidal anti-inflammatory drug-associated gastric ulcers: results of a double-blind, randomized, multicenter study. NSAID-Associated Gastric Ulcer Study Group. Arch Intern Med 2000; 160(10):1455–1461.

97. Goldstein JL, Johanson J, Hawkey C, et al. Comparative healing of gastric ulcers with esomeprazole versus ranitidine in patients taking either continuous COX-2 selective NSAIDs or nonselective NSAIDs. Gastroenterology 2004; 126(4 Suppl 2):A-610.

98. Lee M, Cryer B, Feldman M. Dose effects of aspirin on gastric prostaglandins and stomach mucosal injury. Ann Intern Med 1994; 120(3):184–189.

99. Scheiman JM, Cryer B, Kimmey MB, et al. A randomized, controlled comparison of ibuprofen at the maximal over-the-counter dose compared with prescription-dose celecoxib on upper gastrointestinal mucosal injury. Clin Gastroenterol Hepatol 2004; 2(4):290–295.

100. Lanza FL, Aspinall RL, Swabb EA, et al. Double-blind, placebo-controlled endoscopic comparison of the mucosal protective effects of misoprostol versus cimetidine on tolmetin-induced mucosal injury to the stomach and duodenum. Gastroenterology 1988; 95(2):289–294.

101. Graham DY, Agrawal NM, Roth SH. Prevention of NSAID-induced gastric ulcer with misoprostol: multicentre, double-blind, placebo-controlled trial. Lancet 1988; 2(8623):1277–1280.

102. Yoshida CM, Peura DA. Gastroduodenal mucosal protection. In: Wolfe MM, ed. Gastrointestinal pharmacotherapy. Philadelphia: WB Saunders; 1993:113–117.

103. Zhu X, Hsu BT, Rees DC. Structural studies of the binding of the anti-ulcer drug sucrose octasulfate to acidic fibroblast growth factor. Structure 1993; 1(1):27–34.

104. Graham DY, Smith JL. Gastroduodenal complications of chronic NSAID therapy. Am J Gastroenterol 1988; 83(10):1081–1084.

105. Caldwell JR, Roth SH, Wu WC, et al. Sucralfate treatment of nonsteroidal anti-inflammatory drug-induced gastrointestinal symptoms and mucosal damage. Am J Med 1987; 83(3B):74–82.

106. Agrawal NM, Roth S, Graham DY, et al. Misoprostol compared with sucralfate in the prevention of nonsteroidal anti-inflammatory drug-induced gastric ulcer. A randomized, controlled trial. Ann Intern Med 1991; 115(3):195–200.

107. Miglioli M, Porro GB, Vaira D, et al. Prevention with sucralfate gel of NSAID-induced gastroduodenal damage in arthritic patients. Am J Gastroenterol 1996; 91(11):2367–2371.

108. Robinson MG, Griffin JW Jr, Bowers J, et al. Effect of ranitidine on gastroduodenal mucosal damage induced by nonsteroidal antiinflammatory drugs. Dig Dis Sci 1989; 34(3):424–428.

109. Ehsanullah RS, Page MC, Tildesley G, et al. Prevention of gastroduodenal damage induced by non-steroidal anti-inflammatory drugs: controlled trial of ranitidine. Br J Med 1988; 297(6655):1017–1021.

110. Raskin JB, White RH, Jaszewski R, et al. Misoprostol and ranitidine in the prevention of NSAID-induced ulcers: a prospective, double-blind, multicenter study. Am J Gastroenterol 1996; 91(2):223–227.

111. Koch M, Dezi A, Ferrario F, et al. Prevention of nonsteroidal anti-inflammatory drug-induced gastrointestinal mucosal injury. A meta-analysis of randomized controlled clinical trials. Arch Intern Med 1996; 156(20):2321–2332.

112. Scheiman JM, Behler EM, Loeffler KM, et al. Omeprazole ameliorates aspirin-induced gastroduodenal injury. Dig Dis Sci 1994; 39(1):97–103.

113. Cullen D, Bardhan KD, Eisner M, et al. Primary gastroduodenal prophylaxis with omeprazole for non-steroidal anti-inflammatory drug users. Aliment Pharmacol Ther 1998; 12(2):135–140.

114. Agrawal NM, Campbell DR, Safdi MA, et al. Superiority of lansoprazole vs ranitidine in healing nonsteroidal anti-inflammatory drug-associated gastric ulcers: results of a double-blind, randomized, multicenter study. NSAID-Associated Gastric Ulcer Study Group. Arch Intern Med 2000; 160(10):1455–1461.

115. Walt RP. Misoprostol for the treatment of peptic ulcer and antiinflammatory-drug-induced gastroduodenal ulceration. N Engl J Med 1992; 327(22):1575–1580.

116. Graham DY, White RH, Moreland LW, et al. Duodenal and gastric ulcer prevention with misoprostol in arthritis patients taking NSAIDs. Misoprostol Study Group. Ann Intern Med 1993; 119(4):257–262.

117. Raskin JB, White RH, Jackson JE, et al. Misoprostol dosage in the prevention of nonsteroidal anti-inflammatory drug-induced gastric and duodenal ulcers: a comparison of three regimens. Ann Intern Med 1995; 123(5):344–350.

118. Isaacs P. Misoprostol and NSAID ulcers. Am J Gastroenterol 1996; 91(2):187–188.

119. Hawkey CJ, Tulassay Z, Szczepanski L, et al. Randomised controlled trial of *Helicobacter pylori* eradication in patients on non-steroidal anti-inflammatory drugs: HELP NSAIDs study. Helicobacter Eradication for Lesion Prevention. Lancet 1998; 352(9133):1016–1021.

120. Graham DY, Agrawal NM, Campbell DR, et al. Ulcer prevention in long-term users of nonsteroidal anti-inflammatory drugs: results of a double-blind, randomized, multicenter, active- and placebo-controlled study of misoprostol vs lansoprazole. Arch Intern Med 2002; 162(2):169–175.

121. Chan FK, Graham DY. Review article: prevention of non-steroidal anti-inflammatory drug gastrointestinal complications – review and recommendations based on risk assessment. Aliment Pharmacol Ther 2004; 19(10):1051–1061.

122. Stupnicki T, Dietrich K, Gonzalez-Carro P, et al. Efficacy and tolerability of pantoprazole compared with misoprostol for the prevention of NSAID-related gastrointestinal lesions and symptoms in rheumatic patients. Digestion 2003; 68(4):198–208.

123. Lanza FL, Royer GL Jr, Nelson RS. Endoscopic evaluation of the effects of aspirin, buffered aspirin, and enteric-coated aspirin on gastric and duodenal mucosa. N Engl J Med 1980; 303(3):136–138.

124. Cryer B, Goldschmiedt M, Redfern JS, et al. Comparison of salsalate and aspirin on mucosal injury and gastroduodenal mucosal prostaglandins. Gastroenterology 1990; 99(6):1616–1621.

125. Scheiman JM, Behler EM, Berardi RR, et al. Salicylsalicylic acid causes less gastroduodenal mucosal damage than enteric-coated aspirin. An endoscopic comparison. Dig Dis Sci 1989; 34(2):229–232.

126. Garcia Rodriguez LA. Nonsteroidal antiinflammatory drugs, ulcers and risk: a collaborative meta-analysis. Semin Arthritis Rheum 1997; 26(6 Suppl 1):16–20.

127. Glaser K, Sung ML, O'Neill K, et al. Etodolac selectively inhibits human prostaglandin G/H synthase 2 (PGHS-2) versus human PGHS-1. Eur J Pharmacol 1995; 281(1):107–111.

128. Inman W, Wilton L, Pearce G, et al. Prescription-event monitoring of nabumetone. Pharmaceutical Med 1990; 4:309–317.

129. Schoenfeld P. Gastrointestinal safety profile of meloxicam: a meta-analysis and systematic review of randomized controlled trials. Am J Med 1999; 107(6A):48S–54S.

130. Lanza FL. Gastrointestinal toxicity of newer NSAIDs. Am J Gastroenterol 1993; 88(9):1318–1323.

131. Meade EA, Smith WL, DeWitt DL. Differential inhibition of prostaglandin endoperoxide synthase (cyclooxygenase) isoenzymes by aspirin and other non-steroidal anti-inflammatory drugs. J Biol Chem 1993; 268(9):6610–6614.

132. Laine L, Sloane R, Ferretti M, et al. A randomized double-blind comparison of placebo, etodolac, and naproxen on gastrointestinal injury and prostaglandin production. Gastrointest Endosc 1995; 42(5):428–433.

133. Weideman RA, Kelly KC, Kazi S, et al. Risks of clinically significant upper gastrointestinal events with etodolac and naproxen: a historical cohort analysis. Gastroenterology 2004; 127:1322–1328.

134. Agrawal NM, Caldwell J, Kivitz AJ, et al. Comparison of the upper gastrointestinal safety of arthrotec 75 and nabumetone in osteoarthritis patients at high risk for developing nonsteroidal anti-inflammatory drug-induced gastrointestinal ulcers. Clin Ther 1999; 21(4):659–674.

135. Huang JQ, Sridhar S, Hunt RH. Gastrointestinal safety profile of nabumetone: a meta-analysis. Am J Med 1999; 107(6A):55S–61S; discussion 61S–64S.

136. Singh G, Terry R, Suen R. Comparative GI toxicity of NSAIDs. Arthritis Rheum 1997; 40(suppl 1):S115.

137. Hawkey C, Kahan A, Steinbruck K, et al. Gastrointestinal tolerability of meloxicam compared to diclofenac in osteoarthritis patients. International MELISSA Study Group. Meloxicam Large-scale International Study Safety Assessment. Br J Rheumatol 1998; 37(9):937–945.

138. Wilkins RF. An overview of the long-term safety experience of nabumetone. Drugs 1990; 40(suppl):34–47.

139. Jenner PN. A 12-month postmarketing surveillance study of nabumetone. A preliminary report. Drugs 1990; 40(Suppl 5):80–86.

140. Schattenkirchner M. An updated safety profile of etodolac in several thousand patients. Eur J Rheumatol Inflamm 1990; 10(1):56–65.

141. Schattenkirchner M. The safety profile of sustained-release etodolac. Rheumatol Int 1993; 13(2 Suppl):S31–S35.

142. Roth SH. Endoscopy-controlled study of the safety of nabumetone compared with naproxen in arthritis therapy. Am J Med 1987; 83(4B):25–30.

143. Roth SH. Upper gastrointestinal safety with nabumetone. J Rheumatol 1992;19(Suppl 36):74–79.

144. Roth SH, Tindall EA, Jain AK, et al. A controlled study comparing the effects of nabumetone, ibuprofen, and ibuprofen plus misoprostol on the upper gastrointestinal tract mucosa. Arch Intern Med 1993; 153(22):2565–2571.

145. Lanza F, Rack MF, Lynn M, et al. An endoscopic comparison of the effects of etodolac, indomethacin, ibuprofen, naproxen, and placebo on the gastrointestinal mucosa. J Rheumatol 1987; 14(2):338–341.

146. Vane JR, Botting RM. Mechanism of action of anti-inflammatory drugs. Scand J Rheumatol Suppl 1996; 102:9–21.

147. Distel M, Mueller C, Bluhmki E, et al. Safety of meloxicam: a global analysis of clinical trials. Br J Rheumatol 1996; 35(Suppl 1):68–77.

148. Pairet M, van Ryn J. Experimental models used to investigate the differential inhibition of cyclooxygenase-1 and cyclooxygenase-2 by non-steroidal anti-inflammatory drugs. Inflamm Res 1998; 47(Suppl 2):S93–S101.

149. Pairet M, Churchill L, Trummlitz G, et al. Differential inhibition of cyclooxygenase-1 (COX-1) and -2 (COX-2) by NSAIDs:

consequences of anti-inflammatory activity versus gastric and renal safety. Inflammopharmacology 1996; 4:61–70.

150. Bjarnason I, Macpherson A, Rotman H, et al. A randomized, double-blind, crossover comparative endoscopy study on the gastroduodenal tolerability of a highly specific cyclooxygenase-2 inhibitor, flosulide, and naproxen. Scand J Gastroenterol 1997; 32(2):126–130.

151. Lipsky PE, Isakson PC. Outcome of specific COX-2 inhibition in rheumatoid arthritis. J Rheumatol 1997; 24(Suppl 49):9–14.

152. Vane JR. Inhibition of prostaglandin synthesis as a mechanism of action for aspirin-like drugs. Nat New Biol 1971; 231(25):232–235.

153. Smith JB, Willis AL. Aspirin selectively inhibits prostaglandin production in human platelets. Nat New Biol 1971; 231(25): 235–237.

154. McKenna F. COX-2: separating myth from reality. Scand J Rheumatol Suppl 1999; 109:19–29.

155. Seibert K, Masferrer JL, Fu JY, et al. The biochemical and pharmacological manipulation of cellular cyclooxygenase (COX) activity. Adv Prostaglandin Thromboxane Leukot Res 1991; 21A:45–51.

156. Xie WL, Chipman JG, Robertson DL, et al. Expression of a mitogen-responsive gene encoding prostaglandin synthase is regulated by mRNA splicing. Proc Natl Acad Sci USA 1991; 88(7):2692–2696.

157. O'Banion MK, Sadowski HB, Winn V, et al. A serum- and glucocorticoid-regulated 4-kilobase mRNA encodes a cyclooxygenase-related protein. J Biol Chem 1991; 266(34):23261–23267.

158. Wallace JL. Distribution and expression of cyclooxygenase (COX) isoenzymes, their physiological roles, and the categorization of nonsteroidal anti-inflammatory drugs (NSAIDs). Am J Med 1999; 107(6A):1S–6S; discussion 6S–7S.

159. Feldman M, McMahon AT. Do cyclooxygenase-2 inhibitors provide benefits similar to those of traditional nonsteroidal anti-inflammatory drugs, with less gastrointestinal toxicity? Ann Intern Med 2000; 132(2):134–143.

160. Langman MJ, Jensen DM, Watson DJ, et al. Adverse upper gastrointestinal effects of rofecoxib compared with NSAIDs. JAMA 1999; 282(20):1929–1933.

161. Simon LS, Weaver AL, Graham DY, et al. Anti-inflammatory and upper gastrointestinal effects of celecoxib in rheumatoid arthritis: a randomized controlled trial. JAMA 1999; 282(20):1921–1928.

162. Silverstein FE, Faich G, Goldstein JL, et al. Gastrointestinal toxicity with celecoxib vs nonsteroidal anti-inflammatory drugs for osteoarthritis and rheumatoid arthritis: the CLASS study: A randomized controlled trial. Celecoxib Long-term Arthritis Safety Study. JAMA 2000; 284(10):1247–1255. First study to suggest that celecoxib and possibly other COX-2 selective inhibitors may reduce the risk of ulcers and ulcer complications in individuals receiving NSAIDs.

163. [No authors listed]. Physician advice and individual behaviors about cardiovascular disease risk reduction – seven states and Puerto Rico, 1997. MMWR Morb Mortal Wkly Rep 1999; 48(4):74–77.

164. Weil J, Colin-Jones D, Langman M, et al. Prophylactic aspirin and risk of peptic ulcer bleeding. Br Med J 1995; 310(6983):827–830.

165. Oviedo JA, Wolfe MM. Gastroprotection by coxibs: what do the Celecoxib Long-Term Arthritis Safety Study and the Vioxx Gastrointestinal Outcomes Research Trial tell us? Rheum Dis Clin North Am 2003; 29(4):769–788.

166. Laine L, Harper S, Simon T, et al. A randomized trial comparing the effect of rofecoxib, a cyclooxygenase 2-specific inhibitor, with that of ibuprofen on the gastroduodenal mucosa of patients with

osteoarthritis. Rofecoxib Osteoarthritis Endoscopy Study Group. Gastroenterology 1999; 117(4):776–783.

167. Hawkey C, Laine L, Simon T, et al. Comparison of the effect of rofecoxib (a cyclooxygenase 2 inhibitor), ibuprofen, and placebo on the gastroduodenal mucosa of patients with osteoarthritis: a randomized, double-blind, placebo-controlled trial. The Rofecoxib Osteoarthritis Endoscopy Multinational Study Group. Arthritis Rheum 2000; 43(2):370–377.

168. Cryer B. Second-generation cyclooxygenase-2-specific inhibitors. Clin Perspect Gastroenterol 2002; 5(2):122–128.

169. Harris SI, Kuss M, Hubbard RC, et al. Upper gastrointestinal safety evaluation of parecoxib sodium, a new parenteral cyclooxygenase-2-specific inhibitor, compared with ketorolac, naproxen, and placebo. Clin Ther 2001; 23(9):1422–1428.

170. Goldstein JL, Kivitz AJ, Verburg KM, et al. A comparison of the upper gastrointestinal mucosal effects of valdecoxib, naproxen and placebo in healthy elderly subjects. Aliment Pharmacol Ther 2003; 18(1):125–132.

171. Atherton C, Jones J, McKaig B, et al. Pharmacology and gastrointestinal safety of lumiracoxib, a novel cyclooxygenase-2 selective inhibitor: An integrated study. Clin Gastroenterol Hepatol 2004; 2(2):113–120.

172. Schnitzer TJ, Burmester GR, Mysler E, et al. Comparison of lumiracoxib with naproxen and ibuprofen in the therapeutic arthritis research and gastrointestinal event trial (TARGET), reduction in ulcer complications: randomised controlled trial. Lancet 2004; 364:665–674.

173. Chan FK, Hung LC, Suen BY, et al. Celecoxib versus diclofenac and omeprazole in reducing the risk of recurrent ulcer bleeding in patients with arthritis. N Engl J Med 2002; 347(26):2104–2110.

174. McAdam BF, Catella-Lawson F, Mardini IA, et al. Systemic biosynthesis of prostacyclin by cyclooxygenase (COX)-2: the human pharmacology of a selective inhibitor of COX-2. Proc Natl Acad Sci USA 1999; 96(1):272–277.

175. Mukherjee D, Nissen SE, Topol EJ. Risk of cardiovascular events associated with selective COX-2 inhibitors. JAMA 2001; 286(8):954–959.

176. Patrono C. Aspirin as an antiplatelet drug. N Engl J Med 1994; 330(18):1287–1294.

177. Antithrombotic Trialists Collaborators. Collaborative meta-analysis of randomised trials of antiplatelet therapy for prevention of death, myocardial infarction, and stroke in high risk patients. Br Med J 2002; 324(7329):71–86.

178. Solomon DH, Glynn RJ, Levin R, et al. Nonsteroidal anti-inflammatory drug use and acute myocardial infarction. Arch Intern Med 2002; 162(10):1099–1104.

179. Watson DJ, Rhodes T, Cai B, et al. Lower risk of thromboembolic cardiovascular events with naproxen among patients with rheumatoid arthritis. Arch Intern Med 2002; 162(10):1105–1110.

180. Rahme E, Pilote L, LeLorier J. Association between naproxen use and protection against acute myocardial infarction. Arch Intern Med 2002; 162(10):1111–1115.

181. Bresalier RS, Sandler RS, Quan H, et al. Cardiovascular events associated with rofecoxib in a colorectal adenoma chemoprevention trial. N Engl J Med 2005; 352:1092–1102.

182. Solomon SD, McMurray JJV, Pfeffer MA, et al. Cardiovascular risk associated with celecoxib in a clinical trial for colorectal adenoma prevention. N Engl J Med 2005; 352:1071–1080.

183. Nussmeier NA, Whelton AA, Brown MT, et al. Complications of the COX-2 inhibitors paracoxib and valdecoxib after cardiac surgery. N Engl J Med 2005; 352:1081–1091.

184. Laine L, Maller ES, Yu C, et al. Ulcer formation with low-dose enteric-coated aspirin and the effect of COX-2 selective inhibition: a double-blind trial. Gastroenterology 2004; 127:395–402.

185. Masuda E, Kawano S, Nagano K, et al. Endogenous nitric oxide modulates ethanol-induced gastric mucosal injury in rats. Gastroenterology 1995; 108(1):58–64.

186. Salvemini D, Misko TP, Masferrer JL, et al. Nitric oxide activates cyclooxygenase enzymes. Proc Natl Acad Sci USA 1993; 90(15):7240–7244.

187. Fischer H, Becker JC, Boknik P, et al. Expression of constitutive nitric oxide synthase in rat and human gastrointestinal tract. Biochim Biophys Acta 1999; 1450(3):414–422.

188. Price KJ, Hanson PJ, Whittle BJ. Stimulation by carbachol of mucus gel thickness in rat stomach involves nitric oxide. Eur J Pharmacol 1994; 263(1–2):199–202.

189. Brown JF, Keates AC, Hanson PJ, et al. Nitric oxide generators and cGMP stimulate mucus secretion by rat gastric mucosal cells. Am J Physiol 1993; 265(3 Pt 1):G418–G422.

190. Takeuchi K, Ohuchi T, Okabe S. Endogenous nitric oxide in gastric alkaline response in the rat stomach after damage. Gastroenterology 1994; 106(2):367–374.

191. Wallace JL, Reuter B, Cicala C, et al. A diclofenac derivative without ulcerogenic properties. Eur J Pharmacol 1994; 257(3):249–255.

192. Brown JF, Hanson PJ, Whittle BJ. Nitric oxide donors increase mucus gel thickness in rat stomach. Eur J Pharmacol 1992; 223(1):103–104.

193. Donnelly MT, Stack WA, Courtauld EM. Nitric oxide donating flurbiprofen (HCT 1026) causes less endoscopic damage in healthy volunteers than flurbiprofen (Abstract). Gastroenterology 1998; 114:107.

194. Fiorucci S, Santucci L, Gresele P, et al. Gastrointestinal safety of NO-aspirin (NCX-4016) in healthy human volunteers: a proof of concept endoscopic study. Gastroenterology 2003; 124(3):600–607.

195. Martel-Pelletier J, Lajeunesse D, Reboul P, et al. Therapeutic role of dual inhibitors of 5-LOX and COX, selective and non-selective non-steroidal anti-inflammatory drugs. Ann Rheum Dis 2003; 62(6):501–509.

196. Bias P, Buchner A, Klesser B, et al. The gastrointestinal tolerability of the LOX/COX inhibitor, licofelone, is similar to placebo and superior to naproxen therapy in healthy volunteers: results from a randomized, controlled trial. Am J Gastroenterol 2004; 99(4):611–618.

197. Henry D, Lim LL, Garcia Rodriguez LA, et al. Variability in risk of gastrointestinal complications with individual non-steroidal anti-inflammatory drugs: results of a collaborative meta-analysis. Br Med J 1996; 312(7046):1563–1566.

198. Hernandez-Diaz S, Garcia Rodriguez LA. Association between nonsteroidal anti-inflammatory drugs and upper gastrointestinal tract bleeding/perforation: an overview of epidemiologic studies published in the 1990s. Arch Intern Med 2000; 160(14):2093–2099.

CHAPTER TWENTY

20

Treatment of non-NSAID and non-*H. pylori* gastroduodenal ulcers and hypersecretory states

Yuhong Yuan and Richard H. Hunt

INTRODUCTION

Gastric and duodenal ulcers are mucosal lesions of the stomach and duodenum that result from inflammation and in which gastric acid and pepsin play a major role. Gastric ulcer (GU) and duodenal ulcer (DU) are generally grouped together under the term 'peptic ulcer' because both have many similarities with regard to epidemiology, natural history, pathogenesis, and response to medical treatment. It is now well accepted that *Helicobacter pylori* (*H. pylori*) infection and the consumption of nonsteroidal antiinflammatory drugs (NSAIDs), including aspirin, are the two major causes of peptic ulcer, and together account for up to 90% of gastroduodenal ulcers. In the 1980s *H. pylori* infection was found to be present in more than 90% of duodenal ulcers and 70% of gastric ulcers.[1] The use of NSAIDs accounted for 40–75% of *H. pylori*-negative ulcers,[2-3] and especially in *H. pylori*-negative gastric ulcers[4] and complicated ulcers.[5]

Pathological hypersecretory states such as Zollinger-Ellison syndrome (ZES) and systemic mastocytosis, although rare, must also be considered. Once all known risk factors are excluded, there still remains a group of non-NSAID, non-*H. pylori* related ulcers, usually named 'idiopathic ulcers' in the literature, which are increasingly reported. Currently, gastric and duodenal ulcers are simply and practically classified into four principal categories (Table 20.1).

During the last 4 decades, the prevalence rates of peptic ulcer disease and our understanding of the pathophysiological features have undergone major change. Although treatment strategies have changed dramatically since the discovery of *H. pylori*, inhibition of gastric acid secretion still plays an important role in the management of peptic ulcer disease. This chapter will focus on the traditional treatments of acute gastric and duodenal ulcer and hypersecretory states. Other therapeutic approaches, such as eradication of *H. pylori* infection, the management of NSAID-induced peptic ulcer, treatment of complicated ulcer, and management of gastric neoplasia are discussed in Chapters 18, 19, 21, 22, and 24.

Epidemiology of gastric and duodenal ulcer

The prevalence and incidence of peptic ulcer disease have varied considerably from region to region and from decade to decade. Peptic ulcer disease had a low incidence in the early nineteenth century but an increase, first of GU, and then of DU occurred in

---

Table 20.1 Causes and associations of gastric and duodenal ulcer

***H. pylori* infection**

NSAIDs including aspirin induced ulcer

Acid hypersecretion

Zollinger-Ellison syndrome (ZES) and/or type 1 multiple endocrine neoplasia (MEN-1)

Non-ZES hypersecretory status (rare)

Systemic mastocytosis

Antral G-cell hyperfunction/hyperplasia

Retained gastric antrum syndrome

Duodenal obstruction: congenital bands, annular pancreas

Gastric-outlet obstruction

Short bowel syndrome

Basophilic leukemia

Hyperparathyroidism (some of them associated with MEN-1 syndrome)

Idiopathic ulcers (non-NSAID, non-*H. pylori* ulcers)

Uncommon causes

Stress ulcer: burns, CNS trauma, surgery, acute organ failure

Chronic debilitating diseases: obstructive pulmonary disease, renal failure, cirrhosis, cystic fibrosis, etc.

Drugs other than NSAIDs: KCl, oral bisphosphonates, corticosteroids, immunosuppressive medications, iron, etc.

Crohn's disease

Viral infection: cytomegalovirus (CMV), herpes simplex virus type 1

Other infections: tuberculosis, syphilis, *Helicobacter helimanni*

Alpha-1-antitrypsin deficiency (duodenal ulcer)

Vascular insufficiency (ischemic gastroduodenal injuries)

Radiation induced

Carcinoma, lymphoma

---

the second half of the nineteenth century.[6,7] In the United States, an estimated 1 in 10 people suffered a peptic ulcer at some point in the middle of the twentieth century.[8] Given that eradication of

H. pylori infection has become the mainstay of therapy for ulcer since the 1980s, the incidence and prevalence of peptic ulcer and the ulcer recurrence rate has declined in developed countries and this decrease has occurred in parallel with the declining prevalence of *H. pylori* infection.[9–11] However, peptic ulcer is still common in clinical practice. From a US national survey, 4 million patients visited a physician because of peptic ulcer in 1995, corresponding to a rate of 1500 per 100 000 in the US population.[12]

Epidemiology of non-NSAID and non-H. pylori gastroduodenal ulcer

With the declining prevalence of *H. pylori* infection, the epidemiology of peptic ulcer is also changing. There are studies reporting an increased proportion of non-NSAID, non-*H. pylori* peptic ulcers around the world, especially from the US. In the US, a relatively low prevalence of *H. pylori* infection in peptic ulcer has been reported, even in low socioeconomic areas with a historically high prevalence rate for *H. pylori* infection.[13] Recently, Quan and Talley presented a systematic review of the literature on peptic ulcer disease not related to *H. pylori* infection or NSAIDs from 1995 to 2001.[14] In studies that included more than 100 patients, up to 35% of DU patients[15] and up to 34% of GU patients had idiopathic ulcers.[16] When retrospective studies were excluded, since they underestimate NSAID use, the proportion of idiopathic ulcers was still ≈22% of DU[17] and 11% of GU.[18] When the study sample size was not restricted, idiopathic ulcers accounted for up to half of DU (n=12)[19] and GU (n=36).[15] In contrast, results from Asia, where the prevalence of *H. pylori* infection is high show that non-NSAID, non-*H. pylori* ulcers are very rare.[20,21] These observations have raised questions as to whether the prevalence of non-NSAID, non-*H. pylori* ulcers is really increasing, whether it is a common trend in developed countries or a region-specific phenomenon, and whether the reported increase is associated with a decreasing incidence/prevalence of *H. pylori* infection or the background rate is changing.

Epidemiology of Zollinger-Ellison syndrome and other hypersecretory status

Acid hypersecretion, including Zollinger-Ellison syndrome (ZES), is defined by a basal acid output (BAO) >15 mEq/h.[22] Patients often have refractory duodenal ulcer, often multiple and more frequently beyond the duodenal bulb. Bleeding is common and gastrectomy cannot prevent recurrence of ulceration and other symptoms.[23] Experience from a single center in the US when acid secretion was investigated in all endoscoped DU patients in 1989–1999, 7.4% were found to have acid hypersecretion, in whom approximately three-quarters of acid hypersecretors had ZES (46/63).[24] However, the incidence of ZES is likely much lower in clinical practice.

ZES (see Chapter 31) is caused by the ectopic release of gastrin by a gastrin-producing tumor, which produces hypergastrinemia and gastric acid hypersecretion, resulting in severe peptic ulcer disease, intractable diarrhea and malabsorption.[25] The true incidence and prevalence of ZES is unknown; in the US, the incidence is one per million general population and 0.1–1% in patients with peptic ulcer disease.[26] ZES should be considered in individuals with gastroduodenal ulcers who are *H. pylori* negative and those who do not use NSAIDs, including low-dose aspirin. Up to 25% of patients with acid hypersecretory states do not have ZES and have apparently normal gastrin metabolism. Some are due to other rare diseases, such as systemic mastocytosis and short bowel syndrome (see Table 20.1). In a few, no cause is found, and although *H. pylori* infection is detected in some, the eradication neither reduces acid secretion nor cures the ulcer. They are normally described as having idiopathic hypersecretion.

PATHOGENESIS OF GASTRODUODENAL ULCER

The pathogenesis of gastroduodenal ulcer is complex and involves an imbalance between defensive and aggressive factors that include gastric acid, pepsin, *H. pylori*, and individual factors such as NSAIDs.

Mucosal defensive system

The gastrointestinal (GI) tract has evolved a series of mechanisms that, in concert, create a barrier to protect the mucosa from both exogenous and ingested irritants, including the consequences of microbial colonization. The mechanisms by which the gastric and duodenal mucosa reacts to these stimuli is complex, integrated, and highly dynamic and involves the regulation of intragastric acidity, increased mucus and bicarbonate secretion, maintenance or increase in mucosal blood flow, maintenance of epithelial integrity, rapid cell restitution, cellular repair, and changes in local immune factors.

Gastric acid secretion

Karl Schwarz's often quoted statement in 1910 'No acid, no ulcer' reveals the major mechanism of peptic ulcer and the importance of back-diffusion of acid.[27] Although patients with GU tend to have normal or reduced levels of acid secretion,[28] patients with DU generally secrete more gastric acid than normal controls. Before the discovery of *H. pylori* infection, it was known that patients with DU secrete, when stimulated, about twice as much acid as controls because they have a greater parietal cell mass and a defect in the physiological inhibition of acid secretion.[29] When compared with age-matched controls, DU patients secrete about 70% more acid during the day (meal-stimulated) and about 150% more acid during the night (basal secretion).[30] In DU patients, the increased nocturnal acid secretion amplifies the damaging effect of acid when food in the stomach is absent, thus eliminating any buffering effect.[31] These observations help form the rationale for single nocturnal dosing of H_2-receptor antagonists (H2RAs) in the treatment of DU, which is as effective as multiple-dosing regimens.[32]

However, subsequent studies have shown that the abnormalities in acid secretion seen in patients with DU are primarily due to *H. pylori* infection.[33] The reduced acid secretion in GU patients and elevated secretion in DU patients both normalized after the eradication of *H. pylori* infection.[34] The disturbances seen in acid secretion in *H. pylori*-positive DU patients are due to an increased parietal cell mass with an increased capacity to secrete acid, rather than an increased parietal cell sensitivity, which can slowly resolve after cure of the infection.[35] The attenuated negative feedback inhibition of gastrin release to regulate postprandial gastric acid secretion may also play a role in infected patients with acid hypersecretion.[31] Whether gastric acid hypersecretion, as observed in patients with DU, is a result of infection or the infection promotes the development of ulcer in those who first had acid hypersecretion is still debated. Some studies have found that gastric acid hypersecretion in DU remains after *H. pylori* eradication,[36,37] or that after eradication of *H. pylori* infection, gastric acid hypersecretion per se does not determine the recurrence of DU.[38] The changes in maximum acid output (MAO) varied among DU individuals, suggesting that other factors such as *H. pylori* infection also play a role in ulcer development.

Mechanisms of idiopathic ulcer

The causes of non-NSAID, non-*H. pylori* ulcer remain unclear. After the exclusion of surreptitious NSAID use and false-negative *H. pylori* results, infection may still play a role in a subset of idiopathic ulcers. These patients may still have *H. pylori* infection or an *H. pylori*-associated ulcer history but with the infection eliminated in some way. It has been suggested that a previous infection can weaken the mucosa, which may break down despite bacterial eradication.[14] A meta-analysis in the US found a 20% ulcer recurrence at 6 months even after the successful eradication of *H. pylori* infection and no use of NSAIDs.[39]

Idiopathic ulcer may occur as a result of acid hypersecretion, as pentagastrin-stimulated peak acid output (PAO) was significantly higher in recurrent idiopathic DU.[40] The 24-hour mean intragastric pH in healthy volunteers was lower in those who were *H. pylori* negative than those who were positive.[41] However, in another study, the integrated gastrin response and PAO were comparable in idiopathic DU patients and those with *H. pylori*-positive DU, although higher than *H. pylori*-positive or -negative healthy controls.[19] Less liquid and solid meal is retained in the stomach in idiopathic DU patients, suggesting that the rapid gastric emptying may increase acid exposure in the duodenum and promote ulcer development.[19] Gastric and duodenal prostaglandins decline with aging, which is associated with an increase in gastric acid secretion in some elderly individuals.[42,43] Acid hypersecretion could lead to an increased susceptibility to peptic ulceration in some elderly patients because their mucosal defensive mechanisms are weakened with age-related changes.[44] The presence of concomitant systemic disease may also play a role in the development of idiopathic ulcer, with a 15-times increased risk (95% CI, 8.64–25.9) in a study of 599 active DU patients in Hong Kong.[45]

It is not clear whether diet contributes to any difference in *H. pylori*-negative peptic ulcer prevalence between the United States and European countries. Europeans consume more olive oil than Americans,[46] and studies have indicated that a diet rich in olive oil is associated with a higher GU healing rate and provides a higher resistance against the development of NSAID-induced GU.[47] An in vitro study has suggested that diets high in polyunsaturated fatty acids (PUFAs) may protect against DU, possibly through an increase in the synthesis of prostaglandins or reversion of antioxidant activity.[48] A Russian study in 21 peptic ulcer patients suggested that a fish oil diet promoted more cicatrization of ulcers than a control diet (85% versus 60%); however the sample size was small.[49] More studies are needed to explore the relationship between dietary components and idiopathic ulcer.

Etiological factors

Historically, several factors other than *H. pylori* and NSAIDs have been implicated in the development of gastroduodenal ulcers. Some have been discarded, such as focal infections of the appendix or teeth. Others are thought to have been overestimated, such as stress, race, unbalanced diet, irregular sleeping habits, coffee, alcohol, spices, and smoking. However, several etiological factors may contribute to a subset of the idiopathic ulcers.

Smoking has long been regarded as an important factor in peptic ulcer, particularly before the *H. pylori* era. In a meta-analysis, smoking contributed to 23% of peptic ulcers.[50] Nicotine is harmful to the gastric mucosa and weakens defensive mechanisms, while potentiating the aggressive mechanisms. Epidemiologic studies have shown that the prevalence of peptic ulcer is higher in current smokers, with a dose–response effect to a higher quantity of cigarettes and longer duration of smoking. Data also indicate that once *H. pylori* infection is eradicated, smoking has no effect on ulcer healing and ulcer recurrence, suggesting that smoking is not itself an independent ulcerogen, but rather enhances the harmful effects of *H. pylori* in ulcer development, healing, and recurrence.[51]

The concept of 'stress ulcer' has changed over recent years. Emotional stress and psychic factors were widely considered as causes of peptic ulcer in the early nineteenth century. However, many people experience stress in one form or another in the current era but only a minority develop ulcers and no causal link between psychological stress and idiopathic ulcer has been established. More recently, 'stress ulcer' has been used to refer to acute erosion/ulceration of the gastric or duodenal mucosa following trauma, sepsis, burns, surgery, critical illness, and other serious acute disease processes. Mechanical ventilation and coagulopathy have been identified as the two most important risk factors for stress ulcer bleeding by a meta-analysis of 2252 critically ill patients.[52]

DIAGNOSIS

Diagnosis of Zollinger-Ellison syndrome

A gastrin-producing tumor is not synonymous with the term ZES. Depending on the presence of hypergastrinemia and gastric hypersecretion, ZES is classified as sporadic ZES (without multiple endocrine neoplasia [MEN-1]), ZES with MEN-1, and nonfunctional gastrinoma.[25] Because it is so uncommon and mimics classic peptic ulcer, the diagnosis of ZES is often delayed for 3–6 years from its onset. ZES should be considered in patients with peptic ulcer, particularly when multiple, and when diarrhea is prominent, which is a rare finding in idiopathic peptic ulcer patients.

As stated above, the possibility of ZES should be considered in individuals with non-NSAID, non-*H. pylori* ulcers. The diagnosis of ZES is confirmed when the BAO >15 mEq/h and the basal serum gastrin >1000 pg/mL in the presence of gastric acid secretion with pH<2. If the pH is <2 and the serum gastrin is 100–1000 pg/mL, positive provocative testing with secretin stimulation (an increase of >200 pg/mL post injection) can help make the diagnosis.[26,53] A positive histological diagnosis of gastrinoma, or a combination of signs and symptoms (abdominal pain, secretory diarrhea, steatorrhea, multiple ulcers, etc.) of ZES help to confirm the diagnosis.

Diagnosis of non-ZES hypersecretory states causing ulcer

Systemic mastocytosis

Systemic mastocytosis (SM) is a disorder associated with peptic ulcer, diarrhea, and skin manifestations (pruritus, flushing, or a maculopapular rash). GI symptoms are reported in 14–85% of cases, with a mean frequency of peptic ulcer in 23% (range 5–44%). A few studies investigated gastric acid output in SM patients, with 85–100% of patients having increased histamine production. Basal or stimulated gastric acid secretion was elevated, normal, or decreased, with BAO ranging from 0 to 75 mEq/h. However, some patients can develop gastric hypersecretion secondary to the high histamine levels, in the range seen in patients with ZES.[54] The diagnosis of SM is based on the presence of multifocal dense infiltrates of >15 mast cells in the bone marrow and/or other extracutaneous organs and other minor criteria.[55]

G-cell hyperfunction/hyperplasia

Patients with antral G-cell hyperfunction/hyperplasia may resemble patients with ZES and have intractable peptic ulcer, high BAO, and fasting hypergastrinemia but no evidence of tumor(s). These patients have about 20 times as many as G cells as normal controls.[56] H. pylori infection has been reported in ≈50% of patients, but eradication of H. pylori infection yielded mixed results in normalizing acid secretion.[57,58]

Other causes for non-ZES hypersecretory states are rare and listed in Table 20.1.

Idiopathic gastric acid hypersecretion

The diagnosis of idiopathic acid hypersecretion requires a BAO >15 mEq/h, with a normal plasma gastrin after exclusion of other rare causes of acid hypersecretory states. For patients who have undergone previous gastric acid-reducing surgery and have a normal plasma gastrin, a BAO >10 mEq/h is required to diagnosis acid hypersecretion.[22,24]

MANAGEMENT OF GASTRIC AND DUODENAL ULCER

The goals of management of peptic ulcer are to relieve symptoms, heal the ulcer, prevent ulcer complications, and reduce ulcer recurrence. Peptic ulcer changed from a surgical disease to a medical disease in the latter part of the twentieth century, particularly after the introduction of the histamine H_2-receptor antagonists (H2RAs) in the mid 1970s.[59,60] Treatment for peptic ulcer has been revolutionized since the late 1980s, changing from the traditional suppression of acid alone to combination therapy consisting of an antisecretory agent and antibiotics in a majority of patients with peptic ulcer disease. Yet, antisecretory therapy, especially the use of proton pump inhibitors (PPIs), is still the principal strategy for peptic ulcer therapy in the H. pylori era regardless of whether ulcers are H. pylori- or NSAID-related, non-NSAID non-H.pylori associated, or due to one of the hypersecretory states.

Over the past 3 decades, several classes of pharmacologic agents have proved very effective in the management of peptic ulcer disease. The main strategies include: (1) acid-suppressing agents (e.g., H2RAs, PPIs); (2) agents that increase mucosal defense (e.g., sucralfate, prostaglandins); and (3) antimicrobials that heal ulcers by the eradication of H. pylori infection (e.g., clarithromycin, amoxicillin, metronidazole, tetracycline, bismuth salts, etc.) (Table 20.2). Antacids, which are readily available over the counter, are still used for controlling occasional mild to moderate heartburn or dyspepsia with 'ulcer-like symptoms.' They are seldom used for acute peptic ulcer treatment because of the low ulcer healing efficacy and common unwanted adverse effects.

Numerous studies have assessed the relationship of the inhibition of acid secretion and healing of duodenal or gastric ulcer, and these have been systematically analyzed by our group.[61–63] A dynamic relationship exists between healing of DU or GU and inhibition of intragastric acidity. Three important parameters determine the effect of antisecretory treatment: the degree of suppression of intragastric acidity; the duration of inhibition of acidity during a 24-hour period, and the length of antisecretory treatment. For example, DU healing can be predicted by the proportion of the 24-hour period that intragastric pH is above 3. However, DU can only be 'cured' by H. pylori eradication, after which DU recurrence is <4% at 12 months.[64]

Healing by suppressing acid secretion

H_2-receptor antagonists

H_2-receptor antagonists (H2RAs) were developed specifically to block competitively and reversibly the histamine H_2 receptor on the parietal cell (see Ch. 1). Cimetidine was the first H2RA developed for human use and is more effective than placebo for inhibiting acid secretion and healing peptic ulcers.[65,66] With newer H2RAs, slightly better symptom relief and ulcer healing have been achieved. High doses of H2RAs are also approved for use in pathological hypersecretory conditions such as ZES. The discovery of the H2RAs provided a conceptual and practical means to identify the roles of receptors for secretagogues on the parietal cell. Four H2RAs are available in North America:

Table 20.2 Commonly used agents for the treatment of peptic ulcer diseases

Antisecretory agents (acid suppressing)

H2RA

Cimetidine, ranitidine, famotidine, nizatidine

PPI

Omeprazole, lansoprazole, pantoprozole, rabeprazole, esomeprazole

Mucosal protective agents

Sucralfate

Bismuth compounds

Prostaglandin E analogs: e.g., misoprostol

Antimicrobials

Clarithromycin, metronidazole, amoxicillin, tetracycline, etc.

Antacids

Calcium, magnesium, or aluminum-containing salts

cimetidine (Tagamet®), ranitidine (Zantac®), famotidine (Pepcid®), and nizatidine (Axid®) (Table 20.3). Chemically, the H2RAs resemble histamine but are slightly different in structure (with a substituted imidazole, furan, guanidinothiazole and thiazole ring, respectively), although there are many similarities in pharmacology among them.

Effect on acid and pepsin secretion

H2RAs only partially inhibit gastric acid secretion stimulated by gastrin and are more effective in inhibiting intragastric acidity during periods of basal acid secretion, including the night.[32,67,68] Clinical studies indicate that suppression of nocturnal acid is the most important factor in duodenal ulcer healing, and a dose

Table 20.3 Comparison of four H2RAs used in North American for peptic ulcer diseases and pathological hypersecretory conditions

Variable	Cimetidine (Tagamet)	Ranitidine (Zantac)	Famotidine (Pepcid)	Nizatidine (Axid)
Preparation (may be varied by manufacturers)				
Oral	Tablets, 200 mg, 300 mg, 400 mg, 800 mg; solution, 300 mg/5 mL	Tablets, 150 mg, 300 mg; EFFERdose® tablets, 25 mg, 150 mg; syrup, 15 mg/mL.	Tablets/disintegrating tablets, 20 mg, 40 mg; suspensions, 40 mg/5 mL.	Tablets, 75 mg; capsules, 150 mg, 300 mg; solution, 15 mg/mL
Intravenous injection	300 mg/2 mL	25 mg/mL	10 mg/mL	No
Bioavailability (%)*	60–70	50	40–45	>70
Time to peak plasma concentration (h)*	0.75–1.5	2–3	1–3	0.5–3
Elimination half-life (h)*	2	2.5–3	2.5–3.5	1–2
Effect on gastric acid secretion after dose (h)*				
Nocturnal	8	up to 13	up to 10–12	up to 10
Meal	3–4	up to 3	up to 3–5	up to 4
Excretion of oral dose (%)				
Renal	>48	>50	65–70	>90
Hepatic	<52	<50	30–35	<6
FDA-approved label use of oral preparations for adult peptic ulcer diseases				
Active DU (most heal within 4 wk, rare use up to 6–8 wk)	800 mg h.s., or 400 mg b.i.d., or 300 mg q.i.d. 400 mg h.s.	300 mg h.s. or 150 mg b.i.d.	40 mg h.s. or 20 mg b.i.d.	300 mg h.s. or 150 mg b.i.d.
Maintenance of healed DU#	400 mg h.s.	150 mg h.s.	20 mg h.s.	150 mg h.s.
Active benign GU (most heal within 6 wk, rare use up to 8 wk)	800 mg h.s. or 300 mg q.i.d. up to 8 wks	150 mg b.i.d., up to 6 wk	40 mg h.s. up to 8 wk	150 mg b.i.d. or 300 mg h.s. up to 8 wk
Maintenance of healed GU	Not approved	150 mg h.s.	Not approved	Not approved
Pathological hypersecretory conditions e.g., ZES. Starting dose (Dosage should be adjusted to individual patient needs)	300 mg q.i.d. up to 600 mg q.i.d. has been administrated	150 mg b.i.d. up to 6 g/day has been administered	20 mg q6h up to 160 mg q6h has been administered.	Not approved
Probable side effects	Headache, diarrhea, dizziness, somnolence, reversible confusion states	Headache, constipation, diarrhea	Headache, dizziness, constipation, diarrhea	Headache, dizziness, diarrhea, urticaria

* Average values after an oral dose. # Controlled studies of ranitidine, famotidine, and nizatidine in adults have not extended beyond 1 year. DU, duodenal ulcer; GU, gastric ulcer; q.i.d., four times daily; b.i.d., twice daily; h.s., at bedtime. wk, week

Table 20.3 is summarized from most recently approved individual product monograph/label listed on the Food and Drug Administration (FDA) website (http://www.fda.gov/cder/index.html, accessed on April 2005).

regimen of once-daily H2RA at bedtime is optimal for these drugs for the treatment of DU.[32,69,70]

Although evening dosing regimens provide prolonged nocturnal acid suppression, they are less effective for increasing daytime intragastric pH and cannot overcome food-stimulated acid secretion.[68,71] Some patients do not respond to H2RAs despite increased dosing.[72] Furthermore, H2RAs are less effective in suppressing pepsin secretion.[68]

Suppression of acid secretion and ulcer healing

Cimetidine 800 mg/day showed about 40% inhibition of 24-hour intragastric acidity in patients with duodenal or gastric ulcer, which correlated with a healing rate at 4 weeks of about 70% for patients with DU and 60% for patients with GU (Table 20.4).[61] Increasing the dose of cimetidine to >1 g/day was associated with greater suppression of acidity (67%) and a higher DU healing rate of 80%.[61] Single nighttime dosing of cimetidine 800 mg provided a 73% DU healing rate at 4 weeks together with rapid symptom relief in the majority of patients by the end of the first week. However, increasing the dose of cimetidine to 1600 mg for 4 weeks did not provide a significant improvement in ulcer healing rates over the 800 mg regimen and failed to improve on the early pain relief.[73]

Ranitidine, famotidine, and nizatidine gave slightly better results for ulcer healing and symptom relief since, at the doses marketed, they are more potent than cimetidine in inhibiting acid secretion. In two serial meta-analyses of the relationship between suppression of acid secretion and healing of gastric or duodenal ulcer, ranitidine 300 mg at bedtime or 150 mg twice daily was more effective than various dose regimens of cimetidine for suppressing 24-hour intragastric acidity and healing ulcers (see Table 20.4).[61,63] Ranitidine 300 mg at bedtime heals 84% and 66% of patients with duodenal and gastric ulcers at 4 weeks, respectively. A meta-analysis of 44 trials in over 4300 patients found that ranitidine 150 mg twice daily provided a significantly higher DU healing rate at 4 weeks than cimetidine 400 mg twice daily or 1 g/day with an overall therapeutic gain of 7%.[74] However, multidose regimens have been largely replaced by a single evening-dose regimen equivalent to the total daily dose for DU treatment. Ulcer healing is proportional to the effectiveness of nocturnal acid secretion.[31,32,75]

Famotidine (40 mg h.s.) and nizatidine (150 mg b.i.d. or 300 mg h.s.) are similar to ranitidine in healing DU or GU[76–78] and have a similar recurrence rate.[79] Famotidine 40 mg at bedtime heals 82% and 50% patients with DU and GU, respectively, whereas nizatidine at recommended doses heals 73–75% of patients with DU and 55–65% patients with GU.[61,63,80]

Analysis of intragastric pH data for various dose regimens of H2RAs and omeprazole show that standard doses of H2RAs do not maintain pH above 3.0 for more than 16 hours or pH above 4.0 for more than 10 hours (Fig. 20.1). Studies of nizatidine and famotidine support this finding.[81,82] It is now recommended that all H2RAs be administered after the evening meal or at bedtime, for 4 and 8 weeks of therapy of acute DU and GU, respectively.[31]

Tolerance

Tolerance is a term frequently used in clinical pharmacology but often misunderstood and poorly explained in studies examining the effect of H2RAs in the treatment of peptic ulcer. There is a statistically significant reduction in the antisecretory effect of H2RAs within a few days of starting continuous administration, which is not explained by altered H2RAs pharmacokinetics.[83] By definition, 'tolerance' is a condition in which the body becomes accustomed to a drug so that the previous dose no longer achieves the desired effects and a progressively larger dose is needed to obtain an effect previously observed. This strict definition does not apply to H2RAs for two reasons: (1) increasing the dose of ranitidine does not achieve the same antisecretory effect in the clinical situation or experimentally after chronic oral dosing;[84] and (2) clinical experience with H2RAs during chronic treatment, for example, during the maintenance treatment of DU,

Table 20.4 Suppression of intragastric acidity and ulcer healing at 4 weeks

Treatment	Suppression of acidity (%)			Healing rate (%)	
	24 h	Night	Day	GU	DU
Omeprazole (60 mg)	96	99	94	–	100
Omeprazole (40 mg)	98	99	97	80	98
Omeprazole (30 mg)	96	92	99	77	93
Omeprazole (20 mg)	90	88	92	73	96
Nizatidine (300 mg h.s.)	–	80	–	65	–
Famotidine (40 mg h.s.)	64	95	39	50	82
Ranitidine (300 mg h.s.)	68	90	50	66	84
Ranitidine (150 mg b.i.d.)	68	70	66	63	79
Cimetidine (800 mg h.s.)	48	79	23	–	80
Cimetidine (300 mg q.i.d.)	65	68	63	–	74
Cimetidine (400 mg b.i.d.)	37	54	23	61	72

GU, gastric ulcer; DU, duodenal ulcer; h.s., at bedtime; b.i.d., twice daily; q.i.d., four times daily; t.i.d., three times daily.
Data from Jones DB, Howden CW, Burget DW, et al. Acid suppression in duodenal ulcer: A meta-analysis to define optimal dosing with antisecretory drugs. Gut 1987; 28(9):1120–1127; Howden CW, Hunt RH. The relationship between suppression of acidity and gastric ulcer healing rates. Aliment Pharmacol Ther, 1990; 4(1):25–33.

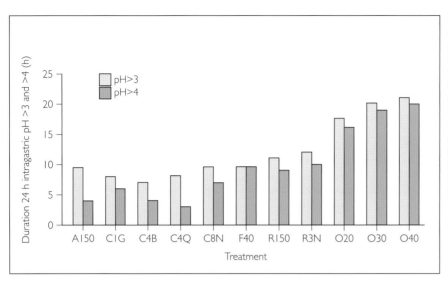

Fig. 20.1 • Duration of 24-hour intragastric pH maintained above 3.0 and 4.0. A150 indicates antacid, 150 mmol 7 times daily; C1G, cimetidine, 200 mg 3 times daily and 400 mg at bedtime; C4B, cimetidine, 400 mg twice daily; C4Q, cimetidine, 400 mg 4 times daily; C8N, cimetidine, 800 mg at bedtime; F40, famotidine, 40 mg at bedtime; R150, ranitidine, 150 mg twice daily; R3N, ranitidine, 300 mg at bedtime; O20, omeprazole, 20 mg daily; O30, omeprazole, 30 mg daily; and O40, omeprazole, 40 mg daily. (Reprinted with permission from Bell and Hunt. Progress with proton pump inhibitors. Yale J Biol Med 1992; 65(6):649–657.)

an increase in the dose of H2RAs is not generally needed to maintain patients in remission.[85] Therefore, the change in response to H2RAs may be better explained by an exaggerated 'first-dose' effect, as has been shown with many types of anti-hypertensive drugs.[84]

Rebound acid hypersecretion

A temporary increase in gastric acid secretion to above pretreatment values after abrupt withdrawal of H2RAs has been reported in many studies in both healthy volunteers[86] and patients with a history of DU.[87] This rebound acid hypersecretion may contribute to a rapid resurgence of ulcer symptoms and ulcer recurrence. Rebound acid hypersecretion is not necessarily associated with hypergastrinemia[88] or *H. pylori* infection.[86] It can be explained as upregulation of gastrin[89] and/or H₂ receptors with enhanced sensitivity of H₂ receptors.[90,91] Increased plasma gastrin stimulates and upregulates the enterochromaffin-like (ECL) cells to produce and release more histamine to stimulate the parietal cell and may increase the parietal cell mass secondary to the chronic use of antisecretory agents.[89] Although rebound acid hypersecretion is a transient phenomenon, the clinical implications should not be ignored.

Adverse events

Side effects of H2RAs are rare and most are of a minor nature and usually rapidly reversible after discontinuation of treatment. Although the total reported adverse events are higher (10.9%) in patients treated with cimetidine, there is no difference when compared with those given placebo.[92] Headache, diarrhea, and dizziness were the most common adverse events (see Table 20.3). Reversible mental confusion has been reported with cimetidine; anemia and urticaria are significantly more common with nizatidine than placebo in clinical trials but with an incidence less than 0.5% (FDA-approved label information).

Drug interactions with cimetidine and other drugs metabolized by cytochrome P450 are seldom of clinical importance because of the wide therapeutic index of these drugs, and their blood levels do not necessarily reflect their pharmacologic effect. However, interactions may be significant with some medications that have a narrow therapeutic–toxic ratio, such as theophylline, phenytoin, and warfarin.[93] In such cases, another H2RA can be substituted. The principle route of excretion of H2RAs is by the kidney, and the risk of toxicity may be increased in patients with impaired renal function, where the dose may need to be adjusted.

Proton pump inhibitors

Proton pump inhibitors (PPIs) are the most effective antisecretory agents currently available; they are all substituted benzimidazoles and have a similar mechanism of action. PPIs bind to the proton pump (H+K+-ATPase) in the canalicular membrane of the parietal cell, inactivating the exchange of hydrogen ions for potassium ions by specific enzyme inhibition. This mechanism prevents the transport of hydrochloric acid across the cell membrane to the lumen of the stomach by blocking the final step of acid production (see Ch. 1). Basal and stimulated acid secretion is inhibited regardless of the stimulus. PPIs provide better pH control than H2RAs.[62] PPIs may also have direct antibacterial activity against *H. pylori*.[94]

The use of omeprazole was approved in 1989 and now five PPIs, omeprazole (Prilosec®, named Losec® in the rest of the world), lansoprazole (Prevacid®), pantoprazole (Protonix®), rabeprazole (Aciphex®), and esomeprazole (Nexium®) are approved for use by the FDA (Table 20.5). Only omeprazole, lansoprazole, and rabeprazole are currently approved for use in the treatment of peptic ulcer disease in the United States; PPIs except esomeprazole are approved for use in pathological hypersecretory conditions; PPIs except pantoprazole are also approved by the FDA for use in treatment regimens for the eradication of *H. pylori* infection in combination with two antibiotics (see Ch. 18). However, off-label use of PPIs is common for the panoply of acid-related disorders, and the recommended indications and dose regimens vary among countries. For example, oral pantoprazole is indicated for the treatment of DU and GU and for the initial treatment of gastroesophageal reflux disease (GERD) in Europe, while its use for peptic ulcer has not been approved in the US.[95] PPIs are now the drugs of first-line choice for most acid-related disorders.

Table 20.5 Comparison of five PPIs used in North America for peptic ulcer diseases and pathological hypersecretory

Variable	Omeprazole	Lansoprazole	Pantoprazole	Rabeprazole	Esomeprazole
Preparation (may be varied by manufacturers)					
Oral	Delayed-release capsules, 10 mg, 20 mg, 40 mg; delayed release tablets, 20 mg	Delayed-release capsules/disintegrating tables, 15 mg, 30 mg; delay released suspensions, 15 mg, 30 mg/packet	Delayed-release tablets, 20 mg, 40 mg	Delayed-release tablets, 20 mg	Delayed-release capsules, 20 mg, 40 mg
Intravenous injection	No	30 mg/vial	40 mg/vial	No	20 mg, 40 mg/vial
Bioavailability (%)*	30–40	>80	77	52	64
Time to peak plasma concentration (h)*	0.5–3.5	1.7	2.5	2–5	1.5
Elimination half-life (h) in normal metabolizers*	0.5–1	1.5	1	1–2	1–1.5
Protein binding (%)	95	97	98	96.3	97
Route of elimination					
Renal	77	33	71	90	80
Billiary/feces	23	66	18	10	20
Metabolic enzymes	CYP2C19	CYP2C19, CYP3A4	CYP2C19, CYP3A4. minor: CYP2D6, 2C9	CYP3A4, CYP2C19	CYP2C19, CYP3A4
FDA-approved label use of oral preparations for adult peptic ulcer diseases					
Active DU	20 mg q.d. for 4 wk, some patients may required another 4 wk	15 mg q.d. for 4 wk	Not approved	20 mg q.d. up to 4 wk	Not approved
Maintenance therapy of DU#	Not approved	15 mg q.d.	Not approved	Not approved	Not approved
Active benign GU	40 mg q.d. for 4–8 wks	30 mg q.d. up to 8 wks for benign GU or NSAID associated GU	Not approved	Not approved	Not approved
Risk reduction of NSAIDs associated GU	Not approved	15 mg q.d. up to 12 wk	Not approved	Not approved	20 mg or 40 mg q.d. up to 6 months

Table 20.5 Comparison of five PPIs used in North American for peptic ulcer diseases and pathological hypersecretory—Cont'd

Variable	Omeprazole	Lansoprazole	Pantoprazole	Rabeprazole	Esomeprazole
Pathological hypersecretory conditions, starting and maintaining dose §	60 mg q.d. Up to 120 mg t.i.d. Some patients have been treated for >5 years	60 mg q.d. Up to 90 mg b.i.d. Some patients have been treated for >4 years	40 mg b.i.d. Up to 240 mg/day. Some patients have been treated for >2 years	60 mg q.d. Up to 60 mg b.i.d. Some patients have been treated for 1 year	Not approved
H. pylori eradication for infectious patients with active DU or DU history					
In triple therapy	20 mg b.i.d. for 10 days	30 mg b.i.d. × 10–14 days	Not approved	20 mg b.i.d. × 7 days	40 mg q.d. × 10 days
In dual therapy	40 mg q.d. for 14 days	30 mg t.i.d. × 14 days	Not approved	Not approved	Not approved
Drug interactions (exclude drugs effect by the change in gastric pH)	Diazepam, phenytoin, warfarin, clarithromycin, sucralfate	Theophylline, sucralfate	None	Clarithromycin	Diazepam clarithromycin

* Average values after an oral dose. # Control studies have not extended beyond 12 months. § Dose should be adjusted to individual patient need. DU, duodenal ulcer; GU, gastric ulcer; q.d., once daily; b.i.d., twice daily; t.i.d., three times daily; h.s., at bedtime; wk, week.
Table is summarized from most recent approved individual product monograph/label listed on the Food and Drug Administration (FDA) website (http://www.fda.gov/cder/index.html, accessed on April, 2005).

Effect on acid and pepsin secretion

PPIs are prodrugs that require protonation to their active moiety. They are activated when the local pH decreases below their respective pKa (≈4 for omeprazole, esomeprazole, lansoprazole, and pantoprazole; ≈5 for rabeprazole).[31,96] The antisecretory effect of PPIs is dose-dependent, and the rapidity of onset of action depends on the bioavailability of the individual PPI.[95,97–101] All PPIs seem comparable with regard to the inhibition of gastric acid secretion, but there are differences in PPI pharmacokinetic and pharmacodynamic profiles that result in differences in the degree of acid suppression and the speed of onset of acid inhibition, which may have clinical implications for symptom relief as well as healing of peptic ulcer and esophagitis.[96]

An in vitro study suggests that rabeprazole produces the most rapid inhibition of H+/K+-ATPase, followed by lansoprazole, omeprazole, then pantoprazole,[102] which may be a result of the pKa of the PPIs and the pH to which they are exposed. Lansoprazole has a high oral bioavailability and achieves maximum effect on pH on day one of dosing.[98] Single comparator studies have shown that lansoprazole,[41] pantoprazole,[103] and rabeprazole,[104] provide significantly higher mean intragastric pH and longer duration of antisecretory effect than omeprazole in healthy subjects. Lansoprazole also produces a faster onset and greater degree of acid inhibition than pantoprazole.[105] In a double-blind, crossover study in 18 *H. pylori*-negative healthy volunteers, the onset of antisecretory action occurred within 2 hours without significant difference for lansoprazole, omeprazole MUPS, omeprazole capsule, pantoprazole, and rabeprazole ($p=0.6$).[106] Rabeprazole and lansoprazole showed significantly greater control of daytime and nighttime pH than comparators (Fig. 20.2). Nonetheless, the slightly more rapid onset of acid inhibition of a given PPI has not been shown to have clinically significant importance in peptic ulcer healing rate.

Compared with omeprazole, esomeprazole, the s-isomer of omeprazole, has increased bioavailability and is metabolized more slowly, and the area under the plasma concentration-time curve (AUC), which is related to the antisecretory effect for esomeprazole 20 mg, is about 180% of that for omeprazole 20 mg. Esomeprazole 20 mg and 40 mg has been shown to provide superior acid suppression when compared with omeprazole 20 mg with regard to consistency among individuals, duration over 24 hours, and overall impact on pH.[107] In addition, the increased dose is correlated with a more rapid onset and greater degree of acid suppression.[101] Crossover studies of gastric pH in GERD patients and healthy volunteers have shown esomeprazole 40 mg once daily is significantly more effective than other PPIs at standard doses on both day 1 and day 5.[101] However, there are no direct comparisons between

esomeprazole and any other PPIs conducted in patients with peptic ulcer, and whether differences between PPIs on day 5 are related to clinical end points relevant to peptic ulcer healing remains unknown.

PPIs are most effective when the parietal cell is activated in response to a meal when the H+K+-ATPase is inserted into the secretory canaliculus. PPIs should therefore be taken ½ to 1 hour before a meal, for example with a first dose before breakfast, and second dose, if and when required, before the evening meal.[31] All the PPIs require accumulation and acid activation, and with the exception of lansoprazole,[98] steady-state is usually not achieved for several days. Once-daily dosing with a PPI achieved 66% of steady-state inhibition of MAO after 5 days, and administration twice daily for the first 2–3 days can provide more rapid maximal acid secretory inhibition.[108] Sporadically taken PPIs are unlikely to provide adequate acid inhibition.[31]

The effect of PPIs on peptic activity can be achieved by direct and indirect mechanisms. PPIs decrease pepsin output and reduce secretory volume, which directly inhibits peptic activity.[109,110] In contrast, increasing intragastric pH to above 4 indirectly eliminates peptic activity because activation of pepsin is highly pH dependent.[111] This effect on pH may partly explain the difference between PPIs and H2RAs in healing peptic ulcer and particularly esophagitis because the intragastric pH achieved with H2RAs over a 24-hour period still allows pepsin to retain proteolytic activity.[111]

Effect on ulcer healing

Despite different recommended doses of PPIs, at equivalent dose, they provide similar healing rates when used for the treatment of peptic ulcer.

Omeprazole was the first PPI and was shown to be superior to H2RAs in suppressing gastric acid secretion, healing peptic ulcers, and relieving symptoms.[61–63,97] Omeprazole, 20 mg in the morning, suppresses 90% of 24-hour intragastric acidity, 88% of nocturnal acidity, and 92% of daytime acidity. The best acid suppression profile achieved with H2RAs is with ranitidine, 300 mg at bedtime, which inhibits 24-hour intragastric acidity by only 68%, nocturnal acidity by 90%, and daytime acidity by 50% (see Table 20.4).[61] Although a reduction in nocturnal acidity is an important determinant for ulcer healing, suppression of 24-hour intragastric acidity has proved to be more critical. If intragastric pH can be maintained above 3 for a period of 18–20 hours of the day, the healing rate of DU approximates 100% at 4 weeks (Fig. 20.3).[62] The length of treatment also plays a critical role. The healing rate achieved with omeprazole, 20 mg daily, at 4 weeks can be approached by H2RAs if the treatment is extended to 8 weeks.[61]

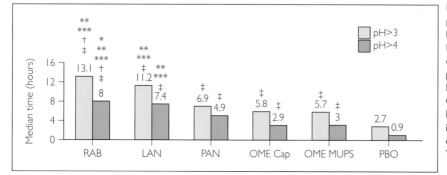

Fig. 20.2 ● Median time (hours) at pH >3, pH >4 of different proton pump inhibitors in healthy volunteers (n=18). RAB, rabeprazole; LAN, lansoprazole; PAN, pantoprazole; OME, omeprazole; Cap: capsule; MUPS, multiple unit pellet system. * $p \leq 0.03$ *vs.* LAN; **, $p \leq 0.03$ *vs.* PAN; ***, $p \leq 0.02$ *vs.* OME Cap; †, $p \leq 0.04$ *vs.* OME MUPS; ‡, $p \leq 0.04$ *vs.* PBO. (Data from Pantoflickova D, Dorta G, Ravic M, et al. Acid inhibition on the first day of dosing: comparison of four proton pump inhibitors. Aliment Pharmacol Ther 2003; 17:1507–1514.)

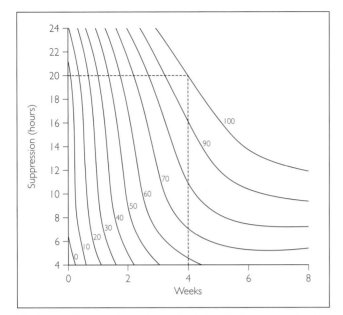

Fig. 20.3 • Contour plot of the duodenal ulcer healing rate predicted by the duration of suppression above a fixed pH threshold and the duration of therapy. Dashed lines indicate that if intragastric pH can be maintained above pH 3 or 4 for a period of ≈20 hours of the day, the healing rate of DU approximates 100% at 4 weeks. (Reprinted from Burget DW et al, Gastroenterology 1990; 99:345–351. © 1990, with permission from The American Gastroenterological Association.)

Omeprazole: Two meta-analyses have shown a clear advantage for omeprazole over various dosing regimens of H2RAs in the healing of peptic ulcers.[78,112] In a meta-analysis of 30 studies, Eriksson and colleagues showed a significant advantage of omeprazole 20 mg over ranitidine and cimetidine at recommended doses in healing DU at 2 and 4 weeks and GU at 4 and 8 weeks.[112] As shown in Table 20.6, 11–12% more duodenal ulcer patients were healed with omeprazole than with H2RAs at 4 weeks, and 7–10% more GU healed at 8 weeks. In addition to rapid ulcer healing, omeprazole provides significantly faster relief of symptoms than H2RAs. After 2 weeks, 9–14% more patients with peptic ulcer were symptom free with omeprazole than with H2RAs.[112] This advantage was more dramatic for daytime than evening symptoms, thus suggesting a pharmacologic difference between these two classes of drugs as discussed previously. Omeprazole 40 mg/day was significantly superior to omeprazole 20 mg/day in healing GU at both 4 and 8 weeks.[113]

Lansoprazole: Lansoprazole has a mechanism of action similar to that of omeprazole but has improved bioavailability, resulting in faster and greater suppression of acid secretion than does omeprazole in approved therapeutic doses. Like omeprazole, studies with lansoprazole show consistent superiority over H2RAs in healing peptic ulcer and relieving symptoms.[114] In a meta-analysis of five randomized clinical trials comparing the effect of lansoprazole 30 mg in the morning with ranitidine 300 mg at bedtime or famotidine, 40 mg at bedtime, for the treatment of acute DU, significantly more ulcers were healed with lansoprazole than with H2RAs.[115] The pooled healing rates were 60% and 85% for lansoprazole at 2 and 4 weeks, respectively, whereas the corresponding figures for the H2RAs were 40% and 75%. Lansoprazole also led to rapid and greater symptom relief of abdominal pain. In patients with GU, lansoprazole is significantly better than H2RAs in comparative clinical trials. Data from a meta-analysis of five published and eight unpublished randomized controlled trials showed that 33% more patients were healed at 4 weeks (RR, 1.33, 95% CI, 1.19–1.49) and 12% more patients healed at 8 weeks (RR, 1.12, 95% CI, 1.06–1.19) with lansoprazole than with H2RAs.[116] Intragastric pH was maintained above 3 for significantly longer in active GU patients treated with lansoprazole than with famotidine.[81]

Lansoprazole has a more rapid onset of action than omeprazole when tested in healthy volunteers.[117] Clinical trials comparing the effect of lansoprazole 30 mg daily with omeprazole 20 mg daily for healing ulcer have shown that they are similar in ulcer healing rate at 4 weeks. In two studies, the DU healing rates were 93.9% and 97.7%, respectively, in the lansoprazole group and were 97.5% and 96.7%, respectively, in the omeprazole group, with similar efficacy in maintenance of ulcer healing over 18 months.[118,119] However, one study showed that at 2 weeks lansoprazole healed significantly more ulcers than omeprazole (71% versus 55%, p=0.045),[120] which is explained by the faster onset of antisecretory effect of lansoprazole[98] and the earlier time point. Faster pain relief was also seen in the lansoprazole group. Lansoprazole 30 mg/day also healed significantly more patients with GU than omeprazole 20 mg/day at 8 weeks (93% versus

Table 20.6 Comparison of omeprazole with ranitidine and cimetidine in healing peptic ulcer

Ulcer	Omeprazole n	%	Ranitidine n	%	Difference (95% CI)	Omeprazole n	%	Cimetidine n	%	Difference (95% CI)
Duodenal										
2 wk	1532	62	1531	47	15 (12–19)*	674	63	689	42	21 (15–26)*
4 wk	1441	88	1448	77	11 (8–14)*	661	86	671	74	12 (8–17)*
Gastric										
4 wk	374	69	369	59	10 (3–17) *	102	73	87	58	15 (2–29)*
8 wk	374	86	369	79	7 (1–12)*	102	85	87	75	10 (–2;21)

Data were analyzed on an intent-to-treat basis. n, total number of patients; CI, confidence interval. * p<0.05.
Data were extracted from Eriksson S, Långström G, Rikner L, et al. Omeprazole and H₂-receptor antagonists in the acute treatment of duodenal ulcer, gastric ulcer and reflux oesophagitis: A meta-analysis. Eur J Gastroenterol Hepatol 1995; 7(5):467–475.

82%) by intent-to-treat analysis, and there was a trend toward better pain relief in the lansoprazole group.[121] In patients with healed DU resistant to H2RAs, lansoprazole 30 mg showed similar efficacy to lansoprazole 15 mg at 12 months of maintenance treatment (85% versus 70%).[122] Lansoprazole is the first PPI approved by the FDA for the prevention of NSAID-related ulcers (see Ch. 19), and also the first PPI to be made available as an orally disintegrating tablet which can be taken with or without water, and of benefit to patients who have difficulty swallowing or are elderly.[123]

Pantoprazole: Structurally and pharmacologically, pantoprazole is similar to omeprazole and lansoprazole. Data suggest that pantoprazole has the prolonged binding to the H+K+-ATPase, which, theoretically, results in a longer half-life of recovery of acid secretion in comparison to other PPIs.[124] Acid inhibition with pantoprazole 40 mg/day is greater than or similar to that with omeprazole 40 mg/day, greater than that with ranitidine 300 mg/day or omeprazole 20 mg/day,[95] less than or similar to that with lansoprazole 30 mg/day[105] or esomeprazole 40 mg/day.[95] In the treatment of peptic ulcer, pantoprazole 40 mg/day is significantly better than ranitidine 300 mg/day. In an analysis combining five clinical trials, the healing rate with pantoprazole was 96% at 4 weeks for DU and 97% at 8 weeks for GU, compared with 84% and 82%, respectively, in patients treated with ranitidine 300 mg/day.[125] When compared with omeprazole, 20 mg/day, in three comparative studies, pantoprazole (91.7% and 87.4%) showed similar results to omeprazole (89.2% and 86.6%) in healing DU,[126,127] and GU (78.5% versus 70%) at 4 weeks,[128] as well as in relieving ulcer symptoms. In a meta-analysis of these three studies, a significant advantage for pantoprazole was seen (RR, 1.07, 95% CI, 1.02–1.13) and no differences were found between omeprazole and lansoprazole or rabeprazole.[129]

Rabeprazole: Although rabeprazole was designed to be more potent than omeprazole in suppressing gastric acid secretion, it appears to dissociate more quickly and completely from the H+K+-ATPase than does omeprazole or lansoprazole, suggesting a partially reversible inhibition of the proton pump.[130] Rabeprazole is more potent than omeprazole for inhibiting the proton pump, with a slightly more rapid onset of acid inhibition than the other PPIs,[106] but the duration of inhibition was shorter than that seen with esomeprazole.[131] As monotherapy for peptic ulcer healing and symptom relief, rabeprazole 10–40 mg/day is superior to ranitidine at 4 and 8 weeks.[100] In two European studies of ulcer healing, rabeprazole 20 mg showed similar efficacy to omeprazole 20 mg for healing DU (98% versus 93%) at 4 weeks and GU (91% versus 91%) at 6 weeks, but provided significantly superior symptom improvement.[132,133] However, this indication has not been approved in North America.

Esomeprazole: Esomeprazole is the first single optical isomer PPI, which generally provides better acid control than current racemic PPIs and has a favorable pharmacokinetic profile relative to its parent, omeprazole. These differences result in increased systemic exposure and less inter-individual variability. Esomeprazole is significantly more effective than other PPIs for controlling intragastric acidity in several studies.[134] Currently, esomeprazole is only approved for *H. pylori* eradication therapy in patients with DU, risk reduction of NSAIDs associated GU and treatment of GERD.[135]

PPIs are also available as components in commercial products designed to enhance ease of use and compliance. For example, PREVPAC® consists of a daily oral administration pack containing two lansoprazole 30 mg capsules, four amoxicillin 500 mg capsules, and two clarithromycin 500 mg tablets, and is indicated for the treatment of patients with *H. pylori* infection and DU to reduce the risk of DU recurrence.[136] Prevacid NapraPAC® is a combination package consisting of 15 mg lansoprazole and an NSAID, naproxen, dosing 250 mg or 375 mg or 500 mg, which is indicated for reduction in the risk of NSAID-associated GU in patients with a history of documented GU who require an NSAID to relieve the signs and symptoms of arthritis.[137] Zegerid®, which is a powder for suspension, consisting of omeprazole 20 mg immediate-release formulation in combination with an antacid (1680 mg sodium bicarbonate) to protect omeprazole from acid degradation. It is indicated for duodenal ulcer and GERD.[138] No proven benefit of zegerid has been demonstrated over the parent compound, omeprazole, or any other PPI in the treatment of peptic ulcer or other acid-related disorders.

Optimum use of proton pump inhibitors in the treatment of peptic ulcer

Like H2RAs, the optimal duration of therapy with PPIs should be 4 and 8 weeks for acute DU and GU, respectively. Lansoprazole, pantoprazole, and rabeprazole are drugs with linear pharmacokinetics; that is, when the dose is doubled, the serum concentration also doubles. However, after doubling the dose of a drug with nonlinear pharmacokinetics, the serum concentrations will be less or greater than the expected doubling seen with linear pharmacokinetics.[96,139] It is not the plasma concentration or maximum plasma concentration (C_{max}) of a PPI which predicts the antisecretory effect, but rather the area under the plasma time curve (AUC) that correlates with the degree of acid suppression.[139] Doses of PPIs currently used in practice seem to induce acid inhibition in the 60–90% range, which are generally at the rectilinear part of their dose–response curve.[140] Therefore, it is difficult to achieve a greater antisecretory effect even when the dose is increased by 25–100%, because little change in the AUC occurs under those conditions. For example, lansoprazole 30–90 mg/day increased mean intragastric pH over 24 hours in a dose-dependent manner, but lansoprazole doses equal to or greater than 120 mg/day provided no greater increase in intragastric pH than did total daily doses of 90 mg/day.[141] Lansoprazole administrates in multiple doses (30 mg t.i.d. or 60 mg b.i.d.) produces significantly greater antisecretory effects than 30 mg daily.[141] These observations are consistent with the finding that significantly more potent and longer acid suppression was seen with rabeprazole 10 mg twice daily than 20 mg once daily.[142] This information can be exploited in conditions such as ZES or refractory ulcer when high-dose PPI is needed (discussed below).

PPIs should not be taken concomitantly with other antisecretory drugs such as H2RAs, as the acid inhibitory effect of the PPI was remarkably reduced in one animal study.[143]

Safety profile of proton pump inhibitors

Proton pump inhibitors are generally well tolerated, and the safety profiles of all PPIs are similar (see Ch. 1). Commonly reported adverse events for PPIs include diarrhea, nausea, headache, abdominal pain, and dizziness, with an incidence of <6% in short-term (≤ 8 weeks) trials and ≤10% in long-term trials.[95,97,100,135,144] Serious adverse reactions to the PPIs are rare.

There have been three major concerns regarding the long-term safety of PPIs: the effects of prolonged hypergastrinemia, the effects of hypochlorhydria, and the possible association with gastric atrophy. There is conflicting evidence as to whether long-term antisecretory therapy accelerates gastric atrophy. An increased prevalence of gastric corpus atrophy and decreased antral atrophy associated with a significantly higher gastrin level was associated with an exacerbated gastric body inflammation in patients with *H. pylori* infection treated with a PPI.[145–147] Therefore, it is suggested that eradication should be considered for all patients receiving long-term antisecretory therapy. However, no studies have shown or reported any significant increase in the prevalence of intestinal metaplasia with long-term PPI therapy.[148] In a long-term safety study of PPIs used for up to 10 years, a general improvement in antral gastritis without relevant changes of atrophy or intestinal metaplasia was reported.[149] In contrast, worsening of gastritis and glandular atrophy was seen in the gastric mucosa of *H. pylori*-infected GERD, but not GU or DU patients.[149] ECL cell hyperplasia was reported in gastric biopsy specimens in a minority of long-term omeprazole users, but no case of ECL cell carcinoids, dysplasia, or neoplasia has been reported in these patients.[147] This observation is consistent with a substantial amount of safety data of long-term PPI therapy regarding neoplastic changes in human stomach. Significant hypergastrinemia occurs only in ≈5% of individuals receiving long-term PPI, and there is no evidence to support a need for serum gastrin measurement in long-term users.[31]

Reduced serum vitamin B_{12} levels have been reported occasionally in selected patient groups during long-term therapy with PPIs or H2RAs, with elderly individuals in particular carrying a fourfold risk for this adverse effect.[150] This complication is now considered to be related to the presence of background atrophic gastritis rather than due to an effect of PPI treatment.[151] Most patients are unlikely to experience a clinically relevant deficiency because of large body stores of vitamin B_{12}. Nevertheless, it might be prudent to monitor vitamin B_{12} levels in patients taking a PPI for longer than 3 years.

In a study of 17 936 patients prescribed omeprazole in the UK, mortality due to all causes was higher in the first year (observed/expected=1.44, 95% CI, 1.34–1.55), but fell to expected population levels by the fourth year. The increased mortality was considered a result of pre-existing illness rather than drug effects because of the wide variety of causes that were also unrelated to the duration of prescription.[152]

No dose adjustment of PPIs is necessary for the elderly or for patients with renal impairment.

Acid rebound

Acid rebound hypersecretion has been documented after discontinuation of treatment with omeprazole at up to 3 months, although not all studies support acid rebound after the withdrawal of PPI treatment.[153] There is no general agreement in the literature as to whether withdrawal of omeprazole therapy results in acid rebound.[153] A current study found that rebound acid secretion after stopping omeprazole (40 mg/day for 8 weeks) is a prolonged phenomenon in *H. pylori*-negative patients lasting for at least 2 months, but no acid rebound is observed in infected subjects; eradicating the infection at the time of stopping omeprazole appears to provoke the rebound phenomenon.[154] The clinical significance of this observation is unclear. No such acid rebound has been investigated with other PPIs, although no rebound was seen after lansoprazole in a short-term study.[155]

Ulcer healing by enhancing mucosal defense

Sucralfate: Sucralfate (aluminum octasulfate) is a site-protective ulcer healing drug, which binds to tissue proteins and forms a protective barrier between the epithelium and luminal damaging agents. It binds to basic fibroblast growth factors, which stimulate the production of granulation tissue, angiogenesis and re-epithelialization; it also appears to reduce parietal cell sensitivity.[156] It may also weakly inhibit *H. pylori* growth.[157] Sucralfate is efficacious in healing both DU and GU with a low recurrence rate,[156] and it is also used for stress ulcer prophylaxis,[158] and has been used for esophagitis, dyspepsia, and colitis.[159] With sucralfate 1 g four times daily, the healing rate for DU ranges from 60% to 90% at 4–6 weeks and up to 90% at 12 weeks for GU.[160] In some patients with ulcer, sucralfate is as effective as H2RAs with respect to healing rates but is less effective than PPIs in both ulcer healing and symptom relief.[78,115] There are no clinical trials of sucralfate for treatment of idiopathic ulcer.

Bismuth compounds: Colloidal bismuth subcitrate (CBS, De-Nol®) and Bismuth subsalicylate (Pepto-Bismol®) have a mucosal protective effect by binding to proteins in the base of an ulcer to prevent further damage[161] and possess antimicrobial effects against *H. pylori* by inhibiting bacterial proteolytic enzyme activity.[162] CBS also inhibits peptic activity and may stimulate local prostaglandin (PG) synthesis.[80] The healing rates of peptic ulcer in comparative trials were similar between bismuth compounds and H2RAs.[161] At a dose of 120 mg four times daily, CBS heals 75–85% of duodenal ulcers at 4 weeks and 85–95% at 6 weeks. Bismuth compounds are also effective in healing ulcers resistant to H2RAs, which may be attributable to its anti-*H. pylori* effect.[161] CBS is widely used worldwide but is not available in North America. Usually, bismuth subsalicylate is prescribed for eradication of *H. pylori* infection in patients with the infection and DU disease (active or past history), in combination with an H_2RA or PPI and two antibiotics (see Ch. 18). Bismuth subcitrate is not used alone for treatment of idiopathic ulcer.

Prostaglandin analogues such as misoprostol (cytotec), arbaprostil, enprostil, trimoprostil, and rioprostil protect the gastric mucosa by increasing mucus and bicarbonate secretion, enhancing mucosal blood flow in the stomach and enhancing epithelial regeneration. They also bind to PG receptors on the parietal cell and inhibit gastric acid secretion. PG analogues are seldom used for the treatment of acute ulcer because of their poor symptom relief and modest healing effect, which is less than with H2RAs. Low-dose misoprostol 25–50 μg four times daily only exerts a cytoprotective effect and is no better than placebo for healing ulcers. At antisecretory doses, misoprostol 100 μg four times daily is more effective than placebo but less effective than H2RAs.[163] Misoprostol is approved only for the prevention of NSAID-induced GU at a dose of 200 μg q.i.d. in patients at high risk of complications from gastric ulcer, based on the fact that NSAIDs inhibit PG synthesis, contributing to mucosal damage (see Ch. 19).[164]

Strategy for acid suppression for Zollinger-Ellison syndrome

As discussed in Chapter 31, the goal of management of patients with Zollinger-Ellison syndrome (ZES) is to control gastric acid hypersecretion and to identify and resect the malignant tumor and its possible metastases. Acid secretion should be controlled rapidly and completely because the complications of hyperacidity can develop rapidly in ZES patients. The long acting and strong acid suppressing effects of PPIs have a clear advantage over the H2RAs and have replaced them as first-line treatment for ZES. PPIs should be used in ZES patients to reduce the BAO to <10 mEq/h for uncomplicated ZES or <5 mEq/h for complicated ZES (e.g., with MEN-1, GERD, or after partial gastrectomy).[26]

The standard dose of PPI is usually insufficient and the dose needs to be individualized. As initial therapy, high daily doses frequently exceed the usual doses for treatment of ulcers (e.g., 60 mg omeprazole, or lansoprazole, or rabeprazole, or 80 mg pantoprazole daily) (see Table 20.5). The only parameter to reliably predict the absence of mucosal injury is the level of acid inhibition rather than epigastric pain relief. Thus, the BAO should be measured (1 hour before the next dose of PPI) every 3–4 weeks or sooner after a steady state has been achieved,[31] and the patient should be evaluated by endoscopy every 3–6 months for 1 year and thereafter at 6–12 months intervals, with dose adjustments made to the PPI accordingly.[26] The goal of therapy is not achlorhydria but rather a BAO of 1–10 mEq/h. If this goal is achieved, the dose of PPI should be decreased by 50% and the patient reassessed, and if the BAO is >10 mEq/h, the dose should be increased incrementally.[165] Previous studies have demonstrated that the dose of omeprazole required to control acid hypersecretion in most ZES patients is between 60 mg and 120 mg/day; around one-third of patients require a divided dose to reach the goal rather than an increased single dose.[97,166,167] Similar to omeprazole, lansoprazole 60 mg once daily as the initial dose produced 95% inhibition of BAO and 65% of pepsin output.[24]

As much as a 6–18-fold increase in dose (e.g., omeprazole 120 mg t.i.d., pantoprazole 240 mg/day) was reported to completely normalize acid secretion and heal the ulcer and other symptoms (see Table 20.5). The PPI should be given in divided doses $\frac{1}{2}$ to 1 hour before breakfast and dinner. For instance, 80 mg/day to 360 mg/day lansoprazole was required to control acid and pepsin secretion in 46 ZES and 17 non-ZES hypersecretors in a long-term 10-year study.[24] The required median dose could not be predicted by the pretreatment acid or pepsin output, serum gastrin, prior PPI dose, or diagnosis, but one-quarter of patients could achieve a dose reduction after acid secretion was controlled.[24] Pantoprazole was used as maintenance therapy for patients with ZES and idiopathic acid hypersecretion, starting from 40 mg twice daily to 240 mg/day and shown to be effective and well tolerated for up to 27 months.[53] Acid output was controlled in 94% of 35 patients with hypersecretory conditions with oral pantoprazole. Intravenous pantoprazole 160–240 mg/day rapidly (within 60 min) and effectively controlled acid output over a 24-hour period (mean 10.9 h) for up to 7 days.[95] Sixteen patients with ZES have been successfully treated with rabeprazole at doses from 60 mg to 120 mg/day for up to 1 year. Gastric acid secretion was satisfactorily inhibited in all patients with complete resolution and prevention of recurrence of signs and symptoms and with good tolerability.[100]

Studies demonstrate that PPIs (except esomeprazole, which is not approved) have a similar long duration of action and produced similar treatment outcomes in patients with ZES.[168] They were found to be safe and effective for years. Once healing and symptom relief has been achieved and effective control of gastric output has been established, the dose of PPI can be reduced in most patients.[26] The need to increase the dose of PPI during long-term therapy is uncommon; the need to increase the dose is likely due to an inappropriate initial dose, rather than the development of drug resistance. In general, the need for an increase in the PPI dose is seen in only ≈10% of patients with ZES.[165]

Intravenous PPIs may be used when patients cannot take oral therapy, particularly at acute presentations (see Ch. 22). Although nearly half of the hypersecretors were *H. pylori* positive, acid and pepsin and serum gastrin were not different between *H. pylori*-positive and -negative patients before or during long-term PPI treatment. Eradication of infection had no significant clinical effects in these acid hypersecretors.[169]

Hypercalcemia due to primary hyperparathyroidism is the most common clinical abnormality in patients with MEN-1 syndrome. Hypercalcemia must be corrected when present because it makes it more difficult to control the gastric acid hypersecretion in patients with ZES.[25] Somatostatin analogues and chemotherapy can be used in a subset of ZES patients. Treatment of the primary tumor is also important in controlling ZES, and all localized gastrinomas should be removed when possible (see Ch. 31).

Treatment of peptic ulcer in systemic mastocytosis

Acid hypersecretion is secondary to hyperhistaminemia in patients with systemic mastocytosis (SM). Numerous studies have demonstrated that standard doses of H2RAs can decrease GI symptoms in SM patients who do not have marked gastric acid hypersecretion. In those who do have hypersecretion (>20–30 mEq/h), higher or more frequent doses of H2RAs are needed to control acid secretion (see Table 20.3). Use of 1.8 g/d of cimetidine and 1.2 g/d of ranitidine were reported to control acid secretion in patients with SM.[54] It appears that a combination regimen of H1RAs, H2RAs, and mast-cell stabilizers gives partial relief to patients with SM symptoms.[170] However, PPIs are more effective in controlling acid secretion than H2RAs, and four PPIs are indicated for pathological hypersecretory conditions including ZES and SM (see Table 20.5). There are no clinical trials comparing the effectiveness of a PPI with an H2RA in patients with SM and an ulcer.

Treatment for non-NSAID, non-*H. pylori*, non-pathological hypersecretory peptic ulcer

Although *H. pylori* infection and NSAIDs are the major causes of peptic ulcer, much remains for us to learn about non-NSAID, non-*H. pylori* ulcer. After exclusion of pathological hypersecretory states, misdiagnosis of *H. pylori* infection, and surreptitious NSAID use, current evidence regarding the optimum treatment for non-NSAID, non-*H. pylori* ulcer is poorly defined. There are no randomized, controlled trials of treatment for idiopathic ulcer. Antisecretory therapy remains the cornerstone of treatment for promoting ulcer healing, as discussed above, since some studies suggest that idiopathic ulcer is characterized by acid hypersecretion. However, there are reports that standard antisecretory therapy is less effective in the absence of *H. pylori* infection.[19,171] It is known that *H. pylori* infection may potentiate the inhibition of gastric acid by PPIs,[172] and *H. pylori* infection itself may produce an antisecretory effect.[173] Alternatively, ulcers refractory to treatment may be caused by an underlying pathophysiology of idiopathic ulcer (e.g., acid hypersecretion and rapid gastric emptying).[19]

Some studies suggest that idiopathic peptic ulcers are associated with more frequent complications and ulcer recurrence that require long-term maintenance therapy.[14] In an Italian study, in non-NSAID users, DU related complication rates were significantly higher in *H. pylori*-negative patients than in those who were positive (29% versus 7.9%, *p*<0.01).[174] These observations corroborate a study from Hong Kong, where more DU bleeding was seen in the idiopathic group, especially in those with more than one concomitant disease.[45] Other studies have not found a difference in ulcer complications.[4,21] Only 4.1% of 977 patients with ulcer bleeding were confirmed to have non-NSAID, non-*H. pylori* ulcers in a prospective study in Hong Kong.[21] In another study from Spain, if NSAID use was excluded, the prevalence of *H. pylori* infection was

nearly 90% in patients with perforated peptic ulcer, which was similar to those with nonperforating ulcers.[175]

Generally, non-NSAID, non-*H. pylori* ulcer patients respond well to conventional acid suppression in both the short and long term. In a randomized study of 276 DU patients, the clinical outcome of long-term omeprazole therapy (20 mg daily for 12 months after ulcer healing) after 2 years in *H. pylori*-negative patients (including NSAID users) was not significantly different compared with *H. pylori*-positive patients.[176] No established evidence supports the need for a longer duration or higher dose of antisecretory therapy in uncomplicated idiopathic ulcer alone, although it may be required in a subset of patients. Patients at low risk for ulcer complications may respond to H2RAs, whereas the use of PPIs is mandatory for the treatment of high-risk patients (Fig. 20.4).[14,177]

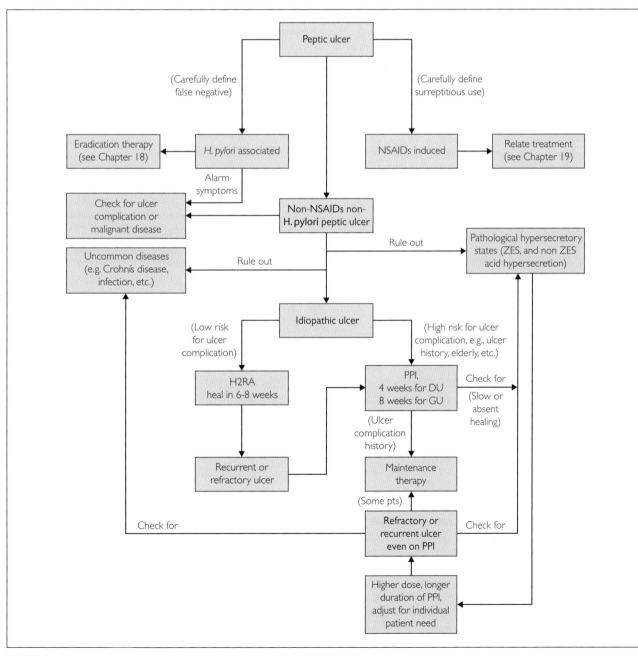

Fig. 20.4 • Treatment algorithm for peptic ulcers.

Patients with a history of an ulcer complication or with frequent recurrences should be placed on long-term maintenance therapy. For prevention of DU recurrence, lansoprazole 15 mg daily provided significantly higher remission rates, longer time to recurrence, and longer symptom-free periods when compared with placebo after 12 months.[178] *H. pylori*-negative ulcer is not an absolute indication for maintenance therapy, but those who fail eradication of infection despite appropriate therapy usually require maintenance therapy, particularly after a complicated ulcer even when *H. pylori* is successfully eradicated. Although the rebleeding rate is low, the risk is not completely abolished, especially if NSAIDs or aspirin are required.

The increased incidence of non-NSAID, non-*H. pylori* ulcer in the population may have important clinical implications for management. If the background rate of *H. pylori* infection is low, the *H. pylori* 'test and treat' strategy is no longer likely to be cost-effective because the positive predictive value of any single test for the infection will fall.[179] Thus, the proportion of patients requiring maintenance acid suppression might increase.

The choice of 'best' PPI and the optimal dose in a particular ulcer patient is an open question. Although variations exist in the rapidity of onset of action and potency of acid inhibition of PPIs at their approved therapeutic doses, their efficacies in ulcer healing and safety profiles are similar. Lansoprazole, the PPI with the most rapid clinical onset, is approved for use for non-*H. pylori* peptic ulcer, although rabeprazole and esomeprazole are not. There is a suggestion that 40 mg/day omeprazole or pantoprazole, or 60 mg/day lansoprazole might be the optimal dose for prompt symptom relief and increased ulcer healing,[140] but these are off-label doses. Alternative dosing formulations (e.g., open capsule or intravenous) may provide an option in selected patients.[180] The decision to select one PPI over another is mostly likely to be based on cost, formulation, FDA-labeled indications, symptomatic response, CYP2C19 genotype, and overall safety profile.

Treatment for *H. pylori*-negative recurrence ulcer after eradication

Treatment of recurrent ulcer after *H. pylori* eradication is a clinically important issue as the gastric and duodenal mucosa is weakened as a result of inflammation from infection. Full-dose PPI therapy should be used after exclusion of any recurrence of infection, and maintenance therapy should be considered. Data are lacking in this group of patients, and further evidence is needed to establish the optimal treatment regimen. For those who have a recurrent ulcer and recurrent *H. pylori* infection, a further course of eradication therapy is needed (see Ch. 18).

Treatment of refractory ulcer

In the era before the PPIs, refractory ulcer was defined as a DU or GU that did not heal with H2RAs within 3 months.[181] Now, a symptomatic, endoscopically proven ulcer >5 mm that does not heal after 6 weeks for DU or 8 weeks for GU treatment with a PPI, or does not heal after full-dose H2RAs within 8 weeks for DU or 12 weeks for GU, is the generally accepted definition for refractory ulcer.[182] Refractory ulcer was common in the 1970s but has declined dramatically with effective treatment. Refractory ulcers occurred in 5–10% of patients in the early 1990s.[181] The incidence of refractory DU declined from 33% in 1976–1978,

to 7% in 1989–1993.[183] The cause of refractory ulcer is seldom identified in practice; however, several factors may contribute to its development, including *H. pylori* infection, the use of NSAIDs and aspirin, poor patient compliance, inadequate suppression of acid secretion or acid hypersecretion, incorrect diagnosis, heavy smoking, impaired gastric emptying, and development of resistance to antisecretory agents such as tachyphylaxis to H2RAs.[182,184]

Refractory peptic ulcers generally respond poorly to extended treatment with H2RAs.[181,185] Although one-third of refractory ulcers after treatment with an H2RA can be healed with a higher dose for 12–18 months, the relapse rate is high (75% of patients) despite maintenance cimetidine up to 3 g daily.[183] However, the majority of ulcers healed with PPI treatment without relapse.[181] Numerous clinical trials confirm that PPIs are very effective in healing resistant ulcers. Nonresponders to PPIs are rare.[181,185] In a randomized clinical trial, 107 patients with DU or GU resistant to 2 month's treatment with cimetidine (0.8–1.0 g daily) or ranitidine (300 mg daily) received either omeprazole 40 mg daily or continued their H2RA for up to 8 weeks. After 4 and 8 weeks, the healing rates were 85% and 96% with omeprazole, respectively, and significantly higher than with H2RA (34% and 57%, respectively). Twenty-one of 22 patients who failed treatment with H2RA healed after 4–8 weeks treatment with omeprazole.[185] Similar results were achieved in patients treated with lansoprazole.[97]

In patients with refractory ulcer, resistant to conventional H2RA therapy, attention should be directed to searching for *H. pylori* infection, surreptitious use of NSAIDs, and other possible factors (see Table 20.1). Any NSAID should be stopped and *H. pylori* infection should be eradicated. Fifteen percent of refractory ulcers are non-NSAID, non-*H. pylori* related,[184] and should be treated with a standard course of PPI. Most will heal in 4–8 weeks. In patients with refractory ulcer resistant to PPI, a double dose of the PPI (e.g., omeprazole 20 mg or lansoprazole 30 mg b.i.d.) should be prescribed for an additional 6–8 weeks. The dose of the PPI can be decreased in some patients after endoscopic confirmation of healing and if the patient is asymptomatic, but most patients will need maintenance treatment. In a study of 12 refractory patients, without *H. pylori* infection or NSAID use, 9 (75%) were healed on high-dose PPI, 4 needed no further therapy, but 5 required maintenance antisecretory therapy (2, omeprazole 20 mg/day; 3, ranitidine 150–300 mg/day) to remain ulcer free. The remaining 3 with persistent ulcer despite PPI therapy were all heavy smokers (1 died of colon cancer).[184]

PPI resistance is a rare phenomenon after eliminating risk factors. The CYP2C19 genotype can impact on the degree of acid suppression achieved with PPIs.[186,187] In clinical practice, the genotype of a patient usually is generally unknown, and an extensive metabolizer may be a nonresponder, who may require a higher dose. Double-dose PPI can achieve ulcer healing in most of these patients. However, the increase in the dose of a PPI does not always lead to a significantly greater acid inhibition because the PPIs are prescribed at the upper range of the dose–response curve (discussed above), which may only lead to a slightly increased effect with a comparably small increment in peptic ulcer healing rate.[140] In such rare cases, if the BAO test supports the diagnosis of acid hypersecretion, a therapeutic strategy based on the treatment of pathological hypersecretory states (discussed above) should be employed, with higher doses and b.i.d. or t.i.d. PPI. In some cases, patients have lower than normal acid output, or have a normal pharmacologic response with decreasing intragastric acidity following antisecretory drugs but may have very low mucosal PG levels. Drugs that enhance mucosal defense, such as misoprostol and sucralfate, may heal the ulcer in such situations.[188] Surgery (e.g., vagotomy plus drainage) may be considered in a minority of patients who fail to achieve symptom relief and ulcer healing with any medications.[184] Caution under such circumstances should be exercised since the best response to surgery is usually observed in those who respond well to antisecretory therapy.

SUMMARY AND CONCLUSION

Although eradicating H. pylori infection heals the majority of peptic ulcers, the pharmacologic reduction of gastric acid secretion plays an important role in the management of patients with ulcers associated with H. pylori infection and NSAID use, and particularly non-NSAID, non-H. pylori ulcers, as well as those with hypersecretory conditions, including Zollinger-Ellison syndrome. PPIs and H2RAs are the most common class of antisecretory drugs to treat peptic ulcer disease and acid-related disorders. PPIs effectively inhibit gastric acid secretion stimulated by all known stimuli and are more potent antisecretory agents with a longer duration of action than H2RAs owing to their ability to block the final step of acid production.

In the treatment of non-NSAID, non-H. pylori peptic ulcer, which appears to be increasingly common, a careful exclusion of a false-negative H. pylori test and surreptitious NSAID or aspirin use is the first step in management. Antisecretory therapy is still the mainstay for treatment of idiopathic ulcer, and there is a dynamic relationship between the suppression of intragastric acidity and ulcer healing. Patients at low risk for an ulcer complication can be considered for an H2RA, which promotes ulcer healing in 70–80% patients after 4–6 weeks. However, the use of a PPI is necessary for high-risk patients and those who need rapid symptom relief. Patients with a history of an ulcer complication or frequent recurrences should continue on maintenance therapy. A search for other possible causes of peptic ulcer, such as ZES, is necessary when ulcers fail to heal after a standard course of treatment with antisecretory agents. PPIs are very effective for the management of patients refractory to H2RAs. Patients with an ulcer refractory to a PPI or who have a pathological hypersecretory state should be treated with higher and more frequent doses for a longer duration, with the dose adjusted for the individual patient (see Fig. 20.4).

Five PPIs are currently available, omeprazole and lansoprazole are approved by the FDA for ulcer treatment, and all PPIs except esomeprazole are approved for pathological hypersecretory conditions. Even though variations do exist among the PPIs with regard to the rapidity of onset of action and the potency of acid inhibition after oral administration at the approved therapeutic doses, the efficacy in ulcer healing and the safety profiles are very similar. PPIs are well tolerated; no dose adjustment of PPI is necessary for the elderly or for patients with renal impairment. Differences in hepatic metabolism related to CYP2C19 may contribute to inter-patient variability in plasma levels of the PPI, consequent acid suppression, and clinical efficacy. The decision to select one PPI over another is most likely to be based on the cost, FDA-labeled indications, choice of formulation, CYP2C19 genotype, previous response to treatment, and overall safety profile.

REFERENCES

1. Marshall BJ, McGechie DB, Rogers PA, et al. Pyloric *Compylobacter* infection and gastroduodenal disease. Med J Aust 1985; 142(8):439–444.

2. Henry A, Batey RG. Low prevalence of *Helicobacter pylori* in an Australian duodenal ulcer population: NSAIDitis or the effect of ten years of treatment? Aust NZ J Med 1998; 28 (3):345.

3. Nensey YM, Schubert TT, Bologna SD, et al. *Helicobacter pylori*-negative duodenal ulcer. Am J Med 1991; 91(1):15–18.

4. Arroyo MT, Forne M, de Argila CM, et al. The prevalence of peptic ulcer not related to *Helicobacter pylori* or non-steroidal anti-inflammatory drug use is negligible in south Europe. Helicobacter 2004; 9(3): 249–254.

   A perspective study from Spain, suggested that non-NSAID non-*H. pylori* ulcer has not increased in Europe, which agrees with other studies that reported a low prevalence of idiopathic ulcer in Europe and Japan.

5. Wolfe MM, Lichtenstein DR, Singh G. Gastrointestinal toxicity of nonsteroidal anti-inflammatory drugs. N Engl J Med 1999; 340(24):1888–1899.

6. Grob GN. Peptic ulcer in twentieth-century America. N Engl J Med 2004; 101(1–2):19–28.

7. Baron JH, Sonnenberg A. Publications on peptic ulcer in Britain, France, Germany and the US. Eur J Gastroenterol Hepatol 2002; 14(7):711–715.

8. Kurata JH. Ulcer epidemiology: an overview and proposed research framework. Gastroenterology 1989; 96(Suppl 2):569–580.

9. Xia HHX, Phung N, Altiparmak E, et al. Reduction of peptic ulcer disease and *Helicobacter pylori* infection but increase of reflux esophagitis in Western Sydney between 1990 and 1998. Dig Dis Sci 2001; 46(12):2716–2723.

10. Loffeld RJ, van der Putten AB. Changes in prevalence of *Helicobacter pylori* infection in two groups of patients undergoing endoscopy and living in the same region in the Netherlands. Scand J Gastroenterol 2003; 38(9) 938–941.

11. Lewis JD, Bilker WB, Brensinger C, et al. Hospitalization and mortality rates from peptic ulcer disease and GI bleeding in the 1990s: relationship to sales of nonsteroidal anti-inflammatory drugs and acid suppression medications. Am J Gastroenterol 2002; 97(10):2540–2549.

12. Munnangi S, Sonnenberg A. Time trends of physician visits and treatment patterns of peptic ulcer disease in the United States. Arch Intern Med 1997; 157(13):1489–1494.

13. Kalaghchi B, Mekasha G, Jack MA, et al. Ideology of *Helicobacter pylori* prevalence in peptic ulcer disease in an inner-city minority population. J Clin Gastroenterol 2004; 38(3):248–251.

14. Quan C, Talley NJ. Management of peptic ulcer disease not related to *Helicobacter pylori* or NSAIDs. Am J Gastroenterol 2002; 97 (12): 2950–2961.

   A systematic literature review of non-*Helicobacter pylori* or non-NSAID related peptic ulcer disease, possible mechanism and management were discussed.

15. Sprung DJ, Apter MN. What is the role of *Helicobacter pylori* in peptic ulcer and gastric cancer outside the big cities? J Clin Gastroenterol 1998; 26(1):60–63.

16. Jyotheeswaran S, Shah AN, Jin HO, et al. Prevalence of *Helicobacter pylori* in peptic ulcer patients in greater Rochester, NY: is empirical triple therapy justified? Am J Gastroenterol 1998; 93(4):574–578.

17. Ciociola AA, McSorley DJ, Turner K, et al. *Helicobacter pylori* infection rates in duodenal ulcer patients in the United States may be lower than previously estimated. Am J Gastroenterol 1999; 94(7):1834–1840.

18. Borody T, Brandl S, Andrews P. et al. *Helicobacter pylori*-negative gastric ulcer. Am J Gastroenterol. 1992; 87(10):1403–1406.

19. McColl KE, EI-Nujumi AM, Chittajallu RS, et al. A study of the pathogenesis of *Helicobacter pylori* negative chronic duodenal ulceration. Gut 1993; 34(6):762–768.

20. Nishikawa K, Sugiyama T, Kato M, et al. Non-*Helicobacter pylori* and non-NSAID peptic ulcer disease in the Japanese population. Eur J Gastroenterol Hepatol 2000; 12(6):635–640.

21. Chan HL, Wu JC, Chan FK, et al. Is non-*Helicobacter pylori*, non-NSAID peptic ulcer a common cause of upper GI bleeding? A prospective study of 977 patients. Gastrointest Endosc 2001; 53(4):438–442.

22. Collen MJ, Sheridan MJ. Definition for idiopathic gastric acid hypersecretion. A statistical and functional evaluation. Dig Dis Sci 1991; 36(10):1371–1376.

23. Hirschowitz BI. Usual and unusual causes of duodenal ulcer. Dig Liver Dis 2003; 35(8):519–522.

24. Hirschowitz BI, Simmons J, Mohnen J. Long-term lansoprazole control of gastric acid and pepsin secretion in ZE and non-ZE hypersecretors: a prospective 10-year study. Aliment Pharmacol Ther 2001; 15(11):1795–1806.

25. Jensen RT. Gastrin-producing tumors. Cancer Treat Res 1997; 89:293–334.

26. Tomassetti P, Salomone T, Migliori M, et al. Optimal treatment of Zollinger-Ellison syndrome and related conditions in elderly patients. Drugs Aging 2003; 20(14):1019–1034.

    A system review of treatment of Zollinger-Ellison syndrome, especially the optimal use of PPI in elderly patients.

27. Schwarz K. Über penetrierende magen-und jejunalgeschwüre. Beitr Klin Chirurgie 1910; 5:96–128.

28. Wolfe MM, Soll AH. The physiology of gastric acid secretion. N Engl J Med 1988; 319(26):1707–1715.

29. Blair AJ, Feldman M, Barnett C, et al. Detailed comparison of basal and food-stimulated gastric acid secretion rates and serum gastrin concentrations in duodenal ulcer patients and normal subjects. J Clin Invest 1987; 79(2):582–587.

30. Feldman M, Richardson CT. Total 24-hour gastric acid secretion in patients with duodenal ulcer: comparison with normal subjects and effects of cimetidine and parietal cell vagotomy. Gastroenterology 1986; 90(3):540–544.

31. Wolfe MM, Sachs G. Acid suppression: optimizing therapy for gastroduodenal ulcer healing, gastroesophageal reflux disease, and stress-related erosive syndrome. Gastroenterology 2000; 118(Suppl1): S9–S31.

    A systematic review of pathophysiology of acid-related disorders, and the rationale of acid secretion and inhibition in disease development and decision making for optimized therapy.

32. Gledhill T, Howard OM, Buck M, et al. Single nocturnal dose of an H_2-receptor antagonist for the treatment of duodenal ulcer. Gut 1983; 24(10):904–908.

33. El-Omar EM, Penman ID, Ardill JE, et al. *Helicobacter pylori* infection and abnormalities of acid secretion in patients with duodenal ulcer disease. Gastroenterology 1995; 109(3): 681–691.

34. Iijima K, Ohara S, Sekine H, et al. Changes in gastric acid secretion assayed by endoscopic gastrin test before and after *Helicobacter pylori* eradication. Gut 2000; 46(1):20–26.

35. Jacobson K, Chiba N, Chen Y, et al. Gastric acid secretory response in *Helicobacter pylori*-positive patients with duodenal ulcer disease. Can J Gastroenterol 2001; 15(1):29–39.

36. Chiba T, Watanabe T, Ito T. *Helicobacter pylori* infection and acid secretion in patients with duodenal ulcer in Japan. Gut 2001; 48(6):871–872.

37. Kato S, Ozawa K, Koike T, et al. Effect of *Helicobacter pylori* infection on gastric acid secretion and meal-stimulated serum gastrin in children. Helicobacter 2004; 9(2):100–105.

38. Capurso G, Martino G, Grossi C, et al. Hypersecretory duodenal ulcer and *Helicobacter pylori* infection: a four-year follow-up study. Dig Liver Dis 2000; 32(2):119–124.

39. Laine L, Hopkins RJ, Girardi LS. Has the impact of *Helicobacter pylori* therapy on ulcer recurrence in the United States been overstated? A meta-analysis of rigorously designed trials. Am J Gastroenterol 1998; 93(9):1409–1415.

40. Harris AW, Gummett PA, Phull PS, et al. Recurrence of duodenal ulcer after *Helicobacter pylori* eradication is related to high acid output. Aliment Pharmacol Ther 1997; 11(2):331–334.

41. Blum RA, Shi H, Karol MD, et al. The comparative effects of lansoprazole, omeprazole, and ranitidine in suppressing gastric acid secretion. Clin Ther 1997; 19(5):1013–1023.

42. Cryer B, Redfern JS, Goldschmiedt M, et al. Effect of aging on gastric and duodenal mucosal prostaglandin concentrations in humans. Gastroenterology. 1992; 102(4 Pt 1):1118–1123.

43. Feldman M, Cryer B, McArthur KE, et al. Effects of aging and gastritis on gastric acid and pepsin secretion in humans: a prospective study. Gastroenterology. 1996; 110(4):1043–1052.

44. Guslandi M, Pellegrini A, Sorghi M. Gastric mucosal defenses in the elderly. Gerontology 1999; 45(4):206–208.

45. Xia HH, Wong BC, Wong KW, et al. Clinical and endoscopic characteristics of non-*Helicobacter pylori*, non-NSAID duodenal ulcers: a long-term prospective study. Aliment Pharmacol Ther 2001; 15(12):1875–1882.

46. Vossen P. Spanish olive oil production. Technical report on the olive oil production tour (11–28 to 12–8, 1997), 1997. *http://cesonoma.ucdavis.edu/HORTIC/spain_olive.pdf.* (Accessed Sep 13, 2004).

47. Alarcon de la Lastra C, Barranco MD, Motilva V, et al. Mediterranean diet and health: biological importance of olive oil. Curr Pharm Des 2001; 7(10):933–-950.

48. Manjari V, Das UN. Effect of polyunsaturated fatty acids on dexamethasone-induced gastric mucosal damage. Prostaglandins Leukot Essent Fatty Acids 2000; 62(2):85–96.

49. Matushevskaia VN, Shakhovskaia AK, Karagodina ZV, et al. Optimization of dietary fat composition in erosive and ulcerative diseases of the gastroduodenal area. Vopr Pitan 1996; 6(6):35–37.

50. Kurata JH, Nogawa AN. Meta-analysis of risk factors for peptic ulcer. Nonsteroidal antiinflammatory drugs, *Helicobacter pylori*, and smoking. J Clin Gastroenterol 1997; 24(1):2–17.

51. Parasher G, Eastwood GL. Smoking and peptic ulcer in the *Helicobacter pylori* era. J Gastroenterol Hepatol 2000; 12(8):843–853.

52. Cook DJ, Fuller HD, Guyatt GH, et al. Risk factors for gastrointestinal bleeding in critically ill patients. Canadian Critical Care Trials Group. N Engl J Med 1994; 330(6):377–381.

53. Metz DC, Soffer E, Forsmark CE, et al. Maintenance oral pantoprazole therapy is effective for patients with Zollinger-Ellison syndrome and idiopathic hypersecretion. Am J Gastroenterol 2003; 98(2):301–307.

54. Jensen RT. Gastrointestinal abnormalities and involvement in systemic mastocytosis. Hematol Oncol Clin North Am 2000; 14(3):579–623.

55. Castells MC. Mastocytosis: classification, diagnosis, and clinical presentation. Allergy Asthma Proc 2004; 25(1):33–36.

56. Polak JM, Stagg B, Pearse AG. Two types of Zollinger-Ellison syndrome: immunofluorescent, cytochemical and ultrastructural studies of the antral and pancreatic gastrin cells in different clinical states. Gut 1972; 13(7):501–512.

57. Kwan CP, Tytgat GN. Antral G-cell hyperplasia: a vanishing disease? Eur J Gastroenterol Hepatol 1995; 7(11):1099–1103.

58. Annibale B, Aprile MR, Ferraro G, et al. Relationship between fundic endocrine cells and gastric acid secretion in hypersecretory duodenal ulcer diseases. Aliment Pharmacol Ther 1998; 12(8):779–788.

59. Burland WL, Hunt RH, Mills JG, et al. Cimetidine – a review. Br J Pharmacol 1979; II (1):24–40.

60. Hunt RH. The use and abuse of the H_2-receptor antagonists. J R Coll Physicians. 1982; 16:33–39.

61. Jones DB, Howden CW, Burget DW, et al. Acid suppression in duodenal ulcer: a meta-analysis to define optimal dosing with antisecretory drugs. Gut 1987; 28(9):1120–1127.

62. Burget DW, Chiverton SG, Hunt RH. Is there an optimal degree of acid suppression for healing of duodenal ulcers? A model of the relationship between ulcer healing and acid suppression. Gastroenterology 1990; 99(2):345–351.

   A model reveals the dynamic relationship between healing of peptic ulcer and inhibition of intragastric acidity. Three important parameters determining the effect of antisecretory drugs were discussed.

63. Howden CW, Hunt RH. The relationship between suppression of acidity and gastric ulcer healing rates. Aliment Pharmacol Ther 1990; 4(1):25–33.

64. O'Brien B, Goeree R, Mohamed AH, et al. Cost-effectiveness of *Helicobacter pylori* eradication for the long-term management of duodenal ulcer in Canada. Arch Intern Med 1995; 155(18):1958–1964.

65. Weberg R, Berstad A, Osnes M. Comparison of low-dose antacids, cimetidine, and placebo on 24-hour intragastric acidity in healthy volunteers. Dig Dis Sci 1992; 37(12):1810–1814.

66. Tatsuta M, Iishi H, Okuda S. Effects of cimetidine on the healing and recurrence of duodenal ulcers and gastric ulcers. Gut 1986; 27(10):1213–1218.

67. Black JW, Duncan WA, Durant CJ, et al. Definition and antagonism of histamine H_2-receptors. Nature 1972; 236(5347):385–390.

68. de Gara CJ, Burget DW, Silletti C, et al. A double-blind randomized study comparing different dose regimens of H_2-receptor antagonists on 24-hour gastric secretion in normal subjects and duodenal ulcer patients. Am J Gastroenterol 1987; 82(1):36–41.

69. Howden CW, Jones DB, Hunt RH. Nocturnal doses of H_2-receptor antagonists for duodenal ulcer. Lancet 1985; 1(8429):647–648.

70. Pounder RE. Degrees of acid suppression and ulcer healing: dosage considerations. Aliment Pharmacol Ther 1991; 5(Suppl 1):5–13

71. Merki HS, Halter F, Wilder-Smith C, et al. Effect of food on H2-receptor blockade in normal subjects and duodenal ulcer patients. Gut. 1990; 31(2):148–150.

72. Gledhill T, Buck M, Hunt RH. Effect of no treatment, cimetidine 1g/day, cimetidine 2g/day and cimetidine combined with atropine on nocturnal gastric secretion in cimetidine non-responders. Gut 1984; 25(11):1211–1216.

73. Young MD, Frank WO, Dickson BD, et al. Determining the optimal dosage regimen for H_2-receptor antagonist therapy – a dose validation approach. Aliment Pharmacol Ther 1989; 3(1):47–57.

74. McIsaac RL, McCanless I, Summers K, et al. Ranitidine and cimetidine in the healing of duodenal ulcer: meta-analysis of comparative clinical trials. Aliment Pharmacol Ther 1987; 1(5):369–381.

75. Hunt RH. Acid suppression and ulcer healing: dichotomy, degree, and dilemma. Am J Gastroenterol. 1988; 83(9):964–966.

76. Khasawneh SM, Affarah HB. Morning versus evening doses in comparison of three H_2-receptor blockers in duodenal ulcer healing. Am J Gastroenterol 1992; 87(9):1180–1182.

77. Naccaratto R, Cremer M, Dammann HG, et al. Nizatidine versus ranitidine in gastric ulcer disease. A European multicentre trial. Scand J Gastroenterol 1987; 136(Suppl):71–78.

78. Di Mario F, Battaglia G, Leandro G, et al. Short-term treatment of gastric ulcer. A meta-analytical evaluation of blind trials. Dig Dis Sci 1996; 41(6):1108–1131.

79. Palmer RH, Frank WO, Karlstadt R. Maintenance therapy of duodenal ulcer with H_2-receptor antagonists – a meta-analysis. Aliment Pharmacol Ther 1990; 4(3):283–294.

80. Freston JW, Bianchi Porro G. The medical treatment of acute peptic ulcer disease. In: Hunt RH, ed. Proton pump inhibitor and acid-related disorders. Osaka, Japan: Adis International; 1995:101–117.

81. Sakaguchi M, Ashida K, Umegaki E, et al. Suppressive action of lansoprazole on gastric acidity and its clinical effect in patients with gastric ulcers: comparison with famotidine. J Clin Gastroenterol 1995; 20(Suppl 2):S27–S31.

82. Savarino V, Mela GS, Zentilin P, et al. Twenty-four-hour control of gastric acidity by twice-daily doses of placebo, nizatidine 150 mg, nizatidine 300 mg, and ranitidine 300 mg. J Clin Pharmacol 1993; 33(1):70–74.

83. Lachman L, Howden CW. Twenty-four-hour intragastric pH: tolerance within 5 days of continuous ranitidine administration. Am J Gastroenterol 2000; 95(1):57–61.

84. Hunt RH, Cederberg C, Dent J, et al. Optimizing acid suppression for treatment of acid-related diseases. Dig Dis Sci 1995; 40(2 Suppl):24S–49S.

   This paper considers the ideal ways of assessing and reporting the pharmacological effectiveness of acid-inhibiting drugs and relating such data to clinical efficacy. These are the degree of suppression of acidity, the duration of suppression of acidity, and the duration of treatment.

85. Kurata JH, Koch GG, Nogawa AN. Comparison of ranitidine and cimetidine ulcer maintenance therapy. J Clin Gastroenterol 1987; 9(6):644–650.

86. El-Omar E, Banerjee S, Wirz A, et al. Marked rebound acid hypersecretion after treatment with ranitidine. Am J Gastroenterol 1996; 91(2):355-359.

87. Fullarton GM, Macdonald AM, McColl KE. Rebound hypersecretion after H_2-antagonist withdrawal – a comparative study with nizatidine, ranitidine and famotidine. Aliment Pharmacol Ther 1991; 5(4):391–398.

88. Fullarton GM, McLauchlan G, Macdonald A, et al. Rebound nocturnal hypersecretion after four weeks treatment with an H_2 receptor antagonist. Gut 1989; 30(4):449–454.

89. Sandvik AK, Brenna E, Waldum HL. Review article: the pharmacological inhibition of gastric acid secretion – tolerance and rebound. Aliment Pharmacol Ther 1997; 11(6):1013–1018.

90. Jones DB, Howden CW, Burget DW, et al. Alteration of H_2 receptor sensitivity in duodenal ulcer patients after maintenance treatment with an H_2 receptor antagonist. Gut. 1988; 29(7):701–703.

91. Takeuchi K, Kajimura M, Kodaira M, et al. Up-regulation of H_2 receptor and adenylate cyclase in rabbit parietal cells during prolonged treatment with H_2-receptor antagonists. Dig Dis Sci 1999; 44(8):1703–1709.

92. Richter JM, Colditz GA, Huse DM, et al. Cimetidine and adverse reactions: a meta-analysis of randomized clinical trials of short-term therapy. Am J Med 1989; 87(3):278–284.

93. Hansten PD. Overview of the safety profile of the H$_2$-receptor antagonists. DICP 1990; 24(Suppl 11):38–41.

94. Peterson WL. The role of antisecretory drugs in the treatment of *Helicobacter pylori* infection. Aliment Pharmacol Ther 1997; 11 (Suppl 1):21–25.

95. Cheer SM, Prakash A, Fauld D, et al. Pantoprazole. An update of its pharmacological properties and therapeutic use in the management of acid-related disorders. Drugs 2003; 63(1):101–132.

96. Robinson M, Horn J. Clinical pharmacology of proton pump inhibitors, what the practising physician needs to know. Drugs 2003; 63(24):2739–2754.

A review compared the clinical pharmacology of five PPIs, including pharmacodynamics, pharmacokinetics, metabolism, clinical consequences and treatment recommendations.

97. Wilde MI, McTavish D. Ompreazole: An update of its pharmacology and therapeutic use in acid-related disorders. Drug 1994; 48(1): 91–132.

98. Bell NJ, Hunt RH. Time to maximum effect of lansoprazole on gastric pH in normal male volunteers. Aliment Pharmacol Ther 1996; 10(6):897–904.

99. Langtry HD, Wilde MI. Lansoprazole. An update of its pharmacological properties and clinical efficacy in the management of acid-related disorders. Drugs 1997; 54(3): 473–500.

100. Carswell CI, Goa KL. Rabeprazole: an update of its use in acid-related disorders. Drugs 2001; 61(15):2327–2356.

101. Hatlebakk JG. Review article: gastric acidity-comparison of esomeprazole with other proton pump inhibitors. Aliment Pharmacol Ther 2003; 17(Suppl 1):10–15.

102. Besancon M, Simon A, Sachs G, et al. Sites of reaction of the gastric H,K-ATPase with extracytoplasmic thiol reagents. J Biol Chem 1997; 272(36):22438–22446.

103. Dammann HG, Burkhardt F. Pantoprazole versus omeprazole: influence on meal-stimulated gastric acid secretion. Eur J Gastroenterol Hepatol 1999; 11(11):1277–1282.

104. Williams MP, Sercombe J, Hamilton MI, et al. A placebo-controlled trial to assess the effects of 8 days of dosing with rabeprazole versus omeprazole on 24-h intragastric acidity and plasma gastrin concentrations in young healthy male subjects. Aliment Pharmacol Ther 1998; 12(11):1079–1089.

105. Huang JQ, Goldwater DR, Thomson AB, et al. Acid suppression in healthy subjects following lansoprazole or pantoprazole. Aliment Pharmacol Ther 2002; 16(3):425–433.

106. Pantoflickova D, Dorta G, Ravic M, et al. Acid inhibition on the first day of dosing: comparison of four proton pump inhibitors. Aliment Pharmacol Ther 2003; 17(12):1507–1514.

107. Dent J. Review article: pharmacology of esomeprazole and comparisons with omeprazole. Aliment Pharmacol Ther 2003; 17(Suppl 1):5–9.

108. Sachs G. Proton pump inhibitors and acid-related diseases. Pharmacotherapy 1997; 17(1):22–37.

109. Kittang E, Aadland E, Schjonsby H. Effect of omeprazole on the secretion of intrinsic factor, gastric acid and pepsin in man. Gut 1985; 26(6):594–598.

110. Brunner G, Hell M, Hengels KJ, et al. Influence of lansoprazole on intragastric 24-hour pH, meal-stimulated gastric acid secretion, and concentrations of gastrointestinal hormones and enzymes in serum and gastric juice in healthy volunteers. Digestion 1995; 56(2):137–144.

111. Hirschowitz BI, Keeling D, Lewin M, et al. Pharmacological aspects of acid secretion. Dig Dis Sci 1995; 40(Suppl 2):3S–23S.

112. Eriksson S, Långström G, Rikner L, et al. Omeprazole and H$_2$-receptor antagonists in the acute treatment of duodenal ulcer, gastric ulcer, and reflux oesophagitis: A meta-analysis. Eur J Gastroenterol Hepatol 1995; 7(5):467–475.

A meta-analysis compared omeprazole with ranitidine or famotidine for the treatment of gastric and duodenal ulcer. Higher healing rate and more freedom from symptoms were seen in patients treated with omeprazole than with H2RAs.

113. Valenzuela JE, Kogut DG, McCullough AJ, et al. Comparison of once-daily doses of omeprazole (40mg and 20mg) and placebo in the treatment of benign gastric ulcer: a multicenter, randomized, double-blind study. Am J Gastroenterol 1996; 91(12):2516–2522.

114. Gremse DA. Lansoprazole: pharmacokinetics, pharmacodynamics and clinical uses. Expert Opin Pharmacother 2001; 2(10): 1663–1670.

115. Poynard T, Lemaire M, Agostini H. Meta-analysis of randomized clinical trials comparing lansoprazole with ranitidine or famotidine in the treatment of acute duodenal ulcer. Eur J Gastroenterol Hepatol 1995; 7(7):661–665.

116. Tunis SR, Sheinhait IA, Schmid CH, et al. Lansoprazole compared with histamine 2-receptor antagonists in healing gastric ulcers: a meta-analysis. Clin Ther 1997; 19(4):743–757.

117. Thoring M, Hedenstrom H, Eriksson LS. Rapid effect of lansoprazole on intragastric pH: a crossover comparison with omeprazole. Scand J Gastroenterol 1999; 34(4):341–345.

118. Dobrilla G, Piazzi L, Fiocca R. Lansoprazole versus omeprazole for duodenal ulcer healing and prevention of relapse: a randomized multicenter, double-masked trial. Clin Ther 1999; 21(8):1321–1331.

119. Ekstrom P, Carling L, Unge P, et al. Lansoprazole versus omeprazole in active duodenal ulcer. Scand J Gastroenterol 1995; 30(3):210–215

120. Petite JP, Slama JL, Licht H, et al. Comparison of lansoprazole (30mg) and omeprazole (20mg) in the treatment of duodenal ulcer. A multicenter double-blind comparative trial. Gastroenterology Clin Biol 1993; 17(5):334–340.

121. Florent C, Audigier JC, Boyer J, et al. Efficacy and safety of lansoprazole in the treatment of gastric ulcer: A multicentre study. Eur J Gastroenterol Hepatol 1994; 6(12):1135–1139.

122. Kovacs TO, Campbell D, Richter J, et al. Double-blinding comparison of lansoprazole 15mg, lansoprazole 30mg and placebo as maintenance therapy in patients with healed duodenal ulcers resistant to H$_2$-receptor antagonists. Aliment Pharmacol Ther 1999; 13(7):959–967.

123. Baldi F, Malfertheiner P. Lansoprazole fast disintegrating tablet: a new formulation for an established proton pump inhibitor. Digestion 2003; 67(1–2):1–5.

124. Sachs G, Shin JM, Pratha V, et al. Synthesis or rupture: duration of acid inhibition by proton pump inhibitors. Drugs Today 2003; 39(Suppl A):11–14.

125. Bader JP, Delchier JC. Clinical efficacy of pantoprazole compared with ranitidine. Aliment Pharmacol Ther 1994; 8(Suppl 1):53–57.

126. Rehner M, Rohner HG, Schepp W. Comparison of pantoprazole versus omeprazole in the treatment of acute duodenal ulceration – a multicentre study. Aliment Pharmacol Ther 1995; 9(4):411–416.

127. Beker JA, Bianchi Porro G, Bigard MA, et al. Double-blind comparison of pantoprazole and omeprazole for the treatment of acute duodenal ulcer. Eur J Gastroenterol Hepatol 1995; 7(5):407–410.

128. Witzel L, Gutz H, Huttemann W, et al. Pantoprazole versus omeprazole in the treatment of acute gastric ulcers. Aliment Pharmacol Ther 1995; 9(1):19–24.

129. Klok RM, Postma MJ, van Hout BA, et al. Meta-analysis: comparing the efficacy of proton pump inhibitors in short-term use. Aliment Pharmacol Ther 2003; 17(10):1237–1245.

130. Prakash A, Faulds D. Rabeprazole. Drug 1998; 52(2):261–267.

131. Miner P Jr, Katz PO, Chen Y, et al. Gastric acid control with esomeprazole, lansoprazole, omeprazole, pantoprazole and rabeprazole: a 5-way crossover study. Am J Gastroenterol 2003; 98(12)2612–2620.

   The first head to head comparative study investigated 5 available PPIs in their gastric acid control efficacy by monitoring 24-hour intragastric pH.

132. Dekkers CP, Beker JA, Thjodleifsson B, et al. Comparison of rabeprazole 20 mg versus omeprazole 20 mg in the treatment of active duodenal ulcer: a European multicentre study. Aliment Pharmacol Ther 1999; 13(2):179–186.

133. Dekkers CP, Beker JA, Thjodleifsson B, et al. Comparison of rabeprazole 20 mg vs. omeprazole 20 mg in the treatment of active gastric ulcer – a European multicentre study. The European Rabeprazole Study Group. Aliment Pharmacol Ther 1998; 12(8):789-795.

134. Johnson DA. Review of esomeprazole in the treatment of acid disorders. Expert Opin Pharmacother 2003; 4(2):253–264.

135. Scott LJ, Dunn CJ, Mallarkey G, et al. Esomeprazole. A review of its use in the management of acid-related disorders. Drugs 2002; 62(10):1503–1538.

136. FDA. 2004; Prevacid. *http://www.accessdata.fda.gov/scripts/cder/drugsatfda/index.cfm?fuseaction=Search.Overview&DrugName=PREVACID.* (accessed July 29, 2004).

137. FDA. 2004; PrevacidNaprapac. http://www.accessdata.fda.gov/scripts/cder/drugsatfda/index.cfm?fuseaction=Search.Overview&DrugName=PREVACID%20NAPRAPAC (accessed July 29, 2004).

138. FDA. 2004; Zegerid. http://www.fda.gov/cder/foi/label/2004/21636_zegerid_lbl.pdf. (accessed July 29, 2004).

139. Yacyshyn BR, Thomson ABR. The clinical importance of proton pump inhibitor pharmacokinetics. Digestion 2002; 66(2):67–78.

140. Hellström PM, Vitols S. The choice of proton pump inhibitors: does it matter? Basic Clin Pharmacol Toxi 2004; 94(3)106–111.

141. Blum RA, Hunt RH, Kidd SL, et al. Dose–response relationship of lansoprazole to gastric acid antisecretory effects. Aliment Pharmacol Ther 1998; 12(4):321–327.

142. Shimatani T, Inoue M, Kuroiwa T, et al. Rabeprazole 10 mg twice daily is superior to 20 mg once daily for night-time gastric acid suppression. Aliment Pharmacol Ther 2004; 19(1):113–122.

143. De Graef J, Woussen-Colle MC. Influence of the stimulation state of the parietal cells on the inhibitory effect of omeprazole on gastric acid secretion in dogs. Gastroenterology 1986; 91(2):333–337.

144. Matheson AJ, Jarvis B. Lansoprazole: an update of its place in the management of acid-related disorders. Drugs 2001; 61(12):1801–1833.

145. Larkin CJ, Watson RGP, Sloan JM, et al. Distribution of atrophy in *Helicobacter pylori*-infected subjects taking proton pump inhibitors. Scand J Gastroenterol 2000; 35(6):578–582.

146. Graham DY, Opekun AR, Yamaoka Y, et al. Early events in proton pump inhibitor-associated exacerbation of corpus gastritis. Aliment Pharmacol Ther 2003; 17(2):193–200.

147. Sanduleanu S, Jonkers D, de Bruïne, et al. Changes in gastric mucosa and luminal environment during acid-suppressive therapy: a review in depth. Dig Liver Dis 2001; 33(8):707–719.

148. Weinstein WM. Proton pump inhibitors and infection: why the concern? Curr Gastroenterol Rep 1999; 1(6):507–510.

149. Lamberts R, Brunner G, Solcia E. Effects of very long (up to 10 years) proton pump blockade on human gastric mucosa. Digestion 2001; 64(4):205–213.

150. Valuck RJ, Ruscin JM. A case-control study on adverse effects: H₂ blocker or proton pump inhibitor use and risk of vitamin B₁₂ deficiency in older adults. J Clin Epidemiol. 2004; 57(4):422–428.

151. Howden CW. Vitamin B₁₂ levels during prolonged treatment with proton pump inhibitors. J Clin Gastroenterol 2000; 30(1):29–33.

152. Bateman DN, Colin-Jones D, Hartz S, et al. Mortality study of 18 000 patients treated with omeprazole. Gut 2003; 52(7):942–946.

153. FDA. 2000; Ome-Mg Briefing Document 20-Oct-00 11511. Rebound of Gastric Acid Secretion. *http://www.fda.gov/ohrms/dockets/ac/00/backgrd/3650b1a_11.pdf.* (accessed July 29, 2004).

154. Gillen D, Wirz AA, McColl KE. *Helicobacter pylori* eradication releases prolonged increased acid secretion following omeprazole treatment. Gastroenterology 2004; 126(4):980–988.

155. Bell N, Karol MD, Sachs G, et al. Duration of effect of lansoprazole on gastric pH and acid secretion in normal male volunteers. Aliment Pharmacol Ther 2001; 15(1):105–113.

156. Korman MG, Bolin TD, Szabo S, et al. Sucralfate: the Bangkok review. J Gastroenterol Hepatol 1994; 9(4):412–415.

157. Banerjee S, El-Omar E, Mowat A, et al. Sucralfate suppresses *Helicobacter pylori* infection and reduces gastric acid secretion by 50% in patients with duodenal ulcer. Gastroenterology 1996; 110(3):717–724.

158. Jung R, MacLaren R. Proton-pump inhibitors for stress ulcer prophylaxis in critically ill patients. Ann Pharmacother 2002; 36(12):1929–1937.

159. Candelli M, Carloni E, Armuzzi A, et al. Role of sucralfate in gastrointestinal diseases. Panminerva Med 2000; 42(1):55–59.

160. Hunt RH. Treatment of peptic ulcer disease with sucralfate: a review. Am J Med 1991; 91(2A):S102–S106.

161. Wagstaff AJ, Benfield P, Monk JP. Colloidal bismuth subcitrate. A review of its pharmacodynamic and pharmacokinetic properties, and its therapeutic use in peptic ulcer disease. Drugs 1988; 36(2):132–157.

162. Sox TE, Olson CA. Binding and killing of bacteria by bismuth subsalicylate. Antimicrob Agents Chemother 1989; 33(12):2075–2082.

163. Lauritsen K, Rask-Madsen J. Prostaglandin analogues. Baillières Clin Gastroenterol 1988; 2(3):621–628.

164. Rostom A, Dube C, Wells G, et al. Prevention of NSAID-induced gastroduodenal ulcers. Cochrane Database Syst Rev 2002; 4:CD002296.

165. Wolfe MM, Jensen RT. Zollinger-Ellison syndrome. Current concepts in diagnosis and management. N Engl J Med 1987; 317(19):1200–1209.

166. Metz DC, Strader DB, Orbuch M, et al. Use of omeprazole in Zollinger-Ellison syndrome: a prospective nine-year study of efficacy and safety. Aliment Pharmacol Ther 1993; 7(6):597–610.

167. Lloyd-Davies KA, Rutgersson K, Solvell L. Omeprazole in the treatment of Zollinger-Ellison syndrome: a 4-year international study. Aliment Pharmacol Ther 1988; 2(1):13–32.

168. Ramdani A, Mignon M, Samoyeau R. Effect of pantoprazole versus other proton pump inhibitors on 24-hour intragastric pH and basal acid output in Zollinger-Ellison syndrome. Gastroenterol Clin Biol 2002; 26(4):355–359.

169. Hirschowitz BI, Simmons J, Mohnen J. Minor effects of *Helicobacter pylori* on gastric secretion and dose of lansoprazole during long-term treatment in ZE and non-ZE acid hypersecretors. Aliment Pharmacol Ther 2002; 16(2):303–313.

170. Mardones P, Moyano C, Pena K, et al. Systemic mastocytosis: clinical case. Rev Med Chil 1998; 126(7):823–827.

171. Gillen D, Wirz AA, Neithercut WD, et al. *Helicobacter pylori* infection potentiates the inhibition of gastric acid secretion by omeprazole. Gut 1999; 44(4):468–475.

172. Labenz J, Tillenburg N, Peitz U, et al. Efficacy of omeprazole one year after cure of *Helicobacter pylori* infection in duodenal ulcer patients. Am J Gastroenterol 1997; 92(4):576–578.

173. Graham DY, Yamaoka Y. *H. pylori* and Cag A: relationships with gastric cancer, duodenal ulcer, and reflux esophagitis and its complications. Helicobacter 1998; 3(3):145–152.

174. Meucci G, Di Battista R, Abbiati C, et al. Prevalence and risk factors of *Helicobacter pylori*-negative peptic ulcer: a multicenter study. J Clin Gastroenterol 2000; 31(1):42–47.

175. Gisbert JP, Legido J, Garcia-Sanz I, et al. *Helicobacter pylori* and perforated peptic ulcer prevalence of the infection and role of non-steroidal anti-inflammatory drugs. Dig Liver Dis 2004; 36(2):116–120.

176. Bytzer P, Teglbjaerg PS, Danish Ulcer Study Group. *Helicobacter pylori*-negative duodenal ulcers: prevalence, clinical characteristics, and prognosis – results from a randomized trial with 2-year follow-up. Am J Gastroenterol 2001; 96(5):1409–1416.

177. Freston JW. Review article: role of proton pump inhibitors in non – related ulcers. Aliment Pharmacol Ther 2001; 15 (Suppl 2):2–5.

178. Lanza F, Goff J, Silvers D, et al. Prevention of duodenal ulcer recurrence with 15mg lansoprazole: a double-blind placebo-controlled study. The lansoprazole Study Group. Dig Dis Sci 1997; 42(12):2529–2536.

179. Vakil N, Vaira D. Non-invasive tests for the diagnosis of infection. Rev Gastroenterol Disord 2004; 4(1):1–6.

180. Johnson DA. Alternative dosing for PPI therapy: rational and options. Rev Gastroenterol Disord 2003; 3(Suppl 4):S10–S15.

181. Bardhan KD. Is there any acid peptic disease that is refractory to proton pump inhibitors? Aliment Pharmacol Ther 1993; 7(Suppl 1):13–24.

182. Lanas AI, Remacha B, Esteva F, et al. Risk factors associated with refractory peptic ulcers. Gastroenterology 1995; 109(4):1124–1133.

183. Bardhan KD, Nayyar AK, Royston C. History in our lifetime: the changing nature of refractory duodenal ulcer in the era of histamine H$_2$ receptor antagonists. Dig Liver Dis. 2003; 35(8):529–536.

184. Lanas A, Remacha B, Sáinz R, et al. Study of outcome after targeted intervention for peptic ulcer resistant to acid suppression therapy. Am J Gastroenterol 2000; 95(2):513–519.

A study of 80 refractory ulcer patients, risk factors leading to refraction, and outcomes were investigated under current antiulcer therapies.

185. Bardhan KD, Naesdal J, Bianchi Porro G, et al. Treatment of refractory peptic ulcer with omeprazole or continued H$_2$ receptor antagonists: a controlled clinical trial. Gut 1991; 32(4):435–438.

186. Furuta T, Shirai N, Sugimoto M, et al. Pharmacogenomics of proton pump inhibitors. Pharmacogenomics 2004; 5(2):181–202.

187. Klotz U, Schwab M, Treiber G. CYP2C19 polymorphism and proton pump inhibitors. Basic Clin Pharmacol Toxi 2004; 95(1):2–8.

188. Arakawa T, Kobayashi K, Dajani EZ. Refractory peptic ulcers. J Assoc Acad Minor Phys 1992; 3(3):95–102.

CHAPTER TWENTY-ONE

21

Upper gastrointestinal bleeding

James Y.W. Lau and Joseph J.Y. Sung

INTRODUCTION

Upper gastrointestinal bleeding (UGIB) is a common medical emergency, accounting for more than 300 000 hospital admissions per annum. The annual rate of hospitalization for upper gastrointestinal (GI) hemorrhage in the United States has been estimated at 102 patients per 100 000 adults of the general population.[1,2] In a population-based National United Kingdom audit conducted a decade ago, the incidence was 103 per 100 000 adults per year.[3] The condition is seen predominantly among the elderly; 68% of the patients were older than 60 years of age and 27% aged over 80. A crude mortality figure of 14% was reported among 4185 patients. When the mortality figure was compared to those from historical series, it had remained unchanged for decades (Table 21.1). Death occurred almost exclusively among elderly patients, often with significant comorbidities. In an increasingly aging population, endoscopic therapy in conjunction with pharmacotherapy should be the mainstay of treatment. However, any reduction in mortality from medical advances is likely to be marginal.

The management of patients with upper GI hemorrhage requires a multidisciplinary approach mandating cooperation among medical and surgical gastroenterologists with access to skills in endoscopic and surgical hemostasis. Endoscopic therapy is often the first treatment in most management algorithms. Institution-specific protocols should be in place for the care of such patients. Approximately 80–85% of upper GI bleeding stops spontaneously and supportive therapy only is required.[4] The remaining 15–20% continues to bleed or develop recurrent bleeding, and these patients constitute the high-risk group with substantially increased morbidity and mortality. Early risk stratification of patients with upper gastrointestinal bleeding based on clinical and endoscopic criteria facilitates the delivery of the appropriate level of care to patients, thereby conferring important resource implications.

This chapter provides details on management of patients with nonvariceal bleeding. These include risk stratification, endoscopic therapy, strategies in the prophylaxis against recurrent bleeding, such as pharmacotherapy and second-look endoscopy, and the role of endoscopic re-treatment versus surgery when bleeding recurs.

Causes of upper gastrointestinal bleeding

The most common cause of upper GI bleeding is peptic ulcer (Table 21.2).[5] The distribution varies with the studied population. In as many as 20% of patients, the diagnosis cannot be ascertained. On the other hand, in around 10% of patients, more than one source of bleeding may be identified.

Table 21.1 Previous British series of upper gastrointestinal bleeding showing age structure, mortality, and age-standardized mortality (Rockall et al. Br Med J 1995; 311:225)

Series	Year	No. of cases	% of cases Age >60	% of cases Age >80	Mortality #	Age standardized mortality ratio (95% CI)
Jones [4]	1940–47	687	33	2	9.9	147 (109–195)
Schiller [5]	1953–67	2149	48	8	8.9	110 (95–126)
Johnston [6]	1967–68	817	49	9	10.6	122 (100–146)
Mayberry [7]	1972–78	583	NA	NA	10.3	–
Katchinski [8]	1984–86	1017	63	18	11.8	91 (73–112)
Rockall [3]	1993	4185	68	27	11.0	100 (reference value)

CI, confidence intervals; NA, Not available; # emergency admissions only.

Table 21.2 Final diagnosis of the cause of upper gastrointestinal bleeding in 2225 patients

Diagnosis	Percentage of total diagnoses (%)
Duodenal ulcer	24.3
Gastric erosions	23.4
Gastric ulcer	21.3
Varices	10.3
Mallory-Weiss tear	7.2
Esophagitis	6.3
Erosive duodenitis	5.8
Neoplasm	2.9
Stomal ulcer	1.8
Esophageal ulcer	1.7
Miscellaneous	6.8

(Reprinted from Silverstein FE et al, Gastrointestinal Endoscopy 1981; 27:73. © 1981, with permission from The American Society for Gastrointestinal Endoscopy.)

INITIAL MANAGEMENT

Patients with acute bleeding should be evaluated immediately on presentation. A rapid assessment should be performed to establish whether: (1) the airway is compromised, (2) there is active bleeding, and (3) the patient is hypovolemic. Orthostatic vital signs can help in the determination of lesser degrees of intravascular volume depletion. Postural hypotension is often present and indicates a 10–20% reduction in blood volume. Fluid resuscitation takes priority in the presence of any of the above signs, and venous access via one or more wide-bore cannulas is essential. Blood is drawn for typing and cross-matching in addition to testing for hemoglobin level, hematocrit, platelet count, and coagulation profiles.

Patients with severe acute bleeding require admission to a high dependency or intensive care unit. Those with significant cardiopulmonary disease are fragile patients and may require intense monitoring that includes central venous pressure measurements. Intravascular volume should be promptly replenished with crystalloid solutions to maintain organ perfusion, and supplemental oxygen should be administered to augment oxygen-carrying capacity of blood. Patients' vital signs, including blood pressure, pulse rate, and urine output, must be closely monitored. After initial volume replacement with crystalloid, unstable vital signs and evidence of ongoing bleeding, such as fresh hematemesis, are requisites for early blood transfusion. Serial hematocrit measurements provide estimates on the dilution of blood. Packed erythrocytes are generally administered, reserving whole-blood transfusion for the unusual circumstances of massive bleeding. Abnormal coagulation profiles require specific correction with fresh-frozen plasma and platelets, as is the case in many patients with liver cirrhosis.

After stabilization with the restoration of intravascular volume, history taking, physical examination, and investigation can proceed in the usual order. A history of chronic liver disease and signs of portal hypertension denote the possibility of variceal bleeding, which requires specific therapy, such as the administration of vasoactive drugs and antibiotics prior to endoscopy. Previous aortic surgery in the presence of massive bleeding raises the concern of an aortoenteric fistula. Those with signs of ongoing bleeding after initial resuscitation, such as fresh hematemesis or fresh hematochezia and hypovolemic shock, should undergo urgent endoscopy to localize the source of bleeding and for possible endoscopic therapy.

Hematemesis indicates that bleeding originates from a site proximal to the ligament of Treitz. A history of fresh hematemesis usually implies a significant bleed. On the other hand, coffee grounds emesis often indicates that active bleeding may have ceased. Melena occurs when hemoglobin is converted to hematin and other hemochromes by bacterial degradation, and the ingestion of as little as 200 mL of blood can produce melenic stool. Although melena generally connotes bleeding proximal to the ligament of Treitz, bleeding from small bowel or proximal colon may also cause melena, especially when colonic transit is slow. A mildly elevated level of blood urea nitrogen (BUN) is another indication of upper GI bleeding, which is due to the absorption of blood via the intestinal tract. Hypovolemia may also account for the transient azotemia.[6]

Massive upper GI bleeding can present as hematochezia, although it is more often a sign of lower GI bleeding. However, 11% of patients with rapid bleeding from an upper GI source pass bright red blood rectally because of rapid GI transit.[7] In a patient with fresh rectal bleeding and hypovolemia, placement of a nasogastric tube or early endoscopic examination should be offered to differentiate bleeding from an upper or a lower GI source.

The routine insertion of a nasogastric tube prior to endoscopy may not be necessary. Nasogastric tube placement with lavage prior to endoscopy is often ineffective, as blood tends to form clots and may thus be difficult to aspirate. Bleeding lesions often locate at the lesser gastric curvature, angular notch, gastric antrum, or bulbar duodenum while blood generally pools in the gastric fundus and corpus. An endoscopic examination is often possible and adequate with suction aspiration and patient positioning. The insertion of a nasogastric tube is associated with a small risk of aspiration, particularly among obtunded patients. In occasions when the source of GI bleeding is uncertain, the insertion of a nasogastric tube can help to confirm an upper GI bleeding source with the presence of gross blood or coffee ground-like substances in the gastric aspirate. In contrast, a clear nasogastric aspirate does not exclude upper GI bleeding inasmuch as bleeding may be episodic or the lesion located distal to the stomach in the presence of a competent pylorus, preventing retrograde reflux of blood from duodenum. In a study by Cuellar and colleagues, only 53% of patients with a positive nasogastric aspirate were actively bleeding when endoscopy was performed, and 20% of patients with a clear aspirate were found to be actively bleeding at endoscopy.[8] Nevertheless, the nature of nasogastric aspirates can serve as a prognostic indicator, as highlighted in the ASGE survey.[9] A clear nasogastric aspirate was associated with a mortality rate of 6%, which increased to 18% when the aspirate was grossly bloody. When both a bloody aspirate and fresh hematochezia are present, the mortality rises to around 30%. Gross blood in the nasogastric aspirate indicates ongoing and often massive bleeding and mandates emergency intervention.

Early endoscopy is usually defined as performance of the examination within 24 hours of patient's admission. This procedure allows risk classification and hence safe and early discharge of patients classified as low risk. In several observational studies[10–14] and randomized controlled trials,[15–17] such an approach reduces resource utilization, such as hospital stay. In high-risk patients, it is logical to believe that the early control of bleeding reduces transfusion requirement and organ dysfunction and generally improves patient outcome.

Risk stratification

In about 80% of patients, bleeding has stopped spontaneously upon presentation.[4] In the remaining 20% of patients, bleeding would continue or recur during their hospitalization. The mortality in this group increases as much as eightfold compared to those without further bleeding. It is therefore mandatory that patients who are at risk be identified.

Several risk stratification schemes with validation have been published. Most are composite scoring systems incorporating both clinical and endoscopic parameters. Such a scheme should aid in the clinical decisions for both (1) the need for urgent intervention as patients must be triaged before endoscopy, and (2) predicting continued or recurrent bleeding in the context of endoscopic therapy. The latter is important as alternate treatment strategies should be readily available to prevent recurrent bleeding. From the National United Kingdom audit, Rockall et al. derived an admission score and postendoscopy scores from 4185 admissions and validated these scores with data from 1625 patients (Table 21.3) in their ability to predict recurrent bleeding and death.[18] The scoring system consists of age, comorbidity, the presence of shock, and endoscopic findings. A total score of 3 or less is associated with an excellent prognosis, while a score 8 or above is associated with a high risk of death.

Blatchford et al. used simple clinical and biochemical parameters to derive a score to predict the need for intervention to control bleeding.[19] The score was modeled on the clinical process rather than treatment outcome. The risk markers of BUN, hemoglobin, systolic blood pressure, pulse rate, the presence of melena or syncope, and evidence of hepatic or cardiac disease with assigned numerical values are used and easy to remember. The full score can be used to determine the required level of care upon the patient's admission and to identify those who may need urgent treatment.

In the Canadian Consensus Conference Statements, Barkun et al. reviewed studies over the last decade that used multivariate analyses to formulate risk schemes.[20] Similar to most scoring systems, they concluded that older age, poor health status or comorbid illness, continued or recurrent bleeding, fresh hematemesis or hematochezia, and the onset of bleeding in hospitalized patients (those admitted for reasons other than upper GI bleeding) represented poor prognostic factors and predicted death. Clinical prognosticators of increased risk for recurrent bleeding are listed in Table 21.4. Of note, endoscopic factors including active bleeding, major stigmata of recent hemorrhage, ulcers greater than 2 cm in size, and location in proximity to large arteries are the factors that predict recurrent bleeding.

Stigmata of hemorrhage

Endoscopic features of an ulcer are important prognostic indicators. The presence of stigmata of recent bleeding in an ulcer confirms the source of bleeding. Three decades ago, Forrest and Finlayson categorized ulcers into those that were actively bleeding, those that showed stigmata of recent bleeding, and those that had a clean base.[21] The nomenclature has since been in widespread use. Forrest class I ulcers are those with active bleeding, which can be either spurting (Forrest class IA) (Fig. 21.1) or oozing (Forrest class IB). Stigmata of recent bleeding belong to Forrest class II: non-bleeding visible vessel, IIA; adherent clots, IIB; and flat pigmented spots, IIC (Figs 21.2, 21.3 , 21.4). Ulcers with a clean base belong to Forrest III (Fig. 21.5). Laine and Peterson summarized endoscopic findings from cohort studies in which endoscopic therapy was not used and correlated the appearance with risk of recurrent bleeding, requirement for surgery, and risk of mortality (Table 21.5).[22] There are, however,

Table 21.3 The Rockall risk score scheme

Variable	0	1	2	3
		Score		
Age (years)	<60	60–79	≥80	
Shock	'No shock,' systolic BP≥100, pulse <100	'Tachycardia,' systolic BP≥100, pulse ≥100	'Hypotension,' systolic BP<100	
Comorbidity	No major comorbidity		Cardiac failure, ischemic heart disease, any major comorbidity	Renal failure, liver failure, disseminated malignancy
Diagnosis	Mallory-Weiss tear, no lesion identified and no SRH	All other diagnoses	Malignancy of upper GI tract	
Major SRH	None or dark spot only		Blood in upper GI tract, adherent clot, visible or spurting vessel	

Maximum additive score prior to diagnosis = 7; maximum additive score following diagnosis = 11.
(Reprinted from Rockall TA et al, Gut 1996; 38:316. © 1996, with permission from British Medical Association.)

Table 21.4 Summary of statistically significant predictors of persistent or recurrent bleeding as assessed by multivariate analyses in studies within the past 10 years*

Risk factor	Odds ratios of increased risk
Clinical factors	
Age >70 years	2.3
Shock (systolic blood pressure <100 mmHg)	1.2–3.6
ASA class 2 or above	1.9–7.6
Erratic mental status	3.2
Ongoing bleeding	3.1
Laboratory factors	
Initial hemoglobin <100 g/L	0.8–3
Coagulopathy (prolonged partial thromboplastin time)	1.96
Presentation of bleeding	
Melena	1.6
Hematochezia	3.8
Blood in gastric aspirate	1.1–11.5
Hematemesis	1.2–5.7
Endoscopic factors	
Active bleeding on endoscopy	2.5–6.5
Endoscopic high-risk stigmata	1.9–4.8
Clot	1.7–1.9
Ulcer size >2 cm	2.3–3.5
Ulcer location	
High lesser curve	2.8
Superior duodenal bulb	13.9
Posterior duodenal bulb	9.2

ASA, American Society of Anesthesiologists.
(Reprinted from Barkun A et al, Annals of Internal Medicine 2003; 139:843–857. © 2003, with permission from American College of Physicians.)

substantial variations in the reported prevalence and associated risks of recurrent bleeding with these stigmata, which may be related to observer variability and the different techniques and vigor in the washing of ulcer floor used.[23–26] Less disagreement exists over those that are actively bleeding. The National Institute of Health Consensus Conference defined a nonbleeding visible vessel as 'protuberant discoloration.'[27] The Consensus Conference statements recommended endoscopic treatment to both actively

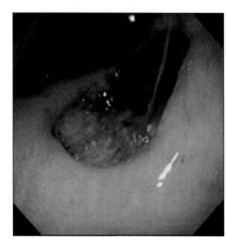

Fig. 21.1 ● A gastric ulcer at the angular notch with pulsatile bleeding.

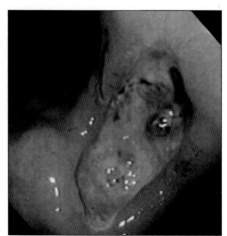

Fig. 21.2 ● A gastric ulcer with a nonbleeding visible vessel defined as a protuberant discoloration.

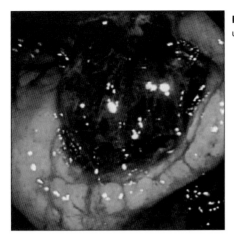

Fig. 21.3 • A gastric ulcer with a clot.

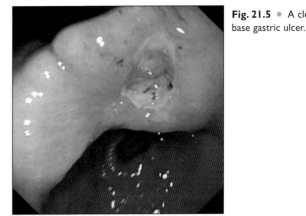

Fig. 21.5 • A clean-base gastric ulcer.

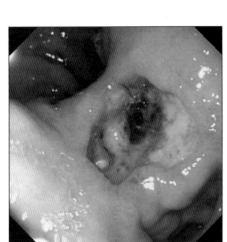

Fig. 21.4 • A gastric ulcer with a flat pigmentation.

bleeding ulcers and ulcers with a visible vessel. Ulcers with flat pigmented spots and clean base are associated with low risks of recurrent bleeding. Endoscopic therapy in these cases is not warranted, and patients can usually be discharged early.

The role of endoscopic treatment of ulcers with adherent clots is not well defined, and the role of endoscopic treatment of nonbleeding ulcers with adherent clots has been controversial. One concern is the possibility of provoking bleeding while elevating the clot. Moreover, the definition of an 'adherent' clot varies with the vigor in which endoscopic washing is applied. Two recent randomized controlled studies supported the lifting of clots overlying an ulcer floor, followed by endoscopic therapy. Jensen et al. randomized 32 patients (17 to medical treatment and 15 to endoscopic therapy) and found that endoscopic therapy completely abolished recurrent bleeding, while 35.3% of patients re-bled on medical therapy alone (OR, 95% CI=17, 0.9–343, p=0.02].[28] Bleau et al. randomized 56 patients (35 to medical therapy and 21 to endoscopic therapy) and reported similar observations.[29] The rate of recurrent bleeding was 34.5 and 4.8 percent, respectively [OR, 95% CI=10, 1.2–87, p=0.02]. However, it must be emphasized that both trials recruited only small numbers of patients. They also differed in their definitions of an adherent clot. Jensen et al. defined an adherent clot as a size of greater than 6 mm in diameter, red in color, and amorphous in texture. In contrast, Bleau et al. defined a clot as a red, maroon, or black protuberance greater than 3 mm in size that could not be dislodged by the forceful irrigation of water. Johnston proposed an evolutionary scheme for the natural history of stigmata of hemorrhage for peptic ulcers (Fig. 21.6).[30] Major bleeding from a peptic ulcer is arterial in origin. A sentinel clot, a term generally used synonymously with a visible vessel, plugs the bleeding point. The clot can initially be contiguous with a larger overlying clot, which will resolve in time. The clot may be variable in color, often initially red and darkening over time, or the color disappears,

Table 21.5 Prevalence and prognosis with stigmata of hemorrhage in bleeding peptic ulcer

Endoscopic characteristics	Prevalence (%)	Further bleeding (%)	Surgery (%)	Mortality (%)
Clean base	42	5	0.5	2
Flat spot	20	10	6	3
Adherent clot	17	22	10	7
Nonbleeding visible vessel	17	43	34	11
Active bleeding	18	55	35	11

(Adapted from Laine L, Peterson WL, New England Journal of Medicine 1994; 331:717–727. © 1994, with permission from Massachusetts Medical Society.)

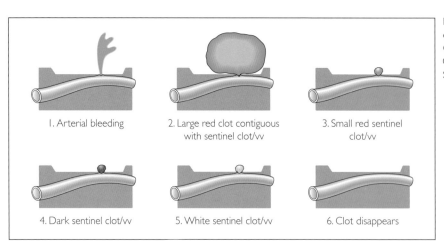

Fig. 21.6 • An evolutionary scheme of stigmata of hemorrhage. (Reprinted from Johnston JH, Gastrointestinal Endoscopy 1990; 36: S16. © 1990, with permission from The American Society for Gastrointestinal Endoscopy.)

leaving a plug of fibrin and platelets. Eventually the plug disappears as the healing process is complete. It is thus often impossible to distinguish the two entities of a nonbleeding visible and an adherent clot.

Endoscopic stigmata should be interpreted along with clinical factors as well as other endoscopic features, including the size and the site of bleeding ulcers. Ulcers at the lesser curvature of the stomach or the posterior duodenal bulb belong to the high-risk ulcers because of their proximity to the left gastric artery and the gastroduodenal artery complex, respectively.

Endoscopic therapy

Endoscopic hemostatic therapy is now widely accepted as the first line of therapy for upper GI bleeding. Numerous clinical trials and two meta-analyses have been published confirming the efficacy of endoscopic therapy.[31,32] The majority of these clinical trials demonstrated a reduction in recurrent bleeding and the need for surgical intervention with the use of endoscopic therapy. Two meta-analyses that included 25 and 30 randomized controlled trials not only showed a significant reduction in the rate of further bleeding (OR, 0.38; 95% CI, 0.32–0.45) and the need for surgery (OR, 0.36, 95% CI, 0.28–0.45), but also a significant reduction in mortality (OR, 0.55; 95% CI, 0.40–0.76). When analyzed separately, thermal contact devices, laser treatment, and injection therapy all decreased further bleeding and surgical intervention rates. Endoscopic therapy can be broadly categorized into injection therapy, thermal coagulation, and mechanical hemostasis. Thermal devices can be further divided into contact and noncontact types. In spite of the large volume of published literature, no single solution for endoscopic injection is superior to another for achieving hemostasis. Similarly, no single method of endoscopic coaptive therapy is superior to others. Combined treatment may represent the best endoscopic therapy – preinjection to stop bleeding, followed by precise coaptive coagulation.

The size of an eroded artery is the critical determinant of the efficacy of endoscopic therapy. In their classic study, Swain et al. examined 27 gastrectomy specimens using postoperative thin barium angiography.[33] Bleeding ulcers were classified as the acute type, with penetration into submucosal arteries only, or as the chronic type, with significant scarring and erosion into serosal arteries. The submucosal arteries were smaller in diameter (0.5 mm) compared to the size of serosal arteries (0.88 mm).

Large chronic ulcers are often transmural, involving the full thickness of the stomach wall. The bleeding artery is technically outside the gut wall and is subserosal in disposition.

Johnston et al. studied the efficacy of thermal devices in securing bleeding using canine mesenteric arteries.[34] At least in animal studies, contact thermocoagulation represents the best method for securing hemostasis. With the use of 3.2 mm contact thermal probes, bleeding can be sealed consistently in arteries up to 2 mm in diameter, although in vivo and clinical conditions are less ideal. It has been suggested that bleeding emanating from arteries greater than 1 mm in diameter cannot be stopped by endoscopic therapies. These arteries often represent the first-generation branch of a larger artery, such as the left gastric artery or part of the gastroduodenal artery complex. Larger chronic ulcers located in proximity to major arterial complexes, such as the lesser curve and posterior bulbar duodenum, often harbor arteries of such size.

Injection therapy

Injection with solutions containing diluted epinephrine is widely used because of its simplicity. A sclerotherapy needle is required and is readily transportable. Chung et al. reported the first randomized trial involving the use of the injection of diluted epinephrine in the treatment of actively bleeding ulcers.[35] Aliquots of 0.5–1 ml are injected around the bleeding point (Fig. 21.7). The principal mechanism of action using diluted epinephrine (1:10 000) solutions is probably volume tamponade, although local vasoconstriction and platelet aggregation represent two of the other suggested mechanisms by which successful hemostasis is likely achieved. Recurrent bleeding after injection with diluted epinephrine alone occurs in around 20% of patients, and epinephrine does not induce thrombosis of the bleeding artery itself. Subsequent to this randomized study, attempts have been made to refine the technique.

One of the newer strategies includes the addition of a sclerosant to induce thrombosis of the artery, such as polidocanol, ethanolamine, and sodium tetradecyl sulfate. Absolute alcohol (98%) causes dehydration of tissues, and in animal experiments, it caused tissue necrosis and ulceration in a dose-dependent manner.[36,37] The acute hemostatic effect of sclerosants was found to be inferior to that of epinephrine. Moreover, the tissue damaging effect of these sclerosants limits the volume that can be

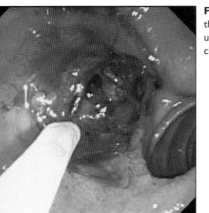

Fig. 21.7 • Injection therapy to a duodenal ulcer with a fresh clot.

until complete fading of bleeding stigmata from ulcer floors.[48] Recurrent bleeding occurred in 18% of 260 patients who received polidocanol injection alone, in 15.8% of 271 who received a single fibrin sealant injection, and in 10% of 274 patients who received repeated fibrin sealants. The differences were statistically significant only between the single polidocanol and the repeated fibrin sealant injection groups ($p=0.01$). The reduction in recurrent bleeding may have been a consequence of the tight surveillance by daily endoscopic examination rather than fibrin sealant itself.

Thermal coagulation

Thermal methods of endoscopic hemostasis can be divided into contact and noncontact ones. Noncontact methods generally refer to laser therapy and argon plasma coagulation. Laser units are difficult to transport and are costly, and as a result, contact probe thermocoagulation has replaced laser treatment. In a canine mesenteric artery model, laser therapy was less effective in sealing larger arteries when compared to contact thermal devices.[34] Argon plasma coagulation is a noncoaptive method of coagulation, which currently is applied to tissues by means of ionized argon gas. Although commonly used to ablate angiodysplasia, few studies have evaluated the efficacy of argon plasma coagulation in the treatment of ulcer hemostasis, and its use in this setting has thus been limited.

Johnston et al. introduced the term 'coaptive thermocoagulation' to refer to the use of contact coagulation probes.[34] The wall of a bleeding artery is compressed together using the mechanical force of a contact probe (Fig. 21.8), which reduces the heat-sink effect from the flowing blood. The activation of heat energy then seals the vessel wall together. In animal experiments, contact thermal devices are superior to noncontact devices and injection therapy in sealing larger arteries up to 2 mm in size Thermocoagulation can be delivered by heater probe, multipolar (gold) probe, and monopolar probes. The differences among these probes in their ability to achieve hemostasis is likely to be small. Most electrodes include built-in irrigation channels, allowing targeted irrigation of the ulcer base. Moreover, they can be applied tangentially without diminishing their effects. Common to all contact thermal probes, their successful applications require: (1) forceful tamponade, (2) the use of a larger (3.2 mm) probe, (3) 15–25 watt

used. Polidocanol incites less tissue damage and a larger volume can thus be used. Soehendra first described the technique of combination treatment, in actively bleeding ulcers, in which 5–10 ml of epinephrine is injected around the bleeding point to produce initial hemostasis.[38] A clear view of the vessel is then possible, thereby allowing the precise injection of a sclerosant. Several comparative trials have examined the benefit of adding a sclerosant to epinephrine.[39–43] In a pooled analysis [treated/control=293/294 patients], the benefit difference was only 2% (95% CI, –4 to 9%, $p=0.47$).[44] However, cases of gastric necrosis associated with the use of sclerosants have been reported, with some leading to fatal outcomes.[45,46] Owing to a lack of additional benefit and the feared complication of sclerosants, the concomitant use of a sclerosant after injection with diluted epinephrine is not recommended.

Human thrombin and the commercially available dual component fibrin sealant are physiological agents that are nontissue damaging and can be used in repeated sessions. The use of these agents is, however, associated with the theoretical risk of transmission of infection from pooled human blood products and intravascular injection leading to systemic thrombosis. Kubba et al. examined the efficacy of a combination of epinephrine plus thrombin extracted from pooled human plasma compared to epinephrine injection alone.[47] This trial represented a single operator experience. In actively bleeding ulcers, preinjection with epinephrine allowed a clear view of the vessel to enable the accurate injection of thrombin. A median volume of 3.5 mL (range 2.8–4.5 mL) of human thrombin suspended in 40 mmol/L of calcium chloride was injected into vessels, representing 600–1000 IU of human thrombin. The combination treatment significantly reduced rebleeding (14/70 versus 3/70, OR 95% CI; 5.9, 1.5–20, $p<0.005$), blood transfusion requirements (297 units versus 219 units, $p=0.041$), and most importantly, mortality (7/70 versus 0/70, OR 95% CI; 16.7, 0.9–297, $p<0.013$). However, this reduction in mortality has not been evident in most clinical trials.

The fibrin sealant is reconstituted by the two components of human thrombin in calcium chloride solution and fibrinogen concentrate in aprotinin. In a multicenter, randomized trial conducted in Europe, 942 patients with bleeding peptic ulcers were randomized to receive endoscopic injection of diluted epinephrine followed by one of three approaches: a single polidocanol injection, a single fibrin sealant injection, or repeated fibrin sealant injections with controlled daily endoscopic examinations

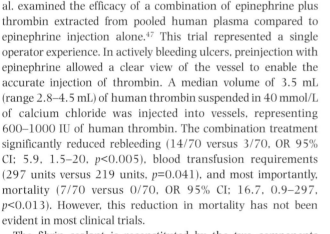

Fig. 21.8 • The concept of 'coaptive thermocoagulation.' The two walls of an artery are firmly pressed together by firm tamponade and sealed by thermocoagulation using a contact probe. Cessation of bleeding reduces the 'heat-sink' effect. (Reprinted from Johnston JH et al, Gastroenterology 1982; 82:904–910. © 1982, with permission from The American Gastroenterological Association.)

setting, and (4) a sustained period of coagulation, consecutive pulses lasting at least 8 seconds.

The only randomized controlled comparison between argon plasma and heater probe coagulation suggested that argon plasma coagulation is equally safe and effective in controlling bleeding.[49] In both groups of patients, epinephrine injection was applied prior to thermal treatment. One hundred and eighty-five cases were analyzed, 97 in the heat probe group and 88 in the argon plasma coagulation group. No significant differences were detected in terms of initial hemostasis (95.9% versus 97.7%), frequency of recurrent bleeding (21.6% versus 17.0%), requirement for emergency surgery (9.3% versus 4.5%), mean number of units of blood transfused (2.4 versus 1.7 units), mean hospital stay (8.2 versus 7.0 days), and hospital mortality (6.2% versus 5.7%).

Injection versus thermal coagulation

Chung et al. compared diluted epinephrine injection to thermo-coagulation using 3.2 mm heater probe in 132 patients with actively bleeding ulcers.[50] Bleeding was initially controlled in 96% of patients treated by epinephrine injection and in 83% by heat probe. No significant differences in outcomes were detected, including transfusion requirement, the need for emergency surgery (20% versus 22%), hospital stay, and mortality (2 versus 4). The accurate placement of a 3.2 mm probe over an actively bleeding vessel can be difficult, especially in certain positions, such as the proximal lesser curvature of the stomach and the posterior wall of the duodenal bulb, which may explain the lower rate of primary control with the use of a larger contact probe.

Choudari et al. randomized 120 patients with major ulcer bleeding to receive injection with epinephrine plus ethanolamine or heat probe treatment.[51] In this study, a small (8-French) probe was used, which proved to be less effective compared to a 10-French probe. Permanent hemostasis was achieved in 87% of the injection group and 85% of the heat probe group. Llach et al. compared epinephrine and polidocanol injection (n=51) to the heater probe (n=53) in patients with major stigmata and found no difference in patient outcomes in either treatment group.[52] Comparative studies of the two treatment methods are thus inconclusive, and the best treatment may be the combination of injection and thermocoagulation.

Hemoclips

Mechanical devices are similar to surgical ligatures and in theory may be ideal for achieving hemostasis. Hemoclips have recently gained popularity in the treatment of ulcer bleeding. In general, 2–5 clips are applied to secure hemostasis (Fig. 21.9). The deployment of hemoclips on fibrotic ulcer floors can, however, be difficult, particularly when they are used tangentially or with the endoscope in a retroflexed position. Ciprolleta and coauthors compared hemoclip (n=56) to heater probe thermocoagulation (n=57) and found a significantly lower rate of recurrent bleeding with the use of hemoclips (1.8% versus 21%).[53] Initial enthusiasm has not, however, been universal as two subsequent trials yielded conflicting results. Lin and colleagues compared hemoclips (n=40) to heater probe coagulation (n=40) and in 6 of 40 patients, hemoclips could not be applied, compared to none of

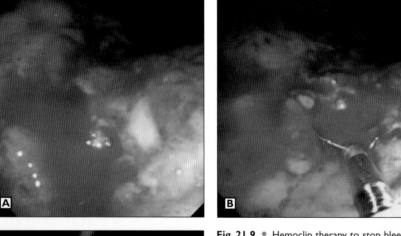

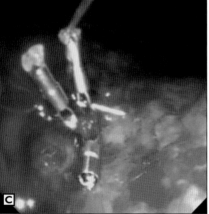

Fig. 21.9 • Hemoclip therapy to stop bleeding from an ulcer with a protruding blood vessel.

40 assigned to heater probe treatment ($p=0.01$).[54] Gevers et al. randomly assigned patients with bleeding ulcers to treatment with hemoclips, injection alone, or both.[55] This study reported a failure rate of 13/35 patients with clips compared to 5 of 34 and 8 of 32 that received injection alone and combined therapy, respectively ($p=0.01$). The efficacy of hemoclips appears limited by difficulty in their successful application, and future studies will be required that assess both successful deployment and the rate of recurrent bleeding after successful clip application.

The combination therapy versus epinephrine injection alone

Many endoscopists favor combined therapy, in which the injection of diluted epinephrine precedes coaptive coagulation. In actively bleeding ulcers, the injection of an ulcer diminishes or even stops bleeding, allowing a clear view of the bleeding vessel, which facilitates accurate coaptive coagulation. The cessation of blood flow may prevent dissipation of thermal energy. Endoscopic treatment end point in the form of a footprint or flattening of the vessel can be better appreciated with the use of a contact probe. Tissue swelling from epinephrine injection may also confer protection against transmural injury.

In a prospective randomized trial recruiting only patients with actively bleeding ulcers, epinephrine alone (n=134) was compared to the combined therapy of epinephrine injection followed by heat probe thermocoagulation using a 3.2 mm probe (n=136).[56] This study did not show any difference in the outcome of the two treatment strategies as measured by rebleeding, the need for surgery, hospital stay, transfusion requirement, mortality, or healing at 4 weeks. However, when the subgroup of spurting ulcers was analyzed separately, rebleeding was less in the combined group (6 transfusion of 27 versus 2 of 31). A reduction in the need for surgery was seen in the combination treatment group (8 of 27 versus 2 of 31, $p=0.03$). Thus, in the severe form of spurting hemorrhage, combined therapy appears to be beneficial.

The benefit of combination therapy has been confirmed in meta-analysis.[57] Calvet and colleagues performed a systemic review to determine whether the addition of a second hemostatic procedure immediately after epinephrine injection improves efficacy at hemostasis or patient outcomes. A total of 16 randomized studies involving 1673 patients were analyzed. The addition of a second procedure reduced the rate of recurrent bleeding from 18.4% to 10.6% (Peto odds ratio 0.53, 95% CI, 0.40–0.69) and emergency surgery from 11.3% to 7.6% (OR, 0.64, 95% CI, 0.46–0.90). Mortality fell from 5.1% to 2.6% (OR, 0.51, 95% CI, 0.31–0.84). Eleven studies used injected substances, such as a sclerosant, tissue adhesive, or thrombin, two studies added hemoclips, and three evaluated the added use of thermal devices. Findings of the meta-analysis suggest that combined therapy is the treatment of choice for high-risk bleeding peptic ulcers. The meta-analysis also confirmed the greater risk of significant complications of perforation and gastric wall necrosis in the combined therapy group (6/558 patients) than in the epinephrine alone group (1/560 patients). Furthermore, the improvement in prognosis seems to be more evident in those with active bleeding (Forrest class I ulcers). Currently, the standard therapy most widely used consists of injection with diluted epinephrine followed by a 3.2 mm heater probe thermocoagulation.

PHARMACOTHERAPY

Rationale for acid suppression

An ulcer stops bleeding when a fibrin or platelet plug blocks the rent in an eroded artery, and importantly, acid suppression prevents clot dissolution. In an in vitro experiment, Green et al. studied platelet aggregation as a function of plasma pH.[58] Platelet aggregation was induced by adding adenosine diphosphate to human plasma, and pH was titrated with dilute sodium hydroxide or hydrochloric acid. When the pH approached neutrality, the percentage of platelet aggregation increased, and conversely, when plasma pH became more acidic, platelet dissolution ensued. This study demonstrated that a plasma pH of >6 is critical for hemostasis. In addition, a pH >4 prevents the conversion of pepsinogen to pepsin and thereby prevents fibrinolysis.

Labenz and coauthors studied intragastric pH in patients with peptic ulcers given either a high-dose infusion of omeprazole (80 mg intravenous bolus followed by 8 mg per hour) or ranitidine (0.25 mg/kg/hour after a bolus of 50 mg) for a period of 24 hours.[59] Both drugs raised the intragastric pH to >6 shortly after drug administration. However, proton pump inhibitors (PPIs) maintain near-neutral pH in the stomach more consistently than H_2-receptor antagonists. The percentage of time intragastric milieu stayed below a pH of 6 was 0.15% with omeprazole and 20.1% with ranitidine ($p=0.001$) in patients with duodenal ulcer, and in patients with gastric ulcer intragastric pH decreased below 6 0.1% of the time with omeprazole and 46.1% with ranitidine ($p=0.002$). Netzer and coauthors compared the antisecretory effect of high-dose omeprazole and ranitidine in both infusion and bolus injections over 72 hours.[60] Omeprazole infusion was superior to all other regimens, maintaining the median pH >6 on each day. Tachyphylaxis of H_2-receptor antagonists led to a rapid loss of antisecretory activity on days 2 and 3. While the overall acid suppressing effects are the same, bolus injections of omeprazole were less effective than an infusion of omeprazole on day 1 in terms of the maintenance of intragastric pH close to neutrality. These studies indicate that in order to maintain an intragastric pH consistently above 6, an infusion of high-dose PPI appears to preferable to H_2-receptor antagonists, which are largely ineffective in this regard.

Clinical studies on the use of H_2-receptor antagonists

Collins and Langman summarized the findings of 27 randomized controlled studies on the efficacy of intravenous H_2-receptor antagonists in the treatment of bleeding peptic ulcers.[61] They concluded that the use of H_2-receptor antagonists reduced the rate of recurrent bleeding, the need for surgery, and death, but only in patients with gastric ulcers. Patients with duodenal ulcer bleeding, who usually have a higher acid output, did not benefit from the use of H_2-receptor antagonists. In another meta-analysis by Levine et al., pooled data from 30 randomized studies comprising 3786 patients showed a remarkably similar finding; i.e., the use of H_2-receptor antagonists was beneficial only in patients with gastric ulcers (absolute risk reduction 7.2%, 6.7%, and 3.2% in the rate of recurrent bleeding, the need for surgery, and death, respectively).[62] H_2-receptor antagonists given as a high-dose infusion were considered superior in controlling intragastric pH. In a multicenter trial involving 67 UK hospitals, Walt et al. randomized 1005 patients with overt signs of upper GI bleeding to receive either famotidine infusion (10 mg intravenous bolus followed by 3.2 mg per hour or placebo).[63] No differences were detected in the rate of recurrent bleeding (23.9 versus 25.5%), the need for surgery (15.5 versus 17.1%), or death (6.2 versus 5.0%) between famotidine and placebo group. Thus, the use of H$_2$-receptor antagonists is not recommended in the management of bleeding peptic ulcer.

Clinical studies on proton pump inhibitors

In the first large-scale study using intravenous omeprazole, 1174 patients with overt signs of upper GI bleeding were randomly assigned to receive omeprazole 80 mg intravenous bolus followed by 40 mg every 8 hours or its equivalent placebo.[64] In this study, no difference was observed between the two treatment groups either on intention-to-treat or per protocol analysis. The difference in death (95% CI) was only 1.6% (−1.2 to 4.4%) on the intention-to-treat analysis. In this particular trial, patients were randomized upon their admissions, and the timing of endoscopic examination was not standardized. The decision to perform endoscopic therapy and its guidelines were not uniform among endoscopists. Endoscopic signs of bleeding, however, were seen less frequently during endoscopy among patients given omeprazole, which suggests that omeprazole might hasten the resolution of endoscopic stigmata of bleeding. Because the proportions of ulcers with specific signs of hemorrhage were not reported, ulcers with minor signs may have been included.

In a study from India, 220 patients were randomized to receive oral omeprazole 40 mg given twice daily or its equivalent placebo for 5 days after documentation of a bleeding peptic ulcer (actively bleeding ulcers or ulcers with nonbleeding visible vessels or clots) at endoscopy.[65] It must be stressed that no endoscopic treatment was given. Patients whose ulcers had a nonbleeding visible vessel (2/17 versus 10/18, p=0.02) or a clot (0/64 versus 13/61, p<0.001) were significantly less likely to have further bleeding. A reduction in recurrent bleeding was not evident in ulcers with spurting or oozing hemorrhage given oral omeprazole. In ulcers that had stopped bleeding spontaneously, acid suppression again appeared to prevent recurrent bleeding, presumably by stabilizing clots.

Two multicenter trials from Scandinavia evaluated the infusion of a high-dose omeprazole (80 mg intravenous bolus followed by 8 mg per hour for 72 hours) in conjunction with endoscopic treatment.[66,67] Both studies reported clinical benefit associated with omeprazole infusion. Both trials, however, lacked discrete outcome variables and used composite end points, which made any interpretation difficult. In the trial by Hasselgren and coauthors, mortality at day 21 was, in fact, higher among those receiving active treatment.

Lin et al. used thermocoagulation to treat 100 patients whose ulcers were actively bleeding or contained a nonbleeding visible vessel.[68] Patients were randomly assigned to receive an infusion of either omeprazole (80 mg intravenous bolus followed by 8 mg per hour for 3 days) or cimetidine infusion (300 mg followed by 1200 mg per day for 3 days). The rebleeding rate in the cimetidine group was 16% at day 3 versus 0% in the omeprazole group (p=0.03); rates at day 14 were 24% and 4%, respectively (p=0.04). In selected patients, intragastric pH was measured, and

omeprazole infusion was better at maintaining pH >6 and superior to H$_2$-antagonist infusion in the prevention of recurrent bleeding after endoscopic control.

Lau et al. adopted the policy of early endoscopic triage and enrolled only patients with actively bleeding ulcers or ulcers with nonbleeding visible vessels into a double-blind placebo-controlled trial.[69] The inclusion of low-risk ulcers, i.e., those with flat pigmentation and clean base, would have diluted the treatment effect associated with the use of omeprazole. These low-risk ulcers constitute 72% of all bleeding ulcers.[70] A high-dose omeprazole infusion was used (80 mg intravenous bolus followed by 8 mg per hour for 72 hours), and a total of 240 patients were randomized. The rate of recurrent bleeding at day 30 was 21.7 and 5.8%, respectively, in those assigned to placebo and omeprazole infusion (RR, 95% CI, 3.7, 1.68–8.23). The study also demonstrated reductions in the need for re-treatment (5 versus 20.8%, p<0.001), blood transfusion (2.7 versus 3.5 units, p=0.04), and trends towards less surgery (3% versus 9%, p=0.14) and death (4.2 versus 10%, p=0.13) among those assigned to omeprazole infusion. This trial provides convincing evidence to support the adjunctive use of high-dose PPI infusion after endoscopic hemostasis.

Two studies further evaluated the use of oral PPI after endoscopic treatment. Javid et al. enrolled 166 patients with peptic ulcers with signs of recent hemorrhage, as confirmed by endoscopy.[71,72] All patients received endoscopic injection sclerotherapy using 1:10 000 epinephrine and 1% polidocanol and were randomly assigned to receive omeprazole (40 mg orally) every 12 hours for 5 days or a placebo identical in appearance. Six (7%) of 82 patients in the omeprazole group had recurrent bleeding, as compared with 18 (21%) in the placebo group (p=0.02). Two patients in the omeprazole group and seven patients in the placebo group needed surgery to control their bleeding (p=0.17). One patient in the omeprazole group and two patients in the placebo group died (p=0.98), while 29 patients (35%) in the omeprazole group and 61 patients (73%) in the placebo group received blood transfusions (p<0.001). The average hospital stay was 4.6±1.1 days in the omeprazole group and 6.0±0.7 days in the placebo group (p<0.001). In a similar study, Kaviani et al. randomized 160 patients with bleeding ulcers after endoscopic injection. The authors showed a lower rate of recurrent bleeding associated with the use of oral omeprazole (12 versus 26, respectively; p=0.022).

The role of acid suppression alone in the management of bleeding peptic ulcer thus remains undefined. Although in the aforementioned study by Khuroo et al., endoscopic treatment was not used,[65] a significant reduction in the rate of recurrent bleeding was observed in ulcers harboring nonbleeding visible vessels or a clot. This trend was not evident among those actively bleeding, suggesting that acid suppression with an oral PPI alone might stabilize clots.

Sung et al. compared the combined endoscopic treatment and adjunct use of PPI infusion to the use of PPI infusion alone in the treatment of ulcers with nonbleeding visible vessels or clots.[73] In those assigned to the combined treatment, recurrent bleeding was seen in 1 of 70 patients, which occurred on day 14 after treatment. In those given intravenous PPI infusion alone, the rate of recurrent bleeding was 11% at day 30. While the results clearly showed that combined therapy was superior in the control of bleeding, the low rate of recurrent bleeding in the PPI infusion alone group would suggest that acid suppression does have a therapeutic role in ulcers with the major stigmata of nonbleeding visible vessel and clot.

In a systemic review including nine trials (1829 patients) with either placebo or H_2-receptor antagonists as control, the use of PPIs was associated with reductions (OR 0.50, 95% CI 0.33–0.77; p=0.002) in the rate of recurrent bleeding and the need for surgery (OR 0.47, 95% CI 0.29–0.77; p=0.003).[74] The use of PPIs also led to a nonsignificant 8% reduction in the odds ratio for death. It can thus be concluded that PPIs are of clear benefit in the management of bleeding peptic ulcer. However, no study has compared high-dose PPI infusion to an oral PPI after endoscopic hemostasis. Intragastric pH control with oral PPI is suboptimal since the oral absorption of a PPI is not always reliable in critically ill patients. Based on the above studies, it would appear that optimal approach to the management of bleeding peptic ulcer should include early endoscopic treatment for patients with high-risk ulcers, followed by a high-dose PPI infusion to prevent recurrent bleeding.

Second-look endoscopy in the prevention of recurrent bleeding

Some endoscopists would routinely schedule patients for a second-look endoscopic examination the next morning, followed by the re-treatment of remaining stigmata of bleeding. However, the value of routinely repeating endoscopic examination has been the subject of debate. Several trials have evaluated this approach and have yielded conflicting results.[75–77] Villaneuva et al. randomized 104 patients with actively bleeding peptic ulcers and ulcers with vessels after injection with epinephrine into two groups; with and without second elective endoscopy and repeated injections.[75] A trend towards better results was noted in the group that received second-look endoscopy: further bleeding, 21% versus 29%; need for emergency surgery, 8% versus 15%; and mortality, 2% versus 4%. Chiu et al. showed a reduction from 14% to 5% in the rate of recurrent bleeding with the use of routine second-look endoscopy in 194 patients.[77] In a meta-analysis, Marmo et al. summarized the findings from four comparative studies and showed a marginal benefit with endoscopic re-treatment (ARR for recurrent bleeding = 6.2%, NNT=16; ARR for surgery = 1.7%, NNT=58; and ARR for death = 1%, NNT=97).[78]

Based on these studies, the use of *routine* second-look endoscopy cannot be recommended for the following reasons: (1) the gain from a second-look endoscopy appears modest as shown from the pooled analysis; (2) most earlier trials used epinephrine injection alone, which may represent a suboptimal index treatment – with improved index therapy, the yield from a second treatment may diminish further; (3) repeat endoscopic treatment, especially with thermocoagulation, increases the risk of perforation; and (4) the use of adjunctive PPI infusion appears to be the dominant strategy after endoscopic control. Nevertheless, it may be logical to consider selective re-endoscopy and re-treatment in cases in which the index endoscopic therapy may have been difficult and suboptimal and in patients with subtle signs of recurrent bleeding. In a small randomized trial, Saeed et al. randomized patients to single treatment or selective re-treatment to those at high risk for recurrent bleeding based on a composite clinical and endoscopic score. In those assigned to re-treatment, recurrent bleeding was completely abolished (0 of 19 versus 5 of 21, p=0.049).[79] The trial, however, consisted of a small sample size, with only 16 of 19 patients assigned to selective re-treatment. This selective approach thus deserves further examination.

The role of surgery

Before the widespread use of endoscopic therapy, surgery represented the only effective means for stopping bleeding. Operative rates of around 20–27% were reported in surgical series. Despite a low overall mortality, an operative mortality of around 20% was generally quoted.[80,81] However, endoscopic therapy has reduced the need for surgery in the acute management of bleeding peptic ulcers. Death among the few patients that require surgery for continued or recurrent bleeding remains high. The National United Kingdom audit revealed an operative rate of 12% among 2071 patients with bleeding peptic ulcers and an associated mortality of 24%.[82]

Although endoscopic therapy has clearly reduced the need for surgical intervention, surgery retains an important role. Indications for emergency surgery include: (1) failure to secure active bleeding by endoscopic or angiographic means, (2) inability to access a bleeding source due to anatomical reasons, (3) rapid exsanguination and the inability to identify a bleeding lesion, and (4) an endoscopic treatment complication, such as a perforation. Many would also recommend surgery after two episodes of recurrent bleeding after initial endoscopic control.

Endoscopic re-treatment versus surgery after recurrent bleeding

At the time of recurrent bleeding, the dilemma often faced by the managing physician is whether to once again attempt endoscopic treatment or to refer the patient directly to surgery. Lau et al. in Hong Kong conducted a randomized trial in patients who re-bled after initial endoscopic control of their bleeding ulcers.[83] In 48 patients who underwent endoscopic re-treatment, long-term hemostasis was achieved in 35 patients. Ulcer perforation occurred in two patients in association with repeat coagulation. In 44 patients assigned to surgery, 22 underwent gastrectomy, which was associated with greater morbidity (7 versus 16, p=0.03). The two groups did not, however, differ with regard to mortality (10% versus 18%, p=0.37). In a logistic regression analysis, ulcers larger than 2 cm in size and hypotension at the time of rebleeding were two independent factors predicting failure with endoscopic re-treatment. In the management of patients with recurrent bleeding after initial endoscopic control, the findings of the Hong Kong study suggest that a selective approach can be adopted based on the local characteristics of the ulcer. Large chronic ulcers should probably be treated by expeditious surgery if recurrent bleeding ensues.

Initial endoscopic hemostasis creates an opportunity for physicians and surgeons to confer and decide the optimal treatment strategy. The role of early elective surgery after endoscopic hemostasis remains undefined. Large ulcers (>2 cm in size) located on the lesser curvature or posterior duodenal bulb in patients who have been in shock are dominant factors that predict adverse outcomes. Unfortunately, patients with such ulcers are often elderly and have significant comorbidites.

Angiographic transcatheter embolization

Angiographic transcatheter embolization is a therapeutic option in patients who do not respond to endoscopic hemostasis and are otherwise poor candidates for surgery. The first description of angiographic transcatheter embolization to a bleeding duodenal ulcer employed the use autologous blood.[84] Subsequently, intra-arterial infusion of vasopressin was introduced. Catheter and guideline technology have evolved significantly during the past few decades, and superselective cannulation using 3–5-French catheters and microcoils is now the standard of transcatheter embolization, with more durable hemostasis and reduced ischemic complications. Considerable skill and expertise are, however, required. Angiographic embolization of a posterior bulbar duodenal ulcer, for instance, requires selective cannulation to the gastroduodenal artery via the celiac trunk and branches of the superior mesenteric artery. Retrograde filling via the inferior pancreaticoduodenal branch via confluence of the superior and inferior arterial arcades becomes possible if the ulcer is approached via the celiac axis alone.[85] The availability of skilled interventional radiologists will limit the general applicability of the technique.

Several anecdotal series have reported a high rate of success in the control of bleeding due to duodenal ulcer hemorrhages,[86–89] although the rate of ischemic necrosis to the pancreas can be as high as 15%. Prospective randomized data comparing transcatheter embolization to surgery are lacking in the literature. In a retrospective comparison of patients who underwent either embolization (n=31) or surgery (n=39) for refractory ulcer bleeding, the rates of recurrent bleeding (29 versus 31%), further surgery (16.1 versus 30.8%) or death (25.8 versus 20.5%) were similar between groups.[90] Those who received embolization were significantly older and had higher incidence of heart disease. Transcatheter embolization and surgery are thus likely to compliment each other in the salvage of patients who fail endoscopic therapy.

TREATMENT OF SPECIFIC CAUSES OF GI HEMORRHAGE

Mallory-Weiss syndrome

Mallory and Weiss first reported a case series of mucosal tears around the gastric cardia in association with vomiting. The mucosal tear was demonstrated to be a fissure-like tear at autopsy studies in four patients.[91] Although initially considered a rare cause for upper GI bleeding, since the advent of endoscopy the condition is diagnosed more frequency and accounts for 3–14% of patients presenting with upper GI bleeding.[92,93] The prognosis of the condition is generally good, with only 5% of patients presenting with hemodynamic instability and a likewise small proportion with hematochezia. Mallory-Weiss tears can also coexist with other bleeding lesions, such as ulcers or varices, which could have caused the bleeding.

A transient increase in the pressure gradient between the intrathoracic and intragastric portion of the gastroesophageal junction, often caused by retching, is thought to cause the tear. In 17–52% of patients with a Mallory-Weiss tear, a hiatal hernia is present;[94] however, whether the presence of a hiatal hernia is etiologic to the tear is not always clear. Retrograde intussusception of the stomach into esophagus has been suggested as a mechanism for pathogenesis of Mallory-Weiss tear. The classic history of a Mallory-Weiss tear is antecedent retching or emesis, initially with clear vomitus followed by hematemesis. Although antecedent retching was previously thought to be prerequisite for the syndrome, it actually occurs in only 30–50% of patients.[95] A significant proportion of these patients report alcohol binge. Mallory-Weiss syndrome may also be associated with a variety of other antecedent events that give rise to an increase in intra-abdominal pressure, such as blunt abdominal trauma, hiccuping, retching during endoscopy, excessive insufflation of air during endoscopy, coughing, parturition, and any other Valsalva maneuver.[96]

Mallory-Weiss tears can be seen clearly on endoscopy as a linear, longitudinal fissure at or below the gastroesophageal junction. The majority of the tears are found on the lesser curvature of the stomach (80%) and less frequently on the greater curvature. Endoscopic stigmata similar to those of ulcers have been described, but their exact significance has not been defined.

The natural history of a Mallory-Weiss tear is to some extent dependent on the initial presentation, endoscopic finding of active bleeding, a visible vessel or clots, and evidence of underlying portal hypertension. At presentation, a low hemoglobin and orthostatic hypotension are two of the proposed adverse prognostic factors. The presence of portal hypertension has been reported to adversely influence the severity and recurrence of an index Mallory-Weiss bleed.[97] Jensen et al. reported a series in which 88% of patients with portal hypertension continued to bleed.[98] During a follow-up period of 11 months, 38% of Mallory-Weiss tears recurred. Active bleeding during endoscopy is associated with a high likelihood that bleeding will continue or recur. In those without evidence of active bleeding, conservative treatment is uniformly successful. Endoscopic treatment is generally indicated for tears with active bleeding and stigmata of bleeding, such as a vessel or a clot analogous to those seen in ulcers.

Laine reported a randomized controlled trial in which multipolar electrocoagulation was used in a small subgroup of 17 patients. Seven of 8 patients that received sham therapy continued to bleed and 4 patients required urgent surgery.[99] Llach et al. compared endoscopic injection sclerotherapy to no treatment in 63 patients suspected of Mallory-Weiss tears.[100] Bleeding recurred in 8 of the control group (25.8%) compared to 2 of the treatment group (6.2%). Endoscopic injection is a useful option in the treatment of Mallory-Weiss tears, and anecdotal reports have described the successful application of other modalities such as hemoclips and band ligation. It must be stressed that the esophagus is a muscular tube with an inner mucosa lining but no serosa. Moreover, the esophageal wall is generally thinner than that of stomach or duodenum, and as a result, coaptive thermocoagulation theoretically carries a higher risk of perforation. Endoscopists should thus be cautioned against forceful probe apposition. A safer choice might be to initially inject diluted epinephrine, followed by gentle tamponade with a 3.2 mm probe at a reduced generator setting (20 Joules at 2–3 pulses). Hemoclips are not tissue damaging and would be ideally suited for tissue approximation in such instances. Their applications are, however, technically demanding.

Dieulafoy's lesion

Dieulafoy's lesion, also known as cirsoid aneurysm or submucosal arterial malformation, is a rare cause of upper GI bleeding. The lesion was named 'exulceratio simplex' by the French surgeon Georges Dieulafoy in 1896.[101] The condition can cause significant bleeding and is often difficult to diagnose. The true incidence is unknown, but in one series, it accounted for 1–5.8% of cases presenting with GI bleeding. Dieulafoy's lesion consists of an abnormally large submucosal artery, a 'caliber-persistent artery,' protruding through a minute 2–5 mm mucosal defect (Fig. 21.10). The diameter of the abnormal and often tortuous artery ranges 1–3 mm, almost 10 times the diameter of normal arteries in the submucosa.[102]

Lee et al. summarized the published series on Dieulafoy's lesions over the last decade, which consisted of 249 cases. Dieulafoy's lesions are found along the entire GI tract, most commonly located in the stomach (74%), duodenum (14%), colon (5%), gastric anastomosis (5%), small bowel (1%), and esophagus (1%). The proximal stomach is by far the most common site, classically described in the proximal lesser curvature within 6 cm of the gastroesophageal junction.[103]

A variety of endoscopic treatments have been described for the treatment of Dieulafoy's lesion. These include injection therapy, thermocoagulation, a combination of both, hemoclips, and even banding ligation.[104–106] Surgery is required when endoscopic therapy fails. Simple plication of the vessel carries high rate of recurrent bleeding, and a wedge excision of the lesion is accordingly recommended. In those that require surgery, mortality approaches 33%. However, the long-term prognosis of patients with Dieulafoy's lesions is usually excellent. In a series of 59 patients treated by endoscopic therapy, who were followed for a mean period of 69 months, none developed recurrent bleeding.[107]

Congestive gastropathy

Congestive gastropathy, also termed portal hypertensive gastropathy, is a cause of chronic blood loss in patients with portal hypertension. McCormack et al. reported the incidence and natural history of macroscopic lesions in 127 consecutive patients with portal hypertension, which mimics gastritis.[108] Histopathologic examinations showed dilated and tortuous submucosal veins and vascular ectasia in the muscle layer. McCormack and colleagues contended that the etiology is due to congestion and suggested the term 'congestive gastropathy.' Portal gastropathy has been described as a diffuse erythematous, reticular, or mosaic pattern of the gastric mucosa. The endoscopic spectrum of portal

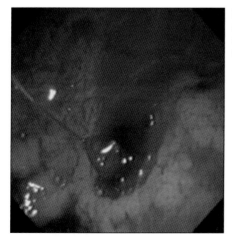

Fig. 21.10 • A Dieulafoy's lesion spurting bleeding in the duodenal bulb.

gastropathy includes a snakeskin appearance, with more severe cases having small areas of intense erythema (e.g., scarlatina rash), frank petechiae, or a granular appearance with multiple bleeding spots. Vascular ectasia may be present throughout the stomach or show an antral predilection, giving the stomach a watermelon appearance. The prevalence of portal gastropathy in patients with cirrhosis is 80%, with acute bleeding occurring in only 2.5% and chronic bleeding in 11%.[109] Patient survival is largely determined by liver function; portal gastropathy is in itself not a prognostic indicator. The reduction of portal venous pressure is the mainstay of treatment for portal gastropathy. Propranolol has been shown to be effective in reducing recurrent bleeding and in improving the severity of gastropathy on endoscopic assessment.[110,111] In refractory cases, portal systemic shunting and a transjugular intrahepatic portal systemic shunt (TIPS) would likely reduce bleeding.

Angiodysplasia

Angiodysplasia occurs mostly in stomach and less frequently in small bowel and colon. It accounts for 5–7% of patients presenting with gastrointestinal bleeding.[112] Often found in patients of advanced age, it has been associated with chronic renal failure, hereditary hemorrhagic telangiectasia (Osler-Weber-Rendu syndrome), and prior radiation therapy. The previous belief of angiodysplasia related to aortic valve disease has been refuted. The diagnosis can be made endoscopically by visualizing small, punctate, bright red, vascular mucosal lesions. Platelet dysfunction associated with chronic renal failure has been postulated as a cause for recurrent bleeding. Most clinicians initially attempt endoscopic coagulation to treat bleeding angiodysplasia, often with contact thermocoagulation. However, the multiplicity and involvement of sites not often accessible, such as the small bowel, make its management difficult. Estrogen-progesterone treatment has been used to prevent recurrent bleeding from angiodysplasia, particularly in the setting of chronic renal insufficiency, but its beneficial effect is questionable. An earlier crossover, randomized trial consisted of only 10 patients.[113] No bleeding occurred in five of six patients who received hormonal therapy, whereas all four patients on placebo needed transfusion. After crossover, all patients previously on hormonal therapy re-bled. No regression of lesion was observed, however. In a more recent multicenter double-blind trial,[114] 72 patients with endoscopic or angiographically confirmed angiodysplasia were randomized to receive a low-dose estrogen-progesterone combination or placebo. No significant differences between the two groups were found with regard to the number of bleeding episodes and transfusion requirement. The role of hormonal therapy remains controversial. More recently, the focus of attention has been the use of capsule endoscopy in the diagnosis of occult lesions.

Osler-Weber-Rendu syndrome is a rare autosomal dominant disorder with characteristic mucocutaneous and visceral vascular malformations.[115] Patients often present during their childhood with recurrent epistaxis followed by chronic GI bleeding, resulting in anemia. The vascular involvement often extends from the stomach and duodenum to the large bowel. In addition to supportive treatment, such as transfusion and iron supplement, ablation of vascular lesions via endoscopy can be considered. Argon plasma thermocoagulation carried out in multiple sessions offers the best endoscopic treatment.

Gastric antral vascular ectasia

Gastric antral vascular ectasia (GAVE), also known as 'watermelon stomach,' is uncommon acquired vascular malformation. The diagnosis is made by a distinctive endoscopic appearance, characterized by longitudinal, angioid, vascular antral folds converging like the spokes or dark stripes of a watermelon onto the pylorus (Fig. 21.11). Most patients present with chronic occult blood loss and often are transfusion dependent. Approximately 30% of patients with GAVE syndrome have cirrhosis, and portal gastropathy can thus be confused for GAVE and visa versa.[116] Antral predilection for GAVE and the diffuse nature of portal gastropathy can sometimes distinguish the two entities. The GAVE syndrome is unrelated to cirrhosis, but may be associated with autoimmune diseases. In a series of 45 consecutive patients with GAVE,[117] 71% were women with a mean age of 73 years, and 62% had signs and symptoms of autoimmune disease, including Raynaud's phenomenon, sclerodactyly, and atrophic gastritis.

The etiology of GAVE remains largely unknown. Although laser thermocoagulation had been used in the past to treat the disorder, the most commonly employed treatment modality at present is argon plasma coagulation, with the therapeutic goal of obliterating as much of the vascular lesion as possible (Fig. 21.12).[118–120] Typically, repeated sessions of endoscopic therapy are required, which generally lead to a reduction in transfusion requirement. GAVE can also present with transient pyloric stenosis from antral edema. Patients who are refractory to endoscopic therapy require surgery in the form of gastric antrectomy. It is important to distinguish GAVE from portal gastropathy as patients with cirrhosis are poor candidates for surgery. In the latter group of patients, therapy should be directed at a reduction of portal venous pressure.

Gastric erosions

The term 'gastritis' should be a histologic diagnosis reserved for the pathologist. Gastric erosions and gastropathy are descriptive changes used by the endoscopist. Gastritis is defined by the presence of an inflammatory cell infiltrate, which may be chronic (i.e., predominantly plasma cells) or acute (i.e., polymorphonuclear cells) together with epithelial distortion. Endoscopically, gastropathy is defined by the gross appearance of mucosal hemorrhages, erythema, and erosions. An erosion is technically a break in the mucosa that does not cross the muscularis mucosae. Practically,

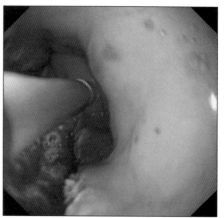

Fig. 21.12 • Gastric antral vascular ectasia treated by argon plasma coagulation.

most endoscopists define an erosion as an area of adherent hemorrhage or a defect in the mucosa with a hematin or necrotic base that is less than 3–5 mm in size. The distinction between an ulcer and an erosion is generally based on the perception that an erosion does not have perceptible depth. Gastric erosions can, however, cause upper GI bleeding and are often associated with specific causes.

Drug-induced gastropathy

Gastropathy induced by aspirin or other NSAIDs is common. In almost all normal volunteers challenged with aspirin, mild hemorrhagic gastropathy develops that involves the proximal or entire stomach within 24 hours. Bleeding is usually, however, clinically insignificant, and adaptation and healing generally ensues. In a small percentage of individuals continually exposed to NSAIDs, chronic erosive gastropathy, predominantly involving the antrum, or frank ulcer disease, may eventually develops. Uneventful healing generally takes place following the withdrawal or abstinence from the offending medication. Bleeding from NSAID-induced gastric erosions is usually mild, while more severe bleeding often arises from concomitant peptic ulcers. Although PPI therapy is effective, the more important issue in the management of NSAID-induced gastropathy is prophylaxis. The approach to the management of NSAID-related upper GI hemorrhage and ulcers is discussed in detail in Chapter 19.

Esophagitis and Esophageal Ulcers

Gastroesophageal reflux disease (GERD) is the primary cause of esophagitis and esophageal ulcers. In the immunocompromised, herpes simplex and *Candida* species can cause esophagitis. Most respond to medical therapy alone. Other unusual causes included pill-induced ulceration and sclerotherapy or band-ligation induced ulcerations. Sucralfate slurries and PPIs have been suggested for the treatment of these ulcers. The approach to GERD and esophageal infections are discussed in detail in Chapters 13 and 6, respectively.

Neoplasms

Neoplasms of the stomach (see Ch. 24), esophagus (see Ch. 17), or duodenum are uncommon causes (2–5%) of upper GI hemorrhage. Bleeding from these lesions is usually self-limited,

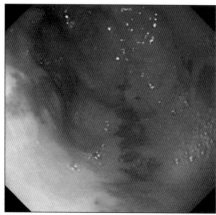

Fig. 21.11 • Gastric antral vascular ectasia (GAVE).

and treatment is ultimately in the hands of the oncologist or surgeon. Endoscopic therapy plays a limited role in the management of bleeding tumors. Bleeding from tumors carries poor prognosis because of underlying malignancy.

Aortoenteric fistula

Most aortoenteric fistulae occur secondarily to prior aortic Dacron graft replacement for aneurysmal or occlusive diseases. Rupture of an atherosclerotic plaque or a mycotic aneurysm may also present with fistulae into duodenum. Aortoenteric fistulae almost always involve the third or fourth portion of the duodenum as the proximal anastomosis lies immediately adjacent to the back wall of duodenum. The graft is occasionally infected and associated with a false aneurysm involving the proximal anastomosis. The classical clinical presentation is a 'herald' bleed that occurs and stops spontaneously hours or occasionally weeks before the exsanguinating hemorrhage. A high index of suspicion is necessary. CT scanning helps to diagnose the condition, showing localized infection around the graft and occasional false aneurysms. In a patient with history of aortic surgery with

Dacron graft placement presenting with upper GI bleeding, the endoscopist should attempt to visualize the third portion of duodenum. A diagnosis of aortoenteric fistula should be presumed until proven otherwise. An opinion from a vascular surgeon should be sought.

Hemobilia and hemosuccus pancreaticus

Hemobilia is defined as hemorrhage into the biliary tree, whereas hemorrhage into the pancreatic duct is called 'hemosuccus pancreaticus,' although in the latter, blood exits through the ampulla of Vater and is considered together with hemobilia. Mortality from the condition is determined by the underlying etiology. The most common cause is biliary tree or hepatic trauma, including iatrogenic trauma resulting from percutaneous liver biopsy and transhepatic cholangiography. In such instances, an aneurysm or a fistula communication between bile ducts and arterial or venous structures is the underlying reasons for bleeding. Angiography can often diagnose the source of bleeding. Angiographic treatment with embolization is usually effective in arresting hemorrhage. Less common causes of hemobilia are

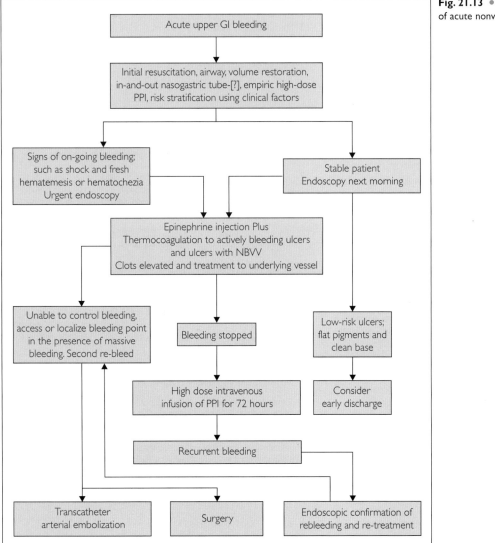

Fig. 21.13 • An algorithm in the management of acute nonvariceal GI bleeding.

extrahepatic or intrahepatic malignancies. Hemosuccus pancreaticus usually occurs in patients with a history of acute or chronic pancreatitis and pseudocysts. Infection weakens arterial walls and causes formation of a pseudoaneurysm. Blood emanates from pseudoaneurysms or veins rupture into pancreatic parenchyma and ducts and present as hemobilia. The diagnosis can be made at endoscopy with visualization of blood coming from the papilla. Treatment is directed at the underlying condition.

SUMMARY

In the management of patients of upper GI hemorrhage, volume resuscitation takes priority. Recurrent or continued bleeding is the single most important adverse prognostic factor. Patients at risk should be identified for early intervention. In general, patients with signs of ongoing bleeding, such as hypotension and fresh hematemesis or hematochezia, should undergo endoscopy after initial stabilization. Early endoscopy localizes the source of bleeding and allows hemostatic therapy to be performed. Endoscopic signs of stigmata of hemorrhage are themselves predictive of recurrent bleeding. Ulcers that are actively bleeding or harbor nonbleeding visible vessels or clots warrant endoscopic treatment. Injection with diluted epinephrine followed by coaptive thermocoagulation is the current standard of therapy to bleeding ulcers. Following initial endoscopic control, evidence in the literature favors the adjunctive use of high-dose proton pump inhibitor usually given in the form of intravenous infusion for 72 hours for clot stabilization. Second-look endoscopy is indicated when there is concern for recurrent bleeding or suboptimal index therapy. If bleeding does recur, a repeat endoscopic examination documents the episode of rebleeding and allows re-treatment, which can often secure hemostasis. The roles of surgery and angiographic therapy have not been fully defined. At index endoscopy, patients with spurting hemorrhage that cannot be stopped by endoscopic therapy warrant surgical or angiographic intervention. After initial endoscopic control, exsanguination in the setting of hypotensive shock and larger ulcers should probably be treated by expedient surgery. Early elective surgery may also be warranted in selected patients with large chronic ulcers and who have had episodes of hypotension. Transcatheter arterial embolization is an option in poor-risk patients refractory to endoscopic hemostasis. See Figure 21.13 for a diagrammatic summary.

REFERENCES

1. Yavorski RT, Wong RKH, Maydonovitch C, et al. Analysis of 3294 cases of upper gastrointestinal bleeding in military medical facilities. Am J Gastroenterol 1995; 90:568.

2. Longstreth GF. Epidemiology of hospitalization for acute upper gastrointestinal hemorrhage: a population-based study. Am J Gastroenterol 1995; 90:206.

3. Rockall TA, Logan RF, Devlin HB, et al. Incidence of and mortality from acute upper gastrointestinal haemorrhage in the United Kingdom. Steering committee and members of the National Audit of Acute Upper Gastrointestinal Haemorrhage. Br Med J; 1995:222–226.

4. Fleischer D. Etiology and prevalence of severe persistent upper gastrointestinal bleeding. Gastroenterology 1983; 84:538.

5. Silverstein FE, Gilbert DA, Tedesco FJ, et al. The national ASGE survey on upper gastrointestinal bleeding. II. Clinical prognostic factors. Gastrointest Endosc 1981; 27:80.

6. Stellato T, Rhodes RS, McDougal WS. Azotemia in upper gastrointestinal hemorrhage. Am J Gastroenterol 1980; 73:486.

7. Jensen DM, Machicado GA. Diagnosis and treatment of severe hematochezia. The role of urgent colonoscopy after purge. Gastroenterology 1988; 95:1569.

8. Cuellar RE, Gavaler JS, Alexander JA, et al. Gastrointestinal tract hemorrhage. The value of a nasogastric aspirate. Arch Intern Med 1990; 150:1381–1384.

9. Silverstein FE, Gilbert DA, Tedesco FJ, et al. The national ASGE survey on upper gastrointestinal bleeding. II. Clinical prognostic factors. Gastrointest Endosc 1981; 27:80.

10. Longstreth GF, Feitellberg SP. Outpatient care of selected patients with acute non-variceal upper gastrointestinal hemorrhage. Lancet 1995; 345:108–111.

11. Hay JA, Maldonado L, Weingarten SR, et al. Prognostic evaluation of a clinical guideline recommending hospital length of stay in upper gastrointestinal tract hemorrhage. JAMA 1997; 278:2151–2156.

12. Lai KC, Hui WM, Wong BC, et al. A retrospective and prospective study on the safety of discharging selected patients with duodenal ulcer bleeding on the same day as endoscopy. Gastrointest Endosc 1997; 45:26–30.

13. Rockall TA, Logan RF, Devlin HG, et al. Selection of patients for early discharge or outpatient care after acute upper gastrointestinal hemorrhage. National Audit of Acute Upper Gastrointestinal Hemorrhage. Lancet 1996; 347:1138–1140.

14. Dulai GS, Gralnek IM, Oei TT, et al. Utilization of health care resources for low-risk patients with acute non-variceal upper GI hemorrhage: a historical cohort study. Gastrointest Endosc 2002; 55:321–7.

15. Cipoletta L, Bianco MA, Rotondano G, et al. Outpatient management for low-risk nonvariceal upper GI bleeding: a randomized controlled trial. Gastrointest Endosc 2002; 55:1–5.

16. Lin HJ, Wang K, Perng CL, et al. Early or delayed endoscopy for patients with peptic ulcer bleeding. A prospective randomized study. J Clin Gastroenterol 1996; 22:267–271.

17. Lee JG, Turnipseed S, Romano PS, et al. Endoscopy-based triage significantly reduces hospitalization rates and costs of treating upper GI hemorrhage: a randomized controlled trial. Gastrointest Endosc 1999; 50:755–761.

18. Rockall TA, Logan RFA, Devlin GB, et al. Risk assessment after upper gastrointestinal haemorrhage. Gut 1996; 38:316.

19. Blatchford O, Murray WR, Blatchford M. A risk score to predict the need for treatment for upper gastrointestinal hemorrhage. Lancet 2000; 356:1318–1321.

20. Barkun A, Bardou M, Marshall J for the Nonvariceal Upper GI Bleeding Consensus Conference Group. Consensus recommendations for managing patients with nonvariceal upper gastrointestinal bleeding. Ann Intern Med 2003; 139:843–857.

21. Forrest JA, Finlayson ND, Shearman DJ. Endoscopy in gastrointestinal bleeding. Lancet 1974; 2:394–397.

22. Laine L, Peterson WL. Bleeding peptic ulcer. N Engl J Med 1994; 331:717–727.

23. Lau JY, Sung JJ, Chan AC, et al. Stigmata of hemorrhage in bleeding peptic ulcers; an interobserver agreement study among international experts. Gastrointest Endosc 1997; 46:33–36.

24. Laine L, Freeman ML, Cohen H. Lack of uniformity in evaluation of endoscopic prognostic features of bleeding ulcers. Gastrointest Endosc 1994; 10:411–417.

25. Laine L, Stein C, Sharma V. A prospective outcome study of patients with clot in an ulcer and the effect of irrigation. Gastrointest Endosc 1996; 43:107–110.

26. Lin HJ, Wang K, Perng CL, et al. Natural history of bleeding peptic ulcers with a tightly adherent clot: a prospective observation. Gastrointest Endosc 1996; 43:470–473.

27. Consensus Development Panel, ASGE. Consensus statement on therapeutic endoscopy and bleeding ulcers. Gastrintest Endosc 1990; 36:S62.

28. Jensen DM, Kovacs TO, Jutabha R, et al. Randomized trial of medical or endoscopic therapy to prevent recurrent ulcer hemorrhage in patients with adherent clots. Gastroenterology 2002; 123:407–413.

29. Bleau BL, Gostout CJ, Sherman KE, et al. Recurrent bleeding from peptic ulcer associated with adherent clot: a randomized study comparing endoscopic treatment with medical therapy. Gastrointest Endosc 2002; 56:1–6.

30. Johnston JH. Endoscopic risk factors for bleeding peptic ulcer. Gastrointest Endosc 1990; 36:S16.

31. Lau J, Sung J, Lee K, et al. Effect of intravenous omeprazole on recurrent bleeding after endoscopic treatment of bleeding peptic ulcers. N Engl J Med 2000; 343:310.

32. Sacks HS, Chalmers TC, Blum AL, et al. Endoscopic hemostasis: an effective therapy for bleeding peptic ulcers. JAMA 1990; 264:494.

33. Swain CP, Storey DW, Bown SG. Nature of the bleeding vessel in recurrently bleeding gastric ulcers. Gastroenterology 1986; 90:595.

34. Johnston JH, Jensen DM, Mautner W. Comparison of endoscopic electrocoagulation and laser photocoagulation of bleeding canine gastric ulcers. Gastroenterology 1982; 82:904–910.

35. Chung SC, Leung JW, Steele RJ, et al. Endoscopic injection of adrenaline for actively bleeding ulcers: a randomized trial. Br Med J 1988; 296:1631–1633.

36. Rutgeerts P, Geboes K, Vantrappen G. Experimental studies of injection therapy for severe nonvariceal bleeding in dogs. Gastroenterology 1989; 97:610–621.

37. Rajgopal C, Lessels A, Palmer KR. Mechanism of action of injection of therapy for bleeding peptic ulcer. Br J Surg 1992; 79:782–784.

38. Soehendra N, Grimm H, Stenzel M. Injection of nonvariceal bleeding lesions of the upper gastrointestinal tract. Endoscopy 1985; 17:129–132.

39. Chung SC, Leung JWC, Leong HT, et al. Adding a sclerosant to endoscopic epinephrine injection in actively bleeding ulcers: a randomized trial. Gastrointest Endosc 1993; 39:611.

40. Lin HJ, Perng CI, Lee SD, et al. Is sclerosant injection mandatory after an epinephrine injection for arrest of peptic ulcer haemorrhage? A prospective, randomised, comparative study. Gut 1993; 34:1182.

41. Villaneuva C, Balanzo J, Espinos JC, et al. Endoscopic injection therapy of bleeding ulcer: a prospective and randomized comparison of adrenaline alone or with polidocanol. J Clin Gastroenterol 1993; 17:195.

42. Choudari CP, Palmer KR. Endoscopic injection for bleeding peptic ulcer: a comparison of adrenaline alone with adrenaline plus ethanolamine oleate. Gut 1994; 35:608.

43. Chung SCS, Leong HT, Chan ACW, et al. Epinephrine or epinephrine plus alcohol for injection of bleeding ulcers: a prospective randomised trial. Gastrointest Endosc 1996; 43:591–595.

44. Rollhauser C, Fleischer D. Current status of endoscopic therapy for ulcer bleeding. Baillière's Best Practice and Research 2000; 14:391–410.

45. Levy J, Khakoo S, Barton R, et al. Fatal injection sclerotherapy of a bleeding peptic ulcer (Letter). Lancet 1991; 337:504.

46. Loperfido S, Patelli G, La Torre L. Extensive necrosis of gastric mucosa following injection therapy of bleeding peptic ulcer (Letter). Endoscopy 1990; 22:285–286.

47. Kubba KA, Murphy W, Palmer KR. Endoscopic injection for bleeding peptic ulcer: a comparison of adrenaline alone with adrenaline plus human thrombin. Gastroenterology 1996; 111:623–628.

48. Rutgeerts P, Rauws E, Wara P, et al. Randomized trial of single and repeated fibrin glue compared with injection of polidocanol in treatment of bleeding peptic ulcer. Lancet 1997; 350:692–696.

49. Chau CH, Siu WT, Law BK, et al. Randomized controlled trial comparing epinephrine injection plus heat probe coagulation versus epinephrine injection plus argon plasma coagulation for bleeding peptic ulcers. Gastrointest Endosc 2003; 57:455–461.

50. Chung SCS, Leung JWC, Sung JY, et al. Injection or heat probe for bleeding ulcer. Gastroenterology 1991; 100:33.

51. Choudari CP, Rajgopal C, Palmer KR. Comparison of endoscopic injection therapy versus the heat probe in major peptic ulcer haemorrhage. Gut 1992; 33:1159–1161.

52. Llach J, Bordas JM, Salmeron JM, et al. A prospective randomized trial of heater probe thermocoagulation versus injection therapy in peptic ulcer hemorrhage. Gastrointest Endosc 1996; 43:117–120.

53. Cipolletta L, Bianco MA, Marmo R, et al. Endoclips versus heater probe in preventing early recurrent bleeding from peptic ulcer: a prospective and randomized trial. Gastrointest Endosc 2001; 53:147–151.

54. Lin HJ, Hsieh YH, Tseng GY, et al. A prospective randomized trial of endoscopic hemoclip versus heater probe thermocoagulation for peptic ulcer bleeding. Am J Gastroenterol 2002; 97:2250–2254.

55. Gevers AM, De Boede E, Simoens M, et al. A randomized trial comparing injection therapy with hemoclip and with injection combined with hemoclip for bleeding ulcers. Gastrointest Endosc 2002; 55:466–469.

56. Chung SCS, Lau JYW, Sung JJY, et al. Randomized comparison between adrenaline injection alone and adrenaline injection plus heat probe treatment for actively bleeding ulcers. Br Med J 1997; 314:1307–1311.

57. Calvet X, Vergara M, Brullet E, et al. Addition of a second endoscopic treatment following epinephrine injection improves outcome in high-risk bleeding ulcers. Gastroenterology 2004; 126:441–450.

58. Green FW, Kaplan MM, Curtis LE, et al. Effect of acid and pepsin on blood coagulation and platelet aggregation. Gastroenterology 1978; 74:38.

59. Labenz J, Peitz U, Leusing C, et al. Efficacy of primed infusions with high dose ranitidine and omeprazole to maintain high intragastric pH in patients with peptic ulcer bleeding: a prospective randomised controlled study. Gut 1997; 40:36–41.

60. Netzer P, Gaia C, Sandoz M, et al. Effect of repeated injection and continuous infusion of omeprazole and ranitidine on intragastric pH over 72 hours. Am J Gastroenterol 1999; 94:351–357.

61. Collins R, Langman M. Treatment with histamine H_2 antagonists in acute upper gastrointestinal hemorrhage. N Engl J Med 1985; 131:660.

62. Levine JE, Leontiadis GI, Sharma VK, et al. Meta-analysis: the efficacy of intravenous H2-receptor antagonists in bleeding peptic ulcer. Aliment Pharmacol Ther 2002; 16(6):1137–1142.

63. Walt RP, Cottrell J, Mann SG, et al. Continuous famotidine for hemorrhage from peptic ulcer. Lancet 1992; 340:1058.

64. Daneshmend TK, Hawkey CJ, Langman MJS, et al. Omeprazole versus placebo for acute upper gastrointestinal bleeding: randomized double-blind controlled trial. Br Med J 1992; 304:143.

65. Khuroo MS, Yattoo GN, Javid G, et al. A comparison of omeprazole and placebo for bleeding peptic ulcer. N Engl J Med 1997; 336:1054.

66. Schaffalitzky de Muckadell OB, Havelund T, Harling H, et al. Effect of omeprazole on the outcome of endoscopically treated bleeding peptic ulcers: randomized double-blind placebo-controlled multicentre study. Scand J Gastroenterol 1997; 32:320–327.

67. Hasselgren G, Lind T, Lundell L, et al. Continuous intravenous infusion of omeprazole in elderly patients with peptic ulcer bleeding: results of a placebo-controlled multicenter study. Scand J Gastroenterol 1997; 32:328-333.

68. Lin HJ, Lo WC, Lee FY, et al. A prospective randomized comparative trial showing that omeprazole prevents rebleeding in patients with bleeding peptic ulcer after successful endoscopic therapy. Arch Intern Med 1998; 158:54–58.

69. Lau J, Sung J, Lee K, et al. Effect of intravenous omeprazole on recurrent bleeding after endoscopic treatment of bleeding peptic ulcers. N Engl J Med 2000; 343:310.

70. Lau JY, Chung SC, Leung JW, et al. The evolution of stigmata of hemorrhage in bleeding peptic ulcers: a sequential endoscopic study. Endoscopy 1998; 30:513–518.

71. Javid G, Masoodi I, Zargar SA, et al. Omeprazole as adjuvant therapy to endoscopic combination injection sclerotherapy for treating bleeding peptic ulcer. Am J Med 2001; 111:280–284.

72. Kaviani MJ, Hashemi MR, Kazemifar AR, et al. Effect of oral omeprazole in reducing rebleeding in bleeding peptic ulcers: a prospective double blind randomized clinical trial. Aliment Pharmacol Ther 2003; 17:211–216.

73. Sung JJY, Chan FK, Lau JY, et al. The effect of endoscopic therapy in patients receiving omeprazole for bleeding ulcers with non-bleeding visible vessels or adherent clots: a randomized comparison. Ann Intern Med. 2003; 139(4):237–243.

74. Zed PJ, Loewen PS, Slavik RS, et al. Meta-analysis of proton pump inhibitors in treatment of bleeding peptic ulcers. Ann Pharmacotherapy 2001; 35:1528–1534.

75. Villanueva C, Balanzo J, Torras X, et al. Value of a second look endoscopy after injection therapy for bleeding peptic ulcer: a prospective and randomized trial. Gastrointest Endosc 1994; 40:34–39.

76. Messmann H, Schaller P, Andus T, et al. Effect of programmed endoscopic follow-up examinations on the rebleeding rate of gastric or duodenal peptic ulcers treated by injection therapy: a prospective, randomized controlled trial. Endoscopy 1998; 30(7):583–589.

77. Chiu PW, Lam CY, Lee SW, et al. Effect of scheduled second therapeutic endoscopy on peptic ulcer rebleeding: a prospective randomised trial. Gut 2003; 52(10):1403–1407.

78. Marmo R, Rotondano G, Bianco MA, et al. Outcome of endoscopic treatment for peptic ulcer bleeding: Is a second look necessary? A meta-analysis. Gastrointest Endosc. 2003 Jan;57(1):62–67.

79. Saeed ZA, Cole RA, Ramirez FC, et al. Endoscopic retreatment after successful initial hemostasis prevents ulcer rebleeding: a prospective randomized trial. Endoscopy 1996; 28:288–294.

80. Hunt PS, Hansky J, Korman MG. Mortality in patients with haematemesis and melaena: a prospective study. Br Med J 1979; 1:1238–1240.

81. Wheatley KE, Snyman JH, Brearley S, et al. Mortality in patients with bleeding peptic ulcer when those aged 60 or over are operated on early. Br Med J 1990; 301(6746):272.

82. Rockall TA. Management and outcome of patients undergoing surgery after acute upper gastrointestinal haemorrhage. Steering Group for the National Audit of Acute Upper Gastrointestinal Haemorrhage. J R Soc Med 1998; 91(10):518–523.

83. Lau JYW, Sung JJY, Lam YH, et al. Endoscopic retreatment compared with surgery in patients with recurrent bleeding after initial endoscopic control of bleeding ulcers. N Engl J Med 1999; 340:751.

84. White RI Jr, Giargiana FA Jr, Bell W. Bleeding duodenal ulcer control. Selective arterial embolization using autologous blood clot. JAMA 1974; 229:546–548.

85. Bell SD, Lau KY, Sniderman KW. Synchronous embolization of the gastroduodenal artery and the inferior pancreaticoduodenal artery in patients with massive duodenal hemorrhage. J Vasc Interv Radiol 1995; 6:531–536.

86. Lang EK. Transcatheter embolization in management of hemorrhage from duodenal ulcer: Long-term results and complications. Radiology 1992; 182:703–707.

87. Toyoda H, Nakano S, Takeda I, et al. Transcatheter arterial embolization for massive bleeding from duodenal ulcers not controlled by endoscopic hemostasis. Endoscopy 1995; 27:304–307.

88. Walsh RM, Anain P, Geisinger M, et al. Role of angiography and embolization for massive gastroduodenal hemorrhage. J Gastrointest Surg 1999; 3:61–66.

89. Defreyne L, Vanlangenhove P, De Vos M, et al: Embolization as a first approach with endoscopically unmanageable acute non-variceal gastro-intestinal hemorrhage. Radiology 2001; 218:739–748.

90. Ripoll C, Banares R, Beceiro I, et al. Comparison of transcatheter arterial embolization and surgery for treatment of bleeding peptic ulcer after endoscopic treatment failure. J Vasc Interv Radiol 2004; 15:447–450.

91. Mallory GK, Weiss S. Hemorrhages from laceration of cardiac orifice of the stomach due to vomiting. Am J Med Sci 1929; 178:506.

92. Graham DY, Schwartz JT. The spectrum of the Mallory-Weiss tear. Medicine 1977; 57:307.

93. Knauer MC. Mallory-Weiss syndrome: characterization of 75 Mallory-Weiss lacerations in 528 patients with upper gastrointestinal hemorrhage. Gastroenterology 1976; 71:5.

94. Sugawa C, Benishek D, Walt AJ. Mallory-Weiss syndrome: a study of 224 patients. Am J Surg 1983; 145:30.

95. Harris JM, DiPalma JA. Clinical significance of Mallory-Weiss tears. Am J Gastroenterol 1993; 88:2056.

96. Lum DF, McQuaid K, Lee JG. Endoscopic hemostasis of nonvariceal non-peptic ulcer hemorrhage. Gastrointest Endosc Clin N Am 1997; 7(4):657–670.

97. Jensen DM, Kovacs TO, Machicado GA, et al. Prospective study of the stigmata of hemorrhage and endoscopic or medical treatment for bleeding Mallory Weiss tears (Abstract). Gastrointest Endosc 1992; 235:38.

98. Jensen DM, Kovacs TO, Machicado GA, et al. Etiology and management of Mallory-Weiss bleeding in patients with and without portal hypertension (Abstract). Gastrointest Endosc 1998; 204:34.

99. Laine L. Multipolar electrocoagulation in the treatment of active upper gastrointestinal tract hemorrhage. N Engl J Med 1987; 316:1613.

100. Llach J, Elizalde JL, Guevara MC, et al. Endoscopic injection therapy in bleeding Mallory-Weiss syndrome: a randomized controlled trial. Gastrointest Endosc 2001; 54:679–681.

101. Dieulafoy G. Exulceratio simplex. Clin med de l' Hotel-Dieu de Paris 1897/98, II; L'intervention chirurgicale dans les hematemeses foudrovantes consecutives a l'exulceration simple de l'estomac [French]. Pr Med 1989; 29–44.

102. Miko TL, Thomazy VA. The caliber persistent artery of the stomach: a unifying approach to gastric aneurysm, Dieulafoy's lesion, and submucosal arterial malformation. Hum Pathol 1988; 19:914–921.

103. Lee YT, Walmsley RS, Leong RW, et al. Dieulafoy's lesion. Gastrointest Endosc 2003; 58:236–243.

104. Baettig B, Haecki W, Lammer F, et al. Dieulafoy's disease: endoscopic treatment and follow up. Gut 1993; 34:1418.

105. Brown GR, Harford WV, Jones WF. Endoscopic band ligation of an actively bleeding Dieulafoy lesion. Gastrointest Endosc 1994; 40:501.

106. D'Imperio N, Papadia C, Baroncini D, et al. N-butyl-2-cyanocrylate in the endoscopic treatment of Dieulafoy ulcer. Endoscopy 1995; 27:216.

107. Romaozinho JM, Pontes JM, Lerias C, et al. Dieulafoy's lesion: management and long-term outcome. Endoscopy 2004; 36:416–420.

108. McCormack TT, Sims J, Eyre-Brook I, et al. Gastric lesions in portal hypertension: inflammatory gastritis or congestive gastropathy. Gut 1985; 26:1226–1232.

109. Gostout CJ, Viggiano TR, Balm RK. Acute gastrointestinal bleeding from portal hypertensive gastropathy. Prevalence and clinical features. Am J Gastroenterol 1993; 88:2030–2033.

110. Hosking SW, Kennedy HJ, Sneddon I, et al. The role of propranolol in congestive gastropathy of portal hypertension. Hepatology 1987; 7:437–441.

111. Perez-Ayuso RM, Pique JM, Bosch J. Beta-blockers in portal hypertension: variation on a theme. Lancet 1991; 337:1431–1434.

112. Quientero E, Pique JM, Bombi JA, et al. Upper gastrointestinal bleeding caused by gastroduodenal vascular malformations: incidence, diagnosis and treatment. Dig Dis Sci 1986; 31:897–905.

113. VanCutsem E, Rutgeerts P, Vantrappen G. Treatment of bleeding gastrointestinal vascular malformations with oestrogen-progesterone. Lancet 1990; 335:953–955.

114. Junquera F, Feu F, Papo M, et al. A multicenter, randomized, clinical trial of hormonal therapy in the prevention of rebleeding from gastrointestinal angiodysplasia. Gastroenterology 2001; 121:1073–1079.

115. Peery WH. Clinical spectrum of hereditary hemorrhagic telangiectasia. Am J Med 1987; 82:989–997.

116. Payen JL, Cales P, Voigt JJ, et al. Severe portal hypertensive gastropathy and antral vascular ectasia are distinct entities in patients with cirrhosis. Gastroenterology 1995; 108:138–144.

117. Gostout CJ, Viggiano TR, Ahlquist DA, et al. The clinical and endoscopic spectrum of the watermelon stomach. J Clin Gastroenterol 1992; 15:256–263.

118. Sebastian S, McLoughlin R, Qasim A, et al. Endoscopic argon plasma coagulation for the treatment of gastric antral vascular ectasia (watermelon stomach): long-term results. Dig Liver Dis 2004; 36:212–217.

119. Pavey DA, Craig PI. Endoscopic therapy for upper-GI vascular ectasias. Gastrointest Endosc 2004; 59:233–238.

120. Romans S, Saurin JC, Dumortier J, et al. Tolerance and efficacy of argon plasma coagulation for controlling bleeding in patients with typical and atypical manifestations of watermelon stomachs. Endoscopy 2003; 35(12):1024–1028.

CHAPTER TWENTY-TWO

22

Gastric outlet obstruction, perforation and other complications of gastroduodenal ulcer

Stephen J. Ferzoco and David I. Soybel

INTRODUCTION

Complications of peptic ulcer disease that are discussed in this chapter include obstruction, perforation, and fistulization to adjacent structures. Optimal care for patients with these complications requires early diagnosis, as well as a systematic approach to fluid, electrolyte, and nutritional imbalances. In addition, for patients with ulcers occurring in the prepylorus or gastric corpus, the clinician must have a continuous regard for the possibility of an underlying malignancy. The surgeon should be consulted when one of these complications of peptic ulcer is recognized. Early consultation between surgeon, gastroenterologist, and primary care physician will lead to early clarification of the goals of medical therapy, and indications and timing of surgical intervention.

GASTRIC OUTLET OBSTRUCTION

In the era before H_2-receptor antagonists and *Helicobacter pylori* were described, it was felt that as many as 10% of patients with chronic duodenal ulcer disease would develop the complication of gastric outlet obstruction.[1,2] The current consensus suggests that obstruction requiring surgery is not as common as suggested by earlier studies. Less than 5% of patients with complicated duodenal ulcer disease and less than 1–2% with complicated gastric ulcer disease[3,4] develop this complication.

Some reports suggest that patients with gastric outlet obstruction due to peptic disease have a higher prevalence of chronic use of nonsteroidal antiinflammatory agents or steroid usage,[2,5] but most cases are not associated with use of these drugs. In addition, *H. pylori* infestation has been associated with certain reversible causes of obstruction,[6,7] but it does not seem to make a special contribution to the chronic scarring and irreversible obstruction seen in the majority of patients.[8] In older surveys,[1,2,9–12] 80% of patients admitted with obstruction have previously been treated for peptic ulcer disease: ~20% have a history of bleeding, ~20% a history of perforation, and 11% a prior episode of obstruction. The average duration of peptic symptoms before development of obstruction is 9–10 years.[2,10] Thus, the appearance of obstruction usually indicates a severe, chronic ulcer diathesis.

Presentation

The symptoms of gastric outlet obstruction are highly predictable: the patient presents with repeated episodes of nausea and vomiting of food and pale yellow gastric juice. The vomitus contains hydrochloric acid and not bile; its taste is sour, not bitter. Blood or 'coffee grounds' in the vomitus is not common, occurring in less than 10% of patients.[9,10] The patient usually reports a chronic history of ulcer pain, which has worsened over the few days prior to presentation. Reflux symptoms of heartburn and regurgitation may also become prominent as the stomach has become distended and the lower esophageal sphincter has lost its competence. A report of weight loss is not uncommon, occurring in up to 40% of patients.[12] With persistent vomiting and dehydration, lethargy and confusion may develop. Tetanus, due to severe alkalosis, occurs rarely.

On physical examination, the mucus membranes are desiccated and the urine is dark and concentrated due to dehydration. The upper abdomen may be distended if the stomach is full, but it is otherwise scaphoid. When the stomach is full, a succussion splash may be audible. When the stomach is empty the bowel sounds are normal. Typical of the laboratory examination are: (1) normal or mildly elevated leukocyte count and hemoconcentration; (2) mild or moderate hyponatremia, marked hypochloremia, moderate or marked hypokalemia, increased serum HCO_3^-, and elevated BUN and creatinine; (3) high arterial pH with normal arterial oxygen levels and saturation; and (4) high urine specific gravity and (paradoxical) aciduria. Abdominal films may reveal a large gastric silhouette and gas bubble, with little or no air in the small intestine or colon.

Differential diagnosis

In Western countries, most cases of gastric outlet obstruction are not attributable to peptic ulcer disease. About two-thirds of patients presenting with symptoms and signs of gastric outlet obstruction have an underlying malignancy of the stomach or duodenum,[13–15] either adenocarcinoma or lymphoma. Gastric outlet obstruction is not usually part of the initial presentation of malignancies of the head of the pancreas.[13–16] However, outlet obstruction eventually appears in 25% of patients with pancreatic cancer that could not be resected for cure.[16] Occasionally, locally advanced retroperitoneal and disseminated ovarian malignancies will present with gastric outlet obstruction. Table 22.1 lists various conditions associated with outlet obstruction.

Within the spectrum of acid-peptic disease, chronic duodenal ulcer and pyloric channel ulceration account for the great majority of cases of obstruction. In Haubrich's 1976 survey,[17] gastric stasis

Table 22.1 The differential diagnosis of gastric outlet obstruction – other than peptic ulcer disease

Benign tumors
  Adenoma
  Lipoma
  Stromal tumors
  Carcinoid

Malignant tumors
  Carcinoma (gastric, pancreatic duodenal, ovarian)
  Lymphoma
  Sarcoma

Inflammatory
  Cholecystitis
  Gallstone (Bouveret's syndrome)
  Acute pancreatitis
  Chronic pancreatitis (duodenal stricturing)
  Crohn's disease
  Behçet's disease
  Eosinophic gastroenteritis
  Systemic lupus

Others causes
  Parasites
  Tuberculosis
  Caustic stricture
  Annular pancreas
  Ectopic pancreas
  Adult hypertrophic pyloric stenosis
  Pyloric/duodenal web or duplications
  Postsurgical scarring
  Autovagotomy (mediastinal tumor encasing the vagi)

AIDS-related
  Lymphoma
  Toxoplasma
  Cryptospiridia
  Tuberculosis
  Kaposi's lesions

was observed in 8.6% of 3027 patients with duodenal ulcer and only 2.1% of 1286 patients with gastric ulcers. The great majority of cases of obstruction associated with gastric ulcers were found in the pyloric channel or in association with duodenal ulcer and scarring. It is very uncommon for the typical benign lesser curve ulcer to cause severe obstruction.[3,18] Rarely, obstruction develops due to an 'hour-glass' deformity, caused by ulceration at the incisura that has elicited chronic scarring and regional muscular spasm.

It has been estimated that >95% of cases of obstructing duodenal ulcer disease are located in the duodenal bulb and <5% are located in the postbulbar region.[1,19–21] However, in one recent report[21] from the tertiary referral practice at the Medical College of Georgia, postbulbar stenosis accounted for 15 of 31 cases of obstruction caused by duodenal ulcer. Postbulbar ulcers are particularly prone to other complications such as bleeding and fistulization to adjacent structures.[19,20] In about one-third of cases, postbulbar ulcers are associated with deformity and scarring more proximally.[20,21] They are indicative of highly aggressive acid-peptic disease and a diagnosis of gastrinoma should be excluded.

Natural history

In 1962, Dworkin and Roth[9] reported a series of 158 patients with gastric outlet obstruction. Of these patients, 85 (53%) had obstruction attributed to chronic fibrosis, 43 (27%) patients had penetrating ulcers causing duodenal deformity, and 30 (19%) had nonpenetrating ulcers without fibrosis surrounding the duodenum. Before the H_2-receptor blocker era, a number of authors suggested that most cases involved active ulcer disease.[22,23] They also suggested that, if treated with comprehensive medical therapies, most cases of gastric outlet obstruction would resolve without operation.

Some more recent reports have suggested this may not be the case. In 1985, Weiland et al.[11] reported a series of 87 patients with gastric outlet obstruction treated at the Minneapolis Veterans Hospital between 1965 and 1979. Thirteen of these patients (14%) were labeled as having acute disease because the obstruction was the initial manifestation of the disease. In long-term follow-up of these patients: 7 ultimately required surgery (4 in the initial hospitalization, 3 in a later hospitalization); 4 resolved without operation; and 2 were lost to follow-up or died. Of 74 patients with a chronic history of peptic symptoms, 45 required surgery because symptoms failed to resolve within 5 days. Twenty-nine went on to discharge without surgery; of these, 20 were ultimately readmitted and required surgery. Thus, 80–90% of these patients ultimately came to surgery for obstructive symptoms. These observations were confirmed by Jaffin and Kaye, who reported that over 80% (60% on first hospitalization; 20% on subsequent hospitalizations) of their 68 patients with acid-peptic gastric outlet obstruction ultimately required surgery.[2] It seems clear that the great majority of patients currently presenting with gastric outlet obstruction complicating peptic ulcer disease will ultimately require operation or some form of intervention to prevent further occurrences.

Diagnostic tests

In most cases, the history and physical examination lead to a clinical diagnosis of gastric outlet obstruction. In a few cases, the important question to be answered by diagnostic testing is whether the patient truly retains gastric contents due to a mechanical gastric outlet obstruction. Additional issues that may be resolved by diagnostic testing and imaging include localization of the obstruction (prepyloric, pyloric, duodenal bulb, postbulbar) and exclusion of malignancy. Thus, the following diagnostic tests may be useful in evaluation of the patient with suspected gastric outlet obstruction.

Confirming the diagnosis of gastric retention

Aspiration of large volumes of gastric content is a seemingly direct approach to a diagnosis of gastric retention. When bile is absent and food particles are present in a volume greater than 400 or 500 cc, it may be concluded that gastric contents are being retained and bile reflux is being prevented. Gastric residuals can be followed serially and are probably as accurate as any other parameter for evaluating the resolution of obstruction. Along these lines, abdominal sonography appears to be capable of detecting abnormally high gastric volume,[24] but the clinical relevance of this imaging technique is not defined.

The saline load test was popularized by Goldstein and Boyle[25] as a means of objectively documenting gastric retention. The test is performed 24–48 hours following admission, when the patient is fully resuscitated (see below) and has undergone nasogastric suction for a sufficient period of time to fully decompress the stomach. After aspiration of the residual gastric volume, 750 mL of warm saline is instilled via the nasogastric tube over a period of 5 minutes, the tube is clamped for 30 minutes, and then the gastric contents are aspirated. Criteria for retention are: *no retention* – less than 200 mL residual; *incomplete retention* – 200 to 400 mL; *near complete or complete retention* – greater than 400 mL.[25,26] Gastric fluid secretion is itself increased in patients with outlet obstruction, contributing to the high volumes under baseline conditions and those measured during the saline load test. However, it has been stated that these higher levels of secretion do not diminish the usefulness of the test.[27]

Imaging techniques that have been used to diagnose gastric retention include the upper gastrointestinal series (barium slurry) and the barium-burger (barium mixed with hamburger). In normal individuals, most of the liquid barium will be emptied by the stomach 2 hours after ingestion, and all of it should be evacuated at 6 hours. When the pylorus is blocked by scarring, a liquid barium study will reveal retention as late as 24 hours. In cases where scarring has severely deformed the duodenum, compromising emptying but not completely occluding the lumen, the liquid barium study may not accurately estimate the degree of gastric retention of solid food. Thus, Pelot et al.[28] have suggested that evaluation of emptying of gastric contents after a solid meal is probably more sensitive for the diagnosis of obstruction than evaluation after liquid barium or saline ingestion. These conclusions are probably still true in the H_2-receptor blocker era, but the issue has not been studied recently.

Efforts to improve diagnosis of gastric retention and delayed gastric emptying in other clinical conditions have led to evaluation of gastric emptying measurements using radionuclides salted into food. The two markers used most commonly in gastric emptying studies are ⁹⁹ᵐTc-DTPA and ⁹⁹ᵐTc-sulfur colloid. However, there have been no reports that have systematically evaluated the role of these techniques in diagnosis of gastric outlet obstruction due to peptic ulcer disease.

Evaluating characteristics of the disease and exclusion of malignancy

Liquid barium studies can play an important role in diagnosing the site of obstruction (Fig. 22.1). Obstruction is rarely so complete that a small column of barium cannot pass into the duodenum. The test is then very useful in detecting deformity and scarring of the duodenum and can provide evidence of malignant infiltration of the gastric and duodenal wall. Nevertheless, endoscopy has become the mainstay for localizing the site of obstruction and evaluating associated pathology. Most reported management strategies indicate that the inability to pass a 9 mm endoscope through the pylorus is a valid criterion for diagnosis of gastric outlet obstruction.[26] In addition, endoscopic biopsy of any abnormal

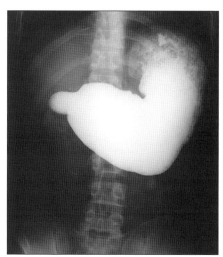

Fig. 22.1 • Barium study in a patient with gastric outlet obstruction. Note rounded cutoff at pylorus, which is more characteristic of benign obstruction than malignancy.

areas can and should be performed in order to exclude underlying malignancy or rare pathology such as Crohn's disease. Because gastric outlet obstruction is now so commonly associated with malignancy, it is helpful to obtain a CT scan with oral contrast prior to endoscopy in order to exclude underlying malignancies and evaluate the pancreas, biliary tree, and retroperitoneum. It is not so uncommon to see evidence for mucinous carcinoma or *linitis plastica* that are clearly identified on CT scan but to have endoscopic biopsies that show no evidence of malignancy. The endoscopic examination can then be directed to any potential areas of concern.

Admission, resuscitation, and evaluation

The patient with symptoms of persistent gastric outlet obstruction is admitted to the hospital. Mild cases may be managed on an outpatient basis, but a patient with disturbances of fluid and electrolyte balance should be hospitalized. Weight loss, hypoalbuminemia, and anemia are not uncommon and contribute to morbidity and mortality. A systematic plan for correcting these abnormalities in the hospital setting permits rapid progression to diagnostic studies and definitive therapy (Fig. 22.2).

The correction of fluid, electrolyte, and pH imbalances requires a detailed understanding of the body's responses to the loss of large quantities of gastric juice by vomiting. The loss of excessive amounts of gastric juice lead to dehydration, decreases in serum Cl^-, K^+ and sometimes Na^+, and an increase in serum HCO_3^- and the arterial pH. Cl^-, the main anion found in gastric juice, is critical for effective absorption of Na^+ in the GI tract and reabsorption of Na^+ in the kidney. The loss of Cl^- makes it impossible for the organism to expand its extracellular volume. The loss of volume, Na^+ and K^+ in the vomited gastric juice, leads the kidney to utilize all mechanisms capable of retaining Na^+. Hence the kidney begins to secrete H^+ into the glomerular filtrate, paradoxically acidifying the urine and preventing renal compensation for systemic alkalosis. K^+ is also sequestered intracellularly and it is also lost in the urine in response to the alkalosis. The loss of K^+ intensifies the loss of H^+ into the urine. If serum Ca^{++} and Mg^{++} levels are lowered by chronic malnutrition, GI losses, and alkalosis, tetanus may result.

The principles of volume and electrolyte resuscitation are: (1) intravenous volume resuscitation with normal (0.95) saline;

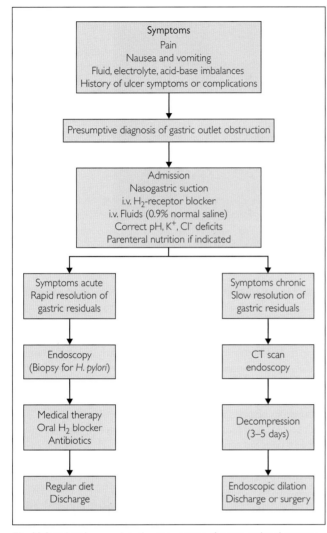

Fig. 22.2 • Initial approach in the management of gastric outlet obstruction. In selected cases, two attempts at endoscopic dilatation may be justified, either to achieve long-term relief of symptoms or as a short-term bridge to improving operative risk.

(2) repletion of K^+ losses with intravenous K^+ supplementation; and (3) serial measurements of electrolytes and arterial pH. Remembering that Cl^- resides largely in the extracellular and vascular spaces, the Cl^- deficit may be calculated as follows:

$$\text{Deficit (mEq/L)} = 0.2 \times \text{weight} \times [Cl^-_{normal} - Cl^-_{observed}] \rightarrow (\text{mEq/L})$$

Potassium losses may be treated aggressively, if the alkalosis is severe, by giving up to 1 mEq/min. This aggressive treatment should only be done in the ICU setting, with appropriate cardiac monitoring in place. The potassium deficit cannot be estimated directly from the serum level because losses reflect shifts into intracellular compartments that will correct as the pH is restored to normal. Close monitoring of serum K^+ is essential during the resuscitation.

The infusion of acidifying solutions is rarely necessary, but it is indicated if arterial pH rises above 7.5. If necessary, ammonium chloride (NH_4Cl) or dilute HCl (0.1 N) can be administered according to the following formula:

$$NH_4Cl \text{ or } HCl \text{ (mEq)} = 0.3 \times \text{body weight} \times \text{base deficit}$$

Ammonium chloride is contraindicated if the patient has renal or hepatic insufficiency. Correction of the alkalosis is permitted to

progress gradually over 24–48 hours; as long as progress is steady, there is no need to hurry it along. Serum K^+ and pH/CO_2 levels should be monitored frequently (2–4 hour intervals) until pH is less than 7.5.

When an episode of gastric outlet obstruction is associated with edema and spasm due to active peptic ulcer disease, the patient usually presents with pain as a prominent component. These patients tend to respond immediately to nasogastric decompression, intravenous fluid hydration with normal saline and potassium supplements, and use of intravenous H_2-receptor blockers. Cases of transient obstruction are suspected when nasogastric outputs decrease rapidly. Barium slurry and the endoscope pass with mild or no difficulty through the pylorus and no other pathology is observed. If edema and gastritis/duodenitis are prominent, testing for *H. pylori* is recommended. If the test is positive, anecdotal observations suggest that antibacterial therapy in the outpatient setting is reasonable.[6,8] As noted above, the pain and gastric hypersecretion in such cases usually resolve quickly, within 48 to 72 hours, and patients are ready to tolerate regular diet within 72 to 96 hours. It is recommended that the trial of the diet begin in the hospital, in order to be sure it is tolerated before discharge.

When chronic symptoms are present and heavy scarring is suspected as the cause of obstruction, the endoscope will not pass easily and barium may be retained for several hours in the stomach. Several days of decompression may be necessary in order to reduce gastric hypersecretion, which may result from gastric distention and hypergastrinemia.[29,30] Despite the inability to tolerate oral feeding, omeprazole given by mouth is not necessarily ineffective. With appropriate decompression of the gastric lumen, however, intravenous H_2-receptor blockers are usually sufficient to control acid secretion in this setting.

After resuscitation and correction of volume, electrolyte, and pH imbalances, a CT scan should be performed to exclude malignancy and to evaluate distal regions of the GI tract. Endoscopy should follow, as the CT may identify areas of the gastric wall or pylorus to be inspected closely and biopsied. A serum gastrin level may be useful if there is postbulbar obstruction, a history of previous, definitive surgical procedure for ulcer disease, or other unusual features to suggest the possibility of gastrinoma. There are not strong reasons to believe that treatment for *H. pylori* will alter the natural history of patients with obstruction due to chronic scarring; thus, testing for *H. pylori* is not likely to be helpful.[31]

Indications for intervention

If the endoscopy and upper GI series strongly suggest that the obstruction is due to heavy scarring or is associated with substantial deformity of the duodenal bulb, some form of intervention will be required. If there is any doubt about the irreversibility of the obstruction, a saline load test may be helpful, but this is rarely necessary. Even in cases where the obstruction seems to have a reversible component, many will ultimately require a definitive ulcer operation.[9,11] The decision to proceed expeditiously to surgery or interventional modalities, as opposed to waiting for another complication, should be individualized. However, definitive intervention would be recommended for any patient with a prior history of obstruction or a patient with long-standing ulcer symptoms or complications and noncompliance with medical regimens. Purely medical management would be preferred for the patient with a first-time episode of obstruction, endoscopic evidence of edema and gastritis, and relatively rapid clearing of obstructive symptoms. In these cases, maximum medical therapy would include oral H_2 blockers or omeprazole, and antibiotics to treat *H. pylori*, if the organisms can be demonstrated in antral biopsies or by Chloe test.[6,7] Follow-up endoscopy should be performed to evaluate the outlet and confirm eradication of *H. pylori*.

Treatment: nonoperative interventional approaches

The irreversibility of obstruction demands dilatation, excision, or bypass of the obstructed segment of pylorus or duodenum. In addition, a definitive approach to prevention of recurrence is recommended, because obstruction represents an unrelenting ulcer diathesis. Pyloric dilatation in the operating room, in conjunction with highly selective vagotomy, was proposed many years ago by Goligher and Johnston[32,33] as a means of addressing the obstructed outlet. In recent years, a number of highly skilled interventional radiologists and endoscopists have evaluated the possibility of dilating the obstruction endoscopically.[12,31,34–43] Early reports indicated that perhaps 60–80% of patients could find relief from obstruction after balloon dilatation of peptic pyloric or duodenal strictures. Recent studies have shown the need for repeated endoscopic balloon dilatations to demonstrate continued response.[37]

The technique for balloon dilatation of the pylorus involves the passage of a dilating balloon via the instrument port of a gastroscope, under direct vision, through the pylorus. Technical variations include size of the balloon, use of a single balloon or sequentially sized balloons, insufflation time, and number of attempts. Dilatation can also be accomplished using fluoroscopy as a guide. It is generally believed that passage under endoscopic control offers the most precise positioning of the balloon and the least likelihood of inadvertent rupture of the pylorus or duodenum.

Subsequent follow-up studies have not been uniform in their agreement about the long-term value of dilatation. In some, the avoidance of surgery was achieved in 60–80% of patients and in others, avoidance of surgery was achieved in less than 50% of patients (Table 22.2). For example, among 42 patients followed for a median 23 months by Perng et al.,[31] 67% were able to avoid surgery. The authors were not able to identify any single factor that would predict failure or only short-term success of balloon dilatation in relief of obstructive symptoms. In contrast, in their 54 patients undergoing balloon dilatation, Lau et al.[12] reported that 49% had long-term relief of symptoms and 51% subsequently required surgery for recurrent obstruction.

At first glance, it might appear that variability in success rates might be due solely to technical variations in the dilatation protocol. However, it seems likely that patient characteristics are more important. Thus, it has been argued[39,41] that the poorer outcomes in Lau's series might have been due to especially intense ulcer diathesis. However, this argument implies that balloon dilatation is often being recommended to patients with less severe forms of ulcer disease. Few of the larger series actually provide details of the criteria for irreversibility of obstruction. In addition, no study has systematically addressed the role of dilatation and intensive medical management for patients with reversible obstruction due to active ulceration. Since intensive medical management is always part of the treatment before proceeding to surgery, it is difficult to know if all of the patients included in these reports would also have been considered as candidates for surgery.

Currently, it seems reasonable to allow a period of intensive resuscitation and medical management before proceeding to surgical or endoscopic intervention. Patients with obstruction that fail an intensive regimen would receive two sessions of endoscopic balloon dilatation before declaring the therapy a failure and recommending surgery (see Fig. 22.2). Management should be individualized, however. Surgery probably should be recommended earlier for patients who have longstanding symptoms and complications or a poor record of compliance with medical regimens. Whether or not symptoms are chronic, severe outlet deformity with complete or near-complete obstruction suggests that surgery should be considered earlier.

Treatment: operative approaches

Surgical approaches to acid-peptic gastric outlet obstruction should be individualized. The goals of therapy are: (1) to reconstruct or dilate the obstructing segment in order to permit normal eating; and (2) to prevent recurrence of life-threatening or disabling ulcer symptoms and complications. The choice of operation takes into consideration the fact that chronic ulceration in the pyloric channel, duodenal bulb, or postbulbar segments may respond differently to standard operations such as highly selective (parietal cell) vagotomy and vagotomy, antrectomy and reconstruction. In addition, the surgeon must be wary of performing extensive dissection and reconstructive procedures when there is severe scarring at the pylorus and duodenal bulb.

Table 22.2 Long-term results of endoscopic dilatation of peptic duodenal or pyloric stricture

Authors	Patients (n)	Follow-up interval	Success (%)	Need for further proc/surgery (%)
Lindor et al. (1985)	23	12 mo (median)	87%	40%
Perng et al. (1996)	42	23 mo (median)	67%	33%
DiSario et al. (1994)	30	15 mo (median)	67%	33%
Misra, Dwivedi (1989)	14	27 mo (median)	50%	50%
Kozarek et al. (1990)	23	30 mo (mean)	70%	30%
Kuwada, Alexander (1995)	19	45 mo (median)	16%	57%
Lau et al. (1996)	54	39 mo (median)	55%	51%

Historically, the initial approaches to pyloric or duodenal dilatation were performed in the operating room, utilizing rigid and successively larger dilators passed through an open gastrotomy.[32,33] Because dilation can now be performed endoscopically, there are currently few indications for attempting this in the operating room. This may change as the indications for combined endoscopic/laparoscopic approaches are evaluated.

Bypass of the obstruction can be accomplished by gastrojejunostomy, in conjunction with some form of selective or nonselective vagotomy or in conjunction with truncal vagotomy and antrectomy. Construction of a gastrojejunostomy in conjunction with vagotomy alone avoids dissection in the region of the scarred pylorus and duodenum entirely. Repair of a tight stricture not amenable to dilatation is also feasible, utilizing a pyloroplasty incision that is repaired transversely (Heinicke-Mickulicz) or using some form of gastroduodenostomy (Jaboulay). The difficulty with both of these methods of pyloric reconstruction is that the duodenum must be mobilized (Kocher maneuver) beyond the stenotic segment, so that it can fold over with minimal tension on the suture line. Heavy scarring at the pylorus and duodenal bulb often precludes this type of mobilization. Critical intraoperative judgment is needed to evaluate whether such a reconstruction is feasible and safe.

The need for a definitive antisecretory operation is based on the recognition that irreversible obstruction is most commonly associated with a prolonged and severe ulcer diathesis.[3,12,19,26] As a rule, vagotomy should be part of the definitive management of obstruction due to peptic ulcer disease.

Antrectomy and vagotomy (usually reconstructed by gastrojejunostomy in this setting) is the most definitive antisecretory operation for chronic duodenal ulcer disease, and the one with the lowest associated risk of recurrence. Traditionally, truncal vagotomy/antrectomy has been recommended for patients with a long-standing history of ulcer symptoms and complications. However, a meticulous dissection of the pylorus and duodenum is necessary for removing the entire antrum. As mentioned above, this dissection is hazardous and poses a risk of devitalizing the duodenal stump.[44,45] Intraoperative judgment is also critical here to determine whether an antrectomy is feasible or whether it is safer to avoid dissection of the pylorus and duodenum altogether.

In this regard, a recent study by Csendes at al.[26] seems to legitimately question the superiority of vagotomy/antrectomy as the procedure of choice for gastric outlet obstruction due to duodenal or pyloric channel ulcer disease. In this study, 90 adult patients with pyloric stenosis due to peptic ulcer disease were randomized to one of three treatments: (1) highly selective vagotomy (HSV) plus gastrojejunostomy (HSV/GJ); (2) HSV plus Jaboulay gastroduodenostomy (HSV/Jab); or (3) selective vagotomy plus antrectomy and Billroth II gastrojejunostomy reconstruction (SV/A). Rigorous criteria for diagnosing irreversible obstruction were utilized, including saline load tests performed after reasonable periods of resuscitation and stabilization. One-third to one-half of patients in each group fulfilled criteria for complete gastric retention, the highest number (one-half) in the HSV/Jab group. In late follow-up (mean 98 months), it appeared that HSV/GJ or SV/A elicited almost equal reductions (90% BAO/73% PAO) in acid secretion, while HSV/Jab was not as effective. Ulcer recurrences were noted only in the HSV/Jab group. Visick grade IV scores were noted in 3 patients in the SV/A group, due to alkaline reflux, none in the HSV/GJ group. Visick grade II/III scores were assigned to 3

patients in the HSV/GJ group, reflecting diarrhea, esophagitis, epigastric discomfort, whereas they were assigned to 4 patients in the SV/A group. Visick grade I was assigned to 80% in the HSV/GJ group, 70% in the HSV/Jab group, and 75% in the SV/A group. On the basis of these results, a gastrojejunostomy plus highly selective vagotomy, which avoids interruption of vagal efferents to the small bowel and gallbladder, gave the best results with the lowest level of long-term side effects. This option could be considered when the surgeon has expertise in performing HSV. If such expertise is not readily available, TV/A would be preferred, and TV/GJ would be recommended if antrectomy and dissection of the pylorus would be too hazardous. Along these lines, a recent retrospective study by Chang et al. looked at 120 patients with complicated duodenal ulcer, including a significant proportion of patients with outlet obstruction. They also found that highly selective vagotomy provided less complications and better weight gain long-term than truncal vagotomy and antrectomy for patients with obstruction duodenal ulcer.[46]

PERFORATION

In developed countries, the incidence and outcomes of perforated peptic ulcer are well documented. A number of reports have emphasized that the incidence of perforation has changed very little over the last 50 years.[47,48] It would appear, however, that perforation is currently observed more commonly among the elderly[49-51] and this may have contributed to a recent upturn in mortality due to peptic ulcer disease.[47] In addition, the proportion of women admitted for ulcer perforation is higher than was observed as recently as 20 years ago, but men still predominate by a ratio of two or three to one.[47,51]

A number of reports have tried to identify specific conditions that might predispose to perforation. H. pylori infestation is present in virtually all cases of duodenal and pyloric channel ulceration, and this is true for cases that are complicated by perforation.[52,53] However, there is no direct evidence that there is a subgroup of patients in whom the response to H. pylori might specifically lead to perforation. Heavy use of nonsteroidal antiinflammatory drugs (NSAIDs) has been documented among patients with perforation.[52-54] Aspirin, indomethacin, ibuprofen, and ketorolac have all been implicated. These observations underscore the ulcerogenic properties of any NSAID.

Acute perforation is also recognized as a complication of acute multiorgan failure and specific forms of stress to the organism. Such an ulcer diathesis is not to be confused with stress erosive gastritis, which is superficial and affects only mucosa and submucosa.[55,56] Classically, perforation has also been recognized as a complication of ulceration due to massive burn injury (Curling's ulcers),[57] or significant neurological insult (Cushing's ulcers).[58,59] In addition, in recent years, a number of acute perforations have been identified in young patients using crack cocaine. It is thought to occur as a result of intense transmural ischemia.[60]

Presentation and evolution of symptoms

Quite commonly, patients describe escalating epigastric pain over several days before the event of perforation. Perforation is marked by sudden, intense upper abdominal pain often occurring within 1 or 2 hours of eating. The pain is constant rather than colicky. It is unrelenting and typically spreads throughout the abdomen.

Nausea and vomiting are not prominent. About one-third to one-half of patients will not have a typically dramatic presentation.[61] This is especially true of patients who are elderly, immunocompromised, or who have neurologic injury (stroke or spinal cord injury).[55–59] A history of peptic ulcer or even of dyspepsia is present in about 50% of patients.[61] As discussed below, symptoms and signs may be indolent or even improving in some patients, due to early sealing of the perforation by the liver edge or a flap of omentum. Occasionally, the leakage is channeled to the right paracolic gutter and the patient may appear to have acute appendicitis.

When the perforation is not quickly sealed or walled off, chemical peritonitis alone may elicit shock and prostration. As time progresses, the peritoneum becomes colonized and infected, and abscess and/or septic shock will develop. On physical examination, the patient often is observed in a recumbent position, with knees flexed. Epigastric tenderness is obvious, and this is associated with involuntary guarding that progresses to board-like rigidity of the abdominal wall musculature. Unlike the localized peritonitis associated with a gangrenous appendix or inflamed gallbladder, the rigidity is usually diffuse and bilateral. The white blood cell count is elevated, usually between 12 000 and 15 000/mm³, but will be higher if it is greater than 12–24 hours since the onset of symptoms. The serum amylase level is often elevated, but not in the range typical of acute pancreatitis.[61] Flat and upright radiographs of the abdomen should be performed, along with an upright chest X-ray. Free air in the peritoneum or under the diaphragm will be found in about 75–85% of cases.[62,63] In elderly patients with a perforated peptic ulcer, the proportion presenting with free air may be a little lower, in the range of 60%.[64] Thus, the absence of free air does not exclude the diagnosis.

Differential diagnosis

The differential diagnosis of perforation is that of acute abdominal pain. As such, a range of diagnoses are in the differential diagnosis. The major considerations include acute cholecystitis, acute pancreatitis (for epigastric and left upper quadrant pain), and acute appendicitis (for right-sided pain). In older patients with a history of atrial fibrillation, recent myocardial infarction or congestive heart failure, mesenteric ischemia may be considered. Free air under the diaphragm can be observed in patients with perforations due to peptic ulcer, diverticulitis, deeply penetrating carcinomas, or granulomatous processes (Crohn's disease or tuberculosis), or gangrenous bowel with perforation (small intestine or appendix). Pneumatosis cystoides intestinalis, a benign condition caused by rupture of gas-filled sacs in the bowel wall, also can produce free intraperitoneal air. In reasonably healthy individuals, it is usually not difficult to estimate the likelihood of perforated ulcer over other diagnoses. However, in the elderly, immuno-compromised, or neurologically impaired patients, diverse diagnoses must be considered. In patients with AIDS, consideration should be given to complicating conditions such as lymphoma, tuberculosis (*M. avium intracellulare*), and cytomegalovirus-induced ulceration.

Diagnostic tests

In the patient presenting with acutely evolving symptoms and signs, the main diagnostic examination is the abdominal film, obtained in both supine and upright positions. In doubtful cases,

a left lateral decubitus film can also be helpful. The key criteria of an adequate upright study is that both sides of the diaphragm must be visible and the film must not be rotated. As a warning about the overall accuracy of the search for free air on plain films, Roh et al.[65] reviewed the records of 89 patients with a diagnosis of pneumoperitoneum or perforated viscus. They found that pneumoperitoneum was detected in 51% of patients with perforated viscus (all causes). Also striking was the finding that 14% (7 patients) with pneumoperitoneum did not have a perforated viscus or intraperitoneal cause for free air under the diaphragm. Pneumoperitoneum in the latter cases was usually due to dissection of air from the pleural cavity caused by positive pressure ventilation in intensive care patients. Pneumoperitoneum, like any other radiographic finding, must be taken in the context of the whole clinical picture before it can be said to have 'made' the diagnosis of perforated viscus. In addition, patients with perforated ulcers may have free air in the lesser sac and not in the subdiaphragmatic space (Fig. 22.3).

In most cases, a presumptive diagnosis of a perforated viscus will be confirmed by plain films or by the acuteness of the clinical presentation. However, there may be a role for other diagnostic studies when the clinical picture is not so acute and plain radiographs cannot confirm the diagnosis. One technique to consider in the emergency room setting is the pneumogastrogram, in which the stomach is insufflated by means of a nasogastric tube positioned in the distal body of the stomach. Lee et al.[66] reported that this maneuver increased the diagnostic sensitivity of plain films from 66% to 91%. The disadvantage of the procedure is that, if the test is positive, insufflation of the stomach causes spitting of gastric contents into the peritoneum and this is usually very uncomfortable for the patient. For this reason, the maneuver is recommended as a last resort or when other modalities are not available.

CT scan is also of use in doubtful cases, because it can detect much smaller amounts of free air than do plain films. CT also may detect other pathologic processes such as diverticulitis or malignancy that would explain the clinical picture. Oral administration of dilute barium or water-soluble contrast material may delineate scarring and deformity of the duodenum or gastric wall and occasionally demonstrate the leakage that proves the diagnosis (Fig. 22.4A). The scan is thus useful for cases in which diagnosis of perforated viscus is in question, and the clinical presentation

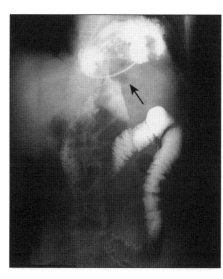

Fig. 22.3 • Barium study showing extraluminal air (arrow) in the lesser sac. (Courtesy of John Braver, M.D., Department of Radiology, Brigham and Women's Hospital.)

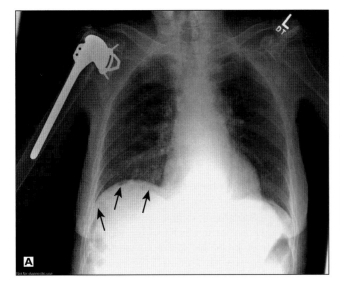

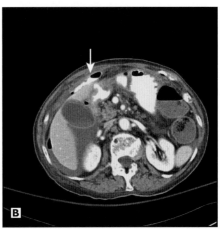

Fig. 22.4 • Imaging of perforated duodenal ulcer. (**A**) Plain film showing sliver of free air (arrows). (**B**) CT scan with oral contrast showing extravasation (arrow).

does not clearly indicate the need for operation.[67] Grassi reported the success of CT scan in identifying perforation due to peptic ulcer disease after negative or equivocal plain radiographs.[68]

Although some clinicians have utilized endoscopy for evaluation in the subacute setting, this cannot be recommended as a safe practice. Likewise, the use of upper GI contrast studies is not recommended as a *routine* means of establishing a diagnosis of perforation. The highest-quality studies utilize barium as the contrast agent of choice and spillage of this material into the peritoneum (if the test is positive) will itself cause a life-threatening peritonitis. As discussed below, however, there are circumstances in which nonoperative management might be contemplated, and in those situations, the upper GI series or CT may play an important role in decision-making.

Natural history of ulcer perforation: early complications and overall outcome

Early complications

Perforation of a peptic ulcer is an acute illness. Patients present in various stages of illness after perforation. Many reports support the conclusion that early presentation, resuscitation, diagnosis, and definitive therapy will reduce morbidity and mortality. At the same time, several studies have attempted to identify clinical factors correlating with severity of illness that could be used to predict outcomes in these very sick patients.[50,69–71] In all of these studies, the main risk factors that would predict worse outcomes are: (1) age above 70; (2) other major medical illness (renal insufficiency, liver failure, cardiac failure, pneumonia, or respiratory failure); (3) shock; and (4) delay in definitive therapy. In addition, it is well recognized that there is a significant difference between mortality of perforation of gastric (20–25%) versus duodenal (6–8%) ulcers.[72–74] Although distinctions have not been clearly drawn between the typical type I benign lesser curve ulcers and ulcers arising in the prepylorus/pyloric channel (type III), the mortality associated with each of these lesions seems worse than that associated with perforation of duodenal lesions.

Long-term outcomes

It is also well recognized that the long-term recurrence rates for perforated peptic ulcers depend on site of perforation and the chronicity of symptoms. The literature describing these differences is difficult to interpret, since it largely reflects studies of patients selected for nondefinitive operations in comparison to patients selected for definitive ulcer operations. Adding to the current confusion, most of these studies were conducted before the introduction of anti-*Helicobacter* therapy and, in many instances, before the introduction of powerful medical antisecretory therapies. Discussed below are some limited conclusions that can be drawn from these studies.

Duodenal ulcer

The recurrence of ulcer symptoms or complications approaches 40% at 3 years' follow-up of patients with perforation of an acute duodenal ulcer when that is defined by the absence of chronic ulcer symptoms or symptoms experienced for less than 3 months.[75–77] If the perforation is simply closed, without definitive ulcer operation or postoperative medical therapy, more than a third of the patients that recur will require reoperation for complications such as bleeding, reperforation, or stenosis.[78] Perforation of a chronic duodenal ulcer, defined by the presence of acid-peptic symptoms for more than 3 months or a prior diagnosis, is associated with a long-term recurrence rate of at least 60%.[76–78] Again, about one-third of these patients would require operation for a life-threatening or disabling complication, if definitive operation is not performed or aggressive postoperative medical management not provided.[76,77]

Gastric ulcer

It is useful to use Johnson's classification scheme[79] for gastric ulcers in evaluating their long-term outcomes. Gastric ulcers can thus be divided into three groups: those occurring in the typical lesser curve location near the junction of the antrum and corpus (type I), those occurring in association with duodenal ulceration (type II) and those occurring in the prepylorus/pyloric channel (type III). Type II ulceration is now quite uncommon and the discussion is restricted to perforations of types I and III.

Type III ulcers comprise the majority of cases of perforated gastric ulcer. These ulcers are, in many respects, similar to duodenal ulcers in pathogenesis and natural history.[61] Perforations of type I gastric ulcers are not as common. Although it is likely that the natural history, in terms of recurrence and complication rates, is not substantially different from gastric ulcers presenting with intractability or bleeding, there are no reliable data on this subject. One retrospective study from Charity Hospital[72] in New Orleans excluded channel ulcers from the analysis. In that report, the long-term rate of reoperation for patients with gastric ulcer perforation (mean interval of follow-up not given) was about 25% if excision/closure and no definitive ulcer operation had been performed at the first operation. With respect to type I gastric ulcer perforation, the clinical importance of acute versus chronic symptoms/complications has not been evaluated systematically.

Management: nonoperative interventional approaches

The diagnosis of a perforated peptic ulcer is usually a presumptive one, based on a suggestive history of the acute event, physical examination, and confirmation of a visceral perforation by the finding of free intraperitoneal air on plain radiographs or CT scan. When the patient's history of past illness is highly suggestive of peptic ulcer disease as a cause of the perforation and there is clear evidence of spreading peritonitis, rapid resuscitation and early operation is the standard of care.

There is, however, a subgroup of patients, that presents with signs and symptoms that suggest the perforation may have sealed and that peritonitis, if present, is localized and limited. As early as 1935, some authors suggested that selected cases might be managed safely without operation.[80,81] Comparing the outcomes of patients treated operatively with those treated nonoperatively, it was even suggested that the majority of patients presenting with perforation should be considered for nonoperative management if they met certain criteria.[81–83] The essential components of the protocol for nonoperative or 'expectant' management of such cases are: (1) a firm clinical diagnosis of perforation, with the clinician's assessment that the perforation is due to peptic ulcer; (2) adequate fluid resuscitation, nasogastric suction, and broad-spectrum intravenous antibiotics; (3) intravenous antisecretory therapy with H-receptor blockers; and (4) serial examinations. A contrast study is also performed, using water-soluble contrast, or even thin barium, to evaluate the presence of leak. In some protocols, leak has been an absolute indication for surgery. In other protocols, it has been a strong but not absolute indication for surgery.[84] In all protocols, improvement in clinical parameters (pulse, temperature, abdominal tenderness, and peritoneal findings) are the key indicators that justify continuation of expectant management.

Berne and Donovan[82] reported 35 patients with duodenal or prepyloric ulcer who were managed according to such a protocol. They represented 12% of all patients with perforated peptic ulcer treated at USC/LA County Hospital during the same period. The ulcer was believed to be acute in three-quarters and chronic in one-quarter of patients. Only one patient required intervention for a complication of intra-abdominal abscess. The mortality rate in this subgroup was 3% compared to the overall mortality of 6.2% in the entire group. Similarly, Cocks et al.[83] reported on 115 patients with perforation managed by a similar protocol. Of these, 15 needed immediate surgery, 12 were judged to require surgery within 6 hours of admission to the protocol, and 8 required surgery during the hospitalization. In all, 71 patients tolerated the protocol of expectant management. The authors concluded that about 75% of cases would seal or improve clinically if given the chance. Mortality was 4% in the group selected for expectant management.

The overall mortality for patients managed by the 'deliberative' policy was 13%, as compared to 18% for a similar group of patients in which operation was the standard of management.

The most compelling report, however, was written by Crofts, Li, and associates from the Prince of Wales Hospital in Hong Kong.[84] They randomized 84 patients to immediate surgery (n=43) versus a policy of expectant management (n=40). Clinical characteristics were similar in both groups. About 27% of patients in the nonsurgical group failed to improve clinically and were taken to surgery. There were two deaths in each group. Hospital stay was prolonged in the nonsurgical group from a mean of 8–12 days and this was statistically significant. One further point of the analysis was that 6 of 9 patients over the age of 70, 5/23 patients between ages 40 and 70, and 0/8 under age 40 failed to respond to expectant management. The authors concluded that the only contraindications to expectant management were doubt about the diagnosis and age over 70.

Three major concerns have been raised about the significance of this report. First, in this study, there was little doubt about the diagnosis of perforated peptic ulcer. In Western countries, where diverticulitis and other diagnoses are just as likely as peptic to be the cause of perforated viscus, there is a higher likelihood of making an incorrect diagnosis. Thus, it is critical to use some sort of contrast study to reliably document a perforated ulcer as the cause of the illness. None of the reports mentioned above precisely described the way in which contrast studies were utilized to verify the diagnosis and exclude other pathology. Second, it is the group over 70 years of age that has the major morbidity following surgery. It is this group in whom expectant management would be most desired. The study by Crofts at al. indicated that younger patients would do well regardless and in fact leave the hospital sooner if they underwent surgery sooner. Third, the studies of nonoperative management reported so far have included mainly patients with perforations of ulcers located in the duodenum or prepyloric channel/pylorus. Based on older studies, it could be argued that perforations of gastric ulcers not only have a higher incidence of associated malignancy, but also do not respond favorably to expectant management.[72] Therefore, one should be cautious in considering expectant management for patients with known type I gastric ulcer.

Taking all of these considerations into account, it can be concluded that patients refusing surgery might have a reasonable expectation of recovery if they meet low-risk criteria, including: (1) age less than 70; (2) location of a sealed ulcer in the duodenum that is confirmed by contrast study; and (3) absence of shock, systemic sepsis, immunocompromise, or poor nutritional status.

A more recent study from Stockton-on-Tees looked at 49 patients who were selected for expectant management.[85] Eight patients (16%) failed and required operation. Complications included abscess formation, pneumonia, and four deaths. Two patients were subsequently found to have cancer on follow-up endoscopy. Adherence to basic study guidelines was noted to be poor and was thought to be the explanation for poor outcomes. This study serves as a warning that application of findings from prospective trials requires that study protocols be used and compliance monitored in order to achieve outcomes reported in those trials.

Treatment: conventional operative approaches

Traditionally, the goals of operation for perforated peptic ulcer have been to: (1) close the perforation; (2) lavage away the contamination;[86] and (3) perform a 'definitive' antiulcer operation that would prevent recurrence of ulcer symptoms and complications. The choice of operation is individualized and based on the following considerations: (1) location of ulcer causing the perforation; (2) presence of shock; (3) associated comorbidities; and (4) estimated time since perforation and extent of peritoneal contamination. It cannot be overemphasized that optimal care of most patients with perforated peptic ulcer requires aggressive fluid resuscitation (with hemodynamic monitoring if necessary), early administration of antibiotics, and expeditious movement to the operating room. It is often helpful to delay, for a short period, to ensure that the resuscitation has corrected hemodynamic instability. In high-risk patients, the operating room itself may be the optimal environment in which to perform that resuscitation. A brief discussion of the operative options follows for perforations occurring in different locations.

Duodenal ulcer

Chronic duodenal ulcers arise in association with increased parietal cell mass and hypersecretion of acid. They are defined as ulcers that have been causing symptoms for 3 months or longer. In contrast, perforated acute ulcers are defined as ulcers that have not been associated with symptoms for more than 3 months prior to presentation. Although the role of *H. pylori* remains incompletely understood, it is reasonable to suppose that *H. pylori* contributes to the lack of healing that leads to perforation of a chronic ulcer. On the other hand, there is no clear evidence of a role of *H. pylori* in pathogenesis of acute perforations; these are often associated with NSAID use.[50,53,54,87]

Based on a number of well-designed, prospective randomized trials, it seems clear that the optimal approach for perforation of a *chronic* duodenal ulcer *in a low-risk setting* would include closure of the perforation and vigorous lavage of the abdomen with warm saline. Definitive ulcer surgery is no longer needed, as ulcer recurrence rates have dropped dramatically due to *H. pylori* eradication and acid-suppressing drugs.[88–90]

There is a rationale for a similar approach to the operative management of *acute* duodenal ulceration and a case can be made for simple closure even in the low-risk setting. As noted above, the recurrence rate for acute duodenal ulcers is no more than 40% and the need for further operation is perhaps only 15%. These outcomes can certainly be improved by oral antisecretory therapy and use of antibiotics if *H. pylori* is present in antral biopsies.[87,88] Pending further information on the role of medical therapy in this setting, it seems reasonable to recommend closure only or, at most, closure plus HSV for simple perforation. Table 22.3 summarizes the outcomes after surgery for simple closure. The highly variable morbidity and mortality speak to the diverse settings in which these patients present, and tend to argue for surgical approaches that avoid unnecessary or complicated approaches to the ulcer diathesis and that, instead, focus solely on the complication requiring surgery, that is, the perforation.

One circumstance that requires a more aggressive surgical approach is when the perforation is accompanied by significant bleeding. This situation usually reflects an anteriorly located perforated ulcer and a posteriorly located bleeding ulcer ('kissing ulcers'). Under these circumstances, it is prudent to perform a definitive antisecretory operation, either HSV or TV and pyloroplasty. The experience of HSV in the setting of acute bleeding is itself difficult to interpret. The authors personally advocate treatment of bleeding duodenal ulcers, in the emergency setting, with TV and pyloroplasty if the patient has a high risk for morbidity and mortality. With minimal spillage and a chronic ulcer history, it would not be unreasonable to perform a truncal vagotomy and antrectomy.

Prepyloric channel/pylorus ulcer

The pathophysiology and factors that impair ulcer healing are similar to those associated with duodenal ulcer. Thus, it is tempting to approach a patient with a perforated PPU as one would approach a patient with a perforated DU. However, in patients undergoing surgery for intractability, it has been noted that pyloric area ulcers have a recurrence rate of 30% when treated by HSV, which is twice the recurrence rate reported for HSV-treated duodenal ulcers.[91] Thus, a number of authors have cautioned against the use of HSV for type III ulcers.

In a preliminary report with some long-term follow-up, however, Jordan and Thornby utilized closure plus HSV in 12 patients with pyloric or juxtapyloric perforations and noted one recurrence during

Table 22.3 Outcomes after simple closure of perforated peptic ulcer

Authors	Site of perf.	No. pts.	Op morb	Op mort
Boey * (1982)	DU	35	0%	0%
Boey # (1987)	DU	183		8%
Feliciano # (1984)	DU,GU	49	31%	27%
Irvin # (1989)	DU,GU	78		41%
Svanes # (1989)	DU,GU	717		8%
Hamby # (1993)	DU,GU		47%	23%
Schein # (1990)	DU	20		30%
	GU	14		57%
Hodnett # (1989)	GU	128		29%
Lau* (1995)	DU	100	12–25%	3%
Lau* (1996)	DU	93	25%	3%

* Indicates placebo group of randomized trial.
\# Indicates treatment arm in retrospective review.

a mean 9-year period of observation.[92] These findings suggested that HSV might be utilized for management of perforations of juxtapyloric perforation with reasonable long-term outcomes. Even if recurrence rates after HSV were not as low as in other settings, HSV could still be performed in this setting, with the expectation that recurrences could be managed with antisecretory and anti-*Helicobacter* therapies. HSV would be especially attractive if there were no chronic history of symptoms, evidence of significant scarring of the pylorus or duodenal bulb, or documented history of other life-threatening or disabling complications (bleeding, obstructive symptoms). With such a history, it would be difficult to recommend HSV as the definitive ulcer procedure. Under these circumstances, truncal vagotomy/drainage or vagotomy and antrectomy should be recommended.

Type I gastric ulcer

Chronic gastric ulcers are thought to arise within a zone of decreased resistance to luminal acid that is located in a 3–4 cm region to either side of the junction of the antrum and corpus.[93] Included in this category are so-called type IV gastric ulcers,[94] which lie high on the lesser curve and probably represent a type I gastric ulcer in a surgically difficult location. The association of *H. pylori* with type I or type III gastric ulcers is not persuasive and these patients secrete levels of acid that are low or normal.

The goals of therapy are: (1) to exclude the presence of malignancy; and (2) to excise the ulcer and its surrounding area, thereby removing the 'locus of decreased resistance.'[88] The difficulties presented by a perforated type I gastric ulcer may be summarized as follows: (1), the patient population tends to be elderly and infirm, with a high likelihood of comorbid illness; (2) partly for anatomic reasons and partly due to delays in presentation, intraperitoneal spillage is often not localized and peritonitis may be more generalized than in the average patient with a duodenal ulcer perforation; and (3) the ulcer and surrounding devitalized area on the lesser curve may be large and not amenable to tension-free primary closure. The major concern for the surgeon is that the magnitude of resection, along with extra time under general anesthesia, might lead to higher levels of morbidity and mortality in this elderly and infirm population.

Over the years, a number of authorities have pointed out that despite the widespread practice of simple closure for perforated gastric ulcers, the data do not justify the fear of increased morbidity and mortality after resection.[72,91,95] In reviewing their 202 cases from the Charity Hospital in New Orleans, Hodnett et al.[72] found that selected patients undergoing resection without vagotomy had a perioperative mortality of 11%, whereas those undergoing closure had a mortality of 23%. Although simple closure was chosen more often for patients who presented in shock or with extensive peritonitis, the few treated by resection did well. In reviewing their 91 patients at Vanderbilt, McGee and Sawyers[95] reported that 51 had undergone excision/closure, with an operative mortality of 29%. Primary gastric resection was performed in 27 patients, with an operative mortality of 15%. In patients with acute perforation, outcomes among patients undergoing closure (n=31, mortality 32%) versus those undergoing resection (n=12, mortality 25%) were not clearly different. There were no obvious differences between the two groups in terms of steroid use, diabetes, preoperative hypotension, or congestive heart failure. The reasons for choosing one operation over another were not systematically addressed in either of these studies.

In contrast, Turner et al.[96] reported outcomes in 107 patients with perforated type I and III gastric ulcers, where the practice was to perform excision/closure (n=96), unless the ulcer crater was so large that resection was unavoidable (n=11). Mortality in the latter group was 45%, while mortality in the former was ≈19%. The outcomes in Turner's series do not necessarily contradict the results of the other reports, since gastric resection was performed in patients with extensive ulceration. It might be predicted that these patients would be sicker than those with smaller perforations and do not reflect outcomes that would be observed if patients with smaller perforations had undergone resection. However, the mortality rate of less than 20% in the overall group compares favorably with the above-mentioned reports.

In summarizing the controversy, it seems fair to point out that the morbidity and mortality of gastrectomy, if routinely performed in this setting, is not known and there seems to be no harm in a routine policy of excision/closure. Thus, simple excision/closure is recommended if the patient is hemodynamically unstable or peritoneal contamination is extensive. Although distal gastrectomy is a reasonable choice for some patients with perforated type I gastric ulcer,[72] more often the practical choice is between ulcer excision with omental reinforcement of the closure versus excision/closure plus a form of vagotomy. In this regard, there is some persuasive evidence that HSV plus wedge excision of the ulcer and its immediately surrounding area is as effective at reducing ulcer recurrence as distal gastric resection without vagotomy, at least in some settings.[97–100] If the patient is deemed stable enough to undergo some form of definitive ulcer operation, excision plus HSV is recommended as the procedure that offers the least physiologic disturbance while providing significant, if not perfect, protection against ulcer recurrence. While truncal vagotomy and drainage (pyloroplasty or gastrojejunostomy) also offer protection against ulcer recurrence, the recurrence rate is not better than that offered by HSV, and the long-term physiologic disturbance is not better than that offered by gastrectomy. Thus, truncal vagotomy with drainage would not be recommended for treatment of perforation of a type I gastric ulcer except in unusual circumstances.

Laparoscopically assisted approaches

The impetus for laparoscopically assisted approaches for peptic ulcer perforation is based on the recognition that patch closure[101] and most forms of vagotomy can be performed with assistance of the laparoscope. These procedures are especially appropriate for ulcers located in the duodenal bulb, where an anteriorly located perforation is easily accessed for sutureless patch closure. In addition, it could be argued that both acute and chronic duodenal ulcers may be safely managed by closure alone, followed by intensive medical therapy that treats hypersecretion of acid and eradicates *H. pylori*.

One of the earliest series on laparoscopic repair of perforated ulcers was published by Druart in 1997.[102] In a study of 100 patients, the laparoscopic approach to perforated peptic ulcer was found to be a feasible alternative. Morbidity, mortality, and length of stay were found to be comparable to published data regarding open repairs. Another early report on laparoscopic ulcer repair stressed the importance of recognizing individuals who presented with signs of shock.[103] Those patients with shock on admission or symptoms for more than 24 hours had a higher conversion rate, but otherwise acceptable morbidity and mortality, compared to historical controls. One of the largest series performed reported a group of 130 patients who were randomized to laparoscopic versus open repairs.[104] In the 63 patients randomized to the laparoscopic approach, nine required conversion to the open procedure. The laparoscopic group had a faster operative time and was noted to have a lower pain score at postoperative days 1 and 3 compared to the open group. In addition, the length of stay was shorter in the laparoscopic group with a faster return to normal activities. Of note, patients in the laparoscopic group were noted to have a higher incidence of reoperation.

The largest experience so far reported, by the group at Prince of Wales Hospital in Hong Kong, suggests that perforations over 1 cm in size cannot be closed safely using current laparoscopic technique.[101] However, the optimal therapy for even small perforations due to duodenal and juxtapyloric ulcers can only be addressed by randomized prospective trials, comparing laparoscopically assisted closure and medical management *versus* closure and some form of selective vagotomy. Such a trial is feasible and awaited. Type I gastric ulcers are somewhat more difficult to manage by closure alone, since excision is needed for definitive management and in order to exclude the presence of malignancy. Laparoscopically assisted wedge excisions of the gastric ulcer with omental flap reinforcement is certainly feasible.[105] Clinical trials will be needed to evaluate laparoscopically assisted excision (with or without selective vagotomy) as an approach for type I gastric ulcer perforation.

FISTULA TO ADJACENT STRUCTURES

The inflammatory response to a deeply penetrating peptic ulcer can lead to the formation of a fistula between the stomach or duodenum and any structure that happens to be in proximity. Rarely, a duodenal ulcer can penetrate to adjoining vascular structures such as the aorta or vena cava. Perforation into pericardium, pleural space, or lung parenchyma and bronchial structures have also been reported as complications of peptic ulcers lying in portions of the stomach that have migrated into the chest as the result of hiatal hernias. Generally, all such complications have an acute presentation and are managed as surgical emergencies.[106–110] The goal of treatment is to separate the source of the ulcer (stomach or duodenum) from the target organ. The ulcer is managed much as a perforated ulcer in the same location would be managed, depending on site of the ulcer, prior history, and medical condition of the patient.

More commonly, fistulae to the pancreatic duct, biliary tract, small intestine, and colon have been described. A fistula arising between the stomach and duodenum, called 'double pylorus' is also a well-recognized complication of peptic ulcer disease. Such fistulae usually present with less acute symptoms, and in some cases represent complex management problems. In each case where a fistula is identified, carcinoma must be considered in the differential diagnosis. Malignancy should be excluded by careful endoscopic evaluation and by appropriate imaging studies.

Double pylorus

When ulcer disease penetrates from the antrum or pyloric channel to distorted and rolled-over first or second portion of the duodenum, a double pylorus results.[111–115] Although such cases are occasionally accompanied by other complications of ulcer disease, such as bleeding or obstruction, they are usually asso-

ciated with recognizable ulcer symptoms. The double channel is not recognized until a contrast study or endoscopy is performed. One study demonstrated that most (75%) fistulous rings were located on the lesser curve of the gastric antrum.[115] In general, the natural history of this complication does not appear to be more or less aggressive than other chronic ulcers.[111] As a result, this lesion tends to heal with correct medical management and is not itself an indication for surgical management. In one report,[114] infestation with *H. pylori* was associated with failure to heal. It seems prudent to evaluate all such cases for *H. pylori*. Other cases have been associated with heavy NSAID ingestion, which should be discontinued, if practical.[111–113]

Fistula to the small intestine

In general, the small intestine is not found in proximity to the stomach or duodenum, protected as it is by the transverse colon and mesocolon. However, fistula to the small intestine has been reported,[116] presenting with standard ulcer symptoms. If the target region of the fistula is very proximal, there is no short-circuiting of gastric contents. If the target site is distal, there may be symptoms and nutritional disturbances similar to those observed with gastrocolic fistula. Management for proximal fistula is similar to that for double pylorus. Indications for surgery are not the fistula per se, but other complications such as free perforation, obstruction, refractory bleeding, or failure to heal with maximum medical therapy and continued symptoms.

Choledochoduodenal fistula

Because of the proximity of the gallbladder and bile duct to the duodenum, fistulae involving these structures can form as a result of peptic ulcer disease (see Fig. 22.4B).[117–121] There are no special symptoms associated with these fistulae. Jaundice and cholangitis are rare, although minor elevations of alkaline phosphatase occur and air in the biliary tract may be observed in plain abdominal x-rays. These fistula are usually detected by upper GI series or CT scan. They are not easily seen by an endoscopist unless there is a high index of suspicion. Although this has not been demonstrated conclusively, there seems to be a relatively aggressive ulcer diathesis associated with these cases. Associated bleeding or pyloric outlet obstruction is not uncommon. Avoidance of NSAIDs, treatment for *H. pylori* (when present) and standard antisecretory medications should lead to healing in most cases. Most authors recommend avoidance of operation except as treatment for such associated complications. If surgery becomes necessary for management of another complication, the scarring that accompanies fistula formation in this region is usually quite formidable. Visualization and protection of the distal common duct is often difficult. For this reason, and because of intense scarring of the duodenal bulb, a vagotomy and antrectomy is generally to be avoided when definitive ulcer operation is required. Depending on the indications for surgery, HSV or TV and gastrojejunostomy are probably safest.

Pancreatic fistula

Fistula to the pancreatic duct most commonly occurs in relation to a benign ulcer located on the posterior gastric wall near the lesser curvature[122–124] and the target is the pancreatic duct in the body of the pancreas. When duodenal ulceration is the source, the bile duct is also usually involved and the pancreatic duct is involved in the head of the pancreas.[124] Such fistulae are usually detected not because of acute pancreatitis, but as incidental findings on CT or upper GI series. Management is similar to that for choledochoduodenal fistula and surgery is rarely indicated for treatment of such a fistula.

Duodenal- or gastrocolic fistula

In duodenal-colic fistula, the target site is the hepatic flexure or proximal transverse colon, whereas in gastrocolic fistula (Fig. 22.5), the target site is more toward the middle or distal portion of the transverse colon. A strong association has been recognized between gastrocolic fistula due to peptic ulcer disease and heavy NSAID use.[125–129] Many of these patients are elderly and require analgesics for treatment of rheumatoid arthritis; others are quite young and could be categorized as NSAID abusers.[125,127]

The major problems presented by fistula from a peptic ulcer to the colon are: (1) dumping of HCl and gastric contents into a defenseless colon; and (2) the short-circuiting of nutrients around the small intestine. Chief presenting symptoms and signs are fecal vomiting, halitosis, weight loss, and anemia. Overt gastrointestinal bleeding is not common, but not rare either.[125] The presentation can be subacute, including fever, dehydration, and alkalosis from vomiting and hypochloremia.[125,128] The differential diagnosis of gastrocolic fistula includes peptic ulcer disease, carcinoma of the stomach or colon, diverticulitis, and Crohn's disease. Diagnosis is usually made by barium given orally or by barium enema. Esophagogastroduodenoscopy (EGD) is indicated in order to evaluate for malignancy. Colonoscopy and/or barium enema are indicated to look for malignancy and to exclude diverticulitis and Crohn's disease.

Treatment almost always requires hospitalization. Initially, the patient is not allowed food by mouth. Fluid and electrolyte imbalances are corrected with intravenous fluids. Antisecretory medications (H_2-receptor blockers) are given intravenously and parenteral nutrition may be indicated. A number of reports have indicated that such patients can be managed medically and that such fistulae can close without surgery once malignancy has been ruled out as the etiology.

Surgery is indicated for patients who do not have endoscopically verified healing of the fistula. It is not necessary to perform surgery until the patient is medically fit and nutritional deficiencies have been addressed. The operative approach usually requires an en-bloc resection of the distal stomach and the transverse colon where the fistula connects them. It is usually feasible to perform a Billroth I gastroduodenostomy in this setting. In some cases where malignancy has been excluded reliably, a less aggressive resection may be reasonable. A vagotomy is not usually necessary, as the source of the fistula is usually a type I gastric ulcer.

SUMMARY

Complications of peptic ulcer disease which necessitate surgical intervention include obstruction, perforation, and fistulization to adjacent structures. It is important that the clinician have a full understanding of the patient's clinical picture before formulating a plan of medical therapy as well as indication for surgical intervention. The current consensus regarding gastric outlet obstruction is that surgery is not always the first line of treatment. Dilation, excision, and bypass of the obstructed segment of pylorus or duodenum represent the main treatment options. Perforation requires immediate recognition and medical support of the patient. Although most are handled with operative intervention, there is a subgroup of patients whom nonoperative or expectant management is appropriate. Finally, the inflammatory response to a deeply penetrating peptic ulcer can lead to the formation of a fistula between the stomach or duodenum and any structure that happens to be in proximity. The goal of the treatment is to separate the source of the ulcer from the target organ. The ulcer is then managed as a perforated ulcer in the same location would be managed, depending on site of the ulcer, prior history, and medical condition of the patient.

REFERENCES

1. Kozoll DD, Meyer KA. Obstructing gastroduodenal ulcers: general factors influence incidence and mortality. Arch Surg 1964; 88:793–799.

2. Jaffin BW, Kaye MD. The prognosis of gastric outlet obstruction. Ann Surg 1985; 201:176–179.

3. Makela JT, Kiviniemi H, Laitinen S. Gastric outlet obstruction caused by peptic ulcer disease: analysis of 99 patients. Hepatogastroenterology 1996; 43:547–552.

4. Paimela H, et al. Peptic ulcer surgery during the H_2-receptor era. Br J Surg 1991; 78:28–31.

5. Weaver GA, et al. Nonsteroidal antiinflammatory drugs are associated with gastric outlet obstruction. J Clin Gastroenterol 1995; 20:196–198.

6. Tursi A, et al. *Helicobacter* eradication helps resolve pyloric and duodenal stenosis. J Clin Gastroenterol 1996; 23:157–158.

7. Gisbert JP, Pajares JM. *Helicobacter pylori* infection and gastric outlet obstruction – prevalence of the infection and role of antimicrobial treatment. Aliment Pharmacol Ther 2002; 16:1203–1208.

8. DeBoer WA, Driessen WM. Resolution of gastric outlet obstruction after eradication of *Helicobacter pylori*. J Clin Gastroenterol 1995; 21:329–330.

9. Dworkin HJ, Roth HP. Pyloric obstruction associated with peptic ulcer: a clinicopathological analysis of 158 surgically treated cases. JAMA 1962; 180:1007–1010.

10. Kreel L, Ellis H. Pyloric stenosis in adults: a clinical and radiological study of 100 consecutive patients. Gut 1965; 6:253–261.

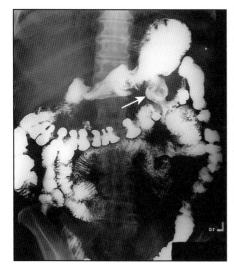

Fig. 22.5 • Imaging of gastrocolic fistula, indicated by arrow. This is the most common location, as the greater curvature of the stomach is most closely associated with the distal transverse colon. (Courtesy of John Braver, M.D., Department of Radiology, Brigham and Women's Hospital.)

11. Weiland D, et al. Gastric outlet obstruction in peptic ulcer disease: an indication for surgery. Am J Surg 1981; 143:90–93.

Eighty-seven patients with duodenal peptic ulcer disease and gastric outlet obstruction were reviewed retrospectively after initial treatment with standard medical regimens. Late follow-up on the entire cohort revealed that 98% of patients with chronic ulcer disease and 64% of patients with acute disease ultimately required an operation.

12. Lau JYW, et al. Through the scope balloon dilation for pyloric stenosis: long-term results. Gastrointest Endosc 1996; 43:98–101.

A retrospective analysis reviewing 54 patients who underwent through-the-scope balloon dilations for pyloric stenosis. While through-the-scope balloon dilation palliated symptoms of obstruction, recurrent obstruction and other ulcer complications were common.

13. Shone DN, et al. Malignancy is the most common cause of gastric outlet obstruction in the era of H$_2$ blockers. Am J Gastroenterol 1995; 90:1769–1770.

14. Khullar SK, DiSario JA. Gastric outlet obstruction. Gastrointest Endosc Clin N Am 1996; 6:585–603.

15. Johnson CD, Ellis H. Gastric outlet obstruction now predicts malignancy. Br J Surg 1990; 77:1023–1024.

16. Meinke WB, et al. Gastric outlet obstruction after palliative surgery for cancer of the head of the pancreas. Arch Surg 1983; 118:550–553.

17. Haubrich W. Complications of peptic ulcer disease. In: Bockus HL, ed. Bockus gastroenterology. 3rd edn. Philadelphia: WB Saunders; 1976:726–762.

18. Adkins RB, et al. The management of gastric ulcers. Ann Surg 1985; 201:741–751.

19. Herrington JL, Sawyers JL, Scott HW. A 25 year experience with vagotomy-antrectomy. Arch Surg 1973; 106:469–474.

20. Scott HW, et al. Definitive surgical treatment in duodenal ulcer disease. Curr Prob Surg 1968; 10:1–56.

21. Bowden TA, Hooks VH, Rogers DA. Role of highly selective vagotomy and duodenoplasty in the treatment of postbulbar duodenal obstruction. Am J Surg 1990; 159:15–19.

22. Brown C. Duodenal ulcer complicated by obstruction. Am J Dig Dis 1959; 4:940–949.

23. Goldstein H, et al. Gastric retention associated with gastroduodenal disease. Am J Dig Dis 1966; 11:887–897.

24. Smithuis RH, Op den Orth JO. Gastric fluid detected by sonography in fasting patients: relation to duodenal ulcer disease and gastric outlet obstruction. AJR Am J Roentgenol 1989; 153:731–733.

25. Goldstein H, Boyle JD. The saline load test: a bedside evaluation of gastric retention. Gastroenterology 1965; 49:375–380.

26. Csendes A, et al. Prospective randomized study comparing three surgical techniques for the treatment of gastric outlet obstruction secondary to duodenal ulcer. Am J Surg 1993; 166:45–49.

A prospective randomized clinical trial was performed in order to evaluate the results of three surgical techniques for the treatment of gastric outlet obstruction secondary to duodenal ulcer. After laparotomy, patients underwent either highly selective vagotomy (HSV) + gastrojejunostomy, HSV + Jaboulay gastroduodenostomy, or selective vagotomy (SV) + antrectomy. There was a significantly better result after HSV + gastrojejunostomy than after Jaboulay anastomosis but not after SV + antrectomy. Study proposed HSV + gastrojejunostomy as the treatment of choice in patients with duodenal ulcer and gastric outlet obstruction.

27. Dobois A, Price SF, Castell DO. Gastric retention in peptic ulcer disease. Am J Dig Dis 1978; 23:993–997.

28. Pelot D. et al. Comparative assessment of gastric emptying by the 'barium-burger' and saline load tests. Am J Gastroenterol 1972; 58:411–416.

29. Hangen D, et al. Marked hypergastrinemia in gastric outlet obstruction. J Clin Gastroenterol 1989; 11:442–444.

30. Omura N, Kashiwagi H, Aoki T. Changes in gastric hormones associated with gastric outlet obstruction. An experimental study in rats. Scand J Gastroenterol 1993; 28:568–572.

31. Perng, C-L, et al. Characteristics of patients with benign gastric outlet obstruction requiring surgery after endoscopic balloon dilation. Am J Gastroenterol 1996; 91:987–990.

32. Johnston D, et al. Highly selective vagotomy without a drainage procedure in the treatment of hemorrhage, perforation, and pyloric stenosis due to peptic ulcer. Br J Surg 1973; 60:790–797.

33. McMahon MJ. et al. Highly selective vagotomy plus dilatation of the stenosis compared with truncal vagotomy and drainage in the treatment of pyloric stenosis secondary to duodenal ulceration. Gut 1976; 17:471–476.

34. DiSario JA, et al. Endoscopic balloon dilation for the ulcer-induced gastric outlet obstruction. Am J Gastroenterol 1994; 89:868–871.

35. Griffin SM, et al. Peptic pyloric stenosis treated by endoscopic balloon dilation. Br J Surg 1989; 76:1147–1148.

36. Misra SP, Dwivedi M. Long-term follow-up of patients undergoing balloon dilation for benign pyloric stenoses. Endoscopy 1996; 28:552–554.

37. Kochhar R, et al. Endoscopic balloon dilatation of benign gastric outlet obstruction. J Gastroenterol Hepatol 2004; 19:418–422.

38. Kozarek RA. Hydrostatic balloon dilation of gastrointestinal stenoses: a national survey. Gastrointest Endosc 1986; 32:15–19.

39. Kozarek RA, Botoman VA, Patterson DJ. Long-term follow-up in patients who have undergone balloon dilation for gastric outlet obstruction. Gastrointest Endosc 1990; 36:558–561.

40. Kozarek RA. Endotherapy for gastric outlet obstruction. Gastrointest Endosc 1996. 43:173–174.

41. Kozarek RA. Dilation therapy for gastric outlet obstruction: are balloons a bust? J Clin Gastroenterol 1997; 17:2–4.

42. Kuwada SK, Alexander GL. Long-term outcome of endoscopic dilation of non-malignant pyloric stenosis. Gastrointest Endosc 1995; 41:15–17.

43. McLean GK, et al. Radiologically guided balloon dilation of gastrointestinal strictures. Radiology 1987; 165:41–43.

44. Soybel DI, Zinner MJ. Stomach and duodenum: operative procedures. In: Zinner MJ, ed. Maingot's abdominal operations. Stamford, CT: Appleton and Lange; 1997:1079–1130.

45. Soybel DI, Zinner MJ. Complications following gastric operations. In: Zinner MJ, ed. Maingot's abdominal operations. Stamford, CT: Appleton and Lange; 1997.

46. Chang TM, et al. Long-term results of duodenectomy with highly selective vagotomy in the treatment of complicated duodenal ulcers. Am J Surg 2001; 181:372–376.

A retrospective analysis was conducted of 120 patients with complicated duodenal ulcer who underwent surgical treatment. Highly selective vagotomy provided less complications than truncal vagotomy and antrectomy for patients with obstruction duodenal ulcer.

47. Kurata JH, Corboy ED. Current peptic ulcer time trends: an epidemiologic profile. J Clin Gastroenterol 1988; 10:259–268.

48. Bardhan KD, et al. Changing pattern of admissions and operations for duodenal ulcer. Br J Surg 1989; 76:230–236.

49. Walt R, et al. Rising frequency of ulcer perforation in elderly people in the United Kingdom. Lancet 1986; I:489–492.

50. Svanes C, et al. A multifactorial analysis of factors related to lethality after treatment of perforated gastroduodenal ulcer. Ann Surg 1989; 209:418–423.

51. Agrez MV, et al. Changing trends in perforated peptic ulcer during the past 45 years. Aust NZ J Surg 1992; 62:729–732.

52. Svanes C, Ovrebo K, Soreide O. Ulcer bleeding and perforation: nonsteroidal anti-inflammatory drugs or *Helicobacter pylori?* Scand J Gastroenterol 1996; Suppl 220:128–131.

53. Ng EKW, et al. High prevalence of *Helicobacter pylori* infection in duodenal ulcer perforations not caused by non-steroidal anti-inflammatory drugs. Br J Surg 1996; 83:1779–1781.

54. Strom BL, et al. Parenteral ketorolac and the risk of gastrointestinal complications and operative site bleeding. JAMA 1996; 275:376–382.

55. Barron PT, Watters JM, Wesley-James T. Perforated ulcers in critical illness. Crit Care Med 1987; 15:584–586.

56. Matthews JB, Tortella BJ, Silen W. Gastroduodenal hemorrhage and perforation in the post-operative period. Surg Gynecol Obstet 1988; 167:389–392.

57. Czaja AJ, McAlhany JC, Pruitt BA. Acute duodenitis and duodenal ulceration after burns. Clinical and pathological characteristics. JAMA 1975; 232:621–624.

58. Chan KH, et al. Factors influencing the development of gastrointestinal complications after neurosurgery. Neurosurgery 1989; 25:378–382.

59. Bar-On Z, Ohry A. The acute abdomen in spinal cord injury individuals. Paraplegia 1995; 33:704–706.

60. Arrillaga A, Sosa JL, Najjar R. Laparoscopic patching of crack-cocaine induced perforated ulcers. Am Surgeon 1996; 62:1007–1009.

61. Horowitz J, Kukora JS, Ritchie WP. All perforated ulcers are not alike. Ann Surg 1989; 209:693–697.

62. Feliciano DV, et al. Emergency management of perforated peptic ulcers in the elderly patient. Am J Surg 1984; 148:764–767.

63. Rogers F. Elevated serum amylase: a review and analysis of findings in 1000 cases of perforated peptic ulcer. Ann Surg 1961; 153:228–240.

64. Kane E, Fried G, McSherry CK. Perforated peptic ulcer in the elderly. J Am Geriatr Soc 1981; 29:222–227.

65. Roh JJ, et al. Value of pneumoperitoneum in the diagnosis of visceral perforation. Am J Surg 1983; 146:830–833.

66. Lee CW, Yip AW, Lam KH. Pneumogastrogram in the diagnosis of perforated peptic ulcer. Aust NZ J Surg 1993; 63:459–461.

67. Jacobs JM, Hill MC, Steinberg WM. Peptic ulcer disease: CT evaluation. Radiology 1991; 178:745–748.

68. Grassi R, et al. Gastro-duodenal perforations: conventional plain film, US and CT findings in 166 consecutive patients. Eur J Radiol 2004; 50:30–36.

    The aim of the study was to report experience in the diagnosis of gastro-duodenal perforation by conventional radiography, US and CT examinations. Grassi reported the success of CT scan in identifying perforation due to peptic ulcer disease after negative or equivocal plain radiograph.

69. Svanes C, et al. Adverse effects of delayed treatment for perforated peptic ulcer. Ann Surg 1994; 220:168–175.

70. Irvin TT. Mortality and perforated peptic ulcer: a case for risk stratification in elderly patients. Br J Surg 1989; 76:215–218.

71. Boey J, et al. Risk stratification in perforated duodenal ulcers. A prospective validation of predictive factors. Ann Surg 1987; 205:22–26.

72. Hodnett RM, et al. The need for definitive therapy in the management of perforated gastric ulcers: review of 202 cases. Ann Surg 1989; 209:36–39.

73. DeBakey ME. Acute perforated gastroduodenal ulceration: statistical analysis and review of the literature. I. Surg 1940; 8:852–883.

74. DeBakey ME. Acute perforated gastroduodenal ulceration: statistical analysis and review of the literature. II. Surge 1940; 8:1028–1057.

75. Boey J, Lee NW, Wong J. Perforations in acute ulcers of the duodenum. Surg Gynecol Obstetr 1982; 155:193–196.

76. Boey J, et al. Immediate definitive surgery for perforated duodenal ulcers: a prospective controlled trial. Ann Surg 1982; 196:338–344.

77. Bornman PC, et al. Simple closure of perforated duodenal ulcer: a prospective evaluation of a conservative management policy. Br J Surg 1990; 77:73–75.

78. Boey J, et al. Proximal gastric vagotomy: the preferred operation for perforations in acute duodenal ulcer. Ann Surg 1988; 208:169–173.

79. Johnson HD. Gastric ulcer: classification, blood group characteristics, secretion pattern, and pathogenesis. Ann Surg 1965; 162:996–1004.

80. Wangensteen OH. Non-operative treatment of localized perforation of the duodenum. Minnesota Med 1935; 18:477–480.

81. Taylor H, The non-surgical treatment of perforated ulcer. Gastroenterology 1957; 33:353–368.

82. Berne TV, Donovan AJ. Nonoperative treatment of perforated duodenal ulcer. Arch Surg 1989; 124:830–832.

83. Cocks JR, et al. Perforated peptic ulcer: a deliberative approach. Aust NZ J Surgery 1989; 59:379–385.

84. Crofts TJ, et al. A randomized trial of non-operative treatment for perforated peptic ulcer. N Engl J Med 1989; 320:970–973.

85. Marshall C, et al. Evaluation of a protocol for the non-operative management of perforated peptic ulcer. Br J Surg 1999; 86:131–134.

86. Sugimoto K, et al. Mechanically assisted intraoperative peritoneal lavage for generalized peritonitis as a result of perforation of the upper part of the gastrointestinal tract. J Am Coll Surgeons 1994; 179:443–448.

87. Reinbach DH, Cruickshank G, McColl KE. Acute perforated duodenal ulcer is not associated with *Helicobacter pylori* infection. Gut 1993; 34:1344–1347.

88. Hulst RWM, et al. Prevention of ulcer recurrence after eradication of *Helicobacter pylori*: a prospective long-term follow-up study. Gastroenterology 1997; 113:S1082–S1086.

    The aim of this study was to determine the long-term outcome of ulcer disease after successful *H. pylori* eradication. Excluding patients taking aspirin or NSAIDs, recurrence of duodenal or gastric ulcers is completely prevented after successful *H. pylori* eradication for up to 9.8 years.

89. Blomgren LGM. Perforated peptic ulcer: long-term results of simple closure in the elderly. World J Surg 1997; 21:412–415.

90. Zittel TT, Jehle EC, Becker HD. Surgical management of peptic ulcer disease today – indication, technique and outcomes. Langenbeck's Arch Surg 2000; 385:84–96.

91. Jordan PH, Morrow C. Perforated peptic ulcer. Surg Clin North Am 1988; 68:315–329.

92. Jordan PH, Thornby J. Perforated pyloroduodenal ulcers. Long-term results with omental patch closure and parietal cell vagotomy. Ann Surg 1995; 221:479–488.

93. Oi M, Oshida K, Sugimura S. The location of gastric ulcer. Gastroenterology 1959; 36:45–56.

94. Csendes A, Braghetto I, Smok G. Type IV gastric ulcer. Surgery 1987; 101:361–366.

95. McGee GS, Sawyers JL. Perforated gastric ulcers: a plea for management by primary resection. Arch Surg 1987; 122:555–561.

96. Turner WW, Thompson WM, Thal ER. Perforated gastric ulcers: a pleas for management by simple closures. Arch Surg 1988; 123:960–964.

97. Emas S, Grupcev G, Eriksson B. Ten-year follow-up of a prospective randomized trial of selective proximal vagotomy with ulcer excision and partial gastrectomy with gastroduodenostomy in the treating corporeal gastric ulcer. Am J Surg 1994; 167:596–600.

98. Reid DA, et al. Late follow-up of highly selective vagotomy with excision of the ulcer compared with Billroth I gastrectomy for treatment of benign gastric ulcer. Br J Surg 1982; 69:605–607.

99. Jordan PH. Type I gastric ulcer treated by parietal cell vagotomy and mucosal ulcerectomy. J Am Coll Surgeons 1996; 182:388–393.

100. Johnson AG. Proximal gastric vagotomy: does it have a place in the future management of peptic ulcer? World J Surg 2000; 24:259–263.

101. Lau W-Y, et al. A randomized study comparing laparoscopic versus open repair of perforated peptic ulcer using suture or suture less technique. Ann Surg 1996; 224:131–138.

102. Druart ML, et al. Laparoscopic repair of perforated duodenal ulcer. A prospective multicenter clinical trial. Surg Endosc 1997; 11:1017–1020.

   Background: A series of 100 consecutive patients with perforated peptic ulcer were prospectively evaluated. Laparoscopic repair was evaluated and found to be technically feasable and carried an acceptable morbidity and mortality rate, compared with conventional surgery.

103. Katkhouda N, et al. Laparoscopic repair of perforated duodenal ulcers: outcome and efficacy in 30 consecutive patients. Arch Surg 1999; 134:845–848.

104. Siu WT, et al. Laparoscopic repair for perforated peptic ulcer: a randomized controlled trial. Ann Surg 2002; 235:320–321.

105. Trus TL, Hunter JG. Minimally invasive surgery of the esophagus and stomach. Am J Surg 1997; 173:242–255.

106. West AB, Nolan N, O'Brian DS. Benign peptic ulcers penetrating pericardium and heart. Gastroenterology 1988; 94:1478–1487.

107. Odze RD, Begin LR. Peptic ulcer-induced aortoenteric fistula. Report of a case and review of the literature. J Clin Gastroenterol 1991; 13:682–686.

108. Soares MA, et al. Fistula between duodenum and portal vein caused by peptic ulcer disease and complicated by hemorrhage and portal vein thrombosis. Am J Gastroenterol 1996; 91:1462–1463.

109. Godwin TA, Mercer G, Holodny AI. Fatal embolization of intestinal contents through a duodenocaval fistula. Arch Pathol Lab Med 1991; 115:93–95.

110. Eisdorfer R, Miskovitz P. Duodenal-caval fistula. Dig Dis Sci 1991; 36:379–380.

111. Einhorn RI, Grace ND, Banks PA. The clinical significance and natural history of the double pylorus. Dig Dis Sci 1984; 29:213–218.

112. Hurwitz J, Friedman L. Pyloroduodenal fistula – a benign complication of peptic ulcer disease. S Af Med J 1987; 72:56–58.

113. Polloni A, et al. Double pylorus. Italian J Gastroenterol 1991; 23:361–363.

114. Hu TH, et al. Double pylorus: report of longitudinal follow-up in two refractory cases with underlying diseases. Am J Gastroenterol 1995; 90:815–818.

115. Hu TH, et al. Clinical characteristics of double pylorus. Gastrointest Endosc 2001; 54:464–470.

   Study demonstrated that most (75%) fistulous rings were located on the lesser curve of the gastric antrum.

116. Phifer TJ, Gladney JD, McDonald JC. Gastrojejunal fistula: a complication of peptic ulcer disease. South Med J, 1986; 79:1015–1017.

117. Feller ER, Warshaw AL, Schapiro RH. Observations on management of choledochoduodenal fistula due to penetrating peptic ulcer. Gastroenterology 1980; 78:126–131.

118. Fowler CL, Sternquist JC. Choledochoduodenal fistula: a rare complication of peptic ulcer disease. Am j Gastroenterol 1987; 82:269–271.

119. Kochhar R, et al. Massive gastrointestinal bleeding due to cholecystoduodenal fistula. Acta Chirurgia Scandinavia 1988; 154:471–472.

120. Iso Y, et al. Choledochoduodenal fistula: a complication of penetrated duodenal ulcer. Hepatogastroenterology 1996; 43:489–491.

121. H'ng MW, Yim HB. Spontaneous choledochoduodenal fistula secondary to long-standing ulcer disease. Singapore Med J 2003; 44:205–207.

122. Hughes JJ, Blunck CE. CT demonstration of gastropancreatic fistula due to penetrating gastric ulcer. J Comput Assist Tomogr 1987; 11:709–711.

123. Meiselman MS, Agha FP. Fistula to the pancreatic duct from a peptic ulcer. J Clin Gastroenterol 1988; 10:537–540.

124. Aitken RJ, Bornman PC, Dent DM. Choledochopancreatoduodenal fistula caused by duodenal ulceration. S Af Med J 1986; 69:707–708.

125. Soybel DI, et al. Gastrocolic fistula as a complication of benign gastric ulcer: report of four cases and update of the literature. Br J Surg 1989; 76:1298–1300.

   A review of the literature regarding gastrocolic fistulas. A strong association was noted due to peptic ulcer disease and heavy NSAID use.

126. Benn M, Nielsen FT, Antonsen HK. Benign duodenocolic fistula. A case presenting with acidosis. Dig Dis Sci 1997; 42:345–347.

127. Levine MS, et al. Gastrocolic fistulas: the increasing role of aspirin. Radiology, 1993; 187:359–361.

128. Tavenor T, Smith S, Sullivan S. Gastrocolic fistula. A review of 15 cases and an update of the literature. J Clin Gastroenterol 1993; 16:189–191.

129. Marschall J, Bigsby R, Nechala P. Gastrocolic fistulae as a consequence of benign gastric ulcer disease. Can J Gastroenterol 2003; 17:441–443.

CHAPTER TWENTY-THREE

23

Treatment of gastric volvulus and diaphragmatic hernias

Jonathan F. Critchlow

INTRODUCTION

'Hiatal hernia' is a common term, but with distinctly different meanings to the various groups of people who use it. To the lay population, it is a description of upper abdominal symptoms such as reflux and dyspepsia. To most practitioners, it represents a sliding hernia, which may or may not be associated with reflux. The sophisticated gastroenterologist or surgeon, however, may recognize the rarer but more serious defects in the diaphragm such as paraesophageal, traumatic, and congenital hernias. Unlike a sliding hernia, the latter may come to attention under urgent circumstances as a result of potentially lethal mechanical complications and could result in death if not diagnosed and treated rapidly.

CLASSIFICATION

The three basic types of hiatal hernia are type I or sliding; type II or paraesophageal; and type III or combined. Hernias containing structures other than the stomach are classified as type IV but are generally considered as subtypes of type II or III. Sliding hernias (type I) are common. They account for more than 90% of all hiatal hernias.[1] Here, a portion of the stomach slides upwards so that the esophagogastric junction lies above the diaphragm (Fig. 23.1A). As a result, the stomach is not contained within a true sac of the peritoneum, but instead a portion of the stomach forms the wall of the sac. A sliding (type I) hernia is often associated with gastroesophageal reflux, which will be discussed elsewhere.

The true paraesophageal hernia (type II) has been said to account for 3–5% of all hiatal hernias.[2] Here, the esophagogastric junction is fixed below the diaphragm in its normal position and the fundus of the stomach 'rolls' upward and into the chest into a true hernia sac (Fig. 23.1B). This true sac allows greater freedom of the stomach and other structures and can thereby lead to potential mechanical complications such as obstruction, incarceration, and volvulus.

A type III, or mixed, hernia is now thought to be more common than the true type II hernia[3] and may be the result of enlargement of the hernia orifice in a type I hernia or stretching the phrenoesophageal ligament over time in a type II hernia (Fig. 23.1C). Patients with combined hernia may experience reflux symptoms, and surgical repair may be more challenging because the esophagus may be shortened and a portion of the sac is adherent to the stomach. Hernias with a very large orifice may have other abdominal viscera or organs in the intrathoracic sac (type IV). These hernias may appear clinically as small bowel or large bowel obstruction.

PARAESOPHAGEAL HERNIA

Clinical manifestations

Paraesophageal hernias are often asymptomatic or may cause minimal symptoms for prolonged periods, which permits them to increase substantially in size.[4] Patients often, however, describe a number of 'non-specific symptoms' that actually do relate to the hernia, such as postprandial discomfort, nausea, dyspnea, palpitations, or chest pain.[2,4] Heartburn is not expected in patients with pure type II hernias, but it is not uncommon in association with the combined type III hernia.

The clinical manifestations of a hernia include anemia, bleeding from ulceration of the herniated stomach, obstruction, and volvulus or gangrene of the stomach or other abdominal viscera that may lie in the sac. Recognition of the actual etiology of some of the symptoms is often difficult because they may mimic ulcer disease, myocardial infarction, or pneumonia.[5] The history of a 'hiatal hernia' is often dismissed because it is assumed that the hernia is a simple sliding one (type I) and not associated with serious acute complications.

Volvulus, obstruction, and strangulation are the most serious complications. The stomach ascends into the hernia sac and then may develop a 180-degree twist of the greater curvature while the duodenum and esophagogastric junction are fixed below the diaphragm.[6] Patients with incarceration or volvulus often have a history of acute or subacute dysphagia and high gastric obstruction. The classical findings described by Borchardt[7] consist of the triad of epigastric pain, retching with inability to vomit, and difficulty in passing a nasogastric tube into the stomach.

DIAGNOSIS

In the patient with appropriate symptoms, a chest radiograph often demonstrates a diagnostic air–fluid level behind the heart.[8] Upper gastrointestinal series are confirmatory and are also helpful in determining the location of the esophagogastric junction, as well as whether gross reflux is present. Rarely, colonic or small bowel gas is seen above the diaphragm and indicates a type

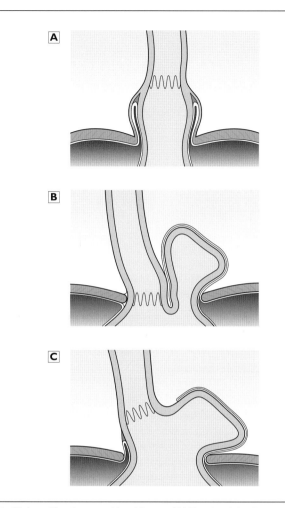

Fig. 23.1 • Classification of hiatal hernia. **(A)** Type I – sliding hernia. **(B)** Type II – paraesophageal hernia; note that the esophagogastric junction is in the normal location. **(C)** Type III – mixed hernia; note the stomach in the thorax and upward migration of the esophagogastric junction. (Reprinted from Trus TL et al, Journal Gastrointestinal Surgery 1997; 1:221–228. © 1997, with permission from the Society for the Surgery of the Alimentary Tract.)

IV hernia, which may also be confirmed by barium enema. The most important step in evaluation of the patient with acute but continued retching is to consider the diagnosis of incarceration or volvulus.

TREATMENT

Acute incarceration

Nonoperative Treatment: In patients with acute symptoms, gentle attempts should be made to decompress the stomach with a nasogastric tube. Successful decompression is signaled by the great release of gas and fluid from the stomach and immediate improvement in symptoms. This maneuver allows time for preoperative resuscitation and preparation of the patient and may avert the need for an emergency operation. Hill[9] reported successful decompression in six of ten patients with acute incarceration, with all surviving surgery. Two of the four patients in whom reduction was not possible died, and the survivors suffered significant morbidity from strangulation and perfora-

tion. Although endoscopy may have a role in the management of volvulus not associated with a hernia (discussed later), its role in the treatment of an acutely incarcerated paraesophageal hernia is limited by the risk of perforation.

Surgical Treatment: In cases of acute incarceration, operative repair may be done via laparotomy or thoracotomy. Either approach should include reduction of the hernia, de-rotation of the volvulus, and resection of gangrenous tissue, if necessary. If the stomach cannot be decompressed preoperatively, some of the diaphragmatic fibers will require division to release the neck of the peritoneal sac for reduction of the hernia. Excision of the hernial sac with primary closure of the hiatus over a large bougie and fixation of the lesser curve of the stomach to the pre-aortic fascia may be all that is required in a pure type II hernia.[2] The author finds a thoracic incision helpful in cases of acute incarceration because the hernia defect and sac are directly visualized and dissection of the sac from the mediastinum can be accomplished easily. Resection of necrotic portions of stomach is also not difficult through the thorax. Many surgeons, however, prefer an abdominal approach because of the more familiar anatomy. Less postoperative respiratory embarrassment and less incisional discomfort are probably associated with the abdominal incision. The hernia sac may be bluntly dissected via the abdomen and excised, and the diaphragmatic defect then repaired. Laparotomy is favored in patients with other abdominal pathology and in those in whom a gastrostomy tube is desired.

Laparoscopic repair of incarcerated paraesophageal hernias has been reported.[10,11] This technique holds even more promise in the chronic or elective situation (see the next section), or may be used in acute cases in which the stomach can be decompressed adequately preoperatively to allow for reduction of the stomach into the abdominal cavity and a primary repair.

ELECTIVE REPAIR

Because of the potentially life-threatening complications that may develop rapidly in patients with paraesophageal hernia, it is generally recommended that all patients with paraesophageal hernia undergo elective surgical repair regardless of the severity of symptoms.[2,5,9,12] This conclusion is based on surgical series that show high rates of incarceration or strangulation up to 30% with resultant significant mortality in patients treated on an emergency basis.[5] It is likely, however, that some of these series are biased by inclusion of a very small percentage of minimally symptomatic patients. The only prospective report is that of Skinner and Belsey[13] who described 21 patients with 'minimal symptoms' over a period of 5 years. Six of these patients died of complications of strangulation, perforation or hemorrhage, after which the remaining 15 patients were treated surgically without an operative mortality. With operative mortality rates of approximately 1%[2,14] it is recommended that all patients with paraesophageal hernias undergo elective surgery if deemed to be acceptable surgical risks. It is also important to note that many of these patients are not truly asymptomatic because symptoms of early satiety, mild discomfort or fullness, or shortness of breath may be discounted or attributed to other disease processes.

Elective surgical repair may be performed via the abdominal or thoracic route. Patients with type III hernia and very shortened esophagus are best approached through the chest because the esophagus may be more adequately mobilized to allow reduction of the stomach below the diaphragm.[15,16] Lengthening procedures (Collis gastroplasty) may also be performed more simply transthoracically. Alternatively, a gastroplasty can be accomplished via the abdomen with the use of circular and linear staplers. Laparoscopic gastroplasty has been successful in very experienced hands[17,18] but is much more difficult. Repair via laparotomy is generally more acceptable to patients with uncomplicated defects because of less postoperative discomfort.

Laparoscopy is becoming accepted as the standard technique in patients without shortened esophagus. The shorter hospital stay and less incisional pain seems to have increased the number of patients referred for repair. Reports of primary repairs with[18-21] and without[10] fundoplication, and repairs with mesh patches[11,22,23] have been described. Only recently are data accumulating to allow some conclusions regarding the proper place for laparoscopic technique. Early attempts at simple patch closure without dissection of the sac have been fraught with recurrence and obstruction. It is generally agreed that the peritoneum over the diaphragmatic defect should be incised where it is most visible so that the sac can be reduced into the abdomen.[24-27] Excessive vigorous attempts at reduction of the stomach itself often result only in laceration and damage to the viscera.[28] It is simpler to reduce the sac than to attempt to reduce the adherent organ itself. Most hernias in recent series seem to be type III hernias (>60%),[3,13,25] with a significant portion of the sac directly attached to the stomach, an anatomical arrangement occasionally causing confusion. After reduction of the sac, it should be removed,[29] allowing a portion of the anterior part of the sac to remain on the stomach to avoid damage to the anterior vagal fibers. After reduction and sac excision, the diaphragmatic defect should be closed posteriorly with permanent sutures over a 50F to 60F bougie (Fig. 23.2). Although anterior repair may seem easier, the posterior repair is more secure and allows for a longer intra-abdominal segment of the esophagus. Closure is almost always achievable by direct repair with sutures. Larger defects may be closed with serial sutures tied extracorporeally and slid down. A

fundoplication (Nissen and Toupet) usually completes the procedure, except in patients with significant motility disorders of the esophagus. The extensive hiatal dissection seems to warrant this additional procedure. Recent reviews of complications after laparoscopic paraesophageal hernia repairs have demonstrated mortality rates of 1–3%, major complication rate of 5–20%, and a recurrence rate of 5–40%. The rate of symptomatic recurrence is substantially lower.[15] Recurrences are more commonly seen in patients with type III hernias and shortened esophagus (>5 cm). Reoperation rates are 3–6%.[30]

Swanstrom found that of the 32 patients in his series 60% had symptomatic reflux. Fundoplication was performed in all patients. Postoperative pH probes were abnormal in 13%, with a number not having symptoms. This procedure requires longer operative times than the open procedure or a more standard antireflux procedure in patients with type I hernias.[26] Complication rates are generally similar to open series of elderly, frail patients. It is recommended that this procedure be attempted only by the experienced laparoendoscopic surgeon.[24,25,28]

Although controversial,[23,31] the use of mesh should generally be avoided for several reasons whatever the chosen operative approach. First, mesh is very rarely required for closure of even large defects. In most series, only 1–2% of patients required mesh.[17,28] Second, it is tempting when using a mesh patch to simply patch the defect and omit complete dissection of the crura and reduction of the sac. This lesser repair, although initially successful, has a tendency towards a higher recurrence rate[5,29] and the development of obstruction.[28,32] Third, a mesh technique results in direct apposition of mesh with esophagus, thus raising the specter of erosion of the prosthesis as seen in other procedures.[33,34] In cases with a great deal of tension on the closure, mesh reinforcement may rarely be required.[17,35] An attractive alternative is the creation of a relaxing incision on the right diaphragm with direct closure of the crura and patch placement over the relaxing incision, which is well away from the esophagus (Fig. 23.3).[36]

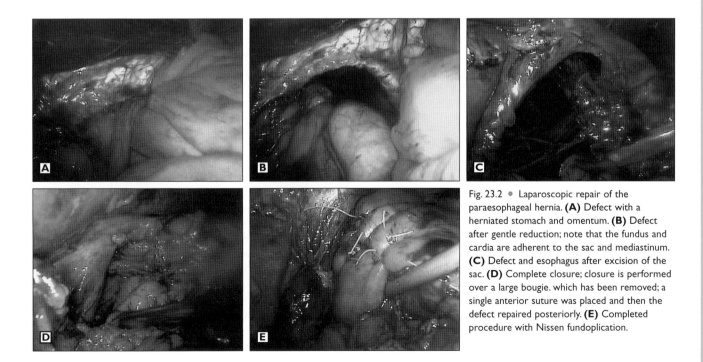

Fig. 23.2 • Laparoscopic repair of the paraesophageal hernia. (A) Defect with a herniated stomach and omentum. (B) Defect after gentle reduction; note that the fundus and cardia are adherent to the sac and mediastinum. (C) Defect and esophagus after excision of the sac. (D) Complete closure; closure is performed over a large bougie. which has been removed; a single anterior suture was placed and then the defect repaired posteriorly. (E) Completed procedure with Nissen fundoplication.

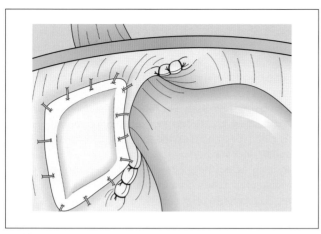

Fig. 23.3 • Use of a relaxing incisio, primary repair, and patch closure of the incision. (Reprinted from Huntington TR, Journal American College of Surgeons 1997; 184:389–400. © 1997, with permission from The American College of Surgeons.)

Although primary repair of the diaphragmatic defect is the gold standard, procedures aimed at preventing volvulus by fixation of the stomach alone may be applicable in selected cases. Rudolph Nissen first described suture fixation of the stomach to the abdominal wall in patients with large hernias not amenable to repair.[37] Because the recurrence rate is high with these procedures (20–40%),[2] placement of a gastrostomy tube or a full-thickness gastropexy done via laparotomy or laparoscopy is thought to provide more secure placement.[2,22,38] Percutaneous endoscopic gastrostomy placement with one or more tubes have been reported with success,[39,40] but this procedure should probably be reserved for a very frail patient unable to withstand formal repair.

ROLE OF ANTIREFLUX OPERATIONS

Antireflux surgery concomitant with repair of esophageal hernias have aroused considerable controversy. The goal of adding an antireflux operation would be to treat reflux in those in whom it was previously present, to prevent reflux in patients in whom it may develop because of extensive dissection of the hiatus, to possibly act as an 'anchor' of the stomach below the diaphragm, and possibly to decrease the redundancy of the stomach in situations in which it is large and floppy and may predispose to an intra-abdominal (mesenteroaxial) volvulus.[21] A reasonable approach would be to study patients, when possible, preoperatively with manometry and pH probe to identify those with pre-existing reflux, though these data are often incomplete due to difficulties in catheter placement.[18] In cases of pure type II hernia without reflux where minimal dissection of the hiatus is performed, such as via thoracotomy, one could omit an antireflux operation.[2] However, when using the abdominal and especially the laparoscopic approach, where extensive dissection of the mediastinum is accomplished with freeing of the esophagus from all of its attachments, one must be very concerned about the development of reflux. To this end, most surgeons, especially those who are performing this procedure laparoscopically, add antireflux procedures, which have been accomplished with minimal morbidity.[24,25]

In the true type II hernia, where the esophagogastric junction is in the normal position and where less dissection of the hiatus may have occurred, it would seem unnecessary to perform antireflux surgery. In a series of 55 patients with paraesophageal hernia studied preoperatively by esophageal manometry, the mean lower esophageal sphincter pressure was 18 mmHg (normal). Closure of the defect with crural repair alone was done in all patients and only one patient experienced reflux symptoms.[2] It was therefore advocated that simple repair is sufficient, which may be especially true in a transthoracic repair. Pearson and colleagues[41] disagree with this approach and noted displacement of the esophagogastric junction in almost all paraesophageal hernias in their series of 53 patients, all of whom where treated with antireflux procedures. Symptomatic gastroesophageal reflux developed in nine of their patients postoperatively. Antireflux surgery is also advocated by Swanstrom, who found 60% of his series to have had symptomatic reflux preoperatively. All received fundoplication. Postoperative pH probe was abnormal in 13%; most were asymptomatic. Dysphagia rate was 6%.[18] In a recent series, 20–40% of patients were found to develop gastroesophageal reflux after paraesophageal hernia repair without fundoplication.[42]

GASTRIC VOLVULUS

Gastric volvulus is an acquired rotation of the stomach of greater than 180 degrees, usually resulting in obstruction. The majority of cases of volvulus have a secondary cause,[43,44] which is most often a paraesophageal hernia.[45] However, volvulus may be associated with other congenital[46] or acquired abnormalities such as traumatic hernia,[47,48] phrenic nerve palsy, or eventration of left diaphragm,[49,50] or be a complication after abdominal operations in which the ligaments of the stomach have been divided,[51–55] or failed antireflux surgery.[56]

The stomach, firmly attached only at the cardia, is suspended by a number of other ligamentous attachments to the diaphragm, spleen, liver, and duodenum. Some relaxation of these attachments, as seen in paraesophageal or diaphragmatic hernias, eventration of the diaphragm, or absence of these ligaments following surgery are prerequisites for volvulus.

The anatomic classification of gastric volvulus may be somewhat confusing. Organoaxial volvulus occurs when the stomach twists around its anatomic axis, which is a line drawn from the cardia to the pylorus. Because the cardia and pylorus are fixed, a closed loop is created as the body and antrum ascend. This type of volvulus is most common and is frequently seen in association with paraesophageal hernias as the 'upside down stomach (Fig. 23.4).'[6,44] A mensenteroaxial volvulus occurs around a line drawn throughout the stomach perpendicular, that is, through the middle of the greater curvature to the lesser curvature of the stomach. Diaphragmatic abnormalities are not usually present with this type of volvulus, and it is more commonly seen in cases following gastric surgery or with severe aerophagia. In these instances, no specific cause can be identified.[57] The esophagogastric junction is usually not obstructed and a nasogastric tube or endoscope may often be passed.

From a practical standpoint, it is often more useful when planning treatment to determine whether the volvulus is associated with a diaphragmatic defect or is due solely to ligamentous laxity.

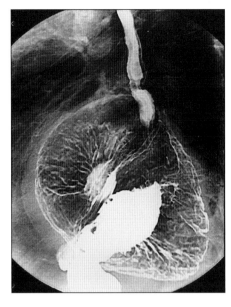

Fig. 23.4 • Paraesophageal hernia with an 'upside-down' stomach.

Clinical manifestations

Acute gastric volvulus associated with a paraesophageal hernia is most common in adults but rare in children. Borschardt's triad (acute onset of severe epigastric pain, retching with inability to vomit, and difficulty passing a nasogastric tube into the stomach) is usually present and may be associated with hematemesis. The patient may be hemodynamically stable or in frank shock, and gastric perforation or rupture may be seen. Acute gastric volvulus may produce a syndrome similar to angina pectoris and chest pain,[58] may radiate into the neck, shoulder or back,[59,60] and be associated with dyspnea. Abdominal findings are usually minimal[45] except in cases of intra-abdominal volvulus occurring post-surgically or idiopathically where the involved segment is not protected from the examiner by the thoracic cage. Chronic volvulus may cause intermittent symptoms of bloating, pain, or discomfort.

Diagnosis

Diagnosis is most readily made when the appropriate clinical picture is recognized in a patient with some predisposing factor such as paraesophageal hernia, recent gastric surgery, or aerophagia. The radiologic signs have been described previously in those patients with incarcerated paraesophageal hernia. In patients with mesenteroaxial volvulus, an erect film of the abdomen may show two air–fluid levels in the left upper quadrant, a 'double bubble sign' that is suggestive of a mesenteroaxial twist. When questionable, barium examination may be necessary to confirm that diagnosis.[12]

Therapy

The therapy of choice in cases of an anatomic defect is repair of that defect.[58] As mentioned earlier, nasogastric decompression may be helpful.

The surgical technique for paraesophageal hernia repair has been discussed. Other diaphragmatic hernias with volvulus should be repaired either via the abdomen or thorax or by laparo-

scopy. Other operative or invasive maneuvers may be necessary in cases of idiopathic volvulus, where the problem is simply that of a massively distended stomach or lax ligamentous attachments. Anterior gastropexy alone has been described but seems to have a significant recurrence rate of 20–40% if anchoring the stomach to the abdominal wall is performed with sutures.[2] Anchoring may be better accomplished with a gastrostomy tube[42] or with full-thickness sutures placed laparoscopically.[2] In cases of diaphragmatic eventration, plication of the diaphragm or colonic transposition has been attempted.[50] Patients with aerophagia and a massively dilated, lax stomach may occasionally require partial gastric resection.

Endoscopic reduction of acute gastric volvulus has been reported.[39,40] Because the esophagogastric junction is not usually obstructed in mesenteroaxial volvulus, endoscopy may play a role in the preoperative care of these patients. Bhasin and colleagues reported endoscopic treatment in seven of ten patients with chronic volvulus.[55] No recurrence was seen after a relatively short follow-up. Although endoscopic correction can be performed successfully and safely in the setting of chronic volvulus, the same is probably not true for acute volvulus. Perforation is a distinct possibility, especially if the esophagogastric junction is closed or if ischemia is present. Endoscopic stabilization of the stomach with percutaneous endoscopic gastrostomy has also been reported,[39,40,61,62] but it should be reserved for selected cases of mesenteroaxial volvulus in which anatomic abnormalities requiring correction are not present, or for the selected patient with a reduced organoaxial volvulus who is not fit for surgery. Ghosh and Palmer[40] reported placement of two percutaneous gastrostomy tubes in the antrum and proximal body of the stomach of a poor-risk patient with chronic volvulus. Laparoscopic detorsion and subsequent placement of three percutaneous gastrostomy tubes has also been reported.[44] It should be noted that several tubes should be placed in situations in which gastric distention and ligamentous laxity are present. Placement of a single gastrostomy tube may lead only to a fixed point around which the remaining floppy stomach can twist and result in recurrent volvulus as illustrated in Figure 23.5.

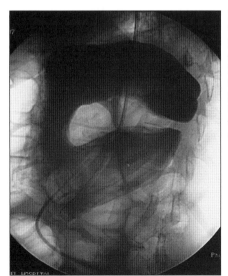

Fig. 23.5 • Recurrent volvulus after placement of a single gastrostomy tube in a patient with aerophagia. Another gastropathy tube and feeding jejunostomy tube were placed after detorsion.

Prognosis

The overall mortality rate of a gastric volvulus involving gastric necrosis approaches 50%.[45] Postoperative morbidity and mortality are high after emergency operation, especially in the presence of strangulation. However, mortality rates following elective surgery should be no more than 1–2%.[1,2,13]

CONGENITAL DIAPHRAGMATIC HERNIA

Foramen of Bochdalek's hernia

Congenital hernias result from abnormalities in formation of the diaphragm during development. The most common abnormality is failure of fusion during the first trimester of gestation that causes a posterior lateral defect without a hernia sac known as Bochdalek's hernia. Because the left side of the diaphragm develops more slowly than the right, these hernias are most often on the left (90%).[35] With this relatively large defect, negative intrathoracic pressure causes herniation of a large portion of the intra-abdominal viscera, along with collapse and hypoplasia of the left lung. Associated disorders of gastrointestinal rotation and other abnormalities may occur.[63] The diagnosis of a congenital diaphragmatic hernia is often made clinically in the neonate with respiratory distress, cyanosis, and a scaphoid abdomen. Plain radiographs of the chest are confirmatory and show gas-filled viscera in the thorax. A small group of patients with this hernia may be seen up to 20 months later with failure to thrive, respiratory symptoms, or volvulus. The treatment of Bochdalek's hernia in infants is surgical repair. Preoperative decompression with a nasogastric tube is helpful in decreasing some symptoms and preventing further respiratory embarrassment. An approach through the abdomen is preferred for the more common left-sided hernia because the surgeon may easily repair the hernia and address other associated intra-abdominal abnormalities.[64] Great care must be taken to avoid overinflation of the hypoplastic lung. Operative mortality is high (40–50%) in the neonate, presenting within 24 hours of birth, and usually is due to respiratory failure secondary to pulmonary insufficiency and persistence of the fetal circulation. Mortality rates have marginally improved over the past decade with careful ventila-tory support, fluid restriction, and the use of vasodilators.[65,66] More recent experience with selective use of extracorporeal membrane oxygenation has resulted in a survival rate of 70%.[67,68] Attempts at repair in utero have been disappointing. Older infants who present with this abnormality have a significantly better prognosis.

Foramen of Morgagni hernia

A retrosternal, or Morgagni, hernia is thought to represent a defect in ventral diaphragmatic fusion. It is assumed to be congenital,[63] although it is only occasionally seen in childhood and is much more common in adults older than 40 years. These hernias are ventrally located and are most often right sided (90%), although occasionally they are bilateral. Most Morgagni hernias contain colon in a well-defined sac, although omentum, stomach, or small bowel may be present. Although these hernias may cause symptoms of colonic obstruction or small bowel obstruction or strangulation, most are minimally symptomatic or are detected incidentally on chest radiography as a loop of transverse colon in the chest. In a number of series, only 15% of adult patients presented acutely, and 30% were totally asymptomatic.[63] The anterior position of the herniated intestine and general lack of gastric involvement distinguish the Morgagni hernia from a type IV paraesophageal hernia on plain film. Because of the concern for obstruction or strangulation, elective repair via the abdomen is recommended because one can deal easily with defects in either or both hemidiaphragms by this approach.

Laparoscopy also affords an excellent view of this area, especially with an angled scope, and primary repairs[69] and mesh placement have been reported.[11,70] As the esophagus is well away from this area, mesh repair would seem to be safer than in paraesophageal hernias, but may not be necessary.

TRAUMATIC DIAPHRAGMATIC HERNIA

Etiology and diagnosis

Diaphragmatic defects following penetrating or blunt injury may be recognized soon afterwards or their complications may present at a later date. Ambrose Pare's description of two cases in the sixteenth century include one patient who died soon after a blunt injury of an acute gastric volvulus. The other developed strangulation of the colon 8 months after a penetrating wound.

Injuries to the diaphragm after blunt trauma occur most often on the left side (66–90%),[48,71] possibly because of weakness of the posterolateral aspect of the left hemidiaphragm or, more likely, because of the protective effect of the liver on the right. With left-sided rupture, the stomach, spleen, or colon may herniate through a large defect. The diagnosis may not be readily apparent, and clinical findings are minimal. Chest radiographs often show only subtle findings such as obscuration of the left diaphragm, or the findings may be misinterpreted as hemothorax, contusion, gastric dilatation, or loculated hemopneumothorax. The true diagnosis may become more obvious on films taken after chest tube placement with visualization of a persistent soft tissue density or a herniated air-filled stomach. A radiograph demonstrating the nasogastric tube in the left side of the chest is a diagnostic but, unfortunately, not an invariable finding. Contrast studies may be required. Because the diagnosis of diaphragmatic rupture is made preoperatively by plain film in only 30–50% of emergency surgery cases,[72,73] thorough exploration to include inspection of the diaphragm must be performed to avoid missing this injury. Unfortunately, computed tomography and peritoneal lavage are also relatively insensitive in the detection of this problem.[74–76]

Penetrating diaphragmatic lacerations are frequently initially asymptomatic, unless associated injuries are present or the hole is unusually large. Only after the defect enlarges over time will symptoms of incarceration or strangulation develop.[47,74] Thoracoscopy has been used successfully to diagnose diaphragmatic injuries[77–79] when the results of other tests have been equivocal. Although thoracoscopy requires a double-lumen tube, it may be especially useful in situations in which a penetrating injury is suspected to be confined to the chest and diaphragm or when pneumothorax or hemothorax is present. Concern over associated intra-abdominal injuries limits its use in blunt injury.[78]

Laparoscopy is quite sensitive in diagnosing diaphragmatic injuries in both blunt and penetrating trauma.[80–82] Invatury and associates identified seven of seven patients with diaphragmatic tears after penetrating trauma with laparoscopy.[81] Its major use may well be to exclude diaphragmatic or peritoneal penetration after stab wounds. The possibility of tension pneumothorax from insufflation through the defect should be considered, and rapid placement of tube thoracostomy may be necessary.

Treatment

Treatment of acute diaphragmatic rupture consists most often of laparotomy and primary repair because the very high incidence of associated injuries, especially to the liver (25%) or spleen (50%),[72,73] are best managed via the abdomen. Primary repair is all that is required because no sac is present and adhesion of the viscera to the mediastinum is not a concern. Thoracoscopic[83] and laparoscopic[84–86] repair has been reported and may be useful in selected cases of penetrating trauma. It is not difficult to suture the diaphragm from either approach, but the major fear is that of missing injuries in the abdomen because of inadequate visualization from the thorax[82] or because of incomplete exploration with the laparoscope.

If the diagnosis is delayed, the thoracic route is often favored because it provides more direct exposure of the defect and any mediastinal adhesions that may be present. Primary repair with nonabsorbable sutures is almost always possible. Because 'missed injuries' are not a concern, directed laparoscopic or thoracoscopic repair with extracorporeally tied sutures may be possible if adhesions are not too severe.[86]

SUMMARY

Recommendations for the management of incarcerated and nonincarcerated hernias are summarized in Figure 23.6.

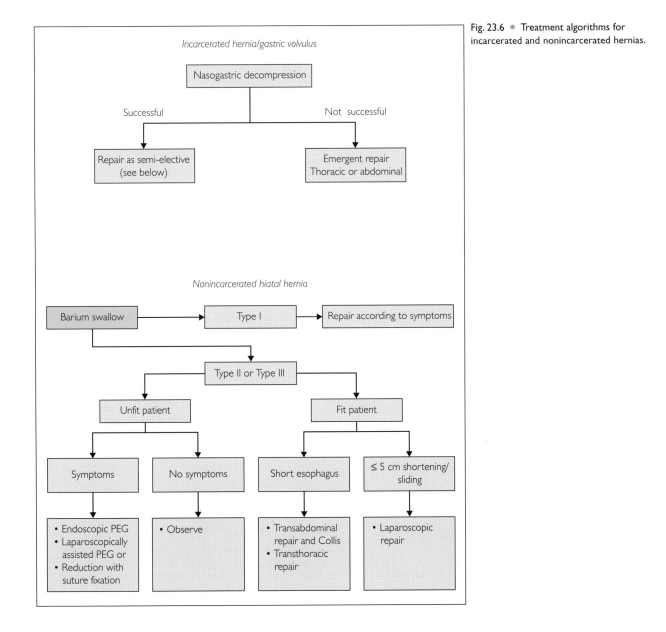

Fig. 23.6 • Treatment algorithms for incarcerated and nonincarcerated hernias.

REFERENCES

1. Woodward ER, Rayl JE, Clark JM. Esophageal hiatus hernia. Curr Prob Surg 1970; Dec:11–62.

2. Ellis FH, Crozier RE, Shea JA. Paraesophageal hiatus hernia. Arch Surg 1986; 121:416–420.

3. Perdikis G, Hinder RA, Filipi C, et al. Laparoscopic paraesophageal hernia repair. Arch Surg 1997; 132:586–591.

4. Hill LD, Tobias JA. Paraesophageal hernia. Arch Surg 1968; 96:735–747.

5. Ozdemir IA, Burke WA, Ikins PM. Paraesophageal hernia: A life threatening disease. Ann Thor Surg 1973; 16:549–554.

6. Wastell C, Ellis H. Volvulus of the stomach: A review with a report of 8 cases. Br J Surg 1971; 58:557–562.

7. Borchardt M. Zun pathologic und therapie des magnervilvulus. Arch Clin Chir 1904; 74:243.

8. Menuch L. Plain film findings of gastric volvulus herniating into the chest. Am J Roengenol 1976; 126:1169–1174.

9. Hill LD. Incarcerated paraesophageal hernia: A surgical emergency. Am J Surg 1973; 126:286–291.

10. Cloyd D. Laparoscopic repair of incarcerated paraesophageal hernias. Surg Endosc 1994; 8:893–897.

11. Franklin ME, Dorman JP, Pharand D. Laparoscopic surgery in acute small bowel obstruction. Surg Laparoscopic Endosc 1994; 4:289–298.

12. Wichterman K, Keha AS, Cahow LE, et al. Giant paraesophageal hernia with intrathoracic stomach and colon: the case for early repair. Surgery 1979; 86:497–506.

13. Skinner DB, Belsy RRH. Surgical management of esophageal reflux and hiatus hernia. Long-term results with 1,010 patients. J Thorac Cardiovasc Surg 1967; 56:33–42.

14. Walther B, DeMeester TR, LaFontaine E, et al. Effect of paraesophageal hernia on sphincter function and its implication on surgical therapy. Am J Surg 1984; 147:111–116.

15. Hashemi M, Peters JH, DeMeester TR, et al. Laparoscopic repair of large type III hiatal hernia: Objective follow-up reveals high recurrence rate. J Am Coll Surg 2000; 190:553–61.

   A review of 54 patients following laparoscopic and open (transthoracic or abdominal) repairs of large type III hernias. There was no difference in symptomatic outcome. Unlike many other series, most patients (80%) had follow-up barium studies, which showed a significant increase in asymptomatic recurrence in the laparoscopic group. This points out the importance of close follow-up and the difficulties in comparing success rates in studies using different endpoints.

16. DeMeester TR. The intrathoracic stomach. J Am Coll Surg: 1998; 187:310–311.

   An editorial written by a teacher in the field of esophageal surgery, emphasizing the importance of a tension-free repair and the significance of a shortened esophagus in large complex hernias. A cautionary tale of the laparoscopic surgeon embarking on the repair of a large type III hernia.

17. Pierre AF, Luketich JD, Fernando HL, et al. Results of laparoscopic repair of giant paraesophageal henias: 200 consecutive patients. Ann Thorac Surg 2002; 76:1909–1916.

18. Swanstrom LL, Jobe BA, Kinzle LR, et al. Esophageal motility and outcomes following laparoscopic paraesophageal hernia repair and fundoplication. Am J Surg 1999; 177:359–364.

19. Cuscheri A. Laparoscopic antireflux surgery and repair of hiatal hernia. World J Surg 1993; 17:40–45.

20. Cuscheri A, Shimi S, Nathanson LK. Laparoscopic reduction, crural repair and fundoplication of large hiatal hernia. Am J Surg 1992; 163:425–432.

21. Willekes CL, Edoga JK, Frezza EE. Laparoscopic repair of paraesophageal hernia. Ann Surg 1997; 25:31–38.

22. Congreve DP. Laparoscopic paraesophageal hernia repair. J Laparosc Surg 1992; 2:45–48.

23. Granerath FA, Kanolz T, Schweiger VM, et al. Laparoscopic re-fundoplication with prosthetic hiatal closure for recurrent hiatal hernia after primary failed anti-reflux surgery. Arch Surg 2003; 138:902–907.

24. Casabella F, Sinanan M, Horgan S, et al. Systematic use of gastric fundoplication in laparoscopic repair of paraesophageal hernias. Am J Surg 1996; 171:485–489.

25. Trus T, Hunter JG. Minimally invasive surgery of the esophagus and stomach. Am J Surg 1997; 173:242–255.

26. Schauer PR, Ikramudden S, McLaughlin R, et al. Comparison of laparoscopic versus open repair of paraesophageal hernia. Am J Surg 1998; 170:659–665.

   A retrospective review of 95 patients undergoing open or laparoscopic repair. Longer operative times and more perforations were seen in the laparoscopic group which had less morbidity and a shorter hospital stay (5 days, which is now quite lengthy). A low rate of symptomatic recurrence is reported but patients were not routinely studied postoperatively. The marked increase in surgical referral for repair since acceptance of laparoscopy is discussed.

27. Horgan S, Eubanks TR, Jacobsen G, et al. Repair of paraesophageal hernia. Am J Surg 1999; 177:354–358.

   This is a report of relatively early experience with laparoscopic repair in 41 patients. There was one death from mesenteric venous thrombosis and two conversations. Excellent descriptive and thoughtful comments about technique and careful symptomatic follow-up.

28. Trus TL, Bax T, Richardson WS, et al. Complications of laparoscopic paraesophageal hernia repair. J Gastrointest Surg 1997; 1:221–228.

29. Edye MB, Camn-Enders J, Gattorno F, et al. Durability of laparoscopic repair of paraesophageal hernia. Ann Surg 1998; 228:528–535.

30. Diaz S, Brint M, Klingensmith M, et al. Laparoscopic paraesophageal hernia repair. A challenging operation: Median term outcome of 116 patients. J Gastrointest Surg 2003; 7:59–67.

31. Carlson MA, Condon RE, Ludwig KA, et al. Management of intrathoracic stomach with polyprophylene mesh prosthesis reinforced transabdominal hiatus hernia repair. J Am Coll Surg 1998; 187:227–230.

32. Edelman DS. Laparoscopic paraesophageal hernia repair with mesh. Surg Laparoscopy Endos 1995; 5:32–37.

33. Subramaryam K, Robbins HT. Erosion of marlex band and silastid ring into the stomach after gastroplasty: endoscopic recognition and management. Am J Gastroenterol. 1989; 84:1319–1321.

34. Smith RS, Chang FC, Hayes KA, et al. Complications of the Anglechik prosthesis. Am J Surg 1985; 150:735–738.

35. McKernon JB, Champion JR. Laparoscopic antireflux surgery. Am J Surg 1995; 61:530–536.

36. Huntington TR. Laparoscopic mesh repair of the esophageal hiatus. J Am Coll Surg 1997; 389–400.

37. Nissen R. Repair of esophageal-hiatal hernia by fixation to the abdominal wall. In: Mulholland JF, Elloon EH, Friesen ST, eds. Current surgical management II. Philadelphia: WB Saunders; 1960:58–59.

38. Johnson PE, Persuad M, Mitchell T. Laparoscopic anterior gastropexy for treatment of paraesophageal hernias. Surg Laparosc Endosc 1994; 4:152–154.

39. Eckhauser ML, Ferron JH. The use of dual percutaneous endoscopic gastrostomy (DPEG) in the management of chronic intermittent gastric volvulus. Gastrointest Endosc 1985; 31:340–342.

40. Ghosh S, Palmer K. Double percutaneous endoscopic gastrostomy fixation: an effective treatment for recurrent gastric volvulus. Am J Gastroenterol 1993; 59:325–328.

41. Pearson FG, Cooper JD, Ilves R, et al. Massive hiatal hernia with incarceration: a report of 53 cases. Ann Thorac Surg 1983; 35:45–51.

42. Williamson WA, Ellis FH, Streitz JM. Paraesophageal hiatal hernia: is an anti-reflux procedure necessary? Ann Thorac Surg 1993; 56:447–452.

43. Wasselle JA, Norman J. Acute gastric volvulus: Pathogenesis, diagnosis, and treatment. Am J Gastroenterol 1993; 88:1780–1784.

44. Koger K, Stone J. Laparoscopic reduction of acute gastric volvulus. Am Surg 1993; 59:325–328.

45. Carter R, Brewer LA, Hinshaw DB. Acute gastric volvulus: A study of 25 cases. Am J 1980; Surg 140:99–106.

46. Cullen ML, Lein MD, Phippart HI. Congenital diaphragmatic hernia. Surg Clin North Am 1985; 65:1115–1138.

47. Ellyson JH, Parks SN. Hernia of Morgagni in a trauma patient. J Trauma 1986; 26:569.

48. Hood RM. Traumatic diaphragmatic hernia. Ann Thorac Surg 1971; 324:311–324.

49. Shreiber H, Flickinger EG, Eichelberger MR, et al. Colonic displacement: Proposed treatment of gastric remnant volvulus due to eventration of the diaphragm. Am J Surg 1980; 139:719–722.

50. McIntyre R, Bensard D, Karer F, et al. The pediatric diaphragm in acute gastric volvulus. J Am Coll Surg 1994; 178:234–238.

51. Festen C. Paraesophageal hernia: A major complication of Nissen's fundoplication. J Pediatr Surg 1981; 16:496–499.

52. Fung K, Rubin S, Scott R. Gastric volvulus complicating Nissen fundoplication. J Pediatr Surg 1990; 25:1242–1243.

53. Casson A, Indulet R, Finley R. Volvulus of the intrathoracic stomach after total esophagectomy. J Thorac Cardiovasc Surg 1990; 100:633–634.

54. Fell S, Kirby T. Volvulus of the intrathoracic stomach after total esophagectomy. J Thorac Cardiovasc Surg 1991; 102:640–641.

55. Bhasin DK, Bagi B, Kochhar R, et al. Endoscopic management of chronic organoaxial volvulus of the stomach. Am J Gastroenterol 1990; 85:1486–1488.

56. Horgan S, Pohl D, Bogetti D, et al. Failed antireflux surgery: What have we learned from reoperations? Arch Surg 1999; 178:541–544.

This nice review of surgical failure after fundoplication includes a useful classification system of postoperative hernias. Careful crural closure and lack of tension are stressed to prevent this difficult problem, which is now more commonly seen.

57. Heldrich F, Kumarasena D, Hakim J, et al. Acute gastric volvulus in children: A rare disorder. Pediatr Emerg Care 1993; 9:221–223.

58. Milne L, Hunter J, Anshus J, et al. Gastric volvulus: Two cases and a review of the literature. J Emerg Med 1994; 12:299–306.

59. Haas O, Rat P, Christoph M, et al. Surgical results of intrathoracic gastric volvulus complicating hiatal hernia. Br J Surg 1990; 77:1379–1381.

60. Hopper T, Lawson R. Volvulus of the stomach, or what cause of pulsus paradoxus. Postgrad Med J 1986; 62:377–379.

61. Kodali V, Maas L. Endoscopic reduction of acute volvulus. J Clin Gastroenterol 1995; 21:331–332.

62. Tsang T, Walker R, Yu D. Endoscopic reductions of gastric volvulus: The alpha-loop maneuver. Gastrointest Endosc 1995; 42:244–248.

63. Baran EM, Housten HE. Foramen of Morgagni's hernias in children. Surgery 1967; 62:1076–1087.

64. Mishalany HG, Nakada K, Wooley MM. Congenital diaphragmatic hernias: Eleven years' experience. Arch Surg 1979; 114:1118–1129.

65. Hendren WH, Lillehei CW. Pediatric surgery. N Engl J Med 1988; 391:86–96.

66. Vacanti JP, Crone RK, Murphy JD, et al. The pulmonary hemodynamic response to perioperative anesthesia in the treatment of high-risk infants with congenital diaphragmatic hernia. J Pediatr Surg 1984; 19:672–679.

67. Reichert GA, Hirschl RB, Atkinson JB, et al. Congenital diaphragmatic hernia survival and use of extracorporeal life support at selected level III nurseries with multimodality support. Surgery 1998; 123(3):305–310.

68. West KW, Bengson K, Rescorla FJ, et al. Delayed surgical repair and ECMO improves survival in congenital diaphragmatic hernia. Ann Surg 1992; 216:454.

69. Kuster GGR, Kline LE, Garzo G. Diaphragmatic hernia through the foramen of Morgagni: Laparoscopic repair case report. J Laparosc Surg 1992; 2:93–100.

70. Ran HG, Schardey HM, Lange V. Laparoscopic repair of Morgagni hernia. Surg Endosc 1994; 8:1439–1442.

71. Beal SL, McKennon M. Blunt diaphragmatic rupture: A morbid injury. Arch Surg 1988; 123:828–832.

72. Pangarello G, Carter J. Traumatic injury to the diaphragm. Timely diagnosis and therapy. J Trauma 1992; 33:194–197.

73. Myers BF, McCabe CJ. Traumatic diaphragm hernia: Occult marker of serious injury. Ann Surg 1993; 218:783–790.

74. Feliciano DV, Cruse PA. Delayed diagnosis of injuries to the diaphragm after penetrating wounds. J Trauma 1989; 28:1135–1142.

75. Chen JC, Wilson SE. Diaphragmatic injuries. Recognition and management in 62 patients. Am J Surg 1991; 57:810–815.

76. Killeen KL, Mirvis SE, Shanuganathan K. Helical CT of diaphragmatic rupture caused by blunt trauma. Am J Roentgenol 1999; 173:1611–1616.

77. Carvillo EH, Heniford BT, Etoch SW, et al. Video-assisted thoracic surgery in trauma patients. J Am Coll Surg 1997; 184:316–324.

78. Ochsner MG, Rozycki GS, Wante F, et al. Prospective evaluation of thoracoscopy for diagnosing diaphragmatic injury in thoracoabdominal trauma: A preliminary report. J Trauma 1993; 34:704–710.

79. Spam JC, Nwarkiaku FE, Walt ME. Evaluation of video-assisted thoracoscopic surgery in the diagnosis of diaphragmatic injuries. Am J Surg 1995; 170:628–630.

80. Falcone RE, Barnes FE. Blunt diaphragmatic rupture diagnosed by laparoscopy. Report of a case. J Laparoendosc Surg 1991; 1:299–302.

81. Ivatury RR, Simon RJ, Weksler B, et al. Laparoscopy in the evaluation of the intrathoracic abdomen after penetrating injury. J Trauma 1992; 33:101–107.

82. Guth AA, Patcher HL. Laparoscopy for penetrating thoracoabdominal trauma. Pitfalls and promises. J Soc Laparoendosc Surg 1998; 2:123–127.

A study of 70 patients showing utility of laparoscopy in assessment of thoracoabdominal trauma. Concern is raised over a 20% missed injury rate for significant thoracic injuries.

83. Koehler RH, Smith RS. Thoracoscopic repair of missed diaphragmatic injury in a penetrating trauma: case report. J Trauma 1994; 36:424–427.

84. Namias N, McKenny M, Sosa JL. Laparoscopic repair of a gunshot wound to the diaphragm: A case report. J Laparoendosc Surg 1995; 5:59–61.

85. Smith CH, Novick TL, Jacobs DG, et al. Laparoscopic management of ruptured diaphragm secondary to blunt trauma. Surg Endosc 2000; 14:1010–1014.

86. Meyer G, Huttle TP, Hatz RA, et al. Laparoscopic repair of traumatic hiatal hernia. Surg Endosc 2000; 14:537–539 (delayed edition).

CHAPTER TWENTY-FOUR

24

Gastric neoplasia

Enders K.W. Ng and Wai K. Leung

INTRODUCTION

The majority of gastric neoplasms are malignant in nature with over 95% being adenocarcinoma. The remainder includes lymphomas, stromal tumors, and rarely neuroendocrine tumors. The approach to treatment of different types of gastric neoplasm varies considerably due to different pathogenic mechanisms and clinical behaviors.

ADENOCARCINOMA OF THE STOMACH

Stomach cancer (adenocarcinoma) is the second most common cause of malignancy related mortality in the world.[1] Over the past few decades, a global declining trend in the overall incidence of gastric cancer has been observed. However, the ratio of proximally to distally located tumors has increased within the same time period. The cause of the gradual decline in stomach cancer incidence is unclear but improvement in environmental hygiene, increase in fresh fruit intake, and decrease in prevalence of *Helicobacter pylori* infection are possible contributing factors. Nonetheless, the change in epidemiology, advance in knowledge of tumor carcinogenesis, and a better understanding of the metastatic mechanisms have important implications on the evolution of a treatment strategy for this malignancy. Figure 24.1 provides an algorithm for the management of gastric adenocarcinoma.

Staging

Preoperative staging is of paramount importance in the planning of management for patients with stomach cancer. Early gastric cancer can be managed with a totally different approach than that needed for locally advanced diseases or for patients who present with metastases. Even for advanced cancer, the treatment plan depends upon tumor staging and other patient factors. It is imperative to incorporate the most cost-effective and accurate preoperative staging tools in the preparatory phase of the treatment program.

Essentially, four major parameters regarding tumor staging should be determined prior to initiation of any specific treatment. They are the depth of tumor invasion (T), the lymph node statuses (N), the presence of distant metastases (M), and the status of peritoneal surface. Being the most complex among all these, the lymph node staging system has evolved drastically over the past few decades. In 1997, the fifth edition of TNM staging

guideline, jointly released by the Union Internationale Contre Le Cancer (UICC) and the American Joint Committee on Cancer (AJCC), had made a substantial revision in the nodal staging of gastric cancer.[2] The previous UICC version classified perigastric lymph nodes into three levels based on their location and distance from the primary lesion, in a way quite similar to that published by the Japanese Research Society for Gastric Cancer (JRSGC).[3] In the fifth edition, the lymph nodes are staged according to the absolute number of nodes being involved by cancer cells, and that includes a prerequisite that at least 15 nodes must be retrieved in order to permit histological assessment. When the number of nodes dissected is smaller than 15, the N-staging becomes unavailable (Nx). Although the new N-staging system has been shown to be more accurate in predicting the long-term outcome of patients, accurate preoperative N-staging is difficult since enlarged nodes detected by any kind of imaging are not necessarily metastatic in nature.

Imaging

Various imaging modalities have been used in preoperative staging of gastric cancer. Ultrasonography (USG) is relatively inexpensive and easily available, but it is highly operator-dependent. In experienced hands, USG can be a useful preoperative investigation for screening of solid organ metastases, enlarged para-aortic and portal lymph nodes, ascites, and pelvic deposits such as Krukenburg tumors of the ovary.

Computed tomography (CT) is widely used in the staging of stomach cancer. It is sensitive in detecting direct invasion of the tumor into adjacent organs and liver metastasis.[4,5] However, its value as a routine preoperative investigation has been questioned because of its inability to differentiate different layers of the gastric wall and its low sensitivity in diagnosing peritoneal metastases. The information generated from CT imaging can actually be obtained using other modalities of investigation. The use of CT scan is therefore mainly recommended for tumors in which T4 invasion or solid organ metastasis is suspected.

Endoscopic ultrasound

Endoscopic ultrasound (EUS) was first introduced in 1980. It allows the placement of the ultrasound probe right on the stomach wall. With the use of high-frequency transponders, it provides excellent spatial resolution and enables the visualization of the five layers of the gastric wall. The ability of EUS to distinguish between mucosa, submucosa, and muscularis mucosa makes

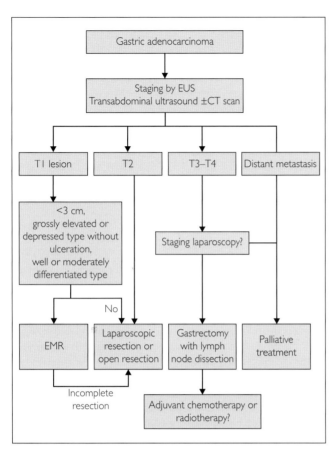

Fig. 24.1 ● Management algorithm of gastric adenocarcinoma.

it the best imaging modality to assess the depth of tumor invasion.[6] It is superior to conventional CT scan with reported accuracy range from 71% to 92% for T-staging, and 55% to 87% for N-staging.[7] In the authors' center, EUS is the routine preoperative staging investigation for all patients with stomach cancer.

Staging laparoscopy

Transcelomic spread happens in about 40% of tumors with serosal involvement (T3 or above). The inability of CT scan to diagnose peritoneal and omental metastases may lead to under-staging of these patients. Staging laparoscopy has been shown to change the management plan of 25–40% of patients who were otherwise deemed to be curable by radical surgery according to other preoperative staging investigations.[8,9]

Surgery

Theodor Billroth performed the first successful distal gastrectomy on a 43-year-old lady who suffered from obstructing antral carcinoma in 1881. The patient died 4 months later from tumor recurrence. Since then, many surgical procedures have been developed with the hope that a modification of operative techniques might confer a better survival outcome for the patients. For many years and even up to now, surgical extirpation has been the mainstay for potentially curing of patients with stomach cancer. Four major issues have to be considered in the management of locally advanced stomach cancer: (1) extent of

gastric resection; (2) extent of lymphadenectomy; (3) mode of reconstruction; and (4) access for the operation.

Extent of gastric resection

Total gastrectomy was, at one time, the recommended surgery for cancers of the stomach regardless of their locations. While the procedure is expected to provide a better loco-regional control of the primary tumor and remove all the remaining at-risk gastric mucosa, the resulting functional disturbance can be disabling. Substantial weight loss and muscle wasting are not uncommon due to a reduction in oral intake and malabsorption. It has been argued that a lesser degree of resection is oncologically reasonable, especially for distal tumors. Two randomized trials conducted in the 1980s showed that the overall survival of patients with antral cancers after subtotal gastrectomy was not inferior to that after total gastrectomy.[10,11] However, because of the lack of quality control regarding lymph node excision in these two trials, total gastrectomy remains a commonly performed procedure, especially in Western countries.

A more recent randomized trial by the Italian Gastrointestinal Tumour Study Group has reinvestigated the issue.[12] A total of 624 patients with distal gastric carcinoma were included: 320 and 304 undergoing subtotal and total gastrectomy, respectively. Both procedures entailed a D2 level of nodal dissection. At 5 years, patients with subtotal gastrectomy had a similar survival probability (65.3%) when compared to those undergoing total gastrectomy (62.4%). However, the nutritional status and quality of life were much better in the subtotal gastrectomy group. Sub-total gastrectomy should therefore be the recommended procedure for distally located tumor with Lauren's intestinal differentiation. For sizable tumor of diffuse subtype or more proximally located lesions, a total gastrectomy is advisable. Tumors involving the esophagogastric junction are better treated with esophago-gastrectomy via a left thoraco-abdominal incision. The macroscopic proximal free resection margin, as recommended by the Japanese Research Society for Gastric Cancer, should be at least 6 cm in order to minimize the risk of microscopic margin involvement.[13] On-table frozen section for the resection margin is desirable but is not a universal practice. Proximal gastrectomy, though being advocated by some, is known to have a high rate of long-term morbidities and is not generally recommended.

Extent of lymph node dissection

Japanese surgeons first advocated the use of extended lymphadenectomy in the 1960s in the hope that it might reduce the chance of nodal recurrence and improve the survival outcome. A different nodal staging system for stomach cancer had been proposed so that the extent of nodal dissection could be performed according to the N-stages. According to the JRSGC, all perigastric lymph nodes are classified into several tiers according to their distance from the primary tumor and the probability of their being involved by the malignancy. In brief, lymph nodes lying along the greater and lesser omentum are classified as N1, while those along the major arteries branching off from the celiac axis and around it are denoted as N2. Nodes further away from N2 stations are labeled as N3. Other nodes such as those in the infracolic compartment or above the diaphragm, if involved by cancer, are classified as metastases. With the current nomenclature system, D1 lymphadenectomy refers to the removal of first tier lymph nodes while D2 means both the first and second tiers are excised en bloc with the stomach. In Japan, the most extensive lymphadenectomy is a D4 dissection which entails the removal of all perigastric lymph nodes as well as para-aortic lymph nodes in both supracolic and infracolic compartments. In addition, the spleen and distal pancreas are resected en bloc with the stomach.

Conceivably, this more extensive lymphatic dissection and organ resection would lead to a higher chance of operative morbidity and mortality. Such an aggressive approach can be justified only if a better survival is attainable. While survival benefit from extended lymph node excision has been repeatedly demonstrated by the Japanese groups, comparable results were not obtained in studies conducted in the West. Two large scale multicenter randomized controlled trials were carried out in three European countries in the early 1990s and, in these studies, the effect of D1 and D2 gastrectomies on patients with stomach cancer was compared.[14,15] No significant improvement in long-term survival was observed from the extended nodal dissection. When compared to D1 lymphadenectomy, D2 lymphadenectomy resulted in significantly more postoperative complications and a higher mortality rate which were mostly related to the concomitant pancreatectomy and splenectomy. These observations, therefore, are not in agreement with those published earlier by the Japanese[16,17] and other centers with high case volume.[18-20] In the D1 versus D2 trial conducted by the Medical Research Council in the United Kingdom, participant institutes were criticized for their low case volume and lack of formal training on D2 resection[14] but, in the Dutch trial, eight surgeons trained by an experienced Japanese surgeon were responsible for all the D2 gastrectomies, and the early postoperative results were still disappointing with high rates of mortality and morbidity.[15] It appears that the early complications after the D2 operation in these randomized trials have offset the potential benefit which might be obtainable from the extended dissection. It remains unclear whether the outcome would be different if such studies had been conducted in Western centers with greater experience.

The evidence regarding the role of nodal dissection in gastric cancer is best summarized in a recently released review by the Cochrane Library database system,[21] in which 2 large-scale randomized trials mentioned above, 2 nonrandomized comparisons of limited (D1) versus extended (D2) node dissection and 11 cohort studies were analyzed. It was concluded that D2 dissection carried higher mortality risks associated with spleen and pancreas resection, probably resulting from inexperience and low case volumes. Although randomized studies showed no evidence of overall survival benefit, there may be possible benefit in T3+ tumors. Gastric surgery for stomach cancer should probably be concentrated and performed in experienced centers if a better outcome is desired.

Mode of reconstruction

Gastrectomy for stomach cancer entails the removal of a large portion of, or even the entire, stomach but how to re-establish the alimentary tract continuity is still a subject of debate. In principle, any reconstruction must restore intestinal transit to provide good nutritional conditions and good quality of life. The food passage is easily restored by simple gastrojejunstomy or oesophago-jejunostomy but persistent weight loss, bilious esophageal reflux, and occasionally severe dumping may seriously affect quality of life. Many technical variants have been suggested, but none is considered entirely satisfactory.

After a subtotal gastrectomy, gastrointestinal continuity can be restored in different ways. The Billroth I style of gastroduodenal anastomosis is widely embraced by Japanese surgeons. By preserving duodenal transit, the Billroth I anastomosis is thought to provide a more physiological outcome and better nutrition. Unfortunately, such a notion lacks support from well-controlled studies. In other parts of the world, the mode of reconstruction generally depends on the discretion of individual surgeons. The most commonly performed reconstruction after a subtotal gastrectomy in the authors' center is the Roux-en-Y procedure, which mainly serves to minimize reflux of bile and pancreatic secretion back into the stomach and esophagus. The recommended length of the Roux loop ranges 40–60 cm. Despite its proclaimed advantages, as many as 30% of patients may develop the so-called Roux stasis syndrome after this procedure.[22] The exact mechanism for this condition remains enigmatic, but detachment of the Roux loop from the intestinal pacemaker located in the proximal duodenum is probably the major culprit.

Patients with total gastrectomy generally have a worse functional outcome when compared to those undergoing subtotal gastrectomy. Bile and pancreatic reflux into the lower esophagus can be notoriously disabling. The lack of a food reservoir following resection of the entire stomach limits food intake and, often, results in malnutrition. Reflux prevention, preservation of duodenal transit and, particularly, the creation of a gastric reservoir to avoid these problems have been the major objective of surgical reconstruction and a variety of techniques have been described. These include a simple Roux-en-Y oesophagojejunostomy, Roux-en-Y anastomosis coupled with an inverted pouch, the use of interposition jejunal loop for preservation of duodenal transit, etc. Lehnert and Buhl reviewed the findings of 19 prospective randomized trials including a total of 866 patients that compared different reconstructions after gastrectomy.[23] Despite the wide variation in endpoints, preservation of duodenal transit was found to have little impact on the oral intake and nutritional outcome of the patients. To the contrary, the construction of a gastric substitute, mostly by a jejunal pouch, was associated with better food intake and weight development, at least in the early postoperative period. Unfortunately, this benefit of a pouch reconstruction seems to diminish with longer follow-up.[24]

Laparoscopic surgery

With the advent of minimal access surgery in the last 2 decades, gastrectomy can now be performed using the laparoscope. Most of the reported series of laparoscopic gastrectomy are confined to cases of early disease for which the demand for extended lymphadenectomy is not as high as that for more advanced diseases.[25,26] In general, laparoscopic gastrectomy takes significantly longer operating time but results in less wound pain in the postoperative period. However, there is no difference in the overall hospital stay and complication rate when compared to the conventional open approach. Whether the laparoscopic method can be adopted for more radical types of gastrectomy remains an uncertainty, but improvement in laparoscopic instruments, including the availability of more precise and potent coagulating and cutting devices, has suggested that laparoscopic surgery may be appropriate for tumors beyond the early stage.

Adjuvant treatment

Chemotherapy

Postoperative systemic chemotherapy has been most widely studied in patients undergoing curative gastrectomy for stomach cancer. While some earlier studies[27,28] reported an increase in the 5-year survival rate, such benefits were not confirmed by subsequent studies. Various combinations such as FAM, FAMTX, FEP, and ECF have been described. As most of these trials have considerable methodological flaws, the actual survival benefit of these regimens remains doubtful.

Earlier meta-analyses based on trials of postoperative adjuvant chemotherapy reported little improvement on the survival of patients receiving systemic chemotherapy.[29,30] However, with more randomized studies, modification of treatment regimens, and introduction of new cytotoxic agents, recent trials have demonstrated better outcome and quality of life with the use of postoperative adjuvant chemotherapy. Meta-analyses published in recent years have often revealed significantly better, albeit small, 5-year survival rates among patients who had systemic chemotherapy after surgery.[31] In the GISCAD study that included 3658 patients and 2180 deaths, 3 studies used single agent chemotherapy, 7 used combination of 5-fluorouracil (5-FU) with anthracyclin, and 10 used combination of 5-FU without anthracyclines.[32] Chemotherapy reduced the risk of death by 18% (hazard ratio 0.82, 95% CI, 0.75–0.89, $p<0.001$). In a more updated meta-analysis by Janunger and others, which includes 21 randomized trials of systemic postoperative chemotherapy for patients with stomach cancer, a significant survival benefit was also identified (odds ratio [OR] 0.84, 95% CI, 0.74–0.96).[33] However, when Western and Asian studies were analyzed separately, there was no survival benefit for patients treated in Western countries (OR 0.96, 95% CI, 0.83–1.12). As commented by most authors of these systematic reviews, the difference in survival based on these pooled data is still strong enough to recommend systemic chemotherapy as a routine postoperative care for patients undergoing curative gastric resection.

Radiotherapy

Gastric carcinoma is relatively resistant to radiotherapy. The British Stomach Cancer Group found that postoperative external beam radiotherapy in addition to surgery did not confer any survival benefit.[34] The 5-year survival in patients receiving surgery plus radiotherapy and surgery alone was 12% and 20%, respectively. On the other hand, intraoperative radiotherapy is frequently given in Japan.[35] Although it has been claimed to prolong survival for patients with stage II and III disease, this therapy needs further evaluation.

Chemo-irradiation

The combination of chemotherapy with radiotherapy has been shown to be effective in reducing local and regional recurrence after curative resection of rectal cancer and pancreatic cancer. This approach has also been explored as a potential option to improve the outcome of patients with gastric cancer. The largest multicenter randomized trial to date evaluating the use of postoperative chemoradiotherapy for patients with gastric cancer was the Intergroup 0116 study in which patients were allocated to receive either surgery alone or surgery plus postoperative radiotherapy and concomitant 5-FU.[36] The 5-year survival rate of the surgery combined with chemoradiotherapy group was significantly greater than the surgery alone group. These data have been used to support the concept that all patients with resectable gastric cancer should receive multimodal adjuvant therapy. On the other hand, the high toxicity of the chemoradiotherapy in the Intergroup 0116 study caused premature termination of the treatment program in 40% of the patients and this has caused some to question the conclusions reached in that study. In addition, the Intergroup 0116 study has also been criticized because of the apparent poor quality of the surgery. Although a D2 dissection had been recommended, only 10% of patients had D2-level nodal clearance and more than half of the patients received only a D0 dissection. In fact, the 5-year survival rate of patients having surgery alone was much poorer than that of patients who had had a good quality D1 or D2 gastrectomy in other series.[15] It has been argued that chemoradiotherapy in the Intergroup 0116 study was beneficial because it compensated for the suboptimal surgery and the effect of undertreatment by surgery has been confirmed by a subsequent regression analysis by the same group.[37] Whether a similar magnitude of survival benefit can be obtained from postoperative chemoradiation therapy after standard nodal clearance remains unclear.

Peritoneal chemotherapy

Transcelomic spread is the most common mode of recurrence after attempted curative surgery for gastric cancer. Whilst the exact mechanism responsible for this phenomenon remains elusive, free-floating cancer cells shed from tumors that breach the serosa are the likely source of seeding. Cytological study of peritoneal washings has revealed a strong correlation between positive cytology and T3 and T4 diseases,[38,39] and it has been shown that patients with microscopic cancer cells in the peritoneal washings have a prognosis equivalent to those with macroscopic peritoneal dissemination. Whether administration of regional treatment can alter the natural history of this subgroup of patients is a subject of debate. In a Japanese trial, 113 patients with serosal invasion who underwent radical gastrectomy were randomized to receive immediate intraperitoneal mitomycin C tagged onto activated charcoal particles or no further treatment.[40] A significantly greater 3-year survival rate was observed for patients who received the peritoneal mitomycin treatment when compared to controls, and there is no increase in mortality or morbidity. However, disappointing abdominal septic complication and mortality rates were observed in a similar trial conducted in Austria.[41]

Hyperthermic intraperitoneal chemotherapy has attracted much attention in recent years. The method was first described and practiced by Spratt et al. in the 1980s on a patient with pseudomyxoma peritonei.[42] The technique had been adopted and applied to other kinds of malignancies with peritoneal dissemination. The concept has evolved over the past 2 decades, and currently cytoreductive surgery followed by hyperthermic intraperitoneal chemoperfusion is being used for the treatment and prevention of transcelomic spread of cancers from several different origins. Most series related to stomach cancer have been reported by Japanese investigators.[43,44] In a recent randomized trial, the use of prophylactic hyperthermic perfusion with mitomycin C following curative resection of stage II and III gastric cancer significantly reduced the peritoneal recurrence rate and improved long-term survival.[44] Nevertheless, lack of efficacy and high perioperative morbidity was reported by other groups.[45,46]

In summary, peritoneal chemotherapy, administered either intraoperatively or in the early postoperative period, should not be used outside an experimental protocol setting. More research and clinical studies are required before it can be more widely accepted and practiced.

Neoadjuvant chemotherapy

Apart from Japan where a mass population screening program is available, most patients with stomach cancer tend to present with locally advanced disease. The prognosis of stage II and III disease is generally poor despite radical surgery and due to the lack of proven efficacy for postoperative systemic or regional adjuvant treatment, a number of studies have been initiated to evaluate the potential value of preoperative therapy in the management of patients with advanced stomach cancer.[47,48] The evidence to date has confirmed both the feasibility and the safety of preoperative chemotherapy. Furthermore, several phase II studies with neo-adjuvant treatment have shown low toxicity and increased R0 resection rate for advanced diseases.[49,50] However, data regarding long-term survival with the combination of neoadjuvant chemo-therapy and surgery are still awaited and large-scale prospective randomized trials are needed before any conclusions can be drawn.

Palliation

Whether to perform palliative gastrectomy for patients with metastatic carcinoma of the stomach remains controversial. The decision to proceed with palliative gastrectomy needs to balance the risks of surgery against the potential benefits of having most of the tumor removed. Palliative gastrectomy could possibly prevent life-threatening tumor complications, such as bleeding or perforation. Moreover, palliative chemotherapy can also be given after a palliative debulking resection. From the available data, palliative resection seems to be associated with a longer median survival and better quality of life but similar morbidity and mortality when compared to laparotomy alone.[51,52] However, most of these series are retrospective comparative studies that carried considerable biases and a prospective comparative study would be extremely difficult to perform, especially when it involves randomizing patients with advanced malignancy.

EARLY GASTRIC CANCER

Early gastric cancer (EGC) is a carcinoma confined to the mucosa and submucosa of the stomach, regardless of nodal status. This entity is more frequently found in countries where screening procedures are widely practiced. Hence, the proportions of EGC range 6–24% in Western countries to 30–50% in Japan.[53]

The overall 5-year survival of EGC is greater than 90% in Japanese series. Despite the successful claim of high cure rate of patients with EGC in Japanese series, there is a considerable difference of opinion regarding the proper histological diagnosis of these 'early cancers'.[54] For example, Japanese pathologists may diagnose gastric carcinoma on nuclear and structural criteria even when invasion is absent. Nonetheless, a recent Japanese study shows that 64% of EGC patients, in whom surgical resection was delayed or not carried out, did progress to more advanced stages during long-term follow-up, suggesting that

these 'early cancers' do, in fact, have invasive potential.[55] The major factor that appears to determine the prognosis of EGC is the presence or absence of lymph node metastasis. Accordingly, endoscopic ultrasound (EUS) plays an instrumental role in delineating the depth of tumor invasion and the risk of lymph node metastasis preoperatively. The accuracy of EUS in T-staging is 71–92% and it is superior to CT.[7] The incidence of nodal metastasis in intramucosal and submucosal cancer is 3% and 20%, respectively.

Treatment of EGC depends on various factors including the depth, the size, the location and macroscopic appearance of the tumor, the histological subtypes, and the lymph node status. Moreover, the clinician's experience has to be taken into consideration. Due to the low incidence of lymph node and distant metastasis, surgical resection of the stomach for EGC is sometimes considered unnecessary. However, there is no randomized control trial comparing the efficacy of endoscopic therapy to surgical treatment. Endoscopic mucosal resection (EMR) was first described by Tada and coworkers[56] and it is widely practiced in Japan as the treatment of choice for cancer confined to the mucosa. The National Cancer Center Hospital of Japan recommends that cancers measuring <3 cm, those that are either grossly elevated or depressed without ulceration, and those that are of histologically well or moderately differentiated type are lesions suitable for EMR.[57] On the other hand, surgical resection is still recommended after EMR when there is submucosal invasion, vessel permeation, or an incomplete resection margin. In a major Japanese series including 479 cancer patients treated by EMR, 69% of tumors were resected with clear margins and a total of 17 (3.5%) local recurrences were detected during subsequent follow-up.[57] There were no gastric cancer-related deaths during the follow-up period (3–120 months) and the risk of missing lymph node metastasis was about 2.5%. A non-randomized study further suggests that eradication of *H. pylori* significantly reduces the risk of subsequent cancer development after endoscopic resection of EGC.[58]

On the other hand, there is no consensus regarding the extent of surgical resection for EGC. Options are largely influenced by the location of the tumor and the suspicion of lymph node metastasis. Limited gastric resection is the preferred option for most patients with EGC. However, the need and extent of lymph node dissection remains unaddressed. There is also recent interest in the use of laparoscopic techniques such as laparoscopic wedge resection and laparoscopy-assisted distal gastrectomy in the treatment of EGC. The use of laparoscopic surgery will certainly hasten patients' recovery as well as improving quality of life.[59]

Although screening for gastric cancer by either contrast study or endoscopy is widely practiced in Japan, formal randomized study that evaluates the effectiveness of this screening strategy is lacking. Given the low incidence of gastric carcinoma in most developed countries, it is unlikely that a similar population-based screening program will have positive results. In contrast, targeted screening of high-risk individuals including those with a family history of gastric cancer or those with intraepithelial neoplasia may be more rewarding.[60]

PRIMARY GASTRIC LYMPHOMA

Although primary gastric lymphoma is a rare malignancy, accounting for less than 5% of all gastric malignancies, it is the commonest form of extranodal lymphoma. It is estimated that approximately 70% of primary gastrointestinal lymphomas arise from the stomach. The majority (80%) of primary gastric lymphomas are B-cell non-Hodgkin's lymphoma, either low-grade mucosa-associated lymphoid tissue (MALT) lymphoma or a high-grade, diffuse, large cell lymphoma. More than 90% of MALT lymphomas are related to chronic *H. pylori* infection.[61]

Although upper gastrointestinal endoscopy is widely used in the diagnosis of gastric lymphoma, multiple and deep gastric biopsies are usually required for accurate histological diagnosis. The Musshoff's modified Ann Arbor staging system is widely used for staging of gastric lymphoma.[62] Stage EI1 refers to infiltration of the mucosa and submucosa only, whereas EI2 lymphomas extend beyond the submucosa. Endoscopic ultrasound is widely used in the staging of gastric lymphoma and it is useful in determination of the depth of tumor infiltration, metastasis to perigastric lymph nodes, and evaluation of treatment response.[63]

Cure of *H. pylori* infection results in long-term cure of low-grade gastric MALT lymphoma in the majority of patients.[64] The overall success of antibiotics in achieving complete remission in stage E1 lymphomas is about 80% with an annual recurrence rate of about 5%.[65] However, the time for complete tumor remission varies and regression may not be apparent until several months after clearance of the organism.[66] Monoclonal B cells, as detected by polymerase chain reaction, may persist for up to several years after cure of *H. pylori* infection or complete histological and endoscopic remission.[67,68] Staging by EUS may be able to predict the response of gastric MALT lymphoma to anti-*Helicobacter* treatment. Patients with stage EI1 disease (confined to mucosa and submucosa) are more likely to have complete regression of the MALT lymphoma after anti-*Helicobacter* therapy.[69,70] Patients should be followed up by endoscopy every 6 months for the first 2 years and then yearly to monitor histological regressions. Other factors associated with a nonresponse to antibacterial therapy include *H. pylori*-negativity and the presence of high-grade lymphoma features. The presence of t(11;18), which results in a chimeric transcript between the API2 and MLT genes, may also predict resistance to antibiotic treatment.[71]

Treatment options for high-grade lymphoma or advanced-stage MALT lymphoma remains controversial. Surgery is particularly useful for localized diseases, such as stages EI and EII, with a favorable 5-year survival of 85–100%.[68] Patients with complete resection or only microscopically residual tumor have significantly better survival rates than those with macroscopically residual tumor.[68] However, aggressive surgery with radical excision is associated with high morbidity and mortality and it is generally considered unnecessary. Recent data also suggested that chemotherapy alone may be as effective as surgery plus chemotherapy in patients with localized disease.[72,73] The combination of cyclophosphamide, doxorubicin, vincristine, and prednisone (CHOP) is the standard regimen used in the treatment of gastric lymphoma. Fears of chemotherapy-related complications such as bleeding or perforation have been overemphasized. For advanced disease (stage III and IV), systemic chemotherapy or combination treatment may be more appropriate. Radiotherapy is usually used as an adjuvant to surgery, chemotherapy, or both. However, radiotherapy alone has been shown to have reasonable outcome.[73–75]

GASTOINTESTINAL STROMAL CELL TUMORS

Gastrointestinal stromal tumors (GIST), previously called smooth muscle tumors, are the most common mesenchymal tumors of the gastrointestinal tract. The stomach is the most frequent site of GIST and the stomach accounts for about 70% of all GIST cases. GISTs are closely related to the interstitial cells of Cajal. Mutations of c-kit that cause constitutive activation of c-kit's tyrosine kinase activity are detectable in most GIST and appear to play a pivotal role in the pathogenesis of these tumors.[76] This can be readily detected by immunohistochemistry against CD117.

The differentiation of benign from malignant GIST can be difficult, and parameters including mitotic activity (>10/high power filed), tumor size (>5 cm), tumor necrosis, histological type/pattern, immunohistochemical profile, staining for proliferation antigens, and ploidy status have been used to predict biological behavior.[77] Surgery is the mainstay of treatment for localized disease. Complete tumor resection can be accomplished in 50–80% of cases.[78] For gastric tumors, limited dissection is known to achieve comparable results to extended resection.[79] Lymphadenectomy is not routinely practiced due to the low incidence of lymph node metastasis, and vital structures should be preserved if gross tumor clearance can be attained. Recently, imatinib (formerly STI571), a selective and competitive inhibitor of ABL tyrosine kinases, was found to be effective in the treatment of metastatic and locally inoperable GIST.[80] Data from phase 1 and 2 trials show a more than 50% partial response to imatinib in advanced GISTs,[81,82] and results from longer-term follow-up are pending.

GASTRIC CARCINOID TUMORS

Gastric carcinoid tumors are rare. They account for about 9% of all gastrointestinal carcinoids.[83] They arise from proliferating enterochromaffin-like cells of the fundus and are associated with chronic atrophic gastritis and pernicious anemia (type I gastric carcinoid), or Zollinger-Ellison syndrome with multiple endocrine neoplasia I (type II gastric carcinoid). In contrast to the type I and type II tumors, the sporadic form (type III gastric carcinoid) is not associated with hypergastrinemia and it usually presents as a single large tumor. This latter type behaves more aggressively with a high tendency of advanced local invasion and metastasis.[84]

Most (53%) gastric carcinoids present as localized disease but 20% have distant metastasis.[83] For small type I and II gastric carcinoids, local removal by endoscopic polypectomy may be adequate. Surveillance endoscopy is recommended at 6-month intervals after initial removal. Antrectomy can be considered in patients with lesions larger than 1 cm, multiple (3–5) lesions, and recurrence after initial removal.[85] This operation could reduce the serum gastrin levels which result in regression of ECL cell carcinoids.[86] For type III gastric carcinoids, a more radical approach, similar to gastric adenocarcinoma, is necessary due to the high malignant potential. Complete or partial gastrectomy with regional lymph node dissection is recommended.[87] Chemotherapy and other adjuvant therapies may be necessary in patients with metastatic disease. Treatment with interferon and/or octreotide may be useful in controlling symptoms associated with carcinoid syndrome.[88]

GASTRIC POLYPS

Gastric polyps are found in 2–3% of all endoscopic examinations.[89] Polyps may occur sporadically or in polyposis syndromes such as familial adenomatous polyposis, Peutz-Jeghers syndrome, Cowden syndrome, and Cronkhite-Canada syndrome. Neoplastic polyps are composed of adenomatous tissue similar to that found in the colon. Non-neoplastic polyps may be of various types – i.e., hyperplastic, hamartomatous, inflammatory or heterotopic. Of various non-neoplastic polyps, fundic gland polyps are the most common gastric polyps followed by hyperplastic polyps.

The recent American Society for Gastrointestinal Endoscopy review suggested that all gastric polyps causing symptoms, such as bleeding and obstruction, and those greater than 2 cm should be removed.[90] Polyps smaller than 2 cm in size can be initially biopsied and excised. If biopsies reveal adenomatous change, endoscopic excision should be considered. Most gastric polyps can be safely removed by snare polypectomy. Complications such as bleeding, perforation, and abdominal pain are rare. Surveillance endoscopy, 1 year after removal, is recommended for patients with adenomatous gastric polyps to assess for any recurrence or development of new polyps.

REFERENCES

1. Jemal A, Tiwari RC, Murray T, et al. Cancer statistics, 2004. CA Cancer J Clin 2004; 54:8–29.

2. Sobin LH, Wittekind Ch, eds. TNM Classification of malignant tumours. 5th edn. New York: Wiley-Liss, Inc.; 1997:59–62.

3. Japanese Gastric Cancer Association. Japanese Classification of Gastric Carcinoma, 2nd English edn. Gastric Cancer 1998; 1(1):10–24.

4. Kuntz C, Herfarth C. Imaging diagnosis for staging of gastric cancer. Semin Surg Oncol 1999; 17:96–102.

5. Davies J, Chalmers AG, Sue-Ling HM, et al. Spiral computed tomography and operative staging of gastric carcinoma: a comparison with histopathological staging. Gut 1997; 41:314–319.

6. Nicholson DA, Shorvon PJ. Review article: endoscopic ultrasound of the stomach. Br J Radiol 1993; 66:487–492.

7. Hohenberger P, Gretschel S. Gastric cancer. Lancet 2003; 362:305–315.

8. Molloy RG, McCourtney JS, Anderson JR. Laparoscopy in the management of patients with cancer of the gastric cardia and oesophagus. Br J Surg 1995; 82:352–354.

9. Lowy AM, Mansfield PF, Leach SD, et al. Laparoscopic staging for gastric cancer. Surgery 1996; 119:611–614.

10. Gouzi JL, Huguier M, Fagniez PL, et al. Total versus subtotal gastrectomy for adenocarcinoma of the gastric antrum. A French prospective controlled study. Ann Surg 1989; 209:162–166.

11. Gennari L, Bozzetti F, Bonfanti G, et al. Subtotal versus total gastrectomy for cancer of the lower two-thirds of the stomach: a new approach to an old problem. Br J Surg 1986; 73:534–538.

12. Bozzetti F, Marubini E, Bonfanti G, et al. Total versus subtotal gastrectomy for gastric cancer: 5-year survival rates in a multicenter randomized Italian trial. The Italian Gastrointestinal Tumor Study Group. Ann Surg 1999; 230:170–178.

13. Arai K, Kitamura M, Miyashita K. Studies on proximal margin in gastric cancer from the standpoint of discrepancy between macroscopic and histological measurement of invasion. Jpn J Gastroenterol Surg 1993; 26:784–789.

14. Cuschieri A, Weeden S, Fielding J, et al. Patient survival after D1 and D2 resections for gastric cancer: long-term results of the MRC randomized surgical trial. Surgical Co-operative Group. Br J Cancer 1999; 79:1522–1530.

15. Bonenkamp JJ, Hermans J, Sasako M, et al. Extended lymph-node dissection for gastric cancer. Dutch Gastric Cancer Group. N Engl J Med 1999; 340:908–914.

A large-scale randomized study comparing D1 versus D2 gastrectomy.

16. Muruyama K, Sasako M, Kinoshita T, et al. Surgical treatment for gastric cancer: the Japanese experience. Semin Oncol 1996; 23:360–368.

17. Noguchi Y, Imada T, Matsumoto A, et al. Radical gastrectomy for gastric cancer. A review of the Japanese experience. Cancer 1989; 64:2053–2062.

18. Hayes N, Ng EK, Raimes SA, et al. Total gastrectomy with extended lymphadenectomy for 'curable' stomach cancer: experience in a non-Japanese Asian center. J Am Coll Surg 1999; 188:27–32.

19. Siewert JR, Bottcher K, Roder JD, et al. Prognostic relevance of systematic lymph node dissection in gastric carcinoma. German Gastric Carcinoma Study Group. Br J Surg 1993; 80:1015–1018.

20. Shiu MH, Moore E, Sanders M, et al. Influence of the extent of resection on survival after curative treatment of gastric carcinoma. A retrospective multivariate analysis. Arch Surg 1987; 122:1347–1351.

21. McCulloch P, Nita ME, Kazi H, et al. Extended versus limited lymph nodes dissection technique for adenocarcinoma of the stomach. Cochrane Database Syst Rev 2003; (4):CD001964.

A comprehensive review of D1 versus D2 gastrectomy.

22. Mathias JR, Fernandez A, Sninsky CA, et al. Nausea, vomiting and abdominal pain after Roux-en-Y anastomosis: Motility of the jejunal limb. Gastroenterology 1985; 88:101–107.

23. Lehnert T, Buhl K. Techniques of reconstruction after total gastrectomy for cancer. Br J Surg 2004; 91:528–539.

24. Svedlund J, Sullivan M, Liedman B, et al. Long-term consequences of gastrectomy for patients' quality of life: the impact of reconstructive techniques. Am J Gastroenterol 1999; 94:438–445.

25. Shimizu S, Uchiyama A, Mizumoto K, et al. Laparoscopically assisted distal gastrectomy for early gastric cancer: Is it superior to open surgery? Surg Endosc 2000; 14:27–31.

26. Weber KJ, Reyes CD, Gagner M, et al. Comparison of laparoscopic and open gastrectomy for malignant disease. Surg Endosc 2003; 17:968–971.

27. Bruckner H, Lokich J, Stablein D. Studies of Baker's antifoil, methotrexate, and razoxane in advanced gastric cancer: A Gastrointestinal Tumor Study Group report. Cancer Treat Rep 1982; 66:1713–1717.

28. Gastrointestinal Tumor Study Group. Controlled trial of adjuvant chemotherapy following curative resection for gastric cancer. Cancer 1982; 49:1116–1122.

29. Hermans J, Bonenkamp JJ, Boon MC, et al. Adjuvant therapy after curative resection for gastric cancer: meta-analysis of randomized trials. J Clin Oncol 1993; 11:1441–1447.

30. Earle CC, Maroun JA. Adjuvant chemotherapy after curative resection for gastric cancer in non-Asian patients: revisiting a meta-analysis of randomized trials. Eur J Cancer 1999; 35:1059–1064.

31. Panzini I, Gianni L, Fattori PP, et al. Adjuvant chemotherapy in gastric cancer: a meta-analysis of randomized trials and a comparison with previous meta-analyses. Tumori 2002; 88:21–27.

32. Mari E, Floriani I, Tinazzi A, et al. Efficacy of adjuvant chemotherapy after curative resection for gastric cancer: a meta-analysis of

published randomised trials. A study of the GISCAD (Gruppo Italiano per lo Studio dei Carcinomi dell'Apparato Digerente). Ann Oncol 2000; 11:837–843.

33. Janunger KG, Hafstrom L, Glimelius B. Chemotherapy in gastric cancer: a review and updated meta-analysis. Eur J Surg 2002; 168:597–608.

34. Hallissey MT, Dunn JA, Ward LC, et al. The second British Stomach Cancer Group trial of adjuvant radiotherapy or chemotherapy in resectable gastric cancer: five-year follow-up. Lancet 1994; 343:1309–1312.

35. Abe M, Nishimura Y, Shibamoto Y. Intraoperative radiation therapy for gastric cancer. World J Surg 1995; 19:544–547.

36. Macdonald JS, Smalley SR, Benedetti J, et al. Chemoradiotherapy after surgery compared with surgery alone for adenocarcinoma of the stomach or gastroesophageal junction. N Engl J Med 2001; 345:725–730.

 A large-scale randomized study comparing the effect of surgery plus postoperative (adjuvant) chemoradiotherapy.

37. Hundahl SA, Macdonald JS, Benedetti J, et al. Surgical treatment variation in a prospective, randomized trial of chemoradiotherapy in gastric cancer: the effect of undertreatment. Ann Surg Oncol 2002; 9:278–286.

38. Hayes N, Wayman J, Wadehra V, et al. Peritoneal cytology in the surgical evaluation of gastric carcinoma. Br J Cancer 1999; 79:520–524.

39. Kaibara N, Iitsuka Y, Kimura A, et al. Relationship between area of serosal invasion and prognosis in patients with gastric carcinoma. Cancer 1987; 60:136–139.

40. Takahashi T, Hagiwara A, Shimotsuma M, et al. Prophylaxis and treatment of peritoneal carcinomatosis: intraperitoneal chemotherapy with mitomycin C bound to activated carbon particles. World J Surg 1995; 19:565–569.

41. Rosen HR, Jatzko G, Repse S, et al. Adjuvant intraperitoneal chemotherapy with carbon-adsorbed mitomycin in patients with gastric cancer: results of a randomized multicenter trial of the Austrian Working Group for Surgical Oncology. J Clin Oncol 1998; 16:2733–2738.

42. Spratt JS, Adcock RA, Muskovin M, et al. Clinical delivery system for intraperitoneal hyperthermic chemotherapy. Cancer Res 1980; 40:256–260.

43. Yonemura Y, Fujimura T, Nishimura G, et al. Effects of intraoperative chemohyperthermia in patients with gastric cancer with peritoneal dissemination. Surgery 1996; 119:437–444.

44. Fujimoto S, Takahashi M, Mutou T, et al. Successful intraperitoneal hyperthermic chemoperfusion for the prevention of postoperative peritoneal recurrence in patients with advanced gastric carcinoma. Cancer 1999; 85:529–534.

45. Kunisaki C, Shimada H, Nomura M, et al. Lack of efficacy of prophylactic continuous hyperthermic peritoneal perfusion on subsequent peritoneal recurrence and survival in patients with advanced gastric cancer. Surgery 2002; 131:521–528.

46. Samel S, Singal A, Becker H, et al. Problems with intraoperative hyperthermic peritoneal chemotherapy for advanced gastric cancer. Eur J Surg Oncol 2000; 26;222–226.

47. Kollmannsberger C, Quietzsch D, Haag C, et al. A phase II study of paclitaxel, weekly, 24-hour continuous infusion 5-fluorouracil, folinic acid and cisplatin in patients with advanced gastric cancer. Br J Cancer 2000; 83:458–462.

48. Gallardo-Rincon D, Onate-Ocana LF, Calderillo-Ruiz G. Neoadjuvant chemotherapy with P-ELF (cisplatin, etoposide, leucovorin, 5-fluorouracil) followed by radical resection in patients with initially unresectable gastric adenocarcinoma: a phase II study. Ann Surg Oncol 2000; 7:45–50.

49. Schuhmacher CP, Fink U, Becker K, et al. Neoadjuvant therapy for patients with locally advanced gastric carcinoma with etoposide, doxorubicin, and cisplatinum. Closing results after 5 years of follow-up. Cancer 2001; 91:918–927.

50. Ott K, Sendler A, Becker K, et al. Neoadjuvant chemotherapy with cisplatin, 5-FU, and leucovorin (PLF) in locally advanced gastric cancer: a prospective phase II study. Gastric Cancer 2003; 6:159–167.

51. Hallissey MT, Alum WH, Roginski C, et al. Palliative surgery for gastric cancer. Cancer 1988; 62:440–444.

52. Monson FR, Donohue JH, Mcllrath DC, et al. Total gastrectomy for advanced cancer: a worthwhile palliative procedure. Cancer 1991; 68:1863–1868.

53. Leung WK, Ng EKW, Sung JJY. Tumors of the Stomach. In: Yamada T, Alpers DH, Kaplowitz N, et al., eds. Textbook of gastroenterology. 5th edn. Philadelphia: Lippincott Williams & Wilkins; 2003:1416–1440.

54. Schlemper RJ, Itabashi M, Kato Y, et al. Differences in diagnostic criteria for gastric carcinoma between Japanese and Western pathologists. Lancet 1997; 349:1725–1729.

 The first study to demonstrate the potential variability in diagnosis of early gastric cancer by Western and Japanese pathologists.

55. Tsukuma H, Oshima A, Narahara H, et al. Natural history of early gastric cancer: a non-concurrent, long term, follow up study. Gut 2000; 47:618–621.

56. Tada M, Shimada M, Murakami F, et al. Development of the strip biopsy. Gastrointest Endosc 1984; 26:833–839.

57. Ono H, Kondo H, Gotoda T, et al. Endoscopic mucosal resection for treatment of early gastric cancer. Gut 2001; 48:225–229.

 The largest series on EMR for EGC.

58. Uemura N, Mukai T, Okamoto S, et al. Effect of Helicobacter pylori eradication on subsequent development of cancer after endoscopic resection of early gastric cancer. Cancer Epidemiol Biomarkers Prev 1997; 6:639–642.

59. Adachi Y, Shiraishi N, Kitano S. Modern treatment of early gastric cancer: Review of the Japanese experience. Dig Surg 2002; 19:333–339.

60. Rugge M, Cassaro M, Di Mario F, et al. The long term outcome of gastric non-invasive neoplasia. Gut 2003; 52:1111–1116.

61. Parsonnet J, Hansen S, Rodriguez L, et al. Helicobacter pylori infection and gastric lymphoma. N Eng J Med 1994; 330:1267–1271.

62. Musshoff K. Klinische Stadieneinteilung der Nicht-Hodgkin-lymphome. Strahlentherapie 1977; 153:218–221.

63. Puspok A, Raderer M, Chott A, et al. Endoscopic ultrasound in the follow up and response assessment of patients with primary gastric lymphoma. Gut 2002; 51:691–694.

64. Fischbach W, Dragosics B, Kolve-Goebeler ME, et al. Primary gastric B-cell lymphoma: results of a prospective multicenter study. The German-Austrian Gastrointestinal Lymphoma Study Group. Gastroenterology 2000; 119:1191–1202

65. Stolte M, Bayerdorffer E, Morgner A, et al. Helicobacter and gastric MALT lymphoma. Gut 2002; 50(Suppl 3):III19–24.

66. Steinbach G, Ford R, Glober G, et al. Antibiotic treatment of gastric lymphoma of mucosa-associated lymphoid tissue. An uncontrolled trial. Ann Intern Med 1999; 131:88–95.

67. Thiede C, Wundisch T, Alpen B, et al. Long-term persistence of monoclonal B cells after cure of Helicobacter pylori infection and complete histological remission in gastric mucosa-associated lymphoid tissue B-cell lymphoma. J Clin Oncol 2001; 19:1600–1609.

68. Fischbach W, Goebeler-Kolve M, Starostik P, et al. Minimal residual low-grade gastric MALT-type lymphoma after eradication of Helicobacter pylori. Lancet 2002; 360:547–548.

69. Nakamura S, Matsumoto T, Suekane H, et al. Predictive value of endoscopic ultrasonography for regression of gastric low grade and high grade MALT lymphoma after eradication of *Helicobacter pylori*. Gut 2001; 48:454–460.

70. Sackmann M, Morgner A, Rudolph B, et al. Regression of gastric MALT lymphoma after eradication of *Helicobacter pylori* is predicted by endosonographic staging. Gastroenterology 1997; 113:1087–1090.

71. Liu H, Ruskon-Fourmestraux A, Lavergne-Slove A, et al. Resistance of t(11;18) positive gastric mucosa-associated lymphoid tissue lymphoma to *Helicobacter pylori* eradication therapy. Lancet 2001; 357:39–40.

72. Binn M, Ruskone-Fourmestraux A, Lepage E, et al. Surgical resection plus chemotherapy versus chemotherapy alone: comparison of two strategies to treat diffuse large B-cell gastric lymphoma. Ann Oncol 2003; 14:1751–1757.

73. Koch P, del Valle F, Berdel WE, et al. Primary gastrointestinal non-Hodgkin's lymphoma: II. Combined surgical and conservative or conservative management only in localized gastric lymphoma – results of the prospective German Multicenter Study GIT NHL 01/92. J Clin Oncol 2001; 19:3874–3883.

74. Kocher M, Muller RP, Ross D, et al. Radiotherapy for treatment of localized gastrointestinal non-Hodgkin's lymphoma. Radiother Oncol 1997; 42:37–41.

75. Tsang RW, Gospodarowicz MK, Pintilie M, et al: Stage I and II MALT lymphoma: results of treatment with radiotherapy. Int J Radiat Oncol Biol Phys 2001; 50:1258–1264.

76. Hirota S, Isozaki K, Moriyama Y, et al. Gain-of-function mutations of c-kit in human gastrointestinal stromal tumors. Science 1998; 279:577–580.

77. Graadt van Roggen JF, van Velthuysen MLF, Hogendoorn PCW. The histopathological differential diagnosis of gastrointestinal stromal tumours. J Clin Pathol 2001; 54:96–102.

78. DeMatteo RP, Lewis JJ, Leung D, et al. Two hundred gastrointestinal stromal tumors: recurrence patterns and prognostic factors for survival. Ann Surg 2000; 231:51–58.

79. Shiu MH, Farr GH, Papachristou DN, et al. Myosarcomas of the stomach: natural history, prognostic factors and management. Cancer 1982; 49:177–187.

80. Joensuu H, Roberts PJ, Sarlomo-Rikala M, et al. Effect of the tyrosine kinase inhibitor STI571 in a patient with a metastatic gastrointestinal stromal tumor. N Engl J Med 2001; 344:1052–1056.

A proof of concept study that demonstrated the effect of imatinib in metastatic GIST.

81. Demetri GD, von Mehren M, Blanke CD. Efficacy and safety of imatinib mesylate in advanced gastrointestinal stromal tumors. N Engl J Med 2002; 347:472–480.

82. van Oosterom AT, Judson I, Verweij J, et al. Safety and efficacy of imatinib (STI571) in metastatic gastrointestinal stromal tumours: a phase I study. Lancet 2001; 358:1421–1423.

83. Modlin IM, Lye KD, Kidd M. A 5-decade analysis of 13,715 carcinoid tumors. Cancer 2003; 97:934–959.

84. Rindi G, Luinetti O, Cornaggia M, et al. Three subtypes of argyrophilic carcinoid and the gastric neuroendocrine carcinoma. A clinicopathological study. Gastroenterology 1993; 104:994–1006.

85. Lauffer JM, Zhang T, Modlin IM. Review article: current status of gastrointestinal carcinoids. Aliment Pharmacol Ther 1999; 13:271–287.

86. Hirschowitz BI, Griffith J, Pellegrin D, et al. Rapid regression of enterochromaffin cell gastric carcinoids in pernicious anemia after antrectomy. Gastroenterology 1992; 102:1409–1418.

87. Davies MG, O'Dowd G, McEntee GP, et al. Primary gastric carcinoids: a view on management. Br J Surg 1990; 77:1013–1014.

88. Granberg D, Wilander E, Stridsberg M, et al. Clinical symptoms, hormone profiles, treatment, and prognosis in patients with gastric carcinoids. Gut 1998; 43:223–228.

89. Dekker W. Clinical relevance of gastric and duodenal polyps. Scand J Gastroenterol Suppl 1990; 178:7–12.

90. American Society for Gastrointestinal Endoscopy. The role of endoscopy in the surveillance of premalignant conditions of the upper gastrointestinal tract. Gastrointest Endosc 1998; 48:663–668.

25

Biliary tract stones

Christopher S. Huang and David R. Lichtenstein

INTRODUCTION

Epidemiology and risk factors

Gallstone disease ranks as one of the most common digestive disorders. Based on large studies in European and American populations, the prevalence of gallstone disease is approximately 5–25%, but varies significantly among different ethnic populations around the world.[1–3] For example, gallstone disease occurs in epidemic proportions in American Indian populations, with prevalence rates of approximately 30% and 64% in men and women, respectively.[4] In general, gallstone disease is more common in western Caucasian, Hispanic and Native American populations, and less common in eastern European, African-American and Asian populations.

Cholesterol gallstones are the predominant type of stone in the Western world. Several risk factors for the development of gallstone disease besides ethnicity have been identified (Table 25.1). The incidence of gallstones increases with age and is considerably higher in females than in males.[5–7] In Caucasian women under age 50, the prevalence of gallstones ranges 5–15%, and approximately 25–30% thereafter, compared to 4–10% and 10–15%, respectively, in men.[6] Other major risk factors for cholesterol stones include parity, obesity, rapid weight loss, ileal disease, and family history. Certain medications have also been implicated, including oral contraceptives, estrogens, octreotide, and clofibrate.

Pigment stones are distinct from cholesterol stones with respect to epidemiology and risk factors (see Table 25.1). Black pigment stones are associated with chronic hemolysis, alcoholism, and cirrhosis. Brown stones, which occur primarily in Asian populations, are strongly associated with biliary stasis and infection with enteric bacteria.

Pathogenesis

Cholesterol stones

The key steps in the pathogenesis of cholesterol gallstones are supersaturation of bile with cholesterol, nucleation of cholesterol monohydrate crystals, and gallbladder hypomotility.

Cholesterol supersaturation can occur as a result of hypersecretion of cholesterol, hyposecretion of bile acids, or a combination of these defects. Free cholesterol is virtually insoluble in water, but is made soluble through packaging with bile salts and phospholipids, forming structures called mixed micelles. Cholesterol is also solubilized by unilamellar vesicles, which are composed of phospholipid bilayers interdigitated with cholesterol. Mixed micelles and unilamellar vesicles are in dynamic equilibrium, depending on the total bile salt and lipid concentration; as cholesterol saturation increases, more cholesterol is carried in the form of vesicles. Vesicles that have a high cholesterol to phospholipid ratio are meta-stable and have a tendency to aggregate and fuse, leading to nucleation of cholesterol monohydrate crystals.

Table 25.1 Risk factors for gallstone disease

Cholesterol stones	Black pigment stones	Brown pigment stones
Age	Age	Age
Female gender	Female gender	Female gender
Hispanic, Native American ethnicity	Chronic hemolysis	Asian ethnicity
Obesity	Alcoholism	Biliary stasis, infection
Multiparity	Cirrhosis	Periampullary duodenal diverticulum
Rapid weight loss		
Ileal disease		
Family history		

This process is promoted by a variety of pronucleating agents, mainly mucin glycoprotein. The final key step in cholesterol stone formation is gallbladder hypomotility, which leads to the formation of biliary sludge (see below) and permits the growth of crystals into macroscopic stones.

Pigment stones

Black pigment stones are composed primarily of polymeric calcium bilirubinate, with lesser amounts of monomeric calcium bilirubinate, calcium carbonate, and calcium phosphate. The secretion of increased amounts of unconjugated bilirubin into bile (as occurs in hemolytic disorders and cirrhosis) leads to the precipitation of calcium bilirubinate. A defect in bile acidification has also been described, permitting the supersaturation and precipitation of calcium carbonate and phosphate.

Brown pigment stones are composed primarily of monomeric calcium bilirubinate. Biliary stasis and anaerobic bacterial infection are believed to be the key steps in the pathogenesis of brown pigment stones. Enteric bacteria produce β-glucuronidase, phospholipase A, and conjugated bile acid hydrolase, which produce unconjugated bilirubin, palmitic stearic acids, and unconjugated bile acids, respectively. These anionic products can then complex with calcium to produce insoluble calcium salts, leading to stone formation.

GALLSTONES

Clinical presentation

Approximately 80% of patients with gallstones are asymptomatic at the time of diagnosis; it is the subgroup of symptomatic patients who are at highest risk for developing complications, such as recurrent biliary colic, acute cholecystitis, pancreatitis, and cholangitis.[8–10] Symptomatic cholelithiasis typically presents with biliary colic: episodic abdominal pain arising from the upper abdomen or right upper quadrant, with radiation to the upper back.[11,12] The pain is typically steady in nature and can persist for several hours, and does not occur in waves as the term 'colic' implies.[12,13] The pain is frequently provoked by food intake (not necessarily fatty foods only) and may be associated with food intolerance, but these symptoms are non-specific and have little discriminative value.[14] Other 'dyspeptic' symptoms apart from upper abdominal pain, such as belching, bloating, and flatulence, are reported with equal frequency by patients with and without gallstones and have no diagnostic value.[12,13]

Acute cholecystitis is the most common severe complication of gallstones, with an annual incidence of 0.3–0.65%.[15] Acute cholecystitis occurs as a result of persistent cystic duct obstruction, resulting in gallbladder inflammation and, commonly, bacterial superinfection. Clinically, patients present with prolonged abdominal pain similar to that of biliary colic, accompanied by nausea, vomiting, abdominal tenderness, and fever.[16] Laboratory abnormalities commonly include leukocytosis, hyperamylasemia and mildly elevated liver function tests (even in the absence of pancreatitis or choledocholithiasis). The classic finding on physical exam is a positive Murphy's sign (pain and arrested inspiration during palpation of the right upper quadrant), which has a sensitivity of 65% and a specificity of 87%.[16,17] Another physical finding specifically associated with acute cholecystitis is the Boas sign, originally referring to point tenderness in the region to the

right of the T10–T12 vertebrae, but more recently described as hyperesthesia to light touch in the right upper quadrant or infrascapular area.[16] However, because no single clinical finding or laboratory test is completely accurate, diagnostic imaging studies are an integral part of the evaluation of patients with suspected gallstone disease.

Diagnostic imaging studies

Abdominal plain films

Although frequently obtained in the initial evaluation of patients with abdominal pain, plain films lack sensitivity and specificity for gallstones. While over 67% of black pigment stones are radiopaque, fewer than 20% of cholesterol stones can be detected on plain films.[18,19] Nonetheless, plain films may be able to detect severe complications of gallstones, such as gallbladder perforation, emphysematous cholecystitis, pneumobilia, and gallstone ileus.

Abdominal ultrasound

Ultrasonography is the diagnostic imaging study of choice for detection of gallstones, offering several advantages: high sensitivity and specificity (>95%), noninvasiveness, portability, lack of radiation exposure, and relatively low cost.[20–22] The three major ultrasonographic characteristics of gallstones are that they (1) appear as echogenic foci, (2) cast acoustic shadows, and (3) seek gravitational dependency.[21,23] The presence of multiple small stones may appear sonographically as an echogenic layer of 'gravel'. When a contracted gallbladder is filled with stones, the resulting appearance is an echogenic double arc, termed the 'wall-echo-shadow' (WES) sign.

In patients with suspected acute cholecystitis, ultrasonography is usually the initial imaging study of choice. The triad of gallstones, positive sonographic Murphy's sign (maximal tenderness elicited by direct pressure of the transducer over the gallbladder) and intramural edema is the best sonographic indicator of acute cholecystitis (Fig. 25.1).[21,23,24] For diagnosing acute cholecystitis, the positive predictive values of gallstones combined with either a positive sonographic Murphy's sign or gallbladder wall thickening are 92% and 95%, respectively.[25] Other signs of acute

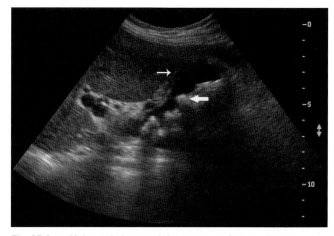

Fig. 25.1 • Abdominal ultrasound demonstrating findings of acute cholecystitis, including diffuse wall thickening (thin arrow), multiple shadowing echogenic gallstones (arrow) and pericholecystic fluid. (Courtesy of Jose Varghese, MD, Boston Medical Center, Boston, MA.)

cholecystitis include pericholecystic fluid, gallbladder distention, and hyperemia of the gallbladder wall.

Cholescintigraphy

Radionuclide cholescintigraphy with [99m]technetium iminodiacetic acid analogues (hydroxyiminodiacetic acid and diisopropyl iminodiacetic acid) is considered a first-line test for diagnosing acute cholecystitis. Cholescintigraphy has a sensitivity of over 95%, specificity of 90–97%, and positive and negative predictive values exceeding 90%.[20,26] The most reliable scintigraphic indicator of acute cholecystitis is nonvisualization of the gallbladder, which implies cystic duct obstruction (Fig. 25.2). The 'rim sign,' referring to increased pericholecystic activity, is also highly predictive of acute cholecystitis.[27] False-positive tests can occur due to prolonged fasting, parenteral nutrition, pancreatitis, and hepatitis. Strategies to reduce the false-positive rate include the adjuvant use of morphine (to induce sphincter of Oddi contraction and promote preferential flow into the gallbladder), or pre-emptying the gallbladder with cholecystokinin (CCK).

Whether abdominal ultrasound or cholescintigraphy is the best test for diagnosing acute cholecystitis remains controversial. Because ultrasound is often performed first for technical or logistical reasons, cholescintigraphy is generally reserved to resolve uncertainty.[26] The diagnosis of acute cholecystitis can be made with certainty if the results of both modalities are concordant, whereas the diagnosis should be reevaluated if discrepancy exists.

Abdominal computed tomography

Computed tomography (CT) has a sensitivity of approximately 75–80% in the detection of gallstones.[28,29] Because stones (particularly cholesterol stones) can have the same radiographic density and attenuation as bile, they may not be well seen on CT. Well-calcified stones, however, are easily detected on CT. Therefore, depending on their composition, stones can have varied appearances on CT, and may be homogeneous or heterogeneous, laminated, rim-calcified, gas-containing, or fissured. Some investigators have advocated the use of CT to predict stone composition during selection of patients for nonsurgical treatment, such as lithotripsy and chemical dissolution.[30]

Although not a first-line test for patients with suspected acute cholecystitis, CT is useful when the clinical presentation is confusing, or when severe complications of gallstone disease are suspected, particularly pericholecystic abscess, emphysematous cholecystitis, hemorrhagic cholecystitis, and gallbladder perforation.[31,32] The most common findings of acute cholecystitis on CT are gallbladder wall thickening, pericholecystic stranding, gallbladder distention, pericholecystic fluid, and subserosal edema (Fig. 25.3). Of these findings, pericholecystic stranding is considered the most specific.[32,33] The sensitivity of CT for diagnosing acute cholecystitis has not been rigorously studied in prospective trials. Therefore, the diagnosis should not be excluded based solely on a normal CT scan.

Oral cholecystography

Although oral cholecystography (OCG) is highly accurate for detecting cholelithiasis, its role has become limited due to the advantages of ultrasonography. When the gallbladder is visualized, the sensitivity and specificity of OCG exceed 90%.[26] Nonvisualization of the gallbladder after two doses of oral contrast is indicative of gallstone disease, but other causes such as intestinal malabsorption and liver disease must be excluded.

TREATMENT OF GALLSTONES

Indications for treatment

The decision to treat should be guided by an understanding of the natural history of gallstone disease, while taking into consideration factors such as risks of treatment, patient preferences, and comorbid conditions. Treatment with cholecystectomy is indicated after an episode of a biliary complication such

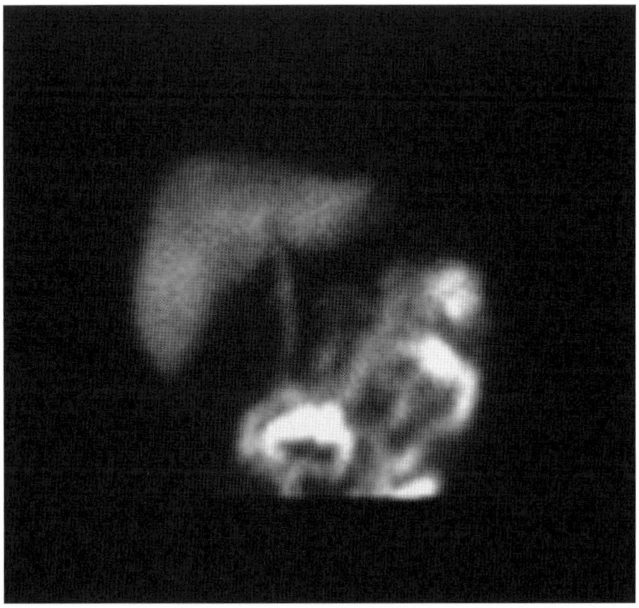

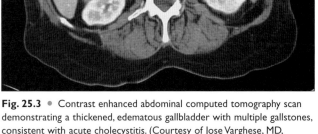

Fig. 25.2 • Radionuclide cholescintigraphy demonstrating nonvisualization of the gallbladder, consistent with acute cholecystitis. (Courtesy of Elizabeth Oates, MD, Boston Medical Center, Boston, MA.)

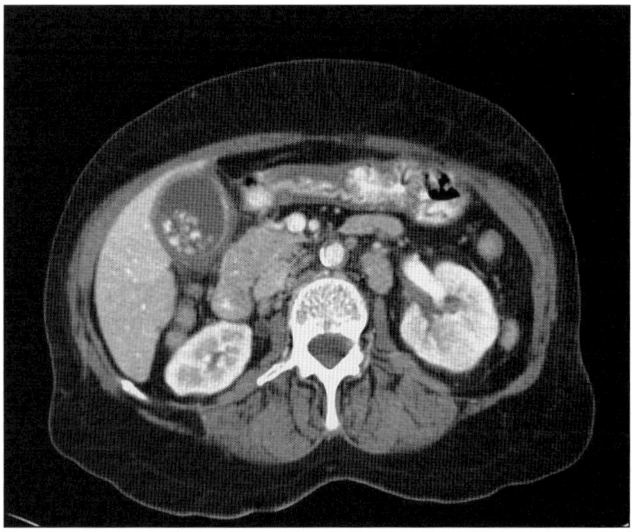

Fig. 25.3 • Contrast enhanced abdominal computed tomography scan demonstrating a thickened, edematous gallbladder with multiple gallstones, consistent with acute cholecystitis. (Courtesy of Jose Varghese, MD, Boston Medical Center, Boston, MA.)

as acute cholecystitis, cholangitis or gallstone pancreatitis, given the high recurrence rate if cholecystectomy is not performed (30% over 3 months).[34,35] Similarly, symptomatic uncomplicated gallstone disease is associated with a high incidence of recurrent pain (40–50% per year), and a 1–3% annual risk of biliary complications.[10,35,36] Elective cholecystectomy is generally recommended in this situation, although studies have shown that life expectancy is extended only a few weeks by surgery, and observation is considered by some to be a safe option.[37,38]

Asymptomatic gallstones appear to have a benign natural history, with symptoms or complications developing in approximately 1–2% per year.[10] Moreover, several studies suggest that in approximately 90% of cases, the initial presentation of previously asymptomatic gallstones is pain, and not a biliary complication.[9,15] Therefore, an expectant approach is appropriate for most of these patients. Certain subgroups of asymptomatic patients may warrant special attention and consideration for prophylactic cholecystectomy, including young patients with sickle cell disease, organ transplant candidates, and those at high risk of gallbladder carcinoma (Pima Indians, patients with large gallstones >3 cm or 'porcelain gallbladder').[39] Whether diabetic patients with asymptomatic gallstones should undergo prophylactic cholecystectomy is discussed below.

Surgical treatment

Cholecystectomy is the treatment of choice for symptomatic or complicated gallstone disease. Laparoscopic cholecystectomy has replaced open cholecystectomy as the 'gold standard' operation for uncomplicated symptomatic gallstones, conferring benefits of lower morbidity and mortality, shorter length of stay, and lower hospital costs.[40,41] Only recently has laparoscopic cholecystectomy become accepted in the treatment of acute cholecystitis.[42–44] In one of the few published prospective, randomized trials comparing laparoscopic versus open cholecystectomy for acute cholecystitis, the laparoscopic approach was associated with a significant reduction in complication rate, duration of hospital stay, and sick leave.[44] However, the rate of conversion to open cholecystectomy was 16%, mainly due to technical difficulties related to unclear anatomy. In contrast, elective surgery for uncomplicated symptomatic gallstone disease has a much lower rate of conversion, generally ranging 4–7%.[45,46] Factors associated with an increased likelihood of conversion to open cholecystectomy in the setting of acute cholecystitis include age >60, male gender, delay in operation (>48 hours from presentation), leukocytosis, obesity, presence of multiple comorbidities, and radiographic evidence of pericholecystic collections or a thickened gallbladder (> 5 mm).[42,46–49]

Patients who are poor candidates for laparoscopic cholecystectomy include those with generalized peritonitis, septic shock from cholangitis, severe acute pancreatitis, end-stage cirrhosis, and gallbladder cancer.[41] Prior upper abdominal surgery can make laparoscopic cholecystectomy more difficult, but is not an absolute contraindication.

Timing of surgery

The optimal timing of cholecystectomy for acute cholecystitis has long been a subject of controversy, recently fueled by the increased acceptance of laparoscopic cholecystectomy in this setting. When open cholecystectomy was the gold standard operation, it was common to allow patients with acute cholecystitis to 'cool down' with medical management, and then operate electively several weeks later. A recent meta-analysis of prospective randomized trials demonstrated no significant difference in rates of operative and perioperative complications between early and delayed cholecystectomy (both open and laparoscopic) for uncomplicated acute cholecystitis.[50] Moreover, early surgery was not associated with an increased risk of choledocholithiasis encountered during surgery or of retained stones post cholecystectomy. Total hospital stay was significantly shorter in the early surgery group, especially for patients undergoing open cholecystectomy. Another important finding from this meta-analysis was that over 20% of patients randomized to delayed surgery failed to respond to medical management or suffered recurrent cholecystitis in the interval period, leading to unplanned urgent surgery in more than 50%. Finally, the conversion rate from laparoscopic to open cholecystectomy was lower in early compared to delayed surgery. Overall, early surgery (within 48–72 hours) should be considered the preferred strategy for patients with uncomplicated acute cholecystitis.[50]

Nonsurgical treatment options

The role for nonsurgical treatment of gallstone disease has decreased in recent years with the advances in laparoscopic cholecystectomy. However, nonsurgical treatment, primarily with oral bile acid therapy, direct contact dissolution, and/or extracorporeal shock wave lithotripsy, remains an effective alternative to cholecystectomy in selected patients with symptomatic gallstone disease who refuse surgery or are not fit for surgery. Percutaneous cholecystostomy as a treatment option for high-risk patients with acute cholecystitis is also discussed in this section.

Oral bile acid therapy

Oral bile acid therapy with chenodeoxycholic acid (CDCA) and ursodeoxycholic acid (UDCA) has been shown to be effective in dissolving cholesterol gallstones. These agents reduce cholesterol saturation and effect dissolution by a number of mechanisms, such as inhibiting biliary secretion of cholesterol, enriching the bile acid pool, promoting liquid crystal formation and transferring cholesterol into micelles and vesicles. A meta-analysis found that UDCA in doses greater than 7 mg/kg/day taken for at least 6 months dissolved radiolucent gallstones in 37% of patients.[51] Long-term use of UDCA has also been shown to reduce the risk of biliary pain and acute cholecystitis in patients with symptomatic gallstones.[52] The effectiveness of oral bile acid therapy is highly dependent on proper patient selection, taking into account gallbladder function and gallstone size, number, and composition. Favorable criteria include small stone size (<1 cm), preserved gallbladder function with a patent cystic duct, and buoyant, radiolucent stones without calcification.[52,53]

Chenodeoxycholic acid therapy is associated with several dose-related side effects, most notably diarrhea and increased serum transaminases and cholesterol levels. Use of low-dose CDCA (5 mg/kg/day) in combination with UDCA has been advocated by some,[54] but it is not clear whether combination therapy is more effective than UDCA alone.[55,56]

Stone recurrence occurs in 50–60% of patients after 11 years of follow-up, with a plateau after 5–9 years.[57,58] The presence of multiple stones before dissolution therapy is associated with a higher risk of recurrence.[58]

Contact dissolution therapy

Direct contact dissolution therapy of cholesterol gallstones can be achieved with the use of a potent organic solvent, methyl tert-butyl ether (MTBE). This therapy requires direct infusion of MTBE into the gallbladder via a catheter placed transhepatically or endoscopically. Successful dissolution (95–100% complete) can be achieved in over 95% of properly selected patients.[59,60] The radiologic selection criteria are similar to those for oral bile acid therapy, although stones of any size or number can be successfully treated with MTBE provided they are radiolucent.

Complications of MTBE therapy include those related to gallbladder cannulation (bleeding, bile leak) and direct toxicity of the solvent. Passage of MTBE into the duodenum can result in duodenitis, and excessive absorption can cause hemolysis, drowsiness, confusion and anesthesia.[61]

Extracorporeal shock wave lithotripsy

Extracorporeal shock wave lithotripsy (ESWL) uses acoustic shock waves to fragment stones into small pieces, which can then pass into the small intestine or be dissolved with oral bile acid therapy. Concomitant use of UDCA is more effective than lithotripsy alone, and equally safe.[62] When combined with oral bile acid dissolution therapy, ESWL results in complete gallstone clearance in 90% of patients by 12–18 months.[63] Eligibility criteria for ESWL include (1) a history of biliary colic in the absence of complications, (2) a solitary radiolucent stone with a diameter of up to 30 mm, or up to 3 stones with a similar total stone mass, (3) normal gallbladder function with a patent cystic duct, and (4) successful positioning of stones in the shock wave focus, avoiding lungs and bone. Contraindications include coagulopathy or platelet abnormalities, cystic or vascular lesions of the liver, pregnancy, and acute gallstone-related complications.

As with the other nonsurgical treatment modalities, stone recurrence after ESWL is a significant problem, occurring in approximately 20–30% of patients within 4–5 years despite concomitant oral bile acid therapy.[64] Moreover, stone recurrence is frequently associated with recurrence of biliary pain. The presence of multiple stones before ESWL, impaired gallbladder function, estrogen intake, number of lithotripsy sessions, and time until stone disappearance are predictive of stone recurrence.[65–67]

Percutaneous cholecystostomy

Percutaneous cholecystostomy is a safe and effective alternative to emergent cholecystectomy in high-risk, critically ill patients with acute cholecystitis who do not respond to medical therapy.[68,69] It is a minimally invasive procedure that can be performed at the bedside, with response rates in the literature of 56–100%.[68] Response rates are higher in patients with clinical symptoms and signs referable to the gallbladder, such as right upper quadrant pain/tenderness or a positive sonographic Murphy's sign, and radiologic findings of pericholecystic fluid.[70,71] Major complications related to percutaneous cholecystostomy occur in <10% of patients, and include bile peritonitis, hemorrhage, catheter dislodgement, vasovagal reaction, and colonic injury.

Percutaneous cholecystostomy is best utilized as a temporizing measure in the setting of acute calculous cholecystitis; interval laparoscopic cholecystectomy is generally recommended following resolution of the acute illness, provided the patient is a surgical candidate.

COMMON BILE DUCT STONES

Choledocholithiasis, or common bile duct (CBD) stones, can be classified as primary (originating within the bile ducts) or secondary (migrating into the bile ducts from the gallbladder). The latter are more common in Western countries, occurring in approximately 8–18% of patients under age 60 years undergoing cholecystectomy, and 15–60% of those over age 60 years.[41,72,73] Choledocholithiasis can be asymptomatic or associated with complications such as obstructive jaundice, cholangitis, and pancreatitis. Secondary biliary cirrhosis due to prolonged obstruction from choledocholithiasis can occur, albeit rarely. Therefore, it is important to identify and treat patients with CBD stones in order to prevent these complications.

Predictors of choledocholithiasis

Several clinical, biochemical, and noninvasive radiographic parameters can predict the presence of choledocholithiasis (Table 25.2), but no single criterion is completely accurate. Presentation with cholangitis or jaundice has positive predictive values (PPVs) of 75–100% and 72%, respectively. Pancreatitis alone is a weaker predictor, with a reported PPV of 10–20% in patients with mild pancreatitis, but as high as 60% in those with severe pancreatitis.[74,75]

Among the biochemical parameters, elevations in serum bilirubin, aspartate aminotransferase, or alkaline phosphatase have been found to be independent predictors of choledocholithiasis.[76,77] The combination of a bilirubin level >3.0 mg/dL and alkaline phosphatase >250 U/L has a PPV of over 75%.[78]

Finally, noninvasive imaging, generally with ultrasonography, is useful in predicting the presence of choledocholithiasis. A CBD stone visualized on ultrasound is highly specific and increases the likelihood of choledocholithiasis over 13-fold;[73] however, this finding has a sensitivity of only 40–50%.[74,79] Ultrasound evidence of CBD dilation is also a strong predictor, increasing the likelihood of choledocholithiasis nearly 7-fold.[73,80] Although not commonly used for this indication, radionuclide cholescintigraphy has been reported to be very accurate in diagnosing CBD obstruction,[81] with a sensitivity and specificity of 83–84% for choledocholithiasis.[74]

Overall, the three most powerful clinical, noninvasive predictors of choledocholithiasis are cholangitis, preoperative jaundice, and identification of common bile duct stones on ultrasound.[73] Since no single test is completely accurate in predicting CBD stones, the decision whether further diagnostic testing is warranted should be based on the integration of clinical, biochemical, and radiographic information.

Diagnostic imaging studies

Endoscopic retrograde cholangiopancreatography

Direct cholangiography is the 'gold standard' diagnostic test for the detection of choledocholithiasis. This can be performed via percutaneous transhepatic cholangiography (PTC), intraoperative

Table 25.2 Predictors of choledocholithiasis

Category	Condition	Sensitivity	Specificity	Positive likelihood ratio
Clinical	Cholangitis	0.11–0.42	0.99	18.3
	Jaundice	0.36–0.69	0.89–0.97	10.1
	Pancreatitis	0.10–0.12	0.95	2.1
	Cholecystitis	0.50	0.76	1.6
Biochemical	Bilirubin	0.69–0.77	0.88	4.8
	Alkaline phosphatase	0.57–0.70	0.86	2.6
	Amylase	0.11	0.95	1.5
Radiographic	CBD stone on ultrasound	0.38–0.50	0.97–1.00	13.6
	Dilated CBD on ultrasound	0.42–0.85	0.82–0.96	6.9
	HIDA scan: partial/complete obstruction	0.83	0.84	–

Data from Abboud 1996[73], and Bose 2001[74].

cholangiography (IOC), or endoscopic retrograde cholangiopancreatography (ERCP). Of these, ERCP is currently the most commonly used; in experienced hands, ERCP has a sensitivity, specificity, and accuracy each exceeding 95%, and can detect stones as small as 2 mm in diameter (Fig. 25.4).[82] An advantage of ERCP is the ability to perform endoscopic sphincterotomy and stone extraction at the time of diagnosis (see below). However, there is a small but significant risk of complications including pancreatitis, hemorrhage, perforation, and cholangitis, as well as adverse reactions to sedatives and cardiopulmonary dysfunction.[83] Most prospective studies report an overall short-term complication rate for ERCP with or without sphincterotomy of 5–10%.[84–86] Therefore, because of these risks, along with recent advances in noninvasive imaging, the use of ERCP in many institutions has become limited to therapeutic, rather than purely diagnostic, indications. It remains the initial test of choice for the treatment of patients with a high likelihood of choledocholithiasis based on clinical, biochemical, and radiographic data.[82] As such, ERCP is the preferred test in patients with cholangitis and/or severe gallstone pancreatitis because these patients benefit from early therapeutic intervention.[87–89]

Magnetic resonance cholangiopancreatography

Since its introduction over a decade ago, magnetic resonance cholangiopancreatography (MRCP) has evolved into a highly accurate, noninvasive method of imaging the biliary tree (Fig. 25.5).[90] Current techniques can image the entire biliary system in a single breath-hold and provide high spatial resolution. Studies examining the performance of MRCP for the diagnosis of choledocholithiasis have generally used ERCP as the reference standard. Recent studies have shown good concordance between the two modalities, with sensitivities and specificities both exceeding 90% for MRCP.[79,91,92] The sensitivity of MRCP varies according to the size of the stone, ranging from approximately 70% for 3–5 mm stones, to 90% for 6–10 mm stones, to 100% for stones larger than 10 mm in diameter.[93]

The major advantages of MRCP are that it is noninvasive and eliminates the risks associated with sedation, instrumentation, contrast administration, and ionizing radiation. Moreover, MRCP can provide complete evaluation of the biliary tree in patients with surgically altered upper gastrointestinal tracts (e.g., Billroth

II anastomosis, Roux-en-Y anastomosis), in whom ERCP may be difficult or impossible. The major limitation of MRCP is that it is a purely diagnostic test and has no therapeutic capability. Therefore, its optimal use is as a screening examination for the detection or exclusion of CBD stones in patients with a low or intermediate probability of harboring stones, sparing such patients a potentially unnecessary ERCP.[90]

Endoscopic ultrasound

Endoscopic ultrasound (EUS) is another alternative to ERCP, with the advantages of being less invasive and having a lower risk of complications.[94] For the diagnosis of choledocholithiasis, EUS is comparable to ERCP and MRCP with respect to sensitivity, specificity, and positive and negative predictive values.[82,95,96] The CBD can also be imaged via intraductal ultrasound (IDUS) using

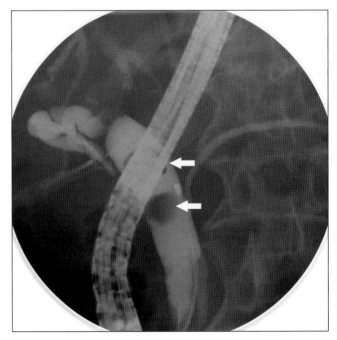

Fig. 25.4 • Endoscopic retrograde cholangiopancreatography demonstrating two large stones in the common bile duct (arrows), corresponding to the images shown in Figure 25.5.

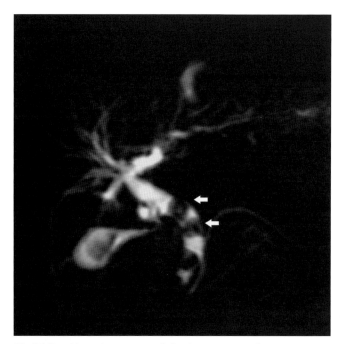

Fig. 25.5 • Magnetic resonance cholangiopancreatography demonstrating multiple common bile duct stones (arrows), which were subsequently confirmed and removed during endoscopic retrograde cholangiopancreatography (Fig. 25.4).

a high-frequency catheter US probe inserted through the accessory channel of a standard endoscope or duodenoscope. In conjunction with ERCP, IDUS significantly increases diagnostic accuracy compared to ERCP alone, especially in the presence of a dilated CBD.[97] Given its safety and excellent negative predictive value, EUS is considered a first-line diagnostic test in patients who are at low or intermediate risk for choledocholithiasis.[82] However, because of limitations in EUS training, experience, and availability, as well as the continued refinement of MRCP technology, EUS has not been widely adopted for this indication.

TREATMENT OF COMMON BILE DUCT STONES

Endoscopic treatment

ERCP with endoscopic sphincterotomy and stone extraction has become the primary therapeutic modality for choledocholithiasis, with success rates exceeding 80% using standard techniques.[98] Advanced techniques for difficult bile duct stones, including mechanical, electrohydraulic, laser, or extracorporeal shockwave lithotripsy, increase the success rate to nearly 100%.[98,99]

Standard techniques for endoscopic treatment of choledocholithiasis include ERCP with sphincterotomy, usually in combination with balloon or wire basket stone extraction. Endoscopic papillary balloon dilation (EPBD) has been proposed as an alternative to sphincterotomy, with a purported benefit of preserving sphincter of Oddi function. EPBD should be considered in selected patients with cirrhosis, coagulopathy, or altered anatomy (e.g., large periampullary diverticulum or Billroth II anatomy).[100] However, endoscopic sphincterotomy remains the preferred technique

because of higher rates of successful stone clearance and possibly lower rates of procedure-induced pancreatitis compared to EPBD.[101]

Endoscopic biliary stenting is an effective temporizing measure in cases of difficult bile duct stones that cannot be extracted by standard techniques. Stenting provides immediate biliary drainage, and occasionally leads to stone resolution or fragmentation, permitting subsequent endoscopic extraction.[102] Stenting has also been used as the sole therapy for difficult CBD stones, but because of the risk of late complications, particularly cholangitis, this should be restricted to highly selected patients unfit for other more definitive treatments.

Surgical treatment

When laparoscopic cholecystectomy replaced open surgery as the preferred treatment of symptomatic gallstones, it was initially unclear whether laparoscopic IOC and LCBDE would be feasible, safe, and cost-effective. Accumulating experience from specialty centers has demonstrated successful duct clearance rates exceeding 90%, with relatively low morbidity rates of approximately 8–10%.[103,104] LCBDE has the advantage of being a one-stage procedure for patients with choledocholithiasis, thereby avoiding the risks of ERCP and sphincterotomy without compromising effectiveness of bile duct clearance, and conferring the additional benefits of shorter hospital stay and reduced costs.[105,106]

Two laparoscopic approaches to LCBDE have been developed: transcystic and transductal (via choledochotomy). The former approach is generally preferred when feasible, because it is less invasive and results in shorter hospital stay than transductal LCBDE.[107] CBD stones documented on laparoscopic IOC can then be retrieved with wire baskets, with or without the use of choledochoscopy or fluoroscopy. Intraoperative electrohydraulic or laser lithotripsy techniques are available but have not been widely used.

If LCBDE is unsuccessful, biliary drainage can be achieved by placing a transcystic duct catheter inserted through a separate abdominal wall puncture, or by placing a standard T tube or biliary stent via choledochotomy. Alternatively, the procedure can be converted to open CBD exploration unless expert endoscopists are available, in which case postoperative ERCP should be performed.

Percutaneous treatment

Percutaneous treatment of CBD stones should be considered when surgical and endoscopic modalities fail, are unavailable, or cannot be safely performed. Several percutaneous methods of duct clearance have been performed with success rates of 75–90%, including basket extraction, mechanical lithotripsy, and ESWL or electrohydraulic lithotripsy under cholangioscopic guidance. Stones smaller than 1 cm can also be pushed through the papilla following transhepatic papillary balloon dilation.[108–110]

A 'rendezvous' procedure can be performed if the ampulla can be reached endoscopically but retrograde cannulation is unsuccessful. In this approach, a guidewire is placed percutaneously into the bile ducts, traversing the papilla into the duodenum. This facilitates localization and cannulation of the papilla, allowing endoscopic sphincterotomy and stone extraction to be safely completed.[111]

SPECIAL CONSIDERATIONS

Gallbladder sludge

Gallbladder sludge is composed of suspension of cholesterol monohydrate crystals, calcium bilirubinate, and other calcium salts embedded in gallbladder mucus. Specific clinical situations commonly associated with sludge formation include pregnancy, rapid weight loss, prolonged fasting, long-term parenteral nutrition, bone marrow or solid organ transplantation, and the use ceftriaxone and octreotide.

Sludge is usually diagnosed on abdominal ultrasound, where it appears as low-level echoes that layer dependently without acoustic shadows. However, the sensitivity of transabdominal ultrasound for sludge is only about 55%.[112] Direct microscopic examination of bile, although less clinically applicable, is more sensitive than ultrasonography, and is considered the diagnostic gold standard.

The natural history of sludge is variable, with three main clinical outcomes: complete resolution, a waxing and waning course, and gallstone formation.[113] Like gallstones, sludge is most often asymptomatic; elimination of precipitating factors and expectant observation are recommended in this situation. However, sludge can also be complicated by biliary colic (in approximately 10% of patients), and less commonly by acute pancreatitis, cholangitis, and cholecystitis. Once symptoms or complications occur, cholecystectomy should be considered as the definitive therapy. Alternatively, oral bile acid dissolution therapy with UDCA can be attempted, although its long-term efficacy has not been proven.

Acute cholangitis

Acute cholangitis occurs as a result of biliary stasis and infection, and is most commonly due to choledocholithiasis. The classic presentation of acute cholangitis is characterized by Charcot's triad of fever, right upper quadrant pain, and jaundice, which is seen in approximately 50–75% of patients.[114] The presence of hypotension and altered mental status (Reynold's pentad) indicates severe infection termed suppurative cholangitis.

All patients with acute cholangitis should be treated with broad-spectrum antibiotics to cover against Gram-negative aerobic enteric organisms (*Escherichia coli*, *Klebsiella*, *Enterobacter*), Gram-positive *Enterococcus*, and anaerobic bacteria (*Bacteroides fragilis*, *Clostridium perfringens*). Urgent biliary decompression is required in patients with suppurative cholangitis and those who fail to respond to antibiotic therapy (approximately 20% of patients), whereas decompression can be safely delayed in patients who respond to antibiotics.[115] Urgent endoscopic decompression should also be considered for patients with adverse prognostic indicators, such as the presence of comorbid medical conditions, thrombocytopenia, azotemia, and hypoalbuminemia. The preferred method of biliary decompression is via ERCP, which has been shown to reduce morbidity and mortality rates compared to surgical therapy.[116]

Gallstone pancreatitis

Gallstone disease is one of the most common causes of acute pancreatitis in North America and Western Europe. Most patients have a mild clinical course and can be conservatively managed with intravenous fluids, bowel rest, and analgesia. Elective cholecystectomy should then be performed once the acute illness has resolved, preferably during the same admission.[117]

Patients with gallstone pancreatitis who have evidence of biliary obstruction, those who deteriorate after an initial mild attack, or those presenting with severe pancreatitis at the outset should be considered for urgent ERCP.[98] Pooled data from four randomized, controlled trials have demonstrated a convincing role for early ERCP and sphincterotomy (within 72 hours of presentation) in patients with *severe* gallstone pancreatitis.[87,89,118,119] A meta-analysis of these trials found statistically significant reductions in overall complications and mortality in patients treated with early ERCP with sphincterotomy compared with those treated conservatively.[120] There is no clear benefit in patients with mild pancreatitis, or in those without obstructive jaundice.[98,118]

Cholecystectomy should be performed following an episode of acute gallstone pancreatitis, but can be safely delayed after sphincterotomy. Endoscopic sphincterotomy is a viable alternative to cholecystectomy for the prevention of recurrent gallstone pancreatitis in high surgical risk patients.[121] Depending on length of follow-up, recurrence rates of gallstone pancreatitis following sphincterotomy with gallbladder in situ are low, ranging 0–5%.[121–123] However, sphincterotomy cannot prevent future episodes of other biliary complications such as recurrent biliary colic and acute cholecystitis if a stone-containing gallbladder remains intact (see below).

Gallbladder in situ

The clinical course of patients with gallbladder in situ following endoscopic sphincterotomy and bile duct clearance is controversial, hence the issue of 'prophylactic' cholecystectomy remains a matter of debate. Several retrospective and nonrandomized prospective studies with varying duration of follow-up have reported symptomatic recurrence or cholecystectomy rates ranging 5–20%, lending support both for and against the need for prophylactic cholecystectomy.[124–127] A recent prospective randomized trial compared a 'wait and see' approach with prophylactic laparoscopic cholecystectomy following endoscopic sphincterotomy in patients with proven gallbladder stones.[128] This study found that after a median follow-up of 30 months, 47% of patients being followed expectantly developed at least one recurrent biliary event, most commonly uncomplicated pain, compared to 2% of patients who underwent cholecystectomy. Acute cholecystitis occurred in 12% of patients in the former group, and 37% required 'on demand' cholecystectomy.

Possible risk factors for recurrence of biliary complications following sphincterotomy with gallbladder in situ include bile duct diameter >15 mm, periampullary diverticula, diabetes, acute cholangitis or gallstone pancreatitis at the time of sphincterotomy, nonfilling of the gallbladder on cholangiography, and brown pigment stones at initial ERCP.[123,124,128–130]

Pregnancy

Alterations in cholesterol secretion and gallbladder motility are thought to contribute to an increased risk of gallstones and biliary sludge during pregnancy. Biliary colic develops in up to a third of pregnant women with gallstones.[131,132] Symptomatic gallstone disease can be managed conservatively in the majority of cases, with definitive therapy deferred until the postpartum period. However, endoscopic and/or surgical therapy are indicated when biliary complications arise, including acute cholecystitis unresponsive to medical therapy, choledocholithiasis, and severe gallstone pancreatitis.[133] With early involvement of the obstetrics team, perioperative fetal monitoring, and the appropriate use of tocolytic agents, laparoscopic cholecystectomy can be safely performed during any stage of pregnancy.[134] Similarly, ERCP and sphincterotomy are safe during pregnancy, but measures should be taken to minimize radiation exposure to the fetus, such as limiting fluoroscopy time or confirming biliary cannulation by bile aspiration into the ERCP catheter (rather than contrast injection), shielding the pelvis with lead, and avoiding hard copy radiographs.[135,136]

Diabetes

Early studies suggested that diabetic patients with gallstones were at increased risk for severe complications from acute cholecystitis, and had higher morbidity and mortality rates from cholecystectomy.[137] Specific complications such as perforation, gangrenous cholecystitis, and emphysematous cholecystitis have been reported to occur in up to 20–40% of diabetics.[138] Increased susceptibility

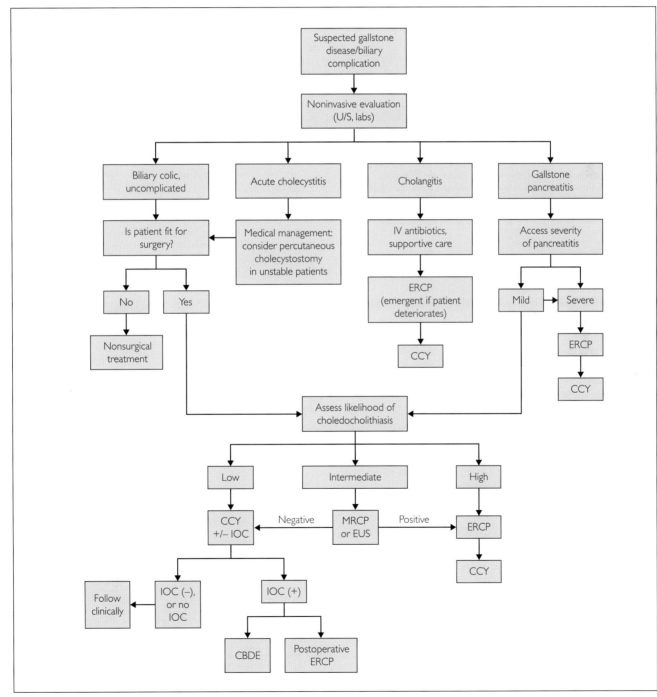

Fig. 25.6 • Algorithm outlining the authors' recommendations for the management of gallstones

Table 25.3 Author's recommendations for the management of gallstones

Gallstones

Ultrasonography is the diagnostic test of choice for cholelithiasis and acute cholecystitis.

Observation is recommended for the vast majority of patients with asymptomatic gallstones.

Laparoscopic cholecystectomy is the treatment of choice for symptomatic cholelithiasis, and can be safely performed for acute cholecystitis by surgeons with expertise in laparoscopic surgery.

Early cholecystectomy (within 48–72 hours) is the preferred treatment approach for patients with acute, uncomplicated cholecystitis.

Common bile duct stones

Cholangitis, jaundice, and identification of common bile duct stones on noninvasive imaging are the best predictors of choledocholithiasis.

ERCP should be reserved for therapeutic indications, but remains the test of choice for treatment of patients with a high likelihood of choledocholithiasis and patients with cholangitis or severe gallstone pancreatitis.

MRCP, EUS, or IOC is recommended when the probability of choledocholithiasis is intermediate. Common bile duct stones can then be removed by pre- or postoperative ERCP, or intraoperatively by LCBDE, depending on local expertise.

to infection, as well as comorbidities commonly associated with diabetes (e.g., cardiovascular and renal disease), are largely responsible for these severe complications. These concerns led to the initial recommendation for prophylactic cholecystectomy in all diabetic patients with gallstones. This recommendation has been challenged by more recent studies showing comparable rates of mortality and serious complications in diabetics undergoing cholecystectomy when compared with appropriate controls.[139–142] Furthermore, the natural history of asymptomatic gallstones in diabetics has been shown to be similar to that in the general population, with approximately 15% of initially asymptomatic patients developing biliary pain or complications over 5 years.[143] Therefore, based on the currently available data, prophylactic cholecystectomy in asymptomatic diabetics with gallstones should not be routinely recommended.[142]

Chronic liver disease

Gallstones (mainly black pigment stones) occur more commonly in cirrhotic patients than in the general population, with prevalence rates of 20–30%.[144–146] A recent case-control study showed that advanced age, female gender, viral etiology of cirrhosis, family history of gallstones, and duration of gallstone disease were risk factors for developing symptomatic gallstones in cirrhotic patients.[147] Elective laparoscopic cholecystectomy can be safely performed in symptomatic patients with compensated cirrhosis (Child Pugh class A or B).[148] Given the high surgical risk in those with decompensated cirrhosis (Child Pugh class C), nonsurgical treatments should be strongly considered in these patients.[149]

SUMMARY

Recommendations for the management of gallstones are summarized in Table 25.3 and in Figure 25.6.

REFERENCES

1. Attili AF, Carulli N, Roda E, et al. Epidemiology of gallstone disease in Italy: prevalence data of the Multicenter Italian Study on Cholelithiasis (MICOL). Am J Epidemiol 1995; 141:158–165.

2. Barbara L, Sama C, Morselli Labate AM, et al. A population study on the prevalence of gallstone disease: the Sirmione Study. Hepatology 1987; 7:913–917.

3. Everhart JE, Khare M, Hill M, et al. Prevalence and ethnic differences in gallbladder disease in the United States. Gastroenterology 1999; 117:632–639.

4. Everhart JE, Yeh F, Lee ET, et al. Prevalence of gallbladder disease in American Indian populations: findings from the Strong Heart Study. Hepatology 2002; 35:1507–1512.

5. Cooper AD, Young HS. Pathophysiology and treatment of gallstones. Med Clin North Am 1989; 73:753–774.

6. Diehl AK. Epidemiology and natural history of gallstone disease. Gastroenterol Clin North Am 1991; 20:1–19.

   This article provides an excellent review on the risk factors for gallstone disease. A short section on the natural history of gallstones is also included, highlighting the differences between silent and symptomatic stones.

7. Bowen JC, Brenner HI, Ferrante WA, et al. Gallstone disease. Pathophysiology, epidemiology, natural history, and treatment options. Med Clin North Am 1992; 76:1143–1157.

8. Browning JD, Horton JD. Gallstone disease and its complications. Semin Gastrointest Dis 2003; 14:165–177.

9. Gracie WA, Ransohoff DF. The natural history of silent gallstones: the innocent gallstone is not a myth. N Engl J Med 1982; 307:798–800.

10. Friedman GD. Natural history of asymptomatic and symptomatic gallstones. Am J Surg 1993; 165:399–404.

11. Diehl AK. Symptoms of gallstone disease. Baillières Clin Gastroenterol 1992; 6:635–657.

12. Diehl AK, Sugarek NJ, Todd KH. Clinical evaluation for gallstone disease: usefulness of symptoms and signs in diagnosis. Am J Med 1990; 89:29–33.

13. Talley NJ. Gallstones and upper abdominal discomfort. Innocent bystander or a cause of dyspepsia? J Clin Gastroenterol 1995; 20:182–183.

14. Berger MY, van der Velden JJ, Lijmer JG, et al. Abdominal symptoms: do they predict gallstones? A systematic review. Scand J Gastroenterol 2000; 35:70–76.

15. Attili AF, De Santis A, Capri R, et al. The natural history of gallstones: the GREPCO experience. The GREPCO Group. Hepatology 1995; 21:655–660.

16. Trowbridge RL, Rutkowski NK, Shojania KG. Does this patient have acute cholecystitis? JAMA 2003; 289:80–86.

17. Adedeji OA, McAdam WA. Murphy's sign, acute cholecystitis and elderly people. J R Coll Surg Edinb 1996; 41:88–89.

18. Trotman BW, Petrella EJ, Soloway RD, et al. Evaluation of radiographic lucency or opaqueness of gallstones as a means of identifying cholesterol or pigment stones. Correlation of lucency or opaqueness with calcium and mineral. Gastroenterology 1975; 68:1563–1566.

19. Dolgin SM, Schwartz JS, Kressel HY, et al. Identification of patients with cholesterol or pigment gallstones by discriminant analysis of radiographic features. N Engl J Med 1981; 304:808–811.

20. Shea JA, Berlin JA, Escarce JJ, et al. Revised estimates of diagnostic test sensitivity and specificity in suspected biliary tract disease. Arch Intern Med 1994; 154:2573–2581.

21. Gore RM, Yaghmai V, Newmark GM, et al. Imaging benign and malignant disease of the gallbladder. Radiol Clin North Am 2002; 40:1307–1323, vi.

22. Bortoff GA, Chen MY, Ott DJ, et al. Gallbladder stones: imaging and intervention. Radiographics 2000; 20:751–766.

23. Zeman RK, Garra BS. Gallbladder imaging. The state of the art. Gastroenterol Clin North Am 1991; 20:127–156.

24. Laing FC, Federle MP, Jeffrey RB, et al. Ultrasonic evaluation of patients with acute right upper quadrant pain. Radiology 1981; 140:449–455.

25. Ralls PW, Colletti PM, Lapin SA, et al. Real-time sonography in suspected acute cholecystitis. Prospective evaluation of primary and secondary signs. Radiology 1985; 155:767–771.

26. Marton KI, Doubilet P. How to image the gallbladder in suspected cholecystitis. Ann Intern Med 1988; 109:722–729.

27. Brachman MB, Goodman MD, Waxman AD. The rim sign in acute cholecystitis. Comparison of radionuclide, surgical, and pathologic findings. Clin Nucl Med 1993; 18:863–866.

28. Barakos JA, Ralls PW, Lapin SA, et al. Cholelithiasis: evaluation with CT. Radiology 1987; 162:415–418.

29. Van Beers BE, Pringot JH. Imaging of cholelithiasis: helical CT. Abdom Imaging 2001; 26:15–20.

30. Brink JA, Kammer B, Mueller PR, et al. Prediction of gallstone composition: synthesis of CT and radiographic features in vitro. Radiology 1994; 190:69–75.

31. Bennett GL, Balthazar EJ. Ultrasound and CT evaluation of emergent gallbladder pathology. Radiol Clin North Am 2003; 41:1203–1216.

32. Paulson EK. Acute cholecystitis: CT findings. Semin Ultrasound CT MR 2000; 21:56–63.

33. Fidler J, Paulson EK, Layfield L. CT evaluation of acute cholecystitis: findings and usefulness in diagnosis. AJR Am J Roentgenol 1996; 166:1085–1088.

34. Jarvinen HJ, Hastbacka J. Early cholecystectomy for acute cholecystitis: a prospective randomized study. Ann Surg 1980; 191:501–505.

35. Ransohoff DF, Gracie WA. Treatment of gallstones. Ann Intern Med 1993; 119:606–619.

36. Thistle JL, Cleary PA, Lachin JM, et al. The natural history of cholelithiasis: the National Cooperative Gallstone Study. Ann Intern Med 1984; 101:171–175.

37. Ransohoff DF, Gracie WA. Management of patients with symptomatic gallstones: a quantitative analysis. Am J Med 1990; 88:154–160.

38. Vetrhus M, Soreide O, Solhaug JH, et al. Symptomatic, non-complicated gallbladder stone disease. Operation or observation? A randomized clinical study. Scand J Gastroenterol 2002; 37:834–839.

39. Schwesinger WH, Diehl AK. Changing indications for laparoscopic cholecystectomy. Stones without symptoms and symptoms without stones. Surg Clin North Am 1996; 76:493–504.

40. Zacks SL, Sandler RS, Rutledge R, et al. A population-based cohort study comparing laparoscopic cholecystectomy and open cholecystectomy. Am J Gastroenterol 2002; 97:334–340.

41. Gallstones and laparoscopic cholecystectomy. NIH Consens Statement 1992; 10:1–28.

42. Prakash K, Jacob G, Lekha V, et al. Laparoscopic cholecystectomy in acute cholecystitis. Surg Endosc 2002; 16:180–183.

43. Lujan JA, Parrilla P, Robles R, et al. Laparoscopic cholecystectomy vs open cholecystectomy in the treatment of acute cholecystitis: a prospective study. Arch Surg 1998; 133:173–175.

44. Kiviluoto T, Siren J, Luukkonen P, et al. Randomised trial of laparoscopic versus open cholecystectomy for acute and gangrenous cholecystitis. Lancet 1998; 351:321–325.

This study, conducted in Finland, is one of the few published randomized trials comparing laparoscopic cholecystectomy with open cholecystectomy in the treatment of acute cholecystitis. Although the study sample size was relatively small, the authors did demonstrate statistically significant reductions in postoperative complication rates and length of hospital stay in patients treated laparoscopically. The rate of conversion from laparoscopic to open surgery was relatively high (16%).

45. Bingener-Casey J, Richards ML, Strodel WE, et al. Reasons for conversion from laparoscopic to open cholecystectomy: a 10-year review. J Gastrointest Surg 2002; 6:800–805.

46. Rosen M, Brody F, Ponsky J. Predictive factors for conversion of laparoscopic cholecystectomy. Am J Surg 2002; 184:254–258.

47. Rattner DW, Ferguson C, Warshaw AL. Factors associated with successful laparoscopic cholecystectomy for acute cholecystitis. Ann Surg 1993; 217:233–236.

48. Brodsky A, Matter I, Sabo E, et al. Laparoscopic cholecystectomy for acute cholecystitis: can the need for conversion and the probability of complications be predicted? A prospective study. Surg Endosc 2000; 14:755–760.

49. Kanaan SA, Murayama KM, Merriam LT, et al. Risk factors for conversion of laparoscopic to open cholecystectomy. J Surg Res 2002; 106:20–24.

50. Papi C, D'Ambrosio L, Capurso L. Timing of cholecystectomy for acute calculous cholecystitis: a meta-analysis. Am J Gastroenterol 2004; 99:147–155.

This meta-analysis pooled the results of twelve randomized trials in order to compare early with delayed cholecystectomy for the treatment of acute cholecystitis. There were no statistically significant differences in the rates of operative complications in early versus late surgery, for both open and laparoscopic cholecystectomy. Total hospital stay was significantly shorter in the early surgery group. The authors also highlighted the fact that over 20% of patients randomized to delayed surgery failed to respond to conservative management or suffered recurrent cholecystitis prior to the planned operation. They concluded that early surgery is the preferred strategy for patients with uncomplicated acute cholecystitis.

51. May GR, Sutherland LR, Shaffer EA. Efficacy of bile acid therapy for gallstone dissolution: a meta-analysis of randomized trials. Aliment Pharmacol Ther 1993; 7:139–148.

52. Tomida S, Abei M, Yamaguchi T, et al. Long-term ursodeoxycholic acid therapy is associated with reduced risk of biliary pain and acute cholecystitis in patients with gallbladder stones: a cohort analysis. Hepatology 1999; 30:6–13.

53. Rubin RA, Kowalski TE, Khandelwal M, et al. Ursodiol for hepatobiliary disorders. Ann Intern Med 1994; 121:207–218.

54. Podda M, Zuin M, Battezzati PM, et al. Efficacy and safety of a combination of chenodeoxycholic acid and ursodeoxycholic acid for gallstone dissolution: a comparison with ursodeoxycholic acid alone. Gastroenterology 1989; 96:222–229.

55. Sackmann M, Pauletzki J, Aydemir U, et al. Efficacy and safety of ursodeoxycholic acid for dissolution of gallstone fragments:

comparison with the combination of ursodeoxycholic acid and chenodeoxycholic acid. Hepatology 1991; 14:1136–1141.

56. Petroni ML, Jazrawi RP, Pazzi P, et al. Ursodeoxycholic acid alone or with chenodeoxycholic acid for dissolution of cholesterol gallstones: a randomized multicentre trial. The British-Italian Gallstone Study Group. Aliment Pharmacol Ther 2001; 15:123–128.

57. O'Donnell LD, Heaton KW. Recurrence and re-recurrence of gall stones after medical dissolution: a longterm follow up. Gut 1988; 29:655–658.

58. Villanova N, Bazzoli F, Taroni F, et al. Gallstone recurrence after successful oral bile acid treatment. A 12-year follow-up study and evaluation of long-term postdissolution treatment. Gastroenterology 1989; 97:726–731.

59. Thistle JL, May GR, Bender CE, et al. Dissolution of cholesterol gallbladder stones by methyl tert-butyl ether administered by percutaneous transhepatic catheter. N Engl J Med 1989; 320:633–639.

60. Leuschner U, Hellstern A, Schmidt K, et al. Gallstone dissolution with methyl tert-butyl ether in 120 patients – efficacy and safety. Dig Dis Sci 1991; 36:193–199.

61. Plaisier PW, van der Hul RL, Terpstra OT, et al. Current treatment modalities for symptomatic gallstones. Am J Gastroenterol 1993; 88:633–639.

62. Schoenfield LJ, Berci G, Carnovale RL, et al. The effect of ursodiol on the efficacy and safety of extracorporeal shock-wave lithotripsy of gallstones. The Dornier National Biliary Lithotripsy Study. N Engl J Med 1990; 323:1239–1245.

63. Sackmann M, Delius M, Sauerbruch T, et al. Shock-wave lithotripsy of gallbladder stones. The first 175 patients. N Engl J Med 1988; 318:393–397.

64. Sackmann M, Niller H, Klueppelberg U, et al. Gallstone recurrence after shock-wave therapy. Gastroenterology 1994; 106:225–230.

65. Ochi H, Tazuma S, Kajihara T, et al. Factors affecting gallstone recurrence after successful extracorporeal shock wave lithotripsy. J Clin Gastroenterol 2000; 31:230–232.

66. Cesmeli E, Elewaut AE, Kerre T, et al. Gallstone recurrence after successful shock wave therapy: the magnitude of the problem and the predictive factors. Am J Gastroenterol 1999; 94: 474–479.

67. Berr F, Mayer M, Sackmann MF, et al. Pathogenic factors in early recurrence of cholesterol gallstones. Gastroenterology 1994; 106:215–224.

68. Akhan O, Akinci D, Ozmen MN. Percutaneous cholecystostomy. Eur J Radiol 2002; 43:229–236.

69. Spira RM, Nissan A, Zamir O, et al. Percutaneous transhepatic cholecystostomy and delayed laparoscopic cholecystectomy in critically ill patients with acute calculus cholecystitis. Am J Surg 2002; 183:62–66.

70. Browning PD, McGahan JP, Gerscovich EO. Percutaneous cholecystostomy for suspected acute cholecystitis in the hospitalized patient. J Vasc Interv Radiol 1993; 4:531–537; discussion 537–538.

71. England RE, McDermott VG, Smith TP, et al. Percutaneous cholecystostomy: who responds? AJR Am J Roentgenol 1997; 168:1247–1251.

72. Ko CW, Lee SP. Epidemiology and natural history of common bile duct stones and prediction of disease. Gastrointest Endosc 2002; 56:S165–S169.

73. Abboud PA, Malet PF, Berlin JA, et al. Predictors of common bile duct stones prior to cholecystectomy: a meta-analysis. Gastrointest Endosc 1996; 44:450–455.

The authors performed a meta-analysis of 22 articles to identify predictors of common bile duct stones. They evaluated 10 indicators that were reported in a common fashion among the articles, and calculated sensitivities, specificities and positive and negative likelihood ratios for each indicator. The indicators with the highest positive likelihood ratios were cholangitis, bile duct stones seen on ultrasound, and preoperative jaundice. The authors reinforced the commonly held perception that no single clinical indicator was completely accurate in predicting choledocholithiasis.

74. Bose SM, Mazumdar A, Prakash VS, et al. Evaluation of the predictors of choledocholithiasis: comparative analysis of clinical, biochemical, radiological, radionuclear, and intraoperative parameters. Surg Today 2001; 31:117–122.

75. Alponat A, Kum CK, Rajnakova A, et al. Predictive factors for synchronous common bile duct stones in patients with cholelithiasis. Surg Endosc 1997; 11:928–932.

76. Onken JE, Brazer SR, Eisen GM, et al. Predicting the presence of choledocholithiasis in patients with symptomatic cholelithiasis. Am J Gastroenterol 1996; 91:762–767.

77. Stain SC, Marsri LS, Froes ET, et al. Laparoscopic cholecystectomy: laboratory predictors of choledocholithiasis. Am Surg 1994; 60:767-771.

78. Saltzstein EC, Peacock JB, Thomas MD. Preoperative bilirubin, alkaline phosphatase and amylase levels as predictors of common duct stones. Surg Gynecol Obstet 1982; 154:381–384.

79. Varghese JC, Liddell RP, Farrell MA, et al. Diagnostic accuracy of magnetic resonance cholangiopancreatography and ultrasound compared with direct cholangiography in the detection of choledocholithiasis. Clin Radiol 2000; 55:25–35.

80. Majeed AW, Ross B, Johnson AG, et al. Common duct diameter as an independent predictor of choledocholithiasis: is it useful? Clin Radiol 1999; 54:170–172.

81. Lecklitner ML, Austin AR, Benedetto AR, et al. Positive predictive value of cholescintigraphy in common bile duct obstruction. J Nucl Med 1986; 27:1403–1406.

82. Canto MI, Chak A, Stellato T, et al. Endoscopic ultrasonography versus cholangiography for the diagnosis of choledocholithiasis. Gastrointest Endosc 1998; 47:439–448.

83. Freeman ML. Adverse outcomes of endoscopic retrograde cholangiopancreatography. Rev Gastroenterol Disord 2002; 2:147–168.

84. Sherman S, Lehman GA. Endoscopic pancreatic sphincterotomy: techniques and complications. Gastrointest Endosc Clin N Am 1998; 8:115–124.

85. Freeman ML, Nelson DB, Sherman S, et al. Complications of endoscopic biliary sphincterotomy. N Engl J Med 1996; 335:909–918.

86. Masci E, Toti G, Mariani A, et al. Complications of diagnostic and therapeutic ERCP: a prospective multicenter study. Am J Gastroenterol 2001; 96:417–423.

87. Neoptolemos JP, Carr-Locke DL, London NJ, et al. Controlled trial of urgent endoscopic retrograde cholangiopancreatography and endoscopic sphincterotomy versus conservative treatment for acute pancreatitis due to gallstones. Lancet 1988; 2: 979–983.

88. Leung JW, Chung SC, Sung JJ, et al. Urgent endoscopic drainage for acute suppurative cholangitis. Lancet 1989; 1:1307–1309.

89. Fan ST, Lai EC, Mok FP, et al. Early treatment of acute biliary pancreatitis by endoscopic papillotomy. N Engl J Med 1993; 328:228–232.

90. Fulcher AS. MRCP and ERCP in the diagnosis of common bile duct stones. Gastrointest Endosc 2002; 56:S178–S182.

91. Soto JA, Alvarez O, Munera F, et al. Diagnosing bile duct stones: comparison of unenhanced helical CT, oral contrast-enhanced CT cholangiography, and MR cholangiography. AJR Am J Roentgenol 2000; 175:1127–1134.

92. Griffin N, Wastle ML, Dunn WK, et al. Magnetic resonance cholangiopancreatography versus endoscopic retrograde cholangiopancreatography in the diagnosis of choledocholithiasis. Eur J Gastroenterol Hepatol 2003; 15:809–813.

93. Sugiyama M, Atomi Y, Hachiya J. Magnetic resonance cholangiography using half-Fourier acquisition for diagnosing choledocholithiasis. Am J Gastroenterol 1998; 93:1886–1890.

94. Sivak MV Jr. EUS for bile duct stones: how does it compare with ERCP? Gastrointest Endosc 2002; 56:S175–S177.

95. Prat F, Amouyal G, Amouyal P, et al. Prospective controlled study of endoscopic ultrasonography and endoscopic retrograde cholangiography in patients with suspected common-bile duct lithiasis. Lancet 1996; 347:75–79.

96. NIH state-of-the-science statement on endoscopic retrograde cholangiopancreatography (ERCP) for diagnosis and therapy. NIH Consens State Sci Statements 2002; 19:1–26.

97. Das A, Isenberg G, Wong RC, et al. Wire-guided intraductal US: an adjunct to ERCP in the management of bile duct stones. Gastrointest Endosc 2001; 54:31–36.

98. Carr-Locke DL. Therapeutic role of ERCP in the management of suspected common bile duct stones. Gastrointest Endosc 2002; 56:S170–S174.

99. Binmoeller KF, Bruckner M, Thonke F, et al. Treatment of difficult bile duct stones using mechanical, electrohydraulic and extracorporeal shock wave lithotripsy. Endoscopy 1993; 25:201–206.

100. Park DH, Kim MH, Lee SK, et al. Endoscopic sphincterotomy vs. endoscopic papillary balloon dilation for choledocholithiasis in patients with liver cirrhosis and coagulopathy. Gastrointest Endosc 2004; 60:180–185.

101. Arnold JC, Benz C, Martin WR, et al. Endoscopic papillary balloon dilation vs. sphincterotomy for removal of common bile duct stones: a prospective randomized pilot study. Endoscopy 2001; 33:563–567.

102. Katsinelos P, Galanis I, Pilpilidis I, et al. The effect of indwelling endoprosthesis on stone size or fragmentation after long-term treatment with biliary stenting for large stones. Surg Endosc 2003; 17:1552–1555.

103. Petelin JB. Laparoscopic common bile duct exploration. Surg Endosc 2003; 17:1705–1715.

104. Dorman JP, Franklin ME Jr, Glass JL. Laparoscopic common bile duct exploration by choledochotomy. An effective and efficient method of treatment of choledocholithiasis. Surg Endosc 1998; 12:926–928.

105. Urbach DR, Khajanchee YS, Jobe BA, et al. Cost-effective management of common bile duct stones: a decision analysis of the use of endoscopic retrograde cholangiopancreatography (ERCP), intraoperative cholangiography, and laparoscopic bile duct exploration. Surg Endosc 2001; 15:4–13.

106. Cuschieri A, Croce E, Faggioni A, et al. EAES ductal stone study. Preliminary findings of multi-center prospective randomized trial comparing two-stage vs single-stage management. Surg Endosc 1996; 10:1130–1135.

107. Petelin JB. Surgical management of common bile duct stones. Gastrointest Endosc 2002; 56:S183–S189.

108. van der Velden JJ, Berger MY, Bonjer HJ, et al. Percutaneous treatment of bile duct stones in patients treated unsuccessfully with endoscopic retrograde procedures. Gastrointest Endosc 2000; 51:418–422.

109. Ogawa K, Ohkubo H, Abe W, et al. Percutaneous transhepatic small-caliber choledochoscopic lithotomy: a safe and effective technique for percutaneous transhepatic common bile duct exploration in high-risk elderly patients. J Hepatobiliary Pancreat Surg 2002; 9:213–217.

110. Moon JH, Cho YD, Ryu CB, et al. The role of percutaneous transhepatic papillary balloon dilation in percutaneous choledochoscopic lithotomy. Gastrointest Endosc 2001; 54:232–236.

111. Shorvon PJ, Cotton PB, Mason RR, et al. Percutaneous transhepatic assistance for duodenoscopic sphincterotomy. Gut 1985; 26:1373–1376.

112. Ko CW, Sekijima JH, Lee SP. Biliary sludge. Ann Intern Med 1999; 130:301–311.

113. Lee SP, Maher K, Nicholls JF. Origin and fate of biliary sludge. Gastroenterology 1988; 94:170–176.

114. Saik RP, Greenburg AG, Farris JM, et al. Spectrum of cholangitis. Am J Surg 1975; 130:143–150.

115. Boender J, Nix GA, de Ridder MA, et al. Endoscopic sphincterotomy and biliary drainage in patients with cholangitis due to common bile duct stones. Am J Gastroenterol 1995; 90:233–238.

116. Lai EC, Mok FP, Tan ES, et al. Endoscopic biliary drainage for severe acute cholangitis. N Engl J Med 1992; 326:1582–1586.

This randomized trial performed in Hong Kong compared surgical decompression of the biliary tract with endoscopic biliary drainage for the treatment of severe acute cholangitis. The study demonstrated significant advantages to endoscopic drainage with respect to complication rate, frequency of residual stones, and mortality rate. These findings strongly support the use of endoscopic drainage as first line therapy for acute cholangitis secondary to choledocholithiasis.

117. Kelly TR, Wagner DS. Gallstone pancreatitis: a prospective randomized trial of the timing of surgery. Surgery 1988; 104:600–605.

118. Folsch UR, Nitsche R, Ludtke R, et al. Early ERCP and papillotomy compared with conservative treatment for acute biliary pancreatitis. The German Study Group on Acute Biliary Pancreatitis. N Engl J Med 1997; 336:237–242.

119. Nowak A, Nowakowska-Dulawa E, Marek T, et al. Final results of the prospective, randomized, controlled study on endoscopic sphincterotomy versus conventional management in acute biliary pancreatitis (Abstract). Gastroenterology 1995; 108:A380.

120. Sharma VK, Howden CW. Metaanalysis of randomized controlled trials of endoscopic retrograde cholangiography and endoscopic sphincterotomy for the treatment of acute biliary pancreatitis. Am J Gastroenterol 1999; 94:3211–3214.

This meta-analysis reviewed data from four published randomized controlled trials comparing ERCP and sphincterotomy with conservative management for acute biliary pancreatitis. This study demonstrated that pooled data from these studies showed a statistically significant reduction in the rate of complications from acute biliary pancreatitis in patients treated with ERCP. Furthermore, there was a statistically significant reduction in mortality in patients treated with ERCP compared with conservative management. The authors predicted that approximately eight patients would need to be treated with ERCP to prevent one complication, and approximately 26 patients would need to be treated to prevent one death.

121. Kaw M, Al-Antably Y, Kaw P. Management of gallstone pancreatitis: cholecystectomy or ERCP and endoscopic sphincterotomy. Gastrointest Endosc 2002; 56:61–65.

122. Uomo G, Manes G, Laccetti M, et al. Endoscopic sphincterotomy and recurrence of acute pancreatitis in gallstone patients considered unfit for surgery. Pancreas 1997; 14:28–31.

123. Davidson BR, Neoptolemos JP, Carr-Locke DL. Endoscopic sphincterotomy for common bile duct calculi in patients with gall bladder in situ considered unfit for surgery. Gut 1988; 29:114–120.

124. Hammarstrom LE, Holmin T, Stridbeck H. Endoscopic treatment of bile duct calculi in patients with gallbladder in situ: long-term outcome and factors. Scand J Gastroenterol 1996; 31:294–301.

125. Yi SY. Recurrence of biliary symptoms after endoscopic sphincterotomy for choledocholithiasis in patients with gallbladder stones. J Gastroenterol Hepatol 2000; 15:661–664.

126. Targarona EM, Ayuso RM, Bordas JM, et al. Randomised trial of endoscopic sphincterotomy with gallbladder left in situ versus open surgery for common bile duct calculi in high-risk patients. Lancet 1996; 347:926–929.

127. Lai KH, Lin LF, Lo GH, et al. Does cholecystectomy after endoscopic sphincterotomy prevent the recurrence of biliary complications? Gastrointest Endosc 1999; 49:483–487.

128. Boerma D, Rauws EA, Keulemans YC, et al. Wait-and-see policy or laparoscopic cholecystectomy after endoscopic sphincterotomy for bile-duct stones: a randomised trial. Lancet 2002; 360:761–765.

   This prospective study of 120 patients addressed the issue of whether patients with gallbladder stones should undergo cholecystectomy following endoscopic sphincterotomy and extraction of common bile duct stones. Patients were randomized to either expectant management or laparoscopic cholecystectomy. The study demonstrated a high rate of recurrent biliary symptoms (47%) among patients managed expectantly, compared to that in patients who underwent cholecystectomy (2%). The authors therefore concluded that cholecystectomy after sphincterotomy and bile duct clearance in patients with gallbladder in situ was the preferred strategy.

129. Pereira-Lima JC, Jakobs R, Winter UH, et al. Long-term results (7 to 10 years) of endoscopic papillotomy for choledocholithiasis. Multivariate analysis of prognostic factors for the recurrence of biliary symptoms. Gastrointest Endosc 1998; 48:457–464.

130. Hill J, Martin DF, Tweedle DE. Risks of leaving the gallbladder in situ after endoscopic sphincterotomy for bile duct stones. Br J Surg 1991; 78:554–557.

131. Maringhini A, Ciambra M, Baccelliere P, et al. Biliary sludge and gallstones in pregnancy: incidence, risk factors, and natural history. Ann Intern Med 1993; 119:116–120.

132. Valdivieso V, Covarrubias C, Siegel F, et al. Pregnancy and cholelithiasis: pathogenesis and natural course of gallstones diagnosed in early puerperium. Hepatology 1993; 17:1–4.

133. Sungler P, Heinerman PM, Steiner H, et al. Laparoscopic cholecystectomy and interventional endoscopy for gallstone complications during pregnancy. Surg Endosc 2000; 14:267–271.

134. Cosenza CA, Saffari B, Jabbour N, et al. Surgical management of biliary gallstone disease during pregnancy. Am J Surg 1999; 178:545–548.

135. Tham TC, Vandervoort J, Wong RC, et al. Safety of ERCP during pregnancy. Am J Gastroenterol 2003; 98:308–311.

136. Tarnasky PR, Simmons DC, Schwartz AG, et al. Safe delivery of bile duct stones during pregnancy. Am J Gastroenterol 2003; 98:2100–2101.

137. Mundth ED. Cholecystitis and diabetes mellitus. N Engl J Med 1962; 267:642–646.

138. Schein CJ. Acute cholecystitis in the diabetic. Am J Gastroenterol 1969; 51:511–515.

139. Shpitz B, Sigal A, Kaufman Z, et al. Acute cholecystitis in diabetic patients. Am Surg 1995; 61:964–967.

140. Ransohoff DF, Miller GL, Forsythe SB, et al. Outcome of acute cholecystitis in patients with diabetes mellitus. Ann Intern Med 1987; 106:829–832.

141. Landau O, Deutsch AA, Kott I, et al. The risk of cholecystectomy for acute cholecystitis in diabetic patients. Hepatogastroenterology 1992; 39:437–438.

142. Aucott JN, Cooper GS, Bloom AD, et al. Management of gallstones in diabetic patients. Arch Intern Med 1993; 153:1053–1058.

143. Del Favero G, Caroli A, Meggiato T, et al. Natural history of gallstones in non-insulin-dependent diabetes mellitus. A prospective 5-year follow-up. Dig Dis Sci 1994; 39: 1704–1707.

144. Del Olmo JA, Garcia F, Serra MA, et al. Prevalence and incidence of gallstones in liver cirrhosis. Scand J Gastroenterol 1997; 32:1061–1065.

145. Acalovschi M, Badea R, Dumitrascu D, et al. Prevalence of gallstones in liver cirrhosis: a sonographic survey. Am J Gastroenterol 1988; 83:954–956.

146. Conte D, Fraquelli M, Fornari F, et al. Close relation between cirrhosis and gallstones: cross-sectional and longitudinal survey. Arch Intern Med 1999; 159:49–52.

147. Acalovschi M, Blendea D, Feier C, et al. Risk factors for symptomatic gallstones in patients with liver cirrhosis: a case-control study. Am J Gastroenterol 2003; 98:1856–1860.

148. Poggio JL, Rowland CM, Gores GJ, et al. A comparison of laparoscopic and open cholecystectomy in patients with compensated cirrhosis and symptomatic gallstone disease. Surgery 2000; 127:405–411.

149. Ishizaki Y, Bandai Y, Shimomura K, et al. Management of gallstones in cirrhotic patients. Surg Today 1993; 23:36–39.

CHAPTER TWENTY-SIX

Primary sclerosing cholangitis

Konstantinos N. Lazaridis and Nicholas F. LaRusso

INTRODUCTION

Primary sclerosing cholangitis (PSC) is a chronic, progressive cholestatic hepatobiliary disease of unknown cause.[1,2] PSC is characterized by concentric, obliterative fibrosis of both the intra- and extrahepatic bile ducts resulting in destruction of the biliary tree and subsequently in biliary cirrhosis.[1,2] PSC is diagnosed after exclusion of secondary sclerosing cholangitis, in which bile duct injury is caused by identifiable etiologies (Table 26.1).

Epidemiology

Over the last 3 decades, the frequency of PSC diagnosis has increased. This is likely because of an enhanced awareness of PSC among physicians in addition to extensive use of endoscopic retrograde cholangiopancreatography (ERCP) in clinical practice. PSC affects primarily young men during their fourth decade of life.[1,2] In the United States, population-based estimates reported an age-adjusted incidence of PSC to be 1.25 and 0.54 per 100 000 person-years in men and women, respectively.[3] From the same study, the prevalence of PSC was calculated to be 20.9 and 6.3 per 100 000 of men and women, respectively.[3] About 75–80% of patients of northern European origin with PSC suffer from inflammatory bowel disease. In this group, chronic ulcerative colitis (CUC) is more common (≈90%) than Crohn's disease (≈10%). Of interest, only 2–6% of patients with CUC have or will develop PSC.[1,2]

Table 26.1 Causes of secondary sclerosing cholangitis

AIDS-associated cholangiopathy

Amyloidosis

Bile duct neoplasm (in the absence of PSC)

Chemicals/drugs (i.e., 5-fluorouracil)

Choledocholithiasis

Congenital bile duct abnormalities (i.e., Caroli's disease)

Iatrogenic biliary strictures/trauma

Ischemic strictures of bile ducts

AIDS, acquired immunodeficiency syndrome.

Pathogenesis

PSC is a heterogeneous disease. To date, the etiopathogenesis of PSC remains elusive. It is believed that the interaction of genetic elements and environmental exposures is pivotal in the pathogenesis of PSC. Figure 26.1 represents a working hypothesis of the environmental and genetic interplay that leads to PSC and may explain the disease's multifactorial etiology and heterogeneous presentation.

Genetic factors

The fact that genetic factors predispose to the development of PSC is evident by reports of familial PSC cases[4,5] and the association of specific HLA haplotypes (i.e., B8, DR3) with PSC patients compared to matched controls.[2] In the last 3 years, additional genetic polymorphisms have been implicated in the pathogenesis of PSC. For example, a functional variant of stromelysin (i.e., matrix metalloproteinase 3) has been shown to affect PSC susceptibility and disease progression;[6] moreover, a functional polymorphism of the MICA gene (major histocompatibility complex [MHC] class I related – MIC gene family) was reported to have a role in PSC susceptibility.[7]

Environmental factors and associated diseases

Environmental elements such as copper and infectious agents (i.e., CMV), have been implicated in the development of PSC. Copper was postulated to participate in the pathogenesis of PSC because of the excessive copper found in the hepatic parenchyma of patients with PSC. Nevertheless, a causative role for copper in PSC development is unlikely given the elevated hepatic copper concentration reported in other chronic cholestatic liver diseases. Moreover, the notion that PSC progresses in spite of a decrease in hepatic copper following chelation therapy with D-penicillamine argues against this hypothesis.[8] Viruses such as cytomegalovirus and reovirus type 3 have also been postulated to cause PSC. To date, however, proven evidence to support involvement of these microorganisms in PSC pathogenesis is lacking.

The association between CUC and PSC has been confirmed by many studies. Nonetheless, the proposal that increased colonic permeability, due to CUC, and the resulting enhanced absorption of luminal contents (i.e., toxins, bacteria, inflammatory mediators) leads to the inflammation of bile ducts in PSC remain unproven. In fact, the development of PSC in the absence of CUC (≈20% of patients) and the failure of proctocolectomy to modify

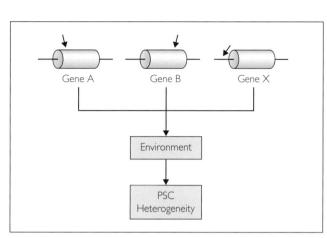

Fig. 26.1 • The interaction of genetic variants located at different loci (arrows) with the environment is proposed to account for the heterogeneity of PSC pathogenesis, clinical presentation and progression.

the natural history of PSC argue against a direct causative mechanism between these two entities.

Humoral and cellular immune abnormalities have been described in patients with PSC implying that altered immunity is involved in its pathogenesis. Whether distorted immunity is linked to PSC causation or is just an epiphenomenon of its pathogenesis remains unclear. Humoral alterations in PSC include: (1) hypergammaglobulinemia with increased serum immunoglobulin M levels; (2) decreased clearance of circulating immune complexes; (3) increased complement activation; and (4) increased titer of autoantibodies (i.e., antineutrophil cytoplasmic antibodies, antinuclear antibodies).[1] Cell-mediated abnormalities of immunity in PSC include: (1) decline of the total number of T cells involving mainly the suppressor/cytotoxic (CD 8) and less frequently the helper (CD 4) T lymphocytes; and (2) aberrant expression of HLA class II antigens by biliary epithelia.[1]

At present, the consensus working hypothesis of PSC pathogenesis proposes that the disease develops in a genetically predisposed individual following exposure(s) to a biliary insult that causes progressive destruction of bile ducts. Moreover, we now know that the cholangiocyte, the epithelial cell that lines the intra- and extrahepatic bile ducts, is the target cell in PSC.

CLINICOPATHOLOGICAL FEATURES AND DIAGNOSIS

Clinicopathological features

Symptoms and signs

The clinical presentation of PSC is heterogeneous. The asymptomatic individual has incidentally detected abnormal liver blood tests. The symptomatic patient presents with signs/symptoms/complications of end-stage hepatic disease. A commonly encountered clinical scenario is a patient with CUC who presents with a cholestatic pattern of liver enzyme changes. Symptomatic patients have fatigue (75%), pruritus (70%), hepatomegaly (55%), jaundice (50%), weight loss (40%), splenomegaly (30%), and skin hyperpigmentation (25%).[1]

Laboratory findings, imaging of the biliary tree, and histologic staging of primary sclerosing cholangitis

The laboratory profile of patients with PSC includes a three- to fourfold elevation of serum alkaline phosphatase of at least 6 months duration. Alanine aminotransferase (ALT), aspartate aminotransferase (AST), and serum bilirubin are mildly elevated and may fluctuate.[1] Serologic tests for antimitochondrial antibodies are generally negative.[9] Serum copper and ceruloplasmin levels, and urine and hepatic copper values may be abnormal. ERCP reveals diffusely distributed, short, annular strictures with intervening segments of dilated ducts (beading) affecting both the intra- and extrahepatic biliary tree (Fig. 26.2). Magnetic resonance cholangiography (MRC) offers comparable accuracy to ERCP, in addition to reduced cost, as the initial test for the diagnosis of PSC.[10] The histologic staging of PSC is shown on Table 26.2.

Diagnosis

The diagnosis of PSC is usually based on the following criteria: (1) elevated serum alkaline phosphatase level of at least 6 months duration; (2) characteristic cholangiographic findings of the bile ducts (see Fig. 26.2); and (3) exclusion of secondary sclerosing cholangitis (see Table 26.1). Liver biopsy is not always necessary for the diagnosis. In a recent study, involving 79 PSC patients who underwent liver biopsy with a previously established PSC diagnosis by cholangiography, the biopsy result itself did not affect the clinical management in 78 out of 79 PSC patients.[11] Nevertheless, liver biopsy is required in PSC patients suspected to have the 'overlap syndrome' (i.e., coexistence of PSC with autoimmune hepatitis) or 'small duct PSC' (i.e., patients with normal ERCP but cholestatic pattern of liver enzymes). Liver biopsy is also indicated for staging PSC prior to entry into therapeutic trials. The differential diagnosis of PSC should include secondary sclerosing cholangitis (see Table 26.1), primary biliary cirrhosis, chronic

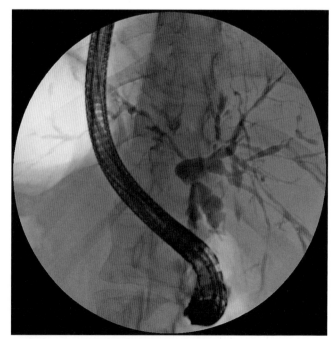

Fig. 26.2 • Typical ERCP findings of PSC. Multifocal stricturing and dilatation of intra- and extrahepatic bile ducts.

Table 26.2 Staging of primary sclerosing cholangitis by liver histology

Portal stage (stage I)	Portal edema, inflammation, ductal proliferation; abnormalities do not extend beyond the limiting plate.
Periportal stage (stage II)	Periportal fibrosis, inflammation with or without ductular proliferation; piecemeal necrosis may be present.
Septal stage (stage III)	Septal fibrosis or bridging necrosis can be identified.
Cirrhotic stage (stage IV)	Biliary cirrhosis.

active hepatitis, idiopathic adulthood ductopenia, and overlap syndrome.

NATURAL HISTORY AND COMPLICATIONS

Natural history

PSC is an insidious and progressive disease. Although some patients with early-stage PSC are asymptomatic, most will advance over time to develop complications of chronic cholestasis and end-stage liver disease. In the absence of liver transplantation, the median survival from the time of diagnosis is about 12 years; even asymptomatic patients have decreased survival compared to matched controls.[12] Children with PSC have a natural history that is comparable to adults. The median survival for children, in the absence of liver transplantation, was reported to be 12.7 years and the overall survival was significantly shorter despite attempted pharmacological treatment.[13]

Prognostic models in PSC have been devised to predict survival, assess efficiency of therapeutic trials, and identify the ideal timing for liver transplantation. In the revised Mayo natural history model for PSC, five independent, reproducible parameters, namely age, bilirubin, albumin, aspartate aminotransferase, and history of variceal bleeding, were used to estimate the survival of patients with PSC.[14] This model's advantage is the avoidance of liver biopsy in estimating patient survival.

Complications

The complications of PSC can be divided into two groups. The first consists of the non-specific complications related to end-stage liver disease and it includes chronic cholestasis and liver failure, steatorrhea and fat-soluble vitamin deficiency, hepatic osteodystrophy, decompensated cirrhosis, and portal hypertension. The second group of complications includes those more directly related to PSC (i.e., cholelithiasis, choledocholithiasis, dominant biliary stricture(s), recurrent bacterial cholangitis, cholangiocarcinoma, and peristomal varices). The latter occurs in patients with coexistent PSC and CUC who have undergone proctocolectomy and ileostomy.

TREATMENT

The management of PSC should be multifaceted. PSC causes chronic, debilitating symptoms and complications of end-stage liver disease. To date, we lack an effective, specific treatment for the underlying disorder. Gastroenterologists are the primary physicians that treat patients with PSC. However, the complexity of the disease requires a team management approach that also involves interventional radiologists and surgeons in order to treat the spectrum of PSC manifestations and complications. Figure 26.3 provides an algorithm for the treatment of PSC.

Medical treatment

The management of PSC should simultaneously focus on: (1) treatment of non-specific PSC complications, (2) therapy of specific PSC complications, and (3) approaches to ameliorate the progression of the underlying hepatobiliary disease.

Treatment of non-specific complications of PSC

Pruritus

Patients with advanced-stage PSC frequently complain of intense pruritus. To alleviate this distressing symptom many medical therapies have been used.[1] Cholestyramine, a nonabsorbable bile acid binding resin, is thought to work by lessening the intestinal absorption of bile acids. The recommended dose of cholestyramine (4 g four times per day) must be given at least 2 hours before or after other medications because their intestinal absorption can be inhibited by this resin. Phenobarbital (120–160 mg per day) have been used in addition to cholestyramine to control nocturnal pruritus. Ursodeoxycholic acid (i.e., ursodiol), a hydrophilic bile acid that likely replaces hydrophobic, toxic bile acids in bile, may also alleviate pruritus in PSC patients at a dose of 13–15 mg per kg of body weight per day, divided in two doses. Antihistamines (i.e., hydroxyzine and diphenhydramine) can be used as supplements to cholestyramine or ursodeoxycholic acid particularly for nocturnal pruritus because of their sedative properties. Rifampin, which works by competing for the hepatocyte uptake of bile acids and by inducing hepatic microsomal enzymes, may also improve pruritus. Rifampin is administered orally at 300–600 mg per day. The potential side effects of rifampin (i.e., drug-induced hepatitis) make it a second-line agent for pruritus. Opiate antagonists such as naloxone, nalmefene, and naltrexone have shown promise in alleviating pruritus.[15] More aggressive treatments for intractable pruritus include the use of plasmapheresis, phototherapy, and orthotopic liver transplantation.

Steatorrhea, fat-soluble vitamin deficiency, and hepatic osteodystrophy

Because prolonged cholestasis results in decreased intestinal bile acid concentration, patients with advanced-stage PSC may develop steatorrhea. However, PSC patients who present with steatorrhea should be evaluated for other concurrent causes of the latter such as pancreatic insufficiency and celiac sprue.[16] Steatorrhea, due to intralumenal bile acid deficiency, may improve by lowering the dietary fat intake to ≈40 g per day, and by substituting medium-chain triglycerides for dietary long-chain triglycerides.

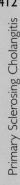

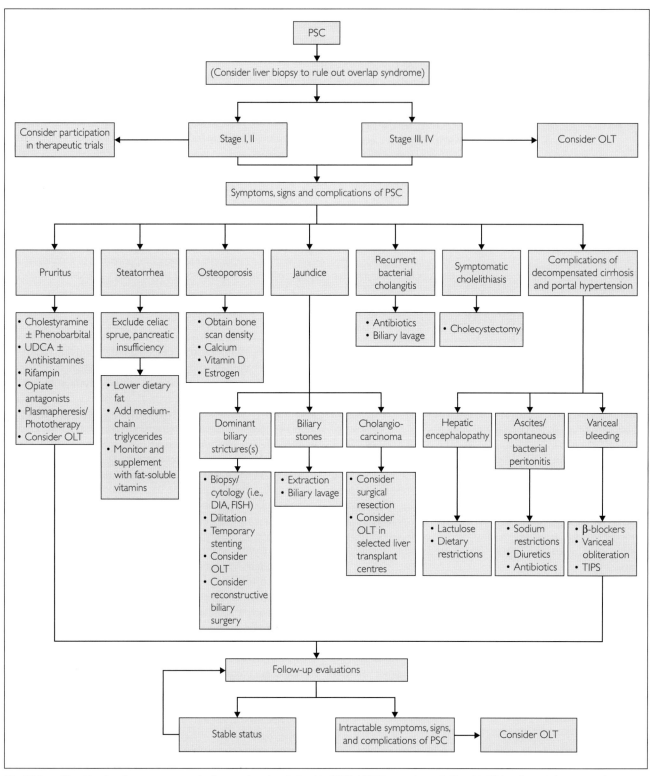

Fig. 26.3 ● Algorithm for the management of primary sclerosing cholangitis (PSC). UDCA, ursodeoxycholic acid; OLT, orthotopic liver transplantation; DIA, digital image analysis; FISH, fluorescence in situ hybridization; TIPS, transjugular intrahepatic portosystemic shunt

Fat-soluble vitamin (i.e., A, D, E, K) deficiencies have been described in PSC.[17] Vitamin A deficiency can cause 'night blindness.' In PSC patients with vitamin A deficiency, oral supplementation with 25 000–50 000 U of vitamin A two to three times per week is recommended. Serum levels of vitamin A must be monitored in treated patients to avoid hepatotoxicity. The main bone disease in patients with PSC is osteoporosis.[18] Special consideration must be given in advanced-stage PSC patients who have moderate to severe osteopenia since about 50% have bone mineral density below the fracture threshold.[18] Patients should receive supportive therapy including: (1) calcium supplements; (2) replenishment with vitamin D (25 000–50 000 U of vitamin D two to three times per week intramuscularly) when low serum levels are detected; and (3) use of estrogens. PSC patients deficient in vitamin K have prolonged prothrombin time. In these cases, a testing oral dose of 10 mg of vitamin K should be administered. If empiric treatment improves prothrombin time, then patients should be started on a maintenance dose of 5–10 mg of water-soluble vitamin K per day. Vitamin E should be replaced if its serum level is reduced. The recommended oral dose of vitamin E is 100–200 mg per day.

Decompensated cirrhosis and portal hypertension
Patients with advanced-stage PSC develop complications of decompensated cirrhosis and portal hypertension including ascites, hepatic encephalopathy, spontaneous bacterial peritonitis, and variceal bleeding. These complications should be managed expectantly as in other end-stage liver diseases. The PSC patient with decompensated cirrhosis and associated complications should receive standard medical therapy (i.e., sodium restriction, lactulose, diuretics, beta blockers) and endoscopic evaluation (i.e., periodic surveillance for esophageal varices and, if needed, variceal obliteration). However, as PSC progresses, these complications become intractable and orthotopic liver transplantation remains the single best therapeutic option.

Treatment of specific complications of PSC
Cholelithiasis and choledocholithiasis
About 30% of PSC patients will develop cholelithiasis and/or choledocholithiasis due to the chronic, progressive nature of intrahepatic and extrahepatic cholestasis. Patients with PSC who present with symptoms and signs of biliary stone disease and a biochemical profile of worsening cholestasis should be evaluated for cholecystitis and/or choledocholithiasis. If the diagnosis of choledocholithiasis is made, ERCP with endoscopic sphincterectomy and removal of biliary stones is the therapeutic intervention of choice.

Symptomatic gallbladder disease in PSC patients should be treated with cholecystectomy. Of note, the presence of a luminal gallbladder mass that cannot be attributed to gallstones needs special attention. In a Mayo Clinic study of 102 patients with PSC who underwent cholecystectomy, 14 of 102 (13.7%) were found to have gallbladder mass of which eight (57%) were malignant (i.e., adenocarcinoma).[19] Therefore, in patients with PSC and suspected gallbladder polyps of any size, cholecystectomy is strongly recommended.

Dominant biliary stricture(s) and recurrent bacterial cholangitis
Dominant biliary stricture(s) develop in 10–20% of PSC patients during the course of their disease. PSC patients with dominant biliary stricture(s) present with acute onset or worsening of jaundice and pruritus. Dominant biliary stricture(s) should be evaluated by ERCP or percutaneous transhepatic cholangiography (PTC) to visualize the biliary tree and permit brushing as well as biopsies of the involved area(s) to exclude cholangiocarcinoma. Biliary aspirate specimens should be sent for standard cytology, digital imaging analysis (DIA), and fluorescence in situ hybridization (FISH). The latter two laboratory tests have improved the diagnostic accuracy for cholangiocarcinoma (see below).

The therapeutic management of dominant biliary stricture(s) and/or recurrent bacterial cholangitis should include a balanced combination of dilatation and stenting interventions, biliary lavage, and the preventive use of antibiotics. The preferred approach of intervention (i.e., ERCP versus PTC) depends on stricture characteristics (i.e., location, length), and availability/local experience with the related procedures. The majority of biliary strictures are amenable to ERCP. Endoscopic cholangioplasty (i.e., balloon dilation) of dominant biliary stricture(s) followed by stenting improves patient symptoms. However, the long-term effect of this approach on disease progression and need for liver transplantation has not been examined. PTC is the suggested method of approaching the biliary tree for mechanical treatment of biliary strictures that affect intrahepatic ducts, in patients with history of Roux-en-Y gastrojejunostomy, and in cases of failed endoscopic approaches. Intravenous antibiotics are strongly recommended immediately prior to mechanical manipulation of the biliary tree and oral antibiotic treatment should be continued for 7–10 days following ERCP or PTC. Ciprofloxacin is the antibiotic that is most frequently used in our practice because of its high biliary secretion and broad spectrum of bacterial coverage. PSC patients with frequent episodes of bacterial cholangitis should also be given ciprofloxacin prophylactically to prevent recurrence or reduce its severity. Recurrent bacterial cholangitis in patients with PSC is not always the result of dominant biliary stricture(s). It has been proposed that edema, inflammatory exudation, and debris in the biliary tree can result in temporary stenosis of bile ducts leading to obstruction and recurrent bacterial cholangitis. Since these events are thought to be transient and more likely reversible, biliary lavage has been devised as an endoscopic modality to flush out potential irritants from the biliary tree. After cannulation of the biliary system, the ducts are irrigated with either saline or with saline plus steroids in an attempt to achieve a topical antiinflammatory effect.

Cholangiocarcinoma
PSC is considered to be a premalignant condition since adenocarcinoma of the bile ducts occurs in 8–15% of patients.[2] The estimated annual incidence of cholangiocarcinoma in patients with PSC is ≈1.5%.[20] The development of cholangiocarcinoma in PSC is frequently heralded by weight loss, abdominal discomfort/pain, and rapid deterioration of liver function tests. The median survival after the diagnosis of cholangiocarcinoma is short (≈6 months). Patients at high risk for this tumor are those with a prolonged history of CUC and advanced-stage PSC. Early detection of cholangiocarcinoma in PSC patients is hampered by the low sensitivity/specificity of diagnostic techniques including fine needle biopsy and brush cytology of bile ducts. CA-19-9, a serum glycoprotein, is a useful marker of cholangiocarcinoma but it may be elevated in pancreatic malignancies and in bacterial cholangitis. In spite of this, periodic testing of CA-19-9 in PSC patients is recommended and a progressive CA-19-9 increase should make one suspect that cholangiocarcinoma has developed. New modalities that may aid in the diagnosis of cholangiocarcinoma include digital imaging analysis (DIA) and fluorescence in situ hybridization (FISH) of bile duct cytology specimens. These two tests have improved the diagnostic yield of cholangiocarcinoma when compared to standard biliary cytology.[20,21]

Liver resection for cholangiocarcinoma is limited to only those few patients who are diagnosed at early stages. Unfortunately, chemotherapy and radiation therapy are not effective in treating cholangiocarcinoma. Liver transplantation for cholangio-carcinoma has had disappointing results with a 5-year survival rate of <20% and frequent tumor recurrence. Nevertheless, liver transplant protocols for cholangiocarcinoma that involve the combination of pretransplantation radiation therapy and chemotherapy for cholangiocarcinoma are offered by selected liver transplant centers. In these centers, promising results, with 5-year actuarial survival of about 80%, have been reported.[22]

Treatment of the primary hepatobiliary disease

For the last 2 decades, multiple medical treatments, aimed at treating the underlying hepatobiliary disease of PSC, have been evaluated. These medical therapies have employed a variety of agents including cupruretics (i.e., D-penicillamine), immuno-suppressive agents (i.e., cyclosporine, azathioprine, budesonide, silymarin), antifibrogenic drugs (i.e., pentoxifylline, colchicine), and choleretic compounds (i.e., ursodeoxycholic acid).

In a well-designed double-blind, randomized, controlled study involving 105 PSC patients, ursodeoxycholic acid (UDCA), at a dose of 13–15 mg/kg of body weight/day failed to demonstrate any clinical benefit in the treatment group compared to control (median follow-up 2.2 years). Indeed, there was no significant difference between the two groups in the time to treatment failure. Of interest, however, two independent, preliminary studies have shown promising effect of high-dose UDCA in PSC. In the first, a double-blind, placebo-controlled study, 26 PSC patients received high-dose (20 mg/kg body weight/day) UDCA or placebo. The high-dose UDCA group demonstrated significant improvement in liver biochemistry, and reduction in progression of cholangiographic appearance and disease staging.[23] In the second study, 30 PSC patients were treated with high-dose (25–30 mg/kg body weight/day) UDCA for 1 year. Improvement of the Mayo PSC risk score at 1 year of therapy and projected survival at 4 years was noted in the high-dose UDCA group compared with that observed in patients randomized to placebo (n=52) or UDCA (n=53) at standard dose (13–15 mg/kg body weight/day).[24] In both studies, the high-dose UDCA was well tolerated. A multicenter, long-term randomized placebo-controlled trial is underway to further evaluate these promising results.

Treatment with UDCA was also shown to affect the frequency of colonic dysplasia or cancer in PSC patients with coexisting CUC. In a cross-sectional study of 59 patients with both PSC and CUC who were undergoing dysplasia surveillance by colonoscopy, UDCA use was associated with decreased prevalence of colonic dysplasia (odds ratio 0.18 [95% CI 0.05–0.61%]; p=0.005).[25] In another randomized, placebo-controlled trial of 52 patients who had both PSC and CUC (total follow-up of 355 person-years) it was reported that those patients who received UDCA had a rela-tive risk of 0.26 for developing colorectal dysplasia or cancer (95% CI, 0.06–0.92; p=0.034).[26] Prospective randomized con-trolled studies are needed to verify the proposed chemopreventive effect of UDCA on colonic mucosa in patients with PSC and CUC.

In conclusion, an effective medical therapy for PSC is currently lacking. Medical therapy is encouraged only in the context of therapeutic trials.

Surgical treatment

Reconstructive biliary surgery

At present, because of the successful outcome of endoscopic manipulations of affected bile ducts and the high survival of PSC patients following liver transplantation (see below), biliary reconstructive surgery is rarely performed. In the past, however, surgery designed to reconstruct the strictured and damaged extrahepatic bile ducts has been performed in an attempt to reduce symptoms and prolong survival.

Proctocolectomy

A retrospective study of patients with a concurrent PSC and CUC found that proctocolectomy did not affect the biochemical/cholangiographic/liver histology findings, clinical progression, or survival of PSC patients.[27] Thus, proctocolectomy in PSC should be performed for established indications related to the CUC and not for the PSC. Moreover, approximately 25–50% of PSC patients who undergo proctocolectomy and ileostomy for CUC will manifest peristomal varices and these varices can often bleed massively. Therapeutic interventions to control bleeding of peristomal varices include revision of the ileostomy, topical sclerotherapy, transjugular intrahepatic portosystemic shunt (TIPS), and orthotopic liver transplantation. Interestingly, patients with PSC and CUC are at higher risk for developing adenocarcinoma of the colon and therefore should have annual surveillance colonoscopy.[28]

Orthotopic liver transplantation

Orthotopic liver transplantation (OLT) is the treatment of choice in patients with advanced-stage PSC. The 5-year survival rate of PSC patients who undergo OLT is 85–90%. Based on the Mayo PSC natural history model, OLT appears to prolong the survival of PSC patients compared to the estimated survival without liver transplantation. Consideration for OLT should be given to patients with intractable symptoms, signs, and complications related to end-stage liver disease that affect their quality of life and shorten survival. The decision of timing for OLT is critical. OLT performed earlier in the natural history of PSC correlates with increased survival compared to OLT carried out later.[29] Of note, the disease recurs in up to 20% of patients transplanted for PSC.[30] However, the clinical significance and long-term implica-tions of the PSC reappearance after OLT remains to be evaluated.

SUMMARY

PSC is an idiopathic, progressive cholestatic hepatobiliary disease. PSC affects mainly young men and demonstrates strong association with CUC. The symptoms and signs of PSC are not specific. This is an insidious disorder that advances over time resulting in ductopenia, end-stage liver disease, and at times development of cholangiocarcinoma. The clinical management of PSC patients should focus on alleviating symptoms of cholestasis and treating complications of end-stage liver disease. To date, no effective medical treatment for the underlying hepatobiliary disorder has been identified. OLT remains the treatment of choice for many patients with advanced-stage PSC and it has proven to extend life. Further basic and clinical studies are required to dissect the genetic and environmental interaction that contributes to the pathogenesis of this devastating disease. Only then will we be in a better position to devise promising novel therapies for PSC.

REFERENCES

1. Angulo P, Lindor KD. Primary sclerosing cholangitis. Hepatology 1999; 30:325–332.

2. Chapman RW. The management of primary sclerosing cholangitis. Curr Gastroenterol Rep 2003; 5:9–17.

   An excellent review on PSC management.

3. Bambha K, Kim WR, Talwalkar J, et al. Incidence, clinical spectrum, and outcomes of primary sclerosing cholangitis in a United States community. Gastroenterology 2003; 125:1364–1369.

   A study of the incidence and prevalence of PSC in the United States.

4. Jorge AD, Esley C, Ahumada J. Family incidence of primary sclerosing cholangitis associated with immunological diseases. Endoscopy 1987; 19:114–117.

5. Quigley EMM, LaRusso NF, Ludwig J, et al. Familial occurrence of primary sclerosing cholangitis and ulcerative colitis. Gastroenterology 1983; 85:1160–1165.

6. Satsangi J, Chapman RW, Haldar N, et al. A functional polymorphism of the stromelysin gene (MMP-3) influences susceptibility to primary sclerosing cholangitis. Gastroenterology 2001; 121:124–130.

7. Norris S, Kondeatis E, Collins R, et al. Mapping MHC-encoded susceptibility and resistance in primary sclerosing cholangitis: the role of MICA polymorphism. Gastroenterology 2001; 120:1475–1482.

8. LaRusso NF, Wiesner RH, Ludwig J, et al. Prospective trial of penicillamine in primary sclerosing cholangitis. Gastroenterology 1988; 95:1036–1042.

9. Angulo P, Peter JB, Gershwin ME, et al. Serum autoantibodies in patients with primary sclerosing cholangitis. J Hepatol 2000; 32:182–187.

10. Talwalkar JA, Angulo P, Johnson CD, et al. Cost-minimization analysis of MRC versus ERCP for the diagnosis of primary sclerosing cholangitis. Hepatology 2004; 40:39–45.

11. Burak KW, Angulo P, Lindor KD. Is there a role for liver biopsy in primary sclerosing cholangitis? Am J Gastroenterol 2003; 98:1155–1158.

12. Wiesner RH, Grambsch PM, Dickson ER, et al. Primary sclerosing cholangitis: natural history, prognostic factors, and survival analysis. Hepatology 1989; 10:430–436.

13. Feldstein AE, Perrault J, El-Youssif M, et al. Primary sclerosing cholangitis in children: a long-term follow-up study. Hepatology 2003; 38:210–217.

14. Kim WR, Therneau TM, Wiesner RH, et al. A revised natural history model for primary sclerosing cholangitis. Mayo Clin Proc 2000; 75:688–694.

15. Beuers U, Spengler U, Kruis W, et al. Ursodeoxycholic acid for treatment of primary sclerosing cholangitis: a placebo-controlled trial. Hepatology 1992; 16:707–714.

16. Hay JE, Wiesner RH, Shorter RG, et al. Primary sclerosing cholangitis and celiac disease: A novel association. Ann Intern Med 1988; 109:713–717.

17. Jorgensen RA, Lindor KD, Sartin JS, et al. Serum lipid and fat-soluble vitamin levels in primary sclerosing cholangitis. J Clin Gastroenterol 1995; 20:215–219.

18. Hay JE, Lindor KD, Wiesner RH, et al. The metabolic bone disease of primary sclerosing cholangitis. Hepatology 1991; 14:257–261.

19. Buckels DC, Lindor KD, LaRusso NF, et al. In primary sclerosing cholangitis, gallbladder polyps are frequently malignant. Am J Gastroenterol 2002; 97:1138–1142.

20. Gores GJ. Cholangiocarcinoma: Current concepts and insights. Gastroenterology 2003; 125:1536–1538.

   A state-of-the-art review on pathogenesis and treatment of cholangiocarcinoma.

21. Baron TH, Harewood A, Rumalla A, et al. A prospective comparison of digital image analysis and routine cytology for the identification of malignancy in biliary tract strictures. J Clin Gastroenterol Hepatol 2004; 2:214–219.

22. Hassoun Z, Gores GJ, Rosen CB. Preliminary experience with liver transplantation in selected patients with unresectable hilar cholangiocarcinoma. Surg Oncol Clin N Am 2002; 11:909–921.

   A promising study using radio-/chemotherapy prior to liver transplantation for treatment of cholangiocarcinoma.

23. Mitchell SD, Bansi DS, Hunt N, et al. A preliminary trial of high-dose ursodeoxycholic acid in primary sclerosing cholangitis. Gastroenterology 2001; 121:900–907.

   A pilot study on the promising therapeutic effect of high-dose UDCA in PSC.

24. Harnois DM, Angulo P, Jorgensen RA, et al. High-dose ursodeoxycholic acid as a therapy for patients with primary sclerosing cholangitis. Am J Gastroenterol 2001; 96:1558–1562.

25. Tung BY, Emond MJ, Haggitt RC, et al. Ursodiol use is associated with lower prevalence of colonic neoplasia in patients with ulcerative colitis and primary sclerosing cholangitis. Ann Intern Med 2001; 134:89–95.

   A promising study on the chemopreventive effect of UDCA on colonic neoplasia in patients with PSC and CUC.

26. Pardi DS, Loftus EV Jr, Kremers WK, et al. Ursodeoxycholic acid as a chemopreventive agent in patients with ulcerative colitis and primary sclerosing cholangitis. Gastroenterology 2003; 124:889–893.

27. Cangemi JR, Wiesner RH, Beaver SJ, et al. Effect of proctocolectomy for chronic ulcerative colitis on the natural history of primary sclerosing cholangitis. Gastroenterology 1989; 96:790–794.

28. Broome U, Lofberg R, Veress B, et al. Primary sclerosing cholangitis and ulcerative colitis: evidence for increased neoplastic potential. Hepatology 1995; 22:1404–1408.

   This study indicated the increased risk of developing colon cancer in patients with both PSC and CUC.

29. Weisner RH. Liver transplantation for primary sclerosing cholangitis: timing, outcome, impact of inflammatory bowel disease and recurrence of disease. Best Pract Res Clin Gastroenterol 2001; 15:667–680.

30. Balan V, Batts KP, Porayko MK, et al. Histologic evidence for recurrence of primary biliary cirrhosis after liver transplantation. Hepatology 1993; 18:1392–1398.

CHAPTER TWENTY-SEVEN

Acute pancreatitis

Michael L. Steer

INTRODUCTION

Acute versus chronic pancreatitis

The distinction between acute and chronic pancreatitis has been the subject of considerable confusion and, as a result, several international meetings devoted to the classification of pancreatic inflammatory diseases have been held.[1–3] A general consensus has emerged and it is now customary to define an attack of acute pancreatitis as one which affects a pancreas that was both structurally and functionally normal prior to the attack and a pancreas which can potentially become normal, once again, after resolution of the attack. In contrast, the pancreas is usually structurally and/or functionally abnormal prior to an attack of chronic pancreatitis and it remains abnormal even after the attack has resolved. Pathologically, acute pancreatitis is characterized by varying degrees of edema and necrosis of parenchymal cells in the presence of an acute inflammatory reaction while, in chronic pancreatitis, there is extensive pancreatic fibrosis, loss of both exocrine and endocrine pancreatic elements, and a chronic inflammatory reaction.

It is important to note that, according to this classification system, the distinction between acute and chronic pancreatitis is not dependent upon the acuteness or chronicity of symptoms, the severity of the attack, or the ultimate development of complications such as pseudocyst and abscess. Rather, it is based entirely upon the functional and structural integrity of the gland before and after the attack. Thus, the acute onset of symptoms can occur in chronic as well as acute pancreatitis, a severe attack can occur in either acute or chronic pancreatitis, and patients with either form of pancreatitis can develop extensive pancreatic necrosis and/or pseudocysts. Morphologic changes of fibrosis and loss of exocrine and/or endocrine elements and clinical evidence of exocrine and/or endocrine pancreatic insufficiency, however, are diagnostic of chronic pancreatitis. This chapter will be focused on issues related to acute pancreatitis and the reader is referred to Chapter 28 for a discussion of chronic pancreatitis.

Etiologies of acute pancreatitis

Some 60–70% of patients with acute pancreatitis develop pancreatitis in association with biliary tract stone disease and, in biliary pancreatitis, the attack is generally triggered by the passage of a stone into or through the terminal biliopancreatic ductal system.[4] Biliary pancreatitis can also be caused by passage of biliary sludge or microcrystals. This mechanism may account for the observation that some patients develop biliary pancreatitis without demonstrable biliary tract stones and those patients' recurrent attacks can frequently be prevented by cholecystectomy or sphincter of Oddi sphincterotomy.[5] Abuse of ethanol is the second most common identifiable cause for acute pancreatitis and, in contrast to the long-standing and chronic abuse of ethanol that is associated with chronic pancreatitis, an attack of ethanol-induced acute pancreatitis is usually associated with a 1–2 day episode of binge drinking. Roughly 10–15% of patients with acute pancreatitis develop their disease without an identifiable cause (i.e., 'idiopathic acute pancreatitis') while another 10–15% of patients develop acute pancreatitis in association with a number of miscellaneous causes. These 'miscellaneous causes' include hyperlipidemia, exposure to certain drugs, pancreatic trauma, pancreatic infections or infestations, the postoperative state, tumors and other lesions causing pancreatic duct outflow obstruction, performance of endoscopic retrograde pancreatography, and performance of sphinctor of Oddi manometry.

PATHOPHYSIOLOGY AND PATHOGENESIS OF ACUTE PANCREATITIS

Studies designed to identify the early events which underlie the development of acute pancreatitis can not be performed using clinical material because, for the most part, the early stages of pancreatitis have passed before the diagnosis of acute pancreatitis is established. Furthermore, access to the pancreas during the early stages of severe pancreatitis is usually not possible. To overcome this problem, most of the studies dealing with the pathophysiology and pathogenesis of acute pancreatitis have employed one or more of the various models of acute pancreatitis in experimental animals. On the basis of those studies, most investigators currently believe that acute pancreatitis evolves in multiple stages.[6] The first stage is characterized by changes that occur within pancreatic acinar cells where the intracellular trafficking of digestive enzyme zymogens such as trypsinogen and lysosomal hydrolases such as cathepsin B is altered. As a result, the two types of enzymes become co-localized within intracellular vacuoles and cathepsin B catalyzes the activation of trypsinogen.[7] Subsequently, trypsin activates the other digestive zymogens leading to acinar cell injury. The next stage of pancreatitis involves the initiation of an intrapancreatic inflammatory response. That response is triggered by the generation, within pancreatic cells, of various proinflammatory factors including chemokines and cytokines.[7] These pancreas-derived chemokines and cytokines cause activation and chemoattraction of inflammatory cells to the pancreas and this, along with increased endothelial permeability, results in an intrapancreatic inflammatory reaction. With further progression of the disease, a third stage evolves during which the pancreatic parenchymal cell injury may worsen and a systemic inflammatory response syndrome (SIRS) may be triggered. In patients with severe pancreatitis, SIRS is typically associated with significant acute lung injury and the adult respiratory distress syndrome (ARDS) may develop.[8]

DIAGNOSIS OF ACUTE PANCREATITIS

History

The classical symptoms of acute pancreatitis are abdominal pain, nausea, and vomiting.[9] Typically, the pain of acute pancreatitis precedes the onset of nausea and vomiting. It begins suddenly and gradually increases in intensity. Pain is usually most severe in the epigastric region of the abdomen but it can be felt elsewhere as well and it often radiates straight through to the mid-back. The pain is usually constant, rather than colicky, and is often described as being 'boring' or 'knife-like' in quality. Many patients find that the pain is reduced by either lying on the side with the knees drawn upward or by sitting upright and leaning forward. The nausea of acute pancreatitis is frequently followed by repeated vomiting but, for the most part, vomiting does not relieve either the nausea or the pain of pancreatitis and those symptoms persist in spite of an emptied stomach.

Physical examination

Patients with severe acute pancreatitis usually appear ill and dehydrated. While they usually have a clear sensorium, they may seem anxious and, on occasion, severe mental status changes are observed. They frequently move about seeking a position of comfort and they often have tachycardia, tachypnea, and fever. Hypotension may also be observed, particularly in patients experiencing a severe attack. Roughly 10–20% of patients with severe acute pancreatitis appear clinically jaundiced but jaundice is unusual in patients with mild pancreatitis in the absence of bile duct obstruction.

Most of the physical findings in acute pancreatitis are confined to the abdomen.[9] It may be soft and only mildly tender but, more commonly, it is markedly tender to palpation, especially in the epigastrium, and there may be localized or diffuse involuntary guarding leading to a 'board-like' abdomen. Other signs of peritoneal irritation, such as tenderness to percussion and pain in response to coughing, are frequently noted. The abdomen may be distended and tympanitic as a result of the associated ileus and there may be a palpable mass, reflecting the inflamed pancreas and peripancreatic tissues, in the upper abdomen. Bowel sounds are usually infrequent or absent. Some patients with severe pancreatitis develop ecchymosis in the periumbilical or flank regions (Cullen's and Grey Turner's signs, respectively) as a result of retroperitoneal bleeding but these signs are not specific to acute pancreatitis and they can be seen in patients with retroperitoneal bleeding from other insults.

The chest examination of patients with severe pancreatitis usually reveals evidence of basilar atelectasis caused by splinting of the diaphragm and of pleural effusions, particularly on the left. Examination of the skin may reveal tender, erythematous nodules resembling those seen in erythema nodosum. They usually result from localized, subcutaneous areas of fat necrosis.

Blood tests

Hyperamylasemia occurs in most, but not all, patients with acute pancreatitis.[10] Usually, the serum amylase level rapidly rises during the initial 2–12 hours of an attack and then gradually declines to the normal level over the next 3–5 days. The magnitude of hyperamylasemia does not correlate with the severity of an attack and it has no prognostic value. The serum level of lipase activity is also elevated in most patients with acute pancreatitis and hyperlipasemia may persist longer than hyperamylasemia. Unfortunately, neither hyperamylasemia nor hyperlipasemia are specific to pancreatitis. The former can be caused by diseases of the salivary glands and both can be triggered by diseases that alter gastrointestinal barrier function (e.g., ischemic bowel, perforated viscus, bowel obstruction, etc.).[11] Both hyperamylasemia and hyperlipasemia can also be observed following pancreatic trauma, endoscopic retrograde cholangiopancreatography (ERCP), or passage of a common bile duct stone even in the absence of pancreatitis. Acute pancreatitis may also cause changes in a number of other blood tests. Usually, the hematocrit is elevated due to hypovolemia and the white blood cell count is increased because of pancreatic inflammation. Calcium levels are often depressed secondary to hypoalbuminemia but true hypocalcemia (i.e., decreased ionized calcium levels) is rare.[12] Mild hyperbilirubinemia along with alkaline phosphatase and transaminase elevations are common in pancreatitis, even in the absence of bile duct obstruction. As a result of prerenal azotemia, elevations in blood urea nitrogen and creatinine can be observed. Hypertriglyceridemia, sometimes with lactescent serum, can occur, particularly in patients with either hyperlipidemia-induced or alcohol-induced pancreatitis.[13] Some patients with severe pancreatitis develop disseminated intravascular coagulation and, as a result, thrombocytopenia along with elevated levels of fibrin degradation products, decreased fibrinogen levels, and prolonged prothrombin and partial thromboplastin times can be noted.

Recently, there has been considerable interest in the possibility that certain urine and blood tests might be useful in predicting the severity of an acute pancreatitis attack. In this regard, urine levels of trypsinogen activation peptide and in serum levels of C-reactive protein, phospholipase-A_2, ribonuclease, polymorphonuclear elastase, and interleukin-6 have each been shown to correlate with the severity of pancreatitis and, as a result, these tests have been used to predict the ultimate morbidity/mortality of an attack.[14–16]

Imaging studies

Routine radiographs of the abdomen may reveal changes indicative of intestinal ileus but, for the most part, they are most helpful in excluding other causes for acute abdominal pain (i.e., bowel obstruction, perforated viscus, etc.). Computed tomography (CT) and magnetic resonance imaging (MRI) are particularly helpful in confirming the presence of suspected pancreatitis and in detecting the presence of acute pancreatitis-associated fluid collections. When performed with rapid administration of contrast material, they can identify regions of diminished pancreatic perfusion and, as a result, they can be used to quantitate the extent of pancreatic necrosis.[17,18]

Differential diagnosis

In its broadest sense, the differential diagnosis of acute pancreatitis, especially that of mild acute pancreatitis, might include almost any process that can cause abdominal pain, nausea, vomiting, and abdominal tenderness. However, the differential diagnosis of severe acute pancreatitis, characterized by severe pain combined with evidence of peritoneal irritation and hypovolemia, is much more narrow. A perforated abdominal viscus, bowel obstruction, mesenteric ischemia/infarction, and cholecystitis/cholangitis are, for the most part, the disease processes which must be considered in the differential diagnosis of patients with suspected severe pancreatitis (Table 27.1), and distinguishing pancreatitis from those processes can usually be made on the basis of history, physical examination, and measurement of the serum amylase or lipase activity. While serum amylase/lipase activities are usually more than twice the upper limit of normal in acute pancreatitis, such high levels are usually not achieved in patients with these other nonpancreatitis diseases. When doubt persists, however, cross-sectional imaging studies (i.e., CT and MRI) may be particularly helpful since the absence of pancreatic and peripancreatic inflammatory changes in patients with suspected severe pancreatitis virtually excludes that diagnosis and, in most of such cases, the absence of changes indicative of acute pancreatitis on cross-sectional imaging studies will prompt exploratory laparotomy.

Natural history

Approximately 80–90% of patients with acute pancreatitis experience a mild attack that resolves within 3–4 days with only supportive treatment. The remaining 10–20% of patients, however, experience a severe attack which, in the past, has been associated with mortality rates that approach 20%. With modern methods of intensive care, however, severe acute pancreatitis is associated with mortality rates of only 7–10%.

Patients who die during the early stages of acute pancreatitis (i.e., 0–2 weeks) usually succumb because of comorbid conditions that reduce their ability to withstand severe illness (e.g., associated coronary artery disease, chronic obstructive lung disease, chronic renal insufficiency, etc.) or as a result of pancreatitis-associated acute lung injury (i.e., ARDS). On the other hand, those that die at later times usually die as a result of pancreatitis-associated infections and multiple organ failure.

Predicting the severity of an acute pancreatitis attack

It is generally believed that the severity of an acute attack is determined by events that occur within the initial stages of pancreatitis

and, consistent with this concept, has been the observation that various clinical, radiographic, and biochemical derangements that occur during the initial 24–48 hours of an attack can be used to predict the ultimate severity of that attack. Ranson and his colleques were the first to develop a prognostic scoring system designed to allow the clinician to predict whether an attack would ultimately be one of mild pancreatitis (i.e., associated with little or no morbidity and a very low likelihood of complications or death) or severe pancreatitis (i.e., associated with marked morbidity, a high likelihood of complications including pseudocyst and abscess formation, and a significant chance of death).[19]

Currently, the three most commonly employed prognostic scoring systems are (1) the Ranson system[19] which is based on a selected group of clinical parameters (Table 27.2), (2) the Balthazar system[20] which is based on a series of CT criteria (Table 27.3), and (3) the APACHE 2 system[21] which is based an a series of physiological criteria. In addition to these predictors of severity, however, pancreatitis severity can also be predicted by other clinical changes[22–24] and by the magnitude of certain biochemical changes including urinary trypsinogen activation peptide levels, serum C-reactive protein levels, and serum IL-6 levels.[14–16] It should be emphasized that none of these predictive systems is designed to establish the diagnosis of pancreatitis and they should not be used for that purpose. Rather, they should be used in triaging patients with predicted severe pancreatitis to care in an intensive care unit and for comparison of various treatment groups in randomized clinical trials.

EARLY TREATMENT OF ACUTE PANCREATITIS

The primary goals of therapy during the initial stages of acute pancreatitis include (1) relief of symptoms including pain, nausea, and vomiting; (2) correction of hypovolemia; (3) prophylaxis

---

Table 27.1 Differential diagnosis of acute pancreatitis

Perforated intra-abdominal viscus
Mesenteric ischemia/infarction
Bowel obstruction
Cholecystitis/cholangitis

Table 27.2 Ranson's prognostic clinical criteria for severe pancreatitis

Admission	Initial 48 hours
Gallstone pancreatitis	
Age >70 yr	Hct fall >10
Glucose >220 mg/100 mL	BUN elevation >2 mg/100 mL
WBC >18 000/mm³	Ca²⁺ >8 mg/100 mL
LDH >40 IU/L	Base deficit >5 mEq/L
AST >250 U/100 mL	Fluid sequestration >4L
Nongallstone pancreatitis	
Age >55 yr	Hct fall >10
Glucose >200 mg/100 mL	BUN elevation >5 mg/100 mL
WBC >16 000/mm³	Ca²⁺ >8 mg/100 mL
LDH >350 IU/L	Base deficit >4 mEq/L
AST >250 U/100 mL	Fluid sequestration >6L
	PaO₂ >55 mmHg

Number of factors	*Mortality*
0–2	<2 %
3–4	17%
5–6	40%
7–8	100%

Adapted from references 19, 59.

Table 27.3 Balthazar's prognostic CT criteria for severe pancreatitis

Inflammation and fluid collections	Score
Normal pancreas	0
Diffuse pancreatic enlargement	1
Stranding around pancreas	2
One fluid collection	3
Two or more fluid collections ± gas in pancreas	4

Necrosis (i.e., nonperfusion)	
None	0
<33%	2
33%–50%	4
>50%	6

Score	Mortality	Morbidity
0–3	3%	7%
4–6	7%	36%
7–10	17%	92%

Adapted from reference 20.

against infection; (4) provision of adequate nutrition; (5) limiting the severity of an attack; and (6) management of acute organ failure. This early stage of acute pancreatitis generally includes the first 10–14 days after the onset of symptoms and it leads to a later stage during which therapy is primarily aimed at maintaining nutritional support and treating the local complications of acute pancreatitis such as pseudocysts, pancreatic ascites, and pancreatic infections.

Management of pain

The pain of an acute pancreatitis attack may be severe, and large doses of narcotic mediations may be needed to control that pain. There appears to be no benefit to any particular narcotic medication over the others in the analgesic management of patients with acute pancreatitis in spite of evidence that certain narcotic medications can cause sphincter of Oddi contraction.[25]

Management of nausea and vomiting

Nausea and repeated vomiting are frequently noted by patients with acute pancreatitis and both symptoms may persist, to some degree, even after the stomach has been emptied by vomiting. On occasion, the vomiting and dry retching of acute pancreatitis can cause Mallory-Weiss tears and upper gastrointestinal bleeding. While considerable symptomatic improvement can usually be achieved by placing a nasogastric tube and keeping the stomach empty, there is no evidence that this alters the eventual course or severity of a pancreatitis attack.

Fluid resuscitation

Patients with severe pancreatitis can develop profound hypovolemia. Gastrointestinal fluid losses caused by vomiting and nasogastric suction contribute to this volume contraction but most of the intravascular fluid loss results from the diffuse capillary leak syndrome that accompanies acute pancreatitis and the localized loss of fluids into the inflamed peripancreatic retroperitoneum. The magnitude of pancreatitis-associated hypovolemia can be estimated by comparing the hematocrit levels noted before and after the onset of the attack but losses in excess of 6–8 liters, prior to the time of hospital admission, are not at all unusual.

Aggressive fluid repletion is often required and gauging the adequacy of fluid resuscitation can be aided by monitoring central filling pressures using a Swan-Ganz catheter. Urine output and systemic blood pressure are unreliable parameters for monitoring the adequacy of resuscitation but the return of an elevated hematocrit to its prepancreatitis level may be of more value. Because the fluid lost during pancreatitis is plasma-like in its composition, the serum electrolytes are usually normal even in the presence of severe volume contraction and replacement with solutions such as Ringer's lactate is appropriate.

Prophylaxis against infection

Pancreatic and peripancreatic infection is the most common cause of death during the later phase of severe pancreatitis and there has been considerable interest in the possibility that early administration of antibiotics to patients with severe pancreatitis might prevent these infections. A number of studies examining this possibility have been reported[26–29] and, in general, they have led to the following conclusions: (1) the value of prophylactic antibiotics is greatest when they are given to patients with severe pancreatitis and/or patients with pancreatic necrosis because most patients with mild pancreatitis recover quickly and without complications even without prophylactic antibiotic therapy; (2) antibiotics which penetrate the pancreas (e.g., imipenem, third-generation cephalosporins, etc.) are of greatest value in preventing pancreatic infections; (3) to be of prophylactic value, antibiotics should be administered within the initial 24–72 hrs after the onset of symptoms and antibiotic administration should be continued for 10–14 days; and (4) in addition to parenterally administered antibiotics, gut decontamination may also help to reduce the incidence of pancreatitis-associated infections. On theoretical grounds, prophylactic administration of antibiotics to patients with severe pancreatitis could favor emergence of resistant bacteria and/or fungi in the areas of pancreatic injury, thus limiting the value of antibiotic prophylaxis but, to date, convincing evidence that this occurs has not been presented.

Nutrition

Most patients are unable to eat during the early stages of acute pancreatitis and worsening of symptoms is frequently associated with attempts to eat. In cases of mild pancreatitis, oral alimentation can generally be resumed once the abdominal pain and tenderness have resolved. This usually occurs during the first week after the onset of an attack and, in patients whose pain and tenderness has resolved, resumption of oral alimentation need not be delayed until radiographic evidence of pancreatic inflammation has disappeared and/or serum amylase levels have returned to normal. In contrast, patients with severe pancreatitis are usually unable to tolerate oral alimentation for longer periods of time and, for those patients, an alternative form of nutritional support must be provided to prevent nutritional depletion.

Traditionally, this has been accomplished by instituting total parenteral nutrition (TPN) within the first several days after the onset of a severe attack but recent studies have suggested that enteral administration of nutrients, achieved by infusing elemental diets through a nasojejunal or nasogastric tube, may offer advantages over TPN by reducing the incidence of septic, catheter-related complications.[30–35] On theoretical grounds, enterally administered nutrients may also exert a trophic effect on the gastrointestinal mucosal barrier and, by this mechanism, reduce the likelihood of bacterial translocation from the gut into areas of pancreatic inflammation.

Limiting the severity of an attack

So-called 'gallstone pancreatitis' is the most common form of acute pancreatitis. It is triggered by passage of biliary tract stones, sludge, or microcrystals into or through the terminal biliopancreatic ductal system. In many instances, a biliary tract stone impacted within the distal duct triggers the attack,[4] and this has led to the suggestion that early removal of such an impacted stone might limit the severity of an attack. Three prospective, randomized clinical trials evaluating the potential benefits of early ERCP and stone clearance in the management of acute pancreatitis have been reported.[36–38] In view of the fact that mild pancreatitis is usually self-limited and associated with little morbidity or mortality, it is not surprising that none of the studies showed a benefit to early ERCP and stone clearance in patients with mild pancreatitis. Beyond this point of agreement, however, there was little agreement among the three studies with regard to the potential benefit of early ERCP in the treatment of patients with severe biliary pancreatitis. One study[36] showed that ERCP and stone clearance performed within the initial 72 hours after the onset of symptoms reduced the morbidity and possibly the mortality rates of severe pancreatitis, while a second study[37] suggested that, because of procedure-related complications, early ERCP and stone clearance might actually worsen the course of severe pancreatitis. Finally, the third study[38] indicated that early ERCP and stone clearance was beneficial but that most of the benefit was observed in jaundiced patients in whom the benefit was primarily related to the early resolution of cholangitis. Taken together, these three studies leave open the question of whether early ERCP and stone clearance should be considered the standard of care for patients with severe biliary pancreatitis. Based on the results of these studies, however, it would seem reasonable to conclude that ERCP and stone clearance is most likely to be of benefit if: (1) it is performed within the initial 48–72 hours after the onset of symptoms; (2) it is performed at centers with high levels of expertise and, therefore, lower likelihood of complications; and (3) it is performed in jaundiced patients or patients suspected of having cholangitis in addition to pancreatitis.

Many other interventions have been advocated for the treatment of acute pancreatitis with the hope that they might limit the severity of an attack and, as a result, reduce the associated morbidity and mortality. Unfortunately, few if any of these therapies have been evaluated in prospective, randomized, and placebo-controlled studies and those that have been subjected to such an evaluation have not been found to be beneficial if instituted after the onset of an attack. Some of these 'unproven' therapies are listed in Table 27.4.

Table 27.4 Pancreatitis therapies of unproven benefit

Nasogastric suction
H_2 blockers
Peritoneal lavage
Indomethacin
Somatostatin
Aprotinin
Thoracic duct drainage
Hypothermia
Antacids
Platelet-activating factor antagonists
Anticholinergic agents
Corticosteroids
Glucagon
Calcitonin
Dextran
Heparin
Chlorophyll-a
Propylthiouricil
Vasopressin

Management of early organ failure

Organ failure during the early stages of severe acute pancreatitis is not uncommon. For the most part, this organ failure involves an acute lung injury leading to the adult respiratory distress syndrome and respiratory failure but other organs, particularly the kidneys, may also be involved. It is likely that organ failure during this early period of pancreatitis reflects the 'cytokine storm' which is triggered by pancreatitis[8] and which is manifest by a systemic immune response syndrome (SIRS) and a hemodynamic picture which is consistent with sepsis.[39] Roughly 60% of patients dying during the initial 2 weeks of pancreatitis succumb to respiratory failure. Unfortunately, specific therapy for these acute inflammatory complications of acute pancreatitis is not currently available and treatment is confined to symptomatic measures such as ventilatory support and hemodialysis. There is, however, considerable investigative interest in developing drugs which might limit the 'cytokine storm' and, thus, abort the systemic inflammatory response to pancreatitis.

DELAYED TREATMENT OF ACUTE PANCREATITIS

The initial phase of pancreatitis is driven, to a great extent, by the cytokine storm and acute inflammatory events triggered by the pancreatitis and it is generally completed within the initial 2 weeks of an attack. Treatment at later times is primarily designed to continue nutritional support as well as support for organ failure. In addition, treatment during the later stages of severe pancreatitis is designed to manage local complications of the disease including acute fluid collections, pseudocysts, pancreatic ascites, infected pseudocysts, pancreatic necrosis, and infected pancreatic necrosis.

Management of acute fluid collections

Acute fluid collections within or around the pancreas are relatively common in patients with severe pancreatitis. In some cases, these fluid collections result from leakage of pancreatic juice from disrupted ducts but, for the most part, the fluid in these acute fluid collections is not pancreatic juice. Rather, it is a transudate/exudate formed in response to the pancreatic inflammation. It is not uncommon for patients to have multiple, apparently discontinuous fluid collections in the retroperitoneum and, in the majority of patients, these collections resolve as the pancreatic inflammation recedes. Acute fluid collections may persist for 4–6 weeks after the onset of pancreatitis but they are usually not the cause of symptoms. In the absence of infection, acute fluid collections in patients with pancreatitis may contain inflammatory cells but Gram-stainable organisms are absent. When infection is present, however, the acute fluid collections around the pancreas usually contain microorganisms and inflammatory cells. Fine needle aspiration of the fluid, usually accomplished with CT guidance, may aid in diagnosing pancreatic infection[40,41] and, when infection is present, debridement of the infected tissue and drainage of the infected fluid is indicated (see below). In the absence of infection, however, no treatment for the acute fluid collection is indicated. The placement of drains into noninfected fluid collections should be discouraged for two reasons: first, because drainage is unnecessary, and second, because placement of an in-dwelling drain may lead to infection of the fluid collection.

Management of pseudocysts

Pancreatic pseudocysts are fluid collections which usually communicate with the pancreatic ductal system and usually contain high concentrations of pancreatic digestive enzymes. They may be intrapancreatic or peripancreatic. Usually, they evolve slowly after the onset of pancreatitis, requiring 4–6 weeks to mature. Their borders are comprised of structures which neighbor the pancreas and their walls are composed of fibrotic and granulation tissue. For reasons that are not clear, pseudocysts generally have a round or oval shape. Asymptomatic pseudocysts require no treatment[42,43] but those that cause pain or obstruction of adjacent structures such as the gastric outlet, duodenum, or colon usually require treatment and many approaches to the treatment of such pseudocysts have been proposed. Percutaneous drainage is simple and safe but often associated with the need for prolonged drainage and a significant chance that the pseudocyst will become secondarily infected. Surgical drainage, achieved by anastomosing the cyst to the stomach, a Roux-en-y limb of jejunum, or duodenum is also simple and relatively safe but it exposes the patient to the morbidity of an open operation.

Currently, the most frequently employed approach involves endoscopic drainage of the pseudocyst into either the stomach or duodenum depending upon the location of the cyst and its proximity to the bowel wall. Safe endoscopic drainage is dependent upon the presence of a relatively well-formed cyst wall, little distance between the cyst and the viscus being used, and the absence of major vessels between the viscus and the cyst. The best results are obtained when endoscopic drainage is employed in the management of cysts that contain little or no debris, since the communication that is created endoscopically, and kept open by placement of a stent, may not be adequate for drainage of cysts containing significant amounts of debris. In those cases, some surgeons have advocated a minimally invasive approach in which a laparoscope is placed, transabdominally, into the gastric lumen and a stapled anastomosis is created that establishes a large opening between the stomach and cyst. Others have taken the position that the presence of debris within the pseudocyst indicates that the cyst would be best treated by laparotomy and surgical cystenterostomy.

Management of pancreatic ascites

Pancreatic ascites develops when a major pancreatic duct or pseudocyst ruptures and the leaking pancreatic juice is not contained by surrounding structures. The leaking pancreatic juice can travel, retroperitoneally, to present in one or both pleural spaces, thus creating a pancreatico-pleural fistula. More commonly, however, the leaking juice is contained within the peritoneal cavity as pancreatic ascites. The diagnosis can be easily made when high amylase levels are detected in pleural or peritoneal fluid. With resolution of pancreatitis, pancreatic ascites and pancreatico-pleural fistulae usually resolve and no specific treatment is required. When they persist, however, the initial approach to treatment should be aimed at reducing pancreatic secretion by eliminating enteral alimentation (i.e., institution of total parenteral nutrition) and administration of somatostatin.[44,45] If this fails, further leakage of pancreatic juice may be prevented by the endoscopic placement of a stent across the point of duct disruption in order to bridge the defect[41] or, alternatively, by surgically establishing internal drainage by anastomosing the disrupted duct to a Roux-en-Y limb of jejunum. For duct disruptions in the pancreatic body or tail of the pancreas, distal pancreatectomy may be simpler and more appropriate.

Management of infected pancreatic pseudocysts

It is not unusual for a pancreatic pseudocyst to become colonized with bacteria and/or fungi. The cyst fluid, under these conditions, contains organisms which can be seen with Gram stain but few inflammatory cells and the patient is usually free of symptoms suggestive of infection. Some patients, however, develop true infection of the pseudocyst, i.e. the fluid contains microorganisms as well as many inflammatory cells, and the patient manifests changes of infection including fever and leukocytosis. No therapeutic intervention is called for simply by the presence of pseudocyst colonization but true infection of the pseudocyst mandates treatment. That treatment usually involves either percutaneous external drainage or endoscopic internal drainage.

Management of sterile pancreatic or peripancreatic necrosis

Most patients with severe pancreatitis and many patients with mild pancreatitis have necrosis of peripancreatic fatty tissues and some have pancreatic necrosis as well. In the past, some clinicians have advocated debridement of these areas of necrosis, particularly in patients who were not doing well clinically.[46–48] More recently, however, the pendulum has swung towards a more conservative approach and a general consensus has emerged by which noninfected necrosis, even if extensive, is rarely considered to be an indication for surgical intervention.[49] It is critical, in these patients, to distinguish noninfected from infected necrosis since the latter may mandate some form of intervention (see below) and CT-guided fine needle aspiration of the involved area and/or associated fluid collection may permit this distinction in patients whose clinical picture suggests the presence of infected necrosis.

Table 27.5 Surgical options for infected pancreatic necrosis.

Debridement
With reoperation at planned intervals
With reoperation when clinically indicated
With no packing
With open packing
With closed packing
With continuous lavage

Management of infected pancreatic or peripancreatic necrosis

The traditional treatment of patients with infected pancreatic or peripancreatic necrosis involves surgical debridement of the infected and necrotic tissue. Several different methods for achieving surgical debridement have been advocated (Table 27.5) but the outcomes appear to be similar regardless of the method employed and the ultimate decision is usually based on the local surgeon's preference. In the past, urgent debridement for all patients with infected necrosis has been the standard of care but several recent reports have indicated that delaying operation, in patients who are tolerating the infection well, may reduce the need for repeated operations, reduce the complications of operation, and improve outcomes.[50,51]

Recent anecdotal reports have suggested that some patients with infected necrosis may be successfully treated nonoperatively with (1) prolonged antibiotic therapy, (2) endoscopic, transpapillary drainage, or (3) percutaneous drainage.[52-56] Minimally invasive methods of achieving drainage and debridement have also been described.[57,58] The ultimate value of these nontraditional approaches to the management of patients with infected necrosis is not known and prospective randomized trials will be needed to resolve this uncertainty.

Prevention of recurrent attacks

It is imperative that the etiology of an acute pancreatitis attack be identified so that efforts can be made to prevent recurrent attacks once the acute attack has resolved. In cases of drug-induced acute pancreatitis, the offending drug must be avoided and alternatives used. In alcohol-induced acute pancreatitis, subsequent abstinence from alcohol is mandatory. The majority of patients, however, have acute pancreatitis that is triggered by biliary tract disease, i.e., either biliary duct stones or sludge. Removal of the gall bladder, in such patients, will usually prevent recurrent attacks and, for these patients, cholecystectomy should be performed after recovery from the attack but before discharge from the hospital. For the most part, attacks of biliary pancreatitis can also be prevented by performance of an endoscopic sphincter of Oddi sphincterotomy and this nonsurgical option may be preferable to cholecystectomy for patients with serious comorbidities who have not experienced

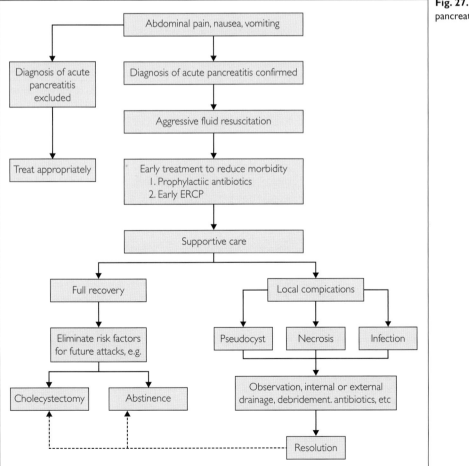

Fig. 27.1 • Algorithm for management of acute pancreatitis.

symptoms of either cholecystitis or biliary colic. Roughly one out of three patients so managed will subsequently experience gallbladder-related symptoms requiring cholecystectomy over the subsequent 3–5 years. The appropriate management of patients with idiopathic acute pancreatitis is somewhat controversial. Roughly half of all patients given the diagnosis of idiopathic acute pancreatitis will not have further attacks if cholecystectomy or sphincter of Oddi sphincterotomy is performed,[5] and this observation might suggest that, in actuality, they had experienced biliary rather than idiopathic pancreatitis. In light of this uncertainty, however, it would seem reasonable to propose that selected patients with 'idiopathic acute pancreatitis' undergo either cholecystectomy or sphincterotomy and that only those who experience recurrent attacks subsequent to this treatment should be considered to have truly idiopathic pancreatitis.

SUMMARY

Acute pancreatitis is a potentially devastating inflammatory disease of the pancreas. While it can be triggered by a number of etiologies, passage of stones or sludge into or through the terminal biliopancreatic ductal system is the most common cause of acute pancreatitis. Most patients present with abdominal pain, nausea, and vomiting (Fig. 27.1). Once the diagnosis of acute pancreatitis is confirmed, aggressive fluid resuscitation is appropriate. Patients with severe pancreatitis should be given prophylactic antibiotics and those with biliary acute pancreatitis may benefit from early endoscopic retrograde cholangiopancreatography with clearance of stones from the biliary tree. Subsequent treatment is primarily supportive and most patients recover uneventfully. For those patients, cholecystectomy and/or abstinence from alcohol are appropriate if future attacks are to be avoided. Roughly 10–20% of patients experience a severe attack of pancreatitis which may be complicated by pancreatic necrosis, infection, and/or formation of a pseudocyst. Management of these local complications of pancreatitis may involve drainage and/or debridement as well as prolonged treatment with antibiotics.

REFERENCES

1. Sarles H. Pancreatitis symposium, Marseille 1963. Basle, New York: S. Karger; 1965.

2. Sarner M, Cotton PB. Classification of pancreatitis. Gut 1984; 25:756–759.

3. Gyr K, Singer MV, Sarles H. Pancreatitis: concepts and classification. Proceedings of the Second International Symposium on the Classification of Pancreatitis in Marseille, France. March 28–30, 1984. Amsterdam: Exerpta Medica; 1984.

4. Opie EL. The etiology of acute hemorrhagic pancreatitis. Johns Hopkins Hosp Bull 1901; 12:182–192.

This classical paper records observations made by a pathologist who performed an autopsy on a patient dying of acute gallstone-induced pancreatitis. The finding of a bile-stained pancreas and a common biliopancreatic channel above an obstructing, impacted stone in the ampulla gave rise to the hypothesis that gallstones trigger pancreatitis by causing bile to reflux, retrogradely, into the pancreatic duct as a result of more distal biliary-pancreatic duct obstruction.

5. Lee SP, Nicholls JF, Park HZ. Biliary sludge as a cause of acute pancreatitis. N Engl J Med 1992; 326:589–593.

This important paper shows that biliary sludge and microcrystals are important causes of so-called idiopathic acute pancreatitis and that the frequency of recurrent attacks of idiopathic acute pancreatitis can be reduced by sphincterotomy and cholecystectomy.

6. Steer ML. The early intraacinar cell events which occur during acute pancreatitis. The Frank Brooks Memorial Lecture. Pancreas 1998; 17:31–37.

This review article summarizes many studies performed both in vivo and in vitro using various models of experimental pancreatitis. Those studies have provided some important insights into the early acinar cell biological events that trigger acute pancreatitis, including the co-localization of digestive zymogens with lysosomal hydrolases and the intracellular activation of zymogens, including trypsinogen.

7. Saluja AK, Bhagat L, Lee HS, et al. Secretagogue-induced digestive enzyme activation and cell injury in rat pancreatic acini. Am J Physiol 1999; 276:G835–G842.

8. Makhija R, Kingsnorth AN. Cytokine storm in acute pancreatitis. J Hepato-Bil-Pancreat Surg 2002; 9:401–410.

9. Steer ML. Exocrine pancreas. In: Sabiston textbook of surgery. Townsend C, Beauchamp R, Evers M, et al., eds. Philadelphia: Elsevier; 2004:1645–1678.

10. Levitt MD, Edkfeldt JH. Diagnosis of acute pancreatitis. In: Go VLW, et al., eds. The exocrine pancreas: biology, pathobiology, and diseases. New York: Raven Press; 1986:481–500.

11. Salt WB, Schenker S. Amylase – its clinical significance: a review of the literature. Medicine (Baltimore) 1976; 55(4):269–290.

12. Imrie CW, Whyte AS. A prospective study of acute pancreatitis. Br J Surg 1975; 62:490–494.

13. Yadav D, Pitchumoni CS. Issues in hyperlipidemic pancreatitis. J Clin Gastroenterol 2003; 36:54–62.

14. Tenner S, Fernandez-del Castillo C, Warshaw A, et al. Urinary trypsinogen activation peptide (TAP) predicts severity in patients with acute pancreatitis. Int J Pancreatol 1997; 21:105–110.

15. Mayer AD, McMahon MJ, Bowen M, et al. C reactive protein: an aid to the assessment and monitoring of acute pancreatitis. J Clin Pathol 1984; 37:207–211.

16. Poulakkainen PA, Valtonen V, Paananen A, et al. C reactive protein and serum phospholipase A2 in the assessment of the severity of acute pancreatitis. Gut 1987; 28:764–771.

17. Runzi M, Raptopoulos V, Saluja A, et al. Evaluation of necrotizing pancreatitis in the opossum by dynamic contrast-enhanced computerized tomography. J Am Coll Surg 1995; 180:673–682.

18. Balthazar EJ. Acute pancreatitis: assessment of severity with clinical and CT evaluation. Radiology 2002; 223:603–613.

19. Ranson JHC, Rifkind KM, Roses DF, et al. Prognostic signs and the role of operative management in acute pancreatitis. Surg Gynecol Obstet 1974; 139:69–81.

This paper reports the first attempts to identify the early characteristics of a pancreatitis attack which might be used to predict the ultimate severity of that attack. In this report, events monitored during the initial 48 hours after hospital admission were used to predict morbidity and death. Many other such prognostic scoring systems have subsequently been described, some of which allow the clinician to predict the severity of an attack within shorter times after hospital admission.

20. Balthazar EJ, Robinson DL, Megibow AJ, et al. Acute pancreatitis: Value of CT in establishing prognosis. Radiology 1990; 174:331–336.

21. Larvin M, McMahon MJ. APACHE II score for assessment and monitoring of acute pancreatitis. Lancet 1989; 2:201–204.

22. Blamey SL, Imrie CW, O'Neill J, et al. Prognostic factors in acute pancreatitis. Gut 1984; 25:1340–1346.

23. Werner J, Hartwig W, Uhl W, et al. Useful markers for predicting severity and monitoring progression of acute pancreatitis. Pancreatol 2003; 3:115–127.

24. Imrie CW. Prognostic indicators in acute pancreatitis. Can J Gastroenterol 2003; 17:325–328.

25. Helm JF, Venu RP, Geenen JE, et al. Effects of morphine on the human sphincter of Oddi. Gut 1988; 29:1402–1407.

26. Pederzoli P, Bassi C, Vesentini S, et al. A randomized multicenter trial of antibiotic prophylaxis of septic complications in acute necrotizing pancreatitis with imipenem. Surg Gynecol Obstet 1993; 176:480–483.

This was one of the first reports to suggest that prophylactic administration of antibiotics might beneficially affect the course of pancreatitis. Benefit was confined to those with necrotizing pancreatitis.

27. Sainio V, Kemppainen E, Poulakkainen P, et al. Early antibiotic treatment in acute necrotising pancreatitis. Lancet 1995; 346:663–667.

28. Ljuiten EJ, Hop WC, Lange JF, et al. Controlled clinical trial of selective decontamination for the treatment of severe acute pancreatitis. Ann Surg 1995; 222:57–65.

29. Bassi C, Larvin M, Villatoro E. Antibiotic therapy for prophylaxis against infection of pancreatic necrosis in acute pancreatitis. Cochrane Database of Systematic Reviews. CD002941, 2003.

30. Kalfarentzos F, Kehagias J, Mead N, et al. Enteral nutrition is superior to parenteral nutrition in severe acute pancreatitis. Br J Surg 1997; 84:1665–1669.

31. McClave SA, Greene LM, Snider HL, et al. Comparison of the safety of early enteral vs parenteral nutrition in mild acute pancreatitis. J Parenter Enteral Nutr 1997; 21:14–20.

32. Windsor AC, Kanwar S, Li AG, et al. Compared with parenteral nutrition, enteral feeding attenuates the acute phase response and improves disease severity in acute pancreatitis. Gut 1998; 42:431–435.

33. Abou-Assi S, Craig K, O'Keefe SJ. Hypocaloric jejunal feeding is better than total parenteral nutrition in acute pancreatitis: results of a randomized comparative study. Am J Gastroenterol 2002; 97:2255–2262.

34. Imrie CW, Carter CR, McKay CJ. Enteral and parenteral nutrition in acute pancreatitis. Best Pract Res Clin Gastroenterol 2002; 16:391–397.

35. Avgerinos C, Delis S, Rizos S, et al. Nutritional support in acute pancreatitis. Dig Dis 2003; 21:214–219.

36. Neoptolemos JF, Carr-Locke D, James D, et al. Controlled trial of urgent endoscopic retrograde cholangiopancreatography and endoscopic sphincterotomy versus conservative treatment for acute pancreatitis due to gallstones. Lancet 1988; 2:979–983.

This controversial study suggests that patients with severe pancreatitis benefit from undergoing ERCP, sphincterotomy, and stone clearance within 72 hours of hospital admission. Some patients appeared to benefit from sphincterotomy even when stones were not found in the ductal system.

37. Folsch UR, Nitsche R, Ludke R, et al. Early ERCP and papillotomy compared with conservative treatment for acute biliary pancreatitis. N Eng J Med 1997; 336:237–242.

38. Fan ST, Lai ECS, Mok FPT, et al. Early treatment of acute biliary pancreatitis by endoscopic papillotomy. N Engl J Med 1993; 328:228–232.

39. Beger HG, Bittner R, Buchler M, et al. Hemodynamic data pattern in patients with acute pancreatitis. Gastroenterology 1986; 90:70.

40. Gerzof SG, Banks PA, Robbins AH, et al. Early diagnosis of pancreatic infection by computed tomography-guided aspiration. Gastroenterology 1987; 93:1315–1320.

This important paper showed that CT-guided percutaneous fine needle aspiration of the pancreas could be safely performed during severe acute pancreatitis and that is was a reliable means of identifying patients with pancreatic infections.

41. Banks PA, Gerzof SG, Langevin RE, et al. CT-guided aspiration of suspected pancreatic infection. Int J Pancreatol 1995; 18:265–270.

42. Vitas GJ, Sarr MG. Selected management of pancreatic pseudocysts: Operative versus expectant management. Surgery 1992; 111:123–130.

43. Yeo CJ, Bastidas JA, Lynch-Nyhan A, et al. The natural history of pancreatic pseudocysts documented by computed tomography. Surg Gynecol Obstet 1990; 170:411–417.

These two frequently cited papers (Vitas and Sarr, and Yeo et al.) challenged the conventional wisdom of the time which argued that a drainage procedure was appropriate for all pancreatic pseudocysts that were greater than 6 cm in diameter and persisted for more than 6 weeks after the onset of an attack. The authors of these two reports showed that many large and persistent pseudocysts eventually resolve without the need for drainage and that those which remain are only infrequently associated with complications.

44. Segal I, Parekh D, Lipschitz J, et al. Treatment of pancreatic ascites and external pancreatic fistulas with a long-acting somatostatin analog (Sandostatin). Digestion 1993; 54S:53–58.

45. Lipsett PA, Cameron JL. Internal pancreatic fistula. Am J Surg 1992; 163:216–220.

46. Beger HG, Buchler M, Bittner R, et al. Necrosectomy and postoperative local lavage in patients with necrotizing pancreatitis: Results of a prospective clinical trial. World J Surg 1988; 255:42.

47. Fernandez-del Castillo C, Rattner DW, Makary MA, et al. Debridement and closed packing for the treatment of necrotizing pancreatitis. Ann Surg 1998; 228:676–684.

48. Warshaw AL. Pancreatic necrosis: to debride or not to debride – that is the question. Ann Surg 2000; 232:627–629.

49. Bradley EL 3rd. Operative vs. nonoperative therapy in necrotizing pancreatitis. Digestion 1999; 1:19–21.

50. Clancy TE, Ashley SW. Current management of necrotizing pancreatitis. Adv Surg 2002; 36:103–121.

51. Hartwig W, Maksan SM, Foitzik T et al. Reduction in mortality with delayed surgical therapy of severe pancreatitis. J Gastrointest Surg 62002; :481–487.

52. Freeney PC, Hauptman E, Althaus SJ, et al. Percutaneous CT-guided catheter drainage of infected acute necrotizing pancreatitis: techniques and results. Am J Roentgenol 1998; 170:969–975.

53. Baron TH, Morgan DE. Endoscopic transgastric irrigation tube placement via PEG for debridement of organized pancreatic necrosis. Gastrointest Endosc 1999; 50:574–577.

54. Zein CO, Baron TH, Morgan DE. Endoscopic pancreaticoduodenostomy for treatment of pancreatic duct disconnection because of severe acute pancreatitis. Gastrointest Endosc 2003; 58: 130–134.

55. Gmeinwieser J, Holstege A, Zirngibl H, et al. Successful percutaneous treatment of infected necrosis of the body of the pancreas associated with segmental disruption of the main pancreatic duct. Gastrointest Endosc 2000; 52:413–415.

56. Horvath KD, Kao LS, Wherry KL, et al. A technique for laparoscopic-assisted percutaneous drainage of infected pancreatic necrosis and pancreatic abscess. Surg Endosc 2001; 15:1221–1225.

57. Kellogg TA, Horvath KD. Minimal-access approaches to complications of acute pancreatitis and benign neoplasms of the pancreas. Surg Endosc 2003; 17:1692–1704.

58. Carter R. Management of infected necrosis secondary to acute pancreatitis: a balanced role for minimal access techniques. Pancreatology 2003; 3:133–138.

59. Ranson JHC. Etiological and prognostic factors in human acute pancreatitis: A review. Am J Gastroenterol 1982; 77:633.

CHAPTER TWENTY-EIGHT

Chronic pancreatitis

Julia Mayerle and Markus M. Lerch

INTRODUCTION

Definition of chronic pancreatitis

Chronic pancreatitis is defined as a continuous or recurrent inflammatory disease of the pancreas characterized by progressive and irreversible morphological changes. It typically causes pain and permanent impairment of pancreatic function. In chronic pancreatitis areas of focal necrosis are typically associated with perilobular and intralobular fibrosis of the parenchyma, by stone formation in the pancreatic duct, and by the development of pseudocysts. Late in the course of the disease a progressive loss of endocrine and exocrine function occurs.[1,2] Several attempts have been undertaken – the last one in the year 2000 – to establish histological and morphological criteria to clearly define chronic pancreatitis. Unfortunately, an exact correlation between clinical symptoms, morphological signs, and histological criteria is still not at hand.[3,4] With an incidence of 8.2, a prevalence of 27.4 per 100 000 population, and a frequency of 0.04–5% in all autopsies performed, chronic pancreatitis represents a common disorder of the gastrointestinal tract.[5,6] Chronic pancreatitis accounts for substantial morbidity and healthcare costs. The annual treatment costs per patient are approximately US$17 000,[4] around 20 000 Americans are admitted to hospital every year with an admission diagnosis of chronic pancreatitis, and about three times as many are discharged with the diagnosis of chronic pancreatitis.[7] The 10-year survival rate of patients suffering from alcohol-induced chronic pancreatitis is 70%, while the 20-year survival rate is 45%. The mortality is thus increased 3.6-fold compared to a cohort without chronic pancreatitis.[8]

PATHOGENESIS

Pathophysiology of chronic pancreatitis

The pathogenesis of chronic pancreatitis is still poorly understood. Alcohol is the leading risk factor and the most common etiology.[9] At present there are four competing hypotheses concerning the pathogenesis of chronic pancreatitis. According to one of these hypotheses,[10] ethanol induces the fatty degeneration of acini similar to that caused by ethanol in the hepatocytes of the liver. This effect of ethanol is either a direct or an indirect toxic effect, mediated by the ethanol metabolite acetaldehyde, on the metabolism of pancreatic acinar cells.[10,11]

According to the second hypothesis,[12–14] ethanol's injurious effects involve the toxic effects of oxygen-derived free radicals on pancreatic acinar cells. Presumably, oxidative stress, caused by nicotine or ethanol, leads to the peroxidation of the lipid bilayer of the cell membrane, ultimately destroying that membrane. According to this hypothesis, an excess of free oxygen radicals would overwhelm the protective, antioxidant mechanisms as shown for some cytochrome P450 enzyme pathways in the liver. This hypothesis has stimulated several clinical studies testing antioxidants in the treatment of chronic pancreatitis and some promising observations have been reported.[12–14] A large European multicenter study testing the effect of antioxidant treatment in patients with idiopathic chronic pancreatitis is presently being launched.

A third hypothesis, proposed by Sarles and Sahel, suggests that protein precipitates in the ductal system causing ductal obstruction that leads to ductal hypertension, and that ductal hypertension ultimately causes destruction of pancreatic acini. This hypothesis asserts that chronic alcohol consumption leads to a decrease in the bicarbonate concentration and volume of pancreatic secretions and that this ultimately leads to the precipitation of protein and calcium crystals within the duct, causing duct obstruction. To avoid stone formation, it would be necessary for the acinar cells to produce a low molecular weight protein called lithostatin which would, in turn, increase the fluidity of pancreatic juice and prevent precipitation of protein plaques and calcite crystals in calcium-supersaturated pancreatic juice. The validity of this hypothesis has been questioned because others have (1) failed to find a decreased concentration of lithostatins in the pancreatic juice of patients with chronic pancreatitis or (2) could not demonstrate an inhibitory function of lithostatins on calcium carbonate precipitation. Nevertheless, the role of duct plugging in cystic fibrosis is unquestioned.[15,16]

The fourth hypothesis, originally proposed by Comfort and colleagues but then revisited by Klöppel and Maillet-Guy argues that chronic pancreatitis is a consequence of recurrent episodes of acute pancreatitis.[17] According to this hypothesis, focal fat necrosis and necrosis of the pancreatic parenchyma leads to the infiltration of lymphocytes, macrophages, and fibroblasts and fibrosis is the consequence of necrosis. This proposed hypothesis would be consistent with the concept that premature intracellular zymogen activation in pancreatic acini is the underlying cause of recurrent bouts of the acute pancreatitis that subsequently lead to the development of chronic pancreatitis. This pathomechanism is also suspected to be the cause of hereditary pancreatitis, which is associated with mutations in the cationic trypsinogen gene.[18] Most of the clinical and experimental evidence suggests that this fourth hypothesis is the one that predicts the pathophysiology of chronic pancreatitis most accurately.

Etiology of chronic pancreatitis

In Western countries alcohol consumption is assumed to be the leading cause (70–90%) of all cases of chronic pancreatitis.[19] According to the studies from Marseilles, the logarithm of the relative risk of chronic pancreatitis increases linearly as a function of the quantity of alcohol and protein consumed. There seems to be no threshold toxicity of alcohol as identified in alcoholic liver damage. Furthermore, the type of alcoholic beverages consumed appears to be less relevant. Patients with chronic pancreatitis and alcohol-induced liver cirrhosis do not differ with regard to their daily intake of alcohol. However the duration of alcohol consumption is shorter in chronic pancreatitis. In most studies the time between the onset of alcohol abuse and first symptoms is 18±11 years. The prevalence of chronic pancreatitis clearly correlates with the alcohol consumption of a given population.[20–27]

The second most common form of chronic pancreatitis, as of today, is so-called idiopathic pancreatitis (25%).[28,29] Patients without an identifiable risk factor for chronic pancreatitis are classified as having idiopathic pancreatitis. This group has constantly decreased since Comfort and Steinberg reported in 1952 an inherited form of chronic pancreatitis following an autosomal dominant inheritance pattern.[30] Hereditary pancreatitis represents a genetic disorder closely associated with mutations in the cationic trypsinogen gene and presents with a disease penetrance of ≈80%.[31] Patients with hereditary pancreatitis develop recurrent bouts of pancreatitis which progress to chronic pancreatitis. Symptoms usually begin in early childhood but, in rare cases, the disease onset can be as late as the sixth decade of life. The severity of the acute attacks in hereditary pancreatitis ranges from mild abdominal discomfort to severe disease complicated by pancreatic necrosis, organ failure, and eventually death, although the latter course is exceedingly rare. Compared to the general population, the risk of developing pancreatic carcinoma is 50–60 times greater in patients suffering from hereditary pancreatitis.[32,33]

As hereditary pancreatitis represents an autosomal dominant disorder, it was suspected that the disease results from a single genetic defect that disrupts a critical component that protects pancreatic function in unaffected individuals. In 1996 Whitcomb et al. identified a single point mutation in the third exon of the cationic trypsinogen gene on chromosome 7 (7q35) that associates with the phenotype of hereditary pancreatitis.[31] This mutation was present in all affected individuals and obligate carriers from five kindreds with hereditary pancreatitis, but not in individuals who married into the family nor in 140 unrelated individuals. This G-to-A transition results in an arginine-(R)-(CGC)-to histidine-(H)-(CAC) substitution, referred to as R122H. It was predicted to eliminate a fail-safe trypsin hydrolysis site that is necessary to initiate the self-destruction of activated trypsin. Since 1996 several more mutations (20 so far) in the trypsinogen gene have been reported, but the R122H mutation is still the most

common.[34–36] As far as the role of premature zymogen activation is concerned, the data from hereditary pancreatitis presently available are inconclusive.[37] Because trypsin activation is an event known to occur in pancreatitis,[38] and because trypsin can activate many other digestive proteases of the pancreas in vitro, previous attempts to interpret the functional consequences of trypsinogen mutations have focused on features that would either allow for premature intracellular activation of trypsinogen or permit an extended intracellular activity of trypsin. Other studies have suggested that trypsin activity may be a critical factor for the degradation of other, much more destructive digestive proteases. Trypsin activity would then have to be regarded as protective factor and hereditary pancreatitis as a disease caused by a loss, rather than a gain, of trypsin function.[34,37] The idea of digestive protease activation dates back a century to when the pathologist Hans Chiari suggested that the pancreas of patients who had died during episodes of acute necrotizing pancreatitis 'had succumbed to its own digestive properties,' and he postulated pancreatic 'autodigestion' as the underlying pathophysiological mechanism of the disease.[39] While the importance of digestive proteases in the onset of pancreatitis is now undisputed, the role of individual serine proteases in that cascade-like event, and that of the different isoforms of trypsin in particular, is still a matter of intense research and debate.[37]

Shortly after the identification of mutations in the trypsinogen gene associated with chronic pancreatitis, another important observation was made by Witt et al.[40] They found mutations in the SPINK-1 gene (encoding the pancreatic secretory trypsin inhibitor, PSTI) to be associated with idiopathic chronic pancreatitis in children. SPINK-1 mutations can frequently be detected in a cohort of patients who do not present with a family history of pancreatitis and are devoid of any classical risk factors for chronic pancreatitis.[41,42] SPINK-1 is believed to form a first line of defense in inhibiting trypsin in the pancreas. The discovery of SPINK-1 mutations therefore provides additional evidence for the role of protease activation in the development of pancreatitis.[43]

Cystic fibrosis is an autosomal recessive disorder, with an estimated incidence of 1:2500, characterized by pancreatic exocrine insufficiency and chronic pulmonary disease. The extent to which the pancreas is affected varies between a complete loss of exocrine and endocrine function to clinically normal pancreatic function. Recurrent episodes of pancreatitis occur in 1–2% of all patients with cystic fibrosis and normal exocrine pancreatic function, and more rarely in patients with exocrine pancreatic insufficiency. Compared to the population of patients without chronic pancreatitis, 16.7–25.9% of patients with idiopathic chronic pancreatitis carry mutations in the cystic fibrosis conductance regulator gene (CFTR). Thus, in addition to chronic lung disease and vas deferens aplasia, chronic pancreatitis represents a third disease entity associated with mutations in the CFTR gene. It is important to note that pancreatic exocrine insufficiency in patients with cystic fibrosis is a completely different disease entity and not to be confused with chronic pancreatitis in the presence of CFTR mutations.[44,45]

Considerable attention, especially in Japan, is nowadays paid to an only recently characterized type of steroid-responsive chronic pancreatitis termed autoimmune pancreatitis. This type of chronic pancreatitis typically presents with an enlargement of the pancreatic gland, diffuse narrowing of the pancreatic duct, elevated serum lipase levels and, in 70–80% of the patients, with obstructive jaundice. For this reason, most patients are initially suspected to have pancreatic carcinoma. The absence of calcification of the gland is regarded as a pathognomonic feature. The gender distribution is 2:1 with a predominance in men. The incidence of autoimmune pancreatitis increases in the second decade of life. Blood tests reveal an increased IgG4 level, nuclear autoantibodies (ANA), autoantibodies directed against lactoferrin as well as against carbonic anhydrase, and elevated serum rheumatic factors. Morphologically, ductal and periductal inflammatory infiltrates, predominantly composed of lymphocytes, plasma cells, and granulocytes, are the most constant histopathological findings. In approximately 60% of cases, the disease is associated with other systemic autoimmune disorders. Endoscopic retrograde cholangiopancreatography (ERCP) examination shows a diffuse irregular narrowing of the main pancreatic duct and narrowing stenoses of the bile duct passing through the head of the pancreas. In contrast to other varieties of chronic pancreatitis, autoimmune pancreatitis responds very well to steroid treatment.[46]

Metabolic disorders associated with hypertriglyceridemia above 1000 mg/dL can be responsible for the development of recurrent episodes of pancreatitis.[47,48] In rare cases chronic calcifying pancreatitis has been reported to be due to hypercalcemia in patients with untreated hyperparathyroidism. This has become a rare cause of pancreatitis today because serum calcium levels are routinely checked and part of most automated clinical chemistry panels. The underlying mechanism of hyperparathyroidism-associated pancreatitis is most likely related to the established role of calcium in the premature, intracellular activation of digestive proteases.[49]

CLINICAL PRESENTATION

The clinical presentation of patients with chronic pancreatitis is highly dependent on the stage of the disease. It varies between severely ill patients with symptoms of acute abdomen, to slowly progressing cachexia. The cardinal symptoms, and often the first signs of the disease which prompt the patient to seek medical help, are beltlike abdominal pain that frequently radiates to the back, loss of body weight (in 80%) and steatorrhea (in less than 50%).[50] Pain is the most commonly encountered symptom in chronic pancreatitis (80–95% of all patients).[51] Some studies which investigated the natural course of the disease showed that with the duration of chronic inflammation the intensity of pain can decline. This observation was termed 'burn out of pain' and correlates frequently with the occurrence of parenchymal calcifications and the loss of endocrine and exocrine function. Pain in chronic pancreatitis can have several causes. It can be caused by inflammatory infiltrates into pancreatic tissue and its perineural sheath. Morphological studies in patients with chronic pancreatitis have demonstrated an increase in diameter and in the number of intrapancreatic nerves, foci of inflammatory cells associated with nerves and ganglia, and damage of the perineural sheath.[52] This disruption of the perineural sheath may allow inflammatory mediators to gain access to the neural elements. It is presently not known whether similar changes within pancreatic nerves also occur among patients without pain.

Several lines of clinical and experimental evidence point to increased pressure within the pancreatic duct or the parenchyma as an important cause of pancreatic pain. Both pancreatic ductal and tissue pressure are often found to be elevated in patients with chronic pancreatitis undergoing surgery for chronic pain.[53,54]

Drainage of the pancreatic duct can lead to an immediate reduction in pressure to normal levels and can be associated with pain relief.[55] Although this mechanism represents an attractive hypothesis it does not explain why decreasing pancreatic secretion with somatostatin analogues results in a reduction of pain in only a minority of patients. Furthermore, there is no predictable correlation between pancreatic duct pressure and duct morphology or between pancreatic duct morphology and clinical symptoms. The mechanism by which increased intrapancreatic pressure causes pain may also involve a decrease in pancreatic blood flow, a decrease in capillary filling, and thus tissue ischemia – not unlike a surgical compartment syndrome.

Gastric or duodenal ulcers as well as meteorism due to bacterial overgrowth in the gut caused by maldigestion must also be considered as a cause of pain in patients with chronic pancreatitis.

More rarely, patients seek medical help because they developed diabetes mellitus, and the loss of endocrine function or cachexia are the initial symptoms of chronic pancreatitis. Some patients who present with symptoms and signs of acute pancreatitis due to alcohol abuse are diagnosed as suffering from chronic pancreatitis only during the hospital admission. The median age at diagnosis of patients with chronic pancreatitis is 37–40 years. Frequently, at that age patients already report a long history of alcohol abuse. At this stage patients often report episodes of pain followed by periods of relative well-being.

DIAGNOSIS

Diagnostic imaging procedures

The diagnosis of chronic pancreatitis is based on clinical data, imaging studies, and laboratory investigations including pancreatic function tests. Unlike liver or inflammatory bowel disease, nonoperative access to tissue for histologic examination is usually not possible for diagnostic purposes. Most patients are therefore subjected to clinical, imaging, and laboratory studies before the diagnosis of chronic pancreatitis is established and, since the results of these studies do not always correlate, their combination is often required (Table 28.1).

Transabdominal ultrasound can provide key information. The procedure is noninvasive and without complications but it is highly dependent on the experience of the examiner. Its diagnostic sensitivity is in the range of 52–68%, while its specificity ranges 95–100%. Most noteworthy is its negative predictive value of above 95%. Nevertheless, the value of this procedure should not be overestimated. A high specificity and sensitivity can only be achieved if the organ can be sufficiently visualized, as is the case in approximately 80% of patients.[56] In 20% of cases overlying bowel gas or adipose tissue prevents adequate visualization. The sensitivity of transabdominal ultrasound can be increased by intravenous application of the secretagogue secretin, at a dose of 100 CU. Three to 5 minutes after the infusion of secretin, the main pancreatic duct in healthy volunteers is found to dilate from a median diameter of 1.07 ± 0.09 mm to 1.9 ± 0.16 mm. In patients with chronic pancreatitis, the diameter of the pancreatic main duct increases only slightly or not at all after application of secretin (unstimulated 3.29 ± 0.79 mm, stimulated 4.14 ± 0.94 mm). The reason for this absence of a dilatation is believed to be the presence of periductular fibrosis, which is found in the chronically inflamed tissue.[57]

Table 28.1 Parameters to be determined at the first visit in patients with suspected chronic pancreatitis

History and clinical examination	Blood test/ fecal test	Imaging studies
Age at onset of symptoms, first episode Frequency of episodes Duration of pain, pain diary, pain medication Steatorrhea, meteorism Weight loss Jaundice, vomiting, fever Smoking habits Etiology: Alcohol abuse Family history for pancreatitis, pancreatic cancer, cystic fibrosis affected relatives or children Hyperparathyroidism Hyperlipidemia Autoimmune disorder, e.g. RA, Sjögren's syndrome	Lipase, Amylase, CRP, Bilirubin, γ-GT, alkaline phosphatase, leukocytes, thrombocytes, red blood count, serum albumin. Blood sugar level, Insulin, C-peptide, HbA1c Triglyceride, Cholesterol Calcium, Phosphate, PTH Carbodeficient transferrin ANA, if positive, autoantibodies against lactoferrin and carboanhydrase II, IgG4. Fecal elastase In case of positive family history or onset below 25 years: genetic testing for trypsinogen mutations Ca-19-9, CEA if cancer is found	Transabdominal ultrasound: depending on the result ERCP Endoscopic ultrasound CT scan MRI/MRCP

Plain abdominal radiography is reasonably specific for the diagnosis of chronic pancreatitis when diffuse pancreatic calcifications are detected. Since calcifications occur relatively late in the natural history of chronic pancreatitis, plain abdominal radiography is inferior to transabdominal ultrasound and, even if it is inexpensive, risk free and widely available, in our opinion, it is today an obsolete procedure for the diagnosis of chronic pancreatitis.

The gold standard of noninvasive imaging in the diagnosis of chronic pancreatitis is contrast enhanced computed tomography. Computed tomography is most accurate in the detection of complications associated with chronic pancreatitis such as pancreatic pseudocysts, thrombosis of the splenic vein, a pancreatic mass, or an acute episode of chronic pancreatitis. The overall sensitivity of CT scans is 74–86%, while its specificity is 98–99%. Chronic pancreatitis is regarded as a risk factor for the development of ductal adenocarcinoma of the pancreas. The lifetime risk of a patient with alcohol-induced chronic pancreatitis for pancreatic cancer is around 4%, but the risk is greatly increased (to a cumulative risk of 40% till the age of 70 years) if the patient suffers from hereditary chronic pancreatitis (even greater if the patient smokes). Contrast enhanced CT appears to be the most accurate and reliable imaging procedure for the detection of early stage, resectable, pancreatic carcinoma (Fig. 28.1).[58,59]

Endoscopic retrograde cholangiopancreatography (ERCP) is generally considered to be the most specific and sensitive test of pancreatic duct morphology. ERCP has become the gold standard for the diagnosis of chronic pancreatitis. The overall sensitivity of ERP is 93–99%, while the specificity is 85–100%. In addition to its accuracy in detecting changes in the main pancreatic duct and its side branches, ERCP can be used to assess the macroscopic appearance of the papilla of Vater and to take biopsies for histological examination. ERCP is not only a diagnostic tool; it also offers the possibility of treatment. Pancreatic pseudocysts, for example, can be drained through the pancreatic duct by insertion of an endoprosthesis and obstructing stones can be endoscopically removed. To uniformly evaluate and accurately diagnose chronic pancreatitis, the so-called Cambridge classification of duct changes on ERCP for patients with chronic pancreatitis was agreed upon in 1984 (Table 28.2). It must be kept in mind that ERCP is an invasive procedure with a complication rate of up to 5% (10% in certain subgroups) and that the procedure is associated with a mortality of 0.1–0.5%.[60–64]

Endoscopic ultrasound has recently emerged as an important tool in the diagnosis of pancreatic disease. Frequently, ERCP-detected changes in the parenchyma of the pancreas precede changes in the pancreatic duct. Endosonography is a sensitive and valuable procedure for the detection of early changes in tissue morphology and it avoids some of the disadvantages of transabdominal ultrasound, i.e., intervening gas in the gut.[62,65,66]

The sensitivity of magnetic resonance cholangiopancreatography (MRCP) varies between 70% and 92% if ERCP is used as the gold standard. The fact that MRCP has a lower complication rate than ERCP and is less investigator dependent than ultrasound will, in the future, lead to its increased use as a diagnostic procedure for chronic pancreatitis in spite of its cost and its inherent lack of therapeutic options (Table 28.3).[60]

Pancreatic function tests

Tests for exocrine and endocrine pancreatic function serve as a second line of diagnostic tools for chronic pancreatitis. Exocrine insufficiency is defined as either global or partial diminution in the pancreatic secretion of amylase, lipase, proteases, and bicarbonate. The most common etiology for this loss of exocrine function in adults is chronic pancreatitis. The human pancreas has a substantial exocrine reserve. Clinical symptoms of exocrine insufficiency do not occur until pancreatic lipase secretion is reduced to less than 10% of normal.[67] A clinically relevant

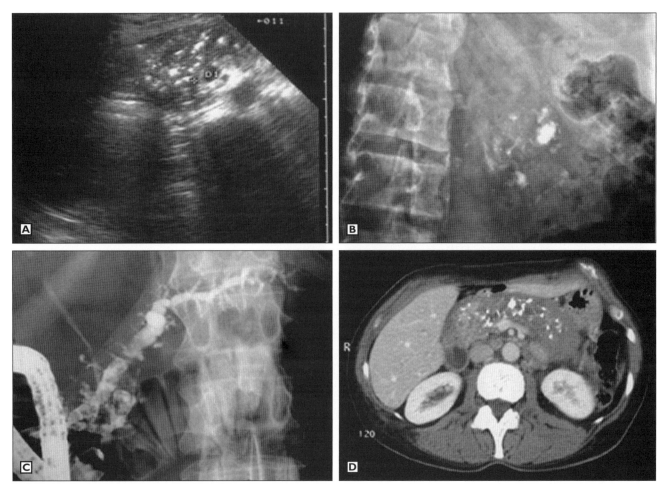

Fig. 28.1 • Typical morphological signs of advanced calcifying chronic pancreatitis. **(A)** Transabdominal ultrasound with numerous calcifications in the pancreatic head. **(B)** Plain abdominal radiography with multiple calcifications. **(C)** Endoscopic retrograde cholangiopancreatography (ERCP) with dilated pancreatic duct and filling defects as well as more than three altered side branches displaying irregularities. In the head of the pancreas a filling defect in the main pancreatic duct can be observed most likely resembling a pancreatic duct stone. **(D)** Contrast enhanced computer-tomography with an enlarged pancreatic gland, dilated pancreatic main duct and numerous calcified spots.

Table 28.2 Classification of chronic pancreatitis according to morphological criteria

	Cambridge classification of ERCP	Ultrasound/CT scan
Normal	No signs of pathological changes	

Grade I, mild	> 3 pathological side branches of the main pancreatic duct	Two of the following pathological findings:
		   Cysts
		   Duct irregularities
		   Focal acute pancreatitis
		   Heterogeneity of the parenchyma
		   Increased echogenity of the ductal wall
		   Intraductal filling defects
		   Gland enlargement

Grade II, moderate	> 3 pathological side branches of the pancreatic duct + dilated main pancreatic duct	All above-mentioned findings

Grade III, severe	Grade II plus one or more of the following findings:
	   Cyst >10 mm
	   Intraductal filling defects
	   Calcification
	   Obstruction or strictures of the pancreatic duct
	   Dilatation of the pancreatic duct as well as irregularities
	Contiguous neighboring organ invasion	

Table 28.3 Sensitivity and specificity of routinely employed techniques for the diagnosis of chronic pancreatitis (after ref. 55)

Diagnostic tool	Sensitivity	Specificity
Transabdominal ultrasound	48–90%	75–90%
Contrast enhanced CT scan	56–95%	85–90%
ERCP	68–93%	89–97%
Endosonography	88–100%	90–100%
Fecal elastase-1	50–93%	62–93%
Serum pancreolauryl test	70–82%	70–87%
Secretin-cholecystokinin test	80–90%	90–95%

The wide range of percentages given for specificity and sensitivity of diagnostic procedures results from a heterogeneous cohort of patients as well as the different mix of severity of cases in the studies used. Furthermore, a gold standard has so far not been defined.

Table 28.4 Direct and indirect pancreatic function tests

Pancreatic function test	
Direct	Secretin-cholecystokinin test
	Endoscopic secretin test
Indirect	Serum tests:
	Pancreolauryl test
	NBT-PABA test (discontinued)
	Fecal tests:
	Fecal elastase-1
	Chymotrypsin
	Stool weight
	Fecal fat quantification

maldigestion can be found in about one-third of all patients with chronic pancreatitis. Reduced exocrine function often precedes morphological changes and, therefore, sensitivity for the detection of early changes is higher for pancreatic function tests than for imaging studies.

Several tests of exocrine pancreatic function are well established in the diagnostic evaluation of patients suspected to have chronic pancreatitis. The approaches can be divided into those that are direct and those that are indirect. When pancreatic function is measured directly, the stimulated secretion of pancreatic juice is collected via a nasoduodenal tube and then the enzymes and bicarbonate are quantitated. Indirect methods detect decreased secretion by measuring the amount of pancreatic enzymes in stool or serum or, alternatively, they evaluate the digestion of synthetic substrates by pancreatic enzymes (Table 28.4). The disadvantage of indirect tests for pancreatic function is that they cannot distinguish between structural or functional abnormalities. The situation after gastrectomy can serve as a good example. In this case, an impaired synchrony of pancreatic secretion and the gastrointestinal passage of food may lead to clinical exocrine insufficiency or abnormal function tests without primary damage of the pancreas (pancreatico-cibale asynchrony).[68]

Direct pancreatic function tests

Secretin-cholecystokinin-test: Pancreatic enzyme activity as well as bicarbonate concentration are measured in the duodenal juice after stimulation with the enterohormones secretin (1 CU/kg, i.v.) and cholecystokinin (CCK 25–100 ng/kg). This requires passing a nasoduodenal tube that has two lumena. The proximal one is used to remove gastric secretions and to prevent gastric juice from stimulating pancreatic secretion. The second lumen is placed beyond the ligament of Treitz and fractions, containing duodenal juice, are aspirated every 15 min. The secretin-cholecystokinin test is the gold standard for pancreatic function testing. Its overall sensitivity and specificity is 90%. Even though the secretin-cholecystokinin test is the most accurate assay for pancreatic function, only few specialized centers routinely use this technique for clinical studies. The cost of testing one patient is about US$150. Furthermore, 2 days of labor by the technician are

required to prepare the test and to do the analysis.[69–71] Some authors use a standardized test meal (Lund test) rather than hormone stimulation of the exocrine pancreas but this more 'physiological' approach is, ultimately, less sensitive in detecting early functional changes and bicarbonate cannot be measured in the collected chyme.

Indirect pancreatic function tests

Fecal elastase-1: Pancreatic elastase accounts for 6% of all proteins in pancreatic juice. Compared to other serine proteases, this enzyme is highly stable during its passage through the gut and can be detected in stool (median concentration of 1200 μg/g). Fecal elastase is measured using an enzyme linked immunoassay (ELISA) and there are polyclonal and monoclonal test kits commercially available. The ELISAs employed have been extensively evaluated for cross-reactivity between species and none has been found. It is therefore not necessary for the patient to discontinue enzyme supplementation treatment with animal-derived enzyme preparations. To measure fecal elastase, only small amounts of stool are required (100 mg) and it is not necessary to test multiple samples because interassay variability is low (8–15%). The overall sensitivity of fecal elastase testing is 63% for mild exocrine insufficiency and it rises to 100% for intermediate and severe exocrine insufficiency if compared to the gold standard of the secretin-cholecystokinin test.[72,73]

Pancreolauryl: The serum pancreolauryl test (PLT) is the most widely accepted oral indirect pancreatic function test for detecting and grading the functional impairment of the gland. The test involves ingestion of fluorescein dilaurate (0.25 mmol) with a standardized breakfast (20 g bread, 20 g butter, and 200 ml tea). The fluorescein dilaurate is cleaved in the duodenum by pancreatic esterases and fluorescein, absorbed from the intestine, can be photometrically measured in the patient's urine or serum after defined time intervals. Before performing this pancreatic function test, the patient must discontinue enzyme supplementation as orally taken enzymes interfere with testing, leading to false-negative results. The pancreolauryl test can also quantify severe exocrine insufficiency via a diminished increase in serum fluorescein or in dialysis fluid of patients with renal insufficiency.[74] The sensitivity is 82% with a specificity of 91% for severe exocrine insufficiency. Mild exocrine insufficiency can only be detected with a sensitivity of 51%. The PLT is regarded as an indirect noninvasive pancreatic function test of high clinical relevance.[75]

Fecal fat: Fecal fat quantification by the classical Van de Kamer (alcohol extraction) technique is the standard for establishing the presence of steatorrhea, i.e., characteristic symptom of reduced exocrine function. The test is performed by collecting stool over 3 days during which oral fat intake is 80–100 g/d. After a 90% loss of exocrine function, fat excretion in stool significantly increases as a sign of fat maldigestion. A mild or intermediate impairment of exocrine function is usually clinically compensated.

Pancreatic endocrine function should be evaluated by fasting and 1 h postprandial blood glucose levels and oral glucose tolerance testing as well as HbA1C according to the guidelines of the WHO for the diagnosis of diabetes mellitus.

In addition to an evaluation of exocrine and endocrine function, considerable attention should be paid to the etiology of the disease. Recent results from molecular and genetic studies suggest that a significant number of patients with chronic pancreatitis suffer from a genetically determined or inherited disease. This is mainly true for patients who were formerly classified as suffering from idiopathic pancreatitis, for patients with an onset of the disease before the age of 25, or for those with a positive family history for chronic pancreatitis or pancreatic cancer. Patients who suffer from chronic pancreatitis due to mutations in the cationic trypsinogen gene are burdened with a 70- to 140-fold increased risk of developing pancreatic cancer, particularly if they smoke. Whether this is also true for patients who carry SPINK-1 or CFTR mutations needs to be determined. Genetic testing for trypsinogen gene mutations can be recommended for chronic pancreatitis patients who have first-degree relatives suffering from pancreatitis or pancreatic cancer, and for patients with chronic pancreatitis or recurrent bouts of acute pancreatitis before the age of 25 years and no identifiable risk factor.[76] Genetic testing for clinically unaffected relatives is not indicated and should only be performed within ethics committee-approved research protocols.

TREATMENT STRATEGIES

The aim of medical treatment of chronic pancreatitis is the compensation of exocrine and endocrine pancreatic insufficiency. It is, therefore, dominated by attempts to control maldigestion, steatorrhea, weight loss, and blood glucose levels and to achieve adequate pain management. The role and prognostic value of psychosocial care with the aim of discontinuing alcohol abuse in patients with chronic pancreatitis should not be underestimated.

Pain management

Following intrapancreatic protease activation or tissue necrosis, inflammatory mediators are locally released. These not only facilitate and sustain the inflammatory process, but they can also exert a direct effect on sensory fibers of the celiac plexus (T5–T9), thus triggering visceral pain, which is a common symptom in patients with chronic pancreatitis. Adequate pain relief is therefore one of the most important and urgent treatment goals. There are several concepts to pain treatment which need to be carefully evaluated on an individual basis. In principle, pain management for chronic pancreatitis follows the guidelines of the WHO for the treatment of chronic pain. The combination of a nonsteroidal analgesic with a centrally active drug should initially be considered. Concerns that morphine analogues may

negatively affect the course of chronic pancreatitis because of their effect on the sphincter of Oddi are unwarranted. Some authors prefer meperidine over other opiates in pancreatitis but this alleged advantage has not been studied in controlled trials. Tramadolsulphate, as an alternative to other opiates, should not be considered in patients with acute or chronic pancreatitis because, according to the authors' personal experience, nausea and vomiting are common side effects in this group of patients. As many patients with chronic pancreatitis are drug addicts, a rigid scheme of pain medication is more effective than medication on demand. Several studies have suggested that enzyme supplementation is associated with pain relief. A randomized, placebo controlled study, however, has not shown such a beneficial effect (Table 28.5).[77,78]

Diabetes mellitus associated with chronic pancreatitis

Diabetes mellitus is an independent predictor of mortality in patients with chronic pancreatitis. Morbidity and mortality due to diabetes mellitus may occur from progressive microangiopathic complications or from more acute complications such as treatment-induced hypoglycemia, particularly in those patients with an inadequate glucagon reserve. Ketoacidosis is relatively unusual. This may be due to the fact that insulin secretion has not entirely ceased when glucagon secretion is already reduced. The underlying pathophysiology of diabetes in chronic pancreatitis is the loss of insulin secretion. Oral antidiabetic agents, therefore, have no role in the treatment of diabetes due to chronic pancreatitis. Control of blood sugar levels should be achieved with exogenous insulin. Guidelines for the treatment and monitoring of the secondary organ failure of type I diabetes mellitus can be used for the treatment of pancreatitis-induced diabetes, but the insulin doses required are usually lower.[79,80]

Nutrition and pancreatic enzyme supplementation

Enzyme supplementation is clinically indicated if patients suffering from chronic pancreatitis lose more than 10% of their body weight, excrete more than 15 g/d fat with their stool, or suffer from clinical symptoms of dyspepsia or meteorism. Treatment of the pain and meteorism associated with chronic pancreatitis and meteorism are two situations in which pancreatic enzymes can be used on an individual basis but there is no conclusive evidence of benefit from controlled trials. Four types of pancreatic enzyme preparation are currently available. Most commercial preparation consists of pancreatin, which is the shock-frozen powdered extract of porcine pancreas containing lipase, amylase, trypsin, and chymotrypsin. Enzyme supplements are not absorbed from the gastrointestinal tract. Rather, they are inactivated by enteral bacterial flora or digestive secretion and fecally eliminated. Administration of acid-stable, encapsulated microspheres or microtablets filled with pancreatic enzymes has greatly increased the efficacy of enzyme supplementation in chronic pancreatitis. Patients with documented exocrine insufficiency should eat three main meals a day and three snacks in between. In general, 25 000 to 50 000 IU of lipase should be ingested simultaneously along with a main meal and 25 000 IU of lipase along with the snacks. They should not be taken either

Table 28.5 Dosage of pain medication in chronic pancreatitis according to the AGA guidelines[77]

Generic	Dosage	Maximal dosage/day
Paracetamol	2–3 × 500–1000 mg	4000 mg
Metamizol	1–4 × 500–1000 mg	4000 mg
Tramadol	4 × 100 mg, 2–3 200 mg (ret)	400 mg (600 mg ret)
Buprenorphin	3–4 × 0.2–0.4 mg	6–9 µg/kg bodyweight
Pentazocin	6–7 ×50 mg	360 mg
Tilidin	3 ×50–200 mg	600 mg
Morphine	Dependent on the effect on pain relief	No maximal dosage given
Levopromazin	3–5 × 10 mg	300 mg
Clomipramin	1 × 50–100 mg	100 mg

before or after the meals. When gastric hyperacidity is present, proton pump inhibitors or H_2 antagonists should be prescribed to delay enzyme inactivation. In cases of progressive maldigestion and steatorrhea, it can be necessary to supplement lipid-soluble vitamins parenterally. In cases of severe exocrine insufficiency, one-third of the daily caloric intake can be met by administration of medium-chain triglycerides, which do not require lipolysis by lipase for absorption. While this is clinically effective, MCT fat is usually disliked by the patients because of its poor taste. The efficacy of enzyme supplementation is demonstrated by the improvement of symptoms and not by laboratory tests.[67,81–85]

Endoscopic therapy

Common bile duct stenting: Many studies which have investigated the natural course of chronic pancreatitis have shown that 30–60% of all patients undergo surgical intervention at some point in the disease process. However, this varies greatly among countries depending whether chronic pancreatitis patients are initially seen by surgeons (e.g., UK, high rate of operations) or physicians (e.g., Switzerland, low rate of operations). Approximately two-thirds of all patients can be managed conservatively or with endoscopic intervention. In 10–40% of patients, a stenosis of the common bile duct occurs that requires either endoscopic or surgical intervention. Either endoscopic or surgical intervention is clinically indicated if the patient presents with jaundice or recurrent bouts of cholangitis, to prevent secondary biliary cirrhosis. It may also allow the clinician to determine whether the common bile duct stenosis in chronic pancreatitis is the cause of pain. Several studies have examined the cost-effectiveness and the outcome of stenting of the common bile duct. They have concluded that endotherapy is initially equivalent to surgery for short-term symptom control and immediate decongestion but that only one-third of patients benefit in the long term. On the other hand, endotherapy is less invasive and is probably associated with less severe complications than surgery. It can thus be offered to patients as initial treatment with an immediate effect and an approximately 30% chance of a long-term benefit. It may be required as an emergency procedure for patients with cholangitis or as the definitive treatment for patients unfit for surgery. However, it needs to be kept in mind that long-term

insertion of biliary stent can also increase the risk of cholangitis and biliary sepsis. For several decades clinicians used antibiotics or ursodeoxycholic acid to prevent clogging of the endoprostheses. Even antibiotic-coated stents were used for this purpose. It has recently been shown that this treatment does not reliably extend the patency of plastic stents. The only way to effectively prevent stent clogging is to insert a large-bore endoprosthesis and to replace the stent at least every three months. The insertion of self-expanding metal wire stents is clinically not indicated for the treatment of benign bile duct strictures in patients with chronic pancreatitis (Table 28.6).[63,86–90]

Stenting of the main pancreatic duct: Whether endoscopic decompression of Wirsung's duct is clinically indicated in the treatment of chronic pancreatitis patients with a dominant stenosis is still a matter of debate. No single prospective randomized controlled trial has shown a beneficial therapeutic effect on the metabolic complications of chronic pancreatitis after ductal decompression by endoprosthesis. The primary outcome of pain relief was addressed in a study by Dite and coworkers. They showed, in a prospective, randomized trial comparing endoscopic and surgical therapy for pain management in chronic pancreatitis, that surgery is superior to endotherapy for long-term pain relief but immediate pain relief can be achieved by endoscopic decompression.[88] A beneficial effect of endoscopic stenting was confirmed by a large retrospective multicenter study enrolling 1000 patients on an intention to treat basis.[90] Pain relief was achieved in this cohort in 65% after endoscopic decompression of the pancreatic duct and patients remained pain-free over the

Table 28.6 Indications for endoscopic biliary stenting

For symptomatic relief of cholestasis and jaundice

To drain infected bile and treat or prevent cholangitis

To gain time for repression of a reversible inflammatory process or pseudocyst

To prevent secondary biliary cirrhosis

To differentiate between pancreatic pain and pain caused by biliary obstruction

observation period of at least 2 years. However, there is evidence that stenting of the pancreatic main duct can damage the ductal epithelium, causing a continuous inflammatory stimulus that subsequently progresses to fibrosis and stricturing of the duct.[88] Due to its low degree of invasiveness and its immediate success in pain management, endotherapy can be offered as a first-line treatment. Surgery could then follow after stent failure or in cases of recurrence.

For patients with intraductal pancreatic stones, a naso-pancreatic drain should be inserted before extracorporeal shock wave lithotripsy of the stones and endoscopic removal of the fragments.[55,91–94] Pancreatic pseudocysts which impress the stomach wall can be drained by endoscopic ultrasound-guided, pigtail drainage into the stomach.

Extracorporal shock wave lithotripsy for pancreatic duct stones: Before the introduction of extracoporal shock wave lithotripsy (ESWL) in 1989, open surgery was the only option for treating pancreatic duct stones which were not accessible to endoscopic removal. Several retrospective studies have since investigated the clincal benefit of ESWL for the treatment of pancreatic duct stones. These studies were not able to demonstrate an advantage for ESWL when compared to surgical intervention. We therefore conclude that ESWL is technically feasible, it is associated with a low complication rate, a low morbidity, and nearly no mortality and it results in an immediate benefit for the patient if technically successful. The results of long-term studies, however, favor surgical intervention.[88,95,96]

Endoscopic treatment of pancreatic pseudocysts: Approximately 25% of patients with chronic pancreatitis develop pancreatic pseudocysts, mainly after an acute episode of the disease. This number is derived from a Swiss longitudinal study investigating the incidence of pseudocysts in a cohort of 245 patients with alcoholic chronic pancreatitis.[1] In the first 6 weeks 40% of pancreatic pseudocysts resolve spontaneously, while in 20% of cases complications such as bacterial superinfection, compression of neighboring organs, hemorrhage, persistent inflammation of the pancreas, or rupture of the pancreatic pseudocyst can occur. If a pseudocyst persists for more than 12 weeks, spontaneous regression is unlikely and the complication rate rises to 60%. Several recent studies have documented that the rate of complications rises when the diameter of the pseudocysts exceeds 5 cm. Smaller cysts and asymptomatic cysts can be safely monitored for at least 12 weeks. When pseudocysts become symptomatic or when they persist for more than 3 months, either surgical or endoscopic decompression should be considered. Endoscopic and surgical drainage procedures have both been shown to be effective in terms of technical feasibility and recurrence rate. In general, endoscopic intervention is used as a first-line treatment because it is less invasive and has a lower morbidity. Endoscopic drainage can be performed via the gastric or intestinal wall or through the pancreatic duct. The lowest complication rate is achieved if the pseudocyst can be drained into the stomach via a pigtail catheter. Although percutaneous pseudocyst drainage was first performed in 1867 and can be safely performed using ultrasound- or CT-guided techniques, it has been more or less abandoned because of the higher risk of secondary infection, the risk of persistent pancreatic fistulas, and the high recurrence rate. The percutaneous complication rate is twice that of internal endoscopic or surgical drainage.[97–99]

Surgical management

Surgical treatment for chronic pancreatitis is clinically indicated if intractable upper abdominal pain is refractory to conservative pain management or when organ complications occur. If pain is the leading symptom and imaging studies exclude other secondary complications of chronic pancreatitis, bilateral thoracoscopic splanchnicectomy can be performed for pain control. In 1943 Mallet-Guy described pancreatic denervation in the treatment of chronic pancreatitis pain. In 1993 the technique was rediscovered and modified as a video-endoscopic-assisted, minimally invasive treatment procedure. In a prospective randomized single-center study, it has been shown that bilateral thoracoscopic splanchnicectomy can lead to effective long-term pain relief with only 7% morbidity in patients who achieve temporary pain relief from peridural analgesia.[100–102]

In addition to refractory pain, the indications for surgery in chronic pancreatitis are closely related to complications that result from an enlarged, inflamed pancreatic head. These include obstruction of the common bile duct, stenosis of the pancreatic duct, obstruction of the duodenal loop and, in rare cases, compression of the portal vein. It should also be noted that in a retrospective analysis the incidence of pancreatic malignancy was 6–14% in a cohort of more than 200 patients with chronic pancreatitis who were originally operated on for an inflammatory mass in the head of the pancreas.[103]

One recent study has shown that early surgical intervention can delay the loss of exocrine and endocrine function in patients with chronic pancreatitis.[104] Surgical procedures include drainage operations, organ preserving procedures, and major pancreatic resections. The classical Kausch-Whipple procedure was long regarded as the standard procedure for chronic calcifying pancreatitis. During the last two decades it has been steadily replaced by more procedures which are more organ-preserving, such as the pylorus-preserving Whipple procedure according to Longmire-Traverso (pp-Whipple), the duodenum preserving pancreatic head resection (DPPHR) according to Beger and, when extended by a longitudinal pancreaticojejunostomy by the so-called Frey procedure.[105]

When deciding upon a suitable surgical procedure, one must distinguish between two different disease manifestations of chronic pancreatitis: large duct disease in which the duct of Wirsung is dilated to more than 7 mm; and small duct disease without a dilated pancreatic duct. In large duct disease, drainage procedures such as the longitudinal pancreaticojejunostomy according to Partington-Rochelle or a Puestow procedure can be performed. Both procedures are employed when pain generation is considered to be the result of increased intrapancreatic ductal and parenchymal pressure. Both include a Roux-en-Y jejunal loop to decompress the pancreatic main duct and the duct of Santorini along with the parenchyma. The procedures are associated with low perioperative morbidity and mortality, but long-term pain relief can be achieved in only 60% of cases.[106]

Because the inflamed pancreatic head is regarded as the pacemaker for the generation of pancreatic pain, and because most pancreatic islets are found in the pancreatic tail, a pancreatic left resection is rarely considered as an option. It is clinically indicated only for persistent or complicated pancreatic pseudocysts or for chronic pancreatitis confined to the tail of the gland.

Classical resective procedures can also be successfully performed in patients with small duct disease. For many years, a pancreaticoduodenectomy (Kausch-Whipple procedure), was regarded as the standard surgical procedure for chronic pancreatitis with complications arising from the pancreatic head, even if the results were burdened with a high perioperative morbidity and mortality rate of up to 44%. More recent studies have shown that hospital mortality has fallen to below 5% and that it may be less than 1% in large specialized centers. Although the classical Kausch-Whipple resection is successful in achieving pain relief in chronic pancreatitis, it is unfortunately associated with a high postoperative morbidity and a poorer long-term surgical result. The Kausch-Whipple procedure is associated with a number of side effects which may alter quality of life. Dysbalanced intestinal motility, including dumping, frequently results from the procedure. Peptic ulcers can arise at the site of the anastomosis as a result of gastrin secretion in the remaining stomach, and reflux of bile occurs due to the removal of the pylorus. Many patients complain about dyspeptic symptoms. In approximately 20% of patients, endocrine function gradually declines after the Kausch-Whipple operation, and the resulting diabetes mellitus is responsible for much of the late postoperative morbidity and mortality. To address the drawbacks of the classical Kausch-Whipple operation, during the last two decades organ-preserving techniques such as the pylorus-preserving Whipple have evolved as an attempt to minimize the disadvantages of the classical procedure. Dumping as well as peptic ulcers and reflux of bile is reduced by the pp-Whipple procedure, and the continuity of the gastrointestinal tract is less affected. Up to 90% of all patients gain weight after the pp-Whipple but up to 50% of patients still suffer from delayed gastric emptying associated with a delayed weight gain and a slightly increased risk of developing cholangitis. However, 45% of patients still lose their remaining exocrine and endocrine function regardless of the operation. Originally, the pp-Whipple procedure was created to treat pancreatic malignancies with adequate oncological radicality. In general, an extended resection, as in the Whipple procedure, is clinically not indicated for a benign disorder such as chronic pancreatitis. In 1972 H.G. Beger established the so-called duodenum preserving pancreatic head resection as a new surgical approach to chronic pancreatitis. With this procedure the anatomical structures of the gastrointestinal tract are not altered and their continuity is not disturbed. In a high-volume single center, duodenum preserving pancreatic head resection was noted to result in pain relief over 5 years in 80% of cases and the perioperative mortality was 0.7%. More than 70% of patients were resocialized into daily work routine and, only in rare cases, the loss of endocrine function progressed.[103] In 1985 Frey and Smith extended the duodenum preserving pancreatic head resection by adding a longitudinal pancreaticojejunostomy and, in this manner, combined the organ preserving surgical procedure with a drainage operation.[107] In a randomized prospective single-center study with a median observation period of 2.5 years, the Beger procedure and the Frey procedure were shown to result in equivalent postoperative outcome.[108]

In 1998 Izbicki suggested a modification of the Frey procedure for the treatment of chronic pancreatitis without a dilatated pancreatic duct.[109] He performed a V-shaped resection of the ventral pancreas to drain the second- and third-order pancreatic ducts via a longitudinal pancreaticojejunostomy. In a small group

of patients and with an observation period of 30 months he was able to show that his modification resulted in complete pain relief in 95% of cases. In 67%, the quality of life increased and the procedure was associated with a low perioperative morbidity rate of 15.4% and no mortality rate.[109] Recently, Büchler et al. modified the Beger procedure to allow the resection of the pancreatic head without transection of the gland over the superior mesenteric vein. In this manner the risk of bleeding complications (especially in patients with portal hypertension) is thought to be minimized while still allowing an excision of the pancreatic head.[110] Future randomized prospective trials will have to evaluate the more recently modified techniques.

It is still a matter of debate whether a prophylactic perioperative application of somatostatin analogues can reduce the rate of leakage from the pancreaticojejunostomy. Leakage at that anastomosis results in an increased mortality and frequently requires interventional treatment. The incidence of leakage at the site of the pancreaticojejunostomy is reported to be 0–30%. In 2001, Li-Ling and Irving demonstrated, in a meta-analysis of all randomized trials, a significant reduction of pancreatic fistulas when a somatostatin analogue was perioperatively administered. The rate of reduction in leakage at the site of anastomosis was as high as 40%.[111] The route of application and the duration required are still being discussed but three doses of 100 μg of sandostatin a day for at least 5–7 days is often regarded as the standard protocol.[112]

In summary, the most widely accepted organ-preserving technique is now the duodenum preserving pancreatic head resection and this procedure should be preferred for the surgical treatment of chronic pancreatitis with complications arising from the pancreatic head.[87,103,104,110]

SUMMARY

With an incidence of 8.2 and a prevalence of 27.4 per 100 000 population, chronic pancreatitis represents a frequent disorder of the gastrointestinal tract. In the past, chronic pancreatitis was considered to be mostly associated with chronic alcohol abuse. During the past two decades idiopathic chronic pancreatitis and, moreover, hereditary pancreatitis have been recognized as distinct disease entities. Hereditary pancreatitis is an autosomal dominant disorder with an 80% penetrance. It is associated with recurrent episodes of pancreatitis starting in early childhood and associated with an increased risk of pancreatic cancer. The pathophysiology of chronic and hereditary pancreatitis is not fully understood. Patients suffering from chronic pancreatitis present with beltlike abdominal pain, weight loss, steatorrhea, and, often, diabetes mellitus. Usually the diagnosis is made by a combination of imaging procedures such as ultrasound and endoscopic retrograde cholangiopancreatography, and exocrine and endocrine function tests. Therapy is presently restricted to symptom control for the lack of a causal treatment strategy. Thirty to 60% of all patients develop disease-associated complications such as persistent pain, strictures of the common bile duct, or pancreatic duct stones that may require either endoscopic or surgical treatment.

Figures 28.2 and 28.3 provide algorithms for the diagnosis of chronic pancreatitis and treatment of chronic pancreatitis, respectively.

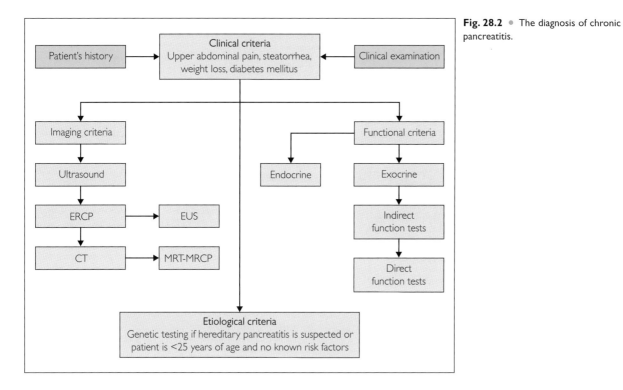

Fig. 28.2 • The diagnosis of chronic pancreatitis.

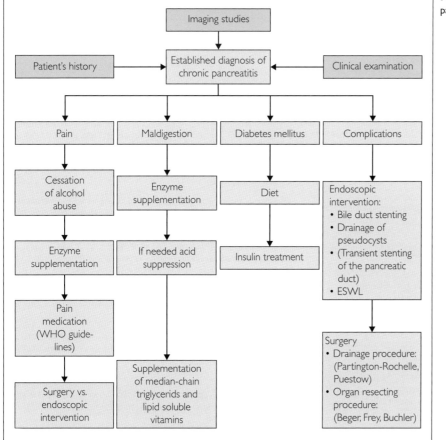

Fig. 28.3 • The treatment of chronic pancreatitis.

REFERENCES

1. Ammann RW, Akovbiantz A, Largiader F, et al. Course and outcome of chronic pancreatitis. Longitudinal study of a mixed medical-surgical series of 245 patients. Gastroenterology 1984; 86:820–828.

   This paper presents the largest longitudinal study ever conducted on the natural course of chronic pancreatitis including 245 patients (163 with alcoholic relapsing pancreatitis); 145 of them with calcific pancreatitis were prospectively studied at regular intervals with particular regard to pain, pancreatic function, calcifications, pancreatic surgery, and survival. The median period of observation in the group with alcoholic relapsing calcific pancreatitis was 10.4 years.

2. Etemad B, Whitcomb DC. Chronic pancreatitis: diagnosis, classification, and new genetic developments. Gastroenterology 2001; 120:682–707.

3. Sarner M, Cotton PB. Classification of pancreatitis. Gut 1984; 25:756–759.

4. Chari ST, Singer MV. The problem of classification and staging of chronic pancreatitis. Proposals based on current knowledge of its natural history. Scand J Gastroenterol 1994; 29:949–960.

5. Andersen BN, Pedersen NT, Scheel J, et al. Incidence of alcoholic chronic pancreatitis in Copenhagen. Scand J Gastroenterol 1982; 17:247–252.

6. Olsen TS. Lipomatosis of the pancreas in autopsy material and its relation to age and overweight. Acta Pathol Microbiol Scand [A] 1978; 86A:367–373.

7. O'Sullivan JN, Nobrega FT, Morlock CG, et al. Acute and chronic pancreatitis in Rochester, Minnesota, 1940 to 1969. Gastroenterology 1972; 62:373–379.

8. Lowenfels AB, Maisonneuve P, Cavallini G, et al. Prognosis of chronic pancreatitis: an international multicenter study. International Pancreatitis Study Group. Am J Gastroenterol 1994; 89:1467–1471.

   This study investigated which factors predict mortality in a cohort of patients with chronic alcoholic and nonalcoholic pancreatitis. They determined the age at diagnosis, smoking status, and drinking habits as the major predictors of mortality in patients with chronic pancreatitis.

9. Ammann RW, Heitz PU, Kloppel G. Course of alcoholic chronic pancreatitis: a prospective clinicomorphological long-term study. Gastroenterology 1996; 111:224–231.

10. Bordalo O, Goncalves D, Noronha M, et al. Newer concept for the pathogenesis of chronic alcoholic pancreatitis. Am J Gastroenterol 1977; 68:278–285.

11. Schoenberg MH, Büchler M, Pietrzyk C, et al. Lipid peroxidation and glutathione metabolism in chronic pancreatitis. Pancreas 1995; 10:36–43.

12. Braganza JM. Pancreatic disease: a casualty of hepatic 'detoxification'? Lancet 1983; 2:1000–1003.

13. Braganza JM, Wickens DG, Cawood P, et al. Lipid-peroxidation (free-radical-oxidation) products in bile from patients with pancreatic disease. Lancet 1983; 2:375–379.

14. Uden S, Bilton D, Nathan L, et al. Antioxidant therapy for recurrent pancreatitis: placebo-controlled trial. Aliment Pharmacol Ther 1990; 4:357–371.

15. Freedman SD, Sakamoto K, Venu RP. GP2, the homologue to the renal cast protein uromodulin, is a major component of intraductal plugs in chronic pancreatitis. J Clin Invest 1993; 92:83–90.

16. Sahel J, Sarles H. Modifications of pure human pancreatic juice induced by chronic alcohol consumption. Dig Dis Sci 1979; 24:897–905.

17. Kloppel G, Maillet B. Pathology of acute and chronic pancreatitis. Pancreas 1993; 8:659–670.

18. Kloppel G. Pathology of chronic pancreatitis and pancreatic pain. Acta Chir Scand 1990; 156:261–265.

19. Ammann RW, Muellhaupt B. Progression of alcoholic acute to chronic pancreatitis. Gut 1994; 35:552–556.

20. Ammann RW, Muellhaupt B, Meyenberger C, et al. Alcoholic nonprogressive chronic pancreatitis: prospective long-term study of a large cohort with alcoholic acute pancreatitis (1976–1992). Pancreas 1994; 9:365–373.

21. Ammann RW, Heitz PU, Kloppel G. The 'two-hit' pathogenetic concept of chronic pancreatitis. Int J Pancreatol 1999; 25:251.

22. Levy P, Mathurin P, Roqueplo A, et al. A multidimensional case-control study of dietary, alcohol, and tobacco habits in alcoholic men with chronic pancreatitis. Pancreas 1995; 10:231–238.

23. Lin Y, Tamakoshi A, Hayakawa T, et al. Associations of alcohol drinking and nutrient intake with chronic pancreatitis: findings from a case-control study in Japan. Am J Gastroenterol 2001; 96:2622–2627.

24. Suda K, Shiotsu H, Nakamura T, et al. Pancreatic fibrosis in patients with chronic alcohol abuse: correlation with alcoholic pancreatitis. Am J Gastroenterol 1994; 89:2060–2062.

25. Whitcomb DC. Genetic predisposition to alcoholic chronic pancreatitis. Pancreas 2003; 27:321–326.

26. Gullo L, Barbara L, Labo G. Effect of cessation of alcohol use on the course of pancreatic dysfunction in alcoholic pancreatitis. Gastroenterology 1988; 95:1063–1068.

27. Somogyi L, Martin SP, Venkatesan T, et al. Recurrent acute pancreatitis: an algorithmic approach to identification and elimination of inciting factors. Gastroenterology 2001; 120:708–717.

28. Comfort MW, Gambrill EE, Baggenstoss AH. Chronic relapsing pancreatitis. A study of twenty-nine cases without associated disease of the biliary or gastro-intestinal tract. Gastroenterology 1968; 54:(Suppl)760–765.

29. Layer P, Yamamoto H, Kalthoff L, et al. The different courses of early- and late-onset idiopathic and alcoholic chronic pancreatitis. Gastroenterology 1994; 107:1481–1487.

30. Comfort MW, Steinberg AG. Pedigree of a family with hereditary chronic relapsing pancreatitis. Gastroenterology 1952; 21:54–63.

31. Whitcomb DC, Gorry MC, Preston RA, et al. Hereditary pancreatitis is caused by a mutation in the cationic trypsinogen gene. Nat Genet 1996; 14:141–145.

   Whitcomb and coworkers reported for the first time a mutation (Arg-His substitution at position 122) in the cationic trypsinogen gene in association with hereditary pancreatitis.

32. Lerch MM, Ellis I, Whitcomb DC, et al. Maternal inheritance pattern of hereditary pancreatitis in patients with pancreatic carcinoma. J Natl Cancer Inst 1999; 91:723–724.

33. Schneider A, Whitcomb DC. Hereditary pancreatitis: a model for inflammatory diseases of the pancreas. Best Pract Res Clin Gastroenterol 2002; 16:347–363.

34. Simon P, Weiss FU, Sahin-Toth M, et al. Hereditary pancreatitis caused by a novel PRSS1 mutation (Arg-122 → Cys) that alters autoactivation and autodegradation of cationic trypsinogen. J Biol Chem 2002; 277:5404–5410.

35. Simon P, Weiss FU, Zimmer KP, et al. Spontaneous and sporadic trypsinogen mutations in idiopathic pancreatitis. JAMA 2002; 288:2122.

   This article demonstrates that cationic trypsinogen mutations and thus hereditary pancreatitis can be diagnosed in patients which do not report to have a family history of pancreatitis (due to de novo mutations or incomplete penetrance in ancestors), particularly if the patient is under 25 years of age at disease onset and has no other risk factors for pancreatitis.

36. Howes N, Lerch MM, Greenhalf W, et al., European Registry of Hereditary Pancreatitis and Pancreatic Cancer (EUROPAC). Clinical and genetic characteristics of hereditary pancreatitis in Europe. Clin Gastroenterol Hepatol 2004; 2:252–261

    The most extensive genotypic and clinical characterization of hereditary pancreatitis (418 European patients) to date.

37. Halangk W, Krüger B, Ruthenbürger M, et al. Trypsin activity is not involved in premature, intrapancreatic trypsinogen activation. Am J Physiol Gastrointest Liver Physiol 2002; 282:G367–G374.

38. Kukor Z, Mayerle J, Krüger B, et al. Presence of cathepsin B in the human pancreatic secretory pathway and its role in trypsinogen activation during hereditary pancreatitis. J Biol Chem 2002; 277:21389–21396.

39. Chiari H. Über die Selbstverdauung des menschlichen Pankreas. Zeitschrift für Heilkunf 1896; 17:69–95.

40. Witt H, Luck W., Hennies HC, et al. Mutations in the gene encoding the serine protease inhibitor, Kazal type 1 are associated with chronic pancreatitis. Nat Genet 2000; 25:213–216.

41. Weiss FU, Simon P, Witt H, et al. SPINK1 mutations and phenotypic expression in patients with pancreatitis associated with trypsinogen mutations. J Med Genet 2003; 40:e40.

42. Witt H, Simon P, Lerch MM. [Genetic aspects of chronic pancreatitis]. Dtsch Med Wochenschr 2001; 126:988–993.

43. Bhatia E, Choudhuri G, Sikora SS, et al. Tropical calcific pancreatitis: strong association with SPINK1 trypsin inhibitor mutations. Gastroenterology 2002; 123:1020–1025.

44. Cohn JA, Friedman KJ, Noone PG, et al. Relation between mutations of the cystic fibrosis gene and idiopathic pancreatitis. N Engl J Med 1998; 339:653–658.

45. Sharer N, Schwarz M, Malone G, et al. Mutations of the cystic fibrosis gene in patients with chronic pancreatitis. N Engl J Med 1998; 339:645–652.

46. Kloppel G, Luttges J, Lohr M, et al. Autoimmune pancreatitis: pathological, clinical, and immunological features. Pancreas 2003; 27:14–19.

47. Toskes PP. Hyperlipidemic pancreatitis. Gastroenterol Clin North Am 1990; 19:783–791.

48. Simon P, Weiss FU, Zimmer KP, et al. Acute and chronic pancreatitis in patients with inborn errors of metabolism. Pancreatology 2001; 1:448–456.

49. Krüger B, Albrecht E, Lerch MM. The role of intracellular calcium signaling in premature protease activation and the onset of pancreatitis. Am J Pathol 2000; 157:43–50.

50. Jensen AR, Matzen P, Malchow-Moller A, et al. Pattern of pain, duct morphology, and pancreatic function in chronic pancreatitis. A comparative study. Scand J Gastroenterol 1984; 19:334–338.

51. Ammann RW, Muellhaupt B. The natural history of pain in alcoholic chronic pancreatitis. Gastroenterology 1999; 116:1132–1140.

    Ammann and coworkers defined in this study the typical pain patterns, correlated pain patterns with the presumptive causes of the pain, and compared the natural history of patients treated conservatively or surgically with respect to pain relief, pancreatic dysfunction, and clinical outcome. They studied in a prospective long-term study a cohort with 207 patients with alcoholic CP (91 without and 116 with surgery for pain relief).

52. Bockman DE, Büchler M, Malfertheiner P, et al. Analysis of nerves in chronic pancreatitis. Gastroenterology 1988; 94:1459–1469.

53. Ebbehoj N, Borly L, Bulow J, et al. Evaluation of pancreatic tissue fluid pressure and pain in chronic pancreatitis. A longitudinal study. Scand J Gastroenterol 1990; 25:462–466.

54. Ebbehoj N, Borly L, Bulow J, et al. Pancreatic tissue fluid pressure in chronic pancreatitis. Relation to pain, morphology, and function. Scand J Gastroenterol 1990; 25:1046–1051.

55. Ponchon T, Bory RM, Hedelius F, et al. Endoscopic stenting for pain relief in chronic pancreatitis: results of a standardized protocol. Gastrointest Endosc 1995; 42:452–456.

56. Glasbrenner B, Kahl S, Malfertheiner P. Modern diagnostics of chronic pancreatitis. Eur J Gastroenterol Hepatol 2002; 14:935–941.

57. Bolondi L, Gaiani S, Gullo L, et al. Secretin administration induces a dilatation of main pancreatic duct. Dig Dis Sci 1984; 29:802–808.

58. Elmas N. The role of diagnostic radiology in pancreatitis. Eur J Radiol 2001; 38:120–132.

59. Rosch T, Schusdziarra V, Born P, et al. Modern imaging methods versus clinical assessment in the evaluation of hospital in-patients with suspected pancreatic disease. Am J Gastroenterol 2000; 95:2261–2270.

60. Sica GT, Braver J, Cooney MJ, et al. Comparison of endoscopic retrograde cholangiopancreatography with MR cholangiopancreatography in patients with pancreatitis. Radiology 1999; 210:605–610.

61. Forsmark CE, Toskes PP. What does an abnormal pancreatogram mean? Gastrointest Endosc Clin N Am 1995; 5:105–123.

62. Catalano MF, Lahoti S, Geenen JE, et al. Prospective evaluation of endoscopic ultrasonography, endoscopic retrograde pancreatography, and secretin test in the diagnosis of chronic pancreatitis. Gastrointest Endosc 1998; 48:11–17.

63. Cremer M, Deviere J, Delhaye M, et al. Endoscopic management of chronic pancreatitis. Acta Gastroenterol Belg 1993; 56:192–200.

64. Menges M, Lerch MM, Zeitz M. The double duct sign in patients with malignant and benign pancreatic lesions. Gastrointest Endosc 2000; 52:74–77.

65. Kahl S, Glasbrenner B, Leodolter A, et al. EUS in the diagnosis of early chronic pancreatitis: a prospective follow-up study. Gastrointest Endosc 2002; 55:507–511.

66. Kahl S, Glasbrenner B, Zimmermann S, et al. Endoscopic ultrasound in pancreatic diseases. Dig Dis Sci 2002; 20:120–126.

67. DiMagno EP, Go VL, Summerskill WH. Relations between pancreatic enzyme outputs and malabsorption in severe pancreatic insufficiency. N Engl J Med 1973; 288:813–815.

    DiMagno described for the first time the substantial exocrine reserve of ≈90% of the human pancreas which needs to be lost before steatorrhea develops in patients with chronic pancreatitis.

68. Chowdhury RS, Forsmark CE. Review article: Pancreatic function testing. Aliment Pharmacol Ther 2003; 17:733–750.

69. Burton P, Evans DG, Harper AA, et al. A test of pancreatic function in man based on the analysis of duodenal contents after administration of secretin and pancreozymin. Gut 1960; 1:111–124.

70. Lankisch PG, Seidensticker F, Otto J, et al. Secretin-pancreozymin test (SPT) and endoscopic retrograde cholangiopancreatography (ERCP): both are necessary for diagnosing or excluding chronic pancreatitis. Pancreas 1996; 12:149–152.

71. Lankisch PG. Function tests in the diagnosis of chronic pancreatitis. Critical evaluation. Int J Pancreatol 1993; 14:9–20.

72. Stein J, Jung M, Sziegoleit A, et al. Immunoreactive elastase I: clinical evaluation of a new noninvasive test of pancreatic function. Clin Chem 1996; 42:222–226.

73. Loser C, Mollgaard A, Folsch UR. Faecal elastase 1: a novel, highly sensitive, and specific tubeless pancreatic function test. Gut 1996; 39:580–586.

74. Lerch MM, Nolte I, Riehl J, et al. Diagnostic value of indirect pancreatic function test in serum of anuric patients with chronic renal failure. Scand J Clin Lab Invest 1994; 54:247–250.

75. Dominguez-Munoz JE, Pieramico O, Büchler M, et al. Clinical utility of the serum pancreolauryl test in diagnosis and staging of chronic pancreatitis. Am J Gastroenterol 1993; 88:1237–1241.

76. Ellis I, Lerch MM, Whitcomb DC, Consensus Committees of the European Registry of Hereditary Pancreatic Diseases, Midwest Multi-Center Pancreatic Study Group, International Association of Pancreatology. Genetic testing for hereditary pancreatitis: guidelines for indications, counselling, consent and privacy issues. Pancreatology 2001; 1:405–415.

77. Mössner J, Secknus R, Meyer J, et al. Treatment of pain with pancreatic extracts in chronic pancreatitis: results of a prospective placebo-controlled multicenter trial. Digestion 1992; 53:54–66.

78. Warshaw AL, Banks PA, Fernandez-Del Castillo C. AGA technical review: treatment of pain in chronic pancreatitis. Gastroenterology 1998; 115:765–776.

79. Donowitz M, Hendler R, Spiro HM, et al. Glucagon secretion in acute and chronic pancreatitis. Ann Intern Med 1975; 83:778–781.

80. Linde J, Nilsson LH, Barany FR. Diabetes and hypoglycemia in chronic pancreatitis. Scand J Gastroenterol 1977; 12:369–373.

81. Layer P, Keller J. Lipase supplementation therapy: standards, alternatives, and perspectives. Pancreas 2003; 26:1–7.

82. Layer P, Holtmann G. Pancreatic enzymes in chronic pancreatitis. Int J Pancreatol 1994; 15:1–11.

83. Haaber AB, Rosenfalck AM, Hansen B, et al. Bone mineral metabolism, bone mineral density, and body composition in patients with chronic pancreatitis and pancreatic exocrine insufficiency. Int J Pancreatol 2000; 27:21–27.

84. Halgreen H, Pedersen NT, Worning H. Symptomatic effect of pancreatic enzyme therapy in patients with chronic pancreatitis. Scand J Gastroenterol 1986; 21:104–108.

85. Isaksson G, Ihse I. Pain reduction by an oral pancreatic enzyme preparation in chronic pancreatitis. Dig Dis Sci 1983; 28:97–102.

86. Cremer M, Deviere J, Delhaye M, et al. Stenting in severe chronic pancreatitis: results of medium-term follow-up in seventy-six patients. Bildgebung 1992; 59(Suppl 1):20–24.

87. Delhaye M, Matos C, Deviere J. Endoscopic technique for the management of pancreatitis and its complications. Best Pract Res Clin Gastroenterol 2004; 18:155–181.

88. Dite P, Ruzicka M, Zboril V, et al. A prospective, randomized trial comparing endoscopic and surgical therapy for chronic pancreatitis. Endoscopy 2003; 35:553–558.

In a prospective, randomized study comparing surgery with endoscopy in 72 patients with painful obstructive chronic pancreatitis surgery was determined to be superior to endotherapy for long-term pain reduction in patients with painful obstructive chronic pancreatitis.

89. Kozarek RA, Traverso LW. Endotherapy for chronic pancreatitis. Int J Pancreatol 1996; 19:93–102.

90. Kozarek RA. Endoscopic treatment of chronic pancreatitis. Indian J Gastroenterol 2002; 21:67–73.

91. Rosch T, Daniel S, Scholz M, et al. Endoscopic treatment of chronic pancreatitis: a multicenter study of 1000 patients with long-term follow-up. Endoscopy 2002; 34:765–771.

92. Dumonceau JM, Deviere J, Le Moine O, et al. Endoscopic pancreatic drainage in chronic pancreatitis associated with ductal stones: long-term results. Gastrointest Endosc 1996; 43:547–555.

93. Renou C, Grandval P, Ville E, et al. Endoscopic treatment of the main pancreatic duct: correlations among morphology, manometry, and clinical follow-up. Int J Pancreatol 2000; 27:143–149.

94. Sherman S, Hawes RH, Savides TJ, et al. Stent-induced pancreatic ductal and parenchymal changes: correlation of endoscopic ultrasound with ERCP. Gastrointest Endosc 1996;44:276–282.

95. Farnbacher MJ, Schoen C, Rabenstein T, et al. Pancreatic duct stones in chronic pancreatitis: criteria for treatment intensity and success. Gastrointest Endosc 2002; 56:501–506.

96. Kozarek RA, Brandabur JJ, Ball TJ, et al. Clinical outcomes in patients who undergo extracorporeal shock wave lithotripsy for chronic calcific pancreatitis. Gastrointest Endosc 2002; 56:496–500.

97. Beckingham IJ, Krige JE, Bornman PC, et al. Long term outcome of endoscopic drainage of pancreatic pseudocysts. Am J Gastroenterol 1999; 94:71–74.

98. Criado E, De Stefano AA, Weiner TM, et al. Long term results of percutaneous catheter drainage of pancreatic pseudocysts. Surg Gynecol Obstet 1992; 175:293–298.

99. Vitas GJ, Sarr MG. Selected management of pancreatic pseudocysts: operative versus expectant management. Surgery 1992; 111:123–130.

100. Gress F, Schmitt C, Sherman S, et al. Endoscopic ultrasound-guided celiac plexus block for managing abdominal pain associated with chronic pancreatitis: a prospective single center experience. Am J Gastroenterol 2001; 96:409–416.

101. Howard TJ, Swofford JB, Wagner DL, et al. Quality of life after bilateral thoracoscopic splanchnicectomy: long-term evaluation in patients with chronic pancreatitis. J Gastrointest Surg 2002; 6:845–852; discussion 853–854.

102. Ihse I, Zoucas E, Gyllstedt E, et al. Bilateral thoracoscopic splanchnicectomy: effects on pancreatic pain and function. Ann Surg 1999; 230:785–790; discussion 790–781.

103. Beger HG, Schlosser W, Friess HM, et al. Duodenum-preserving head resection in chronic pancreatitis changes the natural course of the disease: a single-center 26-year experience. Ann Surg 1999; 230:512–519; discussion 519–523.

This is so far the largest study which presents preoperative and early postoperative data for 504 patients who underwent duodenum-preserving pancreatic head resection (DPPHR) for severe chronic pancreatitis (CP). The authors concluded that in patients with alcoholic chronic pancreatitis in whom an inflammatory mass has developed in the pancreatic head, DPPHR results in a change in the natural course of the disease in terms of pain status, frequency of acute episodes, need for further hospital admission, late death, and quality of life.

104. Nealon WH, Thompson JC. Progressive loss of pancreatic function in chronic pancreatitis is delayed by main pancreatic duct decompression. A longitudinal prospective analysis of the modified Puestow procedure. Ann Surg 1993; 217:458–466

105. Friess H, Berberat PO, Wirtz M, et al. Surgical treatment and long-term follow-up in chronic pancreatitis. Eur J Gastroenterol Hepatol 2002; 14:971–977.

106. Schafer M, Mullhaupt B, Clavien PA. Evidence-based pancreatic head resection for pancreatic cancer and chronic pancreatitis. Ann Surg 2002; 236:137–148.

107. Frey CF, Smith GJ. Description and rationale of a new operation for chronic pancreatitis. Pancreas 1987; 2:701–707.

108. Izbicki JR, Bloechle C, Broering DC, et al. Extended drainage versus resection in surgery for chronic pancreatitis: a prospective randomized trial comparing the longitudinal pancreaticojejunostomy combined with local pancreatic head excision with the pylorus-preserving pancreatoduodenectomy. Ann Surg 1998; 228:771–779.

The first trial that directly compares different surgical approaches to chronic pancreatitis. The authors found no difference between the Beger and the Frey procedures in terms of clinical outcome and pain relief but suggest that the Frey procedure provides a better quality of life.

109. Izbicki JR, Bloechle C, Broering DC, et al. Longitudinal V-shaped excision of the ventral pancreas for small duct disease in severe chronic pancreatitis: prospective evaluation of a new surgical procedure. Ann Surg 1998; 227:213–219.

110. Gloor B, Friess H, Uhl W, et al. A modified technique of the Beger and Frey procedure in patients with chronic pancreatitis. Dig Surg 2001; 18:21–25.

111. Li-Ling J, Irving M. Somatostatin and octreotide in the prevention of postoperative pancreatic complications and the treatment of enterocutaneous pancreatic fistulas: a systematic review of randomized controlled trials. Br J Surg 2001; 88:190–199.

112. Ho HS, Frey CF. The Frey procedure: local resection of pancreatic head combined with lateral pancreaticojejunostomy. Arch Surg 2001; 136:1353–1358.

CHAPTER TWENTY-NINE

Pancreatic cancer

Helmut M. Friess and Markus W. Büchler

EPIDEMIOLOGY

Epidemiological figures

Approximately 200 000 patients are diagnosed worldwide with pancreatic cancer (PCa) each year. Patients often initially present with back pain and are first treated for lumbago or sent for cholecystectomy before a diagnosis of PCa is established. This devastating disease can present with variable non-specific clinical symptoms and therefore its correct diagnosis and appropriate treatment is often delayed. PCa has one of the most abysmal prognoses of all cancers and it is the only cancer in which the mortality rate almost equals its incidence. At present it is the fourth leading cause of cancer-related death in both men (after lung, prostate, colon) and women (after lung, breast, colon) in the US.[1,2] In terms of its prevalence, PCa ranks 11th among all types of cancers.[3] The male:female ratio for the incidence of PCa is 1.5 in industrialized nations and 1.1 in developing countries.[1] The mean age of patients with PCa at diagnosis is 67 years for men and 74 years for women. The incidence of PCa in patients younger than 40 is about 0.3% and 0.1% in patients younger than age 20. PCa is, therefore, primarily a disease of the elderly but it can also occur in younger patients.

Genetic influence

Migration studies in the US have indicated that an immigrant's risk of developing PCa is related to the risk elements of the new home country carried over two generations. This underlines the fact that environmental factors are of importance in the development of PCa. Nevertheless, about 3–10% of all PCa patients have a genetic cause for their disease. These familial PCas can be associated with other cancer syndromes (see Familial/inherited pancreatic cancer, below) but, in most cases, the genetic basis is presently not known.[4,5]

Environmental influence

Many environmental factors have been claimed to be associated with PCa: smoking, high fat intake, diabetes mellitus, obesity, pancreatitis, coffee consumption, alcohol consumption, radiation exposure, occupation, cholecystectomy, allergies and, recently, aspirin.[4,6] However, a causal relationship between these independent factors and PCa cannot be clearly established because multiple factors (e.g., smoking, high fat intake, diabetes, obesity, coffee, and alcohol consumption) are often present at the same time in the same patient.

Smoking and chronic pancreatitis (hereditary chronic pancreatitis in particular) are established risk factors for PCa. However, smoking increases the risk of PCa only modestly (twofold compared to nonsmokers) and the evidence is not as strong for smoking as a risk factor for pancreatic cancer as it is for lung cancer.[4,6] Chronic pancreatitis is generally believed to be a risk factor for PCa but patients with chronic pancreatitis are frequently smokers and consumers of alcohol and the influence of chronic pancreatitis, alone, is not clear.

The incidence of PCa has increased in Japanese and in African-Americans in recent years. Changes in lifestyle, increased smoking and a Western-world diet rich in ω-6 fats are believed to be risk factors for this epidemiologic change. In addition, several epidemiological studies also suggest that obesity is a risk factor for PCa. Furthermore, insulin resistance is related to obesity and type II diabetes mellitus is often seen in these patients. However, the relation of these three factors to PCa is very complex. Not surprisingly, some data suggest diabetes mellitus as a risk factor for PCa while others, including epidemiological data, indicate that diabetes mellitus is a consequence of PCa. Moreover, new data show that patients with type I diabetes mellitus do not develop PCa, suggesting that diabetes mellitus is not really a risk factor for PCa, but rather insulin resistance as a product of obesity predisposes to the development of PCa as well as type 2 diabetes mellitus.[7] Whether aspirin intake increases the risk of developing PCa is still a matter of controversy and both pro and con data have recently been published.[8]

PROGNOSIS

Generally, patients with PCa have a poor prognosis. This poor prognosis is related to the fact that there are few if any effective therapeutic options for the disease and the fact that early diagnosis is usually not possible since the symptoms are non-specific and no early tumor markers have been identified. The overall 5-year survival rate for PCa in all tumor stages is about 3–5% with a median survival time of approximately 6 months. Tumor resection is only possible in about 10–15% of all PCa patients but it is currently the best available treatment option.[9] In patients with resected tumors, median survival is 18–24 months and 5-year survival is around 20%. Adjuvant chemotherapy improves the prognosis following tumor resection.[10] Causes for death are local tumor recurrence or metastatic tumor progression.[10] In advanced pancreatic cancer – i.e., tumors that are locally unresectable or tumors that have distant metastasis – median survival is 4–9 months.

PATHOGENESIS: PATHOLOGY & MOLECULAR ALTERATIONS

Pancreatic tumors comprise a heterogeneous group of neoplasms arising mainly from the exocrine or endocrine components of the pancreas. PCa is the most common and the most clinically relevant of these pancreatic tumors. Molecular research over the last decade has contributed significantly to a better understanding of the aggressive nature of PCa. The observed alterations range from gross chromosomal abnormalities to gene mutations and to epigenetic changes, such as dysregulated expression of a variety of genes which are important in disease progression. These alterations have been identified as representing either early or late steps in pancreatic carcinogenesis, thus suggesting a cancer progression model of histological and molecular changes.

Histologic classification

The normal pancreas consists predominantly of three cell types: acinar cells, ductal cells, and endocrine cells. Tumors arising from the endocrine cells are termed neuroendocrine tumors and are classified depending on their differentiation and their functional status.[11] Rare exocrine tumors that arise from acinar cells include acinar cell carcinoma, acinar cell cystadenocarcinoma, and mixed acinar-endocrine carcinoma. Pancreatic ductal adenocarcinoma, which most likely arises from ductal cells, is the most common form of exocrine pancreatic tumor. Other tumor types that potentially arise from the ductal system and that are far less frequent include serous cystic tumor, mucinous cystic tumor, intraductal papillary-mucinous tumor, invasive papillary-mucinous carcinoma, mucinous noncystic carcinoma, solid pseudopapillary carcinoma, signet ring cell carcinoma, undifferentiated (anaplastic) carcinoma, mixed ductal-endocrine carcinoma, osteoclast-like giant cell tumor, and pancreaticoblastoma.[12]

Precursor lesions

The cell type of origin of PCa has long been a matter of dispute. Trans- and/or dedifferentiating islet cells and acinar cells,[13] as well as ductal cells have been suggested to be the cells of origin for PCa. According to the current model, which is well supported by clinical, histological, and molecular data, a series of histologically defined intraductal lesions termed pancreatic intraepithelial neoplasms (PanINs) are believed to be precursors of PCa.[14] Low-grade PanINs (PanIN-1) display only marginal morphological alterations of the normal cuboidal to low-columnar ductal epithelium. In contrast, high-grade PanINs (PanIN-3) are morphologically similar to invasive PCa, but they are confined to the ducts, thereby constituting in situ carcinomas. Clinical evidence suggests that these PanIN lesions can indeed progress to invasive PCa, and molecular analysis has demonstrated the step-by-step accumulation of certain genetic and epigenetic alterations as the tumor progresses from PanINs to invasive PCa.[15]

Chromosomal alterations

Chromosomal alterations have been identified in virtually all PCas examined. These alterations range from structural abnormalities

such as translocations, breakpoints, and amplifications to whole chromosome gains and losses. Whole chromosome losses have been identified for 6, 12, 13, 17, 18, and Y. More frequently, partial chromosomal losses have been found at 18q, 10q, 8p, and 13q. Whole chromosomal gains have been observed for 7, 11, 20, and commonly gained regions were located on 8q and 3q.[16] In addition, structural abnormalities have been identified frequently at 1p, 2p, 3p, 4q, 6q, 7q, 11q, and 17p. Chromosomal bands 1p32, 1q10, 6q21, 7p22, 8p21, 8q11, 14p11, 15q10-11, and 17q11 are the most common breakpoint sites affected by structural rearrangements. Altogether, the number of breakpoints in PCa ranges from 117 to 608 per case.[16] Furthermore, high copy number amplifications of the chromosomal regions 5p, 8q22-ter, 12p12-cen, 19q12-13.2, and 20q have been identified.

Genetic alterations/mutations

PCas harbor a number of tumor suppressor and oncogene mutations. Tumor suppressor gene mutations result in a loss of function (i.e., control of cellular growth) and might be caused by homozygous deletion or single allelic loss combined with mutation or other alterations in the second allele. On the other hand, oncogene mutations result in a gain of function (i.e., enhanced growth stimulation), caused by mutations, amplification, or overexpression.

The most commonly mutated oncogene in PCa is the K-ras gene (KRAS2) and, as a result of this mutation, the K-ras protein is persistently kept in an active state. Activated K-ras subsequently enhances cell proliferation. K-ras point mutations at codon 12 are present in approximately 85–95% of PCas. They are believed to represent a relatively early event in pancreatic carcinogenesis because they also appear in PanIN lesions surrounding the cancer cells.[17,18]

The most commonly mutated tumor suppressor genes in PCa include p53 (TP53), p16 (CDKN2A), and Smad4 (MADH4). They are involved in cell cycle control and apoptosis. Their mutations result in uncontrolled cell cycle progression and neoplastic transformation. The prevalence of p53 mutations in PCa is about 40–60% and p53 mutations are associated with increased tumor stage, tumor size, worsened tumor grading, the presence of lymph node metastases, and a worsened prognosis following tumor resection. p16 (CDKN2A) is the most frequently inactivated gene in PCa. Inactivation of p16 can be due to its homozygous deletion (40%), to single allelic loss plus mutation in the other allele (40%), or to promoter hypermethylation (15%).[19] The Smad4 gene (MADH4) is inactivated in approximately 55% of PCas either as a result of its homozygous deletion or because of a single allelic loss with a mutation of the second allele. This leads to subsequent decreased growth inhibition and apoptosis due to a disturbance of the TGF-β signaling pathway.[20]

Besides these common and well-characterized gene mutations, PCas also display other tumor suppressor gene mutations, although with lower frequencies. These gene mutations include those of the DCC, APC, FHIT, ARP, BRCA2, MKK4, STK11, EP300, ACVR1B, ACVR2, TβR-I, and TβR-II genes.[21,22]

Epigenetic alterations

PCas not only display a number of alterations at the chromosomal and genetic level, they also exhibit numerous epigenetic alterations, i.e., changes in the expression of other genes that are involved in the pathogenesis of PCa. These genes influence diverse pathways such as those important for cell growth, apoptosis, invasion, and metastasis.[23]

Growth promoting pathways

A number of growth-promoting pathways are activated in PCa (Table 29.1). These include pathways involving the epidermal growth factor receptor family,[24–26] insulin-like growth factor (IGF) receptor,[27] platelet-derived growth factor receptor (PDGFR), and fibroblast growth factor receptor (FGFR).[28–30] In addition to these receptors, the ligands which bind and activate these receptors are also upregulated in PCa cells. As a result, autocrine and paracrine growth stimulation of PCa cells appears to be an important mechanism responsible for the major growth advantage given to pancreatic cancer cells.

Growth inhibiting pathways

Epithelial cells also possess growth factor receptors and ligands, such as the TGF-β pathway (see Table 29.1), which exert growth inhibitory effects.[31,32] Although its signaling receptors (type I and type II) and ligands (TGF-β1-3) are upregulated in PCas, this growth inhibitory pathway has lost its functional effectiveness due to intracellular blockage (smad6, smad7) or mutation of signaling molecules (MADH4).[20,31–34]

Apoptosis pathways

Resistance towards programmed cell death (apoptosis) is one of the hallmarks of malignant growth in PCa. Several genes such as bax, bak and bcl-X_L, etc. which are involved in activation and inhibition of apoptosis are disturbed in PCa cells.[35,36] In addition, TNF-α and its high infinity receptor TNF-R1, as well as Fas ligand (FasL, CD95), TRAIL and its respective high affinity receptors, have lost their functional effectiveness.[37] These changes negatively influence the prognosis of patients with PCa and their response to chemotherapy.

Invasion and metastasis pathways

Tissue invasion and metastasis are other hallmarks of malignant growth of PCa. In PCas, a number of genes which directly or indirectly influence these functions, such as heparanase (an endoglycosidase that digests heparansulfate proteoglycans [HSPGs]),[38] members of the matrix metalloproteinases (MMPs) (MMP-1, MMP-2, MMP-3, MMP-7, MMP-9, MMP-13) as well as their inhibitors (MT1-MMP, TIMP-1, TIMP-2)[39,40] are aberrantly expressed. PCa cells also produce nerve growth factor (NGF) which mediates the spread of cancer cells along pancreatic nerves in which there is enhanced expression of the NGF binding receptor TrkA.[41] In addition, mediators of cell adhesion such as galectin-1 and galection-3,[42] and genes including KAI-1, which directly enhance the ability to form tumor metastases,[43] are dysregulated in PCa.

Table 29.1 Growth factors and growth factor receptors which are involved in PCa pathogenesis

Receptor families		Ligand families	
EGFR	EGFR (HER-1) erbB-2 (HER-2) erbB-3 (HER-3) erbB-4 (HER-4)	EGF	EGF transforming growth factor (TGF)-α betacellulin heparin-binding EGF like growth factor (HB-EGF) amphiregulin neuregulins cripto epiregulin
IGFR	IGF-RI	IGF	IGF-I IGF-II
FGFR	FGF-R1	FGF	FGF-1 FGF-2 FGF-5 FGF-7
PDGFR	PDGF-Rα PDGF-Rβ	PDGF	PDGF-AA PDGF-BB PDGF-AB
Tβ-R	Tβ-R1 Tβ-R2 Tβ-R3 Activin R-IA/B Activin R-IIA/B BMP R-IA/B BMP R-II	TGF-β	TGF-β1 TGF-β2 TGF-β3 Activin Inhibin BMP
Trk	TrkA p75	NGF	NGF BDNF

EGFR, epidermal growth factor receptor; IGFR, insulin-like growth factor receptor; FGFR, fibroblast growth factor receptor; PDGFR, platelet-derived growth factor receptor; Tβ-R, transforming growth factor β receptor; Trk, NGF binding tyrosine kinase receptors.
EGF, epidermal growth factor; IGF, insulin-like growth factor; FGF, fibroblast growth factor; PDGF, platelet-derived growth factor (PDGF); TGF-β, transforming growth factor β; NGF, nerve growth factor; BDNF, brain-derived growth factor; BMP, bone morphogenetic protein.

Familial/inherited pancreatic cancer

Familial/hereditary PCa is associated with a number of different inherited diseases and syndromes and it has considerable heterogenicity. No single mutation which causes familial/hereditary PCa has been identified and the real number of families afflicted by hereditary PCa still remains unclear. No certain criteria or standardized definitions for distinguishing sporadic PCa and familial/hereditary PCa have been established to date. Inherited syndromes that are associated with an increased risk of PCa include: (1) hereditary nonpolyposis colorectal cancer (HNPCC), which is caused by mutations of DNA-mismatch repair enzymes; (2) familial breast cancer syndrome associated with BRCA2 mutations; (3) familial atypical multiple mole melanoma syndrome (FAMMM), which is associated with mutations of the p16 (CSKN2A) gene; (4) familial adenomatosis coli (FAP) with mutations of the APC gene; (5) Peutz-Jeghers syndrome with mutations of the STK1/LKB1 gene; and (6) ataxia-telangiectasia syndrome with mutations of the ATM gene. In addition, hereditary chronic pancreatitis caused by mutations of the cationic trypsinogen (PRSS1), as well as CP associated with cystic fibrosis, represent genetic risk factors for the development of PCa.[44]

CLINICAL PRESENTATION

Most PCa patients are diagnosed in advanced tumor stages due to the lack of specific early symptoms and, in more than 80% of the patients, the tumor has already metastasized before clinical symptoms arise. The initial metastases are to regional lymph nodes and this is followed by distant organ metastasis. Hematogenous metastasis are localized to the liver in 80% and to the lung in 50% of patients.[45]

The symptoms of PCa are, for the most part, non-specific. This sometimes leads to a long delay between the patient's first presentation and the establishment of a diagnosis. Weight loss, jaundice, and pain are the most common early symptoms.[45] Weight loss of more than 10% of the original body weight or 1–2 kg per month can be seen in approximately 90% of the patients at the time of diagnosis. In end stage tumors, cachexia is quite frequent.[46]

Obstructive jaundice is a typical sign of tumors localized in the head of the pancreas and jaundice is present in four out of five of these patients. The obstruction of the bile duct is accompanied by dark urine and acholic stools in 60% and pruritus in 20% of the patients. Obstructive jaundice can be an early symptom of a relatively small tumor, especially in patients with periampullary tumors.

Pain, when it occurs, is usually localized to the upper abdomen and it radiates to the back. Its intensity relates only in part to tumor size and stage. Pain is a sign of tumor infiltration into nerves and tumor cell spread along nerves into the retroperitoneal nerve plexi. The pain of PCa can also be due to an accompanying pancreatitis.[41]

A large tumor mass in the head of the pancreas can cause duodenal obstruction with delayed gastric emptying accompanied by vomiting and nausea in 30–40% of the patients. Reduced appetite is reported by about half of the patients with PCa.

The physical examination can reveal jaundice and, on occasion, a palpable gallbladder caused by bile duct obstruction. The latter is referred to as Courvoisier's sign. A palpable tumor mass at the time of patient presentation is more likely to be present in cystadenomas or neuroendocrine tumors, but can also be present in patients with PCa.

Symptoms related to biliary obstruction are less frequent if the tumor is localized in the body or at the tail of the pancreas. In general, these body and tail tumors cause less severe symptoms than pancreatic head tumors and this may cause a delay in their diagnosis. As a result, patients with PCas of the body and tail are diagnosed at more advanced tumor stages and they have a worsened prognosis compared to cancers in the head of the pancreas.[45] Cancers located in the body and tail of the pancreas often cause splenic vein obstruction, splenomegaly, gastric and esophageal varices, and gastrointestinal hemorrhage.

Laboratory tests may demonstrate increased bilirubin and alkaline phosphatase levels in patients with biliary obstruction or liver metastasis. Tumor markers such as CA 19-9 (sensitivity approximately 80%), CA 50, and CEA may be increased. Twenty-five percent of the patients have elevated glucose levels or a worsening of pre-existing diabetes mellitus within the final few months prior to diagnosis of PCa. This may be related to the secretion, by the tumor, of an antiinsulin hormone referred to as islet amyloid polypeptide (IAPP).[47]

DIAGNOSTICS

Role of tumor markers

CA 19-9 is the tumor marker most frequently used to monitor pancreatic cancer. In a meta-analysis involving 24 different studies, CA 19-9 was found to have a sensitivity of 81% and specificity of 90% for the diagnosis of PCa using a cut-off of 37 U/mL.[48] However, CA 19-9 elevations are also frequently observed in other GI tumors and in benign diseases, such as chronic pancreatitis, liver cirrhosis, cholestasis, and jaundice. Therefore, in patients with jaundice, CA 19-9 is a marker of only limited usefulness. Furthermore, in small pancreatic cancers (<3 cm) CA19-9 is elevated in only 50% of the cases.[49] Other tumor markers such as CEA and CA 50 have no diagnostic advantage over CA 19-9.

Radiological imaging

Radiological imaging plays a central role in the diagnosis and staging of PCa and eventually in the decision to resect these tumors (Fig. 29.1). Multiple imaging techniques, such as abdominal ultrasonography (US), endosonography (EUS), CT scan, MRI, angiography, endoscopic retrograde cholangiopancreatography (ERCP), and positron emission tomography (PET) are currently available.[50]

Abdominal ultrasonography is usually the first test performed when there is clinical suspicion of pancreatic cancer. Its easy availability, low cost, and non-invasiveness makes it a popular screening test for various kinds of abdominal disorders. Its sensitivity (60–100%) and specificity (44–99%) in the diagnosis of pancreatic cancer is, however, highly dependent on the experience of the examiner.[50] Abdominal ultrasonography is useful in patients with biliary obstruction, and it can detect ascites and/or metastatic lesions in the liver which would exclude resection.

EUS was developed to eliminate interference with bowel gas and to reach higher image resolution. The fact that the pancreas is located next to the stomach and duodenum makes EUS an ideal approach for detection of tumors and vessel infiltration. Several studies comparing EUS with spiral CT and MRI have shown the superiority of EUS for detection of small pancreatic tumors (<3 cm)

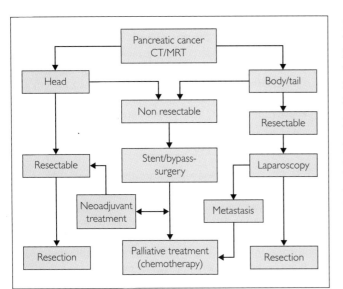

Fig. 29.1 • Treatment algorithm in nonmetastatic pancreatic cancer patients.

and venous infiltration. However, EUS is inferior to CT and MRI for judging arterial involvement and lymph node status.[50]

The rapid evolution of CT scanning in the last two decades has contributed to the earlier tumor detection and to the higher resection rate of PCas today (see Fig. 29.1). To detect tumors in the pancreas, contrast between normal pancreas and the malignant lesion is crucial. In the early venous phase after contrast administration, pancreatic tumors are seen as hypodense lesions. The main role of modern CT techniques (e.g., hydro-CT achieved by filling stomach and duodenum with water) is to evaluate tumor resectability. Most pancreatic surgeons consider a pancreatic tumor to be unresectable if distant metastases are present and/or encasement and infiltration of peripancreatic vessels by the tumor mass has occurred.[51]

In recent years, MRI has developed into the preferred alternative to CT. Although the sensitivity and specificity of both procedures are comparable, MRI is still more costly and complex to perform and takes 4–7 times longer than CT scanning. However, the advantages of MRI are that it uses no radiation and there is the option to combine MRI with pancreatography and angiography (MRCP), allowing the so-called 'one-stop-shopping,' with tumor imaging, angiography, and pancreatic and bile duct visualization.[52]

Although MRCP seems to be an attractive noninvasive technique, ERCP is still the most precise method of imaging the biliary and pancreatic ducts.[53] The pathognomonic sign of PCa is the so called 'double-duct' sign in which both the biliary and the pancreatic ducts are dilated proximal to a stenosis of both ducts in the pancreatic head. The strength of ERCP is its therapeutic potential. At the time of ERCP, stents can be placed in the biliary duct to relieve jaundice. Furthermore, tissue (biopsy) or cells (ductal brushing) from suspicious areas can be collected to aid in diagnosis.

PET scanning is the latest technique to be applied to the diagnosis of pancreatic cancer. It uses the increased glucose metabolism of cancer cells to detect small tumors (<2 cm) and it is, therefore, ideally suited to differentiate benign from malignant tumors in the pancreas.[54] At present, however, it is not widely used. It is costly and has not been shown to be superior to CT or MRI.

Fine needle aspiration

Because of its risk in spreading tumor cells along the needle tract, transabdominal fine needle aspiration (FNA) should be avoided in resectable pancreatic tumors. A negative result does not exclude malignancy and false-negative results of 25–40% have been reported.[55] An attractive alternative to transabdominal FNA is EUS-guided FNA because there is no danger, using EUS-guided FNA, of seeding the peritoneal cavity. Brush biopsies of the tumor, obtained by ERCP, can aid pathologic assessment. On the other hand, the value of cytological examination of pancreatic fluid is a matter of some controversy. FNA is indicated when distant metastases of PCa are present because, in this setting, it can aid in establishing the diagnosis and in planning for neoadjuvant treatment in locally advanced PCas.

Diagnostic laparoscopy

The goal of diagnostic laparoscopy in PCa patients is to avoid unneeded laparotomy when distant metastases have occurred or when the tumor is locally unresectable. Theoretically, laparoscopy could spare the patient an unnecessary operation, speed recovery, and reduce expense. The addition of laparoscopic ultrasound, biopsies, and peritoneal cytology enhances the value of diagnostic laparoscopy by identifying patients who qualify for and will benefit from resection. Twenty years ago, when diagnostic laparoscopy was introduced in PCa, the reported rate of occult metastases, found at the time of laparoscopy, was up to 35%, with a much higher rate in cancers of the pancreatic body or tail compared to pancreatic head carcinomas. However, technical advances in imaging techniques (CT, MRI) have improved staging accuracy of PCa and nowadays only 7–14% of all patients with pancreatic cancer benefit from diagnostic laparoscopy.[56] Whether or not a diagnostic laparoscopy should be performed before a laparotomy is an individual decision. Since cancers of the pancreatic body and tail show occult metastatic disease more often, this patient population benefits most from diagnostic laparoscopy. However, if there is radiological suspicion of distant tumor spread, such as unclear lesions in the liver or peritoneal metastases accompanied by variable amount of ascites, diagnostic laparoscopy is recommended independent of the localization of the tumor.

PALLIATIVE TREATMENT OF PANCREATIC CANCER

Because of local tumor extension and infiltration of arteries (hepatic and/or superior mesenteric) or because of the presence of distant metastases, approximately 80% of all pancreatic cancer patients present with nonresectable disease. In these patients palliative treatment by means of surgical, interventional, or oncological approaches or down-staging is primarily indicated. Palliative treatment for these patients requires an interdisciplinary approach which includes chemotherapy, radiotherapy, or other modalities, and focuses on managing disease-related manifestations such as pain, weight loss, cachexia, depression, fatigue, jaundice, and gastric outlet obstruction.

The role of surgery in the palliative treatment of pancreatic cancer

The final decision for either palliative or curative treatment is often made during surgery for PCa (see Fig. 29.1). It is generally agreed that tumor resection should only be performed in the absence of liver or peritoneal metastasis.[9] A palliative procedure should be considered when distant metastases or local nonresectability are present. The choice of the ideal palliative procedure may be dependent upon the presence of either biliary or duodenal obstruction.

Since 70% of pancreatic cancers are located in the head of the pancreas, obstructive jaundice is either a leading symptom or it develops during the course of the disease in many patients. Thus, performing a biliodigestive anastomosis is a reasonable approach especially in the absence of distant metastases. In case of established gastric outlet obstruction, a gastric bypass procedure should be added. However, the decision to perform or not perform a prophylactic gastric bypass procedure is more complex because only 20% of patients with pancreatic head tumors will develop gastric outlet obstruction before death. Although a prophylactic gastric bypass is not associated with increased morbidity or mortality, whether it is needed or not remains controversial.[57,58]

Relief of jaundice and gastric outlet obstruction can also be achieved by interventional stenting procedures. Patients who present with obstructive jaundice and are unlikely candidates for surgery (e.g., due to liver metastasis) should undergo endoscopic biliary stenting, since it has a higher success rate and a lower complication rate compared to percutaneous transhepatic stenting. In the presence of gastric outlet and duodenal obstruction, expandable metal stents may be an alternative to a surgical bypass, especially in patients with advanced metastatic disease. However, only few data are available on palliation of gastric outlet obstruction by stenting and therefore surgery may be preferred.[59]

Endoscopic stenting, because it is associated with fewer procedure-related complications, may be preferable to surgery in the later stages of PCa but surgery, because it is associated with less cholangitis and less recurrent obstruction, may be preferable to endoscopic stenting in the earlier phases of the disease when life expectancy is longer. Therefore, if life expectancy is >4 months, a surgical bypass should be strongly considered.

Pain management in patients with nonresectable pancreatic cancer

Pain management is a crucial issue in the palliative treatment of PCa patients. About 80% of patients report pain even in the early stages of the disease.[60] Initially, pain may be controllable with nonsteroidal antiinflammatory drugs, Cox-2 inhibitors, or opioids. However, in addition to opioid analgesics, adequate pain control may require intraoperative chemical splanchnicectomy or celiac block (open surgery, laparoscopic approach) or percutaneous celiac block (US, CT, MRI).[61] In addition, thoracoscopic splanchnicectomy can achieve favorable pain relief.[61] Chemotherapy and/or radiotherapy may also decrease pain in PCa. About 24% of patients treated with gemcitabine have pain reduction.[62]

Palliative chemotherapy

In more than 50 phase I, II, and III trials, gemcitabine has shown reproducible antineoplastic activity in advanced pancreatic cancer[62,63] and, therefore, it is currently the benchmark for new anticancer drugs in PCa. At present no newer drug (i.e., Taxanes, Topomerase I Inhibitors, Epirubicin, Cisplatin, Ukrain, etc.) has been shown to be of more benefit than gemcitabine but trials to define

more effective treatment options including gemcitabine-based combinations are ongoing.[63–65] Pharmacokinetic adaptations, such as the use of a fixed-dose infusion rate for gemcitabine, seem to further improve the efficacy of gemcitabine chemotherapy. Furthermore, the combination of gemcitabine and oxaliplatin can prolong the time to progression and increase the response rate but not survival.[64] Unfortunately, they do not improve overall survival.

Palliative radiotherapy

The role of radiotherapy as a palliative treatment option in pancreatic cancer is controversial. Although radiotherapy in patients with advanced disease has some impact, it has no benefit on survival in the adjuvant setting.[10,66] There are emerging techniques, however, including intraoperative radiotherapy (IORT), intensity modulated radiotherapy, interstitial brachytherapy, and radioimmunotherapy which are presently undergoing further evaluation to judge their effectiveness in advanced PCa.

Novel therapies for palliative treatment

Knowledge regarding the molecular background of PCa has increased dramatically over the last few years and, based on this information, new therapies are being developed.[64,65] A variety of different approaches, including tumor vaccines, signal transduction inhibitors (against EGFR, Her-2/neu, c-kit, and others), inhibitors of Ras signaling pathways, and drugs targeting the host microenvironment (antiangiogenesis therapies, matrix metalloproteinase inhibitors, application of antigastrin immunogen) are under investigation. For the most part, however, these novel approaches have not yet become part of the standard treatment for PCa and most of them are still far from integration into the daily routine.

CURATIVE TREATMENT FOR PANCREATIC CANCER

Classical Kausch-Whipple procedure

Partial pancreaticoduodenectomy (also named Kausch-Whipple operation) is the standard operation for resectable cancer of the pancreatic head. It is also the standard operation for ampullary and distal bile duct tumors. The German surgeon Walter Kausch performed the first successful partial duodenopancreatectomy as early as 1909.[67] Because of its high hospital morbidity and mortality, however, it was not widely accepted in the surgical world at that time, and for many years most surgeons avoided pancreatic resection with its accompanying pancreatic anastomosis. In their desire to avoid postoperative anastomosis-related complications, most surgeons favored the simple performance of gastroenterostomy to restore food passage in patients with pancreatic malignancies. Interest in pancreatic resection was renewed, however, when Allen O. Whipple reported three successful duodenopancreatectomies in 1935.[68] In honor of Dr. Whipple, who performed 37 pancreatic resections in his lifetime, the procedure has become known and standardized as the Whipple procedure (Fig. 29.2A, B).

The Kausch-Whipple operation consists of (1) a distal gastrectomy (10–40% of the stomach); (2) resection of the duodenum distal to the transection site and (due to technical reasons) of the first jejunal loop; (3) removal of the gallbladder (if present); (4) removal of the distal common bile duct (from the level of the

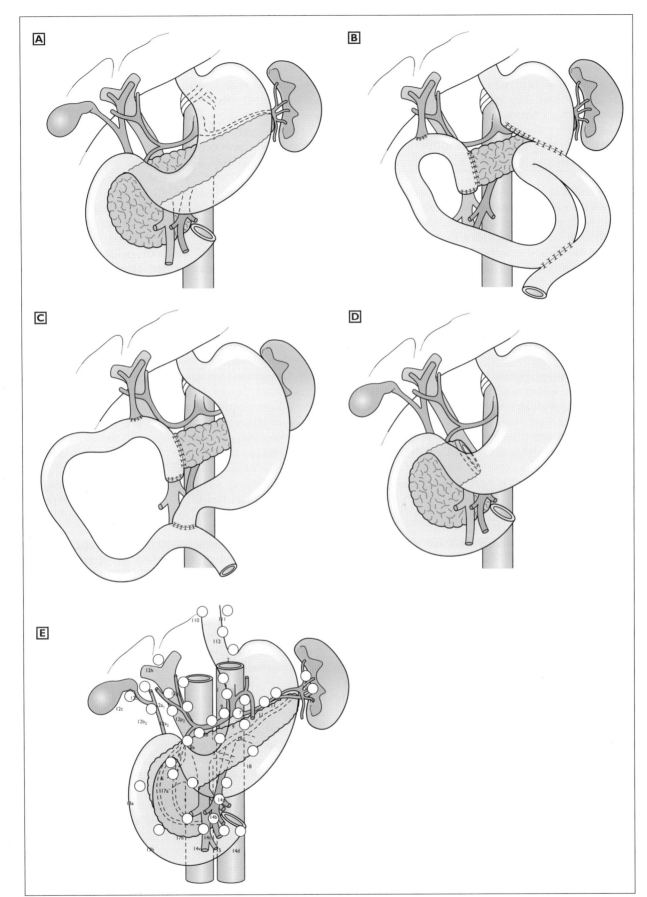

Fig. 29.2 • Surgical approaches in pancreatic cancer. (**A**) Normal abdominal situs. (**B**) Classical Kausch-Whipple procedure. (**C**) Pylorus-preserving Whipple procedure. (**D**) Distal pancreatectomy with splenectomy. (**E**) Regional lymph node stations of the pancreas – lymph node numbering according to the Japanese Society of Pancreatology. Lymph nodes of group 16 are not included in the scheme. They are localized at the anterolateral aspect of the aorta and of the vena cava between the esophagus, celiac axis, superior mesenteric artery, and inferior mesenteric vein.

cystic duct junction distally); and (5) resection of the head of the pancreas, which is divided ventral to the superior mesenteric vein–portal vein axis.

In centers of pancreatic surgery, the Kausch-Whipple procedure is commonly performed today and it is a safe procedure which can be performed with low hospital mortality (≈2%) and morbidity.[69]

Pylorus-preserving pancreaticoduodenectomy (pp-Whipple)

An organ-preserving alternative to the classical Kausch-Whipple procedure is the pylorus-preserving Whipple (Fig. 29.2A,C). This operation was first performed in 1942 by the English surgeon Kenneth Watson for a patient with ampullary cancer.[70] When compared to the classical Kausch-Whipple procedure with distal gastrectomy, the pylorus-preserving Whipple was associated with less postoperative jejunal ulcerations. However, the pylorus-preserving Whipple did not gain widespread acceptance until Longmire and Traverso reintroduced this operative technique 40 years later.[71] The technique itself is similar to the classical Whipple procedure except that the dissection of the duodenum is done 2–4 cm distal to the pylorus. The type of reconstruction differs slightly from the Kausch-Whipple procedure (Fig. 29.2C) and instead of a gastrojejunostomy, a duodenojejunostomy is performed.

The pp-Whipple procedure (Fig. 29.2C) consists of (1) division of the duodenum 2–4 cm distal to the pylorus; (2) resection of the duodenum distal to the transection site and (due to technical reasons) of the first jejunal loop; (3) removal of the gallbladder (if present); (4) removal of the distal common bile duct (from the level of the cystic duct junction distally); and (5) resection of the head of the pancreas, which is divided ventral to the superior mesenteric vein–portal vein axis.

Lymph node dissection in pancreatic cancer

Two different radical approaches to lymph node resection, which differ depending on the extent of lymphadenectomy, have been described.[72,73] The Japanese Society of Pancreatology has developed the most sophisticated of the lymph node classification schemes for PCa (Fig. 29.2E).

Whipple operation with standard lymphadenectomy

Standard lymphadenectomy encompasses regional lymphadenectomy around the duodenum and the resected pancreatic head. The following lymph node groups are resected en bloc with a standard lymphadenectomy (Fig. 29.2E):

Anterior pancreaticoduodenal lymph nodes (station 17 in the Japanese system),

Posterior pancreaticoduodenal lymph nodes (station 13 in the Japanese system),

Lymph nodes in the lower hepatoduodenal ligament (station 12b, 12c),

Lymph nodes along the right lateral aspect of the superior mesenteric artery and vein (14b, 14v.)

Whipple operation with radical (extended) lymphadenectomy

In a radical extended pancreaticoduodenectomy 30–40% of the distal stomach is resected in order to include the lymph node stations 5, 6 and some of 3 and 4. Furthermore, portions of the greater omentum and lesser omentum along the right gastroepiploic artery and right gastric artery are removed. The retroperitoneal lymph node dissection extends from the right renal hilum to the left lateral border of the aorta in the horizontal axis, and from the portal vein to below the third portion of the duodenum in the vertical axis. The inferior-most aspect of the dissection is the origin of the inferior mesenteric artery. The retroperitoneal lymph node dissection harvests lymph nodes from stations 16a2 and 16b1 and samples the celiac lymph node (station 9). This procedure includes the skeletonization of the hepatic arteries, the superior mesenteric artery between aorta and the inferior pancreaticoduodenal and celiac trunk, as well as dissection of the anterolateral aspect of the aorta and vena cava including the Gerota's fascia.

Classical Kausch-Whipple or pylorus-preserving Whipple in pancreatic head cancer?

Several randomized controlled studies have been performed which compare the classical Kausch-Whipple with the pylorus-preserving Whipple in an attempt to determine which is the best operation for patients with resectable cancers of the pancreatic head (Table 29.2). These studies have shown that the pylorus-preserving Whipple procedure achieves the same oncological effectiveness and is as radical as the classical Kausch-Whipple procedure without any major difference in postoperative morbidity or quality of life including delayed gastric emptying.[72,74] As a result, many have adapted pylorus-preserving Whipple as the operation of choice for PCa. On the other hand, in PCa with tumor infiltration of the proximal duodenum or the distal stomach, free margins can be accomplished only by performing a classical Kausch-Whipple operation and, therefore, in those cases, the classical Kausch-Whipple procedure is the operation of choice.

Role of lymphadenectomy in pancreatic head cancer: Standard or extended lymphadenectomy?

Among pancreatic surgeons, there remains considerable controversy regarding how extensive the lymphadenectomy should be. At the time of tumor resection, about 60–80% of the patients have lymph node metastases and most of the resected patients develop locally recurrent disease. This has suggested that a more radical procedure, especially in regard to lymph node dissection, would improve long-term outcome and reduce the rate of local recurrences.[75] However, early anecdotal reports of patients undergoing extended lymphadenectomy were disappointing and randomized, controlled studies were clearly needed. To date, two such studies have been reported – one a multicenter study and one a single-center study.[72,76] The multicenter study showed that the addition of extended lymphadenectomy and retroperitoneal soft-tissue clearance to a pancreaticoduodenectomy does not increase morbidity and mortality rates. Unfortunately, according to this study, addition of the extended lymphadenectomy and soft-tissue clearance also does not improve survival. Only in a subgroup analysis of this study, focusing on the small number of lymph node-positive patients, was a survival benefit for the extended operation noted.[76]

The randomized, controlled single-center study compared pylorus-preserving Whipple with standard lymphadenectomy to the classical Kausch-Whipple with extended retroperitoneal lymphadenectomy. It showed that both groups had similar mortality rates but that

Table 29.2 Classical Kausch-Whipple in comparison to the pylorus-preserving Whipple

		No. of patients	Operation time	Delayed gastric emptying	Operation related morbidity and mortality	Quality of life
Lin et al.[88]	Classical Kausch-Whipple	15	equal	reduced	*equal*	equal
	pp-Whipple	16	equal	increased	*equal*	equal
Wenger et al.[89]	Classical Kausch-Whipple	24	increased	equal	*equal*	reduced
	pp-Whipple	34	reduced	equal	*equal*	increased
Seiler et al.[72]	Classical Kausch-Whipple	51	increased	equal	*equal*	equal
	pp-Whipple	42	reduced	equal	equal	equal

more morbidity (i.e., pancreatic fistulas and delayed gastric emptying) and longer mean postoperative stay was associated with the extended operation. As in the multicenter study, there was no difference in survival between patients with pylorus-preserving Whipple and standard lymphadenectomy compared to patients with the classical Kausch-Whipple and extended lymphadenectomy.

Distal pancreatectomy/pancreatic left resection

The standard surgical therapy for PCa involving the pancreas on the left side of the portal vein (pancreatic corpus and/or tail) is pancreatic left resection with splenectomy (also named distal pancreatectomy). Due to a lack of early symptoms, most patients with PCa involving the pancreas on the left side of the portal/superior mesenteric vein already have distant metastasis or advanced local disease at the time of diagnosis. Even in the absence of distant metastases, these patients frequently have advanced local disease with contiguous organ involvement and/or adherence to the portal-splenic confluence and they would require extensive resection in order to obtain grossly negative resection margins. The level of pancreatic transection is usually located at or to the left of the portal/superior mesenteric vein.[77] However, the individual choice of the resection margin is dependent on the progression and location of the tumor. The closure of the pancreatic stump can be performed in two principal ways: either via simple closure of the stump or via a pancreaticointestinal anastomosis (with the jejunum/stomach). The standard distal pancreatectomy encompasses a regional lymphadenectomy, including lymph node groups at the celiac trunk, the hilum of the spleen, the splenic artery and the inferior border of the body and tail of the pancreas (Fig. 29.2A,D). Elective distal pancreatectomy has a mortality rate of <1%. The survival rate in PCa patients with extended resection of the body or tail is comparable to those undergoing a standard resection. Those patients who can undergo a resection with negative margins have markedly improved long-term survival when compared to those who are considered to be unresectable because of locally advanced disease. Therefore, extended distal pancreatectomy is justified in this small subgroup of patients.

The prognosis of patients undergoing a potentially curative distal pancreatectomy is worse than that of patients with pancreatic head carcinomas. For distal pancreatectomy, the actual 5- and 10-year survival rates are approximately 15–22% and 18%, respectively, following extended resection, 8% and 8% following standard resection, and 0% if no resection was performed due to local nonresectability.[78,79] In general, patients undergoing distal pancreatectomy for PCa have larger tumors but less frequent lymph node metastases and fewer poorly differentiated tumors than those undergoing a pancreaticoduodenectomy for right-sided cancer.[78]

Total pancreatectomy

Total pancreatectomy is usually performed with splenectomy. It combines the standard pancreatoduodenectomy (Whipple procedure) with a pancreatic left resection. The entire pancreas, along with resection of all of the lymph nodes along the left gastric artery, the splenic artery, and the celiac trunk, is removed and the reconstruction is made by an end-to-side hepaticojejunostomy combined with a gastroenterostomy. The first total pancreatectomy was performed by Ross in 1954 and reported in the same year by Porter.[80]

In 1960, Howard reported a perioperative mortality rate of 37% for total pancreatectomy and this led most surgeons to conclude that the procedure was not appropriate for patients with pancreatic cancer. On the other hand, because a similar high mortality was associated with the classical Whipple operation at that time, some surgeons actually came to the opposite conclusion – i.e., that total pancreatectomy might be an appropriate operation for PCa because it is at least as safe as the classical resection and, on theoretical grounds, it might increase the cure rate for PCa. They believed that it might prove to be a safer operation because it avoids the need for a pancreatic anastomosis with its attendant high leak and fistula rate and they reasoned that total pancreatectomy might improve cure rates for pancreatic cancer because it would allow for resection of multicentric pancreatic tumors. Subsequent studies, however, have shown that cure rates following total pancreatectomy are no better than those following the classical Whipple procedure and that the perioperative morbidity/mortality rates for the two procedures are comparable. Total pancreatectomy has many disadvantages when compared to a more limited resection and perhaps the greatest of those disadvantages is the metabolic deterioration which follows. It results in an insulin-dependent diabetes mellitus which is difficult to manage. Furthermore, in the long term, it is associated with an increased incidence of liver diseases and osteopenia.

In an overall sense, therefore, total pancreatectomy results in substantial long-term mortality and morbidity due to uncontrollable diabetes and other metabolic changes without an associated improvement in long-term cure of PCa. Furthermore, improvements in surgical technique have substantially reduced the risk of pancreatic fistula and its associated morbidity following the Whipple procedure. Taken together, therefore, these considerations have led to the abandonment of total pancreatectomy as standard treatment for PCa and, at present, it is performed only when the tumor is expanding over the entire pancreas, when several separate tumors are present, or when a pancreatic anastomosis is not technically feasible.

Adjuvant therapy in resected pancreatic cancer

The value of adjuvant treatment following resection of PCa has been examined in randomized, controlled clinical trials conducted by the Gastrointestinal Tumor Study Group (GITSG) and the European Organization for Research and Treatment of Cancer, Gastrointestinal Tract Cancer Cooperative Group (EORTC). The results of those trials were contradictory. The GITSG trial showed a benefit to adjuvant postoperative radiochemotherapy whereas

Table 29.3 Neoadjuvant therapy for pancreatic adenocarcinoma (selection on recently published studies)

Author	Year	Pts (n)	Therapy	Pretreatment assessment of resectability	Resection rate (%)	Median survival (months) All	Resected
Rich et al.[90]	1985	51	EBRT + 5-FU(± IORT)	Both	30 (59)	NS	19
Jeekel et al.[91]	1991	20	EBRT + 5-FU	Unresectable	2 (10)	10	NS
Evans et al.[92]	1992	28	EBRT + 5-FU (± IORT)	Both	17 (61)	NS	NS
Jessup et al.[93]	1993	16	EBRT + 5-FU	Unresectable	2 (13)	8	NS
Ishikawa et al.[94]	1994	23	EBRT	Both	17 (74)	15	
Coia et al.[95]	1994	27	EBRT + 5-FU/Mit	Both	13 (48)	16	16
Hoffman et al.[96]	1995	34	EBRT + 5-FU +Mit	Resectable	11 (32)		45
Staley et al.[97]	1996	39	EBRT + IORT + 5-FU	Resectable	39 (100)		19
Spitz et al.[98]	1997	91	EBRT + 5-FU (± IORT)	Resectable	41 (45)	19	19.2
Todd et al.[99]	1998	52	5-FU + LV + Mit + DPD	Unresectable	10 (19)	17	24
Hoffman et al.[100]	1998	53	EBRT + 5-FU/Mit	Resectable	24 (45)	9,7	15.7
White et al.[87]	1999	25	EBRT + 5-FU/Mit/Cis	Unresectable	5 (20)	NS	NS
Wanebo et al.[101]	2000	14	EBRT + 5-FU/Cis	Unresectable	9 (64)	9	19
Kastl et al.[86]	2000	27	EBRT + 5-FU + Mit	Unresectable	10 (37)	11	
Snady et al.[102]	2000	68	EBRT + 5-FU/Cis/Strep	Unresectable	20 (29)		32
		(91)*	(± adjuvant chemotherapy ± EBRT)	Resectable	48 Not resected (63 with adjuvant treatment) (28 no adjuvant treatment)		21 16 11
Crane et al.[103]	2001	51	EBRT + Gem	Unresectable	6 (12)	11	17
Mehta et al.[104]	2001	15	EBRT + 5-FU	Unresectable	9 (60)		30
Breslin et al.[105]	2001	(132)	EBRT + 5-FU/Pac/Gem	Resectable	132 (not applicable)		21
Rau et al.[85]	2002	26	EBRT + Gem + 5-FU/Cis	Both	11 (42)	9,8	
Arnoletti et al.[106]	2002	26	EBRT + 5-FU ± Mit/Gem	Both	14 (54)	8	34
Pisters et al.[107]	2002	35	EBRT + Pac (± IORT)	Resectable	20 (57)	12	19
Kim et al.[108]	2002	87	5FU + Gem	Unresectable	3 (3,4)	11	18
Magnin et al.[84]	2003	32	EBRT + 5-FU + Cis	Both	19 (59)	16	30
Al-Sukun et al.[109]	2003	20	PACE (Cis, Cyt, Caf, 5-FU) + EBRT + 5-FU	Unresectable	3 (15)	13,4	18,1

* All patients with resection with no neoadjuvant treatment , but some had adjuvant treatment; EBRT, external beam radiotherapy; IORT, intra-operative radiotherapy; 5-FU, 5-fluorouracil; LV, leucovorin; Mit, mitomycin C; Cis, cisplatin; Strep, streptozocin; Pac, paclitaxel; Gem, gemcitabine; DPD, dipyridamol; Cyt, cytarabine, Caf, caffeine; NI, no information.

the EORTC trial suggested that radiochemotherapy does not prolong survival.[81-83] The largest randomized controlled study, however, was recently reported by the European Study Group for Pancreatic Cancer (ESPAC). That study compared postoperative radiochemotherapy, chemotherapy (5-FU + leucovorin) and a combination of postoperative radiochemotherapy followed by chemotherapy with no adjuvant treatment (observation arm) in patients with R0 or R1 resected PCa.[10] At a median follow-up of 47 months, the overall results of the study showed no benefit for chemoradiation (median survival 15.9 months in 145 patients with chemoradiation versus 17.9 months in 144 patients without, $p=0.05$). There was, however strong evidence of a survival benefit for chemotherapy alone (median survival 20.1 months in 147 patients with chemotherapy versus 15.5 months in 142 patients without, $p=0.009$). The effect was reduced when taking into account whether patients also received chemoradiotherapy ($p=0.01$), indicating that chemoradiotherapy may reduce the overall survival benefit of chemotherapy.

PERSPECTIVES

Neoadjuvant treatment

Since 85–95% of patients with curative resection of PCa develop tumor recurrences and do not survive 5 years postoperatively, it is clear that PCa is usually not a disease that can be cured solely by surgical intervention. Therefore, some clinicians have advocated adding neoadjuvant treatment to the management of patients with PCa. The aim of neoadjuvant treatment in PCa is twofold: first, to down-stage patients who present with unresectable disease and second, to improve the surgical outcome, in regard to tumor control, in patients with resectable tumors. The first report of neoadjuvant radiochemotherapy for PCa appeared in 1986. It involved a group of PCa patients receiving neoadjuvant radiation therapy combined with 5-FU. Since then, a number of other studies, involving the use of drugs either alone or in combination with radiotherapy in the neoadjuvant setting, have been reported (Table 29.3). However, at present, no standard protocol has been defined for neoadjuvant treatment of PCa. Most protocols consist of a fractionated radiation of about 45–54 Gy applied over 5–8 weeks with 1.8 Gy per fraction or 30 Gy at 3.0 Gy per fraction with concomitant infusion chemotherapy of a single drug (5-FU, paclitaxel, gemcitabine, cisplatin, and mitomycin C) or a combination of those drugs. A number of studies conducted in patients with primarily resectable PCa have shown promising results (i.e., a 2-year survival rate of 59.3% and a median survival of 21 months).[84] Other studies have focused on down-staging of patients with primarily nonresectable PCa. These studies have suggested that resectability rates can be increased, but true pathological down-staging appears to be a rare event and no, or only a marginal, improvement in the survival rate occurs.[85-87]

Table 29.3 summarizes the results of recently published neoadjuvant studies in PCa.

New treatment for pancreatic cancer

Treatment of nonresectable and metastatic PCa remains a challenge. Our growing understanding of the molecular background of PCa has led to the exploration of new therapeutic options and several novel strategies are under active investigation. These include attempts to modulate growth factor activity, the use of immunotherapy, and the administration of antiangiogenic factors, vascular inhibitors, and antistromal factors. Together with new chemotherapeutics, these new approaches may improve the prognosis of PCa in the future.

Table 29.4 gives an overview of new agents and approaches being developed and tested in clinical trials. However, at present none of these new drugs has proven to improve the outcome of patients with PCas.

ACKNOWLEDGMENT

We would like to thank Dr. Pascal Berberat, Dr. Peter Büchler, Dr. Lars Fischer, Dr. Rene Hennig, Dr. Jörg Kleeff, Dr. Knut Ketterer, Dr. Beat Künzli, Dr. Marc Martignoni, and Dr. Michael Müller for their contribution in writing this book chapter.

Table 29.4 Novel agents for the treatment of pancreatic adenocarcinoma

Molecular target	Theoretical approach	Trial type	Author	Year
K-RAS	K-RAS Antisense-Oligonucleotide	Phase I	Cunningham et al.[110]	2001
	Farnesyltransferase-Inhibitor (FTI): Tipifarnib (R115777)	Phase II	Cohen et al.[111,112]	2002/2003
		Phase II	Macdonald et al.[113]	2002
		Phase III	Van Cutsem et al.[114]	2002
p53	Adenovirus (Onyx-015) with lytical cycle in p53-deficient cells	Phase I	Mulvihill et al.[115]	2001
EGF-receptor family	Trastuzumab (Herceptin) + Gem	Phase II	Safran et al.[116]	2002
	Cetuximab (IMC-C225 (Erbitux)) + Gem	Phase II	Abbruzzese et al.[117]	2001
VEGF-receptor	Anti-VEGF2-receptor antibody (DC101)	preclinical	Bruns et al.[118]	2002
	Receptortyrosinkinase-inhibitor (PTK787)	preclinical	Solorzano et al.[119]	2001
Metalloproteinase inhibitors (MMPIs)	BAY12-9566	Phase III	Moore et al.[120]	2000
	Marimastat	Phase III	Bramhall et al.[121,122]	2001/2002
Gastrin	Induction of antigastrin-17-antibody	Phase II	Brett et al.[123]	2002

Gem, gemcitabine.

REFERENCES

1. Greenlee RT, Hill-Harmon MB, Murray T, et al. Cancer statistics 2001. CA Cancer J Clin 2001; 51:15.

2. Stat bite. Pancreatic cancer incidence in U.S. blacks and whites, 1973–1999. J Natl Cancer Inst 2002; 94:1742.

3. Datenbank. (2002) World Wide Cancer Statistics der WHO.

4. Lowenfels AB, Maisonneuve P. Epidemiologic and etiologic factors of pancreatic cancer. Hematol Oncol Clin North Am 2002; 16:1.

   Review article on risk factors for pancreatic cancer. Presents the current knowledge on epidemiologic and etiologic factors of pancreatic cancer.

5. Rulyak SJ, Lowenfels AB, Maisonneuve P, et al. Risk factors for the development of pancreatic cancer in familial pancreatic cancer kindreds. Gastroenterology 2003; 124:1292.

6. Mulder I, Hoogenveen RT, van Genugten ML, et al. Smoking cessation would substantially reduce the future incidence of pancreatic cancer in the European Union. Eur J Gastroenterol Hepatol 2002; 14:1343.

7. Hennig R, Ding XZ, Adrian TE, et al. On the role of the islets of Langerhans in pancreatic cancer. Histol Histopathol 2004; 19:999.

8. Schernhammer ES, Kang JH, Chan AT, et al. A prospective study of aspirin use and the risk of pancreatic cancer in women. J Natl Cancer Inst 2004; 96:22.

9. Wagner M, Redaelli C, Lietz M, et al. Curative resection is the single most important factor determining outcome in patients with pancreatic adenocarcinoma. Br J Surg 2004; 91:586.

   Analysis of factors which influence the long-term outcome of patients following resection for pancreatic cancer. Study shows that in a univariate analysis several factors can be identified which influence the long-term prognosis. However, a multivariate analysis shows that an R0 resection is the single most important parameter.

10. Neoptolemos JP, Stocken DD, Friess H, et al. A randomized trial of chemoradiotherapy and chemotherapy after resection of pancreatic cancer. N Engl J Med 2004; 350:1200.

    Largest controlled, randomized trial on adjuvant treatment of pancreatic cancer. Patients were randomized in chemoradiotherapy alone (20 Gy over a two-week period plus fluorouracil), chemotherapy alone (fluorouracil), both chemoradiotherapy and chemotherapy, and to observation. Adjuvant chemotherapy has a significant survival benefit whereas adjuvant chemoradiotherapy has a deleterious effect on survival.

11. Kloppel G. Tumors of the endocrine pancreas. Pathologe 2003; 24:265.

12. Kloppel G, Luttges J. WHO-classification 2000: exocrine pancreatic tumors. Verh Dtsch Ges Pathol 2001; 85:219.

13. Bockman DE, Guo J, Buchler P, et al. Origin and development of the precursor lesions in experimental pancreatic cancer in rats. Lab Invest 2003; 83:853.

14. Hruban RH, Takaori K, Klimstra DS, et al. An illustrated consensus on the classification of pancreatic intraepithelial neoplasia and intraductal papillary mucinous neoplasms. Am J Surg Pathol 2004; 28(8):977.

    Classification for intraductal pancreatic lesions, based on an international consensus. Explains our present understanding of how intraductal pancreatic precursor lesions might progress into pancreatic cancer.

15. Wilentz RE, Iacobuzio-Donahue CA, Argani P, et al. Loss of expression of Dpc4 in pancreatic intraepithelial neoplasia: evidence that DPC4 inactivation occurs late in neoplastic progression. Cancer Res 2000; 60:2002.

16. Gorunova L, Hoglund M, Andren-Sandberg A, et al. Cytogenetic analysis of pancreatic carcinomas: intratumor heterogeneity and nonrandom pattern of chromosome aberrations. Genes Chromosomes Cancer 1998; 23:81.

17. Scarpa A, Capelli P, Villaneuva A, et al. Pancreatic cancer in Europe: Ki-ras gene mutation pattern shows geographical differences. Int J Cancer 1994; 57:167.

18. Lemoine NR, Jain S, Hughes CM, et al. Ki-ras oncogene activation in preinvasive pancreatic cancer. Gastroenterology 1992; 102:230.

19. Gerdes B, Ramaswamy A, Ziegler A, et al. p16INK4a is a prognostic marker in resected ductal pancreatic cancer: an analysis of p16INK4a, p53, MDM2, an Rb. Ann Surg 2002; 235:51.

20. Hahn SA, Schutte M, Hoque AT, et al. DPC4, a candidate tumor suppressor gene at human chromosome 18q21.1. Science 1996; 271:350.

21. Simon B, Bartsch D, Barth P, et al. Frequent abnormalities of the putative tumor suppressor gene FHIT at 3p14.2 in pancreatic carcinoma cell lines. Cancer Res 1998; 58:1583.

22. Su GH, Bansal R, Murphy KM, et al. ACVR1B (ALK4, activin receptor type 1B) gene mutations in pancreatic carcinoma. Proc Natl Acad Sci USA 2001; 98:3254.

23. Friess H, Ding J, Kleeff J, et al. Microarray-based identification of differentially expressed growth- and metastasis-associated genes in pancreatic cancer. Cell Mol Life Sci 2003; 60:1180.

    Example for high throughput gene analysis in pancreatic cancer. Identification of up-regulated and down-regulated genes in pancreatic cancer in comparison to chronic pancreatitis and normal controls.

24. Korc M, Chandrasekar B, Yamanaka Y, et al. Overexpression of the epidermal growth factor receptor in human pancreatic cancer is associated with concomitant increases in the levels of epidermal growth factor and transforming growth factor alpha. J Clin Invest 1992; 90:1352.

25. Friess H, Yamanaka Y, Kobrin MS, et al. Enhanced erbB-3 expression in human pancreatic cancer correlates with tumor progression. Clin Cancer Res 1995; 1:1413.

26. Yamanaka Y, Friess H, Kobrin MS, et al. Overexpression of HER2/neu oncogene in human pancreatic carcinoma. Hum Pathol 1993; 24:1127.

27. Bergmann U, Funatomi H, Yokoyama M, et al. Insulin-like growth factor I overexpression in human pancreatic cancer: evidence for autocrine and paracrine roles. Cancer Res 1995; 55:2007.

28. Yamanaka Y, Friess H, Büchler M, et al. Overexpression of acidic and basic fibroblast growth factors in human pancreatic cancer correlates with advanced tumor stage. Cancer Res 1993; 53:5289.

29. Kleeff J, Ishiwata T, Kumbasar A, et al. The cell-surface heparan sulfate proteoglycan glypican-1 regulates growth factor action in pancreatic carcinoma cells and is overexpressed in human pancreatic cancer. J Clin Invest 1998; 102:1662.

30. Kleeff J, Wildi S, Kumbasar A, et al. Stable transfection of a glypican-1 antisense construct decreases tumorigenicity in PANC-1 pancreatic carcinoma cells. Pancreas 1999; 19:281.

31. Friess H, Yamanaka Y, Büchler M, et al. Enhanced expression of transforming growth factor beta isoforms in pancreatic cancer correlates with decreased survival. Gastroenterology 1993; 105:1846.

32. Friess H, Yamanaka Y, Büchler M, et al. Enhanced expression of the type II transforming growth factor beta receptor in human pancreatic cancer cells without alteration of type III receptor expression. Cancer Res 1993; 53:2704.

33. Kleeff J, Ishiwata T, Maruyama H, et al. The TGF-beta signaling inhibitor Smad7 enhances tumorigenicity in pancreatic cancer. Oncogene 1999; 18:5363.

34. Kleeff J, Maruyama H, Friess H, et al. Smad6 suppresses TGF-beta-induced growth inhibition in COLO-357 pancreatic cancer cells and is overexpressed in pancreatic cancer. Biochem Biophys Res Commun 1999; 255:268.

35. Graber HU, Friess H, Zimmermann A, et al. Bak expression and cell death occur in peritumorous tissue but not in pancreatic cancer cells. J Gastrointest Surg 1999; 3:74.

36. Friess H, Lu Z, Andren-Sandberg A, et al. Moderate activation of the apoptosis inhibitor bcl-xL worsens the prognosis in pancreatic cancer. Ann Surg 1998; 228:780.

37. Ozawa F, Friess H, Kleeff J, et al. Effects and expression of TRAIL and its apoptosis-promoting receptors in human pancreatic cancer. Cancer Lett 2001; 163:71.

38. Koliopanos A, Friess H, Kleeff J, et al. Heparanase expression in primary and metastatic pancreatic cancer. Cancer Res 2001; 61:4655.

39. Ellenrieder V, Adler G, Gress TM. Invasion and metastasis in pancreatic cancer. Ann Oncol 1999; 10(Suppl 4):46.

40. Balaz P, Friess H, Kondo Y, et al. Human macrophage metalloelastase worsens the prognosis of pancreatic cancer. Ann Surg 2002; 235:519.

41. Zhu Z, Friess H, diMola FF, et al. Nerve growth factor expression correlates with perineural invasion and pain in human pancreatic cancer. J Clin Oncol 1999; 17:2419.

42. Berberat PO, Friess H, Wang L, et al. Comparative analysis of galectins in primary tumors and tumor metastasis in human pancreatic cancer. J Histochem Cytochem 2001; 49:539.

43. Guo X, Friess H, Graber HU, et al. KAI1 expression is up-regulated in early pancreatic cancer and decreased in the presence of metastases. Cancer Res 1996; 56:4876.

44. Hansel DE, Kern SE, Hruban RH. Molecular pathogenesis of pancreatic cancer. Ann Rev Genomics Hum Genet 2003; 4:237.

45. Li D, Xie K, Wolff R, et al. Pancreatic cancer. Lancet 2004; 363:1049.

46. Palesty JA, Dudrick SJ. What we have learned about cachexia in gastrointestinal cancer. Dig Dis Sci 2003; 21:198.

47. Permert J, Larsson J, Westermark GT, et al. Islet amyloid polypeptide in patients with pancreatic cancer and diabetes. N Engl J Med 1994; 330:313.

48. European Group on Tumour Markers. Tumour markers in gastrointestinal cancers – EGTM recommendations. Anticancer Res 1999; 19:2811.

49. Duffy MJ. CA 19-9 as a marker for gastrointestinal cancers: a review. Ann Clin Biochem 1998; 35(Pt 3):364.

50. Clarke DL, Thomson SR, Madiba TE, et al. Preoperative imaging of pancreatic cancer: a management-oriented approach. J Am Coll Surg 2003; 196:119.

51. Smith SL, Rajan PS. Imaging of pancreatic adenocarcinoma with emphasis on multidetector CT. Clin Radiol 2004; 59:26.

52. Trede M, Rumstadt B, Wendl K, et al. Ultrafast magnetic resonance imaging improves the staging of pancreatic tumors. Ann Surg 1997; 226:393; discussion 405.

53. Erickson RA. ERCP and pancreatic cancer. Ann Surg Oncol 2004; 11:555.

54. Higashi T, Saga T, Nakamoto Y, et al. Diagnosis of pancreatic cancer using fluorine-18 fluorodeoxyglucose positron emission tomography (FDG PET) – usefulness and limitations in 'clinical reality.' Ann Nucl Med 2003; 17:261.

55. Warshaw AL, Fernandez-del Castillo C. Pancreatic carcinoma. N Engl J Med 1992; 326:455.

56. Hennig R, Tempia-Caliera AA, Hartel M, et al. Staging laparoscopy and its indications in pancreatic cancer patients. Dig Surg 2002; 19:484.

57. Büchler MW, Wagner M, Schmied BM, et al. Changes in morbidity after pancreatic resection: toward the end of completion pancreatectomy. Arch Surg 2003; 138:1310.

58. Povoski SP, Karpeh MS Jr, Conlon KC, et al. Association of preoperative biliary drainage with postoperative outcome following pancreaticoduodenectomy. Ann Surg 1999; 230:131.

59. Soetikno RM, Lichtenstein DR, Vandervoort J, et al. Palliation of malignant gastric outlet obstruction using an endoscopically placed Wallstent. Gastrointest Endosc 1998; 47:267.

60. Molinari M, Helton WS, Espat NJ. Palliative strategies for locally advanced unresectable and metastatic pancreatic cancer. Surg Clin North Am 2001; 81:651.

61. Ihse I, Zoucas E, Gyllstedt E, et al. Bilateral thoracoscopic splanchnicectomy: effects on pancreatic pain and function. Ann Surg 1999; 230:785.

62. Burris HA III, Moore MJ, Andersen J, et al. Improvements in survival and clinical benefit with gemcitabine as first-line therapy for patients with advanced pancreas cancer: a randomized trial. J Clin Oncol 1997; 15:2403.

63. Heinemann V. Gemcitabine in the treatment of advanced pancreatic cancer: a comparative analysis of randomized trials. Semin Oncol 2002; 29:9.

Review on chemotherapy in advanced pancreatic cancer. The paper summarizes current treatment options and underlines that presently gemcitabine is the most effective drug, although also its effects are limited.

64. Ducreux M, Boige V, Malka D. Emerging drugs in pancreatic cancer. Expert Opin Emerg Drugs 2004; 9:73.

65. Shore S, Raraty MG, Ghaneh P, et al. Review article: chemotherapy for pancreatic cancer. Aliment Pharmacol Ther 2003; 18:1049.

66. Ma HB, Di ZL, Wang XJ, et al. Effect of intraoperative radiotherapy combined with external beam radiotherapy following internal drainage for advanced pancreatic carcinoma. World J Gastroenterol 2004; 10:1669.

67. Kausch W. Radical resection of carcinoma of duodenal papilla. Beitr Z Clin Chir 1912; 78:439.

68. Whipple AO, Parsons SB, Mullins CR. Treatment of carcinoma of the ampulla of Vater. Ann Surg 1935; 102:763.

69. Peters JH, Carey LC. Historical review of pancreaticoduodenectomy. Am J Surg 1991; 161:219.

70. Watson K. Carcinoma of the ampulla of Vater. Successful radical resection. Br J Surg 1944; 31:368.

71. Traverso LW, Longmire WP. Preservation of the pylorus in pancreatico-duodenectomy. Surg Gynecol Obstet 1978; 146:959.

72. Yeo CJ, Cameron JL, Lillemoe KD, et al. Pancreaticoduodenectomy with or without distal gastrectomy and extended retroperitoneal lymphadenectomy for periampullary adenocarcinoma, part 2: randomized controlled trial evaluating survival, morbidity, and mortality. Ann Surg 2002; 236:355.

Largest controlled, randomized trial on the benefit of extended lymphadenectomy in pancreatic cancer patients undergoing resection. The study demonstrates that extended lymphadenectomy can be done safely without increased morbidity and mortality. However, there is no survival benefit in the extended lymphadenectomy group.

73. Pedrazzoli S, Beger HG, Obertop H, et al. A surgical and pathological-based classification of resective treatment of pancreatic cancer. Summary of an international workshop on surgical procedures in pancreatic cancer. Dig Surg 1999; 16:337.

74. Seiler CA, Wagner M, Bachmann T, et al. Randomized clinical trial of pylorus-preserving duodenopancreatectomy versus classical Whipple resection-long term results. Br J Surg. 2005; 92:547–56.

   Controlled randomized trial on advantages and disadvantages of classical Whipple versus pylorus-preserving Whipple resection in periampullary cancer. This trial shows, as do similar smaller studies, that the pylorus-preserving Whipple operation is oncological as effective as the classical Whipple operation. Pylorus-preserving Whipple resection offers some minor advantages in the early postoperative period, but not in long-term results.

75. Takada T. Surgery for carcinoma of the pancreas in Japan. Past, present, and future aspects. Digestion 1999; 60(Suppl 1):114.

76. Pedrazzoli S, DiCarlo V, Dionigi R, et al. Standard versus extended lymphadenectomy associated with pancreatoduodenectomy in the surgical treatment of adenocarcinoma of the head of the pancreas: a multicenter, prospective, randomized study. Lymphadenectomy Study Group. Ann Surg 1998; 228:508.

77. Shoup M, Conlon KC, Klimstra D, et al. Is extended resection for adenocarcinoma of the body or tail of the pancreas justified? J Gastrointest Surg 2003; 7:946.

78. Lillemoe KD, Kaushal S, Cameron JL, et al: Distal pancreatectomy: indications and outcomes in 235 patients. Ann Surg 1999; 229:693.

79. Shoup M, Conlon KC, Klimstra D, et al. Is extended resection for adenocarcinoma of the body or tail of the pancreas justified? J Gastrointest Surg 2003; 7:946.

80. Ross DE. Cancer of the pancreas; a plea for total pancreatectomy. Am J Surg 1954; 87:20.

81. Kalser MH, Ellenberg SS. Pancreatic cancer. Adjuvant combined radiation and chemotherapy following curative resection. Arch Surg 1985; 120:899.

82. Lee YT, Tatter D. Carcinoma of the pancreas and periampullary structures. Pattern of metastasis at autopsy. Arch Pathol Lab Med 1984; 108:584.

83. Gastrointestinal Tumor Study Group. Further evidence of effective adjuvant combined radiation and chemotherapy following curative resection of pancreatic cancer. Gastrointestinal Tumor Study Group. Cancer 1987; 59:2006.

84. Magnin V, Moutardier V, Giovannini M-H, et al. Neoadjuvant preoperative chemoradiation in patients with pancreatic cancer. Int J Radiation Oncology Biol Phys 2003; 55:1300.

85. Rau HG, Wichmann MW, Wilkowski R, et al. Surgical therapy of locally advanced and primary inoperable pancreatic carcinoma after neoadjuvant preoperative radiochemotherapy. Chirurg 2002; 73:132.

86. Kastl S, Brunner T, Herrmann O, et al. Neoadjuvant radio-chemotherapy in advanced primarily non-resectable carcinomas of the pancreas. Eur J Surg Oncol 2000; 26:578.

87. White R, Lee C, Anscher M, et al. Preoperative chemoradiation for patients with locally advanced adenocarcinoma of the pancreas. Ann Surg Oncol 1999; 6:38.

88. Lin PW, Lin YJ. Prospective randomized comparison between pylorus-preserving and standard pancreaticoduodenectomy. Br J Surg 1999; 86:603.

89. Wenger FA, Jacobi CA, Haubold K, et al. Gastrointestinal quality of life after duodenopancreatectomy in pancreatic carcinoma. Preliminary results of a prospective randomized study: pancreatoduodenectomy or pylorus-preserving pancreatoduodenectomy. Chirurg 1999; 70:1454.

90. Jeekel J, Treurniet-Donker AD. Treatment perspectives in locally advanced unresectable pancreatic cancer. Br J Surg 1991; 78:1332.

91. Evans DB, Rich TA, Byrd DR, et al. Preoperative chemoradiation and pancreatico-duodenectomy for adenocarcinoma of the pancreas. Arch Surg 1992; 127:1335.

92. Jessup JM, Steele C, Mayer RJ, et al. Neoadjuvant therapy for unresectable pancreatic adenocarcinoma. Arch Surg 1993; 128:559.

93. Rich TA, Lokisch JJ, Chaffey JT. A pilot study of protracted infusion of 5-fluorouracil and concomitant radiation therapy. J Clin Oncol 1985; 3:402.

94. Ishikawa O, Ohigashi H, Imaoka S, et al. Is the long-term survival rate improved by preoperative irradiation prior to Whipple's procedure for adenocarcinoma of the pancreatic head? Arch Surg 1994; 129:1075.

95. Coia L, Hoffman J, Scher R, et al. Preoperative chemoradiation for adenocarcinoma of the pancreas and duodenum. Int J Radiation Oncol Biol Phys 1994; 30:161.

96. Hoffman JP, Weese JL, Solin LJ, et al. A pilot study of preoperative chemo-radiation for patients with localized adenocarcinoma of the pancreas. Am J Surg 1995; 169:71.

97. Staley CA, Lee JE, Cleary KR, et al. Preoperative chemoradiation, pancreatico-duodenectomy, and intraoperative radiation therapy for adenocarcinoma of the pancreatic head. Am J Surg 1996; 171:118.

98. Spitz FR, Abbruzzese JL, Lee JE, et al. Preoperative and postoperative chemoradiation strategies in patients treated with pancreaticoduodenectomy for adenocarcinoma of the pancreas. J Clin Oncol 1997; 15: 28.

99. Todd K, Gloor B, Lane J, et al. Resection of locally advanced pancreatic cancer after downstaging with continuous-infusion 5-fluorouracil, mitomycin-C, leucovorin and dipyridamole. J Gastrointest Surg 1998; 2:159.

100. Hoffman JP, Lipsitz S, Pisansky T, et al. Phase II trial of preoperative radiation therapy and chemotherapy for patients with localized, resectable adenocarcinoma of the pancreas: an Eastern Cooperative Oncology Group Study. J Clin Oncol 1998; 16:317.

101. Wanebo HJ, Glicksman AS, Vezeridis MP, et al. Preoperative chemotherapy, radiotherapy, and surgical resection of locally advanced pancreatic cancer. Arch Surg 2000; 135: 81.

102. Snady H, Bruckner H, Cooperman A, et al. Survival advantages of combined chemoradiotherapy compared with resection as the initial treatment of patients with regional pancreatic carcinoma. Cancer 2000; 89:314.

   Evaluation of preoperative chemoradiotherapy and adjuvant chemotherapy with and without radiotherapy in patients with pancreatic cancer. This study shows significantly improved survival for patients with more advanced pancreatic cancer when initially treated with chemoradiotherapy compared to patients with earlier-stage tumors and immediate resection.

103. Crane CH, Janjan NA, Evans DB, et al. Toxicity and efficacy of concurrent gemcitabine and radiotherapy for locally advanced pancreatic cancer. Int J Pancreatol 2001; 29:2.

104. Mehta VK, Fisher G, Ford JA, et al. Preoperative chemoradiation for marginally resectable adenocarcinoma of the pancreas. J Gastrointest Surg 2001; 5:27.

105. Breslin TM, Hess KR, Harbison DB, et al. Neoadjuvant chemoradiotherapy for adenocarcinoma of the pancreas: treatment variables and survival duration. Ann Surg Oncol 2001; 8:123.

106. Arnoletti JP, Hoffman JP, Ross EA, et al. Preoperative chemoradiation in the management of adenocarcinoma of the body of the pancreas. Am Surg 2002; 68:330.

107. Pisters PW, Wolff RA, Janjan NA, et al. Preoperative paclitaxel and concurrent rapid-fractionation radiation for resectable pancreatic adenocarcinoma: toxicities, histologic response rates, and event-free outcome. J Clin Oncol 2002; 20:2537.

108. Kim HJ, Czischke K, Murray BF, et al. Does neoadjuvant chemoradiation downstage locally advanced pancreatic cancer? J Gastrointest Surg 2002; 6:763.

109. Al-Sukhun S, Zalupski MM, Ben-Josef E, et al. Chemoradiotherapy in the treatment of regional pancreatic carcinoma: a phase II study. Am J Clin Oncol 2003; 26:543.

110. Cunningham CC, Holmlund JT, Geary RS, et al. A phase I trial of H-ras antisense oligonucleotide ISIS 2503 administered as a continuous intravenous infusion in patients with advanced carcinoma. Cancer 2001; 92:1265.

111. Cohen S, Ho L, Ranganathan S, et al. Phase II and pharmacodynamic trial of the farnesyltransferase inhibitor R115777 as initial therapy in patients with metastatic pancreatic adenocarcinoma. Proc Am Soc Clin Oncol 2002; 21:545.

112. Cohen S, Ho L, Ranganathan S, et al: Phase II and pharmacodynamic study of the farnesyltransferase inhibitor R115777 as initial therapy in patients with metastatic pancreatic adenocarcinoma. J Clin Oncol 2003; 21:1301.

113. Macdonald J, Chansky K, Whitehead R, et al. A phase II study of farnesyl transferase inhibitor R115777 in pancreatic cancer. A Southwest Oncology Group study. Proc Am Soc Clin Oncol 2002; 21:548.

114. Van Cutsem E, Karasek P, Oettle H, et al. Phase III trial comparing gemcitabine + R115777 (Zarnestra) versus gemcitabine + placebo in advanced pancreatic cancer. Proc Am Soc Oncol 2002; 21:517.

115. Mulvihill S, Warren R, Venook A, et al. Safety and feasibility of injection with an E1B-55 kDa gene-deleted, replication-selective adenovirus (ONYX-015) into primary carcinomas of the pancreas: a phase I trial. Gene Ther 2001; 8:308.

116. Safran H, Ramanathan R, Schwaltz J, et al. Herceptin and gemcitabine for metastatic pancreatic cancers that overexpress HER2/neu. Proc Am Clin Oncol 2002; 20:517.

117. Abbruzzese J, Rosenberg A, LoBuglio A, et al. Phase II study of anti-epidermal growth factor receptor antibody cetuximab (IMC-C225) in combination with gemcitabine in patients with advanced pancreatic cancer. Proc Am Clin Oncol 2001; 20:518.

118. Bruns CJ, Shrader M, Harbison MT, et al. Effect of the vascular endothelial growth factor receptor-2 antibody DC 101 plus gemcitabine on growth, metastasis and angiogenesis of human pancreatic cancer growing orthotopically in nude mice. Int J Cancer 2002; 102:101.

119. Solorzano CC, Baker CH, Bruns CJ, et al. Inhibition of growth and metastasis of human pancreatic cancer growing in nude mice by PTK 787/ZK222584, an inhibitor of the vascular endothelial growth factor receptor tyrosine kinases. Cancer Biother Radiopharm 2001; 16:359.

120. Moore M, Hamm J, Eisenberg P, et al. A comparison between gemcitabine and the matrix metalloproteinase inhibitor BAY12-9566 in patients with advanced pancreatic cancer. Proc Am Soc Clin Oncol 2000; 19:930.

121. Bramhall SR, Rosemurgy A, Brown PD, et al. Marimastat as first-line therapy for patients with unresectable pancreatic cancer: a randomized trial. J Clin Oncol 2001; 19:3447.

122. Bramhall SR, Schulz J, Nemunaitis J, et al. A double-blind placebo-controlled, randomised study comparing gemcitabine and placebo as first-line therapy in patients with advanced pancreatic cancer. Br J Cancer 2002; 87:161.

123. Brett BT, Smith SC, Bouvier CV, et al. Phase II study of anti-gastrin-17 antibodies, raised to G17DT, in advanced pancreatic cancer. J Clin Oncol 2002; 20:4225.

CHAPTER THIRTY

Cholangiocarcinoma and other biliary tumors

Annette Grambihler and Gregory J. Gores

CHOLANGIOCARCINOMA

Epidemiology and risk factors

Cholangiocarcinoma is the second most common primary liver cancer in the world. It usually occurs over the age of 50 to 60, and slightly more frequently in men than in women. In recent decades, the incidence and mortality of cholangiocarcinoma has risen; the annual incidence in the United States is about 7 per million.[1] Although a number of risk factors for the development of cholangiocarcinoma have been established (Table 30.1), many patients who are diagnosed with this disease have none of these factors in their history. In Western countries, primary sclerosing cholangitis is one of the most important risk factors, and about 10–20% of patients with primary sclerosing cholangitis eventually develop cholangiocarcinoma.[2,3] A second condition predisposing to the development of cholangiocarcinoma is congenital biliary cystic disease in the form of choledochal cysts or Caroli's disease: about 6–10% of patients with cystic abnormalities of the bile ducts will develop cholangiocarcinoma.[4-6] Other established risk factors for cholangiocarcinoma include liver flukes (infection with *Clonorchos sinensis* or *Opisthorchis viverrini*), and chronic hepatolithiasis.[7] In addition, chronic hepatitis C virus infection,[8] nitrosamines in food,[9] and environmental factors such as dioxin, asbestos, and polychlorinated biphenyls have been suggested as causative factors in the pathogenesis of cholangiocarcinoma,[10]

Table 30.1 Factors associated with the development of cholangiocarcinoma
Primary sclerosing cholangitis
Liver flukes
Caroli's disease
Congenital choledochal cysts
Chronic hepatolithiasis
Chronic hepatitis C virus infection?
Dietary habits (nitrosamines)?
Unknown environmental factors
Thorotrast deposition

and recently an association between biliary enteric drainage procedures and ductal cholangiocarcinoma has been postulated.[11]

Pathology

Cholangiocarcinomas are divided into intrahepatic and extrahepatic forms. Extrahepatic cholangiocarcinomas are further grouped into hilar or upper third, middle, and distal third tumors. Hilar adenocarcinomas or Klatskin tumors[12] develop in the main hepatic duct and/or the right or left hepatic duct and represent about 60% of all extrahepatic. Extrahepatic cholangiocarcinomas have also been subclassified based on their gross appearance as either papillary, nodular, or sclerosing.[13] The most common sclerosing tumors cause an annular thickening of the bile duct wall with longitudinal and radial tumor growth as well as infiltration and fibrosis of the periductal tissue. Nodular tumors are characterized by a firm nodule projecting into the bile duct lumen. Tumors featuring characteristics of both nodular and sclerosing forms are relatively frequent. The papillary variant only accounts for approximately 10% and is mostly seen in the distal bile duct.

Intrahepatic cholangiocarcinomas appear as a gray-white scirrhous mass, with an abundance of stroma and mucin secretion, but little vascularization. They may be solitary or multinodular and can be relatively well demarcated or infiltrating, growing along the intrahepatic bile ducts. The Liver Cancer Study Group of Japan has further classified intrahepatic cholangiocarcinoma into three principal types: a mass-forming type that is usually localized with a round shape and distinct borders, a periductal-infiltrating type with diffuse infiltration along the bile ducts, and an intraductal growth type showing intraductal growth.[14] Among these, the mass-forming type is the most frequent, and the intraductal growth type the rarest; overlap, especially between the mass-forming and the periductal-infiltrating type, is very common. This new classification appears to be useful, because the three forms have been shown to differ not only in gross appearance but also in their genetic alterations and prognosis.

Histology

Histologically, most cholangiocarcinomas are well to moderately differentiated tubular adenocarcinomas, with formation of glands and an abundance of dense desmoplastic stroma; calcification may be present. Mucus, but not bile secretion, is observed in the majority of tumors. The glandular lumens are lined by well-differentiated columnar or cuboidal cells with uniform nuclei and small nucleoli. In addition to the most common tubular form of cholangiocellular adenocarcinoma, other variants have been described, such as papillary adenocarcinoma,[15] signet-ring carcinoma,[16] squamous cell or mucoepidermoid carcinoma,[17,18] a spindle cell variant,[19] and a lymphoepithelioma-like form.[20]

Clinical presentation, diagnosis, and staging

Symptoms of intrahepatic cholangiocarcinoma are mostly unspecific symptoms of an intrahepatic mass. Patients may present with abdominal pain, an abdominal mass, anorexia, weight loss, night sweats, and malaise or even be asymptomatic. Because intrahepatic cholangiocarcinoma does not usually involve the large extrahepatic bile ducts, symptoms of cholestasis are rare. In contrast, symptoms of cholestasis such as jaundice, pruritus, pale stools, and dark urine are very important in pointing to the diagnosis of extrahepatic or hilar cholangiocarcinoma. Cholangitis with fever, chills, and abdominal pain is not common in the absence of biliary intervention.

The clinical symptoms of cholestasis in extrahepatic cholangiocarcinoma are associated with a cholestatic biochemical profile. However, even in the absence of clinical symptoms of cholestasis, the serum alkaline phosphatase is usually elevated in both extra- and intrahepatic cholangiocarcinoma. Serum tumor markers including CA19-9, carcinoembryonic antigen (CEA), and CA125 may be elevated. CA19-9 values greater than 100 U/L in the absence of bacterial cholangitis are highly suggestive of cholangiocarcinoma,[21,22] especially in combination with typical imaging studies such as biliary stenosis or a liver mass.

Ultrasound is often the first study performed in patients who present with cholestasis. Although it is not always possible to identify the tumor itself because hilar tumors obstructing bile flow can be quite small, ultrasound is an important tool in excluding other causes of cholestasis, and in localizing the level of obstruction, as usually dilatation of the biliary tree is found above the tumor. Unilobar bile duct obstruction is often associated with atrophy of the affected lobe and hypertrophy of the unaffected lobe, the so-called atrophy-hypertrophy complex;[23] the lobar atrophy can signify vascular encasement of the affected lobe in addition to bile duct obstruction. Further signs of vascular involvement may be found by Doppler ultrasound, with loss of flow in a hepatic artery or portal venous structure. Computed tomography (CT) may also show evidence of a liver mass, dilated intrahepatic bile ducts, atrophy of one liver lobe, or lymphadenopathy; however, lymphadenopathy may also be present in primary sclerosing cholangitis (PSC) and does not necessarily indicate malignancy. Magnetic resonance imaging (MRI) studies have the advantage of providing cross-sectional imaging of the liver and at the same time depicting magnetic resonance cholangiography (MRC) and vascular anatomy (magnetic resonance angiography), and therefore represent the current optimal non-invasive imaging technique for this disease (Fig. 30.1).

Other methods to depict the extra- and intrahepatic bile ducts are endoscopic retrograde cholangiopancreatography (ERCP) and percutaneous transhepatic cholangiography (PTC) (Fig. 30.2). As both are invasive techniques, they carry a risk of infection, bacterial cholangitis being a rather frequent complication especially after ERCP. However, they allow a very detailed examination of the bile duct system, especially if the two methods are combined; while ERCP may often only depict the distal part of a stenosing tumor, PTC can help determine the proximal extent. In contrast to MRC, these invasive techniques also provide the possibility of taking bile samples, brush cytology, or biopsies, and in addition biliary drainage can be achieved by implantation of stents if needed.

If no definite diagnosis can be reached with these techniques, positron emission tomography with [^{18}F]2-deoxy-D-glucose can be useful,[24,25] although false-positive scans have been reported, especially in acute cholangitis.[26] New techniques that so far remain experimental are endoscopic or percutaneous cholangioscopy and intraductal ultrasound as well as radiolabelled ligand imaging.

If possible, the diagnosis of cholangiocarcinoma should be confirmed by histologic or cytologic findings. While it is relatively easy to obtain tissue samples from intrahepatic mass-forming cholangiocarcinoma via ultrasound-guided fine needle aspiration biopsy, there is a risk in performing percutaneous biopsies in patients with potentially curable/resectable disease because of tumor seeding.[7] The pathologic diagnosis of intraductal or extrahepatic cholangiocarcinoma can be challenging because these tumors are often desmoplastic and extend and encircle the bile ducts in the submucosal space. Thus, endoscopic brushings and biopsies are only positive in 40–70% of patients, and negative cytology does not exclude malignancy.[7] New single-cell techniques demonstrating aneuploidy, such as digitized image analysis (DIA) and fluorescent

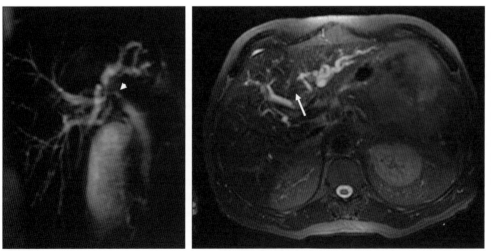

Fig. 30.1 ● MRI images of a cholangiocarcinoma. The panel on the left represents an MRI cholangiogram. The arrow points to a narrowing of the common hepatic duct with proximal bile duct dilitation. The panel on the right represents cross sectional imaging of the liver hilus. The arrow points to a liver mass obstructing the right and left hepatic ducts, although bile duct dilatation is more prominent on the left than the right.

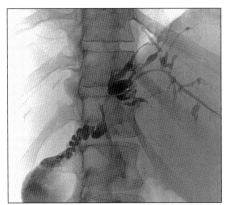

Fig. 30.2 • Percutaneous transhepatic cholangiogram of a cholangiocarcinoma complicating primary sclerosing cholangitis. Note the irregular and saccular dilatation of the obstructed bile ducts in the left lobe of the liver, and the high-grade stricture of the left hepatic duct.

in situ hybridization (FISH), are promising for the diagnosis of cholangiocarcinoma;[27] in one study they doubled the diagnostic yield obtained with routine brush cytology.[28] However, the absence of a tissue diagnosis is common and the diagnosis of cholangiocarcinoma is often based not on pathological criteria, but on a combination of clinical symptoms, laboratory findings and imaging studies, in particular the elevation of serum alkaline phosphatase, CA19-9 greater than 100 U/L, and a malignant-appearing stenosis on imaging studies. A diagnostic approach for evaluating indeterminate strictures is depicted in Figure 30.3.

Clinical staging

The pathologic TNM classifications of biliary cancers are of little value in clinically assessing the hilar and extrahepatic cholangiocarcinomas in particular. Because the prognosis of cholangiocarcinoma strongly depends on its operability, three aims must be achieved by clinical staging:

1. Delineate the proximal and distal extent of the disease. This is necessary to develop a surgical approach and is usually defined using the classification by Bismuth et al.[29] Direct endoscopic and percutaneous transhepatic cholangiography are still the gold standard to define extent of the malignant stricture. However, because the disease can spread submucosally without compromising the biliary lumen, this approach frequently understages the disease. Magnetic resonance studies, in particular with ferredex, permit the identification of submucosal lesions.[30] In patients with PSC, however, MRI studies are not sufficient for the diagnosis and staging of cholangiocarcinoma, and additional invasive endoscopic and percutaneous cholangiography are recommended.

2. Assess vascular involvement, and especially determine if there is vascular encasement involving the contralateral lobe. This is most critical in hilar cancers in which a partial hepatectomy is being considered. Patency of the portal vein and hepatic artery can usually be evaluated by Doppler ultrasound or specific vascular MRI or CT studies.

3. Determine if metastases are present. Cholangiocarcinoma commonly metastasizes to regional lymph nodes, the peritoneum, and the liver surface. It also spreads along the nerves and nerve sheaths, along the bile ducts, and invades adjacent vascular structures. All these metastases can be missed by conventional cross-sectional imaging. To assess regional lymph nodes, endoscopic ultrasound has proved very useful, with the additional benefit of being able to obtain fine needle aspiration biopsies; 15–20% of patients who have no lymphadenopathy on CT scans will have lymph node metastases identified by endoscopic ultrasound.[31] PSC patients often have benign lymphadenopathy and enlarged lymph nodes in this condition should not be automatically ascribed to malignancy without further investigation. To exclude peritoneal involvement and examine the liver surface, many surgeons perform laparoscopy prior to laparotomy.[32]

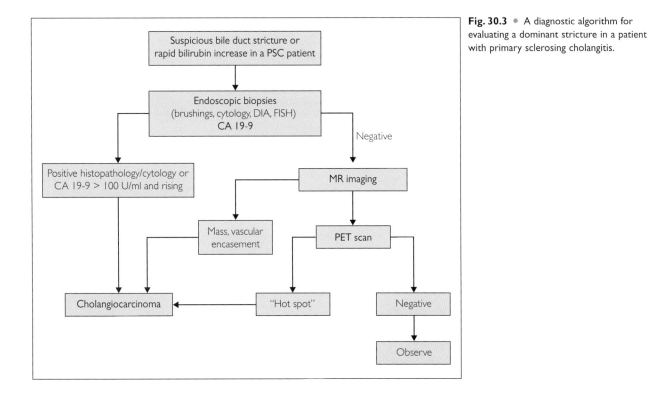

Fig. 30.3 • A diagnostic algorithm for evaluating a dominant stricture in a patient with primary sclerosing cholangitis.

Treatment

Treatment for cholangiocarcinoma is based primarily on extent of the disease and comorbid conditions. The two main aims of therapy are relief of cholestasis and treatment of the cancer. Both approaches are necessary to reduce suffering and extend life. An approach to treatment decisions is depicted in Figure 30.4.

For patients with intra- or extrahepatic cholangiocarcinoma, surgery is the only option by which long-time survival can be obtained.[7] After complete resection of cholangiocarcinoma, 5-year survival rates of 15–50% have been reported.[33] Resectability is determined by the patient's physical condition, comorbidities, and liver function (especially in the case of underlying liver disease such as PSC), as well as by tumor stage and anatomic location. While previously local tumor-related factors such as bilateral bile duct involvement or vascular encasement/occlusion were the most important criteria determining unresectability, with emerging surgical techniques continuously pushing back those frontiers, other patient-related factors and metastasis become more important staging criteria. For intrahepatic cholangiocarcinoma, surgical approaches are the same as for other mass lesions of the liver and will not be discussed in further detail. Three-year survival rates of 40–60% have been reported in patients resected for cure.[34]

Even relatively small cholangiocarcinomas can sometimes be unresectable if they are localized centrally or at the hilum, especially if the patient cannot tolerate an extended liver resection because of pre-existing cirrhosis. Since cholangiocarcinomas, like hepatocellular carcinomas, have little tendency to produce distant metastases early on, orthotopic liver transplantation (OLT) would appear a very attractive alternative for these patients. However, the results of several centers that have attempted OLT as treatment for unresectable cholangiocarcinoma were discouraging, with high recurrence rates and low long-time survival, ranging 13–22% after 5 years.[35] Intraoperative irradiation and adjuvant chemotherapy do not appear to improve survival.[36] Better results were achieved recently through preoperative radiochemotherapy in highly selected patients with early-stage hilar or extrahepatic cholangiocarcinoma;[37,38] with the Mayo Clinic treatment protocol, 5-year survival rates greater than 80% were observed.[38] These favorable results can in part be attributed to the effect of preoperative adjuvant chemotherapy delaying tumor growth and metastasis during the waiting period for transplantation. In addition, careful selection of patients with early-stage disease (TNM stage I or II) and preoperative exploratory laparotomy to examine regional lymph nodes and assess the distal extent of the tumor were probably also responsible for the low rate of tumor recurrence in this study. Thus, it appears that at least for some selected patients with extrahepatic tumors and with careful protocols, OLT might be a promising alternative. Intrahepatic cholangiocarcinoma, however, remains a contraindication for OLT.

Most published studies on systemic chemotherapy for cholangiocarcinoma used 5-fluorouracil (5-FU) with or without leukovorin

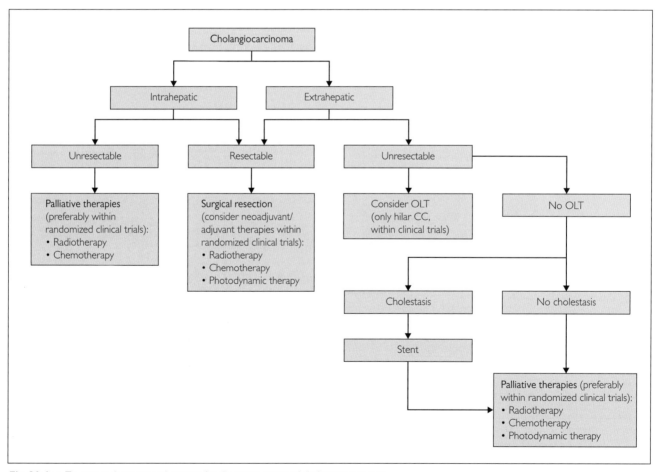

Fig. 30.4 • Treatment decisions and options for the management of cholangiocarcinoma.

as bolus or continuous infusion; with this monotherapy, partial response rates of 10–30% were achieved, and median survival times of up to 9.5 months.[39–41] Similar results were observed using 5-FU in combination with interferon-alpha2b[42] or mitomycin c.[43,44] In one study, the combination of 5-FU with cisplatin achieved partial responses in 34%.[45] Treatment protocols with 5-FU/doxorubicin/mitomycin c or 5-FU/epirubicin/cisplatin showed partial response rates in up to 40%.[46,47] For monotherapy with gemcitabine, partial response rates of up to 36% and median survival times of 11.5 months have been described.[48–50] Gemcitabine in combination with cisplatin achieved 30–50% partial response rates in phase II studies.[50] Overall, the quality of life appears to be improved with systemic chemotherapy, particularly in responders,[51] but there is no proven survival advantage even in responders. Further evaluation of chemotherapeutic treatment in large randomized trials is urgently needed.

Radiotherapeutic approaches to treat unresectable cholangiocarcinoma consist of external beam irradiation and brachytherapy.[52] Significant palliation and occasional long-term survival can be obtained with external beam irradiation (EBRT).[53] However, high doses of EBRT may result in biliary tract injury further confounding the problems associated with bile duct obstruction, and cause unacceptable morbidity because of the presence of dose-limiting organs (liver, stomach, duodenum, kidney). Although advances in imaging techniques now permit the delivery of high-dose EBRT with the aid of three-dimensional treatment planning (conformal irradiation),[54] permanent local control remains uncommon.

Locally administered radiation therapy with ^{192}Ir has been used in an attempt to improve stent patency. Such brachytherapy also allows for combined local and external beam irradiation with doses greater than 50 Gy. Often, 5-FU is given concomitantly for tumor radiosensitization.[55] Following this radiotherapy, plastic or metal stents are placed at the site of biliary stricturing. On the basis of the few studies available, brachytherapy offers a modest survival advantage compared to stents alone.[56]

Biliary drainage

In patients with unresectable cholangiocarcinoma, endoscopic biliary stenting provides fast and effective relief from symptoms of biliary obstruction; a corresponding reduction of cholestasis also improves survival, although survival for more than two years is unusual. Biliary decompression by insertion of plastic or metal stents is successful in up to 97% of patients with cholangiocarcinoma.[57] Stents ideally should not be inserted if curative resection is considered, because this may increase the risk of infection, a major postoperative complication.[58] However, if a hepatic resection is planned and the future remnant lobe is obstructed, biliary drainage is advisable prior to surgery to facilitate recovery and regeneration of the remaining liver.

In patients with complex hilar lesions a study comparing unilateral with bilateral stent placement showed no significant difference between the two approaches.[59] Indeed, the complication rate including cholangitis was higher in patients undergoing stenting of both lobes. Thus, many endoscopists now use preprocedure magnetic resonance cholangiography to make the decision as to which lobe should be stented.

Another issue is whether to use plastic or metal stents. Metal stents remain patent approximately twice as long as plastic stents, and patients with metal stents had 28% fewer cholangiograms.[60] Therefore, metal stents are cost-effective and recommended for patients anticipated to survive less than 6 months. Plastic (polyethylene) stents have median occlusion rates of 4 months, requiring stent replacement; therefore, and also to avoid other complications such as stent dislocation or cholangitis, many endoscopists recommend exchanging plastic stents every 3 months.[7] Antibiotics given before the procedure help minimize the risk of cholangitis, but some patients require long-term antibiotic therapy. The availability of coated stents impregnated with chemotherapeutic agents is eagerly awaited.[61] If endoscopic stenting is not feasible, percutaneous stents are quite successful in obtaining biliary decompression; the frequency of stent occlusion can be minimized by flushing the stent with saline twice daily.

Another endoscopic palliative approach is photodynamic therapy. Photodynamic therapy is accomplished by the systemic administration of a photosensitizer such as a hematoporphyrin derivative that preferentially accumulates in malignant cells. Photoactivation with a red laser light at the time of endoscopic retrograde cholangiography is used to destroy the malignant cells. Although few randomized control trials comparing photodynamic therapy with standard biliary stenting have been reported, pilot studies suggest a survival benefit from this approach in addition to its facilitating biliary decompression.[62] The only randomized trial to date even demonstrated an up to 5 times longer survival with photodynamic therapy plus stenting as compared to stenting alone (493 days versus 98 days).[63]

GALLBLADDER ADENOMAS AND CARCINOMA

Gallbladder adenomas

Adenoma of the gallbladder is relatively frequent. It is found in 3–6% of patients after cholecystectomy. As it is a predisposing factor for the development of gallbladder carcinoma, an adenoma–carcinoma sequence is thought to exist.[64] The prevalence of gallbladder carcinoma increases with polyp size, and polyps of more than 10 mm are more likely to harbor carcinoma than smaller ones, especially if gallstones are present.[65] In patients with primary sclerosing cholangitis and gallbladder polyps, gallbladder carcinoma is present even more frequently, in 40–60% of cases.[66] Indeed, any significant polyp in the presence of underlying primary sclerosing cholangitis is worrisome for the development of cholangiocarcinoma, and serious consideration should be given to performing a cholecystectomy. This recommendation may be tempered if advanced liver disease is present (Childs-Turcotte-Pugh stage B or C). In such patients, the polyp may need to be followed over time to ascertain if growth is occurring – in the absence of growth, observation with frequent imaging studies is reasonable management. If growth is observed, an open cholecystectomy by an experienced hepatobiliary surgeon needs to be considered. In the absence of PSC, polypoid lesions are often detected by ultrasonography, but differentiation of benign from malignant polypoid gallbladder lesions is often difficult. Doppler ultrasonography can be used to help assess indeterminate lesions. If color flow Doppler demonstrates arterialization of the lesion, neoplastic transformation is likely and cholecystectomy is indicated. Endoscopic ultrasound and CT can also be helpful in determining the size and depth of invasion, but a gallbladder polyp greater than 10 mm should be an indication for cholecystectomy; small lesions can be followed by serial imaging studies.

Gallbladder carcinoma

In Western countries, adenocarcinomas of the gallbladder are the sixth most common digestive system malignancies. Autopsy studies revealed a prevalence of gallbladder carcinoma of 0.5–2%.[67] Like cholangiocarcinoma, gallbladder carcinoma is diagnosed most frequently in older adults over the age of 60. It is about three times more common in women than in men, and more common in African and Native Americans than in whites. There are also very important regional differences in the incidence of gallbladder carcinoma: its incidence is especially high in Chile, Poland, Japan, and Israel.[68] Conditions that cause chronic inflammation and/or mechanical irritation can be causative factors in the development of gallbladder carcinoma. The most important risk factor is the presence of gallstones. Indeed, gallstones are found in 74–92% of patients with gallbladder carcinoma.[69–71] The 'porcelain gallbladder,' a calcification of the gallbladder wall that results from chronic cholecystitis, has also been linked to a high risk of gallbladder carcinoma and up to 22% of patients with this condition are diagnosed with gallbladder carcinoma.[72,73] Both cholecystolithiasis and chronic cholecystitis are more common in women than in men, accounting for the higher frequency of gallbladder carcinomas. Finally, gallbladder adenomas have been identified as a risk factor for the development of gallbladder carcinoma, possibly by an adenoma–carcinoma sequence similar to that of colonic polyps.[64]

Microscopically, almost all gallbladder carcinomas are papillary or tubular adenocarcinomas with columnar or cuboidal cells. They have an abundance of stroma, and mucin production and signet-ring cells are also observed frequently. Around 10% of gallbladder cancers are not adenocarcinomas; adenosquamous carcinomas, anaplastic carcinomas, carcinoid tumors, and rhabdomyosarcomas have been described.[69,74]

Gallbladder carcinoma spreads by infiltration of the gallbladder wall and adjacent structures, and by vascular, lymphatic, and perineural invasion. At the time of diagnosis, most patients already have advanced locoregional disease. Direct infiltration of the liver is found in up to 80%, involvement of the biliary tract in 57%, of duodenum, stomach, or transverse colon in 40%, of the pancreas in 23%; encasement of the hepatic artery is found in 15% of cases.[67,75,76] Regional lymph node metastases in the cystic, choledochal, or pancreaticoduodenal lymph nodes are present in 42–70% of patients. Distant metastases are found in the liver in 66%, in the lung in 24%, and in the bone in 12%.[75]

Patients most often present with unspecific symptoms. Right upper quadrant abdominal pain or tenderness are the most frequent complaints. These symptoms are present in up to 97% of patients and they are often attributed to cholecystolithiasis or cholecystitis. Other symptoms include nausea, vomiting, and anorexia in 40–64% of patients; jaundice is seen in around 45%, and significant weight loss in 37–77%.[77]

Even if jaundice is not clinically evident in many patients, 70% present with elevated bilirubin and alkaline phosphatase levels. Liver enzymes such as AST and ALT may be elevated and indicative of advanced hepatic invasion and metastases. The tumor markers CEA and/or CA19-9 are elevated in up to 80% of patients, and high levels usually suggest an advanced tumor stage.[77]

The first imaging study performed is usually ultrasonography; up to 75% of gallbladder carcinomas can be correctly diagnosed by this method.[78] High-resolution ultrasound may detect even early-stage gallbladder carcinoma presenting as a polypoid tumor protruding into the lumen or a focal thickening of the gallbladder wall.[79] In more advanced stages, ultrasonography can demonstrate hepatic invasion and metastases, extra- and intrahepatic bile duct obstruction, and lymphadenopathy at the liver hilus. However, peritoneal dissemination and para-aortic lymphadenopathy cannot be diagnosed accurately. Computed tomography is another effective method for detecting gallbladder carcinoma. CT characteristics of gallbladder carcinoma include diffuse or local gallbladder wall thickness of greater than 0.5 mm, gallbladder wall contrast enhancement, an intraluminal mass, direct invasion of the liver and other gastrointestinal organs, regional lymphadenopathy, concomitant cholelithiasis, and liver metastases. CT will also demonstrate calcification of the gallbladder wall.[80–82] However, the differentiation of gallbladder carcinoma from benign polypoid lesions such as gallbladder adenoma can still be difficult, and because the risk of malignant transformation of adenomas increases with their size, all gallbladder polyps of more than 10 mm should be treated by cholecystectomy.

Surgical resection is the only treatment of gallbladder carcinoma by which long-term survival can be achieved. However, the majority of patients with gallbladder carcinoma have extensive locoregional disease at the time of diagnosis. Thus, curative resection is possible in only 10–30% of cases. The decision about the surgical approach to the treatment of gallbladder carcinoma is dependent in the TNM stage.

Early-stage gallbladder carcinomas are detected in about 1–2% after cholecystectomy performed for presumed benign disease such as cholecystolithiasis or cholecystitis. As laparoscopic cholecystectomy is now performed very frequently, this has raised questions about the risk of tumor dissemination by this method. Thus, if there is any suspicion of cancer before or during laparoscopic surgery, open cholecystectomy should be performed instead. After laparoscopic cholecystectomy, if histologic examination reveals cancer, re-operation is recommended by most authors. If the tumor stage is T1b or higher, if the resection margin is not tumor free, or if there is involvement of the cystic duct, extended cholecystectomy and lymph node dissection should be performed as described below, along with excision or irradiation of the port site.[77,83]

Simple cholecystectomy is sufficient for most patients with tumors confined to the mucosa (T1aN0M0); the 5-year survival rate is 57–100%.[84,85] However, if lymph node dissection is performed, lymph node metastasis is identified in some of these patients. Therefore, some authors suggest extended cholecystectomy with resection of the gallbladder fossa and lymph node dissection. This operation brings about a high mortality and postoperative morbidity, while only around 5% of patients have a survival benefit.[77] Thus, extended cholecystectomy is not recommended for patients with T1aN0M0 tumors by most authors. In contrast, T1b lesions, although classified as AJCC stage I, may indeed benefit from extended cholecystectomy because of the higher incidence of lymphadenopathy compared to T1a lesions.

Lymph node metastasis was identified in 15.6% of patients with T1b gallbladder carcinomas, 56% with T2, and 74% with T3 tumors.[86] Because T3 and T4 tumors often involve the extrahepatic bile ducts, en bloc resection of the hepatic and common bile duct with Roux-en-Y hepaticojejunostomy is recommended along with extended cholecystectomy for these patients as well as for all accidentally diagnosed tumors invading the bile duct.

Sometimes right hepatic lobectomy is necessary due to the tendency of gallbladder carcinoma to grow along the right hepatic bile duct.

Gallbladder carcinoma can only be cured by surgical resection. However, disease recurrence is common, and thus adjuvant and neoadjuvant approaches as well as oncologic treatments for unresectable tumors have been tried. The prognosis of gallbladder carcinoma depends on its resectability as well as the tumor stage. Only complete surgical resection can allow long-term survival for gallbladder carcinoma patients. The 5-year survival rates for patients with T1aN0M0 tumors undergoing simple cholecystectomy range from 57% to 100%.[84,85] For stage II and stage III disease, results are much poorer, and after extended cholecystectomy 5-year survival rates of 7.5–71% have been reported.[77,87] The effect of adjuvant and neoadjuvant treatment approaches is still unknown.

OTHER BILIARY TUMORS

Benign biliary tumors are not very common and account for less than 3% of all neoplasms arising from biliary epithelia.[88] A variety of different benign biliary tumors have been described, including the Von Meyenburg complex or microhamartoma, adenoma, cystadenoma of mucinous or serous type, papilloma and papillomatosis, and granular cell tumors. Benign bile duct tumors are usually incidental findings; they rarely cause symptoms. On imaging studies, benign bile duct tumors may appear as little filling defects, but cannot be easily removed with a balloon or basket catheter during ERCP.[89] The main significance of most of these tumors resides in their possible confusion with carcinomas; cystadenomas and biliary papillomatosis, however, have a tendency to become malignant themselves.

Von Meyenburg complex (microhamartoma)

The von Meyenburg complex is a hamartomatous malformation that is part of the spectrum of fibropolycystic diseases. It is a relatively frequent incidental finding in autopsy studies,[90,91] but causes no symptoms or complications. There is no sex and age predilection. Often, multiple small lesions can be found throughout the liver, and in this case the patient may be considered to have a mild form of adult polycystic liver disease.[88]

Cystadenoma

Cystadenomas most frequently occur in middle-aged women. They can be large and patients may present with symptoms of an abdominal mass or jaundice due to bile duct obstruction. The mucinous type is much more common than the serous type, and it has been suggested that cystadenocarcinomas may arise from mucinous cystadenoma. Therefore, a complete surgical resection is recommended.[92]

Papilloma and papillomatosis

Biliary papilloma and papillomatosis are very rare, but important among the benign biliary tumors as they are considered premalignant conditions.[93] They are seen in older, mostly male patients, and may be symptomatic with recurrent cholangitis, obstructive jaundice, hemobilia, or choledocholithiasis. Complete surgical resection should be performed in suitable patients to avoid those complications and malignant transformation.

Granular cell tumor

Granular cell tumors are benign lesions that most commonly arise in the skin, subcutaneous tissue, tongue, and oral cavity. Granular cell tumors of the biliary tract are rare, and mostly occur in young African-American women.[94] They may appear as hilar strictures mimicking cholangiocarcinoma or PSC, but can be cured by resection.[95]

REFERENCES

1. Patel T. Increasing incidence and mortality of primary intrahepatic cholangiocarcinoma in the United States. Hepatology 2001; 33(6):1353–1357.

2. Bergquist A, Glaumann H, Persson B, et al. Risk factors and clinical presentation of hepatobiliary carcinoma in patients with primary sclerosing cholangitis: a case-control study. Hepatology 1998; 27(2):311–316.

3. Bergquist A, Broome U. Hepatobiliary and extra-hepatic malignancies in primary sclerosing cholangitis. Best Pract Res Clin Gastroenterol 2001;1 5(4):643–656.

4. Lipsett PA, Pitt HA, Colombani PM, et al. Choledochal cyst disease. A changing pattern of presentation. Ann Surg 1994; 220(5): 644–652.

5. Summerfield JA, Nagafuchi Y, Sherlock S, et al. Hepatobiliary fibropolycystic diseases. A clinical and histological review of 51 patients. J Hepatol 1986; 2(2):141–156.

6. Chapman RW. Risk factors for biliary tract carcinogenesis. Ann Oncol 1999; 10(Suppl 4):308–311.

7. Khan SA, Davidson BR, Goldin R, et al. Guidelines for the diagnosis and treatment of cholangiocarcinoma: consensus document. Gut 2002; 51(Suppl 6):VI1–VI9.

8. Kobayashi M, Ikeda K, Saitoh S, et al. Incidence of primary cholangiocellular carcinoma of the liver in Japanese patients with hepatitis C virus-related cirrhosis. Cancer 2000; 88(11):2471–2477.

9. Herrold KM. Histogenesis of malignant liver tumors induced by dimethylnitrosamine. An experimental study in Syrian hamsters. J Natl Cancer Inst 1967; 39(6):1099–1111.

10. Pitt HA, Dooley WC, Yeo CJ, et al. Malignancies of the biliary tree. Curr Probl Surg 1995; 32(1):1–90.

11. Bettschart V, Clayton RA, Parks RW, et al. Cholangiocarcinoma arising after biliary-enteric drainage procedures for benign disease. Gut 2002; 51(1):128–129.

12. Klatskin G. Adenocarcinoma of the hepatic duct at its bifurcation within the porta hepatis. An unusual tumor with distinctive clinical and pathological features. Am J Med 1965; 38:241–256.

13. Weinbren K, Mutum SS. Pathological aspects of cholangiocarcinoma. J Pathol 1983; 139(2):217–238.

14. Liver Cancer Study Group of Japan. Classification of primary liver cancer. 1st English edn. Tokyo: Kanehara-Shuppan; 1997.

15. Nakanuma Y, Sasaki M, Ishikawa A, et al. Biliary papillary neoplasm of the liver. Histol Histopathol 2002; 17(3):851–861.

16. Terada T, Kida T, Nakanuma Y, et al. Intrahepatic cholangiocarcinomas associated with nonbiliary cirrhosis. A clinicopathologic study. J Clin Gastroenterol 1994; 18(4):335–342.

17. Pianzola LE, Drut R. Mucoepidermoid carcinoma of the liver. Am J Clin Pathol 1971; 56(6):758–761.

18. Tomioka T, Tsunoda T, Harada N, et al. Adenosquamous carcinoma of the liver. Am J Gastroenterol 1987; 82(11):1203–1206.

19. Nakajima T, Tajima Y, Sugano I, et al. Intrahepatic cholangiocarcinoma with sarcomatous change. Clinicopathologic and immunohistochemical evaluation of seven cases. Cancer 1993; 72(6):1872–1877.

20. Chen TC, Ng KF, Kuo T. Intrahepatic cholangiocarcinoma with lymphoepithelioma-like component. Mod Pathol 2001; 14(5):527–532.

21. Patel AH, Harnois DM, Klee GG, et al. The utility of CA 19-9 in the diagnoses of cholangiocarcinoma in patients without primary sclerosing cholangitis. Am J Gastroenterol 2000; 95(1):204–207.

22. Nichols JC, Gores GJ, LaRusso NF, et al. Diagnostic role of serum CA 19-9 for cholangiocarcinoma in patients with primary sclerosing cholangitis. Mayo Clin Proc 1993; 68(9):874–879.

Describes the utility of serum CA19-9 determinations for the diagnosis of cholangiocarcinoma unassociated with primary sclerosing cholangitis.

23. Hadjis NS, Adam A, Gibson R, et al. Nonoperative approach to hilar cancer determined by the atrophy-hypertrophy complex. Am J Surg 1989; 157(4):395–399.

24. Kluge R, Schmidt F, Caca K, et al. Positron emission tomography with [(18)F]fluoro-2-deoxy-D-glucose for diagnosis and staging of bile duct cancer. Hepatology 2001; 33(5):1029–1035.

Although the numbers are limited, this paper describes the utility of PET scanning in the diagnosis of cholangiocarcinoma and its limitations in staging this cancer.

25. Keiding S, Hansen SB, Rasmussen HH, et al. Detection of cholangiocarcinoma in primary sclerosing cholangitis by positron emission tomography. Hepatology 1998; 28(3):700–706.

26. Fritscher-Ravens A, Bohuslavizki KH, Broering DC, et al. FDG PET in the diagnosis of hilar cholangiocarcinoma. Nucl Med Commun 2001; 22(12):1277–1285.

27. Gores GJ. Early detection and treatment of cholangiocarcinoma. Liver Transpl 2000; 6(6Suppl 2):S30–S34.

28. Rumalla A, Baron TH, Leontovich O, et al. Improved diagnostic yield of endoscopic biliary brush cytology by digital image analysis. Mayo Clin Proc 2001; 76(1):29–33.

29. Bismuth H, Castaing D, Traynor O. Resection or palliation: priority of surgery in the treatment of hilar cancer. World J Surg 1988; 12(1):39–47.

30. Braga HJ, Imam K, Bluemke DA. MR imaging of intrahepatic cholangiocarcinoma: use of ferumoxides for lesion localization and extension. AJR Am J Roentgenol 2001; 177(1):111–114.

31. Fritscher-Ravens A, Broering DC, Sriram PV, et al. EUS-guided fine-needle aspiration cytodiagnosis of hilar cholangiocarcinoma: a case series. Gastrointest Endosc 2000; 52(4):534–540.

32. Weber SM, DeMatteo RP, Fong Y, et al. Staging laparoscopy in patients with extrahepatic biliary carcinoma. Analysis of 100 patients. Ann Surg 2002; 235(3):392–399.

33. Jarnagin WR. Cholangiocarcinoma of the extrahepatic bile ducts. Semin Surg Oncol 2000; 19(2):156–176.

34. Jarnagin WR, Fong Y, DeMatteo RP, et al. Staging, resectability, and outcome in 225 patients with hilar cholangiocarcinoma. Ann Surg 2001; 234(4):507–517; discussion 517–519.

Well-written paper defining surgical outcomes in a large series of patients with cholangiocarcinoma.

35. Pichlmayr R, Weimann A, Ringe B. Indications for liver transplantation in hepatobiliary malignancy. Hepatology 1994; 20(1 Pt 2):33S–40S.

36. Goldstein RM, Stone M, Tillery GW, et al. Is liver transplantation indicated for cholangiocarcinoma? Am J Surg 1993; 166(6): 768–771; discussion 771–772.

37. Sudan D, DeRoover A, Chinnakotla S, et al. Radiochemotherapy and transplantation allow long-term survival for nonresectable hilar cholangiocarcinoma. Am J Transplant 2002; 2(8):774–779.

38. De Vreede I, Steers JL, Burch PA, et al. Prolonged disease-free survival after orthotopic liver transplantation plus adjuvant chemoirradiation for cholangiocarcinoma. Liver Transpl 2000; 6(3):309–316.

First paper describing successful outcome of liver transplantation for highly selected patients treated in a protocolized manner.

39. Falkson G, MacIntyre JM, Moertel CG. Eastern Cooperative Oncology Group experience with chemotherapy for inoperable gallbladder and bile duct cancer. Cancer 1984; 54(6):965–969.

40. Chen JS, Jan YY, Lin YC, et al. Weekly 24 h infusion of high-dose 5-fluorouracil and leucovorin in patients with biliary tract carcinomas. Anticancer Drugs 1998; 9(5):393–397.

41. Gerhardt T, Mey U, Sauerbruch T, et al. [Palliative therapy of inoperable cholangiocarcinoma]. Dtsch Med Wochenschr 2002; 127(36):1835–1839.

42. Patt YZ, Jones DV Jr, Hoque A, et al. Phase II trial of intravenous fluorouracil and subcutaneous interferon alfa-2b for biliary tract cancer. J Clin Oncol 1996; 14(8):2311–2315.

43. Raderer M, Hejna MH, Valencak JB, et al. Two consecutive phase II studies of 5-fluorouracil/leucovorin/mitomycin C and of gemcitabine in patients with advanced biliary cancer. Oncology 1999; 56(3):177–180.

44. Chen JS, Lin YC, Jan YY, et al. Mitomycin C with weekly 24-h infusion of high-dose 5-fluorouracil and leucovorin in patients with biliary tract and periampullar carcinomas. Anticancer Drugs 2001; 12(4):339–343.

45. Taieb J, Mitry E, Boige V, et al. Optimization of 5-fluorouracil (5-FU)/cisplatin combination chemotherapy with a new schedule of leucovorin, 5-FU and cisplatin (LV5FU2-P regimen) in patients with biliary tract carcinoma. Ann Oncol 2002; 13(8):1192–1196.

46. Harvey JH, Smith FP, Schein PS. 5-Fluorouracil, mitomycin, and doxorubicin (FAM) in carcinoma of the biliary tract. J Clin Oncol 1984; 2(11):1245–1248.

47. Ellis PA, Norman A, Hill A, et al. Epirubicin, cisplatin and infusional 5-fluorouracil (5-FU) (ECF) in hepatobiliary tumours. Eur J Cancer 1995; 31A(10):1594–1598.

48. Kubicka S, Rudolph KL, Tietze MK, et al. Phase II study of systemic gemcitabine chemotherapy for advanced unresectable hepatobiliary carcinomas. Hepatogastroenterology 2001; 48(39):783–789.

49. Penz M, Kornek GV, Raderer M, et al. Phase II trial of two-weekly gemcitabine in patients with advanced biliary tract cancer. Ann Oncol 2001; 12(2):183–186.

50. Scheithauer W. Review of gemcitabine in biliary tract carcinoma. Semin Oncol 2002; 29(6Suppl 20):40–45.

51. Hejna M, Pruckmayer M, Raderer M. The role of chemotherapy and radiation in the management of biliary cancer: a review of the literature. Eur J Cancer 1998; 34(7):977–986.

52. Todoroki T. Radiotherapy as a component of multidisciplinary treatment of bile duct cancer: a surgeon's perspective. J Hepatobiliary Pancreat Surg 2001; 8(2):130–136.

53. Shinchi H, Takao S, Nishida H, et al. Length and quality of survival following external beam radiotherapy combined with expandable metallic stent for unresectable hilar cholangiocarcinoma. J Surg Oncol 2000; 75(2):89–94.

54. Gunderson LL, Haddock MG, Foo ML, et al. Conformal irradiation for hepatobiliary malignancies. Ann Oncol 1999; 10(Suppl 4):221–225.

55. Foo ML, Gunderson LL, Bender CE, et al. External radiation therapy and transcatheter iridium in the treatment of extrahepatic bile duct carcinoma. Int J Radiat Oncol Biol Phys 1997; 39(4):929–935.

56. Eschelman DJ, Shapiro MJ, Bonn J, et al. Malignant biliary duct obstruction: long-term experience with Gianturco stents and combined-modality radiation therapy. Radiology 1996; 200(3):717–724.

57. Banerjee B, Teplick SK. Nonsurgical management of primary cholangiocarcinoma. Retrospective analysis of 40 cases. Dig Dis Sci 1995; 40(3):701–705.

58. Gores GJ. Cholangiocarcinoma: current concepts and insights. Hepatology 2003; 37(5):961–969.

Concise review on the etiopathogenesis, molecular biology, clinical, and therapeutic aspects of cholangiocarcinoma.

59. De Palma GD, Galloro G, Siciliano S, et al. Unilateral versus bilateral endoscopic hepatic duct drainage in patients with malignant hilar biliary obstruction: results of a prospective, randomized, and controlled study. Gastrointest Endosc 2001; 53(6):547–553.

Demonstrates that unilateral stenting is as efficacious as bilateral staging and fraught with fewer complications.

60. Davids PH, Groen AK, Rauws EA, et al. Randomised trial of self-expanding metal stents versus polyethylene stents for distal malignant biliary obstruction. Lancet 1992; 340(8834–8835):1488–1492.

61. Baron TH. Chemotherapy impregnated plastic biliary endoprostheses: one small step for man(agement) of cholangiocarcinoma. Hepatology 2000; 32(5):1170–1171.

62. Berr F, Wiedmann M, Tannapfel A, et al. Photodynamic therapy for advanced bile duct cancer: evidence for improved palliation and extended survival. Hepatology 2000; 31(2):291–298.

63. Ortner ME, Caca K, Berr F, et al. Successful photodynamic therapy for nonresectable cholangiocarcinoma: a randomized prospective study. Gastroenterology 2003; 125(5):1355–1363.

Randomized, controlled trial demonstrating a survival benefit for patients with unresectable cholangiocarcinoma receiving photodynamic therapy.

64. Aldridge MC, Bismuth H. Gallbladder cancer: the polyp-cancer sequence. Br J Surg 1990; 77(4):363–364.

65. Kozuka S, Tsubone N, Yasui A, et al. Relation of adenoma to carcinoma in the gallbladder. Cancer 1982; 50(10):2226–2234.

66. Buckles DC, Lindor KD, Larusso NF, et al. In primary sclerosing cholangitis, gallbladder polyps are frequently malignant. Am J Gastroenterol 2002; 97(5):1138–1142.

A unique paper emphasizing that gall bladder polyps in primary sclerosing cholangitis are frequently malignant.

67. Piehler JM, Crichlow RW. Primary carcinoma of the gallbladder. Surg Gynecol Obstet 1978; 147(6):929–942.

68. Lazcano-Ponce EC, Miquel JF, Munoz N, et al. Epidemiology and molecular pathology of gallbladder cancer. CA Cancer J Clin 2001; 51(6):349–364.

69. Nagorney DM, McPherson GA. Carcinoma of the gallbladder and extrahepatic bile ducts. Semin Oncol 1988; 15(2):106–115.

70. Khan ZR, Neugut AI, Ahsan H, et al. Risk factors for biliary tract cancers. Am J Gastroenterol 1999; 94(1):149–152.

71. Chow WH, Johansen C, Gridley G, et al. Gallstones, cholecystectomy and risk of cancers of the liver, biliary tract and pancreas. Br J Cancer 1999; 79(3–4):640–644.

72. Polk HC Jr. Carcinoma and the calcified gall bladder. Gastroenterology 1966; 50(4):582–585.

73. Berk RN, Armbuster TG, Saltzstein SL. Carcinoma in the porcelain gallbladder. Radiology 1973; 106(1):29–31.

74. Sumiyoshi K, Nagai E, Chijiiwa K, et al. Pathology of carcinoma of the gallbladder. World J Surg 1991; 15(3):315–321.

75. Fahim RB, McDonald JR, Richards JC, et al. Carcinoma of the gallbladder: a study of its modes of spread. Ann Surg 1962; 156:114–124.

76. Ohtsuka M, Miyazaki M, Itoh H, et al. Routes of hepatic metastasis of gallbladder carcinoma. Am J Clin Pathol 1998; 109(1):62–68.

77. Curley SA. Gallbladder and bile duct cancer. In: eds. Holland-Frei Cancer medicine. 6th edn. Hamilto, Ont.: BC Decker: 2003.

78. Soiva M, Aro K, Pamilo M, et al. Ultrasonography in carcinoma of the gallbladder. Acta Radiol 1987; 28(6):711–714.

79. Koga A, Yamauchi S, Izumi Y, et al. Ultrasonographic detection of early and curable carcinoma of the gallbladder. Br J Surg 1985; 72(9):728–730.

80. Thorsen MK, Quiroz F, Lawson TL, et al. Primary biliary carcinoma: CT evaluation. Radiology 1984; 152(2):479–783.

81. Wilbur AC, Sagireddy PB, Aizenstein RI. Carcinoma of the gallbladder: color Doppler ultrasound and CT findings. Abdom Imaging 1997; 22(2):187–189.

82. Furukawa H, Kosuge T, Shimada K, et al. Small polypoid lesions of the gallbladder: differential diagnosis and surgical indications by helical computed tomography. Arch Surg 1998; 133(7):735–739.

83. Orth K, Beger HG. Gallbladder carcinoma and surgical treatment. Langenbecks Arch Surg 2000; 385(8):501–508.

84. Shirai Y, Yoshida K, Tsukada K, et al. Inapparent carcinoma of the gallbladder. An appraisal of a radical second operation after simple cholecystectomy. Ann Surg 1992; 215(4):326–331.

85. Shimada H, Endo I, Togo S, et al. The role of lymph node dissection in the treatment of gallbladder carcinoma. Cancer 1997; 79(5): 892–899.

86. Ogura Y, Mizumoto R, Isaji S, et al. Radical operations for carcinoma of the gallbladder: present status in Japan. World J Surg 1991; 15(3):337–343.

87. Ouchi K, Owada Y, Matsuno S, et al. Prognostic factors in the surgical treatment of gallbladder carcinoma. Surgery 1987; 101(6):731–737.

88. Colombari R, Tsui WM. Biliary tumors of the liver. Semin Liver Dis 1995; 15(4):402–413.

89. Baillie J. Tumors of the gallbladder and bile ducts. J Clin Gastroenterol 1999; 29(1):14–21.

90. Chung EB. Multiple bile-duct hamartomas. Cancer 1970; 26(2): 287–296.

91. Thommesen N. Biliary hamartomas (von Meyenburg complexes) in liver needle biopsies. Acta Pathol Microbiol Scand [A] 1978; 86(2):93–99.

92. Devaney K, Goodman ZD, Ishak KG. Hepatobiliary cystadenoma and cystadenocarcinoma. A light microscopic and immunohistochemical study of 70 patients. Am J Surg Pathol 1994; 18(11):1078–1091.

93. Neumann RD, LiVolsi VA, Rosenthal NS, et al. Adenocarcinoma in biliary papillomatosis. Gastroenterology 1976; 70(5 Pt.1): 779–782.

94. Butler JD Jr, Brown KM. Granular cell tumor of the extrahepatic biliary tract. Am Surg 1998; 64(11):1033–1036.

95. te Boekhorst DS, Gerhards MF, van Gulik TM, et al. Granular cell tumor at the hepatic duct confluence mimicking Klatskin tumor. A report of two cases and a review of the literature. Dig Surg 2000; 17(3):299–303.

CHAPTER THIRTY-ONE

31

Zollinger-Ellison syndrome and other neuroendocrine tumors

John Del Valle

INTRODUCTION

Endocrine tumors of the pancreas are rare neoplasms characterized by cells that synthesize and autonomously secrete a large array of biologically active peptides. The actions of these peptides on a distinct target often lead to a constellation of signs and symptoms that can vary from frank neuroglycopenia associated with insulinomas to the indolent signs (rash, diarrhea) of a glucagon-producing tumor. More recently, it has become evident that these tumors can be silent from the hormonal standpoint and instead be manifested as a pancreatic mass. The last several decades have witnessed steady growth in the understanding and diagnosis of these rare neoplasms. Advances have led to the development of novel therapeutic modalities aimed at ameliorating the signs and symptoms of these unusual tumors. Despite these inroads, surgical resection provides the only opportunity for cure. The primary focus of this chapter will be to review the therapeutic modalities available for the control of signs, symptoms, and growth of these rare tumors. In an effort to place treatment in perspective, a brief overview of the clinical aspects of several endocrine neoplasms including insulinoma, Zollinger-Ellison syndrome or *gastrinoma*, VIPoma (Verner-Morrison syndrome), glucagonoma, somatostatinoma, GRFoma, and nonfunctioning tumors will be presented.

CLINICAL FEATURES

Definition and epidemiology

Pancreatic endocrine tumor was first described in 1927 by Wilder and colleagues in a patient with severe hypoglycemia resulting from metastatic islet cell carcinoma.[1] Subsequently, many clinical syndromes resulting from hypersecretion of one or more peptides by neoplastic lesions of the pancreas have been discovered (Table 31.1). More recently, it has become apparent that these neoplasms may be silent from the hormonal standpoint but present instead with signs and symptoms of a pancreatic mass.

The reported frequency of symptomatic endocrine tumors is less than 1 per 100 000 population,[2] with insulinomas and gastrinomas being the most common neoplasms detected. Of interest, despite this very low incidence of symptomatic tumors, prevalence of endocrine tumors in unselected autopsy cases approximate 0.5–1.5% of cases.[3] More recent studies demonstrate that 20–30% of all pancreatic endocrine neoplasms are asymptomatic.[4] The high incidence of neoplasms that remain undetected or are asymptomatic may be due to low hormone secretion rates, presence of inactive precursors, or the release of peptides with subtle biological effects.[4]

Table 31.1 Functioning neuroendocrine tumors of the pancreas

Tumor	Clinical manifestations	Location (%)	Malignancy rate (%)
Insulinoma	Hypoglycemia	Pancreas	5–10
Gastrinoma	Peptic diathesis, diarrhea	Pancreas (66) Duodenum (30) Other	>60
VIPoma	Secretory diarrhea, hypokalemia, alkalosis	Pancreas (90) Other (10)	>60
Glucagonoma	Necrolytic migratory erythema, weight loss, diarrhea, thromboembolic phenomena	Pancreas	50–80
Somatostatinoma	Diabetes, cholelithiasis, diarrhea	Pancreas (56) Small bowel (44)	>70

Adapted from Jensen RT, Norton JA[11] and Arnold R, et al.[26]

Pancreatic neuroendocrine tumors may be sporadic (non-familial) or develop as part of the MEN I syndrome.[5–9] MEN I (Werner's syndrome) is inherited as an autosomal dominant disorder with a high degree of penetrance. It is characterized by neoplasms or hyperplasia involving the parathyroid glands, pancreas, pituitary and, less commonly, the adrenal cortex and thyroid gland. Gastrinomas are the most frequent tumor associated with MEN I. The genetic defect predisposing to MEN I has been mapped to the long arm of chromosome 11 (11q11-q13). Establishing the diagnosis of MEN I (strong family history, multiple organ involvement) is essential since family screening is mandatory in this disorder. The gene responsible for MEN I has been cloned[10] and will ultimately facilitate genetic screening for this disorder. The presence of MEN I will impact the surgical approach to the patient, as will become evident when the treatment of gastrinomas is reviewed below.

Awareness of the signs and symptoms associated with these rare tumors in addition to a high level of suspicion by the clinician provides the elements needed for the establishment of an early diagnosis. Early detection will enhance the likelihood of definitive surgical therapy, which is particularly important when one considers that the likelihood of these tumors being malignant exceeds 50%. A detailed review of the clinical features of pancreatic endocrine tumors is beyond the scope of this chapter, and several comprehensive reviews of this subject are available.[4,5,11–14] The following is a brief summary of several salient clinical features of these rare syndromes.

Specific syndromes

Zollinger-Ellison syndrome

Severe peptic ulcer diathesis secondary to gastric acid hypersecretion due to autonomous gastrin release from a non-β cell endocrine tumor (gastrinoma) defines the components of the Zollinger-Ellison syndrome.[5,6] Early on, Zollinger-Ellison syndrome was typified by aggressive and refractory ulceration in which total gastrectomy provided the only chance for enhancing survival. Advances in medical and surgical approaches have converted Zollinger-Ellison syndrome into a disease that, if identified early, can be cured by surgical resection in up to 30–34% of patients with sporadic (non-MEN I related) disease. The true incidence of gastrinoma is unknown, but in the United States it is estimated to be present in 0.1–1% of individuals with peptic ulcer disease. There is a slight predominance of males over females, and the majority of patients are diagnosed between the age of 30 and 50 years. Gastrinomas are classified into sporadic tumors (60–80%) and those associated with multiple endocrine neoplasia type I (MEN I, see below).[9]

Greater than 80% of these neoplasms are found within the hypothetical gastrinoma triangle, defined as the confluence of the cystic and common bile ducts superiorly, junction of the second and third portions of the duodenum inferiorly, and junction of the neck and body of the pancreas medially (Fig. 31.1).[15] Duodenal tumors constitute the most common nonpancreatic lesions, with recent studies suggesting that as many as 50% of gastrinomas are found in this location. In excess of 60–80% of tumors are considered malignant, with up to 30–50% of patients having multiple lesions or metastatic disease at presentation.[6]

Peptic ulcer is the most common clinical manifestation, occurring in over 90% of gastrinoma patients. Suspicion of a gastrinoma

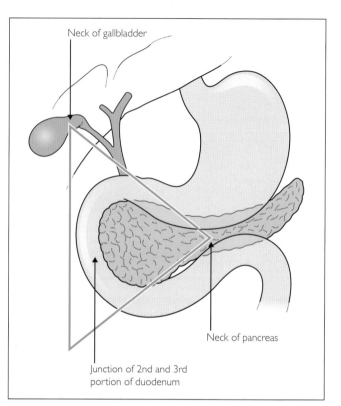

Fig. 31.1 • Gastrinoma triangle. This hypothetical triangle is defined as the confluence of the cystic and common bile ducts superiorly, junction of the second and third portions of the duodenum inferiorly and junction of the neck and body of the pancreas medially. Adapted with permission from Stabile BE, et al.[15]

should arise in patients with ulcers in unusual locations (second part of the duodenum and beyond), ulcers refractory to standard medical therapy, ulcer reoccurrence after acid reducing surgery, or ulcers presenting with frank complications (bleeding, obstruction, and perforation). Symptoms of esophageal origin are present in up to two-thirds of Zollinger-Ellison patients, with a spectrum ranging from mild esophagitis to frank ulceration with stricture and Barrett's mucosa.

Diarrhea is the next most common clinical manifestation, being present in as many as 50% of patients, with the etiology being multifactorial, resulting from marked volume overload to the small bowel, pancreatic enzyme inactivation and bile salt precipitation by acid overload, and mild damage of the intestinal epithelial surface by acid.

Gastrinomas can develop in the presence of MEN I syndrome in approximately 25% of patients.[9] An additional distinguishing feature in Zollinger-Ellison patients with MEN-I is the higher incidence of gastric carcinoid tumor development (as compared to patients with sporadic gastrinomas). Moreover, gastrinomas tend to be smaller, multiple, and located in the duodenal wall more often then what is seen in patients with sporadic disease. Establishing the diagnosis of MEN I is critical not only from the standpoint of providing genetic counseling to the patient and his/her family, but also from the surgical approach recommended (see below).

Recent success in controlling gastric acid hypersecretion in this group of patients (see Ch. 20) has shifted emphasis of therapy towards providing a surgical cure. Detecting the primary tumor and excluding metastatic disease is critical in view of this paradigm shift.

Insulinoma

Insulinomas are the most common symptomatic endocrine tumor of the pancreas.[11–14,16] The clinical features are secondary to hypoglycemia resulting from the autonomous release of insulin from the neoplasm. Symptoms are frequently associated with fasting and are most commonly of the neuroglycopenic variety (mild personality changes, confusion, drowsiness, visual disturbance, coma) as opposed to the signs and symptoms related to compensatory catecholamine release (diaphoresis, pallor, tachycardia). Insulinomas are generally solitary benign tumors of the pancreas (70–80%) that are often amenable to resection. The diagnosis requires documenting hypoglycemia in the presence of inappropriately elevated plasma insulin levels. An in-hospital fast (up to 72 hours) coupled with monitoring of blood glucose and insulin levels is the most effective way of establishing the diagnosis. This test is positive for insulinoma if serum insulin levels are stable or increase during hypoglycemia (blood sugar <50 mg/dL) or the insulin (in mU/L) to glucose (in mg/dL) ratio is greater than 0.3. The differential diagnosis of fasting hypoglycemia is extensive.[16] The use of proinsulin and C-peptide levels may assist in establishing the diagnosis.

VIPoma (Verner-Morrison syndrome)

The clinical manifestations of Verner-Morrison syndrome are most commonly due to the excessive release of vasoactive intestinal polypeptide from a neoplasm most often found in the pancreas.[4,11–14] Other bioactive substances have been implicated in the pathogenesis of this syndrome including secretin, gastrin inhibitory polypeptide (GIP), pancreatic polypeptide (PP), and prostaglandins. Clinical features include profuse (large volume, 1–6 L/day) watery diarrhea (100%) in association with symptoms of hypokalemia (90–100%), and dehydration. Achlorhydria (70%) has also been added to the syndrome, thus the acronym, WDHA syndrome (watery diarrhea, hypokalemia, and achlorhydria). Other associated signs and symptoms include hyperglycemia (25–50%), hypercalcemia (25%), and flushing (20%). VIPomas tend to be large tumors (≈5 cm) and are primarily located in the pancreas (>90%), with more than 60% being malignant. The diagnosis depends on establishing the presence of secretory diarrhea (>700 mL/day, which persists during fasting and is isotonic) in association with elevated plasma VIP levels (normal levels = 0–170 pg/mL).

Glucagonoma

Excessive release of glucagon from a pancreatic neoplasm account for the signs and symptoms associated with this syndrome.[4,11–14,17–19] Clinical manifestations include a characteristic rash (migratory necrolytic erythema, 70–85%), glucose intolerance or diabetes (85%), hypoaminoacidemia (80–90%), weight loss (85%), anemia (85%), diarrhea (15%), thromboembolic phenomena (20%), and glossitis (15%). The rash progresses over 7–14 days from erythematous macules to fluid-filled bullae followed by central necrosis, scaly eczematoid lesions, and central clearing and scaling. The lesions occur most commonly in areas of friction, as well as on the face and distal extremities. The mechanism for rash development is unclear. Glucagonomas occur almost exclusively in the pancreas (body and tail) and are large (>5 cm), with the majority

having evidence of metastasis (liver) at the time of presentation. Delay in diagnosis is probably related to the insidious signs and symptoms. Diagnosis depends on the presence of elevated plasma glucagon level (normal levels = 0–150 pg/mL) in the appropriate clinical scenario. Several causes of increased glucagon levels have been described (diabetes mellitus, renal failure, cirrhosis, acute injury, bacteremia, and Cushing's syndrome), and thus a plasma glucagon level should exceed 500 pg/mL for the diagnosis of this endocrine neoplasm.

Somatostatinoma

Release of somatostatin from an endocrine neoplasm originating from either the pancreas or the small intestine typifies this syndrome.[4,11–14] The variable clinical presentation has led to some controversy regarding the existence of a distinct somatostatinoma syndrome. The triad of symptoms most frequently encountered in pancreatic somatostatinoma patients includes gallstones (95%), diabetes mellitus (95%), diarrhea (92%). Other manifestations include weight loss (90%), hypochlorhydria (85%), and steatorrhea (80%). With intestinal neoplasms, weight loss (70%), gallbladder disease (40%), and diarrhea (38%) are the most commonly encountered clinical manifestations with diabetes (20%), hypochlorhydria (17%), and steatorrhea (12%) following thereafter. As with gastrinomas, somatostatinomas are frequently found in extrapancreatic sites (44% small intestine) as well as in the pancreas (56%, usually head of pancreas). Similar to VIP and glucagon producing tumors, somatostatinomas are large (≈5 cm in diameter) at the time of diagnosis. The diagnosis requires a high level of suspicion (clinical triad: gallstone, diabetes, and diarrhea) coupled with an elevated plasma somatostatin level.

GRFoma

This more recently described neoplasm (1982) usually originates in the pancreas and secretes high levels of growth hormone-releasing factor (GRF).[4,11–14] The most common clinical manifestations are those associated with acromegaly (large extremities, coarsening of facial features, oily skin, malodorous perspiration, hypertrichosis, voice changes, visceral hypertrophy, and glucose intolerance). Forty percent of these cases have been associated with Zollinger-Ellison syndrome, and approximately 30% are associated with MEN I syndrome. Patients frequently have a large pancreatic mass (>5 cm) with evidence of metastasis to the liver at the time of presentation in approximately one-third of the cases. The diagnosis depends on identifying an elevated plasma GRF level in a patient with the appropriate clinical presentation.

A summary of the salient clinical features corresponding to the different endocrine neoplasms is outlined in Table 31.1.

THERAPY

As is the case with solid tumors in general, the only chance at curing these indolent neoplasms is through surgical resection. Despite this concept, additional considerations must be brought to light when approaching the treatment of individuals with these rare neoplasms. Specifically, the clinician needs to ameliorate the potentially life-threatening sequelae and often incapacitating symptoms related to hormone overproduction. This principle will be critically important in managing the patient who is awaiting localization studies while anticipating surgery, and in individuals who are deemed unresectable because of metastatic disease. Recent work demonstrating the direct impact of tumor extent on survival,[20–24] coupled with the limited success of medical therapy in controlling progression of metastatic disease, serves to further reinforce the importance of early diagnosis, localization, and surgical resection of these indolent, yet often relentless, neoplasms.

The following section will review the medical and surgical management of endocrine tumors of the pancreas. In view of the potential applicability of somatostatin analogues to the diagnosis and therapy of the majority of these tumors, the first portion of this section will review the pharmacology of these novel compounds. Subsequent sections will focus on the medical and surgical therapy of specific syndromes.

Somatostatin analogues

Understanding the biology of peptide hormone receptors expressed on neuroendocrine tumors has ushered in an exciting paradigm for the treatment of these rare neoplasms.[24] For example, development of stable somatostatin analogues (see below) has revolutionized the therapy of functional endocrine tumors. Over 80% of neuroendocrine tumors (with the exception of insulinomas) express somatostatin receptors. Octreotide[24–28] and lanreotide[28,29] are two examples of analogues that have reached clinical utility. The former is available in the United States and has been used extensively for the therapy of functioning secretory tumors.

Somatostatin was first isolated as a 14-amino-acid peptide from ovine hypothalamus by Brazeau and colleagues during their search for a factor involved in regulating pituitary growth hormone release. Subsequent to this discovery, somatostatin was found distributed throughout the body in areas extending from the nervous system to the gastrointestinal tract. Moreover, five subtypes of somatostatin receptors have been described and cloned, each having a characteristic structure, distribution, and biological function.[24,28] Somatostatin is unique because it exerts a wide array of inhibitory actions on multiple physiologic functions (Fig. 31.2). Early studies using native somatostatin for the therapy of secretory diarrhea were promising, but the peptide's short half-life (approximately 2 minutes) limited its practical utility. Advances in peptide hormone biochemistry have facilitated the engineering of the chemically stable analogue of somatostatin, octreotide.

Octreotide is a synthetic eight-amino-acid peptide designed on the basis of the structural components of somatostatin that are essential for its biological activity (see Fig. 31.2).[25,26,28] In addition to retaining biological activity, octreotide has a longer plasma half-life than its native counterpart (90 minutes as compared to 2 minutes). Octreotide exerts its action by binding to the somatostatin receptor subtype 2.[24] Due to its poor intestinal absorption, this analogue must be administered parenterally, reaching peak plasma levels approximately one hour after subcutaneous injection, with maximal clinical efficacy noted 2 hours after administration. Initial reports suggest that hepatic extraction can account for 30–40% of octreotide metabolism, while approximately 11–30% of the parent compound is recovered from the urine and less than 2% appears unchanged in feces. Prolonged plasma clearance of octreotide has been demonstrated in patients with renal failure on hemodialysis, and the dose should thus be adjusted accordingly.

From the standpoint of its biological activity, in vitro studies have demonstrated that the inhibitory effect of octreotide on cellular function is equal to or slightly greater than that of native

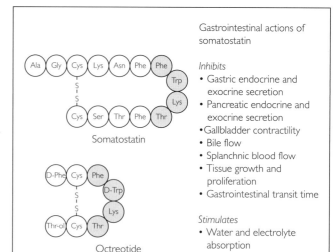

Fig. 31.2 ● Structure and gastrointestinal actions of somatostatin and octreotide. Shaded amino acids are important for biological activity. (Reprinted from Maton PN, Gardner JD, Jensen RT, Digestive Disorder Science, 1989; 34:285. © 1989 with permission from Springer Science and Business Media.)

somatostatin. In contrast, in vivo studies reveal that the stable analogue is three times, 23 times, and 80 times more potent than somatostatin in mediating inhibition of insulin, glucagon, and gastric acid secretion, respectively. The enhanced potency of octreotide in vivo is most likely due to its prolonged stability in plasma.

A large number of clinical trials have demonstrated the efficacy of octreotide in ameliorating the signs and symptoms of several pancreatic neuroendocrine tumors of the pancreas (see below). Moreover the potential antiproliferative effects of this compound have led to its use as an antitumoral agent. The recent development of radiolabeled octreotide has added a new dimension to this compound as a diagnostic/staging tool and more interestingly as a nuclear probe for tumor therapy.[24]

A consensus statement regarding dosing schedules for octreotide has been published.[30] In the case of VIPoma and other secretory diarrhea related to neuroendocrine tumors, octreotide should be started at a dose of 100–150 μg/day and increased to 200 μg every 8 hours if the response is not adequate. If the patient is still refractory, 100 μg increments per dose can be administered to a maximum 1500 μg per day. If control of symptoms is achieved, a gradual decrease in the dose after 2–3 weeks of therapy can be initiated. The dose should be decreased by 25 μg/injection per week. In patients with severe or life threatening signs and symptoms, the initial dose (100 μg) can be administered intravenously followed by a continuous infusion of 50 μg/hour. Once symptoms are controlled, a change to subcutaneous octreotide should be initiated. A long-acting form of octreotide has been developed and is presently available for use in the United States and Europe.[28,31] The compound (Sandostatin LAR®) consists of octreotide prepared in a slow-release formulation that can be administered as an intramuscular depot injection once per month. Early studies in patients with carcinoid tumors suggest that symptom control is achieved by 7–14 days of administration.[31] The compound is available in 10-, 20- and 30-mg doses (as compared to microgram dosing for octreotide). One suggested approach to using this compound is to begin the patient on short-acting octreotide as outlined above and then administer a 20-mg dose of the long-acting formulation within 1–2 weeks of the patient taking the short-acting compound and continuing the latter for an additional 1–2 weeks until a therapeutic level has been reached with the depot form. The short-acting compound can then be used for breakthrough symptoms. The dose of the depot formulation can subsequently be adjusted the following month according to the amount of breakthrough symptoms the patient experiences.

Adverse effects related to octreotide therapy have been relatively infrequent and of minor consequence.[25,26,28,31] Less than 10% of reported cases experience nausea, injection site pain, diarrhea, abdominal discomfort, loose stools, or vomiting. Gastrointestinal side effects with the short-acting formulation may be diminished by avoiding meals around the time of drug administration. Early studies demonstrate that the depot form of octreotide is very well tolerated. Injection site pain with the short-acting form can be reduced by decreasing the volume of drug administered and by warming the solution to room temperature. Injection of the depot formulation is a bit more involved and should be administered by a trained staff member. Although diarrhea/steatorrhea is felt to be related to octreotide-mediated inhibition of pancreatic secretion, the role of pancreatic enzyme replacement to reverse this side effect has not been assessed.

Cholelithiasis has been reported to develop in 20–30% of patients on long-term octreotide therapy.[25,28] The rate of gallstone formation may be even higher, based on a recent report by Trendle and coworkers.[32] An overall incidence of 52.3% for cholelithiasis/sludge was reported in 44 patients receiving octreotide for treatment of malignant neuroendocrine tumors of the pancreas or carcinoid syndrome. The incidence was higher (61.9%) in individuals receiving high-dose therapy (1500 μg/day, 21 patients) as compared to those receiving low-dose octreotide (450 μg/day, 17 patients), in whom the incidence was 35.3%. The overall incidence of symptomatic gallbladder disease requiring cholecystectomy was 6.8%, which was not predictable by the dose of octreotide administered. Based on these data, it is clear that patients on long-term octreotide (>2 months) should be monitored for gallstone development. The low rate of symptomatic disease does not warrant prophylactic cholecystectomy, but may be a consideration in patients undergoing surgery for a different reason (debulking, etc.).

Medical therapy of specific syndromes

Zollinger-Ellison syndrome

The cornerstone to the therapy of gastrinoma patients is aggressive control of gastric acid secretion.[4,20,33] Prior to the advent of inhibitors of gastric acid secretion (histamine H_2-receptor antagonists, proton pump inhibitors), the only option for these patients was total gastrectomy. The advent of potent antisecretory agents, in particular proton pump inhibitors (PPIs), has dramatically changed the approach to these patients.[4,33,34] (See Chapters 1 and 20 for a review on the treatment of Zollinger-Ellison syndrome with inhibitors of gastric acid secretion.) In general, therapy is aimed at decreasing basal acid secretion to <10 mmol per hour immediately prior to the next dose. PPI therapy is generally instituted at a dose of 40 mg once daily of omeprazole (or equivalent doses of other PPIs) and increased by increments of 20 mg daily until acid secretion is sufficiently suppressed. If the daily dose exceeds 80 mg, twice daily dosing

is generally instituted. *Intravenous pantoprazole is effective in controlling gastric acid hypersecretion in patients who are not able to take the PPI orally.*[35] It must be emphasized that symptom relief does not predict sufficient acid suppression, and basal acid output determination should be performed to ensure adequate antisecretory therapy. Octreotide therapy is reserved for those individuals with somatostatin receptor-positive tumors (established by somatostatin receptor scintigraphy) who are refractory or progressing despite maximal acid suppression.

Insulinomas

Insulinomas are one of the two most common types of functional neuroendocrine tumors (up to 50%).[14] In contrast to the majority of other neuroendocrine tumors, surgical resection can be successful in 70–90% of cases.[16] Management of patients with documented insulinoma who are awaiting surgery or are deemed unresectable must be targeted for controlling the potentially life-threatening complications of hypoglycemia. Dietary maneuvers should be the first line of therapy. Increasing the frequency of meals (up to 6 meals/day) and the ingestion of carbohydrates that are slowly absorbed (breads, potatoes, rice, starches) should be initiated.[14]

Several pharmacological agents are available for the therapy of insulinoma-related hypoglycemia, the most commonly used agent being diazoxide.[14,15,36] This benzothiadiazine directly decreases insulin levels by inhibiting release of secretory granules from normal pancreatic β-islet cells and tumor tissues and by stimulating α-adrenergic receptors on normal pancreatic β-cells. Diazoxide also induces hyperglycemia by inhibiting cAMP phosphodiesterase activity, resulting in enhanced glycogenolysis. Dosing will vary among patients, but the range extends from 25 mg twice to 200 mg three times per day.[37] The dose should be adjusted to the patient's response or the development of side effects (see below). Response rates vary, but approximately two-thirds of patients should improve with this agent.[38] Several untoward effects have been attributed to diazoxide therapy, including nausea, sodium retention, hirsutism, and, less commonly, bone marrow suppression.[36] The addition of a mild diuretic and salt restriction may ameliorate the side effects related to sodium retention. Additional drugs reported to be useful in the management of hypoglycemia include phenytoin, the calcium channel blockers verapamil and diltiazem,[39] mithramycin, propranolol, and octreotide. These drugs should be reserved for patients refractory or not tolerant to diazoxide. The overall success rate of calcium channel blockers and phenytoin has been limited.[14] Moreover, the potential for beta-blockers to mask the signs and symptoms of hypoglycemia make this drug class potentially dangerous. The efficacy of octreotide in ameliorating insulinoma related hypoglycemia has also met with varying results. Reports indicate that between 30% and 50%[40–44] of patients may experience a decrease in insulin levels and an improvement in hypoglycemic symptoms. The relatively low response rates in insulinoma patients may be due to heterogeneous expression of somatostatin receptors in tumor tissue.[45] In fact, octreotide-induced hypoglycemia in insulinoma patients has been documented.[14]

VIPoma (Verner-Morrison syndrome)

The clinical hallmark of this syndrome is profuse watery diarrhea (1–6 liters/day) associated with signs and symptoms of dehydration, hypokalemia, and achlorhydria (WDHA syndrome).[46] The first line of therapy must be aimed at correcting the fluid and electrolyte abnormalities since these can be quite severe and potentially fatal. Subsequently, control of the large-volume diarrhea is essential. A host of therapeutic modalities have been used in an effort to decrease high stool outputs related to VIPoma. These options have included high-dose prednisone (>60 mg/day),[47–49] which has been shown to decrease the diarrhea in a significant percentage of patients. Other agents reserved for patients that are intolerant to prednisone have included indomethacin,[50,51] clonidine, lithium,[52] phenothiazines,[53] propranolol,[54] and loperamide. Unfortunately, patients are not uniformly responsive to any one of these drugs. Octreotide has also proven most useful in ameliorating the signs and symptoms related to VIPoma. Early studies demonstrated significant improvement in patient's diarrhea after treatment with native somatostatin administered by continuous infusion, but the short plasma half-life limited its practical utility.[55–58] Subsequent studies have confirmed that octreotide can decrease diarrhea in over 80% of VIPoma patients.[59–62] Of interest, there have been several patients who improved symptomatically with octreotide and continued to have elevated plasma VIP levels. Some have suggested that synthesis of VIP in the tumor may have been altered such that a biologically less active molecular form was released from the neoplasm.[63] This observation also reinforces the concept that the inhibitory effect of somatostatin is multifactorial and is not limited to its effect on secretogogue release from the neoplasm.

In summary, over 80% of VIPoma patients treated with octreotide have experienced significant symptomatic improvement. The dosage utilized has ranged from 100 to 1500 μg/day, and the duration of therapy for some has been as long as 38 months.[64] These observations indicate that octreotide is the most effective drug available for the treatment of this disorder. Experience with the long-acting form of octreotide in patients with VIPoma, as well as the subsequent tumors reviewed in this chapter, is limited, but the anticipation is that it will also provide a useful addition to the treatment of these patients.

Glucagonomas

The presentation of glucagonoma patients can be quite indolent and escape detection for many years, with more than 60% being metastatic at the time of diagnosis. As in the case of other neuroendocrine tumors, surgical resection provides the only possibility for cure. Unfortunately, surgery is not often feasible in view of metastatic disease being present at diagnosis. A surgical procedure will often be recommended, and preoperative correction of hypoaminoacidemia (malnutrition) and anemia seem warranted. Some have described improvement of the severe rash with total parenteral nutrition and zinc replacement, although this approach remains controversial. Thirty percent of patients may present with thromboembolic phenomena including pulmonary emboli,[17,18,65] and measures should thus be taken to prevent venous thrombosis, especially if the patient is awaiting surgery. These measures should include low-dose subcutaneous heparin and/or compression stockings.[13] If distal pancreatectomy with splenectomy is contemplated, a pneumococcal vaccine should be administered.[13] Both native somatostatin and octreotide have been utilized in the treatment of glucagonoma patients with some success. Over 17 glucagonoma patients have been treated with the stable analogue in doses ranging 50–450 μg per day,[66–68] with greater than 50% experiencing resolution of the rash and greater

than 60% of subjects having a reduction in plasma glucagon levels. Approximately one-half of these patients received octreotide for more than 6 months. Of note, octreotide had little effect on tumor size and diabetes.

Somatostatinoma, GRFoma

The indolent and variable presentation of somatostatinomas make medical therapy difficult to generalize. The most common clinical sequelae related to pancreatic lesions that will often lead to medical attention include diabetes mellitus (95%), gallbladder disease, and diarrhea. Each of these may be managed prior to establishing an association with a somatostatin-producing tumor. The role of octreotide has not been examined extensively in this disorder.

GRFomas most often present with signs and symptoms of acromegaly. It is important to consider this type of tumor in patients with peptic ulcer disease and acromegaly in view of the known association with Zollinger-Ellison syndrome. In such cases, acid suppressive therapy will be critical in the management of these individuals (see Ch. 20). Octreotide has been utilized successfully in patients with GRFomas, decreasing plasma levels of GRF, and reducing symptoms[70–73] in 100% of a small number of patients treated. Although limited, the data available suggest that octreotide is the drug of choice in patients with this neoplasm.

Surgical therapy of nonmetastatic disease

As outlined throughout this chapter, the only possibility for long-term cure in patients with neuroendocrine tumors is surgical resection of the neoplasm. The potential for curative resection will vary according to the specific tumor type. In addition, the presence of MEN I will impact the surgical approach taken. The rare incidence of these neoplasms, coupled with the fact that these tumors may be small, multiple, and in difficult areas to locate, makes it imperative that the procedure be performed by a surgeon experienced in the resection of neuroendocrine tumors.

The last decade has witnessed a steady increase in the tools available to assist in the preoperative localization of these sometimes difficult to find tumors. A review of these modalities and their application to the different tumor types is beyond the scope of this chapter. The advent of endoscopic ultrasonography (EUS) (Fig. 31.3)[74,75] and somatostatin receptor scintigraphy (Octreoscan®) (Fig. 31.4)[76–78] has complemented and even supplanted the more traditional modalities, including extracorporeal ultrasound, CT scanning, nuclear magnetic resonance imaging (MRI), and angiography. Somatostatin receptor scintigraphy should generally be the first modality utilized to localize gastrinomas since it is more sensitive than CT scanning, ultrasound, MRI, and angiography *combined* in localizing primary tumors and as sensitive as all these

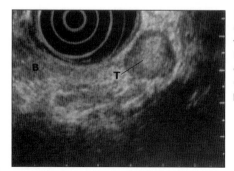

Fig. 31.3 • Endoscopic ultrasound in a patient with the Zollinger-Ellison syndrome demonstrating a tumor (T) in the head of the pancreas.

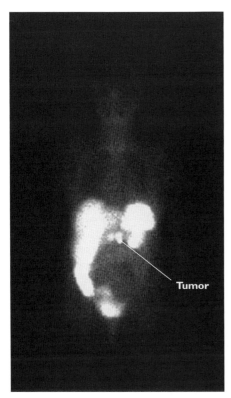

Fig. 31.4 • Octreoscan in a patient with the Zollinger-Ellison syndrome demonstrating a tumor within the gastrinoma triangle.

Tumor

modalities in detecting metastatic disease. EUS has been found to be as accurate as somatostatin receptor scintigraphy in localizing gastrinomas and more sensitive in localizing insulinomas. EUS is often used to confirm and more specifically localize gastrinomas after localization by initial somatostatin receptor scintigraphy. A summary of the sensitivity of the various modalities used for localizing insulinomas and gastrinomas is summarized in Table 31.2. It is essential that all patients with documented biochemical evidence of a neuroendocrine tumor undergo detailed evaluation in an effort to localize the tumor and determine the extent of involvement (metastatic versus nonmetastatic).

As discussed above, the tumor with greatest potential for surgical cure is an insulinoma. Between 75% and 95% of insulinoma patients can be cured with surgery.[11–16] As in the case of insulinomas, the ultimate goal of surgery in gastrinoma patients is to provide a definitive cure. No longer is total gastrectomy routinely required in these patients. Early attempts at resection of the under-

lying neoplasm lead to cure rates below 10%. Recent advances in early tumor detection and improved understanding of tumor distribution has led to 10-year disease-free intervals as high as 34% in sporadic gastrinoma patients undergoing surgery.[79] A positive outcome is highly dependent on the experience of the surgical team treating these rare tumors. Surgical therapy of gastrinoma patients with MEN I remains controversial and is related to the difficulty in rendering these patients disease free with surgery. In contrast to the encouraging postoperative results observed in patients with sporadic disease, only 6% of MEN I patients are disease free 5 years after an operation. Some groups suggest surgery only if a clearly identifiable, nonmetastatic lesion is documented by structural studies. Others advocate a more aggressive approach, where all patients free of hepatic metastasis are explored and all detected tumors in the duodenum resected, followed by enucleation of lesions in the pancreatic head, with a distal pancreatectomy to follow. The outcome of the two approaches has not been clearly established. In contrast to insulinomas and gastrinomas, greater than 50% of glucagonomas have metastasized by the time of diagnosis,[19] with an even greater percentage having extensive disease at the time of operation. Similar odds of having metastatic disease holds true for VIPoma, somatostatinoma, GRFoma, and nonfunctioning tumors, and the long-term benefit of surgical resection has thus not been clearly established in these patients.

Therapy of metastatic disease

Despite the steady advances made in the diagnosis, localization, and therapeutic modalities pertinent to neuroendocrine tumors of the pancreas, issues regarding the approach to unresectable or metastatic disease remain unresolved. The reasons include the rarity with which these tumors develop, their slow-growing nature and the somewhat limited information available regarding the natural history of these tumors. The advent of effective therapy for the control of symptoms and potential-life threatening complications of neuroendocrine tumors has now shifted the emphasis of treatment towards controlling the growth of metastatic disease, since mortality presently appears more directly related to the latter. Grama and coworkers[80] retrospectively examined 85 patients with functional pancreatic neuroendocrine neoplasms. The tumor types and the corresponding median survival are summarized in Table 31.3. Forty-eight percent (41/85) had metastatic disease at the time of diagnosis. Of these, two-thirds died from tumor progression. Although there appears to be some differences in overall 5- and 10-year survival for individual tumors, the survival rates for all malignant tumors was 54% and 28%, respectively.

With regard to gastrinoma patients, 5- and 10-year survival rates vary between 62–75% and 47–53%, respectively, for all patients.[5,33] Individuals with the entire tumor resected or those with a negative laparotomy have 5- and 10-year survival rates in excess of 90%. Patients with incompletely resected tumors have a 5- and 10-year survival of 43% and 25%, respectively. Finally, survival in patients with hepatic metastasis is less than 20% survival at 5 years. Characteristics considered to be favorable prognostic indicators include primary duodenal wall tumors, isolated lymph node tumor, undetectable tumor upon surgical exploration, and possibly the presence of MEN I. Poor prognostic indicators include hepatic metastasis or the presence of Cushing's syndrome

	Sensitivity (%)	
Imaging procedure	**Gastrinoma**	**Insulinoma**
EUS	11/14 (79)	13/14 (93)
SRS	12/14 (86)	2/14 (14)
CT	4/14 (29)	3/14 (21)
US	4/14 (29)	1/14 (7)
MRI	4/14 (29)	1/14 (7)

Table 31.2 Sensitivity of multiple imaging modalities in detecting primary gastrinomas and insulinomas

Adapted from Zimmer T, et al. Gut 1996; 39:562–568.

Table 31.3 Survival estimates for patients with malignant endocrine pancreatic tumors

Diagnosis	Survival (%)		Median survival (months)
	5-year	10-year	
Insulinoma	50	50	151
Gastrinoma	47	18	51
VIPoma	88	25	103
All malignant tumors*	54	28	68

* Including glucagonoma and somatostatinoma.
Adapted from Grama D, et al.[78]

in a sporadic gastrinoma patient.

The approach to patients with metastatic neuroendocrine tumors will vary somewhat according to the type of neoplasm. First, the control of signs and symptoms related to hormone excess is essential, as discussed above, and reversing or controlling tumor growth should follow. Unfortunately, the success rates of traditional chemoradiation therapeutic approaches have been highly variable and often of limited success in altering survival. The reason for poor outcome is unclear, but may be related to the relatively well-differentiated state of these tumor cells, making them less vulnerable to agents that depend on high cell proliferative rates for success. Moreover, the relatively prolonged survival of these patients (in comparison to adenocarcinoma of the pancreas), coupled with the rarity of these tumors and inconsistencies in defining response to treatment, makes the available data difficult to interpret. The limited success rates associated with classic cytotoxic agents in conjunction with the relatively high side effect profile associated with these agents has led to a host of relatively novel approaches to the therapy of patients with metastatic endocrine tumors. These have extended from the use of hormonal agents, such as octreotide, to liver transplantation. The approach will depend to some extent on the tumor type and to a significant extent on the clinical state of the patient in terms of signs, symptoms, and tumor growth. Most patients will qualify for a step-wise approach in which a combination of therapies will be utilized in an effort to ameliorate signs and symptoms of hormone excess and tumor growth. The following sections will summarize both medical and surgical approaches that have been utilized in the therapy of metastatic neuroendocrine tumors of the pancreas.

Medical therapy

Hormonal therapy

The expression of somatostatin receptors on a large number of neuroendocrine tumors,[24,81] coupled with experimental data suggesting that this peptide has antiproliferative effects,[82–86] led to the utilization of stable somatostatin analogues as antitumoral agents.[14,27,35] Early reports using octreotide demonstrating tumor shrinkage were encouraging.[87–90] Unfortunately, subsequent larger-scale studies have not been as convincing of the antitumoral effect of somatostatin analogues. In a retrospective report of 94 patients by Maton and colleagues,[91] it was observed that tumor

size decreased, stabilized, or progressed in 13%, 63%, and 24% of patients, respectively. More recent prospective studies have documented modest tumor shrinkage and stabilization of the neoplasm.[92] Arnold and coworkers[26] prospectively examined 47 patients with documented tumor progression who were treated with octreotide (200 µg twice daily). Initial stabilization of tumor growth was observed in 40% of patients, and the disease state remained stable in 25% and 13% of patients for 12 and 36 months, respectively. The authors did not, however, observe tumor shrinkage in any of the patients tested. It has been postulated that the lack of antiproliferative effects of octreotide may have been due to the relatively low dose tested. A recent prospective multicenter trial addressed this question by examining the effect of octreotide at either 500 µg (23 patients) or 1000 µg three times daily (35 patients) in 58 patients with metastatic neuroendocrine tumors.[27] Therapy was continued until evidence of tumor progression was noted. The majority of patients had carcinoid tumors, with only 12 individuals having other hormonal neoplasms. Although the population was heterogeneous, only two carcinoid patients showed an objective decrease in tumor size, with duration of response of 10 and 14 months, respectively. Tumor stabilization for 6 months was observed in 27 patients (22%). Of note, all of these patients had either carcinoid tumors or medullary thyroid carcinomas. In addition, the beneficial effects were not related to the octreotide dose utilized. The median overall survival was 22 months, but for the noncarcinoid tumor patients, survival was only 12 months.

Lanreotide has also been utilized, in a preliminary fashion, as an antiproliferative agent in the treatment of metastatic neuroendocrine tumors.[93] Faiss and colleagues report observing cessation of tumor growth in 46% of all patients with high-dose Lanreotide (5 mg three times daily). Unfortunately, the tumor types examined and the duration of response were not outlined in this preliminary report.

In summary, it appears that stable analogues of somatostatin will not provide a significant antitumoral effect in patients with metastatic neuroendocrine tumors. At best, it appears that tumor stabilization is achievable at high doses, but the major benefit appears to be for carcinoid tumor patients.

A novel therapeutic approach attempting to capitalize on the high level of somatostatin receptor expression on neuroendocrine tumors has recently been reported. In a phase I trial, Krenning and co-workers[94] treated six end-stage neuroendocrine tumor patients with octreotide radionuclide therapy. These investigators utilized [^{111}In-DTPA-D-Phe^1] octreotide in cumulative doses as high as 53 GBq per patient. The group studied was heterogeneous, consisting of two pancreatic neuroendocrine tumors (one glucagonoma, one insulinoma), two medullary thyroid carcinomas, one carcinoid tumor, and one glomus tumor. No major side effects were reported (2-year follow-up) and a decrease in tumor size was observed in 3/6 patients (both neuroendocrine tumor patients). More recent studies utilizing [^{111}In-DTPA°] octreotide in 20 patients with advanced disease demonstrated a decrease (30%) or stabilization (40%) of the tumor. Additional radioligands being piloted include ^{90}Y-labeled octreotide and ^{177}Lu-DOTA-Tyr^3-octreotide. The potential of targeting therapy to metastatic endocrine tumors is an exciting modality with potential future applicability, but the overall impact, efficacy, and safety of this therapeutic approach requires treatment of a larger number of patients.[12,95]

Interferon

The limited success of octreotide and chemotherapy (see below) in the therapy of metastatic endocrine tumors has led to studies examining the potential benefits of α-interferon in this clinical setting. Initially described as antiviral agents, these naturally occurring substances have been shown to inhibit cell proliferation and modulate an immune response in several systems. The initial report examining the effect of α-interferon in patients with carcinoid tumor was encouraging, showing a decrease in bioactive hormone production, but no effect on tumor size.[96] Subsequent studies were more encouraging, suggesting not only a beneficial effect on hormone release, but in addition an antiproliferative effect.[97-99] Oberg and coworkers performed a meta-analysis of available data obtained in 310 patients treated with α-interferon. They observed a partial remission (decrease in tumor size by >50%) and a biochemical response in 11% and 42% of patients, respectively. Unfortunately, the heterogeneous patient population examined and the variable dose of interferon utilized led to difficulty in deriving a definite conclusion from this analysis. When examining a population of patients with metastatic neuroendocrine tumors of the pancreas, a reduction in tumor size was observed in 12% of patients, while tumor stabilization was seen in 24% of individuals treated with 5 million units of interferon-α three times per week.[98] Unfortunately, these encouraging results were not observed in two reports examining the efficacy of interferon-α in patients with VIPoma[100] and Zollinger-Ellison syndrome.[101] In these reports, no beneficial effect of interferon on tumor growth was detected.

In summary, the efficacy of interferon in the therapy of neuroendocrine tumors of the pancreas is still somewhat controversial. It appears that the antiproliferative effect of these agents is rather limited and comparable to that observed with octreotide. The major disadvantage of the former is related to the potential adverse side effects, such as flu-like symptoms, neutropenia, and depression.[96-101]

The marginal benefit of interferon or octreotide alone on tumor growth, coupled with the observation that these compounds exert a biological response via different mechanisms,[103] has led to several small trials examining the combination of these two agents. Nold and coworkers[104] observed a partial response in one patient, stable disease in three, and progressive disease in three of seven patients with neuroendocrine tumors of the pancreas. These are preliminary results that are difficult to interpret due to the small number of patients examined, and the potential benefit of combination therapy thus awaits further trials.

In view of the modest benefit of α-interferon and octreotide as inhibitors of tumor growth, additional combination therapies have been attempted. Saltz and coworkers undertook a phase II trial of α-interferon in combination with 5-fluorouracil (5-FU) in patients with advanced carcinoid (14 patients) and neuroendocrine tumors (7 patients).[105] Of the neuroendocrine tumor patients, one had a partial response (8 months' duration) and four patients had stable disease for a median of 13 months. Unfortunately, significant drug toxicity developed with 14 of 21 patients, requiring reduction in the interferon dose. This degree of toxicity was much higher than that observed with interferon alone or interferon in combination with octreotide. Therefore, these results do not support the use of combination interferon and 5-FU for the routine therapy of neuroendocrine tumors.

Chemotherapy

More than 26 studies examining over a dozen possible chemotherapeutic regimens for pancreatic endocrine tumors have been published. The large number of studies is in part a reflection of the difficulty in treating this type of metastatic disease. A detailed review of these reports is beyond the scope of this chapter, and reference is made to a recent thorough review of the subject by Jensen and Norton.[11] Evaluating the efficacy of these different regimens is made difficult by the heterogeneous group of neoplasms included in each study. As is the case when assessing other treatment modalities, the relatively slow growth rate of these tumors, coupled with a somewhat limited understanding of their biology and natural history, limits to some extent interpretation of the available data. Despite these limitations, several general observations can be made regarding the use of chemotherapy in the therapy of metastatic neuroendocrine tumors of the pancreas.

Multiple agents have been used with varying results. The most often used agent with the greatest success rate is the nitrourea antibiotic streptozotocin.[106-112] As a single agent, this drug has been associated with an objective response in over 30% to as high as 60% of patients. The only additional single agent with this response rate is the analogue of streptozotocin, chlorozotocin.[113,114] Combination therapy has been utilized in an effort to improve response rates. Moertel and coworkers compared streptozotocin plus doxorubicin to the former and 5-FU or to chlorozotocin alone in patients with metastatic pancreatic endocrine tumors.[112] These investigators observed a response rate of 69% for streptozotocin plus doxorubicin, 45% for streptozotocin plus 5-FU, and 30% for chlorozotocin alone. Moreover, a significant improvement in survival with the strepto/doxo (2.2 versus 1.4 years) combination was observed when evaluating 105 patients treated. A significant advantage of combination therapy over single-agent treatment was also observed with streptozotocin plus 5-FU. Unfortunately, others[115,116] have not observed similar response rates in gastrinoma patients, a discrepancy possibly due to inherent differences in the patients examined. Variation in response rates to chemotherapy may hold true for different neuroendocrine tumor types. For example, based on the above data, it appears that the combination of streptozotocin and doxorubicin would be the regimen of choice for the therapy of metastatic neuroendocrine tumors of the pancreas. Yet, when evaluating selected subgroups, a heterogeneous response can be observed. Metastatic VIPomas are reported to have response rates as high as 90% to streptozotocin.[46] Dacarbazine, an agent with marginal benefit in several neuroendocrine tumors, has been reported to be extremely effective in the therapy of glucagonomas,[117-121] leading to complete remission in selected cases.

Side effect profiles will also vary among the different agents utilized. Nausea and vomiting are commonly observed in patients treated with streptozotocin or its derivative. Renal insufficiency occasionally leading to chronic renal failure (5–7%) has also been described with these compounds.

In summary, it appears that streptozotocin in combination with doxorubicin may represent the best chemotherapeutic agents for the therapy of metastatic neuroendocrine tumors. In view of the more favorable toxicity profile of 5-FU, some recommend using this agent in place of doxorubicin.[93] In patients with glucagonoma, dacarbazine may represent the best selection.

Hepatic artery embolization

In light of the limited benefit of the above-listed therapies and the inevitable recurrence of signs and symptoms observed in these patients, alternative therapeutic options have been developed. One such option for neuroendocrine tumor patients with liver metastasis is hepatic artery occlusion.[122–125] The rationale for this approach is based on several factors. Hepatic metastasis of neuroendocrine tumors tends to be highly vascular[126,127] and predominantly supplied by the hepatic artery. Normal liver parenchyma receives 75–80% of its blood supply from the portal vein, thus protecting it from ischemic damage if one hepatic artery were to be occluded. The largest experience with this technique has been in patients with metastatic carcinoid tumor, but several studies have included metastatic pancreatic neuroendocrine tumor patients as well. Marlink and colleagues observed a prompt decrease in symptoms related to hormone secretion and a decrease in tumor size for varying intervals in 6/6 patients with metastatic pancreatic neuroendocrine tumors treated with this modality.[125] Hepatic artery occlusion has also been combined with chemotherapy, achieving a complete symptomatic response in over 60% of patients treated.[128] Ruszniewski et al.[129] performed a prospective phase II study examining the efficacy of chemoembolization with doxoribicin in 24 patients with metastatic neuroendocrine tumors. Of these, five had pancreatic primaries (gastrinomas). Although results achieved with carcinoid patients were somewhat promising, only a minor response or tumor stabilization was observed in three of the pancreatic tumor patients. More encouraging results were achieved by Mavligit and coworkers,[130] who observed >50% tumor regression, lasting 8–44 months in four of five patients treated with hepatic artery chemoembolization with cisplatin, followed by intra-arterial infusion of vinblastine. Complications related to hepatic artery embolization can vary from transient abdominal pain, nausea, and fever in greater than 90% of patients to hormonal crisis and renal insufficiency in a smaller percentage of patients. Death has been reported in <3% of cases.[131,132]

More recently, 111 patients (carcinoid and pancreatic neuroendocrine tumors) were treated with systemic chemotherapy in addition to chemoembolization,[133] with an overall response rate of 80%. Of note, a 60% response rate in this series was achieved with chemoembolization alone. Hepatic artery embolization has also been combined with α-interferon in the therapy of metastatic carcinoid tumors with some success (60% response rate, 75% 5-year survival).[134]

In summary, hepatic artery embolization with or without cytotoxic drugs appears to be a feasible alternative for the palliation of pancreatic endocrine tumors that have metastasized to the liver and are progressing in size and/or are associated with refractory symptoms despite hormonal and/or systemic chemotherapy. Whether this therapeutic option will replace more standard treatment modalities is presently unclear.

Surgical therapy

Surgical intervention in pancreatic neuroendocrine tumors is not limited to curative resection. The slow-growing nature of these neoplasms and the tendency to metastasize to upper abdominal lymph nodes and liver have led some to explore whether aggressive removal of tumor tissue (debulking) can impact signs, symptoms, and survival in these patients. More recently, hepatic transplantation has also been attempted in patients with metastatic neuroendocrine tumors.

Debulking

Multiple reports have outlined the potential benefit of debulking procedures in the therapy of metastatic neuroendocrine tumors of the pancreas.[135–147] Symptom control has been reported with debulking procedures in patients with VIPoma,[147,148] glucagonoma,[135,136] and somatostatinoma.[149] In a retrospective analysis (20 years), Thompson and colleagues[136] observed that 51% of patients with metastatic neuroendocrine tumors experienced an improvement in symptoms, with a mean duration of 39 months after aggressive surgery. More recently, it was observed that 50% of patients were cured (no residual disease) and 90% experienced complete symptom relief after hepatic resection.[147] Although encouraging, both of these reports are limited by the fact that they are retrospective in nature. More recently, Carty and coworkers[146] prospectively evaluated this surgical approach in 17 patients with metastatic pancreatic neuroendocrine tumors. Five-year survival was achieved in over 75% of patients with tumors that were amenable to complete resection. Others have observed similar encouraging results[150,151] Unfortunately, only a minority of patients (<10%) would be candidates for this therapeutic approach. Based on the available literature, some advocate aggressive debulking procedures in patients with metastatic glucagonoma and VIPoma in an effort to facilitate medical control of severe symptoms and perhaps prolong survival.

Although these data are encouraging, indicating a potential role for aggressive debulking in patients with severe symptoms that are difficult to control medically, the benefit of this approach in patients with metastatic disease that have stable tumor size and well-controlled symptoms is not established.

Liver transplantation

In view of the slow-growing nature of these tumors and the propensity to metastasize to liver, orthotopic liver transplantation

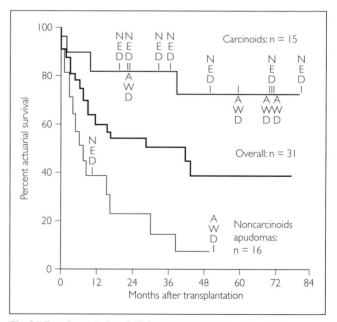

Fig. 31.5 • Survival after OLT for metastatic neuroendocrine tumors. NED, no evidence of disease; AWD, alive with disease. Carcinoid versus noncarcinoid tumors, $p<0.001$. Reprinted with permission from Le Treut, et al.[156]

(OLT) has been attempted as a therapeutic option. The poor response to other treatment modalities, the observation that hepatic metastases are multifocal and bilateral in 90% of cases,[152] and the limited number of individuals amenable to debulking procedures have served as the rationale for this extreme therapeutic approach.[153-156] LeTreut et al. recently reviewed the French experience for OLT in metastatic neuroendocrine tumors.[156] The outcome of OLT in 15 patients with carcinoid tumor and 16 individuals with neuroendocrine tumors of the pancreas (eight nonfunctioning tumors) were retrospectively reviewed. These data were accumulated in 11 centers between 1989 and 1994. Primary tumor was removed by upper abdominal exenteration in seven patients and by a Whipple procedure in three individuals. Overall actuarial survival was 59%, 47%, and 36% at 1, 3, and 5 years, respectively. Of note, survival rates were significantly higher for metastatic carcinoid tumors (69% at 5 years) than for neuroendocrine tumors of the pancreas (8% at 4 years)

(Fig. 31.5). These authors conclude that although OLT may be an option for patients with carcinoid tumors that have refractory symptoms or following resection of the primary tumor, it does not appear to be useful for patients with neuroendocrine tumors of the pancreas.

Future treatment options

As indicated by the preceding sections, the therapy of metastatic neuroendocrine tumors of the pancreas is fraught with great limitations. Under the best of circumstances, only a partial response, which is often limited, is achievable with the host of treatment modalities outlined. A search for more effective therapy of this unfortunate disease continues. Targeted radiotherapy with somatostatin or other peptide analogues may be promising.[94] The use of monoclonal antitumor antibody[157] and immunoendocrine therapy with low-dose interferon-α and melatonin[158] are additional options being explored.

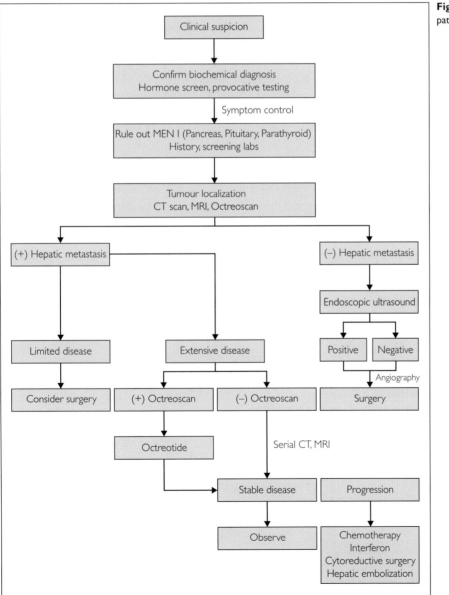

Fig. 31.6 • Algorithm for the approach to the patient with a neuroendocrine tumor.

SUMMARY: TREATMENT OF NEUROENDOCRINE TUMORS

Neuroendocrine tumors of the pancreas are rare neoplasms that are slow growing, often escaping detection by the clinician for years. Clinical suspicion and prompt diagnosis are critical. Control of potentially life-threatening sequelae is essential in patients with functioning neoplasms. Localization of the primary tumor with resection is the only chance for cure. Despite advances in the diagnostic and therapeutic modalities available for these patients, once metastatic, these tumors are relentless despite extreme therapeutic measures. Novel and exciting targeted therapy may change the future outlook for patients with metastatic disease.

At present, the only chance for cure in patients with neuroendocrine tumors is early diagnosis and resection of the primary lesion. The first step in making the diagnosis of these rare neoplasms is clinical suspicion, which can be a challenge in light of the at times subtle manifestations of the syndromes (Fig. 31.6). Biochemical confirmation with hormone screening and provocative testing (if needed) should follow. Presence of signs and symptoms will require targeted therapy that will extend from dietary manipulations to PPIs or octreotide depending on the tumor type. Medical therapy should continue during the time that tumor localization and extent is being established and while awaiting surgery (if indicated). Next, it must be determined whether the tumor is sporadic or occurring as part of the MEN I syndrome by focusing on the presence of other organ involvement and family history. A clinical suspicion of MEN I warrants additional screening of the parathyroid and pituitary gland. Establishing tumor location and extent of disease should follow utilizing somatostatin receptor scintigraphy, CT scanning, and MRI. If hepatic metastases are excluded, EUS should be performed in an effort to examine the pancreas and surrounding structures in greater detail. In the case of a sporadic tumor, surgical exploration by an expert team should then follow independent of the EUS results. If the EUS is negative, the surgical team may use intraoperative ultrasound and or duodenal transillumination (depending on the local expertise) to find the lesion. A consensus regarding the surgical approach to a patient with nonmetastatic disease and MEN I has not been developed. The approach may extend from exploring all patients independent of the structural studies to operating only on those individuals with a clearly delineated tumor. If hepatic metastases are identified and the disease is limited in a patient who is otherwise healthy, some would consider local resection. Despite the list of treatment modalities that have been considered for the therapy of neuroendocrine tumors, there is still a lack of consensus regarding the timing of medical or surgical therapy in patients with metastatic disease. Some advocate using chemotherapy or combination therapy when refractory symptoms develop. Others await evidence of tumor progression by size before initiating treatment.

ACKNOWLEDGMENTS

Thanks to Carolyn Wurster for help in preparing this manuscript.

REFERENCES

1. Wilder RM, Allan FN, Power MN, et al. Carcinoma of the islands of the pancreas. Hyperinsulinism and hypoglycemia. JAMA 1927; 89:348.

2. Schein PS, DeLellis RA, Kahn CR, et al. Islet cell tumors. Current concepts and management. Ann Int Med 1973; 79:239.

3. Grimelius L, Hultquist GT, Steinkiuist B. Cytological differentiation of asymptomatic pancreatic islet cell tumors in autopsy material. Virchows Arch Pathol Anat 1975; 365:275.

4. Kaltsas GA, Besser GM, Grossman AB. The diagnosis and medical management of advanced neuroendocrine tumors. Endocr Rev 2004; 25(3):458.

   This is a timely and state-of-the-art review of the topic.

5. Jensen RT. Carcinoid and pancreatic endocrine tumors: recent advances in molecular pathogenesis, localization, and treatment. Curr Opin Oncol 2000; 12:368.

   Excellent review of the molecular pathways involved in the pathophysiology of neuroendocrine tumors.

6. Del Valle J, Scheiman JM. Zollinger-Ellison syndrome. In: Yamada T, ed. Textbook of gastroenterology. Philadelphia: JB Lippincott; 2004:1377.

7. Brandi ML. Multiple endocrine neoplasia type 1: General features and new insights into etiology. J Endocrinol Invest 1991; 14:61.

8. Trump D, Farren B, Wooding C, et al. Clinical studies of multiple endocrine neoplasia type 1 (MEN I). Q J Med 1996; 89(9):653.

9. Gibril F, Schumann M, Pace A, et al. Multiple endocrine neoplasia type 1 and Zollinger-Ellison syndrome. Medicine 2004; 83(1):43.

   Most comprehensive and up-to-date review of the relationship of Zollinger-Ellison syndrome and MEN I.

10. Chandrasekharappa S, Guru S, Manickam P, et al. Positional cloning of the gene for multiple endocrine neoplasia 1. Science 1997; 276:404.

    Original description of the cloning of the MEN I gene.

11. Jensen RT, Norton JA. Endocrine tumors of the pancreas. Pancreas 1993; sec. VI, ch. 83, 1965.

12. Jensen RT. Endocrine tumors of the pancreas. In: Yamada T, ed. Textbook of gastroenterology. Philadelphia: JB Lippincott; 2004:2108.

13. Bieligk S, Jaffee BM. Islet cell tumors of the pancreas. Surg Clin North Am 1995; 75:1025.

14. Perry RR, Vinik AI. Endocrine tumors of the gastrointestinal tract. Annu Rev Med 1996; 47:57.

15. Stabile BE, Morrow DJ, Passaro E. The gastrinoma triangle: operative implications. Am J Surg 1984;107:334.

16. Comi R, Gorden P, Doppman JL. Insulinoma. In: Go VLW, DiMagno EP, Gardner JD, et al., eds. The pancreas: biology, pathobiology, and diseases. 2nd edition. New York: Raven Press; 1993:979.

17. Leichter S. Clinical and metabolic aspects of glucagonoma. Medicine 1980; 59:100.

18. Bloom SR, Polak JM. Glucagonoma syndrome. Am J Med 1987; 82:25.

19. Wermers RA, Fatourechi V, Wynne AG, et al. The glucagonoma syndrome: Clinical and pathologic features in 21 patients. Medicine 1996; 75:53.

    Largest series of glucagonoma patients described in the literature.

20. Jensen RT, Gardner JD. Gastrinoma. In: Go VLW, DiMagno EP, Gardner JD, et al., eds. The pancreas: biology, pathobiology, and diseases. 2nd edition. New York: Raven Press; 1993:931.

21. Norton JA, Levin B, Jensen RT. Cancer of the endocrine system. In: DeVita VT, Hellman S, Rosenberg SA, eds. Cancer: principles and practice of oncology. 4th edition, vol. II. Philadelphia: JB Lippincott; 1993:1333.

22. Stabile BE, Passaro E Jr. Benign and malignant gastrinoma. Am J Surg 1985; 149:144.

23. Norton JA, Doppman JL, Jensen RT. Curative resection in patients with Zollinger-Ellison syndrome: results of a 10-year prospective study. Ann Surg 1992; 215:8.

24. Reubi JC. Peptide receptors as molecular targets for cancer diagnosis and therapy. Endocr Rev 2003; 24(4):389.

    Comprehensive, state-of-the-art review outlining the bench-to-bedside relationship between peptide hormones, their receptors, and neuroendocrine tumors.

25. Del Valle J. Application of somatostatin and its analogue octreotide in the therapy of gastrointestinal disorders. In: Wolfe MM, ed. Gastrointestinal pharmacotherapy. Philadelphia: WB Saunders; 1993:275.

26. Arnold R, Frank M, Kajdan U. Management of gastroenteropancreatic endocrine tumors: The place of somatostatin analogues. Dig Dis Sci 1994; 55:107.

27. Di Bartolomeo M, Bajetta E, Buzzoni R, et al. Clinical efficacy of octreotide in the treatment of metastatic neurodendocrine tumors. Cancer 1996; 77:402.

28. Lamberts SWJ, van der Lely A, de Herder W, et al. Octreotide. N Eng J Med 1996; 334(4):246.

    Comprehensive review of somatostatin and its analogue octreotide.

29. Ruszniewski P, Ducreux M, Chayvialle JA, et al. Treatment of the carcinoid syndrome with the long-acting somatostatin analogue lanreotide: a prospective study in 39 patients. Gut 1996; 39(2):279.

30. Harris AG, O'Dorisio TM, Woltering EA, et al. Consensus statement: Octreotide dose titration in secretory diarrhea. Diarrhea management consensus development panel. Dig Dis Sci 1995; 40:1464.

31. Garland J, Buscombe JR, Bouvier C, et al. Sandostatin LAR (long acting octreotide acetate) for malignant carcinoid syndrome: a 3 year experience. Aliment Pharmacol Ther 2003; 17:437.

32. Trendle MC, Moertel CG, Kvols LK. Incidence and morbidity of cholelithiasis in patients receiving chronic octreotide for metastatic carcinoid and malignant islet cell tumors. Cancer 1997; 79(4):830.

32. Van Heerden JA, Edis AJ, Service FJ. The surgical aspects of insulinomas. Ann Surg 1979; 189:677.

33. Tomassetti P, Salomone T, Migliori M, et al. Optimal treatment of Zollinger-Ellison syndrome and related conditions in elderly patients. Drugs Aging 2003; 20(14):1019.

34. Maton PN, Vinayek R, Frucht H, et al. Long term efficacy and safety of omeprazole in patients with Zollinger-Ellison syndrome: a prospective study. Gastroenterology 1989; 97:827.

35. Lew EA, Pisegna JR, Starr JA, et al. Intravenous pantoprazole rapidly controls gastric acid hypersecretion in patients with Zollinger-Ellison syndrome. Gastroenterology 2000; 118:696.

36. Ehrlich RM, Martin JM. Diazoxide in the management of hypoglycemia in infancy and childhood. Am J Dis Child 1969; 117:411.

37. Arnold R. Therapeutic strategies in the management of endocrine GEP tumors. Eur J Clin Invest 1990; 20(Suppl 1):S82.

38. Aomi R, Gorden P, Doppman JL. Insulinoma. In: Go VLW, Dimango EP, Gardner JD, et al., eds. The pancreas: biology, pathobiology, and diseases. 2nd edition. New York: Raven Press; 1993:979.

39. Ulbrecht JS, Schneltz R, Aarons JH, et al. Insulinoma in a 94 year old woman: long term therapy with verapamil. Diabetes Care 1986; 9:186.

40. Vinik AI, Moattari AR. Treatment of endocrine tumors. Endocrinol Metab Clin North Am 1989; 18:483.

41. Maton PN, Gardner JD, Jensen RT. Use of long-acting somatostatin analogue SMS 201-995 in patients with pancreatic islet cell tumors. Dig Dis Sci 1989; 34:285.

42. Wynick D, Bloom SR. Clinical review 23: The use of long-acting somatostatin analog octreotide in the treatment of gut neuroendocrine tumors. J Clin Endocrinol Metab 1991; 57:1590.

43. Boden G, Ryan IG, Shuman CR. Ineffectiveness of SMS 201-995 in severe hyperinsulinemias. Diabetes Care 1988; 11:664.

44. Kvols LK, Buck M, Moertel CG. Treatment of metastatic islet cell carcinoma with a somatostatin analogue (SMS 201-995). Ann Intern Med 1987; 107:162.

45. Kubota A, Yamada Y, Kagimoto S, et al. Identification of somatostatin receptor subtypes and an implication for the efficacy of somatostatin analogue SMS 201-995 in treatment of human endocrine tumors. J Clin Invest 1994; 93:1321.

46. Kraft AR, Tompkins RK, Zollinger RM. Recognition and management of the diarrheal syndrome caused by nonbeta islet cell tumors of the pancreas. Am J Surg 1970; 119:163.

47. O'Dorisio TM, Mekhjian HS. VIPoma syndrome. In: Cohen S, Soloway RD, eds. Hormone producing tumors of the pancreas. New York: Churchill-Livingstone; 1985:101.

48. O'Dorisio TM, Mekhjian HS, Gaginella TS. Medical therapy of VIPomas. Endocrinol Metab Clin North Am 1989; 18:545.

49. Charney AN, Donowitz M. Prevention and reversal of cholera enterotoxin-induced intestinal secretion by methyl prednisolone induction of Na^+/K^+-ATPase. J Clin Invest 1976; 57:1590.

50. Jaffe BM, Kopen DF, DeSchryver-Kecskemeti K, et al. Indomethacin-responsive pancreatic cholera. N Engl J Med 1977; 297:817.

51. Alburquerque RH, Owens CWI, Bloom SR. A study of vasoactive intestinal polypeptide (VIP) stimulated intestinal fluid secretion in rat and its inhibition by indomethacin. Experientia 1979; 35:1496.

52. Pandol SJ, Korman LY, McCarthy DM, et al. Beneficial effects of oral lithium carbonate in the treatment of pancreatic cholera syndrome. New Engl J Med 1980; 302:1403.

53. Smith PL, Field M. In vitro antisecretory effects of trifluoroperazine and other neuroleptics in rabbit and human small intestine. Gastroenterology 1980; 78:1545.

54. Powell DW, Field M. Pharmacological approaches to treatment of secretory diarrhea. In: Field M, Fordtran JS, Schultz SG, eds. Secretory diarrhea. Baltimore: Waverly Press; 1980:187.

55. Long RG, Barnes AJ, Adrian TE, et al. Suppression of pancreatic endocrine tumor secretion by long-acting somatostatin analogue. Lancet 1979; II:764.

56. Lennon JR, Sircus W, Bloom SR, et al. Investigation of a recurrent VIPoma. Gut 1975; 16:821.

57. Ruskone A, Rene E, Chayvialle JA, et al. Effect of somatostatin on diarrhea and on small intestinal water and electrolyte transport in a patient with pancreatic cholera. Dig Dis Sci 1982; 27:459.

58. Adrian TE, Barnes AJ, Long RG, et al. The effect of somatostatin analogs on secretion of growth, pancreatic and gastrointestinal hormones in man. J Clin Endocrinol Metab 1981; 53:675.

59. Anderson JV, Bloom SR. Neuroendocrine tumors of the gut: long term therapy with the somatostatin analogue SMS 201-995. Scand J Gastroenterol 1986; 21:115.

60. Maton PH, O'Dorisio TM, Howe BA, et al. Effect of a long-acting somatostatin analogue (201-995) in a patient with pancreatic cholera. N Engl J Med 1985; 312:17.

61. Santangelo WC, O'Dorisio TM, Kim JG, et al. Pancreatic cholera syndrome: effect of a synthetic somatostatin analogue on intestinal water and ion transport. Ann Intern Med 1985; 103:363.

62. Yoshioka M, Sakazume M, Fukawaka M, et al. A case of the watery diarrhea hypokalemia achlorhydria syndrome: successful preoperative treatment of watery diarrhea with a somatostatin analogue. J Clin Oncol (Japan) 1989; 19:294.

63. Maton PN, O'Dorisio TM, O'Dorisio MS, et al. Successful therapy of pancreatic cholera with long-acting somatostatin analogue SMS 201-995. Scan J Gastroenterol 1986; 21:181.

64. Battershill PE, Clisold SP. Octreotide. A review of its pharmacological and pharmacokinetic properties and therapeutic potential in conditions associated with excessive peptide secretion. Drugs 1989; 38:658.

65. Mozell E, Stenzel P, Woltering E, et al. Functional endocrine tumors of the pancreas: Clinical presentation, diagnosis and treatment. Curr Probl Surg 1980; 27:303.

66. Boden G, Ryan IG, Eisenschmid BL, et al. Treatment of inoperable glucagonoma with the long-acting somatostatin analogue SMS 201-995. N Engl J Med 1986; 314:1686.

67. Altimiri AF, Bhoopalam N, O'Dorisio TM, et al. Use of a somatostatin analog (SMS 201-995) in the glucagonoma syndrome. Surgery 1986; 100:989.

68. Blanchin M, Deidier AJ, Chauner-Riffaud D, et al. Utilisation de l'octreotide dans les tumeurs endocrines digestives: etude Francaise multicentreque. Presse Med 1992; 21:697.

69. Moller DE, Moses AC, Jones K, et al. Octreotide suppresses both growth hormone (GH) and GH-releasing hormone (GHRH) in acromegaly due to ectopic GHRH secretion. J Clin Endocrin Metab 1989; 68:499.

70. Von Werder K, Losa M, Stalla FK, et al. Long-term treatment of a metastasizing GRFoma with a somatostatin analogue (SMS 201-995) in a girl with gigantism. Scand J Gastroenterol 1986; 21:338.

71. Lambers SWJ. Non-pituitary actions of somatostatin: A review on the therapeutic role of SMS 201-995 (Sandostatin). Acta Endocrinol (Copenh) 1986; 276:41.

72. Wilson DM, Hoffman AR. Reduction of pituitary size by the somatostatin analogue SMS 201-995 in a patient with an islet cell tumour secreting growth hormone releasing factor. Acta Endocrinol (Copenh) 1986; 113:23.

73. Melmed S, Ziel FH, Braunstein GD, et al. Medical management of acromegaly due to ectopic production of growth hormone-releasing hormone by a carcinoid tumor. J Clin Endocrinol Metab 1988; 67:395.

74. Rösch T, Lightdale CJ, Botet JF, et al. Localization of pancreatic endocrine tumors by endoscopic ultrasonography. N Engl J Med 1992; 326:1721.

75. Thompson NW, Czako PF, Fritt LL, et al. Role of endoscopic ultrasonography in the localization of insulinomas and gastrinomas. Surgery 1994; 116(6):1131.

76. Krenning EP, Breeman WAP, Kooij PPM, et al. Localization of endocrine related tumors with radiodinated analogue of somatostatin. Lancet 1989; 1:242.

77. Gibril F, Reynolds JC, Doppman JL et al. Somatostatin receptor scintigraphy: its sensitivity compared with that of other imaging methods in detecting primary and metastatic gastrinomas. A prospective study. Ann Intern Med 1999; 125:26.

78. Chayvialle J. A comparison of imaging techniques for the localisation of gastro-enteropancreatic neuroendocrine tumors. Digestion 1996; 57(Suppl 1):54.

79. Norton JA, Jensen RT. Current surgical management of Zollinger-Ellison syndrome (ZES) in patients without multiple endocrine neoplasia-type 1 (MEN 1). Surg Oncol 2003; 12:145.

Most recent review on the surgical management of gastrinoma by two world-renowned experts in the field.

80. Grama D, Eriksson B, Martensson H, et al. Clinical characteristics, treatment and survival in patients with pancreatic tumors causing endocrine hormonal syndromes. World J Surg 1992; 16:632.

81. Reubi JC, Hacki WH, Lamberts WS. Hormone-producing gastrointestinal tumours contain high density of somatostatin receptors. J Clin Endocrinol Metab 1987; 65:1127.

82. Redding TW, Schally AV. Inhibition of growth of pancreatic carcinomas in animal models by analogs of hypothalamic hormones. Proc Natl Acad Sci USA 1984; 84:248.

83. Kvols LK, Moertel CG, O'Connell MJ. Treatment of the malignant carcinoid syndrome: evaluation of a long-acting somatostatin analogue. N Engl J Med 1986; 315:663.

84. Lamberts SW, Reubi JC, Uitterlinden P, et al. Studies on the mechanism of action of the inhibitory effect of the somatostatin analogue SMS 201-995 on the growth of the PRL/ACTH pituitary tumor 7135 a. Endocrinology 1986; 118:2188.

85. Kraenzin ME, Ch'ng JLC, Wood SM, et al. Long term treatment of a VIPoma with somatostatin analogue resulting in remission of symptoms and possible shrinkage of metastases. Gastroenterology 1985; 88:185.

86. Gorden PH. NIH Conference: somatostatin and somatostatin analogue (SMS 201-995) in treatment of hormone-secreting tumors of the pituitary and gastrointestinal tract and non-neoplastic diseases of the gut. Ann Int Med 1989; 110:35.

87. Kraenzlin ME, Ch'ng ILC, Wood SM, et al. Long-term treatment of a VIPoma with somatostatin analogue resulting in remission of symptoms and possible shrinkage of metastases. Gastroenterology 1985; 88:185.

88. Clements D, Elias E. Regression of metastatic VIPoma with somatostatin analogue SMS 201-995. Lancet 1985; I:874.

89. Shepherd JJ, Senator GB. Regression of liver metastases in patients with gastrin-secreting tumour treated with SMS 201-995. Lancet 1986; I:574.

90. Wiedenmann B, Rath U, Radsch R, et al. Tumour regression of an ileal carcinoid under the treatment with the somatostatin analogue SMS 201-995. Klin Wochensch 1988; 66:75.

91. Maton PN. Octreotide and islet cell tumors. Gastroenterol Clin North Am 1989; 18:897.

92. Shujamanesh H, Gibril F, Louie A, et al. Prospective study of the antitumor efficacy of long-term octreotide treatment in patients with progressive metastatic gastrinoma. Cancer 2002; 94(2):331.

93. Faiss S, Scherubl H, Riecken EO, et al. Drug therapy in metastatic neuroendocrine tumors of the gastroenteropancreatic system. Recent Results in Cancer Research 1996; 142:193.

94. Krenning EP, Kooij PPM, Pauwel S, et al. Somatostatin receptor: Scintigraphy and radionuclide therapy. Dig Dis Sci 1996; 57:57.

95. Buscombe JR, Caplin ME, Hilson JW. Long-term efficacy of high-activity ^{111}In-pentetreotide therapy in patients with disseminated neuroendocrine tumors. J Nuclear Med 2003; 44(1):1.

96. Oberg K, Lindstron H, Alm G. Effects of leukocyte interferon on clinical symptoms and hormone levels in patients with mid-gut carcinoid tumors and carcinoid syndrome. N Engl J Med 1983; 309:129.

97. Oberg K, Norheim I, Lind E, et al. Treatment of malignant carcinoid tumors with human leukocyte interferon: long-term results. Cancer Treat Rep 1986; 11:1297.

98. Eriksson B, Oberg K. An update of medical treatment of malignant endocrine pancreatic tumors. Acta Oncol 1993; 32:203.

99. Oberg K. Chemotherapy and biotherapy in neuroendocrine tumors. Curr Opin Oncol 1993; 5:110.

100. Anderson JV, Bloom SR. Treatment of malignant endocrine tumors with human leukocyte interferon. Lancet 1987; 1:97.

101. Pisegna JR, Slimak GG, Doppman JL, et al. An evaluation of human recombinant alpha interferon in patients with metastatic gastrinoma. Gastroenterology 1993; 105:1179.

102. Erikkson B, Obert K, Alm G, et al. Treatment of malignant endocrine pancreatic tumours with human leukocyte interferon. Lancet 1986; II:1307.

103. Creutzfeldt W, Bartsch HH, Jacubaschke U. Treatment of gastrointestinal endocrine tumours with interferon-α and octreotide. Acta Oncologica 1991; 30:529.

104. Nold R, Frank M, Kajdan U, et al. Kombinierte behandlung metastasierter neuroendokriner tumoren des gastrointestinaltrakts mit octreotid und interferon alpha. Z. Gastroenterol 1994; 32:193.

105. Saltz L, Kemeny N, Schwartz G, et al. A phase II trial of alpha-interferon and 5-fluorouracil in patients with advanced carcinoid and islet cell tumors. Cancer 1994; 74:958.

106. Herr RR, Jahnke HK, Argoudelis AD. The structure of streptozotocin. J Am Chem Soc 1967; 98:4808.

107. Moertel CG, Hanley JA, Johnson LA. Streptozotocin alone compared with streptozotocin plus fluorouracil in the treatment of advanced islet-cell carcinoma. N Engl J Med 1980; 303:1189.

108. Broder LE, Carter SK. Pancreatic islet cell carcinoma. II. Results of therapy with streptozotocin in 52 patients. Ann Intern Med 1973; 79:108.

109. Buchanan KD, O'Hare MMT, Russel CJF, et al. Factors involved in the responsiveness of gastrointestinal apudomas to streptozotocin. Dig Dis Sci 1986; 31:551S.

110. Moertel CG. An odyssey in the land of small tumors. J Clin Oncol 1987; 5:1503.

111. Bonfils S, Ruszniewski P, Haffar S, et al. Chemotherapy of hepatic metastases (HM) in Zollinger-Ellison syndrome (ZES): report of a multicentric analysis. Dig Dis Sci 1986; 31:WS51.

112. Moertel CG, Leikopoulo M, Lipsitz S, et al. Streptozotocin-doxorubicin, streptozotocin-fluorouracil, or chlorozotocin in the treatment of advanced islet cell carcinoma. N Engl J Med 1992; 326:519.

113. Hoth P, Woolley P, Green D, et al. Phase I studies on chlorozotocin. Clin Pharmacol Ther 1978; 23:712.

114. Kovach JS, Moertel CS, Schutt AJ, et al. A phase I study of chlorozotocin. Cancer 1979; 43:2189.

115. Ruszniewski PH, Hochlaf S, Rougier P, et al. Chimio-therapie intraveineuse par streptozotocin et 5-fluoro-uracile des metastases hepatiques du syndrome de Zolinger-Ellison etude prospective multicentrique chez 21 patients. Gastroenterol Clin Biol 1991; 15:393.

116. Von Schrenck T, Howard JM, Doppman JL, et al. Prospective study of chemotherapy in patients with metastatic gastrinoma. Gastroenterology 1988; 94:1326.

117. Kvols LK, Buck M. Chemotherapy of the metastatic carcinoid and islet cell tumors: A review. Am J Med 1987; 82:77.

118. Kessinger A, Lemon HM, Foley JF. The glucagonoma syndrome and its management. J Surg Oncol 1977; 9:419.

119. Prinz RA, Budrinath K, Banerji M, et al. Operations and chemotherapeutic management of malignant glucagon producing tumors. Surgery 1981; 90:713.

120. Awrich AE, Peetz M, Fletcher WS. Dimethyltriazenomidazole carboxamide therapy of islet cell carcinomas of the pancreas. J Surg Oncol 1981; 17:321.

121. Kurose T, Seino Y, Ishida LT, et al. Successful treatment of metastatic gastrinoma with dacarbazine. Lancet 1984; 1:621.

122. Valette PJ, Souquet JC. Pancreatic islet cell tumors metastatic to the liver; treatment by hepatic artery chemo-embolization. Horm Res 1989; 32:77.

123. Nesovic M, Civic J, Radojkovic S, et al. Improvement of metastatic endocrine tumors of the pancreas by hepatic artery embolization. J Endocrinol Invest 1992; 15:543.

124. Ajani JA, Carrasco CH, Charnsangavej C. Islet cell tumors metastatic to the liver: effective palliation by sequential hepatic artery embolization. Ann Intern Med 1988; 108:340.

125. Marlink RG, Lokich JJ, Robins HR. Hepatic arterial embolization for metastatic hormone-secreting tumors. Cancer 1990; 65:2227.

126. Breedis C, Young G. The blood supply of neoplasms in the liver. Am J Pathol 1954; 30:969.

127. Bierman HR, Byron RL, Kelly KH, et al. Studies on the blood supply of tumors in man: vascular patterns of the liver by hepatic arteriography in vivo. J Natl Cancer Inst 1951; 12:107.

128. Moertel CG, May GR, Martin JK, et al. Sequential hepatic artery occlusion and chemotherapy for metastatic islet carcinoid tumor and islet cell carcinoma. Proc Am Soc Clin Oncol 1985; 4:80.

129. Ruszniewski PH, Rougier P, Roche A, et al. Hepatic arterial chemoembolization in patients with liver metastases of endocrine tumors. Cancer 1993; 71:2624.

130. Mavligit GM, Pollock RE, Evans HL, et al. Durable hepatic tumor regression after arterial chemoembolization-infusion in patients with islet cell carcinoma of the pancreas metastatic to the liver. Cancer 1993; 72:375.

131. Allison DJ, Jordan H, Hennessy O. Therapeutic embolization of the liver: A review of 75 procedures. Lancet 1985; I:595.

132. Clouse ME, Lee RF. Management of the posthepatic embolization syndrome. Radiology 1984; 152:238.

133. Moertel CG, Johnson CM, McKusick MA, et al. The management of patients with advanced carcinoid tumors and islet cell carcinomas. Ann Intern Med 1994; 120:302.

134. Hansen LE, Schrumpf E, Kolbenstvedt AN, et al. Treatment of malignant metastatic midgut carcinoid tumors with recombinant human-2β interferon with or without prior hepatic artery embolization. Scand J Gastroenterol, 1989; 24:787.

135. Legaspi A, Brennan MF. Management of islet cell carcinoma. Surgery 1988; 104:1018.

136. Thompson GB, van Heerden JA, Grant CS, et al. Islet cell carcinomas of the pancreas: A twenty-year experience. Surgery 1988; 104:1011.

137. Ajani JA, Levin B, Wallace S. Systemic and regional therapy of advanced islet cell tumors. Gastroenterol Clin North Am 1989; 18:923.

138. Dial PF, Brasch JW, Rossi RL, et al. Management of nonfunctioning islet ccll tumors of the pancreas. Surg Clin North Am 1985; 65:291.

139. Danforth DN, Gordon P, Brennan MF. Metastatic insulin secreting carcinoma of the pancreas: clinical course and role of surgery. Surgery 1984; 96:1027.

140. Montenegro F, Lawrence GD, Macon W, et al. Metastatic glucagonoma – improvement after debulking. Am J Surg 1980; 139:424.

141. Thompson NW. Pancreatic islet cell tumors. In: Current surgical therapy. Cameron JL, ed. Philadelphia: BC Decker: 1985.

142. North JA, Sugarbaker PH, Doppman JL, et al. Aggressive resection of metastatic disease in selected patients with malignant gastrinoma. Ann Surg. 1986; 203:325.

143. Brennan MF, McDonald JS. Cancer of the endocrine system: treatment. In: Cancer – principle and practice in oncology. Devita VT, Hellman S, Rosenberg SA, eds. Philadelphia: JB Lippincott; 1985.

144. McEntee GP, Nagorney DM, Kwols LK, et al. Cytoreductive hepatic surgery for neuroendocrine tumors. Surgery 1990; 108:1091.

145. Murray FT, Nakhood AF, Rae L, et al. Remission of hypoglycemia after partial resection of a metastatic islet cell tumor. Am J Surg 1978; 135:846.

146. Carty SE, Jensen RT, Norton JA. Prospective study of aggressive resection of metastatic pancreatic endocrine tumors. Surgery 1992; 112:1024.

147. McEntee GP, Nagorney DM, Kvols LK, et al. Cytoreductive hepatic surgery for neuroendocrine tumors. Surgery 1990; 108:1091.

148. O'Dorisio TM, Mekhjian HS. VIPoma syndrome. In: Cohen S, Soloway RD, eds. Contemporary issues in gastroenterology. New York: Churchill Livingstone; 1984.

149. McFadden D, Jaffe BN. Surgical approaches to endocrine producing tumors of the gastrointestinal tract. In: Cohen S, Soloway RD, eds. Hormone producing tumors of the gastrointestinal tract. New York: Churchill-Livingstone, 1985:139.

150. Nagorney DM, Que FG. Cytoreductive hepatic surgery for metastatic gastrointestinal neuroendocrine tumors. Front Gastrointest Res 1995; 23:416.

151. Azoulay D, Bismuth H. Role of liver surgery and transplantation in patients with hepatic metastases from pancreatic endocrine tumors. Front Gastrointest Res 1995; 23:461.

152. Ihse I, Persson B, Tibblin S. Neuroendocrine metastases of the liver. World J Surg 1995; 19:76.

153. Pichlmayr R, Weimann A, Ringe B. Indications for liver transplantation in hepatobiliary malignancy. Hepatology 1994; 20:33S.

154. Routley D, Ramage JK, Peake JC, et al. Orthotopic liver transplantation in the treatment of metastatic neuroendocrine tumors of the liver. Liver Transplant Surg 1995; 1:118.

155. Alessiani M, Tzakis A, Todo S, et al. Assessment of five-year experience with abdominal cluster transplantation. J Am Coll Surg 1995; 180:1.

156. Le Treut YP, Delpero JR, Dousset B, et al. Results of liver transplantation in the treatment of metastatic neuroendocrine tumors. Ann Surg 1997; 225:355.

157. Juhlin C, Papanicolaou V, Arnberg H. Clinical and biochemical effects in vivo of monoclonal antitumor antibody in Verner-Morrison's syndrome. Cancer 1994; 73:1346.

158. Lissoni P, Barni S, Tancini G, et al. Immunoendocrine therapy with low-dose subcutaneous interleukin-2 plus melatonin of locally advanced or metastatic endocrine tumors. Oncology 1995; 52:163.

Section

6Six

Management of hepatic disorders

CHAPTER THIRTY-TWO

32

Treatment of hereditary hemochromatosis, Wilson disease, and other metabolic disorders of the liver

Carl L. Berg, Maureen M. Jonas and Bruce R. Bacon

INTRODUCTION

This chapter will focus on the medical and, in some cases, surgical management of the more common metabolic disorders of the liver. In addition to a discussion of the management of patients whom we see in our clinical practices, recommendations are provided for screening of asymptomatic family members when appropriate. The reader is referred also to Chapter 46, which outlines the approach to neonatal jaundice. Several of the metabolic diseases of the liver are primarily manifested as jaundice during infancy, so these topics are not repeated in this chapter. In addition, a number of metabolic diseases that persist through childhood and into adulthood (e.g., Gilbert syndrome, Crigler-Najjar syndrome type II) are also covered in Chapter 46 and will not be further reviewed in this section. The material that follows will focus on treatment of the specific diseases described and not on clinical manifestations of liver disease that are common to advanced liver disease in general (e.g., portal hypertension, ascites, spontaneous bacterial peritonitis). The reader is referred to the specific chapters that cover these topics individually for a thorough review of management of these conditions.

HEREDITARY HEMOCHROMATOSIS

Pathophysiology

Hereditary hemochromatosis (HH) represents one of the most common metabolic diseases of the liver. In populations of northern European descent, HH has been found to occur in about 1 in 250 individuals.[1–5] Undiagnosed and untreated, the disorder of total body iron overload may result in cirrhosis, hepatocellular cancer (HCC), congestive heart failure, diabetes mellitus, arthropathy, endocrinopathies, and premature death.[6,7] The mechanisms underlying the pathogenesis of the disease remain incompletely defined, although identification of the *HFE* gene[8] and its strong association with phenotypic expression of HH is resulting in an enhanced understanding of the pathogenesis of the disease.

In HH, the balance between intestinal uptake of iron and total body stores of iron is disrupted. In normal subjects, intestinal absorption of iron is upregulated in the face of iron deficiency or anemia. However, in individuals who have HH, iron absorption is increased, even in the face of elevated total body iron stores. In hemochromatosis, the initial site of excess iron deposition is in parenchymal cells of the liver,[9] where cellular injury is postulated to be the result of free radical-mediated injury and lipid peroxidation.[10] Hepatocellular injury, fibrosis, cirrhosis, and ultimately HCC may ensue. Additional iron deposition in the heart, joints, pancreas, pituitary, skin, and other organs may lead to extrahepatic manifestations of the disease.[2,11]

Epidemiology and genetics

HFE-linked HH is responsible for about 85–90% of cases of HH.[2,11] The other inherited forms of iron overload which do not involve mutations in *HFE* include juvenile HH,[12] iron overload resulting from mutations in transferrin receptor-2,[13] or ferroportin-1,[14] and African iron overload.[15] Juvenile hemochromatosis is caused either by mutations in hemojuvelin[16] or in the hepcidin gene.[17] It must be recognized that there are several other clinically distinct syndromes of iron overload that should be distinguished from the inherited syndromes of iron overload. These other disorders are grouped as secondary iron overload where there is an increase in absorption of intestinal iron that is promoted by an underlying condition other than HH.[18] Examples of such underlying conditions are syndromes of ineffective erythropoiesis such as in thalassemia, aplastic anemia, and sideroblastic anemia. Many patients with various types of chronic liver disease have mild to moderate degrees of secondary iron overload. Transfusional or parenteral iron overload can occur following blood transfusions as treatment for anemia, in the absence of blood loss. Neonatal iron overload is a rare disorder that has been recognized over the last 15–20 years which is thought to be caused by an intrauterine hepatic viral infection resulting in an excessive uptake of iron into the fetal liver (Table 32.1).[19]

HFE-linked HH is inherited as an autosomal recessive disorder whose phenotypic expression is dependent on diet, gender, and other as yet unidentified factors (probably genetic). Given the frequency of heterozygosity for C282Y of approximately 1 in 10 in the US population, an affected individual is often the offspring of two heterozygotes rather than two homozygotes or a heterozygote and a homozygote. This observation has some implications with regard to the screening of asymptomatic family members of a proband.

The gene for *HFE*-linked HH was identified in 1996.[8] *HFE* encodes for a major histocompatibility complex (MHC) class 1-like molecule that requires interaction with β2-microglobulin (β2M) for normal presentation on the surface of cells. The protein

Table 32.1 Iron overload syndromes

Iron overload syndromes

Hereditary hemochromatosis
- *HFE*-related (Type 1)
  - C282Y/C282Y
  - C282Y/H63D
  - Other *HFE* mutations
- Non-*HFE*-related
  - Juvenile HH
    - *HJV*-Hemojuvelin (Type 2, subtype A)
    - *HAMP*-Hepcidin (Type 2, subtype B)
  - *TfR*-2-related HH (Type 3)
  - Ferroportin 1-related HH (Type 4)
  - African iron overload

Secondary iron overload
- Iron-loading anemias
  - Thalassemia major
  - Sideroblastic anemia
  - Chronic hemolytic anemia
  - Aplastic anemia
  - Pyruvate kinase deficiency
  - Pyridoxine-responsive anemia
- Parenteral iron overload
  - Red blood cell transfusions
  - Iron-dextran injections
  - Long-term hemodialysis
- Chronic liver disease
  - Porphyria cutanea tarda
  - Hepatitis C
  - Hepatitis B
  - Alcoholic liver disease
  - Nonalcoholic steatohepatitis
  - Following portocaval shunt
- Dysmetabolic iron overload syndrome

Miscellaneous
- Neonatal iron overload
- Aceruloplasminemia
- Congenital atransferrinemia

has a single peptide binding domain, an immunoglobulin-like domain, a single transmembrane region, and a short cytoplasmic tail. At least three missense mutations have been identified in *HFE*. One results in a change of cysteine to tyrosine at position 282 (C282Y); a second results in a change in histidine to aspartate at amino acid position 63 (H63D); and the third results in a change of serine to cysteine at amino acid position 65 (S65C) Homozygosity for the C282Y mutation has been identified in approximately 90% of individuals who have typical phenotypic HH.[20] The clinical impact of the H63D and S65C mutations is small.

Family screening and population screening

It is recommended that all first-degree relatives of an identified proband be screened for HH, including siblings, parents, and children. Certainly, this recommendation could be extended to include aunts, uncles, and cousins as well (Fig. 32.1). Genetic testing with *HFE* mutation analysis has replaced HLA-typing and is now used as the preferred method for family screening. Many physicians obtain transferrin saturation, ferritin, and *HFE* mutation analysis all at the same time. If there is an elevated ferritin level indicating increased iron stores in a C282Y homozygote or a compound heterozygote (C282Y/H63D), it is reasonable to proceed to therapeutic phlebotomy to deplete excess iron stores without a liver biopsy as long as liver enzymes are normal and the ferritin is less than 1000 ng/mL.[21,22]

Similarly, when patients are identified by a positive genetic test outside of the context of a family history, when there is an elevated transferrin saturation or ferritin, they should be treated accordingly. If there is an increased ferritin level in the absence of elevated liver enzymes, patients should be offered treatment with therapeutic phlebotomy. A liver biopsy is not needed in this situation. It has been debated as to whether genetic testing should be used as a general population screening technique.[23] Several recent studies have shown that when *HFE* mutation analysis as well as iron studies have been done prospectively in large general populations, the prevalence of phenotypic expression in C282Y homozygotes has been around 50% (Table 32.2).[20,24] Thus, a plan to screen the entire population would identify many individuals and 'label' them as C282Y homozygotes with the 'potential' for iron overload, which might never be realized. Theoretically, this could lead to genetic discrimination with possible psychological and/or economic consequences. At present, there are no recommendations for generalized population screening

Treatment of hereditary hemochromatosis

Once the diagnosis of HH is fully established, physicians must turn their responsibility to insuring that patients are adequately treated and that family screening (see above) is performed. Treatment is simple, effective, inexpensive, and safe. Patients should be encouraged to have weekly therapeutic phlebotomy of 500 mL of whole blood. This is equivalent to approximately 200 to 250 mg of iron, depending upon the hemoglobin concentration of the blood removed. Some patients can tolerate twice-weekly phlebotomy, and reports from older literature describe patients who tolerated phlebotomy three times per week; however, this is tedious and often inconvenient. Monthly phlebotomy should not be recommended unless patients cannot tolerate phlebotomy more frequently. Therapeutic phlebotomy should be performed until patients develop iron-limited erythropoiesis, which is identified by the failure of the hemoglobin or hematocrit level to recover before the next phlebotomy. It is reasonable to monitor transferrin saturation and ferritin levels periodically to predict the return to normal iron stores and to provide a method of encouragement to patients who are undergoing phlebotomy. However, some physicians treat patients until they are anemic and then reorder iron studies. Therapeutic phlebotomy is continued until the transferrin saturation is less than 50% and serum ferritin levels are less than 50 ng/mL; some clinicians recommend bringing the ferritin level down to less than 20 ng/mL. It is not necessary for patients

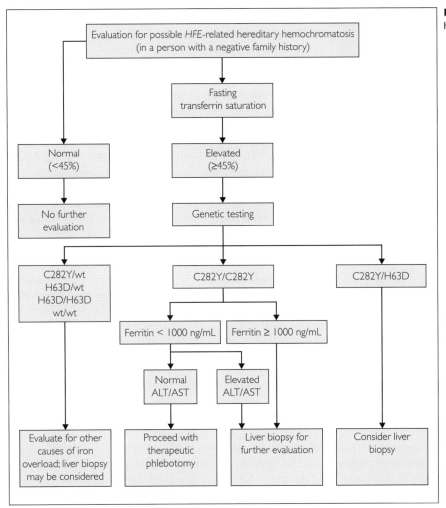

Fig. 32.1 • Evaluation for possible *HFE*-related hereditary hemochromatosis.

to become anemic; rather, the desired end point is for them to be depleted of their excess iron stores. Most patients tolerate therapeutic phlebotomy quite well and actually have a sense of improved well-being after the initial phlebotomies have been completed. If liver enzymes have been abnormal, they will characteristically return to normal once iron stores have been depleted; however, established cirrhosis does not reverse.[25] There are some reports of portal fibrosis improving with phlebotomy therapy. Other benefits of therapeutic phlebotomy include: reduction of skin pigmentation, improvement in cardiac function, reduction of insulin

requirements in those patients who are diabetic, reduction in portal hypertension in those patients who are cirrhotic, reduction in abdominal pain, and an improved energy level and sense of well-being (Table 32.3). Conditions that characteristically do not reverse with phlebotomy include testicular atrophy, established cirrhosis, and arthropathy.

Once the initial therapeutic phlebotomy has been completed, and patients have been successfully depleted of their excess iron stores, most patients will require maintenance phlebotomy of one unit of blood to be removed every 2–3 months. Because most

Table 32.2 Prevalence of C282Y homozygotes without iron overload in screening studies

Population sample	Country	Number	C282Y homozygotes	C282Y homozygotes with a normal ferritin (%)
Electoral roll	New Zealand	1,064	1 in 213	40
Primary care	USA	1,653	1 in 276	50
Epidemiological survey	Australia	3,011	1 in 188	25
Blood donors	Canada	4,211	1 in 327	81
General public	USA	41,038	1 in 270	33
Total		50,977	1 in 255	46

Table 32.3 Response to phlebotomy therapy in hereditary hemochromatosis

Reduction of excessive tissue iron stores

Improved survival, if diagnosis and treatment before development of cirrhosis and diabetes

Improved sense of well-being, energy level

Improved cardiac function

Improved control of diabetes

Reduction in abdominal pain

Reduction in skin pigmentation

Normalization of elevated liver enzymes

Reversal of hepatic fibrosis (approximately 30% of cases)

No reversal of established cirrhosis

Reduction in portal hypertension in cirrhotics

No (or only minimal) improvement in arthropathy

No reversal of testicular atrophy

patients with HH absorb approximately 2–3 milligrams of iron per day in excess of their daily requirement, they will accumulate an excess of approximately 250 mg of iron over a 3-month period. This is balanced by the 250 mg of iron that is removed from a single phlebotomy; thus, maintenance phlebotomy every 3 months is usually adequate. Some patients absorb more than the 2–3 mg of iron per day and thus require maintenance phlebotomy more often. It is unusual for patients to require maintenance phlebotomy more often than every 2 months. Occasionally, a few patients who have been accurately diagnosed (i.e., homozygosity for the C282Y mutation) do not reaccumulate iron for reasons that are unclear. These patients are usually older and the presumption is that their efficiency of iron absorption has been diminished with age; however, when this situation occurs, patients should be evaluated for occult blood loss from the gastrointestinal tract.

Iron chelating agents

In circumstances in which phlebotomy is not appropriate or rapid iron depletion is contraindicated, the drug most commonly used for iron chelation in patients with HH (and other conditions resulting in iron overload, such as thalassemia), has been deferoxamine mesylate. This agent is capable of preferentially chelating parenchymal iron stores. The drug enters cells such as hepatocytes, complexes with iron that is reductively released from ferritin and hemosiderin, and is then excreted from the cell in the form of feroxamine.[26] The chelated iron is excreted from the body primarily in urine, although some enhanced iron excretion may also occur via bile and is eliminated in feces.[26]

Deferoxamine is not orally active and must be administered parenterally. The plasma half-life of the intravenously administered drug is measured in minutes, and thus the compound is typically given by slow overnight subcutaneous infusion. Doses of 1–2 g of deferoxamine per day, infused subcutaneously over a period of 8–12 hours, are frequently used,[27] although more recent studies also support experience with higher dosages of up to 50 mg/kg/day.[28] If administered intravenously, slow infusion is

necessary to avoid hypotension. Daily iron depletion of 20–30 mg can be expected. The disadvantages of the use of deferoxamine relate to its cumbersome mode of administration, which often leads to patient noncompliance, the high cost of therapy (≈US$40 000 per year for home treatment), the relatively modest amount of iron removed each day, and reported side effects. Some controversy exists about whether deferoxamine predisposes to bacterial and/or fungal infections or whether the occurrence of these infections in such patients is related to their underlying iron overload.[29–33] Ocular and auditory abnormalities have also been noted in patients treated with deferoxamine, particularly with high-dose chronic chelation.[34] Fortunately, these abnormalities have typically been reversible with cessation of therapy. Periodic testing of visual acuity, slit lamp examination for cataracts, and audiometric testing are recommended for patients receiving long-term therapy. Further, base-line examinations of visual and auditory acuity should be done prior to initiating therapy in order to have a frame of reference.

Given the drawbacks of deferoxamine therapy, it is not surprising that significant research efforts have been directed towards the development of alternative iron chelating agents. Specifically, the availability of an orally active compound would greatly simplify therapy for patients with anemia and secondary iron overload.[35] One such compound, a hydroxypyrid-4-one, has been investigated in Europe, Canada, and India.[28,36–39] Daily iron losses in response to this drug are similar to those observed with deferoxamine;[28] however, enthusiasm regarding the use of this class of compounds has been restrained as recognition of side effects has emerged.[39] Adverse effects include neutropenia, agranulocytosis, arthralgias, and the development of systemic lupus erythematosus-like syndrome.[40,41] Ongoing research involving related orally effective agents continues, and it is likely that one or more of these agents will ultimately prove to be efficacious.[35]

Given the relative disadvantage of these chelating agents and their limited ability to remove large amounts of systemic iron, these compounds will continue to play a relatively limited role in the management of HH. In patients with concomitant cardiomyopathy or a cardiac arrhythmia secondary to hemochromatosis, one may consider deferoxamine therapy as an adjunct to phlebotomy to enhance the rate of initial iron depletion and to potentially detoxify cellular 'free' iron. In addition, in the rare patient with hemochromatosis who has anemia as a result of chronic liver disease, renal failure, or other systemic conditions, iron chelation may be an important option for iron reduction.

Orthotopic liver transplantation

Orthotopic liver transplantation (OLT) is a management option for some patients for whom HH is diagnosed late in the course of their disease. It is uncommon for patients with decompensated cirrhosis resulting from HH to regain significant hepatic function in the setting of successful iron depletion. Thus, patients in whom HH is diagnosed in the setting of decompensated cirrhosis should be evaluated for liver transplantation. In addition to the usual assessment of general medical fitness for transplantation, which is standard for all patients, particular emphasis should be directed to assessment of cardiac disease, which may increase post-transplant morbidity and mortality in these patients. Historical evidence suggesting the presence of arrhythmias should be sought, and it is the practice of some clinicians to obtain an assessment of left ventricular function in *all* patients with HH independent of clinical symptoms of heart failure when being considered for liver transplantation. Although few data exist regarding the role of iron depletion in patients awaiting a liver transplant for hemochromatosis, it is important to reduce the frequency of post-transplant infections and cardiac complications.

Even though recurrent disease in the allograft does not appear to develop in patients with HH, these patients nonetheless have diminished survival rates in comparison to patients who undergo liver transplantation for most other forms of liver disease.[42–46] The principal reasons for this diminished survival are usually related to unrecognized cardiac disease and an increased propensity for infections in patients who were untreated prior to transplant.[43] Patients who are successfully de-ironed prior to transplant have a successful outcome comparable to transplant for other disorders. Patients with HH and cirrhosis have a significantly increased risk of HCC. In one series, HCC was identified in the explant organs of 27% of patients who received transplants for HH.[42] Although the presence of such tumors did not affect survival 1 year post-transplant, thorough preoperative screening for HCC is important in HH patients being evaluated for liver transplantation.

WILSON DISEASE

Pathophysiology

Wilson disease, a disorder of excessive hepatic copper overload, is distributed worldwide and has a disease prevalence of approximately 1 in 30 000 live births. It has long been recognized that the primary defect in this disease is associated with excessive copper accumulation in the liver. Advances in the molecular genetics of Wilson disease have resulted in the identification of a gene on chromosome 13, designated *ATP7b*.[47,48] The gene encodes a cation-transporting P-type adenosinetriphosphatase (Wilson disease ATPase) that is expressed in the liver, kidney, and placenta.[47,48] mRNA for the protein is also present to a lesser degree in the heart, brain, lung, muscle, and pancreas.[49] Mutations in ATP7b result in disordered export of copper from the liver into bile, with resultant accumulation of the cation in hepatocytes. The ATP7b protein is present primarily in the trans-Golgi,[50,51] where it is critical for excretion of copper into bile, as well as providing appropriate copper for binding to ceruloplasmin. Lack of a functional ATP7b limits the availability of copper for ultimate incorporation into ceruloplasmin. When copper is not available for binding to ceruloplasmin, an apoprotein is secreted from the hepatocytes that is rapidly degraded in the plasma,[52] resulting in the hallmark of the condition, diminished circulating ceruloplasmin levels.

Screening of family members

To date, more than 200 different mutations in the Wilson gene have been identified,[53] in marked contrast to the limited mutations in *HFE* (see earlier). In this circumstance, confirmation of the diagnosis in a proband patient must still rely on standard biochemical testing (e.g., serum ceruloplasmin, quantitative hepatic copper determination, urinary copper determination, etc.). Once a proband case has been definitively identified as having Wilson disease, it may be possible to screen siblings on the basis of genetic analysis, although this technology is not widely

available. As an autosomal recessive disorder, one in four siblings may be expected to be homozygous for the gene defect. Genetic testing of siblings requires the sequencing of both alleles of the ATP7b gene in the proband and then subsequent comparison of those alleles to the ATP7b alleles in siblings.[54,55] The ATP7b allele sequences in affected siblings should be identical to those in the proband patient.

Treatment of Wilson disease

Dietary therapy

Dietary therapy plays only a minor role in the management of Wilson disease. The ubiquitous presence of copper in food makes complete elimination of copper from the diet impractical. Nonetheless, it is reasonable to limit the ingestion of foods that are particularly high in dietary copper, such as shellfish, legumes, nuts, mushrooms, chocolate, and liver. Vegetarians with Wilson disease should be counseled regarding the copper content of their diet inasmuch as ingestion of large amounts of legumes in such a diet may lead to considerable copper ingestion. It has also been suggested that the copper content of a patient's drinking water supply be analyzed, although few firm data support this recommendation. If testing is performed, deionized or distilled water may be recommended if the copper content of the drinking water exceeds 1 ppm.[53] Domestic water softeners should be avoided because they may substantially increase the copper content of drinking water.[56]

Copper chelating agents
D-penicillamine

Since its introduction as a therapeutic agent for the medical management of Wilson disease by Walshe in 1956,[57] D-penicillamine has remained the first-line pharmacologic agent (Table 32.4), although recent practice guidelines have recognized the role of trientine as an alternative first-line chelating agent.[58] In the setting of Wilson disease, the primary long-term mechanism of action of D-penicillamine appears to be hepatic 'decoppering' related to the chelating properties of the drug.[59] The marked enhancement of cupuresis, resolution of Kayser-Fleischer rings, and diminution of hepatic copper content in the majority of patients with Wilson disease treated with this agent support this mode of action.[60,61] However, identification of a series of patients treated with D-penicillamine in whom no significant reduction in hepatic copper concentration occurred despite up to 18 years of therapy[62] led to the investigation of other potential mechanisms of copper detoxification. These postulated mechanisms include sequestration of toxic hepatocellular copper in an innocuous form, either by the formation of copper complexes directly with D-penicillamine or by the induction of metallothionein in hepatocytes, a protein capable of sequestering intracellular copper.[63,64] Other potential mechanisms of action include inhibition of collagen cross-linking,[65] suppression of inflammation,[66] and enhancement of intracellular reduced glutathione levels.[67]

The usual dose of D-penicillamine for the initial treatment of Wilson disease is 1–2 g given daily in two divided doses, although as much as 3 g/day may be administered to critically ill patients for brief periods. The medication is best administered on an empty stomach since food reduces its systemic absorption. It should always be given in conjunction with 25 mg of pyridoxine daily

Table 32.4 Pharmacologic therapy for Wilson disease

Therapeutic agent	Typical adult dosage	Mechanism of action
D-penicillamine	1–2 g in 2 divided doses	Chelation of copper Induction of metallothionein
Trientine hydrochloride	1–2 g in 3 divided doses	Chelation of copper
Zinc sulfate/acetate	150 mg Zn in 3 divided doses between meals	Induction of metallothionein
Tetrathiomolybdate	60–100 mg in 2 divided doses	Chelation of copper

because penicillamine has an antipyridoxine effect. The majority of excess hepatic copper will be mobilized within the first year of therapy,[60] and typical urinary copper excretion during this initial 'decoppering' period should measure 2–4 mg/day. Some patients will respond dramatically within weeks of beginning D-penicillamine therapy, whereas others will exhibit no clinical improvement for some months. Complete reversal or alleviation of hepatic, neurologic, and psychiatric abnormalities can be anticipated in patients treated early in the course of their disease. After completion of at least several years of D-penicillamine treatment, once symptoms have largely abated and a stable clinical course has been achieved, the maintenance dose of D-penicillamine may be reduced to 0.5 g twice per day. It is anticipated that urinary copper concentrations at this point in a patient's course will fall within the range of 0.3–1.0 mg/day. Even with complete resolution of symptoms and normalization of biochemical abnormalities related to Wilson disease, it is essential to continue uninterrupted, lifelong therapy because acute hepatic deterioration, which may be fatal, has been noted in patients in whom D-penicillamine therapy has been discontinued for some months.[68] As noted below, however, there is a trend among experts to convert some patients from a chelating agent such as D-penicillamine to chronic zinc therapy once stabilization has occurred.[58]

An important caveat regarding the initiation of D-penicillamine therapy for the treatment of Wilson disease is the recognition of an uncommon syndrome of acute neurologic deterioration, which has been reported in some patients with pre-existing neurologic abnormalities and in presymptomatic individuals.[69,70] Neurologic deterioration, if it occurs, typically develops within the first 4 weeks of therapy.[70] One approach to the management of such a deterioration is reduction of the dose of D-penicillamine. The dose may then be increased progressively by 250 mg/day every 4–7 days until a 24-h urinary copper excretion of at least 2 mg is attained.[70] Alternatively, trientine may be employed in such a circumstance as it has been less frequently associated with neurologic decompensation.

D-penicillamine therapy for Wilson disease is generally well tolerated and serious complications are infrequent (Table 32.5). In up to 20% of patients, however, sensitivity reactions may develop within the first month of therapy.[63] These reactions typically include fever, malaise, pruritus, rash, and less often, lymphadenopathy, leukopenia, or thrombocytopenia.[71,72] Historically, discontinuation of the medication, followed by its reinstitution in low doses (250 mg/day), occasionally in conjunction with steroids, has been recommended as this will generally lead to desensitization. The dose of D-penicillamine may then be increased gradually over a 1-month period. With increasing experience with other chelating agents such as trientine, it is now recommended that in the setting of D-penicillamine hypersensitivity, conversion to trientine should be contemplated.[58] Other reactions to D-penicillamine, which may occur in 5–7% of patients,[63] include penicillamine dermatopathy,[73] lupus, pemphigus, agranulocytosis, aplastic anemia, arthralgias, neuromyotonia, a Goodpasture-like syndrome, depression of serum IgA levels, and aphthous ulcerations.[71] Loss of taste for sweet and salt has also been documented.[74] Thus, continued clinical follow-up in conjunction with routine urinalysis and blood counts is recommended, even in stable patients receiving chronic D-penicillamine therapy. Successful pregnancy has been described in women treated with D-penicillamine for Wilson disease,[75,76] and the drug should be continued during pregnancy, particularly in light of the potential hazards associated with its discontinuation, as noted earlier.

Triethylene tetramine dihydrochloride (trientine)

In patients who develop side effects to D-penicillamine or in patients for whom chelating therapy is being initiated, consideration may be given to the therapeutic agent triethylene tetramine dihydrochloride, or trientine (Syprine).[68,77,78] The mechanism of action of this oral chelator, which was approved by the Food and Drug Administration in 1985, remains uncertain,[77] although the drug appears to be capable of promoting cupuresis and reducing the intestinal absorption of copper. Administered in dosages of 750–1500 mg/day in two or three divided doses, the drug has been used continuously in some patients for up to 16 years.[77]

Table 32.5 Potential side effects of D-penicillamine therapy

Acute sensitivity reaction

Penicillamine dermatopathy

Systemic lupus erythematosus

Aplastic anemia

Agranulocytosis

Arthralgias

Neuromyotonia

Diminished serum IgA levels

Aphthous ulceration

Goodpasture-like syndrome

Loss of taste

Maintenance dosing consists of 750–1000 mg/day in divided doses. Administration 1 hour prior to, or 2 hours after, meals is recommended to enhance absorption. Adequacy of therapy is monitored by 24-hour urine collection, with urinary copper levels in the setting of adequate therapy reaching 200–500 μg/d. Side effects have been minimal and consist primarily of mild anemia (described variously as secondary to iron deficiency[78] or as a sideroblastic anemia[68]). Administration with iron should be avoided as the iron-trientine complex may be toxic.[58] Although long-term clinical follow-up of patients with Wilson disease treated with triethylene tetramine dihydrochloride is available, other data regarding hepatic copper concentration in treated patients remain incomplete. After conversion from D-penicillamine to trientine therapy in patients experiencing D-penicillamine side effects, the majority of the side effects will resolve. The exception to this statement regards elastosis perforans serpiginosa, an acneiform papular skin lesion that may progress in patients despite conversion to trientine therapy. As outlined above, therapy with trientine should be continuous, without interruption. Conversion to zinc monotherapy may be considered after extensive chelation has occurred.

Zinc

Oral zinc therapy has been proposed as a therapeutic modality for the management of Wilson disease and was approved by the FDA for such an indication in 1997. At least two mechanisms may be responsible for the reported mitigation of copper toxicity by zinc. The first putative mechanism of action, based on data derived from animal models, is related to the induction of metallothionein synthesis in intestinal epithelial cells. Metallothionein is a protein capable of sequestering copper (and other selected metals) and may thus diminish the absorption of copper from the intestinal tract.[79] A second mechanism of action has been postulated from studies in cultured hepatocytes.[80] Zinc pretreatment has been demonstrated to markedly improve hepatocyte viability in the presence of copper, probably as a consequence of enhanced hepatocyte metallothionein synthesis with a concomitant reduction in free copper toxicity.[80]

Despite these experimental studies of the effect of zinc on hepatic copper toxicity and metabolism, experience with this medication as first-line therapy for Wilson disease remains somewhat limited.[81–88] Based on the ability of 50 mg of zinc given either as zinc sulfate or, preferably, zinc acetate orally three times per day between meals to maintain neutral or negative copper balance, a role certainly exists for zinc supplementation in a previously decoppered patient. Thorough documentation of hepatic copper concentrations after long-term zinc therapy, however, remains incomplete, and several reports have suggested increasing hepatic copper levels when zinc administration was the sole mode of therapy.[60,81,84] The role of zinc monotherapy as initial and sole therapy for the treatment of the newly diagnosed Wilson disease patient remains somewhat controversial. Recent AASLD practice guidelines recommend chelation therapy as the primary treatment regimen, but recognize the potential role for zinc monotherapy in the asymptomatic or pre-symptomatic patient. The largest group of such patients studied have tended to have neurologic disease where concerns about progression of neurologic dysfunction with chelation have been appropriately raised. In this setting, zinc therapy may be as effective as D-penicillamine, with fewer side effects.[89,90] Additionally, oral zinc therapy may

serve as an adjunct to standard chelation treatment with D-penicillamine or trientine, although at least one report has raised theoretical concerns regarding the formation of zinc-penicillamine complexes, which may diminish or abolish the therapeutic effectiveness of both drugs when used in combination.[91] When employed as an adjunct to chelation therapy, several hours between zinc and chelation treatment dosing should be recommended. Treatment of patients with hepatic decompensation with a combination of a trientine and zinc has been successful in a limited number of patients, and was followed by conversion to zinc monotherapy after 4 or more months.[92]

Tetrathiomolybdate

Tetrathiomolybdate is an agent that has been studied in a limited number of patients with Wilson disease, and is not commercially available for use in North America.[60,93] Its use in copper overload has been based on the observation that dietary molybdenum results in a state of copper deficiency in ruminants.[94] Thiomolybdates appear to lower systemic copper levels by complexing with intestinal copper, thereby interfering with intestinal absorption of copper. In addition, tetrathiomolybdate may form complexes with copper in the blood[93] and thereby render systemic copper nontoxic. When compared with metallothionein in vitro, the thiomolybdates exhibit a higher affinity for copper, which suggests that these drugs may be capable of removing even bound copper from hepatocytes. Use of tetrathiomolybdate has been demonstrated to result in diminished hepatic copper concentrations,[60,94] thus supporting the aforementioned putative mechanisms of action. Tetrathiomolybdate administered in doses of 60–100 mg/day as ammonium tetrathiomolybdate in two divided doses has been used in the clinical studies reported to date. Of note, tetrathiomolybdate has been used successfully in patients with neurologic Wilson disease without precipitation or worsening of neurologic signs or symptoms.[95] Although the drug is generally well tolerated, at least two cases of bone marrow suppression have been documented.[96] Further clinical trials are thus needed before tetrathiomolybdate may join D-penicillamine, trientine, and zinc as primary therapies for Wilson disease.

Orthotopic liver transplantation

Despite advances in medical therapy and improved clinical recognition of Wilson disease, fulminant hepatic failure will still develop in a number of patients,[97] either as an initial manifestation of the disease or as a consequence of noncompliance with medical therapy. An additional smaller subset of patients will have cirrhosis and hepatic decompensation unresponsive to the medical interventions just outlined. In such patients, OLT should be considered. In a review of 55 patients undergoing liver transplantation for Wilson disease, the 1-year survival rate was found to be 79%.[98] Replacement of the affected liver expressing mutant *ATP7b* with a donor organ that expresses the normal Wilson gene protein product can be expected to correct the defect in hepatic copper metabolism. Thus, the allograft is not susceptible to ongoing copper accumulation. Resolution of the extrahepatic manifestations of Wilson disease after OLT, however, has been less than universal.[99,100] Thus, transplantation in the absence of decompensated liver disease and solely for management of extrahepatic disease such as neurologic deficits is not routinely recommended.

α_1-ANTITRYPSIN DEFICIENCY

Pathophysiology

α_1-Antitrypsin deficiency results in diminished serum levels of the major serum inhibitor of neutrophil elastase, α_1-antitrypsin. More than 75 allelic variants of this protein are known and are named according to the position of migration of the α_1-antitrypsin molecule on isoelectric focusing gels.[101] The common 'normal' alleles are designated M, and the most common 'at risk' alleles are designated Z and S and confer increased risk for the development of emphysema in the homozygous state. Chronic liver disease is also clearly recognized to develop in individuals who are homozygous for the Z or Null$_{Hong Kong}$ alleles. The mechanisms involved in the development of liver disease in ZZ homozygotes have been at least partially delineated. The Z mutation involves a single-base substitution in exon V of the normal M1 allele causing a Glu 342 Lys substitution in the α_1-antitrypsin molecule.[102] This amino acid substitution reduces the stability of α_1-antitrypsin in the monomeric form and favors the generation of α_1-antitrypsin polymers within the endoplasmic reticulum of hepatocytes (and other cells) where α_1-antitrypsin is synthesized.[103,104] Accumulation of this mutant α_1-antitrypsin molecule results in liver damage by undefined mechanisms. Recent studies have demonstrated that in addition to carrying the ZZ mutation, individuals with this mutation in whom significant liver disease develops may also have a lag in endoplasmic reticulum degradation of the mutant α_1-antitrypsin molecules that confers susceptibility to subsequent liver injury.[105]

Whether individuals with an MZ Pi type are at increased risk for liver disease remains controversial. Although periodic acid-Schiff-positive, diastase-resistant globules, which are characteristic of α_1-antitrypsin, may be seen on histologic examination of livers from MZ patients, the majority of these patients will not have clinically significant liver disease.

Treatment of α_1-antitrypsin deficiency

Enzyme replacement therapy

Although enzyme replacement therapy has been used in an attempt to decrease the impact of α_1-antitrypsin deficiency on the progression of pulmonary disease, no data suggest that this approach has any effect on progression of the associated liver disease. Based on the observation that liver disease develops only in patients with α_1-antitrypsin mutations that lead to the accumulation of α_1-antitrypsin globules within the hepatocyte, it is reasonable to postulate that systemic enzyme replacement would not have any impact on the development of progressive liver disease.[105]

Orthotopic liver transplantation

OLT has been performed successfully in patients with α_1-antitrypsin deficiency. Survival rates and complications have been similar to those reported for OLT in general.[92] Obviously, careful assessment of pulmonary function must be undertaken in patients with α_1-antitrypsin deficiency who are being evaluated for OLT. The precise timing at which such transplant evaluation should be performed remains controversial inasmuch as the reported natural history of liver disease associated with α_1-antitrypsin deficiency may be quite variable.[105,106] However, careful monitoring of hepatic function is recommended, with consideration of referral to a transplant center once abnormal bilirubin levels and prothrombin times have been identified.

Gene therapy

At the present time, only a conceptual framework for the prevention or definitive treatment of α_1-antitrypsin deficiency-associated liver disease exists. With enhanced understanding of the mechanisms that control the production of mutant α_1-antitrypsin molecules, as well as the folding of such molecules and their degradation, it may become possible to prevent the development of liver disease in patients with α_1-antitrypsin deficiency. Successful strategies in this regard may involve manipulation of hepatocellular α_1-antitrypsin synthesis (e.g., by manipulating the SEC receptor,[105] avoidance of pyrexia[104]), prevention of abnormal protein folding by peptide delivery to the endoplasmic reticulum,[104,105] or regulation of mutant protein degradation.[105]

HEREDITARY TYROSINEMIA (TYROSINEMIA TYPE I)

Pathophysiology and clinical features

Tyrosinemia is an inborn error of amino acid metabolism caused by a deficiency of fumarylacetoacetate hydrolase (FAH), an enzyme required for tyrosine degradation. Although tyrosine and its early metabolites have no significant toxicity, the metabolic products immediately preceding FAH, fumarylacetoacetate and its derivatives succinylacetoacetate (SAA) and succinylacetone (SA), have known biologic toxicity. Clinical manifestations of tyrosinemia include severe hepatic dysfunction in infancy (early cirrhosis, ascites, coagulopathy), renal disease (Fanconi's syndrome, nephromegaly), and neurologic crises typical of acute intermittent porphyria; these adverse effects are caused by inhibition of porphobilinogen synthase by SA, which allows 5-aminolevulinic acid to accumulate. The mechanism of hepatic disease has not been elucidated, but direct tissue injury by SAA and SA is postulated. Tyrosinemia carries a very high risk of HCC beginning around the age of 3 years; by age 5, HCC has developed in about 36% of affected children.[107]

Tyrosinemia is an autosomal recessive disorder. The human gene for FAH has been sequenced and mapped to chromosome 15q23-q25.[108] The incidence of tyrosinemia is approximately 1 in 100 000 to 120 000 live births, and it has been reported in many ethnic groups. In some populations of Quebec, rates as high as 1 in 2000 have been observed as the result of a founder effect. The diagnosis of tyrosinemia should be suspected in infants or children with unexplained cirrhosis and coagulopathy, renal tubular dysfunction, or neurologic symptoms. It is most easily demonstrated by the presence of SA in plasma or in urine (hypertyrosinemia itself is not diagnostic because it may be associated with all forms of hepatic dysfunction or other inborn errors). Serum alpha-fetoprotein levels are often markedly elevated. FAH activity may be assayed in lymphocytes, erythrocytes, or liver tissue.

Treatment of hereditary tyrosinemia

Dietary therapy

The principles of dietary therapy for tyrosinemia are twofold: (1) restriction of tyrosine and its precursor phenylalanine to minimize the amount degraded to toxic metabolites, and (2) provision of adequate calories to avoid catabolism and the release of endogenous tyrosine and phenylalanine, especially under conditions of metabolic stress. This goal is accomplished with high-carbohydrate, low-protein formulas. Other amino acids and micronutrients must be provided in amounts necessary to support growth. Once the high plasma levels of tyrosine and methionine typical of this disease begin to improve, tyrosine and phenylalanine intake is titrated to achieve a normal plasma tyrosine level.

Although neurologic symptoms and renal dysfunction may improve with dietary therapy, its effect on hepatic disease is less certain. Liver dysfunction may begin prenatally, even when the placenta maintains amino acid levels in the physiologic range.[109] In addition, progression of hepatic disease despite adequate dietary management is well documented.[110] Thus, dietary treatment alone is insufficient for the management of this disorder.

Metabolic therapy

Treatment of hereditary tyrosinemia has been revolutionized by the use of a metabolic inhibitor that acts early in the tyrosine degradation pathway (inhibiting 4-hydroxyphenylpyruvate dioxygenase) to prevent formation of the toxic intermediates SAA and SA. This inhibitor, called NTBC (2-{2-nitro-4-trifluoromethylbenzolyl]-1,3-cyclohexanedione), was first used in 1992 in five children with tryosinemia.[111] After 7–9 months, these patients had normal liver enzymes and coagulation studies, a decrease in alpha-fetoprotein levels, and no SA excretion. No toxicity was demonstrated. This report has led to widespread clinical trials that have largely reproduced the original experience, and more than 300 children with tyrosinemia have been treated, with subsequent stabilization of hepatic and renal function, improvement in growth and nutritional parameters, and delay or avoidance of liver transplantation. This drug has been licensed as nitisinone (trade name Orfadin®). Although enthusiasm for this treatment has been somewhat tempered by the demonstration that NTBC administration corrects the hepatic and renal abnormalities in knockout mice deficient in FAH activity but does not prevent all of the SA accumulation or the development of HCC,[112] it is considered the standard of care for the treatment of hereditary tyrosinemia, in addition to the dietary measures discussed above.[113] At the present time, the most prudent therapy for tyrosinemia is the institution of nitisinone and dietary therapy at the time of diagnosis. One milligram/kilogram (mg/kg) daily is recommended initially in two divided doses. Subsequent dose adjustments should be based on monitoring of erythrocyte porphobilinogen synthase activity, urine succinylacetone, and urinary 5-aminolevulinic acid, with the goal of normalizing porphyrin metabolism (reflected by normal erythrocyte porphobilinogen synthase activity and urine 5-ALA) and producing undetectable levels of urine succinylacetone. Close medical and radiographic monitoring is suggested for hepatic nodules that may herald early HCC, since a small percentage of children begun on therapy late in the course of disease have developed HCC despite treatment.[114]

Liver transplantation

Liver transplantation is considered the definitive therapy for hereditary tyrosinemia. Hepatic replacement not only cures the chronic hepatic dysfunction and obviates the concern about HCC

but also reverses the renal and central nervous system abnormalities.[115] However, the optimal timing of hepatic transplantation has not been clearly defined, especially in view of the metabolic therapy that has become available. As further data on long-term outcome of metabolic therapy become available, it may become apparent that some children never require liver transplantation. However, although some children will have normal growth and no hepatic nodules for years, they must be monitored closely by a transplant center. If hepatic nodules consistent with HCC are detected before transplantation, death from recurrent tumor may ensue.[115,116] Thus, hepatic transplantation should be performed before macroscopic malignancy is detected. In addition, there is a role for transplantation in the management of the small percentage of infants and children who do not respond to nitisinone treatment in the acute setting.[117]

Gene therapy

One report documents stable correction of the enzyme defect in fibroblasts from patients with tyrosinemia by retrovirus-mediated transfer[118] of the human wild-type gene. Hence, gene therapy for this inborn error may eventually become feasible.

GLYCOGEN STORAGE DISEASES

Pathophysiology and clinical features

Glycogen, the primary storage form of glucose, is found predominantly in liver and muscle tissue. Degradation of glycogen is the process by which free glucose is released to maintain normal blood concentrations during fasting and sustain normal intracellular concentrations. Although 12 different glycogen storage diseases (GSDs) resulting from deficiencies of the various enzymes involved in glycogen degradation have been described, only three types have primary hepatic involvement.

GSD I, also known as von Gierke's disease, is the most common glycogen storage disease and represents about 25% of cases. GSD I results from absence of the activity of glucose-6-phosphatase. Two major (and a few minor) subtypes have been described: Patients with type Ia completely lack enzyme activity, whereas those with type Ib have a defect in the transport protein T_1 that interferes with the transport of glucose-6-phosphatase across the microsomal membrane. Both types are characterized by hepatomegaly, short stature, hypoglycemia after brief periods of fasting, metabolic acidosis, lactic acidemia, hyperuricemia, hyperlipidemia, and nephromegaly. In addition, patients with type Ib GSD have variable degrees of neutropenia and an increased incidence of infection. GSD I does not cause hepatic failure or cirrhosis. The major long-term consequence of the disease is the frequent development of hepatic adenomas, usually beginning in early adolescence. Rarely, HCC may develop within an adenoma. The diagnosis may be suspected in infants and young children with marked hepatomegaly and the metabolic derangements described. It is further suggested by monitoring blood glucose and lactate levels during a controlled fasting period. The diagnosis is confirmed by assay of enzyme activity in fresh liver tissue, which may be obtained by percutaneous biopsy.

GSD III is a deficiency of the glycogen debranching enzyme amylo-1,6-glucosidase. It is also known as Forbes' disease. In this disorder, abnormal glycogen accumulation is noted in both liver and muscle tissue. Several subtypes have been defined by tissue distribution and residual enzymatic activity. The clinical manifestations are similar to those of GSD I, but much milder. Patients with GSD III have hepatomegaly, fasting hypoglycemia, and hyperlipidemia, but lactic acidosis and hyperuricemia are not seen. In infants and children, hepatomegaly and growth failure predominate. Liver disease may progress to fibrosis and cirrhosis in some affected individuals. In older patients, GSD III is primarily manifested as progressive muscle weakness and atrophy. The diagnosis may be suggested by an elevated serum creatinine kinase concentration and is confirmed by assay of enzyme activity in liver or muscle tissue.

GSD IV, or Andersen's disease, is a deficiency of the branching enzyme 1,4-glucan-6-glycosyltransferase; this disorder is also known as amylopectinosis. GSD IV is characterized by hepatomegaly, failure to thrive, hypotonia, and muscular atrophy, often seen within the first year or two of life. Cardiac failure secondary to amylopectin deposition in cardiac muscle may occur. Hypoglycemia and lactic acidemia are not evident. Progression of hepatic involvement to cirrhosis is common, and most patients with liver disease succumb by 3 years of age. A few adults with myopathy but no liver disease have been described. The diagnosis, which may be suspected in an infant or young child with hepatomegaly, hepatic dysfunction, growth failure, hypotonia, or heart disease, is confirmed by assay of the branching enzyme in muscle, leukocytes, or fibroblasts.

Treatment of glycogen storage disease

Dietary therapy

Early reports of correction of many of the metabolic derangements of GSD I by provision of nutrients directly into the systemic circulation by total parenteral nutrition or by portacaval shunting gave important clues to its pathogenesis and therapy. Subsequently, it was demonstrated that maintenance of blood glucose levels greater than 70–90 mg/dL obviated most of the clinical manifestations of GSD I.[119] The presumed mechanism of action for this therapy is reduction of the stimulus for glycogenolysis and prevention of the abnormal compensatory metabolic pathways leading to lactate accumulation, lipid synthesis, purine synthesis, and subsequent hyperuricemia. The neutropenia of GSD Ib is not corrected by glucose homeostasis.

Originally, maintenance of blood glucose was accomplished by continuous enteral feeding of infants with nasogastric or gastrostomy tubes. Alternatively, it has been shown that frequent daytime feedings (every 2–3 h) of a high-starch diet can be combined with continuous nighttime tube feedings with the same effects. However, as children become older, this regimen is more difficult to maintain and is altered to include daytime meals supplemented with raw cornstarch. Cornstarch undergoes slow degradation to glucose by α-amylase and, when given at a dose of 2 g/kg every 6 h, steadily releases sufficient glucose into the system.[120] This cornstarch supplementation can be combined with continuous nighttime feedings until the children are through the period of rapid growth and their glucose requirement decreases to the point that cornstarch supplements alone are sufficient for metabolic control.[121]

As patients with GSD I approach late adolescence, the tendency for hypoglycemia decreases and some investigators believe that less rigorous dietary therapy is required. However, treatment of the secondary complications of the disease with agents such as allopurinol for hyperuricemia or lipid-lowering agents for the prevention of cardiovascular disease and pancreatitis may be necessary. Renal insufficiency of unclear etiology may develop in some older individuals and require non-specific management.

A long-term complication of GSD I for which no definitive therapy has been established is hepatic adenoma. It is believed that adenomas develop because of chronic stimulation of the liver by glucagon and other trophic agents produced in response to chronic or recurrent hypoglycemia. Although some authors have reported regression of adenomas with aggressive dietary therapy,[122] many patients who have received this treatment since infancy or early childhood are just now reaching adulthood and adenomas are a common finding in this group. Currently, a major challenge in the management of patients with GSD I is the prevention, detection, and management of these lesions, as well as the development of a strategy for early detection of the rare transformation of adenomas into malignant lesions. In addition, a link between the hepatic adenomas and the normocytic anemia that often accompanies this disorder has been made. Hepcidin was found in abundance in the adenomas in GSD Ia, and resection of the adenomas has resulted in normalization of the hematologic parameters and iron studies.[123] Recent guidelines regarding monitoring of adenomas have been published, suggesting abdominal ultrasounds and measurement of serum alpha-fetoprotein and carcinoembryonic antigen every 3 months, as well as CT scan or magnetic resonance imaging in the case of growth or blurring of the margins of the lesions.[124]

Therapy for GSD III and IV is less clearly defined. Dietary therapy has been used in a few patients with GSD III,[125] but there is no indication for its implementation in patients with GSD IV. At the present time, treatment is primarily targeted to symptoms.

The progress in metabolic management has improved the prognosis for patients with the hepatic glycogen storage diseases. An increasing number of patients are surviving into adulthood in better health, but careful evaluation of these patients reveals numerous medical issues that require study and intervention.[126] These include disturbances in bone mineralization and renal function, hepatic tumors, and lipid abnormalities in GSD I, and derangement of cardiac function in GSD III. Females over the age of 5 years with GSD I, III, VI, and IX often have morphologically polycystic ovaries. These disorders involve multiple systems; therefore, there is need for careful long-term follow-up.

Liver transplantation

Liver transplantation has been used in patients with GSD I refractory to dietary management[127,128] or those with complications associated with hepatic adenomas such as bleeding or malignant degeneration. The role of hepatic replacement in GSD III or IV is less apparent inasmuch as it is not expected to correct the metabolic disturbances in other tissue such as skeletal or cardiac muscle.

CYSTIC FIBROSIS

Pathophysiology and clinical features

Cystic fibrosis (CF) is one of the most common serious inherited diseases in white populations. The median survival has increased to more than 30 years, and the proportion reaching adulthood has increased. The overall prevalence of overt liver disease in patients with CF is 4–5%, with clinically apparent cirrhosis in

2–10%. However, as the general care of patients with CF has continued to improve, the relative importance of liver disease has increased.[129] The incidence of liver disease rises steadily with age, and liver disease peaks in the adolescent years. However, it is rare for liver disease to have its onset after 20 years of age. Although the reasons for this decline are unclear, two hypotheses have been offered: (1) liver disease increases mortality selectively so that individuals without liver disease are more likely to survive into adult life, or (2) a cohort effect 10–15 years previously increased the likelihood of liver disease, and current adolescent prevalence reflects that increase.[130] A 3:1 male preponderance of liver disease is seen in patients with CF, especially during the adolescent years.[131] Although liver disease is most common in patients with steatorrhea, it may occur in those with intact pancreatic exocrine function.[132] Genotype analysis has not revealed a specific mutation in the CF gene that correlates with the existence of liver disease. One study has suggested an association with particular histocompatibility antigens, thus implicating a possible role for altered immune responses in patients with CF and liver disease.[133] A more recent study demonstrated an association of a specific polymorphism of glutathione S-transferase with liver disease in CF patients.[134]

The etiology of the hepatobiliary lesions in CF has not been fully elucidated. The description of the gene product cystic fibrosis transmembrane regulator in the apical domain of bile duct epithelial cells[135] suggests that altered ductular secretion results in concentrated viscous bile with subsequent plugging and inflammation.

Several forms of liver disease are seen in patients with CF. Neonatal cholestasis occurs in 2–20% of affected infants and may persist for several months. It is generally attributed to viscous bile with sludging. Hepatic steatosis is common, but its cause has not been clearly elucidated. Micronodular cirrhosis is evident in only 2–5% of patients and may be multifactorial in etiology. Focal biliary cirrhosis, a lesion virtually unique to CF, is seen in up to 10–20% of individuals. Focal biliary cirrhosis begins with accumulation of amorphous material in intrahepatic ducts, which causes focal obstruction, edema, and chronic inflammation. Subsequently, bile duct proliferation and fibrosis evolve into biliary cirrhosis. This lesion occurs most often without signs or symptoms until portal hypertension and its complications ensue. Results of standard biochemical tests may be normal or nearly normal. Patients with CF also have a high incidence of biliary tract disease, including hypoplastic gallbladders, gallstones and/or sludge, common bile duct strictures, common bile duct obstruction from severe pancreatic fibrosis, and a cholangiopathy indistinguishable from primary sclerosing cholangitis.

The optimal method for detection of liver disease in CF has not been established, but several studies have documented the utility of serial ultrasonography in discovery of abnormalities such as steatosis, heterogeneity in echotexture, nodularity, and evidence of portal hypertension, often in the absence of biochemical abnormalities.

Treatment of cystic fibrosis associated liver disease

Dietary therapy

Because of pancreatic insufficiency and steatorrhea, most patients with CF should receive supplements of fat-soluble vitamins. However, infants with cholestasis or older patients with severe liver disease may require these supplements in higher dosages because of the additional fat malabsorption associated with low intestinal luminal bile salt concentrations. Because taurine deficiency has been demonstrated in some patients with CF as a result of excessive losses, some authors recommend that supplemental taurine be provided to CF patients treated with ursodeoxycholic acid (UDCA) (i.e., based on the theoretical concern of excessive consumption of this conjugating amino acid induced by large amounts of the unconjugated bile acid.[136] However, in clinical trials, no significant effect of taurine supplementation is documented. Other than the supportive role of nutritional management for chronic liver disease, no other specific dietary therapies are known.

Drug therapy

Ursodeoxycholic acid (UDCA), a hydrophilic bile acid with choleretic activity, has shown promise in the management of hepatobiliary disease in patients with CF. Several studies have documented improvement in clinical, biochemical, and nutritional parameters in children and adults with CF treated with UDCA for 6–12 months.[136–138] A more recent study documented therapeutic effects over the long term as well.[139] Mechanisms postulated for this beneficial effect include displacement of potentially toxic endogenous hydrophobic bile acids, immunomodulation, and decreased bile viscosity because of the presence of the hydrophilic bile acid. A dose–response study demonstrated that a UDCA dose of 20 mg/kg/day, somewhat higher than that administered for gallstone dissolution or other chronic cholestatic liver diseases, was required to achieve favorable biochemical effects in patients with CF.[140] This amount is usually divided into two doses.

Portal hypertension

End-stage liver disease associated with hepatic insufficiency is uncommon in CF. The most common life-threatening manifestation of cirrhosis in CF is portal hypertension and its complications. Therapies typically applied in this setting, including surgical and transjugular portosystemic shunts, splenectomy and splenic embolization, have all been used in patients with CF, with varying degrees of success.

Liver transplantation

Liver transplantation has been performed in children and adults with end-stage liver disease associated with CF.[141,142] Special attention needs to be given to pulmonary function and infection, medication dosages in the setting of malabsorption, and blood glucose control because of a higher incidence of diabetes mellitus in patients with CF. Nonetheless, survival rates in this group are approximately 75%. Pulmonary function either remains the same or improves in survivors of liver transplantation. Some authors recommend early liver transplantation in this setting, to avoid complications from advanced lung disease and infection.[143] For CF patients with severe pulmonary disease in conjunction with complications of cirrhosis, combined lung/liver or heart/lung/liver transplantation may be an option.[144,145]

INBORN ERRORS OF METABOLISM CAUSING HYPERAMMONEMIA

Pathophysiology and clinical features

In addition to fulminant hepatic failure of varied etiology, many congenital and acquired disorders are associated with hyperammonemia and encephalopathy.[146] Although most of these disorders occur during infancy or childhood, some such as heterozygous ornithine transcarbamylase deficiency (a urea cycle defect) may occur in adolescence or adulthood. Others may occur in association with adult disorders such as very long-chain acyl coenzyme A (CoA) dehydrogenase deficiency, a disorder of fatty acid metabolism, in infants born to women with acute fatty liver of pregnancy or the HELLP syndrome (hemolytic anemia, elevated liver enzymes, and low platelets). A list of conditions associated with hyperammonemia is presented in Table 32.6.

Excess dietary protein and nitrogen derived from cell turnover are metabolized immediately to energy and the byproduct ammonia. Ammonia is converted to urea within the liver; urea is then excreted via the kidney. *Urea cycle defects* disrupt this process and lead to recurrent episodes of hyperammonemia, neurobehavioral changes, and vomiting. In older children and young adults affected with milder forms, clinical manifestations include 'recurrent Reye's syndrome,' cyclic vomiting, psychiatric disturbances, and intermittent hepatomegaly. Aminotransferase levels may be normal or mildly elevated. Hepatic histology may be normal or demonstrate microvesicular steatosis. Other disorders that involve defects in the transport of amino acids result in insufficient substrate for the generation of urea; clinical manifestations of these disorders may be similar to those described earlier.

Organic acidemias are defects in the catabolism of branched-chain amino acids; the resultant accumulation of propionyl-CoA inhibits several important metabolic pathways, including lactate and pyruvate metabolism, some urea cycle enzymes, and organic and fatty acid degradation enzymes. These abnormalities are in turn responsible for episodes of hyperammonemia, vomiting, lethargy or obtundation, acidosis, and ketosis. Milder defects that may occur in older patients cause episodic vomiting and ataxia. Hepatomegaly with hepatocellular steatosis is common. Diagnosis of the organic acidemias is accomplished by urine organic acid analysis during symptomatic episodes.

Defects in the mitochondrial metabolism of fatty acids, that is, *fatty acid oxidation disorders*, interrupt the gluconeogenesis, ketogenesis, and generation of acetyl-CoA necessary for glucose homeostasis during fasting. In addition, the fatty acid acyl-CoA compounds that accumulate inhibit other metabolic pathways. Affected infants may have hypoketotic hypoglycemia, lethargy, and coma after fasting. Older children, adolescents, and adults may manifest cardiac arrhythmias, muscle weakness or pain, or rhabdomyolysis. Hyperammonemia is modest and probably caused by accelerated protein breakdown. Variable aminotransferase levels, a mildly prolonged prothrombin time, hepatomegaly with hepatic steatosis, and non-specific mitochondrial changes characterize these disorders. Typically, total plasma carnitine levels are low, but esterified carnitine is increased, an effect of the accumulation of acyl-CoA. The diagnosis of a fatty acid oxidation disorder is suggested by biochemical and organic acid analyses during hypoglycemic episodes and confirmed by measurement of enzyme activities in skin fibroblasts.

Reye's syndrome is an acquired disorder of unclear etiology manifested by hepatocellular injury, coagulopathy, and hyperammonemia with encephalopathy. The degree of hyperammonemia correlates inversely with the likelihood of survival. Histologic examination of the liver reveals microvesicular steatosis; mitochondria are swollen with abnormal cristae. Biochemical analysis indicates impaired fatty acid oxidation.

Treatment of hyperammonemia

Dietary therapy

The first step in management of the hyperammonemic syndromes is the elimination of exogenous protein intake by supplying calories in the form of carbohydrate and lipid. This type of diet can be achieved for only brief periods because essential amino acids must be provided. Once the hyperammonemic crises have passed, maintenance protein intake should be restricted but given in a quantity sufficient to allow normal growth. It is also critical to prevent endogenous ammonia production secondary to protein catabolism. This goal is accomplished by providing sufficient calories at baseline, as well as during periods of stress, and the avoidance of fasting.

Medical therapy

The goal of medical therapy is reduction in ammonia level. Principles of treatment or urea cycle defects include minimizing endogenous ammonia production and protein catabolism, restricting nitrogen intake, administering substrates of the urea cycle, administering compounds that facilitate the removal of ammonia through alternative pathways, and, in severe cases, dialysis therapy. Lactulose or antibiotics may be given to decrease the ammonia produced by colonic flora. Ammonia excretion can be facilitated by the administration of sodium benzoate or phenylacetate.[147] Benzoate becomes conjugated with glycine to form hippurate. Phenylacetate is conjugated with glutamine to form phenylacetyl-glutamine. Both hippurate and phenylacetylglutamine are rapidly

---

Table 32.6 Metabolic diseases associated with hyperammonemia

Urea cycle defects

Ornithine transcarbamylase

Carbamoyl phosphate synthetase

Argininosuccinate synthetase

Argininosuccinate lyase

Arginase

Urea cycle substrate transport defects

Lysinuric protein intolerance

Hyperammonemia-hyperornithinemia-homocitrullinuria

Organic acidemias

Propionicacidemias

Methylmalonicacidemia

Isovalericacidemia

Multiple carboxylase deficiency

Fatty acid oxidation defects

Medium-chain acyl-CoA dehydrogenase

Long-chain 3-hydroxyacyl-CoA dehydrogenase

Carnitine transport defects

Miscellaneous

Reye's syndrome

Congenital portosystemic shunts

excreted by the kidney, with the result being a net loss of nitrogen. Sodium benzoate and phenylacetate may be given to any patient during episodes of hyperammonemia. They are also commonly administered as prophylactic therapy to children with urea cycle disorders to improve protein tolerance and growth and to prevent some neurologic sequelae. The potential for benzoate toxicity is diminished by the concomitant administration of L-carnitine, which results in esterification to form benzoylcarnitine. Because secondary carnitine deficiency has been described in many of these disorders, supplemental L-carnitine is often given prophylactically to children with urea cycle defects and fatty acid oxidation defects. Some urea cycle defects lead to substrate deficiencies that are amenable to exogenous supplementation with arginine or citrate.

Hyperammonemia is less profound and only one of the metabolic disturbances in fatty acid oxidation defects. Early diagnosis is key to prevent developmental disabilities from recurrent episodes of hypoglycemia and hyperammonemia. Preventive measures should be taken to ensure that affected individuals do not go without food for extended periods of time (12–16 hours). These measures may include awakening a child at night for feeding (i.e., intravenous or parenteral). A low-fat diet may be of benefit to some individuals. During periods of fasting, oral cornstarch may be used to prevent hypoglycemia. During episodes of hypoglycemia, intravenous fluids containing 10% dextrose should be administered promptly. Genetic counseling will be of benefit for affected individuals and their families. Other treatment is symptomatic and supportive.

In infants or young children with severe hyperammonemia, rapid removal of ammonia may be necessary to prevent neurologic injury. Initiation of dialysis in the encephalopathic patient with hyperammonemia is indicated if the ammonia blood level is greater than three to four times the upper limit of normal.[148] Continuous hemofiltration and peritoneal dialysis may also be effective in reducing blood ammonia levels.

A comprehensive strategy for management of infants and children with urea cycle defects has been presented as a consensus statement.[149]

Liver transplantation

OLT has been successful in correction of the metabolic abnormalities of urea cycle defects. However, it should be reserved for disorders in which the likelihood of neurologic injury is high and for which medical therapy does not provide stable metabolic control. It is not usually necessary for fatty acid oxidation defects, since these can usually be managed with strict dietary and medical measures. Death from Reye's syndrome is most often due to uncontrolled intracranial hypertension rather than hepatic failure per se, so liver transplantation is not indicated.

Gene therapy

Preliminary experiments have demonstrated the feasibility of virally mediated transfer of urea cycle enzyme genes into animal models, human hepatocytes, and human fibroblasts from affected individuals, which raises the possibility of effective gene therapy for these disorders in the near future.

ADDITIONAL READING

A detailed review with focus on pathophysiology of A1AT deficiency is provided by D. H. Perlmutter (Alpha-1-antitrypsin deficiency. Semin Liver Dis 1998;18:217–225). The limited discussion of treatment options reflects lack of recognized therapies for treatment of liver disease.

REFERENCES

1. Bacon BR, Powell LW, Adams PC, et al. Molecular medicine and hemochromatosis: At the crossroads. Gastroenterology 1999; 116:193–207.

2. Harrison SA, Bacon BR. Hereditary hemochromatosis: Update for 2003. J Hepatol 2003; 38(Suppl 1):S14–S23.

3. Pietrangelo A. Hereditary hemochromatosis: A new look at an old disease. N Engl J Med 2004; 350:2383–2397.

4. Beutler E, Felitti VJ, Koziol JA, et al. Penetrance of 845G→A (C282Y) HFE hereditary haemochromatosis mutation in the USA. Lancet 2002; 359:211–218.

5. Asberg A, Hveem K, Thorstensen K, et al. Screening for hemochromatosis: High prevalence and low morbidity in an unselected population of 65,238 persons. Scand J Gastroenterol 2001; 36:1108–1115.

6. Milder MS, Cook JD, Stray S, et al. Idiopathic hemochromatosis, an interim report. Medicine (Baltimore) 1980; 59:34–49.

7. Edwards CQ, Cartwright GE, Skolnick MH, et al. Homozygosity for hemochromatosis: Clinical manifestations. Ann Intern Med 1980; 93:519–525.

8. Feder JN, Gnirke A, Thomas W, et al. A novel MHC class 1-like gene is mutated in patients with hereditary hemochromatosis. Nat Genet 1996; 13:399–408.

9. Powell LW. Hereditary hemochromatosis. Pathology 2000; 32:24–36.

10. Bacon BR, Britton RS. The pathophysiology of iron overload: A free radical-mediated process? Hepatology 1990; 11:127–137.

11. Bacon BR. Diagnosis and management of hemochromatosis. Gastroenterology 1997; 113:995–999.

12. Papanikolaou G, Samuels ME, Ludwig EH, et al. Mutations in HFE2 cause iron overload in chromosome 1q-linked juvenile hemochromatosis. Nat Genet 2004; 36:77–82.

13. Camaschella C, Roetto A, Cali A, et al. The gene TFR2 is mutated in a new type of haemochromatosis mapping to 7q22. Nat Genet 2000; 25:14–15.

14. Pietrangelo A, Montosi G, Totaro A, et al. Hereditary hemochromatosis in adults without pathogenic mutations in the hemochromatosis gene. N Engl J Med 1999; 341:725–732.

15. Gordeuk VR. African iron overload. Semin Hematol 2002; 39:263–269.

16. Pietrangelo A. Non-HFE hemochromatosis. Hepatology 2004; 39:21–29.

17. Roetto A, Papanikolaou G, Politou M, et al. Mutant antimicrobial peptide hepcidin is associated with severe juvenile hemochromatosis. Nat Genet 2003; 33:21–22.

18. Bottomley SS. Secondary iron overload disorders. Semin Hematol 1998; 35:77–86.

19. Knisely AS, Mieli-Vergani G, Whitington PF. Neonatal hemochromatosis. Gastroenterol Clin North Am 2003; 32:877–889.

20. Bacon BR, Britton RS. Hereditary hemochromatosis. In: Feldman M, Scharschmidt BF, Sleisenger MH, eds. Sleisenger & Fordtran's gastrointestinal and liver disease. 8th edn. Philadelphia: WB Saunders 2006; (in press).

21. Bacon BR, Olynyk JK, Brunt EM, et al. HFE genotype in patients with hemochromatosis and other liver diseases. Ann Intern Med 1999; 130:953–962.

22. Guyader D, Jacquelinet C, Moirand R, et al. Noninvasive prediction of fibrosis in C282Y homozygous hemochromatosis. Gastroenterology 1998; 115:929–936.

23. Galhenage SP, Viiala CH, Olynyk JK. Screening for haemochromatosis: patients with liver disease, families, and populations. Curr Gastroenterol Rep 2004; 6:44–51.

24. Bacon BR, Hereditary hemochromatosis. In: Bacon BR, O'Grady J, Di Bisceglie AM, Lake J. Comprehensive clinical hepatology. 2nd edn. Oxford, UK: Elsevier; 2006; 341–351.

25. Bacon BR, Sadiq SA. Hereditary hemochromatosis: Presentation and diagnosis in the 1990s. Am J Gastroenterol 1997; 92:784–789.

26. Huebers H. Iron overload: Pathogenesis and treatment with chelating agents. Blut 1983; 47:61–67.

27. Mossey R, Wielopolski L, Bellucci A, et al. Reduction in liver iron in hemodialysis patients with transfusional iron overload by deferoxamine mesylate. Am J Kidney Dis 1988; 12:40–44.

28. Olivieri N, Koren G, Hermann C, et al. Comparison of oral iron chelator L1 and deferoxamine in iron-loaded patients. Lancet 1990; 2:1275–1279.

29. Seifert A, Von Herrath D, Schaefer K. Iron overload, but not treatment with desferrioxamine favours the development of septicemia in patients on maintenance hemodialysis. Q J Med 1987; 65:1015–1024.

30. Tielemans C, Lenclud C. Respective role of haemosiderosis and desferrioxamine therapy in the risk of infection of haemodialysed patients. Q J Med 1988; 68:573–574.

31. Boelaert J, van Landuyt H, Valcke Y, et al. The role of iron overload in *Yersinia enterocolitica* and *Yersinia pseudotuberculosis* bacteremia in hemodialysis patients. J Infect Dis 1987; 156:384–387.

32. Goodill J, Abuelo J. Mucormycosis – A new risk of deferoxamine therapy in dialysis patients with aluminum or iron overload (Letter). N Engl J Med 1987; 317:54.

33. Windus D, Stokes T, Julian B, et al. Fatal *Rhizopus* infections in hemodialysis patients receiving deferoxamine. Ann Intern Med 1987; 107:678–680.

34. Marciani M, Cianciulli P, Stefani N, et al. Toxic effects of high-dose deferoxamine treatment in patients with iron overload: An electrophysiological study of cerebral and visual function. Haematologica 1991; 76:131–134.

35. Porter J, Hider R, Huehns E. Update on the hydroxypyridone oral iron-chelating agents. Semin Hematol 1990; 27:95–100.

36. Tondury P, Kontoghiorghes G, Ridolfi-Luthy A, et al. L1 (1,2-dimethyl-3-hydroxypyrid-4-one) for oral iron chelation in patients with beta-thalassemia major. Br J Haematol 1990; 76:550–553.

37. Agarwal M, Viswanathan C, Ramanathan J, et al. Oral iron chelation with L1 (Letter). Lancet 1990; 1:601.

38. Kontoghiorghes G, Bartlett A, Hoffbrand A, et al. Long-term trial with the oral iron chelator 1,2-dimethyl-3-hydroxypyrid-4-one (L1). Br J Haematol 1990; 76:295–300.

39. Olivieri NF. Orally active chelators in the treatment of iron overload. Curr Opin Hematol 1996; 3:125–130.

40. Mehta J, Singhal S, Revankar R, et al. Fatal systemic lupus erythematosus in patient taking oral iron chelator L1. Lancet 1991; 1:298.

41. [Anonymous]. Oral iron chelators. Lancet 1989; 2:1016–1017.

42. Kowdley KV, Hassanein T, Kaur S, et al. Primary liver cancer and survival in patients undergoing liver transplantation for hemochromatosis. Liver Transpl Surg 1995; 1:237–241.

43. Farrel FJ, Nguyen M, Woodley S, et al. Outcome of liver transplantation in patients with hemochromatosis. Hepatology 1994; 20:404–410.

44. Poulos JE, Bacon BR. Liver transplantation for hereditary hemochromatosis. Dig Dis 1996; 14:316–322.

45. Grace ND. Liver transplantation for hemochromatosis: An ironic dilemma. Liver Transpl Surg 1995; 1:234–236.

46. Brandhagen DJ, Alvarez W, Therneau TM, et al. Iron overload in cirrhosis: *HFE* genotypes and outcome after liver transplantation. Hepatology 2000; 31:456–460.

47. Petrukhin K, Fisher SG, Pirastu M, et al. Mapping, cloning, and genetic characterization of the region containing the Wilson disease gene. Nat Genet 1993; 5:338–343.

48. Tanzi RE, Petrukhin K, Chernov I, et al. The Wilson disease gene is a copper transporting ATPase with homology to the Menkes disease gene. Nat Genet 1993; 5:344–350.

49. Gollan JL, Gollan TJ. Wilson disease in 1998: Genetic, diagnostic and therapeutic aspects. J Hepatol 1998; 28(Suppl 1):28–36.

50. Schaefer M, Hopkins R, Failla M, et al. Hepatocyte-specific localization and copper-dependent trafficking of the Wilson's disease protein in the liver. Am J Physiol 1999; 276:G639–G646.

51. Schaefer M, Roelofsen H, Wolters H et al. Localization of the Wilson's disease protein in human liver. Gastroenterology 1999; 117:1380–1385.

52. Sato M, Gitlin JD. Mechanisms of copper incorporation during the biosynthesis of human ceruloplasmin. J Biol Chem 1991; 266:5128–5134.

53. Gitlin JD. Wilson disease. Gastroenterology 2003; 125:1868–1877.

54. Schilsky ML. Identification of the Wilson's disease gene: Clues for disease pathogenesis and the potential for molecular diagnosis. Hepatology 1994; 20:529–533.

55. Maier-Dobersberger T, Mannhalter C, Rack S, et al. Diagnosis of Wilson's disease in an asymptomatic sibling by DNA linkage analysis. Gastroenterology 1995; 109:2015–2018.

56. Nagano K, Nakamura K, Urakami KI, et al. Intracellular distribution of the Wilson's disease product (ATPase7B) after in vitro and in vivo expression in hepatocytes from the LEC rat, an animal model of Wilson's disease. Hepatology 1998; 27:799–807.

57. Walshe J. Wilson's disease: New oral therapy. Lancet 1956; 1:25–26.

58. Roberts EA, Schilsky ML. A practice guideline on Wilson disease. Hepatology 2003; 37:1475–1492.

   This recently published AASLD practice guideline provides a thorough overview of diagnosis and treatment options for patients with Wilson disease. Formal recommendations are rated based on the strength of evidence-based medicine underlying the recommendation. Comprehensively referenced with 208 citations.

59. Joyce D. D-Penicillamine pharmacokinetics and pharmacodynamics in man. Pharmacol Ther 1989; 42:405–427.

60. Gibbs K, Walshe J. Liver copper concentrations in Wilson's disease: Effect of treatment with 'anti-copper' agents. J Gastroenterol Hepatol 1990; 5:420–424.

61. Marecek Z, Heyrovsky A, Volek V. The effect of long term treatment with penicillamine on the copper content in the liver in patients with Wilson's disease. Acta Hepatogastroenterol 1975; 22:292–296.

62. Scheinberg I, Sternlieb I, Schilsky M, et al. Penicillamine may detoxify copper in Wilson's disease (Letter). Lancet 1987; 2:95.

63. Sternlieb I. Perspectives on Wilson's disease. Hepatology 1990; 12:1234–1239.

64. Heilmaier H, Jiang J, Griem H, et al. D-Penicillamine induces rat hepatic collagen. Toxicology 1986; 42:23–31.

65. Nimni M. Mechanism of inhibition of collagen cross-linking by penicillamine. Proc R Soc Med 1977; 70(Suppl 3):65–72.

66. Davis G, Czaja A, Ludwig J. Development and prognosis of histologic cirrhosis in corticosteroid-treated hepatitis B surface antigen negative chronic active hepatitis. Gastroenterology 1984; 87:1222–1227.

67. Munthe E, Guldal G, Jellum E. Increased intracellular glutathione during penicillamine treatment for rheumatoid arthritis. Lancet 1979; 2:1126–1127.

68. Scheinberg I, Jaffe M, Sternlieb I. The use of trientine in preventing the effects of interrupting penicillamine therapy in Wilson's disease. N Engl J Med 1987; 317:209–213.

69. Glass J, Reich S, DeLong M. Wilson's disease: Development of neurologic disease after beginning penicillamine therapy. Arch Neurol 1990; 47:595–596.

70. Brewer G, Terry C, Aisen A, et al. Worsening of neurologic syndrome in patients with Wilson's disease with initial penicillamine therapy. Arch Neurol 1987; 44:490–493.

71. Lipsky M, Gollan J. Treatment of Wilson's disease: In D-penicillamine we trust – What about zinc? Hepatology 1987; 7:593–595.

72. Marsden C. Wilson's disease (Editorial). Q J Med 1987; 65:959–966.

73. Iozumi K, Nakagawa H, Tamaki K. Penicillamine-induced degenerative dermatoses: Report of a case and brief review of such dermatoses. J Dermatol 1997; 24:458–465.

74. Knudsen L, Weismann K. Taste dysfunction and changes in zinc and copper metabolism during penicillamine therapy for generalized scleroderma. Acta Med Scand 1978; 204:75–79.

75. Scheinberg I, Sternlieb I. Pregnancy in penicillamine-treated patients with Wilson's disease. N Engl J Med 1975; 293:1300–1302.

76. Walshe J. Pregnancy in Wilson's disease. Q J Med 1977; 46:73–83.

77. Dubois R, Rodgerson D, Hambridge K. Treatment of Wilson's disease with triethylene tetramine hydrochloride (trientine). J Pediatr Gastroenterol Nutr 1990; 10:77–81.

78. Walshe J. Treatment of Wilson's disease with trientine (triethylene tetramine) dihydrochloride. Lancet 1982; 1:643–647.

79. Brewer G, Hill G, Prasad A, et al. Oral zinc therapy in Wilson's disease. Ann Intern Med 1983; 99:314–320.

80. Schilsky M, Blank R, Czaja M, et al. Hepatocellular copper toxicity and its attenuation by zinc. J Clin Invest 1989; 84:1562–1568.

81. Rossaro L, Sturniolo G, Giacon G, et al. Zinc therapy in Wilson's disease: Observations in five patients. Am J Gastroenterol 1990; 85:665–668.

82. Marrella M, Milanino R, Moretti U, et al. One year of oral zinc therapy in a child with Wilson's disease. Pharmacol Res 1989; 21:489–490.

83. Brewer G, Hill G, Dick R, et al. Treatment of Wilson's disease with zinc: Prevention of reaccumulation of hepatic copper. J Lab Clin Med 1987; 109:526–531.

84. Stremmel W, Strohmeyer G. Oral zinc therapy is not always effective for treatment of Wilson's disease (Abstract). Hepatology 1988; 8:1335.

85. Milanino R, Marrella M, Moretti U, et al. Oral zinc sulfate as primary therapeutic intervention in a child with Wilson disease. Eur J Pediatr 1989; 148:654–655.

86. Hoogenraad T, Van Hattum J, Van der Hamer C. Management of Wilson's disease with zinc sulphate. Experience in a series of 27 patients. J Neurol Sci 1987; 77:137–146.

87. Hill G, Brewer G, Prasad A, et al. Treatment of Wilson's disease with zinc. I. Oral zinc therapy regimens. Hepatology 1987; 7:522–528.

88. Brewer GJ, Dick RD, Johnson VD, et al. Treatment of Wilson's disease with zinc. XV. Long-term follow-up studies. J Lab Clin Med 1998; 132:264–278.

This manuscript is one in an ongoing series published by Brewer and colleagues in J Lab Clin Med regarding the use of zinc for the management of Wilson disease. This report is notable for the duration of follow-up and serves as an excellent guide for the clinician contemplating the use of zinc therapy either after chelation therapy is complete, or in isolation.

89. Czlonkowska A, Gajda J, Rodo M. Effects of long-term treatment in Wilson's disease with D-penicillamine and zinc sulphate. J Neurol 1996; 243:269–273.

90. Brewer GJ. Practical recommendations and new therapies for Wilson's disease. Drugs 1995; 50:240–249.

91. Scheinberg I, Sternlieb I. The efficacy of oral zinc therapy as an alternative to penicillamine for Wilson's disease. N Engl J Med 1988; 318:323.

92. Askari FK, Greenson J, Dick RD, et al. Treatment of Wilson's disease with zinc: XVIII. Initial treatment of hepatic decompensation presentation with trientine and zinc. J Lab Clin Med 2003; 142:385–390.

93. Brewer G, Dick R, Yuzbasiyan-Gurkin V, et al: Initial therapy of patients with Wilson's disease with tetrathiomolybdate. Arch Neurol 1991; 48:42–47.

94. Bremner I, Mills C. The copper-molybdenum interaction in ruminants: Involvement of thiomolybdates. In: Scheinberg I, Walshe J, eds. Orphan diseases and orphan drugs. London: Manchester University Press; 1986:69–75.

95. Brewer GJ, Johnson V, Dick RD, et al. Treatment of Wilson's disease with ammonium tetrathiomolybdate. II. Initial therapy in 33 neurologically affected patients and follow-up with zinc therapy. Arch Neurol 1996; 53:1017–1025.

96. Walshe J. Wilson's disease patients can be decoppered (Letter). Lancet 1989; 2:228.

97. [Anonymous]. Case records of the Massachusetts General Hospital. Weekly clinicopathological exercises. Case 1-1997. A 23-year-old man with fulminant hepatorenal failure of uncertain cause. N Engl J Med 1997; 336:118–125.

98. Schilsky ML, Scheinberg IH, Sternlieb I. Liver transplantation for Wilson's disease: Indications and outcome. Hepatology 1994; 19:583–587.

99. Schumacher G, Platz KP, Mueller AR, et al. Liver transplantation: Treatment of choice for hepatic and neurological manifestations of Wilson's disease. Clin Transplant 1997; 11:217–224.

100. Guarino M, Stracciari A, D'Alessandro R, et al. No neurologic improvement after liver transplantation for Wilson's disease. Acta Neurol Scand 1995; 92:405–408.

101. Crystal RG. α_1-Antitrypsin deficiency, emphysema, and liver disease. J Clin Invest 1990; 85:1343–1352.

102. Brantly M, Nukiwa T, Crystal RG. Molecular basis of α_1-antitrypsin deficiency. Am J Med 1988; 84:13–31.

103. Yu M-H, Lee KN, Kim J. The Z type variation of human α_1-antitrypsin causes a protein folding defect. Nat Struct Biol 1995; 2:363–367.

104. Lomas DA, Evans DL, Finch JT, et al. The mechanism of Z α_1-antitrypsin accumulation in the liver. Nature 1992; 357:605–607.

105. Teckman J, Perlmutter DH. Conceptual advances in the pathogenesis and treatment of childhood metabolic liver disease. Gastroenterology 1995; 108:1263–1279.

106. Ibarguen E, Gross CR, Savik SK, et al. Liver disease in α_1-antitrypsin deficiency: Prognostic indicators. J Pediatr 1990; 117:864–870.

107. Russo P, O'Regan S. Visceral pathology of hereditary tyrosinemia type I. Am J Hum Genet 1990; 47:317–324.

108. Phaneuf D, Lambert M, Laframboise R, et al. Type 1 hereditary tyrosinemia. Evidence for molecular heterogeneity and identification of a causal mutation in a French Canadian patient. J Clin Invest 1992; 90:1185–1192.

109. Hostetter MK, Levy HL, Winter HS, et al. Evidence for liver disease preceding amino acid abnormalities in hereditary tyrosinemia. N Engl J Med 1983; 308:1265–1267.

110. Paradis K, Weber A, Seidman EG, et al. Liver transplantation for hereditary tyrosinemia: The Quebec experience. Am J Hum Genet 1990; 47:338–342.

111. Lindstedt S, Holme E, Lock EA, et al. Treatment of hereditary tyrosinaemia type I by inhibition of 4-hydroxyphenylpyruvate dioxygenase. Lancet 1992; 340:813–817.

112. Grompe M, Lindstedt S, al-Dhalimy M, et al. Pharmacological correction of neonatal lethal hepatic dysfunction in a murine model of hereditary tyrosinaemia type I. Nat Genet 1995; 10:453–460.

113. Grompe M. Pathophysiology and treatment of hereditary tyrosinemia type 1. Semin Liv Dis 2001; 21:563–571.

114. Holme E, Lindstedt S. Tyrosinaemia type I and NTBC (2-2 nitro-4-trifluoromethylbenzoyl)-1,3-cyclohexanedione). J Inherit Metab Dis 1998; 21:507–517.

115. Freese DK, Tuchman M, Schwarzenberg SJ, et al. Early liver transplantation is indicated for tyrosinemia type I. J Pediatr Gastroenterol Nutr 1991; 13:10–15.

116. Mieles LA, Esquivel CO, VanThiel DH, et al. Liver transplantation for tyrosinemia. A review of 10 cases from the University of Pittsburgh. Dig Dis Sci 1990; 35:153–157.

117. Holme E, Lindstedt S. Nontransplant treatment of tyrosinemia. Clin Liv Dis 2000; 4:805–814.

118. Phaneuf D, Hadchouel M, Tanguay RM, et al. Correction of fumarylacetoacetate hydrolase deficiency (type I tyrosinemia) in cultured human fibroblasts by retroviral-mediated gene transfer. Biochem Biophys Res Commun 1995; 208:957–963.

119. Moses SW. Pathophysiology and dietary treatment of the glycogen storage diseases. J Pediatr Gastroenterol Nutr 1990; 11:155–174.

120. Chen YT, Cornblath M, Siudbury JB. Cornstarch therapy in type I glycogen-storage disease. N Engl J Med 1984; 310:171–175.

121. Chen YT, Bazzarre CH, Lee MM, et al. Type I glycogen storage disease: Nine years of management with cornstarch. Eur J Pediatr 1993; 152(Suppl):56–59.

122. Parker P, Burr I, Slonim A, et al. Regression of hepatic adenomas in type Ia glycogen storage disease with dietary therapy. Gastroenterology 1981; 81:534–536.

123. Weinstein DA, Roy CN, Fleming MD, et al. Inappropriate expression of hepcidin is associated with iron refractory anemia: implications for the anemia of chronic disease. Blood 2002; 100:3776–3781.

124. Rake JP, Visser G, Labrune P, et al. Guidelines for management of glycogen storage disease type I – European Study on Glycogen Storage Disease Type I (ESGSD I). Eur J Pediatr 2002; 161:S112–S119.

125. Borowitz SM, Greene HL. Cornstarch therapy in a patient with type III glycogen storage disease. J Pediatr Gastroenterol Nutr 1987; 6:631–634.

126. Lee PJ, Leonard JV. The hepatic glycogen storage diseases – problems beyond childhood. J Inher Metabol Dis 1995; 18(4):462–472.

127. Malatack JJ, Finegold DN, Iwatsuki S, et al. Liver transplantation for type I glycogen storage disease. Lancet 1983; 1:1073–1075.

128. Sokal EM, Lopez-Silvarrey A, Buts JP, et al. Orthotopic liver transplantation for type I glycogenosis unresponsive to medical therapy. J Pediatr Gastroenterol Nutr 1993; 16:465–467.

129. Cystic Fibrosis Foundation, Patient Registry 1999 Annual Data Report. Bethesda, MD, September 2000.

130. Williams SGJ, Westaby D, Tanner MS, et al. Liver and biliary problems in cystic fibrosis. Br Med Bull 1992; 48:877–892.

131. Scott-Jupp R, Lama M, Tanner MS. Prevalence of liver disease in cystic fibrosis. Arch Dis Child 1991; 66:698–701.

132. Waters DL, Dorney SFA, Gruca MA, et al. Hepatobiliary disease in cystic fibrosis patients with pancreatic sufficiency. Hepatology 1995; 21:963–969.

133. Duthie A, Doherty DG, Donaldson PT, et al. The major histocompatibility complex influences the development of chronic liver disease in male children and young adults with cystic fibrosis. J Hepatol 1995; 23:532–537.

134. Henrion-Claude A, Flamant C, Roussey M, et al. Liver disease in pediatric patients with cystic fibrosis is associated with glutathione S-transferase P1 polymorphism. Hepatology 2002; 36:913–917.

135. Cohn JA, Strong TV, Picciotto MR, et al. Localization of the cystic fibrosis transmembrane conductance regulator in human bile duct epithelial cells. Gastroenterology 1993; 105:1857–1864.

136. Colombo C, Battezzati PM, Podda M, et al. Ursodeoxycholic acid for liver disease associated with cystic fibrosis: A double-blind multicenter trial. Hepatology 1996; 23:1484–1490.

137. Cotting J, Lentze MJ, Reichen J. Effects of ursodeoxycholic acid treatment on nutrition and liver function in patients with cystic fibrosis and longstanding cholestasis. Gut 1990; 31:918–921.

138. Galabert C, Montet JC, Lengrand D, et al. Effects of ursodeoxycholic acid on liver function in patients with cystic fibrosis and chronic cholestasis. J Pediatr 1992; 121:138–141.

139. Nousai-Arvanitakis S, Foutoulaki M, Economou H, et al. Long-term prospective study of the effect of ursodeoxycholic acid on cystic fibrosis-related liver disease. J Clin Gastroenterol 2001; 23:324–328.

140. Colombo C, Crosignani A, Assaisso M, et al. Ursodeoxycholic acid therapy in cystic fibrosis-associated liver disease: A dose-response study. Hepatology 1992; 16:924–930.

141. Cox KL, Ward RE, Furgiuele TL, et al. Orthotopic liver transplantation in patients with cystic fibrosis. Pediatrics 1987; 80:571–574.

142. Mack DR, Traystman MD, Colombo JL, et al. Clinical denouement and mutation analysis of patients with cystic fibrosis undergoing liver transplantation for biliary cirrhosis. J Pediatr 1995; 127:881–887.

143. Milkiewicz P, Skiba G, Kelly D, et al. Transplantation for cystic fibrosis: outcome following early liver transplantation. J Gastroenterol Hepatol 2002; 17:208–213.

144. Couetil JP, Houssin DP, Soubrane O, et al. Combined lung and liver transplantation in patients with cystic fibrosis. A 4 $\frac{1}{2}$ year experience. J Thorac Cardiovasc Surg 1995; 110:1415–1422.

145. Couetil JP, Soubrane O, Houssin DP, et al. Combined heart-lung-liver, double lung-liver, and isolated liver transplantation for cystic fibrosis in children. Transpl Int 1997; 10:33–39.

146. Treem WR. Inherited and acquired syndromes of hyperammonemia and encephalopathy in children. Semin Liver Dis 1994; 14:236–258.

147. Batshaw ML, Monahan PS. Treatment of urea cycle disorders. Enzyme 1987; 38:242–250.

148. Mathias RS, Kostiner D, Packman S. Hyperammonemia in urea cycle disorders: role of the nephrologists. Am J Kid Dis 2001; 37(5):1069–1080.

149. Consensus statement from a Conference for the Management of Patients With Urea Cycle Disorders. Urea Cycle Disorders Conference Group. J Pediatr 2001; 138(1 Suppl):S1–S5.

CHAPTER THIRTY-THREE

33

Prophylaxis and treatment of viral hepatitis

Gary L. Davis

INTRODUCTION

The management of hepatitis can be divided into measures aimed at primary prevention of disease (prophylaxis), primary therapy for established disease, and management of disease complications. The purpose of this chapter is to review immunoprophylaxis and primary therapy for viral hepatitis. Management of complications of chronic viral hepatitis and cirrhosis are discussed elsewhere in this book. Comments on viral hepatitis will be restricted to hepatitis A, B, C, and D. Although there are many other viral agents that may cause hepatic injury, they are uncommon, and specific pharmacotherapy is not available. An exception is cytomegalovirus (CMV). This virus is a major clinical pathogen in immunosuppressed patients, particularly transplant recipients, and is not discussed here.

Immunoprophylaxis can be divided into attempts to convey passive immunity by transfer of protective antibody or active immunity induced by vaccination with virus or viral antigens. Both of these strategies are well established for most forms of viral hepatitis. Passive protection against hepatitis A and B virus infections has been available for many years.[1–3] Immunoglobulin preparations with potential activity against hepatitis C are being studied in clinical trials. Vaccines against hepatitis B have been available for more than a decade.[4,5] Hepatitis A vaccines have proven extremely efficacious. An aggressive approach to immunization and immunoprophylaxis against infectious diseases has long been the standard of care in pediatrics.[6] Universal vaccination of newborns against hepatitis B is already a standard practice in many parts of the world where the infection is highly endemic. In the United States, the Centers for Disease Control (CDC) have recommended universal hepatitis B vaccination for children.[7] Control of viral hepatitis is unlikely to occur unless immunoprophylaxis is applied universally and high-risk life styles can be modified in those who either fail to respond or refuse to comply with immunoprophylactic regimens.

Treatment of acute hepatitis is usually not an issue since most cases of acute viral hepatitis are asymptomatic and go unrecognized. Furthermore, there is little need to consider therapy for most cases of acute hepatitis, particularly viral hepatitis A and B, since these typically resolve spontaneously. However, treatment of acute hepatitis should be considered for hepatitis C virus infection since it frequently progresses to chronic infection and results in liver disease.

Most data on the therapy of viral hepatitis is in patients with chronic hepatitis. The need for therapy in cases of chronic viral hepatitis is often decided based upon the severity of illness, risk of progressive injury, availability of agents, and likelihood of response. Specific antiviral therapy is available and necessary only for hepatitis B, C, and D.

HEPATITIS A

Hepatitis A virus infection is the most common cause of acute hepatitis in the United States, accounting for nearly half of cases. Of the estimated 125 000 to 200 000 acute cases, 100 develop fulminant hepatitis while the remainder recover spontaneously. However, infection is associated with considerable morbidity. After a short incubation period of 15–50 days, symptomatic and icteric infection may occur. In children under age 14 years, infection is usually asymptomatic and anicteric. In contrast, 70–80% of adults have icteric infection that is often associated with severe clinical symptoms. Case mortality also increases with age and is particularly high among patients with other forms of liver disease.[8]

Although virus is present in blood during acute infection, the main route of infection is fecal–oral. Hepatitis can be prevented by immune globulin or vaccine, but the risk of infection can also be reduced by avoiding exposure to infected individuals and by following strict hygienic practices when in endemic areas. Infected persons generally remain most infectious during the week after onset of symptoms and peak aminotransferase levels, but fecal shedding of virus may continue, at least intermittently, for much longer in some patients. When in endemic areas, drinking water should be boiled and uncooked fruits and vegetables should be avoided. Undercooked shellfish should also be avoided.

Immunoprophylaxis

Immune serum globulin

Immune serum globulin (ISG) is the only preparation available for the prevention of hepatitis A. ISG is not protective against hepatitis B virus infection and has unproven and unlikely efficacy in preventing hepatitis C or hepatitis E.[6] ISG contains normal human immunoglobulins (predominantly IgG) isolated by Cohn ethanol fractionation from the pooled plasma of multiple (>1000) paid donors and brought to a concentration of 16.5%.[9] The preparation is stabilized in glycine and preserved with thimerosal. ISG is not specific for hepatitis A, but contains multiple antibodies, some at high titers. Thus, ISG may interfere with live, attenuated vaccines such as measles, mumps, rubella, and varicella, and these vaccines should not be administered within several months before or after receiving globulin. The anti-HAV titer varies considerably between lots since anti-HAV could not be tested when ISG standards were first developed.[2] Anti-HAV is usually present at titers of >1:1000 (range 1:500–1:4000 by hemagglutination testing).[10] Low titers of anti-HBs are present, but HBsAg has not been present since initiation of donor screening in 1972.[10] Likewise, screening of donors has resulted in a progressive fall in antibodies to HCV. Recent donor screening policies also eliminated the possibility of anti-HIV being present.[11] Blood-borne transmission of hepatitis A virus has never been documented from administration of commercially available ISG.[1,6,11] Adverse effects following ISG administration, primarily rash, fever, and arthralgia, are rare (<1% of recipients).[12] The preparation available is for intramuscular (i.m.) use only. The intravenous form (ISG) used in immunodeficient patients is not intended for prophylaxis because of the risk of anaphylaxis.[9] ISG is safe for use in pregnant and lactating women.[1,6]

Indications for pre- and postexposure passive immunoprophylaxis against hepatitis A virus infection are listed in Table 33.1. The dosage regimen is outlined in Table 33.2. Peak antibody concentrations occur 48–72 hours after administration, but protection persists for a few months. Immune serum globulin given before exposure or during the incubation period is protective against clinical illness.[2,3] This prophylactic value is greatest (80–90%) when ISG is given early in the incubation period (within 2 weeks of exposure) and declines thereafter.[3]

Since the hepatitis A vaccine has become widely available, ISG is no longer indicated for pre-exposure prophylaxis in travelers to areas in which hepatitis A infection is endemic unless travel will occur within a few weeks. ISG continues to be indicated for postexposure prophylaxis following contact by susceptible individuals to HAV, but vaccine should also be considered in such cases. Since hepatitis A cannot be reliably diagnosed on clinical presentation alone, serologic confirmation of index cases by detection of IgM

Table 33.1 Indications for hepatitis A prophylaxis with immune globulin

Pre-exposure prophylaxis

International travelers to developing areas when insufficient time for vaccination exists

Postexposure prophylaxis

Home and sexual contacts of index case

All contacts of patient in day-care attended by children in diapers[a]

Classroom contacts of patient in day-care with no children in diapers[a]

Institutional personnel and occupants during an outbreak of hepatitis A

Coworkers of an infected food handler

Exposed individuals in a point-source epidemic, e.g. food source[b]

[a] Children and employees.
[b] Only if hepatitis cases are documented. In the absence of such cases, administration to patrons of establishments where an infected food handler has been identified is usually not necessary.

Table 33.2 Immune globulin prophylaxis for hepatitis A virus

Pre-exposure prophylaxis[a]

0.02 mL/kg i.m. if exposure is <3 months duration

0.06 mL/kg i.m. every 5 months if exposure is >3 months duration

Postexposure prophylaxis[b]

0.02 mL/kg i.m. immediately after exposure[c]

[a] For travelers.
[b] Serologic assessment of the exposed subject not required (see text).
[c] Must be given within 2 weeks of exposure.

---

anti-HAV is suggested before postexposure prophylaxis is considered. The serologic screening of contacts for anti-HAV prior to the administration of ISG is not recommended since screening is more costly than ISG, most individuals in the United States will not be immune, and such testing would only delay ISG administration.[13]

Hepatitis A vaccines

The ultimate control of hepatitis A infections hinges upon the development of an effective vaccine that can be incorporated into childhood vaccination programs.[14] The ability to grow hepatitis A in cell culture has made the development of hepatitis A vaccines possible.[15] Inactivated virus and live attenuated virus can now be produced in culture and are the most reliable approaches for vaccine development. Both of these forms of the HAV vaccine are well tolerated and highly immunogenic.[16,17] Almost all vaccinees develop high-titer anti-HAV antibodies.[16,17] In animal studies, this antibody response is protective against either oral or parenteral challenge with wild-type HAV.[18] Inactivated virus vaccines have now completed human trials and are clinically available.[19–22] These inactivated vaccines must be administered in 2 or 3 doses depending on the formulation.[16,19] Protective antibody appears early and is about 95% efficacious in preventing infection.[19–22] Thus, these inactivated HAV vaccines should replace ISG as preexposure prophylaxis when sufficient time exists before travel.

Indications for active immunoprophylaxis (vaccination) against hepatitis A virus infection are listed in Table 33.3. These indications include those at higher risk of acquiring infection as well as those at increased risk of complications of infection. Acute hepatitis A infection is associated with high mortality in persons

---

Table 33.3 Recommendations for hepatitis A vaccination

Travelers to intermediate and high HAV-endemic countries[a]

Homosexual and bisexual men

Drug users

Persons with chronic liver disease

Communities with high rates of hepatitis A (e.g. Alaskan natives and American Indians)

[a] If travel is to occur within 4 weeks, ISIG is recommended instead (see Table 33.1).

with chronic liver diseases, particularly chronic hepatitis C or alcoholic liver disease.[23,24] The dosage regimen is outlined in Table 33.4. Recently, a vaccine that combines antigens for hepatitis A and B has been approved (Twinrix).[25] Few data currently exist for vaccine use or response in children less than 2 years of age, but one study suggests that it is safe and effective in infants.[26] Prevaccination testing for anti-HAV is usually not indicated unless previous infection is suspected. In addition, serologic testing delays vaccination and may impact compliance. In general, prevaccine screening is not cost-effective unless there is a high prevalence of previous infection in the population. Thus, prevaccination testing should usually only be considered in adults who were born or resided in highly endemic areas, adults older than 50 years, and persons at or beyond adolescence in certain groups such as American Indians, Alaskan natives, and Pacific Islanders. Postvaccination anti-HAV testing is not necessary because of the high response rate.

Treatment of disease

Acute hepatitis A resolves spontaneously after several weeks in most symptomatic patients. Chronic hepatitis does not occur. Thus, only supportive comfort therapy is necessary in most patients. Rarely, a prolonged and relapsing course of cholestatic hepatitis may persist for several months. Bile salt binding resins such as cholestyramine may help pruritus in such patients. Corticosteroid treatment has been reported to decrease jaundice in a few patients. A single case of successful interferon treatment of vasculitis and angioedema associated with hepatitis A is reported.[27] Fulminant hepatitis occurs rarely. Liver transplantation should be considered in such cases. Clinical recurrence of hepatitis A following liver transplantation has been reported[28] and it would seem prudent to consider ISG administration following liver transplantation, though the pharmacokinetics of immunoglobulins in the post-transplant setting are significantly altered and repeated administration may be necessary.

HEPATITIS B

Hepatitis B virus infection accounts for approximately one-third of the cases of acute hepatitis in the United States. The estimated incidence of acute hepatitis B has fallen dramatically over the last 20 to 25 years. The incidence fell from 8.5 per 100 000 population in 1990 to 2.8 per 100 000 in 2002, which is approximately equivalent to 8000 new cases per year.[29] The decline in the incidence of acute hepatitis is attributable to vaccination of children and adolescents.[30] Since 30–90% of children who are acutely infected when less than age 5 years of age will develop chronic infection (as compared to only 2–5% among healthy adults), this reduction in acute infections will significantly reduce the prevalence of chronic HBV infection in the general population. Recovery and convalescence from infection is indicated by the presence of anti-HBs, while those who develop chronic infection have persistence of HBsAg. It is estimated that approximately 1.2 million persons in the United States are chronically infected with the hepatitis B virus.[31] Of these, 15–25% will have premature mortality due to their liver disease or associated hepatocellular carcinoma.

The hepatitis B virus is present in blood, serum, wound exudates, semen, vaginal fluid, and saliva. The major routes for acquiring infection are heterosexual contact (41%), injecting drug use (15%), homosexual activity (9%), household contacts (2%), and healthcare worker exposure (1%). A source is not apparent in approximately 30% of cases. Perinatal infection may also occur but is no longer common in the United States because of maternal screening for infection and appropriate treatment of infants born to infected mothers.

Immunoprophylaxis

Hepatitis B immune globulin

Hepatitis B immune globulin (HBIG) is prepared from pooled plasma preselected to contain high titers of anti-HBs, the antibody which confers protective immunity to HBV infection. The ethanol fractionation process used to prepare HBIG effectively eliminates both HBsAg and HIV from the vaccine.[13] Commercial preparations of HBIG have an anti-HBs titer of at least 1:100 000. By contrast, ISG has a titer of anti-HBs between 1:100 and 1:1000 and therefore has no role in the treatment of hepatitis B infections.[13,32] HBIG provides temporary, passive protection and is indicated for discrete postexposure situations. Indications for postexposure prophylaxis are listed in Table 33.5, though the need for HBIG in some of these situations will gradually decline as more of the 'at-risk' population is routinely vaccinated. The suggested dosing regimens for HBIG are outlined in Table 33.6. Perinatal transmission of HBV from a HBsAg-positive mother to her child is

---

Table 33.4 Recommended dosages of hepatitis A vaccine

Age (years)	Vaccine	Dose units (ml)	No. doses	Schedule (months)
2–8	HAVRIX[a]	360 ELU (0.5)	3	0, 1, and 6–12
		720 ELU (0.5)	2	0, 6–12
	VAQTA[b]	25 Units (0.5)	2	0, 6–18
>18	HAVRIX	1440 ELU (1.0)	2	0, 6–12
	VAQTA	50 Units (1.0)	2	0, 6–12

[a] HAVRIX (Smith-Kline, Beecham) is currently licensed in 3 formulations. The formulation and dose differs according to age. Doses of the formulations are expressed in enzyme-linked immunosorbent assay units (ELU).
[b] VAQTA (Merck, Sharp and Dohme) is licensed in 2 formulations. The formulation and dose differs according to age. Doses of the formulations are expressed in vaccine units which are not comparable to the other vaccine preparations.

Table 33.5 Indications for postexposure prophylaxis against HBV

Infant born to HBsAg-positive mother

Accidental percutaneous or permucosal exposure to HBsAg-positive blood

Sexual exposure to HBsAg-positive partner

Household exposure of infant to primary care provider with acute hepatitis B

reduced by 85–95% when HBIG is administered within 24 hours of birth and followed by a course of hepatitis B vaccination initiated within 7 days. By comparison, hepatitis B vaccine administered without HBIG is only 70–89% effective in preventing infection.[4,14] For persons experiencing accidental percutaneous exposure, HBIG is 75% effective.[30] HBIG is also 75% effective in preventing infection following sexual exposure, if administered within 14 days of exposure.[33] Immunologic testing of the exposed individual to evaluate susceptibility is indicated only if this time period will not be exceeded. Hepatitis B vaccine should be administered to susceptible persons at the same time in order to confer long-term protection.[13] Household contacts of chronic carriers of the virus should all be given HBV vaccine. Prophylaxis for household contacts of patients with acute hepatitis B is not indicated unless blood exposure is suspected. Potential routes for blood exposure in this setting include sharing of hygiene items such as toothbrushes or razors.[13]

Prophylaxis of persons experiencing accidental percutaneous or mucosal exposure to blood depends on the HBsAg status of the blood (if available), the exposed individual's vaccination history, and the response to any previously administered course of hepatitis B vaccine.[13]

Hepatitis B vaccine

Hepatitis B vaccine development began in the early 1970s using plasma derived from HBV carriers. Partial protection was demonstrated after the administration of boiled plasma.[1] Subsequent vaccines were developed from plasma concentrates of free viral envelope lipoprotein, the 22 nm spherical HBsAg particles.[5] Although the surface protein is itself noninfectious, the preparations underwent extensive thermal or chemical steps to inactivate any possible contaminating live viruses.[34] The resulting vaccine was highly immunogenic and effective if given at or before exposure to the virus. It was first licensed for clinical use in the United States in 1981 and was highly efficacious.[5,14] These are still the most popular vaccines worldwide since they can be produced at extremely low cost in developing countries. However, in Western countries, the declining availability of suitable plasma donors and concerns over safety and liability prompted a search for alternate sources of vaccines for HBV. Advances in genetic engineering in the 1980s culminated in production of recombinant HBsAg vaccines.[35,36] The gene encoding for production of the HBsAg protein, which is the major protein constituent of the spherical HBsAg particle, was incorporated into a plasmid and expressed in either bacteria or yeast.[35] The immunogenicity, efficacy, and safety profile of the recombinant vaccines proved comparable to the plasma-derived preparation.[14]

Four hepatitis B vaccines have been licensed for use in the United States. The plasma-derived Heptavax (Merck, Sharp and Dohme) was the first available (1982), but has recently been withdrawn from the market in favor of recombinant forms of vaccine. Recombivax (Merck, Sharp and Dohme), the first recombinant vaccine, has been available since 1986 and Engerix-B (GlaxoSmithKline), another recombinant preparation, has been available since 1989. Twinrix (GlaxoSmithKline) combines antigens for both hepatitis A and B into a single vaccine preparation. The indications for pre-exposure prophylaxis are listed in Table 33.7. The need for universal vaccination against hepatitis B is controversial. Such an approach is likely to be most cost-effective when the incidence or risks of infection are great. Thus, universal vaccination of newborns is the standard of care in many parts of the Far East. Universal vaccination of all children has recently been recommended in the United States.[7] However, in areas of low endemicity, the cost and societal benefit of universal vaccine has been questioned. Nonetheless, the incidence of acute infection in the United States has fallen dramatically since initiation of vaccine policies in children and adolescents.[30]

Prevaccination testing for anti-HBs to document immunity to hepatitis B virus is only cost-effective in populations in endemic areas and in groups at high risk. Either anti-HBc or anti-HBs can be used for screening; however, in low-risk groups, anti-HBc is frequently falsely positive. Obviously, no screening is necessary when vaccinating infants.

The recommended age-specific dosing schedules for each vaccine are listed in Table 33.8. Hepatitis B vaccine must be given into the deltoid muscle of adults and children in order to elicit optimum anti-HBs responses. Intradermal administration, using lower doses of vaccine (1 μg or 2μg), may elicit similar antibody titers, but response is erratic and this route should not be used routinely.[13] The vaccine series is given as 3 doses. The first two priming doses are given 1 month apart. The two priming doses induce detectable antibody in 70–80% of healthy recipients, but the titers are low (50–300 milli-International units (mIU/mL)). Delaying the second dose until 3–4 months after the first does not adversely affect the overall antibody response.[37,38] If the recom-

Table 33.6 Postexposure prophylaxis of HBV

| HBIG | Recommended vaccine | | Recommended exposure | |
	Dose (i.m.)	Timing	Dose (i.m.)	Timing
Perinatal	0.5 mL	Within 12 hrs of birth	0.5 mL	Within 12 hrs of birth[a]
Sexual	0.06 mL/kg	Within 14 days of sexual contact	1.0 mL single dose	Time of HBIG[a]

[a] First dose at the same time as the HBIG, but in a different site.

Table 33. 7 High risk indications for pre-exposure prophylaxis against HBV

Occupational risk to blood or blood products

Clients and staff in institutions for the developmentally disabled

Hemodialysis patients

Sexually active homosexual and bisexual men

Users of illicit injectable drugs

Recipients of pooled blood products[a]

Household and sexual contacts of HBV carriers

Adoptees, immigrants, and refugees from countries of high HBV endemicity

Populations with high endemicity of HBV infection[b]

Inmates of long-term correctional facilities

Persons with chronic liver disease

Sexually active heterosexual persons[c]

International travelers to endemic areas[d]

NOTE: The CDC has recommended universal vaccination for HBV
[a] Hemophiliacs should be vaccinated subcutaneously, not intramuscularly.
[b] Alaskan Natives, Pacific Islanders.
[c] Prostitutes, >1 sexual partner in previous 6 months, recent STD.
[d] Visit exceeds 6-months duration, blood or sexual contact anticipated.

mended schedule is interrupted after the first dose, no change in vaccine efficacy results if the second and third doses are administered with an interval of 3–5 months between them. A third dose is usually given 6 months after the first and is essential. It optimizes the antibody response by boosting the titer and thereby ensuring long-term persistence of this response.[5,13,14,36] The final dose induces antibody titers of 1000–3000 mIU/mL in 90–95% of healthy adults.[39] Higher titers are usually achieved in children. Delaying the third dose until 12 months after the first may induce even higher levels of antibody. No clear evidence exists that the four-dose regimen vaccine is more efficacious.

A response to hepatitis B vaccine is defined as development of levels detectable by the enzyme-linked immunosorbent assay (ELISA) or >10 sample ratio units (SRU) by radioimmunoassay (RIA) (approximately 10 mIU/mL using the international standard). Complete protection is afforded in 82–98% of vaccinees receiving 3 doses.[39] Anti-HBs titers decline progressively over time following successful vaccination. Between 15% and 40% of responders have titers <10 mIU/mL after 5–10 years.[40–42] However, protection against viremic infection and clinical disease appears to persist for at least 10 years after successful vaccination.[40–44] Evidence of infection (either HBsAg or anti-HBc) after more than 5 years of follow-up has been noted in only about 2% of vaccine recipients who were at high risk of infection (CDC, personal communication). No cases of chronic hepatitis B have been documented in vaccine responders. Despite loss of detectable anti-HBs in a proportion of patients, most retain cellular immune reactivity to the virus and have a rapid amnestic response to virus exposure or booster vaccine doses. Thus, data out to 16 years do not support either serial monitoring of anti-HBs levels or for booster doses of vaccine following successful hepatitis B vaccination.[13,14,43] However, it may be prudent for individuals with repeated exposure to the virus to document protective levels of anti-HBs.

Suboptimal anti-HBs levels (<10 mIU/mL) after the initial course of vaccine fortunately occur in only a small minority of patients, but this response is not protective against infection.[14] Low levels of antibody tend not to persist.[13,14,21] Such individuals may respond to an extra dose of vaccine.[14] Nonresponders may respond to one or more additional doses, or administration of a different preparation. Any patient who has undetectable or a poor response after receiving vaccine into the buttocks (not a recommended site of vaccine administration), should receive a course of the vaccine into the deltoid muscle.[13,45]

Although the hepatitis B vaccines are effective in most patients, results are disappointing in the elderly, the obese, and those with chronic diseases such as renal failure, cirrhosis, diabetes, and HIV infection. Age is the most important factor influencing the response to vaccination.[5,13,14] Response rates are greater than 95% in people below 19 years of age, 90% in young adults, and 50–70%

Table 33.8 Dosing schedules for hepatitis B vaccines

	Heptavax-B[b] Dose (μg) (mL)	Vaccine[a] Recombivax HB Dose (μg) (mL)	Energix-B[c] Dose (μg) (mL)
Infants of HBV-carrier mothers	10 (0.5)	5 (0.5)	10 (0.5)
Other infants and children <11 years	10 (0.5)	2.5 (0.25)	10 (0.5)
Children and adolescents 11–19 years	20 (1.0)	5 (0.5)	20 (1.0)
Adults >19 years	20 (1.0)	10 (1.0)	20 (1.0)
Dialysis or immune compromised persons	40 (2.0)[d]	40 (1.0)[e]	40 (2.0)[d,f]

[a] Three doses at 0, 1, and 6 months.
[b] Available only for hemodialysis and immunocompromised patients, and patients with known allergy to yeast.
[c] Alternative schedule: four doses at 0, 1, 2, and 12 months.
[d] Two 1.0 mL doses given at different sites.
[e] Special formulation for dialysis patients.
[f] Four-dose schedule recommended: 0, 1, 2, and 6 months.

in those persons greater than 60 years of age. Only 60–70% of hemodialysis and HIV patients respond to hepatitis B vaccine.[14,46,47] Additional doses or double doses are recommended in hemodialysis patients. Ideally, vaccination should be completed prior to the initiation of hemodialysis or renal transplantation in hope of improving the response rate. Hemodialysis patients who respond to vaccine usually have low titers and may require booster doses to maintain protection.[13,14,46] Titers should be checked yearly, and boosters administered if levels are below 10 mIU/mL. Although postvaccination testing of antibody levels is not necessary in immunocompetent persons, it may be helpful in patients with a predisposition to suboptimal antibody responses.[13]

The hepatitis B vaccines are safe. Pain at the injection site is the most common complaint and occurs in up to 20% of vaccine recipients.[13] There are no side effects that preclude hepatitis B vaccination of eligible persons.[14] Most initial concerns regarded the potential for transmission of blood-borne viruses, especially HIV, by the plasma-derived vaccine. These concerns proved unfounded.[34] Postlicensure surveillance by the CDC and FDA also documented a low incidence of Guillain-Barré syndrome after the first dose of plasma-derived vaccine (risk, 0.5/100 000 vaccinees).[48] Plasma-derived vaccines are no longer produced in the United States. Their use in this country is limited to hemodialysis patients, other immunocompromised hosts, and persons with allergies to yeast.[13] There are no postmarketing data regarding side effects for the recombinant hepatitis B vaccines to indicate any serious adverse effects.[14] They are safe in pregnant women.[13] Although administration of hepatitis vaccine to chronic hepatitis B carriers or persons with anti-HBs is neither helpful nor indicated, its inadvertent use has not been associated with adverse effects.[13] Hepatitis B vaccines do not interfere with other simultaneously administered vaccines.[13] Finally, concerns regarding the potential health hazards of the trace amounts of thimerosal (mercury) in infant vaccines have not been resolved though its risk, if any, is probably quite small.[49]

Treatment of acute and chronic infection

Treatment of acute hepatitis B is rarely indicated, since the risk of chronicity is relatively low. On the other hand, treatment of chronic hepatitis B is justified by infectivity and the natural history of the disease, namely propensity to development of cirrhosis or hepatocellular carcinoma.[50] The benefits of treating chronic hepatitis B are well established and therapy has evolved rapidly in recent years. Therapy is directed at those patients in the high-replication phase of infection (HBV-DNA >10^5 copies per mL by a sensitive assay or positive by an unamplified [non-PCR] method such as dot blot, solution hybridization, or bDNA; HBeAg is usually present). The goal of therapy is eradication of the virus, but sustained reduction of hepatitis B virus (HBV) replication (10^5 copies/mL or lower) is currently more realistic. Since the decision as to whether or not to treat is usually based upon biochemical and virologic markers, liver biopsy is not necessary for this purpose in many patients although it may provide other clinical information. When successful, treatment should be followed by the loss of HBeAg, HBsAg, reduction in the serum HBV-DNA level to at least less than 10^5 copies per mL (negative by unamplified HBV DNA assays), and the normalization of serum aminotransferase activities.[50] The treatment response in patients who have high levels of HBV replication but are HBeAg negative, as a result of mutations in the precore or core promoter region of the virus genome, is determined by persistent reduction of the HBV DNA levels below 10^5 copies per mL and normalization of serum aminotransferase activity.

Table 33.9 summarizes the current treatment recommendations of patients with chronic hepatitis B as developed by the American Association for the Study of Liver Disease (AASLD), European Association for the Study of the Liver (EASL), and the Asian-Pacific Association for the Study of the Liver (APASL).[51–53] In general, the decision about whether or not to treat the patient with a high level of HBV replication is not influenced by whether or not the patient has the HBeAg-positive or HBeAg-negative form of chronic hepatitis B, though the selection of therapeutic agents may differ (see text below; Table 33.10). Several treatment options are available and the choice of agent must consider several issues including goal of therapy, safety, patient preference, and cost. The advantages and disadvantages of currently available agents are listed in Table 33.11 and described below.

Interferons

Interferons are a heterogeneous family of proteins grouped according to structure, antiviral effects, and immunomodulatory properties. The alpha-interferons have a variety of biological effects which might explain their activity in viral hepatitis.[54,55] They inhibit the replication of a wide spectrum of RNA and DNA viruses by interfering with viral attachment and uncoating, inducing intracellular proteins and ribonucleases which convey antiviral properties to the cell, reducing viral RNA and protein

---

Table 33.9 Indications for interferon treatment in chronic hepatitis B

Serum ALT level	HBV DNA	Recommendations
Normal or ≤2 × ULN	< 10^5 copies/mL	No treatment; monitor for ALT or HBV DNA change
Normal	> 10^5 copies/mL	No treatment; monitor
≤2 × ULN	> 10^5 copies/mL	Treat if biopsy shows moderate or severe inflammation or advanced fibrosis
>2 × ULN	> 10^5 copies/mL	Treat; may observe HBeAg-positive patients for 3–6 months for spontaneous seroconversion. Treat immediately for decompensation or worsening

Modified from the recommendations of the American Association for the Study of Liver Disease, European Association for the Study of the Liver, and the Asian-Pacific Association for the Study of the Liver.[51–53]

Table 33.10 Selection of treatment agents for chronic hepatitis B

Condition	Recommendation[a,b]
HBeAg positive, HBV DNA >10⁵ copies/mL	Pegylated IFN, LAM, or ADV[c]
HBeAg negative, HBV DNA >10⁵ copies/mL	Pegylated IFN or ADV preferred[c]
Compensated cirrhosis	Pegylated IFN, LAM, or ADV[c]
Decompensated cirrhosis	LAM or ADV[c]
IFN nonresponder or IFN contraindication	LAM or ADV[c]

[a] Modified from the recommendations of the American Association for the Study of Liver Disease.
[b] IFN, interferon; LAM, lamivudine; ADV, adefovir.
[c] Entecavir would also be an alternative when FDA approved.

Table 33.11 Advantages and disadvantages of currently available agents for treatment of chronic hepatitis B

Agent	Advantages	Disadvantages
Standard interferon	Short course High seroconversion rate Durable response HBsAg loss common	Side effects Optimal duration unknown Less if ALT normal or patient immunosuppressed May cause decompensation in patients with advanced cirrhosis
Pegylated interferon	1 year duration High seroconversion rate Good response in HBeAg-negative chronic hepatitis B Durable response HBsAg loss common	High cost (though course short) Side effects Less if ALT normal or patient immunosuppressed May cause decompensation in patients with advanced cirrhosis
Lamivudine	Oral Well tolerated Inexpensive Safe/effective despite advanced liver disease or immune suppression	Low seroconversion rate Drug resistance common Requires long-term treatment HBsAg loss not common
Adefovir	Oral Well tolerated Lower drug resistance Active against lamivudine-resistant HBV Safe/effective despite advanced liver disease or immune suppression	Low seroconversion rate Not as potent as lamivudine Requires long-term treatment HBsAg loss not common
Entacavir	Oral Well tolerated Active against lamivudine-resistant HBV	Low seroconversion rate Requires long-term treatment
Tenofovir[a]	Oral Well tolerated Extremely potent antiviral activity Active against lamivudine-resistant HBV	Low seroconversion rate Requires long-term treatment
Emtricitabine[a]	Oral Well tolerated No de novo resistance to date (except in patients already resistant to lamivudine)	Low seroconversion rate Not as potent as lamivudine Requires long-term treatment

[a] Commercially available for HIV; no approved labeling for HBV.

synthesis, and amplifying specific (cytotoxic T lymphocyte) and non-specific (natural killer cell) immune responses to viral proteins.[54–57]

Alpha-interferons was the first agent that was shown to have efficacy in the treatment of chronic viral hepatitis and several recombinant forms, including pegylated forms of the parent compounds, are commercially available. Standard alpha-interferon was first shown to be effective for the treatment of chronic HBV infection about 15 years ago. Short courses (16–24 weeks) of subcutaneous recombinant interferon-alfa-2b administered as 5 million units daily or ten million units administered three times per week appeared to be optimal and were equally effective, although the daily dosing regimen appeared to be better tolerated.[50,55,58] Serum HBV DNA levels declined by as much as 75% during treatment.[59] Serum ALT levels usually remained unchanged for the first 8–10 weeks of treatment, but there was often a flare in ALT activity between 10 and 16 weeks in about 70% of responding patients and this was frequently followed by the disappearance of HBV DNA by the older dot-blot hybridization techniques, loss of HBeAg, and normalization of serum ALT, in that order.[50,58] Thus, it is important to recognize that an abrupt elevation of serum ALT during treatment is not an indication to adjust interferon dose or prematurely terminate therapy.[58] Entry into the phase of low replication is thought to represent immune-mediated clearance of the bulk of HBV-infected hepatocytes.[55] It is worth noting an important change in terminology between the literature describing these early trials and more recent studies. These early studies utilized rather insensitive dot-blot hybridization techniques to detect HBV DNA and commonly described loss of HBV DNA on treatment and entry into a nonreplicative phase of infection. It is now clear that low levels of HBV replication, generally less than 10^{4-5} copies per milliliter by the sensitive DNA amplification methods employed today, persist in such patients and therefore the term *low replicative phase* is preferable to *no-replicative phase*. Using this newer terminology, HBV DNA levels fell into the low replication range in approximately half of the patients treated with standard interferon.[55] About 10% of these responders subsequently lost HBsAg within 6 months of seroconversion.[58] Long-term follow-up studies demonstrated that about two-thirds of patients who responded to interferon eventually lost HBsAg and become HBV DNA negative by PCR;[60] this is a feature unique to interferon treatment and not common with nucleosides (see below). Although patients who lose HBsAg and detectable HBV DNA might appear to be clinically cured, small amounts of integrated HBV DNA sequences remain sequestered in either the liver or extrahepatic sites in some of these individuals.[61,62] Whether these are clinically relevant is not known.

Pegylation of interferons has decreased clearance of the parent drug allowing for once per week dosing and more consistent plasma drug levels. Pegylated interferons have been approved for treatment of chronic hepatitis C (see below). Two recent trials examined the effectiveness of 48 weeks of treatment with peginterferon-alfa-2a (180 micrograms once per week) with or without the nucleoside lamivudine in patients with HBeAg-negative chronic hepatitis B and wild-type infection.[63,64] Among the HBeAg-positive patients, HBeAg seroconversion occurred in 32% of subjects treated with pegylated interferon alone (27% if combined with lamivudine).[63] HBV DNA decreased to and remained less than 100 000 copies per milliliter in 32%. Among HBeAg-negative subjects, HBV DNA decreased to and remained less than 20 000 copies per milliliter in 43% of subjects treated pegylated interferon alone (44% if combined with lamivudine).[64] Loss of HBsAg and development of anti-HBs occurred in 2–3% of interferon-treated subjects within 6 months.

Several factors influence the response to interferon therapy. Those who respond best include those with low levels of HBV replication (less than 200 pg/mL by the Abbott Genostics assay; note that available HBV DNA assays are not compared to a common standard and therefore their use for selecting patients for treatment based on viral levels is limited) and high serum ALT levels (>100 IU/L).[50] Side effects occur in most patients who receive interferon.[65] These are usually confined to flu-like side effects such as fever, chills, myalgia, arthralgia, and headache. Tachyphylaxis to these symptoms generally occurs after the first few doses, but in some cases these side effects may persist at a low level throughout the treatment course.[65] A mean weight loss of 2.5 kg, and a consistent 15% reduction in white cell and platelet counts has also been described.[66] Leukopenia, granulocytopenia, and thrombocytopenia generally reach their nadir during the first 4 weeks of treatment. Thus, it is advisable to monitor these laboratory tests weekly during the first month and monthly thereafter during therapy. In general, interferon is well tolerated. About 10–20% of patients treated with standard interferons required temporary discontinuation of treatment or dose reductions because of side effects, usually leukopenia or thrombocytopenia, and 2–10% had to discontinue treatment altogether.[65–67] Pegylated interferon appears to be similarly tolerated.[63,67] It is interesting to note that intolerance is much less common in patients with chronic hepatitis B than in those with chronic hepatitis C, though the doses are similar.[68]

Contraindications to interferon therapy are relative. Treatment of patients with decompensated cirrhosis (coagulopathy, hypoalbuminemia, encephalopathy, ascites, or jaundice) requires considerable caution.[69] Side effects include significant cytopenia and bacterial infections. Worsening hepatic failure due to the interferon-mediated flare in hepatitis may require timely liver transplantation. Interferon therapy in this high-risk population should similarly be carried out only by experienced clinicians with ready access to a liver transplant program. Caution should also be used when considering treatment in patients with autoimmune disorders, pre-existing cytopenia, severe depression or other psychiatric conditions, severe congestive cardiac diseases, poorly controlled diabetes, seizure disorders, an organ transplant, and autoimmune or potentially immune-mediated diseases including but not limited to rheumatoid arthritis, systemic lupus, inflammatory bowel disease, or neuropathy. The drug should not be used in pregnant women.

Despite the gratifying viral responses reported with interferon treatment, the cost and associated side effects have hindered its acceptance as the preferred therapy. Thus, interferon was quickly replaced by well-tolerated oral reverse transcriptase inhibitors such as lamivudine and adefovir when these became commercially available.

Nucleoside analogues

Nucleoside analogues are compounds that are thought to impair viral replication by competing with the natural substrate for binding to cellular DNA polymerases, thereby becoming incorporated into the nascent DNA chain and terminating DNA chain synthesis. Most nucleosides are phosphorylated by cytoplasmic enzymes to nucleoside 5′-triphosphates. However, the unique metabolic and pharmacologic properties of each nucleoside analogue make it difficult to predict their mechanisms of action, toxicity, or efficacy.

A variety of nucleoside analogues have been studied as potential treatment for chronic hepatitis B. Many of these drugs have only been studied in small, controlled clinical trials. Adenine arabinoside (Ara-A) and its aqueous monophosphate derivative (Ara-AMP) are potent DNA polymerase inhibitors, but both agents were withdrawn from investigative use in the United States and western Europe because of neuromuscular toxicity and limited efficacy.[70,71] Acyclovir and the more absorbable prodrug, 6-deoxyacyclovir, are appreciably safer compounds, but clinical experience has indicated that neither has significant activity against HBV.[72,73] Ganciclovir may have more antiviral activity against hepatitis B.[74] Famciclovir appears to have similar effects, but has the advantage of being orally administered. Dideoxy-nucleosides such as DDI have proven to be potent inhibitors of duck hepatitis B virus, a virus closely resembling the human hepatitis B virus.[75] However, early studies in humans did not demonstrate activity. Ribavirin is a weak inhibitor of HBV replication. Fialuridine (FIAU), a fluoridated uracil which acts as a thymidine analogue, showed significant activity against HBV in cell culture and early short-term human trials. Unfortunately, the agent was associated with lethal toxicity when treatment was extended beyond 1 month. The relative potencies of the agents that are currently approved or under study are listed in Table 33.12, although potency alone does not determine their attractiveness as clinical agents.

Lamivudine

Lamivudine (3TC), a cytosine analogue, is a potent in vitro inhibitor of HBV. Initial human trials showed dramatic reductions in HBV DNA levels in all recipients of a single daily dose of 100 mg or more.[76] In contrast to interferon therapy, lamivudine is also associated with a relatively simultaneous fall in HBV DNA levels and serum ALT. As with all of the nucleoside analogues, the effects of short-term treatment with lamivudine are transient with detectable viral replication reappearing shortly after the drug is stopped.[76] However, longer treatment duration (several hepatocyte half-lives) with lamivudine was associated with sustained suppression of virus in most patients. For example, HBeAg to anti-HBe seroconversion was 12%, 17%, 21%, and 40% after 3, 12, 18, and 36 months of treatment, respectively.[76–79] HBV DNA suppression with HBeAg seroconversion is usually permanent, with 64% being maintained 3 years later and some of these patients may even lose HBsAg.[80] Prolonged treatment-related suppression of virus results in histologic improvement and even loss of fibrosis in some patients.[81] Lamivudine has an excellent safety record.[82] The major drawback of the drug is the development of drug resistance which results in loss of response and, eventually, histologic progression.[79,81,83] The likelihood of drug resistance is related to treatment duration increasing from 14% to 24% at one year, to 38% after 2 years, and to nearly 60% after 3 years.[79,84]

Adefovir dipivoxil

Drug resistance to lamivudine results in HBV DNA breakthrough and can result in loss of any previously obtained benefit. Thus, it is important to have other agents that are active against the lamivudine-resistant strains of the virus. Adefovir dipivoxil is an orally bioavailable prodrug of adefovir, a phosphonate nucleotide analogue of adenosine monophosphate.[85] It was originally developed for treatment of HIV but was associated with nephrotoxicity at the doses required to efficiently inhibit HIV.[86] It is active against HBV at lower doses that do not result in renal injury, although its ability to inhibit HBV is not as great as lamivudine or the nucleosides discussed below (see Table 33.12). The major attraction of adefovir is its ability to inhibit lamivudine-resistant mutants of HBV.[85]

Large multicenter randomized controlled trials of adefovir compared to placebo have been conducted in patients with chronic hepatitis B.[87,88] A 10 mg daily dose of adefovir for 48 weeks decreased HBV DNA levels by 3.52 and 3.91 logs from baseline for those with treatment naïve HBeAg-positive and HBeAg-negative chronic hepatitis B, respectively.[87,88] The drug was well tolerated without evidence of renal or other toxicity at this dose. Although no breakthrough drug resistance was seen in these studies, substitutions within the polymerase coding region develop at low frequency.[89] A small number of cases of drug resistance ($\approx$2% after 2 years of treatment) have now been reported.[85]

Thus, it appears that the major advantage of adefovir is its ability to inhibit HBV DNA in patients with lamivudine-resistant mutations of the virus. However, the antiviral effect of adefovir can be inconsistent in such patients, especially those with high viral loads, so other antiviral agents such as tenofovir or entecavir might be preferable.[90] It does not appear to have an advantage over lamivudine as primary therapy in treatment naïve patients and may not be as potent an antiviral agent. Nonetheless, some have recommended it over lamivudine since drug resistance is less common and the patients may not require monitoring of their virus levels as frequently. It is likely, however, that other antiviral agents will eventually replace adefovir.

Entecavir

Entecavir is a cyclopentyl guanosine analogue that is a potent inhibitor of the HBV polymerase. In contrast to both lamivudine and adefovir, it is a selective inhibitor of HBV and has no activity against HIV or other DNA viruses.[91] It is effective against both wild-type and lamivudine-resistant HBV, but is most effective against wild-type.[92,93] It appears to be about 30 times more potent than lamivudine.[94] It is highly bioavailable and administered once daily. A recent phase 3 multicenter study compared 48 weeks of entecavir at a dose of 0.5 mg per day to 100 mg of lamivudine in subjects with HBeAg-positive chronic hepatitis B.[95] Among entecavir-treated subjects, the median fall in HBV DNA was almost 7 logs, HBV DNA became undetectable in 69%, and seroconversion occurred in 21% compared to 5.5 logs, 38%, and 18%, respectively, for lamivudine. An identically designed study compared 48 weeks of entecavir at a dose of 0.5 mg per day to 100 mg of lamivudine in subjects with HBeAg-negative chronic hepatitis B.[96] HBV DNA decreased to less than 200 copies per milliliter

Table 33.12 Relative antiviral potencies of nucleosides and nucleotides available or under study

Drug	Drug status	log decrease HBV DNA
Pegylated interferon	Approved	3.5
Lamivudine (3TC)	Approved	4.4
Adefovir	Approved	3.5
Entecavir	Approved	4.6
Tenofovir	Approved (HIV only)	6.6
Emtricitabine (FTC)	Approved (HIV only)	3.0
Telbivudine (LdT)	Investigational	6.1

in 89% of entecavir-treated subjects compared to 70% of lamivudine-treated. Entecavir-resistant mutations of HBV have not been identified yet in nucleoside-naïve patients, but emerged in 6% of lamivudine-resistant patients who received the drug.[97] Entecavir was approved for use in chronic hepatitis B by the Food and Drug Administration in 2005.

Other antiviral agents

Several other nucleosides with activity against HBV are currently under study and show promise.[91] Tenofovir disoproxil fumarate is a nucleotide analogue, similar to adefovir, that is currently approved for the treatment of HIV but also has potent activity against HBV. Like adefovir, it is active against both wild-type and lamivudine-resistant HBV.[98] However, in contrast to adefovir, tenofovir results in rapid and consistent early viral suppression even in patients with advanced liver disease or HIV coinfection.[90] Emtricitabine (ETC) is a cytosine nucleoside analogue that is currently approved for use against HIV and has moderate (3 log) inhibitory activity against HBV. Resistance may limit its use as a single agent. Clevudine (L-FMAU) is a pyrimidine analogue that has selective inhibitory activity against HBV. Long-term dosing studies are underway. Telbivudine (LdT), an L-nucleoside thymidine analogue, is a member of a new class of natural β-L configured nucleosides. It is a very potent and selective HBV inhibitor; most treated patients achieve a 4-log reduction in HBV DNA. Interestingly, studies in woodchucks suggest that combinations of β-L-nucleosides (e.g. LdC and LdT) may have additive or even synergistic inhibitory effects. Development of these and other agents will continue and it is likely over the next few years that some of these agents will join the list of nucleosides approved for use in patients with chronic hepatitis B.

Selection of therapeutic agents for chronic hepatitis B

The approach to deciding whether to treat a patient with chronic hepatitis B is discussed above and summarized in Table 33.9. Although clinical trials have made a point to distinguish HBeAg-positive and HBeAg-negative patients with replicative chronic hepatitis B, this distinction is much less important in practice. Rather, the levels of HBV DNA and ALT, and sometimes the degree of histologic injury, are critical in making the decision to proceed with therapy (see Table 33.10). A possible exception might be to use a nucleoside with less chance of resistance when treating patients with HBeAg-negative chronic hepatitis B since therapy is often prolonged and resistance is likely with lamivudine; this remains controversial. The advantages and disadvantages of the available agents with efficacy in hepatitis B are listed in Table 33.11. Although interferons are attractive because of the finite duration of therapy, durability of response, and high clearance rate for HBsAg, the initial cost, and significant side effects of interferons have limited their acceptance. This may change with pegylated interferons. In contrast, nucleosides such as lamivudine, adefovir, and entecavir have been quickly accepted because of their ease of administration and lack of significant side effects. The major frustrations with these agents are the uncertain duration of use and the need to serially monitor for drug resistance. Fortunately, the latter has not limited

acceptance since a variety of active nucleosides are now available.

HEPATITIS D

Hepatitis D virus (delta agent) infection occurs only in patients infected with the hepatitis B virus. Thus, protection against HBV is protective against hepatitis D. However, most cases of hepatitis D occur as superinfection in patients already infected with HBV. There is currently no effective passive or active immunoprophylaxis to protect the HBV-infected patient against this infection. HBIG will not confer protection against HDV superinfection in carriers of HBsAg. Since HDV is a viroid consisting of unenveloped single-stranded RNA, i.e. it does not have a viral protein envelope, it is unlikely that vaccines will be easily developed. Fortunately, delta infection is becoming uncommon.

Treatment options

Interferons

Early studies suggested that interferon had a limited role in the treatment of HDV infection. Interferon does not inhibit HDV replication,[99] but conveys any benefit to the patient through inhibition of HBV. The antiviral effects are usually transient, i.e. are dependent upon ongoing therapy, and require high doses (9 MU three times per week for one year) for long periods of time.[100,101] Interestingly, about half of treated patients have persistent ALT normalization and histologic improvement, despite persistent HDV viremia.[99,101] Recently, the results of long-term follow-up of these biochemical responders were reported. Surprisingly, half of the patients with normal ALT levels after treatment still had normal ALT levels 14 years later and some had resolution of fibrosis.[102] Both HBV and HDV replication decreased, or even ceased, in some of these patients. Thus, long-term (1 year) high-dose interferon is currently the only effective therapy for chronic hepatitis D. The goal of therapy is ALT normalization, but this may eventually result in viral clearance and histologic improvement. No data with pegylated interferons are available to date.

HEPATITIS C

Hepatitis C virus infection currently accounts for only about 15% of cases of acute hepatitis in the United States. The estimated incidence of acute hepatitis C has fallen dramatically over the last two decades and it is now estimated that less than 30 000 new cases occur per year in the United States.[103] However, chronic infection (persistent viremia) occurs in 50–90% of acutely infected individuals and chronic hepatitis (abnormal liver tests) develops in 60–70%. There are nearly 4 million chronically infected persons in the United States.[104] Chronic hepatitis C is the most common cause of liver disease and the most common indication for liver transplantation.

The hepatitis C virus is present in blood, and therefore it is most efficiently transmitted by parenteral routes. At present, injection drug use is the most common route of transmission, accounting for 60% of cases. Blood transfusion, a common source of infection in the past, is no longer a common route of acquisition. Hepatitis C can also be transmitted sexually and perinatally, though these routes are not as efficient as they are with hepatitis B.

Immunoprophylaxis

Immune globulin

Studies evaluating the efficacy of immunoglobulin administration in preventing HCV have yielded conflicting results.[9] Three studies conducted in the 1970s examined the ability of immune globulin to reduce post-transfusion non-A, non-B hepatitis.[105–107] Although two of these studies significantly reduced the incidence of icteric hepatitis, the overall risk of hepatitis was not changed.[106,107] Several points regarding these studies must be emphasized. First, the risk of post-transfusion hepatitis was very high during the 1970s because of the use of commercial blood donors. It would be unlikely that any effect of immune globulin could be seen with the low rate of post-transfusion hepatitis that now exists since institution of voluntary blood donation and screening tests to eliminate HCV infection from the blood donor pool. Second, in one of these two studies, immune globulin was given before transfusion and its results are therefore not applicable to discussions of postexposure immunoprophylaxis.[106] Finally, it must be recognized that extrapolation of post-transfusion studies to other types of exposure to HCV, e.g. needlestick injuries, is probably inappropriate since the risk of infection by other routes is only 2–3%.[108] In short, there are currently no data to justify administration of immune globulin in hopes of preventing hepatitis C infection. Furthermore, current criteria for selecting plasma donors (anti-HCV negative) virtually guarantee that the titer of antibodies to HCV in IG preparations will be negligible. Some continue to recommend IG for post-exposure prophylaxis since the risk of its use is low;[6,13] however, the Advisory Committee on Immunization Practices has stated unequivocally that … IG does not protect against infection with HCV. Thus, available data do not support the use of IG for post-exposure prophylaxis of hepatitis C.

In contrast to ISG, a high titer anti-HCV immunoglobulin preparation has been shown to delay the onset of HCV infection in chimpanzees.[109] Such preparations do not appear to prevent infection, however. A recent clinical trial of high-titer polyclonal anti-HCV prepared from pooled plasma did not prevent HCV reinfection of grafts following liver transplantation of patients with chronic hepatitis C.[110]

Based on the current lack of an effective immune globulin, persons with percutaneous exposure to HCV should be closely monitored for infection. At a minimum, this requires serial testing of serum ALT and anti-HCV. Serial HCV RNA determinations by PCR might be a more effective means of monitoring and would be expected to identify acute infection earlier, when it would be more amenable to interferon treatment (see below).[111]

Hepatitis C vaccines

Development of an effective vaccine against HCV faces several obstacles. Most importantly, neutralizing antibodies against the hypervariable envelope proteins are isolate specific and therefore likely to provide only partial, if any, protection against a heterogeneous virus such as HCV.[92] Furthermore, clinical testing of an HCV vaccine would be difficult since the current risk of infection is extremely low except in active injection drug users. These limitations in mind, several efforts toward developing hepatitis C vaccines have been undertaken. Several prototype HCV vaccines have been developed in an effort to prevent primary infection. Envelope glycoprotein vaccines can produce high titers of neutralizing antibodies and prevent primary infection in chimpanzees

challenged with low doses of the homologous strain of HCV and perhaps even with some heterologous strains.[112,113] However, the heterogeneity of the viral envelope proteins is a major obstacle to making an effective envelope vaccine. Efforts to create a more effective vaccine using the relatively well-conserved HCV nucleocapsid (core) have been disappointing.[114] Vaccination with HCV genes in plasmid or viral expression vectors induces a humoral immune response to core and cytotoxic T-lymphocyte activity in mice, but neutralizing antibodies are not produced.[115–118] At this time, there are no promising candidates for a traditional vaccine for hepatitis C.

An alternative approach is development of therapeutic vaccines aimed at improving or resolving established infection. Several companies are active in therapeutic vaccine research. Repeated courses of a recombinant HCV E1 vaccine over 3 years resulted in increased anti-E1 antibody levels, E1-specific T-cell responses, decreased serum ALT levels, and lack of histologic progression, though no change in HCV RNA was observed.[119] This study was not controlled. Another study using a synthetic vaccine comprised of 5 peptides containing HLA-restricted cytotoxic T-helper epitopes of HCV and a T-cell adjuvant, poly-L-arginine, found that gamma interferon producing cytotoxic and helper T cells were induced in vaccine recipients but not in controls.[120] Clinical response data are not yet available.

Treatment of acute and chronic infection

The major goal of treatment of HCV infection is to prevent development of decompensated liver disease and death. This can be accomplished by preventing new infections, reducing the chance of acute infection progressing to chronic hepatitis, or effectively treating chronic infection. The goals in treating chronic hepatitis should include eradication or prolonged suppression of virus replication, reduction of hepatic inflammation, and, ultimately, slowing of the rate of progressive liver injury. Not all of these goals may be achievable in an individual patient.

Interferon in acute hepatitis C

The goal of treating patients with acute hepatitis is termination of infection, thereby eliminating the risk of progressing to chronic infection or liver disease. Several studies have examined the role of IFN in patients with acute hepatitis C.[121–124] Of these, four were randomized, controlled trials (three using recombinant alpha IFN for 3 months[121–123] and one using beta IFN for 1 month).[124] A recent meta-analysis of these studies demonstrated complete ALT response at the end of treatment in 69% of patients receiving IFN but only 29% of controls.[125] Sustained response 12 months after completion of treatment was seen in 53% of IFN-treated patients and only 32% of untreated controls.[125] Furthermore, serum HCV RNA was undetectable at the last follow-up in 41% of treated patients but only 4% of untreated controls. Thus, even a short course of IFN at standard doses reduces the proportion of patients developing chronic HCV infection (HCV RNA positive) from 96% to 59% and chronic hepatitis (elevated ALT) from 68% to 47%. Pegylated interferon either alone or in combination with ribavirin for 6 months cleared infection in 80–85% of cases compared to 36% of controls.[126]

While these results are encouraging, treatment of patients with acute HCV infection must be considered in the proper perspective. The incidence of acute hepatitis C in the United States has fallen dramatically to about 28 000 infections per year.[127] Only a small proportion of these cases are symptomatic and recognized by either the patient or physician. Furthermore, there is no test to distinguish acute from chronic infection. Nonetheless, when acute hepatitis C is suspected, treatment should be strongly considered.

Interferon for chronic hepatitis C

Interferon is the foundation of therapy for chronic hepatitis C. The efficacy of IFN in patients with chronic non-A, non-B hepatitis was first described in 1986, 3 years before the identification of HCV.[128] Several subsequent reports confirmed that low doses of IFN-α improved liver tests and histology in patients with chronic hepatitis C.[129-133] Over the last decade, interferon-based treatment regimens have become increasingly effective, and sustained viral response or clearance can now be achieved in approximately 55% of treated patients.[134] Sustained viral response (SVR) is defined by undetectable HCV RNA by a sensitive amplification method, such as polymerase chain reaction (PCR) or transcription-mediated amplification (TMA), 6 months after completion of therapy. SVR is durable[135] and associated with histologic improvement[136,137]

All patients with chronic hepatitis C should be considered for possible interferon treatment. If contraindications to therapy are not present (see below), then a quantitative HCV RNA level and viral genotype should be done (Table 33.13). At the present time, a pretreatment liver biopsy remains important in determining the degree of underlying liver injury because neither serum ALT, HCV RNA, nor symptoms correlate well with histologic activity.[138,139] Liver biopsy provides an estimation of prognosis and is helpful in counseling the patient about the need and urgency for therapy. The National Institutes of Health Consensus Development Conference on Hepatitis C concluded that the need for treatment

in patients with chronic hepatitis of moderate or severe histologic activity with or without fibrosis was unequivocal, while patients with mild activity and those with decompensated cirrhosis need to be considered on an individual basis after weighing such factors as projected prognosis, age, comorbid factors, and pre-existing cytopenia.[140] However, as the efficacy of treatment regimens improves, it is likely the role of liver histology in helping determine the need for treatment will decrease.

Initial therapy for chronic hepatitis C in the early 1990s consisted of standard interferon administered thrice weekly. SVR rates were low, averaging 6% to 16% for 6 to 12 months of therapy, respectively.[125] The addition of the oral nucleoside ribavirin increased SVR rates to 33% and 44% for 6 and 12 months, respectively.[141,142] Current therapy consists of pegylated interferon administered once per week plus daily ribavirin therapy.[143,144] Overall SVR rates now average above 50%. The current recommendation for dose and duration have evolved from the large randomized studies of pegylated interferon and ribavirin[143,144] and from a more recent study that examined a shorter duration of treatment and lower doses of ribavirin.[138] The current recommendation for genotype 1, which accounts for about 70% of cases in the United States, is 12 months of pegylated interferon and ribavirin, the latter at a dose of 1000 mg for a subject weighing less than 75 kg and 1200 mg for those who weigh more. Genotypes 2 and 3 are more sensitive to interferon-based therapy and they require only 6 months of treatment and 800 mg of ribavirin per day.

The typical response to interferon therapy is a rapid fall in serum ALT and HCV RNA.[129] With current treatment regimens, HCV RNA levels decrease by at least 2 logs after 12 weeks of treatment in approximately 80% of patients (70% for genotype 1, 96% for genotypes 2 or 3) and are undetectable by PCR in most of these cases.[139] Patients who do not decrease their HCV RNA level by at least 2 logs during the first 12 weeks of treatment (termed early viral response or EVR) will not respond to treatment and therapy can be stopped (Fig. 33.1).[139] A fall in the serum ALT level typically occurs in parallel with the virologic response, and ALT often normalizes between 4 and 12 weeks after initiation of treatment.[140,145,146] These biochemical and virologic changes are accompanied by histologic improvement.[129,143,144,147] Once the prescribed duration of therapy has been completed, drugs should be stopped; there is currently no evidence that a longer course of therapy is helpful. Serum ALT and HCV RNA should be repeated 6 months after treatment is completed to determine whether an SVR has been achieved. SVR should be confirmed by HCV RNA testing again 1 year after completing therapy and yearly thereafter for at least 2 years in order to confirm a durable response.

About half of patients with chronic hepatitis C who are treated with IFN fail to respond.[125,129,143,144] Nonresponse is usually evident early in the treatment course as described above. It is important to recognize that not all nonresponders are the same in terms of their sensitivity to interferon-based regimens; HCV RNA may fall significantly and become nearly undetectable or may not change at all.[129,146,148] The degree of initial interferon sensitivity probably provides a good estimate of the likelihood of response when new and more effective therapies are developed. It has long been noted that some patients without a complete virologic response will nevertheless show some histologic improvement.[125,129] This appears to depend upon the ability of interferon to at least decrease the viral level since no such histologic

---

Table 33.13 Selection of patients with chronic hepatitis C for treatment

Indications

Documented HCV infection (anti-HCV and HCV RNA positive)
No contraindications to therapy

Contraindications

For interferon
  Significant cytopenia (relative)
  Major depression or other psychiatric disease
  Autoimmune diseases

For ribavirin
  Inability to tolerate acute fall in hemoglobin
  Chronic anemia or hemolytic anemia
  Severe cardiac or pulmonary disease
  Elderly patients, particularly with risk factors for coronary disease
  Patients of childbearing potential not using adequate contraception

Baseline assessment

Quantitative HCV RNA
HCV genotype
Liver biopsy (optional)

Note: See text for discussion of optimal treatment regimen.
ALT, alanine aminotransferase; HCV, hepatitis C virus.

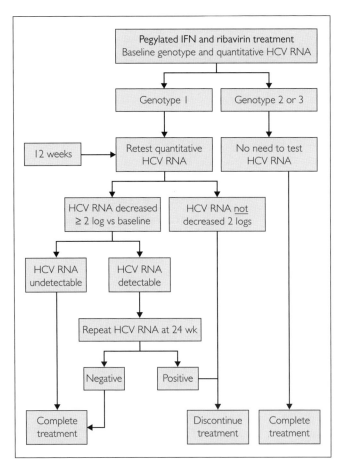

Fig. 33.1 • Algorithm for monitoring antiviral treatment in patients with chronic hepatitis C.

improvement is seen in those who fail to suppress virus by at least 2 logs during therapy.[148,149] Thus, there has been great interest in continuing therapy or retreating patients with histologically advanced disease, i.e. fibrosis or cirrhosis, in hopes of preventing disease progression. Certainly, all nonresponders, particularly those who decreased viral levels with their initial course of treatment, should be considered for re-treatment if advances in therapy, such as a new agent, evolve and are proven to be effective. However, re-treatment with the same regimen is not effective and should not be considered in such patients. Very high doses of interferons or prolongation of therapy may improve overall outcomes, but these studies have not been controlled and require confirmation.[150,151] Most interest recently has focused on maintenance interferon therapy. Several studies are underway to assess whether maintenance therapy with long-term, low-dose interferon is of benefit to patients with chronic hepatitis C and fibrosis who have failed to eradicate HCV with conventional antiviral therapy. These studies include the NIH-sponsored HALT-C trial, the international EPIC trial, and the COPILOT study. Only the COPILOT study has reported data so far.[152] A 2-year interim analysis reported no difference between interferon-treated and control groups for death, hepatocellular carcinoma, or need for transplantation. However, by Kaplan-Meier analysis, the annual risk of variceal bleeding was 13.5% in the control group and 5% in the interferon group. These preliminary findings are the first data to suggest that low-dose maintenance interferon may be useful in preventing complications of cirrhosis, but the benefit appears to be confined to

reducing the complications of portal hypertension, and the rate of variceal bleeding in the control group appears to be high considering that they were supposed to be adequately beta blocked. However, another recent report suggests that interferon may decrease portal pressure and this might explain the observations in the COPILOT study.[153] The results of other similar interferon maintenance studies will be of great interest in confirming these important observations and determining whether pegylated interferon maintenance might be an option in cirrhotic patients who fail to eradicate HCV with interferon-based therapies.

Factors that influence treatment response

Viral genotype is the most important factor influencing response to combination treatment (Table 33.14). In recent trials that evaluated a year of pegylated interferon and ribavirin in previously untreated patients, SVR was achieved in 41–42% of patients infected with genotype 1 and 66–75% of those with genotype 2 or 3.[143,144] This led to a study to define the optimal dose of ribavirin and duration of therapy according to genotype.[138] Patients with genotype 1 had the highest SVR with 48 weeks of therapy (51% versus 41% with 24 weeks at full-dose ribavirin) at a dose of 1000 to 1200 mg of ribavirin per day (51% versus 40% with a lower dose of ribavirin for 1 year). In contrast, patients with genotype 2 or 3 did as well with just 6 months of treatment and 800 mg per day of ribavirin (73% to 78% for all doses and durations studied). Preliminary reports from ongoing studies suggest that patients with genotype 2 or 3 who lose detectable HCV RNA after 4 weeks can be treated for just 14–16 weeks,[154,155] but this needs confirmed in other trials before becoming standard clinical practice.

The effect of HCV RNA before treatment influences response, but not to the same degree as viral genotype does. The effect is observed mainly in patients with genotype 1 infection. Those with pretreatment HCV RNA levels greater than 2 million copies per milliliter have an SVR of 30–39% compared to SVR of 56–68% in patients with lower levels of viremia.[143,144] One study recently suggested that patients with genotype 3 and high viral loads had a poor response and should be treated with 48 weeks instead of 24 weeks of therapy,[156] but analysis of larger clinical databases has failed to confirm the value of this suggestion.[157]

Table 33.14 Influence of pretreatment and treatment factors on response to pegylated interferon and ribavirin

Increased SVR	Decreased SVR
Genotype 2 or 3	Genotype 1
HCV RNA <2 million copies/mL	HCV RNA >2 million copies/mL
Young	Bridging fibrosis or cirrhosis
Female gender	Male gender
Short duration of infection	Obesity
Early viral response	Hepatic steatosis
	Alcohol intake
	Poor adherence
	Early dose reductions

Fibrosis or cirrhosis, known to reduce the response to interferon alone, does not appear to reduce the sustained response quite as much with combination therapy (41–44% SVR in stage 3–4 disease versus 54–55% with stage 0–2).[141–144,158] This is an important observation since these patients are at the greatest risk for developing hepatic decompensation if not treated.[159]

SVR is reduced, though to a far lesser extent than with the factors discuss above, by age, weight, alcohol use, and hepatic steatosis.[143,144,160,161] SVR is not significantly influenced by ALT level (including normal ALT). There are currently no data to suggest that the response rates are significantly different with the two forms of pegylated interferon or with different brands of ribavirin.

SVR is reduced in African-Americans and patients coinfected with HIV. Since African-Americans are predominantly infected with genotype 1, they might be expected to have lower SVR than the general population. However, even among those with genotype 1 the SVR in this group is lower than in non-Hispanic whites (19–26% versus 39–52%).[162,163] The explanation for this difference in response remains elusive and may be related to genetic polymorphisms that influence immune responsiveness. Patients coinfected with HIV also have lower SVR than HIV-negative patients when treated with combination therapy. Three large clinical trials have clearly shown that SVR after a year of treatment with pegylated interferon and ribavirin is reduced compared to patients infected with HCV alone (27–40% overall; 14–29% in genotype 1).[164–166] Somewhat surprisingly, patients infected with genotype 2 or 3 did quite well with SVR ranging from 43% to 73%.

Side effects of interferon and ribavirin

The side effects of interferon, regardless of the formulation used, are dose-dependent and include initial flu-like symptoms, fatigue, depression, and cytopenia. These have been well described (see above in Hepatitis B).[129] Overall, about 10% of patients in clinical trials have discontinued therapy because of these symptoms or laboratory changes. It is important to recognize the side effects of therapy and manage them appropriately (Table 33.15). When safe and possible, side effects should be managed while therapy continues since inappropriate dose reductions and discontinuations may significantly compromise the chance of response.[139,167]

In general, the addition of ribavirin to the treatment regimen does not usually increase the clinically perceived side effects of treatment. However, ribavirin causes hemolysis at currently recommended doses. The hemoglobin fall occurs during the first 8 weeks of treatment and remains relatively stable thereafter. Rapid and significant drops may occur in a short period of time and therefore careful monitoring is required during the first few weeks of combination therapy. The mean fall in hemoglobin of 2.5–3.7 gm/dL depending on the dose of ribavirin used.[143,144,168–171] About 10% develop hemoglobin levels less than 10 g/dL.[143,144] Ribavirin dose reductions are required in 10–20% of cases. Although the fall in hemoglobin is accompanied by a reticulocytosis, interferon may partially block this, and reduction of the ribavirin dose alone may sometimes be insufficient to arrest the drop in hemoglobin. Hemoglobin levels typically return to baseline within 4 weeks of the end of therapy. It is clear from the side effect profile of ribavirin that combination therapy is not indicated for every patient. It should be used with great caution or not at all in patients with pre-existing anemia or hemolytic

Table 33.15 Management of drug toxicity in the treatment of chronic hepatitis C

Drug-related problem	Management options[a]
Flu-like symptoms	Dose in evening Acetaminophen Oral fluids Activity
Nausea ± vomiting	Metaclopramide Phenothiazines Serotonin HT3 receptor antagonist
Fatigue	Treat anemia and depression Exercise SSRIs with stimulatory properties (e.g. flouxetine, sertaline) Bupropion Modafinil
Depression	SSRIs Counseling if poorly controlled
Anxiety	SSRI with sedating properties (e.g. low-dose venlafaxine)
Mania	Stop interferon and all antidepressants Emergency referral to psychiatry
Insomnia	Sleep hygiene Take second dose of ribavirin in early evening, not before bed Avoid stimulating SSRIs Diphenhydramine Short-acting hypnotics (e.g. zolpidem, zaleplon)
Anemia	Stop ribavirin if Hgb <8.5 g/dL or symptomatic; transfuse as required Ribavirin dose reduction if Hgb <10 g/dL Consider slight ribavirin dose reduction if Hgb <11–12 Consider erythropoietin (lag time until effect)
Neutropenia[a]	Observe ANC weekly when ANC <750 Dose reduce interferon for ANC <500 Consider G-CSF if ANC <500 and dose reduction fails
Thrombocytopenia[a]	Reduce interferon when platelets <30 000–50 000 or bleeding
Rash	Avoid sun exposure No therapy for mobilliform rash unless pruritic Antihistamines or topical hydrocortisone for urticarial or pruritic rash Discontinue interferon and ribavirin for rare Stevens-Johnson syndrome, but otherwise can usually continue therapy despite rash

[a] These suggestions may differ from package insert instructions and are based on the author's clinical experience. They are neither recommendations nor guidelines. Clinicians should treat within their comfort level.

disorders, coronary artery disease, or hypoxia. Careful consideration to the potential effects of anemia should be given for each patient in whom combination treatment is considered. Because of its embryotoxic and teratogenic effects in animals, it should not be used in patients (male or female) of child-bearing potential.

Decreases in white blood cell and absolute neutrophil count (ANC) are similar in patients treated with interferons alone or with ribavirin.[143,144,171] Neutropenia (ANC <750 cells/mm³) is more common with pegylated interferons (15–20%) than with standard interferons. The fall usually occurs within the first 2–3 weeks and stabilizes thereafter. Although package labeling for the interferons defines dose reduction guidelines, these are based on infection risks in neutropenic oncology patients. In fact, interferon-related neutropenia in hepatitis patients has not been shown to increase the risk of infection, but neutropenia does merit closer patient observation.[172] Platelet counts decline with both treatment regimens, but the decline is less with combination therapy as the result of a relative reactive thrombocytosis due to anemia.[171] Discontinuation of treatment is more common with combination therapy than with interferon alone (10% versus 5%). The most common laboratory reason for dose reduction or interruption is anemia, though this probably contributes to symptoms such as fatigue and depression as well.[171]

Neuropsychiatric symptoms are common and perhaps the most distressing to patient and physician. Depressed mood occurs in up to 60% of patients when prospectively sought by symptom surveys.[173] Other symptoms such as irritability, anxiety, loss of concentration, malaise, and disturbed sleep are also quite common. While any of these can be problematic, the most significant is depression. Suicidal ideation may occur in up to 10% of cases.[173] Neither age nor a previous history of depression is predictive for the development of depression during interferon therapy.[174] However, the presence of depressive or anxiety symptoms at the time treatment is started is highly predictive of worsening during the course of therapy.[174] Pretreatment of such patients with a selective serotonin reuptake inhibitor (SSRI) is quite effective in reducing treatment interruptions related to depression.[174] In some cases, it is helpful to have the patient followed by a psychiatrist during the course of therapy. If either suicidal ideation or mania occurs during treatment, both drugs should be stopped and consultation with a psychiatrist should be obtained emergently.

Other treatment options

Several agents or maneuvers including ursodeoxycholic acid, indomethacin, N-acetycysteine, amatidine, thymosin, and phlebotomy have been reported to be useful adjuncts to IFN treatment, but none has been consistently shown to be effective in randomized, controlled trials.

Direct inhibitors of HCV replication

Direct inhibition of the replicative mechanism of a virus has proven to be an effective therapeutic strategy in patients with chronic infections with other viruses such as HIV or HBV. However, this has been a much more elusive strategy to implement with chronic hepatitis C. The viral targets including the serine protease, helicase, and RNA-dependent RNA polymerase have been difficult to inhibit with small molecules. Furthermore, some molecules that are active in the in vitro HCV replicon system have not always been shown to have activity in vivo. Despite these obstacles, several agents have entered or soon will enter clinical trials. A protease

inhibitor showed potent antiviral activity with 2 days of administration, but animal toxicity prevented further development of the drug.[175] Nonetheless, this report was an important proof of concept. Several other agents are in trial and at least some of these will likely become adjuncts to our current regimen in coming years.

Viramidine, a prodrug of ribavirin, is metabolized in the liver thereby reducing systemic levels of ribavirin and, hopefully, the development of anemia. Preliminary trials suggest that reduction of HCV RNA during therapy is similar to patients treated with ribavirin, and dose-limiting anemia is almost eliminated.[176] Whether SVR will be the same as with the parent drug remains to be proven, but this drug might reduce much of the treatment-related morbidity.

Nonprescription agents used for chronic hepatitis

In the United States, it is likely that more patients with chronic hepatitis C use nonprescription agents of unproven effectiveness than use interferon. Several agents such as alpha-tocopherol, bayberry, blessed thistle, milk thistle, blue flag, dandelion root, fringetree bark, gentian, yellow dock, and various Chinese herbal remedies have been touted in the lay literature; however, there are no reliable data available to support their use. On the other hand, at this time there is little evidence that these agents do any harm when used for short periods of time. However, all herbal and nonprescription agents should be used with extreme caution, especially preparations with multiple or unknown ingredients, since the safety profiles of these remedies have not been critically studied.

All herbals should be avoided in patients with advanced liver disease.

Milk thistle is perhaps the most popular of the nonprescription agents used for chronic hepatitis C. Its active ingredients are the flavonoid silymarin, and its main structural component silybin. Animal and cell culture studies have demonstrated that these compounds inhibit the lipoxygenase pathway and have antioxidant properties that diminish toxicity induced by a variety of hepatotoxins.[177,178] Both silymarin and silybin have been shown to induce cell damage in cell culture systems.[179] A single small, controlled trial of a 1-week course of silybin in patients with chronic hepatitis (type unspecifed) has been reported.[180] Liver enzymes decreased slightly, but remained abnormal, in treated patients. A pilot study with another antioxidant, alpha-tocopherol, showed no effect on serum ALT or HCV RNA.[181]

SUMMARY

Hepatitis A is a self-limited illness that is now preventable by vaccine administration. No therapy is necessary for infected individuals, though vaccine or immune globulin should be considered for contacts.

Hepatitis B is a common worldwide problem. Widespread use of the hepatitis B vaccine has already resulted in a striking reduction of new cases and disease-related morbidity and mortality. Chronic infection can be treated with a variety of effective drugs. The selection of the appropriate method of therapy, if necessary, depends upon the level of replication and degree of liver injury. Ongoing suppression appears to reduce the chance of progressive liver injury and can reverse established fibrosis in some cases.

Hepatitis C is the most common cause of chronic viral hepatitis in the United States. Most cases are asymptomatic and unrecognized. Treatment consists of pegylated interferon and ribavirin.

Eradication of virus is possible in more than half of treated cases and this alone justifies treatment of most patients with chronic infection who do not have contraindications to this form of therapy.

REFERENCES

1. Krugman S, Overby LR, Mushawar IK, et al. Viral hepatitis type B: studies on natural history and prevention re-examined. N Engl J Med 1979; 200:101–106.

2. Mosley JW, Reisler DM, Brachott D, et al. Comparison of two lots of immune serum globulin for prophylaxis of infectious hepatitis. Am J Epidemiol 1968; 87:539–550.

3. Kluge I. Gamma-globulin in the prevention of viral hepatitis: a study of the effect of medium-size doses. Acta Med Scand 1963; 174:469–477.

4. Beasley RP, Hwang LY, Lee GC, et al. Prevention of perinatally transmitted hepatitis B virus infections with hepatitis B immune globulin and hepatitis B vaccine. Lancet 1983; 2:1099–1102.

5. McLean AA, Hilleman MR, McAleer WJ, et al. Summary of worldwide experience with H-B-Vax (B, MSD). J Infect 1983; 7(Suppl):95–104.

6. American College of Physicians Task Force on Adult Immunization. Guide for adult immunization. 2nd edn. Philadelphia: American College of Physicians Task Force on Adult Immunization; 1990.

7. [No authors listed]. Hepatitis B virus: A comprehensive strategy for eliminating transmission in the United States through universal childhood immunization: Recommendations of the Immunization Practices Advisory Committee. MMWR 1991; 40:1–25.

8. Vento S, Garofano T, Renzini C, et al. Fulminant hepatitis associated with hepatitis A virus superinfection in patients with chronic hepatitis C. N Engl J Med 1998; 338:286–290.

9. Seeff LB. Diagnosis, therapy and prognosis of viral hepatitis. In: Zakim D, Boyer TD, eds. Hepatology: a textbook of liver disease. 2nd edn. Philadelphia: WB Saunders; 1989:958–1025.

10. Hoofnagle JH, Waggoner JG. Hepatitis A and B virus markers in immune serum globulin. Gastroenterology 1980; 78:259–263.

11. Centers for Disease Control. Safety of therapeutic immune globulin preparations with respect to transmission of human T-lymphotropic virus type III/lymphadenopathy-associated virus infection. MMWR 1986; 35:231–233.

12. National Transfusion Hepatitis Study. Risk of post-transfusion hepatitis in the United States – a prospective comparative study. JAMA 1972; 220:692–701.

13. Centers for Disease Control. Protection against viral hepatitis Recommendations of the Immunization Practices Advisory Committee (ACIP): MMWR 1990; 39 (Suppl 2):1–26.

14. Hadler SC. Vaccines to prevent hepatitis B and hepatitis A virus infections. Infect Dis Clin North Am 1990; 4:29–46.

15. Lemon SM. Type A viral hepatitis. New developments in an old disease. New Engl J Med 1985; 313:1059–1061.

16. Wiederman G, Ambrosch F, Kollaritsch H, et al. Safety and immunogenicity of an inactivated hepatitis A candidate vaccine in healthy adult volunteers. Vaccine 1990; 8:581–584.

17. Midthun K, Ellerbeck E, Gershman K, et al. Safety and immunogenicity of a live attenuated hepatitis A virus vaccine in seronegative volunteers. J Infect Dis 1991; 163:735–739.

18. Provost PJ, Banker FS, Wadsworth CW, et al. Further evaluation of a live hepatitis A vaccine in marmosets. J Med Virol 1991; 34:227–231.

19. Van Damme P, Thoelen S, Cramm M, et al. Inactivated hepatitis A vaccine: reactogenicity, immunogenicity, and long-term antibody persistence. J Med Virol 1994; 44:446–451.

20. Muller R, Chriske H, Dienhardt F, et al. Hepatitis A vaccination: schedule for accelerated immunization. Vaccine 1992; 10 (Suppl 1):S124–S125.

21. Innis BL, Snitbhan R, Kunasol P, et al. Protection against hepatitis A by an inactivated vaccine. JAMA 1994; 271:1328–1334.

22. Werzberger A, Mensch B, Kuter B, et al. A controlled trial of formalin-inactivated hepatitis A vaccine in healthy children. N Engl J Med 1992; 327:453–457.

23. Vento S. Fulminant hepatitis associated with hepatitis A virus superinfection in patients with chronic hepatitis C. J Viral Hepat 2000; 7(Suppl 1):7–8.

24. Feller A, Uchida T, Rakela J. Acute viral hepatitis superimposed on alcoholic liver cirrhosis: clinical and histopathologic features. Liver 1985; 5:239–246.

25. Van Damme P, Van Herck K. A review of the efficacy, immunogenicity and tolerability of a combined hepatitis A and B vaccine. Expert Rev Vaccines 2004; 3:249–267.

26. Shapiro CN, Letson GW, Kuehn D, et al. Effect of maternal antibody on immunogenicity of hepatitis A vaccine in infants (Abstract). Interscience Conference on Antimicrobial Agents and Chemotherapy; 1995; September 17–20. San Francisco, CA: American Society for Microbiology; 1995:90.

27. Matteson EL. Interferon alpha 2a therapy for urticarial vasculitis with angioedema apparently following hepatitis A infection. J Rheumatol 1996; 23:382–384.

28. Gane E, Sallie R, Saleh M, et al. Clinical recurrence of hepatitis A following liver transplantation for acute liver failure. J Med Virol 1995; 45:35–39.

29. [No authors listed]. Incidence of acute hepatitis B – United States, 1990–2002. MMWR Morb Mortal Wkly Rep. 2004; 52:1252–1254.

30. Centers for Disease Control (CDC). Acute hepatitis B among children and adolescents – United States, 1990–2002. MMWR Morb Mortal Wkly Rep. 2004; 53(43):1015–1018.

31. Custer B, Sullivan SD, Hazlet TK, et al. Global epidemiology of hepatitis B virus. J Clin Gastroenterol 2004; 38(10 Suppl):S158–S168.

32. Kaneko S, Miller RH, Di Bisceglie AM, et al. Detection of hepatitis B virus DNA in serum by polymerase chain reaction. Application for clinical diagnosis. Gastroenterology 1990; 99:793–798.

33. Centers for Disease Control. Immunization Practices Advisory Committee: Recommendations for protection against viral hepatitis. MMWR 1985; 24:313–335.

34. Francis DP, Feorino PM, McGougal JS, et al. The safety of the hepatitis B vaccine: Inactivation of the AIDS virus during routine vaccine manufacture. J Amer Med Assoc 1986; 256: 869–872.

35. Emini EA, Ellis RW, Miller WJ, et al. Production and immunological analysis of recombinant hepatitis B vaccine. J Infect 1986; 13(Suppl A):3–9.

36. Zajac BA, West DJ, McAleer WJ, et al. Overview of clinical studies with hepatitis B vaccine made by recombinant DNA. J Infect 1986; 13(Suppl):36–45.

37. Jilg W, Schmidt M, Deinhardt F. Vaccination against hepatitis B: Comparison of three different vaccination schedules. J Infect Dis 1989; 160:766–769.

38. Hadler SC, Monzon MA, Lugo DR, et al. Effect of timing of hepatitis B vaccine doses on response to vaccine in Yucpa Indians. Vaccine 1989; 7:106–110.

39. Szmuness W, Stevens CE, Harley EJ, et al. Hepatitis B vaccine: demonstration of efficacy in a controlled clinic trial in a high risk population in the United States. New Engl J Med 1980; 303:833–838.

A landmark study that documented the efficacy of the plasma-derived hepatitis B vaccine in a large controlled trial of high-risk men.

40. Hadler SC, Francis DP, Maynard JE, et al. Long-term immunogenicity and efficacy of hepatitis B vaccine in homosexual men. N Engl J Med 1986; 315:209–212.

41. Floreani A, Baldo V, Cristofoletti M, eet al. Long-term persistence of anti-HBs after vaccination against HBV: an 18 year experience in health care workers. Vaccine 2004; 22:607–610.

42. Young BW, Lee SS, Lim WL, et al. The long-term efficacy of plasma-derived hepatitis B vaccine in babies born to carrier mothers. J Viral Hepat 2003; 10:23–30.

43. Banatvala J, Van Damme P, Oehen S. Lifelong protection against hepatitis B: the role of vaccine immunogenicity in immune memory. Vaccine 2000; 19:877–885.

44. Wang RX, Boland GJ, van Hattum J, et al. Long-term persistence of T cell memory to HBsAg after hepatitis B vaccination. World J Gastroenterol 2004; 10:260–263.

45. Ukena T, Esber H, Bessette R, et al. Site of injection and response to hepatitis B vaccine (Letter). N Engl J Med 1985; 313:579–580.

46. Stevens CE, Alter J, Taylor PE, et al. Hepatitis B vaccine in patients receiving hemodialysis. Immunogenicity and efficacy. N Engl J Med 1984; 311:496–501.

47. Collier AC, Corey L, Murphy VL, et al. Antibody to human immunodeficiency virus (HIV) and suboptimal response to hepatitis B vaccination. Ann Intern Med 1988; 109:101–105.

48. Shaw FE, Graham DJ, Guess HA, et al. Postmarketing surveillance for neurologic adverse events reported after hepatitis B vaccination. Experience of the first 3 years. Am J Epidemiol 1988; 127:337–352.

49. Clements CJ. The evidence for the safety of thiomersal in newborn and infant vaccines. Vaccine 2004; 22:1854–1861.

50. Perrillo RP. Treatment of chronic hepatitis B with interferon: Experience in Western countries. Semin Liver Dis 1989; 9:240–248.

51. Lok AS, McMahon BJ, and Practice Guidelines Committee, American Association for the Study of Liver Diseases (AASLD). Chronic hepatitis B: update of recommendations. Hepatology 2004; 39:857–861.

The practice guidelines for management of chronic hepatitis B developed by the American Association for the Study of Liver Diseases.

52. de Franchis R, Hadengue A, Lau GK, et al. Proceedings of the EASL International Consensus Conference on Hepatitis B. J Hepatol 2003; 39(Suppl 1):S3–S35.

53. Liaw YF, Leung N, Guan R, et al, and Asian-Pacific Consensus Working Parties on Hepatitis B. Asian-Pacific consensus statement on the management of chronic hepatitis B: an update. J Gastroenterol Hepatol 2003; 18:239–245.

54. Peters M, Davis GL, Dooley JS, et al. The interferon system in acute and chronic viral hepatitis. Prog Liver Dis 1986; 8:453–467.

55. Davis GL, Hoofnagle JH. Interferon in viral hepatitis: Role in pathogenesis and treatment. Hepatology 1986; 6:1038–1041.

56. Peters M. Mechanism of action of interferons. Semin Liver Dis 1989; 9:235–239.

57. Galabru J, Katze MG, Robert N, et al. The binding of double stranded RNA and adenovirus VAI RNA to the interferon induced protein kinase. Eur J Biochem 1989; 178:581–589.

58. Perrillo RP, Schiff ER, Davis GL, et al. A Randomized, controlled study of interferon alfa-2b alone and after prednisone withdrawal for the treatment of chronic hepatitis B. N Engl J Med 1990; 323:295–301.

59. Dooley JS, Davis GL, Peters M, et al. Pilot study of recombinant human alpha interferon for chronic type B hepatitis. Gastroenterology 1986; 90:150–157.

60. Korenman J, Baker B, Waggoner J, et al. Long term remission of chronic hepatitis B after alpha-interferon therapy. Ann Intern Med 1991; 114:629–634.

61. Perrillo RP, Brunt EM. Hepatic histologic and immunohistochemical changes in chronic hepatitis B after prolonged clearance of hepatitis B e antigen and hepatitis B surface antigen. Ann Int Med 1991; 115:113–115.

62. Mason A, Yoffe B, Noonan C, et al. Hepatitis B virus DNA in peripheral blood mononuclear cells in chronic hepatitis B after HBsAg clearance. Hepatology 1992; 16:36–41.

63. Lau G, Piratvisuth T, Luo KX, et al. Peginterferon alfa-2a (40 kD) (Pegasys) monotherapy and in combination with lamivudine is more effective that lamivudine monotherapy in HBeAg-positive chronic hepatitis B: Results of a large multinational study. Hepatology 2004; 40 (Suppl 1):171A.

64. Marcellin P, Lau GK, Bonino F, et al. Peginterferon alfa-2a HBeAg-negative chronic hepatitis B study group. Peginterferon alfa-2a alone, lamivudine alone, and the two in combination in patients with HBeAg-negative chronic hepatitis B. N Engl J Med 2004; 351:1206–1217.

A well-designed study demonstrating the efficacy of pegylated interferon in chronic hepatitis B. Although this study is in patients with the HBeAg-negative (pre-core) mutation of the virus, the results are similar to wild-type infection (reference 63).

65. Davis GL, Balart LA, Schiff ER, et al. Treatment of chronic hepatitis C with recombinant interferon alfa: A multicenter randomized, controlled trial. N Engl J Med 1989; 321:1501–1506.

The first study demonstrating the efficacy of interferon in patients with chronic hepatitis C.

66. DiBisceglie AM, Martin P, Kassianides C, et al. Recombinant interferon alfa therapy for chronic hepatitis C. A randomized, double-bind, placebo-controlled trial. N Engl J Med 1989; 1321:1506–1510.

67. Perrillo RP, Schiff ER, Davis GL, et al. A randomized, controlled study of interferon alfa-2b alone and after prednisone withdrawal for the treatment of chronic hepatitis B. N Engl J Med 1990; 323:295–301.

68. Fried MW, Shiffman ML, Reddy R, et al. Peg-interferon alfa-2a plus ribavirin for chronic hepatitis C virus infection. N Engl J Med 2002; 347:975–982.

69. Kassianides C, Di Bisceglie AM, Hoofnagle JH, et al. Alpha interferon therapy in patients with decompensated chronic type B hepatitis. In: Zuckerman AJ, ed. Viral hepatitis and liver disease. New York: Alan R Liss; 1988:840–843.

70. Garcia G, Smith CI, Weissberg JI, et al. Adenine arabinoside monphosphate (vidarabine phosphate) in combination with human leukocyte interferon in the treatment of chronic hepatitis B: a randomized double blinded, placebo-controlled trial. Ann Int Med 1987; 107:278–285.

71. Hoofnagle JH, Hanson RG, Minuk GY, et al. Randomized controlled trial of edenosine arabinoside monophosphate for chronic type B hepatitis. Gastroenterology 1984; 86:150–157.

72. Alexander GJM, Fagan EA, Hegarty JE, et al. Controlled clinical trial of acyclovir in chronic hepatitis B virus infection. J Med Virol 1987; 21:21–27.

73. Weller IVD, Tedder RS, Karayiannis P, et al. A pilot study of BW A515U (6-deoxyacyclovir) in chronic hepatitis B virus infection. J Hepatology 1986; 3(Suppl): S119–S122.

74. Gish RG, Keefe EB, Fang JWS, et al. Ganciclovir treatment of recurrent hepatitis B virus infection in orthotopic liver transplant recipients. Gastroenterology 1994; 106:899A.

75. Kassianides C, Hoofnagle JH, Miller RH, et al. Inhibition of duck hepatitis B virus replication by 2′,3′-dideoxycytidine: a potent inhibitor of reverse transcriptase. Gastroenterology 1989; 97:1275–1280.

76. Dienstag JL, Perrillo RP, Schiff ER, et al. Double-blind randomized three-month dose-ranging trial of lamivudine for chronic hepatitis B. Hepatology 1994; 20:199A.

77. Dienstag JL, Schiff ER, Mitchell M, et al. Extended lamivudine retreatment for chronic hepatitis B: maintenance of viral suppression after discontinuation of therapy. Hepatology 1999; 30:1082–1087.

78. Dienstag JL, Schiff ER, Wright TL, et al. Lamivudine as initial treatment for chronic hepatitis B in the United States. N Engl J Med 1999; 341:1256–1263.

79. Leung NW, Lai CL, Chang TT, et al. Extended lamivudine treatment in patients with chronic hepatitis B enhances hepatitis B e antigen seroconversion rates: results after 3 years of therapy. Hepatology 2001; 33:1527–1532.

    Demonstration of the long-term efficacy of HBV suppression with nucleosides. This study also documented the high rate of drug resistance to lamivudine and the consequences of that event.

80. Dienstag JL, Cianciara J, Karayalcin S, et al. Durability of serologic response after lamivudine treatment of chronic hepatitis B. Hepatology 2003; 37:748–755.

81. Dienstag JL, Goldin RD, Heathcote EJ, et al. Histological outcome during long-term lamivudine therapy. Gastroenterology 2003; 124:105–117.

82. Lok AS, Lai CL, Leung N, et al. Long-term safety of lamivudine treatment in patients with chronic hepatitis B. Gastroenterology 2003; 125:1714–1722.

83. Lai CL, Dienstag J, Schiff E, et al. Prevalence and clinical correlates of YMDD variants during lamivudine therapy for patients with chronic hepatitis B. Clin Infect Dis 2003; 36:687–696.

84. Liaw YF, Leung NW, Chang TT, et al. Effects of extended lamivudine therapy in Asian patients with chronic hepatitis B. Gastroenterology 2000; 119:172–180.

85. Dusheiko G. Adefovir dipivoxil for the treatment of HBeAg-positive chronic hepatitis B: a review of the major clinical studies. J Hepatol 2003; 39:S116–S123.

86. Izzedine H, Hulot JS, Launay-Vacher V, et al. Renal safety of adefovir dipivoxil in patients with chronic hepatitis B: two double-blind, randomized, placebo-controlled studies. Kidney Int 2004; 66:1153–1158.

87. Marcellin P, Chang TT, Lim SG, et al. Adefovir dipivoxil for the treatment of hepatitis B e antigen-positive chronic hepatitis B. N Engl J Med 2003; 348:808–816.

88. Hadziyannis SJ, Tassopoulos NC, Heathcote EJ, et al. Adefovir dipivoxil for the treatment of hepatitis B e antigen-negative chronic hepatitis B. N Engl J Med 2003; 348:800–807.

89. Westland CE, Yang H, Delaney WE, et al. Week 48 resistance surveillance in two phase 3 clinical studies of adefovir dipivoxil for chronic hepatitis B. Hepatology 2003; 38:96–103.

90. van Bommel F, Wunsche T, Mauss S, et al. Comparison of adefovir and tenofovir in the treatment of lamivudine-resistant hepatitis B virus infection. Hepatology 2004; 40:1421–1425.

91. Buti M, Estaban R. Entecavir, FTC, L-FMAU, LdT and others. J Hepatol 2003; 39:S139–S142.

92. Yamanaka G, Wilson T, Innaimo S, et al. Metabolic studies on BMS-200475, a new antiviral compound active against hepatitis B virus. Antimicrob Agents Chemother 1999; 43:190–193.

93. Sherman M, Yurdaydin C, Sollano J, et al. Entecavir is superior to continued lamivudine for the treatment of lamivudine-refractory HBeAg-positivie chronic hepatitis B: Results of phase III study ETV-026. Hepatology 2004; 40:664A.

94. Marion PL, Salazar FH, Winters MA, et al. Potent efficacy of entecavir in a duck model of hepatitis B virus replication. Antimicrob Agents Chemother 2002; 46:81–88.

95. Chang TT, Gish R, de Man R, et al. Entecavir is superior to lamivudine for the treatment of HBeAg-positive chronic hepatitis B: Results of phase III study ETV-022 in nucleoside-naïve patients. Hepatology 2004; 40:193A.

96. Shouval D, Lai CL, Cheinquer H, et al. Entecavir demonstrates superior histologic and virologic efficacy over lamivudine in nucleoside naïve HBeAg negative chronic hepatitis B: Results of a phase III trial. Hepatology 2004; 40:728A.

97. Colonno RJ, Rose R, Levine SM, et al. Emergence of entecavir resistant hepatitis B virus after one year of therapy in phase II and III studies is only observed in lamivudine refractory patients. Hepatology 2004; 40:661A.

98. Kuo A, Dienstag JL, Chung RT. Tenofovir disoproxil fumarate for the treatment of lamivudine-resistant hepatitis B. Clin Gastroenterol Hepatol 2004; 2:266–272.

99. Rizzetto M, Rosina F. Hepatitis D treatment. In: Zuckerman AJ, Thomas HC, eds. Viral hepatitis. Edinburgh: Churchill Livingstone; 1997:387–393.

100. Rosina F, Rizzetto M. Treatment of chronic type D (Delta) hepatitis with alpha interferon. Semin Liver Dis 1989; 9:264–266.

101. Farci P, Mandas A, Coiana A, et al. Treatment of chronic hepatitis C with interferon alfa-2a. N Engl J Med 1994; 330:88–94.

102. Farci P, Chessa L, Peddis G, et al. Influence of alpha interferon on the natural history of chronic hepatitis D: dissociation of histologic and virologic response. Hepatology 2000; 32:222A.

103. Alter MJ, Sampliner RE. Hepatitis C and miles to go before we sleep. N Engl J Med 1989; 321:1538–1540.

104. Alter MJ. Epidemiology of hepatitis C in the West. Sem Liver Dis 1995; 15:5–14.

105. Kuhns WJ, Prince AM, Brotman B, et al. A clinical and laboratory evaluation of immune serum globulin from donors with a history of hepatitis: attempted prevention of post-transfusion hepatitis. Am J Med Sci 1976; 272:255–261.

106. Knodell RG, Conrad ME, Ginsberg AL, et al. Efficacy of prophylactic gamma globulin in preventing non-A, non-B post-transfusion hepatitis. Lancet 1976; 1:557–561.

107. Seeff LB, Zimmerman HJ, Wright EC, et al: A randomized, double-blind, controlled study of the efficacy of immune serum globulin for the prevention of post-transfusion hepatitis. A Veterans Administration cooperative study. Gastroenterology 1977; 72:111–121.

108. Kiyosawa K, Sodeyama T, Tanaka E, et al. Hepatitis C in hospital employees with needlestick injuries. Ann Int Med 1991; 15:367–369.

109. Krawczynski K, Alter MJ, Tankersley DL, et al. Effect of immune globulin on the prevention of experimental hepatitis C virus infection. J Inf Dis 1996; 173:822–828.

110. Davis GL, Nelson DR, Terrault N, et al. A randomized, open-label study to evaluate the safety and pharmacokinetics of human hepatitis C immune globulin (Civacir™) in liver transplant recipients. Liver Transpl 2005; in press.

111. Schiff ER. Hepatitis C among health care providers: risk factors and possible prophylaxis [Editorial]. Hepatology 1992; 16:1300–1301.

112. Choo QL, Kuo G, Ralston R, et al. Vaccination of chimpanzees against infection by the hepatitis C virus. PNAS USA 1994; 91:1294–1298.

113. Rosa D, Campagnoli S, Moretto C, et al. A quantitative test to estimate neutralizing antibodies to the hepatitis C virus: cytofluorimetric assessment of envelope glycoprotein 2 binding to target cells. PNAS USA 1996; 93:1759–1763.

114. Major ME, Vitvitski L, Mink MA, et al. DNA-based immunization with chimeric vectors for the induction of immune responses against the hepatitis C virus nucleocapsid. J Virol 1995; 69:5798–5805.

115. Lagging LM, Meyer K, Hoft D, et al. Immune response to plasmid DNA encoding the hepatitis C virus core protein. J Virol 1995; 69:5859–5863.

116. Saito T. IX Triennial International Symposium on Viral Hepatitis and Liver Disease, Rome: April, 1996.

117. Tokushiga K, Wakita T, Pachuk C, et al. Expression and immune response to hepatitis C virus core DNA-based vaccine constructs. Hepatology 1996; 24:14–20.

118. Makimura M, Miyaka S, Akino N, et al. Induction of antibodies against structural proteins of hepatitis C virus in mice using recombinant adenovirus. Vaccine 1996; 14:28–34.

119. Nevens F, Roskams R, van Vlierberghe H, et al. Improvement in liver histology after 3 years of E1 therapeutic vaccination in 23 patients with chronic hepatic C. Hepatology 2004; 40:250A.

120. Manns M, Berg T, Wedemeyer H, et al. Immunization with the therapeutic hepatitis C virus peptide vaccine IC41 in 66 chronic hepatitis C non-responder patients. Hepatology 2004; 40:251A.

121. Viladomiu L, Genescà J, Esteban JI, et al. Interferon-alpha in acute posttransfusion hepatitis C: a randomized controlled trial. Hepatology 1992; 15:767–769.

122. Lampertico R, Rumi M, Romeo R, et al. A multicenter randomized controlled trial of recombinant interferon alpha-2b in patients with acute transfusion-associated hepatitis C. Hepatology 1994; 19:19–22.

123. Hwang SJ, Lee SC, Chan CY, et al. A randomized controlled trial of recombinant interferon a2b in the treatment of Chinese patients with acute post-transfusion hepatitis C. J Hepatol 1994; 21:831–836.

124. Omata M, Yokosuka O, Takano S, et al. Resolution of acute hepatitis C after therapy with natural beta interferon. Lancet 1991; 338:914–915.

125. Poynard T, Leroy V, Cohard M, et al. Meta-analysis of interferon randomized trials in the treatment of viral hepatitis C: Effects of dose and duration. Hepatology 1996; 24:778–789.

126. Kamal SM, Ismail A, Graham CS, et al. Pegylated interferon alpha therapy in acute hepatitis C: relation to hepatitis C virus-specific T cell response kinetics. Hepatology 2004; 39:1721–1731.

127. Alter MJ. The epidemiology of acute and chronic hepatitis C. Clin Liver Dis 1997; 1(3):559–568.

128. Hoofnagle JH, Mullen KD, Jones DB, et al. Treatment of chronic non-A, non-B hepatitis with recombinant human alpha interferon: A preliminary report. N Engl J Med 1986; 315:1575–1578.

129. Davis GL, Balart LA, Schiff ER, et al. Treatment of chronic hepatitis C with recombinant interferon alfa: a multicenter randomized controlled trial. New Engl J Med 1989; 321:1501–1506.

130. DiBisceglie AM, Martin P, Kassianides C, et al. Recombinant interferon alfa therapy for chronic hepatitis C. A randomized, double-bind, placebo-controlled trial. New Engl J Med 1989; 321:1506–1510.

131. Marcellin P, Boyer N, Giostra E, et al. Recombinant human alpha-interferon in patients with chronic non-A non-B hepatitis: a multicenter randomized controlled trial from France. Hepatology 1991; 13:393–397.

132. Causse X, Godinot H, Ouzan D, et al. Comparison of 1 or 3 MU of interferon alfa-2b and placebo in patients with chronic non-A non-B hepatitis. Gastroenterology 1991; 101:497–502.

133. Weiland O, Schvarcz R, Wejstal R, et al. Therapy of chronic post-transfusion non-A, non-B hepatitis with interferon alfa-2b: Swedish experience. J Hepatol 1990; 11(Suppl 2):557–562.

134. Saadeh S, Davis GL. Treatment of chronic hepatitis c: a decade later. Cleveland Clinic J Med 2004; 71(Suppl 3): S1–S9.

135. McHutchison J, Davis GL, Esteban-Mur R, et al. Durability of sustained virologic response in patients with chronic hepatitis C after treatment with interferon alfa-2b alone or in combination with ribavirin . Hepatology 2001;34:244A.

136. Marcellin P, Boyer N, Gervais A, et al. Long-term histologic improvement and loss of detectable intrahepatic HCV RNA in patients with chronic hepatitis C and sustained response to interferon-alpha therapy. Ann Intern Med 1997;127:875–881.

137. Shindo M, Di Bisceglie AM, Hoofnagle JH. Long-term follow-up of patients with chronic hepatitis C treated with alpha-interferon. Hepatology 1992;15:1013–1016.

138. Hadziyannis SJ, Sette H, Morgan TR, et al. Peginterferon-alpha2a and ribavirin combination therapy in chronic hepatitis C: a randomized study of treatment duration and ribavirin dose. Ann Intern Med 2004; 140:346–355.

An important study looking at the effect of ribavirin dose and treatment duration on outcome according to viral genotype.

139. Davis GL, Wong JB, McHutchison JG, et al. Early virologic response to treatment with pegylated interferon alfa-2b plus ribavirin in patients with chronic hepatitis C. Hepatology 2003; 38:645–652.

Documentation of the predictive value of failure to suppress virus during the first months of therapy. This study is the basis for the current 12-week stopping rule for treatment of chronic hepatitis C.

140. Chayama K, Saitoh S, Arase Y, et al. Effect of interferon administration on serum hepatitis C virus RNA in patients with chronic hepatitis C. Hepatology 1991; 13:1040–1043.

141. McHutchison JG, Gordon SC, Schiff ER, et al. Interferon alpha-2b alone or in combination with ribavirin as initial treatment for chronic hepatitis C. N Engl J Med 1998; 339:1485–1492.

142. Poynard T, Marcellin P, Lee SS, et al. Randomised trial of interferon alpha2b plus ribavirin for 48 weeks or for 24 weeks versus interferon alpha2b plus placebo for 48 weeks for treatment of chronic infection with hepatitis C virus. International Hepatitis Interventional Therapy Group (IHIT). Lancet 1998; 352:1426–1432.

143. Manns MP, McHutchison JG, Gordon S, et al. Peginterferon alpha-2b plus ribavirin compared to interferon alpha-2b plus ribavirin for the treatment of chronic hepatitis C: a randomized trial. Lancet 2001; 358:958–965.

One of the two large international clinical studies that demonstrated the efficacy of pegylated interferon and ribavirin for chronic hepatitis C. This is now the standard of care.

144. Fried MW, Shiffman ML, Reddy R, et al. Peginterferon alpha-2a plus ribavirin for chronic hepatitis C virus infection. N Engl J Med 2002; 347:975–982.

One of the two large international clinical studies that demonstrated the efficacy of pegylated interferon and ribavirin for chronic hepatitis C. This is now the standard of care.

145. Brillanti S, Garson JA, Tuke PW, et al. Effect of alpha-interferon therapy on hepatitis C viremia in community-acquired chronic non-A, non-B hepatitis: a quantitative polymerase chain reaction study. J Med Virol 1991; 34:136–141.

146. Shindo M, DiBisceglie AM, Hoofnagle JH. Long-term follow-up of patients with chronic hepatitis C treated with alpha-interferon. Hepatology 1992; 15:1013–1016.

147. Schvarcz R, Glaumann H, Weiland O, et al. Histological outcome in interferon alpha-2b treated patients with chronic posttransfusion non-A, non-B hepatitis. Liver 1991; 11:30–38.

148. Shiffman ML, Hofmann CM, Thompson EB, et al. Relationship between biochemical, virological, and histological response during interferon treatment of chronic hepatitis C. Hepatology 1997; 26:780–785.

149. Davis GL. Treatment of chronic HCV: Should we stop treating non-responders (Reply to comment). Gastroenterology 2004; 126:1485–1487.

150. Leevy C, Chalmers C, Blatt LM. Comparison of African American and non-African American patient end-of-treatment response for Peg-IFN alfa-2 and weight-based ribavirin non-responders retreated with IFN Alfacon-1 and weight-based ribavirin. Hepatology 2004; 40:240A.

151. Sanchez-Tapias JM, Diago M, Escartin P, et al. Longer treatment duration with peginterferon Alfa-2a (40KD) (Pegasys®) and ribavirin (Copegus®) in naïve patients with chronic hepatitis C and detectable HCV RNA by week 4 of therapy: final results of the randomized, multicenter TERAVIC-4 study. Hepatology 2004; 40:218A.

152. Afdhal N, Freilich B, Levine R, et al. Colchicine versus Peg-Intron long term (COPILOT) trial: Interim analysis of clinical outcomes at year 2. Hepatology 2004; 40:239A.

153. Rincón D, Bañares R, Ripoll C, et al. Antiviral therapy decreases hepatic venous pressure gradient in patients with chronic hepatitis C and fibrosis stage 3 or 4. Hepatology 2004; 40:248A.

154. Dalgard O, Bjøro K, Hellum K, et al. Short (14 weeks) treatment with pegylated interferon alpha-2b and ribavirin in patients with hepatitis C genotype 2/3 virus infection and early virological response. Hepatology 2004; 40:252A.

155. von Wagner M, Huber M, Berg T, et al. Randomized multicenter study comparing 16 versus 24 weeks of combination therapy with peginterferon alfa-2a plus ribavirin in patients chronically infected with HCV genotype 2 or 3. Hepatology 2004; 40:725A.

156. Zeuzem S, Hultcrantz R, Bourliere M, et al. Peginterferon alfa-2b plus ribavirin for treatment of chronic hepatitis C in previously untreated patients infected with HCV genotypes 2 or 3. J Hepatol 2004; 40: 993–999.

157. Rizzetto M, Hadziyannis SJ, Ackrill AM. Sustained virological response (SVR) to peginterferon alfa-2a (40kd) (Pegasys®) plus ribavirin (Copegus®): comparison of outcomes in patients infected with HCV genotype 2 and 3. Hepatology 2004; 40:252A.

158. Davis GL, Esteban-Mur R, Rustgi V, et al. Recombinant interferon alfa-2b (Intron A®) alone or in combination with ribavirin (Rebetol) for retreatment of interferon relapse in chronic hepatitis C. N Engl J Med 1998; 339:1493–1499.

159. Davis GL. Interferon treatment of cirrhotic patients with chronic hepatitis C: a logical intervention. Am J Gastroenterol 1994; 89:658–660.

160. Harrison SA, Brunt EM, Oliver DA, et al. The presence of severe steatosis or steatohepatitis impairs response to antiviral therapy in patients with chronic hepatitis C. Hepatology 2003; 38(Suppl 1):626A.

161. Peters MG, Terrault NA. Alcohol use and hepatitis C. Hepatology 2002; 36(Suppl 1):S220–S225.

162. Jeffers LJ, Cassidy W, Howell CD, et al. Peginterferon alfa-2a (40 kd) and ribavirin for black American patients with chronic HCV genotype 1. Hepatology 2004; 39:1702–1708.

Clearly shows the lower response rate to pegylated interferon and ribavirin in African-American patients with chronic hepatitis C.

163. Muir AJ, Bornstein JD, Killenberg PG. Peginterferon alfa-2b and ribavirin for the treatment of chronic hepatitis C in blacks and non-Hispanic whites. N Engl J Med 2004; 350:2265–2271.

164. Carrat F, Bani-Sadr F, Pol S, et al. Pegylated interferon alfa-2b vs standard interferon alfa-2b, plus ribavirin, for chronic hepatitis C in HIV-infected patients: a randomized controlled trial. JAMA 2004; 292:2839–2848.

165. Chung RT, Andersen J, Volberding P, et al. Peginterferon Alfa-2a plus ribavirin versus interferon alfa-2a plus ribavirin for chronic hepatitis C in HIV-coinfected persons. N Engl J Med 2004; 351:451–459.

Best study of pegylated interferon and ribavirin in patients coinfected with HIV and HCV.

166. Torriani FJ, Rodriguez-Torres M, Rockstroh JK, et al. Peginterferon Alfa-2a plus ribavirin for chronic hepatitis C virus infection in HIV-infected patients. N Engl J Med 2004; 351:438–450.

167. McHutchison JG, Manns M, Patel K, et al. Adherence to combination therapy enhances sustained response in genotype-1-infected patients with chronic hepatitis C. Gastroenterology 2002; 123:1061–1069.

168. Bodenheimer HC, Lindsay K, Davis GL, et al. Tolerance and safety of oral ribavirin treatment of chronic hepatitis C: a multicenter trial. Hepatology 1997; 26:473–477.

169. Reichard O, Andersson J, Schvarcz R, et al. Ribavirin treatment for chronic hepatitis C. Lancet 1991; 337:1058–1061.

170. Di Bisceglie AM, Shindo M, Fong TL, et al. A pilot study of ribavirin therapy for chronic hepatitis C. Hepatology 1992; 16:649–654.

171. Schalm SW, Hansen BE, Chemello L, et al. Ribavirin enhances the efficacy but not the adverse effects of interferon in chronic hepatitis C: Meta-analysis of individual patient data from European centers. J Hepatol 1997; 26:961–966.

172. Soza A, Everhart JE, Ghany MG, et al. Neutropenia during combination therapy of interferon alfa and ribavirin for chronic hepatitis C. Hepatology 2002; 36:1273–1279.

173. Capuron L, Gumnick JF, Musselman DL, et al. Neurobehavioral effects of interferon-alpha in cancer patients: phenomenology and paroxetine responsiveness of symptom dimensions. Neuropsychopharmacology 2002; 26:643–652.

174. Musselman DL, Lawson DH, Gumnick JF, et al. Paroxetine for the prevention of depression induced by high-dose interferon alfa. N Engl J Med 2001; 344:961–966.

175. Benhamou Y, Hinrichsen H, Sentjens R, et al. Safety tolerability and antiviral effect of BILN 2061. A novel HCV serine protease inhibitor, after oral treatment over 2 days in patients with chronic hepatitis C, genotype 1, with advance liver fibrosis. Hepatology 2002; 36:304A.

176. Gish RG, Arora S, Nelson DR, et al. End-of-treatment response in therapy-naive patients treated for chronic hepatitis C with viramidine in combination with pegylated interferon alfa-2a. Hepatology 2004; 40:388A.

177. Shear NH, Malkiewicz IM, Klein D, et al. Acetaminophen-induced toxicity to human epidermoid cell line A431 and hepatoblastoma cell line Hep G2, in vitro, is diminished by silymarin. Skin Pharmacol 1995; 8:279–291.

178. Dehmlow C, Erhard J, de Groot H. Inhibition of Kupffer cell functions as an explanation for the hepatoprotective properties of silibinin. Hepatology 1996; 23:749–754.

179. Miguez MP, Anundi I, Sainz-Pardo LA. Hepatoprotective mechanism of silymarin: no evidence for involvement of cytochrome p450 2E1. Chem Biol Interact 1994; 91:51–63.

180. Buzzelli G, Moscarella S, Giusti A, et al. A pilot study on the liver protective effect of silybin-phosphatidylcholine complex (IdB1016) in chronic active hepatitis. Int J Clin Pharmacol Ther Toxicol 1993; 31:456–460.

181. Houglaum K, Venkataramani A, Lyche K, et al. A pilot study of the effects of d-alpha-tocopherol on hepatic stellate cell activation in chronic hepatitis C. Gastroenterology 1997; 113:1069–1073.

CHAPTER THIRTY-FOUR

34

Autoimmune hepatitis

Edward L. Krawitt and Gilda Porta

INTRODUCTION

Autoimmune hepatitis (AIH) is a progressive, sometimes fluctuating chronic hepatitis which occurs in children and adults of all ages.[1,2] Although of unknown etiology, its pathogenesis is believed to be based at least in part on aberrant autoreactivity. A high percentage of cases responds to antiinflammatory/immunosuppressive therapy, even if cirrhosis is present.[3]

The diagnosis of AIH and other autoimmune liver diseases, such as primary biliary cirrhosis (PBC) and primary sclerosing cholangitis (PSC) is based on histologic changes,[4] characteristic clinical and biochemical findings, circulating autoantibodies, and abnormalities of serum globulins, in the absence of evidence of viral or drug-induced disease. Overlap or variant syndromes of autoimmune liver diseases, however, may obscure the classic clinical and seroimmunologic boundaries of these disorders and create diagnostic and therapeutic dilemmas.[5–7]

PATHOGENESIS

A commonly used paradigm for the pathogenesis of AIH is that an environmental agent triggers a cirrhosis-producing process in a genetically predisposed individual, resulting in a loss of tolerance to self-antigens. Infectious organisms and drugs have been suggested as triggering agents but none has been unequivocally identified. Drug-induced toxicity does not appear to result in AIH, although may unmask the disease. Most of the information regarding genetic predisposition to disease expression and progression and treatment response has involved the major histocompatibility complex.[8] In particular, the serotypes HLA DR3 and DR4 are associated with AIH, but associations are being sought for other loci on chromosome 6 and on other chromosomes.

The tolerogenic mechanisms are incompletely understood but the B-cell responses, including circulating autoantibodies, are considered to be merely 'footprints of disease' and uninvolved in pathogenesis. The T-cell responses are thought to lead to presently undefined cascades important in pathogenesis. Implicit in this hypothesis is that self-reactive T cells, responsible for ongoing inflammation and necrosis, escape normal suppression. Early studies of immune regulation suggested that CD8 positive, so-called T-suppressor cells were inhibited. Recent evidence suggests that a subset of CD4 positive CD25 positive T-regulatory cells may be involved.[9]

CLASSIFICATION

AIH occurs in all age groups but, more commonly, in young women and girls. It is characterized by a heterogeneity of clinical features, histologic findings, immunogenetic phenotypes, serologic abnormalities, and treatment responses. Although classification can be based on a number of features, the differences in circulating autoantibody patterns are most often used to classify the disease into two major forms (Table 34.1). An international group of experts has agreed upon criteria for the diagnosis of autoimmune hepatitis to help eliminate confusion about the diagnosis.[10]

Type 1 autoimmune hepatitis

The form of AIH presently known as type 1, or classic, was originally called active chronic hepatitis and subsequently lupoid hepatitis, plasma cell hepatitis, and most frequently autoimmune chronic active hepatitis; now it is referred to simply as AIH. Although much less common than chronic viral hepatitis, it does occur in both adults and children. Circulating antibodies to nuclei (ANA) and/or to smooth muscle (SMA), the latter thought to be reflective of more specific antibodies to actin,[11,12] occur in over 90% of patients, the exact percentage depending on the titer specified for positivity. It should be noted, however, that although ANA and SMA are characteristic of AIH, they are not specific and may be seen in other liver diseases including chronic viral hepatitis and nonalcoholic fatty liver disease. A subset of antibodies to neutrophilic cytoplasmic antigens (atypical pANCA) are also

Table 34.1 Classification of autoimmune hepatitis	
Disorder	**Autoantibody**
Type 1 (classic) AIH	ANA (antinuclear) SMA (smooth muscle) ANCA (antineutrophil cytoplasmic) Anti SLA/LP (antisoluble liver antigen/liver-pancreas antigen)
Type 2 AIH	ALKM-1 (antiliver/kidney microsome-1) Anti-LC-1 (liver cytosol-1)

frequently seen in type 1 AIH.[13] Antibodies to the soluble liver antigen/liver pancreas protein (anti SLA/LP), although uncommon, are rather specific and are found in 10–30% of patients with type 1 AIH.[14,15]

Type 2 autoimmune hepatitis

Type 2 AIH is a distinct form of autoimmune disease that is uncommon and seen most often in girls and young women. It is characterized by the presence of antibodies to cytochrome P-450 2D6, also known as CYP2D6, and liver/kidney microsome type 1 (ALKM-1); it is referred to as type 2 or ALKM-1 AIH. Patients with this type of AIH may have antiliver cytosol antibodies (ALC-1) either exclusively or in conjunction with ALKM-1.

Overlap syndromes

In addition to type 1 and type 2 AIH, patients may have clinical and serologic features also suggesting the presence of PBC or PSC, resulting in disorders referred to as overlap syndromes and variant forms (Table 34.2).[7] One method of viewing the overlap syndromes of AIH and PBC is to consider them as a spectrum extending from AIH to PBC. AIH/PSC overlap syndromes occur in patients who have serologic and histologic features of AIH but have cholangiographic abnormalities.[6,7,16] This overlap should be suspected in patients with pruritus, inflammatory bowel disease, histologic bile duct abnormalities and cholestatic laboratory changes, particularly elevations of alkaline phosphatase and gamma glutamyltranspeptidase. Evolution from AIH to PSC has been reported.[17] The disease in children may differ from that in adults and has been referred to as autoimmune sclerosing cholangitis.

TREATMENT IN ADULTS

Treatment of AIH

Despite the striking clinical heterogeneity of AIH and our incomplete understanding of its pathogenesis, the disease in adults generally responds to antiinflammatory/immunosuppressive treatment. Although azathioprine may be used as a steroid-sparing agent, initial induction regimens in adults should include glucocorticosteroids. The response rate in AIH is better than that suggested in early trials which involved more patients with severe disease and antedated our ability to test for hepatitis B and C. The remission rate induced by initial therapy, including patients with cirrhosis, is approximately 80%. The survival rate for treated patients is now considered to be over 90%, 10 years after diagnosis. The 20-year survival, however, is closer to 80% in patients without cirrhosis and less than 40% in those with cirrhosis at presentation (Fig. 34.1).[18]

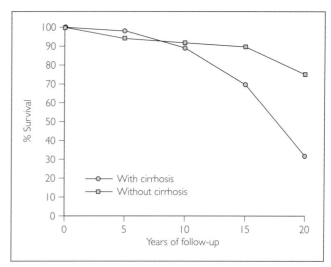

Fig. 34.1 • Survival of patients with classic autoimmune hepatitis. Death and liver transplantation were used as end points to compare survival in patients with cirrhosis (circles) and without cirrhosis (squares) at initial examination. (Reprinted data from Roberts SK et al, Gastroenterology 1996; 110:848–857. © 1996, with permission from The American Gastroenterological Association.)

Initial treatment with prednisone, alone or in combination with azathioprine, should be instituted in almost all patients, in whom the histologic findings include interface hepatitis, with or without fibrosis or cirrhosis. In patients with portal inflammatory infiltrates only, the decision to treat is often determined by symptoms. Asymptomatic patients and those with portal inflammation but no fibrosis may be observed without institution of treatment, but their clinical status, including liver biopsy appearance, should be monitored carefully for evidence of progression of disease, while keeping in mind the sometimes fluctuating nature of AIH.

In most patients, treatment can be initiated with 20–30 mg of prednisone or prednisolone per day (Table 34.3). Higher doses may sometimes be needed, especially in younger patients with severe disease, but the use of higher doses increases the risk of major side effects. The use of lower doses (10–15 mg/day) initially, with subsequent incremental increases if a satisfactory response does not occur, is not generally recommended, as this approach may not control the disease adequately in many cases and may prolong the period of ongoing liver damage.

Initial treatment with a combination of prednisone and azathioprine may be instituted to avoid or mitigate the side effects of steroid treatment, particularly in diabetics and postmenopausal women. An alternative is to wait until remission is achieved before initiating steroid sparing with azathioprine (see Table 34.3).

Table 34.2 Overlap/variant syndromes	
AIH/PBC overlap syndrome	AMA positive with histologic findings characteristic of AIH; generally steroid responsive.
Autoimmune cholangitis	AMA negative, often ANA and SMA positive; histologic findings suggestive of PBC; generally not steroid responsive.
AIH/PSC overlap syndrome	AMA negative with or without other autoantibodies and histologic and/or cholangiographic evidence suggestive of PSC; generally not steroid responsive.

Table 34.3 Treatment of autoimmune hepatitis in adults

Regimen	Single-drug therapy	Combination therapy
Initial	Prednisone 20–40 mg daily	Prednisone 15–30 mg daily and Azathioprine 50–100 mg daily
Maintenance	Prednisone 5–15 mg daily or Azathioprine 100–200 mg daily	Prednisone 5–10 mg daily and Azathioprine 50–150 mg daily

One issue of treatment that has been of particular interest in adults, as well as children (see below), is that of toxicity and intolerance to azathioprine and/or 6-mercaptopurine (6-MP). Azathioprine is a prodrug for 6-MP. The methylation of 6-MP and 6-thioguanosine 5′-monophosphate is catalyzed by thiopurine methyltransferase (TPMT). The genes encoding TPMT are highly polymorphic. Homozygosity for a mutation in TMPT genes results in loss of activity in approximately 1 to 300 people, and patients accumulate high levels of thioguanine nucleotides in bone marrow cells, leading to toxicity.[19–21] Patients who are homozygous for a mutation of TPMT which results in inadequate enzyme activity are at high risk for severe toxicity, including death. Patients who are heterozygous for the TPMT gene probably have an intermediate risk of toxicity, leading to the suggestion that prior to placing patients on azathioprine or 6-MP, TPMT phenotyping be performed. It is also known, however, that patients who are intolerant to azathioprine may take 6-MP without side effects, indicating that toxicity is not all due to TPMT deficiency.[22] Despite reliable methods for measurement of TPMT genotyping, its assessment in the clinical management of AIH is not established.[23] Measuring 6-MP metabolite levels is also under investigation and may prove more helpful.

Liver tests, in particular serum aminotransferases (alanine aminotransferase [ALT] and aspartate aminotransferase [AST]) and total globulins (or gamma globulin), should be monitored at least monthly, initially. When the ALT level has fallen by at least 50%, the steroid dose may be reduced to 15 mg/day in decrements of 5 mg/day every 2 to 4 weeks. Alternatively, at this point azathioprine may be introduced at 1 mg/kg/day (50–100 mg/day) while reducing the steroid dose to 10–15 mg/day in the same fashion. If the ALT or AST and globulin levels plateau, the steroid dose should not be tapered further. If ALT or AST levels rise, steroid doses should be increased by 5 mg/day weekly until the aminotransferase level falls again. At that point an attempt may again be made to reduce the steroid dosage.

Biochemical response, as measured by reductions in enzyme and globulin levels, is generally seen within a few months, but in a small percentage of patients a biochemical response may occur only after years of treatment. Histologic response lags behind biochemical response, and clinical remission does not necessarily mean histologic resolution. Although some patients will remain in remission when drug treatment is withdrawn, the majority requires long-term maintenance therapy. In general, the response is better with milder disease. Patients with cirrhosis at the time of initial biopsy rarely stay in remission when treatment is withdrawn and will almost always require lifelong maintenance therapy.

Most patients who achieve remission (normal ALT and globulin levels) can be maintained with low doses of prednisone alone (5–15 mg/day) or with a combination of 5–10 mg of prednisone and 50–150 mg of azathioprine, or with azathioprine alone (Fig 34.2).[24] Patients who are being maintained with azathioprine alone may require daily doses as high as 2 mg/kg body weight. Using azathioprine either as a steroid-sparing agent or alone involves weighing the long-term glucocorticosteroid side effects against those of azathioprine. Patients treated with azathioprine alone frequently have arthralgia.[24] In patients intolerant or unresponsive to azathioprine, 6-mercaptopurine may sometimes be successfully substituted.[22]

Because of severe glucocorticosteroid side effects, partial suppression may be preferable and can be achieved with low doses rather than conventional doses of prednisone in patients who suffer multiple relapses.[25] This practice results in a significant reduction in side effects without apparently affecting the rates of development of cirrhosis or mortality when compared with the rates in conventionally treated patients. This approach of less strict control seems particularly appropriate for postmenopausal women in whom osteoporosis is of great concern, for patients with diabetes, and for those intolerant of other glucocorticosteroid side effects.

No firm guidelines exist for decisions regarding withdrawal or reduction of medication, primarily because histologic changes may lag behind biochemical changes; levels of autoantibodies do not parallel disease activity; and a quiescent histologic

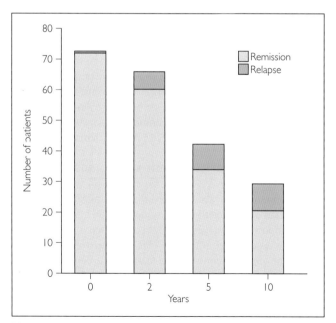

Fig. 34.2 • Response to azathioprine for long-term maintenance of remission in autoimmune hepatitis. (Data from Johnson PJ, McFarlane IG, Williams R. Azathioprine for long term maintenance of remission in autoimmune hepatitis. N Engl J Med 1995; 333:958–963.)

appearance while patients are still receiving therapy is not necessarily predictive of maintenance of remission after discontinuance of treatment. Traditionally, the histologic end points of response have been normal aminotransferase levels or levels equal to 2 times normal and histologic inactivity or mild activity with confinement of inflammatory changes to the portal areas.

Some patients stay in remission for months to years before the disease flares. These patients may enjoy long periods during which they do not require antiinflammatory therapy, but they should still be monitored with liver tests every 3–6 months; therapy should be reinstated when disease reactivates.

The first indication of relapse may be increasing fatigue, anorexia, and general malaise with or without arthralgias (other than associated with steroid withdrawal), with little or no change in biochemical liver test results. On the other hand, some patients remain asymptomatic despite increases in AST and/or ALT. Early identification is important because without intervention relapses can become severe, even uncontrollable, and deaths can occur when appropriate treatment is not given promptly. Management of relapse depends on its severity. In cases of severe relapse, it may be necessary to again use high levels of steroids to induce remission, whereas in less severe cases, lower doses of steroids may be adequate. Patients who relapse while taking azathioprine alone may require combination maintenance therapy for life. Patients who relapse after complete withdrawal of all therapy should subsequently be treated as though they were being treated for the first time; it may be possible eventually to wean patients from steroids and maintain remission with azathioprine alone.

The precise roles of budesonide, cyclosporine, tacrolimus, methotrexate, cyclophosphamide, and mycophenolate mofetil in adult patients unresponsive or intolerant to established regimens has not been defined, as data on efficacy and tolerability are limited.[3,26–30]

Despite antiinflammatory therapy, treatment failures occur. They are more common in patients with cirrhosis; in those in whom disease develops at a younger age, in patients who have a long duration of disease before therapy is instituted, in patients with type 2 AIH, and in those with an HLA-B8 or HLA-DR3 phenotype.

Sustained activity results in the development and/or worsening of cirrhosis and decompensation may occur. Despite management of complications, liver transplantation may be required. Patient and graft survival after orthotopic transplantation is comparable to that seem in other autoimmune liver diseases, but disease recurrence may occur after liver transplantation.[31]

Treatment of overlap/variant syndromes

In autoimmune liver disease, as in other areas of medicine, appreciation of the heterogeneity of disease and advances in our understanding of pathogenesis have contributed to a blurring of previously established criteria or classifications of diseases. To resolve the apparent contradictive features, the concept of overlap syndromes or variants has been adopted (see Table 34.2). No trials have been performed on which to base the treatment of overlap/variant syndromes.

In one AIH/PBC overlap syndrome described, histologic findings are most consistent with AIH despite the presence of AMA, directed toward enzymes in the 2-oxoacid dehydrogenase family, identical to those found in PBC.[32] The therapeutic decision in these cases is clear, i.e., treatment is identical to that outlined above for AIH, although higher doses of azathioprine may be required. In some cases, therapy may eventually be withdrawn without subsequent relapse.

In another AIH/PBC variant, circulating AMA is not detectable, although the histologic features are more reminiscent of PBC. This syndrome, in which ANA or SMA may be present, has been referred to by a variety of terms, including autoimmune cholangitis, immune cholangitis, autoimmune cholangiopathy, and immune cholangiopathy.[7,33,34] Some feel it may simply be AMA-negative primary biliary cirrhosis. Reports of efficacy of glucocorticosteroids in these cases have been conflicting. Although ursodeoxycholate may reduce liver enzymes, it is not known whether it mitigates the necroinflammatory process and/or retards the progression of disease. A therapeutic trial of steroids with or without ursodeoxycholate may be required before determining a long-term therapy regimen.[33,35]

The existence of an overlap syndrome of AIH and PSC in adults has been proposed.[36–38] Gohlke and colleagues have had limited success with a regimen combining glucocorticosteroids, azathioprine, and ursodeoxycholate.[36] In some cases PSC appears to evolve in the face of AIH.[17] Treatment data available are insufficient to make firm recommendations regarding treatment.

TREATMENT IN CHILDREN

Treatment of AIH

Although uncommon, AIH is an important cause of progressive inflammatory liver disease in children. Reported series of the treatment of autoimmune hepatitis in children are scanty, and the results are similar to those obtained in adults, with reported clinical and biochemical improvement rates of approximately 80% and remission in 60–80% of patients.[1,39]

At the onset of the disease, AIH is treated with regimens which employ monotherapy or a combination of prednisone and azathioprine (Table 34.4). With prednisone monotherapy the doses are high for prolonged periods of time and potential complications such as cushingoid facies, hypertension, reduced growth velocity, osteoporosis, cataracts, opportunistic infections, psychiatric problems, glucose intolerance, and striae may occur.

Combination therapy leads to fewer adverse effects and the response is usually rapid, as measured by clinical and biochemical improvement. Prednisone is usually given orally at a dosage of 1–2 mg/kg/day (maximum 60 mg/day) and azathioprine at doses 1.5–2 mg/kg/day (see Table 34.4).

Azathioprine should be administered carefully because the cytotoxic activity achieved by interfering with protein synthesis and nucleic acid metabolism may damage rapidly proliferating cells and impair an antigen-mediated immune response. As noted, azathioprine is a prodrug for 6-MP. TPMT deficiency may lead to toxicity in children as well as in adults (see above); Rumbo et al. found that azathioprine metabolite testing in children with AIH is useful in identifying medication toxicity and nonadherence.[40] We recommend monitoring leukocyte and platelet counts in patients every 15 days during the first month of treatment and subsequently when liver tests are determined.

The biochemical response to treatment should be monitored by measuring circulating aminotransferases, bilirubin, prothrombin time, albumin, and gamma globulin values. Patients should be

Table 34.4 Treatment of autoimmune hepatitis in children

Regimen	Single-drug therapy	Combination therapy
Initial	Prednisone 1–2 mg/kg of body weight daily	Prednisone 1–2 mg/kg of body weight daily and azathioprine 1.5–2 mg/kg of body weight daily
Maintenance	Prednisone 1 mg/kg of body weight daily or azathioprine 1.5–2 mg/kg of body weight	Prednisone 0.5–1 mg/kg of body weight daily and azathioprine 1.5–2 mg/kg of body weight daily

assessed at 4–6-week intervals until clinical and biochemical remission is achieved and then at 3-month intervals during the first year of treatment. If the patient continues in clinical and biochemical remission, follow-up should be at 4-month intervals for 2 years of treatment. At that time we recommend a repeat liver biopsy to help in the decision of whether or not to discontinue therapy. In patients with type 1 AIH, the improvement in aminotransferase levels often precedes other measures. Gamma globulin reduction may take several months or as long as 2–4 years to achieve acceptable values. Corticosteroid side effects occur frequently at the beginning of treatment but generally do not reflect activity or completely resolve after dose reduction. Each patient appears to have a critical level of immunosuppression below which relapse occurs; therefore, although doses are variable, attempts should be made to use the lowest possible dose of steroids compatible with biochemical control. In general, we taper prednisone at each clinical evaluation until a dose of 0.25 mg/kg/day is achieved.

No universal guidelines are available regarding timing of withdrawal of immunosuppressive therapy. The frequency of relapse in children is often more difficult to assess because of the problem of noncompliance. A general guide is to attempt withdrawal only in patients with type 1 AIH, when laboratory values (aminotransferases, albumin, prothrombin time) are persistently normal for at least 2 years and in the absence of necroinflammatory changes in the liver biopsy. Interruption of therapy is possible only in a minority of type 1 AIH patients and almost never in type 2 AIH. Maggiore et al.[41] were able to stop therapy in only 2 of 15 children and adolescents, whereas Vegnente et al.[42] were able to discontinue therapy in 8 of 28 children. In the series reported by Gregorio et al.[1] discontinuation of therapy was possible in 6 of 32 children with type 1 AIH but in none of 15 children with type 2 AIH disease. Porta's observations were similar to those of Gregorio; discontinuation of therapy was achieved in only 18 of 92 patients, and remission was achieved in 11. All of those who relapsed responded to reintroduction of therapy.[39]

In some patients the combination of prednisone and azathioprine is not tolerated or fails to induce remission. Treatment failures in children usually require high doses of corticosteroids or combination of other immunosuppressive drugs with different modes of action such as the calcineurin inhibitors cyclosporine, and tacrolimus.

Cyclosporine has been reported to be effective in small numbers of adult AIH patients who failed to respond to conventional therapy. The data in children are sparse.[43–45] Two major publications on treatment of children with cyclosporine, which were done with the aim of inducing a biochemical remission at onset of disease, have been reported. A multicenter prospective study[44] used a 6-month cyclosporine protocol in a pilot study which demon-

strated that cyclosporine can induce a biochemical remission of AIH in children with relatively few and well-tolerated side effects. The initial dosage in this study was 4 mg/kg of body weight, daily, divided into three doses. The authors observed an increase in growth velocity and height. After 6 months of treatment, cyclosporine was given concurrently with, then replaced by, relatively low doses of prednisone (0.3–0.5 mg/kg of body weight, daily) and azathioprine (1.5 mg/kg of body weight, daily). Thirty of 31 treated children had normal aminotransferase levels at the end of the first year of treatment, and no relapses were observed during follow-up. The second publication was a retrospective study limited to children with type 2 AIH.[45] Both studies showed good efficacy in inducing remission, with minimal side effects. Recently Sciveres et al.[46] reviewed the records of 12 patients with AIH treated with cyclosporine. The mean duration of therapy was 35.6 months, and mean follow-up was 6.5 years. All patients achieved complete remission in a median period of 4.5 weeks. No treatment withdrawal due to side effects occurred and the tolerance was excellent. Cyclosporine may therefore be considered as alternative therapy.

Other drugs sometimes used in adults such as budesonide, mycophenolate mofetil, cyclophosphamide, and methotrexate have not been reported in treatment of children. Orthotopic liver transplantation should be considered in children with fulminant hepatic failure and in those unresponsive to immunosuppressive therapy who progress to end-stage disease.

Treatment of overlap/variant syndrome

When children with AIH undergo immunosuppressive treatment and aminotransferase levels decrease to normal values but alkaline phosphatase or gammaglutamyl transpeptidase levels remain persistently abnormal, cholangiography is indicated to search for the overlap syndrome of AIH and PSC, often referred to as autoimmune sclerosing cholangitis (ASC). However, published pediatric series have shown cholangiography to be abnormal at presentation in children with clinical, biochemical, and histological manifestations of AIH,[16] and some pediatric hepatologists recommend cholangiography in all children who present with a picture suggesting AIH.

The features of ASC in children are highly variable with prevalence as high as of 27–35% among AIH pediatric patients.[6,16] Since AIH and ASC are similar in their mode of presentation, and their response to treatment varies, the only clear difference may be the involvement of the biliary tree in ASC.

No reports of controlled trials to treat ASC in children have been reported. Standardized treatment protocols for overlap/variant syndromes have not yet been established. Options include immunosuppressive, choleretic and/or antifibrotic drugs, but data regarding efficacy are conflicting. Gregorio et al.[6] found biochemical and clinical responses in 23 children with ASC, treated with prednisolone and azathioprine. However, follow-up cholangiography was unchanged; none showed regression and eight had a progression of cholangiopathy. Their results contrast with the disappointing results reported by others,[15,47–49] possibly because, at the time of diagnosis, the children had more advanced disease.

SUMMARY

Autoimmune hepatitis (AIH) is a progressive, sometimes fluctuating chronic hepatitis which occurs in children and adults of all ages. Although of unknown etiology, its pathogenesis is believed to be based at least in part on aberrant autoreactivity. The diagnosis is based on histologic changes, characteristic clinical and biochemical findings, circulating autoantibodies, and abnormalities of serum globulins, in the absence of evidence of viral or drug-induced disease. Despite the striking clinical heterogeneity of AIH and our incomplete understanding of its pathogenesis, the disease in adults and children generally responds to antiinflammatory/immunosuppressive treatment. Initial therapy in most cases involves prednisone alone or in combination with azathioprine. No firm guidelines exist for decisions regarding withdrawal or reduction of medication, primarily because histologic changes may lag behind biochemical changes, levels of autoantibodies do not parallel disease activity, and a quiescent histologic appearance while patients are still receiving therapy is not necessarily predictive of maintenance of remission after discontinuance of treatment. Lifetime maintenance therapy may be required, especially for patients with type 2 AIH and for those who have cirrhosis at presentation. Liver transplantation has been successful in patients who do not respond to medical treatment. No trials have been performed on which to base the treatment of overlap/variant syndromes.

REFERENCES

1. Gregorio GV, Portmann B, Reid F, et al. Autoimmune hepatitis in childhood: a 20-year experience. Hepatology 1997; 25:541–547.

    A detailed analysis of a large number of young patients followed at a King's College Hospital in London, UK.

2. Schramm C, Kanzler S, zum Buschenfelde KH, et al. Autoimmune hepatitis in the elderly. Am J Gastroenterol 2001; 96:1587–1591.

    A discussion of the clinical characteristics of patients ages 65 and over in comparison with those of younger patients seen at the Johannes Gutenberg University in Mainz, Germany.

3. Heneghan MA, McFarlane IG. Current and novel immunosuppressive therapy for autoimmune hepatitis. Hepatology 2002; 35:7–13.

4. Batts KP, Ludwig J. Histopathology of autoimmune liver disease. In: Krawitt EL, Wiesner RS, Nishioka M, eds. Autoimmune liver diseases 2nd edn. Amsterdam: Elsevier Science; 1998:115–140.

    A detailed discussion of histopathology of autoimmune liver diseases based on an extensive database of the Mayo Clinic population.

5. Czaja AJ, Manns MP, McFarlane IG, et al. Autoimmune hepatitis: the investigational and clinical challenges. Hepatology 2000; 31:1194–1200.

    The summary of a single-topic conference convened in 1999 and attended by experts in autoimmunity and autoimmune hepatitis.

6. Gregorio GV, Portmann B, Karani J, et al. Autoimmune hepatitis/sclerosing cholangitis overlap syndrome in childhood: a 16-year prospective study. Hepatology 2001; 33:544–553.

7. Woodward J, Neuberger J. Autoimmune overlap syndromes. Hepatology 2001; 33:994–1002.

8. Donaldson PT, Albertini RJ, Krawitt EL. Immunogenetic studies of autoimmune hepatitis and primary sclerosing cholangitis. In: Krawitt EL, Wiesner RS, Nishioka M, eds. Autoimmune liver diseases. 2nd edn. Amsterdam: Elsevier Science; 1998:141–165.

    An overview of the genetic organization of the HLA region, the structure and function of class I and II molecules, and immunogenetic studies of autoimmune hepatitis and primary sclerosing cholangitis.

9. Yun M, Longhi MS, Bogdanos DP, et al. Functional impairment of CD25+CD4+regulatory T-cells characterizes autoimmune hepatitis type 2 (Abstract). Hepatology 2003; 38:1634

10. Alvarez F, Berg PA, Bianchi FB, et al. International autoimmune hepatitis group report: review of criteria for diagnosis of autoimmune hepatitis. J Hepatol 1999; 31:929–938.

11. Czaja AJ. Behavior and significance of autoantibodies in type 1 autoimmune hepatitis. J Hepatol 1999; 30:394–401.

12. Czaja AJ, Cassani F, Cataleta M, et al. Frequency and significance of antibodies to actin in type 1 autoimmune hepatitis. Hepatology 1996; 24:1068–1073.

13. Roozendaal C, de Jong MA, van den Berg AP, et al. Clinical significance of anti-neutrophil cytoplasmic antibodies (ANCA) in autoimmune liver diseases. J Hepatol 2000; 32:734–741.

14. Wies I, Brunner S, Henninger J, et al. Identification of target antigen for SLA/LP autoantibodies in autoimmune hepatitis. Lancet 2000; 355:1510–1515.

15. Ballot E, Homberg JC, Johanet C. Antibodies to soluble liver antigen: an additional marker in type 1 autoimmune hepatitis. J Hepatol 2000; 33:208–215.

16. Feldstein AE, Perrault J, El-Youssif M, et al. Primary sclerosing cholangitis in children: A long-term follow-up study. Hepatology 2003; 38:210–217.

17. Abdo AA, Bain VG, Kichian K, et al. Evolution of autoimmune hepatitis to primary sclerosing cholangitis: a sequential syndrome. Hepatology 2002; 36:1393–1399.

18. Roberts SK, Therneau TM, Czaja AJ. Prognosis of histological cirrhosis in type 1 autoimmune hepatitis. Gastroenterology 1996; 110:848–857.

19. Marshall E. Preventing toxicity with gene test. Science 2003; 302:588–590.

20. Lennard L. Clinical implications of thiopurine metyltransferase – optimization of drug dosage and potential drug interactions. Ther Drug Monit 1998; 20:527–531.

21. Yates CR, Krynetski EY, Loennechem T, et al. Molecular diagnosis of thiopurine metyltransferase deficiency: genetic bases for azathioprine and mercaptopurine intolerance. Am Int Med 1997; 6:608–614.

22. Pratt DS, Flavin DP, Kaplan MM. The successful treatment of autoimmune hepatitis with 6-mercaptopurine after failure with azathioprine. Gastroenterology 1996; 110:271–274.

23. Langley PG, Underhill J, Tredger JM, et al. Thiopurine methyltransferase phenotype and genotype in relation to azathioprine therapy in autoimmune hepatitis. J Hepatol 2002; 37:441–447.

24. Johnson P, McFarlane IG, Williams R. Azathioprine for long-term maintenance of remission in autoimmune hepatitis. N Engl J Med 1995; 333:958–963.

25. Czaja AJ. Low-dose corticosteroid therapy after multiple relapses of severe HBsAg-negative chronic active hepatitis. Hepatology 1990; 11:1044–1049.

26. Czaja AJ, Lindor KD. Failure of budesonide in a pilot study of treatment-dependent autoimmune hepatitis. Gastroenterology 2000; 119:1312–1316.

27. Fernandes NF, Redeker AG, Vierling JM, et al. Cyclosporine therapy in patients with steroid resistant autoimmune hepatitis. Am J Gastroenterol 1999; 94:241–248.

28. Van Thiel DH, Wright H, Carroll P, et al. Tacrolimus: a potential new treatment for autoimmune chronic active hepatitis: results of an open-label preliminary trial. Am J Gastroenterol 1995; 90: 771–776.

29. Burak KW, Urbanski SJ, Swain MG. Successful treatment of refractory type 1 autoimmune hepatitis with methotrexate. J Hepatol 1998; 29:990–993.

30. Richardson PD, James PD, Ryder SD. Mycophenolate mofetil for maintenance of remission in autoimmune hepatitis in patients resistant to or intolerant of azathioprine. J Hepatol 2002; 33:371–375.

31. Faust TW. Recurrent primary biliary cirrhosis, primary sclerosing cholangitis, and autoimmune hepatitis after transplantation. Liver Transplant 2001; 7:S99–S108.

32. Davis PA, Leung P, Manns M, et al. M4 and M9 antibodies in the overlap syndrome of primary biliary cirrhosis and chronic active hepatitis: epitopes or epiphenomena. Hepatology 1992; 16:1128–1136.

33. Chazouilleres O, Wendum D, Serfaty L, et al. Primary biliary cirrhosis-autoimmune hepatitis overlap syndrome: clinical features and response to therapy. Hepatology 1998; 28:296–301.

34. Lohse AW, zum Buschenfelde KH, Franz B, et al. Characterization of the overlap syndrome of primary biliary cirrhosis (PBC) and autoimmune hepatitis: evidence for it being a hepatitic form of PBC in genetically susceptible individuals. Hepatology 1999; 29:1078–1084.

35. Joshi S, Cauch-Dudek K, Wanless IR, et al. Primary biliary cirrhosis with additional features of autoimmune hepatitis: response to therapy with ursodeoxycholic acid. Hepatology 2002; 35:409–413.

36. Gohlke F, Lohse AW, Dienes HP, et al. Evidence for an overlap syndrome of autoimmune hepatitis and primary sclerosing cholangitis. J Hepatol 1996; 24:699–705.

37. McNair AN, Moloney M, Portmann BC, et al. Autoimmune hepatitis overlapping with primary sclerosing cholangitis in five cases. Am J Gastroenterol 1998; 93:777–784.

38. van Buuren HR, van Hoogstraten JF, Terkivatan T, et al. High prevalence of autoimmune hepatitis among patients with primary sclerosing cholangitis. J Hepatol 2000; 33:543–548.

39. Porta G. Hepatite auto-imune na infância. Análise clínico-laboratorial, histológica e evolutiva. São Paulo. Tese (Livre-Docência) – Faculdade de Medicina: Universidade de São Paulo; 1993:189.

40. Rumbo C, Emerick KM, Emre S, et al. Azathioprine metabolite measurements in the treatment of autoimmune hepatitis in pediatric patients: a preliminary report. J Pediatr Gastroenterol Nutr 2002; 35(3):391–398.

41. Maggiore G, Bernard O, Hadchouel M, et al. Treatment of autoimmune chronic hepatitis in childhood. J Pediatr 1984; 104:838–844.

42. Vegnente A, Larcher VF, Mowat AP, et al. Duration of chronic active hepatitis and the development of cirrhosis. Arch Dis Child 1984; 59:330–335.

43. Sherman KE, Narkewicz M, Pinto PC. Cyclosporine in the management of corticosteroid-resistant type 1 autoimmune chronic active hepatitis. J Hepatol 1994; 21:1040–1047.

44. Alvarez F, Ciocca M, Canero-Velasco C, et al. Short-term cyclosporine induces a remission of autoimmune hepatitis in children. J Hepatol 1999; 30(2):222–227.

45. Debray D, Maggiore G, Girardet JP, et al. Efficacy of cyclosporine A in children with type 2 autoimmune hepatitis. J Pediatr 1999; 135(1):111–114.

46. Sciveres M, Caprai S, Palla G, et al. Effectiveness and safety of cyclosporine as therapy for autoimmune diseases of the liver in children and adolescents. Aliment Pharmacol Ther 2004; 1519(2):209–217.

47. Wilschanski M, Chait P, Wade JA, et al. Primary sclerosing cholangitis in 32 children: clinical, laboratory, and radiographic features, with survival analysis. Hepatology 1995; 22(5):1415–1422.

48. Floreani A, Zancan L, Melis A, et al. Primary sclerosing cholangitis (PSC): clinical, laboratory and survival analysis in children and adults. Liver 1999; 19(3):228–33.

49. el-Shabrawi M, Wilkinson ML, Portmann B, et al. Primary sclerosing cholangitis in childhood. Gastroenterology 1987; 92(5Pt1):1226–1235.

CHAPTER THIRTY-FIVE

35

Bacterial, fungal and granulomatous diseases of the liver

David P. Nunes

INTRODUCTION

Over the last few decades the incidence and spectrum of liver infections has changed, primarily as a result of an increase in immunosuppressed populations with the advent of HIV infections, organ transplantation, and cancer chemotherapy. Early identification and treatment is essential to minimize both the morbidity and mortality associated with liver infections. The clinician should also recognize that abnormalities in liver blood tests are not unusual in patients with systemic infection. These abnormalities are related to functional changes in the liver and do not indicate hepatic infection. Management of these patients consists of the treatment of the underlying infection and associated hemodynamic abnormalities, if present.

BACTERIAL INFECTIONS

Pyogenic liver abscess

The incidence of liver abscesses had been rising during the last century, with an apparent reduction more recently (Fig. 35.1). During this time there has also been an increase in mean age, proportion with diabetes mellitus, and in the number of cases related to immunosuppression, including liver transplantation as well as instrumentation of the liver.[1]

Infection of the liver with the development of liver abscesses may occur as a result of: (1) direct extension from adjacent structure, e.g., as a complication of empyema of the gallbladder or perforated viscus;[1-4] (2) seeding from the systemic circulation; (3)

spread via the portal venous system from an intra-abdominal source, e.g., diverticulitis or appendiceal abscess (pylophlebitis); (4) ascending biliary infection; or (5) following trauma or instrumentation of the liver. In most cases there is a slight predilection for the right lobe of the liver, related to the greater volume of the right lobe and perhaps to a streaming effect of portal venous blood flow.[4] Some series have suggested that ascending biliary infection is now the most common cause in adults and is more frequently associated with multiple abscesses.[1,5] Abscesses occurring as a result of portal venous infection are more commonly single, or few in number. Liver abscesses may also occur as a complication of liver tumors, cysts, or biliary duct abnormalities such as Caroli's disease, or following chemoembolization or percutaneous ablation of liver tumors.[6] Abscesses resulting from hepatic artery thrombosis after liver transplantation are also becoming more common.

The causative bacteria and changing pattern of bacterial infections is shown in Figure 35.2. The bacteria isolated depends upon the mechanism of infection, host immune status, as well as local and regional factors. Polymicrobial infection, with Gram-negative organisms and anaerobes is most frequent in those with ascending biliary tract, intra-abdominal infection, or extension from an adjacent site.[7] Overall, anaerobes are identified in as many as 45–60% of all cases.[8] With ascending biliary infection, *E. coli* and *Klebsiella* species are commonest and often occur in association with enterococcus.[8] Where there has been spread from an intra-abdominal infection, the same pattern of bacteria may be isolated but with a higher incidence of *Bacteroides*. A single organism, often a streptococcal, staphylococcal, or Gram-negative organism

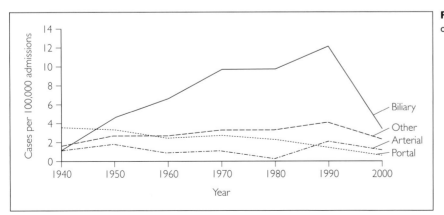

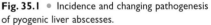

Fig. 35.1 • Incidence and changing pathogenesis of pyogenic liver abscesses.

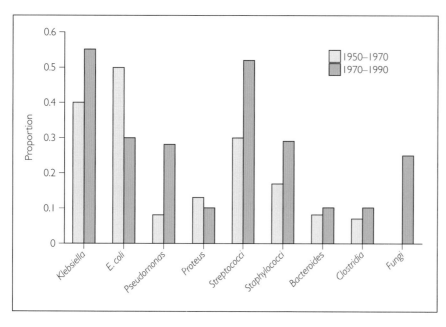

Fig. 35.2 • Proportion of bacterial isolates responsible for pyogenic abscess, 1950–1970 and 1970–1990.

is commonest in those with hematogenous spread. Of the *Strep. viridans* species, *Strep. milleri* is by far the most frequent, usually indicating hematogenous spread to the liver.[9] *Yersinia enterocolitica* may be the cause in individuals with iron overload states (hemochromatosis and thalassemia) and diabetes.[10,11] Individuals with indwelling stents and underlying malignancy appear to be at high risk of mixed fungal and bacterial infections and carry a poor prognosis. *Candida* abscesses occur in those who have been neutropenic for prolonged periods, usually in association with systemic chemotherapy.[12]

Clinical presentation

The clinical presentation can be quite variable. Most have a relatively slow-onset illness with low-grade fever, right-upper quadrant pain, poor appetite, and fatigue. Those with biliary disease may present more acutely with features of ascending cholangitis, severe pain, high fever, rigors, jaundice and may progress rapidly to septicemic shock. There is usually a leukocytosis with a left shift and an increased erythrocyte sedimentation rate. The liver blood tests are often increased, most typically with a cholestatic pattern.[1] However, normal, atypical, or minimally elevated liver blood tests do not exclude the diagnosis.[4]

On chest X-ray, the right hemidiaphragm may be elevated, with or without a pleural effusion or basal pulmonary infiltrate. Abscesses are seen on ultrasound in over 80% of cases, while the diagnostic accuracy of CT and MRI scans approaches 100%.[4,13] Blood cultures are positive in 40–60% while direct aspiration is positive in 70–80%.[4,8] The differential diagnosis includes necrotic tumors, hydatid disease, amebic abscess, and polycystic disease of the liver. Each of these conditions can rarely be complicated by secondary bacterial infection.

Treatment

Management of a hepatic abscess should address the abscess, as well as identifying and treating the underlying cause. The initial evaluation should include a careful clinical history and examination seeking evidence for a source. Intra-abdominal, biliary, and distant foci of infection should be sought. Blood cultures and

aspiration of the abscess with Gram stain and culture should be performed since the results are crucial for guiding therapy as well as pointing to a possible source.[14]

Both antibiotic therapy and drainage of the abscess are usually required. Percutaneous drainage has largely supplanted the surgical approach.[8] However, surgery should be considered where the abscess(es) cannot be drained adequately by the percutaneous route, due to their number, location, or viscosity of their contents. Surgery is also indicated when the primary cause of the abscess requires surgical management, e.g., an appendiceal or diverticular abscess, or empyema with extension into the liver. Recent studies have shown that the laparoscopic approach is safe and effective and can be used in selected cases.[15] Drainage of the biliary system and sometimes the abscess can be achieved by endoscopic retrograde cholangiopancreatography (ERCP).

Percutaneous drainage of single or multiple abscesses can be achieved by simple aspiration and/or placement of a percutaneous catheter.[8,16] A recent comparative study has shown that aspiration alone is simpler, more cost-effective, and gives results equivalent to the placement of a percutaneous drain.[16] However, selection of the most appropriate technique depends upon local expertise, condition of the patient, and the ability to obtain adequate drainage by aspiration.

Antibiotics should be selected to treat the likely pathogen(s). Unless there is a known bacterial source, initial therapy should consist of broad-spectrum antibiotics aimed at covering aerobic Gram-negative organisms, as well as Gram-positives including streptococci, enterococcus, and anaerobes. Gram-negative coverage can be achieved with a third-generation cephalosporin, a quinolone such as levofloxacin, an aminoglycoside, piperacillin/tazobactam, or imipenem/cilastatin. Caution should be used in giving aminoglycosides to jaundiced patients because of the increased risk of renal toxicity. Anaerobes, particularly *Bacteroides*, should be treated with metronidazole or clindamycin. Depending on the regimen selected, some authorities would add amoxicillin to treat enterococcus and other Gram-positive organisms. Antibiotic choice should be adjusted based upon Gram stain and culture results, as they become available. There are no controlled studies to guide the exact duration and route of antibiotic administration. Two weeks of parenteral antibiotics followed by 4 weeks or longer of oral antibiotics has been shown to be adequate in most cases.[17] Follow-up imaging either by CT scan or ultrasound should be performed regularly to confirm treatment response. Antibiotics should be continued until resolution of the abscess has been demonstrated radiologically. In those high-risk patients, (e.g., diabetes, immunosuppressed, postinstrumentation) with a poor response to drainage and antibiotic therapy, a mixed fungal infection should be considered and a trial of antifungal therapy is often warranted.

Outcome

The overall case fatality rate of hepatic abscesses has fallen over the last few decades.[2] Much of this decline has been attributed to earlier diagnosis, as a result of improved liver imaging. This improvement in survival has occurred despite the increasing age and number of comorbid diseases observed in more recent series. Overall case fatality rates are now between 5% and 20%.[4,5,8] The best prognosis is seen in those with benign biliary disease, while the outcome is poorer in those with severe infection, multiple abscesses, malignant disease, cirrhosis, and mixed fungal and bacterial infections.[2,5,18]

Mycobacterial infections

HIV infection and the use of potent immunosuppressives, including reports of reactivation of tuberculosis with the use of TNFα blockers for the treatment of autoimmune disease, have resulted in an increased incidence of both *Mycobacterium tuberculosis* and atypical mycobacterial infections.[19–21] Hepatic involvement is a common feature of disseminated infection with almost all mycobacteria and is a commoner cause of granulomatous liver disease.[19] As a result, all liver biopsies performed for suspected granulomatous hepatitis should be sent for mycobacterial culture.

Mycobacterium tuberculosis

Liver involvement by *Mycobacterium tuberculosis* most often presents as a granulomatous hepatitis, but less common presentations include 'tuberculoma,' TB abscess, and biliary tract disease.[22] In most cases there is evidence of extrahepatic disease but isolated liver involvement is well recognized.[23] Extrapulmonary tuberculosis is more common in those with HIV infection, cirrhosis of the liver, and in the African-American population.[24]

Granulomatous disease results from secondary tuberculous infection. The granulomas are usually small, located in the lobules, and in over 50% of cases there is no evidence of caseation. Similar-appearing granulomatous disease can follow BCG vaccination or intravesicle instillation of BCG for the treatment of bladder tumors.[25,26] Clinical presentation of granulomatous TB is variable. Most present with features of extrahepatic disease including pulmonary disease, fever, night sweats and weight loss. Liver involvement is suggested by abnormal liver function tests, usually a cholestatic pattern.[27,28]

The majority of patients with miliary tuberculosis have liver involvement. In rare cases there may be massive infection of the liver causing right-upper quadrant pain and jaundice. There have even been reports of hepatic failure.[29] Tuberculomas and tuber-

cular abscesses often present indolently with one or more masses or abscesses.[22,30] Biliary involvement is very rare, but can present with bile duct obstruction[31] or gallbladder disease.[32] Obstruction may also occur as a complication of pancreatic tuberculosis or tubercular adenitis at the hilum of the liver.[33]

The diagnosis of hepatic tuberculosis may be difficult and is based upon clinical presentation, a high index of suspicion, and demonstration of infection in the liver or extrahepatic site. It should be noted that up to 50% of patients with miliary disease have a negative tuberculin skin test. If the diagnosis is made at an extrahepatic site it is usually not necessary to confirm hepatic disease unless there are atypical hepatic features or the liver disease does not respond to therapy. Furthermore, staining of liver biopsies for acid-fast bacilli is only positive in about 20% of cases and the organism will be cultured in only 50%. PCR-based diagnosis of clinical specimens, including liver biopsy tissue, is becoming more widely available, but has not been fully validated and standardized.[34,35] Where there is hematogenous spread, blood cultures using the lysis centrifugation technique may be useful, though these are most often positive in immunosuppressed populations with higher levels of bacteremia.[36]

Current recommendations for the treatment of hepatic tuberculosis are the same as for pulmonary disease.[37,38] Empiric treatment should commence with a four-drug regimen consisting of rifampin, isoniazid, ethambutol, and pyrazinamide. If after 8 weeks of therapy the organism has been shown to be sensitive to pyrazinamide, isoniazid, and rifampin, then ethambutol and pyrazinamide may be stopped and treatment continued for a further 18 weeks. In the event that the organism is resistant to pyrazinamide, or if pyrazinamide is not used during the initial 8 weeks, rifampin and isoniazid should be continued for a total of 9 months. This is because regimens that include pyrazinamide have been shown to have lower failure rates and result in earlier elimination of mycobacteria. If rapid sensitivity results show that the isolate is sensitive to both isoniazid and rifampin then the ethambutol can be stopped prior to week 8. Less frequent dosing regimens are also available, but must be given as directly observed therapy. While there are no good controlled data, patients with HIV disease, high bacterial loads, lymphadenitis, a large hepatic abscess, bone or joint involvement, or a slow clinical response, should be considered for more prolonged therapy. Specific recommendations for the management of individuals with neurological disease are beyond the scope of this contribution.

The treatment of tuberculosis in HIV-infected individuals poses special problems, but is nevertheless very effective.[39] The major problem is the interaction between rifampin and the HIV protease inhibitors as well as some of the non-nucleoside reverse transcriptase inhibitors.[40] In this situation most practitioners use rifabutin in place of rifampin, but dose adjustments may still be necessary, e.g., the dose of daily rifabutin should be reduced in individuals receiving indinavir, amprenavir, and nelfinavir, while the dose of rifabutin should be increased in those receiving efavirenz. Rifabutin should not be used without adjusting the dose of saquinavir or delaviridine. HIV RNA levels should be measured to assess the efficacy of the antiretroviral regimen and patients should be followed for evidence of rifabutin toxicity.

The management of tubercular liver abscesses is problematic, with no good data to guide treatment. While standard TB therapy is indicated in all cases, the role of percutaneous drainage and surgery is less clear.[22,30] Large abscesses with features suggestive of impending rupture should probably be drained percutaneously or surgically.

Atypical mycobacterial infections

Prior to the advent of HIV infection, atypical mycobacterial infections of the liver were extremely uncommon. The most significant of these problems has been the emergence of *Mycobacterium avium* complex (MAC) in immunosuppressed patients, particularly those with HIV infection, hematological malignancies, and following organ transplantation.[41,42] There are also rare case reports of other opportunistic mycobacterial infections of the liver including *M. lentiflavum*,[19] *M. kansasii*,[43] and *M. gordona*.[44]

In HIV-infected individuals, MAC occurs when the CD4 count has fallen below 100 cell/mm³. The disease often presents with systemic features, including fevers, weight loss, diffuse lymphadenopathy, and multiorgan involvement, particularly pulmonary disease, bone marrow involvement, and gastrointestinal disease. Hepatic disease is common and presents with hepatomegaly and increased alkaline phosphatase.[41] The diagnosis can be made in up to 70% of cases by centrifuge lysis blood culture, a rate similar to liver and bone marrow biopsy.[45,46] Liver and bone marrow biopsies are thus reserved for patients with atypical features, where blood cultures are negative or the response to empiric therapy is poor. Bone marrow biopsy is preferred because of the lower risk. Liver biopsies show small poorly formed granulomas, which usually contain numerous acid-fast bacilli.[47]

In HIV-positive individuals chemoprophylaxis for MAC should be commenced at a CD4 count of less than 50 cells/mm³ L. Studies have shown that treatment with a macrolide, either azithromycin 1200 mg once weekly or clarithromycin 500 mg b.i.d. are effective and reduce the cost of HIV management.[48,49] With the advent of effective antiretroviral therapy, prophylactic therapy is probably not necessary if there is no evidence of disease and a rapid recovery in CD4 count is expected. Those who commence chemoprophylaxis should have their treatment continued until the CD4 count exceeds 100 cells/mm³ L.[50,51]

The treatment of MAC is based upon correction of the immune suppression and use of appropriate antibiotics.[52] Effective drugs include the macrolides, ethambutol, rifabutin, and streptomycin. Combination therapy is preferred to prevent resistance. This normally consists of a macrolide and one of the other agents, usually rifabutin or ethambutol.[53-55] Examples of effective therapies include azithromycin 250 mg daily with rifabutin 300 mg daily, or clarithromycin 500 mg twice daily and rifabutin 300 mg daily. Of note, clarithromycin has a higher affinity for cytochrome P450 than azithromycin and is thus subject to important drug–drug interactions, including increasing serum levels of rifabutin.[56,57] For this reason clarithromycin is most often used in combination with ethambutol.[58,59] Ethambutol is given at a dose of 25 mg/kg for 2 months followed by 15 mg/kg. Streptomycin is also active against atypical mycobacteria and may be considered for inclusion during the first 8 weeks of therapy.[60] The availability of alternative oral regimens has meant that streptomycin is used only where other regimens have proven ineffective or not tolerated. The treatment of MAC is associated with a fairly rapid resolution of constitutional symptoms and overall clinical improvement. In HIV-positive individuals treatment should be continued for 3–6 months, and long-term suppression is needed only if the CD4 count remains below 100 cells/mm³ L.[50]

Uncommon liver infections

A variety of bacteria can cause liver infection. Many of these infections are relatively rare and liver involvement is usually not the primary site of infection, such that the clinical presentation is frequently with extrahepatic or systemic manifestations. The histological presentation of these infections is dependent on both etiology and stage of infection. Acute and subacute disease often results in liver abscess formation, as is seen with *Yersinia* and *Borrelia* infection. Chronic conditions such as syphilis, brucellosis, Whipple's disease, and coxiella are important causes of granulomatous liver disease. The management of many of the rarer causes of hepatic infection is summarized in Table 35.1.

Leptospirosis

Leptospirosis is a zoonosis caused by the spirochete *Leptospira interrogans* and its various serovars and is endemic worldwide. The organism is excreted in the urine of infected animals where it can survive in stagnant soil and water. Infection is acquired via defects in the skin or mucous membranes and is most common in those who work or undertake recreational activities in a contaminated environment, e.g., sewage workers, fresh water swimming, etc.

Leptospirosis presents as an acute febrile illness with associated nausea, vomiting, diarrhea, abdominal and bone pain, sore throat, and cough.[61] Hepatosplenomegaly, a diffuse rash, muscle tenderness with rigidity, and conjunctival suffusion are characteristic of this illness.[62,63] The most severe form of the condition is Weil's disease in which the patient also has jaundice and renal dysfunction.[64] As the disease progresses, cardiac failure or arrhythmias as well as a bleeding diathesis, including gastrointestinal bleeding, epistaxis, subconjunctival hemorrhage, skin petechiae, and ecchymoses may occur. This severe form of the disease is associated with the *L. icterohemorrhagica* serovar. Laboratory findings include leukocytosis and increased liver enzymes. Serum aminotransferase levels may be 5–10 times the upper limit of normal and there is often marked conjugated hyperbilirubinemia. Urinalysis is usually positive for blood, protein, and leukocytes. Creatinine kinase levels are frequently elevated. A positive antibody response or blood culture confirms the diagnosis.

Leptospira are sensitive to the aminoglycosides, penicillins, tetracyclines, cephalosporins, macrolides, and chloramphenicol.[65,66] Treatment with doxycycline and penicillin has been shown to shorten the clinical illness and duration of urinary shedding. The effectiveness of treatment in more severe disease is unclear, but a trial of therapy may be warranted.[67] In this situation intravenous penicillin or ceftriaxone are probably the drugs of choice.[65,67] As with other spirochetes, treatment has been associated with the Jarisch-Herxsheimer reaction.[68] In one series the mortality from severe icteric leptospirosis was 11% despite antibiotic therapy.[67] However, those who survive the illness have an excellent prognosis without sequelae.

Bartonella

Bartonella henselae infection of the liver results in a number of clinical syndromes, including an acute hepatitis-like illness, granulomatous hepatitis, and bacillary peliosis.[69] Disseminated 'cat-scratch disease' can result in an acute hepatitis- like illness in fewer than 1% of cases, but is most common in those with immune suppression, particularly that associated with HIV infection.[70,71]

Table 35.1 Bacterial infections of the liver

Infection	Characteristic features	Treatment	Comments
Treponema pallidum[122]			
Secondary	Abnormal liver blood tests associated with secondary syphillis. Rarely RUQ pain, hepatomegaly and jaundice. Hepatic granulomas	Benzathine penicillin 2.4 million units i.m.	Doxycycline 200 mg b.i.d. × 14 days
Tertiary	Usually asymptomatic. Liver nodular, may mimic cirrhosis on metastatic disease on CT imaging.	Benzathine penicillin 2.4 million units i.m. weekly for 3 weeks	Doxycycline 200 mg b.i.d. for 30 days
Leptospirosis[65]	Jaundice, acute hepatitis-like illness renal failure, muscle injury. Liver enlargement with acute zone III injury, hepatocyte swelling, apoptosis with prominent mitotic activity.	Doxycycline 100 mg p.o. b.i.d. Or Penicillin 6 million units daily	Consider ceftriaxone in severe disease
Francisella tularensis (tularemia)[123]	Liver involvement with bacteremic disease. Microabscess formation and coagulative necrosis.	Streptomycin 10 mg/kg for 7–10 days	Sensitive to gentamicin, fluoroquinolones, chloramphenicol, tetracyclines.
Perihepatitis (*Neisseria gonorrhoeae*, and/or *Chlamydia trachomatis*)[124]	Fever and right upper quadrant pain. Associated pelvic inflammatory disease. Perihepatic adhesion formation. (Lysis leads to pain resolution).	Levofloxacin 500 mg b.i.d. × 14 days Or Ceftriaxone 250 mg × 1 then doxycycline 100 mg b.i.d. for 14 days	Consider adding metronidazole 500 mg b.i.d.
Relapsing fever			
Louse borne (*B. recurrentis*)[125] Tick borne (*B. hermsii* and *turicatae*)	Acute onset febrile illness. Hepatomegaly and jaundice frequent. Non-specific hepatitis with hepatocyte necrosis	Tetracycline 500 mg × 1 Or Erythromycin 500 mg × 1 Doxycycline 100 mg b.i.d. × 10 days Or Erythromycin 500 mg q.i.d. × 10 days	Neurological disease high dose Penicillin G or ceftriaxone
Brucellosis[126]	Fever, arthralgia, bone pain. Lymphadenopathy hepatosplenomegaly. Granulomatous hepatitis: occasionally caseating. Rarely abscess formation, may be due to reactivation of latent infection.	Doxycycline 100 mg b.i.d. plus rifampin 600–900 mg daily for 3–6 weeks Or Doxycycline 100 mg b.i.d. plus streptomycin 1 g daily.	Ciprofloxacin may be used in place of tetracycline Co-trimoxazole is an alternative in children
Bartonella[71] Cat-scratch disease	Liver involvement rare, associated with immune suppression. Three clinical syndromes: acute hepatitis, granulomatous hepatitis, peliosis hepatis. Peliosis: vascular lesions with eosinophilic aggregates positive for *Bartonella* on silver stain	Erythromycin 500 mg p.o. q.i.d. Or Doxycycline 100 mg p.o. b.i.d.	Consider adding rifampin in severe disease. Add ceftriaxone or aminoglycoside with endocarditis[81]
Yersinia[127]	Acute disseminated disease Multiple liver abscesses Granulomatous reaction reported	Mild disease: ciprofloxacin 500 mg b.i.d. Severe disease: Ceftriaxone 1–2 g daily ± gentamicin	Doxycline and cotrimoxazole also effective. Iron chelation therapy should be stopped[128]

Continued

Table 35.1 Bacterial infections of the liver—cont'd

Infection	Characteristic features	Treatment	Comments
Q fever: *Coxiella burnetti*	Acute infection: non-specific hepatitis Chronic infection: fibrin ring granulomas	Doxycycline 100 mg b.i.d. × 2 weeks	Ofloxacin 400 mg t.i.d. A course of prednisone should be considered in patients with granulomatous hepatitis not responding to antibiotics
Whipple's disease (*Tropheryma whiplii*)	Rare cause of a granulomatous hepatitis. PAS-positive macrophages	Co-trimoxazole 960 mg p.o. b.i.d. for 1 year Severe disease initiate treatment with ceftriaxone or penicillin plus streptomycin for first 2 weeks.	Treatment with tetracycline is an alternative but associated with higher relapse rate.
Actinomycosis	Rare disease. Occurs in immune competent patients, usually a single hepatic abscess	Penicllin G i.v. 12–24 million units daily for 4–6 weeks, followed by oral amoxicillin	

Liver biopsy demonstrates necrotizing granulomas.[72,73] The diagnosis is confirmed by culture of the organism from involved tissues. Serological studies including ELISA and indirect immunofluorescent assays are available but have limited sensitivity. PCR assays are in development.[74] Treatment of uncomplicated cat-cratch disease in nonimmunosuppressed patients is a 5-day course of azithromycin 500 mg on day 1, followed by 250 mg daily for 4 days.[75] Alternatives include co-trimoxazole or a quinolone antibiotic.[76] Disseminated disease including acute liver disease requires treatment for 2 months or longer.

Immunosuppressed individuals, especially those with HIV infection, can develop bacillary angiomatosis and peliosis of the liver and spleen. Bacillary angiomatosis-peliosis refers to vascular lesions that can involve the skin, CNS, bone, lymph nodes, liver, respiratory, and gastrointestinal tracts. These conditions are caused by both *B. henselae* and *B. quintana*, but liver disease is much more commonly due to *B. henselae*.[77] CT scan of the abdomen shows vascular enhancement of liver and spleen, as well as any involved lymph nodes.[78,79] On biopsy, bacillary peliosis hepatis and splenitis are characterized by dilated vascular spaces with eosinophilic aggregates that stain positive for *Bartonella* using a silver stain.[80]

Treatment of bacillary angiomatosis-peliosis in immunosuppressed patients is empiric and based upon clinical experience rather than randomized controlled trials. Treatment is with prolonged courses of erythromycin (500 mg four times daily) or doxycycline 100 mg b.i.d.[71,81] In those with associated endocarditis, addition of a bactericidal agent such as ceftriaxone or an aminoglycoside is recommended for the first 2–3 weeks of therapy.[81] The newer macrolides are probably equally effective, though experience with these is more limited.[82] Rifampin is sometimes added to the treatment regimen in those with severe disease.[71] The duration of treatment for visceral infection requires treatment for 4 months or longer.

FUNGAL INFECTIONS

Introduction

Fungal infections of the liver usually occur following hematogenous spread in at-risk individuals. The more common causes of fungal liver diseases are summarized in Table 35.2. They may be classified into the pathogenic fungi such as *Histoplasma capsulatum*, coccidiomycosis, paracoccidiomycosis, and blastomycosis, or opportunistic fungi such as *Candida albicans*, *Cryptococcus neoformans*, *Aspergilla* species, and mucormycosis. More recently, infection with the opportunistic fungus, *Penicillium marmeffei*, has been described in HIV-positive individuals in the Far East.[83]

Treatment of systemic fungal infections has largely relied upon two drug classes, the azoles (fluconazole, itraconazole, and the more recently introduced voriconazole[84]) and amphotericin B. The widespread availability and increased use of azoles has resulted in more azole resistance, with the increased need for, and availability of, in vitro testing for fungal resistance.[85,86] A new class of agent, the echinocandins, has recently been introduced.[87] These agents inhibit the glucan synthase complex, necessary for the synthesis of fungal cell walls. Because of their novel mechanism of action they have proven useful in the management of serious *Candida* and *Aspergillus* infections.[84,87–89]

Candida

Candida is a normal commensal of the mouth, gastrointestinal tract, and vagina with higher rates of carriage in immunosuppressed populations. In the case of *Candida albicans* conversion to a pathogenic form is characterized by the appearance of hyphal forms. Risk factors for systemic *Candida* infection include neutropenia, HIV infection, lymphoma, diabetes, antibiotic therapy, nutritional deficiencies, intravenous lines, and injection drug use. Recent epidemiological data have shown that there has been a

Table 35.2 Fungal infections of the liver

Fungus	Characteristic features	Treatment	Comments
Opportunistic fungi			
Candidiasis[94]	Liver disease associated with neutropenia, diabetes, bacterial abscess formation and liver instrumentation. Hepatic abscess(es) or infiltrative process.	Amphotericin B 0.5–1.0 mg/kg i.v. Or Fluconazole 400 mg daily	Echinocandins and voriconazole have good activity Consider combination therapy in severe disease
Aspergillosis[129,130]	Liver abscess Invasion of necrotic tissue Aspergilloma (rare)	Amphotericin 1.0–1.5 mg/kg i.v. Or Itraconazole 200 mg p.o. b.i.d.	Voriconazole and the echinocandins have good activity
Cryptococcus[131]	Occurs in disseminated infection, liver involvement usually incidental.	Mild disease Fluconazole 200–400 mg daily Itraconazole 200 mg b.i.d. Severe disease Amphotericin 0.3–0.6 mg/kg i.v. plus flucytosine 150 mg/kg × 2 weeks then fluconazole 100–200 mg p.o. daily	Voriconazole good activity against cryptococcus
Mucormycosis[132]	Very rare, associated with DM, liver transplantation and chemotherapy.	Amphotericin B 0.5–1.0 mg/kg i.v.	
Penicillinosis[133]	Associated with HIV infection (SE Asia). Granulomatous hepatitis.	Amphotericin B 0.6–1.0 mg/kg i.v. then itraconazole 200 mg p.o. b.i.d.	
Pathogenic fungi			
Histoplasmosis[134]	Acute: Lymphohistiocytic inflammation of the liver. 20% have granulomas. Histoplasma numerous on biopsy. Chronic: Granulomatous inflammation, Histoplasma: scant or absent on fungal stains.	Amphotericin B 0.7–1.0 mg/kg i.v. then itraconazole 200 mg p.o. b.i.d.	Itraconazole or fluconazole may be used initially in mild disease. Voriconazole has good in vitro activity
Paracoccidioidomycosis[135]	Granulomas or diffuse infiltration Biliary involvement not uncommon	Itraconazole 100–200 mg PO daily for 6 months	Amphoteracin B Ketoconazole
Coccidioidomycosis[136]	Granulomas or diffuse infiltration	Itraconazole 200 mg p.o. b.i.d. or Fluconazole 400 p.o. mg daily	Amphotericin B and Voriconazole have good activity

Doses of amphotericin B are for standard preparations. Liposomal preparations require higher doses. p.o., orally; i.v., intravenously; b.i.d., twice daily; q.i.d., four times daily.

shift away from *C. albicans* to other candidal species as the cause of systemic candidiasis.[90,91] These findings have significance since not all *Candida* species are equally sensitive to the available antifungal agents.

The clinical presentation of systemic candidiasis is that of a systemic infection or sepsis syndrome in an at-risk individual. Disseminated candidiasis should be considered in neutropenic patients on appropriate antibiotics whose condition is otherwise deteriorating. Liver involvement is not usually a prominent clinical feature, but right-upper quadrant pain and hepatomegaly may be present.[92]

The term hepatosplenic candidiasis has been used to describe a specific syndrome most commonly observed in individuals with hematological malignancies who have been neutropenic for prolonged periods.[93] In this condition the liver and spleen are the primary sites of infection and blood cultures are frequently negative since it is believed that the *Candida* gains access to the liver and spleen via the GI tract. Infected individuals present with spiking fevers and right-upper quadrant pain. Laboratory studies show an elevated alkaline phosphatase consistent with an infiltrative process. On imaging, there is often quite subtle evidence of an infiltrative process, but in more severe cases multiple small abscesses in the liver and/or spleen can be seen.[12] Confirmation of the diagnosis often depends on liver biopsy. Biopsy early in the course usually shows acute necrotizing inflammation with numerous candidal organisms. In the later stages, and in those who have received therapy, biopsy often reveals granulomas with few or no organisms present.[12]

Treatment

The management of systemic *Candida* infections should include removal of intravenous catheters, restoration of immune function, and the administration of a systemic anticandidal agent(s). Selection of the most appropriate agent depends on the clinical situation. The majority of *Candida* species are sensitive to amphotericin B, the azoles, including the second-generation agents (e.g., voriconazole) as well as the echinocandins such as caspofungin or micafungin.[94] Because of long clinical experience and proven efficacy, amphotericin B remains the agent of first choice in severe infections. However, its use is associated with significant toxicity as well as treatment failures. Liposomal forms of amphotericin B permit higher doses of amphotericin and may improve clinical responses with lower toxicity.[95,96] More recent comparative studies have shown that both intravenous fluconazole and caspofungin are equivalent to amphotericin B for the treatment of systemic and invasive candidiasis and may be reasonable alternatives.[97–100] Furthermore, there has been at least one report of a patient responding to caspofungin after failing amphotericin B.[101]

Amphotericin B, with or without one of the other agents, is still recommended as the agent of choice for severe hepatosplenic candidiasis. However, fluconazole is often preferred for stable patients, though some authors still suggest an initial 1–2 week course of amphotericin B.[102] Treatment should continue until resolution of the lesions and during periods of immune suppression.[94] Caspofungin may also be effective in this scenario.[101]

There is a growing literature on the use of prophylactic antifungal agents in the primary prevention of systemic fungal infection in neutropenic patients undergoing chemotherapy and for organ transplantation. While some studies have suggested good efficacy others have been less convincing.[79,102,104]

GRANULOMATOUS LIVER DISEASE

The differential diagnosis of granulomatous liver disease is shown in Table 35.3. This includes a wide variety of infections, many of which have been reviewed above, but also includes a number of viral and parasitic infections including hepatitis C, Epstein-Barr virus, and cytomegalovirus, as well as schistosomiasis. Granulomas may also be a feature of both Hodgkin's and non-Hodgkin's lymphoma and a variety of immune-mediated diseases including primary biliary cirrhosis, sarcoidosis, inflammatory bowel disease, and idiopathic granulomatous hepatitis. A large number of drugs have also been associated with granulomatous liver disease, some of which are listed in Table 35.3. Other miscellaneous conditions include chronic bile duct obstruction, fat granulomas as well as foreign body reactions as seen in those with berylliosis, as well as those who self-inject illicit drugs contaminated with talc and other foreign bodies. Foreign body granulomas may be recognized by the presence of birefringent material on polarizing light microscopy.

Reviews of liver biopsy series from developed countries have shown that primary biliary cirrhosis, sarcoidosis, mycobacterial infections, and drugs are the most common causes of granulomatous liver disease.[28,105,106] Prior fungal infections with histoplasmosis or coccidioidomycosis are common causes in endemic areas. In these larger case series, between 10% and 50% of cases were deemed idiopathic. In underdeveloped countries tuberculosis and other infections are the most common causes. Since many of these conditions have already been discussed or are discussed in more detail elsewhere, only sarcoidosis and idiopathic granulomatous hepatitis will be discussed here. The treatment of

Table 35.3 Causes of granulomatous liver disease

Bacterial

Tuberculosis, atypical mycobacteria, *Treponema pallidum*, brucellosis, *Bartonella*, *Coxiella*, syphillis, listeria, *Brucella*, *Salmonella*, *Yersinia*, *Burkholderia pseudomallei* (melioidosis), *Francisella tularensis* (tularemia), Whipple's disease

Viral

CMV, HCV, EBV

Parasites

Leishmania, toxoplasma, schistosoma, toxocara, fasciola, ascariasis

Immune mediated

Primary biliary cirrhosis, sarcoidosis, idiopathic granulomatous hepatitis, Crohn's disease, Wegener's granulomatosis, polymyalgia rheumatica

Medications

Allopurinol, carbamazepine, gold, hydralazine, methyl dopa, nitrofurantoin, phenytoin, procainamide, sulfonamides, sulfonylureas

Neoplastic

Hodgkin's lymphoma, non-Hodgkin's lymphoma, renal cell carcinoma

Miscellaneous

BCG, large duct obstruction, fatty liver disease, berylliosis, talc

drug-induced disease is removal of the offending agent. There is no evidence that corticosteroids improve clinical outcome.

Sarcoidosis

Liver involvement with sarcoid is very common. Approximately 60% of individuals with pulmonary sarcoid have liver disease[107] and liver involvement may occur in the absence of lung disease.[108] Furthermore extrapulmonary sarcoidosis is more common in patients of African than European descent.[109] Hepatic sarcoidosis is usually asymptomatic, the only manifestation being mildly abnormal liver blood tests usually with elevation in serum alkaline phosphatase levels. Between 2% and 6% of patients are thought to have clinically significant liver disease.[110] Most clinical cases present with features of portal hypertension or cholestasis.[63,111,112] Cirrhosis is only rarely reported. Histological examination of the liver reveals periportal granulomas and occasionally portal fibrosis. Disturbance of normal portal venous blood flow as a result of granulomatous injury is thought to be the basis of the development of portal hypertension.[113] Rarer complications include vascular involvement which can lead to the Budd-Chiari syndrome or nodular hyperplasia of the liver.[107] Cholestasis can occur as a result of granulomatous inflammation of the intrahepatic biliary radicles. Histologically, this can mimic primary biliary cirrhosis or sclerosing cholangitis.[114]

The diagnosis is easily made in the setting of a patient with known sarcoidosis and abnormal liver blood tests. In this situation liver biopsy is seldom indicated. Occasionally, the diagnosis of sarcoidosis is first raised when an individual with abnormal liver blood tests is found to have numerous sarcoid-like granulomas on liver biopsy. Since the differential diagnosis of granulomatous liver disease is so large, and serum angiotensin converting enzyme levels are non-specific, it is our practice to exclude other causes of granulomatous liver disease and to seek evidence of extrahepatic sarcoidosis before making a firm diagnosis.

Treatment of hepatic sarcoidosis is seldom needed and there are no controlled trials of the treatment of hepatic sarcoidosis.[112,115] In particular, there is no good evidence in the literature demonstrating that steroids alter the natural history of the disease. A trial of corticosteroids may be warranted in patients with significant constitutional symptoms, those with evidence of progressive portal hypertension, biliary obstruction, or with painful hepatomegaly. A dose of 40–60 mg of prednisone followed by a slow taper in those showing a clinical response is warranted. As in patients with other cholestatic liver diseases, management should include evaluation and treatment of osteoporosis and hyperlipidemia where applicable. A trial of ursodeoxycholic acid or steroids is warranted in individuals with the cholestatic form of the illness.[116]

Idiopathic granulomatous disease of the liver

Idiopathic granulomatous liver disease is a rare cause of liver granulomas. The diagnosis accounts for between 10% and 50% of patients in liver biopsy series of granulomatous hepatitis[28,105,106] It is usually associated with granulomas in many other sites, including the spleen, bone marrow, and lymph nodes.[117] The diagnosis should only be made after careful exclusion of other causes of granulomatous liver diseases. The clinical presentation is with fever, weight loss, anorexia, and increased liver enzymes, usually a cholestatic pattern.[118,119]

There are no good clinical studies to direct therapy. Treatment is indicated in patients with marked constitutional symptoms and those with evidence of significant hepatic dysfunction. In this setting corticosteroids are the first line of treatment. In one retrospective series of 17 patients with idiopathic disease, 7 resolved spontaneously, 3 responded to a short course of steroids or indomethacin, and the remaining 7 required long-term steroid therapy.[120] In steroid-nonresponsive cases, other immunosuppressives, including cyclophosphamide and methotrexate have been used with varying success.[117,121]

REFERENCES

1. Wong WM, Wong BC, Hui CK, et al. Pyogenic liver abscess: retrospective analysis of 80 cases over a 10-year period. J Gastroenterol Hepatol 2002;17:1001–1007.

2. Huang CJ, Pitt HA, Lipsett PA, et al. Pyogenic hepatic abscess. Changing trends over 42 years. Ann Surg 1996; 223:600–607; discussion 607–609.

3. Perera MR, Kirk A, Noone P. Presentation, diagnosis and management of liver abscess. Lancet 1980; 2:629–632.

4. Mohsen AH, Green ST, Read RC, et al. Liver abscess in adults: ten years experience in a UK centre. Q J Med 2002; 95:797–802.

5. Alvarez Perez JA, Gonzalez JJ, Baldonedo RF, et al. Clinical course, treatment, and multivariate analysis of risk factors for pyogenic liver abscess. Am J Surg 2001; 181:177–186.

6. Huang SF, Ko CW, Chang CS, et al. Liver abscess formation after transarterial chemoembolization for malignant hepatic tumor. Hepatogastroenterology 2003; 50:1115–1118.

7. Filice C, Brunetti E, Dughetti S. Diagnostic yield of abscess drainage. Dig Dis Sci 1995; 40:1582.

8. Hansen PS, Schonheyder HC. Pyogenic hepatic abscess. A 10-year population-based retrospective study. APMIS 1998; 106:396–402.

9. Corredoira J, Casariego E, Moreno C, et al. Prospective study of *Streptococcus milleri* hepatic abscess. Eur J Clin Microbiol Infect Dis 1998; 17:556–560.

10. Bergmann TK, Vinding K, Hey H. Multiple hepatic abscesses due to *Yersinia enterocolitica* infection secondary to primary haemochromatosis. Scand J Gastroenterol 2001; 36:891–895.

11. Wang SC, Lin KH, Chern JP, et al. Severe bacterial infection in transfusion-dependent patients with thalassemia major. Clin Infect Dis 2003; 37:984–988.

12. Thaler M, Pastakia B, Shawker TH, et al. Hepatic candidiasis in cancer patients: the evolving picture of the syndrome. Ann Intern Med 1988; 108:88–100.

13. Chan JH, Tsui EY, Luk SH, et al. Diffusion-weighted MR imaging of the liver: distinguishing hepatic abscess from cystic or necrotic tumor. Abdom Imaging 2001; 26:161–165.

14. Chemaly RF, Hall GS, Keys TF, et al. Microbiology of liver abscesses and the predictive value of abscess Gram stain and associated blood cultures. Diagn Microbiol Infect Dis 2003; 46:245–248.

15. Wang W, Lee WJ, Wei PL, et al. Laparoscopic drainage of pyogenic liver abscesses. Surg Today 2004; 34:323–325.

16. Yu SC, Ho SS, Lau WY, et al. Treatment of pyogenic liver abscess: prospective randomized comparison of catheter drainage and needle aspiration. Hepatology 2004; 39:932–938.

Randomized study comparing catheter drainage to simple aspiration of pyogenic abscesses. Study demonstrates equivalent, with a trend to improved, results with simple needle aspiration and concomitant antibiotic therapy.

17. Ng FH, Wong WM, Wong BC, et al. Sequential intravenous/oral antibiotic vs. continuous intravenous antibiotic in the treatment of pyogenic liver abscess. Aliment Pharmacol Ther 2002; 16:1083–1090.

Comparison of continuous intravenous antibiotics or 2 weeks of oral followed by intravenous antibiotics for the management of pyogenic liver abscess. The intravenous regimen showed equal efficacy at lower cost compared to the oral regimen.

18. Molle I, Thulstrup AM, Vilstrup H, et al. Increased risk and case fatality rate of pyogenic liver abscess in patients with liver cirrhosis: a nationwide study in Denmark. Gut 2001; 48:260–263.

19. Tortoli E, Bartoloni A, Erba ML, et al. Human infections due to *Mycobacterium lentiflavum*. J Clin Microbiol 2002; 40:728–729.

20. Wallis RS, Broder MS, Wong JY, et al. Granulomatous infectious diseases associated with tumor necrosis factor antagonists. Clin Infect Dis 2004; 38:1261–1265.

21. Mohan AK, Cote TR, Block JA, et al. Tuberculosis following the use of etanercept, a tumor necrosis factor inhibitor. Clin Infect Dis 2004; 39:295–299.

22. Oliva A, Duarte B, Jonasson O, et al. The nodular form of local hepatic tuberculosis. A review. J Clin Gastroenterol 1990; 12:166–173.

23. Huang WT, Wang CC, Chen WJ, et al. The nodular form of hepatic tuberculosis: a review with five additional new cases. J Clin Pathol 2003; 56:835–839.

24. Gonzalez OY, Adams G, Teeter LD, et al. Extra-pulmonary manifestations in a large metropolitan area with a low incidence of tuberculosis. Int J Tuberc Lung Dis 2003; 7:1178–1185.

25. Bodurtha A, Kim YH, Laucius JF, et al. Hepatic granulomas and other hepatic lesions associated with BCG immunotherapy for cancer. Am J Clin Pathol 1974; 61:747–752.

26. Gottke MU, Wong P, Muhn C, et al. Hepatitis in disseminated bacillus Calmette-Guerin infection. Can J Gastroenterol 2000; 14:333–336.

27. Essop AR, Posen JA, Hodkinson JH, et al. Tuberculosis hepatitis: a clinical review of 96 cases. Q J Med 1984; 53:465–477.

28. Sartin JS, Walker RC. Granulomatous hepatitis: a retrospective review of 88 cases at the Mayo Clinic. Mayo Clin Proc 1991; 66:914–918.

29. Hussain W, Mutimer D, Harrison R, et al. Fulminant hepatic failure caused by tuberculosis. Gut 1995; 36:792–794.

30. Rahmatulla RH, al-Mofleh IA, al-Rashed RS, et al. Tuberculous liver abscess: a case report and review of literature. Eur J Gastroenterol Hepatol 2001; 13:437–440.

31. Bearer EA, Savides TJ, McCutchan JA. Endoscopic diagnosis and management of hepatobiliary tuberculosis. Am J Gastroenterol 1996; 91:2602–2604.

32. Abu-Zidan FM, Zayat I. Gallbladder tuberculosis (case report and review of the literature). Hepatogastroenterology 1999; 46:2804–2806.

33. Desai DC, Swaroop VS, Mohandas KM, et al. Tuberculosis of the pancreas: report of three cases. Am J Gastroenterol 1991; 86:761–763.

34. Akcan Y, Tuncer S, Hayran M, et al. PCR on disseminated tuberculosis in bone marrow and liver biopsy specimens: correlation to histopathological and clinical diagnosis. Scand J Infect Dis 1997; 29:271–274.

35. Marchetti G, Gori A, Catozzi L, et al. Evaluation of PCR in detection of *Mycobacterium tuberculosis* from formalin-fixed, paraffin-embedded tissues: comparison of four amplification assays. J Clin Microbiol 1998; 36:1512–1517.

36. Esteban J, de Gorgolas M, Santos-O'Connor F, et al. *Mycobacterium tuberculosis* bacteremia in a university hospital. Int J Tuberc Lung Dis 2001; 5:763–768.

37. American Thoracic Society. Medical Section of the American Lung Association: Treatment of tuberculosis and tuberculosis infection in adults and children. Am Rev Respir Dis 1986; 134:355–363.

American Thoracic Society guidelines for the management of tuberculosis in adults and children.

38. Davies PD, Yew WW. Recent developments in the treatment of tuberculosis. Expert Opin Investig Drugs 2003; 12:1297–1312.

39. Aaron L, Saadoun D, Calatroni I, et al. Tuberculosis in HIV-infected patients: a comprehensive review. Clin Microbiol Infect 2004; 10:388–398.

40. [No authors listed]. Updated guidelines for the use of rifabutin or rifampin for the treatment and prevention of tuberculosis among HIV-infected patients taking protease inhibitors or nonnucleoside reverse transcriptase inhibitors. Centers for Disease Control and Prevention. MMWR Morb Mortal Wkly Rep 2000; 49:185–189.

41. Poles MA, Dieterich DT, Schwarz ED, et al. Liver biopsy findings in 501 patients infected with human immunodeficiency virus (HIV). J Acquir Immune Defic Syndr Hum Retrovirol 1996; 11:170–177.

42. Neau-Cransac M, Dupon M, Carles J, et al. Disseminated *Mycobacterium avium* infection after liver transplantation. Eur J Clin Microbiol Infect Dis 1998; 17:744–746.

43. Smith MB, Molina CP, Schnadig VJ, et al. Pathologic features of *Mycobacterium kansasii* infection in patients with acquired immunodeficiency syndrome. Arch Pathol Lab Med 2003; 127:554–560.

44. den Broeder AA, Vervoort G, van Assen S, et al. Disseminated *Mycobacterium gordonae* infection in a renal transplant recipient. Transpl Infect Dis 2003; 5:151–155.

45. Akpek G, Lee SM, Gagnon DR, et al. Bone marrow aspiration, biopsy, and culture in the evaluation of HIV-infected patients for invasive mycobacteria and histoplasma infections. Am J Hematol 2001; 67:100–106.

46. Kilby JM, Marques MB, Jaye DL, et al. The yield of bone marrow biopsy and culture compared with blood culture in the evaluation of HIV-infected patients for mycobacterial and fungal infections. Am J Med 1998; 104:123–128.

47. Farhi DC, Mason UG 3rd, Horsburgh CR Jr. Pathologic findings in disseminated *Mycobacterium avium-intracellulare* infection. A report of 11 cases. Am J Clin Pathol 1986; 85:67–72.

48. Phillips P, Chan K, Hogg R, et al. Azithromycin prophylaxis for *Mycobacterium avium* complex during the era of highly active antiretroviral therapy: evaluation of a provincial program. Clin Infect Dis 2002; 34:371–378.

49. Sendi PP, Craig BA, Meier G, et al. Cost-effectiveness of azithromycin for preventing *Mycobacterium avium* complex infection in HIV-positive patients in the era of highly active antiretroviral therapy. The Swiss HIV Cohort Study. J Antimicrob Chemother 1999; 44:811–817.

50. Liao CH, Chen MY, Hsieh SM, et al. Discontinuation of secondary prophylaxis in AIDS patients with disseminated non-tuberculous mycobacteria infection. J Microbiol Immunol Infect 2004; 37: 50–56.

51. El-Sadr WM, Burman WJ, Grant LB, et al. Discontinuation of prophylaxis for *Mycobacterium avium* complex disease in HIV-infected patients who have a response to antiretroviral therapy. Terry Beirn Community Programs for Clinical Research on AIDS. N Engl J Med 2000; 342:1085–1092.

52. Benson CA, Williams PL, Cohn DL, et al. Clarithromycin or rifabutin alone or in combination for primary prophylaxis of *Mycobacterium avium* complex disease in patients with AIDS:

A randomized, double-blind, placebo-controlled trial. The AIDS Clinical Trials Group 196/Terry Beirn Community Programs for Clinical Research on AIDS 009 Protocol Team. J Infect Dis 2000; 1 81:1289–1297.

53. Gordin FM, Sullam PM, Shafran SD, et al. A randomized, placebo-controlled study of rifabutin added to a regimen of clarithromycin and ethambutol for treatment of disseminated infection with *Mycobacterium avium* complex. Clin Infect Dis 1999; 28:1080–1085.

54. Benson CA, Williams PL, Currier JS, et al. A prospective, randomized trial examining the efficacy and safety of clarithromycin in combination with ethambutol, rifabutin, or both for the treatment of disseminated *Mycobacterium avium* complex disease in persons with acquired immunodeficiency syndrome. Clin Infect Dis 2003; 37:1234–1243.

55. Dunne M, Fessel J, Kumar P, et al. A randomized, double-blind trial comparing azithromycin and clarithromycin in the treatment of disseminated *Mycobacterium avium* infection in patients with human immunodeficiency virus. Clin Infect Dis 2000; 31:1245–1252.

56. Kuper JI, D'Aprile M. Drug–drug interactions of clinical significance in the treatment of patients with *Mycobacterium avium* complex disease. Clin Pharmacokinet 2000; 39:203–214.

57. Apseloff G, Foulds G, LaBoy-Goral L, et al. Comparison of azithromycin and clarithromycin in their interactions with rifabutin in healthy volunteers. J Clin Pharmacol 1998; 38:830–835.

58. Ward TT, Rimland D, Kauffman C, et al. Randomized, open-label trial of azithromycin plus ethambutol vs. clarithromycin plus ethambutol as therapy for *Mycobacterium avium* complex bacteremia in patients with human immunodeficiency virus infection. Veterans Affairs HIV Research Consortium. Clin Infect Dis 1998; 27:1278–1285.

59. Wright J. Current strategies for the prevention and treatment of disseminated *Mycobacterium avium* complex infection in patients with AIDS. Pharmacotherapy 1998; 18:738–747.

Review on the current management of *Mycobacterium avium* complex in patients with HIV.

60. Wallace RJ Jr., Brown BA, Griffith DE, et al. Clarithromycin regimens for pulmonary *Mycobacterium avium* complex. The first 50 patients. Am J Respir Crit Care Med 1996; 153:1766–1772.

61. Christova I, Tasseva E, Manev H. Human leptospirosis in Bulgaria, 1989–2001: epidemiological, clinical, and serological features. Scand J Infect Dis 2003; 35:869–872.

62. Bishara J, Amitay E, Barnea A, et al. Epidemiological and clinical features of leptospirosis in Israel. Eur J Clin Microbiol Infect Dis 2002; 21:50–52.

63. James DG. Life-threatening situations in sarcoidosis. Sarcoidosis Vasc Diffuse Lung Dis 1998;15:134–139.

64. Leblebicioglu H, Sencan I, Sunbul M, et al. Weil's disease: report of 12 cases. Scand J Infect Dis 1996; 28:637–639.

65. Faucher JF, Hoen B, Estavoyer JM. The management of leptospirosis. Expert Opin Pharmacother 2004; 5:819–827.

66. Hospenthal DR, Murray CK. In vitro susceptibilities of seven *Leptospira* species to traditional and newer antibiotics. Antimicrob Agents Chemother 2003; 47:2646–2648.

67. Panaphut T, Domrongkitchaiporn S, Vibhagool A, et al. Ceftriaxone compared with sodium penicillin G for treatment of severe leptospirosis. Clin Infect Dis 2003; 36:1507–1513.

68. Leblebicioglu H, Sunbul M, Esen S, et al. Jarisch-Herxheimer reaction in leptospirosis. Eur J Clin Microbiol Infect Dis 2003; 22:639; author reply 640.

69. Cotell SL, Noskin GA. Bacillary angiomatosis. Clinical and histologic features, diagnosis, and treatment. Arch Intern Med 1994; 154:524–528.

70. Ahsan N, Holman MJ, Riley TR, et al. Peloisis hepatis due to *Bartonella henselae* in transplantation: a hemato-hepato-renal syndrome. Transplantation 1998; 65:1000–1003.

71. Liston TE, Koehler JE. Granulomatous hepatitis and necrotizing splenitis due to *Bartonella henselae* in a patient with cancer: case report and review of hepatosplenic manifestations of *Bartonella* infection. Clin Infect Dis 1996; 22:951–957.

72. Ventura A, Massei F, Not T, et al. Systemic *Bartonella henselae* infection with hepatosplenic involvement. J Pediatr Gastroenterol Nutr 1999; 29:52–56.

73. Margileth AM, Wear DJ, English CK. Systemic cat scratch disease: report of 23 patients with prolonged or recurrent severe bacterial infection. J Infect Dis 1987; 155:390–402.

74. Agan BK, Dolan MJ. Laboratory diagnosis of *Bartonella* infections. Clin Lab Med 2002; 22:937–962.

75. Bass JW, Freitas BC, Freitas AD, et al. Prospective randomized double-blind placebo-controlled evaluation of azithromycin for treatment of cat-scratch disease. Pediatr Infect Dis J 1998; 17:447–452.

76. Windsor JJ. Cat-scratch disease: epidemiology, aetiology and treatment. Br J Biomed Sci 2001; 58:101–110.

77. Santos R, Cardoso O, Rodrigues P, et al. Bacillary angiomatosis by *Bartonella quintana* in an HIV-infected patient. J Am Acad Dermatol 2000; 42:299–301.

78. Moore EH, Russell LA, Klein JS, et al. Bacillary angiomatosis in patients with AIDS: multiorgan imaging findings. Radiology 1995; 197:67–72.

79. Koh LP, Kurup A, Goh YT, et al. Randomized trial of fluconazole versus low-dose amphotericin B in prophylaxis against fungal infections in patients undergoing hematopoietic stem cell transplantation. Am J Hematol 2002; 71:260–267.

80. Perkocha LA, Geaghan SM, Yen TS, et al. Clinical and pathological features of bacillary peliosis hepatis in association with human immunodeficiency virus infection. N Engl J Med 1990; 323:1581–1586.

81. Ohl ME, Spach DH. *Bartonella quintana* and urban trench fever. Clin Infect Dis 2000; 31:131–135.

82. Guerra LG, Neira CJ, Boman D, et al. Rapid response of AIDS-related bacillary angiomatosis to azithromycin. Clin Infect Dis 1993; 17:264–266.

83. Duong TA. Infection due to *Penicillium marneffei*, an emerging pathogen: review of 155 reported cases. Clin Infect Dis 1996; 23:125–130.

84. Wong-Beringer A, Kriengkauykiat J. Systemic antifungal therapy: new options, new challenges. Pharmacotherapy 2003; 23: 1441–1462.

85. Masia Canuto M, Gutierrez Rodero F. Antifungal drug resistance to azoles and polyenes. Lancet Infect Dis 2002; 2:550–563.

86. Hospenthal DR, Murray CK, Rinaldi MG. The role of antifungal susceptibility testing in the therapy of candidiasis. Diagn Microbiol Infect Dis 2004; 48:153–160.

87. Denning DW. Echinocandin antifungal drugs. Lancet 2003; 362:1142–1151.

Review on the newly released echinocandins in the treatment of fungal infection.

88. Cesaro S, Toffolutti T, Messina C, et al. Safety and efficacy of caspofungin and liposomal amphotericin B, followed by voriconazole in young patients affected by refractory invasive mycosis. Eur J Haematol 2004; 73:50–55.

89. Kontoyiannis DP, Hachem R, Lewis RE, et al. Efficacy and toxicity of caspofungin in combination with liposomal amphotericin B as primary or salvage treatment of invasive aspergillosis in patients with hematologic malignancies. Cancer 2003; 98:292–299.

90. Baran J Jr, Muckatira B, Khatib R. Candidemia before and during the fluconazole era: prevalence, type of species and approach to treatment in a tertiary care community hospital. Scand J Infect Dis 2001; 33:137–139.

91. Trick WE, Fridkin SK, Edwards JR, et al. Secular trend of hospital-acquired candidemia among intensive care unit patients in the United States during 1989–1999. Clin Infect Dis 2002; 35:627–630.

92. Haron E, Feld R, Tuffnell P, et al. Hepatic candidiasis: an increasing problem in immunocompromised patients. Am J Med 1987; 83:17–26.

93. Sallah S, Semelka RC, Wehbie R, et al. Hepatosplenic candidiasis in patients with acute leukaemia. Br J Haematol 1999; 106:697–701.

94. Pappas PG, Rex JH, Sobel JD, et al. Guidelines for treatment of candidiasis. Clin Infect Dis 2004; 38:161–189.

Guidelines for the management of Candida infection, including the use and selection of some of the newer agents.

95. Patel R. Amphotericin B colloidal dispersion. Expert Opin Pharmacother 2000; 1:475–488.

96. Brogden RN, Goa KL, Coukell AJ. Amphotericin-B colloidal dispersion. A review of its use against systemic fungal infections and visceral leishmaniasis. Drugs 1998; 56:365–383.

97. Rex JH, Bennett JE, Sugar AM, et al. A randomized trial comparing fluconazole with amphotericin B for the treatment of candidemia in patients without neutropenia. Candidemia Study Group and the National Institute. N Engl J Med 1994; 331:1325–1330.

98. Phillips P, Shafran S, Garber G, et al. Multicenter randomized trial of fluconazole versus amphotericin B for treatment of candidemia in non-neutropenic patients. Canadian Candidemia Study Group. Eur J Clin Microbiol Infect Dis 1997; 16:337–345.

98. Mora-Duarte J, Betts R, Rotstein C, et al. Comparison of caspofungin and amphotericin B for invasive candidiasis. N Engl J Med 2002; 347:2020–2029.

100. Villanueva A, Arathoon EG, Gotuzzo E, et al. A randomized double-blind study of caspofungin versus amphotericin for the treatment of candidal esophagitis. Clin Infect Dis 2001; 33:1529–1535.

101. Sora F, Chiusolo P, Piccirillo N, et al. Successful treatment with caspofungin of hepatosplenic candidiasis resistant to liposomal amphotericin B. Clin Infect Dis 2002; 35:1135–1136.

102. Edwards JE Jr, Bodey GP, Bowden RA, et al. International conference for the development of a consensus on the management and prevention of severe candidal infections. Clin Infect Dis 1997; 25:43–59.

103. Kaptan K, Ural AU, Cetin T, et al. Itraconazole is not effective for the prophylaxis of fungal infections in patients with neutropenia. J Infect Chemother 2003; 9:40–45.

104. Kelsey SM, Goldman JM, McCann S, et al. Liposomal amphotericin (AmBisome) in the prophylaxis of fungal infections in neutropenic patients: a randomised, double-blind, placebo-controlled study. Bone Marrow Transplant 1999; 23:163–168.

105. McCluggage WG, Sloan JM. Hepatic granulomas in Northern Ireland: a thirteen year review. Histopathology 1994; 25:219–228.

106. Guckian JC, Perry JE. Granulomatous hepatitis. An analysis of 63 cases and review of the literature. Ann Intern Med 1966; 65:1081–1100.

107. James DG, Sherlock S. Sarcoidosis of the liver. Sarcoidosis 1994; 11:2–6.

108. Thanos L, Zormpala A, Brountzos E, et al. Nodular hepatic and splenic sarcoidosis in a patient with normal chest radiograph. Eur J Radiol 2002; 41:10–11.

109. Baughman RP, Teirstein AS, Judson MA, et al. Clinical characteristics of patients in a case control study of sarcoidosis. Am J Respir Crit Care Med 2001; 164:1885–1889.

110. Lynch JP 3rd, Sharma OP, Baughman RP. Extrapulmonary sarcoidosis. Semin Respir Infect 1998; 13:229–254.

111. Pereira-Lima J, Schaffner F. Chronic cholestasis in hepatic sarcoidosis with clinical features resembling primary biliary cirrhosis. Report of two cases. Am J Med 1987; 83:144–148.

112. Valla D, Pessegueiro-Miranda H, Degott C, et al. Hepatic sarcoidosis with portal hypertension. A report of seven cases with a review of the literature. Q J Med 1987; 63:531–544.

113. Ishak KG. Sarcoidosis of the liver and bile ducts. Mayo Clin Proc 1998; 73:467–472.

114. Devaney K, Goodman ZD, Epstein MS, et al. Hepatic sarcoidosis. Clinicopathologic features in 100 patients. Am J Surg Pathol 1993; 17:1272–1280.

115. Mueller S, Boehme MW, Hofmann WJ, et al. Extrapulmonary sarcoidosis primarily diagnosed in the liver. Scand J Gastroenterol 2000; 35:1003–1008.

116. Becheur H, Dall'osto H, Chatellier G, et al. Effect of ursodeoxycholic acid on chronic intrahepatic cholestasis due to sarcoidosis. Dig Dis Sci 1997; 42:789–791.

117. Knox TA, Kaplan MM, Gelfand JA, et al. Methotrexate treatment of idiopathic granulomatous hepatitis. Ann Intern Med 1995; 122:592–595.

118. Simon HB, Wolff SM. Granulomatous hepatitis and prolonged fever of unknown origin: a study of 13 patients. Medicine (Baltimore) 1973; 52:1–21.

119. Telenti A, Hermans PE. Idiopathic granulomatosis manifesting as fever of unknown origin. Mayo Clin Proc 1989; 64:44–50.

120. Zoutman DE, Ralph ED, Frei JV. Granulomatous hepatitis and fever of unknown origin. An 11-year experience of 23 cases with three years' follow-up. J Clin Gastroenterol 1991; 13:69–75.

121. Friedland JS, Weatherall DJ, Ledingham JG. A chronic granulomatous syndrome of unknown origin. Medicine (Baltimore) 1990; 69:325–331.

122. Pao D, Goh BT, Bingham JS. Management issues in syphilis. Drugs 2002; 62:1447–1461.

123. Enderlin G, Morales L, Jacobs RF, et al. Streptomycin and alternative agents for the treatment of tularemia: review of the literature. Clin Infect Dis 1994; 19:42–47.

124. [No authors listed]. National guideline for the management of Chlamydia trachomatis genital tract infection. Clinical Effectiveness Group (Association of Genitourinary Medicine and the Medical Society for the Study of Venereal Diseases). Sex Transm Infect 1999; 75(Suppl 1):S4–S8.

125. Butler T, Jones PK, Wallace CK. Borrelia recurrentis infection: single-dose antibiotic regimens and management of the Jarisch-Herxheimer reaction. J Infect Dis 1978; 137:573–577.

126. Solera J, Martinez-Alfaro E, Espinosa A. Recognition and optimum treatment of brucellosis. Drugs 1997; 53:245–256.

127. Gayraud M, Scavizzi MR, Mollaret HH, et al. Antibiotic treatment of Yersinia enterocolitica septicemia: a retrospective review of 43 cases. Clin Infect Dis 1993; 17:405–410.

128. Green NS. *Yersinia* infections in patients with homozygous beta-thalassemia associated with iron overload and its treatment. Pediatr Hematol Oncol 1992; 9:247–254.

129. Linden PK, Coley K, Fontes P, et al. Invasive aspergillosis in liver transplant recipients: outcome comparison of therapy with amphotericin B lipid complex and a historical cohort treated with conventional amphotericin B. Clin Infect Dis 2003;3 7:17–25.

130. Boogaerts M, Maertens J. Clinical experience with itraconazole in systemic fungal infections. Drugs 2001; 61(Suppl 1):39–47.

131. Saag MS, Graybill RJ, Larsen RA, et al. Practice guidelines for the management of cryptococcal disease. Infect Dis Soc America. Clin Infect Dis 2000; 30:710–718.

132. Eucker J, Sezer O, Graf B, et al. Mucormycoses. Mycoses 2001; 44:253–260.

133. Sirisanthana T, Supparatpinyo K, Perriens J, et al. Amphotericin B and itraconazole for treatment of disseminated *Penicillium marneffei* infection in human immunodeficiency virus-infected patients. Clin Infect Dis 1998; 26:1107–1110.

134. Wheat LJ, Cloud G, Johnson PC, et al. Clearance of fungal burden during treatment of disseminated histoplasmosis with liposomal amphotericin B versus itraconazole. Antimicrob Agents Chemother 2001; 45:2354–2357.

135. Negroni R, Palmieri O, Koren F, et al. Oral treatment of paracoccidioidomycosis and histoplasmosis with itraconazole in humans. Rev Infect Dis 1987; 9(Suppl 1):S47–S50.

136. Galgiani JN, Ampel NM, Catanzaro A, et al. Practice guideline for the treatment of coccidioidomycosis. Infect Dis Soc America. Clin Infect Dis 2000; 30:658–661.

Alcoholic and nonalcoholic fatty liver disease

Aijaz Ahmed, Emmet B. Keeffe and Sherif Saadeh

ALCOHOLIC LIVER DISEASE

Alcohol is used by three-quarters of Americans, and alcohol abuse and dependence are common. Approximately 10% of Americans who drink will experience alcohol-related problems. Alcoholic liver disease is one of the most serious medical consequences of alcohol abuse and remains the most common cause of cirrhosis in the Western world. Once a threshold level of consumption is exceeded (estimated to be 80 g/day for men and 20 g/day for women), the risk of alcoholic liver disease increases. This chapter reviews the pathophysiology, diagnosis, and treatment of alcoholic liver disease.

Pathophysiology of alcoholic liver disease

The cytokine-mediated hepatocellular injury resulting from alcohol can be evident as a wide spectrum of pathological changes including varying degree of steatosis, inflammation and fibrosis. In order to optimize the management of alcoholic liver disease, it is important to define the mechanism of hepatocellular injury.

Mechanism and pathogenesis of alcoholic liver disease

Both cell-mediated and humoral responses play a pivotal role in the immune-mediated hepatocyte inflammation associated with excessive use of alcohol.[1-3] It has been demonstrated in experimental models of alcohol-induced liver injury that cytokine-mediated pathway is responsible for hepatic damage.[1-3] Cytokines that are proinflammatory in nature, such as tumor necrosis factor-alpha (TNF-α), interleukin-1 (IL-1), IL-6, and IL-8 are activated and secreted by Kupffer cells and other inflammatory cells (neutrophils and macrophages) following exposure to alcohol.[4-10] The generation of free radicals from NADPH oxidase in Kupffer cells is crucial in the pathogenesis of alcohol-induced hepatitis by activating and secreting cytotoxic TNF-α.[1-3] Free radicals and protein adducts that are induced by cytokine-mediated pathways are responsible for oxidative stress on hepatocytes.[11-13] The persistence of oxidative stress will result in failure of defensive mechanisms and lead to apoptosis and cellular necrosis. Alcohol, and its derivative acetaldehyde, can disrupt epithelial tight junctions and increase paracellular permeability.[2,3] Alcohol-induced altered intestinal permeability results in endotoxemia and plays a role in the pathogenesis of alcoholic liver disease.[3] Alterations in the humoral immune system include increased levels of circulating immunoglobulins, the presence of various autoantibodies, and the development of antibodies against neoantigens, i.e., proteins altered by reaction to acetaldehyde and various radicals.[1-3]

Histopathology of alcoholic liver disease

The histological damage induced by alcohol can be divided into the following three categories: alcoholic fatty liver (steatosis), alcoholic hepatitis, and alcoholic cirrhosis.[14-19] In patients with alcohol-induced damage, fatty liver may be associated with evidence of mild inflammation and absence of fibrosis. In others, fibrosis may be advanced and prominent. In most patients, features of alcohol-induced fatty liver, inflammation, and fibrosis coexist.

Alcohol-induced hepatic fatty liver is associated with alterations in lipid metabolism, with an excessive accumulation of reducing equivalents favoring metabolic pathways that lead to the accumulation of intracellular lipid.[14] The excess lipid is stored in large droplets within individual hepatocytes. Fatty liver resulting as a consequence of alcohol-induced oxidative stress is typically benign and reversible, but can rarely lead to lobular or perivenular fibrosis and death.[15-17]

Alcoholic hepatitis is characterized by a wide spectrum of coexisting histologic damage including steatosis, acute inflammation, hepatocellular necrosis, and fibrosis. The characteristic eosinophilic fibrillar material (Mallory's hyaline bodies) may be present in ballooned hepatocytes. Although characteristic of alcoholic hepatitis, Mallory's bodies are not specific and also seen in other forms of chronic liver disease. The acute inflammation in alcoholic hepatitis is characteristically focal intense lobular infiltration of polymorphonuclear leukocytes, which distinguishes alcoholic hepatitis from other types of hepatitis in which the inflammatory infiltrate is predominantly composed of mononuclear cells.

Alcoholic cirrhosis is associated with longstanding hepatic injury secondary to alcohol. Alcoholic liver damage is typically associated with the deposition of collagen around the terminal hepatic vein and along the sinusoids, resulting in a 'chicken-wire' pattern of fibrosis typical of alcoholic liver disease. Chronic alcohol use interferes with the regenerative process in response to hepatocellular necrosis, typically resulting micronodular cirrhosis in patients actively using alcohol on a long-term basis. On the other hand, alcoholic cirrhotics who are abstinent may develop macronodular cirrhosis in the absence of antiproliferative actions of alcohol.

Diagnosis of alcoholic liver disease

A history of chronic heavy use of alcohol suggests that alcohol is the cause of liver disease, but the non-specific nature of clinical and laboratory findings in alcoholic liver disease mandate that appropriate serological, virological, immunological, and genetic tests be performed to exclude viral, autoimmune, or genetic liver conditions. The clinical features associated with alcoholic liver damage are non-specific and rarely useful in predicting predominant liver histology.[20] However, hepatic decompensation (jaundice, coagulopathy, fluid retention, and hepatic encephalopathy) is commonly associated with cirrhosis, less frequently with alcoholic hepatitis, and only rarely with alcoholic steatosis.

It is may be helpful to confirm the diagnosis of alcoholic liver disease with a liver biopsy for several reasons. First, as many as 20% of patients initially suspected of alcoholic liver disease may have evidence of nonalcoholic causes of liver disease on liver biopsy.[21] This, of course, may be dependent on the nature of the referral population and a more recent study showed that 34 of 35 patients with clinically suspected alcoholic liver disease were confirmed on biopsy.[22] Second, patients who are suspected of having severe alcoholic hepatitis based on clinical manifestations may, in fact, be infected with a virus, have drug-induced liver injury, or have liver failure due to alcoholic cirrhosis. Therefore, liver biopsy in this patient population is strongly encouraged to confirm alcoholic hepatitis before starting corticosteroid therapy. In patients with coagulopathy, biopsy may need to be performed via the transjugular route. Third, liver biopsy may help determine the prognosis and reversibility of liver disease since clinical and biochemical indices are not always able to characterize the extent and severity of underlying liver disease.[21,22]

Treatment of alcoholic liver disease

The treatment of alcoholic liver disease is dependent on a variety of factors including abstinence, nutritional state, psychosocial status, predominant hepatic histology, severity of clinical complications, and coexisting comorbid medical illnesses.

Behavioral treatment

Abstinence

Abstinence is essential to optimize management of patients with alcoholic liver disease. Alcohol-induced liver damage may be reversible with abstinence.[23] The evidence supporting the role of abstinence in patients with alcoholic liver damage is based on retrospective analyses and nonrandomized trials.[24–27] The 5-year survival rate for patients with compensated alcoholic cirrhosis is 63–90% with abstinence compared to 41–70% in those with continued alcohol use.[25,26] In addition, 6 months of documented abstinence from alcohol is needed before liver transplantation can be considered in a patient with decompensated alcoholic cirrhosis.

Despite the necessity of abstinence for improving the outlook of patients with alcoholic liver injury, the data on maintenance of abstinence from alcohol use are not encouraging.[28] Therefore, several agents that may help maintain abstinence have been studied. Alcohol use results in the stimulation of excitatory amino acids and net neuronal hyperexcitability.[29] Naltrexone, an opioid antagonist, may reduce the amount of alcohol consumption by inhibiting the central nervous system center for alcohol craving.[30] Acamprosate (acetylhomotaurine), which structurally resembles the excitatory amino acids, may also block the neuronal hyperexcitability pathway.[31–33] Further controlled studies are needed to confirm the efficacy of these agents.

Nutritional treatment

Nutrition replacement therapy

Protein-calorie malnutrition (PCM) has been associated with both alcoholic hepatitis and alcoholic cirrhosis, particularly those cases with jaundice or hepatic encephalopathy, and many of these patients require nutritional support.[34,35] Nutritional PCM score is a tool that integrates eight parameters for nutritional evaluation to predict the nutritional status and is as reliable as standard biochemical testing.[36] The prevalence of PCM is directly related to the severity of hepatic decompensation (Child-Turcotte-Pugh score).[36] PCM is a poor prognostic sign and reflects on short-term and long-term mortality, and survival following liver transplantation.[37,38]

PCM results from anorexia, poor dietary habits and compliance, and a hypercatabolic state resulting in an increased need for basic estimated energy requirements (EERs).[4–6,39] The mean EER in patients with alcoholic liver disease can increase to 2500 kcal/day reflecting at least a 150% rise in basic metabolic needs of a person who is already malnourished.[35] Patients with alcoholic hepatitis and/or cirrhosis are usually unable to meet the caloric requirements without nutritional support.

Numerous clinical trials have been conducted to evaluate the effects of nutritional replacement therapy.[35,40–44] However, due to the variability of the study populations in terms of severity of hepatic decompensation and degree of malnutrition, comparison is difficult.[40–42] In general, the degree of malnutrition is clearly associated with the response to nutritional replacement therapy. Patients with mild to moderate PCM demonstrated a poor response to nutritional replacement (17% improved survival; p=NS) compared to those with severe malnutrition (70% improved survival; p=0.002).[35] Therefore, patients with severe hepatic decompensation and PCM are candidates for aggressive nutritional replacement therapy.[35] Nonetheless, though some of these studies have shown improvement in biochemical tests and nutritional status, only a few have demonstrated survival benefit.[43,44]

Branched-chain amino acids

The use of specific supplements, in particular branched-chain amino acids (BCCA), has produced encouraging results.[45–47] The rationale for using BCCA in patients with alcoholic cirrhosis is to provide protein calories that can be metabolized outside of the liver. Thus, BCCA may improve nutritional status and decrease the risk of hepatic encephalopathy. BBCA do indeed fulfill the metabolic needs and may allow nutritional benefit without increasing the risk of hepatic encephalopathy.[45] However, results have been mixed with only one of many studies clearly demonstrating a beneficial effect of BCCA on hepatic encephalopathy.[46] In another study, BCCA supplementation improved nutritional status, hepatic function, and short-term survival.[47] Despite the rationale for BCCA, it does not appear that they offer an advantage in most patients. Furthermore, clinicians should not routinely restrict protein intake even in the setting of hepatic encephalopathy.[48] Only the encephalopathy worsens on a protein-rich diet despite lactulose treatment should BCCA supplementation be considered.[48]

Pharmacological treatment

Corticosteroids

The rationale for using corticosteroids in alcoholic hepatitis is to reduce the inflammatory response that may perpetuate hepatocyte injury.[1,2] Corticosteroids suppress cytokine production, interfere with protein-acetaldehyde adduct formation, and directly inhibit collagen production.[49,50]

Numerous clinical trials have addressed the role of corticosteroids in alcoholic hepatitis.[34,51-63] Unfortunately, the results are conflicting and not definitive. Few clinical trials have demonstrated improved survival compared to placebo.[51-55] The two largest clinical trials, VA Cooperative Study[34] with 180 patients and the Copenhagen Study Group for Liver Disease[56] with 99 patients, were among the studies that demonstrated no improvement in outcomes compared to the control group. The lack of uniformity in the studies can be explained by differences in patient population included in these clinical trials. A meta-analysis analyzed 11 randomized clinical trials with a total number of 562 patients.[63] These combined data demonstrated that corticosteroid therapy provided survival benefit only in the subset of patients with hepatic encephalopathy without gastrointestinal bleeding.[51-55] Patients without hepatic encephalopathy did not benefit from corticosteroid use.[34,57-62] In a retrospective review, a multivariate regression analysis assessed the effect of Maddrey's discriminant function of alcoholic hepatitis severity on 30-day survival in patients receiving corticosteroids versus placebo.[44] A beneficial effect of corticosteroids was noted in patients with a discriminant function between 35 and 54.[51,52] The short-term survival at 1 month was significantly higher in patients with alcoholic hepatitis with a discriminant function greater than 32.[44] It was demonstrated that survival benefit can be extended to as long as 1 year in patients with severe alcoholic hepatitis who are treated with corticosteroids.[64] Adverse effects resulting from corticosteroid therapy in this setting may include infection, gastrointestinal bleeding, pancreatitis, glucose intolerance, and psychoses. Based on pharmacologic properties, prednisolone 40 mg per day for 4 weeks followed by a taper over 2–4 weeks is recommended.

In summary, a few practical guidelines can be suggested based on these studies.[44,51-55] First, patients with hepatic encephalopathy or a discriminant function greater than 32 in the setting of severe alcoholic hepatitis are candidates for corticosteroid therapy. Importantly, exogenous and readily correctable causes of hepatic encephalopathy such as fluid and electrolyte alterations, sedatives, infections, or gastrointestinal bleeding should be ruled out and treated. These causes of encephalopathy should not compel steroid use. Second, it is crucial to confirm the diagnosis of alcoholic hepatitis with a liver biopsy before committing to steroid therapy. Approximately one-fifth of patients who are suspected to have alcoholic hepatitis based on clinical manifestations may not have histologic evidence of the disease on liver biopsy. Third, it is important to recognize that despite a 25% reduction in the risk of mortality with corticosteroid use, there is still a high mortality in patients receiving steroids.[63] Fourth, up to seven patients must be treated with corticosteroids to prevent one death.[63] Therefore, it is important to select patients carefully and only if they meet the criteria for corticosteroid use. Patients with active infections and other comorbid conditions may need to be managed conservatively even if they meet the criteria for corticosteroid use.

There are no data supporting the role of corticosteroids in alcoholic cirrhosis. Retrospective data from two controlled clinical trials were unable to demonstrate a clinical benefit.[56]

Anabolic steroids

Anabolic steroids have been proposed as a way to reverse the hypercatabolic state in patients with severe alcoholic hepatitis and/or alcoholic cirrhosis and thereby improve PCM and prognosis. Initial experience with anabolic steroids, such as testosterone propionate in patients with alcoholic cirrhosis, demonstrated beneficial effects.[65] These encouraging reports led to numerous controlled clinical trials in patients with alcoholic hepatitis and cirrhosis.[66-72] Several different anabolic steroids have been studied including testosterone propionate,[66,67,69,70] micronized free testosterone,[71] methenolone enanthate,[67] mesterolone,[68] and oxandrolone.[35,72] Some of these trials included patients with severe hepatic decompensation with mortality rates ranging from 20% to 60% at 1 month and demonstrated survival benefit.[34,35,66,67] However, a large controlled clinical trial using testosterone administered at 200 mg three times a day for a median of 28 months showed no benefit in patients with alcoholic cirrhosis.[71] Approximately half of these patients also had evidence of alcoholic hepatitis. The trial was eventually terminated due to a lack of benefits and an increased risk of complications in the treatment arm. There was no improvement in hepatic function or survival. Furthermore, a higher incidence of portal vein thrombosis was noted in the treated group. In another study, the effects of short-term use of oxandrolone, 80 mg/day for 1 month failed to demonstrate a survival benefit in patients with moderate to severe alcoholic hepatitis with or without cirrhosis.[34]

The combination of anabolic steroids with nutritional replacement therapy has demonstrated benefits in certain subpopulations of patients with alcoholic hepatitis.[35,51,73] The patients were treated with oxandrolone, 80 mg/day for 30 days followed by 40 mg/day for an additional 60 days. Oxandrolone is a potent anabolic steroid with minimal androgenic activity and high nitrogen retaining activity. Nutritional replacement therapy included a high-calorie, high-protein diet, including BCCA. There was no overall survival benefit on intention-to-treat analysis. However, in the subpopulation of patients with moderate malnutrition who were able to maintain caloric intake of 2500 kcal/day, oxandrolone was associated with significant improvement in survival with reduction in 6-month mortality from 28% to 4%. In the subset of patients with severe malnutrition, adequate caloric intake was associated with a significant decline in mortality rate from 51% to 19%, but oxandrolone did not appear to offer any additional survival benefit.[35,51,73]

Pentoxifylline

Pentoxifylline reduces the production of TNF-α by modifying the gene transcription.[74] A randomized, double-blind, placebo-controlled trial of pentoxifylline, 400 mg orally three times a day versus placebo was conducted in 101 patients with severe alcoholic hepatitis, defined by a Maddrey discriminant functions score greater than 32.[75] A survival benefit was observed in the treated group during the initial hospitalization (mortality 25% versus 46% in placebo). Hepatorenal syndrome was the most common cause of mortality (50% deaths in treated and 92% deaths in placebo). This study suggests that pentoxifylline may reduce renal failure in severe acute alcoholic hepatitis, but it requires confirmation.

Propylthiouracil

Acute alcoholic hepatitis is associated with a hypermetabolic state resulting in net catabolic effect and increased hepatic oxygen consumption.[39,76,77] Alcoholic hepatitis may resemble hypoxemia-related hepatic injury involving the perivenular area, or zone 3. Propylthiouracil (PTU) decreases metabolic activity and oxygen consumption, and may have direct vasodilator and antioxidant properties.[78,79] Experiments in animal model demonstrated that PTU provided protection from hypoxemia-related hepatic injury.[80] Later, patients with alcoholic liver disease were randomized to PTU 300 mg/day or placebo for 46 days.[81] There was no survival benefit during the short-term 6-week period, although patients receiving PTU showed significant clinical improvement compared to the placebo group.

Subsequently, several clinical trials have been conducted to assess the role of PTU in alcoholic hepatitis.[82–85] One of these studies has demonstrated a significant survival benefit after 2 years with PTU treatment.[83] However, a recent meta-analysis which included 710 patients with varying severity of alcoholic liver disease was unable to demonstrate any clinical or survival benefit from PTU therapy.[86]

Insulin and glucagon

Data from animal studies have suggested a role of insulin and glucagon in stimulating hepatic regeneration.[87] Nonetheless, human studies have shown conflicting results.[88–91]

Colchicine

The rationale for the use of colchicine in patients with alcoholic cirrhosis is its antifibrotic properties.[92–97] Colchicine inhibits inflammation and granulocyte migration,[92–94] blocks the synthesis and secretion of collagen,[92] and induces collagenase production.[95–100] Based on these properties, it has been suggested that colchicine might retard and even reverse hepatic fibrosis.

In 1979, Kershenobich and colleagues[101] reported improved survival with colchicine in patients with cirrhosis, mostly attributable to alcohol. They later published their long-term experience in 100 patients with treatment extending as long as 14 years (mean 4.6 years).[102] The study demonstrated 74% survival at 5 years in the colchicine arm compared to only 34% survival in placebo recipients ($p=0.001$). The survival benefit persisted at 10 years as well. However, the study was flawed by a high dropout rate and the results have therefore not been widely accepted. Other trials in alcoholic hepatitis have not demonstrated a survival benefit.[103,104] A meta-analysis of 14 randomized clinical trials with 1150 patients showed no improvement in clinical parameters and survival benefit with colchicine use.[105] Furthermore, there was a significantly higher incidence of adverse effects with colchicine therapy.

Phosphatidylcholine

Phosphatidylcholine[106–110] is a derivative of polyunsaturated lecithin which may have some hepatoprotective properties due to its incorporation into hepatocyte membranes, inactivation of stellate cells, stimulation of collagenase activity, inhibition of cytochrome P450 2E1, affect on TNF-α activity, and other antioxidant activities.[111–116] Experiments in the baboon model of alcoholic liver disease have suggested that phosphatidylcholine might retard the rate of fibrosis progression.[117] Two small studies,

one in patients with chronic hepatitis and the other in patients with alcoholic hepatitis, appeared to confirm the results in primates.[118,119] This prompted a randomized, prospective, double-blind trial in 789 men with fibrotic (not cirrhotic) alcohol liver disease at 20 VA sites.[120] Patients were treated with phosphatidyl-choline or placebo for 24 months. There was no evidence of histological benefit in patients treated with phosphatidylcholine.

Surgical treatment

Liver transplantation

Liver transplantation is the treatment of choice for patients with end-stage liver disease secondary to alcoholic cirrhosis.[121,122] Patients with alcoholic cirrhosis can be considered for liver transplantation if they meet the minimal listing criteria for transplantation, demonstrate at least 6 months of sobriety, and have no medical and/or psychosocial contraindications. The duration of pretransplant abstinence is a poor predictor of post-transplant sobriety.[123–125] Following liver transplantation for alcoholic cirrhosis, up to 15% patients will resume heavy alcohol use and 20–50% will report at least occasional use of alcohol.[35,126] Short-term survival at 1 year following transplant surgery is greater than 70%. The survival rates at 5–10 years following transplantation is comparable to other indications despite significant relapse. In addition, liver transplantation is more cost-effective than prolonged medical management of end-stage liver disease secondary to alcoholic cirrhosis.[127]

Review of data from Liver Transplant Registry at UNOS with over 16 000 adults who underwent liver transplantation between 1988 and 1995 demonstrate comparable host and graft survival in patients with alcoholic liver disease compared to those transplanted for nonalcoholic liver disease.[128] The 1- and 5-year survival rate post-transplant for alcoholic cirrhosis was 80% and 70%, respectively. In a separate review, analyses of the National Institute of Diabetes and Digestive and Kidney Diseases Liver Transplantation database demonstrated a comparable 3-year graft survival for patients transplanted for alcoholic cirrhosis or nonalcoholic liver disease; however, patient survival was lower in recipients transplanted for alcoholic liver disease.[129] This analysis found that patients with alcoholic cirrhosis generally had more advanced liver failure than others at the time of transplantation, which may have explained the reduced survival. These observations may no longer be valid, however, because priority for transplantation has since changed to a disease severity score instead of time on the waiting list.

Future treatment

As previously mentioned, TNF-α may play a role in the pathogenesis of alcoholic hepatitis. Monoclonal anti-TNF-α (infliximab) has been compared to placebo in patients with alcoholic hepatitis managed with corticosteroids.[130] The infliximab group demonstrated significant improvement in the Maddrey discriminant score after 4 weeks, but there was no improvement in histology. Mortality data were not available. A small uncontrolled, open-label study of infliximab in 12 patients with alcoholic hepatitis showed inhibition of IL-8, a cytokine regulated by TNF-α, after 4 weeks.[131] Follow-up of these studies and encouraging reports with other agents that might interfere with hepatic injury from alcohol are needed.[132–142]

Summary

In summary, abstinence is the most crucial step in the treatment of alcoholic liver disease (Fig. 36.1; Table 36.1). Nutritional support improves the efficacy of other interventions, particularly in patients who are suffering from moderate to severe malnutrition. Patients with alcoholic steatosis usually require no further intervention. Patients who develop severe alcoholic hepatitis can be considered for corticosteroid therapy with or without pentoxifylline. Lastly, patients with alcoholic cirrhosis should be considered for liver transplantation if they can remain abstinent for at least 6 months, meet the minimal listing criteria, and have no other contraindications to transplantation. In addition, numerous experimental agents and therapies have demonstrated promising preliminary results, and may become available in the near future.

NONALCOHOLIC FATTY LIVER DISEASE

Introduction

Nonalcoholic fatty liver disease (NAFLD) is a common cause of chronic liver disease. The pathological picture resembles that of alcohol-induced liver injury, but it occurs in patients who do not abuse alcohol.[143–147] NAFLD is more common among patients with evidence of insulin resistance, such as that observed in adults with obesity and type 2 diabetes mellitus.[143–154] However, with the rising prevalence of obesity in the population, NAFLD is even considered a significant health issue for obese children and adolescents.[155–157] Since NAFLD was first described by Ludwig and colleagues[143] in 1980, it has become increasingly recognized as a common condition that may occasionally progress to cirrhosis and liver failure. Other terminologies that were used for this disease entity include pseudoalcoholic hepatitis, alcohol-like hepatitis, nonalcoholic Laennec's disease, fatty liver hepatitis, steatonecrosis, diabetic hepatitis, and nonalcoholic steatohepatitis (NASH), the latter now being recognized as a distinct subset of NAFLD.[145,146] Recently, the acronym NAFLD has been used to describe a wide spectrum of fatty liver diseases ranging from simple steatosis (fat without inflammation, fibrosis, or other hepatocyte changes) to NASH (fat with hepatocyte changes, inflammation, and possibly fibrosis). Progression to advanced fibrosis and cirrhosis is thought to occur in the subset with NASH.[145–147] The diagnostic criteria for NAFLD continue to evolve and rely on a liver biopsy with the histologic finding of steatosis. Other findings that may be present

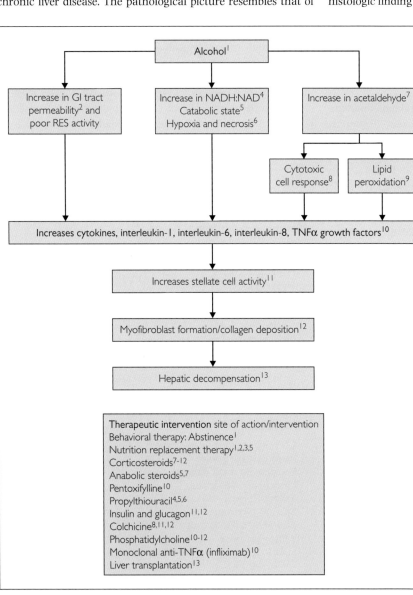

Fig. 36.1 • Pathways of alcohol-induced cell injury and site of therapeutic intervention.

Table 36.1 Management of alcoholic liver disease

Discontinuation of alcohol consumption

Treatment of extrahepatic complications of alcoholism

Withdrawal syndromes
Poor nutrition
Electrolyte abnormalities
Cardiac dysfunction
Pancreatitis
Infection

Specific treatment of alcoholic hepatitis

Corticosteroids (prednisone or prednisolone 40 mg/d, or its equivalent, × 4 weeks, followed by a taper over 2–4 weeks) in selected patients (with clinically severe disease defined by a discriminant function >32 and no evidence of infection or gastrointestinal bleeding)

Pentoxifylline (400 mg t.i.d. × 4 weeks) in selected patients (possibly those with evidence of renal dysfunction) either alone or with corticosteroids

Management of the sequelae of cirrhosis

Ascites
Portal hypertensive bleeding
Hepatic encephalopathy

Consideration of liver transplantation in the abstinent patient

include hepatocellular injury (portal or periportal inflammation, hepatocyte ballooning, Mallory hyaline bodies), and the pattern of fibrosis. Fibrosis often has a distinctive pericellular or 'chicken-wire' pattern before developing into confluent septae. Insulin resistance and oxidative stress have critical roles in the pathogenesis of NAFLD. No effective pharmacologic therapy yet exists for patients with NAFLD. However, lifestyle modifications including weight reduction and exercise may improve the spectrum of the disease. Liver transplantation remains a therapeutic alternative for some patients with decompensated end-stage liver disease, but NAFLD may recur after liver transplantation.[158]

Epidemiology and risk factors

NAFLD is thought to be very common and the prevalence of fatty liver of any degree in the general population is estimated to range from 13% to 18%.[159–161] Studies of liver biopsies of unselected autopsies or living donors for liver transplant indicate that the prevalence of steatohepatitis (NASH) is less common and ranges from 2% to 4%.[162,163] NAFLD can affect any age group and is reported increasingly in pediatric population, including 2.6% of children overall and up to 53% of obese children and adolescents.[164–166] The spectrum of histologic injury in this pediatric group clearly includes cirrhosis.[155] It is now suspected that there is an even distribution of NAFLD among men and women although there may be gender variation among the specific classes. Series of patients with more advanced disease have generally had more women, suggesting a more aggressive course.[167] Surveys have also suggested ethnic variation, with the disease being relatively uncommon among African-Americans as compared with European and Hispanic Americans. This may represent variation in referral patterns, genetic differences in body fat distribution, or metabolic

thermogenesis.[168–175] Clustering within kindreds also has been described, further suggesting that genetic factors predispose to the development of NAFLD.[176,177]

Associated conditions

The most common risk factor associated with NAFLD is the presence of the metabolic syndrome,[178] which is defined by the presence of three or more of the following criteria: (1) increased waist circumference, (2) hypertriglyceridemia, (3) hypertension, (4) high fasting glucose, and (5) a low level of high-density lipoprotein (HDL) (Table 36.2). Therefore, NAFLD is now recognized to be the hepatic manifestation of the metabolic syndrome. However, it is important to note that all of the individual clinical components of the metabolic syndrome are strongly associated with obesity and it is obesity itself that has the strongest association with NAFLD. Obesity is defined as a body mass index (BMI) >30 kg/m².[179] The more obese the patient, the greater is the likelihood of fatty liver. Thirty percent of patients who are obese have fatty liver, as do up to 80% of morbidly obese patients (BMI >35).[180,181] However, NAFLD is not confined to the obese. An increasing number of patients have been described who have a normal BMI, although these individuals may have central adiposity and occult insulin resistance.[145,147]

In addition to the association with the components of the metabolic syndrome described above,[145,147,178] NAFLD can also be associated with many other conditions (see Table 36.2) including peroxisomal diseases,[182] polycystic ovarian disease,[145] mitochondrialopathies,[183] Weber-Christian disease,[184] jejunoileal bypass,[145–147] Mauriac syndrome,[185] Made-lung's lipomatosis,[186] Wilson's disease,[187] industrial solvent exposure,[188] celiac disease,[189] abetalipoproteinemia,[190] and medications (including amiodarone,

Table 36.2 Causes of nonalcoholic fatty liver disease

Metabolic syndrome

Obesity
Type 2 diabetes mellitus
Hyperlipidemia
Hypertension

Medications

Glucocorticoids
Methotrexate
Amiodarone
Tamoxifen
Synthetic estrogens
Calcium channel blockers
Nucleoside analogues

Miscellaneous

Chronic hepatitis C, genotype 3
Peroxisomal diseases
Polycystic ovarian disease
Mitochondrialopathies
Weber-Christian disease
Mauriac syndrome
Made-lung's lipomatosis
Wilson's disease
Industrial solvent exposure
Celiac disease
Abetalipoproteinemia

tamoxifen, perhexiline maleate, glucocorticoids, synthetic estrogens, calcium channel blockers, nucleoside analogues, methotrexate).[145–147,191–194] Many of these disorders have in common either abnormal fat metabolism and/or mitochondrial injury or dysfunction. NAFLD can also be associated with hyperuricemia.

Pathogenesis

The pathogenesis of NAFLD remains incompletely understood though many theories have been formulated to explain the observed sequence of events in the disease (Fig. 36.2). The critical feature in NAFLD associated with the metabolic syndrome is the presence of insulin resistance. It is still unknown why simple steatosis develops in only some of the patients at risk, and furthermore why steatohepatitis and progressive disease develops in others. A 'two-hit' hypothesis has been proposed, whereby steatosis (first hit) sensitizes the liver to a variety of metabolic injuries (second hit) that lead to necrosis, inflammation, and fibrosis.[195,196] Differences in body fat distribution or host antioxidant systems, possibly in the context of a genetic predisposition, may be among the explanations.[145,147] The net retention of lipids within hepatocytes, mostly in the form of triglycerides, is a prerequisite for the development of NAFLD. The primary metabolic processes leading to lipid accumulation are not yet well understood, but probably relate to alterations of the pathways of uptake, synthesis, degradation, or secretion in hepatic lipid metabolism resulting from insulin resistance.[197] The molecular pathogenesis of insulin resistance seems to be multifactorial. Several molecular targets involved in the inhibition of insulin action have been identified and may serve as targets for therapeutic agents in the future. These include Rad (ras associated with diabetes),[198] which inter-

feres with essential cell functions (growth, differentiation, vesicular transport, and signal transduction); PC-1 (a membrane glycoprotein that has a role in insulin resistance),[199] which reduces insulin-stimulated tyrosine kinase activity; leptin,[200] which induces dephosphorylation of insulin-receptor substrate-1; fatty acids,[201] which inhibit insulin-stimulated peripheral glucose uptake; and tumor necrosis factor alpha,[202] which downregulates insulin-induced phosphorylation of insulin-receptor substrate-1 and reduces the expression of the insulin-dependent glucose-transport molecule Glut4. Insulin resistance leads to fat accumulation in hepatocytes by two main mechanisms: lipolysis and hyperinsulinemia.[145] Clinically significant amounts of dicarboxylic acids, which are potentially cytotoxic, can be formed by microsomal oxidation. This pathway of fatty acid metabolism is closely related to mitochondrial beta-oxidation and peroxisomal beta-oxidation. Deficiency of the enzymes of peroxisomal beta-oxidation has been recognized as an important cause of microvesicular steatosis and steatohepatitis.[203] In particular, deficiency of acyl-coenzyme A oxidase disrupts the oxidation of very-long-chain fatty acids and dicarboxylic acids, leading to extensive microvesicular steatosis and steatohepatitis. Loss of this enzyme also causes sustained hyperactivation of peroxisome-proliferator-activated receptor-α (PPAR-α), leading to transcriptional upregulation of PPAR-α-regulated genes.[203] PPAR-α has been implicated in promoting hepatic synthesis of uncoupling protein-2, which is expressed in the liver of patients with NAFLD.[204] Increased intrahepatic levels of fatty acids provide a source of oxidative stress, which may in large part be responsible for the progression from steatosis to steatohepatitis to cirrhosis. Mitochondria are the main cellular source of reactive oxygen species, which may trigger steatohepatitis and fibrosis by three main mechanisms: lipid peroxidation, cytokine induction, and induction of Fas ligand. Patients with steatohepatitis have ultrastructural mitochondrial lesions, including linear crystalline inclusions in megamitochondria.[183] This mitochondrial injury is absent in most patients with simple steatosis and in healthy subjects.[205] Patients with steatohepatitis slowly resynthesize adenosine triphosphate (ATP) in vivo after a fructose challenge, which causes acute hepatic ATP depletion.[206] This impaired ATP recovery may reflect the mitochondrial injury found in patients with steatohepatitis.[183,205]

Diagnosis

NAFLD is usually suspected in patients with asymptomatic elevations of serum aminotransferase levels, unexplained hepatomegaly, or the incidental discovery of findings suggestive of fatty liver on imaging studies.[145–150] However, the clinical presentation varies from patient to patient. Most are asymptomatic or minimal non-specific complaints such as malaise or abdominal discomfort. Hepatomegaly, if present, is the only physical finding in most patients.[145–147]

Serum aminotransferase levels are elevated in more than 90% of patients with NAFLD.[145,149] These elevations are typically mild, usually 2–3 times the upper limit of normal.[145–147] The ALT level is more elevated than the AST level, with an AST/ALT ratio of less than 1 (in contrast to alcoholic liver disease).[207] However, this ratio increases in the presence of fibrosis so it is usually not helpful in diagnosing NAFLD.[208] The alkaline phosphatase and gamma-glutamyltransferase are usually within normal limits or only slightly above the normal range. Other abnormalities including

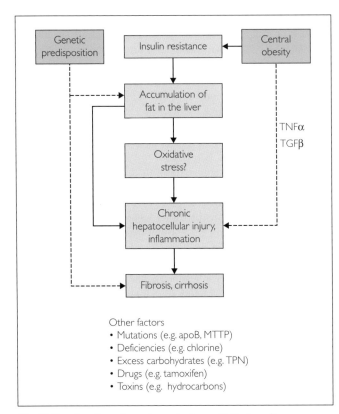

Fig. 36.2 • Putative pathogenic mechanisms of fatty liver disease.

hyperbilirubinemia, hypoalbuminemia, or a prolonged pro-thrombin time may be found in patients with advanced cirrhosis.[145–147] Elevated serum ferritin and transferrin saturation are found in up to 50% of the patients; however, these represent an acute-phase response to inflammation and not iron over-load.[166,208] Although the hepatic iron index and hepatic iron levels are normal, some have suggested that heterozygosity for the hemochromatosis gene (HFE) may be increased in NAFLD and that accumulation of hepatic iron may lead to more progressive liver injury.[145,209] This remains to be confirmed. Low-titer anti-nuclear antibody positivity is present in up to 20% of patients with NAFLD but is non-specific and probably not different from age and gender matched patients without fatty liver disease. Nonetheless, a liver biopsy should exclude autoimmune hepatitis, as long-term management will differ.[146] Taken together, the clinical presentation and liver tests have poor predictive value with respect to histologic involvement.[145,147,210] Thus, the confi-dent diagnosis of NAFLD requires histologic confirmation in the absence of excessive alcohol intake; a daily intake as low as 20 grams of alcohol in females and 30 grams in males may be sufficient to cause alcohol-induced liver disease in some patients.[211] Other causes of elevated liver enzymes including viral hepatitis, autoimmune responses, metabolic or hereditary factors, and drugs or toxins should always be excluded though these rarely present with hepatic fat.[145–147]

Imaging studies

Radiological modalities such as ultrasonography, computerized tomography, and magnetic resonance imaging may show increased fat accumulation (steatosis) in the hepatic parenchyma.[145–147] However, none of these imaging techniques can reliably detect hepatic fat content less than 25–30%.[212] Furthermore, radio-logical features of NAFLD may be non-specific, leading to a significant variability in their interpretation between different radiologists. On ultrasonography, fatty infiltration of the liver produces a diffuse increase in echogenicity as compared with that of the kidneys, but steatosis can often not be distinguished from fibrosis.[212,213] Fatty infiltration of the liver produces a low-density hepatic parenchyma on computerized tomographic scanning.[212] Steatosis is usually diffuse, but occasionally is focal and can suggest the presence of a mass.[214] In such cases, magnetic resonance imaging can distinguish space-occupying lesions from focal fatty infiltration or sparing.[215] Magnetic resonance spectroscopy is a promising modality that allows a quantitative assessment of fat content in fatty liver.[147,216] Importantly, no imaging study can distinguish fat alone from steatohepatitis and none is able to reliably identify or quantitate (stage) fibrosis.[212]

Role of liver biopsy and histology

The question of whether a liver biopsy is required in every person suspected of having NAFLD is controversial. However, liver biopsy remains the gold standard and the best diagnostic tool for confirming and staging NAFLD.[145–147,212] It also provides impor-tant prognostic information. It may also be useful in determining the effect of medical treatment, given the poor correlation between histologic findings and laboratory tests or imaging studies.[145] Liver biopsy should be considered in patients with persistent elevation of serum aminotransferase levels regardless of whether

treatment is considered, especially if the patient is obese or has diabetes mellitus.[146] The role of the liver biopsy in assessing patients with liver abnormalities while using statin drugs has yet to be established; however, it is usually difficult to distinguish NAFLD from hepatotoxicity on clinical grounds in such patients. Interpretation and classification of liver biopsy findings in this disease is evolving. The degree of sampling error and the significance of occasional apoptotic bodies have not been studied adequately.[147] The histologic features of NAFLD may be indis-tinguishable from those of alcoholic fatty liver disease, and clinical correlation with careful history of alcohol consumption may be mandatory to distinguish between both groups.[145–147] Unlike other forms of chronic liver disease, no consensus currently exists regarding the grading and staging of NAFLD.[145–147,217] The grade indicates the activity of steatohepatitis (inflammation), while the stage reflects the degree of fibrosis. Although the interobserver variability is relatively low in terms of diagnosing steatosis, cyto-logic ballooning, and perisinusoidal fibrosis, there is considerable variability with regard to the assessment of inflammatory changes.[217] A scoring system has been proposed by Brunt and colleagues[218] in which individual parameters indicative of necroinflammatory activity (cytologic ballooning, steatosis, and inflammation) are scored separately and then a composite score is derived to indicate the grade of steatohepatitis (Table 36.3). This approach also includes a staging system to assess hepatic fibrosis, which is comprised of components for perisinusoidal fibrosis, portal fibrosis, and bridging fibrosis. A finding of fibrosis in NAFLD suggests more advanced and severe liver injury. According to a number of cross-sectional studies including a total of 673 liver biopsies,[143,145,166,208,217,219,220] some degree of fibrosis is found in up to 66% of patients with NASH at the time of diagnosis, whereas severe fibrosis (septal fibrosis or cirrhosis) is found in 25% and well-established cirrhosis is found in 14%. Once cirrhosis develops, the amount of steatosis and cytologic ballooning may decrease or disappear completely, making the diagnosis difficult to make.[145–147,166,217] Many such cases are labeled as cryptogenic cirrhosis or 'burned-out' NASH. In these settings, the diagnosis can only be suspected from the clinical profile of the patient and the presence of risk factors for NAFLD.[217,218]

Natural history and clinical course

The natural history of NAFLD has not been well defined. The existing literature is almost entirely based on retrospective studies. An important study by Matteoni and colleagues[217] provided some assistance in predicting the clinical course of patients with NAFLD. In this study, subjects were grouped into four categories based on their initial liver histology as follows: (1) fatty liver alone; (2) fatty liver and lobular inflammation; (3) fatty liver and ballooning degeneration; and (4) fatty liver and ballooning and Mallory's hyaline or fibrosis. The overall death rates over 18 years of follow-up were 33%, 30%, 26%, and 44%, respectively. Subjects in group 3 and 4 had the highest number of liver-related deaths, and liver-related diseases were the second most common cause of death, with cancer being the first cause.

The frequency and rates of progression from fat alone to steato-hepatitis and fibrosis are not known. Risk factors for progression have also not been well described. However, cross-sectional studies suggest that age greater than 40–50 years, degree of obesity, diabetes mellitus, or hyperlipidemia (especially hypertrigly-

Table 36.3 Grading and staging the histopathological lesions of NAFLD

Grading for steatosis
Grade 1: <33% of hepatocytes affected
Grade 2: 33–66% of hepatocytes affected
Grade 3: >66% of hepatocytes affected

Grading for steatohepatitis

Grade 1, mild
Steatosis: predominantly macrovesicular, involves up to 66% of lobules
Ballooning: occasionally observed; zone 3 hepatocytes
Lobular inflammation: scattered and mild acute inflammation (polymorphonuclear cells) and occasional chronic inflammation (mononuclear cells)
Portal inflammation: none or mild

Grade 2, moderate
Steatosis: any degree; usually mixed macrovesicular and microvesicular
Ballooning: obvious and present in zone 3
Lobular inflammation: polymorphonuclear cells may be noted in association with ballooned hepatocytes; pericellular fibrosis; mild chronic inflammation may be seen
Portal inflammation: mild to moderate

Grade 3, severe
Steatosis: typically involves >66% of lobules (panacinar); commonly mixed steatosis
Ballooning: predominantly zone 3; marked
Lobular inflammation: scattered acute and chronic inflammation; polymorphonuclear cells may be concentrated in zone 3 areas of ballooning and perisinusoidal fibrosis
Portal inflammation: mild to moderate

Staging for fibrosis
Stage 1: zone 3 perivenular, perisinusoidal, or pericellular fibrosis; focal or extensive
Stage 2: as above, with focal or extensive periportal fibrosis
Stage 3: bridging fibrosis, focal or extensive
Stage 4: cirrhosis

ceridemia), and a ratio of aspartate aminotransferase to alanine aminotransferase of 1 or greater are strong indicators of advanced stages of liver fibrosis.[159,208,221] The relatively increased prevalence of females among series with more advanced disease suggest that female gender may be a risk factor for progression, but this not a consistent finding in reported series.[145,166,167,208] A recent study by Fassio and colleagues[222] found that progression of fibrosis was present in one-third of NASH patients 4.3 years after the first liver biopsy, and obesity and body mass index were the only factors associated with progression. Patients found to have pure steatosis on liver biopsy seem to have the best prognosis within the spectrum of NAFLD.[145,160] Other cross-sectional series have shown that 30–40% of patients have advanced liver fibrosis at the time of presentation,[166,220,223] whereas 10–15% of them may have established cirrhosis.[143,166,224] Three studies have found that patients with cryptogenic cirrhosis have a higher prevalence of diabetes, obesity, or both than those with cirrhosis from other causes, thereby suggesting that cryptogenic cirrhosis may represent 'burned-out' NASH.[225–227] Furthermore, some patients who undergo liver transplantation for cryptogenic cirrhosis develop steatosis and/or NASH in the graft during follow-up.[158,228]

Hepatocellular carcinoma has been reported in NASH patients, but the magnitude of this risk is not known.[229] Two large series of patients with hepatocellular carcinoma reported that 7–13% of patients carried a diagnosis of cryptogenic cirrhosis and had a clinical phenotype of NASH.[230]

Management

Resolution of histologic abnormalities as determined by liver biopsy remains the goal of treatment in patients with NAFLD. Common surrogate markers include normalization of serum aminotransferases and loss of fat as detected by radiologic imaging,[145–147,166] though these are probably insensitive, as discussed above.

General considerations

It is not known whether alcohol use should be prohibited or restricted in patients with NAFLD. Lacking data, a pragmatic approach is to tailor this to the liver biopsy findings and recommend abstinence if either inflammation or fibrosis is present.[147] The concomitant use of medications that are associated with steatohepatitis, as stated earlier, requires weighing of the individual's risks and benefits. Certainly, the benefits of controlling diabetes or hyperlipidemia exceed the small potential for hepatotoxity, and such therapy may even result in improvement of the liver disease (see below). An increasingly common but little-explored issue is workplace exposure to hydrocarbon solvents.[231]

Exercise and diet

Exercise and diet continue to be the cornerstones of therapy.[232] Although typically recommended together, the concept of the fit fat individual (i.e., relatively well-conditioned but obese) is relevant and suggests a benefit of exercise even in the absence of weight loss.[233] Exercise alters insulin sensitivity and substrate use in skeletal muscle, although only about one-third of patients achieve target levels of exercise,[234,235] and obese individuals may be resistant to these changes. A small number of studies of diet and exercise therapy have been reported in both adults and children. These typically demonstrate improvement of biochemical measures but variable changes in histology.[155,236–241] Histologic exacerbation has been observed when the rate of weight loss exceeds 1.6 kilograms per week. High-intensity exercise regimens are probably more effective in producing significant metabolic changes than low-intensity regimens or diet alone.[242]

Specific diets and weight loss surgery

The effects of many popular diets on hepatic steatosis are not known. A pragmatic approach is to recommend a reduced calorie, balanced diet such as that endorsed by the American Heart Association or, as proposed by Spieth and colleagues in pediatric patients, the low glycemic index diet that emphasizes dietary composition.[243] Increased polyunsaturated fats (fish, flax seed oils) alter insulin sensitivity and prostaglandin metabolism, may increase uncoupling protein expression, and may promote lipid peroxidation, but the net effect in steatohepatitis is not known.[244–247] Appetite-suppressing agents have lost favor due to their side effects.[248] Recent data suggest a role for orlistat, a lipase inhibitor, as an adjunct to weight loss.[249] Several studies have reported beneficial effects of bariatric surgery,[180,250,251] although precipitous weight loss has the potential to exacerbate steatohepatitis and may lead to liver failure. Pretreatment with cytoprotective or antioxidant agents in this setting has not been tested. Older studies of the now abandoned jejunoileal intestinal bypass procedure supported a role for antibiotics and amino acid supplementation for patients who experienced decompensation.[252,253]

Cytoprotective agents

These agents combine an attractive safety profile, few drug interactions, and a plausible mechanism of action at the cellular or subcellular level. Ursodeoxycholic acid (UDCA) has been suggested to be of benefit based on open-label studies.[254–257] However, a recent prospective multicenter randomized clinical study reported by Lindor and colleagues[258] reported that 2 years of therapy with UDCA at a dose of 13–15 mg/kg/day was no better than placebo for patients with NASH. Although safe and well tolerated, this treatment did not improve either liver biochemistries or histology as compared to untreated controls.[258]

Antioxidant agents and iron reduction therapy

The suggestion that oxidative stress is involved in the pathogenesis of NASH has led to recent studies to examine the potential role of antioxidants in the treatment of NAFLD. Three studies have evaluated the effects of vitamin E in NASH patients. Two studies, one in children and one in adults, were uncontrolled, pilot trials. Lavine[259] demonstrated improvement in aminotransferase levels in children with NASH, but did not evaluate the effect on histology. Hasegawa and colleagues[260] showed improvement in both hepatic inflammation and fibrosis in five of nine NAFLD patients who lost weight and then were treated with vitamin E (300 mg/day) for 6 months. Recently, a prospective, randomized trial of vitamin E and vitamin C (1000 IU and 1000 mg, respectively) in 49 patients demonstrated a significant improvement in fibrosis in the vitamin-treated group. Diabetic patients with fibrosis appeared to have the greatest improvement.[261] The activated form of methionine, S-adenosyl-L-methionine (SAME), is involved in several key hepatic metabolic pathways involved in gene expression and membrane fluidity and the generation of glutathione.[262] SAME has been shown to reduce liver injury in several animal models. Betaine is a drug that serves as a methyl donor in the generation of methionine from homocysteine, increases SAME levels, and would be anticipated to have a similar effect. Indeed, betaine resulted in improvement in histology and serum aminotransferase levels in a pilot study in 10 NASH patients.[263] Silymarin, a popular milk thistle extract, is commonly used by patients with liver disease though there are no published data to support its use in NAFLD.[264] Iron may increase oxidative injury. Serial phlebotomy for iron reduction in 17 patients with NAFLD and normal iron levels led to improvement in liver enzyme levels and insulin sensitivity in a small pilot study.[265]

Antidiabetic and insulin-sensitizing agents

Neither insulin therapy, sometimes recommended early in the course of type 2 diabetes,[266] nor sulfonylureas have been adequately studied as treatment of fatty liver disease.[147] On the other hand, the thiazolidinediones have been studied and show promise.[267–273] These agents activate the PPAR-α nuclear transcription factor,[274] alter skeletal muscle glucose uptake (through increased Glut4 activity),[275] decrease central adiposity,[276] promote adipocyte differentiation, alter mitochondrial mass,[277] and alter thermogenesis.[278] The efficacy of troglitazone in lipodystrophy suggests a primary effect on lipid metabolism.[279] Similarly, metformin has undergone limited study in NAFLD.[280–283] It down-regulates hepatic gluconeogenesis and also appears to divert fatty acids from triglyceride production to mitochondrial beta oxidation.[284] Other candidate agents include acarbose (an α-glucosidase inhibitor),[285] acipimox (inhibits lipolysis),[286] and d-chiro-inositol.[287]

Antihyperlipidemic agents

Fibrates alter lipoprotein metabolism through the PPAR-α receptor but early studies demonstrated no benefit.[254] However, bezafibrate showed benefit in tamoxifen-associated steatohepatitis.[288] Basaranoglu and colleagues[289] showed improvement in liver enzyme levels in patients treated with gemfibrozil, but histology was not measured. Atorvastatin, an HMG-CoA reductase inhibitor, resulted in improvement in biochemical and histologic parameters in a small pilot study.[290] However, a recent report showed no significant histologic differences between controls and patients with various statin drugs.[291] Recent reports of subclinical skeletal muscle toxicity characterized by formation of ragged red fibers and mediated by mitochondrial injury are justifiable cause for concern for the use of these drugs in NAFLD.[292]

Liver transplantation

Patients with liver failure from NAFLD are often poor candidates for transplantation due to comorbid conditions such as obesity, coronary artery disease, hypertension, and complications of diabetes. Both recurrence of NAFLD in patients with previously established NAFLD and de novo occurrence of NAFLD after transplantation for cryptogenic cirrhosis have been reported.[158,293–295] Progression to cirrhosis may develop in some patients who develop NAFLD after liver transplantation, but predictive factors have not been identified and treatment has not been studied in this setting. Immunosuppression, particularly the use of corticosteroids, could play a role in recurrence and progression due to the promotion of fatty liver and diabetes. Cyclosporine might promote fatty liver disease through direct effects on mitochondria.[296]

Summary

There is currently no effective therapy for NAFLD, although several agents show promise in early studies. However, it is likely that new therapeutic targets will become available as our understanding of the pathogenesis of this disease evolves. For the present time, rigorous control of risk factors for NAFLD such as obesity, diabetes, and hyperlipidemia seems appropriate. Lifestyle modifications including weight reduction and steady regular exercise may improve the spectrum of the disease. Currently, with the possible exception of vitamin E, pharmacotherapy for NAFLD should be undertaken in the setting of clinical trials to assess the efficacy of therapy in a formal fashion. There remain insufficient data to justify the use of insulin-sensitizing agents in patients with insulin resistance but no diabetes. However, such therapies may be shown to be useful if ongoing clinical trials confirm a benefit. Other agents that have not been studied are antihypertensive agents such as angiotensin II receptor blockers and probiotics to reduce bacterial endotoxin levels seem possible.

Additionally, the combination of specific diets that improve insulin resistance coupled with pharmacotherapy to reduce oxidative stress and improve insulin might be an attractive option.

REFERENCES

1. Hoek JB, Pastorino JG. Ethanol, oxidative stress, and cytokine-induced liver cell injury. Alcohol 2002; 27:63–68.

   Cytokine-mediated cell–cell interactions play an important role in the onset of alcohol-induced liver damage.

2. Kono H, Rusyn I, Yin M, et al. NADPH oxidase-derived free radicals are key oxidants in alcohol-induced liver disease. J Clin Invest 2000; 106:867–872.

3. Rao RK, Seth A, Sheth P. Recent advances in alcoholic liver disease I. Role of intestinal permeability and endotoxemia in alcoholic liver disease. Am J Physiol Gastrointest Liver Physiol 2004; 286:G881-G884.

4. Felver FE, Mezey E, McGuire M, et al. Plasma tumor necrosis factor α predicts decreased long-term survival in severe alcoholic hepatitis. Alcohol Clin Exp Res 1990; 14:225–259.

5. McClain CJ, Cohen DA. Increased tumor necrosis factor production by monocytes in alcoholic hepatitis. Hepatology 1989; 9:349–351.

6. Khoruts A, Stahnke L, McClain CJ, et al. Circulating tumor necrosis factor, interleukin-1 and interleukin-6 concentrations in chronic alcoholic patients. Hepatology 1991; 13:267–276.

7. Hill DB, Marsano LS, McClain CJ. Increased plasma interleukin-8 concentrations in alcoholic hepatitis. Hepatology 1993; 18:576–580.

8. Kakumu S, Leevy CM. Lymphocyte cytotoxicity in alcoholic hepatitis. Gastroenterology 1997; 72:594–597.

9. Si L, Whiteside TL, Schade RR, et al. Lymphocyte subsets studied with monoclonal antibodies in liver tissues of patients with alcoholic liver disease. Alcohol Clin Exp Res 1983; 1:431–435.

10. Chedid A, Mendenhall CL, Moritz TE, et al. Cell-mediated hepatic injury in alcoholic liver disease. Gastroenterology 1993; 105:254–266.

11. Smith SL, Jennett RB, Sorrel MF, et al. Acetaldehyde substoichiometrically inhibits bovine neurotubulin polymerization. J Clin Invest 1989; 84:337–341.

12. DiLuzio NR. Antioxidants, lipid peroxidation and chemical-induced liver injury. Fed Proc 1973; 32:1875–1881.

13. Comporti M, Hartman A, DiLuzio NR, et al. Effect of in vivo and in vitro ethanol administration on liver lipid peroxidation. Lab Invest 1967; 16:616–624.

14. Lieber CS, DeCarli LM. Metabolic effects of alcohol on the liver. In: Lieber CS, ed. Metabolic aspects of alcoholism. Baltimore: University Park Press; 1977:31–80.

15. Caulet S, Fabre M, Schoevaert D, et al. Quantitative study of centrolobular hepatic fibrosis in alcoholic disease before cirrhosis. Arch Pathol Anat 1989; 416:11–17.

16. Sorensen TIA, Bentsen KD, Eghoje K, et al. Prospective evaluation of alcohol abuse and alcoholic liver injury in men as predictors of development of cirrhosis. Lancet 1984; 2:242–245.

17. Nakano M, Worner TM, Lieber CS. Perivenular fibrosis in alcoholic liver injury: Ultrastructure and histologic progression. Gastroenterology 1982; 83:777–785.

18. Deaciuc IV, Fortunato F, D'Souza NB, et al. Chronic alcohol exposure of rats exacerbates apoptosis in hepatocytes and sinusoidal endothelial cells. Hepatol Res 2001; 19:306–324.

19. McClain CJ, Hill DB, Song Z, et al. Monocyte activation in alcoholic liver disease. Alcohol 2002; 27:53–61.

20. Christoffersen P, Nielson K. Histologic changes in liver biopsies from chronic alcoholics. Acta Pathol Microbiol Scand 1972; 80:557–565.

21. Levin DM, Baker AL, Riddell RH, et al. Nonalcoholic liver disease. Overlooked causes of liver injury in patients with heavy alcohol consumption. Am J Med 1979; 66:429–434.

    Only 80% of patients with clinically suspected alcoholic liver disease had the diagnosis confirmed by liver biopsy; 20% of patients had alternative liver disorders.

22. Talley NJ, Roth A, Woods J, et al. Diagnostic value of liver biopsy in alcoholic liver disease. J Clin Gastroenterol 1988; 10:647–650.

    Liver biopsy may not always be necessary for the confirmation of alcoholic liver disease; the prebiopsy diagnosis of alcoholic liver disease was confirmed in all but one of 35 patients.

23. Teli MR, Day CP, Burt AD, et al. Determinants of progression to cirrhosis or fibrosis in pure alcoholic fatty liver. Lancet 1995; 346:987–990.

24. Brunt PW, Kew MC, Scheuer PJ, et al. Studies in alcoholic liver disease in Britain. I. Clinical and pathological patterns related to natural history. Gut 1974; 15:52–58.

25. Powell WJ Jr, Klatskin G. Duration of survival in patients with Laennec's cirrhosis. Influence of alcohol withdrawal, and possible effects of recent changes in general management of the disease. Am J Med 1968; 44:406–420.

26. Alexander JF, Lischner MW, Galambos JT. Natural history of alcoholic hepatitis. II. The long-term prognosis. Am J Gastroenterol 1971; 56:515–525.

27. Galambos JT. Natural history of alcoholic hepatitis. 3. Histological changes. Gastroenterology 1972; 63:1026–1035.

28. Karman JF, Sileri P, Kamuda D, et al. Risk factors for failure to meet listing requirements in liver transplant candidates with alcoholic cirrhosis. Transplantation 2001; 71:1210–1213.

29. Zeise ML, Kasparov S, Capogna M, et al. Acamprosate (calcium acetylhomotaurinate) decreases postsynaptic potentials in the rat neocortex: possible involvement of excitatory amino acid receptors. Eur J Pharmacol 1993; 231:47–52.

30. Volpicelli JR, Clay KL, Watson NT, et al. Naltrexone in the treatment of alcoholism: predicting response to naltrexone. J Clin Psychiatry 1995; 56(Suppl 7):39–44.

31. Lhuintre JP, Moore N, Tran G, et al. Acamprosate appears to decrease alcohol intake in weaned alcoholics. Alcohol Alcohol 1990; 25:613–622.

32. Brasser SM, McCaul ME, Houtsmuller EJ. Alcohol effects during acamprosate treatment: a dose-response study in humans. Alcohol Clin Exp Res 2004; 28:1074–1083.

33. Paille FM, Guelfi JD, Perkins AC, et al. Double-blind randomized multicentre trial of acamprosate in maintaining abstinence from alcohol. Alcohol Alcohol 1995; 30:239–247.

34. Mendenhall CL, Anderson S, Garcia PP, et al. Short-term and long-term survival in patients with alcoholic hepatitis treated with oxandrolone and prednisolone. N Engl J Med 1984; 311:1464–1470.

35. Mendenhall CL, Moritz TE, Roselle GA, et al. A study of oral nutritional support with oxandrolone in malnourished patients with alcoholic hepatitis: Results of a Department of Veterans Affairs Cooperative Study. Hepatology 1993; 17:564–576.

36. Mendenhall CL, Tosch T, Weesner RE, et al. Veterans Administration Cooperative Study on Alcoholic Hepatitis II. Prognostic significance of protein-calorie malnutrition. Am J Clin Nutr 1986; 43:213–218.

37. Porayko MK, DiCecco S, O'Keefe SJD. Impact of malnutrition and its therapy on liver transplantation. Semin Liver Dis 1991; 11:305–314.

38. Nompleggi DJ, Bonkovsky HL. Nutritional supplementation in chronic liver disease: an analytical review. Hepatology 1994; 19:518–533.

39. John WJ, Phillips R, Ott L, et al. Resting energy expenditure in patients with alcoholic hepatitis. J Parenter Enteral Nutr 1989; 13:124–127.

40. Bonkovsky HL, Singh RH, Jafri IH, et al. A randomized controlled trial of treatment of alcoholic hepatitis with parenteral nutrition and oxandrolone. II. Short-term effects on nitrogen metabolism, metabolic balance and nutrition. Am J Gastroenterol 1991; 86:1209–1218.

41. Naveau S, Pelletier G, Poynard T, et al. A randomized clinical trial of supplementary parenteral nutrition in jaundiced alcoholic cirrhotic patients. Hepatology 1986; 6:270–274.

42. Diehl AM, Boitnott JK, Herlong HF, et al. Effect of parenteral amino acids supplementation in alcoholic hepatitis. Hepatology 1985; 5:57–63.

43. Cabre E, Gonzalez-Huiz F, Abad-Lacruz A, et al. Effect of total enteral nutrition on the short-term outcome of severely malnourished cirrhotics. Gastroenterology 1990; 98:715–720.

44. Mendenhall CL, Roselle GA, Gartside P, et al. Relationship of protein calorie malnutrition to alcoholic liver disease: A reexamination of data from two VA Cooperative Studies. Alcohol Clin Exp Res 1995; 19:635 641.

45. Fabbri A, Magrini N, Bianchi G, et al. Overview of randomized clinical trials of oral branched-chain amino acid treatment in chronic hepatic encephalopathy. J Parenter Enteral Nutr 1996; 20:159–164.

46. Marchesini G, Dioguardi FS, Bianchi GP, et al. Long-term oral branched-chain amino acid treatment in chronic hepatic encephalopathy. A randomized double-blind casein-controlled trial. The Italian Multicenter Study Group. J Hepatol 1990; 11:92–101.

47. Yoshida T, Muto Y, Moriwaki H, et al. Effect of long-term oral supplementation with branched-chain amino acid granules on the prognosis of liver cirrhosis. Gastroenterol Jpn 1989; 24:692–698.

48. Orrego H, Israel Y, Blake JE, et al. Assessment of prognostic factors in alcoholic liver disease: toward a global quantitative expression of severity. Hepatology 1983; 3:896–905.

49. Tome S, Lucey MR. Review article: current management of alcoholic liver disease. Aliment Pharmacol Ther 2004; 19:707–714.

The current management of alcoholic liver disease is concisely reported in this recent review article.

50. Sherman DI, Williams R. Liver damage: mechanisms and management. Br Med Bull 1994; 50:124–138.

51. Maddrey WC, Boitnott JK, Bedine MS, et al. Corticosteroid therapy of alcoholic hepatitis. Gastroenterology 1978; 75:193–199.

52. Carithers RJ, Herlong HF, Diehl AM, et al. Methylprednisolone therapy in patients with severe alcoholic hepatitis. A randomized multicenter trial. Ann Intern Med 1989; 110:685–690.

53. Helman RA, Temko MH, Nye SW, et al. Alcoholic hepatitis: Natural history and evaluation of prednisolone therapy. Ann Intern Med 1971; 74:311–321.

54. Lesesne HR, Bozymski EM, Fallon JH. Treatment of alcoholic hepatitis with encephalopathy. Comparison of prednisolone with caloric supplements. Gastroenterology 1978; 74:169–173.

55. Ramond MJ, Poynard T, Rueff B, et al. A randomized trial of prednisolone in patients with severe alcoholic hepatitis. N Engl J Med 1992; 326:507–512.

56. Schlicting P, Juhl E, Poulsen H, et al. Alcoholic hepatitis superimposed on cirrhosis. Clinical significance and effect of long-term prednisone treatment. Scand J Gastroenterol 1976; 11:305–312.

57. Porter HP, Simon FR, Pope CE, et al. Corticosteroid therapy in severe alcoholic hepatitis. N Engl J Med 1971; 284:1350–1355.

58. Campra JL, Namlin EM, Dirshbaum RJ, et al. Prednisone therapy of acute alcoholic hepatitis. Ann Intern Med 1973; 79:625–631.

59. Blitzer BL, Mutchnick MG, Joshi PH, et al. Adrenocorticosteroid therapy in alcoholic hepatitis. Dig Dis Sci 1977; 22:477–484.

60. Shumaker JB, Resnick RH, Galambos JT, et al. A controlled trial of 6-methylprednisolone in acute alcoholic hepatitis. With a note on published results in encephalopathic patients. Am J Gastroenterol 1978; 69:443–449.

61. Depew W, Boyer T, Omata M, et al. Double-blind controlled trial of prednisolone therapy in patients with severe acute alcoholic hepatitis and spontaneous encephalopathy. Gastroenterology 1980; 78:524–529.

62. Theodossi A, Eddleston AL, Williams R. Controlled trial of methylprednisolone therapy in severe acute alcoholic hepatitis. Gut 1982; 23:75–79.

63. Imperiale TF, McCullough AJ. Do corticosteroids reduce mortality from alcoholic hepatitis? A meta-analysis of the randomized trials. Ann Intern Med 1990; 113:299–307.

This meta-analysis demonstrated that corticosteroids reduce short-term mortality in patients with acute alcoholic hepatitis who have hepatic encephalopathy in the absence of gastrointestinal bleeding; corticosteroids were of no benefit in patients without hepatic encephalopathy.

64. Mathurin P, Duchatelle V, Ramond MJ, et al. Survival and prognostic factors in patients with severe alcoholic hepatitis treated with prednisolone. Gastroenterology 1996; 110:1847–1853.

65. Rosenak BD, Moser RH, Kilgore B Jr. Treatment of cirrhosis of the liver with testosterone propionate. Gastroenterology 1947; 9:695–704.

66. Well R. Prednisolone and testosterone proprinate in cirrhosis of the liver: A controlled trial. Lancet 1960; 2:1416–1419.

67. Fenster LF. The nonefficacy of short-term anabolic steroid therapy in alcoholic liver disease. Ann Intern Med 1966; 65:738–744.

68. Figueroa RB. Mesterolone in steatosis and cirrhosis of the liver. Acta Hepatogastroenterol (Stuttg) 1973; 20:282–290.

69. Islam N, Islam A. Testosterone propionate in cirrhosis of the liver. Br J Clin Pract 1973; 27:125–128.

70. Puliyel MM, Vyas GP, Mehta GS. Testosterone in the management of cirrhosis of the liver – a controlled study. Aust NZ J Med 1977; 7:17–30.

71. Copenhagen Study Group for Liver Disease. Testosterone treatment of men with alcoholic cirrhosis: A double-blind study. Hepatology 1986; 6:807–813.

72. Bonkovsky HL, Fiellin DA, Smith GS, et al. A randomized, controlled trial of treatment of alcoholic hepatitis with parenteral nutrition and oxandrolone. I. Short-term effects on liver function. Am J Gastroenterol 1991; 86:1200–1208.

73. Gill R, Zieve L, Logan G. Severe alcoholic hepatitis improved by combined treatment with prednisolone, testosterone and an amino acid supplement. Hepatology 1984; 4:1013(A26).

74. Strieter RM, Remick DG, Ward PA, et al. Cellular and molecular regulation of tumor necrosis factor-alpha production by pentoxifylline. Biochem Biophys Res Commun 1988; 155:1230–1236.

75. Akriviadis E, Botla R, Briggs W, et al. Pentoxifylline improves short-term survival in severe acute alcoholic hepatitis: a double-blind, placebo-controlled trial. Gastroenterology 2000; 119:1637–1648.

76. Heymsfield SB, Waki M, Reinus J. Are patients with chronic liver disease hypermetabolic. Hepatology 1990; 11:502–505.

77. Vachiery F, Moreau R, Hadengue A, et al. Hypoxemia in patients with cirrhosis: Relationship with liver failure and hemodynamic alterations. J Hepatol 1997; 27:492–495.

78. Rojter S, Tessler J, Alvarez D, et al. Vasodilatory effects of propylthiouracil in patients with alcoholic cirrhosis. J Hepatol 1995; 22:184–188.

79. Hicks M, Wong LS, Day RO. Antioxidant activity of propylthiouracil. Biochem Pharmacol 1992; 43:439–444.

80. Israel Y, Kalant H, Orrego H, et al. Experimental alcohol-induced hepatic necrosis: Suppression by propylthiouracil. Proc Natl Acad Sci USA 1975; 72:1137–1141.

81. Orrego H, Kalant H, Israel Y, et al. Effect of short-term therapy with propylthiouracil in patients with alcoholic liver disease. Gastroenterology 1979; 76:105–115.

82. Peirrugues R, Blanc P, Barneon C, et al. Short-term therapy with propylthiouracil for alcoholic hepatitis. A clinical, biochemical and histological randomized trial [Abstract]. Gastroenterology 1989; 96:644.

83. Orrego H, Blake J, Blendis L, et al. Long-term treatment of alcoholic liver disease with propylthiouracil. N Engl J Med 1987; 317:1421–1427.

84. Halle P, Pare P, Kaptein E, et al. Double-blind, controlled trial of propylthiouracil in patients with severe acute alcoholic hepatitis. Gastroenterology 1982; 82:925–931.

85. Serrano-Cancino H, Botero R, Jeffers L, et al. Treatment of severe alcoholic hepatitis with propylthiouracil. Am J Gastroenterol 1981; 76:194.

86. Rambaldi A, Gluud C. Meta-analysis of propylthiouracil for alcoholic liver disease – a Cochrane Hepato-Biliary Group Review. Liver 2001; 21:398–404.

87. Bucher NLR, Swaffield MN. Regulation of hepatic regeneration in rats by synergistic action of insulin and glucagons. Proc Natl Acad Sci USA 1975; 72:1157–1160.

88. Feher J, Cornides A, Romany A, et al. A prospective multicenter trial study of insulin and glucagon infusion therapy in acute alcoholic hepatitis. J Hepatol 1987; 5:224–231.

89. Baker AL, Jaspan JB, Haines NW, et al. A randomized clinical trial of insulin and glucagon infusion for treatment of alcoholic hepatitis. Progress report in 50 patients. Gastroenterology 1981; 80:1410–1414.

90. Bird G, Lau JY, Koskinas J, et al. Insulin and glucagon infusion in acute alcoholic hepatitis. A prospective randomized controlled trial. Hepatology 1991; 14:1097–1101.

91. Trinchet JC, Balkau B, Poupon RE, et al. Treatment of severe alcoholic hepatitis by infusion of insulin and glucagon: A multicenter sequential trial. Hepatology 1992; 15:76–81.

92. Mourelle M, Amezcua JL, Hong E. Effect of rioprostil and colchicine on CCl₄ – acute liver damage in rats. Relationship with plasma membrane lipids. Prostaglandins 1987; 33:869–877.

93. Mourelle M, Meza MA. Colchicine prevents D-galactosamine-induced hepatitis. J Hepatol 1989; 8:165–172.

94. Leoni S, Spagnuolo S, Conti Devergilis L, et al. Effect of colchicine on rat liver plasma membrane. Biochim Biophys Acta 1980; 596:451–455.

95. Bauer EA, Valle KJ. Colchicine-induced modulation of collagenase in human skin fibroblast cultures. Stimulation of enzyme synthesis in normal cells. J Invest Dermatol 1982; 79:398–402.

96. Erlich HP, Ross R, Bornstein P. Effects of antimicrotubular agents on the secretion of collagen. J Cell Biol 1974; 62:390–405.

97. Fell HB, Lawrence CE, Bagga MR, et al. The degradation of collagen in pig synovium in vitro and the effect of colchicine. Matrix 1989; 9:116–126.

98. Floridi A, Fini C, Palmerini CA, et al. Experimental liver cirrhosis: Effects of low and high doses of colchicine [Abstract]. Gastroenterology 1983; 84:1371.

99. Rojkind M, Kershenobich D. Effect of colchicine on collagen, albumin and transferrin synthesis by cirrhotic rat liver slices. Biochim Biophys Acta 1975; 378:415–423.

100. Rojkind M, Uribe M, Kershenobich D. Colchicine and the treatment of liver cirrhosis. Lancet 1973; 1:38–39.

101. Kershenobich D, Uribe M, Suarez GI, et al. Treatment of cirrhosis with colchicine. Gastroenterology 1979; 77:532–536.

102. Kershenobich D, Vargas F, Garcia-Tsao G, et al. Colchicine in the treatment of cirrhosis of the liver. N Engl J Med 1988; 318:1709–1713.

This randomized, double-blind, placebo-controlled study, which has been criticized because of a high dropout rate, showed that patients with cirrhosis had an improved survival with therapy with colchicine 1 mg/day for 5 days per week.

103. Akriviadis EA, Steindel H, Pinto PC, et al. Failure of colchicine to improve short-term survival in patients with alcoholic hepatitis. Gastroenterology 1990; 99:811–818.

104. Trinchet JC, Meargrand M, Callard P, et al. Treatment of alcoholic hepatitis with colchicine: Results of a randomized double blind trial. Gastroenterol Clin Biol 1989; 13:551–555.

105. Rambaldi A, Gluud C. Colchicine for alcoholic and non-alcoholic liver fibrosis and cirrhosis. Cochrane Database Syst Rev 2001; 3:CD002148.

106. Wallnofer H, Hanusch M. Essential phospholipids for therapy in liver diseases. Med Monatsschr 1973; 27:131–136.

107. Fassati P, Horejsi J, Fassati M, et al. Essential choline phospholipids and their effect on HBsAg and selected biochemical tests in cirrhosis of the liver. Cas Lek Cesk 1981; 120:56–70.

108. Giammona G, Marano P, Patti F. Polyunsaturated phosphatidylcholine in combination with vitamin B complex in the treatment of liver diseases in drug addicts. Clin Ter 1986; 119:373–377.

109. Lazzara A, Mauceri G, Costanzo V, et al. Use of polyunsaturated phosphatidylcholine associated with a vitamin B complex in the treatment of hepatic injuries caused by antitubercular agents. Clin Ter 1986; 118:423–426.

110. Kuntz E. Pilotstudie mit Polyenylphosphatidylcholin bei schwerer Leberinsuffizienz. Med Welt 1989; 40:1327–1329.

111. Aleynik SI, Leo MA, Ma X, et al. Polyenylphosphatidylcholine prevents carbon tetrachloride-induced lipid peroxidation while it attenuates liver fibrosis. J Hepatol 1997; 27:554–561.

112. Lieber CS, Robbins SJ, Li J-J, et al. Phosphatidylcholine protects against fibrosis and cirrhosis in the baboon. Gastroenterology 1994; 106:152–159.

113. Li J-J, Kim C-I, Leo MA, et al. Polyunsaturated lecithin prevents acetaldehyde-mediated hepatic collagen accumulation by stimulating collagenase activity in cultured lipocytes. Hepatology 1992; 15:373–381.

114. Lekim D, Graf E. Tierexperimentelle Studien zur Pharmakokinetik der 'essentiellen' Phospholipide (EPL). Drug Res 1976; 26:1772–1782.

115. Lieber CS. Alcoholic liver disease: new insights in pathogenesis lead to new treatments. J Hepatol 2000; 32:113–128.

116. Cao Q, Mak KM, Lieber CS. Dilinoleoylphosphatidylcholine decreases acetaldehyde-induced TNF-alpha generation in Kupffer cells of ethanol-fed rats. Biochem Biophys Res Commun 2002; 299:459–464.

117. Lieber CS, DeCarli LM, Mak KM, et al. Attenuation of alcohol-induced hepatic fibrosis by polyunsaturated lecithin. Hepatology 1990; 12:1390–1398.

118. Jenkins PJ, Portmann BP, Eddleston AL, et al. Use of polyunsaturated phosphatidylcholine in HBsAg negative chronic active hepatitis: Results of a prospective double blind control trial. Liver 1982; 2:77–81.

119. Panos MZ, Polson R, Johnson R, et al. Polyunsaturated phosphatidylcholine for acute alcoholic hepatitis: A double-blind, randomized, placebo-controlled trial. Eur J Gastroenterol Hepatol 1990; 2:351–355.

120. Lieber CS, Weiss DG, Groszmann R, et al. for the Veterans Affairs Cooperative Study 391 Group. II. Veterans Affairs Cooperative Study of polyenylphosphatidylcholine in alcoholic liver disease. Alcohol Clin Exp Res 2003; 27:1765–1772.

121. Starzl TE, Van Thiel D, Tzakis AG, et al. Orthotopic liver transplantation for alcoholic cirrhosis. JAMA 1988; 260:2542–2544.

122. Cowling T, Jennings LW, Goldstein RM, et al. Societal reintegration after liver transplantation: findings in alcohol-related and non-alcohol-related transplant recipients. Ann Surg 2004; 239:93–98.

123. Howard L, Fahy T, Wong P, et al. Psychiatric outcome in alcoholic liver transplant patients. Q J Med 1994; 87:731–736.

124. Vaillant GE. What can long-term follow-up teach us about relapse and prevention of relapse in addiction? Br J Addict 1988; 83:1147–1157.

125. Iasi MS, Vieira A, Anez CI, et al. Recurrence of alcohol ingestion in liver transplantation candidates. Transplant Proc 2003; 35:1123–1124.

126. Mendenhall CL, Seeff L, Diehl AM, et al. Antibodies to hepatitis B virus and hepatitis C virus in alcoholic hepatitis and cirrhosis: their prevalence and clinical relevance. The VA Cooperative Study Group (No. 119). Hepatology 1991; 14:581–589.

127. Pageaux GP, Souche B, Perney P, et al. Results and cost of orthotopic liver transplantation for alcoholic cirrhosis. Transplant Proc 1993; 25:1135–1136.

128. Belle SH, Beringer KC, Detre KM. Liver transplantation for alcoholic liver disease in the United States: 1988 to 1995. Liver Transpl Surg 1997; 3:212–219.

129. Wiesner RH, Lombardero M, Lake JR, et al. Liver transplantation for end-stage alcoholic liver disease: an assessment of outcomes. Liver Transpl Surg 1997; 3:231–239.

Patients undergoing liver transplantation for alcoholic liver disease had decreased survival, but this appeared to be related to the performance of transplantation at a later stage in their disease.

130. Spahr L, Rubbia-Brandt L, Frossard JL, et al. Combination of steroids with infliximab or placebo in severe alcoholic hepatitis: a randomized controlled pilot study. J Hepatol 2002; 37:448–455.

In this interesting pilot study comparing prednisone 40 mg/d and either infliximab 5 mg/kg i.v. or placebo at day 0 for severe alcoholic hepatitis, infliximab was well tolerated and the discriminant function significantly improved in patients treated with prednisone and infliximab, but not prednisone alone, at day 28.

131. Tilg H, Jalan R, Kaser A, et al. Anti-tumor necrosis factor-alpha monoclonal antibody therapy in severe alcoholic hepatitis. J Hepatol 2003; 38:419–425.

132. Bykov I, Jarvelainen H, Lindros K. L-carnitine alleviates alcohol-induced liver damage in rats: role of tumour necrosis factor-alpha. Alcohol Alcohol 2003; 38:400–406.

133. Minagawa M, Deng Q, Liu ZX, et al. Activated natural killer T cells induce liver injury by Fas and tumor necrosis factor-alpha during alcohol consumption. Gastroenterology 2004; 126:1387–1399.

134. Enomoto N, Takei Y, Hirose M, et al. Thalidomide prevents alcoholic liver injury in rats through suppression of Kupffer cell sensitization and TNF-alpha production. Gastroenterology 2002; 123:291–300.

135. Ronis MJ, Korourian S, Zipperman M, et al. Dietary saturated fat reduces alcoholic hepatotoxicity in rats by altering fatty acid metabolism and membrane composition. J Nutr 2004; 134:904–912.

136. Baltaziak M, Skrzydlewska E, Sulik A, et al. Green tea as an antioxidant which protects against alcohol induced injury in rats – a histopathological examination. Folia Morphol (Warsz) 2004; 63:123–126.

137. Tapiero H, Townsend DM, Tew KD. The role of carotenoids in the prevention of human pathologies. Biomed Pharmacother 2004; 58:100–110.

138. Tomita K, Azuma T, Kitamura N, et al. Pioglitazone prevents alcohol-induced fatty liver in rats through up-regulation of c-Met. Gastroenterology 2004; 126:873–885.

139. Lieber CS, Leo MA, Cao Q, et al. Silymarin retards the progression of alcohol-induced hepatic fibrosis in baboons. J Clin Gastroenterol 2003; 37:336–339.

140. Gueguen S, Pirollet P, Leroy P, et al. Changes in serum retinol, alpha-tocopherol, vitamin C, carotenoids, zinc and selenium after micronutrient supplementation during alcohol rehabilitation. J Am Coll Nutr 2003; 22:303–310.

141. Jablonska-Kaszewska I, Swlatkowska-Stodulska R, Lukaslak J, et al. Serum selenium levels in alcoholic liver disease. Med Sci Monit 2003; 9:15–18.

142. You M, Crabb DW. Recent advances in alcoholic liver disease II. Minireview: molecular mechanisms of alcoholic fatty liver. Am J Physiol Gastrointest Liver Physiol 2004; 287:G1–G6.

143. Ludwig J, Viggiano TR, McGill DB, et al. Nonalcoholic steatohepatitis: Mayo Clinic experiences with a hitherto unnamed disease. Mayo Clin Proc 1980; 55:434–438.

First recent study to describe NAFLD as a distinct pathological entity.

144. Schaffner F, Thaler H. Nonalcoholic fatty liver disease. Prog Liver Dis 1986; 8:283–298.

145. Angulo P. Nonalcoholic fatty liver disease. N Engl J Med 2002; 346(16):1221–1231.

146. Saadeh S, Younossi ZM. The spectrum of nonalcoholic fatty liver disease: From steatosis to nonalcoholic steatohepatitis. Cleve Clin J Med 2000; 67(2):96–104.

147. Neuschwander-Tetri BA, Caldwell SH. Nonalcoholic steatohepatitis: Summary of an AASLD single topic conference. Hepatology 2003; 37:1202–1219.

Excellent recent comprehensive review of all important clinical trials that addresses all important aspects of NAFLD from diagnosis to pathogenesis to management.

148. Mathiesen UL, Franzen LE, Fryden A, et al. The clinical significance of slightly to moderately increased liver transaminase values in asymptomatic patients. Scand J Gastroenterol 1999; 34:85–91.

149. Daniel S, Ben-Menachem T, Vasudevan G, et al. Prospective evaluation of unexplained chronic liver transaminase abnormalities in asymptomatic and symptomatic patients. Am J Gastroenterol 1999; 94:3010–3014.

150. Clark JM, Brancati FL, Diehl AM. Nonalcoholic fatty liver disease. Gastroenterology 2002; 122:1649–1657.

151. Sorbi D, McGill DB, Thistle JL, et al. An assessment of the role of liver biopsies in asymptomatic patients with chronic liver test abnormalities. Am J Gastroenterol 2000; 95:3206–3210.

153. Byron D, Minuk GY. Clinical hepatology: profile of an urban, hospital based practice. Hepatology 1996; 24:813–815.

153. Hilden M, Christoffersen P, Juhl E, et al. Liver histology in a 'normal' population: examination of 503 consecutive fatal traffic casualties. Scand J Gastroenterol 1977; 12:593–597.

154. Bellentani S, Saccoccio G, Masutti F, et al. Prevalence of and risk factors for hepatic steatosis in Northern Italy. Ann Intern Med 2000; 132:112–117.

155. Rashid M, Roberts EA. Nonalcoholic steatohepatitis in children. J Pediatr Gastroenterol Nutr 2000; 30:48–53.

156. Strauss RS, Barlow SE, Dietz WH. Prevalence of abnormal serum aminotransferase values in overweight and obese adolescents. J Pediatr 2000; 136:727–733.

157. Manton ND, Lipsett J, Moore DJ, et al. Non-alcoholic steatohepatitis in children and adolescents. Med J Aust 2000; 173:476–479.

158. Contos MJ, Cales W, Sterling RK, et al. Development of nonalcoholic fatty liver disease after orthotopic liver transplantation for cryptogenic cirrhosis. Liver Transpl 2001; 7:363–373.

159. Anderson T, Christoffersen P, Gluud C. The liver in consecutive patients with morbid obesity: a clinical morphological and biochemical study. Int J Obesity 1984; 8:107–115.

160. Teli MR, James OF, Burt AD, et al. The natural history of nonalcoholic fatty liver: a follow-up study. Hepatology 1995; 22:1714–1719.

161. Nasrallah SM, Wills CE Jr, Galambos JT. Hepatic morphology in obesity. Dig Dis Sci 1981; 26:325–327.

162. Marcos A, Fisher RA, Ham JM, et al. Selection and outcome of living donors for adult to adult right lobe transplantation. Transplantation 2000; 69:2410–2415.

163. Ground KEV. Prevalence of fatty liver in healthy adults accidentally killed. Aviat Space Environ Med 1984; 55:59–61.

164. Tominaga K, Kurata JH, Chen YK, et al. Prevalence of fatty liver in Japanese children and relationship to obesity: an epidemiological ultrasonographic survey. Dig Dis Sci 1995; 40:2002–2009.

165. Franzese A, Vajro P, Argenziano A, et al. Liver involvement in obese children: ultrasonography and liver enzyme levels at diagnosis and during follow-up in an Italian population. Dig Dis Sci 1997; 42:1428–1432.

166. Bacon BR, Farahvash MJ, Janney CG, et al. Nonalcoholic steatohepatitis: an expanded clinical entity. Gastroenterology 1994; 107:1103–1109.

167. Lee RG. Nonalcoholic steatohepatitis: tightening the morphological screws on a hepatic rambler. Hepatology 1995; 21:1742–1743.

168. Dulloo AG. Biomedicine. A sympathetic defense against obesity. Science 2002; 297:780–781.

169. Bachman ES, Dhillon H, Zhang CY, et al. betaAR signaling required for diet-induced thermogenesis and obesity resistance. Science 2002; 297:843–845.

170. Caldwell SH, Harris DM, Patrie JT, et al. Is NASH underdiagnosed among African Americans? Am J Gastroenterol 2002; 97:1496–1500.

171. Santos L, Molina EG, Jeffers LJ, et al. Prevalence of nonalcoholic steatohepatitis among ethnic groups. Gastroenterology 2001; 120:A117.

172. Squires RH, Lopez MJ. Steatohepatitis is a serious condition in Hispanic children. Hepatology 2000; 32:A418.

173. Kemmer NM, McKinney KH, Xiao S-Y, et al. High prevalence of NASH among Mexican American females with type II diabetes mellitus. Gastroenterology 2001; 120:A117.

175. Weston SR, Leyden WA, Murphy R, et al. Racial/ethnic distribution of newly diagnosed non-alcoholic fatty liver among participants of the chronic liver disease surveillance study. Hepatology 2002; 36:A405.

175. Perry AC, Applegate EB, Jackson ML, et al. Racial differences in visceral adipose tissue but not anthropometric markers of health-related variables. J Appl Physiol 2000; 89:636–643.

176. Struben VMD, Hespenheide EE, Caldwell S. Nonalcoholic steatohepatitis and cryptogenic cirrhosis within kindreds. Am J Med 2000; 108:9–13.

177. Willner IR, Waters B, Patil SR, et al. Ninety patients with nonalcoholic steatohepatitis: insulin resistance, familial tendency, and severity of disease. Am J Gastroenterol 2001; 96:2957–2961.

178. National Institutes of Health. Third report of the national cholesterol education program expert panel on detection, evaluation and treatment of high blood cholesterol in adults (Adult treatment panel III). 2001; NIH publication available at <http://www.nhlbi.nih.gov/guidelines/cholesterol/atp3full.pdf >.

179. Lyznicki JM, Young DC, Riggs JA, et al. Council on Scientific Affairs AM. Obesity: assessment and management in primary care. Am Fam Physician. 2001; 63:2185–2196.

180. Luyckx FH, Desaive C, Thiry A, et al. Liver abnormalities in severely obese subjects: effect of drastic weight loss after gastroplasty. Int J Obes Relat Metab Disord 1998; 22:222–226.

181. Anderson T, Gluud C. Liver morphology in morbid obesity: a literature study. Int J Obesity 1984; 8:97–106.

182. De Craemer D, Pauwels M, Van den Branden C. Alterations of peroxisomes in steatosis of the human liver: a quantitative study. Hepatology 1995; 22:744–752.

183. Caldwell SH, Swerdlow RH, Khan EM, et al. Mitochondrial abnormalities in non-alcoholic steatohepatitis. J Hepatol 1999; 31:430–434.

184. Wasserman JM, Thung SN, Berman R, et al. Hepatic Weber-Christian disease. Semin Liver Dis 2001; 21:115–118.

185. Van Steenbergen W, Lanckmans S. Liver disturbances in obesity and diabetes mellitus. Int J Obes Relat Metab Disord 1995; 19:S27–S36.

186. Vila MR, Gamez J, Solano A, et al. Uncoupling protein-1 mRNA expression in lipomas from patients bearing pathogenic mitochondrial DNA mutations. Biochem Biophys Res Commun 2000; 278:800–802.

187. Mansouri A, Gaou I, Fromenty B, et al. Premature oxidative aging of hepatic mitochondrial DNA in Wilson's disease. Gastroenterology 1997; 113:599–605.

188. Cotrim HP, Andrade ZA, Parana R, et al. Nonalcoholic steatohepatitis: a toxic liver disease in industrial workers [see comments]. Liver 1999; 19:299–304.

189. Cassagnou M, Boruchowicz A, Guillemot F, et al. Hepatic steatosis revealing celiac disease: a case complicated by transitory liver failure [Letter]. Am J Gastroenterol 1996; 91:1291–1292.

190. Partin JS, Partin JC, Schubert WK, et al. Liver ultrastructure in abetalipoproteinemia: evolution to micronodular cirrhosis. Gastroenterology 1974; 67:107–118.

191. Simon JB, Manley PN, Brien JF, et al. Amiodarone hepatotoxicity simulating alcoholic liver disease. N Engl J Med 1984; 311:167–172.

192. Cai Q, Bensen M, Greene R, et al. Tamoxifen-induced transient multifocal hepatic fatty infiltration. Am J Gastroenterol 2000; 95:277–279.

193. Cote HC, Brumme ZL, Craib KJ, et al. Changes in mitochondrial DNA as a marker of nucleoside toxicity in HIV-infected patients. N Engl J Med 2002; 346:811–820.

194. Dahl MG, Gregory MM, Scheuer PJ. Liver damage due to methotrexate in patients with psoriasis. Br Med J 1971; 1:625–630.

195. James O, Day C. Non-alcoholic steatohepatitis: another disease of affluence. Lancet 1999; 353:1634–1636.

Important study that shed light on the 'two-hit' hypothesis in the pathogenesis of NAFLD.

196. Day CP. Non-alcoholic steatohepatitis (NASH): where are we now and where are we going? Gut 2002; 50:585–588.

197. Marchesini G, Brizi M, Morselli-Labate AM, et al. Association of nonalcoholic fatty liver disease with insulin resistance. Am J Med 1999; 107:450–455.

198. Reynet C, Kahn CR. Rad: a member of the Ras family overexpressed in muscle of type II diabetic humans. Science 1993; 262:1441–1444.

199. Maddux BA, Sbraccia P, Kumakura S, et al. Membrane glycoprotein PC-1 and insulin resistance in non-insulin-dependent diabetes mellitus. Nature 1995; 373:448–451.

200. Cohen B, Novick D, Rubinstein M. Modulation of insulin activities by leptin. Science 1996; 274:1185–1188.

201. Boden G. Role of fatty acids in the pathogenesis of insulin resistance and NIDDM. Diabetes 1997; 46:3–10.

202. Hotamisligil GS, Peraldi SP, Budavari A, et al. IRS-1-mediated inhibition of insulin receptor tyrosine kinase activity in TNF-alpha- and obesity-induced insulin resistance. Science 1996; 271:665–668.

203. Fan C-Y, Pan J, Usuda N, et al. Steatohepatitis, spontaneous peroxisome proliferation and liver tumors in mice lacking peroxisomal fatty acyl-CoA oxidase: implications for peroxisome proliferator-activated receptor alpha natural ligand metabolism. J Biol Chem 1998; 273:15639–15645.

204. Chavin KD, Yang SQ, Lin HZ, et al. Obesity induces expression of uncoupling protein-2 in hepatocytes and promotes liver ATP depletion. J Biol Chem 1999; 274:5692–5700.

205. Sanyal AJ, Campbell-Sargent C, Mirshahi F, et al. Nonalcoholic steatohepatitis: association of insulin resistance and mitochondrial abnormalities. Gastroenterology 2001; 120:1183–1192.

206. Cortez-Pinto H, Chatham J, Chacko VP, et al. Alterations in liver ATP homeostasis in human nonalcoholic steatohepatitis: a pilot study. JAMA 1999; 282:1659–1664.

207. Itoh S, Yougel T, Kawagoe K. Comparison between nonalcoholic steatohepatitis and alcoholic hepatitis. Am J Gastroenterol 1987; 82:650–654.

208. Angulo P, Keach JC, Batts KP, et al. Independent predictors of liver fibrosis in patients with nonalcoholic steatohepatitis. Hepatology 1999; 30:1356–1362.

Important work on the predictors of fibrosis in patients with NAFLD.

209. Bonkovsky HL, Jawaid Q, Tortorelli K, et al. Non-alcoholic steatohepatitis and iron: increased prevalence of mutations of the HFE gene in nonalcoholic steatohepatitis. J Hepatol 1999; 31:421–429.

210. Van Ness MM, Diehl AM. Is liver biopsy useful in the evaluation of patients with chronically elevated liver enzymes? Ann Intern Med 1989; 111:473–478.

211. Becker U, Deis A, Sorensen TI, et al. Prediction of risk of liver disease by alcohol intake, sex, and age: a prospective population study. Hepatology 1996; 23:1025–1029.

212. Saadeh S, Younossi ZM, Remer EM, et al. The utility of radiological imaging in nonalcoholic fatty liver disease. Gastroenterology 2002; 123:745–750.

First prospective study to evaluate the utility of the 3 most used imaging studies in the diagnosis of NAFLD.

213. Joseph AE, Saverymuttu SH, al-Sam S, et al. Comparison of liver histology with ultrasonography in assessing diffuse parenchymal liver disease. Clin Radiol 1991; 43:26–31.

214. Debaere C, Rigauts H, Laukens P. Transient focal fatty liver infiltration mimicking liver metastasis. J Belge Radiol 1998; 81:174–175.

215. Mitchell DG. Focal manifestations of diffuse liver disease at MR imaging. Radiology 1992; 185:1–11.

216. Longo R, Pollesello P, Ricci C, et al. Proton MR spectroscopy in quantitative in vivo determination of fat content in human liver steatosis. J Magn Reson Imaging 1995; 5:281–285.

217. Matteoni CA, Younossi ZM, Gramlich T, et al. Nonalcoholic fatty liver disease: a spectrum of clinical and pathological severity. Gastroenterology 1999; 116:1413–1419.

This retrospective study was the first to show the risk of progression of NAFLD to more advanced fibrosis and cirrhosis, thereby, conflicting with the earlier belief that NAFLD had a benign course.

218. Brunt EM, Janney CG, Di Bisceglie AM, et al. Nonalcoholic steatohepatitis: a proposal for grading and staging the histological lesions. Am J Gastroenterol 1999; 94:2467–2474.

Comprehensive study of a pathological scoring system of grading and staging the various histopathological lesions of NAFLD.

219. Pinto HC, Baptista A, Camilo ME, et al. Nonalcoholic steatohepatitis: clinico-pathological comparison with alcoholic hepatitis in ambulatory and hospitalized patients. Dig Dis Sci 1996; 41:172–179.

220. Lee RG. Nonalcoholic steatohepatitis: a study of 49 patients. Hum Pathol 1989; 20:594–598.

221. Dixon JB, Bhathal PS, O'Brien PE. Nonalcoholic fatty liver disease: predictors of nonalcoholic steatohepatitis and liver fibrosis in the severely obese. Gastroenterology 2001; 121:91–100.

222. Fassio E, Alvarez E, Dominguez N, et al. Natural history of nonalcoholic steatohepatitis: A longitudinal study of repeat liver biopsies. Hepatology 2004; 40:820–826.

223. Sanyal AJ, American Gastroenterological Association. AGA technical review on nonalcoholic fatty liver disease. Gastroenterology 2002; 123:1705–1725.

224. Powell EE, Cooksley WGE, Hanson R, et al. The natural history of nonalcoholic steatohepatitis: a follow-up study of forty-two patients for up to 21 years. Hepatology 1990; 11:74–80.

225. Caldwell SH, Oelsner DH, Iezzoni JC, et al. Cryptogenic cirrhosis: clinical characterization and risk factors for underlying disease. Hepatology 1999; 29:664–669.

226. Poonawala A, Nair SP, Thuluvath PJ. Prevalence of obesity and diabetes in patients with cryptogenic cirrhosis: a case-control study. Hepatology 2000; 32:689–692.

227. Sakugawa H, Nakasone H, Nakayoshi T, et al. Clinical characteristics of patients with cryptogenic liver cirrhosis in Okinawa, Japan. Hepatogastroenterology 2003; 50:2005–2008.

228. Ong J, Younossi ZM, Reddy V, et al. Cryptogenic cirrhosis and posttransplantation nonalcoholic fatty liver disease. Liver Transpl 2001; 7:797–801.

229. Shimada M, Hashimoto E, Taniai M, et al. Hepatocellular carcinoma in patients with non-alcoholic steatohepatitis. J Hepatol 2002; 37:154–160.

230. Bugianesi E, Leone N, Vanni E, et al. Expanding the natural history of nonalcoholic steatohepatitis from cryptogenic cirrhosis to hepatocellular carcinoma. Gastroenterology 2002; 123:134–140.

231. Brodkin CA, Daniell W, Checkoway H, et al. Hepatic ultrasonic changes in workers exposed to perchloroethylene. Occup Environ Med 1995; 52:679–685.

232. Saksena S, Johnson J, Ouiff SP, et al. Diet and exercise: important first steps in therapy of NASH. Hepatology 1999; 30:A436.

233. Bertram SR, Venter I, Stewart RI. Weight loss in obese women – exercise v. dietary education. S Afr Med J 1990; 78:15–18.

234. Tuomilehto J, Lindstrom J, Eriksson JG, et al. Prevention of type 2 diabetes mellitus by changes in lifestyle among subjects with impaired glucose tolerance. N Engl J Med 2001; 344:1343–1350.

235. Jones NL, Killian KJ. Exercise limitation in health and disease. N Engl J Med 2000; 343:632–641.

236. van Baak MA. Exercise training and substrate utilisation in obesity. Int J Obes Relat Metab Disord 1999; 23:S11–S17.

237. Ueno T, Sugawara H, Sujaku K, et al. Therapeutic effects of restricted diet and exercise in obese patients with fatty liver. J Hepatol 1997; 27:103–107.

238. Palmer M, Schaffner F. Effect of weight reduction on hepatic abnormalities in overweight patients. Gastroenterology 1990; 99:1408–1413.

239. Drenick EJ, Simmons F, Murphy JF. Effect on hepatic morphology of treatment of obesity by fasting, reducing diets and small bowel bypass. N Engl J Med 1970; 282:829–834.

240. Andersen T, Gluud C, Franzmann M-B, et al. Hepatic effects of dietary weight loss in morbidly obese subjects. J Hepatol 1991; 12:224–229.

241. Vajro P, Franzese A, Valerio G, et al. Lack of efficacy of ursodeoxycholic acid for the treatment of liver abnormalities in obese children. J Pediatr 2000; 136:739–743.

242. Kraus WE, Houmard JA, Duscha BD, et al. Effects of the amount and intensity of exercise on plasma lipoproteins. N Engl J Med 2002; 347:1483–1492.

243. Spieth LE, Harnish JD, Lenders CM, et al. A low-glycemic index diet in the treatment of pediatric obesity. Arch Pediatr Adolesc Med 2000; 154:947–951.

244. Vessby B. Dietary fat and insulin action in humans. Br J Nutr 2000; 83:S91–S96.

245. Kurihara T, Adachi Y, Yamagata M, et al. Role of eicosapentaenoic acid in lipid metabolism in the liver, with special reference to experimental fatty liver. Clin Ther 1994; 16:830–837.

246. Nanji AA, Sadrzadeh SM, Yang EK, et al. Dietary saturated fatty acids: a novel treatment for alcoholic liver disease. Gastroenterology 1995; 109:547–554.

247. Lanza-Jacoby S, Smythe C, Phetteplace H, et al. Adaptation to a fish oil diet before inducing sepsis in rats prevents fatty infiltration of the liver. J Parenter Enteral Nutr 1992; 16:353–358.

248. Kolanowski J. A risk-benefit assessment of anti-obesity drugs. Drug Safety 1999; 20:119–131.

249. Harrison SA, Fincke C, Helinski D, et al. Orlistat treatment in obese, non-alcoholic steatohepatitis patients: a pilot study. Hepatology 2002; 36:A406.

250. Mun EC, Blackburn GL, Matthews JB. Current status of medical and surgical therapy for obesity. Gastroenterology 2001; 120:669–681.

251. Silverman EM, Sapala JA, Appelman HD. Regression of hepatic steatosis in morbidly obese persons after gastric bypass. Am J Clin Pathol 1995; 104:23–31.

252. Ackerman NB. Protein supplementation in the management of degenerating liver function after jejunoileal bypass. Surg Gynecol Obstetr 1979; 149:8–14.

253. Drenick EJ, Fisler J, Johnson D. Hepatic steatosis after intestinal bypass – prevention and reversal by metronidazole, irrespective of proteincalorie malnutrition. Gastroenterology 1982; 82:535–548.

254. Laurin J, Lindor KD, Crippin JS, et al. Ursodeoxycholic acid or clofibrate in the treatment of non-alcohol-induced steatohepatitis: a pilot study. Hepatology 1996; 23:1464–1467.

255. Guma G, Viola L, Thome M, et al. Ursodeoxycholic acid in the treatment of nonalcoholic steatohepatitis: results of a prospective clinical controlled trial. Hepatology 1997; 26:A387.

256. Ceriani R, Bunati S, Morini L, et al. Effect of ursodeoxycholic acid plus diet in patients with nonalcoholic steatohepatitis. Hepatology 1998; 28:A386.

257. Mendez-Sanchez N, Gonzalez V, Pichardo-Bahena R, et al. Weight reduction and ursodeoxycholic acid in subjects with nonalcoholic fatty liver disease: a randomized, double-blind, placebo-controlled trial. Hepatology 2002; 36:A412.

258. Lindor KD, Kowdley KV, Heathcote EJ, et al. Ursodeoxycholic acid for treatment of nonalcoholic steatohepatitis: results of a randomized trial. Hepatology 2004; 39(3):770–778.

A multicenter randomized clinical trial that addressed the role of UDCA in the management of NAFLD.

259. Lavine JE. Vitamin E treatment of nonalcoholic steatohepatitis in children: a pilot study. J Pediatr 2000; 136:734–738.

260. Hasegawa T, Yoneda M, Nakamura K, et al. Plasma transforming growth factor-β1 level and efficacy of α-tocopherol in patients with non-alcoholic steatohepatitis: a pilot study. Aliment Pharmacol 2001; 15:1667–1672.

261. Harrison SA, Torgerson S, Ward J, et al. Vitamin E and vitamin C treatment improves fibrosis in patients with nonalcoholic steatohepatitis. Am J Gastroenterol 2003; 98:2485–2490.

262. Lu SC. S-adenosylmethionine. Int J Biochem Cell Bio 2000; 32:391–395.

263. Abdelmalek MF, Angulo P, Jorgensen RA, et al. Betaine, a promising new agent for patients with nonalcoholic steatohepatitis: results of a pilot study. Am J Gastroenterol 2001; 96:2711–2717.

264. Venkataramanan R, Ramachandran V, Komoroski BJ, et al. Milk thistle, a herbal supplement, decreases the activity of CYP3A4 and uridine diphosphoglucuronosyl transferase in human hepatocyte cultures. Drug Metab Dispos 2000; 28:1270–1273.

265. Facchini FS, Hua NW, Stoohs RA. Effect of iron depletion in carbohydrate-intolerant patients with clinical evidence of nonalcoholic fatty liver disease. Gastroenterology 2002; 122:931–939.

266. DeFronzo RA. Pharmacologic therapy for type 2 diabetes mellitus. Ann Intern Med 1999; 131:281–303.

267. Caldwell SH, Hespenheide EE, Redick JA, et al. A pilot study of a thiazolidinedione, troglitazone, in nonalcoholic steatohepatitis. Am J Gastroenterol 2001; 96:519–525.

268. Acosta RC, Molina EG, O'Brien CB, et al. The use of pioglitazone in nonalcoholic steatohepatitis. Gastroenterology 2001; 120:A546.

269. Neuschwander-Tetri BA, Brunt EM, Bacon BR, et al. Histological improvement in NASH following increased insulin sensitivity with the PPAR-α ligand rosiglitazone for 48 weeks. Hepatology 2002; 36:A379.

270. Galli A, Crabb DW, Ceni E, et al. Antidiabetic thiazolidinediones inhibit collagen synthesis and hepatic stellate cell activation in vivo and in vitro. Gastroenterology 2002; 122:1924–1940.

271. Azuma T, Tomita K, Kato S, et al. A pilot study of a thiazolidinediones, pioglitazone, in nonalcoholic steatohepatitis. Hepatology 2002; 36:A406.

272. Sanyal AJ, Contos MJ, Sargeant C, et al. A randomized controlled pilot study of pioglitazone and vitamin E versus vitamin E for non-alcoholic steatohepatitis. Hepatology 2002; 36:A382.

273. Promrat K, Lutchman G, Uwaifo GI, et al. A pilot study of pioglitazone treatment for nonalcoholic steatohepatitis. Hepatology 2004; 39:188–196.

274. Vamecq J, Latruffe N. Medical significance of peroxisome proliferator activated receptors. Lancet 1999; 354:141–148.

275. Ribon V, Johnson JH, Camp HS, et al. Thiazolidinediones and insulin resistance: peroxisome proliferator-activated receptor α activation stimulates expression of the CAP gene. Proc Natl Acad Sci USA 1998; 95:14751–14756.

276. Kelly IE, Han TS, Walsh K, et al. Effects of a thiazolidinedione compound on body fat and fat distribution of patients with type 2 diabetes. Diabetes Care 1999; 22:288–293.

277. Lenhard JM, Kliewer SA, Paulik MA, et al. Effects of troglitazone and metformin on glucose and lipid metabolism: alterations of two distinct molecular pathways. Biochem Pharmacol 1997; 54:801–808.

278. Aubert J, Champigny O, Saint-Marc P, et al. Up-regulation of UCP-2 gene expression by PPAR agonists in preadipose and adipose cells. Biochem Biophys Res Commun 1997; 238:606–611.

279. Arioglu E, Duncan-Morin J, Sebring N, et al. Efficacy and safety of troglitazone in the treatment of lipodystrophy syndromes. Ann Intern Med 2000; 133:263–274.

280. Lin HZ, Yang SQ, Chuckaree C, et al. Metformin reverses fatty liver disease in obese, leptin-deficient mice. Nat Med 2000; 6:998–1003.

281. Coyle WJ, Delaney N, Yoshihashi A, et al. Metformin treatment in patients with nonalcoholic steatohepatitis normalizes LFTs and improves histology. Gastroenterology 1999; 116:A1198.

282. Urso R, Visco-Comandini U. Metformin in non-alcoholic steatohepatitis [Letter]. Lancet 2002; 359:355–356.

283. Marchesini G, Brizi M, Bianchi G, et al. Metformin in non-alcoholic steatohepatitis [Letter]. Lancet 2001; 358:893–894.

284. Zhou G, Myers R, Li Y, et al. Role of AMP-activated protein kinase in mechanism of metformin action. J Clin Invest 2001; 108: 1167–1174.

285. Chiasson JL, Josse RG, Gomis R, et al., for the Stop-NIDDM Trial Research Group. Acarbose for prevention of type 2 diabetes mellitus: the STOP-NIDDM randomised trial. Lancet 2002; 359:2072–2077.

286. Santomauro AT, Boden G, Silva ME, et al. Overnight lowering of free fatty acids with acipimox improves insulin resistance and glucose tolerance in obese diabetic and nondiabetic subjects. Diabetes 1999; 48:1836–1841.

287. Nestler JE, Jakubowicz DJ, Iuorno MJ. Role of inositolphosphoglycan mediators of insulin action in the polycystic ovary syndrome. J Pediatr Endocrinol 2000; 13:1295–1298.

288. Saibara T, Onishi S, Ogawa Y, et al. Bezafibrate for tamoxifen-induced non-alcoholic steatohepatitis [Letter]. Lancet 1999; 353:1802.

289. Basaranoglu M, Acbay O, Sonsuz A. A controlled trial of gemfibrozil in the treatment of patients with nonalcoholic steatohepatitis [Letter; Comment]. J Hepatol 1999; 31:384.

290. Horlander JC, Kwo PY, Cummings OW, et al. Atorvastatin for the treatment of NASH. Gastroenterology 2001; 120:A544.

291. Nair S, Wiseman M. HMG-CoA reductase inhibitors in non-alcoholic fatty liver disease: is their potential hepatotoxicity an issue in these patients? A case control study based on histology. Hepatology 2002; 36:A409.

292. Phillips PS, Haas RH, Bannykh S, et al. Statin-associated myopathy with normal creatine kinase levels. Ann Intern Med 2002; 137: 581–585.

293. Czaja AJ. Recurrence of nonalcoholic steatohepatitis after liver transplantation [Editorial]. Liver Transplant Surg 1997; 3:185–186.

294. Molloy RM, Komorowski R, Varma RR. Recurrent nonalcoholic steatohepatitis and cirrhosis after liver transplantation. Liver Transplant Surg 1997; 3:177–178.

295. Kim WR, Poterucha JJ, Porayko MK, et al. Recurrence of nonalcoholic steatohepatitis following liver transplantation. Transplantation 1996; 62:1802–1805.

296. Cassarino DS, Swerdlow RH, Parks JK, et al. Cyclosporine A increases resting mitochondrial membrane potential in SY5Y cells and reverses the depressed mitochondrial membrane potential of Alzheimer's disease cybrids. Biochem Biophys Res Commun 1998; 248:168–173.

CHAPTER THIRTY-SEVEN

37

Drug-induced hepatic injury (prevention)

Geoffrey C. Farrell and Shivakumar Chitturi

INTRODUCTION

Definition and sources of hepatotoxins

Drug-induced liver disease encompasses hepatotoxicity resulting from chemicals ingested for therapeutic, nutritional or recreational purposes. It therefore includes drugs of abuse, herbal remedies as well as industrial, agricultural and household hepatotoxins.[1,2] This review will focus primarily on liver injury related to medically prescribed agents, emphasizing aspects of prevention and management. For an in-depth discussion of pathogenesis and details of liver toxicity associated with individual drugs and other hepatotoxins, the reader is referred to recent reviews and monographs on the subject.[1,3–6]

The phrase *drug-induced hepatic or liver injury* is preferred to *drug-induced liver disease* because liver histology is lacking in many cases. An international consensus meeting classified hepatic drug reactions based on changes in conjugated bilirubin, serum alanine aminotransferase (ALT), aspartate aminotransferase (AST), and alkaline phosphatase (SAP). In application to define patterns of liver injury, these liver tests are expressed as multiples of the upper limit of their normal range (ULN).[7] Liver injury is defined *either* by an ALT increase of two to three times above ULN, *or* by conjugated bilirubin increase twofold above ULN, *or* alternatively by raised AST, bilirubin, or SAP (one of these indices should be twice above ULN). Hepatic injury is further subdivided into 3 categories: *hepatocellular* (ALT $>2 \times$ ULN with normal SAP and/or ALT/SAP ratio $=5 \times$ ULN), *cholestatic* (SAP $>2 \times$ ULN and/or ALT/SAP ratio $=2$), or *mixed* (both ALT and SAP raised, ALT/SAP ratio between 2 and 5).[7]

Clinical and general significance

Hepatotoxicity constitutes only 6% of all adverse drug reactions. However, it is disproportionately represented among instances of serious drug toxicity, and case fatality rates exceed those attributable to other liver diseases of similar pathology.[8] For example, the mortality from severe isoniazid hepatitis ($\approx$10%) is considerably higher than that associated with hepatitis A virus infection (less than 1%).[9]

Currently, medication-related liver injury has surpassed viral hepatitis as a major cause of acute liver failure in many countries.[10] In the United States, acetaminophen hepatotoxicity (39%) is the leading cause of acute liver failure (ALF group); other idiosyncratic drug reactions accounted for 13% of cases of acute liver failure.[10]

Incorrect recognition of drug toxicity can lead to errors in management. For instance, a patient presenting with right hypochondrial pain due to erythromycin-related acute cholestatic hepatitis may be subjected to a needless laparotomy on the presumption of gallbladder disease.[2] Likewise, failure to appreciate drug-induced acute liver injury in a person known to have quiescent chronic viral hepatitis could lead to commencement of potentially long, hazardous, and expensive antiviral therapy. Finally, from the perspective of manufacturers, if a new drug shows proclivity for liver injury, then approval by regulatory agencies is usually withheld; additional clinical trial data are sought, and this often leads to restrictions in prescribing indications after approval.[11] Liver toxicity remains the principal cause for drug withdrawal after marketing.[11] Recent examples include troglitazone, trovafloxacin, fialuridine, bromfenac, ebrotidine, tolcapone, and nefazodone.[12–18]

Clinicopathologic syndromes

The diversity of clinicopathologic expression of drug-induced liver disease is displayed in Table 37.1. Only the predominant mode of liver injury associated with an individual drug is represented. It is noteworthy that while 'signature patterns' of clinical and laboratory features may be noteworthy for many drug reactions, more than one pattern of hepatotoxicity can occur with any particular drug. Likewise, other liver diseases may present with similar syndromes, emphasizing the need for careful clinicopathologic consideration of all possible etiologies. Although the clinicopathologic syndromes caused by drug-induced liver injury have remained unchanged, the most common causative agents at any time mirror those currently used in society and clinical practice. For example, hepatic veno-occlusive disease was archetypically associated with pyrrolizidine alkaloid toxicity (from drinking bush teas and crop contamination).[2,19] More recently, chemotherapeutic agents have been implicated as a major cause of this reaction.[20] Likewise, currently, liver injury from halothane and chlorpromazine (very commonly incriminated agents in the 1960s) is now far less common than antibiotic or nonsteroidal antiinflammatory drug-associated hepatitis.[21]

Hepatocellular injury is by far the most common type of hepatic adverse drug reaction. Further clinicopathologic classification is possible, based on the duration of liver injury (acute or chronic),

Table 37.1 Clinicopathologic classification of drug-induced liver disease

Category	Description	Examples
Hepatic adaptation	No symptoms; raised GGT and SAP (occasionally ALT) Hyperbilirubinemia	Phenytoin Rifampin
Dose-dependent hepatotoxicity	Short latent period; zonal, bridging or massive hepatic necrosis; marked rise in ALT	Acetaminophen, nicotinic acid
Other cytopathic, acute steatosis	Microvesicular steatosis, lactic acidosis	Valproic acid, didanosine, HAART, L-asparaginase
Acute hepatitis	Onset 1–20 weeks; hepatitis symptoms, ALT >5 × ULN; occasional hypersensitivity features	Isoniazid, sulfonamides, halothane, ketoconazole, terbinafine, troglitazone
Chronic hepatitis	Duration >3 months; interface hepatitis, bridging necrosis, cirrhosis; occasional autoantibodies	Diclofenac, nitrofurantoin, mesalamine, minocycline
Granulomatous hepatitis	Hepatic granulomas, raised liver enzymes especially SAP, GGT	Allopurinol, carbamazepine, quinine, hydralazine
Steatohepatitis	Steatosis, ballooning change, Mallory's hyaline, pericellular or perisinusoidal fibrosis, cirrhosis	Amiodarone, perhexiline, tamoxifen
Cholestasis	See Table 37.4	
Vascular disorders	Dilated sinusoids, peliosis hepatis, noncirrhotic portal hypertension, nodular regenerative hyperplasia, sinusoidal obstruction syndrome (veno-occlusive disease)	Anabolic steroids, oral contraceptives, cancer chemotherapy agents
Liver tumors	Focal nodular hyperplasia, hepatic adenoma, hepatocellular carcinoma, angiosarcoma	Anabolic steroids, oral contraceptives, vinyl chloride, arsenic, 6-thioguanine

GGT, gamma glutamyl transpeptidase; SAP, serum alkaline phosphatase; ALT, alanine aminotransferase; ULN, upper limit of normal; HAART, highly active antiretroviral therapy.

special features on liver biopsy (microvesicular steatosis, steatohepatitis, or granulomatous hepatitis), or characteristics of dose-dependency. Likewise, cholestatic drug reactions are grouped together based on duration (acute or chronic) or on histology ('bland cholestasis,' cholestatic hepatitis with or without significant bile duct injury) (Table 37.2). Syndromes of chronic cholestatic syndromes can closely mimic either primary biliary cirrhosis or sclerosing cholangitis.

The range of hepatic lesions resulting from vascular injury includes hepatic sinusoidal dilatation, peliosis hepatis, through to sinusoidal obstruction syndrome (or veno-occlusive disease), nodular regenerative hyperplasia, and portal fibrosis with non-cirrhotic portal hypertension. Finally, prolonged use of certain drugs can promote formation of hepatic neoplasms such as hepatic adenoma and, rarely, hepatocellular carcinoma and angiosarcoma (see Table 37.1).

Epidemiology

Previous pharmacoepidemiological studies have estimated the incidence of drug-induced hepatitis at approximately 8.9 to 406 per million persons per year.[21] The methodologies of these studies have been criticized for their retrospective design, lack of follow-up, and insufficient detail about viral hepatitis testing. Further, some of these reports have preceded the discovery of the hepatitis C virus. Contemporary estimates based on two prospective population-based French and Spanish studies cite lower figures, between 7.4 to 8 per million persons exposed per year.[21,22]

It is estimated that only about 10% of cases of serious liver injury are reported; the figures for milder reactions could be even lower (2–4%).[23] Regional differences in spontaneous drug reaction reporting also account for the heterogeneity in population-based estimates of hepatotoxicity. For example, when assessed from voluntary adverse reaction reports, the annual incidence of drug hepatotoxicity is 2.2 and 0.9 per 100 000 persons for Sweden and France, respectively.[24]

The occurrence of hepatic adverse reactions is nonlinear with time; most reactions occur within 6 months of drug ingestion, and most reports of hepatic adverse drug reactions are made within 2 years of approval of the new drug. Therefore, conventional indices such as incidence or prevalence are less meaningful than the risk of liver injury for an individual drug. This is expressed as *frequency* of reactions per persons exposed to a particular compound.[25] For the majority of drugs, the risk of hepatotoxicity ranges from 1 in 1000 to 1 in 100 000 per persons exposed. The risk is even lower with drugs such as minocycline (1 in a million).[8] However, these figures are only crude estimates. What is more important clinically is that hepatotoxicity can occur at greater frequencies (0.1–2%) in persons with particular sets of demographic, medical, and environmental risk factors (see below).

PATHOGENESIS

Dose-dependent hepatotoxins

Unlike several industrial compounds, only a small proportion of current drugs operate as *dose-dependent* hepatotoxins.[2,3] Examples include acetaminophen, cancer chemotherapeutic agents such as busulfan and cyclophosphamide, and the antimalarial, amodiaquine. Dose-dependent hepatic injury occurs after a short

Table 37.2 Syndromes of drug-induced cholestasis

Syndrome	Clinical and biochemical features	Typical examples	Recent additions
Acute			
Cholestasis without hepatitis	Pruritus, SAP >3 × ULN, transient increase in ALT; bilirubin < 12 mg/dl	Estrogens, anabolic steroids	Infliximab Fosinopril
Cholestasis with hepatitis	Right upper quadrant or generalized abdominal pain; jaundice; can simulate acute cholangitis; SAP >3 × ULN in 70%, ALT 2–5 × ULN	Chlorpromazine, other phenothiazines, macrolides, amoxicillin-clavulanate, sulindac, oxypenicillins, azathioprine	Ticlopidine, irbesartan, gatifloxacin, levofloxacin, risperidone, glimepiride, pyritinol, rofecoxib
Cholestasis with bile duct injury	Features simulate acute cholangitis	Dextropropoxyphene, flucloxacillin	Terbinafine, ramipril, ciprofloxacin
Chronic			
Vanishing bile duct syndrome	Resembles primary biliary cirrhosis; antimitochondrial antibodies absent	Chlorpromazine, flucloxacillin, oxypenicillins	Ramipril
Large bile duct strictures	Resembles primary sclerosing cholangitis	Floxuridine, intralesional scolicidal agents (absolute alcohol, 2% formaldehyde, hypertonic saline)	

latent period, usually within 1 to 5 days. Typical ALT values exceed 1000 IU/L and liver histology shows zonal, bridging, or massive hepatic necrosis. Dose-dependent toxins are endowed with 'intrinsic hepatotoxic potential,' implying that the circumstances in which they cause liver injury are predictable.[3] Thus, hepatotoxicity occurs when their chemically reactive metabolites exceed a predetermined threshold. However, host factors can profoundly influence the formation of these metabolites, as well as 'tissue resistance' to their accumulation (such as antioxidant reserves).

Acetaminophen (APAP) hepatotoxicity is a model of dose-dependent hepatotoxicity. In keeping with this paradigm, liver injury occurs when a threshold dose is exceeded (150 mg/kg body weight). Onset of toxicity is rapid (24–48 hours) and marked elevation of ALT is characteristic. However, patients with a history of chronic alcohol excess are more likely to develop hepatotoxicity, sometimes with intake of regular (several days) doses regarded as within the therapeutic range (2–4 g/day).[26] The actual risk of heightened susceptibility to paracetamol among alcoholics has been questioned by Prescott,[26a] but contemporary hepatologic practice supports a real association between excessive alcohol intake and instances of paracetamol induced severe liver injury, occasionally due to "therapeutic misadventure".

APAP undergoes metabolism to glucuronide and sulfate conjugates, which are excreted in the urine (Fig. 37.1). A reactive metabolite, N-acetyl-p-benzoquinoneimine (NAPQI), is also formed by cytochrome P450 (CYP)-mediated oxidation, particu-larly CYP2E1 and CYP3A4. NAPQI is readily detoxified by hepatic glutathione (GSH). Therefore, circumstances which favor NAPQI accumulation include hepatic GSH depletion (e.g., prolonged fasting) or induction of CYP2E1 (by fasting, isoniazid, chronic alcohol intake) and CYP3A4 (by anticonvulsants). Depletion of glucuronide or sulfate stores (fasting, intake of some other drugs) reduces the capacity to conjugate APAP, again favoring the CYP-mediated oxidation pathway to form NAPQI.

NAPQI alters hepatocyte membrane proteins directly or generates oxidative stress, leading to mitochondrial injury with cell death (whether by necrosis or apoptosis).[27] The host innate immune system may also be involved in the pathogenesis of APAP liver injury.[28] Replenishing intracellular GSH by administering thiol donors such as N-acetylcysteine (NAC) and methionine is the cornerstone of antidote therapy in management of patients with APAP hepatotoxicity.[29]

Idiosyncratic drug reactions

Other than a few dose-dependent and some partial dose-dependent hepatotoxins (e.g., tacrine, dantrolene), the majority (over 95%) of drug-induced liver diseases are dose-independent or 'idiosyncratic' by nature. Broadly, idiosyncratic drug reactions are considered to have either a metabolic or an immunoallergic basis.

Metabolic idiosyncrasy refers to liver injury resulting from drug or drug metabolite accumulation as a consequence of altered metabolic pathways (e.g., in persons with polymorphisms of drug

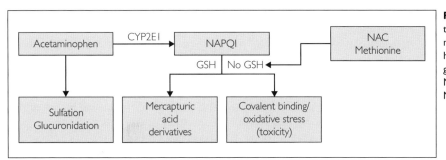

Fig. 37.1 • Metabolism of acetaminophen and the role of NAPQI in liver injury. NAC and methionine ameliorate acetaminophen hepatotoxicity by replenishing hepatic glutathione. GSH, reduced hepatic glutathione; NAPQI, N-acetyl-p-benzoquinoneimine; NAC, N-acetylcysteine.

metabolizing enzymes). In turn, there is activation of cell death pathways by mitochondrial injury, covalent binding to macro-molecules, induction of oxidative stress, or interference with canalicular transporter functions. Both hepatocytes and hepatic nonparenchymal cells (e.g., Kupffer cells, endothelial cells, liver lymphocytes, stellate cells) may be involved.

Troglitazone hepatotoxicity is a contemporary paradigm for likely metabolic idiosyncrasy. Like acetaminophen, troglitazone is principally conjugated with glucuronide and sulfate and also forms a potentially reactive quinone metabolite. However, in com-parison with the parent compound, the quinone metabolite is less toxic.[30,30a] Troglitazone-associated mitochondrial injury, culminating in cell death (apoptosis or necrosis), has been suggested as a possible pathway to liver injury,[30] but the evidence to support this suggestion has been challenged.[30b] Associated inhibition of the bile salt export pump could also induce apoptosis by promoting accumulation of bile salts (well known to cause apoptosis). Certain host factors may underlie troglitazone toxicity. Thus, those at risk were obese persons with type 2 diabetes, which are risk factors for nonalcoholic steato-hepatitis but there is no convincing evidence that preexisting steatohepatitis with its associated oxidative stress and possible energy depletion, rendered the liver more susceptible to troglitazone-induced injury.[30b] Drug–drug interactions could also have con-tributed to severe liver injury; co-administration of cholestasis-inducing drugs (e.g., glibenclamide) could have aggravated troglitazone-induced bile salt retention,[30] but direct evidence in favour of his proposition is also lacking.[30b]

Immunoallergic idiosyncrasy has been implicated in some hepatic drug reactions, typically those accompanied by other allergic mani-festations such as fever, skin rash, neutrophilia, and eosinophilia. The anticonvulsant hypersensitivity syndrome is a well-studied example of this pattern of toxicity. More recently, the term *reactive metabolite syndrome* has been preferred to emphasize the pathogenic role of drug metabolites in its development.[31] Other drugs which have been associated with this syndrome include sulfonamides, allopurinol, dapsone, and minocycline. The clinical presentation is characterized by short latency (2–6 weeks), high-grade fever, pharyngitis, facial edema, lymphadenopathy, and skin reactions ranging from an exanthematous eruption to Stevens-Johnson syndrome and toxic epidermal necrolysis. Visceral involvement can occur; this includes interstitial nephritis, encephalitis or aseptic meningitis, pneumonitis, atypical lymphocytosis or cytopenias, and vasculitis. Cross-reactivity with similar drugs that can produce reactive metabolites and a positive family history of similar drug reactions (in 25%) indicate the genetic basis for this syndrome.

It is hypothesized that drug metabolites form adducts with cellular proteins. The ensuing protein-adducts then provide a target for the host immune response that culminates in liver injury. However, drugs such as acetaminophen, which readily produce reactive metabolites, do not evoke such an immune response. Further, demonstration of a damage-inducing cytotoxic T-cell response has not been easy. A modified concept is the 'danger hypothesis,' which proposes that an immune (or tissue-specific inflammatory) response occurs only if the reactive metabolite also elicits danger signals by producing intracellular oxidative stress or necrosis.[31]

Drug-induced cholestasis

Molecular characterization of hepatobiliary transport processes has provided insights into the pathogenesis of drug-induced cholestasis.[32,33] Thus, cholestasis could result from cis- or trans-inhibition of the bile salt export pump by such agents as cyclosporine A, rifampicin, estradiol, and troglitazone. Alterna-tively, drugs or their metabolites could cause covalent modifi-cation of canalicular transport proteins (e.g., diclofenac) or alter membrane fluidity. Individuals with genetic defects in transporter proteins, such as those with progressive familial cholestasis (defects in multidrug resistance protein-3) can develop cholestasis with drugs such as estrogens that inhibit the bile salt export pump or multidrug resistance-related protein (MRP)-2 (formerly known as canalicular multispecific organic anion transporter-cMOAT) function. The pathogenesis of chronic forms of cholestasis is unknown but immune mechanisms may be involved. This is supported by the observation that Stevens-Johnson syndrome, a disorder with an immunological basis has accompanied some cases of vanishing bile duct syndrome.[34]

Individual risk factors

Underlying host and disease variables which influence the expres-sion and severity of drug-induced hepatic injury are listed in Table 37.3. Overall, children are less susceptible to drug hepato-toxicity with the exceptions of valproic acid toxicity, Reye's syndrome with aspirin, and cholestatic hepatitis caused by ery-thromycin estolate. The restriction of aspirin use for febrile illness in this age group has led to a dramatic decline in the incidence of Reye's syndrome.[35] By contrast, older patients are vulnerable to hepatic injury by way of increased exposure, altered drug disposi-tion, and often drug–drug interactions due to polypharmacy. The reason for gender differences in hepatic drug reactions is unclear and cannot be explained merely by increased exposure. Women are over-represented in reports of drug-induced hepatitis, par-ticularly in cases of chronic hepatitis. On the other hand, amoxicillin-clavulanate and azathioprine toxicity are more com-mon in males. Both undernutrition and obesity can predispose to hepatotoxicity. Undernutrition is an independent risk factor for antituberculous therapy; dose recommendations are now strictly by body weight.[36] On the other hand, obese individuals are more susceptible to halothane and methotrexate toxicity. In the case of methotrexate, the underlying nonalcoholic steatohepatitis may be important in the pathogenesis of the liver injury.[37] Central obesity may also be a risk factor for tamoxifen-induced fatty liver disorders.[38]

The impact of underlying liver disease on hepatotoxicity is also illustrated by the interactions between chronic hepatitis B and antituberculous therapy (ATT) and of highly active antiretroviral therapy (HAART) with chronic hepatitis B (HBV) and C virus (HCV) infection. In a study from Taiwan, persons infected with HBV were more likely (35% versus 9%, respectively) to develop an ALT rise with ATT as compared to persons without HBV infection.[39] Further, among those who developed liver injury, coinfected individuals had higher histological severity scores than those without HBV infection. By multiple logistic regression analysis, only age and hepatitis B surface antigen positivity were independent risk factors for liver injury (odds ratio 5.5, 95% CI, 2.1–14.3).[39] Likewise, in some studies, a proportion of HAART recipients coinfected with HBV or HCV were at an increased risk of hepatotoxicity.[40] In one study, the presence of chronic viral hepatitis B and C was associated with an increased risk of severe hepatotoxicity, especially among patients prescribed regimens

Table 37.3 Risk factors for increased incidence and severity of drug-induced liver diseases

Risk factors	Representative agents	Importance
Age	Isoniazid, troglitazone, halothane, nitrofurantoin Valproic acid, salicylates	Age >60 increases frequency and severity of liver injury More common in children
Gender	Halothane, diclofenac, nitrofurantoin, dextropropoxyphene Azathioprine, amoxicillin-clavulanic acid	More common in women More common in men
Dose	Acetaminophen, salicylates Anticancer drugs, perhexiline, tacrine, oxypenicillins, dantrolene Methotrexate, vitamin A	Toxicity correlates with drug levels Partial relationship to dose Total dose, frequency, and duration of exposure correlate with fibrosis risk
Genetic factors	Halothane, phenytoin, sulfonamides Amoxicillin-clavulanic acid Valproic acid	Family history of similar reactions; in vitro susceptibility tests in lymphocytes Strong HLA association Associated with inherited mitochondrial enzyme deficiencies
Cross-sensitivity	Isoflurane, enflurane, halothane; erythromycin and other macrolides; diclofenac and ibuprofen	Relevant to prevention of drug-induced liver disease
Multiple drug therapy (polypharmacy) including drug interactions	Acetaminophen and isoniazid, zidovudine or phenytoin	Lower hepatotoxic dose threshold
Excessive alcohol use	Acetaminophen Isoniazid, methotrexate	Lower hepatotoxic dose threshold Increased risk of liver injury, fibrosis
Nutritional status Obesity Fasting	 Halothane, troglitazone, tamoxifen, methotrexate Acetaminophen	 Increased risk of liver injury, NASH or hepatic fibrosis Increased risk of liver injury
Liver disease	Pemoline Viral hepatitis B or C	Increased risk of liver injury Increased risk with HAART, antituberculosis treatment, ibuprofen
Other diseases		
Diabetes mellitus	Methotrexate	Increased risk of hepatic fibrosis
Osteoarthritis	Diclofenac	Increased risk of liver injury
HIV/AIDS	Sulfonamides (cotrimoxazole)	Increased risk of liver injury
Renal failure	Methotrexate	Increased risk of liver injury, fibrosis
Rheumatoid arthritis, SLE	Salicylates	Increased risk of liver injury
NASH	Methotrexate	Increased risk of liver fibrosis
Pregnancy	Intravenous tetracycline	Increased risk of acute fatty liver of pregnancy
Organ and bone marrow transplantation	Azathioprine, thioguanine, busulfan	Increased risk of vascular toxicity

HLA, human leukocyte antigen; NASH, nonalcoholic steatohepatitis; HAART, highly active antiretroviral therapy; HIV/AIDS, human immunodeficiency virus, acquired immunodeficiency syndrome; SLE, systemic lupus erythematosus.

which excluded ritonavir (odds ratio, 3.7; 95% CI, 1.0–11.8); overall, around 12% of patients receiving a protease inhibitor developed liver injury.[41] One suggested strategy to minimize hepatotoxicity associated with HAART includes use of a published algorithm based on ALT monitoring, signs and symptoms of hepatitis and/or mitochondrial toxicity.[42] The other approach to this problem is to consider pretreatment of chronic viral hepatitis in HIV-infected patients prior to administration of HAART.[43]

Pharmacogenetics

Genetic factors are estimated to account for 20–95% of variations in drug disposition and effects.[44,45] In more extreme examples, this may manifest as polymorphisms of drug metabolizing enzymes, drug receptors, or transporters.[44] Pharmacogenetics deals with these variations in drug response with reference to single-gene or genome-based approaches to pharmacology (pharmacogenomics) or toxicology (toxicogenomics). With reference to drug-induced liver

Table 37.4 Genetic polymorphisms and drug-induced liver disease

Polymorphism	Phenotype	Drugs associated with increased hepatotoxicity
CYP2D6	Poor metabolizer	Perhexiline maleate
CYP2C19	Poor metabolizer	Atrium
CYP 2C9*3	Poor metabolizer	Leflunomide
CYP2E1	c1/c1 phenotype associated with increased CYP2E1 activity	Isoniazid
Glutathione S-transferase	Poor metabolizer (combined GST M1-T1 phenotype only)	Tacrine
Glutathione S-transferase	Poor metabolizer (GST M1 phenotype only)	Isoniazid
N-acetyl transferase 2	Slow acetylator status; other studies have shown fast acetylators to be at greater risk	Isoniazid
HLA associations	Absence of HLA-DQA1*0102 (OR 4.0) and presence of HLA-DQB1*0201	Antituberculous drugs
	HLA-DRB1*1501, DRB5*0101, DQB1*0602	Amoxicillin-clavulanate
	HLA-A33/B44/DR6	Tiopronin

injury, those polymorphisms that have been implicated in hepatotoxic reactions are listed in Table 37.4.[46–49] However, the practical significance of these associations within the community has not been defined. One of the problems is the population-specific variation of each polymorphism; thus, independent validation is needed across different ethnic groups. Variations in immune response genes have been linked to certain forms of drug allergy. Again, reanalysis of putative preliminary associations in different populations or in larger studies has given rise to conflicting reports. Given these limitations, as well as cost considerations, the routine application of pharmacogenetic methods cannot yet be widely recommended.

DIAGNOSIS

Clinical suspicion, causality assessment, scoring systems

In the absence of confirmatory tests, the diagnosis of drug-induced liver disease is based on circumstantial evidence (Table 37.5).[8] Key diagnostic points include the temporal profile of drug use, the response to drug withdrawal (dechallenge) and rechallenge. Generally, reactions occurring within 1–12 weeks of commencing

Table 37.5 Clinical features raising suspicion of drug-induced liver disease

New drug introduced (within 1 to 6 months)

Extrahepatic involvement; hypersensitivity features

'Idiopathic' acute hepatitis

Chronic hepatitis without antibodies or hyperglobulinemia

Mixed hepatocellular-cholestatic biochemical profile

Cholestasis with normal biliary tract imaging

Suggestive histologic features (see Table 37.6)

Complex medical situations (e.g., intensive care unit), special risk categories (see Table 37.3)

Concurrent herbal drug intake

a drug are considered most likely to represent drug toxicity. Latent periods of 12 weeks to 1 year are still compatible with drug toxicity, but are considered less likely. Other than certain forms of delayed toxicity, such as development of chronic hepatitis (e.g., minocycline), cirrhosis (e.g., methotrexate, arsenic) or hepatic neoplasia (e.g., oral contraceptives, anabolic steroids, arsenic), reactions occurring beyond 1 year of use are very unlikely to be medication-related. By contrast, re-exposure to the drug in previously sensitized persons may produce hepatotoxicity within hours or days. Such rechallenge, whether deliberate or inadvertent, is regarded as the gold standard when assigning causality to a particular agent. However, ethical considerations usually prevent its application because safer therapeutic alternatives may be available, and, more importantly, re-exposure can provoke severe reactions and even fatalities with drug reactions of an immunoallergic nature. Therefore, emphasis is placed on observation of the 'dechallenge,' i.e., the response to drug withdrawal. Accordingly, hepatocellular reactions may be categorized as 'very suggestive' or 'suggestive' if the liver enzymes decrease by 50% of excess above ULN within 8 days or 30 days, respectively. The time frame for improvement for 'suggestive' cholestatic reactions is extended to 180 days.[50]

Scoring systems to assign causality have been developed by consortia of experts in this field. Two such systems, the detailed CIOMS and a simpler modification, the clinical diagnostic scale (CDS) are in use.[50,51] The components of these scores include: time to onset from drug commencement or drug discontinuation, course of the reaction after drug cessation, concomitant treatment, complete exclusion of non-drug-related causes, previous track record of the suspected drug, extrahepatic manifestations and response to rechallenge. Comparisons between the two systems showed poor concordance, with agreement in only 31% of cases.[52] Agreement was better for hypersensitivity cases (perhaps due to the emphasis on extrahepatic features of drug hypersensitivity) but the overall performance of the CIOMS was better. The CDS has been criticized for its heavier weighting towards hypersensitivity reactions, bias towards recent drugs (<5 years in use) and exoneration of drug toxicity if the latent period exceeded 15 days after stopping a drug.[53] Both systems rely on follow-up. Thus, there is no preliminary tool available for a clinician confronted with a possible drug reaction. Discrepancies also exist between a physician's (global) assessment of drug reactions, and achievement of a diagnosis through application of scoring systems.[54] In one French study, complete agreement was observed in only 6% of the cases. Physicians were more likely to score reactions as 'likely or very likely' (60%), whereas causality was considered 'likely' in only 10% of the same case mix when the scoring system was used.[54] Therefore, the exact place of scoring systems is not defined. Although they can be used as research tools and their use is being increasingly encouraged in case reports, individual assessment on a case-by-case basis remains critical.

Exclusion of other liver disorders

Appropriate serologic, virologic, immunologic, biochemical, and hepatobiliary imaging studies are mandatory to exclude viral hepatitis, endemic infectious agents (if recent travel is involved), metabolic, autoimmune and infiltrative/neoplastic hepatobiliary liver disorders. Persons presenting with cholestasis should first be assessed for possible extrahepatic biliary obstruction by hepatobiliary sonography. If the clinical suspicion is strong (abdominal pain, older age, gradual onset), more sensitive modalities such as computerized tomography, magnetic resonance cholangiography, endoscopic retrograde cholangiography, or endoscopic ultrasound should be considered. Drug-induced chronic hepatitis (e.g., nitrofurantoin) can closely mimic autoimmune hepatitis by sharing the same gender (female), serologic (raised immunoglobulin G, antinuclear antibodies, and/or smooth muscle antibodies), and histologic features. Such cases may initially respond well to corticosteroids.

Hepatic injury can result from systemic disorders, including severe Gram-positive and Gram-negative infections, paraneoplastic syndromes, and disorders of diffuse inflammatory responses (sarcoidosis, vasculitis, systemic lupus erythematosus). This is an important consideration in patients admitted to tertiary care centers where extrahepatic sepsis, benign postoperative cholestasis, and ischemic (or ischemic reperfusion) hepatopathy are encountered more often than in ambulatory care settings. The importance of excluding other disorders is underscored by a retrospective survey in one English healthcare region of all suspected hepatic drug reactions; an alternative diagnosis for the liver disease was found in more than 50% of cases.[55]

Table 37.6 Liver histologic changes suggestive of drug-induced liver disease

Zonal lesions, including steatosis and necrosis

Necrotic lesions disproportionate to clinical severity

Microvesicular steatosis

Mixed hepatitis and cholestasis

Prominent neutrophils and (later stages) eosinophils (>25% of cells in infiltrate)

Bile duct injury

Granulomas, vascular lesions

Features of severe steatohepatitis

Presence of vitamin A deposits (autofluorescence)

Indications for liver biopsy

Many instances of drug-induced liver injury are self-limiting. Liver biopsy is not usually performed in these individuals, particularly when improvement is evident or there is only a minor alteration in liver biochemical tests. However, liver biopsy may be useful in borderline cases to exclude other liver disorders or to provide corroborative evidence of drug toxicity; the latter may assume greater importance when a new pharmacologic or complementary/alternative medicine (CAM) agent not previously associated with liver injury is the most likely cause. Although a specific diagnosis can be rarely made, several histologic features raise the suspicion of a drug etiology (Table 37.6). The prognosis of drug injury can also be inferred in some instances. For example, detection of severe bile duct injury in cases of acute cholestatic hepatitis foreshadows the development of ductopenia and the possibility of prolonged cholestasis,[56] while bridging or zonal necrosis is indicative of a surprisingly severe form of hepatocellular injury. Liver biopsy plays an important role in patients with risk factors for other forms of liver injury such as metabolic causes of fatty liver, in whom methotrexate is being considered. The risk–benefit ratio for liver biopsy needs to be assessed carefully for each individual, and informed consent is clearly essential.

GOALS OF PREVENTION

Pharmacologic principles, patient and professional education, appreciation of special risk categories

Preventing drug hepatotoxicity is a moral, ethical, and legal responsibility of every prescribing doctor. Since serious drug reactions are infrequent and often idiosyncratic, individual experience with dealing with such cases will be limited. Further, recognizing medication errors may not be sufficiently stressed during medical training; in one American survey, only 16% of interns received formal training during their clerkship.[57]

At the level of the prescriber, minimizing harm requires attention to core pharmacologic principles: appropriate drug, appropriate dose, considering safer alternatives (especially nonpharmacologic), avoid polypharmacy and appreciation of host and drug factors which heighten the influence of adverse drug effects (see Table 37.3). As discussed below, protocol ALT monitoring has its limitations and should never replace patient and physician education about drug toxicity. The increasing availability of drug information software (e.g., ePocrates®) on personal digital assistants in clinical practice or drug alerts in hospital network systems is an interesting contemporary trend; it could be hoped that such applications will help reduce prescribing errors and consequent drug toxicity, but this remains to be seen. From a hospital perspective, implementation of an automated computer-assisted laboratory result monitoring system is feasible.[58,59] In a pilot project, 91% of all adverse reactions were identified, but the specificity of this computer-generated alert was low (23%), rendering the process of reaction identification ineffective. However, specificity of the computer-generated alert could be improved upon (to 76%) by incorporation of specific laboratory algorithms. Governmental initiatives may also have an impact on preventing or reducing drug-induced liver injury. For example, in the UK, restrictions on pack sizes of acetaminophen, and restricting sales (in 1998) changing the mode of packing, have been associated contemporaneously with reduced requirement for liver transplantation (by 66%) and mortality (by 21%) after acetaminophen overdose although the contribution of the 1998 regulations to the reduction is unclear.[60,60a]

Drug screening, post-marketing surveillance

The elaborate drug development process includes extensive toxicologic preclinical testing in animal models, followed by dose-ranging studies, phase II and finally phase III trials.[11,11a] Despite this, identification of idiosyncratic drug reactions is not always possible. This is because the number of participants in prerelease clinical trials (2000–3000) is much lower than typical frequencies of drug hepatotoxicity (1 in 10 000 above). The troglitazone story highlights this shortcoming.[12a] Thus, although approximately 2% of clinical trial recipients of troglitazone developed raised aminotransferases, no cases of acute liver failure were observed. Nonetheless, in the 5 years following its launch, over 90 cases of serious liver injury were reported to the FDA, leading to its ultimate withdrawal. Based on current estimates of troglitazone hepatotoxicity (50 per 220 per million person-years), it is obvious that such events could not have been adequately predicted from phase III trials.[12,12a,30b]

The troglitazone experience underscores the importance of post-marketing surveillance. Prescribers are encouraged to report unusual or serious adverse events to drug licensing authorities (e.g., MEDWATCH database maintained by the Food and Drug Administration, USA). The information sought extends beyond prescribed drugs to other hepatotoxins, and in particular, to the hepatic reactions with some nutritional supplements (e.g., Lipokinetix)[61] and CAM.[62,63] Standardization, better documentation of efficacy, and similar procedures for approval as for other drugs has been suggested for these compounds.[64]

Protocol ALT monitoring

Routine monitoring of liver tests (especially ALT) is often recommended for persons receiving long courses of treatment (>4 weeks). This is an established practice for drugs with an established track record of hepatotoxicity, such as isoniazid, methotrexate, etretinate, and other synthetic retinoids, ketoconazole and anticancer drugs. However, drugs that have low hepatotoxic potential cause a conundrum for patients and prescribers; in the case of the widely prescribed "statins" (3-hydroxy-3-methylglutarhyde coenzyme-A reductase inhibitors), the usefulness of this approach has been seriously questioned.[66a,66b] Several caveats apply to protocol ALT screening. Progression to acute liver failure can be rapid with certain drugs (e.g., troglitazone). Thus, monthly monitoring of ALT did not identify 19 (20%) of 94 cases of troglitazone-associated liver failure.[12] Second, the threshold at which 'injury' occurs is not well defined. Raised aminotransferases more often occur transiently during drug intake, representing true 'hepatic adaptation.' Thus, liver test abnormalities may resolve without stopping treatment. Third, liver enzyme changes (outside of the stated 'normal range', the definition of which is controversial[65]) are also observed in persons receiving placebo during clinical trials. Finally, the cost-effectiveness of such monitoring has never been documented, but has been questioned.[66] In this context, recommendations of manufacturers for monitoring ALT (or AST) with drugs like minocycline and the statins is hard to endorse.

Common practice is to recommend drug withdrawal when ALT levels exceed 5 times ULN (roughly 250–300 IU/L). Alterations in bilirubin, prothrombin time, and onset of non-specific symptoms (nausea, anorexia, malaise, hepatic discomfort), jaundice or other signs of liver injury are much more important. Above all, educating the patient (and practitioners) about symptoms of hepatotoxicity is critical because the goal is to stop the offending drug as early as possible. The progressive nature and poor outcome of drug-induced liver injury, when patients continue their medications after the onset of symptoms, is a recurring theme in publications on drug hepatotoxicity. Other methods of monitoring for early detection of liver problems include performing liver biopsies to assess hepatic fibrosis (for methotrexate), and annual ultrasound examination of the liver to screen for hepatic adenoma formation (for danazol).[67] Guidelines for performing liver biopsy in long-term methotrexate recipients have been published.[68–70] Liver histology is obtained at baseline only in persons at risk, and particularly those with history of chronic excessive ethanol intake, baseline abnormalities of ALT, or strong risk factors for nonalcoholic fatty liver disease. For others, liver biopsy is considered when a cumulative amount of 1.5 grams is reached and for every 1–1.5 grams thereafter according to the result of the first liver biopsy. Aithal and colleagues have called for a revision in these guidelines. In their study, only 2.6% of recipients receiving a cumulative amount of 4 grams showed significant hepatic fibrosis.[71] Further, the risk–benefit ratio of liver biopsy appeared unfavorable with complication rates of 4% in this cohort; notwithstanding that such a high rate of liver biopsy complications is not in accord with that currently accepted,[72] the authors have suggested a higher threshold (cumulative dose, 5 grams) before liver biopsy.[71] We partially agree with this view, with the exception of those with the aforementioned risk factors.

MANAGEMENT

In mild cases, early recognition of drug toxicity and prompt withdrawal of the offending drug usually leads to a rapid and uneventful clinical recovery. Conversely, resolution (especially at the biochemical level) can be protracted in cholestatic reactions, and also with drugs that have a long half-life (amiodarone, vitamin A, ketoconazole, etretinate). A more variable set of outcomes pertains to individuals who develop severe liver injury. In some such cases, prolonged intensive support may be needed. Patients fulfilling standard criteria for liver transplantation[73] should be considered for referral to a liver transplant center. Early discussion with transplant centers is critical, to facilitate transfer before an irretrievable clinical situation is reached and to allow time for obtaining a donor liver, assessing comorbidity and psychosocial issues.

Dose-dependent hepatotoxins

In cases of dose-dependent hepatotoxicity, approaches to management include gastric lavage to remove unabsorbed drug (for acetaminophen, metals, and toxic mushrooms). Drug levels should be measured (acetaminophen, salicylates, metals).

Acetaminophen (APAP) hepatotoxicity is the only form of drug-induced liver disease for which a specific antidote is available.[74] NAC is administered either orally (USA) or intravenously (Australia, Europe), but only the oral form of NAC is approved by the FDA. An inhalant preparation of NAC can also be used for intravenous administration.[75] Although the hepatotoxic dose of APAP is 150 mg/kg, APAP levels should be obtained within 24 hours in all patients who present. Physicians should consult a treatment nomogram (Rumack-Mathew, Prescott) in which the plasma APAP level is plotted against time since ingestion.[76,77] NAC is commenced if plasma levels exceed the standard treatment line (drawn joining a level of 200 mg/L at 4 hours and 30 mg/L at 15 hours). The threshold for treatment is lowered in certain *high-risk* patient groups, such as those receiving enzyme-inducing drugs (carbamazepine, phenytoin) or under conditions of hepatic glutathione depletion (fasting, anorexia nervosa, cancer cachexia). For these patients, a lower threshold treatment line is used (joining plasma APAP levels over 100 mg/L at 4 hours and 15 mg/L at 15 hours). The nomograms are less reliable after 15 hours of APAP ingestion and also in persons presenting with staggered overdoses or continued ingestion of APAP at moderately high levels for more than 48 hours. In these cases, treatment is initiated if the total dose of APAP exceeds 150 mg/kg or in any cases of doubt. The 4-hour APAP levels may be below treatment threshold with extended-release APAP overdoses; repeat measurement at 8 hours is suggested in these cases.[78]

The benefits of continuing NAC in late-presenters (beyond 24 hours of ingestion) are controversial.[79,80] Improved cerebral outcome due to stabilization of vascular tone has been reported[79] but others have refuted this.[81] However, current practice in many liver units around the world is to continue NAC till recovery or liver transplantation.

Dosing schedule for N-acetylcysteine

Oral N-acetylcysteine

Oral dosing is an initial dose of 140 mg/kg, 70 mg/kg 4 hours later, and subsequent doses of 70 mg/kg every 4 hours for 17 doses. The unpleasant odor and flavor of NAC can be masked by administering it with fruit juice and by dilution of NAC to a 5% solution.

Intravenous N-acetylcysteine

An initial loading dose of 150 mg/kg of NAC is given in 200 mL of 5% dextrose over 15 minutes, followed by 50 mL/kg in 500 mL of 5% dextrose over 4 hours. The maintenance dose is 100 mL/kg in 1 liter of 5% dextrose over 16 hours. Newer protocols include a 48-hour intravenous and a 20-hour oral protocol.[82] The latter has been evaluated only in early presenters (within 8 hours of APAP ingestion).

All regimens appear to be equally effective. Anaphylactoid reactions (flushing, wheezing, urticaria, rarely angioedema) are observed in 6–15% of intravenous NAC recipients. However, these reactions are usually mild, and rarely lead to treatment discontinuation. Minor reactions require no additional treatment (for flushing) or antihistaminics (for pruritus). The NAC infusion is temporarily discontinued if angioedema and respiratory distress develop. After antihistaminics are administered, the infusion can usually be resumed after 1 hour. Bronchial asthma is not an absolute contraindication to use of NAC. However, caution is advised because such persons are more likely to develop other adverse effects that can rarely be fatal.[83–85]

Oral methionine can also be used in early cases (within 10 hours) of APAP overdose. However, methionine can cause vomiting and is now usually restricted to persons with NAC hypersensitivity.

Idiosyncratic drug reactions

Corticosteroids

No controlled data are available for the role of corticosteroids in drug-induced liver disease. However, patients receiving corticosteroids for systemic hypersensitivity reactions (e.g., with allopurinol) have also shown improvement in biochemical and clinical manifestations of the coexisting liver injury. Likewise, corticosteroids have been used with apparent benefit in some cases of acute and chronic hepatitis due to diclofenac, piroxicam, methyldopa, minocycline, and the sulfa drugs.[86–90] The literature abounds with instances of 'corticosteroid-whitewash' in cases of drug-induced jaundice, especially with cholestatic hepatitis; conversely, a partial response could mask another disorder (e.g., occult cholangiocarcinoma). Based on these considerations, the use of corticosteroids may be considered on a case-by-case basis based on the severity and duration of illness and careful assessment of comorbidity (diabetes mellitus, active sepsis, and other relative contraindications to steroid use). Further, the adequacy (complete or otherwise) of any response and the post-biopsy course all need to be considered with unusual diligence.

Ursodeoxycholic acid in the treatment of chronic cholestasis

As with corticosteroids, controlled trials of efficacy for ursodeoxycholic acid (UDCA) are lacking. Anecdotally, UDCA has been used with success in predominantly cholestatic reactions with drugs such as cyclosporine in heart transplant recipients, amoxicillin-clavulanate, flutamide, flucloxacillin, and ticlopidine.[91–95] Therefore, it may be considered in protracted cases of cholestasis.

Liver transplantation

Patients fulfilling standard liver transplant criteria (developed at King's College Hospital, London) (Table 37.7) have a poor outcome and should be considered for liver transplantation.[73,96,97] Other additions and modifications to these criteria have been suggested, but further appraisal is necessary (Table 37.8).[98–101] Artificial liver support systems based on molecular adsorbent recirculating systems have shown benefit in uncontrolled studies, but remain investigational.[102]

Short-term transplant-free survival for acute liver failure induced by acetaminophen was significantly better than for nonacetaminophen-related cases (68% versus 25%, respectively).[103] Of those undergoing liver transplantation, 75% could be discharged from hospital; 66% were alive at a median of 37 months (range 1–72 months).[96]

Table 37.7 Criteria for liver transplantation in acetaminophen-induced acute liver failure

Arterial pH <7.3 after adequate fluid resuscitation

or

Serum creatinine >300 μmol/L

Prothrombin time >100 seconds (international normalized ratio >6.5)

Grade III/IV encephalopathy (if all 3 of these occur within a 24-hour period)

Table 37.8 Other predictors of poor outcome in acetaminophen-induced liver failure

Criteria	Significance	Comment
Blood lactate levels[96]	Poor outcome if blood lactate levels >3.5 mmol/L after early fluid resuscitation or if blood lactate levels >3.0 mmol/L after adequate fluid resuscitation	Timing of testing is critical. The significance of hyperlactatemia in a center accepting only late referrals may be different from a unit dealing with early cases. Independent validation is needed.
Acute physiology and chronic health evaluation (APACHE II) score[97]	Highest positive and lowest negative likelihood ratio in assessing need for liver transplantation	Single study only
Serum phosphate[98–101]	Hyperphosphatemia was found to be a predictor of nonsurvival	Sensitivity questioned. Addition to King's College Hospital criteria[73] improved sensitivity but decreased specificity, positive predictive value and accuracy.
Galactose elimination capacity[102]	Predictor of hepatic encephalopathy	Good sensitivity but low specificity

FUTURE DIRECTIONS

Newer strategies include improvement of methods used in assessing the hepatotoxic potential of new compounds, using sophisticated monitoring tools once the drug is marketed, and also advances in the management of patients with drug-induced liver disease. High-throughput assays examining multiple cellular functions appear promising in efforts to predict hepatotoxicity at an early stage of drug development.[104] Sophisticated tools to monitor specific organelle injury (e.g., mitochondrial injury with HAART) are being explored. Likewise, the role of noninvasive serum markers in estimating hepatic fibrosis is an area of study. Vector analysis of liver tests can detect early biochemical trends during clinical trials.[105] The development of antibodies to drug-cell adducts may facilitate diagnosis in cases of acute liver failure of uncertain cause.[106] For example, in cases of APAP overdosage, such antibodies are present up to 1 week later when APAP levels are undetectable.[106]

An important spin-off from the Human Genome project is to accurately identify disease-producing genes in various populations. Polymorphisms of drug-metabolizing enzymes that promote drug toxicity will be increasingly sought before treatment is initiated. Such strategies are already in place for some drug reactions (e.g., thiopurine methyltransferase assays in persons receiving azathioprine to prevent marrow suppression but not liver reactions). At present, abrogating drug-induced liver injury is limited to drugs such as APAP. Potential newer targets include inhibition of apoptosis (caspase inhibitors).[107] Global organ shortage has provided an impetus to developing temporary liver support systems, which allow sufficient time for recovery of the native liver. They provide extracorporeal hepatic support or act as filtering devices (e.g., molecular adsorbent recirculating system, MARS) to remove circulating hepatic toxins.[102]

SUMMARY

Drug-induced liver injury remains an underrecognized, underreported, occasionally fatal form of adverse drug reaction. Numerous host-related factors can influence the risk and severity

of drug hepatotoxicity. Diagnosis is still based on circumstantial evidence and appropriate exclusion of other liver diseases. Use of scoring systems can facilitate uniformity in comparisons but are of little if any practical clinical value in diagnosis. Preventing liver injury relies on attention to pharmacologic principles, and patient and professional education. Spontaneous reporting of drug reactions to regulatory authorities is critical in collating evidence of drug toxicity. Protocol monitoring of liver tests should not and cannot replace patient education of hepatotoxic symptoms. Other than N-acetylcysteine for acetaminophen overdose, the management of drug hepatotoxicity is largely supportive. Liver transplantation may be required in severe cases, while ursodeoxycholic acid may have beneficial effects in some cases of severe and prolonged cholestasis.

See Table 37.9 for the authors' summary of recommendations for the management of drug-induced liver injury.

Table 37.9 Authors' recommendations on management of drug-induced liver injury

Early recognition and prompt discontinuation of the offending drug is critical to minimize progressive liver injury.

All patients need baseline and continued monitoring for signs of acute liver failure.

Oral or intravenous N-acetylcysteine is the preferred treatment for acetaminophen hepatotoxicity.

Anecdotal evidence supports the use of corticosteroids in persons with coexisting hypersensitivity manifestations and liver injury. Uncontrolled data favor the use of ursodeoxycholic acid in severe and protracted cholestatic drug reactions.

Supportive care is critical for all patients with drug-induced hepatic injury. Early liaison with liver transplant centers is encouraged in cases of acute liver failure.

Providing temporary support to the failing liver with extracorporeal liver support devices is yet to be FDA approved, but appears to be a promising future strategy.

REFERENCES

1. Chitturi S, Farrell GC. Drug-induced liver disease. In: Schiff E, Davis GL, Maddrey WC, eds. Schiff's diseases of the liver. Philadelphia: Lippincott Williams and Wilkins; 2002:1059–1127.

2. Farrell GC. Drug-induced liver disease. Edinburgh: Churchill Livingstone; 1994.

3. Zimmerman HJ. Hepatotoxicity: The adverse effects of drugs and other chemicals on the liver. 2nd edn. Philadelphia: Lippincott Williams and Wilkins; 1999.

4. Kaplowitz N, DeLeve LD, eds. Drug-induced liver disease. New York: Marcel Dekker; 2003.

5. Farrell GC, Liddle C, eds. Hepatotoxicity in the twenty-first century. Semin Liv Disease 2002; 22:115–210.

   Theme issue on drug hepatotoxicity with discussions of epidemiology, regulation of hepatic drug metabolism, pathophysiology, with an updated account of liver injury associated with contemporary drugs.

6. Black M, ed. Drug induced liver disease. Clin Liver Dis 2003; 7:295–512.

   Theme issue featuring clinical hepatotoxicity associated with major drug classes.

7. Benichou C. Criteria for drug-induced liver disorder. Report of an international consensus meeting. J Hepatol 1990; 11:272–276.

8. Larrey D. Epidemiology and individual susceptibility to adverse drug reactions affecting the liver. Semin Liver Dis 2002; 22:145–155.

9. Black M, Mitchell JR, Zimmerman HJ, et al. Isoniazid-associated hepatitis in 114 patients. Gastroenterology 1975; 69:289–302.

10. Lee WM. Acute liver failure in the United States. Semin Liver Dis 2003; 23:217–226.

11. Ballet F. Hepatotoxicity in drug development: detection, significance and solutions. J Hepatol 1997; 26(Suppl 2):26–36.

11a. Peters TS. Do preclinical testing strategies help predict human hepatotoxicity potentials. Toxicol Pathol 2005; 33:146–154.

12. Graham DJ, Green L, Senior JR, et al. Troglitazone-induced liver failure: a case study. Am J Med 2003; 114:299–306.

   A review of cases presented to the FDA, highlighting the failure of monthly ALT monitoring in identifying patients progressing rapidly to acute liver failure.

12a. Watkins PB. Insight into hepatotoxicity: The troglitazone experience. Hepatology 2005; 41:229–230.

13. Anonymous. Trovafloxacin and alatrofloxacin – suspension and warnings: hepatotoxicity. WHO Inform Exchange Syst 1999; 86:1.

14. McKenzie R, Fried MW, Sallie R, et al. Hepatic failure and lactic acidosis due to fialuridine (FIAU), an investigational nucleoside analogue for chronic hepatitis B. N Engl J Med 1995; 26:1099–1105.

15. Fontana RJ, McCashland TM, Benner KG, et al. Acute liver failure associated with prolonged use of bromfenac leading to liver transplantation. The Acute Liver Failure Study Group. Liver Transpl Surg 1999; 5:480–484.

16. Anonymous. Withdrawal of medicinal products containing ebrotidine: liver toxicity. WHO Inform Exchange Syst 1998; 72:1.

17. Committee on Safety of Medicines/Medicines Control Agency. Withdrawal of tolcapone (Tasmar). Curr Probl Pharmacovigil 1999; 25:2.

18. Choi S. Nefazodone (serzone) withdrawn because of hepatotoxicity. CMAJ 2003; 169:1187.

19. Chojkier M. Hepatic sinusoidal-obstruction syndrome: toxicity of pyrrolizidine alkaloids. J Hepatol 2003; 39:437–446.

20. Wadleigh M, Ho V, Momtaz P, et al. Hepatic veno-occlusive disease: pathogenesis, diagnosis and treatment. Curr Opin Hematol 2003; 10:451–462.

21. Ibanez L, Perez E, Vidal X, et al. Prospective surveillance of acute serious liver disease unrelated to infectious, obstructive, or metabolic diseases: epidemiological and clinical features, and exposure to drugs. J Hepatol 2002; 37:592–600.

22. Sgro C, Clinard F, Ouazir K, et al. Incidence of drug-induced hepatic injuries: a French population-based study. Hepatology 2002; 36:451–455.

   The above 2 studies are prospective community-based studies on the incidence of drug-induced liver disease.

23. Gluud C. Acute, serious drug-induced liver injury. J Hepatol 2002; 37:675–677.

24. Olsson R, Brunlof G, Johansson ML, et al. Drug-induced hepatic injury in Sweden. Hepatology 2003; 38:531–532.

25. Farrell GC. Liver disease caused by drugs, anesthetics, and toxins. In: Gastrointestinal disease. Feldman M, Scharschmidt BF, Sleisenger MH, eds. Philadelphia: Saunders; 2002:1403–1447.

26. Zimmerman HJ, Maddrey WC. Acetaminophen (paracetamol) hepatotoxicity with regular intake of alcohol: analysis of instance of therapeutic misadventure. Hepatology 1995; 22:767–773.

26a. Prescott LF. Paracetamol, alcohol and the liver. Br J Clin Pharmacol 2000; 49:291–301.

27. Kon K, Kim J-S, Doyal E. Role of the mitochondrial permeability transition in acetaminophen-induced necrotic and apoptotic cell death to cultured mouse hepatocytes. Hepatology 2003; 34(Suppl.1):271A.

28. Liu Z-X, Kaplowitz N. Innate immune system determines acetaminophen (APAP) hepatotoxicity (Abstract). Hepatology 2003; 34(Suppl.1):250A.

29. Routledge P, Vale AJ, Bateman D, et al. Paracetamol (acetaminophen) poisoning: No need to change current guidelines to accident departments. Br Med J 1998; 317:1609–1610.

30. Smith MT. Mechanisms of troglitazone hepatotoxicity. Chem Res Toxicol 2003; 16:679–687.

30a. Park BK, Kitteringham NR, Maggs JL, et al. The role of metabolic cultivation in drug-induced hepatotoxicity. Annu Rev Pharmacol Toxicol 2005; 45:174–202.

30b. Chojkier M. Troglitazone and liver injury: insearch of answers/ Hepatology 2005; 41:229–230.

31. Knowles SR, Uetrecht J, Shear NH. Idiosyncratic drug reactions: the reactive metabolite syndromes. Lancet 2000; 356:1587–1591.

32. Bohan A, Boyer JL. Mechanisms of hepatic transport of drugs: implications for cholestatic drug reactions. Semin Liver Dis 2002; 22:123–136.

33. Stieger B, Fattinger K, Madon J, et al. Drug- and estrogen-induced cholestasis through inhibition of the hepatocellular bile export pump (Bsep) of rat liver. Gastroenterology 2000; 118:422–430.

34. Srivastava M, Perez-Atayde A, Jonas MM. Drug-associated acute-onset vanishing bile duct and Stevens-Johnson syndromes in a child. Gastroenterology 1998; 115:743–746.

35. Autret-Leca E, Jonville-Bera AP, Llau ME, et al. Incidence of Reye's syndrome in France: a hospital-based survey. J Clin Epidemiol 2001; 54:857–862.

36. Pande JN, Singh SP, Khilnani GC, et al. Risk factors for hepatotoxicity from antituberculosis drugs: a case-control study. Thorax 1996; 51:132–136.

37. Langman G, Hall PM, Todd G. Role of non-alcoholic steatohepatitis in methotrexate-induced liver injury. J Gastroenterol Hepatol 2001; 16:1395–1401.

38. Farrell GC. Drugs and steatohepatitis. Semin Liver Dis 2002; 22:185–194.

39. Wong WM, Wu PC, Yuen MF, et al. Antituberculosis drug-related liver dysfunction in chronic hepatitis B infection. Hepatology 2000; 31:201–206.

40. den Brinker M, Wit FW, Wertheim-van Dillen PM, et al. Hepatitis B and C virus co-infection and the risk for hepatotoxicity of highly active antiretroviral therapy in HIV-1 infection. AIDS 2000; 14:2895–2902.

41. Sulkowski MS, Thomas DL, Chaisson RE, et al. Hepatotoxicity associated with antiretroviral therapy in adults infected with human immunodeficiency virus and the role of hepatitis C or B virus infection. JAMA 2000; 283:74–80.

42. Sulkowski MS, Thomas DL. Hepatitis C in the HIV-infected person. Ann Intern Med 2003; 138:197–207.

   Guidelines for treatment of HCV/HIV coinfected patients and strategies to deal with abnormal liver tests in these patients.

43. Uberti-Fopa C, De Bona A, Morsica G, et al. Pretreatment of chronic active hepatitis C in patients coinfected with HIV and hepatitis C virus reduces the hepatotoxicity associated with subsequent antiretroviral therapy. J Acquir Immune Defic Syndr 2003; 33:146–152.

44. Givens RC, Watkins PB. Pharmacogenetics and clinical gastroenterology. Gastroenterology 2003; 125:240–248.

   A review of the possible applications of pharmacogenetics in minimizing gastrointestinal drug toxicity.

45. Evans WE, McLeod HL. Pharmacogenomics – drug disposition, drug targets, and side effects. N Engl J Med 2003; 348:538–549.

46. Larrey D, Pageaux GP. Genetic predisposition to drug-induced hepatotoxicity. J Hepatol 1997; 26(suppl 2):12–21.

47. Roy B, Chowdhury A, Kundu S, et al. Increased risk of antituberculosis drug-induced hepatotoxicity in individuals with glutathione S-transferase M1 'null' mutation. J Gastroenterol Hepatol 2001; 16:1033–1037.

48. Huang YS, Chern HD, Su WJ, et al. Polymorphism of the N-acetyltransferase 2 gene as a susceptibility risk factor for antituberculosis drug-induced hepatitis. Hepatology 2002; 35:883–889.

49. Sharma SK, Balamurugan A, Saha PK, et al. Evaluation of clinical and immunogenetic risk factors for the development of hepatotoxicity during antituberculosis treatment. Am J Respir Crit Care Med 2002; 166:916–919.

50. Danan G, Benichou C. Causality assessment of adverse reactions to drugs–I. A novel method based on the conclusions of international consensus meetings: application to drug-induced liver injuries. J Clin Epidemiol 1993; 46:1323–1330.

51. Maria VA, Victorino RM. Development and validation of a clinical scale for the diagnosis of drug induced hepatitis. Hepatology 1997; 26:664–669.

52. Lucena MI, Camargo R, Andrade RJ, et al. Comparison of two clinical scales for causality assessment in hepatotoxicity. Hepatology 2001; 33:123–130.

   Poor correlation of these two scales in causality assessment except in patients with associated hypersensitivity features.

53. Kaplowitz N. Causality assessment versus guilt-by-association in drug hepatotoxicity. Hepatology 2001; 33:308–310.

54. Miremont G, Haramburu F, Begaud B, et al. Adverse drug reactions: physicians' opinions versus a causality assessment method. Eur J Clin Pharmacol 1994; 46:285–289.

55. Aithal GP, Rawlins MD, Day CP. Accuracy of hepatic adverse drug reaction reporting in one English health region. Br Med J 1999; 319:1541.

   An alternative liver disorder was observed in more than 50% of cases labeled as having drug-induced liver disease.

56. Degott C, Feldmann G, Larrey D, et al. Drug-induced prolonged cholestasis in adults: a histological semiquantitative study demonstrating progressive ductopenia. Hepatology 1992; 15:244–251.

57. Rosebraugh CJ, Honig PK, Yasuda SU, et al. Formal education about medication errors in internal medicine clerkships. JAMA 2001; 286:1019–1020.

58. Dormann H, Criegee-Rieck M, Neubert A, et al. Implementation of computer-assisted monitoring system for the detection of adverse drug reactions in gastroenterology. Aliment Pharmacol Ther 2004; 19:303–309.

   A pilot attempt at identifying adverse drug reactions in hospitalized patients by computer-generated alerts.

59. Azaz-Livshits T, Levy M, Sadan B, et al. Computerized surveillance of adverse drug reactions in hospital: pilot study. Br J Clin Pharmacol 1998; 45:309–314.

60. Hawton K, Townsend E, Deeks J, et al. Effects of legislation restricting pack sizes of paracetamol and salicylate on self poisoning in the United Kingdom: before and after study. Br Med J 2001; 322:1203–1207.

60a. Morgan O, Grifiths C, Majeed A. Impact of paracetamol pack size restrictions on poisoning from paracetamol in England and Wales: an observational study. J Public Health 2005; 27:19–24.

61. Favreau JT, Ryu ML, Braunstein G, et al. Severe hepatotoxicity associated with the dietary supplement LipoKinetix. Ann Intern Med 2002; 136:590–595.

62. Chitturi S, Farrell GC. Herbal hepatotoxicity: an expanding but poorly defined problem. J Gastroenterol Hepatol 2000; 15:1093–1099.

63. Stedman C. Herbal hepatotoxicity. Semin Liver Dis 2002; 22:195–206.

64. Lewis JD, Strom BL. Safety of dietary supplements with the free market. Ann Intern Med 2002; 136:616–618.

   Calls for stricter regulation of complementary/alternative medicines.

65. Kaplan MM. Alanine aminotransferase levels: what's normal? [Editorial]. Ann Intern Med 2002; 137:49–51.

66. Tolman KG. The liver and lovastatin. Am J Cardiol 2002; 89:1374–1380.

66a. Smith CC, Bernstein LI, Dains RB, et al. Screening for statin-related toxicity: the yield of transaminase and creatine kinase measurement in a primary care setting. Arch Intern Med 2003; 163:688–692.

66b. Chalasami N, Statins and hepatotoxicity: focus on patients with fatty liver. Hepatology 2005; 41:690–695.

67. Bork K, Pitton M, Harten P, et al. Hepatocellular adenomas in patients taking danazol for hereditary angio-oedema. Lancet 1999; 353:1066–1067.

68. Kremer JM, Alarcon GS, Lightfoot RW Jr, et al. Methotrexate for rheumatoid arthritis: suggested guidelines for monitoring liver toxicity. Arth Rheum 1994; 7:316–328.

69. Roenigk HH, Auerbach R, Maibach HI, et al. Methotrexate in psoriasis: revised guidelines. J Am Acad Dermatol 1988; 19:145–156.

70. Said S, Jeffes EW, Weinstein GD. Methotrexate. Clin Dermatol 1997; 15:781–797.

71. Aithal GP, Haugk B, Das S, et al. Monitoring methotrexate-induced hepatic fibrosis in patients with psoriasis: are serial liver biopsies justified? Aliment Pharmacol Ther. 2004; 19:391–399.

72. Bravo AA, Sheth SG, Chopra S. Liver biopsy. N Engl J Med 2001; 344:495–500.

73. O'Grady JG, Alexander GJ, Hayllar KM, et al. Early indicators of prognosis in fulminant hepatic failure. Gastroenterology 1989; 97:439–445.

74. Chitturi S, Farrell GC. Drug-induced liver disease. Current treatment options in gastroenterology. Gastroenterology 2000; 3:457–462.

75. Dribben WH, Porto SM, Jeffords BK. Stability and microbiology of inhalant N-acetylcysteine used as an intravenous solution for the treatment of acetaminophen poisoning. Ann Emerg Med 2003; 42:9–13.

76. Rumack BH, Matthew H. Acetaminophen poisoning and toxicity. Pediatrics 1975; 55:871–876.

77. Prescott LF, Illingworth RN, Critchley JAJH, et al. Intravenous N-acetylcysteine: the treatment of choice for paracetamol poisoning. Br Med J 1979; 2:1097–1100.

78. Zed PJ, Krenzelok EP. Treatment of acetaminophen overdose. Am J Health Syst Pharm 1999; 56:1081–1093.

79. Keays R, Harrison PM, Wendon JA, et al. Intravenous acetylcysteine in paracetamol induced fulminant hepatic failure: a prospective controlled trial. Br Med J 1991; 303:1026–1029.

80. Pajoumand A, Jalali N, Abdollahi M, et al. Successful treatment of acetaminophen overdose associated with hepatic failure. Hum Exp Toxicol 2003; 22:453–458.

81. Walsh TS, Hopton P, Philips BJ. The effect of N-acetylcysteine on oxygen transport and uptake in patients with fulminant hepatic failure. Hepatology 1998; 27:1332–1340.

82. Dargan PI, Jones AL. Management of paracetamol poisoning. Trends Pharmacol Sci 2003; 24:154–157.

83. Yip L, Dart RC, Hurlbut KM. Intravenous administration of oral N-acetylcysteine. Crit Care Med 1998; 26:40–43.

84. Appelboam AV, Dargan PI, Knighton J. Fatal anaphylactoid reaction to N-acetylcysteine: caution in patients with asthma. Emerg Med J 2002; 19:594–595.

85. Schmidt LE, Dalhoff K. Risk factors in the development of adverse reactions to N-acetylcysteine in patients with paracetamol poisoning. Br J Clin Pharmacol 2001; 51:87–91.

86. Iveson TJ, Ryley NG, Kelly PMA, et al. Diclofenac associated hepatitis. J Hepatol 1990; 10:85–89.

87. Shalev O, Mosseri M, Ariel I, et al. Methyldopa-induced immune hemolytic anemia and chronic active hepatitis. Arch Intern Med 1983; 143:592–593.

88. Gough A, Chapman S, Wagstaff K, et al. Minocycline induced autoimmune hepatitis and systemic lupus erythematosus-like syndrome. Br Med J 1996; 312:169–172.

89. Mitnick PD, Klein WJ Jr. Piroxicam-induced renal disease. Arch Intern Med 1984; 144:63–64.

90. Sterling MJ, Kane M, Grace ND. Pemoline-induced autoimmune hepatitis. Am J Gastroenterol 1996; 91:2233–2234.

91. Kallinowski B, Theilmann L, Zimmermann R, et al. Effective treatment of cyclosporine-induced cholestasis in heart-transplanted patients treated with ursodeoxycholic acid. Transplantation 1991; 51:1128–1129.

92. Katsinelos P, Vasiliadis T, Xiarchos P, et al. Ursodeoxycholic acid (UDCA) for the treatment of amoxicillin-clavulanate potassium (Augmentin)-induced intra-hepatic cholestasis: report of two cases. Eur J Gastroenterol Hepatol 2000; 12:365–368.

93. Kojima M, Kamoi K, Ukimura O, et al. Clinical utility of ursodeoxycholic acid in preventing flutamide-induced hepatopathy in patients with prostate cancer: a preliminary study. Int J Urol 2002; 9:42–46.

94. Piotrowicz A, Polkey M, Wilkinson M. Ursodeoxycholic acid for the treatment of flucloxacillin-associated cholestasis. J Hepatol 1995; 22:119–120.

95. Leone N, Giordanino C, Baronio M, et al. Ticlopidine-induced cholestatic hepatitis successfully treated with corticosteroids: a case report. Hepatol Res 2004; 28:109–112.

96. Bernal W, Wendon J, Rela M, et al. Use and outcome of liver transplantation in acetaminophen-induced acute liver failure. Hepatology 1998; 27:1050–1055.

97. Bernal W, Donaldson N, Wyncoll D, et al. Blood lactate as an early predictor of outcome in paracetamol-induced acute liver failure: a cohort study. Lancet 2002; 359:558–563.

98. Schmidt LE, Dalhoff K. Serum phosphate is an early predictor of outcome in severe acetaminophen-induced hepatotoxicity. Hepatology 2002; 36:659–665.

99. Bernal W, Wendon J. More on serum phosphate and prognosis of acute liver failure. Hepatology 2003; 38:533–534.

100. Gow PJ, Sood S, Angus PW. Serum phosphate as a predictor of outcome in acetaminophen-induced fulminant hepatic failure. Hepatology 2003; 37:711–712.

101. Schmidt LE, Ott P, Tygstrup N. Galactose elimination capacity as a prognostic marker in patients with severe acetaminophen-induced hepatotoxicity: 10 years' experience. Clin Gastroenterol Hepatol 2004; 2:418–424.

102. Koivusalo AM, Yildirim Y, Vakkuri A, et al. Experience with albumin dialysis in five patients with severe overdoses of paracetamol. Acta Anaesthesiol Scand 2003; 47:1145–1150.

Preliminary experience with an albumin-based dialysis in drug-induced acute liver failure.

103. Ostapowicz G, Fontana RJ, Schiodt FV, et al. Results of a prospective study of acute liver failure at 17 tertiary care centers in the United States. Ann Intern Med 2002; 137:947–954.

104. Sussman NL, Kelly JH. High throughput screening for drug-induced liver disease-investigative and preemptive toxicology (Abstract). Hepatology 2003; 34(Suppl.1):702A.

105. Trost DC, Freston JW. Use of vector analysis of liver function tests to detect an early signal of hepatotoxicity of a drug in early clinical trials (Abstract). Hepatology 2003; 34(Suppl.1):698A.

106. Davern TJ, James LP, Fontana RJ, et al. Serum acetaminophen adducts reliably distinguish acetaminophen toxicity from other causes of acute liver failure (Abstract).Hepatology 2003; 34(Suppl.1):538A.

107. Hoglen NC, Fisher CD, Hirakawa BP, et al. IDN-6556, the first anti-apoptotic caspase inhibitor: preclinical efficacy and safety (Abstract). Hepatology 2003; 34(Suppl.1):579A.

Primary biliary cirrhosis

Jayant A. Talwalkar and Keith D. Lindor

INTRODUCTION

Primary biliary cirrhosis (PBC) is a chronic cholestatic liver disease of unknown etiology. The disease is characterized histologically by the presence of portal inflammation and necrosis of the interlobular and septal bile ducts. Progressive bile duct destruction is associated with the development of cirrhosis and end-stage liver disease requiring transplantation. The etiology of PBC remains unknown although evidence for an interaction between host and environmental factors is likely. PBC is commonly diagnosed among women in the fifth and sixth decade of life with a majority being asymptomatic at initial presentation. Serum antimitochondrial antibody (AMA) is present in 90–95% of affected patients. Medical therapy with ursodeoxycholic acid (UDCA) can halt disease progression in selected individuals and improves survival free of liver transplantation.

EPIDEMIOLOGY AND NATURAL HISTORY

Primary biliary cirrhosis affects all races and has no specific geographic predilection. Women are primarily affected with a female to male ratio of 9:1. The median age of disease onset is 50 years but varies between 20 and 90 years. The annual incidence of PBC ranges between 2 and 24 cases per million population.[1,2] Prevalence estimates range from 19 to 402 cases per million population.[2–5] Potential risk factors for the development of PBC include cigarette smoking, history of extrahepatic autoimmune disease, history of urinary tract infection, and previous tonsillectomy.[6,7] The risk for developing PBC among first-degree relatives of an index case is at least 10 times higher when compared to the general population risk, especially among daughters of affected women.[8]

For asymptomatic patients at diagnosis, the cumulative risk for developing symptoms is 50% at 5 years and 95% at 20 years of follow-up.[9] The median time from serum AMA positivity to persistent serum liver test elevations is 5.6 years.[10] Among patients with normal liver biochemistries and detectable serum AMA at diagnosis, a 40% rate of histologic disease progression is observed over a median of 11.4 years.[10] Death from liver disease is less frequent in asymptomatic versus symptomatic patients.[9] However, a lower overall median survival for asymptomatic patients is observed when compared to an age- and sex-matched healthy population in the absence of treatment.[9,11] Disease progression to end-stage liver failure is more likely to occur among symptomatic patients. Independent predictors of mortality for all patients include age, total bilirubin, albumin, prothrombin time, and severity of edema.[12]

PATHOGENESIS

The major finding associated with immune system dysregulation in PBC is recognition of the antimitochondrial antibody. Serum AMA is directed against the E2 subunit of the pyruvate dehydrogenase complex (PDC-E2) along the inner surface of biliary epithelial mitochondrial membrane.[13] The reason for developing AMA specifically directed against inner mitochondrial membrane proteins of small intrahepatic bile ducts rather than other tissues is unknown. Furthermore, the occurrence of PBC in patients without AMA seropositivity remains incompletely understood.[14] Arguments against direct cytotoxic activity from AMA include: (1) the persistence of antibody after liver transplantation without immediate disease recurrence; (2) the absence of correlation between serum antibody titer and hepatic involvement; (3) the absence of AMA in some patients with histologic confirmation of PBC; and (4) the ability to induce AMA by administration of recombinant PDC-E2 protein in animal models without causing PBC.[15]

The concept of 'molecular mimicry' wherein microbial infection induces cross-reactivity with self-antigens has been proposed as an underlying mechanism for PBC.[16] A number of infectious agents including *Escherichia coli* (*E. coli*), *Helicobacter* species, *Chlamydia pneumoniae*, and retroviruses have been implicated yet findings to date remain non-specific to PBC.[17,18] Evidence for an underlying viral infection is supported by electron microscopy of cholangiocytes and the increased frequency of serum antibodies to retroviral antigens in PBC.[19] Alternate explanations for the development of PBC include fetal microchimerism,[20] selenium deficiency,[21] and impaired sulfoxidation of endogenous bile acids.[22]

DIAGNOSIS (Figure 38.1)

Biochemical features

The most characteristic biochemical abnormality in PBC is an elevated serum alkaline phosphatase (usually 3–4 times the upper limit of normal).[23] Subjects with a positive serum AMA and histology compatible with PBC may rarely have normal serum

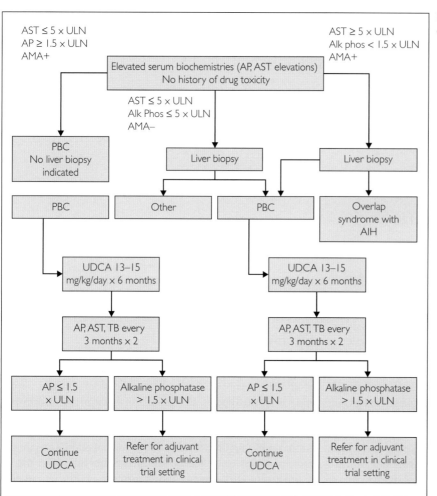

Fig. 38.1 • Proposed clinical algorithm for the diagnosis and treatment of PBC.

alkaline phosphatase levels.[10] No association exists between the level of serum alkaline phosphatase elevation and prognosis prior to initiation of medical therapy. Modestly increased values for alanine aminotransferase (ALT) and aspartate aminotransferase (AST) are common, but significant elevations (greater than 200 U/L) requires the exclusion of superimposed viral or drug-induced hepatic injury. Serum total bilirubin levels often rise during disease progression but are commonly within normal limits at the time of diagnosis. Levels reaching 20 mg/dL are unusual but can be associated with advanced hepatic disease. Elevations in serum total bilirubin, hypoalbuminemia, and prolongations in prothrombin time are associated with poor clinical outcomes and often justify consideration for liver transplantation. Hypercholesterolemia is observed in up to 85% of cases at diagnosis. Serum IgM levels and bile acids (cholic acid, chenodeoxycholic acid) are also elevated in patients with PBC.[23]

Serologic features

Between 90% and 95% of patients with the diagnosis of PBC have positive serum AMA in titers greater than or equal to 1:40.[24] Although the AMA assay that is widely commercially available is not organ-specific, a titer at or above 1:40 remains highly sensitive (98%) as a diagnostic test.[25] Of note, an estimated 8–10% of cases with autoimmune hepatitis[26] and a small proportion of PSC

cases are AMA seropositive. PBC patients may also exhibit serum antinuclear antibody (ANA) and/or smooth muscle antibody (SMA) in 35–66% of cases.[23] Some of these patients exhibit features of AMA-negative PBC (see below and also Chapter 34 for a description of overlap syndromes).[27] Serum anticentromere antibodies in patients with scleroderma or the CREST syndrome occur in 10–15% of PBC cases.[28] Other autoantibodies in PBC patients include rheumatoid factor (70%), antithyroid antibodies (40%), and anti-sp-100 antibodies (25%).[23]

Histologic features

While the biochemical and serologic presentation described above usually confirms the diagnosis of PBC, a liver biopsy is needed for determining the stage of histologic disease at the time of diagnosis.[29] Stage I PBC is associated with portal tract inflammation from predominantly lymphoplasmacytic infiltrates resulting in the destruction of septal and interlobular bile ducts up to 100 μm in diameter. Focal duct obliteration with granuloma formation has been termed the 'florid duct lesion' and is considered almost pathognomonic for PBC when present. Stage II PBC is consistent with an extension of portal tract infiltrates with associated lymphocytic cholangitis and interface hepatitis. Stage III PBC is dominated by the existence of septal or bridging fibrosis. The inflammatory features described with stage II disease are often present as well. Ductopenia (defined as the loss of >50% of interlobular bile ducts) becomes more common, resulting in progressive cholestasis. Stage IV disease is consistent with biliary cirrhosis. Nodular regeneration with extensive ductular proliferation resembling a 'garland-shaped' appearance is characteristic of advanced PBC.[30,31]

Overlap syndrome with autoimmune hepatitis

Selected patients with PBC may also have clinical and histologic features compatible with autoimmune hepatitis. An 'overlap' syndrome has been described in this situation with original estimates of frequency as high as 20%. Refinement of diagnostic criteria, however, has reduced the prevalence rate of this condition to <5%. No long-term data regarding prognosis with overlap syndrome compared to patients with typical PBC are reported.[32]

TREATMENT OF DISEASE-RELATED COMPLICATIONS (Tables 38.1 & 38.2)

Fatigue

Natural history and controlled trial investigations have reported the presence of fatigue variably ranging from 0% to 76% of affected patients.[33] Referral bias, extent of disease, and the extent of patient evaluation to document fatigue are likely responsible for this discrepancy. For asymptomatic patients at diagnosis, the cumulative risk for developing fatigue over a 5-year period is substantial at nearly 50%.[34] Further investigation reveals that fatigue is independent of severity of hepatic disease severity, sleep disturbance, or depression. Fatigue is not significantly improved with ursodeoxycholic acid therapy.[35] Alterations in central neurotransmission[36] and impaired corticotrophin-releasing hormone response[37] have been hypothesized as mechanisms of fatigue in PBC.

Attempts to identify effective medical treatment for fatigue in PBC patients have only recently been made. Antioxidant therapy has no effect on fatigue scores in a randomized, crossover trial

Table 38.1 Symptoms and therapeutic options in PBC

Symptoms	Therapy
Fatigue	None
Sicca syndrome	Artificial tears Oral sialagogues
Pruritus	Antihistamines UDCA Cholestyramine Rifampin Naltrexone/naloxone
Metabolic bone disease	Calcium Vitamin D HRT* Oral bisphosphonates
Steatorrhea	Pancreatic enzymes Gluten free diet Rotating antibiotics

* HRT, hormone replacement therapy.

Table 38.2 Monitoring of patients with PBC

History and physical exam every 6–12 months

Serum liver biochemistries and prothrombin time every 3–6 months

Serum TSH at diagnosis and yearly thereafter

Serum vitamin A, D, and E levels at diagnosis

Liver ultrasound at diagnosis and yearly

Bone mineral density test at diagnosis and 2 years later if therapy initiated

Ultrasound and serum alpha-fetoprotein every 6–12 months with cirrhosis

Screening endoscopy for esophageal varices if Mayo risk score greater than 4 or cirrhosis present

setting.[38] In a recent abstract, fatigue severity in patients with PBC was improved by ondansetron (Zofran) as compared to placebo.[39] While implying that altered serotoninergic neurotransmission may influence fatigue, the use of selective serotonin reuptake inhibitors was ineffective in two small randomized trials.[40,41]

Pruritus

Pruritus is reported in 25–70% of patients affected by PBC. Increased serum alkaline phosphatase levels and Mayo risk score are independently associated with pruritus, but symptom severity is independent of histologic stage.[42] The underlying pathogenesis of pruritus in PBC remains obscure. Recent hypotheses include the accumulation of serum bile acids and an increased release of endogenous opioids.[43]

Antihistamines and phenobarbital have marginal clinical efficacy in the treatment of pruritus of PBC.[44] Cholestyramine (a bile-acid binding resin) decreases the intensity of pruritus to an acceptable level in most patients, but rarely leads to complete symptom resolution.[45] Among subjects with intact gallbladders, the use of 4 g of cholestyramine before and/or after breakfast is thought to maximize bile acid sequestration resulting in symptom improvement. The use of divided doses of cholestyramine spaced several hours apart from other medications (including ursodeoxycholic acid) is recommended to prevent reduction in gastrointestinal absorption of other drugs.[23] The oral antibiotic rifampin (150–450 mg daily) is highly effective for the treatment of moderate to severe pruritus.[46] Although well tolerated, this medication is also associated with liver injury in 15% of cases and bone marrow aplasia on rare occasions.[47] Parenteral naloxone[48] and oral nalmefene[49] can result in symptomatic improvement. Novel therapies requiring further testing include flumenicol, stanozolol, propofol, ondansetron, S-adenosylmethionine (SAMe), and sertraline.[50,51] Among patients with pruritus refractory to medical therapy, liver transplantation is the most effective therapeutic option.

Keratoconjunctivitis sicca

While receiving less attention in the literature compared to fatigue and pruritus, the symptoms from keratoconjunctivitis sicca is reported in over 70% of patients (unpublished data) and can be extremely problematic. Both dry eyes and dry mouth are observed in patients with PBC. Secondary involvement of salivary and lacrimal glands with inflammation is thought to be the underlying cause. The majority of patients, however, do not satisfy criteria for the diagnosis of Sjögren's syndrome. In contrast, patients with classical features of Sjögren's syndrome and serum AMA positivity often develop PBC at a later date.[52] Treatment is directed at symptomatic improvement using artificial tears and oral sialagogues as first-line agents. Topical cyclosporine for keratoconjunctivitis has not been tested in PBC.[53] Oral pilocarpine and cemeviline, which have been used in patients with primary Sjögren's syndrome, have not been extensively tested in PBC.[54,55]

Dyslipidemia

Hypercholesterolemia and hyperlipidemia are present in up to 85% of patients with PBC. In early-stage disease, there is a marked elevation in high-density lipoprotein (HDL) rather than low-density lipoprotein (LDL), but this ratio is reversed with histologic disease progression. Total serum cholesterol levels tend to be markedly elevated early in the disease and may fall to low levels once end-stage liver disease has developed. There is no clear correlation between xanthelasma formation and serum cholesterol levels.[56] Dietary fat restriction and cosmetic surgery to eliminate xanthomas are ineffective. A reduction in serum cholesterol and LDL levels with improvement in xanthelasma formation is associated with ursodeoxycholic acid therapy.[57] Statin-based therapy is effective for dyslipidemia in PBC, yet no large experience has been reported to date and there does not currently appear to be a strong justification for its use. Two published investigations have independently concluded there is no increased risk of death from cardiovascular disease in PBC patients with severe hypercholesterolemia compared to the general population.[56,58]

Metabolic bone disease

Metabolic bone disease in PBC is related to osteopenia rather than osteomalacia (defective bone mineralization). While a number of chronic liver diseases have recently been associated with osteopenia, the greater involvement in PBC is likely associated with cholestasis and the predilection of PBC for females who are independently at risk for metabolic bone disease. Potential etiologies include defective osteoblast activity in premenopausal women, increased osteoclast activity in pre- and postmenopausal women, polymorphisms of vitamin D metabolism which predispose to bone disease, and cigarette smoking which reduces serum vitamin D levels.[59]

Approximately one-third of patients with PBC have osteopenia and 11% have osteoporosis defined by a Z score <−2.5 by lumbar spine bone mineral densitometry testing. The increased risk for osteoporosis from PBC remains controversial, however, as other studies observe similar rates of bone loss when compared to age-matched healthy postmenopausal women. Risk factors for metabolic bone disease in PBC include age, body mass index, and stage 3 or 4 histologic disease.[60]

First-line therapy for metabolic bone disease includes weight-bearing exercise, oral calcium (1000–1200 mg daily), sun exposure, and vitamin D replacement (25 000 to 50 000 IU two to three times weekly) when low serum levels are documented.

Hormone replacement therapy (HRT) is safe and effective among postmenopausal patients with PBC.[61] If HRT is to be used, a repeat serum liver biochemical evaluation at 2-week intervals for 8 weeks is advised to exclude worsening cholestasis. The use of oral bisphosphonates is associated with improvements in lumbar spine BMD, but no data are available regarding the effect of treatment on reducing incident fractures.[62,63]

Fat-soluble vitamin deficiency

Malabsorption of fat-soluble vitamins from cholestasis and impaired bile acid delivery to the small intestine is common among PBC patients. Symptomatic vitamin A deficiency (manifested as night blindness) is successfully treated with 25 000 IU to 50 000 IU two to three times weekly. As discussed previously, vitamin D deficiency may also occur and is the next most common fat-soluble vitamin deficiency. Vitamin E deficiency is rarely observed but can be responsible for ataxia. Oral replacement therapy at 400 IU daily is recommended for these patients. Increased serum prothrombin time can be associated with vitamin K deficiency as well as end-stage liver disease. Daily oral doses of 5–10 mg daily should be initiated.[64]

Steatorrhea

Steatorrhea in PBC may be attributed to a number of potential causes. Impairment of bile acid delivery with insufficient critical micellar concentration in the small intestine is the most common etiology. Oral replacement with median-chain triglycerides may be helpful in this situation. Associated, but undiagnosed or poorly controlled celiac disease may also be a cause of steatorrhea. Adherence to a gluten-free diet should result in symptomatic improvement. Exocrine pancreatic insufficiency and bacterial overgrowth syndrome (in patients with scleroderma) should also be kept in mind. Pancreatic enzyme replacement therapy and rotating empiric antibiotic use, respectively, are the treatments of choice.

DISEASE MODIFYING THERAPIES

Immunosuppressive agents

Corticosteroids

Improvements in symptoms, serum hepatic biochemistries, and histology occurred with the use of corticosteroids in 36 patients in a 1-year placebo-controlled trial.[65] However, no improvement in mortality was observed even after an additional 2 years of treatment.[66] Furthermore, there is concern that chronic use of steroids would accelerate bone loss and be detrimental. Larger randomized controlled trials will be required to determine treatment safety and efficacy. On the other hand, anecdotal reports suggest that patients with AIH-PBC overlap syndromes may enjoy biochemical and histological improvement with corticosteroids.[32]

Azathioprine

Despite the successful use of azathioprine in autoimmune hepatitis, similar benefits have not been observed in PBC. Despite a preliminary report to the contrary, no improvements in symptoms, serum hepatic biochemistries, histology, or survival have been reported in two studies.[67,68]

Cyclosporine

A randomized trial including 19 subjects receiving cyclosporine (4 mg/kg/day) and 10 subjects receiving placebo appeared to show improved symptoms and hepatic biochemistries after 1 year.[69] However, a large, randomized controlled trial of 346 patients with a median follow-up of 2.5 years failed to reveal any histologic benefit despite biochemical improvement.[24] Significant renal toxicity and hypertension were noted in both studies.

Methotrexate

Oral methotrexate in patients with PBC showed some biochemical and histologic benefit in early uncontrolled reports.[70,71] One placebo-controlled trial using a low dose of methotrexate (7.5 mg/week) resulted in biochemical improvement (not including total bilirubin) without an increase in survival. However, the study enrolled a high proportion of patients with early histologic stage disease.[72] Interstitial pneumonitis has been observed in 15% of PBC patients who receive methotrexate (compared to 3–5% in patients with rheumatologic disease), raising safety concerns for long-term clinical use.[73]

Antifibrotic agents

D-penicillamine

Based on abnormalities in copper excretion and the presence of significant concentrations in hepatic tissue, a number of clinical trials using d-penicillamine for PBC were performed. No substantial benefits among a total of 748 patients given the drug have been observed. In the largest study reported (312 subjects),[74] as many as 20% of patients developed serious drug-related side effects including membranous glomerulonephritis and death in a few instances.

Colchicine

Improvements in serum hepatic biochemical parameters were noted in a study examining a dose of 1.2 mg/day. An increase in liver-related survival was also observed at 4 years of follow-up but only after all placebo-treated patients were crossed over to colchicine.[75] A recent meta-analysis failed to confirm either a beneficial or detrimental effect from colchicine based on limitations in study methodological quality.[76]

Ursodeoxycholic acid

Ursodeoxycholic acid monotherapy

Ursodeoxycholic acid (UDCA) is safe and has been shown to be of benefit in PBC patients. UDCA therapy has several effects that may lead to benefit in PBC. In addition to promoting endogenous bile acid secretion with membrane stabilization, UDCA also inhibits apoptosis and mitochondrial dysfunction.[77] Five well-powered, randomized, controlled trials have provided extensive information regarding the effectiveness of UDCA in PBC.[78–82] Improvements in symptom and hepatic biochemical parameters were demonstrated in all five studies. A combined analysis of three studies using UDCA at doses of 13–15 mg/kg/day revealed improvements in survival free of liver transplantation among patients receiving active drug.[83,84] UDCA may also stabilize or improve histopathological lesions in early-stage PBC, but this requires prospective confirmation.[85] Nonetheless, the positive effects of UDCA on disease progression and survival free of liver

transplantation have been questioned in a recent meta-analysis.[86] The majority of identified studies were recognized with follow-up periods of 2 years or less, which may reduce the ability of UDCA to demonstrate its total effect over this short duration. Among the five large randomized trials with greater than 2 years' follow-up, UDCA is associated with a 32% risk reduction in death or the need for liver transplantation.[87] Extended follow-up of an original study also suggests that long-term administration of UDCA may translate into a survival benefit.[83] Finally, it should be noted that higher doses do not appear to offer a greater potential for benefit. Indeed, doses of UDCA above 20 mg/kg/day do not appear to uniformly improve serum liver biochemistries despite optimal bile enrichment, and lower doses were not effective.[88,89]

Between 50% and 70% of patients treated with UDCA do not completely normalize serum hepatic biochemistries within 6 months and even go on to develop cirrhosis in some cases (incomplete response).[90] A recent Markov model described a 17–27% risk for cirrhosis over 10 years in patients with early-stage histological disease treated with UDCA. Predictors of incomplete response leading to cirrhosis include higher levels of serum alkaline phosphatase, serum total bilirubin, and lower serum albumin levels prior to therapy.[91] A number of factors must be considered as possibly contributing to an incomplete response to UDCA. These include medication noncompliance, inappropriate dosing by weight, concomitant use of cholestyramine impairing UDCA absorption, or concomitant disease, e.g., autoimmune hypothyroidism, celiac disease, or overlap syndrome, as a cause of elevated serum liver enzymes.

Combination therapies with ursodeoxycholic acid

Two randomized controlled trials of UDCA plus corticosteroids showed reductions in serum hepatic biochemistry values and mixed results involving histologic improvement. Follow-up in both trials was short, ranging from 9 to 12 months.[92,93] One study included the use of azathioprine at 50 mg/day.[93] The use of oral budesonide in combination with UDCA has been variably associated with biochemical improvements.[94,95] A recent investigation, however, demonstrated preliminary safety and efficacy in patients with early-stage compared to advanced PBC given budesonide.[96]

No significant benefit from combination therapy with UDCA and colchicine has been demonstrated. Short durations of treatment (less than 2 years) and low doses of colchicine (approximately 1 mg/day) have been proposed as limitations. A recent investigation, however, reported reductions in the number of treatment failures, slower progression of Mayo risk score, and improvement in hepatic histology from UDCA with colchicine compared to patients receiving UDCA monotherapy.[97] Confirmation of these results is awaited.

Despite improvements in biochemical parameters from an open-label investigation,[98] no overall benefit has been reported from other studies using UDCA and methotrexate. Results from two long-term, multicenter, randomized, control trials comparing UDCA with combination therapy also showed no additional benefit with methotrexate.[99,100]

Novel agents

Malotilate

Malotilate is a compound that improves hepatic protein metabolism. In a randomized, multicenter trial of 101 PBC patients given malotilate (n=52) or placebo (n=49), improvements in biochemical parameters occurred in the active treatment arm compared to placebo.[101] However, no impact on disease progression or survival at the end of 2 years' treatment was noted.

Chlorambucil

A randomized trial of 24 PBC patients using doses of chlorambucil 0.5–4 mg/day showed no significant improvement in biochemical or histologic parameters after 2–6 years of follow-up.[102] Significant bone marrow suppression required chlorambucil discontinuation in four subjects.

Thalidomide

Thalidomide is a derivative of glutamic acid, which selectively inhibits tumor necrosis factor-alpha (TNF-α) production by monocytes. No improvements in biochemical or histologic parameters were observed in PBC patients given thalidomide (n=10) or placebo (n=8) in a small pilot trial.[103] Side effects including sedation and fatigue caused two patients to discontinue active treatment.

Silymarin

Silymarin is an antioxidant drug that is the active ingredient in milk thistle. It has reportedly been associated with hepatoprotective effects in experimental and clinical studies, especially among patients with alcoholic liver disease. Among patients with an incomplete response to UDCA monotherapy, the use of silymarin with UDCA was not associated with significant benefits in an open-label, pilot investigation.[104]

Bezafibrate

Bezafibrate is a hypolipidemic medication that stimulates the canalicular phospholipid pump MDR3 via binding and activation of transcription factor peroxisome-proliferator-activated receptor-alpha (PPAR-α). This results in an increased biliary secretion of phospholipids that are cytoprotective against the proinflammatory effects of bile salts. Bezafibrate alone or in combination with UDCA[105,106] has been associated with improvements in serum hepatic biochemical values in patients with PBC. Long-term studies, however, are required to confirm these early positive results.

Sulindac

Increased bile acid transport is associated with the use of sulindac in experimental animal models. The combination of sulindac (100–300 mg/day) with UDCA (10–15 mg/kg/day) resulted in significant biochemical improvement in 11 PBC patients without complete response to UDCA compared to 12 patients remaining on UDCA monotherapy.[107] However, patients in the UDCA monotherapy group had more advanced histological stage at baseline compared to the combination therapy group.

Simvastatin

An open-label pilot investigation focusing on the lipid-lowering abilities of simvastatin (a 3-hydroxy-3-methylglutaryl coenzyme A reductase inhibitor) studied six patients with PBC for 2 months with doses of 5–20 mg daily.[108] Significant reductions in serum alkaline phosphatase, immunoglobulin M levels, and serum lipid levels were observed. Further study is required to determine if this class of agents will be useful for adjuvant therapy.

Tetracycline

Tetracycline was recently studied for PBC because of the suggestion that *Chlamydia pneumoniae* might play a role in the development of PBC.[18] Fifteen patients received tetracycline 1 g twice a day for 3 weeks, but this was not associated with significant biochemical improvement. Liver histology in this pilot investigation was not a study endpoint.[109]

Pyruvate dehydrogenase

The concept of oral tolerance induction was tested using purified bovine pyruvate dehydrogenase complex (PDC) in six patients with early-stage PBC. After 6 months of therapy, no significant change in liver biochemistries or serum AMA titers was observed.[110]

Liver transplantation (Table 38.3)

The most effective therapeutic alternative for patients with end-stage PBC is liver transplantation. Indications for referral include accepted criteria required for all hepatic disease etiologies as well as refractory complications of portal hypertension. Severe fatigue, intractable pruritus, and disabling pain from vertebral body compression fractures may also be considered indications for liver transplantation. PBC remains among the top five most frequent indications for liver transplantation in the United States. Patient and graft survival rates, however, remain excellent at 90–95% and 80–85% at 1-year and 5-year intervals, respectively.[111,112] Hepatic retransplantation occurs in less than 10% of patients with PBC.[113]

Previously considered a controversial topic, the recurrence of PBC following liver transplantation has now been accepted.[114] The estimated cumulative incidence rates for developing recurrent PBC are 15% at 3 years and 30% at 10 years with prospective follow-up.[115] Serum AMA status does not influence the recurrence risk. A shorter time to recurrence with tacrolimus rather than cyclosporine as primary immunosuppression has recently been described.[116] While UDCA has empirically been administered to selected patients with recurrent PBC, there is no information regarding the efficacy of UDCA in halting disease progression.

SUMMARY

Primary biliary cirrhosis is an important hepatic disease, which affects middle-aged women. While data regarding its pathophysiology continue to emerge, much remains unknown about the interaction between host factors and immune system

Table 38.3 Indications for liver transplant referral in PBC

Child-Turcotte-Pugh score ≥7
Recurrent variceal bleeding
Ascites
Hepatic encephalopathy
Spontaneous bacterial peritonitis
Hepatopulmonary syndrome
Hepatocellular carcinoma (1 lesion ≤5 cm or 3 lesions ≤3 cm each)
Intractable pruritus

dysregulation in this condition. Disease-specific complications including fatigue, pruritus, sicca syndrome, and metabolic bone disease are important to recognize and treat appropriately. The natural history of PBC is usually indolent but often accelerates once advanced histologic stages are reached. Among various medical therapies intended to halt disease progression, only UDCA has been associated with an increase in transplant-free survival. Liver transplantation is an effective therapeutic modality for patients with end-stage liver disease.

AUTHORS' RECOMMENDATIONS

1. The diagnosis of PBC should be considered when the following clinical features are present:
   Cholestatic serum liver profile,
   Serum AMA positivity,
   Liver histology compatible with PBC.
2. Liver biopsy is not indicated for the diagnosis of PBC in the following circumstances:
   Serum alkaline phosphatase level ≥1.5 times the upper limit of normal,
   Serum AST level ≤5 times the upper limit of normal,
   Serum AMA positivity.
3. Initial therapy with UDCA at 13–15 mg/kg/day for a minimum treatment period of 6 months is recommended. Treatment goal is to achieve reduction in serum alkaline phosphatase level ≤1.5 times the upper limit of normal (complete response).
4. If a complete response to UDCA therapy is not observed, consider adjuvant therapy in the setting of ongoing clinical trials.

REFERENCES

1. Remmel T, Remmel H, Uibo R, et al. Primary biliary cirrhosis in Estonia. With special reference to incidence, prevalence, clinical features, and outcome. Scan J Gastroenterol 1995; 30:367–371.

2. Metcalf JV, Bhopal RS, Gray J, et al. Incidence and prevalence of primary biliary cirrhosis in the city of Newcastle upon Tyne, England. Int J Epidemiol 1997; 6:830–836.

3. Watson RG, Angus PW, Dewar M, et al. Low prevalence of primary biliary cirrhosis in Victoria, Australia. Melbourne Liver Group. Gut 1985; 36:927–930.

4. Kim WR, Lindor KD, Locke GR, et al. Epidemiology and natural history of primary biliary cirrhosis in a U.S. community. Gastroenterology 2000; 119:1631–1636.

   The only population-based epidemiologic study of PBC from the continental United States.

5. Witt-Sullivan H, Heathcote J, Cauch K, et al. The demography of primary biliary cirrhosis in Ontario, Canada. Hepatology 1990; 12:98–105.

6. Howel D, Fischbacher CM, Bhopal RS, et al. An exploratory population-based case-control study of primary biliary cirrhosis. Hepatology 2000; 31:1055–1060.

7. Parikh-Patel A, Gold EB, Worman H, et al. Risk factors for primary biliary cirrhosis in a cohort of patients from the United States. Hepatology 2001; 33:16–21.

8. Jones DEJ, Watt FE, Metcalf JV, et al. Familial primary biliary cirrhosis reassessed: a geographically based population study. J Hepatol 1999; 10:402–407.

   Population-based study describing a 6.4% prevalence rate of PBC among first-degree relatives of index cases.

9. Prince MI, Chetwynd A, Craig WL, et. al. Asymptomatic primary biliary cirrhosis: clinical features, prognosis, and symptom progression in a large population based cohort. Gut 2004; 53:865–870.

10. Mitchison HC, Bassendine MF, Hendrick A, et al. Positive antimitochondrial antibody but normal alkaline phosphatase: is this primary biliary cirrhosis? Hepatology 1986; 6:1279–1284.

11. Springer J, Cauch-Dudek K, O'Rourke K, et al. Asymptomatic primary biliary cirrhosis: a study of its natural history and prognosis. Am J Gastroenterol 1999; 94:47–53.

12. Dickson E, Grambsch PM, Fleming TR, et al. Prognosis in primary biliary cirrhosis: model for decision making. Hepatology 1989; 10:1–7.

13. Leung PSC, Chuang DT, Wynn RM, et al. Autoantibodies to BCOADC-E2 in patients with primary biliary cirrhosis recognize a conformational epitope. Hepatology 1995; 22:505–513.

14. Tsuneyama K, Van De Water J, Van Thiel DH, et al. Abnormal expression of PDC-E2 on the apical surface of biliary epithelial cells in patients with antimitochondrial antibody negative primary biliary cirrhosis. Hepatology 1995; 22:1440–1446.

15. Krams SM, Surh CD, Coppel RI, et al. Immunization of experimental animals with dehydrolipoamide acyltransferase, as a purified recombinant polypeptide, generates mitochondrial autoantibodies but not primary biliary cirrhosis. Hepatology 1989; 9:411–416.

16. Burroughs AK, Butler P, Sternberg MJE, et al. Molecular mimicry in liver disease. Nature 1992; 358:377–378.

17. Haydon GH, Neuberger J. PBC: an infectious disease? Gut 2000; 47:586–588.

18. Abdulkarim AS, Petrovic LM, Kim WR, et al. Primary biliary cirrhosis: an infectious disease caused by *Chlamydia pneumoniae*? J Hepatol 2004; 40(3):380–384.

19. Xu L, Shen Z, Guo L, et al. Does a betaretrovirus infection trigger primary biliary cirrhosis? Proc Natl Acad Sci USA 2003;100(14): 8454–8459

20. Corpechot C, Barbu V, Chazouilleres O, et al. Fetal microchimerism in primary biliary cirrhosis. J Hepatol 2000; 33:696–700.

21. Thuluvath PJ, Triger DR. Selenium in primary biliary cirrhosis. Lancet 1987; 2:219.

22. Olomu AB, Vickers CR, Waring RH, et al. High incidence of poor sulfoxidation in patients with primary biliary cirrhosis. N Eng J Med 1988; 318:1089–1092.

23. Talwalkar JA, Lindor KD. Primary biliary cirrhosis. Lancet 2003; 362(9377):53–61

24. Lombard M, Portmann B, Neuberger J, et al. Cyclosporine A treatment in primary biliary cirrhosis: Results of a long-term placebo controlled trial. Gastroenterology 1993; 104:519–526.

   Large randomized placebo-controlled trial, which failed to demonstrate clear benefit in the absence of drug toxicity.

25. Walker JG, Doniach D, Roitt IM, et al. Serologic tests in diagnosis of primary biliary cirrhosis. Lancet 1965; 1:827.

26. Kenny RP, Czaja AJ, Ludwig J, et al. Frequency and significance of antimitochondrial antibodies in severe chronic active hepatitis. Dig Dis Sci 1986; 31:705–711.

27. Goodman ZD, McNally PR, Davis KR, et al. Autoimmune cholangitis: A variant of primary biliary cirrhosis: Clinicopathologic and serologic correlations in 200 cases. Dig Dis Sci 1995; 40:1232–1242.

28. Bernstein RM, Callendar ME, Neuberger JM, et al. Anticentromere antibody in primary biliary cirrhosis. Ann Rheum Dis 1982; 41:612–614.

29. Zein CO, Angulo P, Lindor KD. When is liver biopsy needed in the diagnosis of primary biliary cirrhosis? Clin Gastroenterol Hepatol 2003; 1(2):89–95.

30. Ludwig J, Dickson ER, McDonald GS. Staging of chronic non-suppurative destructive cholangitis (syndrome of primary biliary cirrhosis). Virchows Arch 1978; 379:103.

31. Scheuer PJ. Primary biliary cirrhosis: Chronic non-suppurative destructive cholangitis. Am J Pathol 1965; 46:387.

32. Talwalkar JA, Keach JC, Angulo P, et al. Overlap of autoimmune hepatitis and primary biliary cirrhosis: an evaluation of a modified scoring system. Am J Gastroenterol 2002; 97(5):1191–1197.

33. Leuschner U. Primary biliary cirrhosis – presentation and diagnosis. Clin Liver Dis 2003; 7(4):741–758

34. Prince M, Chetwynd A, Newman W, et al. Survival and symptom progression in a geographically based cohort of patients with primary biliary cirrhosis: follow-up for up to 28 years. Gastroenterology 2002; 1044:51–123.

    Large cohort study of primarily untreated patients documenting the natural history of symptom and hepatic disease progression.

35. Cauch-Dudek K, Abbey S, Stewart DE, et al. Fatigue in primary biliary cirrhosis. Gut 1998; 43(5):705–710.

36. Jones EA, Yurdaydin C. Is fatigue associated with cholestasis mediated by altered central neurotransmission? Hepatology 1997; 25:492–494.

37. Swain MG, Maric M. Defective corticotrophin-releasing hormone mediated neuroendocrine and behavioral responses in cholestatic rats: implications for cholestatic liver disease-related sickness behaviors. Hepatology 1995; 22:1560–1564.

38. Prince MI, Mitchison HC, Ashley D, et al. Oral antioxidant supplementation for fatigue associated with primary biliary cirrhosis: results of a multicenter randomized, placebo-controlled, cross-over trial. Aliment Pharmacol Ther 2003; 17:137–1 43.

39. Theal J, Toosi MN, Girlan LM, et al. Ondansetron ameliorated fatigue in patients with primary biliary cirrhosis (PBC). Hepatology 2002; 36(Part 2):296A.

40. Talwalkar JA, Jorgensen RA, Keach JC, et al. Fluoxetine for the treatment of fatigue in primary biliary cirrhosis. Dig Dis Sci 2004 (in press)

41. Ter Borg PC, Van Os E, Van Den Broek WW, et al. Fluvoxamine for fatigue in primary biliary cirrhosis and primary sclerosing cholangitis: a randomized controlled trial BMC. Gastroenterol 2004; 134(1):13

42. Talwalkar JA, Souto E, Jorgensen RA, et al. Natural history of pruritus in primary biliary cirrhosis. Clin Gastroenterol Hepatol. 2003; 1(4):297–302

43. Jones EA, Bergasa NV. The pruritus of cholestasis: from bile acids to opiate agonists. Hepatology 1990; 11:884–887.

44. Bloomer JR, Boyer JL. Phenobarbital effects in cholestatic liver diseases. Ann Intern Med 1975; 82:310–317.

45. Gillespie DA, Vickers CR. Pruritus and cholestasis: therapeutic options. J Gastroenterol Hepatol 1993; 8(2):168–173

46. Ghent CN, Carruthers SG. Treatment of pruritus in primary biliary cirrhosis with rifampin. Results of a double blind, crossover, randomized trial. Gastroenterology 1988; 94:488–493.

47. Prince MI, Burt AD, Jones DE. Hepatitis and liver dysfunction with rifampicin therapy for pruritus in primary biliary cirrhosis. Gut 2002; 50(3):436–439.

48. Bergasa NV, Alling DW, Talbot TL, et al. Naloxone ameliorates the pruritus of cholestasis: results of a double blind, randomized placebo controlled trial. Ann Intern Med 1995; 123:161.

49. Bergasa NV, Alling DW, Talbot TL, et al. Oral nalmefene therapy reduces scratching activity due to the pruritus of cholestasis: a controlled study. J Am Acad Derm 1999; 41:431–434.

50. Bergasa NV, Mehlman JK, Jones EA. Pruritus and fatigue in primary biliary cirrhosis. Best Prac Res Clin Gastro 2000; 14:643–655.

51. Browning J, Combes B, Mayo MJ. Long-term efficacy of sertraline as a treatment for cholestatic pruritus in patients with primary biliary cirrhosis. Am J Gastroenterol 2003; 98(12):2736–2741.

52. Csepregi A, Szodoray P, Zeher M. Do autoantibodies predict autoimmune liver disease in primary Sjögren's syndrome? Data of 180 patients upon a 5 year follow-up. Scand J Immunol 2002; 56(6):623–629.

53. Sall K, Stevenson OD, Mundorf TK, et al. Two multicenter, randomized studies of the efficacy and safety of cyclosporine ophthalmic emulsion in moderate to severe dry eye disease. CsA Phase 3 Study Group. Ophthalmology 2000; 107(4):631–639

54. Vivino FB, Al-Hashimi I, Khan Z, et al. Pilocarpine tablets for the treatment of dry mouth and dry eye symptoms in patients with Sjögren syndrome: a randomized, placebo-controlled, fixed-dose, multicenter trial. P92-01 Study Group. Arch Intern Med 1999; 159(2):174–181.

55. Petrone D, Condemi JJ, Fife R, et al. A double blind, randomized, placebo-controlled study of cevimeline in Sjögren's syndrome patients with xerostomia and keratoconjunctivitis sicca. Arthritis Rheum 2002; 46(3):748–754.

56. Crippin JS, Lindor KD, Jorgensen RA, et al. Hypercholesterolemia and atherosclerosis in primary biliary cirrhosis: what is the risk? Hepatology 1992; 15:858–862.

57. Balan V, Dickson ER, Jorgensen RA, et al. Effect of ursodeoxycholic acid on serum lipids of patients with primary biliary cirrhosis. Mayo Clin Proc 1994; 69:923–929.

58. Longo M, Crosignani A, Battezzati PM, et al. Hyperlipidemic state and cardiovascular risk in primary biliary cirrhosis. Gut 2002; 51(2):265–269.

59. Rouillard S, Lane NE. Hepatic osteodystrophy. Hepatology 2001; 33(1):301–307.

60. Menon KV, Angulo P, Weston S, et al. Bone disease in primary biliary cirrhosis: independent indicators and rate of progression. J Hepatol 2001; 35(3):316–323.

61. Pereira SP, O'Donohue J, Moniz C, et al Transdermal hormone replacement therapy improves vertebral bone density in primary biliary cirrhosis: results of a 1-year controlled trial. Aliment Pharmacol Ther 2004; 19(5):563–570.

62. Guanabens N, Pares A, Monegal A, et al. Etidronate versus fluoride for treatment of osteopenia in primary biliary cirrhosis: preliminary results after 2 years. Gastroenterology 1997; 113:219–224.

63. Guanabens N, Pares A, Ros I, et al. Alendronate is more effective than etidronate for increasing bone mass in osteopenic patients with primary biliary cirrhosis. Am J Gastroenterol 2003; 98(10):2268–2274.

64. Levy C, Lindor KD. Management of osteoporosis, fat-soluble vitamin deficiencies, and hyperlipidemia in primary biliary cirrhosis. Clin Liver Dis 2003; 7(4):901–910.

65. Mitchison HC, Bassendine MF, Malcolm AJ, et al. A pilot, double blind controlled 1-year trial of prednisolone treatment in primary biliary cirrhosis. Hepatic improvement but greater bone loss. Hepatology 1989; 10:420–429.

66. Mitchison HC, Palmer JM, Bassendine MF, et al. A controlled trial of prednisolone treatment in primary biliary cirrhosis: Three-year results. J Hepatol 1992; 15:336–344.

67. Crowe J, Christensen E, Smith M, et al. Azathioprine in primary biliary cirrhosis: A preliminary report of an international trial. Gastroenterology 1980; 78:1005–1010.

68. Christensen E, Neuberger J, Crowe J, et al. Beneficial effect of azathioprine and prediction of prognosis in primary biliary cirrhosis: Final results of an international trial. Gastroenterology 1985; 89:1084–1091.

69. Wiesner RH, Ludwig J, Lindor KD, et al. A controlled trial of cyclosporine in the treatment of primary biliary cirrhosis. N Eng J Med 1990; 322:1419–1424.

70. Kaplan MM, Knox TA, Arora S. Primary biliary cirrhosis treated with low-dose oral pulse methotrexate. Ann Intern Med 1988; 109:429–431.

71. Kaplan MM, Knox TA. Treatment of primary biliary cirrhosis with low-dose weekly methotrexate. Gastroenterology 1991; 101:1332–1338.

72. Hendrickse MT, Rigney E, Giaffer MH, et al. Low-dose of methotrexate is ineffective in primary biliary cirrhosis: long-term results of a placebo-controlled trial. Gastroenterology 1999; 117:400–407.

73. Sharma A, Provenzale D, McKusick A, et al. Interstitial pneumonitis after low-dose methotrexate therapy in primary biliary cirrhosis. Gastroenterology 1994; 107:266–270.

74. Dickson ER, Fleming TR, Wiesner RH, et al. Trial of penicillamine in advanced primary biliary cirrhosis. N Engl J Med 1985; 312:1011–1015.

75. Kaplan MM, Alling DW, Zimmerman HJ, et al. A prospective trial of colchicine for primary biliary cirrhosis. N Engl J Med 1986; 215:1448–1454.

76. Gong Y, Gluud C. Colchicine for primary biliary cirrhosis. Cochrane Database Syst Rev. 2004; (2):CD004481.

77. Guicciardi ME, Gores GJ. Ursodeoxycholic acid cytoprotection: dancing with death receptors and survival pathways. Hepatology 2002; 35(4):971–973.

78. Lindor KD, Dickson ER, Baldus WP, et al. Ursodeoxycholic acid in the treatment of primary biliary cirrhosis. Gastroenterology 1994; 106:1284–1290.

79. Poupon RE, Balkan B, Eschwege E, et al. A multicenter, controlled trial of ursodiol for the treatment of primary biliary cirrhosis. N Eng J Med 1991; 324:1548–1554.

80. Heathcote EJ, Cauch-Dudek K, Walker V, et al. The Canadian multicenter, double blind, randomized controlled trial of ursodeoxycholic acid in primary biliary cirrhosis. Hepatology 1994; 19:1149–1156.

81. Combes B, Carithers RL, Maddrey WC, et al. A randomized, double blind, placebo-controlled trial of ursodeoxycholic acid in primary biliary cirrhosis. Hepatology 1995; 22:759–766.

82. Pares A, Caballeria L, Rodes J, et al. Long-term effects of ursodeoxycholic acid in primary biliary cirrhosis: results of a double-blind, controlled multicentric trial: the UDCA-Cooperative Group from the Spanish Association for the Study of the Liver. J Hepatol 2000; 32:561–566.

83. Poupon RE, Poupon R, Balkau B, et al. Ursodiol for the long-term treatment of primary biliary cirrhosis. N Engl J Med 1994; 330:1342–1347.

84. Poupon RE, Lindor KD, Cauch-Dudek K, et al. Combined analysis of randomized controlled trials of ursodeoxycholic acid in primary biliary cirrhosis. Gastroenterology 1997; 113:884–890.

Combined analysis of three large single-center investigations which support the efficacy of UDCA for improving survival free of liver transplantation in PBC.

85. Poupon RE, Lindor KD, Pares A, et al. Combined analysis of the effect of treatment with ursodeoxycholic acid on histologic progression in primary biliary cirrhosis. J Hepatol 2003; 39(1):12–16.

86. Goulis J, Leandro G, Burroughs AK. Randomized controlled trials of ursodeoxycholic acid therapy for primary biliary cirrhosis: a meta-analysis. Lancet 1999; 354:1053–1060.

87. Poupon RE. Ursodeoxycholic acid for primary biliary cirrhosis: lessons from the past – issues for the future. J Hepatol 2000; 32:685–688.

88. Combes B, Luketic VA, Peters MG, et al. Prolonged follow-up of patients in the U.S. multicenter trial of ursodeoxycholic acid for primary biliary cirrhosis. Am J Gastroenterol 2004; 99(2):264–268.

89. Angulo P, Dickson ER, Therneau TM, et al. Comparison of three doses of ursodeoxycholic acid in the treatment of primary biliary cirrhosis: a randomized trial. J Hepatol 1999; 30:830–835.

90. Leuschner M, Dietrich CF, You T, et al. Characterization of patients with primary biliary cirrhosis responding to long-term ursodeoxycholic acid treatment. Gut 2000; 46:121–126.

91. Corpechot C, Carrat F, Poupon R, et al. Primary biliary cirrhosis: incidence and predictive factors of cirrhosis development in ursodiol-treated patients. Gastroenterology 2002; 122(3):652–658

92. Leuschner M, Gultdutuna S, You T, et al. Ursodeoxycholic acid and prednisolone versus ursodeoxycholic acid and placebo in the treatment of early stages of primary biliary cirrhosis. J Hepatol 1996; 25:49–57.

93. Wolfhagen FHJ, van Hooganstraten HJF, van Buuren HR, et al. Triple therapy with ursodeoxycholic acid, prednisone, and azathioprine in primary biliary cirrhosis: a 1-year, randomized placebo-controlled study. J Hepatol 1998; 29:736–742.

94. Leuschner M, Maier K-M, Schlichting J, et al. Oral budesonide and ursodeoxycholic acid for the treatment of primary biliary cirrhosis: results of a prospective, double-blind trial. Gastroenterology 1999; 117:918–925.

95. Angulo P, Smith C, Jorgensen R, et al. Oral budesonide in the treatment of patients with primary biliary cirrhosis with suboptimal response to ursodeoxycholic acid. Hepatology 2000; 31(2):318–323.

96. Hempfling W, Grunhage F, Dilger K, et al. Pharmacokinetics and pharmacodynamic action of budesonide in early- and late-stage primary biliary cirrhosis. Hepatology 2003; 38(1):196–202.

97. Almasio PL, Floreani A, Chiaramonte M, et al. Multicenter randomized placebo-controlled trial of ursodeoxycholic acid with or without colchicine in symptomatic primary biliary cirrhosis. Alim Pharm Ther 2000; 14:1645–1652.

98. Bonis PAL, Kaplan MM. Methotrexate improves biochemical tests in patients with primary biliary cirrhosis who respond incompletely to ursodiol. Gastroenterology 1999; 117:395–399.

99. Bach N, Bodian C, Bodenheimer H, et al. Methotrexate therapy for primary biliary cirrhosis. Am J Gastroenterol 2003; 98(1): 187–193.

100. Combes B, Emerson SS, Flye NL. The primary biliary cirrhosis ursodiol plus methotrexate or its placebo study – a multicenter randomized trial. Hepatology 2003; 38(S1):210A.

Large multicenter study which failed to show additional benefit from methotrexate and UDCA compared to UDCA alone.

101. European Multicenter Study Group. The results of a randomized double blind controlled trial evaluating malotilate in primary biliary cirrhosis. J Hepatol 1993; 17:227–235.

102. Hoofnagle JH, Davis GL, Schafer DF, et al. Randomized trial of chlorambucil for primary biliary cirrhosis. Gastroenterology 1986; 91:1327–1334.

103. McCormick PA, Scott F, Epstein O, et al. Thalidomide as therapy for primary biliary cirrhosis: a double-blind placebo controlled pilot study. J Hepatol 1994; 21:496–499.

104. Angulo P, Patel T, Jorgensen RA, et al. Silymarin in the treatment of patients with primary biliary cirrhosis with a suboptimal response to ursodeoxycholic acid. Hepatology 2000; 32:897–900.

105. Kunihara T, Nimi A, Maeda A, et al. Bezafibrate in the treatment of primary biliary cirrhosis: comparison with ursodeoxycholic acid. Am J Gastroenterol 2000; 95:2990–2992.

106. Miyaguchi S, Ebinuma H, Imaeda H, et al. A novel treatment for refractory primary biliary cirrhosis? Hepatogastroenterology 2000; 47:1518–1521.

107. Leuschner M, Holtmeier J, Ackermann H, et al. The influence of sulindac on patients with primary biliary cirrhosis that responds incompletely to ursodeoxycholic acid: a pilot study. Eur J Gastroenterol Hepatol 2002; 14:1369–1376.

108. Ritzel U, Leonhardt U, Nather M, et al. Simvastatin in primary biliary cirrhosis: effects on serum lipids and distinct disease markers. J Hepatol 2002; 36:454–458.

109. Maddala YK, Jorgensen RA, Angulo P, et al. Open-label pilot study of tetracycline in the treatment of primary biliary cirrhosis. Am J Gastroenterol 2004; 99:566–567.

110. Suzuki A, Van de Water J, Gershwin ME, et al. Oral tolerance and pyruvate dehydrogenase in patients with primary biliary cirrhosis. Dev Immunol 2002; 9:55–61.

111. Neuberger J. Liver transplantation for primary biliary cirrhosis. Autoimmun Rev 2003; 2:1–7.

112. Kim WR, Wiesner RH, Therneau TM, et al. Optimal timing of liver transplantation for primary biliary cirrhosis. Hepatology 1998; 28:33.

113. Kim WR, Wiesner RH, Poterucha JJ, et al. Hepatic retransplantation in cholestatic liver disease: impact of the interval to retransplantation on survival and resource utilization. Hepatology 1999; 30:395.

114. Hubscher SG, Elias E, Buckels JAC, et al. Primary biliary cirrhosis: Histological evidence of disease recurrence after liver transplantation. J Hepatol 1993; 18:173.

115. Liermann Garcia RF, Evangelista Garcia C, McMaster P, et al. Transplantation for primary biliary cirrhosis: retrospective analysis of 400 patients in a single center. Hepatology 2001; 33:22–27.

Large single-center study which documents a cumulative incidence rate of 30% at 10 years for recurrent PBC.

116. Neuberger J, Gunson B, Hubscher S, et al. Immunosuppression affects the rate of recurrent primary biliary cirrhosis after liver transplantation. Liver Transpl 2004; 10:488–491.

CHAPTER THIRTY-NINE

Variceal hemorrhage

Arun J. Sanyal

INTRODUCTION

Cirrhosis of the liver causes nearly 32 000 deaths and a loss of more than 20 million workdays annually in the United States. Much of this morbidity and mortality is directly related to the development of portal hypertension and its complications. While the existence of portal hypertension was speculated upon by Banti in the nineteenth century, the term portal hypertension was only coined in 1906. Thompson and colleagues first measured portal pressures and defined normal levels of portal pressure which formed the basis of their subsequent definition of portal hypertension. The normal portal vein pressure is less than 5 mmHg (7 cm H_2O). Portal hypertension is a syndrome of hemodynamic abnormalities and is defined as an increase in the portal pressure gradient (hepatic vein minus portal vein pressure) above 5 mmHg. The principal consequences of portal hypertension include the development of varices, variceal hemorrhage, and/or ascites which are the major complications of cirrhosis. Given the contribution of portal hypertension to the outcome of cirrhosis, appropriate management of portal hypertension is a cornerstone of the management of cirrhosis. In this chapter, the management of portal hypertension and variceal hemorrhage are discussed.

ANATOMY OF PORTAL SYSTEM AND GASTROESOPHAGEAL VARICES

The portal vein is formed by the confluence of tributaries draining blood from the stomach (left gastric vein), small and large intestines (superior and inferior mesenteric veins), spleen (splenic vein), and the pancreatic bed. These drainage beds communicate with other veins that directly drain in to the systemic circulation. These sites are (as shown in Table 39.1): (1) at the transition zones between the squamous and glandular epithelium, i.e., at the lower end of esophagus and gastric cardia via the extrinsic and intrinsic veins, at the anal canal via anastomoses between the superior and the middle hemorrhoidal veins, and the ileostomy sites; (2) in the falciform ligament via recanalization of the para-umblical veins; (3) in the splenic venous bed and the left renal vein or adrenal vein; (4) sites of previous abdominal surgery or intra-abdominal trauma; and (5) in the retroperitoneum where the somatic surface is in contact with the area not covered with the peritoneum. While these porta-systemic venous communications are normally not functional, they allow blood to the systemic circulation when portal pressures rise, thereby decompressing the portal circulation. This is accompanied by enlargement of these collaterals which become varicose and sometimes bleed.

The gastroesophageal collaterals are the most important of all these due to their propensity to bleed. The gastro-esophageal varices divert portal venous inflow by accommodating blood diverted from the left gastric vein and the splenic hilus through the short gastric veins. The veins that drain the esophagus are classified as intrinsic, extrinsic, and vena comitantes of the vagus. The intrinsic veins of the gastroesophageal junction have been divided into four well-defined zones (Fig. 39.1) by Vianna and colleagues: (1) gastric zone, (2) palisade zone, (3) perforating zone, and (4) truncal zone. The perforating veins penetrate from the sub-mucosa at random intervals to drain into the extrinsic veins.

To compensate for portal hypertension by increasing porta-systemic shunting via gastroesophageal collaterals, the valves in the perforating veins become incompetent, allowing a reverse flow from the extrinsic to the intrinsic veins. The intrinsic veins at the gastroesophageal junction become dilated and tortuous, forming the so-called gastroesophageal varices occurring in four patterns: (1) fundal varices that are fed by short gastric veins but may also be fed by the left gastric vein; (2) gastric and palisade zone varices are the most commonly seen varices in the clinical practice; (3) varices in the perforating zone; and (4) paraesophageal varices that involve the extrinsic veins and are not at risk for bleeding.

PATHOPHYSIOLOGY OF PORTAL HYPERTENSION

The pressure in the portal vein is a product of the portal venous inflow and resistance to outflow and can be represented mathematically by the following expression (Ohm's law):

$$P = Q \times R$$

where P is the pressure in the portal vein, Q is the blood flow and R is the resistance to the outflow. The initiating event in the development of portal hypertension is an increase in the resistance to the portal venous outflow. The most common cause of portal hypertension is cirrhosis, where the resistance is at the level of the sinusoids primarily due to the architectural changes associated with cirrhosis.

Clincally, portal pressure is measured from the hepatic venous pressure gradient (HVPG) which is defined by:

$$HVPG = WHVP - FHVP$$

Table 39.1 Sites for porto-systemic collaterals

Squamo-glandular transition zones	Gastroesophageal varices Recto-anal varices
Falciform ligament (recanalization of fetal circulation)	Paraumbilical veins Umbilical veins
Splenic venous bed	Spontaneous lieno-renal/ adrenal shunts
Retroperitoneal	Spleen and liver Duodenum Descending and ascending colon Sigmoid colon
Previous abdominal surgery/ intra-abdominal trauma	Stomal varices Ileostomy Colostomy

Modified from Table 21.1 Zakim

where the wedged hepatic vein pressure (WHVP) reflects the sinusoidal pressure and the free hepatic venous pressure (FHVP) is the correction for the intra-abdominal pressure. The HVPG most closely reflects the portal pressure when the portal vein is patent. It is normal when the portal vein is occluded and cirrhosis is not present.

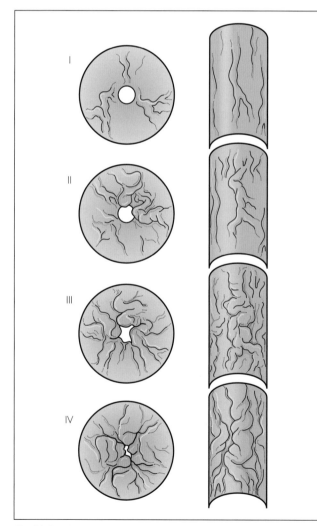

Fig. 39.1 • Pacquet's grading of esophageal varices.

Increased vascular resistance

Large variations in the portal blood flow are accommodated with only minor variations in the portal pressure owing to the high compliance of the porto-hepatic circulation. A decrease in compliance of the porto-hepatic circulation causes the outflow resistance to increase. In patients with cirrhosis, this occurs due to both dynamic changes in the vasculature and fixed changes in the hepatic architecture. The architectural changes in the cirrhotic liver are produced by collagen deposition in the perisinusoidal space (capillarization of the sinusoids), compression by the regenerative nodules, hepatic inflammation, sclerosis of terminal hepatic venules (e.g., in alcoholic liver disease, radiation or cytotoxic chemotherapy-induced injury to the liver), enlarged and swollen hepatocytes (e.g., in hepatic steatosis, storage disorders), and compression of sinusoids by granulomas (e.g., in primary biliary cirrhosis, schistosomiasis).

In addition to the fixed changes in hepatic vasculature, the hepatic stellate cells that surround the hepatic sinusoids also play an active role in modifying the resistance to the hepatic blood flow. These cells exhibit a contractile response to vasoconstrictors such as endothelin (ET), levels of which are increased in the blood and liver tissue of patients with cirrhosis.[1,2] In addition, a relative deficiency of the vasodilator (nitric oxide) in the intrahepatic circulation has also been found and can lead to worsening of the intrahepatic vasoconstriction.[3] The circulating levels of noradrenaline, angiotensin II, and vasopressin, three highly vasoconstrictive substances, are elevated in cirrhosis, and can also potentially contribute to the increased intrahepatic vascular resistance.

Increased portal venous inflow

Increased portal venous inflow also contributes to the development and aggravation of portal hypertension in patients with cirrhosis due to the splanchnic arteriolar dilatation. This is part of a hemodynamic syndrome associated with cirrhosis which is characterized by systemic arterial vasodilation. The consequent increase in vascular capacity and decreased systemic vascular resistance produces a hyperdynamic circulatory state the hallmarks of which include an increased cardiac index, increased absolute circulatory volume, and a decrease in effective circulating volume.

Role of endogenous vasoactive mediators

There is now sufficient evidence to support the role of a variety of vasoactive mediators in the pathophysiology of portal hypertension. Several humoral factors such as nitric oxide (NO), glucagon, eicosanoids, adenosine, bile salts, platelet activating factor (PAF), and gamma-aminobutyric acid (GABA) have been postulated to be involved in the hyperdynamic circulation in cirrhosis. The exact mechanism of increase of these factors is unclear, but decreased clearance by the liver and increased production are the possible factors involved. Glucagon has been considered as a key humoral factor that causes splanchnic vasodilation by impairing the systemic vascular sensitivity to noradrenaline. Inhibition of hyperglucagonemia by administration of somatostatin or octreotide produces splanchnic vasoconstriction.

NO is a vascular endothelium-derived relaxant factor and a very potent vasodilator. NO is synthesized by two distinct enzyme pathways: a constitutively expressed NO synthetase (cNOS), and an inducible NO synthetase (iNOS). There are two forms of cNOS termed eNOS and nNOS. NO is believed to play a role in the hyperdynamic circulation seen in patients with cirrhosis.[4] NO relaxes the vascular smooth muscle by activating soluble guanylate cyclase. Cirrhotic patients have been shown to have high serum, urinary and breath concentrations of nitrites and nitrates, the metabolic products of NO. Inhibition of NO synthesis restores the splanchnic vascular reactivity to vasoconstrictors, and also ameliorates the systemic hemodynamic changes seen in animal models of portal hypertension. Also, the administration of methylene blue, which is known to block NO action, increases blood pressure and improves oxygenation in hepato-pulmonary syndrome. High levels of NO result from increased activity of eNOS in the splanchnic vascular bed and pulmonary endothelium. Increased flow and shear stress are the factors probably responsible for increased eNOS activity.

ENDOSCOPIC CLASSIFICATION OF GASTROESOPHAGEAL VARICES

Esophageal varices

Esophageal varices are classified on the basis of their endoscopic appearance, location, and size in the esophageal and gastric lumen. Pacquet originally proposed a classification of esophageal varices and graded them as grade 1 through 4 (see Fig. 39.1). The main limitation of this classification is the poor interobserver concordance for grades 1–2 and 3–4. Another classification proposed by the North Italian Endoscopy Club is simple and classifies varices into: F1: small straight varices; F2: enlarged tortuous varices occupying less than one-third of esophageal lumen; F3: large, coil-shaped varices occupying more than one-third of the esophageal lumen. This classification has an interobserver concordance ranging from fair to good agreement (kappa index 0.52) to excellent agreement (kappa index 0.95).[5]

Gastric varices

Gastric varices are classified on the basis of their location in the stomach and their relationship with the esophageal varices (Fig. 39.2) as: (1) Gastroesophageal varices (GOV) are those that extend from the esophagus to the stomach. They are further subclassifed as: (i) type 1 (GOV 1) when they extend from the esophagus to the lesser curve of the stomach for 2–5 cm below the gastroesophageal junction; and (ii) type 2 (GOV 2) when the varices are long and tortuous, extending from the esophagus towards the fundus of the stomach. (2) Isolated gastric varices (IGV) are those that are not directly continuous with esophageal varices. These are also subclassified as: type 1 (IGV 1) when the varices are located in the fundus and are tortuous and complex in shape; and type 2 (IGV 2) when the varices are located in the body, antrum or around the pylorus.[6]

Portal hypertensive gastropathy

Portal hypertensive gastropathy (PHG) is classified as mild when mosaic-like pattern (MLP) of mild degree is present (without redness at the areola), and severe when MLP is superimposed by any red signs.

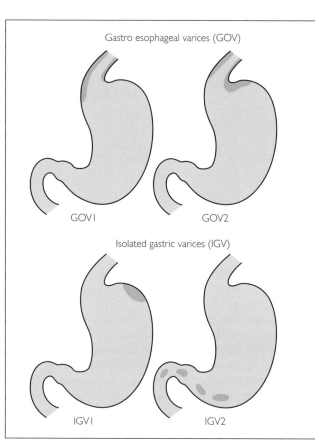

Gastro esophageal varices (GOV)

GOV1 GOV2

Isolated gastric varices (IGV)

IGV1 IGV2

Fig. 39.2 • Classification of gastric varices.

Natural history of gastroesophageal varices

Varices are known to develop eventually in most patients with cirrhosis if followed long enough. Gastroesophageal varices are seen in 50–60% of cirrhotic patients at presentation with large varices in 20%.[7] In those without varices, it has been reported that varices develop at the highly variable rates of 5–15% annually[8] Small varices enlarge into large varices at a rate of 4–10% per annum. Another study showed that over a follow-up of 16 months, small varices resolved in 16%, remained the same in 42%, and increased in size in the remaining 42% patients.[8] Almost one-third (25–35%) of cirrhotic patients with gastroesophageal varices bleed within 2 years of diagnosis of varices.[5,9,10] The risk of initial variceal bleeding is greatest within a 6–12-month period of the detection of the varices.

Predictive factors for variceal bleeding

Varices do not develop and hence cannot bleed when the HVPG is <12 mmHg. Although varices develop when the HVPG is ≥12 mmHg, there is a poor correlation between portal pressure (as measured by HVPG) and risk of variceal bleeding.[11,12] It has, however, been observed that once bleeding occurs, those with a HVPG >20 mmHg are more likely to continue to bleed and fail first-line therapy.[13] The intravariceal pressure as measured by a pressure-sensitive gauge has also been correlated with the risk of bleeding which approaches 50% when the variceal pressure exceeds 15 mmHg (Table 39.2).[14] It has also been shown that the

Table 39.2 Intravariceal pressure and risk of variceal bleeding

Variceal pressure (mmHg)	Incidence of variceal bleeding (%)
≤13.0	0
13.1–14.0	9
14.1–15.0	17
15.1–16.0	50
>16.0	72

Data from Nevens et al.

patients who had bled had a higher variceal pressure than the patients who have not bled, even though the HVPG in the two subgroups was similar.[15]

The frequency of bleeding from large varices is 50–53% as compared to 5–18% with small varices.[5,16] The presence of red color signs seen during endoscopy, as *red weal marks* (longitudinal red streaks on the varices), *cherry red spots* (discrete cherry-colored flat spots on the varices), and *hematocystic spots* (raised discrete red spots on varices resembling blisters) and the severity of cirrhosis predict the probability of variceal bleeding fairly reliably (Table 39.3).[5] The probability of bleeding from varices in a patient with Child's class C who has large-sized varices in the presence of red color signs is nearly 76% within the first year of diagnosis. On the other hand, the probability of bleeding from the varices in a patient in Child's class A, with small varices and no red color signs, is less than 10%.

Spontaneous cessation of bleeding occurs in around 50% of the patients. However, the patients with Child's class C cirrhosis and who are actively bleeding on endoscopy are unlikely to have a spontaneous cessation of bleeding. After the index bleeding episode, the risk of rebleeding is high within the first 6 weeks.[10,17] Over 50% of such rebleeding episodes occur within 3–4 days from the time of admission for the bleeding.[10,18,19] The risk factors for early rebleeding are severe initial bleeding as defined by a hemoglobin <8 g/dL, gastric variceal bleeding, thrombocytopenia, encephalopathy, alcohol-related cirrhosis, large varices, active bleeding during endoscopy, and a high hepatic venous pressure gradient (HVPG).[6,18–20] In the long term, approximately 70% of subjects

experience further variceal hemorrhage and have a similar risk of mortality within the first year.[21] Age greater than 60 years, large esophageal varices, severity of liver disease, continued alcoholism, renal failure, and presence of a hepatoma increase the risk of rebleeding (Table 39.4).[17]

Gastric varices have a higher (nearly 25%) frequency of bleeding and the risk of bleeding is related to their location.[6] Although GOV 1 constitutes more than 70% of the gastric varices, bleeding occurs in only 11%. On the other hand, IGV 1 constitutes only 8% of the gastric varices, but bleeding occurs in almost 80% of these varices.[6] The overall frequency of bleeding from the gastric varices is much less than from the esophageal, but the former bleed more severely than the latter. After the obliteration of the esophageal varices by sclerotherapy, GOV 1 spontaneously regress in about 60% of the cases. The risk of rebleeding among those in whom the GOV 1 do not regress after esophageal variceal obliteration is higher (28% versus 2%) than in those where varices do regress. Esophageal variceal obliteration has no effect on the GOV 2. In the case of IGV 1, the risk of variceal bleeding is directly proportional to the variceal size (>10 mm), severity of liver disease, and presence of red color signs on the varices.

MANAGEMENT OPTIONS FOR VARICEAL BLEEDING

Screening for varices

All patients with cirrhosis must undergo screening endoscopy to identify varices that are at risk of bleeding. Some variables such as a low platelet count <88 000/mm³, prothrombin activity of <70%, splenomegaly, and a portal vein diameter of ≥13 mm on ultrasonography correlate with the presence of varices. However, the predictive values of these parameters is not sufficient to be useful in clinical practice. The standard of care remains routine screening endoscopy in all subjects with cirrhosis.

Patient with no varices on screening endoscopy should be screened every 2 years if they have stable liver functions, and yearly if liver function deterioration occurs.[8,22] Those with small varices at screening should be rescreened on a yearly basis.[8,22]

Goals of management

The goals of management depend on where a given patient is in the natural history of varices and may be considered in three

Table 39.3 Prediction of variceal bleeding by the NIEC index

Red weal marks	Child's class								
	A			B			C		
	F1	F2	F3	F1	F2	F3	F1	F2	F3
−	6	10	15	10	16	26	20	30	42
+	8	12	19	15	23	33	28	38	54
+++	16	23	34	28	40	52	44	60	76

F1, F2, F3 are progressively larger varices.
Data from deFranchis et al.

Table 39.4 Risk factors for rebleeding in esophageal varices

Early rebleeding (<6 weeks)	Late rebleeding (>6weeks)
Age >60 years	Severity of liver failure
Severity of initial bleed	Ascites
Ascites	Hepatoma
Active bleeding on endoscopy	Active alcoholism
Red color signs	Red color signs
Platelet clot on varices	
Renal failure	

phases: (1) primary prophylaxis, (2) control of acute bleeding episode, and (3) prevention of a rebleeding. A variety of management tools are available to accomplish these goals and are considered below.

Principles and techniques of various therapeutic modalities

A large number of therapeutic modalities have been developed for the treatment of variceal hemorrhage. These either attempt to correct portal hypertension or provide local treatment for varices.

Pharmacologic therapy

Various pharmacologic agents have been studied and used in the prevention and management of variceal bleeding. While a large number of drugs have been studied, only a few are currently in routine clinical use.

Nonselective beta-blockers

Nonselective beta-blockers are the most widely used and studied drug in the prevention of the first variceal bleeding episode. Portal venous inflow is an important determinant of the portal pressure and is related to the resistance in the mesenteric arteriolar bed. The β-adrenergic antagonists block β-adrenergic receptor-mediated vasodilation of the mesenteric arterioles and promote unopposed α-receptor-mediated vasoconstriction, thereby decreasing the portal venous inflow and ultimately the portal pressure. At high doses, β-blockers decrease the blood pressure and cardiac output, further decreasing the portal venous inflow and hence the portal pressures.[23,24] Propranolol and nadolol are the two nonselective β-blockers that have been studied in most of the trials.

The oral or intravenous administration of propranolol produces a decrease in the HVPG ranging 9–31%.[23–26] Propranolol abolishes the nocturnal peak in the portal venous inflow in cirrhotic patients,[27] prevents the rise in portal pressure related to modest physical exercise, and attenuates the meal-related rise in the portal pressures. There is considerable heterogeneity in the portal pressure response to propranolol in different individuals, with around 50% showing a less than a 10% decrease in portal pressures following acute administration. Nearly 50–70% of the patients receiving propranolol fail to decrease HVPG below 12 mmHg, or sustain a decrease in portal pressures by 20% of the baseline portal pressure.[23,28–30] Tachyphylaxis results from: (1) an increase in the collateral resistance that negates the hypotensive effects of decreased portal inflow, and (2) an increase in the hepatic arterial flow to maintain sinusoidal perfusion and thereby increase WHVP. Moreover, there is poor correlation between the site of portal obstruction, severity, and etiology of cirrhosis, baseline hemodynamics, plasma propranolol levels, and heart rate response to the portal hypotensive effects of β-blockers. Propranolol does not prevent the progression in the size of varices from small to large as published in one randomized controlled trial.[31]

When the dosage is titrated to the heart rate, the dose requirements of each patient for propranolol and nadolol vary due to variable first-pass effects and the influence of extensive portosystemic shunting and degree of liver failure upon bioavailability. The dose of propranolol required for adequate β-receptor blockade varies from 80 to 160 mg/day, usually given in 2 divided doses, whereas that for nadolol varies from 40 to 80 mg given as a single dose every day.

The dose of drug is titrated to achieve a target resting heart rate of 55–60 beats/min or a 25% decrease in the resting basal heart rate. In those who are unable to achieve these targets, the dose is titrated to maximal tolerated doses. However, none of the above targets correlates well with portal pressures. The patients who develop a decrease in the HVPG below 12 mmHg or a drop in HVPG by 25% have a high probability of remaining free of variceal bleeding.[28,29] This has been the basis for recommendations to monitor HVPG as a way to assess the success of pharmacologic treatment. HVPG measurement is an invasive procedure and the medical work force is, in general, inadequately trained in this technique. Moreover, the cost-effectiveness of this procedure has not been demonstrated and its utility in routine clinical practice remains to be completely defined. The direct measurement of variceal pressure by a pressure-sensitive endoscopic gauge was evaluated as an alternative to assess the effectiveness of the β-blocker therapy to this technique. A 20% decline or more in the variceal pressure as measured by the endoscopic gauge 4 months after the initiation of the propranolol was associated with a very low risk of variceal bleeding over a follow-up period of 28 months.[32] Carvedilol, which possesses both nonselective beta-antagonist and alpha1-receptor antagonist activity, also presents a potential option for lowering portal pressures and has been reported to be associated with mean reductions of 16–43% in HVPG after single and multiple doses.

Beta-blocker therapy is associated with many side effects including bronchospasm, development of heart failure, and sexual dysfunction. These side effects are responsible for discontinuation of therapy in around 20% of patients.[12] There is no impairment of the normal hemodynamic response to an acute bleeding episode in the patients receiving β-blocker therapy. There are many clinical trials where β-blockers have been used for the prevention of first variceal bleeding and prevention of recurrent bleeding, and these are discussed in detail below. On discontinuation of β-blocker therapy, the risk of variceal bleeding returns to the same level as in an untreated patient. However, the mortality after discontinuation of the β-blocker therapy is increased compared to those who continue treatment, highlighting the need for a lifelong commitment to therapy.[33]

Vasodilators

Vasodilating agents acting at various sites have also been found to decrease portal pressures and have been tried in many clinical trials. Isosorbide di-nitrate (ISDN), isosorbide 5-mononitrate (ISMN), and nitroglycerine (NTG) are the most studied vasodilators for portal hypertension. Nitrates are predominantly systemic venous dilators at usual doses and decrease the cardiac output by decreasing the venous return. Systemic venous dilation decreases the postsinusoidal resistance and thereby decreases portal pressure. At high doses, there is arterial dilation and systemic hypotension that triggers a splanchnic arterial constriction, further decreasing the portal blood inflow and decreasing the portal pressures. In addition, the nitrate-mediated baroreceptor reflexes in the pulmonary capillary bed also trigger the splanchnic vasoconstriction and contribute towards decreased portal venous inflow. Nitrates may decrease the portal and collateral outflow resistance by venodilation, further decreasing portal and variceal pressure.

The nitro-vasodilator group of drugs activates the NO pathways and produce vasodilation in the target beds. Acute administration of nitrates (NTG, ISMN, or ISDN) decreases the HVPG by up to 44%,[34] portal blood flow by 30%,[35] and azygous blood flow by 15%. The dose of the nitrates required to ensure an adequate decrease in the portal pressure in cirrhotic patients is not easily titrated. This limits the use of nitrates as a single agent in the management of variceal bleeding. Tachyphylaxis is known to occur with nitrates and the long-term effects on the degree of HVPG reduction are variable. Nitrate use is associated with increased sympathetic activity, a tendency to retain sodium, tissue hypoxia, and increased lactate levels. Nitrates reduce portal-collateral resistance and counteract the increased portal-collateral resistance associated with the usage of β-blockers.

Vasopressors

Vasopressin Vasopressin (ADH) is a powerful vasoconstrictor and is one of the most widely studied drugs in the management of acute variceal bleeding for the last three decades. The ability of vasopressin to control variceal bleeding is due to powerful splanchnic arteriolar vasoconstriction, which decreases the portal inflow and thus the portal pressure. In addition to the effects on the splanchnic circulation and portal system, vasopressin causes profound systemic vasoconstriction with increased peripheral resistance, reduced cardiac output, heart rate, and coronary blood flow. These are responsible for causing myocardial ischemia and/or infarction, cardiac arrhythmias, mesenteric ischemia, extremity ischemia, and cerebrovascular accidents. Fatal complications due to vasopressin have also been reported.[30] The systemic vasoconstrictive side effects of vasopressin may be minimized by the concomitant use of nitrates. The nitrates, in addition to preventing the complications due to systemic vasoconstriction, also have a synergistic effect with vasopressin in decreasing the portal pressures. Vasopressin is rarely used in the management of variceal bleeding due to its side effect profile.

Terlipressin (glypressin) The large number of complications associated with use of vasopressin has led to the development of a relatively safer analogue. Triglycyl-lysl-vasopressin (terlipressin), a synthetic analogue of vasopressin is itself inactive but is activated after the glycyl residue is cleaved. The intrinsic activity of terlipressin causes immediate vasoconstriction which is followed by a more prolonged vasoconstriction related to the slow release of the active metabolite by transformation in vivo into vasopressin by enzymatic cleavage of the triglycyl residues. Terlipressin has a longer biological half-life and is administered every 4 hours. Terlipressin does not increase plasminogen activator activity, as is seen with vasopressin, but has similar effects on the coronary vasculature.

Somatostatin and analogues

Somatostatin is a naturally occurring peptide originally named for its growth hormone inhibiting properties. Somatostatin causes an increase in splanchnic vascular resistance by causing vasoconstriction. The portal hypotensive effects of somatostatin are therefore due to a decrease in the portal blood inflow. The vasoconstriction is mediated by inhibiting the release of splanchnic vasodilator hormones such as glucagon and vasoactive intestinal peptide.[36,37] Somatostatin has a short half-life and is rapidly cleared from the blood. Somatostatin decreases azygous blood flow, indicating a decrease in collateral blood flow.

Synthetic analogues of somatostatin, namely octreotide and vapreotide, have also been used in various clinical trials in the management of acute variceal bleeding and have a longer duration of action. Octreotide produces a modest decline in the WHVP, a variable effect on the intravariceal pressure, and significantly decreases the azygous blood flow. Somatostatin and its analogues are used mainly for the treatment of active hemorrhage. It has an excellent safety profile in the absence of the systemic circulatory side effects, as seen with vasopressin.

Endoscopic therapy

Endoscopic therapy is now the cornerstone of the management of variceal bleeding. Endoscopy is necessary both to identify the source of bleeding and to provide therapy. The two principal forms of endoscopic treatment of esophageal varices: endoscopic sclerotherapy (EST) and endoscopic variceal band ligation (EVL).

Endoscopic sclerotherapy

Endoscopic sclerotherapy is based upon the principle of variceal thrombosis and scarring by injection of a sclerosing agent. Various types of sclerosing agents are used and there are still insufficient data to decide about the best sclerosant for EST. Tissue adhesives such as N-butyl-2-cyanoacrylate (tissue glue) have been used successfully in the sclerosis of gastric varices.[38] The immediate hemostatic effect is mostly due to sealing off of the bleeding spot by edema with subsequent thrombosis of the varix.

EST is performed using a freehand technique and injections are directed at the bleeding sites in an acutely bleeding patient. Both intravariceal and paravariceal injections are effective. However, the intravariceal injection of the sclerosant is the most widely practiced technique. Variceal injections are started at the gastroesophageal junction and usually restricted to the distal 5 cm of the esophagus. There is controversy about the optimal volume of sclerosant to be injected during a single EST session. The volume of sclerosant injected at each site is usually around 1–2 mL and a total of 10–15 mL per session seems optimal and effective.

Once hemostasis has been achieved with emergency EST, the next session is performed within a week and later at 3-weekly intervals to achieve eradication of varices. Although variceal eradication can be achieved faster with weekly regimens, it is balanced by a higher risk of rebleeding from EST-induced mucosal lesions. Variceal recurrence has been observed in 50–70% of individuals after initial obliteration.[39]

EST is associated with local as well as systemic complications.[40] Complications including retrosternal pain, transient dysphagia, fever, and small pleural effusions are common but usually not life threatening. Although esophageal ulcers are seen in about 90% of patients on the day following EST and in 70% after a week from EST, the risk of bleeding from mucosal ulceration is only 20%.[41] Esophageal strictures leading to dysphagia are seen in approximately 15% of patients, although the frequency and severity of this complication vary widely based on the definitions used to diagnose this condition. Proton pump inhibitors are probably the most widely used agent for the prevention and treatment for EST ulcers. EST has also been associated with an increased risk of bacterial peritonitis, esophageal perforation, mediastinitis, and rarely, portal vein thrombosis.

Endoscopic variceal band ligation

Endoscopic variceal band ligation was introduced in the 1980s as an alternative to EST. EVL works by mechanically occluding the varices and variceal flow. An elastic band is used to strangulate the varix producing thrombosis, inflammation, necrosis, and finally sloughing of the mucosa which heals with formation of a mural scar that is restricted to the mucosa and submucosa. EVL is currently performed using one of several multiband ligators that are commercially available.

The banding device consists of a cylinder preloaded with elastic bands. This cylinder is attached to the tip of the endoscope and the trigger wire responsible for deploying the bands on the varices passes through the biopsy channel of the endoscope. The varix to be ligated is suctioned into the cylinder and when a complete 'red out' occurs, the band is released by the trigger wire. The bands are applied circumferentially, starting from the gastroesophageal junction. Five to 10 bands are applied in each session. EVL in the actively bleeding patient can be challenging as the plastic cylinder carrying the bands at the tip of the endoscope limits the operator's field of vision.

EVL is associated with fewer complications than EST. Systemic complications with EVL are rare. Esophageal strictures, bleeding from EVL-induced ulcers, pulmonary infection, bacterial peritonitis, and death have all been reported less commonly with EVL than with EST. However, in a meta-analysis of the EVL-related trials, only the reduced frequency of esophageal strictures reached statistical significance.[42] Mucosal ulceration is seen in 90% of the patients 1 week after EVL.

Balloon tamponade

Most of the variceal blood flows through the gastroesophageal junction. Balloon tamponade is based on the principle of mechanical occlusion of the variceal blood flow. Balloon tamponade can effectively control active bleeding in more than 90% of cases. Rebleeding occurs in a high proportion of patients once the balloon is deflated. Balloon tamponade may result in serious complications including esophageal perforation, aspiration pneumonia, necrotic ulcers at the site of compression, asphyxiation, and mortality (up to 20%).[43] Several types of balloon devices with esophageal and gastric balloons and suction channels are commercially available. There is no strong evidence that one is better than another. Endotracheal intubation should be done for airway protection before insertion of the tube. The gastric balloon should be fully inflated only after radiographic confirmation of the position of the partly inflated gastric balloon. Continuous patient monitoring should be done, and the tube should be removed at the earliest possible time, with continuous inflation for no more than 24 hours. Due to the high rate of rebleeding when the balloon is deflated, as well as the high rate of complications, balloon tamponade is currently used as a temporizing measure in patients who have active, life-threatening hemorrhage refractory to endoscopic and pharmacologic therapy.

Shunts

Transjugular intrahepatic portosystemic shunt

Transjugular intrahepatic portosystemic shunt (TIPS) is a low-resistance intrahepatic communication between a hepatic vein and an intrahepatic branch of the portal vein which is kept patent by deployment of a metal stent across this tract. This procedure is performed by an interventional radiologist and does not require general anesthesia or major surgery. The ability to decompress the portal vein via this tract without general anesthesia or surgery has led to its rapid incorporation in to routine clinical practice. Preliminary data on its use for variceal hemorrhage were not encouraging. The use of a self-expandable metal stent to ensure long-term patency led to the improvement in the results and finally the widespread use of this procedure (Table 39.5).

A preprocedure Doppler sonogram should be performed to document the patency of the portal venous system. The right internal jugular vein is punctured percutaneously, and a vascular sheath is advanced into the inferior vena cava and finally into a hepatic vein. A Colapinto transjugular needle is advanced through the sheath caudally and anteriorly into the liver parenchyma. Contrast or CO_2 is injected as the needle is withdrawn to identify the portal vein. After the portal vein is identified, a wire is inserted into the main portal vein over which an angioplasty catheter is introduced and the needle withdrawn. Portal pressure is measured after a branch of the portal venous system is entered and portal venography is performed. The tract between the hepatic and portal veins is dilated and an 8–10 mm diameter expandable metallic stent is then deployed across the tract. Portal venography is repeated, and post-TIPS portal and vena caval pressures are determined. Newer stents that are coated with polytetrafluoroethylene (PTFE) reduce the risk of thrombosis or TIPS.

Table 39.5 Indications and contraindications of TIPS

Indications

Well accepted
  Refractory variceal bleeding
  Recurrent variceal bleeding despite endoscopic treatment
  Prevention of recurrent variceal bleeding in patients awaiting transplant
  Bleeding isolated gastric varices in fundus
  Refractory ascites
  Refractory hepatic hydrothorax
  Budd-Chiari syndrome

Highly experimental but insufficient data
  Hepatorenal syndrome
  Veno-occlusive disease
  Bleeding portal gastropathy
  Thrombocytopenia due to hypersplenism

Others
  Bleeding ectopic varices
  Protein-losing enteropathy due to portal hypertension

Contraindications

Absolute
  Right heart failure
  Severe pulmonary artery hypertension
  Polycystic liver disease
  Severe hepatic failure
  Portal vein thrombosis with cavernoma

Relative
  Severe hepatic encephalopathy poorly controlled on medical therapy
  Biliary obstruction
  Active infection (local/systemic)
  Portal vein thrombosis without cavernoma

It is not necessary to decrease the HVPG to values less than 12 mmHg to obtain clinical benefits in those who are bleeding. A 25–50% decrease in HVPG is usually seen after a 10 mm shunt is placed and is associated with control of active bleeding in over 90% of cases. In one study,[44] a 50% drop in HVPG was associated with negligible rebleeding. These data are also compatible with the well-established paradigm that a sustained drop in HVPG by 25% virtually always prevents variceal hemorrhage. It must also be remembered that increasing the shunt diameter beyond 10 mm increases the degree of shunting considerably and may worsen encephalopathy and liver failure. Based on these considerations, an initial shunt diameter of 10 mm appears to be the best target diameter for a TIPS. Embolization of the left gastric vein along with TIPS is rarely required and is indicated only when active bleeding persists after an adequate TIPS.[45] Doppler ultrasonography should be performed within the first week after TIPS, mainly to exclude shunt thrombosis.

TIPS is associated with many complications. Technical complications are generally seen in 10% of the patients after TIPS. The technique-related mortality ranges from 0% to 2%. Puncture of the liver capsule with resulting hemoperitoneum or inadvertent puncture of the biliary tree with resulting hemobilia are two potentially life-threatening complications. The 30-day mortality ranges 7–55% and reflects the differences in patient selection in various studies.[46,47] The 1-year mortality after TIPS varies 10–52% when used to control variceal bleeding, and 24–54% in those with refractory ascites.[48–51] Various prognostic models have been designed to evaluate the outcome of patients after TIPS.

Hepatic encephalopathy occurs in 20–30% of subjects after TIPS. Complete diversion of portal flow as well as a proportion of hepatic arterial blood flow into the shunt (hepatofugal flow) are responsible for hepatic encephalopathy.[52–54] The encephalopathy can be managed medically in most cases. Clinically significant increases in serum bilirubin or alanine aminotransferase levels or prolongation of the prothrombin time are seen in over one-fourth of patients after TIPS. Although this deterioration is transient, accelerated liver failure can also occur in up to 5% patients and is probably related to diversion of nutrient portal blood flow away from the hepatic parenchyma. A pre-TIPS bilirubin of 3 mg/dL or higher is a risk factor for accelerated liver failure after TIPS. Accelerated liver failure can also contribute to the development of encephalopathy. TIPS is also associated with complications including mild self-limited hemolysis, contrast-induced renal failure, heart failure, stent migration, fever, infection, transient arrhythmias, and inadvertent puncture of the gallbladder or other organs adjacent to the liver.

Stenosis or occlusion of the shunt is a major problem that has limited the long-term utility of TIPS. TIPS stenosis occurred in 50–70% of the patients within the first year in early studies. The actuarial probability of development of shunt insufficiency ranges from 30% to 50% at 12 months and over 80% at 24 months.[54,55] Shunt thrombosis is usually an early event.[54,56] While European centers often use anticoagulation to prevent shunt thrombosis, the incidence of this complication is so low in US centers that it is rarely used for prophylaxis of thrombosis. Pseudo-intimal hyperplasia is responsible for a chronic stenosis or occlusion of TIPS stents. This is the most common cause of significant shunt insufficiency after TIPS. Recurrence of variceal hemorrhage or ascites is seen in around 30–50% of cases of shunt insufficiency. This necessitates routine monitoring of shunt patency after TIPS.

Doppler sonography is the most widely used method for evaluation of shunt patency. It is noninvasive and relatively inexpensive. Doppler ultrasound findings suggestive of shunt insufficiency include a reduction in mean peak flow velocity in the TIPS, reversal of previous hepatofugal flow to hepatopetal flow, and reversal of flow in the stented hepatic vein. It is important to realize that the specificity and sensitivity of TIPS flow velocity for diagnosis of shunt stenosis depend on the specific cutoffs used (Table 39.6).[57] Thus, depending on the cutoff used, stenosis may be present despite a radiologic reading of a patent TIPS.[58] Venography is the gold standard for evaluation of TIPS patency but is expensive and invasive. Narrowing of the lumen by 50% or more or a rise in pressure gradient across the shunt by 20% or to values greater than 15 mmHg are often arbitrarily used as angiographic criteria for stenosis. In clinical practice, Doppler sonography is used to monitor shunt patency and venography is reserved for those cases where there is clinical or radiologic evidence for recurrent portal hypertension.[54,59] Reappearance of varices by endoscopy also accurately predicts shunt insufficiency.

Surgical treatment

A large body of literature on the surgical management of variceal hemorrhage exists. Bleeding is effectively controlled in 90–95% of the patients. The outcome in recent studies are better than earlier reports, probably reflecting both better patient selection and perioperative care.[22]

Surgical shunts

Different types of shunts have been created to achieve variceal decompression. The different shunts are: (1) *Total portosystemic shunts* that divert all the portal blood from the liver into the inferior vena cava.[60] End-to-side portacaval shunts involve the transection of the portal vein at its bifurcation and creation of an anastomosis between the end of the portal vein and the side of the inferior vena cava, thereby diverting all portal flow. Side-to-side portacaval shunts involve a communication between the adjacent aspects of the portal vein and inferior vena cava. Hepatic arterial steal is an important complication of the side-to-side portacaval shunts because they encourage reversal of portal venous flow, with diversion of part of the hepatic arterial blood flow, into the vena cava. Hepatic arterial steal is responsible for the high frequency of encephalopathy (20–50%) and hepatic decompensation with these types of shunts. Interposition

Table 39.6 Correlation of TIPS flow velocity and shunt stenosis

Peak stent flow velocity (cm/s)	Sensitivity	Specificity
>50	78	99
60	84	89
70	89	83
80	92	60
90	93	55
100	98	4

Feldstein et al.

prosthetic H-grafts have also been used as alternative surgical approaches to the side-to-side shunt.[61] Mesocaval shunt is an interposition shunt performed by creating an anastomosis between the superior mesenteric vein and the inferior vena cava. This shunt avoids the hepatic hilum and preserves the portal vein, which may be important in potential liver transplantation candidates. (2) *Partial portosystemic shunts*, e.g., a small-diameter portacaval H-graft, are created in an attempt to lower the portal pressure below the threshold for bleeding and, at the same time, maintain some portal flow. Decreasing the diameter of the portacaval H-graft from 16 mm or 20 mm to 8 mm maintains portal perfusion in most patients and reduces the frequency of encephalopathy.[61] (3) The *selective shunts* selectively decompress variceal flow, while preserving portal blood flow. The distal splenorenal shunt (DSRS) was designed to avoid the high rate of encephalopathy seen with total shunts.[62–64] It involves separation of the splanchnic circulation in to a relatively portal hypertensive venous circulation which maintains antegrade flow into the liver and a decompressed variceal compartment where blood flow is diverted away from varices via the short gastric veins and splenic veins into the left renal vein. While the literature uniformly support their efficacy in controlling hemorrhage, the data related to encephalopathy are less consistent.[41]

Devascularization surgery

Surgical devascularization of the lower esophagus and stomach is an alternative method to control variceal bleeding which does not increase the risk of encephalopathy. These procedures have been used extensively in Japan and favorable results have been reported from other parts of Asia and Europe as well.[65] Surgical variceal ligation with esophageal transection is an effective means of controlling acute variceal bleeding, but bleeding frequently recurs as additional varices develop. The Sugiura operation involves a more extensive procedure consisting of transthoracic paraesophageal devascularization, esophageal transection, splenectomy, esophagogastric devascularization, pyloroplasty, and vagotomy, and is associated with an improved long-term control of bleeding.[65] However, the experience with the rest of the world is less favorable, with increased rebleeding and mortality. This procedure is performed when surgery is required in a patient with extensive thrombosis of the splanchnic bed precluding a portal decompressive procedure.

PRIMARY PROPHYLAXIS OF VARICEAL BLEEDING

Nonselective β-adrenergic receptor antagonists (propranolol and nadolol) and nitrates are the mainstay of therapy in the prevention of a first variceal bleeding episode. The role of EVL as a modality for the primary prophylaxis is very promising, but needs further confirmation.

Pharmacologic therapy

A large number of studies have examined the utility of nonselective β-adrenergic receptor antagonists for the primary prophylaxis of variceal hemorrhage. Seven trials have used propranolol while two used nadolol (Fig. 39.3).[41,66] A meta-analysis of nine randomized, controlled trials concluded that the use of nonselective β-adrenergic receptor antagonists decreases the risk of

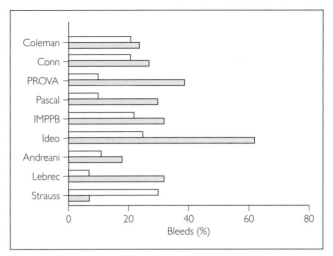

Fig. 39.3 • Clinical trials of the effects of nonselective β-adrenergic receptor antagonists with controls in the primary prophylaxis of variceal bleeding.

initial hemorrhage in patients with cirrhosis and gastroesophageal varices.[41] These trials included a total of 996 patients (489 treated and 507 controls) with four studies focused on those with large varices. Five studies included varices of any size with a portal pressure gradient >10–12 mmHg. Only two trials had a double-blinded design. A decreased risk of variceal bleeding was observed in seven trials, and was statistically significant in four of these trials. The risk of bleeding was reported to increase in only one of these nine clinical trials, which was only published as an abstract. The odds ratio for death was decreased (less than 1.0) in seven of the nine trials, and reached statistical significance in one trial.[67] These data have been corroborated by two recent meta-analyses.[68,69] These meta-analyses confirm that nonselective β-blockers reduce the incidence of initial variceal bleeding by 45% and decrease the bleeding related mortality by 50%. Also, propanolol is the most cost-effective therapy for primary prophylaxis of variceal bleeding in cirrhotic patients who have esophageal varices regardless of their Child's class and the risks of bleeding.[70] As most of the studies conducted have been in the patients with medium to large varices, these results cannot be extrapolated for using these agents in small varices.

Various randomized, controlled trials have evaluated the role of nitrates for primary prophylaxis of variceal hemorrhage.[34,71–76] These studies suggest that the potential for a beneficial or detrimental effect of nitrates depends on the stage of liver disease and the extension of portal collaterals. Thus, in the early stages of cirrhosis, it would be desirable to target nitrates to the liver microvasculature, while in a later stage, nitrates could be deleterious by aggravating the hyperdynamic syndrome through the expansion of the vascular bed. While ISMN monotherapy is as effective as nadolol in preventing variceal hemorrhage,[75] it was associated with a higher mortality, especially in those over 51 years of age. A combination of ISMN and nadolol has been shown to be superior to nadolol alone (12% versus 29% bleeding) for the primary prophylaxis of variceal bleeding.[71] The mortality was similar across the study groups. The current role of nitrates is restricted to combination therapy along with a nonselective betablocker in selected individuals with high-risk varices who have relatively preserved liver functions.

Endoscopic sclerotherapy

The role of endoscopic sclerotherapy (EST) as a modality for primary prophylaxis of variceal bleeding has been evaluated in several clinical trials and subjected to meta-analysis. Sclerotherapy trials were highly heterogeneous as regards to the treatment effects on both bleeding (pooled odds ratio, 0.6; CI, 0.49–0.74) and mortality (pooled odds ratio, 0.76; CI, 0.61–0.94).[77,78] There was also heterogeneity in the rate of bleeding in the untreated groups. Favorable results of sclerotherapy were obtained in trials with high bleeding rates among controls and several of these trials had a low quality score.[79] A large prospective study had to be terminated due to a significantly higher mortality in the EST group as compared to controls.[80] EST should therefore not be used for primary prophylaxis of variceal hemorrhage. Primary prophylaxis of variceal bleeding with β-blockers is also more cost-effective than EST.[70]

Endoscopic variceal band ligation

Esophageal varices are obliterated more rapidly with EVL compared to EST. Also, EVL is associated with fewer complications.[81] EVL has been reported to be superior to no therapy in the prevention of the index variceal bleed and also has a survival benefit.[82–84] While a single study has found EVL to be superior to propranolol for primary prophylaxis,[84] other studies have failed to confirm this.[85] Moreover, the bleeding rates associated with the propranolol group were higher than those reported with placebo in another study published by the same group in the same time period. Currently, the β-blocker therapy remains the first-line modality of primary prophylaxis, and EVL should be used in the patients with contraindications or side effects to these medications.

Shunts

Several studies evaluated the role of shunt surgery for primary prophylaxis in the 1960s to 1970s. Even though the rate of bleeding was very low, this modality of primary prophylaxis of variceal bleeding was abandoned due to the high rates of hepatic encephalopathy. TIPS is not indicated for primary prophylaxis because there are no data or a priori reasons to support this concept.

Summary

It is recommended that all patients with cirrhosis undergo screening endoscopy.[22] Those with no varices should have repeat endoscopy performed at 2–3 year intervals while those with small varices should have endoscopy repeated in a year. Those with normal liver function (Child's class A) and medium to large varices or those with advanced liver failure and varices of any size should be considered for primary prophylaxis with a nonselective beta-blocker. The dose should be titrated to achieve a resting heart rate of about 55–60 beats/min. Ideally, HVPG measurements should be done 4–8 weeks after initiation of therapy to identify nonresponders (HVPG >12 mmHg or a nonsustained drop in HVPG by 25%). Such individuals, along with those who are intolerant of therapy, may be considered for EVL. Nitrates may be used in combination with a nonselective beta-blocker in selected cases of young cirrhotics with well-preserved liver function,

particularly if they are hemodynamic nonresponders to beta-blockade alone.

MANAGEMENT OF ACUTE VARICEAL BLEEDING

According to the Baveno II consensus conference,[86] an acute variceal bleeding episode is clinically significant when there is: blood transfusion requirement of β2 units, and a systolic pressure <100 mmHg, or a postural drop of 20 mmHg and/or pulse rate >100/min, at the time of hospital admission for the bleed. The goals of management include hemodynamic resuscitation, prevention and treatment of complications, and control of bleeding.

Resuscitation

Hemodynamic resuscitation should be started immediately after ensuring a protected airway and estimation of blood loss. After the initial assessment of blood loss, the next step is volume replacement with crystalloids and blood products. Care should be taken to replace the lost blood by packed cells to avoid overtransfusion, as it can lead to rebound increase of portal pressure and precipitate early rebleeding.[87] The hematocrit should be maintained around the low 30% range. Replacement of clotting factors and platelets, when <50 000/mm³, should be done when required as the cirrhotic patients are often found to have both these abnormalities. A recent study has shown that the use of recombinant factor VII with endoscopic treatment is associated with improved hemostasis rates compared to endoscopic treatment alone but did not impact survival.

Management of complications

The prevention and treatment of complications associated with variceal bleeding are also important in the management and should be carefully addressed, and are highlighted in Table 39.7.

Table 39.7 Supportive measures in the management of an acute variceal bleeding

Airway protection
Endotracheal intubation if altered mental status or unconscious

Gastric aspiration
Hemodynamic resuscitation
Crystalloids and blood transfusion
Correction of coagulopathy and thrombocytopenia

Antibiotic prophylaxis for spontaneous bacterial peritonitis
Renal support
Urine output above 50 mL per hour
Avoid nephrotoxic drugs

Metabolic support
Injectable thiamine when indicated
Monitoring and treating delerium tremens
Monitoring and treating acid base and electrolyte disturbances
Monitoring blood glucose level

Neurologic support
Monitoring mental state
Avoid sedation

Role of antibiotics

Bacterial sepsis is a major complication associated with cirrhosis, particularly during an episode of variceal bleeding. Systemic antibiotics or selective intestinal decontamination with an oral nonabsorbable antibiotic reduce the risk of Gram-negative infections after gastrointestinal hemorrhage. Antibiotic prophylaxis in the patients with gastrointestinal hemorrhage improves survival and decreases the amount of blood transfused, as infections increase the risk of early rebleeding.[88]

Initial treatment options for acute variceal bleeding

Pharmacologic therapy

Theoretically, the pharmacotherapy is the most ideal therapy for management of acutely bleeding varices as it is readily available, easy to administer, can be started immediately, and is relatively inexpensive.

Vasopressin and analogues

The clinical efficacy of vasopressin has been extensively studied in various clinical trials. The clinical utility of vasopressin is compromised by its extensive side effect profile. Terlipressin, a synthetic analogue of vasopressin has been shown to be superior to placebo,[89] and equivalent to balloon tamponade and vasopressin[90] in three different clinical trials. There were significantly lower side effects with the use of terlipressin compared to the combination of vasopressin and NTG. The efficacy of terlipressin in controlling an acute variceal bleeding episode is comparable to somatostatin and its analogue, octerotide.[89,91] Terlipressin is the only pharmacologic agent that has shown a survival benefit when used in the patients with active variceal bleeding.[92] This agent was recently approved in the United States for type 1 hepatorenal syndrome, but has not yet received approval for use in variceal hemorrhage.

Somatostatin and analogues

Somatostatin was found to be as effective as vasopressin in terms of controlling active variceal bleeding and reducing early rebleeding, with fewer side effects.[30,89] Somatostatin has also been shown to be as effective as EST in controlling acute variceal bleeding and preventing early rebleeding, with similar mortality.[93,94] In another trial, by Avgerinos et al., somatostatin was shown to be as effective as balloon tamponade and EST and more effective than placebo.[95] It was concluded at a consensus conference that somatostatin is more effective in controlling acute variceal bleeding than a placebo or vasopressin and has fewer side effects.

Octreotide, a longer-acting synthetic analogue of somatostatin, has become a more widely used pharmacologic agent in the control of acute variceal bleeding. It has been reported to be superior to a placebo, and similar to vasopressin, used with or without NTG, in arresting an active bleed.[91] Octreotide is as effective as EST in controlling an active variceal bleeding.[96] Octreotide, used along with either EST or EVL, improves 5-day control of bleeding without affecting mortality.[97,98] These results have not, however, been corroborated in other trials. Subcutaneously administered octreotide does not add to the benefits of EST alone on the outcomes of an acute variceal bleed.[99] Presently, octreotide is the pharmacologic agent of choice for controlling an acute variceal bleeding episode in the United States.

A meta-analysis of the 15 randomized, controlled trials comparing the vasoactive treatment with the endoscopic treatment in achieving hemostasis was performed where vasopressin (α NTG), somatostatin, octreotide, and terlipressin were compared with the endoscopic therapy (EST). It was concluded that these drugs add to the effects of endoscopic treatment and should be used in combination with endoscopic treatment. It has been reported that early use of these drugs improve the field of vision during subsequent endoscopy and should therefore be started in those with a suspected variceal bleed even before diagnostic endoscopy is performed.[100]

Endoscopic therapy

Endoscopic treatment has revolutionized the care of patients with cirrhosis and variceal hemorrhage and is currently the first line of treatment for an acute variceal bleeding episode. EST is capable of stopping variceal bleeding in 80–90% of the patients. EST has been compared with no therapy (one study), vasopressin and its analogues (five studies), somatostatin and octreotide (four studies),[93,96,97] balloon tamponade (five studies), and surgery (five studies).[101–103] EST is either superior to no treatment, balloon tamponade alone, vasopressin alone or in combination with balloon tamponade, and equivalent to somatostatin or octreotide in achieving hemostasis, prevention of early rebleeding, and survival (Fig. 39.4). Cyanoacrylate is a tissue adhesive and is used for injection sclerotherapy of bleeding gastric varices. Uncontrolled clinical trials have shown that cyanoacrylate is an effective modality to control gastric variceal bleeding.[104,105]

EVL was introduced as an alternative to EST due to the high rate of complications with the latter. Randomized trials of patients with acute variceal bleeding have shown that EVL is as effective as EST in achieving initial hemostasis. EVL has been shown to control bleeding in 80–94% of patients.[81,106] EVL is associated with fewer complications compared to EST.[81,107] In an acute bleeding episode the visualization of the endoscopic field might be impaired by the band ligating device. Recurrent bleeding from the post-EVL ulcers may occur in up to 10% of cases.[81]

Balloon tamponade

Balloon tamponade successfully achieves hemostasis in most of the patients with acute variceal bleeding. Balloon tamponade is only a temporary rescue measure due to a high rate of complications associated with this technique, and rebleeding once the

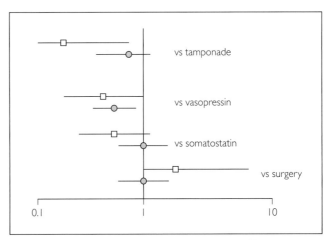

Fig. 39.4 ● Comparative data on the meta-analysis of EST and other treatment modalities in controlling acute variceal bleeding.

balloon is deflated. Moreover, this technique can be used only by experienced physicians, further limiting its availability and ease of use.

Surgical shunts

There are limited controlled data on the use of esophageal transection or devascularization procedures. Esophageal resection can achieve similar results as a portacaval shunt at a lower risk of encephalopathy.[102] There is a higher short-term mortality and a greater cost involved with staple transection, and moreover the 2-year survival is similar to that with EST. Esophageal devascularization is generally performed only when surgery is indicated in a subject with extensive splanchnic thrombosis precluding the use of a portal decompressive procedure.

Porta-systemic decompressive shunts are a second-line treatment of variceal bleeding when the endoscopic and vasoactive drug treatment has failed. The overall mortality associated with surgical treatment of variceal hemorrhage is approximately 50%. A landmark study, performed in the mid-eighties, showed that the 30-day outcomes were similar with EST and surgical portacaval shunts in patients with Child's class C cirrhosis and active variceal hemorrhage.[103] In another important study, it was shown that the best approach was initial treatment with endoscopic therapy, reserving distal splenorenal shunts for refractory bleeding.[108] A very high incidence (40–50%) of post-shunt encephalopathy has also led to the decline in use of these modalities. Based on these data, surgical therapy is reserved as a second-line treatment for those who fail first-line endoscopic and pharmacologic treatment.

Transjugular intrahepatic portosystemic shunts

Transjugular intrahepatic portosystemic shunt (TIPS) has evolved as an effective salvage therapy for uncontrolled variceal bleeding.[45,46,109] TIPS is more effective than EST in preventing variceal rebleeding if performed early after the commencement of the bleeding. The advantage of TIPS over shunt surgery is that TIPS can be done in patients with advanced liver failure, sepsis, renal failure, deep coma, or other severe comorbid conditions where there is a high risk (>90%) of death related to the shunt surgery. In a subgroup of patients with severe active variceal bleeding who were considered to be at a high risk of dying after shunt surgery,[109] TIPS was effective in achieving hemostasis in all the patients with a 6-week mortality of 50%. Also, TIPS is very effective in controlling gastric variceal bleeding.[110]

Summary

Figure 39.5 shows an algorithm for the management of an acute variceal bleeding. After starting the initial resuscitative measures, vasoactive therapy with terlipressin, somatostatin, or octreotide should be started immediately. The bleeding varices are treated with EVL, or EST if EVL is not available. Failure to control bleeding with these measures is an indication for TIPS or surgery.

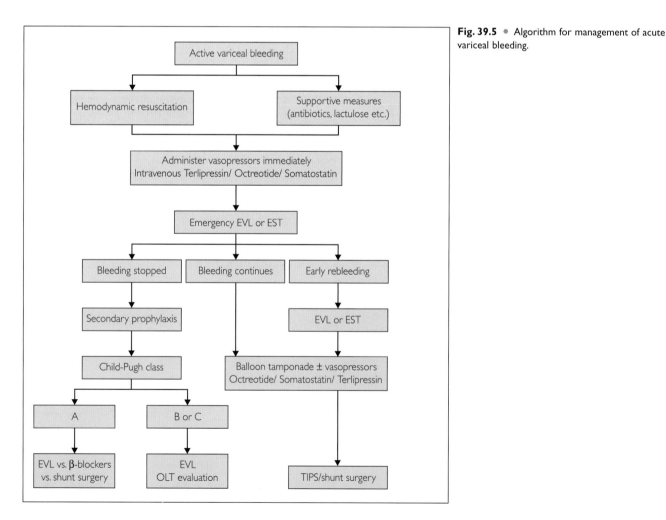

Fig. 39.5 • Algorithm for management of acute variceal bleeding.

Balloon tamponade is often used as a temporary way to control bleeding and stabilize the patient before TIPS is performed. If bleeding occurs more than 48 hours after the initial episode, a second-look endoscopy with another attempt to control the bleeding with EVL or EST may be done. However, it is imperative not to delay institution of definitive second-line treatment in order to control bleeding before life-threatening complications set in.

SECONDARY PROPHYLAXIS OF VARICEAL BLEEDING

All patients who survive an index bleed are at a very high risk for rebleeding, therefore necessitating secondary prophylactic therapy. The various options for a secondary prophylaxis are discussed below.

Pharmacologic therapy

Nonselective β-blockers are the most studied pharmacologic agents for the secondary prophylaxis of a variceal bleeding. The role of nonselective β-blockers was assessed in eleven clinical trials, wherein 428 patients received β-blockers, and 400 received placebo.[21,111,112] While seven trials showed improved rebleeding rates with β-blockers, four studies could not demonstrate such an effect (Fig. 39.6).[21,112] Overall, there was a 40% decreased risk of bleeding and a 20% decreased risk of death.[68,113] Poor prognostic indicators associated with rebleeding in patients receiving propranolol are the presence of hepatocellular carcinoma, poor patient compliance, lack of persistent decrease in pulse, and continued alcohol use.[114] Acute hemodynamic changes after the initiation of propranolol did not predict long-term outcome.[115] However, a sustained decline in the portal pressure for 1 month after initiation of therapy has been shown to decrease the risk of rebleeding.

EST has been compared to β-blocker therapy in various clinical trials.[41,116–118] The data are difficult to summarize given the heterogeneity among trials. Overall, EST is somewhat superior to β-blockers for prevention of rebleeding, but does not confer a survival advantage.[41] The combination of ISMN and nadolol was superior to EST as well as EVL with respect to the incidence of

rebleeding, but the mortality rate among the two groups was not significantly different.[116]

The combination of pharmacologic therapy (nadolol or propranolol) and EST has been compared to EST alone in many clinical trials. In a meta-analysis, 10 clinical trials comparing the two treatment options showed that the combination is better than EST alone. However, when an outlier trial in the EST alone group showing exceedingly high rebleeding rate (75%) was excluded, there was no difference in the rebleeding rates between the two groups, and the mortality rate was similar (Fig. 39.7).[41] The combination of EST and propranolol was found to be superior to propranolol alone in decreasing the rebleeding rate and risk of death.[117] A recent randomized trial comparing the combination of EVL, sucralfate, and nadolol versus EVL alone showed that the combination is better than EVL alone in preventing a rebleeding (23% versus 47%).[118] The preliminary results of a controlled trial comparing TIPS with EST and β-blockers showed lower rebleed rates in the TIPS subgroup.

Endoscopic therapy

The role of EST in the secondary prophylaxis of variceal bleeding has been extensively evaluated. Compared to placebo, EST decreases both the rebleeding risk (from 70% to 40–50%), and risk of death (from 50–75% to 30–60%).[112,119–121] EVL has been shown to be superior to EST for the prevention of rebleeding and has fewer complications (see Fig. 39.7). Also, the number of sessions required to achieve variceal obliteration were less with EVL as compared to EST.[41] However, the recurrence of varices was higher in the patients who received EVL rather than EST. Patients with paraesophageal varices larger than 5 mm in diameter are more likely to develop recurrent varices.[122,123] Combined EVL and EST, when compared to EST alone, showed similar efficacy (80% versus 85%) in achieving variceal obliteration. However, the complication rate (3% versus 20%), and rebleeding rate (3% versus 16%) was lower with the combination therapy. However, several other clinical trials have demonstrated a higher incidence of complications in the combination group,[124] without reducing the number of sessions required to eradicate varices. Recently,

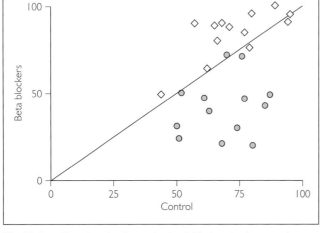

Fig. 39.6 • Clinical trials of nonselective β-blockers in the secondary prophylaxis of variceal bleeding.

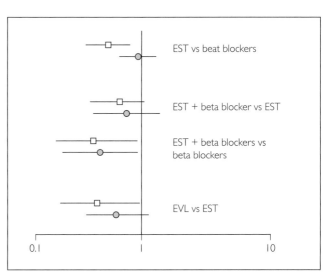

Fig. 39.7 • Clinical trials comparing EVL alone, EST alone, and EST plus pharmacologic therapy in the secondary prophylaxis of variceal bleeding.

argon plasma coagulation of the esophageal mucosa has been used to reduce the risk of recurrent varices; its role in routine practice remains to be defined. EVL is therefore the preferred endoscopic intervention for secondary prophylaxis.

Transjugular intrahepatic portosystemic shunts

Transjugular intrahepatic portosystemic shunts (TIPS) is more effective than the endoscopic therapy for prevention of recurrent variceal bleeding with a cumulative risk of bleeding at 1 year being 8–18%.[56,125,126] A total of 12 randomized clinical trials have been published comparing TIPS with endoscopic treatment with or without β-blockers (Fig. 39.8). While TIPS was associated with better long-term control of bleeding, there was no survival benefit with TIPS. The risk of encephalopathy was significantly higher in patients with TIPS as new or worsened encephalopathy occurred in 25–33% of the patients after TIPS.[52] Advanced age, liver failure, shunt diameter, and a history of encephalopathy before TIPS were the risk factors for worsening of encephalopathy post-TIPS.[52] The role of TIPS as a first-line modality for the secondary prophylaxis of variceal bleeding has been offset by the lack of survival benefit and high morbidity. TIPS is used as a salvage therapy in the patients with bleeding refractory to endoscopic therapy.[45] A single clinical trial found better long-term control of bleeding with small-diameter H surgical grafts compared to TIPS.[127] The results of this trial are not easily generalizable because of the high failure rates associated with TIPS.

Shunt surgery

Surgical shunt is an excellent option to prevent recurrent variceal bleeding in patients who have failed on endoscopic or pharmacologic therapies, particularly when hepatic synthetic capacity is well preserved. There are four published trials comparing DSRS (307 patients) with EST,[62,108,128] and three trials comparing central portal-caval shunts.[103] Shunt surgery when compared to the EST significantly reduced the incidence of rebleeding (OR, 0.18; 95% CI, 0.12–0.28), but failed to show a survival benefit and significantly increased the incidence of hepatic encephalopathy (OR,

2.11; 95% CI, 1.1–4.0). Recurrent bleeding after shunt occurs in 10–20% of the patients, the highest risk being in the first month after surgery.[62] Devascularization procedures are usually considered in the patients with contraindications to shunts as splanchnic vascular thrombosis and should preferably be performed by the experienced surgeons. The choice of surgical procedure should be individualized and must take into account the severity of the liver disease and the local expertise in the procedure.

REFERENCES

1. Pinzani M, Gentilini P. Biology of hepatic stellate cells and their possible relevance in the pathogenesis of portal hypertension in cirrhosis. Semin Liver Dis 1999; 19(4):397–410.

2. Asbert M, Gines A, Gines P, et al. Circulating levels of endothelin in cirrhosis. Gastroenterology 1993; 104(5):1485–1491.

3. Rockey DC, Chung JJ. Reduced nitric oxide production by endothelial cells in cirrhotic rat liver: endothelial dysfunction in portal hypertension. Gastroenterology 1998; 114(2):344–351.

4. Vallance P, Moncada S. Hyperdynamic circulation in cirrhosis: a role for nitric oxide? Lancet 1991; 337:776.

5. [No authors listed]. Prediction of the first variceal hemorrhage in patients with cirrhosis of the liver and esophageal varices. A prospective multicenter study. The North Italian Endoscopic Club for the Study and Treatment of Esophageal Varices. N Engl J Med 1988; 319(15):983–989.

   Identified Child's class, variceal size, and the presence of red weal markings as risk factors for variceal bleeding and developed a prognostic index that enabled identification of a subset of patients with a 1-year incidence of bleeding exceeding 65%.

6. Sarin SK, Lahoti D, Saxena SP, et al. Prevalence, classification and natural history of gastric varices: a long-term follow-up study in 568 portal hypertension patients. Hepatology 1992; 16(6):1343–1349.

7. Burroughs AK, Mezzanotte G, Phillips A, et al. Cirrhotics with variceal hemorrhage: the importance of the time interval between admission and the start of analysis for survival and rebleeding rates. Hepatology 1989; 9(6):801–807.

8. Cales P, Desmorat H, Vinel JP, et al. Incidence of large oesophageal varices in patients with cirrhosis: application to prophylaxis of first bleeding. Gut 1990; 31(11):1298–1302.

9. Gores GJ, Wiesner RH, Dickson ER, et al. Prospective evaluation of esophageal varices in primary biliary cirrhosis: development, natural history, and influence on survival. Gastroenterology 1989; 96(6):1552–1559.

10. Graham DY, Smith JL. The course of patients after variceal hemorrhage. Gastroenterology 1981; 80(4):800–809.

11. Viallet A, Marleau D, Huet M, et al. Hemodynamic evaluation of patients with intrahepatic portal hypertension. Relationship between bleeding varices and the portohepatic gradient. Gastroenterology 1975; 69(6):1297–1300.

    Identified the relationship between the portal pressure gradient and the risk of variceal hemorrhage.

12. Garcia-Tsao G, Groszmann RJ, Fisher RL, et al. Portal pressure, presence of gastroesophageal varices and variceal bleeding. Hepatology 1985; 5(3):419–424.

13. Moitinho E, Escorsell A, Bandi JC, et al. Prognostic value of early measurements of portal pressure in acute variceal bleeding. Gastroenterology 1999; 117(3):626–631.

14. Nevens F, Bustami R, Scheys I, et al. Variceal pressure is a factor predicting the risk of a first variceal bleeding: a prospective cohort study in cirrhotic patients. Hepatology 1998; 27(1):15–19.

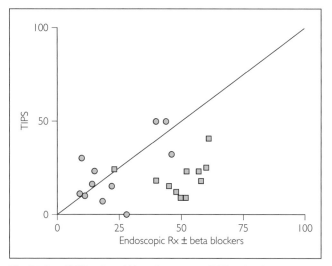

Fig. 39.8 ● L'Abbe plot of 12 trials comparing TIPS and endoscopic treatment ± β-blockers for prevention of recurrent variceal bleeding.

15. Rigau J, Bosch J, Bordas JM, et al. Endoscopic measurement of variceal pressure in cirrhosis: correlation with portal pressure and variceal hemorrhage. Gastroenterology 1989; 96(3):873–880.

16. Zoli M, Merkel C, Magalotti D, et al. Evaluation of a new endoscopic index to predict first bleeding from the upper gastrointestinal tract in patients with cirrhosis. Hepatology 1996; 24(5):1047–1052.

17. Smith JL, Graham DY. Variceal hemorrhage: a critical evaluation of survival analysis. Gastroenterology 1982; 82(5 Pt 1):968–973.

18. de Franchis R, Primignani M. Why do varices bleed? Gastroenterol Clin North Am 1992; 21(1):85–101.

19. McCormick PA, Jenkins SA, McIntyre N, et al. Why portal hypertensive varices bleed and bleed: a hypothesis. Gut 1995; 36(1):100–103.

20. Ready JB, Robertson AD, Goff JS, et al. Assessment of the risk of bleeding from esophageal varices by continuous monitoring of portal pressure. Gastroenterology 1991; 100(5 Pt1):1403–1410.

21. Burroughs AK, Jenkins WJ, Sherlock S, et al. Controlled trial of propranolol for the prevention of recurrent variceal hemorrhage in patients with cirrhosis. N Engl J Med 1983; 309(25):1539–1542.

22. Grace ND, Groszmann RJ, Garcia-Tsao G, et al. Portal hypertension and variceal bleeding: an AASLD single topic symposium. Hepatology 1998; 28(3):868–880.

23. Bosch J, Masti R, Kravetz D, et al. Effects of propranolol on azygous venous blood flow and hepatic and systemic hemodynamics in cirrhosis. Hepatology 1984; 4(6):1200–1205.

24. Lebrec D, Hillon P, Munoz C, et al. The effect of propranolol on portal hypertension in patients with cirrhosis: a hemodynamic study. Hepatology 1982; 2(5):523–527.

   Demonstrated the role of beta adrenergic antagonists in lowering portal pressure and the risk of variceal bleeding.

25. Garcia-Tsao G, Grace ND, Groszmann RJ, et al. Short-term effects of propranolol on portal venous pressure. Hepatology 1986; 6(1):101–106.

26. Westaby D, Bihari DJ, Gimson AE, et al. Selective and non-selective beta receptor blockade in the reduction of portal pressure in patients with cirrhosis and portal hypertension. Gut 1984; 25(2):121–124.

27. Alvarez D, Golombek D, Lopez P, et al. Diurnal fluctuations of portal and systemic hemodynamic parameters in patients with cirrhosis. Hepatology 1994; 20(5):1198–1203.

28. Groszmann RJ, Bosch J, Grace ND, et al. Hemodynamic events in a prospective randomized trial of propranolol versus placebo in the prevention of a first variceal hemorrhage. Gastroenterology 1990; 99(5):1401–1407.

29. Feu F, Garcia-Pagan JC, Bosch J, et al. Relation between portal pressure response to pharmacotherapy and risk of recurrent variceal haemorrhage in patients with cirrhosis. Lancet 1995; 346(8982):1056–1059.

30. Kravetz D, Bosch J, Teres J, et al. Comparison of intravenous somatostatin and vasopressin infusions in treatment of acute variceal hemorrhage. Hepatology 1984; 4(3):442–446.

31. Cales P, Oberti F, Payen JL, et al. Lack of effect of propranolol in the prevention of large oesophageal varices in patients with cirrhosis: a randomized trial. French-Speaking Club for the Study of Portal Hypertension. Eur J Gastroenterol Hepatol 1999; 11(7):741–745.

32. Escorsell A, Bordas JM, Castaneda B, et al. Predictive value of the variceal pressure response to continued pharmacological therapy in patients with cirrhosis and portal hypertension. Hepatology 2000; 31(5):1061–1067.

33. Abraczinskas DR, Ookubo R, Grace ND, et al. Propranolol for the prevention of first esophageal variceal hemorrhage: a lifetime commitment? Hepatology 2001; 34(4):1096–1102.

34. Navasa M, Chesta J, Bosch J, et al. Reduction of portal pressure by isosorbide-5-mononitrate in patients with cirrhosis. Effects on splanchnic and systemic hemodynamics and liver function. Gastroenterology 1989; 96(4):1110–1118.

35. Zoli M, Marchesini G, Brunori A, et al. Portal venous flow in response to acute beta-blocker and vasodilatatory treatment in patients with liver cirrhosis. Hepatology 1986; 6(6):1248–1251.

36. Reichlin S. Somatostatin. N Engl J Med 1983; 309(24):1495–1501.

37. Reichlin S. Somatostatin (second of two parts). N Engl J Med 1983; 309(25):1556–1563.

38. Binmoeller KF, Soehendra N. 'Superglue': the answer to variceal bleeding and fundal varices? Endoscopy 1995; 27(5):392–396.

39. Rivero M, Sanchez E, Fabrega E, et al. Variceal ligation compared with endoscopic sclerotherapy for variceal hemorrhage: prospective randomized trial. Gastrointest Endosc 1999; 49(4 Pt 1):417–423.

40. Kahn D, Jones B, Bornman PC, et al. Incidence and management of complications after injection sclerotherapy: a ten-year prospective evaluation. Surgery 1989; 105(2 Pt 1):160–165.

41. D'Amico G, Pagliaro L, Bosch J. The treatment of portal hypertension: a meta-analytic review. Hepatology 1995; 22(1):332–354.

42. Laine L, Cook D. Endoscopic ligation compared with sclerotherapy for treatment of esophageal variceal bleeding. A meta-analysis. Ann Intern Med 1995; 123(4):280–287.

43. Panes J, Teres J, Bosch J, et al. Efficacy of balloon tamponade in treatment of bleeding gastric and esophageal varices. Results in 151 consecutive episodes. Dig Dis Sci 1988; 33(4):454–459.

44. Rossle M, Siegerstetter V, Olschewski M, et al. How much reduction in portal pressure is necessary to prevent variceal rebleeding? A longitudinal study in 225 patients with transjugular intrahepatic portosystemic shunts. Am J Gastroenterol 2001; 96(12):3379–3383.

45. Rossle M, Haag K, Ochs A, et al. The transjugular intrahepatic portosystemic stent-shunt procedure for variceal bleeding. N Engl J Med 1994; 330(3):165–171.

46. Ring EJ, Lake JR, Roberts JP, et al. Using transjugular intrahepatic portosystemic shunts to control variceal bleeding before liver transplantation. Ann Intern Med 1992; 116(4):304–309.

47. Freedman AM, Sanyal AJ, Tisnado J, et al. Complications of transjugular intrahepatic portosystemic shunt: a comprehensive review. Radiographics 1993; 13(6):1185–1210.

48. Chalasani N, Clark WS, Martin LG, et al. Determinants of mortality in patients with advanced cirrhosis after transjugular intrahepatic portosystemic shunting. Gastroenterology 2000; 118(1):138–144.

49. Jalan R, Elton RA, Redhead DN, et al. Analysis of prognostic variables in the prediction of mortality, shunt failure, variceal rebleeding and encephalopathy following the transjugular intrahepatic portosystemic stent-shunt for variceal haemorrhage. J Hepatol 1995; 23(2):123–128.

   Patients with severe liver disease, hyponatremia, and encephalopathy have poor survival and should only undergo TIPS as a bridge to transplantation. Patients with a TIPS gradient of >18 mmHg require close supervision. Encephalopathic patients should have smaller shunts and prophylactic measures to prevent worsening encephalopathy.

50. Malinchoc M, Kamath PS, Gordon FD, et al. A model to predict poor survival in patients undergoing transjugular intrahepatic portosystemic shunts. Hepatology 2000; 31(4):864–871.

51. Patch D, Nikolopoulou V, McCormick A, et al. Factors related to early mortality after transjugular intrahepatic portosystemic shunt for failed endoscopic therapy in acute variceal bleeding. J Hepatol 1998; 28(3):454–460.

52. Sanyal AJ, Freedman AM, Shiffman ML, et al. Portosystemic encephalopathy after transjugular intrahepatic portosystemic shunt: results of a prospective controlled study. Hepatology 1994; 20(1 Pt 1):46–55.

53. Somberg KA, Riegler JL, LaBerge JM, et al. Hepatic encephalopathy after transjugular intrahepatic portosystemic shunts: incidence and risk factors. Am J Gastroenterol 1995; 90(4):549–555.

54. LaBerge JM, Somberg KA, Lake JR, et al. Two-year outcome following transjugular intrahepatic portosystemic shunt for variceal bleeding: results in 90 patients. Gastroenterology 1995; 108(4):1143–1151.

55. McCormick PA, Dick R, Panagou EB, et al. Emergency transjugular intrahepatic portasystemic stent shunting as salvage treatment for uncontrolled variceal bleeding. Br J Surg 1994; 81(9):1324–1327.

56. Jalan R, Forrest EH, Stanley AJ, et al. A randomized trial comparing transjugular intrahepatic portosystemic stent-shunt with variceal band ligation in the prevention of rebleeding from esophageal varices. Hepatology 1997; 26(5):1115–1122.

57. Feldstein VA, Patel MD, LaBerge JM. Transjugular intrahepatic portosystemic shunts: accuracy of Doppler US in determination of patency and detection of stenoses. Radiology 1996; 201(1):141–147.

58. Sanyal AJ, Freedman AM, Luketic VA, et al. The natural history of portal hypertension after transjugular intrahepatic portosystemic shunts. Gastroenterology 1997; 112(3):889–898.

59. LaBerge J, Feldstein VA. Ultrasound surveillance of TIPS – why bother? Hepatology 1998; 28(5):1433–1434.

60. Orloff MJ, Orloff MS, Orloff SL, et al. Three decades of experience with emergency portacaval shunt for acutely bleeding esophageal varices in 400 unselected patients with cirrhosis of the liver. J Am Coll Surg 1995; 180(3):257–272.

61. Sarfeh IJ, Rypins EB. The emergency portacaval H graft in alcoholic cirrhotic patients: influence of shunt diameter on clinical outcome. Am J Surg 1986; 152(3):290–293.

62. Spina GP, Henderson JM, Rikkers LF, et al. Distal spleno-renal shunt versus endoscopic sclerotherapy in the prevention of variceal rebleeding. A meta-analysis of 4 randomized clinical trials. J Hepatol 1992; 16(3):338–345.

63. Henderson JM, Gilmore GT, Hooks MA, et al. Selective shunt in the management of variceal bleeding in the era of liver transplantation. Ann Surg 1992; 216(3):248–254.

64. Warren WD, Zeppa R, Fomon JJ. Selective trans-splenic decompression of gastroesophageal varices by distal splenorenal shunt. Ann Surg 1967; 166(3):437–455.

65. Idezuki Y, Kokudo N, Sanjo K, et al. Sugiura procedure for management of variceal bleeding in Japan. World J Surg 1994; 18(2):216–221.

66. Andreani T, Poupon RE, Balkau BJ, et al. Preventive therapy of first gastrointestinal bleeding in patients with cirrhosis: results of a controlled trial comparing propranolol, endoscopic sclerotherapy and placebo. Hepatology 1990; 12(6):1413–1419.

67. Pascal JP, Cales P. Propranolol in the prevention of first upper gastrointestinal tract hemorrhage in patients with cirrhosis of the liver and esophageal varices. N Engl J Med 1987; 317(14):856–861.

68. Poynard T, Cales P, Pasta L, et al. Beta-adrenergic-antagonist drugs in the prevention of gastrointestinal bleeding in patients with cirrhosis and esophageal varices. An analysis of data and prognostic factors in 589 patients from four randomized clinical trials. Franco-Italian Multicenter Study Group. N Engl J Med 1991; 324(22):1532–1538.

A reanalysis of the individual data from four randomized controlled trials. Propranolol and nadolol were both effective in preventing first bleeding and reducing the mortality rate associated with gastrointestinal bleeding in patients with cirrhosis, regardless of severity.

69. Cheng JW, Zhu L, Gu MJ, et al. Meta-analysis of propranolol effects on gastrointestinal hemorrhage in cirrhotic patients. World J Gastroenterol 2003; 9(8):1836–1839.

70. Teran JC, Imperiale TF, Mullen KD. Primary prophylaxis of variceal bleeding in cirrhosis: a cost-effectiveness analysis. Gastroenterology 1997; 112(2):473–482.

71. Merkel C, Marin R, Sacerdoti D, et al. Long-term results of a clinical trial of nadolol with or without isosorbide mononitrate for primary prophylaxis of variceal bleeding in cirrhosis. Hepatology 2000; 31(2):324–329.

72. Merkel C, Marin R, Enzo E, et al. Randomised trial of nadolol alone or with isosorbide mononitrate for primary prophylaxis of variceal bleeding in cirrhosis. Gruppo-Triveneto per L'ipertensione portale (GTIP). Lancet 1996; 348(9043):1677–1681.

73. Garcia-Pagan JC, Feu F, Navasa M, et al. Long-term haemodynamic effects of isosorbide-5-mononitrate in patients with cirrhosis and portal hypertension. J Hepatol 1990; 11(2):189–195.

74. Garcia-Pagan JC, Navasa M, Bosch J, et al. Enhancement of portal pressure reduction by the association of isosorbide-5-mononitrate to propranolol administration in patients with cirrhosis. Hepatology 1990; 11(2):230–238.

75. Angelico M, Carli L, Piat C, et al. Effects of isosorbide-5-mononitrate compared with propranolol on first bleeding and long-term survival in cirrhosis. Gastroenterology 1997; 113(5):1632–1639.

76. Angelico M, Carli L, Piat C, et al. Isosorbide-5-mononitrate versus propranolol in the prevention of first bleeding in cirrhosis. Gastroenterology 1993; 104(5):1460–1465.

77. Witzel L, Wolbergs E, Merki H. Prophylactic endoscopic sclerotherapy of oesophageal varices. A prospective controlled study. Lancet 1985; 1(8432):773–775.

78. Piai G, Cipolletta L, Claar M, et al. Prophylactic sclerotherapy of high-risk esophageal varices: results of a multicentric prospective controlled trial. Hepatology 1988; 8(6):1495–1500.

79. Pagliaro L, D'Amico G, Sorensen TI, et al. Prevention of first bleeding in cirrhosis. A meta-analysis of randomized trials of nonsurgical treatment. Ann Intern Med 1992; 117(1):59–70.

80. The Veterans Affairs Cooperative Variceal Sclerotherapy Group. Prophylactic sclerotherapy for esophageal varices in men with alcoholic liver disease: A randomized single-blind, multicenter clinical trial. N Engl J Med 1991; 324:1779.

81. Stiegmann GV, Goff JS, Michaletz-Onody PA, et al. Endoscopic sclerotherapy as compared with endoscopic ligation for bleeding esophageal varices. N Engl J Med 1992; 326(23):1527–1532.

82. Lay CS, Tsai YT, Teg CY, et al. Endoscopic variceal ligation in prophylaxis of first variceal bleeding in cirrhotic patients with high-risk esophageal varices. Hepatology 1997; 25(6):1346–1350.

83. Lo GH, Lai KH, Cheng JS, et al. Prophylactic banding ligation of high-risk esophageal varices in patients with cirrhosis: a prospective, randomized trial. J Hepatol 1999; 31(3):451–456.

84. Sarin SK, Lamba GS, Kumar M, et al. Comparison of endoscopic ligation and propranolol for the primary prevention of variceal bleeding. N Engl J Med 1999; 340(13):988–993.

85. Lui HF, Stanley AJ, Forrest EH, et al. Primary prophylaxis of variceal hemorrhage: a randomized controlled trial comparing band ligation, propranolol, and isosorbide mononitrate. Gastroenterology 2002; 123(3):735–744.

86. de Franchis R. Developing consensus in portal hypertension. J Hepatol 1996; 25(3):390–394.

87. Kravetz D, Sikuler E, Groszmann RJ. Splanchnic and systemic hemodynamics in portal hypertensive rats during hemorrhage and blood volume restitution. Gastroenterology 1986; 90(5 Pt 1):1232–1240.

88. Goulis J, Armonis A, Patch D, et al. Bacterial infection is independently associated with failure to control bleeding in cirrhotic patients with gastrointestinal hemorrhage. Hepatology 1998; 27(5):1207–1212.

89. Walker S, Stiehl A, Raedsch R, et al. Terlipressin in bleeding esophageal varices: a placebo-controlled, double-blind study. Hepatology 1986; 6(1):112–115.

90. Freeman JG, Cobden I, Record CO. Placebo-controlled trial of terlipressin (glypressin) in the management of acute variceal bleeding. J Clin Gastroenterol 1989; 11(1):58–60.

91. Silvain C, Carpentier S, Sautereau D, et al. Terlipressin plus transdermal nitroglycerin vs. octreotide in the control of acute bleeding from esophageal varices: a multicenter randomized trial. Hepatology 1993; 18(1):61–65.

92. Dagradi AE. The natural history of esophageal varices in patients with alcoholic liver cirrhosis. An endoscopic and clinical study. Am J Gastroenterol 1972; 57(6):520–540.

93. Planas R, Quer JC, Boix J, et al. A prospective randomized trial comparing somatostatin and sclerotherapy in the treatment of acute variceal bleeding. Hepatology 1994; 20(2):370–375.

94. Escorsell A, Bordas JM, del Arbol LR, et al. Randomized controlled trial of sclerotherapy versus somatostatin infusion in the prevention of early rebleeding following acute variceal hemorrhage in patients with cirrhosis. Variceal Bleeding Study Group. J Hepatol 1998; 29(5):779–788.

Continuous somatostatin infusion is as effective as sclerotherapy in preventing early variceal rebleeding and maintaining low mortality after the initial variceal bleed. Somatostatin has a lower complication rate than sclerotherapy.

95. Avgerinos A, Armonis A, Raptis S. Somatostatin or octreotide versus endoscopic sclerotherapy in acute variceal haemorrhage: a meta-analysis study. J Hepatol 1995; 22(2):247–248.

96. Jenkins SA, Shields R, Davies M, et al. A multicentre randomised trial comparing octreotide and injection sclerotherapy in the management and outcome of acute variceal haemorrhage. Gut 1997; 41(4):526–533.

97. Sung JJ, Chung SC, Yung MY, et al. Prospective randomised study of effect of octreotide on rebleeding from oesophageal varices after endoscopic ligation. Lancet 1995; 346(8991–8992):1666–1669.

98. Besson I, Ingrand P, Person B, et al. Sclerotherapy with or without octreotide for acute variceal bleeding. N Engl J Med 1995; 333(9):555–560.

The combination of sclerotherapy and octreotide is more effective than sclerotherapy alone in controlling acute variceal bleeding, but there is no difference between the overall mortality rates associated with the two approaches to treatment.

99. Primignani M, Andreoni B, Carpinelli L, et al. Sclerotherapy plus octreotide versus sclerotherapy alone in the prevention of early rebleeding from esophageal varices: a randomized, double-blind, placebo-controlled, multicenter trial. New Italian Endoscopic Club. Hepatology 1995; 21(5):1322–1327.

100. D'Amico G, Pietrosi G, Tarantino I, et al. Emergency sclerotherapy versus vasoactive drugs for variceal bleeding in cirrhosis: a Cochrane meta-analysis. Gastroenterology 2003; 124(5):1277–1291.

101. Teres J, Baroni R, Bordas JM, et al. Randomized trial of portacaval shunt, stapling transection and endoscopic sclerotherapy in uncontrolled variceal bleeding. J Hepatol 1987; 4(2):159–167.

102. Burroughs AK, Hamilton G, Phillips A, et al. A comparison of sclerotherapy with staple transection of the esophagus for the emergency control of bleeding from esophageal varices. N Engl J Med 1989; 321(13):857–862.

103. Cello JP, Grendell JH, Crass RA, et al. Endoscopic sclerotherapy versus portacaval shunt in patient with severe cirrhosis and acute variceal hemorrhage. Long-term follow-up. N Engl J Med 1987; 316(1):11–15.

104. Huang YH, Yeh HZ, Chen GH, et al. Endoscopic treatment of bleeding gastric varices by N-butyl-2-cyanoacrylate (histoacryl) injection: long-term efficacy and safety. Gastrointest Endosc 2000; 52(2):160–167.

105. Vargas L, Ovalle L, Estay R, et al. [Esophagogastric varix hemorrhage. Experience with cyanoacrylate and polidocanol in 68 patients with active hemorrhage]. Rev Med Chil 1999; 127(6):685–692.

106. Lo GH, Lai KH, Cheng JS, et al. A prospective, randomized trial of sclerotherapy versus ligation in the management of bleeding esophageal varices. Hepatology 1995; 22(2):466–471.

107. Lo GH, Lai KH, Cheng JS, et al. Emergency banding ligation versus sclerotherapy for the control of active bleeding from esophageal varices. Hepatology 1997; 25(5):1101–1104.

108. Henderson JM, Kutner MH, Millikan WJ Jr, et al. Endoscopic variceal sclerosis compared with distal splenorenal shunt to prevent recurrent variceal bleeding in cirrhosis. A prospective, randomized trial. Ann Intern Med 1990; 112(4):262–269.

109. Sanyal AJ, Freedman AM, Luketic VA, et al. Transjugular intrahepatic portosystemic shunts for patients with active variceal hemorrhage unresponsive to sclerotherapy. Gastroenterology 1996; 111(1):138–146.

110. Chau TN, Patch D, Chan YW, et al. 'Salvage' transjugular intrahepatic portosystemic shunts: gastric fundal compared with esophageal variceal bleeding. Gastroenterology 1998; 114(5):981–987.

111. Lebrec D, Poynard T, Bernuau J, et al. A randomized controlled study of propranolol for prevention of recurrent gastrointestinal bleeding in patients with cirrhosis: a final report. Hepatology 1984; 4(3):355–358.

112. Rossi V, Cales P, Burtin P, et al. Prevention of recurrent variceal bleeding in alcoholic cirrhotic patients: prospective controlled trial of propranolol and sclerotherapy. J Hepatol 1991; 12(3):283–289.

113. Hayes PC, Davis JM, Lewis JA, et al. Meta-analysis of value of propranolol in prevention of variceal haemorrhage. Lancet 1990; 336(8708):153–156.

114. Poynard T, Lebrec D, Hillon P, et al. Propranolol for prevention of recurrent gastrointestinal bleeding in patients with cirrhosis: a prospective study of factors associated with rebleeding. Hepatology 1987; 7(3):447–451.

115. Valla D, Jiron MI, Poynard T, et al. Failure of haemodynamic measurements to predict recurrent gastrointestinal bleeding in cirrhotic patients receiving propranolol. J Hepatol 1987; 5(2):144–148.

116. Villanueva C, Balanzo J, Novella MT, et al. Nadolol plus isosorbide mononitrate compared with sclerotherapy for the prevention of variceal rebleeding. N Engl J Med 1996; 334(25):1624–1629.

117. Ink O, Martin T, Poynard T, et al. Does elective sclerotherapy improve the efficacy of long-term propranolol for prevention of recurrent bleeding in patients with severe cirrhosis? A prospective multicenter, randomized trial. Hepatology 1992; 16(4):912–919.

118. Lo GH, Lai KH, Cheng JS, et al. Endoscopic variceal ligation plus nadolol and sucralfate compared with ligation alone for the prevention of variceal rebleeding: a prospective, randomized trial. Hepatology 2000; 32(3):461–465.

119. Westaby D, Macdougall BR, Williams R. Improved survival following injection sclerotherapy for esophageal varices: final analysis of a controlled trial. Hepatology 1985; 5(5):827–830.

120. The Copenhagen Esophageal Varices Sclerotherapy Project. Sclerotherapy after first variceal hemorrhage in cirrhosis. N Engl J Med 1984; 311:1594.

121. Terblanche J, Bornman PC, Kahn D, et al. Failure of repeated injection sclerotherapy to improve long-term survival after oesophageal variceal bleeding. A five-year prospective controlled clinical trial. Lancet 1983; 2(8363):1328–1332.

122. Lo GH, Lai KH, Cheng JS, et al. Prevalence of paraesophageal varices and gastric varices in patients achieving variceal obliteration by banding ligation and by injection sclerotherapy. Gastrointest Endosc 1999; 49(4 Pt 1):428–436.

123. Leung VK, Sung JJ, Ahuja AT, et al. Large paraesophageal varices on endosonography predict recurrence of esophageal varices and rebleeding. Gastroenterology 1997; 112(6):1811–1816.

124. Saeed ZA, Stiegmann GV, Ramirez FC, et al. Endoscopic variceal ligation is superior to combined ligation and sclerotherapy for esophageal varices: a multicenter prospective randomized trial. Hepatology 1997; 25(1):71–74.

125. Sanyal AJ, Freedman AM, Luketic VA, et al. Transjugular intrahepatic portosystemic shunts compared with endoscopic sclerotherapy for the prevention of recurrent variceal hemorrhage. A randomized, controlled trial. Ann Intern Med 1997; 126(11):849–857.

126. Rossle M, Deibert P, Haag K, et al. Randomised trial of transjugular-intrahepatic-portosystemic shunt versus endoscopy plus propranolol for prevention of variceal rebleeding. Lancet 1997; 349(9058): 1043–1049.

127. Rosemurgy AS, Goode SE, Zwiebel BR, et al. A prospective trial of transjugular intrahepatic portasystemic stent shunts versus small-diameter prosthetic H-graft portacaval shunts in the treatment of bleeding varices. Ann Surg 1996; 224(3):378–384.

128. Teres J, Bordas JM, Bravo D, et al. Sclerotherapy vs. distal splenorenal shunt in the elective treatment of variceal hemorrhage: a randomized controlled trial. Hepatology 1987; 7(3):430–436.

CHAPTER FORTY

40

Ascites and spontaneous bacterial peritonitis

Andrés Cárdenas, Pere Ginés Gibert and Juan Rodés

INTRODUCTION

Ascites is the accumulation of free fluid in the peritoneal cavity. This entity was first described by the ancient Egyptians and Greeks; however it was Erasitratus of Cappadoccia, circa 300 BC,[1] that first described hardness of the liver as a risk factor for ascites formation. A celebrated figure with ascites and cirrhosis was Ludwig van Beethoven who was treated with serial large-volume paracentesis and died of liver failure in the early nineteenth century.[2]

In the natural history of cirrhosis, patients may develop significant complications of renal function manifested by impaired sodium and solute-free water excretion, and renal vasoconstriction. These are responsible for fluid accumulation in the form of ascites, dilutional hyponatremia, and hepatorenal syndrome, respectively. Ascites is the most common complication of cirrhosis resulting in poor quality of life, increased risk for infections, renal failure, and mortality. Nearly 60% of patients with compensated cirrhosis develop ascites within 10 years of the disease.[3] The development of ascites in cirrhosis is a poor prognostic feature and it has been estimated that half of these patients will die within 2 years without liver transplantation.[4] Thus, the onset of ascites in a cirrhotic patient is an indication to consider liver transplantation. Dilutional hyponatremia and hepatorenal syndrome are events that occur later and carry a very poor prognosis. Patients with cirrhosis and ascites are at risk of developing infections, particularly infection of the ascitic fluid, which is known as spontaneous bacterial peritonitis (SBP). This chapter will focus on the evaluation, diagnostic approach, and management of ascites, dilutional hyponatremia, and spontaneous bacterial peritonitis. The evaluation and management of hepatorenal syndrome is discussed in Chapter 42.

PATHOPHYSIOLOGY OF ASCITES

Most patients with advanced cirrhosis have impaired ability to maintain extracellular fluid volume within normal limits. This results in increased total extracellular fluid volume and subsequent accumulation of fluid in the peritoneal and/or pleural cavities and interstitial tissue.[5-9] The main factor responsible for this increase in extracellular fluid volume is an abnormal increase in renal sodium reabsorption.[6] Although the exact pathogenesis of abnormal fluid regulation in cirrhosis is not completely known, a large body of evidence indicates that it is secondary to arterial splanchnic vasodilation with a subsequent decrease in effective arterial blood volume (the volume sensed by arterial and cardiopulmonary receptors).[5-9] The accumulation of fluid and the abnormalities in renal function are the consequence of the homeostatic activation of vasoconstrictor and antinatriuretic factors triggered to compensate for the relative arterial underfilling (Fig. 40.1). A detailed review of the pathogenesis of ascites may be found elsewhere.[6-9]

DIAGNOSIS AND EVALUATION OF PATIENTS WITH CIRRHOSIS AND ASCITES

In most cases, ascites develops insidiously over the course of weeks to months. The main symptoms are an increase in abdominal girth often accompanied by lower extremity edema. In patients with a large amount of ascites, respiratory function and physical activity may be impaired. Dyspnea in these patients may occur as a consequence of increasing abdominal distention and/or accompanying pleural effusions. Other common manifestations of patients with ascites include dull abdominal pain, anorexia, malaise, weakness, malnutrition, jaundice, and spider nevi or telangiectasias. Increased intra-abdominal pressure may favor the development of abdominal hernias in patients with cirrhosis and long-standing ascites.[10] Umbilical hernias increase in size if ascites is not treated and occasionally cause complications such as strangulation or rupture. Inguinal hernias can also be problematic in patients with ascites.[10]

The current classification of ascites divides patients in three groups.[8] In grade 1 ascites, fluid is detected only by ultrasound; in grade 2, ascites is moderate with symmetrical distention of the abdomen; and in grade 3, ascites is large or tense with marked abdominal distention.[8] Besides a complete physical examination, evaluation of cirrhotic patients with ascites should include standard electrolyte, renal, hematology, coagulation (prothombin time or INR), liver tests (aminotransferases, bilirubin, albumin, total protein, alkaline phosphatase, serum alpha-fetoprotein) and an abdominal ultrasonography to rule out hepatocellular carcinoma and evaluate patency of portal venous system.[9] In addition, an upper gastrointestinal endoscopy to assess the presence and characteristics of esophageal and gastric varices or portal hypertensive gastropathy should be performed since these may require prophylaxis to reduce the risk of hemorrhage (Table 40.1). In patients without previously documented liver disease, the

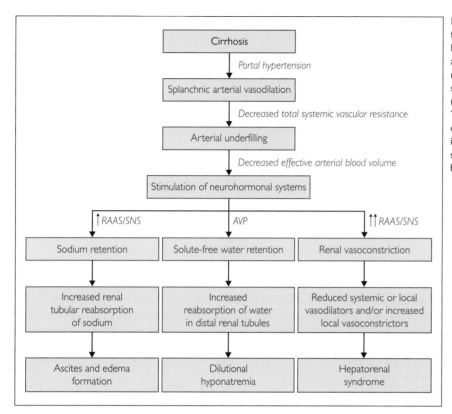

Fig. 40.1 • The pathogenesis of ascites formation, dilutional hyponatremia, and hepatorenal syndrome in patients with cirrhosis and ascites. The neurohormonal systems are represented by the renin-angiotensin-aldosterone system (RAAS), sympathetic nervous system (SNS), and arginine vasopressin (AVP). The neurohumoral effects of these systems on the systemic circulation and renal function in cirrhosis with ascites are responsible for sodium and water retention as well as hepatorenal syndrome.

Table 40.1 Evaluation of patients with cirrhosis and ascites

General evaluation

Complete history and physical examination
Arterial blood pressure, heart rate, and pulse oxymetry
Standard hematology, coagulation, liver tests, and alpha-fetoprotein
Abdominal ultrasonography and Doppler flow (including the kidneys)
Upper gastrointestinal endoscopy
Liver biopsy (selected cases)

Evaluation of ascitic fluid

Total protein and albumin measurement
Cell count
Culture in blood culture bottles

Evaluation of renal function*

24-h urine sodium
Diuresis after water load (5% dextrose i.v., 20 mL/kg)**
Serum electrolytes, serum blood urea nitrogen, and serum creatinine
Urine sediment and protein excretion

Evaluation of circulatory function*

Arterial pressure
Plasma renin activity and plasma noradrenaline concentration***

* Renal and circulatory function should be assessed with the patient maintained on a low-sodium diet without diuretic therapy for at least 5 days.
** May provide important information when an accurate estimate of prognosis is required.
*** In clinical research setting.

diagnosis of cirrhosis should be confirmed either histologically or by a combination of clinical (cutaneous stigmata), ultrasonographic (diffuse parenchymal heterogeneity, nodular liver edge, or signs of portal hypertension), and endoscopic findings (presence of gastro-esophageal varices). When indicated, percutaneous liver biopsy should be performed preferably after the resolution of ascites inasmuch as the presence of intra-abdominal fluid may increase the risk of complications. In patients with significant coagulation disturbances, liver biopsy may be performed through a trans-jugular approach.

Renal and circulatory function should be carefully evaluated in patients with cirrhosis and ascites because of its key importance in the assessment of prognosis and design of therapy (see later).[11-14] Evaluation of renal function should be performed in conditions of low sodium intake (approximately 80 mEq/day) and at least 4 days after diuretic withdrawal.[9] Parameters to be measured include 24-hour urine volume and sodium excretion, serum electrolytes, and serum creatinine. A strong prognostic marker in cirrhotic patients with ascites is the ability to handle water by means of a water load test. In this test a patient receives 20 mL/kg of intravenous 5% dextrose and following this the renal excretion of water is measured. Impaired ability to excrete the water load (urine volume of <8 mL/min) is associated with a poor prognosis.[14] In patients with renal failure (serum creatinine greater than 1.5 mg/dL), urine sediment and 24-hour urine protein should be assessed and the kidneys examined by ultra-sonography. Evaluation of circulatory function should include measurement of arterial pressure in conditions of bed rest, low sodium diet, and no diuretic therapy. Finally, measurement of plasma renin activity and plasma noradrenaline concentration, though perhaps not clinically required, provide an index of the activity of the renin-angiotensin system and sympathetic nervous system, respectively, that may be of prognostic value.[11–13]

Diagnostic paracentesis (approximately 30 mL of fluid) is required in all patients presenting with ascites de novo, requiring hospitalization, and those with any evidence of clinical deterioration such as fever, abdominal pain, gastrointestinal bleeding, hepatic encephalopathy, or hypotension. Basic parameters to be determined in ascitic fluid are cell count, culture in blood culture bottles (10 mL of fluid injected at the bedside), albumin, and total protein. Most patients with cirrhosis have a total ascitic fluid protein concentration lower than 1.0 g/dL. However, values greater than 1.0 g/dL are not uncommon.[15] Patients with a protein concentration in ascitic fluid lower than 1.0–1.5 g/dL seem to have a greater risk of SBP than do patients with higher ascitic fluid protein levels.[15–17] The difference between the serum albumin concentration and ascites albumin concentration (serum-ascites albumin gradient; SAAG) in patients with cirrhosis and ascites is usually greater than 1.1 g/dL.[18] Values lower than 1.1 g/dL suggest a cause of ascites other than cirrhosis (e.g., peritoneal carcinomatosis, tuberculosis, pancreatitis). The red blood cell count in ascitic fluid is usually low in patients with cirrhosis (below 1000 cells/mm³), although bloody ascites (more than 50 000 red blood cells/mm³) may be observed. Superimposed hepatocellular carcinoma should be excluded in such patients. In bloody ascites a correction factor of 1 polymorphonuclear (PMN) cell per 250 red blood cells is recommended.[19]

In most cases, the ascitic fluid white blood cell count is less than 500/mm³ with a predominance of mononuclear cells (>75%) and a very low number of PMN cells. An increased number of white blood cells with predominance of PMNs is usually indicative of peritoneal infection. The diagnosis of SBP is made when the fluid sample has a PMN count greater than 250/mm³.[19,20] The use of reagent strips or 'urine dipsticks' has been proposed for the rapid diagnosis of SBP.[21] Although this test has a sensitivity of 96% and a specificity of 89% in diagnosing SBP,[21] a drawback of this method is that there is no cell count number or differential; therefore, it is prudent to also obtain a concomitant cell count and differential if the reagent strips are going to be used. A low proportion of patients may have a positive ascitic fluid culture without increased PMN cell count. This condition is known as bacterascites.[19,22] Conversely, as indicated above, many patients with a high PMN count suggestive of peritoneal infection may have a negative ascitic fluid culture. This condition is known as culture-negative SBP and should be managed as culture-positive SBP.[19,23]

TREATMENT OF ASCITES

Therapeutic methods

Liver transplantation

The most important aspect in the management of all patients with cirrhosis and ascites is an evaluation for liver transplantation. Early referral is recommended due to the short survival of patients once they develop this complication. Although there are no established prognostic models for patients with cirrhosis and ascites, predictive factors related to renal and circulatory function that are useful in identifying candidates for liver transplantation have been known for years. These factors include dilutional hyponatremia, low arterial blood pressure, serum creatinine >1.2 mg/dL,

and intense sodium retention (urine sodium less than 10 meq/ day) (Table 40.2).[4,12] However, the easiest way to identify patients in need of liver transplantation is to recognize those with severe renal functional abnormalities such as refractory ascites or hepatorenal syndrome. Interestingly, in patients with ascites, parameters of renal function and systemic hemodynamics are better predictors of prognosis than liver tests, such as albumin, bilirubin, and prothrombin time.

Sodium restriction

Because the amount of exogenous fluid retained as ascites or edema depends on the balance between sodium intake and excretion, a reduction in sodium intake helps achieve negative sodium balance. The response of patients to sodium restriction may be predicted by measuring baseline (i.e., without diuretics) urinary sodium excretion.[24] Patients with marked sodium retention (urine sodium excretion less than 10 mEq/day) will have a markedly positive sodium balance even under conditions of sodium restriction of 80 mEq/day. The daily gain of sodium in these patients will range between 70 and 80 mEq/day, which is equivalent to an increase of approximately 500 mL/day of extracellular fluid (average increase in body weight of 500 g/day). In these patients, ingestion of greater amounts of sodium with the diet will proportionally increase the gain in extracellular fluid and

Table 40.2 Prognostic factors in cirrhotic patients with ascites

Parameter	Median survival (mo)
Urine sodium (mEq/day)	
≥10	46
<10	17
Diuresis after water load* (mL/min)	
>8	39
3–8	17
<3	5
Serum creatinine (mg/dL)	
<1.2	25
1.2–1.5	11
≥1.5	4
Hyponatremia (≤130 mEq/L)	
No	27
Yes	7
Mean arterial pressure (mmHg)	
>80	36
≤80	12
Plasma renin activity	
Normal	57
Increased	16
Plasma noradrenaline	
Normal	23
Increased	13

Median survival times were calculated from a series of 216 cirrhotic patients with ascites. All parameters were measured with patients maintained on a low-sodium diet without diuretic therapy, p<0.02 for all parameters. (Reprinted from Llach J et al, Gastroenterology, 1988; 94: 482–487. © 1988, with permission from The American Gastroenterological Association.)
* Five percent dextrose, 20 mL/kg body weight. Normal values in healthy subjects are greater than 8 mL/min.

result in larger accumulations of ascites or edema. Once ascites and edema disappear or are markedly reduced, sodium intake may be increased progressively in patients who had moderate sodium retention before treatment. By contrast, patients with marked baseline sodium retention must usually be maintained on a sodium-restricted diet to prevent ascites recurrence. Conversely, patients with a baseline urine sodium greater than 10 mEq/day will have a sodium balance ranging from slightly positive to negative when maintained on a sodium-restricted diet (80 mEq/day). Consequently, the response to sodium restriction in these patients is less predictable.

Diuretic therapy

The treatment of ascites for many years has been based exclusively on the administration of diuretics, which are drugs that increase sodium excretion by reducing the tubular reabsorption of sodium. The aim of diuretic therapy for ascites is to achieve a negative sodium balance (urine sodium excretion greater than sodium intake). The diuretic most commonly used in patients with cirrhosis and ascites is spironolactone (25–400 mg/day), a drug that inhibits sodium reabsorption by binding to the mineralocorticoid receptor in the renal collecting tubules, thus blocking the effects of aldosterone.[20,25] Spironolactone is frequently given in combination with loop diuretics, especially furosemide (20–160 mg/day), which act by inhibiting the Na^+-K^+-$2Cl^-$ cotransporter in the loop of Henle.[25] The response to diuretic therapy in cirrhotic patients should be evaluated regularly by measuring body weight, urine volume, and sodium excretion. Inadequate sodium restriction is a common cause of failure of diuretic therapy. This situation should be suspected when body weight and ascites do not decrease despite natriuresis higher than the prescribed sodium intake. Approximately 10–20% of patients with ascites either do not respond to diuretic therapy or have diuretic-induced complications that prevent the use of high doses of these drugs. This condition is known as refractory ascites (see later).[26] Complications of diuretic therapy in patients with cirrhosis include hepatic encephalopathy, hyponatremia, renal impairment, potassium disturbances, gynecomastia, and muscle cramps.[20,25] A reduction in serum sodium concentration is a common finding in patients treated with diuretics. In most cases, only a minor reduction is observed. A reduction of more than 10 mEq/L to a level lower than 120–125 mEq/L is usually an indication to stop diuretic therapy. Treatment may be reintroduced when serum sodium increases. The classic type of impairment in renal function during diuretic therapy is usually intravascular volume depletion, which occurs in patients with a positive response and is rapidly reversible after dose reduction or discontinuation of diuretic therapy. Nevertheless, impairment in renal function may develop in some patients in the absence of a negative sodium balance, and this complication may preclude the use of an effective diuretic dosage.[26] These patients should also be considered for alternative therapies (see later). Mild increases in serum potassium (less than 6 mEq/L) are common in cirrhotic patients on diuretic therapy. Severe hyperkalemia (greater than 6 mEq/L) is an uncommon complication of diuretic therapy in patients with ascites without renal failure, but it may develop when patients with renal failure are treated with moderate or high doses of spironolactone. Therefore, serum potassium should be monitored closely in patients with renal impairment (serum creatinine, >1.5 mg/dL) who are treated with spironolactone. Hypokalemia

may occur only in patients treated with loop diuretics alone. Painful gynecomastia is a common complication of chronic spironolactone therapy. However, in most cases pain is mild and does not require discontinuation of the drug. In selected cases, tamoxifen (20 mg p.o. b.i.d.) may be useful to decrease pain, but clinical experience is limited.[27] Finally, muscle cramps, sometimes severe, are frequent in patients treated with diuretics and may require a reduction in diuretic dosage. Quinidine (quinidine sulfate, 400 mg/day),[28] intravenous albumin administration (25 g/week),[29] or oral zinc have been shown to reduce the frequency and intensity of muscle cramps in some cirrhotic patients with ascites treated with diuretics.

Therapeutic paracentesis

Therapeutic paracentesis is the treatment of choice in the management of grade 3 ascites.[8,9,30] Complete removal of ascites in one tap in combination with intravenous albumin (6–8 g per liter tapped) has been shown to be quick, effective, and associated with a lower number of complications than conventional diuretic therapy.[30] After a therapeutic tap, a postparacentesis circulatory dysfunction may develop; this is a circulatory derangement with marked activation of the renin-angiotensin system that occurs 24–48 hours after the procedure.[31] This disorder is clinically silent, not spontaneously reversible, and associated with hyponatremia, renal impairment, decreased survival, and may be prevented with the administration of plasma expanders.[32] When less than 5 L of ascites are removed, artificial plasma expanders and albumin are equally effective. However, when more than 5 L is removed, albumin is the plasma expander of choice (Fig. 40.2).[33] Albumin is administered at a dose of 6–8 grams per liter of ascites removed. It is recommended that 50% of the total amount is given immediately after the procedure and 50% 2–4 h later. The recommended doses of dextran 70 and polygeline are 8 g and 150 mL per liter of ascites removed, respectively. Patients with a known history of cirrhosis and without any complications of ascites or paracentesis can be managed as outpatients. However, patients in

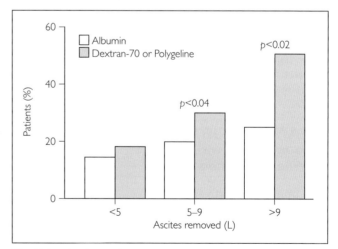

Fig. 40.2 • Incidence of postparacentesis circulatory dysfunction, as defined by marked activation of the renin-angiotensin system, according to the plasma expander used and the amount of ascites fluid removed. *p=0.04 and **p=0.02 with respect to patients receiving albumin. (Reprinted from Gines A et al, Gastroenterology, 1996; 111: 1002–1110. © 1996, with permission from The American Gastroenterological Association.)

whom tense ascites is the first manifestation of cirrhosis or those with associated hepatic encephalopathy, gastrointestinal bleeding, or bacterial infections require hospitalization. Since most of these patients have marked sodium retention, they need to be started or continued on relatively high doses of diuretics after paracentesis together with a low sodium diet in order to avoid positive sodium balance and re-formation of ascites.

Other therapeutics methods

Peritoneovenous shunting was commonly used in the past in the treatment of refractory ascites. However, its use has appropriately been abandoned due to severe side effects (shunt occlusion, vena cava thrombosis, hemolysis, peritoneal fibrosis), its limited long-term effectiveness, and the introduction of alternative therapies such as therapeutic paracentesis.[34,35] Transjugular intrahepatic portosystemic shunts (TIPS) is a nonsurgical method of portal decompression that acts as a side-to-side portocaval shunt reducing portal pressure and decreasing ascites and diuretic requirements in some patients with refractory ascites.[36] The main disadvantage with TIPS is frequent obstruction of the prosthesis, which precipitates rapid reaccumulation of ascites in some patients.[36,37] Other major side effects associated with TIPS include a 30% chance of hepatic encephalopathy, congestive heart failure, hemolytic anemia, and impairment in liver function.[36] The main advantage of TIPS over surgical portosystemic shunts is a reduction in operative mortality.

TREATMENT STRATEGIES

In the following sections, management of different clinical situations that may occur in patients with cirrhosis and ascites is described separately in clinical profiles. In general, these profiles represent the clinical expression of changes in renal function that occur during the evolution of cirrhosis. Patients with grade 1 ascites (only detected by ultrasound) do not appear to require any specific treatment; however, reduction of sodium intake is probably beneficial.

Profile A: grade 2 or moderate ascites

This clinical profile usually corresponds to patients with moderate sodium retention, no solute-free water retention, and normal renal perfusion. Consequently, urine sodium is low relative to sodium intake, but serum sodium, blood urea nitrogen, and serum creatinine are within normal limits. In some patients, ascites, with or without peripheral edema, is the only sign of decompensation of cirrhosis. In other patients, mild or moderate ascites develops after an episode of gastrointestinal hemorrhage or is the consequence of a superimposed alcoholic hepatitis. Most patients belonging to this profile can be managed as outpatients with sodium restriction (approximately 80 mEq/day of sodium) and spironolactone (50–200 mg/day as a single dose) (Table 40.3). Low doses of furosemide (20–40 mg/day) may also be added to increase the natriuretic effect. However, loop diuretics should never be the first-line diuretic and should be used with caution in these patients because they may cause excessive diuresis and subsequent renal failure due to volume depletion. Response to therapy should be evaluated by monitoring body weight and urine sodium. The goal of treatment should be to achieve a weight loss of 300–500 g/day in patients without peripheral edema and

800–1000 g/day in patients with peripheral edema. In most cases, this approach is enough to eliminate ascites and peripheral edema. In the exceptional case of a negative response, the dose of diuretics should be increased stepwise every 7–10 days up to 400 mg/day of spironolactone and 160 mg/day of furosemide. As previously discussed, lack of compliance with the low-sodium diet or treatment is a common cause of therapy failure, especially in alcoholic patients. Once ascites has been reduced, the dose of diuretics should be decreased to approximately half and kept as maintenance therapy to prevent ascites recurrence. If ascites or edema does not recur, sodium intake may be increased progressively while maintaining a low dose of diuretics. Because the goal of treatment at this stage is to maintain neutral sodium balance, this latter approach has an efficacy similar to that of suppression of diuretics and maintenance of a strict low-sodium diet but is better accepted by patients.

Profile B: grade 3 or tense ascites

This clinical profile usually corresponds to patients with marked sodium retention (urine sodium excretion less than 10 mEq/day), although grade 3 ascites may also develop in some patients with less avid sodium retention when sodium intake is sufficiently high to cause a markedly positive sodium balance. Intense sodium retention is commonly associated with impaired renal capacity to excrete solute-free water, but this latter disorder may be overlooked in clinical practice unless water excretion is measured under conditions of a water load.[14] Despite this abnormality, most patients have normal serum sodium concentrations in baseline conditions because they are able to handle their normal daily fluid intake (1500–2000 mL/day), but dilutional hyponatremia (serum sodium below 130 mEq/L) may develop when fluid intake is increased over these limits (for example, during the administration of intravenous fluids in hospitalized patients). A minority

---

Table 40.3 Treatment strategy for profile A: patients with grade 2 or moderate ascites

1. Start with low-sodium diet (approx. 80 mEq/day) and spironolactone (50–200 mg/day as a single dose). Monitor body weight daily and urine sodium weekly. Ideal weight loss should be 300–500 g/day in patients without peripheral edema and 800–1000 g/day in patients with peripheral edema. Outpatients should be instructed to reduce the diuretic dosage in case of greater weight loss.

2. Low doses of loop diuretics (furosemide 20–40 mg/day) may be used in combination with spironolactone to increase the natriuretic effect. Patients should be monitored closely to prevent excessive diuresis.

3. If no response is seen, check compliance with treatment and low-sodium diet. Increase the dose of diuretics stepwise every 7–10 days up to 400 mg/day of spironolactone and 160 mg/day of furosemide.

Maintenance therapy

1. Maintain sodium restriction and reduce the diuretic dosage approximately in half.

2. If ascites or edema does not recur, increase sodium intake progressively and maintain a low dose of diuretics.

of patients have marked impairment in water excretion and may develop dilutional hyponatremia despite normal fluid intake. Most patients with severe ascites have normal or only moderately reduced renal perfusion and glomerular filtration rate. From a clinical standpoint, some patients may have severe ascites without any other sign of decompensation, whereas other patients have associated conditions such as gastrointestinal bleeding, hepatic encephalopathy, SBP, hepatocellular carcinoma, or alcoholic hepatitis.

The treatment of choice for patients with severe and tense ascites is total or large volume paracentesis plus intravenous albumin (Table 40.4).[8,9,20,30,32–34] If albumin is not available, patients may be treated with partial (up to 5 L) paracentesis plus dextran 70 or polygeline.[33] Patients with ascites and a known history of cirrhosis and without any associated complications can be managed as outpatients. However, patients in whom tense ascites is the first manifestation of cirrhosis or those with associated hepatic encephalopathy, gastrointestinal bleeding, or bacterial infections require hospitalization. Patients with massive peripheral edema may require a second paracentesis shortly after the first tap because of a rapid shift of fluid from interstitial tissue to the abdominal cavity. After paracentesis, all patients must receive diuretics to increase sodium excretion and prevent the re-formation of ascites.[38] Because of the intense sodium retention usually associated with severe ascites, patients should initially receive relatively high doses of diuretics (e.g., spironolactone, 200 mg/day, with or without furosemide, 40 mg/day) after paracentesis together with a low-sodium diet. Diuretics should then be adjusted according to individual responses.

Profile C: refractory ascites

The definition and diagnostic criteria of refractory ascites are listed in Table 40.5. The great majority of patients with refractory ascites have very intense sodium retention and a severely impaired capacity to excrete solute-free water, the latter resulting in dilutional hyponatremia in a significant proportion of cases.[8,26] Moreover, most patients have a reduction in renal plasma flow and glomerular filtration rate. The difference between profiles B and C is that in the former group of patients, sodium excretion may be increased with the use of diuretics, whereas in the latter, sodium retention cannot be overcome pharmacologically either because patients do not respond to high doses of diuretics or because side effects develop and preclude the use of an effective diuretic dosage.

Current treatment strategies include repeated therapeutic paracentesis plus intravenous albumin, TIPS, or liver transplantation. Therapeutic paracentesis is the most accepted initial therapy for refractory ascites. Patients generally require a tap every 2–4 weeks and the majority may be treated as outpatients. This approach is therefore easy to perform and cheap.[39] TIPS, although very effective in relieving ascites, is commonly complicated by obstruction of the prosthesis within the first year.[36] However, this is less frequent with larger shunts and newer polytetrafluoroethylene-covered prostheses.[40] Clinical trials comparing TIPS to repeated paracentesis show that TIPS is associated with a

---

Table 40.4 Treatment strategy for profile B: patients with grade 3 or tense ascites

1. Total paracentesis plus intravenous albumin (8 g/L of ascites removed).

Maintenance therapy

1. Low-sodium diet (approx 80 mEq/day) associated with diuretic therapy.

2. If the patient was not taking diuretics before the development of severe ascites, start with spironolactone (100–200 mg/day as a single dose) with or without loop diuretics (furosemide 20–40 mg/day) and then adjust the dose to maintain the patient with mild or no ascites or edema. Check body weight daily and urine sodium weekly. Closely monitor the patient during the first weeks of therapy.

3. If the patient was taking diuretics before the development of severe ascites, start with a dose slightly higher than the dose taken before paracentesis.

4. If ascites or edema increases, check compliance with treatment and the low-sodium diet. Increase the dose of diuretics stepwise every 7–10 days up to 400 mg/day of spironolactone and 160 mg/day of furosemide. Patients should be asked to reduce their physical activity.

5. If ascites or edema does not recur, a balance should be maintained between sodium intake and diuretic therapy.

Table 40.5 Definition and diagnostic criteria for refractory ascites in cirrhosis

Diuretic-resistant ascites: Ascites that cannot be mobilized or the early recurrence of which cannot be prevented because of a lack of response to sodium restriction and diuretic treatment.

Diuretic-intractable ascites: Ascites that cannot be mobilized or the early recurrence of which cannot be prevented because of the development of diuretic-induced complications that preclude the use of an effective diuretic dosage.

Requisites

1. Treatment duration: Patients must be on intensive diuretic therapy (spironolactone 400 mg/day and furosemide 160 mg/day) for at least 1 week and on a salt-restricted diet of less than 80 mmoles/day.

2. Lack of response: Mean weight loss of <0.8 kg over 4 days and urinary sodium output less than the sodium intake.

3. Early ascites recurrence: Reappearance of grade 2 or 3 ascites within 4 weeks of initial mobilization.

4. Diuretic-induced complications: Diuretic-induced hepatic encephalopathy is the development of encephalopathy in the absence of any other precipitating factor. Diuretic-induced renal impairment is an increase of serum creatinine by >100% to a value >2 mg/dL in patients with ascites responding to treatment. Diuretic-induced hyponatremia is defined as a decrease of serum sodium by >10 mmol/L to a serum sodium of <125 mmol/L. Diuretic induced hypo- or hyperkalemia is defined as a change in serum potassium to <3 mmol/L or >6 mmol/L despite appropriate measures.

Modified with permission from Moore KP, Wong F, Ginès P, et al. The management of ascites in cirrhosis: report on the consensus conference of the International Ascites Club. Hepatology 2003; 38:258–266,

lower rate of ascites recurrence.[39,41–43] Yet, hepatic encephalopathy was seen in 30–50% of patients treated with TIPS.[39,42,43] Although one study showed a survival benefit with TIPS,[42] two studies demonstrated no difference.[39,43] Finally, the cost of treating patients with refractory ascites with TIPS was higher than the cost of repeated paracentesis plus albumin.[39] Therefore, large-volume paracentesis appears to be the treatment of choice because of its wider applicability and lower cost and fewer side effects when compared to TIPS. TIPS placement should be evaluated on case-by-case basis and probably reserved for patients with preserved liver function, without hepatic encephalopathy, with loculated fluid, or those unwilling to undergo repeated taps.[8,9,20] The recommendations for treatment of refractory ascites are outlined in Table 40.6.

Profile D: dilutional hyponatremia

Dilutional hyponatremia in cirrhotic patients is defined as serum sodium <130 mEq/L.[44] This type of hyponatremia occurs in the setting of increased total body water and dilution of extracellular fluid volume. Dilutional hyponatremia is associated with sodium retention and increased total body sodium and should be distinguished from true hyponatremia caused by sodium depletion which, although less common, may develop in cirrhotic patients on high doses of diuretics. In most patients hyponatremia is asymptomatic, but in some it may be associated with symptoms such as anorexia, headache, poor concentration, lethargy, nausea, vomiting, and occasionally seizures. The clinical implications of dilutional hyponatremia are not well known; however, it appears that in some patients there may be an association with hepatic encephalopathy.[45,46] The pathogenesis of impairment of solute-free water excretion in cirrhosis is complex and involves a reduced delivery of filtrate to the ascending limb of the loop of Henle, reduced renal synthesis of prostaglandins, and most importantly, increased nonosmotic secretion of arginine vasopressin (antidiuretic hormone).

Presently, there is no pharmacological therapy for dilutional hyponatremia. Water restriction of 1 liter per day prevents the progressive decrease in serum sodium concentration but does not correct hyponatremia.[47] The administration of hypertonic saline solutions is not recommended because it leads to further expansion of extracellular fluid volume and accumulation of ascites and edema.[44] Clinical studies show that antagonists of the V2 receptor of antidiuretic hormone in the distal collecting duct increase solute-free water excretion and improve serum sodium concentration in hyponatremic patients with cirrhosis and ascites.[47,48] These drugs selectively antagonize the water-retaining effect of antidiuretic hormone in the cortical collecting duct. Phase II–III studies are being conducted in the aim of learning more about the safety and efficacy of these agents.

TREATMENT AND PROPHYLAXIS OF SPONTANEOUS BACTERIAL PERITONITIS

Definition and pathogenesis

Spontaneous bacterial peritonitis (SBP) is a common and severe complication of cirrhotic patients with ascites characterized by infection of ascitic fluid in the absence of any intra-abdominal source of infection.[19,49] The prevalence of SBP in hospitalized cirrhotic patients ranges between 10% and 30%. Aerobic Gram-negative bacteria are responsible for nearly 80% of cases and *Escherichia coli* accounts for most of them. Aerobic Gram-positive bacteria, mostly *Streptococcus viridans*, *Staphylococcus aureus*, and *Enterococcus fecalis*, are isolated in approximately 20% of cases.[50] Anaerobic and microaerophilic organisms, although very abundant in gut flora, rarely cause SBP. The pathogenesis of SBP relates to passage of bacteria from the intestinal lumen to the systemic circulation, bacteremia secondary to the impairment of the reticuloendothelial system (RES) phagocytic activity, and infection due to poor opsonization and defective bactericidal activity of ascitic fluid.[51] The clinical spectrum of SBP is quite variable and ranges from a full-blown picture of peritonitis to complete absence of symptoms. Patients with SBP can present with fever, chills, abdominal pain, encephalopathy, and/or rebound abdominal tenderness. However, they are often asymptomatic in the initial stages and the diagnosis relies on a high index of suspicion and examination of peritoneal fluid. For this reason and because of the high prevalence of SBP in patients with ascites, diagnostic paracentesis should be performed routinely in all cirrhotic patients admitted to the hospital with ascites and in hospitalized patients with systemic or local signs suggestive of SBP (e.g., fever, leukocytosis, shock, abdominal pain, rebound tenderness, ileus) or hepatic encephalopathy. Important clinical features of SBP are the frequent development of renal function impairment during the infection and the high recurrence rate.[52,53] Cirrhotic patients with hydrothorax may also acquire a spontaneous infection of pleural fluid that seems to be pathogenetically similar to SBP. Patients with this complication should be managed just as those with SBP.[19]

Therapy and prognosis

Antibiotic therapy should be initiated in patients with a polymorphonuclear count in ascitic fluid greater than 250/mm^3 before fluid culture results are obtained.[19,51] Empiric antibiotic therapy with an intravenous third-generation cephalosporin (cefotaxime 2 g every 8–12 hours; ceftriaxone 1 g/24 hours) for at least 5 days, is required after the diagnosis is confirmed.[19,51]

Table 40.6 Treatment strategy for profile C: patients with refractory ascites

Initial therapy

1. Total paracentesis plus intravenous albumin (6–8 g per liter of ascites removed).

Maintenance therapy

1. Maintain a low-sodium diet (80 mmol/day) constantly.
2. In patients taking the highest doses of diuretics, check urinary sodium. If less than 30 mEq/day, stop diuretic therapy.
3. Total paracentesis plus intravenous albumin when necessary (approximately every 2–3 weeks).
4. Consider use of TIPS in patients with preserved hepatic function, no hepatic encephalopathy, either with loculated fluid or unwilling to have repeated paracentesis.

Ofloxacin (400 mg every 12 h orally), a quinolone rapidly absorbed with high diffusion into ascitic fluid and very active against Gram-negative and Gram-positive bacteria, is as effective as cefotaxime in terms of resolution of infection and survival.[54] Nevertheless, in severely affected patients (e.g., septic shock) or patients with complications that may impair the oral absorption of drugs (gastrointestinal hemorrhage or ileus), intravenous third-generation cephalosporins should be the treatment of choice. Therapy modification depends on results from cultures. Responses to therapy include frequent clinical evaluation and repeat diagnostic paracentesis 2–3 days after beginning antibiotics. In case of treatment failure (worsening infection or no decrease in PMN count), antibiotic therapy should be revised and appropriately changed. Patients should be treated until the complete disappearance of all signs of infection (fever, abdominal pain, normalization of blood PMN count) and decrease of PMN count in ascitic fluid less than 250/mm³.[19]

SBP resolves in approximately 90% of cases if treated with the above regimens.[19] However, hospital mortality remains near 30%, because most of these patients have advanced liver failure and complications such as gastrointestinal bleeding, renal failure, and hepatic encephalopathy.[51–53] The most important predictor of survival in patients with SBP is the development of renal failure during the infection. Renal failure is triggered by an impairment of circulatory function with activation of the vasoconstrictor systems.[52] The administration of albumin at a dose of 1.5 g/kg at the diagnosis of the infection and 1 g/kg 48 hours later prevents renal failure and improves survival in patients with SBP.[53] Recommendations for the management of SBP are summarized in Table 40.7. Recurrence is common, nearly 70% in 1 year, and constitutes a major cause of death in these patients.[55] Long-term prognosis of patients with SBP is very poor, and therefore patients should be evaluated for liver transplantation once they have recovered from SBP (Fig. 40.3).[55]

Prophylaxis

Unfortunately, life expectancy after an episode of SBP is short, with a 1-year probability of survival of 30–50% if antibiotic prophylaxis is not given (Fig. 40.3).[56] Conditions associated with an increased risk of SBP include: gastrointestinal bleeding, low-protein concentration in ascitic fluid, advanced liver failure (high serum bilirubin and/or markedly prolonged prothrombin time), and a past history of SBP.[19] Because most episodes of SBP are caused by Gram-negative bacteria present in the normal intestinal flora, the approach used for the prophylaxis of SBP has been based on the administration of antibiotics, usually quinolones such as norfloxacin or ciprofloxacin, that produce selective decontamination of the gastrointestinal tract with reduction of aerobic Gram-negative bacteria. The efficacy of this approach has been demonstrated in patients with gastrointestinal hemorrhage[57–60] and patients who have recovered from the first SBP episode,[61] and has been recommended recently by a panel of experts in an International Consensus Conference on SBP.[19]

In patients with gastrointestinal hemorrhage, the short-term administration of norfloxacin reduces the incidence of SBP or bacteremia as compared with patients not receiving prophylactic antibiotics.[57–60] The results of a recent meta-analysis indicate that antibiotic prophylaxis in patients with gastrointestinal bleeding not only prevents infection but also improves survival.[56] Long-

Table 40.7 Recommendations for the management and prevention of spontaneous bacterial peritonitis

Therapy

1. After diagnosis of peritonitis has been made (>250 polymorphonuclear cells/mm³ in ascitic fluid), start with third-generation cephalosporins (i.e., cefotaxime 2 g/12 h i.v. or ceftriaxone 1g/24 h i.v.).[19]

2. Infuse albumin (1.5 g/kg at diagnosis of the infection and 1 g/kg 48 hours later).[53]

3. Maintain antibiotic therapy until disappearance of signs of infection or for at least 5 days. Patients should be evaluated daily to assess signs of infection and at least one follow-up paracentesis should be performed to determine polymorphonuclear cell count. If there is a reduction of less than 25% of polymorphonuclear cells compared to the basal levels, the presence of a secondary peritonitis and/or bacteria resistant to antibiotic therapy should be suspected and treatment changes made accordingly.

4. After resolution of infection, start long-term norfloxacin 400 mg/day p.o.

Prevention

1. Patients with gastrointestinal hemorrhage:[19,56]
   1. Norfloxacin 400 mg/12 h orally or per gastric tube, for 7 days.
   2. Alternative regimens include combination of systemic antibiotics (ciprofloxacin, amoxicillin-clavulanic acid, ofloxacin).

2. Patients with ascites with a previous episode of SBP:[19,61]
   1. Norfloxacin 400 mg/day indefinitely.
   2. Consider liver transplantation.

3. Patients with ascites without a previous episode of SBP:
   1. Low ascitic fluid protein concentration (<10 g/liter): no consensus on the use of prophylactic antibiotics.

term norfloxacin administration is very effective in the prevention of SBP recurrence (secondary prophylaxis).[57] Patients treated with norfloxacin show a markedly lower probability of developing

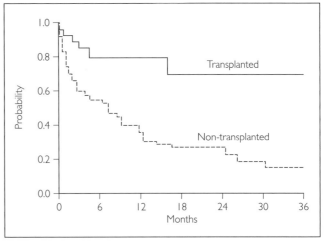

Fig. 40.3 • Probability of survival in patients with spontaneous bacterial peritonitis (SBP) submitted and not submitted to liver transplantation. (Modified with permission from Titó L, Rimola A, Ginès P, et al. Recurrence of spontaneous bacterial peritonitis in cirrhosis. Frequency and predictive factors. Hepatology 1988; 8:27.)

SBP recurrence caused by Gram-negative bacteria compared to that of patients not receiving norfloxacin, while the risk of developing SBP by Gram-positive bacteria remains unchanged. Whether this decrease in SBP recurrence rate results in an improved survival has not been assessed but appears likely on the basis of the high mortality rate associated with SBP.

Antibiotic prophylaxis (norfloxacin, ciprofloxacin, or trimethoprim-sulfamethoxazole) also appears to be effective in the prevention of SBP (primary prophylaxis) in patients with low ascitic fluid protein (<10–15 g/L), who are at high risk of developing the first episode of SBP, but no definitive conclusions can be obtained from published studies because either they include a low number of patients, have a short-follow-up, or are not placebo-controlled.[62] Recommendations for prophylaxis of SBP are summarized in Table 40.7.

In recent years, Gram-negative bacteria resistant to quinolones have been isolated with an increasing frequency from fecal flora of patients under chronic quinolone therapy. While early studies in cirrhosis did not show the appearance of bacterial resistance to quinolones in the fecal flora,[61] later studies have demonstrated that bacteria resistant to these antibiotics (either Gram-negative or Gram-positive bacteria) are a common finding in fecal flora of patients under chronic treatment.[50] In some patients, this colonization of intestinal flora by resistant bacteria may result in bacterial infections and it may well be that in years to come more episodes of microorganisms resistant to quinolones may complicate the clinical course of cirrhotic patients with previous episodes of SBP.

SUMMARY

Nearly 60% of patients with compensated cirrhosis develop ascites within 10 years. The development of ascites in cirrhosis is a poor prognostic feature and it has been estimated that half of these patients will die within 3 years without liver transplantation. Thus, evaluation for possible liver transplant should be initiated when ascites develops. The mainstays of therapy include sodium restriction and diuretic therapy including spironolactone with or without a loop diuretic for patients with moderate ascites and LVP for patients with large ascites. For more difficult to manage cases such as those who develop recurrent side effects from, or are refractory to, diuretic therapy, either repeated large volume paracenteses or a transvenous intrahepatic porto-systemic shunt (TIPS) is an option. Spontaneous bacterial peritonitis is a common and severe complication in cirrhotic patients with ascites. Recognition and rapid treatment is imperative. The diagnosis is made by documenting a polymorphonuclear count in ascitic fluid greater than $250/mm^3$. Antibiotic therapy should consist of an intravenous third-generation cephalosporin or a quinolone initiated empirically after the diagnostic paracentesis and before culture results are available. Generally, albumin is also administered and this may reduce the risk of hepatorenal syndrome and improve survival. Prophylactic antibiotics, generally a quinolone, are useful in patients with a previous episode of SBP or an ascites protein less than 10–15 g/L.

REFERENCES

1. Dawson A. Historical notes on ascites. Gastroenterology 1960; 39:790–791.

2. Reuben A. Out came copious water. Hepatology 2002; 36:261–264.

3. Ginès P, Quintero E, Arroyo V, et al. Compensated cirrhosis: natural history and prognostic factors. Hepatology 1987; 7:122–128.

4. Ginès P, Fernández-Esparrach G. Prognosis of ascites. In: Arroyo V, Ginès P, Rodés J, et al., eds. Ascites and renal dysfunction in liver disease. Malden: Blackwell Science; 1999:431–441.

5. Schrier RW, Arroyo V, Bernardi M, et al. Peripheral arterial vasodilation hypothesis: a proposal for the initiation of renal sodium and water retention in cirrhosis. Hepatology 1988; 8:1151–1157.

   Description of the physiology of renal water and sodium handling in the patient with cirrhosis as this relates to formation of ascites.

6. Cardenas A, Arroyo V. Mechanisms of water and sodium retention in cirrhosis and the pathogenesis of ascites. Best Pract Res Clin Endocrinol Metab 2003; 17:607–622.

7. Arroyo V, Colmenero J. Ascites and hepatorenal syndrome in cirrhosis: pathophysiological basis of therapy and current management. J Hepatol 2003; 38(Suppl 1):S69–S89.

8. Moore KP, Wong F, Ginès P, et al. The management of ascites in cirrhosis: report on the consensus conference of the International Ascites Club. Hepatology 2003; 38:258–266.

   Guidelines on the management of ascites as developed by a group of hepatologists from the United States and Europe.

9. Ginès P, Cardenas A, Arroyo V, et al. Management of cirrhosis and ascites. N Engl J Med 2004; 350:1646–1654.

   A detailed review of the pathogenesis and treatment of ascites related to cirrhosis.

10. Belghiti J, Durand F. Abdominal wall hernias in the setting of cirrhosis. Semin Liver Dis 1997; 17:219–226.

11. Arroyo V, Bosch J, Gaya J, et al. Plasma renin activity and urinary sodium excretion as prognostic indicators in nonazotemic cirrhosis with ascites. Ann Intern Med 1981; 94:198–201.

12. Llach J, Ginès P, Arroyo V, et al. Prognostic value of arterial pressure, endogenous vasoactive systems, and renal function in cirrhotic patients admitted to the hospital for the treatment of ascites. Gastroenterology 1988; 94:482–487.

13. Ginès A, Escorsell A, Ginès P, et al. Incidence, predictive factors, and prognosis of the hepatorenal syndrome in cirrhosis with ascites. Gastroenterology 1993; 105:229–236.

14. Fernandez-Esparrach G, Sanchez-Fueyo A, Ginès P, et al. A prognostic model for predicting survival in cirrhosis with ascites. J Hepatol 2001; 34:46–52.

15. Cárdenas A, Bataller R, Arroyo V. Mechanisms of ascites formation. Clin Liver Dis 2000; 4:447–465.

16. Runyon B. Low-protein-concentration ascitic fluid is predisposed to spontaneous bacterial peritonitis. Gastroenterology 1986; 91:1343–1346.

17. Llach J, Rimola A, Navasa M, et al. Incidence and predictive factors of first episode of spontaneous bacterial peritonitis in cirrhosis with ascites. Relevance of ascitic fluid protein concentration. Hepatology 1992; 16:742–747.

18. Runyon BA, Montano AA, Akriviadis EA, et al. The serum-ascites albumin gradient is superior to the exudate-transudate concept in the differential diagnosis of ascites. Ann Intern Med 1992; 117:215–220.

19. Rimola A, Garcia-Tsao G, Navasa M, et al. Diagnosis, treatment and prophylaxis of spontaneous bacterial peritonitis: a consensus document. International Ascites Club. J Hepatol 2000; 32:142–153.

20. Runyon B. Management of adult patients with ascites due to cirrhosis. Hepatology 2004; 39:841–856.

21. Castellote J, Lopez C, Gornals J, et al. Rapid diagnosis of spontaneous bacterial peritonitis by use of reagent strips. Hepatology 2003; 37: 893–896.

22. Runyon BA. Monomicrobial nonneutrocytic bacterascites: A variant of spontaneous bacterial peritonitis. Hepatology 1990; 12:710–715.

23. Runyon BA, Hoefs JC. Culture-negative neutrocytic ascites: A variant of spontaneous bacterial peritonitis. Hepatology 1984; 4:1209–1211.

24. Arroyo V, Rodés J. A rational approach to the treatment of ascites. Postgrad Med J 1975; 51:558–562.

25. Pérez-Ayuso RM, Arroyo V, Planas R, et al. Randomized comparative study of efficacy of furosemide versus spironolactone in nonazotemic cirrhosis with ascites. Relationship between the diuretic response and the activity of the renin-aldosterone system. Gastroenterology 1983; 84:961–968.

26. Arroyo V, Ginès P, Gerbes A, et al. Definition and diagnostic criteria of refractory ascites and hepatorenal syndrome in cirrhosis. Hepatology 1996; 23:164–176.

    Definition of criteria for diagnosing refractory ascites and hepatorenal syndrome, both important complications of ascites.

27. Li CP, Lee FY, Hwang SJ, et al. Treatment of mastalgia with tamoxifen in male patients with liver cirrhosis: a randomized crossover study. Am J Gastroenterol 2000; 5:1051–1055.

28. Lee FY, Lee SD, Tsai YT, et al. A randomized controlled trial of quinidine in the treatment of cirrhotic patients with muscle cramps. J Hepatol 1991; 12:236–240.

29. Angeli P, Albino G, Carraro P, et al. Cirrhosis and muscle cramps: evidence of a causal relationship. Hepatology 1996; 23:264–273.

30. Ginès P, Arroyo V, Quintero E, et al. Comparison of paracentesis and diuretics in the treatment of cirrhotics with tense ascites. Results of a randomized study. Gastroenterology 1987; 93:234–241.

    Compares options for managing patients with advanced ascites.

31. Ruiz-del-Arbol L, Monescillo A, Jiménez W, et al. Paracentesis-induced circulatory dysfunction: mechanism and effect on hepatic hemodynamics in cirrhosis. Gastroenterology 1997; 113:579–586.

32. Ginès P, Tito L, Arroyo V, et al. Randomized comparative study of therapeutic paracentesis with and without intravenous albumin in cirrhosis. Gastroenterology 1988; 94:1493–1502.

    Compares options for managing patients with advanced ascites.

33. Ginès A, Fernández-Esparrach G, Monescillo A, et al. Randomized trial comparing albumin, dextran 70, and polygeline in cirrhotic patients with ascites treated by paracentesis. Gastroenterology 1996; 111:1002–1010.

    Compares options for managing volume maintenance following large volume paracentesis.

34. Ginès P, Arroyo V, Vargas V, et al. Paracentesis with intravenous infusion of albumin as compared with peritoneovenous shunting in cirrhosis with refractory ascites. N Engl J Med 1991; 325:829–835.

35. Ginès A, Planas R, Angeli P, et al. Treatment of patients with cirrhosis and refractory ascites by LeVeen shunt with titanium tip. Comparison with therapeutic paracentesis. Hepatology 1995; 22:124–131.

36. Boyer T. Transjugular intrahepatic portosystemic shunt: current status. Gastroenterology 2003; 124:1700–1710.

37. Casado M, Bosch J, Garcia-Pagan JC, et al. Clinical events after transjugular intrahepatic portosystemic shunt: correlation with hemodynamic findings. Gastroenterology 1998; 114:1296–1303.

38. Fernández-Esparrach G, Guevara M, Sort P, et al. Diuretic requirements after therapeutic paracentesis in non-azotemic patients with cirrhosis. A randomized double-blind trial of spironolactone versus placebo. J Hepatol 1997; 26:614–620.

39. Ginès P, Uriz J, Calahorra B, et al. Transjugular intrahepatic portosystemic shunting versus paracentesis plus albumin for refractory ascites in cirrhosis. Gastroenterology 2002; 123:1839–1847.

40. Bureau C, Garcia-Pagan JC, Otal P, et al. Improved clinical outcome using polytetrafluoroethylene-coated stents for TIPS: results of a randomized study. Gastroenterology 2004; 126:469–475.

41. Lebrec D, Giuily N, Hadengue A, et al. Transjugular intrahepatic portosystemic shunts: comparison with paracentesis in patients with cirrhosis and refractory ascites: a randomized trial. J Hepatol 1996; 25:135–144.

42. Rossle M, Ochs A, Gulberg V, et al. A comparison of paracentesis and transjugular intrahepatic portosystemic shunting in patients with ascites. N Engl J Med 2000; 342:1701–1707.

43. Sanyal A, Genning C, Reddy RK, et al. The North American study for treatment of refractory ascites. Gastroenterology 2003; 124:634–641.

44. Cárdenas A, Ginès P. Pathogenesis and treatment of dilutional hyponatremia in cirrhosis. In: Arroyo V, Forns X, Garcia-Pagan JC, et al., eds. Progress in the treatment of liver diseases. Barcelona: Ars Medica; 2003:31–42.

45. Hausinger D. Hepatic encephalopathy in chronic liver disease: a clinical manifestation of astrocyte swelling and low-grade cerebral edema? J Hepatol 2000; 32:1035–1038.

46. Restuccia T, Gómez-Ansón B, Guevera M, et al. Effect of dilutional hyponatremia on brain organic osmolytes and water content in patients with cirrhosis. Hepatology 2004; 39:1613–1622

47. Gerbes AL, Gulberg V, Ginès P, et al., and VPA Study Group. Therapy of hyponatremia in cirrhosis with a vasopressin receptor antagonist: a randomized double-blind multicenter trial. Gastroenterology 2003; 124:933–939.

48. Wong F, Blei AT, Blendis LM, et al. A vasopressin receptor antagonist (VPA-985) improves serum sodium concentration in patients with hyponatremia: a multicenter, randomized, placebo-controlled trial. Hepatology 2003; 37:182–191.

49. Fernandez J, Bauer TM, Navasa M, et al. Diagnosis, treatment and prevention of spontaneous bacterial peritonitis. Baillières Best Pract Res Clin Gastroenterol 2000; 14:975–990.

50. Fernández J, Navasa M, Gómez J, et al. Bacterial infections in cirrhosis: epidemiological changes with invasive procedures and norfloxacin prophylaxis. Hepatology 2002; 35:140–148.

51. Garcia-Tsao G. Bacterial infections in cirrhosis. Can J Gastroenterol 2004; 18:405–406.

52. Follo A, Llovet JM, Navasa M, et al. Renal impairment after spontaneous bacterial peritonitis in cirrhosis: Incidence, clinical course, predictive factors and prognosis. Hepatology 1994; 20:495–501.

53. Sort P, Navasa M, Arroyo V, et al. Effect of intravenous albumin on renal impairment and mortality in patients with cirrhosis and spontaneous bacterial peritonitis. N Engl J Med 1999; 341:403–409.

54. Navasa M, Follo A, Llovet JM, et al. Randomized, comparative study of oral ofloxacin versus intravenous cefotaxime in spontaneous bacterial peritonitis. Gastroenterology 1996; 111:1011–1017.

55. Tító L, Rimola A, Ginès P, et al. Recurrence of spontaneous bacterial peritonitis in cirrhosis. Frequency and predictive factors. Hepatology 1988; 8:27.

56. Bernard B, Grangé JD, Nguyen K, et al. Antibiotics prophylaxis in cirrhotic patients with gastrointestinal bleeding: a meta-analysis. Hepatology 1999; 29:1655–1661.

57. Toledo C, Salmerón JM, Rimola A, et al. Spontaneous bacterial peritonitis in cirrhosis: predictive factors of infection resolution and survival in patients treated with cefotaxime. Hepatology 1993; 17:251–257

58. Soriano G, Guarner C, Tomás A, et al. Norfloxacin prevents bacterial infection in cirrhotics with gastrointestinal hemorrhage. Gastroenterology 1992; 103:1267–1272.

59. Blaise M, Pateron D, Trinchet JC, et al. Systemic antibiotic therapy prevents bacterial infections in cirrhotic patients with gastrointestinal hemorrhage. Hepatology 1994; 20:34–38.

60. Rimola A, Bory F, Terés J, et al. Oral, nonabsorbable antibiotics prevent infection in cirrhotics with gastrointestinal hemorrhage. Hepatology 1995; 5:463–467.

61. Ginès P, Rimola A, Planas R, et al. Norfloxacin prevents spontaneous bacterial peritonitis recurrence in cirrhosis: Results of a double-blind, placebo-controlled trial. Hepatology 1990; 12:716–724.

62. Ginès P, Navasa M. Antibiotics prophylaxis for spontaneous bacterial peritonitis: How and whom? J Hepatol 1998; 29:490–494.

CHAPTER FORTY-ONE

Hepatic encephalopathy

Srinivasan Dasarathy and Kevin D. Mullen

INTRODUCTION

Hepatic encephalopathy (HE) is a term used to describe the wide spectrum of neuropsychiatric abnormalities in patients with liver diseases.[1] The causal link between liver disease and the encephalopathy is based on the clinical setting and temporal course in addition to excluding other causes of encephalopathy including primary neurological disorders. There now exists a consensus classification system for HE dividing it into 3 main categories: type A or acute liver failure associated HE; type B, which is encephalopathy in patients with major portosystemic bypass of blood without intrinsic liver disease; and type C, which is encephalopathy associated with chronic liver disease/cirrhosis (Table 41.1)[1]

There are significant differences in the neurological syndromes of encephalopathy in acute liver failure (type A) and chronic liver disease/portosystemic shunt associated HE (types B and C) (Table 41.2). Type C, and the less common type B, HE is now subcategorized into episodic, persistent, and minimal HE. This change in terminology was necessary because of confusion created by the previous terms acute and chronic HE.[1,2] Typically, episodic HE is defined by a distinct period of time (less than 4 weeks) with altered sensorium with the potential for total recovery. This is usually precipitated by specific events, but can occur spontaneously. When multiple episodes of HE occur with intervening periods of normal mental status, the term recurrent is applied. Persistent HE is defined by continuous alterations in mental status lasting longer than 4 weeks.[1] There may or may not be precipitating events underlying a fluctuation in intensity of the persistent HE. Minimal HE refers to patients with basically normal overall mental status, but subnormal performance in psycho-metric test performance.[3] Minimal HE has also been referred to as subclinical encephalopathy in the past.

Types B and C HE occur in patients with cirrhosis, alcoholic hepatitis, venous outflow obstruction, and idiopathic portal hypertension especially after creation of decompressive shunts.[4–6] Circulatory bypass of the liver alone is probably insufficient to result in encephalopathy, as evidenced by reports of the infrequency of occurrence of overt or minimal HE in patients with extrahepatic portal venous obstruction even after portacaval shunts.[7] Even though pure type B HE is uncommon, it is worthy of its own classification because some case reports of its occurrence are well described in the literature.[8,9] In addition to the abnormalities in the hepatic parenchymal circulation in patients with HE, the development of neurological manifestations is mediated by a number of putative toxins.[10] No single agent has been proven to result in the syndrome of HE, and the lack of consensus in this has resulted in various management options being developed. Why some patients with major portosystemic shunts develop HE but the majority do not may be an important key to our understanding of HE. To date, there is little understanding of this phenomenon.

A unifying concept of all types of HE is the idea that brain edema is a component of all three types of HE.[11,12] Patients with acute liver failure (type A) associated HE are at major risk for the development of cerebral edema and resulting intracranial hypertension.[13] Alterations in blood flow may partially underly this phenomenon but pericapillary astrocyte swelling appears to be an early change in HE.[14–16] This in large part is caused by generation of glutamine in astrocytes as a detoxification mechanism to handle increased brain penetration of ammonia.[17]

In contrast to the rapidly evolving edema in acute liver failure, the brain osmolytes show adaption in patients with chronic liver disease. As glutamine and other osmolytes are generated in brain astrocytes, myoinositiol is released, partially improving astrocyte volumes.[18] However, sometimes this compensatory system is overwhelmed and overt cerebral edema and intracranial hypertension are seen in chronic liver disease patients with HE.[12] Generally, a more subtle degree of cerebral edema is observed using a variety of techniques.[19,20] This disappears with successful liver transplantation.[20]

PATHOGENESIS

There are many hypotheses concerning the pathogenesis of HE (Table 41.3).[21] Undoubtedly, precise elucidation of the

---

Table 41.1 The spectrum of hepatic encephalopathy

Type A	Acute liver failure associated encephalopathy (fulminant hepatitis) (ALFA)
Type B	Bypass of hepatic circulation resulting in encephalopathy
Type C	Chronic liver disease related encephalopathy Episodic encephalopathy Recurrent encephalopathy Persistent encephalopathy Minimal encephalopathy

Table 41.2 Acute liver failure and hepatic encephalopathy: differences

	Acute liver failure	Hepatic encephalopathy
Underlying liver disease	Acute <8 weeks	Chronic (over 6 months)
Precipitating factors	Uncommon	Usual
Pathophysiology	Acute hepatic insufficiency	Chronic hepatic insufficiency and circulatory bypass
Animal model	Galactosamine rabbit	Portacaval anastomosis rat
Implicated agents	GABA ? Ammonia	Ammonia False neurotransmitters Amino acid imbalances Benzodiazepines
Documented prior hepatic disease	No	Yes/usual
Nutritional state	Normal	Cachexia, muscle loss
Collateral vessels	Very rare	Usual
Treatment strategy	Hepatic support (acute)	Hepatic support (acute and chronic) Avoid ppt factors Treat ppt factors
Outcome of survivors	Excellent	Survivors need long-term management of underlying liver disease
Residual neuropsychiatric sequelae	Unusual/never	Not uncommon
Follow-up liver function	Excellent, no residual disease	Abnormal, persistent liver disease

GABA, gamma amino butyric acid; ppt, precipitating.

fundamental molecular mechanism responsible for this syndrome would help greatly in management.[10,22,23] In the interim, for the vast majority of clinicians, the ammonia hypothesis is ideal.[24] It is simple and it explains the mechanism of benefit of virtually all currently available therapy. However, from a scientific standpoint, the fact that ammonia administration to cirrhotics failed to induce HE in the only controlled trials ever performed is of concern.[25,26] Nonetheless, a more recent study of inducing hyperammonemia in stable cirrhotic patients using an amino acid mixture, based on the components of hemoglobin, lends support to the role of ammonia in the pathogenesis of hepatic encephalopathy.[27] Two very deleterious aspects of this hypothesis in the past have been: (1) the insistence of its

proponents that no other mechanisms could be involved in HE; and (2) perpetuation of the myth that measurement of blood ammonia levels is a key component in the diagnosis and management of HE. Ammonia has toxic effects on the neurons and astrocytes and, despite many limitations, is still considered to be the most favored hypothesis.[22] The background support for the various hypotheses is beyond the scope of this chapter. Selected citations are given for the interested reader.[16,24,28] Future research on this issue will require open minds and application of more rigorous study design. The advent of transjugular intrahepatic portosystemic shunts (TIPS) has resparked interest in this syndrome because it is frequently responsible for development of HE and ensures continuing interest in the pathogenesis of HE.[29]

CLINICAL APPROACH TO DIAGNOSIS

The establishment of liver disease and alteration in mental status without organic neurological disease with a relation between the two are essential to diagnose HE. When HE occurs in chronic liver disease, it may not always be evident by clinical or laboratory investigations that significant liver disease is present. At times, one may have to depend on the clinical presentation – cirrhosis of liver is chronic even if the patient's complaints are only for a few weeks. Histological documentation is very helpful, but often is not available in patients with HE. In such a situation, one depends on clinical evidence for chronic liver disease such as pedal edema, ascites, gynecomastia, loss of secondary sexual characters, and jaundice.[30] Evidence of portal hypertension includes collateral veins over the abdominal wall and splenomegaly. These findings can be supported by biochemical and imaging criteria for the diagnosis of cirrhosis.[31] The alterations in mental status in HE may

Table 41.3 Putative agents implicated in pathogenesis of hepatic encephalopathy

1. Ammonia
2. Gamma amino butyric acid
3. Endogenous benzodiazepines
4. False neurotransmitters
5. Altered amino acid ratios in plasma
6. Tryptophan and its metabolites (including serotonin)
7. Zinc deficiency
8. Manganese toxicity
9. Opioid system alterations
10. Glutaminergic system alterations

vary from clinically subtle changes in memory or personality to overt coma. A metabolic cause of the encephalopathy is suggested by the lack of persistent localizing or lateralizing neurological signs and a fluctuating consciousness.[32] Occasional exceptions to this rule have appeared.[33]

A number of clinical dilemmas are encountered in patients with HE. Diagnostic problems include: demonstrating underlying liver disease, establishing a causal link between liver disease and encephalopathy, and excluding organic primary neurological disorders such as encephalitis, meningitis, cerebrovascular accidents, or dementia. Management issues include assessment of hepatic function and grade of the encephalopathy as well as a search for precipitating factors that resulted in the encephalopathy. Management of other complications of decompensated hepatic function, if they are present, is an important factor in therapy of these patients. The desired goals of therapy include recovery from coma to full arousal or previous baseline mental state, control of the precipitating factors that resulted in the encephalopathy, and survival.

The clinical features of HE are not specific. It is essential to exclude other causes of altered sensorium in a patient with chronic liver disease (Table 41.4). Asterixis has been considered fairly specific for HE but has been observed in patients with other metabolic encephalopathies (e.g., azotemia, hypoxia, chronic severe congestive heart failure, and advanced chronic obstructive airway disease).[34] The arterial ammonia level have been suggested to be of diagnostic help but it has limitations, especially in cirrhotic patients with portosystemic shunting.[24] This is even more true of venous ammonia levels that are of little clinical use. Other causes of metabolic encephalopathy need to be excluded by biochemical screens, intracranial disorders by cranial CT, MRI, or a lumbar puncture depending on the clinical setting. Alcohol

may be the cause of the liver disease, but the neurotoxic effect of alcohol needs to be considered in the evaluation of patients with HE.[35]

Episodic HE

In a clinically stable patient with chronic liver disease, HE does not usually develop unless some definite precipitating event occurs.[36–38] Prompt identification and control of these precipitating events is one of the major goals of therapy. The commonly encountered precipitating factors and possible treatment options are shown in Table 41.5. Precipitating factors may be overt and easily identified on clinical and laboratory evaluation, or covert and not obvious and these need a high index of suspicion for detection.

Identification and control of the precipitating factors is critical in therapy because their continued presence worsens the encephalopathy and prognosis of the patients. Unexplained development of new-onset or worsening encephalopathy in a previously stable patient with chronic liver disease should suggest a precipitating event. These include: ongoing gastrointestinal (GI) bleed, occult sepsis, overdiuresis, constipation, marked dehydration, hypokalemia, dietary indiscretions with excessive ingestion of animal proteins, unintentional sedative ingestion especially as part of over-the-counter medications, or incorrect prescriptions and progressive renal or hepatic dysfunction.

The major precipitating factor is gastrointestinal bleeding which may present as either hematemesis or melena. However, the clinical challenge lies in the identification of occult bleeding that may present as unexplained tachycardia, or an unexplained drop in hematocrit and a rising blood urea nitrogen. Nasogastric tube drainage, inspection of the stool, and a guaiac test may be necessary to document the bleeding. Bleeding is usually from the upper gastrointestinal tract but this can also be in the small intestine or the colon. Potential sources include: esophageal and gastric varices, portal hypertensive gastropathy, ectopic (not gastroesophageal) varices, duodenal ulcer, and gastric and duodenal erosions. Bleeding may be exacerbated by the coagulopathy of advanced liver disease that usually accompanies HE. Gastrointestinal bleeding may precipitate or perpetuate HE as a result of a number of pathophysiological alterations that include hepatic hypoperfusion, azotemia (renal hypoperfusion, diffusion of urea into the gut and bacterial urealysis, ammoniagenesis in the gastrointestinal tract from the blood load), hypoxia, cerebral hypoperfusion, and a large load of protein with a high ammoniagenic potential in the gut.[39] Sepsis, especially pneumonitis, urinary tract infection, cellulitis. and bacterial peritonitis need to be specifically evaluated.[38,40] Pneumonitis may be the precipitating factor or secondary to aspiration during the course of encephalopathy resulting in additional morbidity and mortality. Spontaneous bacterial peritonitis is a complication in comatose patients with ascites that may be clinically inapparent. Diagnosis may need a high index of suspicion with a low threshold for diagnostic paracentesis. Gastrointestinal bleeding may precipitate an infection that maintains the encephalopathy unless identified and treated.[41] Electrolyte abnormalities and hypovolemia, secondary to vomiting, diarrhea, vigorous diuresis, or overenthusiastic paracentesis may also be direct or contributing factors for encephalopathy. Some of the factors that used to be considered important to either the development or progression of HE have now been questioned with the availability of more objective randomized trials.[42] For

---

Table 41.4 Differential diagnosis of hepatic encephalopathy

Metabolic encephalopathies

Hypoxia
Hypercapnia
Hypoglycemia
Hyponatremia
Azotemia
Diabetic coma (ketoacidosis, hyperosmolar coma)

Intracranial disorders

Cerebrovascular disorders: intracerebral hemorrhage, thrombosis
Subarachnoid hemorrhage
Intracranial tumors
Intracranial infections: meningitis, encephalitis, cerebral abscess
Seizure disorders
Subdural hematoma

Toxins

Alcohol
Drugs
Hypnotics
Tranquilizers
Analgesics
Heavy metals: lead, manganese, mercury

Table 41.5 Precipitating factors for HE and their therapy

I	GI bleed	Variceal	Sclerotherapy Vasopressin Somatostatin Emergency TIPS Emergency surgery – devascularization
		Non-variceal	H_2RA, PPI, blood transfusion
II	Sepsis	Pneumonia Cellulitis, SBP	Identify site Antibiotics
III	Electrolyte abnormality	Hypokalemia Hyponatremia	Stop diuretics Modify intravenous fluids Potassium supplementation Adjust lactulose dose if diarrhea
IV	Exogenous sedatives	Narcotics Benzodiazepines	Discontinue
V	Dietary proteins	Animal protein	Discontinue animal proteins* Daily dietary protein not to exceed 40 g initially
VI	Constipation		Cathartics Bowel wash/enemas
VII	Azotemia	Nephrotoxic agents Diuretics Sepsis	Discontinue nephrotoxic Antibiotics and NSAIDs Volume replacement Control sepsis

H_2RA, Histamine 2 receptor antagonists; PPI, proton pump inhibitors; SBP, spontaneous bacterial peritonitis; NSAIDs, nonsteroidal antiinflammatory drugs; TIPS, transjugular intrahepatic portosystemic stent.
* Recent studies question the role of dietary protein restriction in the immediate and postrecovery phase of encephalopathy.

example, ingestion of a high-protein meal is no longer felt to be an important precipitant. A recent trial has shown that restricting dietary proteins is not of benefit in the development, progression, or outcome after HE.[43] Finally, identification of one precipitating factor for HE does not exclude the presence of others. Often, several factors contribute simultaneously or develop during the course of a single episode of HE, and a high index of suspicion is necessary to identify and treat the same.[44]

Biochemical assays and imaging studies may support the presence of liver disease, identify other causes of metabolic encephalopathy, or establish the diagnosis of other neurological disorders. Blood and urine analyses for drugs and alcohol should form part of the diagnostic panel. Alcohol may be responsible for neurological signs and symptoms in the absence of liver disease. Blood ammonia, both venous and arterial, have been used in the past with varying degrees of confidence. Recent studies have suggested that in view of the variability in the collection, transportation, and assay for ammonia, this test is not clinically helpful and should not be used except in the setting of clinical trials. We would therefore be left with the need to establish the diagnosis of HE by a combination of positive clinical findings in the absence of objective evidence of other causes of neurological disorders. This does not suggest that HE is a diagnosis of exclusion; far from it, it is a positive diagnosis that requires both a high index of suspicion and a high level of clinical acuity.

Persistent HE

The second group of patients with HE are those with persistent HE who have persistent neuropsychiatric manifestations in the absence of a continuing presence of a precipitating factor. The major reasons for this clinical course are portacaval shunt, including TIPS, and advanced chronic liver disease.[6,45] In such patients, the causes are endogenous or persistent, and there may be an initial reversible component followed by a later phase of irreversible neurological abnormalities. These potentially irreversible changes include demyelination, changes in astrocyte number and function, and deposition of heavy metals such as manganese in the central nervous system.[46] Even though persistent HE results from loss of hepatic function or diversion of hepatic blood flow through large collaterals or exogenous shunts, the putative mediators are the same as those for all types of HE. Thus, the treatment strategies are similar to those in episodic HE.

TREATMENT STRATEGIES

The initial goal in the management of HE is to reverse the change in mental status. The long-term goal is to manage the underlying liver disease to prevent the recurrence of HE. The neuropsychiatric manifestations of episodic HE are usually reversible.[47] Recurrent exacerbation or persistent mental and motor function abnormalities may be encountered in the setting of persistent HE.

The altered state of consciousness of HE is itself associated with an increased morbidity and mortality. The duration of this loss of consciousness correlates with the outcome because of poor nutrition, aspiration pneumonia, stress ulceration and gastrointestinal bleeding, pressure sores, and nosocomial infections. Although the recommendations for standard treatment vary, there are no established standards of care or controlled assessment of the efficiency of one or more of these interventions. This makes interpretation of published studies difficult and at times confusing.[48] We will try to establish these standards in the following section based on objective evidence and in situations where this is lacking by logical interpretation of the existing data. The consensus of most investigators in this field is that rapid reversal of HE is essential. The differences in the management of patients with episodic and persistent HE are shown in Table 41.6.

Episodic HE

Treatment of episodic HE focuses on the different pathogenic factors that have been implicated in the development of HE. These are shown in Table 41.7. Despite the fairly vocal arguments, both favoring and opposing ammonia as the pathogenic factor for HE, one key observation has stood the test of time: measures that have been directed towards lowering ammonia in patients with HE are clinically effective. We will therefore focus on these measures and will then address the alternative treatment strategies and their current role in the treatment of episodic and persistent HE.

Decrease in ammonia substrate

The major source of ammonia is from the metabolism of dietary and endogenous protein in the gastrointestinal tract by the urealytic and proteolytic bacteria as well as the metabolism of small intestinal enterocyte glutaminase.[28,49,50] Gut protein (both endogenous and dietary) and urea that diffuses into the small intestine and colon serve as substrates for ammoniagenesis.[51] Removal of this substrate is achieved by a combination of reduction of dietary intake of protein, and catharsis or enema.

Catharsis induced by lactulose is orally administered, clinically effective, and esthetically acceptable. However, its disadvantages include the time lag between administration and catharsis, and risks of dehydration, and electrolyte abnormalities induced during the course of therapy. Enemas are also effective and easy to control. They are, however, usually not administered correctly, need mildly acidic solutions, and may cause trauma to the rectum and anal canal if administered inappropriately.[52] For an effective enema, volumes of 100–250 mL of an acidic solution (pH 4.5) of lactose, lactulose, or lactitol solutions are administered rectally.[53] The patient is turned through supine, left lateral, prone, and right lateral position, each position lasting at least 5 minutes before emptying the bowels. This is difficult at best and especially so in a comatose patient. An alternative mechanism of action of enemas

could be the effect of rectal distention on colonic motility which may allow colonic contents to be expelled without the actual need for colonic acidification. This needs to be evaluated, though the data from one trial had suggested that plain water enemas are not as effective as acidic enemas.[52]

On the basis of available data, mildly acidic enemas are effective in treating HE.

Dietary protein restriction

Animal and human studies have shown an increase in blood ammonia levels and worsening of encephalopathy after dietary protein ingestion.[54,55] Animal proteins have been considered more ammoniagenic and encephalopathogenic than vegetable proteins.[56,57] The beneficial effects of vegetable proteins on nitrogen metabolism in cirrhotics has been suggested to be due to the higher fiber content and elimination of nitrogen in fecal bacteria.[58] This hierarchy of encephalopathogenic proteins has been used in restricting the protein administration during the acute episode and subsequent management of HE. However, complete avoidance of dietary proteins may result in obligatory endogenous protein breakdown, especially from skeletal muscle.[42,59,60] This is the equivalent of animal protein intake. Any reduction in caloric intake would also result in an exaggerated protein breakdown to provide for calories from amino acids.[61] A protein intake of at least 0.8–1 g/kg per day may be necessary to maintain nitrogen balance (see Ch. 5). This amount of protein has been considered to be poorly tolerated by patients with episodic HE in the past. The traditional recommendation has been the initial administration of only 40 g/day of protein with this being increased by 10–15 g every 3–4 days as tolerated. Recently, this concept of restricting proteins in HE has been questioned[62] and a recent controlled trial has shown that protein tolerance after recovery from the episodic coma may be much higher than previously suspected.[43]

Dietary protein in patients with episodic HE should begin as soon as oral feeding is tolerated and should initially consist of 40 g of protein, preferably vegetable protein. Protein intake should be increased by 10–15 g every 3–4 days as tolerated. Long-term protein restriction is not advised and can be detrimental.

Antibiotics

Gut ammoniagenesis is dependent on the substrate (protein/urea) and the bacteria that generate it.[63] Suppression or elimination of these bacteria would be effective in decreasing ammoniagenesis and possibly other compounds including false neurotransmitters, and benzodiazepines. Anaerobic, Gram-negative bacteria such as bacteroides may be a major contributor to intestinal ammoniagenesis.[64] Neomycin, metronidazole, vancomycin, and rifaximin have been subjected to randomized trials in the therapy of HE.[65-68] They have been shown to be effective in suppressing intestinal flora, reducing blood ammonia levels, and improving mental status in patients with HE. Initial uncontrolled reports and later randomized trials have established neomycin as a standard treatment in HE.[69] Doses vary from 2 g to 8 g daily in divided doses given orally. About 70–80% of patients improve on neomycin therapy. Traditionally, neomycin has been considered to be nonabsorbable. However, when used in large doses such as those discussed above, the 1–5% of absorbed drug may cause oto- and nephrotoxicity.[70] The other potential disadvantages of neomycin include development of staphylococcal enterocolitis, *Clostridium*

Table 41.6 Hepatic encephalopathy: episodic versus persistent

Episodic HE	Persistent HE
Control precipitating factor	Reverse encephalopathy
Reverse encephalopathy	Avoid recurrence
Hospital/in-patient therapy	Home/out-patient therapy
Maintain supportive measures	Supportive measures, manage persistent neuropsychiatric manifestations, hepatic support
Expect normal mentation after recovery	High prevalence of abnormal mentation following recovery from exacerbation

Table 41.7 Treatment strategies in a patient with episodic hepatic encephalopathy

Management of a patient in encephalopathy

Nutrition
Fluid and electrolyte maintenance
Bladder and bowel function
Intravenous catheter care
Avoid aspiration pneumonitis
Prevent sepsis
Avoid/treat pressure sores

Identify and treat precipitating factors

	Precipitating factors	*Possible causes*
A	GI bleed	Variceal; nonvariceal
B	Infection	Pneumonitis, urinary tract infection, bacterial peritonitis
C	Hypokalemia, alkalosis	Diuretics, fluid/electrolyte management problems
D	Sedatives, tranquilizers	Narcotics
E	Dietary proteins	Animal protein
F	Azotemia	Drug (NSAID, others) induced dysfunction, catabolic state (sepsis, others) Hepatorenal syndrome GI bleed, hypovolemia
G	Acute hepatic injury	Hepatotoxic drugs Reactivation/super infection of hepatotropic virus Progressive hepatic dysfunction

Treatment strategies based on putative toxins

A Ammonia
    Decrease ammonia substrate
      Clearance of intestinal tract
        Cathartics
        Enema
      Decreased protein intake
    Decrease ammoniagenesis
      Gut bacterial suppression (antibiotics)
      Nonabsorbable disaccharides
        Lactulose, lactitol, lactose
      Modify proteolytic gut bacteria
    Biochemical neutralization of ammonia
      L glutamic acid
      Sodium benzoate
      Ornithine L aspartate
      Keto analogues of amino acids
      Acidifying enemas

B False neurotransmitters (octopamine, phenylethanolamine)
    Suppress gut bacterial flora
    L-dopa
    Bromocriptine

C Altered amino acid balance
    Branched-chain amino acid infusion
    Substitute vegetable protein for animal protein

D Endogenous benzodiazepenes
    Flumezanil

Treatment of associated problems

    Ascites
    Variceal bleed
    Hepatotropic viral infection
    Hepatic support
      Acute
    Liver transplantation

difficile colitis, resistance to neomycin by colonic bacterial, and steatorrhea.[71] It is, therefore, suggested that neomycin be used as an adjunct to lactulose and not be administered for more than 1 month. Other antibiotics that have been studied have been used only in a small numbers of patients for short durations. They may be considered in special situations when even the minimal risk of neomycin toxicity is considered unacceptable. Metronidazole is an alternative to neomycin with good success reported in the treatment of episodic HE. Recently, interest has been growing in the use of rifaximin, an orally administered nonabsorbable analogue of rifampicin. Randomized, controlled trials have shown that rifaximin is well tolerated, has a high success rate in improving HE and a low incidence of adverse effects.[69] A number of trials have subsequently shown that rifaximin is an effective and well-tolerated treatment for HE and may soon replace the traditionally used neomycin.[65,72]

Antibiotics are considered to be standard therapy in HE, though their use is typically confined to short duration as an adjunct to lactulose. The choice of antibiotics used (neomycin, metronidazole, or rifaximin) would, however, depend on clinical situation.

Nonabsorbable disaccharides

Nonabsorbable disaccharides pass largely unchanged to the colon and are acted upon by colonic bacteria.[63] The two major disaccharides used in clinical practice are lactulose and lactitol (not yet approved by FDA).[73,74] These compounds have also been used as enemas to allow direct delivery to the colon. A total of 34 trials (26 randomized) to evaluate the efficacy of lactulose have been published.[69] Significant improvement in clinical parameters was observed in 54 (85.7%) of patients with episodic HE in cirrhosis. It was as effective as neomycin alone or catharsis, but acts more rapidly and has a lower therapeutic risk compared to neomycin.

The suggested mechanism of action of nonabsorbable disaccharides include removal of dietary and endogenous ammonia-genic substrates from the intestinal lumen by osmotic cathartic action, lowering the growth of urealytic and proteolytic bacteria, and facilitation of growth of saccharolytic bacteria.[64,75] The lowering of colonic pH reduces absorption of ammonia by non-ionic diffusion and promotes movement of ammonia from blood to the gut.[76] Lactulose is effective when administered appropriately. The dose of lactulose is titrated to allowing the passage of 1–2 semi-formed stools per day.[76] Therapeutic benefit has been reported to be maximal with a stool pH of 6.0 or less. Stool pH is not routinely checked unless the response to therapy is less than optimal. The average dose of lactulose required to achieve therapeutic response has been 45–90 mL/day. Limitations of lactulose include its liquid nature, sickly sweet taste, and a sensation of bloating and diarrhea if the dose is not adjusted appropriately.

Lactitol is an alternative to lactulose and has a similar mechanism of action. Its advantages over lactulose include its crystalline powder state and better tolerance because of its sugar-like taste without the sickly sweet taste of lactulose. The results of lactitol in episodic HE has been evaluated in two randomized, controlled trials comparing lactitol and lactulose.[77,78] Significant improvement was observed in nearly 85% in each group. Lactitol showed a quicker response and had higher improvement in the first 24 hours of therapy though the overall improvement was similar in the two groups. In another study comparing lactitol to rifaximin, similar efficacy was observed but rifaximin resulted in

a greater decrease in some clinical manifestations of encephalopathy.[65] A recent Cochrane systematic review of all published randomized trials of nonabsorbable disaccharides concluded that there was insufficient evidence to support or refute their use in hepatic encephalopathy.[79] It was also observed that antibiotics were superior to nonabsorbable disaccharides and this group of compounds should not be used as a control arm in future therapeutic trials. Enemas containing lactulose, lactitol, or lactose may be used if oral or nasogastric administration is not possible.[53] The recently developed, non-sweet krystallose is an alternative to the syrupy lactulose or the sweet lactitol.

Lactulose in doses adjusted to produce 1–2 semi-formed stools per day is the standard therapy for episodic HE. The non-sweet solid formulation, krystallose, should be considered an alternate in patients who are unable to tolerate the taste of lactulose.

Combination of antibiotics and nonabsorbable disaccharides

Published data to date have demonstrated that nonabsorbable disaccharides and antibiotics are equally effective in the therapy of episodic and persistent hepatic encephalopathy. They work by different mechanisms of controlling bacterial metabolism generating ammonia.[63,80,81] The beneficial effects of antibiotics depend on inhibiting luminal bacterial activity while disaccharides need to be metabolized by colonic bacteria. Thus, combination therapy may be effective in patients with HE refractory to either agent alone. Alternatively, antibiotics that inhibit the growth of disaccharide metabolizing bacteria, though effective on their own, might lower or abolish the efficacy of disaccharides.[82]

Studies published to date to evaluate the combination of disaccharides and antibiotics have used only neomycin combined with lactulose or lactitol.[83–85] These studies suggest that lactulose and possibly lactitol continue to be metabolized after neomycin administration, but they do not demonstrate a clear clinical advantage of combination therapy. A reduction in blood ammonia does not necessarily mean improvement in HE, but based on the ammonia hypothesis for HE it is likely to be useful.

The combination of neomycin and disaccharides may be instituted in patients when either does not seem to be effective or there is an inadequate response to single-agent therapy. Monitoring of stool pH maybe needed if clinical benefits are not noted in 48 hours. A rise in stool pH may warrant discontinuation of combination therapy.

Modifying gut bacteria

Replacement of ammoniagenic bacteria may result in lowering blood ammonia levels and as a consequence clinical benefit.[86] *Lactobacillus acidophilus* and *Enterococcus faecium SF68* have been used in patients with persistent HE.[87,88] Buffered *Lactobacillus acidophilus* milk in 2 patients and freeze-dried preparation of *Lactobacillus acidophilus* in 10 patients have been reported to be beneficial in HE. Limitations include the difficulty of maintaining an unnatural fecal flora for prolonged time periods, unacceptable taste of sour milk, and the confounding effect of neomycin coadministration with the freeze-dried preparation. *Enterococcus faecium SF68* is a lactic acid producing, urease-negative bacterium resistant to several antibiotics, which inhibits the growth of other intestinal flora. In a randomized study, it was as effective as lactulose in therapy of persistent HE without adverse effects. Therapy could be interrupted for up to 2 weeks without loss of clinical benefit.[89]

Modification of colonic flora remains an investigational therapy especially in HE.

Alternative methods of ammonia removal

Molecular adsorbents recirculating system

This is one form of liver assist device that has been studied as a possible tool in the management of episodic encephalopathy of acute on chronic liver failure.[90] Episodic hepatic encephalopathy is one component of acute on chronic liver failure.[91] Liver support devices such as the molecular adsorbents recirculating system (MARS) system have the overall aim of removing putative toxins that cause encephalopathy. Reports to date are anecdotal and this must be considered as experimental therapy until well-designed controlled trials have been performed.

L ornithine L aspartate

Hepatic ammonia removal occurs at two sites: the periportal hepatocytes involved in ureagenesis and perivenous hepatocytes in glutamine synthesis.[92,93] Ureagenesis is impaired in cirrhosis and the alternative pathway can be employed for ammonia removal by aspartate, glutamate, or ornithine, especially in the setting of acute and persistent hepatic diseases. These dicarboxylates serve as a carbon source for glutamine synthase in perivenous hepatocytes. Ornithine also stimulates ornithine carbamoyl transferase and carbamoyl phosphate synthase in addition to serving as a substrate for the first step in ureagenesis.[94] Initial animal studies followed by uncontrolled trials in humans showed that ornithine, aspartate, and their salt, L-ornithine aspartate (OA), reduced blood ammonia levels.[95] The four randomized clinical trials of OA in HE have all included patients with latent or early HE (grade I or II) and in patients who had undergone the TIPS procedure.[95–98] In these studies, OA was effective in reducing venous ammonia, time to complete number connection tests (a measure of subtle encephalopathy), and the grade of HE. Data for use of OA in more advanced HE are not yet available.

Sodium benzoate

Hepatic metabolism of ammonia for ureagenesis can be bypassed using sodium benzoate, a commonly used food preservative. Ammonia is bound to benzoate extrahepatically to form a dialyzable compound hippurate, which is nontoxic. Sodium benzoate in a dose of 10 g/day has been shown to be as effective as lactulose in episodic HE.[99,100] Its oral bioavailability, absence of effect on GI motility, and lack of hepatic metabolism make it an attractive treatment option. Recently, concern has been expressed about its use in cirrhotic patients because plasma ammonia levels rose after a glutamine challenge while on sodium benzoate.[101]

Alfa keto analogues of amino acids

Amino acids have been restructured and deaminated to generate keto compounds, which then combine with the nitrogen in ammonia.[102]

While this is theoretically an attractive therapeutic avenue to pursue, there have been only limited studies and the compounds are difficult to obtain.

Zinc replacement

Zinc deficiency is common in patients with cirrhosis and may be associated with neurological dysfunction.[103] In experimental studies, zinc depletion results in hyperammonemia. This could be due to the zinc dependency of 2 of the 5 enzymes involved in the ureagenesis cycle. Published trials of long-term zinc replacement in subjects with mild persistent HE have shown improved psychometric testing and blood ammonia levels.[104] However, others have not shown a beneficial effect of zinc replacement.[105,106] Due to the time required for the effect, it is unlikely to be of short-term benefit in episodic HE.

Urease inhibition

Urease is an enzyme not found in mammals that can cause breakdown of the urea synthesized by the cirrhotic liver back to ammonia. Gastric *Helicobacter pylori* and intestinal bacteria have been demonstrated in human and animal studies to possess urease activity.[107] Antibiotics, immunization against purified urease, and biochemical or bacterial urease inhibitors have been tried in animals. Uncontrolled studies have suggested a benefit in reducing blood ammonia and increasing tolerance to protein load.[108] This is an interesting form of therapy but it needs critical clinical evaluation before recommendations can be made. Eradication of *H. pylori*, however, has not been shown to consistently improve HE in prospective studies though it may reduce plasma ammonia levels.[109]

Prebiotics and probiotics

Recently there is increasing interest in the use of prebiotics and probiotics in patients with hepatic encephalopathy.[110,111] Probiotics have been defined as viable microbial food supplements which beneficially influence the health of the host.[112] Prebiotics are food ingredients that are largely undegraded in the small bowel and are thought to be of potential benefit to the host by selectively stimulating the growth and/or activity of one or a limited number of gut bacteria.[112] At the present time, there is no convincing evidence to support the use of pre- and probiotics in HE. That being said, nonabsorbable disaccharides, *Lactobacillus* and SF68 might be considered by some to be probiotic therapy.

Altered cerebral neurotransmitter levels

Branched-chain amino acids

False neurotransmitters are neuroactive compounds derived in vivo from aromatic amino acids and they have been proposed as one mechanism for encephalopathy.[113] If this is true, then exogenous replacement by amino acid preparations rich in branched-chain amino acids (BCAA) and poor in aromatic amino acids might be beneficial in patients with the HE.[69] There have been eight randomized trials of parental BCAA in the therapy of episodic HE. These studies are quite different with respect to inclusion criteria, control therapy, supplemental therapy with BCAA, time of randomization, and status at inclusion. Two reviews that analyzed the data in these trials have reached conflicting conclusions about the effectiveness of BCAA.[114,115] A recent Cochrane systematic review of 11 randomized trials of BCAA did not find convincing evidence of a beneficial role for these in the treatment of hepatic encephalopathy.[116]

Dopaminergic agonists

Decreased dopaminergic neurotransmission has been suggested to play a role in the pathogenesis of HE. Measures to increase cerebral dopamine using L-dopa or bromocriptine have been tried with benefit in uncontrolled trials. Intraventricular infusion of dopamine in animal experiments was ineffective. Controlled clinical trials also failed to demonstrate beneficial effects of dopaminergic modifiers in HE. The Cochrane systematic review of the published trials on the use of dopaminergic agonists suggested that they should not be used in the therapy of hepatic encephalopathy.[117]

Benzodiazepine antagonists

Flumazenil is the only commercially available and approved benzodiazepine antagonist. To date, 13 prospective trials have been published on the use of flumazenil in HE in cirrhotic patients. In 10 of the studies, flumazenil was beneficial while in three, there was no difference compared to placebo. The negative studies had included patients with subclinical or mild encephalopathy. The limitations of flumazenil include its highly variable efficacy ranging from 17–78%, high cost, short duration of action, and parenteral route of administration. Its major role at present seems to be to reverse coma precipitated by exogenous benzodiazepine administration. A Cochrane systematic review of published trials on the use of benzodiazepine antagonists suggested that flumazenil had a beneficial effect on short-term improvement of HE in patients with cirrhosis.[118] However, the drug did not have any benefit on the recovery or survival in these patients.

Portacaval shunt-related HE

Aggravation of HE has been reported in cirrhotic patients who undergo surgical or transjugular intrahepatic portosystemic (TIPS) shunts.[119,120] Episodic or less commonly persistent HE is a problem in the absence of precipitating factors in this group of patients.[121] This may be related to a heightened sensitivity to precipitating factors for HE in shunted than in nonshunted patients.[122] More of these shunted patients are likely to be diagnosed to have a spontaneous episodic HE compared to the nonshunted patient. This may be related to mild alteration in hemodynamics, electrolyte abnormalities or other precipitating factors that may result in rapid development of coma. The acute management of these patients is similar to that of other patients with episodic HE. Various factors have been suggested to predict postsurgical shunt HE and similar factors may be operative in patients who have had placement of TIPS (Table 41.8).[119,121,123] Alteration in hepatic arterial blood flow after TIPS has not been shown to protect against HE following the procedure. Following placement of TIPS, 13–44% are likely to have new onset or worsening of existing HE.[124]

Table 41.8 Predictors of postshunt/post-TIPS encephalopathy

Residual hepatic functional reserve (hypoalbuminemia)

Preoperative portosystemic shunting

Age >65 years

Postprocedure portahepatic gradient

Preshunting episodes of encephalopathy

Etiology of cirrhosis (nonalcoholic)

Sex of the patient (female sex at greater risk)

Shunt age

Hepatic arterial buffer

Type of shunt performed

Doppler-predicted loss of hepatic perfusion

Surgical shunt procedures are also associated with the development of HE. A meta-analysis of the randomized trials of portosystemic shunt surgery in cirrhotic patients demonstrated a lower risk for early development of HE after distal splenorenal shunt compared to central or total portacaval shunts.[125,126] The majority of cases of postshunt-associated HE respond well to conservative medical measures. However, frequent episodes of episodic HE or debilitating episodic HE may warrant intervention to reduce the shunt diameter or actually occlude the shunt. In TIPS, a time-dependent spontaneous narrowing of the shunt occurs over the first 3 months and decisions to occlude the shunt should take this into account.[127] If patients continue to have major limitations related to HE after 3 months, interventional procedures using gel foam or balloon occlusion of the shunt or placement of a smaller stent can be considered.[122,128] However, occlusion or reduction of shunt diameter may cause reoccurrence of the original complication (e.g., GI bleeding, ascites, etc.). A recent study of the use of the expanded polytetraflouroethylene-covered stent grafts for TIPS has shown them to be well tolerated with a low incidence of shunt narrowing or occlusion.[129] While HE was unusual in these studies, it was likely related to patient selection rather than to the shunt itself.[129] Finally, a small portion of patients will develop refractory HE after shunt surgery or TIPS and it may not improve even after complete shunt occlusion. This is probably due to progressive hepatic failure, perhaps related in some cases to shunt-induced alteration in hepatic blood flow. Orthotopic liver treatment may be the transplantation option for these patients.

Persistent HE

The definition of persistent HE is not clear yet in terms of the time-frame needed to classify a patient in this category, but most favor a duration of encephalopathy more than 28 days. The therapeutic options available to these patients are similar to those previously discussed for episodic HE. However, the goal of therapy in these patients is to prevent recurrent exacerbations of encephalopathy. Most studies in patients with chronic or persistent HE were, in fact, conducted on patients with episodic HE, so their findings should not be considered to be conclusive.[69]

Supportive measures in patients with persistent HE include correction of anemia, control of infection, mobilization of ascites, adjustment of the dose of diuretics, and social support. The treatment modalities for persistent HE are shown in Table 41.9. Since the rationale of therapeutic options in episodic and persistent HE are similar, these will not be discussed again.

Nonabsorbable disaccharides

At least 21 prospective studies have been published on the efficacy of lactulose in persistent HE. Four were randomized and 10 were controlled studies. A total of 362 patients with persistent HE were treated with lactulose and improvement occurred in 280 (77.3%). Lactitol has been used in 58 patients in 5 prospective trials and clinical improvement observed in 30 patients (51%).[69]

Antibiotics

Neomycin and metronidazole have been evaluated in the therapy of persistent HE and shown to be beneficial.[130] Prolonged administration of broad-spectrum antibiotics may alter the bacterial flora

Table 41.9 Therapeutic strategies for persistent HE

Decrease ammonia content

Substrate reduction
Protein restriction
Regular diet
Vegetable proteins
Oral BCAA (?)
Bowel movements – cathartics

Decrease ammonia production

Antibiotics
Nonabsorbable disaccharides
Bacterial replacement

Convert ammonia to nontoxic products

Sodium benzoate
L ornithine L aspartate
Keto analogues of BCAA (?)

Improve hepatic perfusion

Shunt narrowing/obliteration
TIPS narrowing

Benzodiazepine antagonists

Long-term flumazenil/alternatives

Hepatic support

Artificial liver
Hepatocyte transplantation
Liver transplantation

BCAA: Branched chain amino acids.

of the gut and result in spread of resistance amongst residual or superinfecting flora. The dose schedules of antibiotics, especially neomycin, need to be evaluated further in view of potential renal and cochlear toxicity. Lower doses of neomycin may be safer than the high dose recommended in earlier literature. A dose of 1–2 g/day for 6–12 months is thought to be relatively safe, but this is unproven.[131]

Combination of antibiotics and disaccharides

A combination of neomycin and lactulose in mild encephalopathy (Grade I) showed clinical benefit in 10 patients in two centers.[132]

Amino acids

Long-term administration of enteral preparations of BCAA, dietary supplementation with BCAA, or protein hydrolysates enriched with BCAA might be useful in the treatment of persistent HE. The limitations of these studies are similar to those already discussed for BCAA infusion in persistent HE. In six of the nine studies published, no beneficial effects were observed.[133] Long-term BCAA supplementation orally may be superior to casein therapy alone in persistent HE. In protein-intolerant patients, oral BCAA may allow increased dietary protein intake without worsening of HE.[133]

Branched-chain keto analogues

Branched-chain keto analogues (BCKA) have been used in persistent HE in alcoholic cirrhotics in two randomized, controlled trials.[102,134] In the first study on eight patients, they were beneficial compared to branched-chain amino acids. In a second trial on 12 patients, no difference between BCKA and placebo was noted. No further studies have been published and the results would need evaluation before recommendations can be made.

Dietary therapy

In patients with chronic liver disease, nutritional support is needed to ameliorate malnutrition and hypoalbuminemia, to maintain hepatic function, and to promote hepatic regeneration. Protein intolerance is a major limitation in the dietary management of HE and protein excess may precipitate HE. Tolerance of protein loads differs in patients. Impaired glucose and fat tolerance occur due to the hormonal alterations in patients with chronic liver disease. Various factors may modify the course of HE. These include: the degree of hepatic decompensation, portosystemic shunting, nutritional status, GI motility, enzymatic and functional status of the gut, normal intestinal flora, and hormonal response to food. In view of the large number of factors that influence the effect of diet on HE, it is difficult to accurately evaluate the influence of diet in altering the course of HE. Dietary factors that may modify the course of HE include dietary protein content, source of the protein, zinc content, vitamins and dietary fibers. A patient with grade 2 or deeper coma cannot eat regular food. Most studies have therefore been conducted in patients with mild persistent HE and these may be helpful in managing a patient with episodic HE once diet can be introduced in the management program. There have been 10 controlled trials comparing vegetable and animal proteins in cirrhotic patients with persistent HE.[69] Nine of these showed better tolerance of vegetable proteins and improvement in indices of encephalopathy.

Dietary fiber also seems to favorably alter the course of persistent HE.[58] Colonic acidification and provision of substrate for colonic bacterial metabolism in lieu of urea and protein have been suggested.[135] Improvement in mental status and HE after fiber supplementation seemed independent of the amino acid profiles in cirrhotic patients with HE. Fiber supplementation may be a useful adjunct in the long-term management of persistent HE, especially due to negligible adverse effects and potential benefits on other systems in the body.

Zinc

The role of zinc therapy has already been discussed in the section of episodic HE. There may be a case for zinc replacement in persistent HE in a dose of 600 mg oral zinc sulfate daily for 3 months.[103]

Manganese

Deposition of manganese in the basal ganglia of cirrhotic patients has been suggested to contribute to the pathogenesis of HE.[136] No prospective studies of manganese chelation on the course of persistent HE are available.

Other treatment options

Other treatment options include L-ornithine-L-aspartate that seem to be beneficial in mild persistent HE. Long-term use of sodium benzoate in persistent HE that is refractory to conventional treatment options has been suggested but must be viewed with caution because of lack of long-term safety and benefits reported in this group of patients.

Surgical procedures

In persistent hepatic encephalopathy, colonic exclusion procedures were performed in the past. With the advent of OLT, these procedures have been abandoned.

Orthotopic liver transplantation

Transplantation allows one to manage end-stage liver disease when all other treatment modalities have failed.[137] Onset of HE generally implies a poor prognosis in patients with cirrhosis. However, the symptoms can usually be well controlled with medical therapy and the presence of HE per se does not increase the priority for acquiring a donor organ.[137,138] It therefore does not seem likely that these patients will often come to transplant unless they develop other complications of liver disease.

Minimal HE

The treatment of minimal HE may become important in devising new treatment options due to their stability and response to treatment. Nonetheless, there are currently no guidelines for the treatment of patients with minimal (subclinical) hepatic encephalopathy. Indeed, it is debatable whether such treatment is even necessary at all. There are no data to support the need for therapy in these patients even though there is evidence to suggest eventual progression of these patients to overt hepatic encephalopathy.[3] Long-term treatment trials are required to demonstrate a beneficial role of treating these patients with the goal of prevention of overt HE.

Table 41.10 Treatment protocol considerations in HE

Standard therapy
- Lactulose/disaccharides
- Neomycin
- i.v. fluids
- Control precipitating factors
- Protein restriction

Alternative therapy (considered beneficial)

Indications
- Controlled clinical trial
- Setting of HE refractory/resistant to standard therapy
- L ornithine – L aspartate
- Sodium benzoate
- Flumazenil/alternative BZ antagonists
- Vegetable proteins
- Zinc supplementation

Therapy of doubtful/no value
- Branched-chain amino acid infusions
- L-dopa
- Bromocriptine
- *Lactobacillus acidophilus*

Therapy that holds promise but poorly evaluated to date
- Melatonin
- Opioid antagonists
- Serotonin antagonists
- Keto analogues of BCAA

BZ, benzodiazepine; BCAA, branched chain amino acids.

Table 41.11 Troubleshooting tips in therapy of episodic HE

Diagnosis: Is it hepatic encephalopathy?

Demonstrate evidence of liver disease
- Clinical
- Biochemical
- Histological
- Sonographic (?)
- Endoscopic

Demonstrate encephalopathy

Attend sensorium/neural function

No primary neurologic disease that could explain clinical profile

Acute liver failure versus episodic HE (in chronic liver disease)

Grade of coma, associated complications, severity of underlying liver disease

Therapy

Precipitating factors

Covert	Overt
Dietary indiscretions	GI bleed
Over-the-counter medications	SBP
Diagnosis incorrect: meningitis, subdural hematoma, stroke, brain tumor, demyelination disease (MS)	Pneumonitis

Treatment protocol: standard therapy instituted

No/adequate response to therapy

Continuing precipitating factor

Incorrectly administered therapy

Severe, advanced liver disease

Cause of coma other than advanced liver disease

Inadvertent drug interactions

Sepsis	Resistant organisms
Hypokalemia	Low total body potassium
Azotemia	HRS, renal tubular injury persists
Drugs	Long-acting sedatives

SBP, spontaneous bacterial peritonitis; MS, multiple sclerosis.

SUMMARY OF PRACTICAL ISSUES IN MANAGEMENT OF HE

Hepatic encephalopathy is an important clinical complication in patients with cirrhosis. The diagnosis is clinical and usually straightforward. Laboratory tests are usually not necessary and some, such as plasma ammonia levels, are neither reliable nor helpful. Management consists of seeking and treating precipitating factors such as GI bleeding, infection, dehydration, or electrolyte abnormalities (Table 41.10). Treatment is centered on nonabsorbable disaccharides (lactulose or lactitol) with or without the short-term administration of a nonabsorbable antibiotic such as neomycin. It is important to reiterate that the different clinical manifestations of HE are probably mediated by similar mechanisms, but need different treatment approaches. A guide to the various practical difficulties in the management of HE and a brief outline of various troubleshooting strategies is shown in the flowchart provided (Table 41.11).

REFERENCES

1. Ferenci P, Lockwood A, Mullen K, et al. Hepatic encephalopathy – definition, nomenclature, diagnosis, and quantification: final report of the working party at the 11th World Congresses of Gastroenterology, Vienna, 1998. Hepatology 2002; 35(3):716–721.

   This is the definitive paper that deals with the current classification and the issues emphasizing the difficulties of interpreting treatment trials published in the past. A must read for anyone interested in the field of HE.

2. Dasarathy S, Mullen KD. Hepatic encephalopathy. Curr Treat Options Gastroenterol 2001; 4(6):517–526.

3. Weissenborn K. Minimal hepatic encephalopathy: a permanent source of discussion. Hepatology 2002; 35(2):494–496.

4. Klempnaue J, Schrem H. Review: surgical shunts and encephalopathy. Metab Brain Dis 2001; 16(1–2):21–25.

5. Mullen KD. Interplay of portal pressure, portal perfusion and hepatic arterial inflow in modulating expression of hepatic encephalopathy in patients with spontaneous or artificially created portosystemic shunts. Indian J Gastroenterol 2003; 22(Suppl 2):S25–S27.

6. Madoff DC, Wallace MJ, Ahrar K, et al. TIPS-related hepatic encephalopathy: management options with novel endovascular techniques. Radiographics 2004; 24(1):21–36.

7. Bismuth H, Franco D, Alagille D. Portal diversion for portal hypertension in children. The first ninety patients. Ann Surg 1980; 192(1):18–24.

8. Pocha C, Maliakkal B. Spontaneous intrahepatic portal-systemic venous shunt in the adult: case report and review of the literature. Dig Dis Sci 2004; 49(7-8):1201–1206.

9. Ohnishi K, Sato S, Saito M, et al. Clinical and portal hemodynamic features in cirrhotic patients having a large spontaneous splenorenal and/or gastrorenal shunt. Am J Gastroenterol 1986; 81(6):450–455.

10. Butterworth RF. Pathogenesis of hepatic encephalopathy: update on molecular mechanisms. Indian J Gastroenterol 2003; 22(Suppl 2):S11–S16.

11. Cordoba J, Alonso J, Rovira A, et al. The development of low-grade cerebral edema in cirrhosis is supported by the evolution of (1)H-magnetic resonance abnormalities after liver transplantation. J Hepatol 2001; 35(5):598–604.

12. Donovan JP, Schafer DF, Shaw BW Jr, et al. Cerebral oedema and increased intracranial pressure in chronic liver disease. Lancet 1998; 351(9104):719–721.

   This illustrates that overt cerebral edema does occur in patients with chronic liver disease, needs to be identified, and may require treatment.

13. Bhatia V, Batra Y, Acharya SK. Prophylactic phenytoin does not improve cerebral edema or survival in acute liver failure – a controlled clinical trial. J Hepatol 2004; 41(1):89–96.

14. Larsen FS, Gottstein J, Blei AT. Cerebral hyperemia and nitric oxide synthase in rats with ammonia-induced brain edema. J Hepatol 2001; 34(4):548–554.

15. Del Piccolo F, Sacerdoti D, Amodio P, et al. Central nervous system alterations in liver cirrhosis: the role of portal-systemic shunt and portal hypoperfusion. Metab Brain Dis 2002; 17(4):347–358.

16. Ahl B, Weissenborn K, van den HJ, et al. Regional differences in cerebral blood flow and cerebral ammonia metabolism in patients with cirrhosis. Hepatology 2004; 40(1):73–79.

17. Blei AT. Pathophysiology of brain edema in fulminant hepatic failure, revisited. Metab Brain Dis 2001; 16(1–2):85–94.

18. Cordoba J, Gottstein J, Blei AT. Glutamine, myo-inositol, and organic brain osmolytes after portocaval anastomosis in the rat: implications for ammonia-induced brain edema. Hepatology 1996; 24(4):919–923.

19. Haussinger D, Kircheis G, Fischer R, et al. Hepatic encephalopathy in chronic liver disease: a clinical manifestation of astrocyte swelling and low-grade cerebral edema? J Hepatol 2000; 32(6):1035–1038.

   This paper comes from the originator of the concept that cerebral edema occurs in all forms of liver disease and illustrates the importance of astrocytes in the pathophysiology of HE.

20. Rovira A, Cordoba J, Raguer N, et al. Magnetic resonance imaging measurement of brain edema in patients with liver disease: resolution after transplantation. Curr Opin Neurol 2002; 15(6):731–737.

21. Lizardi-Cervera J, Almeda P, Guevara L, et al. Hepatic encephalopathy: a review. Ann Hepatol 2003; 2(3):122–130.

22. Butterworth RF. Role of circulating neurotoxins in the pathogenesis of hepatic encephalopathy: potential for improvement following their removal by liver assist devices. Liver Int 2003; 23(Suppl 3):5–9.

23. Vaquero J, Chung C, Cahill ME, et al. Pathogenesis of hepatic encephalopathy in acute liver failure. Semin Liver Dis 2003; 23(3):259–269.

24. Ong JP, Aggarwal A, Krieger D, et al. Correlation between ammonia levels and the severity of hepatic encephalopathy. Am J Med 2003; 114(3):188–193.

   This paper finally puts to rest the correlation between severity of HE and blood ammonia levels. This studies shows a correlation between severity of HE and arterial and venous ammonia levels.

25. Cohn R, Castel D. The effects of acute hyperammonemia on the electroencephalogram. Lab Clin Med 1968; 68:189–205.

26. Eichler M, Bessman S. A double blind study of the effect of ammonium infusion on psychological functioning in cirrhotic patients. J Nerv Ment Dis 1962; 134:539–562.

27. Balata S, Damink SW, Ferguson K, et al. Induced hyperammonemia alters neuropsychology, brain MR spectroscopy and magnetization transfer in cirrhosis. Hepatology 2003; 37(4):931–939.

28. Jalan R, Shawcross D, Davies N. The molecular pathogenesis of hepatic encephalopathy. Int J Biochem Cell Biol 2003; 35(8):1175–1181.

29. Maleux G, Nevens F, Wilmer A, et al. Early and long-term clinical and radiological follow-up results of expanded-polytetrafluoroethylene-covered stent-grafts for transjugular intrahepatic portosystemic shunt procedures. Eur Radiol 2004; 14(10):1842–1850.

30. Sherlock S, Dooley J. Hepatic cirrhosis. diseases of the liver and biliary system 10th edn. Blackwell, Oxford. 1992:371–384.

31. Brown JJ, Naylor MJ, Yagan N. Imaging of hepatic cirrhosis. Radiology 1997; 202(1):1–16.

32. Chen R, Young GB. Metabolic encephalopathies. Baillières Clin Neurol 1996; 5(3):577–598.

33. Cadranel JF, Lebiez E, Di M, et al. Focal neurological signs in hepatic encephalopathy in cirrhotic patients: an underestimated entity? Am J Gastroenterol 2001; 96(2):515–518.

34. Lockwood A. Clinical and laboratory features of hepatic encephalopathy. Hepatic Encephalopathy, Butterworth-Heinemann, Boston. 11–32. 1992.

35. McIntosh C, Chick J. Alcohol and the nervous system. J Neurol Neurosurg Psychiatry 2004; 75(Suppl 3):iii16–iii21.

36. Strauss E, da Costa MF. The importance of bacterial infections as precipitating factors of chronic hepatic encephalopathy in cirrhosis. Hepatogastroenterology 1998; 45(21):900–904.

This paper established clearly the importance of sepsis, especially bacterial peritonitis in the precipitation of HE, by a very experienced investigator in this field.

37. Faloon WW, Evans GL. Precipitating factors in genesis of hepatic coma. NY State J Med 1970; 70(23):2891–2896.

One of the most widely quoted abstracts in HE.

38. Strauss E, Gomes de Sa Ribeiro MDE. Bacterial infections associated with hepatic encephalopathy: prevalence and outcome. Ann Hepatol 2003; 2(1):41–45.

39. Tromm A, Griga T, Greving I, et al. Orthograde whole gut irrigation with mannite versus paromomycine + lactulose as prophylaxis of hepatic encephalopathy in patients with cirrhosis and upper gastrointestinal bleeding: results of a controlled randomized trial. Hepatogastroenterology 2000; 47(32):473–477.

40. Navasa M, Rimola A, Rodes J. Bacterial infections in liver disease. Semin Liver Dis 1997; 17(4):323–333.

41. Carbonell N, Pauwels A, Serfaty L, et al. Improved survival after variceal bleeding in patients with cirrhosis over the past two decades. Hepatology 2004; 40(3):652–659.

42. Mullen KD, Dasarathy S. Protein restriction in hepatic encephalopathy: necessary evil or illogical dogma? J Hepatol 2004; 41(1):147–148.

43. Cordoba J, Lopez-Hellin J, Planas M, et al. Normal protein diet for episodic hepatic encephalopathy: results of a randomized study. J Hepatol 2004; 41(1):38–43.

A study by an experienced group of investigators that boldly have addressed the issues of dietary management of HE and reemphasizes the controversies that have surrounded this area. The editorial along with this manuscript illustrates the changes in approach to nutritional management of HE.

44. Bleichner G, Boulanger R, Squara P, et al. Frequency of infections in cirrhotic patients presenting with acute gastrointestinal haemorrhage. Br J Surg 1986; 73(9):724–726.

45. Henderson JM. The timing and role of non-transplant surgery in management of variceal bleeding. Gastrointest Endosc Clin N Am 1999; 9(2):331–345.

46. Martin H, Voss K, Hufnagl P, et al. Morphometric and densitometric investigations of protoplasmic astrocytes and neurons in human hepatic encephalopathy. Exp Pathol 1987; 32(4):241–250.

47. Abou-Assi S, Vlahcevic ZR. Hepatic encephalopathy. Metabolic consequence of cirrhosis often is reversible. Postgrad Med 2001; 109(2):52–60, 63.

48. Sanaka MR, Ong JP, Mullen KD. Challenges of designing hepatic encephalopathy treatment trials. Hepatology 2003; 38(2):527–528.

49. Dejong CH, Deutz NE, Soeters PB. Intestinal glutamine and ammonia metabolism during chronic hyperammonaemia induced by liver insufficiency. Gut 1993; 34(8):1112–1119.

50. Plauth M, Roske AE, Romaniuk P, et al. Post-feeding hyperammonaemia in patients with transjugular intrahepatic portosystemic shunt and liver cirrhosis: role of small intestinal ammonia release and route of nutrient administration. Gut 2000; 46(6):849–855.

51. Wrong OM, Vince AJ, Waterlow JC. The contribution of endogenous urea to faecal ammonia in man, determined by 15N labelling of plasma urea. Clin Sci (Lond) 1985; 68(2):193–199.

52. Uribe M, Campollo O, Vargas F, et al. Acidifying enemas (lactitol and lactose) vs. nonacidifying enemas (tap water) to treat acute

portal-systemic encephalopathy: a double-blind, randomized clinical trial. Hepatology 1987; 7(4):639–643.

53. Ratnaike RN, Hicks EP, Hislop IG. The rectal administration of lactulose. Aust NZ J Med 1975; 5(2):137–140.

54. Amodio P, Caregaro L, Patteno E, et al. Vegetarian diets in hepatic encephalopathy: facts or fantasies? Dig Liver Dis 2001; 33(6):492–500.

55. Seymour CA, Whelan K. Dietary management of hepatic encephalopathy. Br Med J 1999; 318(7195):1364–1365.

56. Rudman D, Galambos JT, Smith RB III, et al. Comparison of the effect of various amino acids upon the blood ammonia concentration of patients with liver disease. Am J Clin Nutr 1973; 26(9):916–925.

57. Rudnan D, Smith RB III, Salam AA, et al. Ammonia content of food. Am J Clin Nutr 1973; 26(5):487–490.

58. Weber FL Jr, Minco D, Fresard KM, et al. Effects of vegetable diets on nitrogen metabolism in cirrhotic subjects. Gastroenterology 1985; 89(3):538–544.

59. Russell DM, Walker PM, Leiter LA, et al. Metabolic and structural changes in skeletal muscle during hypocaloric dieting. Am J Clin Nutr 1984; 39(4):503–513.

60. Leiter LA, Marliss EB. Survival during fasting may depend on fat as well as protein stores. JAMA 1982; 248(18):2306–2307.

61. Biolo G, Declan Fleming RY, Wolfe RR. Physiologic hyperinsulinemia stimulates protein synthesis and enhances transport of selected amino acids in human skeletal muscle. J Clin Invest 1995; 95(2):811–819.

62. Soulsby CT, Morgan MY. Dietary management of hepatic encephalopathy in cirrhotic patients: survey of current practice in United Kingdom. Br Med J 1999; 318(7195):1391.

63. Dasarathy S. Role of gut bacteria in the therapy of hepatic encephalopathy with lactulose and antibiotics. Indian J Gastroenterol 2003; 22(Suppl 2):S50–S53.

64. Vince AJ, Burridge SM. Ammonia production by intestinal bacteria: the effects of lactose, lactulose and glucose. J Med Microbiol 1980; 13(2):177-191.

65. Mas A, Rodes J, Sunyer L, et al. Comparison of rifaximin and lactitol in the treatment of acute hepatic encephalopathy: results of a randomized, double-blind, double-dummy, controlled clinical trial. J Hepatol 2003; 38(1):51–58.

A well-conducted study demonstrating similar efficacy for nonabsorbable antibiotic rifaximin and lactitol. Possibly the last study to use the PSE index.

66. Strauss E, Tramote R, Silva EP, et al. Double-blind randomized clinical trial comparing neomycin and placebo in the treatment of exogenous hepatic encephalopathy. Hepatogastroenterology 1992; 39(6):542–545.

One of the few randomized, placebo-controlled trials in the treatment of HE that actually showed that neomycin was not superior to placebo in HE.

67. Morgan MH, Read AE, Speller DC. Treatment of hepatic encephalopathy with metronidazole. Gut 1982; 23(1):1–7.

68. Tarao K, Ikeda T, Hayashi K, et al. Successful use of vancomycin hydrochloride in the treatment of lactulose resistant chronic hepatic encephalopathy. Gut 1990; 31(6):702–706.

69. Mullen K, Dasarathy S. Hepatic encephalopathy. In: Schiff E, Sorrell MF, Maddrey W, eds. Diseases of the liver. 10th edn. New York: Lippincott Raven; 1999.

70. Berk DP, Chalmers T. Deafness complicating antibiotic therapy of hepatic encephalopathy. Ann Intern Med 1970; 73(3):393–396.

71. Curioso WH, Monkemuller KE. Neomycin should not be used to treat hepatic encephalopathy. Br Med J 2001; 323(7306):233.

72. Williams R, James OF, Warnes TW, et al. Evaluation of the efficacy and safety of rifaximin in the treatment of hepatic encephalopathy: a double-blind, randomized, dose-finding multi-centre study. Eur J Gastroenterol Hepatol 2000; 12(2):203–208.

73. Camma C, Fiorello F, Tine F, et al. Lactitol in treatment of chronic hepatic encephalopathy. A meta-analysis. Dig Dis Sci 1993; 38(5):916–922.

74. Blanc P, Daures JP, Rouillon JM, et al. Lactitol or lactulose in the treatment of chronic hepatic encephalopathy: results of a meta-analysis. Hepatology 1992; 15(2):222–228.

75. Patil DH, Westaby D, Mahida YR, et al. Comparative modes of action of lactitol and lactulose in the treatment of hepatic encephalopathy. Gut 1987; 28(3):255–259.

76. Price JB Jr, Sawada M, Voorhees AB Jr. Clinical significance of intraluminal pH in intestinal ammonia transport. Am J Surg 1970; 119(5):595–598.

77. Morgan MY, Hawley KE. Lactitol vs. lactulose in the treatment of acute hepatic encephalopathy in cirrhotic patients: a double-blind, randomized trial. Hepatology 1987; 7(6):1278–1284.

78. Heredia D, Caballeria J, Arroyo V, et al. Lactitol versus lactulose in the treatment of acute portal systemic encephalopathy (PSE). A controlled trial. J Hepatol 1987; 4(3):293–298.

79. Als-Nielsen B, Gluud LL, Gluud C. Non-absorbable disaccharides for hepatic encephalopathy: systematic review of randomised trials. Br Med J 2004; 328(7447):1046.

This review suggests that there is no convincing evidence that lactulose is effective in HE. Therefore, it should not be used as a comparator in any clinical treatment trials unless its efficacy is proven.

80. Clausen MR, Mortensen PB. Lactulose, disaccharides and colonic flora. Clinical consequences. Drugs 1997; 53(6):930–942.

81. Conn H. Complications of portal hypertension. Current hepatology. New York: John Wiley and Sons; 1984:225–226.

82. Bird SP, Hewitt D, Ratcliffe B, et al. Effects of lactulose and lactitol on protein digestion and metabolism in conventional and germ free animal models: relevance of the results to their use in the treatment of portosystemic encephalopathy. Gut 1990; 31(12):1403–1406.

83. Weber FL Jr, Fresard KM, Lally BR. Effects of lactulose and neomycin on urea metabolism in cirrhotic subjects. Gastroenterology 1982; 82(2):213–217.

84. Mann NS, Borkar BB, Narenderan KP, et al. Effect of lactulose, neomycin and antacid on colonic pH recorded continuously with an implanted electrode. Am J Gastroenterol 1979; 72(2):141–145.

85. Weber FL Jr. Lactulose and combination therapy of hepatic encephalopathy: the role of the intestinal microflora. Dig Dis Sci 1996; 14(Suppl 1):53–63.

86. Garcia-Tsao G, Wiest R. Gut microflora in the pathogenesis of the complications of cirrhosis. Best Pract Res Clin Gastroenterol 2004; 18(2):353–372.

87. Fenton JC, Knight EJ, O'Grady FW. Treatment of hepatic encephalopathy by alteration of intestinal flora with *Lactobacillus acidophilus*. Lancet 1965; 17:764.

88. Macbeth WA, Kass EH, Mcdermott WV Jr. Treatment of hepatic encephalopathy by alteration of intestinal flora with *Lactobacillus acidophilus*. Lancet 1965; 191:399–403.

89. Loguercio C, Abbiati R, Rinaldi M, et al. Long-term effects of *Enterococcus faecium SF68* versus lactulose in the treatment of patients with cirrhosis and grade 1–2 hepatic encephalopathy. J Hepatol 1995; 23(1):39–46.

90. Khuroo MS, Khuroo MS, Farahat KL. Molecular adsorbent recirculating system for acute and acute-on-chronic liver failure: a meta-analysis. Liver Transpl 2004; 10(9):1099–1106.

91. Sen S, Williams R, Jalan R. The pathophysiological basis of acute-on-chronic liver failure. Liver 2002; 22(Suppl 2):5–13.

92. Haussinger D. Nitrogen metabolism in liver: structural and functional organization and physiological relevance. Biochem J 1990; 267(2):281–290.

93. Stoll B, McNelly S, Buscher HP, et al. Functional hepatocyte heterogeneity in glutamate, aspartate and alpha-ketoglutarate uptake: a histoautoradiographical study. Hepatology 1991; 13(2):247–253.

94. Zieve L, Lyftogt C, Raphael D. Ammonia toxicity: comparative protective effect of various arginine and ornithine derivatives, aspartate, benzoate, and carbamyl glutamate. Metab Brain Dis 1986; 1(1):25–35.

95. Kircheis G, Wettstein M, Dahl S, et al. Clinical efficacy of L-ornithine-L-aspartate in the management of hepatic encephalopathy. Metab Brain Dis 2002; 17(4):453–462.

96. Staedt U, Leweling H, Gladisch R, et al. Effects of ornithine aspartate on plasma ammonia and plasma amino acids in patients with cirrhosis. A double-blind, randomized study using a four-fold crossover design. J Hepatol 1993; 19(3):424–430.

97. Kircheis G, Nilius R, Held C, et al. Therapeutic efficacy of L-ornithine-L-aspartate infusions in patients with cirrhosis and hepatic encephalopathy: results of a placebo-controlled, double-blind study. Hepatology 1997; 25(6):1351–1360.

98. Rees CJ, Oppong K, Al Mardini H, et al. Effect of L-ornithine-L-aspartate on patients with and without TIPS undergoing glutamine challenge: a double blind, placebo-controlled trial. Gut 2000; 47(4):571–574.

99. Mendenhall CL, Rouster S, Marshall L, et al. A new therapy for portal systemic encephalopathy. Am J Gastroenterol 1986; 81(7):540–543.

100. Sushma S, Dasarathy S, Tandon RK, et al. Sodium benzoate in the treatment of acute hepatic encephalopathy: a double-blind randomized trial. Hepatology 1992; 16(1):138–144.

This a comprehensive study established that a nonenzymatic ammonia disposal pathway can be effectively utilized in the treatment of HE, lending further support to the role of ammonia in the pathogenesis of HE.

101. Efrati C, Masini A, Merli M, et al. Effect of sodium benzoate on blood ammonia response to oral glutamine challenge in cirrhotic patients: a note of caution. Am J Gastroenterol 2000; 95(12):3574–3578.

102. Walker S, Gotz R, Czygan P, et al. Oral keto analogs of branched-chain amino acids in hyperammonemia in patients with cirrhosis of the liver. A double-blind crossover study. Digestion 1982; 24(2):105–111.

103. Marchesini G, Fabbri A, Bianchi G, et al. Zinc supplementation and amino acid-nitrogen metabolism in patients with advanced cirrhosis. Hepatology 1996; 23(5):1084–1092.

104. Reding P, Duchateau J, Bataille C. Oral zinc supplementation improves hepatic encephalopathy. Results of a randomised controlled trial. Lancet 1984; 2(8401):493–495.

105. Riggio O, Ariosto F, Merli M, et al. Short-term oral zinc supplementation does not improve chronic hepatic encephalopathy. Results of a double-blind crossover trial. Dig Dis Sci 1991; 36(9):1204–1208.

106. Bresci G, Parisi G, Banti S. Management of hepatic encephalopathy with oral zinc supplementation: a long-term treatment. Eur J Med 1993; 2(7):414–416.

107. Dasani BM, Sigal SH, Lieber CS. Analysis of risk factors for chronic hepatic encephalopathy: the role of *Helicobacter pylori* infection. Am J Gastroenterol 1998; 93(5):726–731.

108. Summerskill WH, Thorsell F, Feinberg JH, et al. Effects of urease inhibition in hyperammonemia: clinical and experimental studies with acetohydroxamic acid. Gastroenterology 1968; 54(1):20–26.

109. Zullo A, Hassan C, Morini S. Hepatic encephalopathy and *Helicobacter pylori*: a critical reappraisal. J Clin Gastroenterol 2003; 37(2):164–168.

110. Solga SF, Diehl AM. Gut flora-based therapy in liver disease? The liver cares about the gut. Hepatology 2004; 39(5):1197–1200.

111. Marteau P, Boutron-Ruault MC. Nutritional advantages of probiotics and prebiotics. Br J Nutr 2002; 87(Suppl 2):S153–S157.

112. Schrezenmeir J, de Vrese M. Probiotics, prebiotics, and synbiotics – approaching a definition. Am J Clin Nutr 2001; 73(2 Suppl): 361S–364S.

113. Zieve L. Pathogenesis of hepatic encephalopathy. Metab Brain Dis 1987; 2(3):147–165.

114. Naylor CD, O'Rourke K, Detsky AS, et al. Parenteral nutrition with branched-chain amino acids in hepatic encephalopathy. A meta-analysis. Gastroenterology 1989; 97(4):1033–1042.

115. Erikkson LS, Conn HO. Branched-chain amino acids in hepatic encephalopathy. Gastroenterology 1990; 99(2):604–607.

116. Als-Nielsen B, Koretz RL, Kjaergard LL, et al. Branched-chain amino acids for hepatic encephalopathy. Cochrane Database Syst Rev 2003; (2):CD001939.

117. Als-Nielsen B, Gluud L, Gluud C. Dopaminergic agonists for hepatic encephalopathy. Cochrane Database Syst Rev 2004; (4):CD003047.

118. Als-Nielsen B, Gluud LL, Gluud C. Benzodiazepine receptor antagonists for hepatic encephalopathy. Cochrane Database Syst Rev 2004; (2):CD002798.

119. Hassoun Z, Deschenes M, Lafortune M, et al. Relationship between pre-TIPS liver perfusion by the portal vein and the incidence of post-TIPS chronic hepatic encephalopathy. Am J Gastroenterol 2001; 96(4):1205–1209.

120. Sachdev A, Duseja A. Decompressive shunts and hepatic encephalopathy. Indian J Gastroenterol 2003; 22(Suppl 2):S21–S24.

121. Malinchoc M, Kamath PS, Gordon FD, et al. A model to predict poor survival in patients undergoing transjugular intrahepatic portosystemic shunts. Hepatology 2000; 31(4):864–871.

122. Nolte W, Wiltfang J, Schindler C, et al. Portosystemic hepatic encephalopathy after transjugular intrahepatic portosystemic shunt in patients with cirrhosis: clinical, laboratory, psychometric, and electroencephalographic investigations. Hepatology 1998; 28(5):1215–1225.

123. Riggio O, Merlli M, Pedretti G, et al. Hepatic encephalopathy after transjugular intrahepatic portosystemic shunt. Incidence and risk factors. Dig Dis Sci 1996; 41(3):578–584.

Discusses the risks of HE after TIPS. With the increasing use of TIPS in HE, this paper is a must for all practicing hepatologists who are likely to deal with patients who need or have been subjected to a TIPS.

124. Rossle M, Piotraschke J. Transjugular intrahepatic portosystemic shunt and hepatic encephalopathy. Dig Dis Sci 1996; 14(Suppl 1):12–19.

125. Pomier-Layrargues G, Huet PM, Infante-Rivard C, et al. Prognostic value of indocyanine green and lidocaine kinetics for survival and chronic hepatic encephalopathy in cirrhotic patients following elective end-to-side portacaval shunt. Hepatology 1988; 8(6):1506–1510.

126. Maffei-Faccioli A, Gerunda GE, Neri D, et al. Selective variceal decompression and its role relative to other therapies. Am J Surg 1990; 160(1):60–66.

127. Rossle M, Siegerstetter V, Huber M, et al. The first decade of the transjugular intrahepatic portosystemic shunt (TIPS): state of the art. Liver 1998; 18(2):73–89.

128. Cox MW, Soltes GD, Lin PH, et al. Reversal of transjugular intrahepatic portosystemic shunt (TIPS)-induced hepatic encephalopathy using a strictured self-expanding covered stent. Cardiovasc Intervent Radiol 2003; 26(6):539–542.

129. Hausegger KA, Karnel F, Georgieva B, et al. Transjugular intrahepatic portosystemic shunt creation with the Viatorr expanded polytetrafluoroethylene-covered stent-graft. J Vasc Interv Radiol 2004; 15(3):239–248.

130. Morgan MY. The treatment of chronic hepatic encephalopathy. Hepatogastroenterology 1991; 38(5):377–387.

131. Last PM, Sherlock S. Systemic absorption of orally administered neomycin in liver disease. N Engl J Med 1960; 262:385–389.

132. Weber FL Jr. Combination therapy with lactulose or lactitol and antibiotics. Hepatic encephalopathy. Bloomington, IL: MediEd Press; 1996:285–297.

133. Fabbri A, Magrini N, Bianchi G, et al. Overview of randomized clinical trials of oral branched-chain amino acid treatment in chronic hepatic encephalopathy. J Parenter Enteral Nutr 1996; 20(2):159–164.

134. Herlong H, Maddrey W, Walser M. Treatment of portal systemic encephalopathy with ornithine salts of branched chain ketoacids; a comparative trial. Walser M, Williamson J, eds. Metabolism and clinical implications of branched chain amino and keto acids. Amsterdam, Holland: Elsevier; 1981:141–148.

135. Pomare EW, Branch WJ, Cummings JH. Carbohydrate fermentation in the human colon and its relation to acetate concentrations in venous blood. J Clin Invest 1985; 75(5):1448–1454.

136. Morgan MY. Cerebral magnetic resonance imaging in patients with chronic liver disease. Metab Brain Dis 1998; 13(4):273–290.

137. Blei AT, Cordoba J. Hepatic encephalopathy. Am J Gastroenterol 2001; 96(7):1968–1976.

138. Kamath PS, Wiesner RH, Malinchoc M, et al. A model to predict survival in patients with end-stage liver disease. Hepatology 2001; 33(2):464–470.

CHAPTER FORTY-TWO

42

Hepatorenal syndrome

Vicente Arroyo Perez and Pere Ginés Gibert

INTRODUCTION

Hepatorenal syndrome (HRS) is a common complication in patients with cirrhosis, severe hepatic failure, and portal hypertension. It is characterized by renal vasoconstriction, very low renal perfusion, and glomerular filtration rate (GRF), and intense reduction of the kidney's ability to excrete sodium and free water[1,2] in the absence of significant histological renal lesions sufficient to justify the impairment in renal function.

HRS is the extreme expression of the circulatory dysfunction of cirrhosis. The circulatory dysfunction observed in cirrhosis has traditionally been considered to be the consequence of an arterial vasodilation in the splanchnic circulation. However, recent data suggest that impairment of cardiac function may also play a role. These patients typically have arterial hypotension and intense stimulation of antidiuretic hormone, the renin-angiotensin axis, and the sympathetic nervous system. Nonazotemic cirrhotic patients with ascites, increased renin-angiotensin and sympathetic nervous system activity, intense sodium retention, and dilutional hyponatremia are especially susceptible to HRS.

The syndrome may develop spontaneously during the natural course of the disease or be precipitated by factors that induce renal hypoperfusion such as bacterial infections. The annual incidence of HRS in patients with cirrhosis and ascites has been estimated to be 8%.[3] Since HRS is a functional type of renal failure, there is no specific diagnostic marker for HRS.[2,4,5] Thus, diagnosis relies on the exclusion of other causes of renal insufficiency.[6] HRS is the complication of cirrhosis associated with the worst prognosis and, for many years, it has been considered as a terminal event of the disease. However, effective treatment modalities have recently been introduced that appear to improve survival, and a significant number of patients also now benefit from liver transplantation.

DIAGNOSIS AND CLINICAL TYPES OF HEPATORENAL SYNDROME

Diagnosis

The first step in the diagnosis of HRS is the demonstration of a reduced GFR, and this is not easy in advanced cirrhosis.[7,8] The muscle mass, and therefore the release of creatinine, is considerably reduced in these patients and they often have normal serum creatinine concentrations even in the setting of a very low GFR.

Similarly, urea is synthesized by the liver and may be reduced as a consequence of hepatic insufficiency. Therefore, it is not uncommon to miss the diagnosis of HRS because the serum creatinine is normal.[9,10] The consensus is that the diagnosis of HRS cannot be established until the serum creatinine has risen above 1.5 mg/dL or the creatinine clearance has decreased to less than 40 ml/min.

The second step in the diagnosis is to differentiate HRS from other causes of renal failure. For many years this was based on the traditional criteria used by nephrologists to distinguish functional renal failure (oliguria, low urine sodium concentration and urine-to-plasma osmolality ratio greater than unity, normal fresh urine sediment and no proteinuria). However, acute tubular necrosis in patients with cirrhosis and ascites may also present with oliguria, low urine sodium concentration, and urine osmolality greater than plasma osmolality.[11] To further complicate the diagnosis, relatively high urinary sodium concentrations have been reported in some patients with HRS.[12]

Because of the lack of specific tests, the diagnosis of HRS should be based on the exclusion of other disorders that can cause renal failure in cirrhotic patients (Table 42.1).[13] Prerenal causes of renal failure due to renal (diuretics) or extrarenal fluid losses (diarrhea, GI blood loss) should be investigated. If renal failure is secondary to volume depletion, renal function improves rapidly after volume expansion, whereas no improvement occurs in HRS. Even if there is no history of fluid loss, renal function should be assessed after diuretic withdrawal and volume replacement (1.5 liters of isotonic saline) in order to rule out any subtle reduction in plasma volume as the cause of renal failure. The presence of shock before the onset of renal failure points towards a diagnosis of acute tubular necrosis. Cirrhotic patients with infections may develop transient renal failure, which resolves after resolution of the infection. Therefore, in the cirrhotic patient with a bacterial infection, the diagnosis of HRS should only be made in the absence of septic shock and if renal failure persists following resolution of infection. Cirrhotic patients have a high risk of renal failure when treated with aminoglycosides, nonsteroidal antiinflammatory drugs, and vasodilators (renin-angiotensin system inhibitors, prazosin, nitrates). Therefore, evidence of treatment with these drugs in the days preceding the diagnosis of renal failure should be sought. Finally, patients with cirrhosis can develop renal failure due to intrinsic renal diseases, particularly glomerulonephritis. These cases can be recognized by the presence of proteinuria, hematuria, or both.

Table 42.1 International Ascites Club's diagnostic criteria of hepatorenal syndrome[38]

Major criteria
Chronic or acute liver disease with advanced hepatic failure and portal hypertension
Low glomerular filtration rate, as indicated by serum creatinine of >1.5 mg/dL or 24-h creatinine clearance <40 mL/min
Absence of shock, ongoing bacterial infection, and current or recent treatment with nephrotoxic drugs. Absence of gastrointestinal fluid losses (repeated vomiting or intense diarrhea) or renal fluid losses (weight loss >500 g/day for several days in patients with ascites without peripheral edema or 1000 g/day in patients with peripheral edema)
No sustained improvement in renal function (decrease in serum creatinine to 1.5 mg/dL or less or increase in creatinine clearance to 40 mL/min or more) following diuretic withdrawal and expansion of plasma volume with 1.5 L of isotonic saline
Proteinuria <500 mg/dL and no ultrasonographic evidence of obstructive uropathy or parenchymal renal disease
Additional criteria
Urine volume <500 mL/day
Urine sodium <10 mEq/L
Urine osmolality greater than plasma osmolality
Urine red blood cells <50 per high-power field
Serum sodium concentration <130 mEq/L

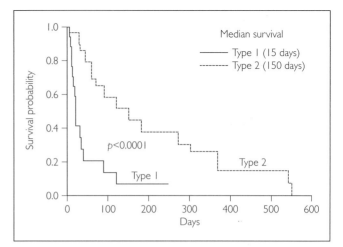

Fig. 42.1 • Survival of patients with cirrhosis after the diagnosis of type-1 or type-2 HRS (unpublished data).

Types of hepatorenal syndrome

There are two types of HRS.[13] Type-1 HRS is characterized by severe and rapidly progressive renal failure, which has been defined as a doubling of serum creatinine, reaching a level greater than 2.5 mg/dL in less than two weeks. Although type-1 HRS may arise spontaneously it frequently occurs proximate to a precipitating factor such as a severe bacterial infection, gastrointestinal hemorrhage, a major surgical procedure, or acute hepatitis superimposed on cirrhosis. The association of HRS and spontaneous bacterial peritonitis has been well documented.[14–16] Type-1 HRS develops in approximately 25% of patients with spontaneous bacterial peritonitis despite rapid resolution of the infection with non-nephrotoxic antibiotics. Patients with intense inflammatory response and high cytokine levels in plasma and ascitic fluid are particularly prone to develop type-1 HRS after the infection. Patients with type-1 HRS secondary to spontaneous bacterial peritonitis typically shows signs of severe liver insufficiency (jaundice, coagulopathy and hepatic encephalopathy) and circulatory dysfunction (arterial hypotension, very high plasma levels of renin and noradrenaline [norepinephrine]) that worsen with the impairment in renal function. Type-1 HRS is the most ominous complication of cirrhosis and has a very poor prognosis with a median survival time of only 2 weeks (Fig. 42.1).[3]

Type-2 HRS is characterized by a moderate and steady decrease in renal function, but a serum creatinine lower than 2.5 mg/dL. Patients with type-2 HRS show signs of liver failure and arterial hypotension, but in general to a lesser degree than patients with

type-1 HRS. The dominant clinical feature is marked ascites with poor or no response to diuretics (a condition known as refractory ascites). Patients with type-2 HRS have a particularly high risk of developing type-1 HRS following infections or other precipitating events.[10–12] Median survival of patients with type-2 HRS (6 months) is worse than that of nonazotemic patients with cirrhosis and ascites.[17]

PATHOGENESIS

Peripheral arterial vasodilation

Cirrhotic portal hypertension is associated with decreased systemic vascular resistance and vasodilation in the splanchnic arterial circulation due to the local release of nitric oxide and other vasodilatory substances including calcitonin gene-related peptide, substance P, carbon monoxide, and endogenous canabinoids.[18–23] Early in the course of the disease, this decrease in systemic vascular resistance is compensated by the development of a hyperdynamic circulation (increased heart rate and cardiac output).[24–26] However, as the disease progresses and arterial vasodilation increases, the hyperdynamic circulation is insufficient to correct the effective arterial hypovolemia.[27] Arterial hypotension develops, leading to activation of high-pressure baroreceptors, reflex stimulation of the renin-angiotensin axis and sympathetic nervous system, increase in arterial pressure to normal or near normal levels, sodium and water retention and, eventually, ascites formation. The stimulation of antidiuretic hormone, which is less sensitive to arterial hypovolemia than the renin-angiotensin response or sympathetic nervous system, occurs later during the course of the disease. Patients then develop water retention and dilutional hyponatremia. At this stage of the disease the renin-angiotensin and sympathetic nervous systems are markedly stimulated and arterial pressure is critically dependent upon the vascular effects of sympathetic nervous activity, angiotensin II, and antidiuretic hormone. Since the splanchnic arterial circulation is resistant to the effect of these endogenous vasoconstrictors,[28,29] the maintenance of arterial pressure is due to vasoconstriction in extrasplanchnic vascular beds such as the kidneys, muscle, skin, and brain.[30–33] HRS develops at the latest phase of the disease when there is an extreme deterioration in effective arterial blood volume and severe arterial hypotension. The homeostatic stimulation of the renin-angiotensin system, the sympathetic nervous system, and antidiuretic hormone is very intense, leading to renal vasoconstriction, marked decrease in renal perfusion and GFR, azotemia, and increased serum creatinine concentration (Fig. 42.2).

Cardiac dysfunction

Most hemodynamics studies in cirrhotics have been performed in patients without HRS and their findings have been extended to the entire population of patients with decompensated cirrhosis. Based on these data, it has been assumed that HRS develops in the setting of the hyperdynamic circulation typically seen in patients with portal hypertension. However, in the few hemodynamic studies assessing cardiovascular hemodynamics in patients with HRS or refractory ascites, cardiac output was significantly reduced comparing to patients without HRS.[34,35] In some cases, cardiac output was even lower than in normal subjects, suggesting that circulatory dysfunction associated with HRS is due to both arterial vasodilation and impaired cardiac function. A recent study in patients with spontaneous bacterial peritonitis confirms this observation (Table 42.2).[36] Since effective arterial blood volume, as estimated by the plasma levels of renin and noradrenaline (norepinephrine), and cardiac output improves following plasma volume expansion in patients with HRS, the most likely explanation of the reduced cardiac function is a central hypovolemia secondary to a decreased venous return.

Regional hemodynamics

Patients with HRS have reduced brachial and femoral blood flow, indicating an increased resistance in the cutaneous and muscular arterial vascular beds.[32] The resistive index in the cerebral artery is also increased in these patients, indicating cerebral vasoconstriction.[33] These three measurements correlate directly with the

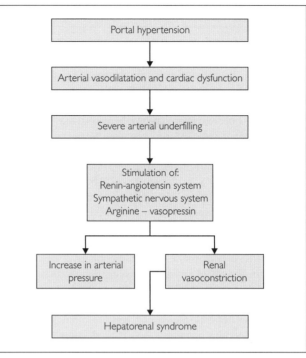

Fig. 42.2 • Pathogenesis of hepatorenal syndrome.

plasma levels of renin in patients with decompensated cirrhosis. In patients with spontaneous bacterial peritonitis, the development of circulatory dysfunction and HRS is associated with a reduction in hepatic blood flow (Ruiz del Arbol, unpublished observations) and an increase in portal pressure, and this also correlates directly with the plasma levels renin and noradrenaline (norepinephrine) (see Table 42.2).[36] Therefore, in addition to renal vasoconstriction, circulatory dysfunction in HRS is related to vasoconstriction in other organs (liver, brain, muscle, and skin) and to an increased resistance to portal venous flow.

Table 42.2 Renal function, neurohormonal measurements and cardiovascular hemodynamics at diagnosis of infection and following resolution of infection in patients with SBP who did and did not develop renal failure during treatment[36]

	Group with renal failure		Group without renal failure	
	Diagnosis of infection	Resolution of infection	Diagnosis of infection	Resolution of infection
Serum creatinine (mg/dL)	1.3 ± 0.6	2.5 ± 0.4‡	1.0 ± 0.3	0.9 ± 0.2
Serum sodium (mmol/L	132 ± 3	127 ± 2‡	135 ± 4	136 ± 4
Plasma renin activity (ng/mL/h)	18 ± 11*	28 ± 12‡	4 ± 4	3 ± 4
Plasma aldosterone (ng/dL)	149 ± 107*	252 ± 157‡	28 ± 11	20 ± 20
Plasma norepinephrine (pg/mL)	797 ± 227*	1290 ± 415‡	316 ± 173	317 ± 195
Mean arterial pressure (mmHg)	83 ± 7	73 ± 8†	83 ± 10	83 ± 8
Cardiac output (L/min)	5.7 ± 0.9**	4.6 ± 0.7‡	7.4 ± 1.9	6.8 ± 2
Systemic vascular resistance (dyn. sec/cm⁵)	1137 ± 220**	1268 ± 320	893 ± 196	968 ± 226

* $p < 0.001$ vs values at diagnosis of infection of group without renal failure
** $p < 0.025$ vs values at diagnosis of infection of group without renal failure
‡ $p < 0.01$ vs values following resolution of infection of group without renal failure
† $p < 0.025$ vs values following resolution of infection of group without renal failure

Renal dysfunction

HRS develops during advanced liver disease, when patients already have severe circulatory dysfunction, arterial hypotension, marked activation of the renin-angiotensin-aldosterone system, sympathetic nervous system and antidiuretic hormone response, significant renal sodium and water retention/ascites, and impairment in free water excretion. The mechanism(s) that lead to renal vasoconstriction and HRS are complex. Since renal vascular resistance in decompensated cirrhosis correlates closely with the activity of the renin-angiotensin and sympathetic nervous systems,[30,31,37–40] HRS is thought to be related to the extreme activation of these systems. The urinary excretion of prostaglandin E2, 6-keto prostaglandin F1a (a prostacyclin metabolite), and kallikrein is decreased in patients with HRS, which is compatible with reduced renal production of these substances.[41,42] Renal failure in HRS may therefore be the consequence of an imbalance between the activity of systemic vasoconstrictor systems and the renal production of vasodilators. Finally, renal hypoperfusion may be amplified by the stimulation of intrarenal vasoconstrictors. For example, renal ischemia increases generation of angiotensin II by the juxtaglomerular apparatus, boosts production of adenosine which acts as a renal vasoconstrictor, and also potentiates the vascular effect of angiotensin II, and augments the synthesis of endothelin. Other intrarenal vasoconstrictors, such as leukotrienes and F2-isoprostanes, have also been implicated in HRS.[43]

Although clinicians often believe that the clinical differences in type-1 and type-2 HRS reflect degrees of severity of a common pathogenetic chain of events, this is in fact not the case. Renal failure in type-1 HRS is severe and progressive, whereas in type-2 it is moderate and relatively stable over time. Circulatory dysfunction with a significant decrease in cardiac output is characteristic of type-1 HRS and usually progressive, whereas circulatory function is usually well maintained in type-2 HRS.[36] Type-1 HRS is frequently associated to a precipitant event, while type-2 HRS is not. Finally, the main clinical consequence of type-1 HRS is severe hepatorenal failure and death, whereas in type-2 HRS it is refractory ascites. It is possible that type-2 but not type-1 HRS represents the extreme expression of the circulatory dysfunction that occurs in cirrhosis secondarily to the progression of portal hypertension.

Patients with type-1 HRS present features of multiorgan failure including impairment in cardiac function, aggravation of liver failure and portal hypertension, and encephalopathy. As in some other causes of acute renal failure, there are also data suggesting that renal failure in type-1 HRS is related to intrarenal mechanisms such as impaired synthesis of intrarenal vasodilators, increased production of intrarenal vasoconstrictors, or both.[44] The progressive nature of renal failure in type-1 HRS could therefore be related not only with the progressive nature of the circulatory dysfunction but also with the development of a vicious intrarenal cycle of hypoperfusion leading to a vasoactive imbalance leading in turn to more vasoconstriction.[44] The demonstration of a clear temporal dissociation between the improvement in circulatory function and the increase in renal perfusion and GFR in patients with type-1 HRS treated with albumin infusion and vasoconstrictors is in keeping with this concept.[45] This treatment normalizes plasma renin activity and noradrenaline (norepinephrine) concentration within 3 days. In contrast, a significant increase in renal perfusion and GFR do not occur until 1 week later. The longer time required to deactivate the intrarenal mechanisms may account for this delay.

Type-2 HRS is associated with an extremely low urinary sodium excretion. The renal ability to excrete free water is also markedly reduced, and most patients present significant hyponatremia. Sodium retention in patients with HRS is due to decreased filtered sodium and increased sodium reabsorption in the proximal tubule. The amount of sodium reaching the loop of Henle and distal nephron, the site of action of furosemide and spironolactone, respectively, is very low. The delivery of furosemide and spironolactone to the renal tubules is also reduced due to the renal hypoperfusion. It is, therefore, not surprising that patients with type-2 HRS respond poorly to diuretics.[46] The mechanism of the impaired renal water metabolism is multifactorial.[47] The generation of free water, which is the result of the reabsorption of sodium chloride without a concomitant reabsorption of water in the loop of Henle, is reduced in HRS due to the low distal delivery of filtrate. On the other hand, the plasma levels of antidiuretic hormone are markedly elevated and the renal synthesis of prostaglandin E2, the physiologic antagonist of this hormone, may be reduced.[48]

TREATMENT OF TYPE-1 HEPATORENAL SYNDROME (SEE ALGORITHM 1)

Volume expansion and vasoconstrictors

The rationale for treatment is based on the concept of interrupting specific steps in the current concept of the pathogenesis of type-1 HRS (Fig. 42.3). Volume expansion is meant to improve venous return and cardiac output. Vasoconstrictors are given to reverse the splanchnic arterial vasodilation. Vasopressin analogues (ornipressin and terlipressin) were the initial drugs used for the treatment of type-1 HRS due to their preferential effect on the splanchnic circulation. Terlipressin, which is marketed in many countries for control of acute variceal bleeding, has been extensively studied. Ornipressin is also effective but, like vasopressin, must be given by constant intravenous infusion and frequently produces ischemic complications. Terlipressin (0.5–2 mg intravenously every 4–6 hours) reduces serum creatinine to below 1.5 mg/dL in 50–75% of patients treated (Fig. 42.4).[49–53] This is associated with marked suppression of renin and noradrenaline (norepinephrine) (Fig. 42.5) and a significant increase in mean arterial pressure. There is a lag between suppression of endogenous neurohormonal systems, which occurs within the first 3 days of treatment, and the decrease in serum creatinine that begins 2–4 days later. Despite normalization of serum creatinine, renal function does not return to a normal level and there is persistence of low GFR, which ranges 30–50 ml/min in most cases (normal: 120 ml/min). In most studies, treatment with terlipressin has been maintained until serum creatinine decreased to below 1.5 mg/dL or for a maximun of 15 days. It is not known whether the continued administration of terlipressin after the end point of 1.5 mg/dL of serum creatinine has been reached would result in a greater increase in glomerular filtration rate. In patients who respond to terlipressin, there is an improvement in urine volume within the first 24 hours. In some, but not all patients, treatment also causes an increase in sodium excretion and improvement of the serum sodium concentration.[49–53] This latter effect is remarkable given that terlipressin is a V2 vasopressin agonist. It suggests that impairment in free water clearance in type-1 HRS is more related to abnormalities in intrarenal sodium handling than to nonosmotic hypersecretion of antidiuretic hormone. It should

Fig. 42.3 • Algorithm treatment of HRS.

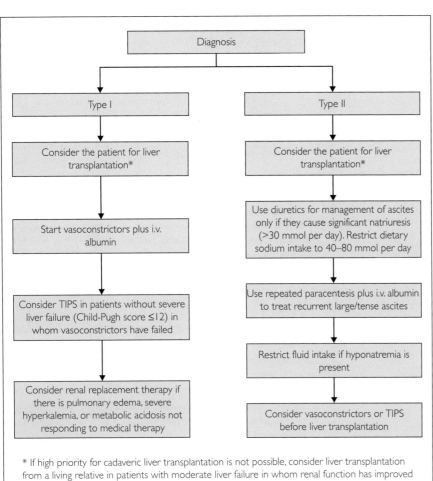

Diagnosis

Type I

Consider the patient for liver transplantation*

Start vasoconstrictors plus i.v. albumin

Consider TIPS in patients without severe liver failure (Child-Pugh score ≤12) in whom vasoconstrictors have failed

Consider renal replacement therapy if there is pulmonary edema, severe hyperkalemia, or metabolic acidosis not responding to medical therapy

Type II

Consider the patient for liver transplantation*

Use diuretics for management of ascites only if they cause significant natriuresis (>30 mmol per day). Restrict dietary sodium intake to 40–80 mmol per day

Use repeated paracentesis plus i.v. albumin to treat recurrent large/tense ascites

Restrict fluid intake if hyponatremia is present

Consider vasoconstrictors or TIPS before liver transplantation

* If high priority for cadaveric liver transplantation is not possible, consider liver transplantation from a living relative in patients with moderate liver failure in whom renal function has improved after therapy

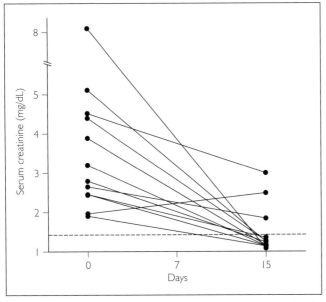

Fig. 42.4 • Individual values of serum creatinine in patients treated with terlipressin and i.v. albumin. (Reprinted from Uriz, Journal Hepatology 2000. © 2000, with permission from The European Association for the Study of the Liver.)

be noted that albumin was administered intravenously in all studies with terlipressin. This is critical to the response to terlipressin. Indeed, there are now data indicating that the therapeutic response to terlipressin is very poor without concomitant albumin.[51,53] The recommended schedule for albumin administration is 1 g/kg of body weight during the first day followed by 20–40 g/day thereafter.[53] The administration of albumin is interrupted if central venous pressure increases above 18 cm of water. Predictors of poor response to terlipressin include old age, advanced liver failure (Child-Pugh score greater than 13), or failure to administer albumin.[51,53] Recurrence of type-1 HRS after discontinuation of treatment is uncommon (approximately 15% of patients), but re-treatment of HRS is usually effective. The incidence of an ischemic side effect requiring discontinuation of terlipressin is low (5–10%), although it has to be considered that most studies excluded high-risk patients with ischemic heart or artery diseases.[49–53] The probability of survival in patients with type-1 HRS responding to terlipressin has been estimated as 50% at 3 months and 30% at 1 year (Fig. 42.6).[51] This is comparable to the reported survival in patients with type-2 HRS and considerably longer than survival in untreated patients with type-1 HRS. Indeed, a significant proportion of patients with type-1 HRS treated with terlipresin and albumin survive to reach liver transplantation.

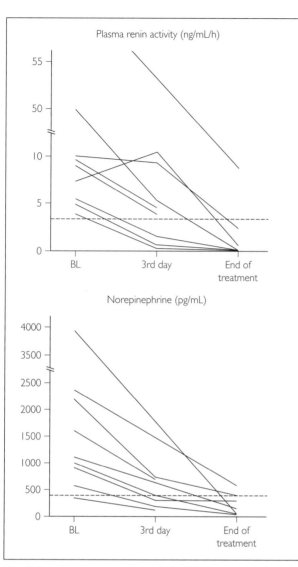

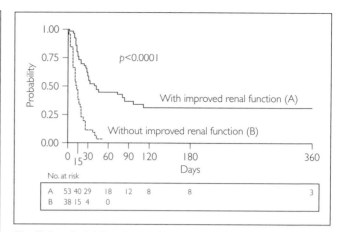

Fig. 42.6 • Probability of survival in patients with type-1 HRS who had improvement in renal function during terlipressin therapy and in those who did not. (Reprinted from Moreau, Gastroenterology 2002 © 2002, with permission from The American Gastroenterological Association.)

Fig. 42.5 • Plasma renin activity and plasma concentration of noradrenaline (norepinephrine) in patients treated with terlipressin and i.v. albumin in baseline conditions (BL), at day 3 and the end of treatment (reversal of HRS or for a maximum of 15 days). (Reprinted from Uriz, Journal Hepatology 2000. © 2000, with permission from The European Association for the Study of the Liver.)

Catecholamines are also effective for the treatment of HRS. Midrodrine (an oral α-adrenergic agonist) was given by Angeli et al.[54] in association with intravenous albumin and subcutaneous octreotide (to suppress glucagon) to five patients with type-1 HRS. The dose of midrodrine (7.5–12.5 mg every 8 hours) was adjusted to increase mean arterial pressure by 15 mmHg or more. Patients received treatment for at least 20 days in hospital and continued treatment at home. There was a marked improvement in renal perfusion and glomerular filtration rate. Renin, noradrenaline (norepinephrine), and antidiuretic hormone levels were suppressed to normal or near normal levels in all cases. A recent study assessing the effects of octreotide on systemic hemodynamics, neurohormonal systems, and renal function in patients with HRS showed no significant effect. Therefore, the therapeutic efficacy in the study of Angeli et al. cannot be attributed to octreotide and is likely related exclusively to the vasoconstrictor effect of midrodrine and the expansion of the central blood volume by albumin. Duvoux and

colleagues[55] treated 12 patients with type-1 HRS with intravenous albumin and noradrenaline (norepinephrine) (0.5–3.0 mg/h) for a minimum of 5 days. Reversal of HRS was observed in 10 patients in association with an increase in mean arterial pressure and a marked reduction in renin and aldosterone. There was an episode of reversible myocardial hypokinesia. Three patients were transplanted and four other cases had prolonged survival (over 6 months).

Transjugular intrahepatic portocaval shunt

Since portal hypertension is the initial event of circulatory dysfunction in cirrhosis, the decrease of portal pressure by portacaval anastomosis is a rational approach for the treatment of HRS. There are several case reports showing reversal of HRS following surgical portacaval shunt.[56,57] However, the applicability of major surgical procedures in patients with HRS is small. The development of the transjugular intrahepatic portocaval shunt (TIPS) has reintroduced the idea of treating HRS by reducing portal pressure.

Four studies assessing TIPS in the management of type-1 HRS have been reported[58–61] and recently reviewed by Brensing et al.[62] In total, 30 patients were treated. In two series no liver transplantation was performed, whereas in the other two series three out of nine patients were transplanted 7, 13 and 35 days after TIPS. TIPS insertion was technically successful in all patients. Only one patient died as a consequence of the procedure. GFR improved markedly 1–4 weeks after TIPS and stabilized thereafter. In one study specifically investigating the neurohormonal response to TIPS, improvement in GFR and serum creatinine was related to a marked suppression of the plasma levels of renin and antidiuretic hormone.[59] Plasma noradrenaline (norepinephrine) was not suppressed as much as renin, a feature also observed in refractory ascites treated by TIPS. Follow-up of hepatic function was reported in 21 patients. De novo hepatic encephalopathy or deterioration of pre-existing hepatic encephalopathy occurred in nine patients, but in five it could be controlled with lactulose Survival rates based on the 27 patients without early liver transplantation were 81%, 59%, and 44% at 1 month, 3 months, and 6 months, respectively. These studies strongly suggest that TIPS is useful in the management of type-1 HRS. Studies comparing TIPS with pharmacological treatment in type-1 HRS are needed.

It remains intriguing that low GFR persists despite marked suppression of renin and noradrenaline (norepinephrine), indicating a significant improvement in circulatory function, in patients with type-1 HRS who receive vasoconstrictors and albumin. The reason for the failure to normalize GFR is not known. Perhaps there is a component of renal failure unresponsive to changes in circulatory function or, alternatively, effective arterial blood volume is not improved to a point that allows return of function. A recent study of Wong et al.[63] is consistent with this hypothesis. The addition of TIPS in patients responding to pharmacological treatment (midodrine, octreotide, and albumin) was associated to normalization of GFR in most cases. Whether the effect of TIPS in the normalization of GFR was due to the correction of the arterial vasodilation, to an increase in cardiac preload and ventricular function, or to both, remains to be investigated.

Liver transplantation

Liver transplantation is the treatment of choice of HRS.[64–68] Immediately after transplantation, GFR may deteriorate even further and many patients require temporary hemodialysis (35% of patients with HRS as compared with 5% of patients without HRS).[64] Because cyclosporine or tacrolimus may contribute to this early impairment in renal function, it has been recommended that these drugs should not be used until recovery of renal function is noted, usually 48–72 hours after transplantation. GFR generally starts to improve thereafter and reaches an average of 30–40 mL/min by 1–2 months postoperatively. This moderate renal failure persists during follow-up, is more marked than that observed in transplantation patients without HRS, and is probably due to a greater nephrotoxicity of cyclosporine or tacrolimus in patients with renal impairment prior to transplantation.[64] The hemodynamic and neurohormonal abnormalities associated with HRS disappear within the first month after the operation and the patients regain a normal ability to excrete sodium and free water.[69]

Patients with HRS who undergo transplantation have more complications, spend more days in the intensive care unit, and have a higher in-hospital mortality rate than transplantation patients without HRS.[64–68,70] The long-term survival of patients with HRS who undergo liver transplantation is good, however, with a 3-year probability of survival of 60%. This survival rate is only slightly reduced compared with that of transplantation in patients without HRS (which ranges between 70% and 80%).[64–70]

The main problem of liver transplantation in type-1 HRS is logistics. Patients with type-1 HRS have extremely short survival and most patients die before transplantation. The recent introduction of the MELD score, which includes serum creatinine as a component, as the basis for organ priority has improved the outlook for patients with HRS since they achieve higher MELD scores. Treatment of HRS with vasoconstrictors and albumin increases survival in a significant proportion of patients and, therefore, may improve access to cadaveric transplantation or open the option of elective living donor transplantation. Treatment of HRS prior liver transplantation is desirable since reversal of HRS decreases early morbidity and mortality after transplantation and prolongs the long-term survival.[71]

Other therapeutic options

Hemodialysis is used in the management of type-1 HRS in many centers, particularly in patients who are candidates for liver transplantation, with the aim of preventing the complications associated with renal failure and maintaining patients alive until transplantation. However, the beneficial effects of this procedure in type-1 HRS have not been convincingly demonstrated.[72] Complications during hemodialysis in these patients are common and include arterial hypotension, bleeding, and infections. On the other hand, clinical or biochemical features indicating the need for renal replacement therapy, such as heart or respiratory failure, severe acidosis, or severe hyperkalemia, are uncommon in type-1 HRS.

Drugs other than vasoconstrictors have been used for many years in the management of HRS despite their unproved efficacy. This holds true for drugs with renal vasodilator effect, such as dopamine or prostaglandins.[73] Several isolated reports suggested a beneficial effect of octreotide alone, a drug that inhibits the production of several vasodilator peptides of splanchnic origin, especially glucagon. However, a recent randomized, controlled study with a 50 µg/h infusion showed no benefit.[74] Finally, N-acetyl-cysteine showed efficacy in a short series of patients at a dose of 300 mg/12 h, but these results require confirmation in larges series.[75]

Molecular adsorbent recirculating system

Extracorporeal albumin dialysis, a system that uses an albumin-containing dialysate that is recirculated and perfused through charcoal and anion-exchanger columns, has been reported to improve renal function and survival in a small series of patients with HRS. Mitzner[76] performed a prospective controlled trial to comparing molecular adsorbent recirculating system (MARS) to standard supportive therapy (intravenous fluids, dopamine and, if necessary, vasoconstrictors) in patients with type-1 HRS and severe hepatic failure (bilirubin level ≥ 15 mg/dL). Thirteen patients were included, all Child's class C (mean CTP score, 12.4±1), United Network for Organ Sharing status 2A, and mean total bilirubin values of 25.7±14 mg/dL. A significant decrease in bilirubin and creatinine levels ($p<0.01$) and increase in serum sodium level and prothrombin activity ($p<0.01$) were observed in the MARS group. Mortality rates were 100% in the control group and 62.5% in the MARS group at day 7, and 100% and 75%, respectively, at day 30 ($p<0.01$). Further studies are required on this therapy.

MANAGEMENT OF PATIENTS WITH TYPE 2 HEPATORENAL SYNDROME

Survival of patients with type-2 HRS is better than with type-1 HRS and many cases are able to survive until liver transplantation. The main clinical problem in these patients is refractory ascites. Total therapeutic paracentesis along with albumin infusion is the treatment of choice. It is rapid, effective, and safe, though patients reaccumulate ascites rapidly. However, paracentesis can be done as an outpatient or single-day hospitalization as frequently as required. TIPS is another option and there are four randomized, controlled trials comparing this treatment with refractory ascites.[77–80] TIPS markedly reduces the number of days with ascites compared to patients treated by paracentesis, but it increases the frequency of hepatic encephalopathy and does not improve survival. TIPS dysfunction and the high cost of this treatment were also important issues. The LeVeen shunt for refractory ascites has been abandoned in most centers. Although effective, it is also associated to serious complications including shunt obstruction, infection, superior vena cava thrombosis, and plastic peritonitis.

There is limited information on the use of vasoconstrictors in the treatment of patients with type-2 HRS, but some reports suggest that vasoconstrictors and albumin improve renal function in these patients.[53,81] However, and in contrast to type-1 HRS, renal failure recurs in most patients after stopping therapy.

PREVENTION OF HEPATORENAL SYNDROME

Two large randomized, controlled studies have shown that HRS can be prevented in certain clinical settings. In the first study,[82] administration of albumin (1.5 g/kg at presentation and 1 g/kg 48 hours later) to patients with cirrhosis and spontaneous bacterial peritonitis markedly reduced the incidence circulatory dysfunction and type-1 HRS (10% versus 33% in the control group). Hospital mortality rate (10% versus 29%) and the 3-month mortality rate (22% versus 41%) were also lower in patients receiving albumin (Fig. 42.7). In a second study,[83] the administration of the tumor necrosis factor inhibitor pentoxyfilline (400 mg 3 times a day) to patients with severe acute alcoholic hepatitis reduced the occurrence of HRS (8% versus 35% in the placebo group) and the hospital mortality (24% versus 46%). Because bacterial infections and acute alcoholic hepatitis are important precipitating factors of type-1 HRS, these prophylactic measures may decrease the incidence of this complication.

SUMMARY

HRS is a common and ominous complication of advanced cirrhosis. It is characterized by renal failure and major abnormalities in the systemic circulatory function. Renal failure is caused by intense renal vasoconstriction. The syndrome is probably the final consequence of an extreme underfilling of the arterial circulation secondary to vasodilatation in the splanchnic vascular bed and a decrease in cardiac output due to central hypovolemia. The diagnosis of HRS is based on the exclusion of other causes of renal failure. The survival of patients with HRS is very poor, particularly when there is rapidly progressive renal failure (type-1 HRS). Liver transplantation is the best therapeutic option but it is sometimes difficult to do, given the rapid course. Two effective therapeutic options for HRS have recently been reported: vasoconstrictor agents (vasopressin analogues, α-adrenergic agonists) in conjunction with intravenous albumin, and TIPS. They improve circulatory function, normalize serum creatinine, and increase survival. Sequential treatment with vasoconstrictors plus albumin followed by TIPS is attractive since this may result in better recovery of GFR. Finally, plasma volume expansion with albumin in patients with spontaneous bacterial peritonitis and administration of pentoxiphilline in patients with severe alcoholic hepatitis appear to significantly reduce the chance of developing type-1 HRS.

REFERENCES

1. Ginès P, Rodés J. Clinical disorders of renal function in cirrhosis with ascites. In: Arroyo V, Ginès P, Rodés J, Schrier RW, eds. Ascites and renal dysfunction in liver disease: pathogenesis, diagnosis, and treatment. Malden: Blackwell Science; 1999:36–62.

2. Hecker R, Sherlock S. Electrolyte and circulatory changes in terminal liver failure. Lancet 1956; 271:1121–1125.

3. Ginès A, Escorsell A, Ginès P, et al. Incidence, predictive factors, and prognosis of the hepatorenal syndrome in cirrhosis with ascites. Gastroenterology 1993; 105:229–236.

4. Koppel MH, Coburn JW, Mims MM, et al. Transplantation of cadaveric kidneys from patients with hepatorenal syndrome. Evidence for the functional nature of renal failure in advanced liver disease. N Engl J Med 1969; 280:1367–1371.

5. Iwatsuki S, Popovtzer MM, Corman JL et al. Recovery from 'hepatorenal syndrome' after orthotopic liver transplantation. N Engl J Med 1973; 289:1155–1159.

6. Ginès P, Guevara M, Arroyo V, et al. Hepatorenal syndrome. Lancet 2003; 362:1819–1827.

7. Orr TG, Helwing FC. Liver trauma and the hepatorenal syndrome. Ann Surg 1939; 110:683–692.

8. Hecker R, Sherlock S. Electrolyte and circulatory changes in terminal liver failure. Lancet 1956; 2:1221–1225.

9. Papadakis MA, Arieff AI. Unpredictability of clinical evaluation of renal function in cirrhosis: a prospective study. Am J Med 1987; 82:845–852.

10. Caregaro L, Menon F, Angeli P, et al. Limitations of serum creatinine level and creatinine clearance as filtration markers in cirrhosis. Arch Intern Med 1994; 154:201–205.

11. Cabrera J, Arroyo V, Ballesta AM, et al. Aminoglycoside nephrotoxicity in cirrhosis. Value of urinary B2-microglobulin to discriminate functional renal failure form acute tubular damage. Gastroenterology 1982; 82:97–105.

12. Dudley FJ, Kanel GC, Wood LJ, et al. Hepatorenal syndrome without avid sodium retention. Hepatology 1986; 6:248–251.

13. Arroyo V, Ginès P, Gerbes A, et al. Definition and diagnostic criteria of refractory ascites and hepatorenal syndrome in cirrhosis. Hepatology 1996; 23:164–176.

14. Toledo C, Salmerón JM, Rimola A, et al. Spontaneous bacterial peritonitis in cirrhosis: predictive factors of infection resolution and survival in patients treated with cefotaxime. Hepatology 1993; 17:251–257.

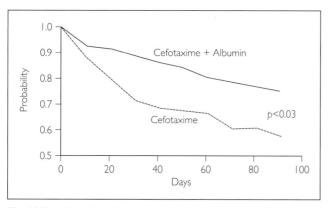

Fig. 42.7 • Probability of patient survival 3 months after spontaneous bacterial peritonitis episode. (Sort, N Engl J Med 1999.)

15. Follo A, Llovet JM, Navasa M, et al. Renal impairment following spontaneous bacterial peritonitis in cirrhosis. Incidence, clinical course, predictive factors and prognosis. Hepatology 1994; 20:1495–1501.

This is the first study showing that bacterial infections in decompensated cirrhosis are a precipitating factor of type-1 hepatorenal syndrome.

16. Navasa M, Follo A, Filella X, et al Tumor necrosis factor and interleukin-6 in spontaneous bacterial peritonitis in cirrhosis: relationship with the development of renal impairment and mortality. Hepatology 1998; 27:1227–1232.

17. Rodés J, Arroyo V, Bosch J. Clinical types and drug therapy of renal impairment in cirrhosis. Postgrad Med J 1975; 51:492–497.

18. Goyal RK, Irano I. The enteric nervous system. N Engl J Med 1996; 334:1106–1115.

19. Gupta S, Morgan TR, Gordan GS. Calcitonin-gene related peptide in hepatorenal syndrome. J Clin Gastroenterol 1992; 14:122–126.

20. Bendtsen F, Schifter S, Henriksen JH. Increased circulation of calcitonin-gene related peptide (CGRP) in cirrhosis. J Hepatol 1991; 12:118–123.

21. McNiol PL, Lin G, Shulkes A, et al. Vasoactive intestinal peptide and calcitonin-gene related peptide and hemodynamics during human liver transplantation. Transplant Proc 1993; 25:1830–1831.

22. Moller S, Bendtsen F, Schifter S, et al. Relation of calcitonin gene-related peptide to systemic vasodilation and central hypovolaemia in cirrhosis. Scand J Gastroenterol 1996; 31:928–933.

23. Hori N, Okaneve T, Sawa Y, et al. Role of calcitonine gene-related peptide in the vascular system on the development of the hyperdynamic circulation in conscious cirrhotic rats. Hepatology 1997; 26:111–119.

24. Benoit JN, Granger DN. Splanchnic hemodynamics in chronic portal hypertension. Semin Liver Dis 1986; 6:287–298.

25. Vorobioff J, Bredfeldt JE, Groszmann RJ. Increased blood flow through the portal system in cirrhotic rats. Gastroenterology 1984; 87:1120–1126.

26. Vorobioff J, Bredfeldt JE, Groszmann RJ. Hyperdynamic circulation in portal hypertensive rat model: a primary factor for maintenance of chronic portal hypertension. Am J Physiol 1983; 244:G52–G57.

27. Schrier RW, Arroyo V, Bernardi M, et al. Peripheral arterial vasodilation hypothesis: a proposal for the initiation of renal sodium and water retention in cirrhosis. Hepatology 1988; 8:1151–1157.

The article reports the conclusion of a consensus meeting held in Barcelona in 1987 proposing the most accepted theory on the pathogenesis of circulatory and renal dysfunction in cirrhosis.

28. Lee FY, Albillos A, Colombato LA, et al. The role of nitric oxide in the vascular hyporesponsiveness to methoxamine in portal hypertensive rats. Hepatology 1992;1 6:1043–1048.

29. Sieber C, López-Talavera JC, Groszmann RJ. Role of nitric oxide in the in vitro splanchnic vascular hyporeactivity in ascitic cirrhotic rats. Gastroenterology 1993; 104:1750–1754.

30. Maroto A, Gines A, Salo J, et al. Diagnosis of functional renal failure of cirrhosis by Doppler sonography. Prognostic value of resistive index. Hepatology 1994; 20:839–844.

31. Fernández-Seara J, Prieto J, Quiroga J, et al. Systemic and regional hemodynamics in patients with liver cirrhosis and ascites with and without functional renal failure. Gastroenterology 1989; 97:1304–1312.

32. Maroto A, Gines P, Arroyo V, et al. Brachial and femoral artery blood flow in cirrhosis: relationship to kidney dysfunction. Hepatology 1993; 17:788–793.

This article first reports the development of arterial vasoconstriction in the cutaneous and muscular vascular beds in patients with hepatorenal syndrome.

33. Guevara M, Bru C, Ginés P, et al. Increased cerebral vascular resistance in cirrhotic patients with ascites. Hepatology 1998; 28:39–44.

This article first describes the development of cerebral vasconstriction in patients with advanced cirrhosis and ascites.

34. Tristani FE, Cohn JH. Systemic and renal hemodynamics in oliguric hepatic failure: Effect of volume expansion. J Clin Invest 1967; 46:1894–1906.

35. Lebrec D, Kotelansku B, Cohn JH. Splanchnic hemodynamic factors in cirrhosis with refractory ascites. J Lab Clin Med 1979; 93:301–309.

36. Ruiz-del-Arbol L, Urman J, Fernandez J, et al. Systemic, renal, and hepatic hemodynamic derangement in cirrhotic patients with spontaneous bacterial peritonitis. Hepatology 2003; 38(1)210–218.

This study first reports that type-1 HRS is not only due to arterial vasodilation but also to a decreased cardiac output.

37. Schroeder ET, Eich RH, Smulyan H, et al. Plasma renin levels in hepatic cirrhosis. Relationship to functional renal failure. Am J Med 1970; 49:186–191.

38. DiBona GF. Renal nerve activity in hepatorenal syndrome. Kidney Int 1984; 25:841–853.

39. Henriksen JH, Ring-Larsen H. Hepatorenal disorders: role of the sympathetic nervous system. Sem in Liver Dis 1994; 116:446–455.

40. Dudley FJ, Esler MD. The sympathetic nervous system in cirrhosis. In: Arroyo V, ed. Ascites and renal dysfunction in liver disease. Malden (MA): Blackwell Science; 1999;198–219.

41. Arroyo V, Planas R, Gaya J, et al. Sympathetic nervous activity, renin-angiotensin system and renal excretion of prostaglandin E2 in cirrhosis. Relationship to functional renal failure and sodium and water excretion. Eur J Clin Invest 1983; 13:271–278.

42. Rimola A, Ginés P, Arroyo V, et al. Urinary excretion of 6-keto-prostaglandin F1-alpha, thromboxane B2 and prostaglandin E2 in cirrhosis with ascites. Relationship to functional renal failure (hepatorenal syndrome). J Hepatol 1986; 3:111–117.

43. Moore KP. Arachidonic acid metabolites and the kidney in cirrhosis. In: Arroyo V, ed. Ascites and renal dysfunction in liver disease. Malden (MA): Blackwell Science; 1999:249–272.

44. Arroyo V, Jimenez W. Complications of cirrhosis. Renal and circulatory dysfunction: lights and shadows in an important clinical problem. J Hepatol 2000; 32(1):157–170.

45. Guevara M, Gines P, Fernandez-Esparrach G, et al. Reversibility of hepatorenal syndrome by prolonged administration of ornipressin and plasma volume expansion. Hepatology 1998; 27:35–41.

This is the first study proving that hepatorenal syndrome is reversible if circulatory dysfunction is corrected by plasma volume expansion and vasoconstrictors.

46. Arroyo V, Epstein M, Gallus G, et al. Refractory ascites in cirrhosis. Mechanism and management. Gastroenterol Int 1982; 2:195–207.

47. Ginés P, Berl T, Bernardi M, et al. Hyponatremia in cirrhosis: from pathogenesis to treatment. Hepatology 1998; 28:851–864.

48. Pérez-Ayuso RM, Arroyo V, Camps J, et al. Evidence that renal prostaglandins are involved in renal water metabolism in cirrhosis. Kidney Int 1984; 26:72–80.

49. Uriz J, Ginès P, Cardenas A, et al. Terlipressin plus albumin in an effective and safe therapy of hepatorenal syndrome. J Hepatol 2000; 33:43–48.

50. Mulkay JP, Louis H, Donckter V, et al. Long-term terlipressin administration improves renal function in cirrhotic patients with type 1 hepatorenal syndrome: a pilot study. Acta Gastroenterol Belg 2001; 64:15–19.

51. Moreau R, Durand F, Poynard T, et al. Terlipressin in patients with cirrhosis and type y HRS: a retrospective multicenter study. Gastroenterology 2002; 122:923–930.

52. Colle I, Durand F, Pessione F et al. Clinical course, predictive factors and prognosis in patients with cirrhosis and type 1 hepatorenal syndrome treated with Terlipressin: A retrospective analysis. J Gastroenterol Hepatol, 2002; 17: 882–888.

53. Ortega R, Ginès P, Uriz J, et al. Terlipressin therapy with and without albumin for patients with hepatorenal syndrome: results of a prospective, non-randomized study. Hepatology 2002; 36:941–948.

54. Angeli P, Volpin R, Gerunda G, et al. Reversal of type 1 HRS with the administration of midodrine and octreotide. Hepatology 1999; 29:1690–1697.

55. Duvoux C, Zanditenas D, Hezode C, et al. Effects of noradrenaline and albumin in patients with type 1 hepatorenal syndrome: a pilot study. Hepatology 2002; 36:374–380.

56. Schroeder ET, Numann PJ, Chamberlain BE. Functional renal failure in cirrhosis. Recovery after portacaval shunt. Ann Intern Med 1970; 72:293–298.

57. Ariyan S, Sweeney T, Kerstein MD. The hepatorenal syndrome: recovery after portacaval shunt. Ann Surg 1975; 181:847–849

58. Brensing KA, Textro J, Perz J, et al. Long-term outcome after transjugular intrahepatic portosystemic stent-shunt in non-transplant patients with hepatorenal syndrome: a phase II study. Gut 2000; 47:288–295.

This is the first study showing that TIPS is effective for some as treatment of type-I HRS.

59. Guevara M, Ginès P, Bandi JC, et al. Transjugular intrahepatic portosystemic shunt in hepatorenal syndrome: effects on renal function and vasoactive systems. Hepatology 1998; 28:416–422.

60. Alam I, Bass NM, LaBerge JM, et al. Treatment of hepatorenal syndrome with the transjugular intrahepatic shunt (TIPS) (abstract). Gastroenterology 1995; 108:A1024.

61. Ochs A, Rössle M, Haag K, et al. TIPS for hepatorenal syndrome. Hepatology 1994; 20:114A.

62. Brensing KA, Perz J, Sauerbruch T. TIPS in hepatorenal syndrome. In: Arroyo V, ed. Treatment of liver diseases. Barcelona: Masson; 1999:53–59.

63. Wong F, Pantea L, Sniderman K. Midodrine, octreotide and albumin followed by tranjugular intrahepatic portosystemic shunt in selected patients with cirrhosis and type 1 hepatorenal syndrome. Hepatology 2004; 40:55–64.

64. Gonwa TA, Morris CA, Goldstein RM, et al. Long-term survival and renal function following liver transplantation in patients with and without hepatorenal syndrome – experience in 300 patients. Transplantation 1991; 91:428–430.

65. Lerut J, Goffette P, Laterre PF, et al. Sequential treatment of hepatorenal syndrome and posthepatic cirrhosis by intrahepatic portosystemic shunt (TIPS) and liver transplantation. Hepatogastroenterology 1995; 42:985–987.

66. Gonwa TA, Klintmalm GB, Jennings LS, et al. Impact of pretransplant renal function on survival after liver transplantation. Transplantation 1995; 59:361–365.

67. Seu P, Wilkinson AH, Shaked A, et al. The hepatorenal syndrome in liver transplant recipients. Am Surg 1991; 57:806–809.

68. Rimola A, Gavaler JS, Schade RR, et al. Effects of renal impairment on liver transplantation. Gastroenterology 1987; 93:148–156.

69. Navasa M, Feu F, Garcia-Pagan JC, et al. Hemodynamic and humoral changes after liver transplantation in patients with cirrhosis. Hepatology 1993; 17:355–360.

70. Nair S, Verma S, Thuluvath PJ. Pretransplant renal function predicts survival in patients undergoing orthotopic liver transplantation. Hepatology 2002; 35:1179–1185.

71. Restuccia T, Ortega R, Guevara M, et al. Effects of treatment of hepatorenal syndrome before transplantation on posttransplantation outcome. A case-control study. J Hepatol 2004; 40(1):140–146.

72. Perez GO, Golper TA, Epstein M, et al. Dialysis, hemofiltration, and other extracorporeal techniques in the treatment of renal complications of liver disease. In: Epstein M, ed. The kidney in liver disease, 4th edn. Philadelphia: Hanley & Belfus; 1996: 517–528.

73. Arroyo V, Bataller R, Guevara M. Treatment of hepatorenal syndrome in cirrhosis. In: Arroyo V, Ginès P, Rodés J, et al, eds. Ascites and renal dysfunction in liver disease. Pathogenesis, diagnosis and treatment. Malden: Blackwell Science; 1999: 492–510.

74. Pomier-Layrargues G, Paquin SC, Hassoun Z, et al. Octreotide in hepatorenal syndrome: a randomized, double blind, placebo controlled, crossover study. Hepatology 2003; 38:238–243.

75. Holt S, Goodier D, Marley R, et al. Improvement in renal function in hepatorenal syndrome with N-acetyl-cysteine. Lancet 1999; 353:294–295.

76. Mitzner SR, Stange J, Klammt S, et al. Improvement of hepatorenal syndrome with extracorporeal albumin dialysis MARS: results of a prospective randomized, controlled clinical trial. Liver Transpl 2000; 6:277–286.

77. Ginès P, Uriz J, Calahorra B, et al. Transjugular intrahepatic portosystemic shunting versus paracentesis plus albumin for refractory ascites in cirrhosis. Gastroenterology 2002; 123: 1839–1847.

78. Rossle M, Ochs A, Gulberg V, et al. A comparison of paracentesis and tranjugular intrahepatic portosystemic shunting in patients with ascites. N Engl J Med 2000; 342:1701–1707.

79. Lebrec D, Giuily N, Hadengue A, et al. Transjugular intrahepatic portosystemic shunts: comparison with paracentesis in patients with cirrhosis and refractory ascites: a randomized trial. French Group of Clinicians and a Group of Biologists. J Hepatol. 1996; 25:135–144.

80. Sanyal AJ, Genning C, Reddy KR, et al. North American Study for the Treatment of Refractory Ascites Group. The North American Study for the Treatment of Refractory Ascites. Gastroenterology. 2003; 124:634–641.

81. Alessandria C, Debernardi W, Marzano A, et al. Renal failure in cirrhotic patients: role of terlipressin in clinical approach to hepatorenal syndrome type 2. Eur J Gastroenterol Hepatol 2002; 14:1363–1368.

82. Sort P, Navasa M, Arroyo V. et al. Effect of plasma volume expansion on renal impairment and mortality in patients with cirrhosis and spontaneous bacterial peritonitis. N Engl J Med 1999; 341:403–409.

This important clinical study demonstrates that circulatory support with i.v. albumin reduces the incidence of type-I HRS by 60% in patients with spontaneous bacterial peritonitis (SBP).

83. Akriviadis E, Botla R, Briggs W, et al. Pentoxyfilline improves short-term survival in severe acute alcoholic hepatitis: a double-blind, placebo-controlled trial. Gastroenterology 2000; 119:1637–1648.

CHAPTER FORTY-THREE

43

Fulminant hepatic failure

Tram T. Tran and Paul Martin

INTRODUCTION

Fulminant hepatic failure (FHF), also referred to as acute liver failure, is the onset of hepatic encephalopathy within 8 weeks of initial onset of symptoms of liver disease or alternatively, coagulopathy and encephalopathy in a patient wihout cirrhosis and an illness of less than 26 weeks duration. The absence of a history of antecedent liver disease implies that there is the potential for spontaneous recovery. Although relatively rare, with approximately 2000 cases recognized in the United States annually,[1] the significance of FHF lies with its high mortality rate and frequent need for liver transplantation (OLT). Fulminant hepatic failure occurs as a result of massive liver cell necrosis and therefore typically presents with coagulopathy and jaundice, in addition to encephalopathy. In an effort to better identify patients most likely to succumb without OLT, a number of refinements in the definition have been proposed, including characterization into hyperacute (encephalopathy within 1 week), acute (1–4 weeks), and subacute or subfulminant (5–26 weeks).[2] Subfulminant hepatic failure may reflect an acute presentation of a chronic liver disease such as Wilson disease or autoimmune hepatitis. These patients may already have portal hypertension and they generally have a worse prognosis. Encephalopathy develops later in the course and cerebral edema is less frequent. All of the definitions include hepatic encephalopathy, which is the precursor to the most frequently lethal complication of FHF, cerebral edema. Paradoxically, the more rapid the development of encephalopathy, the greater the likelihood of spontaneous recovery.

ETIOLOGY

Etiologies for FHF vary greatly by the era of published study and their geographic origin. Although viral hepatitis remains the most common cause worldwide, acetaminophen hepatotoxicity is the predominant cause in the United States and Great Britain, accounting for nearly 75% of cases.[3] The US Acute Liver Failure Study Group prospectively studied cases of FHF identified in 1998 and 2001.[4] In this report from 17 centers throughout the United States, acetaminophen toxicity accounted for 120 of 308 cases of FHF (39%). Other frequent causes were idiosyncratic drug reactions (13%), hepatitis B (7%), and hepatitis A (4%) (Fig. 43.1). The cause of FHF could not be identified despite extensive evaluation in a large number of patients in this study (20%). Subsequent study of sera from these patients suggested that some cases were

due to occult hepatitis B infection only detected with highly sensitive PCR-based assays.[5] Other less frequent causes of FHF included Wilson disease, autoimmune hepatitis, acute Budd-Chiari syndrome, and acute fatty liver of pregnancy.

Hepatitis B is the most common cause of FHF worldwide, especially in Asia. Death from acute hepatitis B infection occurs in 1.0–1.2% of infected individuals and a fulminant presentation of HBV can occur in chronically infected patients who have spontaneous reactivation of infection or reactivation induced by therapeutic immunosuppression or chemotherapy. Hepatitis D infection (HDV) occurs in individuals concurrently infected with hepatitis B and is a cofactor in 50% or FHF cases attributed to hepatitis B. HDV infection can occur as a coinfection at the same time at HBV transmission, or as a superinfection in an individual already chronically infected with HBV. Acute hepatitis A (HAV) causes 75 000 cases of icteric hepatitis annually in the United States with a case fatality rate of 0.2–0.4%. Individuals at greatest risk to develop FHF as a result of acute HAV infection include those with chronic liver disease (particularly alcoholic cirrhosis), intravenous drug users, and the elderly, in whom mortality approaches 3%. Hepatitis C rarely, if ever, causes FHF. Hepatitis E is endemic in areas with poor sanitation and affects pregnant women in the third trimester, with high mortality estimated at 20%. Other viral causes of FHF include cytomegalovirus in the immunosuppressed, herpes simplex, herpes zoster, and parvovirus B19.

Drug hepatotoxicity may be due to either an intrinsic and dose-dependent mechanism, as in the case of acetaminophen, or by idiosyncratic mechanism. Intrinsic toxicity can then be further divided into direct or indirect injury at the subcellular level with subsequent steatosis, necrosis, or both. Direct cellular injury occurs in carbon tetrahydrochloride and phosphorus poisoning. Indirect toxicity is injury to metabolic pathways, such as in acetaminophen toxicity, where the formation of a toxic metabolite, N-acetyl-p-benzoquinone-imine (NAPQI) causes perturbations in mitochondrial membrane integrity. Acetaminophen toxicity, by both suicidal intention and therapeutic misadventure, is most often seen with ingestion of at least 4 grams of drug within 24 hours in adults. In the ALF study the median ingested dose was 13 grams in a day; however, lower doses can be hepatotoxic in alcoholics or fasting individuals. Therapeutic misadventures leading to FHF are common since acetaminophen is contained in many prescriptions, and over-the-counter analgesic preparations which are sometimes taken simultaneously.

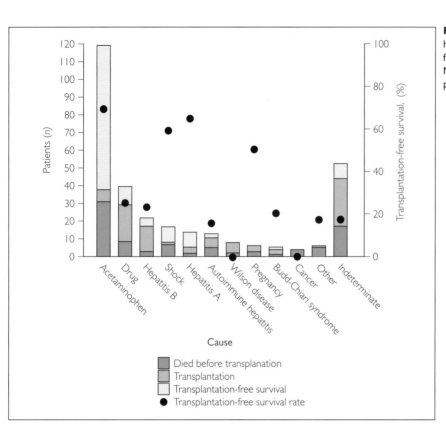

Fig. 43.1 • Causes and outcomes of fulminant hepatic failure in the United States. (Reprinted from Ostapowicz GA et al, Annals of Internal Medicine, 2002; 137: 947–954. © 2002, with permission from American College of Physicians.)

Autoimmune hepatitis is a less frequent cause of FHF, presenting most often as a subfulfilment subfulminant hepatitis, and recognition is important because treatment with immunosuppression may arrest the course, obviating the need for transplantation. Hypergammaglobulinemia and the presence of autoantibodies in the absence of other causes of liver disease may facilitate prompt diagnosis. Autoimmune hepatitis, like Wilson disease, may also present with clinical clues suggesting preexisting chronic liver disease.

The exact pathophysiologic mechanism(s) that result in development of FHF is unknown. However, it is likely that no single mechanism is responsible. Hypoxia, endotoxemia, and immunemediated injury have been proposed and each is supported by evidence in certain etiologic groups. Regardless of the responsible mechanism of hepatic injury, each results in a similar clinical outcome of encephalopathy, jaundice, and coagulopathy.

CLINICAL PRESENTATION AND DIAGNOSIS

The initial symptoms of FHF are typically non-specific, e.g., malaise, anorexia, and nausea. However, once patients present, progression to outright hepatic decompensation is typically rapid. Jaundice may not be present early in the clinical course, and the non-specific complaints may be overlooked. Subsequently, jaundice and the mental status changes of encephalopathy become apparent. The recognition of encephalopathy is essential to the diagnosis of FHF, and degree of alteration is graded in stages 1 through 4 (Table 43.1). Physical examination is usually notable for a lack of stigmata of chronic liver disease or portal hypertension (spider angioma, splenomegaly, hepatomegaly, ascites); however, in a protracted subfulminant course, ascites associated with renal

failure may be present. The liver size may decrease as hepatocellular necrosis and collapse occur with FHF.

When the diagnosis of FHF is suspected, a thorough history and examination, as well as expedited biochemical and serological laboratory testing, are necessary. A complete history should elicit a careful drug ingestion history including all narcotics and pain medications, over-the-counter medications, and herbal preparations. Alcohol consumption, recent travel, sexual or other exposures, time course of events, and previous medical problems should also be elicited. A confirmatory history of drug and substance abuse should be obtained from a family member, especially if the patient is already somnolent. Laboratory tests should include a standard biochemistry panel including aminotransferases, bilirubin, alkaline phosphatase, albumin, prothrombin time, lactate dehydrogenase (which may be elevated in infiltrative diseases), and blood gas for pH (Table 43.2). A prolonged prothrombin time, elevated aminotransferases generally greater than 10 times normal, elevated bilirubin, and moderately elevated alkaline phosphatase

Table 43.1 Stages of encephalopathy	
Stage	**Mental status**
1	Altered sleep cycle, dysphoria, mild confusion, forgetfulness
2	Drowsiness, inappropriate behavior, decreased mental acuity, asterixis
3	Stuporous but arousable, inability to perform mental tasks, speech uninterpretable, marked confusion
4	Deep coma, unarousable, little or no reaction to painful stimuli

Table 43.2 Diagnostic testing in suspected fulminant hepatic failure

Complete blood count

Serum biochemistries: comprehensive metabolic panel
   including:
    Aminotransferases
    Bilirubin, direct and indirect
    Alkaline phosphatase
    Lactate dehyrogenase
    Serum electrolytes: sodium, potassium, magnesium,
      phosphorus
    Creatinine
Prothrombin time
Arterial blood gas
Serum and urine toxicology panel
Acetaminophen level

Hepatitis serologies:
   Hepatitis A IgM
   Hepatitis B anti-core IgM
   Hepatitis B s Ag
   Hepatitis B DNA
   Hepatitis C antibody
   Hepatitis C RNA
   Hepatitis D IgM
   Hepatitis E IgM
Ceruloplasmin
Blood cultures
Glucose
Serum autoantibodies (antinuclear antibody, smooth muscle
   antibody)

is a typical biochemical picture. Acetaminophen toxicity can result in markedly elevated aminotransferases >10 000 IU/mL, and alkaline phosphatase can be normal or only minimally elevated in fulminant Wilson's disease.

Initial serologies ordered should include: hepatitis A IgM, hepatitis B surface antigen, hepatitis B core IgM, hepatitis C RNA (antibodies may not have developed yet in acute infection), delta antibody, and hepatitis E antibody. Autoimmune markers including antinuclear antibody, smooth muscle antibody, and immunoglobulin levels should be done. Wilson's disease should be ruled out by serum ceruloplasmin and copper level, and a 24-hour urine quantification for copper. Urine or plasma toxicology panels and acetaminophen levels should be ordered as clinically indicated, recognizing that drug histories may be misleading.

A prompt Doppler ultrasound is necessary to assess vascular patency and exclude Budd-Chiari or other processes such as massive tumor infiltration. Steatosis may be detected by ultrasound in acute fatty liver of pregnancy.

Once the diagnosis of FHF is suspected, prompt referral to a liver transplant center is appropriate since rapid clinical decline can occur over a matter of hours, making later transfer more hazardous and even precluding transplantation as an option.

PROGNOSIS

An estimation of prognosis is critical in the early assessment of FHF to identify patients who are less likely to spontaneously recover in the absence of liver transplantation. Before the era of liver transplantation, mortality due to FHF was nearly 90%. Earlier recognition and better specialized care in intensive care units has improved survival rates to between 20% and 50%, depending on the etiology. The most widely used prognostic scoring system was proposed by O'Grady et al. in 1989 based on an analysis of 588 patients and divided into acetaminophen and nonacetaminophen etiology (Table 43.3).[6] The sensitivity of these King's College Hospital (KCH) criteria is 50–80% and the specificity is 86–96% with a positive predictive value of about 80%. However, prognostic criteria such as the King's College criteria, the Acute Physiology and Chronic Health Evaluation (APACHE) which uses a combination of clinical and laboratory assessments, and factor V levels are still controversial in their ability to accurately predict complications of FHF in individual patients. Other prognostic criteria including group specific (Gc) protein, liver biopsy, liver volume, alpha-fetoprotein, and human hepatocyte growth factor levels have also been described, but these have not been as easy to apply in practice or have not been validated. Late-onset or subacute hepatic failure, with a prolonged prodrome prior to onset of encephalopathy, is a particulary bad predictor of outcome and is associated with a poor survival rate (14%).[2]

Hypophosphatemia has been noted in patients with acetaminophen-induced hepatotoxicity and correlates with the severity of liver damage.[7] Schmidt et al. recently measured serum phosphate levels in 125 patients with severe acetaminophen toxicity and found that a phosphate level greater than 1.2 mmol/L at 48–96 hours after overdose predicted death with a sensitivity of 89%, specificity of 100%, positive predictive value of 100%, and negative predictive value of 98%.[8] The phosphate criteria had higher sensitivity, accuracy, and positive and negative predictive values than the KCH criteria. Hyperphosphatemia correlated with acute renal insufficiency and absence of hepatic regeneration. Subsequent comparison of phosphate levels to previously studied cases at King's College confirmed improved sensitivity in predicting nonsurvival as compared to the King's College criteria; however, specificity, accuracy, and positive predictive value were not as good.[9]

Ultimately, the rapid and frequent assessment of the individual patient's clinical and biochemical status at a transplant center, maximizing current knowledge of management, is more important than any single prognostic indicator.

MANAGEMENT

Effective management of FHF depends in part on the etiology of liver failure. For example, specific treatment for acute fatty liver of pregnancy is delivery of the infant and therapy for ACM overdose

Table 43.3 King's College criteria

Acetaminophen toxicity	Nonacetaminophen etiology
pH <7.3 (independent of degree of encephalopathy) OR	Prothrombin time >100 seconds OR
Prothrombin time >100 seconds and creatinine > 3.4 with grade 3 or 4 encephalopathy	Any three of the following: Age <10 or >40 Prothrombin time >50 sec Bilirubin >17.5 Duration of jaundice before encephalopathy >7 days

is N-acetylcysteine. However, fulminant Wilson disease progresses despite initiation of the copper chelation therapy, which is effective in nonacute presentations.

When an overdose of acetaminophen is suspected, measurement of the blood acetaminophen level and establishment of the potential risk of FHF based on the published nomogram relating time after ingestion to serum acetaminophen level should be performed since patient reporting of amount and timing of ingestion, as well as concurrent medications and alcohol that may impact drug disposition, may be inaccurate. Gastric lavage, prompt initiation of N-acetylcysteine (NAC) given as a loading dose 140 mg/kg followed by 17 doses at 70 mg/kg every 4 hours is standard. NAC is most efficacious if administered within the first 24 hours of ingestion; however, it is safe and may still be effective if given after 24 hours.[10,11] The King's College criteria should be applied upon admission and clinical and biochemical parameters followed during hospitalization. Most cases will recover, but early consideration of transplantation should be given, particularly if hepatic function continues to decline.

Irrespective of the etiology of FHF in a particular patient, general management should focus on the prevention of complications while awaiting hepatic regeneration with spontaneous recovery or liver transplantation. These measures include prevention of infection, management of cerebral edema, nutritional support, and management of multiorgan system failure. Given the complexity of the FHF patient, an intensive care unit experienced in the management of FHF is the best environment for these patients.

Neurologic management

The key manifestation of FHF is the development of hepatic encephalopathy. The pathophysiology of encephalopathy in FHF is still controversial and has been attributed to a variety of mechanisms including hyperammonemia and alterations in GABA, serotonin, or dopamine neurotransmission. Astrocyte swelling is also believed to be a component.[12,13] Altered mental status may be subtle in stage 1 encephalopathy with only mild confusion or mania and excitation. Stage 2 encephalopathy is characterized by asterixis (not always present) and obtundation; however, the patient is usually arousable. Rapid progression to coma may occur. Once stage 3 or 4 encephalopathy occurs, cerebral edema is present in up to 80% of patients and is the most common cause of death in FHF. Clinical signs and symptoms such as papilledema and systemic hypertension may be absent or late. Thus, if a patient is a transplant candidate, accurate assessment and monitoring of intracranial pressure is warranted. CT scanning is not particularly sensitive and evidence of cerebral edema may be delayed, but CT is indicated to exclude intracerebral hemorrhage in the face of rapid neurological deterioration. Epidural transducers to monitor intracranial pressure (ICP), although less accurate, have lower morbidity (3.8%) from intracranial hemorrhage than subdural or intraparenchymal monitors (20%).[14,15] The goal should be to keep cerebral perfusion pressure (CPP) above 50 mmHg to prevent brain hypoperfusion. Cerebral perfusion pressure is the difference between the mean arterial pressure (MAP) and the intracranial pressure (ICP). The use of ICP monitoring may also avoid the transplantation of an individual with refractory intracranial hypertension who may not only have higher operative mortality, and irreversible neurologic sequelae (Fig. 43.2). Preventative measures to reduce intracranial hypertension

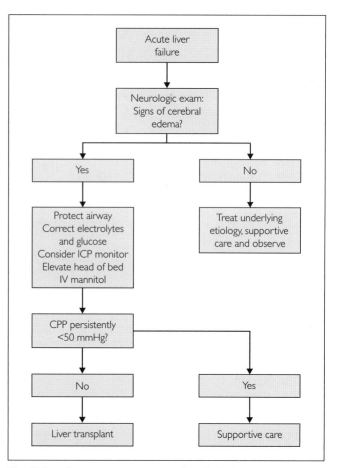

Fig. 43.2 • Appropriate management of cerebral edema is essential to the outcome of patients with acute liver failure awaiting liver transplant. Neurologic examination with any early signs of neurologic compromise should be quickly identified and intracranial pressure monitor considered for diagnosis and treatment of cerebral perfusion pressure.

include minimization of external stimulation and elevation of the head of the bed to no higher than 20 degrees, as this may result in increased CPP.[16] Administration of mannitol as an osmotic agent (0.5–1 g/kg over 5 minutes), repeated every hour until serum osmolality reaches 310 mOsm/L can acutely control elevations of ICP. Hyperventilation may also work as a short-term maneuver to decrease ICP; however, many patients with FHF already spontaneously hyperventilate. If ICP does not respond to these short-term measures, induction of a pentobarbital or thiopental coma may be considered (3–5 mg/kg loading dose, followed by continuous infusion 0.5–1 mg/kg/h), though caution is warranted to avoid systemic hypotension with a resulting reduction in CPP. Standard measures, such as protein restriction or lactulose, to treat the more typical hepatic encephalopathy seen in cirrhotics have little effect in the encephalopathy associated with FHF.

Respiratory management

Pulmonary complications including adult respiratory distress syndrome, pulmonary edema, hypoxemia, pneumonia, and hyperventilation are frequent in advanced FHF. In patients with grade 3 or 4 encephalopathy, special attention to prevent aspiration pneumonia is warranted and protection of the airway is essential.

Elective, controlled endotracheal intubation and ventilatory support is preferred, with careful attention to pulmonary toilet. The use of positive end-expiratory pressure (PEEP) may increase intracranial pressure and reduce cardiac output, and it should therefore be employed only after careful consideration. Hypoxemia and impaired oxygen consumption results in increased anaerobic metabolism and lactic acidosis, portending a poor prognosis. Hyperventilation may be a clue to increased intracranial pressure and this should be evaluated as described above.

Circulatory/hemodynamic management

Hypotension is commonly seen and may reflect sepsis or hemodynamic changes due to FHF. Central hemodynamic monitoring with a Swan-Ganz catheter and an arterial line are helpful and often confirm a hyperdynamic state with low peripheral vascular resistance, increased cardiac output, and low mean arterial pressure. Proinflammatory cytokines such as TNF-alpha and vasodilators such as nitric oxide may play a role in this process. Low oxygen delivery state results in tissue hypoxia and lactic acidosis, which is a poor prognostic indicator. If blood pressure cannot be maintained with fluid and colloid resuscitation, then vasopressor support may be required to increase cardiac output and increase systemic vascular resistance.

Infectious complications

Infectious complications, common in FHF, reflect a myriad of factors including macrophage dysfunction, poor opsonization, low levels of serum complement, and defective lymphocyte function. Bacterial infection can occur as early as 2 days after presentation, although fungal infections generally occur 1 week or more following hospitalization. Up to 80% of FHF patients have bacterial infection when routine cultures are obtained,[17] and fungal infections eventuate in more than 30%.[18] The most common organisms are Gram-positive *Staphylococcus aureus* and *Candida* species. Despite infection, fever and leukocytosis may be absent in the FHF patient, so careful observation for mental status change, deteriorating hepatic or renal function, or changes in ventilatory or oxygenation requirements is essential and changes should raise suspicion for infection. Controversy exists in the current literature about whether prophylactic antibiotics, either systemically administered or as intestinal decontamination, are beneficial. Once infection is suspected, broad-spectrum antibiotics, with consideration for antifungal coverage, should be initiated. Due to high rates of renal dysfunction in FHF, aminoglycosides should be avoided, as in any patient with liver disease.

Nutritional and electrolyte management

A prolonged hospital course may necessitate parenteral nutrition in the encephalopathic patient. Minimal protein restriction (40 g/d) may be beneficial early in the clinical course, but branched-chain amino acid formulations have shown no additional benefit. Hypoglycemia due to impaired hepatic gluconeogenesis is common, and continuous 10% i.v. glucose should be administered with frequent glucose monitoring once frank encephalopathy is present. Hyperkalemia in the setting of renal failure can also occur.

Renal complications

The hemodynamic changes associated with FHF, including low peripheral vascular resistance, result in activation of the renin-angiotensin-aldosterone system with sodium retention and renal failure in more than 50% of patients, and up to 75% of those with acetaminophen toxicity.[19,20] Early renal failure is associated with 95% mortality without liver transplantation in acetaminophen-induced FHF. Acute tubular necrosis, hyperkalemia, hypophosphatemia, and metabolic acidosis may result, requiring hemodialysis. The King's College criteria state that acidosis (pH <7.3) indicates a need for OLT regardless of degree of encephalopathy. Acute hemodialysis must be performed carefully since changes in systemic blood pressure may cause increases in ICP and reduction in CPP. Thus, continuous veno–veno hemoperfusion or hemodiafiltration may be preferred.

Coagulopathy

Coagulopathy in FHF reflects decreased hepatic production of coagulation factors as well as disseminated intravascular coagulation. Serial measurement of prothrombin time and factor V helps assess whether spontaneous recovery is occurring and helps make clinical decisions in regards to proceeding with transplantation. Administration of fresh-frozen plasma or other clotting factors prevents monitoring of prothrombin time and factor V levels, and should therefore be avoided unless bleeding is suspected or a necessary invasive procedure is planned. Likewise, transfusion of platelets is not required unless clinically indicated by bleeding, as spontaneous bleeding occurs uncommonly.

Gastrointestinal complications

Gastrointestinal hemorrhage can occur especially in the setting of coagulopathy and thrombocytopenia. Most often, the source of bleeding is erosive gastritis or esophagitis, and risk may be reduced by H_2 blocker or proton pump inhibitor administration. Serious hemorrhage is uncommon.

TRANSPLANTATION FOR FULMINANT HEPATIC FAILURE

Spontaneous survival without liver transplantation in the FHF patient has been reported to be between 10% and 25%, but varies widely by etiology.[21,22] With transplantation, survival rates range between 60% and 90% with significant variability in patient selection between transplant centers.[23–25] More recent series generally report better survival following OLT for FHF, reflecting more effective patient selection, precluding candidates with irreversible neurological injury. The national waiting list for orthotopic liver transplantation in the US now exceeds 17 000 patients, while only 5 315 patients received a liver transplant in 2002. The Model for End Stage Liver Disease score is now used to prioritize patients for cadaveric organ allocation and has reduced the number of deaths on the waiting list.[26] Recognizing the high mortality in the absence of OLT and the favorable outcomes with transplantation, patients with FHF receive the highest priority as Status 1. Kremer et al. recently published a review of the 836 adult patients listed by the United Network for Organ Sharing (UNOS) as Status 1 from November 1999 to March 2002. The majority of patients fell into four groups divided by etiology: acetaminophen, nonacetaminophen, primary nonfunction of a transplanted liver, and hepatic artery thrombosis. This analysis showed that patients with FHF of a nonacetaminophen etiology had the poorest survival while awaiting OLT, which correlated well with their MELD score, and had the best overall improvement in outcome with OLT (58% survival without to 91% survival with OLT).[27] Overall, liver transplantation remains the definitive treatment for acute liver failure with acceptable survival rates as compared to medical management only.

Living donor liver transplantation (LDLT) has been attempted in patients with FHF and is not recommended. Liu et al. reported eight children transplanted for FHF with a mean follow-up period of 13 months. Actuarial graft and patient survival were 50% and 62.5%, respectively, compared to 89% graft and patient survival in a non-LDLT cohort.[28] Other small series in adult LDLT have reported variable success, but with short-term follow-up.[29–31] In the United States, LDLT has been reported in severely decompensated cirrhotics with resulting graft and patient survival rates of only 43%.[32] Thus, given the tempered enthusiasm for LDLT since adverse outcomes have been described, LDLT has been reserved for the well-compensated cirrhotic, and the role in FHF needs to be further evaluated.

Supportive care to bridge the FHF patient to liver transplant remains the mainstay of management. However, development of extracorporeal liver support systems holds ongoing promise. A prospective, randomized, controlled study on an extracorporeal cell-based liver support system (BAL) comprised of porcine hepatocytes housed within a bioreactor has recently been reported and showed survival benefit in the fulminant/subfulminant group as compared to the control group (44% reduction in mortality).[33]

SUMMARY

Fulminant hepatic failure, although uncommon, has a poor outcome without prompt, aggressive medical management. Initial efforts should include concerted efforts to determine the etiology to direct specific therapy when possible (see Table 43.2). For example, specific treatment for acute fatty liver of pregnancy is delivery of the infant and therapy for ACM overdose is N-acetylcysteine. Intensive monitoring of multisystemic organ dysfunction including neurologic, infectious, and metabolic complications is an important component of potential spontaneous recovery and has significantly improved outcomes in recent years. Early recognition of poor prognostic indices and clinical deterioration can lead to successful recovery with timely liver transplantation.

REFERENCES

1. Lee WM. Acute liver failure. N Engl J Med. 1993; 329(25): 1862–1872.

   A thorough review of the causes, course, and outcomes of fulminant hepatic failure.

2. O'Grady JG, Schalm SW, Williams R. Acute liver failure: redefining the syndromes. Lancet 1993; 342(8866):273–275.

3. Bernal W. Changing patterns of causation and the use of transplantation in the United Kingdom. Semin Liver Dis 2003; 227–237.

4. Ostapowicz GA, Fontana RJ, Schiodt FV, et al. Results of a prospective study of acute liver failure at 17 tertiary care centers in the United States. Ann Internal Med 2002; 137:947–954.

   This is the initial report of the United States Acute Liver Failure Study Group. Acetaminophen overdose and idiosyncratic drug reactions were the most frequent causes of acute liver failure. Cause and coma grade were associated with outcome. Liver transplantation improved patient survival, but was unavailable or unnecessary for most patients.

5. Teo EK, Ostapowicz GA, Hussain M, and the US ALF Study Group. Hepatitis B infection in patients with acute liver failure in the United States. Hepatology 2001; 33:972–976.

6. O'Grady JG, Alexander GJM, Hayllar KM, et al. Early indications of prognosis in fulminant hepatic failure. Gastroenterology 1989; 97(2):439–445.

   The classic King's College criteria of estimating prognosis in patients with fulminant hepatic failure due to acetaminophen, other drugs, or virus-induced liver injury.

7. Dawson DJ, Babbs C, Warnes TW, et al. Hypophosphatemia in acute liver failure. Br Med J 1987; 295(6609):1312–1313.

8. Schmidt LE, Dalhoff K. Serum phosphate is an early predictor of outcome in severe acetaminophen-induced hepatotoxicity. Hepatology 2002; 36(3):659–665.

9. Bernal W, Wendon J. More on serum phosphate and prognosis of acute liver failure (Letter). Hepatology 2003; 38(2):533–534.

10. Parker D, White JP, Paton D, et al. Safety of late acetylcysteine treatment in paracetamol poisoning. Hum Exp Toxicol 1990; 9(1):25–27.

   Description of N-acetylcysteine for acetaminophen hepatotoxicity. Incidence of hepatotoxicity was decreased by more than half.

11. Keays R, Harrison PM, Wendon JA, et al. Intravenous acetylcysteine in paracetamol induced fulminant hepatic failure: a prospective controlled trial. Br Med J 1991; 303(6809):1026–1029.

12. Butterworth RF. Molecular neurobiology of acute liver failure. Semin Liv Disease 2003; 23(3):251–258.

13. Vaquero J, Chung C, Cahill M, et al. Pathogenesis of hepatic encephalopathy in acute liver failure. Semin Liv Dis 2003; 23(3):259–269.

14. Keays RT, Alexander GJ, Williams R. The safety and value of extradural intracranial pressure monitors in fulminant hepatic failure. J Hepatol 1993; 18(2):205–209.

15. Lidofsky SD, Bass NM, Prager MC, et al. Intracranial pressure monitoring and liver transplantation for fulminant hepatic failure. Hepatology 1992; 16(1):1–7.

16. Davenport A, Will EJ, Davison AM. Effect of posture on intracranial pressure in patients with fulminant hepatic failure after acetaminophen self-poisoning. Crit Care Med 1990; 18(3)286–289.

17. Rolando N, Harvey F, Brahm J, et al. Prospective study of bacterial infection in acute liver failure: an analysis of fifty patients. Hepatology 1990; 11(1):49–53.

18. Rolando N, Harvey F, Brahm J, et al. Fungal infection: a common, unrecognized complication of acute liver failure. J Hepatology 1991; 12(1):1–9.

19. Ring-Larsen H, Palazzo U. Renal failure in fulminant hepatic failure and terminal cirrhosis: a comparison between incidence, types and prognosis. Gut 1981; 22(7):585–591.

20. Makin A, Williams R. The current management of paracetamol overdosage. Br J Clin Pract 1994; 48(3):144–148.

21. Ritt DJ, Whelan G, Werner DJ, et al. Acute hepatic necrosis with stupor or coma. An analysis of thirty-one patients. Medicine 1969; 48:151–172.

22. Schiodt FV, Atillasoy E, Shakil AO, et al. Etiology and outcome for 295 patients with acute liver failure in the United States. Liver Transpl Surg 1999; 5:29–34.

23. Bismuth H, Samuel D, Castaing D, et al. Orthotopic liver transplantation in fulminant and subfulminant hepatitis. The Paul Brousse experience. Ann Surg 1995; 222(2):109–119.

Experience with liver transplantation for fulminant hepatic failure. Overall 1-year survival including use of partial and marginal donor grafts was 68%.

24. Emond JC, Aran PP, Whitington PF, et al. Liver transplantation in the management of fulminant hepatic failure. Gastroenterology 1989; 96:1583–1588.

25. Ascher NL, Lake JR, Emond JC, et al. Liver transplantation for fulminant hepatic failure. Arch Surg 1993; 128:677–684.

26. Freeman RB, Weisner RH, Edwards E, et al. Results of the first year of the new liver allocation plan. Liver Transpl 2004; 10(1):7–15.

27. Kremers WK, Van J Peren M, Kim WR, et al. MELD score as a predictor of pretransplant and posttransplant survival in OPTN/UNOS status 1 patients. Hepatology 2004; 39(3):764–769.

28. Liu CL, Fan ST, Lo CM, et al. Live donor liver transplantation for fulminant hepatic failure in children. Liver Transpl 2003; 9(11):1185–1190.

29. Matsunami H, Makuuchi M, Kawasaki S, et al. Living-related liver transplantation in fulminant hepatic failure. Lancet 1992; 340(8832):1411–1412.

30. Sugawara Y, Kaneko J, Imamura H, et al. Living donor liver transplantation for fulminant hepatic failure. Transplant Proc 2002; 34(8):3287–3288.

31. Miwa S, Hashikura Y, Mita A, et al. Living-related liver transplantation for patients with fulminant and subfulminant hepatic failure. Hepatology 1999; 30(6):1521–1526.

32. Testa G, Malago M, Nadalin S, et al. Right-liver living donor transplantation for decompensated end-stage liver disease. Liver Transpl 2002; 8(4):340–346.

33. Demetriou AA, Brown RS, Busuttil RW, et al. Prospective, randomized, multicenter, controlled trial of a bioartificial liver in treating acute liver failure. Ann Surg 2004; 239(5):660–670.

CHAPTER FORTY-FOUR

44

Long-term care of the liver transplant recipient

Consuelo Soldevila-Pico and David R. Nelson

INTRODUCTION

Long-term management of liver transplant recipients relies on the coordinated involvement of the liver transplant center, the primary care physician, and the referring gastroenterologist. As more patients survive beyond the first decade after the transplant procedure, the need for proactive interventions to minimize the adverse consequences of immunosuppression and disease recurrence need to be promoted. These interventions have to be carefully tailored to promote immune tolerance with the graft and to avoid the complications and comorbid conditions that are either newly developed or present at the time of transplant. Many medical issues require special considerations after transplantation, particularly those related to diabetes mellitus, hypertension, drug interactions, renal dysfunction, bone disease, and neuropsychiatric syndromes. The gastroenterologist, internist, or local family physician is frequently called upon to identify and treat these postoperative complications in conjunction with physicians at the transplant center. This chapter reviews these issues in detail, and suggestions are offered to aid in the management of medical complications encountered after liver transplantation.

EARLY MANAGEMENT

Allograft rejection

Approximately two-thirds of liver transplant recipients will develop acute cellular rejection in the early post-transplant course, though the majority of these episodes are mild and easily controlled with medication. Typically, immune suppression medications are decreased with time as the risk of rejection lessens. However, patients transplanted for primary sclerosing cholangitis, primary biliary cirrhosis, and autoimmune hepatitis may be at increased risk of acute cellular rejection or disease recurrence, leading many transplant centers to maintain a higher level of immunosuppression in these cases.[1,2] With time, the incidence of rejection decreases, while mechanical problems, de novo or recurrent viral infections, and drug-induced abnormalities enter into the differential of liver test abnormalities. Furthermore, recurrent liver disease, particularly recurrent viral hepatitis or primary biliary cirrhosis, may resemble rejection on liver biopsy and lead to confusion.

Infections

Infectious complications are still a significant cause of morbidity and mortality in liver transplant recipients. The risk of infection is largely determined by three factors: the net state of immunosuppression, the epidemiologic exposure the patient encounters, and the consequences of the invasive procedures to which the patient is subjected.[3] Most infectious complications occur early after liver transplantation, due to the relatively high level of immune impairment. Fever is a common event in organ transplant recipients and most commonly indicates infection, but can also occur in patients with acute cellular rejection. Infections occurring in the first 4 weeks after transplantation are primarily nosocomial, related to surgical or technical complications of transplantation. Bacterial infections are by far the most common infections to occur in the first 4 weeks after transplantation. The most common sources are vascular catheter-related infections, nosocomial pneumonia, and wound or surgical site infections. Gram-positive bacteria (staphylococci and enterococci) have emerged as the predominant pathogens at most transplant centers, along with a marked increase in the prevalence of antibiotic resistant strains. Another dangerous but uncommon pathogen that is seen in the first 4 weeks is fungal infections (aspergillous, cryptococcus, and candida). A poorly functioning hepatic allograft and renal dysfunction significantly increase the risk for more invasive fungal infections, especially aspergillosis,[4] but clinical benefit of prophylaxis is still unproven and invasive fungal infections fortunately remain infrequent.

Cytomegalovirus (CMV) has historically been the predominant infectious origin of fever occurring 4–8 weeks post transplant. Although CMV-associated morbidity has declined significantly due to the advent of reliable early diagnostic assays and effective antiviral therapy, it still remains a significant threat to organ transplant recipients. Prophylactic antiviral and antibiotics therapies have markedly decreased the early incidence of previously common infections such as CMV and *Pneumocystis carinii*. CMV disease had been reported in as many as 35% of liver transplant patients, but has recently decreased to less than 5% with aggressive prophylaxis strategies.[5] The preferred strategy toward the prevention of CMV is the preemptive approach targeting patients with high risk for serious disease. Most commonly, prophylactic oral ganciclovir is given for 3–4 months in high-risk patients (based on donor and recipient CMV status).[6] Other strategies involve close monitoring for CMV disease and treating those upon detection of CMV in the serum.[7] CMV antigenemia (pp65-antigen assay), leukocyte PCR, and quantitative human CMV-DNA assays are all used as diagnostic tools for CMV detection.[8] CMV disease should be suspected in high-risk patients who develop fever, leukopenia, hepatitis, or pneumonitis. Another common post-transplant infection is *Pneumocystis carinii*, which historically occurred in 3–11% of liver transplant recipients who do not receive prophylaxis, leading to the widespread use of trimethoprim-sulfamethoxazole. Since the incidence of PCP following solid organ transplantation during the first year is eight times higher than during subsequent years, it is common practice to discontinue PCP prophylaxis after 1 year.[9] Rarely, reactivation of latent infections (herpes simplex or HHV-6) may also present in the early post-transplant period. Once patients have reached more than 6 months after transplantation, most have achieved a good outcome and are primarily at risk from community acquired respiratory viruses or recurrent viral hepatitis.

Biliary tract complications

Biliary tract complications are a very common cause of abnormal liver function tests after transplantation, occurring in 10–34% of cases, with biliary strictures occurring most frequently.[10] Biliary strictures are usually related to either technical (anastomotic) or ischemic (anastomotic or diffuse intrahepatic) causes. Evaluation of the biliary tract should be considered after liver transplantation in patients with recurrent fevers or rising gamma glutamyl transpeptidase, alkaline phosphatase, or bilirubin levels. Fluctuating calcineurin inhibitor drug levels without a change in dosage also raises suspicion for a biliary tract abnormality. Other reasons to investigate the biliary tract include evidence of cholangitis on liver biopsy or hepatic artery thrombosis, which

predisposes to both intrahepatic and extrahepatic stricturing. Although Doppler ultrasonography provides excellent initial screening for vascular and biliary abnormalities, cholangiography is essential to rule out biliary complications. Most anastomotic or simple strictures are amenable to percutaneous or endoscopic dilation with or without the use of biliary endoprostheses. Patients who do not respond to these conservative measures should be considered for biliary reconstructive surgery.

CHRONIC MEDICAL MANAGEMENT

Immunosuppressive therapy dominates much of the medical management that accompanies liver transplantation, as side effects are almost universal and may result in several long-term health issues that require attention. Calcineurin inhibitors are usually the foundation of maintenance immunosuppression protocols and play a direct role in the development of hypertension, diabetes, renal dysfunction, and hyperlipidemia. Prednisone is used in almost all immunosuppression protocols and is associated with early onset of post-transplant diabetes, hypertension, hyperlipidemia, and weight gain. It is even more likely to cause these problems when used chronically and therefore most centers attempt to discontinue corticosteroid use after the first few months. The level of maintenance immunosuppression is dictated according to the rejection history of the patient, underlying liver disease, comorbidities, and philosophical bias of the transplant program. Although many strategies exist, the common goal is to maintain the patient at the lowest level of immunosuppression necessary to avoid rejection and minimize the occurrence of immunosuppression-related side effects. The pharmacokinetics, drug interactions, side effects, and toxicities of the immunosuppressive agents are summarized in Tables 44.1 and 44.2 and form the basis for medical management after transplant.

Table 44.1 Current drugs used in maintenance immunosuppression

Drug	Strength	Frequency	Drug interactions	Side effects
Tacrolimus	0.5 mg, 1 mg, 5 mg	Twice daily	Numerous interactions Grapefruit juice elevates levels	Nausea, vomiting, diarrhea, headache, hair loss, HTN, tremors, hyperglycemia, hypomagnesemia, hyperkalemia, renal insufficiency
Cyclosporine	25 mg, 100 mg	Twice daily	Numerous interactions Grapefruit juice elevates levels	Hypertrichosis, tremors, headaches, gingival hyperplasia, HTN, nausea, vomiting, diarrhea, hyperkalemia, renal insufficiency
Sirolimus	1 mg, 2 mg	Once daily	CsA and ketoconazole markedly increase levels	Hyperlipidemia, leukopenia, thrombocytopenia, anemia, HSV infection
Mycophenolate mofetil	250 mg, 500 mg	Twice daily	Acyclovir, antacids with Mg or Aluminum, cholestyramine, Probenecid	Nausea, vomiting, diarrhea, headaches, leukopenia
Azathioprine	50 mg, 100 mg	Once daily	Allopurinol, ACE inhibitors	Nausea, vomiting, diarrhea, leukopenia, thrombocytopenia
Prednisone	1 mg, 2.5 mg, 5 mg, 10 mg, 20 mg, 50 mg	Once daily		Nausea, vomiting, stomach irritation, weight gain, fluid retention, mood swings, hyperglycemia, light sensitivity, *Candida*, cataracts, bone loss.

Table 44.2 Common drug interactions with immunosuppression drugs

Drug	Transplant medication	Effect on medication
Antibiotics: erythromycin, clarithromycin, ceftazidime, doxycycline	Calcineurin inhibitor	Increase levels of cyclosporine or tacrolimus
Anti-fungals: ketoconazole, fluconazole, clotrimazole, itraconazole		
Anti-hypertensives: diltiazem, nicardipine, verapamil, ace inhibitors		
Miscellaneous: metroclopramide cimetidine, quinolones, warfarin, phenobarbital, isoniazid, carbamezapine, barbiturate, phenytoin, rifampin, nafcillin and valproic acid	Calcineurin inhibitor	Decrease levels of cyclosporine or tacrolimus
Miscellaneous: allopurinol and ACE inhibitors	Azathioprine	May potentiate bone marrow suppression. May increase creatinine
Warfarin	Azathioprine	May decrease anticoagulation effect
Acyclovir	Mycophenolate	May increase acyclovir levels
Antacids/cholestyramine	Mycophenolate	Decrease absorption of mycophenolate

Neurologic and psychiatric complications

Patients who undergo a liver transplant may present with various neurologic manifestations that are often attributed to immunosuppression. These can be divided into three broad categories: intercurrent disease (mass lesion, neoplasm, abscess, allograft failure, and central pontine myelinolysis), immunosuppressant vasoconstriction (ischemia), or immunosuppressant pharmacodynamic effect (stroke, impaired neurocircuitry, encephalopathy, seizure).[11] Early symptoms related to immunosuppression commonly include tremors, headaches, parasthesias, insomnia, confusion, agitation, delirium, or seizures. Most of these symptoms will resolve with adjustment of immunosuppression. Use of SSRI agents should be discontinued in patients who experience post-transplant delirium and tremors as these drugs may worsen the neuronal serotonin depletion thought to be responsible for this presentation. Less common early CNS events that need to be considered include strokes, infections, leukoencephalopathy, central pontine myelinolysis, or malignancy.[12–15] Late symptoms include migraine-like headaches which may affect the ability to sleep, concentrate, or work. The treatment of headaches requires a step-wise approach and often includes reduction of immunosuppressant dose, beta blockers, caffeine-containing preparations, tylenol-based anlagesics, or serotonin agonists. Initial management should try to avoid aspirin, NSAIDs, or phenobarbital-like preparations such as fioricet which contains butalbital that may decrease calcineurin inhibitor drug levels by inducing the p450 system. The treatment of insomnia may include modification of medication schedule or use of sleep aides. Treatment of depression should be continued in those patients previously on medication, or initiated if significant depression ensues after transplant.

Gastrointestinal complications

Gastrointestinal (GI) symptoms are very common after liver transplantation. These can be a direct side effect of the immunosuppression or secondary to postoperative conditions. The most frequent GI symptom after transplantation is diarrhea, which has many potential causes. Timing of diarrhea can help distinguish the etiology. If early in the post-transplant course it likely can be attributed to immunosuppression. Other early causes include *Clostridium difficile* toxin-induced pseudomembranous colitis, bacterial overgrowth, antibiotic-induced diarrhea, or diarrhea as a consequence of other medications, such as magnesium supplements, proton pump inhibitors, or antimetabolites. Later-onset diarrhea (after 1 month) should raise the suspicion for other pathogens such as *Pneumocystis carinii*, *Listeria monocytogenes*, *Aspergillus*, and CMV. Parasites including *Strongyloides stercoralis* and *Giardia lamblia* can also be present under immunosuppression. Late (after 6 months) infectious causes include community acquired pathogens such as *Salmonella* and *Campylobacter*.

By far, the most common cause of diarrhea after transplantation is drug-induced. Steroids can cause diarrhea via mucosal injury, which can be prevented with H_2 blockers or proton pump inhibitors. Diarrhea is more common with tacrolimus and can lead to dehydration. Both tacrolimus and sirolimus have been associated with prokinetic effects.[16,17] Similarly, sirolimus by itself or in combination with cyclosporine can induce diarrhea. This diarrhea usually responds to lowering the dose of tacrolimus or sirolimus.[18] Mycophenolic acid (MPA) is also a common cause of GI symptoms and these may limit its clinical use in up to 20% of patients. Other GI complications include intestinal perforation and pancreatitis, which require urgent diagnosis and management. The etiology of these perforations is often unclear but cofactors to be considered include NSAID use, high-dose steroids, CMV infection, or diverticular disease.

Hypertension

Hypertension (HTN) is very prevalent in the transplant population, occurring in up to 50% of patients within the first year after transplant.[19,20] It is related to the use of calcineurin inhibitors and corticosteroids.[21] Consequences of prolonged and uncontrolled HTN are serious and include left ventricular hypertrophy, microangiopathic hemolysis, renal disease, and seizures. Additional risk factors for hypertension include chronic renal insufficiency, diabetes, alcohol intake, and obesity. Treatment of hypertension in transplant recipients should be based on the likely cause and the choice of antihypertensive agents may be influenced by coexistent medical conditions. The most common problems that affect the choice of antihypertensive therapy include renal dysfunction, hyperkalemia, and hypomagnesemia. Current recommendations for treatment thresholds of hypertension are based on updated guidelines (Table 44.3).[22] Diuretics may control mild hypertension or fluid-related hypertension. Diuretics may also be needed to control resulting peripheral edema in some patients. Furosemide should be used with caution due to its potential nephrotoxicity in association with cyclosporine. Calcium channel blockers are the first line of treatment of moderate HTN in the post-transplant setting. Calcium channel blockers cause smooth muscle dilatation and may counteract calcineurin inhibitor-induced afferent constriction. The usual drug regimen is long acting nifedipine (Procardia XL or Adalat CC, 30–90 mg/day). Nifedipine, isradipine, amlodipine and felodipine have no effects on calcineurin inhibitor drug levels, while verapamil, nicardipine and diltiazem increase levels and require close monitoring. Other agents that may be used include angiotensin-converting enzyme (ACE) inhibitors and angiotensin II antagonists (ARB), particularly if the patient has diabetes with proteinuria. Close monitoring of potassium and creatinine is required in patients on ACE inhibitors as calcineurin inhibitors may impair potassium and hydrogen ion secretion causing hyperkalemic metabolic acidosis. A rise in the creatinine up to 35% in patients with already compromised renal function is acceptable while using these drugs, provided that hyperkalemia does not develop. Beta blockers remain an alternate choice provided there is no contraindication for their use. Lifestyle changes are also important in the management of hypertension and should include weight reduction, exercise, salt restriction, and avoidance of alcohol.

Renal dysfunction

Azotemia, renal insufficiency, or hyperkalemia are not uncommon after liver transplantation. Up to a 30% decrease in creatinine clearance may develop in the first 6 months after transplant though renal function usually remains relatively stable thereafter in most patients. Nonetheless, the 5-year risk of chronic renal failure after liver transplantation is 18%.[23] The cause is multi-factorial and related to pre-existing diabetes or hypertension, immunosuppressive medications, or antihypertensives such as ACE inhibitors or ARB.[24] Calcineurin inhibitor therapy has been implicated as a principal cause of post-transplant renal dysfunction.[25]

Current definitions for chronic kidney disease are outlined in Table 44.4[26] Careful attention should be made to identify potentially reversible causes of renal insufficiency. However, creatinine values should be interpreted with caution, as they may not accurately reflect the underlying renal function. Since normal-range creatinine may give a false sense of security about the lack of renal problems, a 24-hour urine collection or other assessment of glomerular filtration rate is often required to define the degree of renal impairment.

Hyperlipidemia

Prior to transplantation, patients with parenchymal liver disease often have diminished cholesterol synthesis and esterification. In contrast, patients with chronic cholestatic disorders may have marked hyperlidemia due to production of protein X and impaired biliary secretion of cholesterol and phospholipids. Between 16%

Table 44.3 Classification of hypertension and treatment recommendations

Blood pressure	Systolic	Diastolic	Therapy
Normal	<120	<80	None
Prehypertensive	120–139	80–89	Treat if diabetic or CRD
Stage 1 hypertensive	140–159	90–99	Diuretics unless special disease*
Stage 2 hypertensive	>160	>100	2 drugs for most patients

*ACE/ARB are indicated in patients with DM, CAD, CKD (Cr >1.5 mg/dL), and heart failure. Beta blockers are indicated in CAD.

Table 44.4 Clinical practice guidelines for chronic kidney disease

Stage	Description	GFR (mL/min/1.73 m²)
1	Kidney damage*, normal or increased GFR	>90
2	Kidney damage with mild decrease GFR	60–89
3	Moderate decrease GFR	30–59
4	Severe decrease GFR	15–29
5	Kidney failure	<15 (or dialysis)

* Kidney damage is defined by pathologic abnormalities or markers of damage, including abnormalities in blood or urine tests or imaging studies.

and 43% of liver transplant recipients have elevated cholesterol and 40% have hypertrygliceridemia. Type 2a and 2b hyperlipidemia is one of the most common abnormalities observed after liver transplantation.[27] The causes are multifactorial and include excessive weight gain (average 30% post transplant), use of corticosteroids and cyclosporine, diabetes, hypothyroidism, and genetic susceptibility. Other contributing factors include increasing age, renal dysfunction, pretransplant hyperlipidemia, dietary factors and drugs such as beta blockers, diuretics, contraceptives, and alcohol. Patients who are hyperlipidemic may tolerate higher levels of cyclosporine, as it binds to lipoproteins. In contrast, patients with low cholesterol may show more side effects, even while maintaining low to therapeutic levels.

It is unclear whether sustained post liver transplant hyperlipidemia leads to atherosclerotic cardiovascular disease (ASCVD). A significant risk reduction has been shown in kidney transplant recipients and in the general population, but limited data are available in liver transplant recipients.[28] However, based on the known association of hyperlipidemia with atherosclerotic disease, it is reasonable to treat hyperlipidemia aggressively in this setting. An initial approach would be to encourage weight loss with diet modification and regular exercise. HTN and DM should be controlled and oral contraceptives should be avoided. When possible, modification of steroid or CSA doses may improve the abnormality. Several studies indicate that immunosuppression with tacrolimus is associated with less hyperlipidemia than with cyclosporine-based regimens. If these measures are unsuccessful, drug therapy should be utilized according to the guidelines published by the National Cholesterol Education Program Adult Treatment Panel III as outlined in Table 44.5.[29] Some general comments regarding the use of common agents in transplant recipients are important. Cholestyramine interferes with lipid-soluble drugs and may increase the triglycerides, limiting its use in this setting. If used, it should be given either 1 h before or 4 h after other medications. Nicotinic acid has potential hepatotoxic effects, but can be useful with mixed hyperlipidemia. HMG-CoA reductase inhibitors are potent inhibitors of cholesterol synthesis and form the basis of most medical intervention.[30] Rarely, these drugs can cause myopathy, rhabdomyolysis, constipation, asthenia, abdominal pain, nausea, and abnormal liver tests, mandating a careful monitoring schedule. Currently available drugs in this category such as atorvastatin, rosuvastatin, simvastatin, and pravastatin may also increase levels of calcineurin inhibitors.

Hyperglycemia

The prevalence of hyperglycemia after liver transplantation has been reported to be as high as 50%.[31] Development of post-transplant diabetes is related to multiple factors including the lack of reversal of insulin resistance after liver transplant, persistence of pancreatic insulin secretory failure,[32] and the diabetogenic effects of obesity and medications such as steroids and calcineurin inhibitors.[33–36] Calcineurin inhibitors are believed to cause diabetes via islet cell toxicity, diminished insulin synthesis or release, and decreased peripheral insulin sensitivity. They may also potentiate the hyperglycemic effects of corticosteroids.[37] Treatment of hyperglycemia in the post-transplant period is no different than in nontransplant patients and should initially include diet modification, weight loss, and increased activity. Medical therapy can include insulin, oral hypoglycemic agents such as sulfonylureas, or a biguanide such as metformin. The selection of a specific agent should be based on the baseline renal and hepatic function, which if impaired may not favor the selection of the oral agents which are mostly excreted by the kidney after metabolism occurs in the liver. Increased drug accumulation of metformin in the setting of renal dysfunction may contribute to lactic acidosis. In contrast to the pretransplant setting, more than 90% of post-transplant diabetics are insulin dependent, especially in the early post-transplant period.[38] However, with decreasing immunosuppression, the prevalence of insulin use decreases from 27% at 1 year after transplant to 7% at 3 years post transplant.[39] Compliance with current ADA guidelines should be encouraged, which include glucose levels less than 100 mg/dL, HgA$_1$ levels <6, and weight reduction to achieve a BMI below obesity.

Hyperuricemia

Elevated uric acid is very common after solid organ transplantation, but acute gout attacks are not common in liver transplant

Table 44.5 Cholesterol treatment guidelines

Risk category	LDL-C value	Intervention	LDL-C goal
Very high: CVD plus DM, HBP and cigarette smoking or metabolic syndrome	>100	Lifestyle changes and drug therapy	<70
High: CVD, DM or multiple risk factors with 20% chance of MI in 10 yr	>100	Lifestyle changes and drug therapy	<100
Moderately high: 2 or more risk factors with 10–20% chance of MI in 10 yr	>130 (100–129)	Lifestyle changes and drug therapy	<130 (<100)
Moderate: 2 or more risk factors; <10–20% chance of MI in 10 yr	>130 >160	Lifestyle changes Drug therapy	<130
Low: 0–1 risk factor	>160 >190	Lifestyle changes Drug Therapy	<160

recipients. Patients more likely to develop acute gout attacks are usually older, male, and have a history of either diabetes or hypertension, both conditions associated with decreased renal function. Hyperuricemia is felt to result from impaired GFR and decreased proximal tubular reabsorption of uric acid. Medications that can precipitate or exacerbate an attack include diuretics and aspirin. Hyperuricemia is more common with cyclosporine-based immunosuppression as the result of a drug-related decrease in uric acid clearance. Occasionally, uric acid crystals deposit within joint spaces and cause painful attacks of gouty arthritis. Treatment strategies available include a renal-modified dose of allopurinol, after initial acute treatment with colchicine. NSAIDs need to be used with caution, due to the potential worsening of renal function. Sulfinpyrazone can also be considered, but its use may be limited in patients with renal impairment. Intra-articular steroid injections, systemic steroids, or switching from cyclosporine- to tacrolimus-based immunosuppression have been used with some success.[40,41]

Thyroid abnormalities

Patients with liver disease may show subtle abnormalities in their thyroid tests which may reflect subclinical hypothyroidism. Understanding thyroid tests in the background of liver conditions can be complicated as both T_4 and T_3 are bound to protein predominantly via thyroxine-binding globulin (70%), albumin (15–20%), and transthyretin (10–15%). Commonly used medications that displace thyroid hormones from thyroid-binding globulins include furosemide, aspirin, NSAIDs, phenytoin, carbamezapine, and heparin. Medications such as iron, bile acid-binding resins, soy products, sucralfate, aluminum-containing antacids, and calcium may inhibit absorption of levothyroxine.[42]

Screening for hypothyroidism should be triggered by common symptoms such as fatigue, weight gain, constipation, dry skin, cold intolerance, or bradycardia. Less frequent symptoms include muscle cramps, infertility, menstrual irregularities, depression, sleep apnea, elevated LDL-cholesterol, hyperlipidemia, hypertension, or carpal tunnel syndrome. A significant background of autoimmune disease, prior treatment with interferon in those patients with viral hepatitis, or head and neck irradiation should also prompt screening. The guidelines that define this entity include elevated TSH, paired with a low free T_4. Normal values for TSH can range from 0.5 to 5.0 µU/ml, but the mean value in the normal population is 1.5 µU/ml.[43] Replacement can be calculated on 1.6 µg/kg/day.[44] Initial replacement therapy can be as low as 25–50 µg and can be raised every 6–8 weeks until a TSH level of 0.5–2 µU/ml is reached.[45] Once this goal is achieved the testing frequency can be spread to 6–12 months. Iatrogenic hyperthyroidism is defined by a very low TSH with a normal free T_4. A decrease in the thyroxine dose is indicated for these patients, since abnormalities in bone density[46] and cardiac function[47] have been described.

Obesity

Most patients experience weight gain after liver transplant. This is due to the general improvement in their health, increase in appetite, use of steroids, and fluid retention.[48,49] By 1 year, 40–70% of liver transplant recipients are overweight or obese.[50] The use of tacrolimus as the baseline immunosuppression may result in less weight gain than cyclosporine-based regimens.[51] Obesity is a major contributing factor in the development of other comorbidities after liver transplantation, including arterial hypertension, hyperlipidemia, diabetes mellitus, coronary artery disease, and osteoporosis. Thus, patients with pretransplant obesity should be encouraged to initiate treatment for their obesity in preparation for their transplant because pretransplant obesity is a risk factor for increased weight gain after transplantation.[52] In the post-transplant setting, it is important to encourage patients to exercise, avoid excessive weight gain, and limit corticosteroid use.

Osteoporosis

Bone loss is a common problem after transplantation and up to 30% of patients may sustain a fracture during transplant recovery, particularly if they are chronically bed ridden or have limited activity. Bone loss is worsened by immunosuppression, as both cyclosporine and tacrolimus may contribute to decreased osteoclast formation and steroids may worsen bone loss. Risk characteristics that should prompt a more aggressive screening strategy should include prior history of fractures, long-term use of steroids, postmenopausal state, hypogonadism, small body size or low body weight, history of smoking, excessive alcohol consumption, medication use such as anticonvulsants, heparin or corticosteroids, or medical conditions such as primary biliary cirrhosis, autoimmune hepatitis, alcoholic cirrhosis, hyperparathyroidism, hematopoietic disorders, chronic renal failure, malabsorption, gastrectomy, or celiac disease.

Strategies to lessen the consequences of this problem start with establishing a baseline bone density with a dexa scan, either preceding transplantation or in the months following it. Medication and lifestyle changes can be catered to the degree of loss with the aim of restoring the bone balance and preventing future fractures. T-scores between −1 and −2.5 define osteopenia, and values above −2.5 define osteoporosis. These values, along with the location of the bone loss (spine versus hip), should be used to decide on the choice of treatment modality. Available medications for treatment of osteoporosis are outlined in Table 44.6 and include weekly biphosphonates,[53] which bind to bone mineral and inhibit osteoclastic bone resorption. Raloxifene is a selective estrogen receptor modulator that has estrogen effects in the bone and blocks estrogen effects in the breast and uterus. Raloxifene increases bone mass and decreases vertebral fractures in postmenopausal women. Parathyroid hormone stimulates bone formation and increases bone mass, likely by decreasing apoptosis of osteoblasts. Teriparatide works by stimulating osteoblastic bone formation and markedly increases bone mass and reduces fractures.[54] It should not be used for longer than 2 years as there is some concern for development of osteosarcoma. All these medications should be supplemented with daily calcium (1000–1500 mg/d). Exercise that promotes bone strengthening, such as weight-bearing activity or low weight-bearing aerobic exercise, and control of obesity should also be promoted.

Other skeletal conditions which can occur with liver disease or after transplant include osteonecrosis and foot pain. Osteonecrosis often affects the femoral head and its presentation is characterized by acute pain and can be diagnosed with MRI. Treatment may include hip replacement in severe cases. Non-specific foot pain can be caused by calcineurin inhibitors and MRI may show

Table 44.6 Medications for the treatment of osteoporosis

Medication	Dose	Frequency	Route	Special concerns
Alendronate (Fosamax)	35–70 mg	Week	Oral	GI irritation, bone pain
Risedronate (Actonel)	35 mg	Week	Oral	GI irritation, bone pain
Raloxifene (Evista)	60 mg	Day	Oral	Thromboembolic events Hot flashes
Teriparatide (Forteo)	20 μg	Day	Sq	Osteosarcoma

bone marrow edema. Lowering drug levels may improve this complaint.

Reproductive function: contraception and pregnancy

After successful transplantation, young female patients usually recover their menses and regain normal sexual function with the potential of becoming pregnant. It is recommended that the female recipient wait between 6 months and a year before attempting pregnancy in order to optimize the immunosuppressive regimen and minimize rejection.[55] The selected contraceptive method remains the individual's choice but insertion of an IUD should be avoided as it has the potential for infection. Successful pregnancy is well documented among transplant recipients, but all such pregnancies should be monitored as high risk.[56] Possible complications include miscarriage (up to 40%), small for gestational age infants, hypertension, diabetes, infection, and rejection. No teratogenic effects have been reported secondary to immunosuppression and the dose should only be adjusted according to the transplant center's immunosuppressive protocol.

HEALTH MAINTENANCE

Immunizations and antibiotic prophylaxis

Despite evidence that vaccinations are safe and effective among immunosuppressed patients, most vaccines are underutilized in these patients.[57] Liver transplant recipients should receive influenza vaccination each fall and a pneumococcal primary immunization prior to transplantation and booster doses every 2–5 years.[58] All patients without pre-existing immunity should be vaccinated for hepatitis A and B prior to transplant. However, response is poor in patients with liver failure. The immune response to standard-dose HBV vaccine in the setting of patients awaiting liver transplantation is only 16–28%.[59] In order to overcome these poor responses, different strategies for hepatitis B vaccination have been utilized, including accelerated schedule, increased doses, and repeated vaccinations.[60,61] HBV vaccination is also becoming increasingly important for prophylaxis against reactivation in patients who receive a hepatitis B surface antigen negative and core antibody positive donor graft. Monitoring of titers should be considered after liver transplantation, with potential booster doses given when antibody levels fall below 10 mIU/ml.[62]

Consideration should be given to vaccination of pediatric and adolescent liver transplant candidates who have not had prior varicella infection and do not have detectable varicella-zoster

virus (VZV) IgG antibody.[63] However, the routine use of varicella vaccine in adult liver transplant recipients remains controversial, due to the small risk of reactivation of a live attenuated virus and development of zoster.[64] Thus, no recommendation can be given at this time. Liver transplant recipients indirectly exposed to VZV require only close monitoring, not active or passive immunization. For direct exposures, patients who are VZV IgG negative should be given varicella-zoster immune globulin (VZIG) prophylaxis within 96 hours of initial contact.[65]

Bacteremia arising from invasive procedures also represents a significant potential risk in the immunocompromised host, and premedication is usually recommended despite the lack of any controlled trials in this population.[66] Adherence to the current American Heart Association guidelines[67] that recommend a single-dose premedication regimen is most often utilized in an effort to minimize the risk of adverse drug reactions. Amoxicillin (2 g orally) is most often given 1 hour before the procedure, with clindamycin (600 mg) being used for those with a penicillin allergy.

CANCER SURVEILLANCE

Screening for cancer is important in the post-transplant setting, given the increased risk for certain malignancies due to the immunosuppressive regimen. De novo tumors are the leading cause of late death among liver transplant recipients with an incidence of 5–15%, which is significantly greater than the general population.[68] Screening for common cancers should adhere to current recommendations for colon, breast, cervical, and prostate screening.[69] Screening colonoscopy should start at age 50 or earlier if a clinical indication such as family history, guaiac-positive stool, or change in bowel habits is present.[70] Increased frequency of colonoscopy is recommended in patients who were transplanted for primary sclerosing cholangitis (PSC) and who have ulcerative colitis.[71,72] The recommendation of elective colectomy post transplant in patients with ulcerative colitis has been challenged by several studies,[73] but colectomy should certainly be undertaken if high-grade dysplasia is documented on any given screening biopsy.

Skin cancers are the most common malignancy in liver transplant recipients, eventually occurring in up to half of Caucasian recipients. Close surveillance is certainly warranted. The incidence of skin cancers is proportional to the level of immunosuppression,[74] and is increased in liver transplant recipients.[75] Rejection events and higher need for immunosuppression may increase the risk of skin cancer. However, sirolimus may confer a lower risk of cancer than standard therapy.[76,77] The most common skin cancer in transplant patients is squamous cell carcinoma and it occurs up to 250 times more frequently than in the general population. In contrast, basal cell carcinomas occur less commonly in the post-transplant setting (squamous to basal cell cancer ratio, 4:1) although the risk is still 10-fold higher than in the population at large.[78] UV light induces mutations in the p53 tumor suppressor gene and serves as the major risk factor for skin cancer.[79] Thus, areas exposed to the sun are more susceptible to the formation of cancer and the most common sites in young people (<40 years) are the dorsum of the hands, forearms, and upper trunk. In older patients (>60 years), lesions often develop on the head. Time of appearance of tumors after transplant is dependent on age, with an earlier appearance in patients over 60. In those who develop a skin cancer, recurrence can be as high as 25% at 1 year and 50% by 3.5 years, mandating close skin surveillance.

Other cancers that need to be surveyed include cancers in the anogenital region which tend to occur later after transplant, and for cancers of the vulva and perineum. Risk factor for the development of these cancers include multiple sexual partners, HPV infection, history of herpes genitalis, heavy smoking, the presence of skin cancers elsewhere, and a high level of immuno-suppression.[80,81] Lesions can be multiple, appearing as pigmented papular lesions with histological features of Bowen's disease. Persistent refractory wartlike lesions should therefore be examined histologically as the extent of the lesions can be as little as in situ carcinoma or involve lymph node metastasis. Treatment options include laser therapy, electrocautery, and topical fluorouracil. Invasive tumors require surgical excision and adjuvant therapy which may include radiotherapy and chemotherapy.[82] Tapering of immunosuppression to its lowest level is also a routinely recommendation.

Lymphomas affect up to 5% of transplant recipients and a relationship between immunosuppression and the development of post-transplant lymphoproliferative disorders (PTLDs) is well known.[83] They may be associated to EBV[84] or HHV-8.[85] These lesions most commonly involve sites such as lymph nodes, adenotonsillar region, allograft, gastrointestinal tract, or central nervous system.[86] Opelz et al. studied more than 50 000 solid organ transplants in Europe and North America and the incidence of PTLD was increased in the first year of transplantation when the degree of immunosuppression was highest.[87] B-cell lymphomas are by far the most common form of PTLD (90%). As for T-cell lymphomas, the majority of patients presented after 5 years, with less than 10% presenting in the first year. Compared with B-cell PTLD, T-cell lymphomas tend to manifest as mycosis fungoides, erythroderma, or hemorrhagic lesions, usually with generalized lymphadenopathy.[88] They also have a worse prognosis than B-cell lymphomas. Early detection is important for successful management, and patients with localized disease have been shown as a group to have the best prognosis.[89]

The outcome of PTLD has been correlated to clinical presentation. Patients with an infectious mononucleosis-like illness do well with reduction of immune suppression with or without other therapies. Patients with fulminant, disseminated, systemic disease that clinically resembles septic shock do poorly despite therapy. The majority of PTLD patients present with lymphomatous lesions (localized or disseminated) that are often extranodal. Although reduction of immune suppression may be sufficient in controlling the disease, patients who do not tolerate reduction of immune suppression (i.e., graft rejection), or do not respond to immune suppression reduction, require more aggressive therapy and have a much poorer prognosis, with a mortality reported to be as high as 50–90%.[90] Antiviral agents (acyclovir or ganciclovir) and/or i.v. immunoglobulin have been used extensively for prophylaxis and treatment of PTLD, but the efficacy of antivirals in treating PTLD is uncertain because antivirals are seldom used without other interventions (e.g., reduction of immunosuppression).[91] Other treatment approaches include local control with surgery and/or radiotherapy, which are very effective in curing localized disease, but this represents only a small percentage of patients. IFN has been used to treat PTLD that was refractory to immune suppression reduction with a complete remission rate of about 70%, but death caused by relapse, allograft rejection, and infection have been problematic, resulting in disease-free survival of less than 50%.[92] Successful treatment of PTLD necessitates controlling the inherent B-cell proliferation and facilitating the development of an appropriate EBV-CTL response. Immuno-therapy for PTLD using anti-B-cell antibodies was first attempted using anti-CD21 and anti-CD24 with a 55% long-term disease-free survival. More recently, a murine humanized chimeric anti-CD20 monoclonal antibody (Rituximab, Roche; typically, four to six doses are administered i.v. weekly) has been used, which usually depletes CD20+ B cells for over 12 months. Two phase II studies were completed and indicated that Rituximab was effective and well tolerated with few side effects.[93,94] The overall response was very good, complete remission was observed in 40–60% of patients, and a partial response observed in most other patients. For patients who fail reduction of immune suppression or anti-CD20+ therapy by not resolving the PTLD and/or developing rejection, cytotoxic chemotherapy is attractive because it will treat both processes. A low-dose chemotherapy regimen of Cy/Pred has been associated with good remission rates and allograft survival (>80%), and treatment-related toxicity was low (5%). The 2-year survival was 73%, but disease-free survival was only 58%.[95]

Recurrence of disease

Viral hepatitis, cholestatic diseases, metabolic diseases, and auto-immune hepatitis may all recur after liver transplantation. Primary biliary cirrhosis (PBC) and primary sclerosing cholangitis (PSC) may show classic lesions in allograft liver biopsies suggesting recurrent disease and are both associated with greater risk of developing acute and chronic rejection.[96] Rates of recurrence for PSC and PBC have been as high as 40%, but the indolent course observed in the majority of these patients does not appear to impact survival. Although no data are available on efficacy in the transplant population, ursodeoxycholic acid is often used for disease recurrence of PBC and PSC. Bile duct changes are not always related to recurrent PSC and the possibility of secondary changes from recurrent cholangitis or hepatic artery thrombosis should be considered.

Autoimmune hepatitis (AIH) commonly recurs post transplant and may be severe enough to require retransplant. Prior to considering a possible recurrence of this disease post transplant, other etiologies for abnormal aminotransferases need to be ruled out, including drug-induced and viral causes, as well as acute cellular rejection. Recurrence of AIH is diagnosed in almost one-third of patients based upon the presence of autoantibodies, increased gamma globulins, steroid dependency, and histological evidence of chronic hepatitis. Patients with AIH have a higher frequency of acute cellular rejection[97] and are often maintained on somewhat higher levels of immunosuppression long term.

Management of viral hepatitis in the transplant setting remains a very challenging issue. The strongest predictor of recurrence of HBV infection post transplant is the presence of pretransplant high level of HBV replication characterized by a serum HBV DNA level greater than 10^5 copies per milliliter with or without HBeAg. Patients with these markers appear to have a higher risk for reinfection than those with lower levels of HBV replication before transplant, although prophylaxis with hepatitis B immune globulin (HBIG) may override this predictive factor to a large degree.[98] In those patients who are persistently HBsAg-negative post transplant, overall survival is similar to that of patients transplanted for other diseases. Immunoprophylaxis with HBIG long-term in the post-transplant period (10 000 U i.v. q.d. × 7 days followed by 10 000 U i.v. q month thereafter to maintain the anti-HBs level 100–200 mIU/mL) has resulted in a decreased HBV recurrence rate (from 80–100% to 10–20%) and an increased survival.[99] Many centers are exploring the long-term use of lamivudine in combination with HBIG,[100] and the use of the intramuscular rather than intravenous route of administration of lower doses of HBIG.[101] Nucleoside analogues such as lamivudine or adefovir can usually control the progression of breakthrough post-transplant HBV infection.[102]

Although patients undergoing transplantation for HCV have been reported to have patient and graft survival comparable to most other indications[103,104] recurrence of hepatitis C is a substantial source of morbidity, mortality, and graft loss.[105,106] In a recent retrospective cohort study of over 11 000 transplant recipients, HCV infection as an indication for liver transplant was associated with significantly impaired patient and allograft survival.[107] Viral recurrence occurs universally; however, recurrence is apparent histologically in only about 50% of HCV-infected grafts and progression to allograft failure leading to death or graft loss occurs in approximately 10% by the fifth postoperative year.[108–110] When recurrent HCV leads to decompensated cirrhosis, retransplantation is now often denied due to very poor survival.[111] HCV-related disease progression is accelerated in immunocompromised compared to immunocompetent patients with a progressive increase in patients who have recently undergone LT, although the reasons for this worsening outcome are under question.[112] Possible reasons for this disturbing trend include the use of more potent immunosuppressive agents and more marginal donors (older).[113] Most transplant centers have employed surveillance liver biopsies on a yearly basis post-LT to allow clinicians to identify those recipients at increased risk for fibrosis progression and may allow better targeting of antiviral therapy.[114] Unfortunately, it is often difficult to distinguish recurrent HCV infection in the allograft histologically from that of acute cellular rejection. Thus, the diagnosis of recurrent hepatitis C post transplant may be challenging and requires an experienced liver pathologist.

Once recurrent HCV infection has been documented, it is reasonable to reduce immunosuppression in an attempt to decrease viral replication and subsequent hepatitis in the allograft. To date, however, there has been no good correlation between post-transplant serum HCV RNA levels and the degree of histologic viral hepatitis in the allograft. Recent studies are demonstrating effectiveness of combination antiviral therapy with interferon or peginterferon and ribavirin, with sustained loss of HCV RNA in 15–30% of patients, but when to initiate therapy remains uncertain. Treatment options after liver transplant include either early, empiric therapy in all patients or withholding treatment until there is histologic evidence of disease recurrence. When interferon-based therapy is started soon after liver transplantation, patients are typically taking high doses of immunosuppressive drugs, adverse side effects are high, and treatment discontinuation is common.[115] Although results have been mixed, some studies show that a proportion of patients can benefit from interferon-based therapy started within the first few weeks following transplantation. More commonly, HCV treatment is initiated months or years after liver transplantation, once signs of damage to the new liver are apparent. By this time, patients are usually healthier overall and taking lower doses of immunosuppressive drugs, enabling them to better tolerate HCV therapy. In general, studies have found sustained viral response (SVR) rates for this population to approach 30% using interferon plus ribavirin.[116] Although SVR rates for transplant recipients are lower than those seen in nontransplant patients, treatment can keep HCV under control in some individuals, and those who respond may experience decreased fibrosis progression. Caution is necessary, however, because interferon therapy may increase the risk of liver rejection. Further study is needed to determine the optimal timing for antiviral therapy.

SUMMARY

The continuing success of liver transplantation and the organ shortage has placed a premium on the long-term care of these patients. When a patient leaves the hospital, attention needs to focus on both routine and transplant-related comorbidities. Many medical issues require special considerations after transplantation, particularly those related to diabetes mellitus, hypertension, drug interactions, renal dysfunction, bone disease, and disease recurrence. A team approach between the allograft recipient, transplant physicians, and primary care provider continues to be the most effective strategy to ensure optimal patient care.

REFERENCES

1. Vogel A, Heinrich E, Bahr MJ, et al. Long-term outcome of liver transplantation for auotoimmune hepatitis. Clin Transplant 2004; 18(1):62–69.

2. Neuberger J. Liver transplantation for cholestatic liver disease. Curr Treat Options Gastroenterol 2003; 6(2):113–121.

   Good summary of transplant issues related to PBC and PSC.

3. Rubin RH, Schaffner A, Speich R. Introduction to the immunocompromised host society consensus conference on epidemiology, prevention, diagnosis, and management of infections in solid-organ transplant patients. Clin Infect Dis 2001; 33:S1–S4.

   Overview of medical complications arising in long-term management of liver transplant patients.

4. Patterson DL, Singh N. Invasive aspergillosis in transplant recipients. Medicine 1999; 78:123–132.

5. Gane E, Saliba F, Valdecasas GJC, et al. Randomized trial of safety and efficacy of oral ganciclovir in the prevention of cytomegalovirus disease in liver-transplant recipients. Lancet 1997; 350:1729–1733.

6. Singhal S, Khan OA, Bramble RA, et al. Cytomegalovirus disease following liver transplantation: an analysis of prophylaxis strategies. J Infect 2003; 47:104–109.

7. Paya CV, Wilson JA, Espy MJ, et al. Preemptive use of oral ganciclovir to prevent cytomegalovirus infection in liver transplant patients: a randomized, placebo-controlled trial. J Infect Dis 2002; 185:854–860.

8. Seehofer D, Meisel H, Rayes N, et al. Prospective evaluation of the clinical utility of different methods for the detection of human cytomegalovirus disease after liver transplantation. Am J Transplant 2004; 4:1331–1337.

9. Gordon SM, LaRosa SP, Kalmadi S, et al. Should prophylaxis for Pneumocystis carinii pneumonia in solid organ transplant recipients ever be discontinued? Clin Infect Dis 1999; 28:240–246.

10. Donovan J. Nonsurgical management of biliary tract disease after liver transplantation. Gastroenterol Clin North Am 1993; 22:317.

11. Beresford TP. Neuropsychiatric complications of liver and other solid organ transplantation. Liver Transplant 2001; 11:S36–S45.

12. Bonham CA, Dominguez EA, Fukui MB, et al. Central nervous system lesions in liver transplant recipients. Transplantation 1998; 66(12):1596–1604.

13. Adams DH, Ponsford S, Gunson B, et al. Neurological complications following liver transplant. Lancet 1987; 1(8539):949–951.

14. Singh N, Yu VL, Gayowski T. Central nervous system lesions in adult liver transplant recipients: Clinical review with implications for management. Medicine (Baltimore) 1994; 73(2):110–118.

15. Ferreiro JA, Robert MA, Townsend J, et al. Neuropathologic findings after liver transplantation. Acta Neuropathol (Berl) 1992; 84(1):1–14.

16. Maes BD, Vanwalleghem J, Kuypers D, et al. Differences in gastric motor activity in renal transplant recipients treated with FK-506 versus cyclosporine. Transplantation 1999; 68:1482–1485.

17. Maes B et al. Steroid-free immunosuppression during and after liver transplantation – a 3-yr follow-up report. Clinical Transplant 2003; 17:171–176.

18. Maes BD, Lemahieu W, Kuypers D, et al. Differential effect of diarrhea on FK 506 versus cyclosporine A trough levels and resultant prevention of allograft rejection in renal transplant recipients. Am J Transplant 2002; 2:989–992.

19. Stegall MD, Everson G, Schroter G, et al. Metabolic complications after liver transplantation: diabetes, hypercholesterolemia, hypertension and obesity. Transplantation 1995; 60(9)1057–1060.

20. Sheiner PA, Magliocca JF, Bodian CA, et al. Long-term medical complications in patients surviving > or =5 years after liver transplant. Transplantation 2000; 69(5):781–789.

   Overview of medical complications arising in long-term management of liver transplant patients.

21. Textor SC, Canzanello VJ, Taler SJ, et al. Cyclosporine-induced hypertension after transplantation. Mayo Clin Proc 1994; 69(12):1182–1193.

22. Chobanian AV, Bakris GL, Black HR, et al. The Seventh Report of the Joint National Committee on Prevention, Detection, Evaluation, and Treatment of High Blood Pressure: the JNC 7 report. JAMA 2003; 289:2560–2572.

   Current algorithm for HTN management.

23. Ojo AO, Held PJ, Port FK, et al. Chronic renal failure after transplantation of a nonrenal organ. N Engl J Med 2003; 349(10):931–940.

24. Lin J, Valeri AM, Markowitz GS, et al. Angiotensin converting enzyme inhibition in chronic allograft nephropathy. Transplantation 2002; 73:783–788.

25. Bennett WM, De Mattos A, Meyer MM, et al. Chronic cyclosporine nephropathy: the Achilles' heel of immunosuppressive therapy. Kidney Int 1996; 50:1089–1100.

26. National Kidney Foundation (NKF) Kidney Disease Outcome Quality Initiative clinical practice guidelines for chronic kidney disease, evaluation, classification, and stratification: Kidney Disease Oucome Quality Initiative. Am J Kidney Dis 2002; 39(Supple 2):S1–S246.

27. Munoz S, Deems R. Hyperlipidemia and obesity after liver transplantation. Transplant Proc 1991; 23:1480–1483.

28. Del Castillo D, Cruzado JM, Manel Diaz J, et al. The effects of hyperlipidaemia on graft and patient outcome in renal transplantation. Nephrol Dial Transplant 2004; 19(Suppl 3): iii67–71.

29. Grundy SM, Cleeman JI, Bairey Merz CN, et al. Implications of Recent Clinical Trials for the National Cholesterol Education Program Adult Treatment Panel III Guidelines. Circulation 2004; 110:227–239.

30. Wierzbicki AS. The role of lipid lowering in transplantation. Int J Clin Pract 1999; 53:54–59.

31. Trail KC, McCashland TM, Larsen JL, et al. Morbidity in patients with post transplant diabetes mellitus following orthotopic liver transplantation. Liver Transpl Surg 1996; 276–283.

32. Perseghin G, Mazzaferro V, Sereni LP, et al. Contributions of reduced insulin sensitivity and secretion to the pathogenesis of hepatogenous diabetes: Effect of liver transplantation. Hepatology 2000; 31:694–703.

33. Yale JF, Chamelian M, Courchesne S, et al. Peripheral insulin resistance and decreased insulin secretion after cyclosporine A treatment. Transplant Proc 1988; 20(Suppl 3):985–988.

34. Alejandro R, Feldman EC, Bloom AD, et al. Effects of cyclosporine on insulin and C-peptide secretion in healthy beagles. Diabetes 1989; 38:698–703.

35. Jindal RM, Sidner RA, Milgrom ML. Post transplant diabetes mellitus. The role of immunosuppression. Drug Safety 1997; 16:242–257.

36. Jain AB, Kashyap R, Rakela J, et al. Primary adult liver transplantation under tacrolimus: More than 90 months actual follow-up survival and adverse events. Liver Transpl Surg 1999; 5:114–150.

37. Chilcott JB, Witby SM, Moore R. Clinical impact and health economic consequences of posttransplant type 2 diabetes mellitus. Transplant Proc 2001; 33 (Suppl 5A):3S.

38. Trail KC, Stratta RJ, Larsen JL, et al. Results of liver transplantation in diabetic recipients. Surgery 1993; 114:650.

39. Navasa M, Bustamante J, Martoni C, et al. Diabetes mellitus after liver transplantation: Prevalence and predictive factors. J Hepatol 1996; 25:64–71.

40. Pilmore HL, Faire B, Dittmer I. Tacrolimus for the treatment of gout in renal transplantation: two case reports and a review of the literature. Transplantation 2001; 72(10):1703–1705.

41. Shibolet O, Elinav E, Ilan Y, et al. Reduced incidence of hyperuricemia, gout and renal failure following liver transplantation in comparison to heart transplantation: a longitudinal follow-up study. Transplantation 2004; 77:1576–1580.

42. Surks MI, Sievert R. Drugs and thyroid function. N Engl J Med 1995; 333:1688–1694.

43. Hollowell JG, Staehling NW, Flanders WD, et al. Serum TSH, T4, and thyroid antibodies in the United States population (1988 to 1994): National Health and Nutritional Examination Survey (NHANES III). J Clin Endocrinol Metab 2002; 87:489–499.

44. Franklin JA, Daykin J, Betteridge J, et al. Thyroxine replacement therapy and circulating lipid concentrations. Clin Endocrinol 1993; 38:453–459.

45. McDermott MT, Haugen BR, Lezotte DC, et al. Management practices among primary care physicians and thyroid specialists in the care of hypothyroid patients. Thyroid 2001; 11:757–764.

46. Bauer DC, Ettinger B, Nevitt MC, et al. Risk for fracture in women with low serum levels of thyroid-stimulating hormone. Ann Intern Med 2001; 134:561–568.

47. Biondi B, Palmieri EA, Lombardi G, et al. Effects of subclinical thyroid dysfunction on the heart. Ann Intern Med 2002; 137:904–914.

48. Palmer M, Schaffner F, Thung SN. Excessive weight gain after liver transplantation. Transplantation 1991; 51:797–800.

49. Hasse J. From malnutrition to obesity: Changes in nutritional status associated with liver transplantation. Nutrition 1999; 15:507–508.

50. Munoz SJ, Deems RO, Moritz MJ, et al. Hyperlipidemia and obesity after orthotopic liver transplantation. Transpl Proc 1991; 23:1480.

51. Canzanello VJ, Textor SC, Taler SJ, et al. Evolution of cardiovascular risk after liver transplantation: A comparison of cyclosporine A and tacrolimus. Liver Transpl Surg 1997; 3:1.

52. Keefe EB, Gettys C, Esquivel CO. Liver transplantation in patients with severe obesity. Transplantation 1994; 57:309.

53. Cranney A, Tugwell P, Wells G, et al. Meta-analysis of therapies for post-menopausal osteoporosis. I. Systematic review of randomized trials in osteoporosis: introduction and methodology. Endocr Rev 2002; 23:496–507.

54. Neer RM, Arnaud CD, Zanchetta JR, et al. Effect of parathyroid hormone (1-34) on fractures and bone mineral density in post-menopausal women with osteoporosis. N Engl J Med 2001; 344:1434–1441.

55. Riley CA. Contraception and pregnancy after liver transplantation. Liver Transplant 2001; 11:S74–S76.

56. Laifer SA. Guido RS. Reproductive function and outcome of pregnancy after liver transplantation in women. Mayo Clin Proc 1995; 70:388–394.

57. Henning KJ, White MH, Sepkowitz KA, et al. A national survey of immunization practices following allogeneic bone marrow transplantation. JAMA 1997; 277:1148–1151.

58. Duchini A, Goss JA, Karpen S, et al. Vaccinations for adult solid-organ transplant recipients: current recommendations and protocols. Clin Microbiol Rev 2003; 16:357–364.

Recommendations for vaccinations in transplant recipients.

59. Chalasani N, Smallwood G, Halcomb J, et al. Is vaccination against hepatitis B indicated in patients waiting for or after orthotopic liver transplantation? Liver Transpl Surg 1998; 4:128–132.

60. Dominguez M, Barcena R, Garcia M, et al. Vaccination against hepatitis B virus in cirrhotic patients on liver transplant waiting list. Liver Transpl 2000; 6:440–442.

61. Kallinowski B, Benz C, Bucholz L, et al. Accelerated schedule of hepatitis B vaccination in liver transplant candidates. Transplant Proc 1998; 30:797–799.

62. Hibberd PL, Rubin RH. Approach to immunization in the immunosuppressed host. Infect Dis Clin North Am 1990; 4:123–142.

63. Broyer M, Tete MJ, Guest G, et al. Varicella and zoster in children after kidney transplantation: long term results of vaccination. Pediatrics 1997; 99:35–39.

64. Krause P, Klinman DM. Efficacy, immunogenicity, safety, and use of live attenuated chickenpox vaccine. J Pediatr 1995; 127:518–525.

65. Levitsky J, Te HS, Faust TW, et al. Varicella infection following varicella vaccination in a liver transplant recipient. Am J Transplan 2002; 2:880–882.

66. Cohen D, Galbraith C. General health management and long term care of the renal transplant recipient. Am J Kidney Dis 2001; 38:S10–S24.

67. Dajani AS, Taubert KA, Wilson W, et al. Prevention of bacterial endocarditis: recommendations by the American Heart Association. JAMA 1997; 277:1794–1801.

68. Rubio E, Moreno JM, Turrion VS, et al. De novo malignancies and liver transplantation. Trans Proc 2003; 35:1896–1897.

69. US Preventive Services Task Force. Guide to clinical preventive services. 2nd edn. Baltimore: Williams & Wilkins; 1996.

70. Fleischer DE, Goldberg SB, Browning TH, et al. Detection and surveillance of colorectal cancer. JAMA 1989; 261:580–585.

71. Narumi S, Roberts JP, Emond JC, et al. Liver transplantation for sclerosing cholangitis. Hepatology 1995; 22:451–457.

72. Knechtle SJ, D'Alessandro AM, Harms BA, et al. Relationship between sclerosing cholangitis, inflammatory bowel disease, and cancer in patients undergoing liver transplantation. Surgery 1995; 118:615–620.

73. Loftus EV, Aguilar HI, Sandborn WJ, et al. Risk of colorectal neoplasia in patients with primary sclerosing cholangitis and ulcerative colitis following orthotopic liver transplantation. Hepatology 1998; 27:685–690.

74. Bouwess-Bavinck JN, Hardie DR, Green A, et al. The risk of skin cancer in renal transplant recipients in Queensland, Australia: a follow-up study. Transplantation; 1996; 61:715–712.

75. Frezza EE, Fung JJ, van Thiel DH. Non-lymphoid cancer after liver transplantation. Hepatogastroenterology 1997; 4:1172–1181.

76. Guba M, von Breienbuch P, Steinbauer M, et al. Rapamycin inhibits primary and metastatic tumor growth by antiangiogenesis: involvement of vascular endothelial growth factor. Nat Med 2002; 8:128–135.

77. Luan FL, Hojo M, Maluccio M, et al. Rapamycin blocks tumor progression: unlinking immunosuppression from antitumor efficacy. Transplantation 2002; 73:1565–1572.

78. Euvard S, Kanitakis J, Claudy A. Skin cancers after organ transplantation. N Engl J Med 2003; 348:1681–1691.

79. McGregor JM, Berkhout RJM, Rsozyck M, et al. P53 mutations implicate sunlight in post-transplant skin cancer irrespective of human papillomavirus status. Oncogene 1997; 15:1737–1740.

80. Arends MJ, Benton EC, McLaren KM, et al. Renal allograft recipients with high susceptibility to cutaneous malignancy have an increased prevalence of human papillomavirus DNA in skin tumours and a greater risk of anogenital malignancy. Br J Cancer 1997; 75:722–728.

81. Euvard S, Kanitakis J, Chardonnet Y, et al. External anogenital lesions in organ transplant recipients: a clinicopathologic and virologic assessment. Arch Dermatol 1997; 133:175–178.

82. Sillman FH, Sentovich S, Shaffer D. Anogenital neoplasia in renal transplant recipients. Ann Transplant 1997; 2:59–66.

83. Starzl TE, Nalesnik MA, Porter KA, et al. Reversibility of lymphomas and lymphoproliferative lesions developing under cyclosporine-steroid therapy. Lancet 1984; 1(8337): 583.

84. DeCarlis L, Slim A, De Gasperi A, et al. Posttransplant lymphoproliferative disorders: report from a single center. Transplant Proc 2001; 33:2815–2816.

85. Kapelushnik J, Ariad S, Benharroch D, et al. Post renal transplantation human herpesvirus 8-associated lymphoproliferative disorder and Kaposi's sarcoma. Br J Haematol 2001; 113:425–428.

86. Cohen JI. Epstein-Barr virus lymphoproliferative disease associated with acquired immunodeficiency. Medicine 1991; 70:137.

87. Opelz G, Henderson R. Incidence of non-Hodgkin lymphoma in kidney and heart transplant recipients. Lancet 1993; 342: 1514–1516.

88. Euvrard S, Pouteil Noble C, Kanitakis J, et al. Successive occurrence of T-cell and B-cell lymphomas after renal transplantation in patients with multiple cutaneous squamous-cell carcinomas. N Engl J Med 1992; 327:1924–1926.

89. Leblond V, Dhedin N, Mamzer Bruneel MF, et al. Identification of prognostic factors in 61 patients with posttransplantation lymphoproliferative disorders. J Clin Oncol 19: 772, 2001.

90. Benkerrou M, Jais JP, Leblond V, et al. Anti-B-cell monoclonal antibody treatment of severe posttransplant B-lymphoproliferative disorder: prognostic factors and long-term outcome. Blood, 1998; 92:3137–3147.

91. Cohen JI. Epstein-Barr virus lymphoproliferative disease associated with acquired immunodeficiency. Medicine (Baltimore) 1991; 70:137–160.

92. Davis CL, Wood BL, Sabath DE, et al. Interferon-α treatment of posttransplant lymphoproliferative disorder in recipients of solid organ transplants. Transplantation (Baltimore) 1998; 66:1770–1779.

93. Rehwald U, Schulz H, Reiser M, et al. Treatment of relapsed CD20+ Hodgkin lymphoma with the monoclonal antibody rituximab is effective and well tolerated: results of a phase 2 trial of the German Hodgkin Lymphoma Study Group. Blood 2003; 101:420–424.

94. Ekstrand BC, Lucas JB, Horwitz SM, et al. Rituximab in lymphocyte-predominant Hodgkin disease: results of a phase 2 trial. Blood 2003; 101:285–289.

95. Gross TG, Hinrichs SH, Winner J, et al. Treatment of post-transplant lymphoproliferative disease (PTLD) following solid organ transplantation with low-dose chemotherapy. Ann Oncol 1998; 9:339–340.

96. Neuberger J. Liver transplantation for cholestatic liver disease. Curr Treat Options Gastroenterol 2003; 6:113–121.

97. Vogel A, Heinrich E, Bahr MJ, et al. Long-term outcome of liver transplantation for autoimmune hepatitis. Clin Transplant 2004; 18:62–69.

98. McGory RW, Ishitani MB, Oliveira WM, et al. Improved outcome of orthotopic liver transplantation for chronic hepatitis B cirrhosis with aggressive passive immunization. Transplantation 1996; 61:1358–1364.

99. Kruger M. European hepatitis B immunoglobulin trials: prevention of recurrent hepatitis B after transplantation. Clin Transplant 2000; 14:14–19.

100. Markowitz JS, Martin P, Conrad AJ, et al Prophylaxis against hepatitis B recurrence following liver transplantation using combination lamivudine and hepatitis B immune globulin. Hepatology 1998; 28:585–589.

    Article showing benefit of most commonly applied strategy for HBV prophylaxis.

101. Faust D, Rabenau HF, Allwinn R, et al. Cost-effective and safe ambulatory long-term immunoprophylaxis with intramuscular instead of intravenous hepatitis B immunoglobulin to prevent reinfection after orthotopic liver transplantation. Clin Transplant 2003; 17:254–258.

102. Lo CM, Fan ST, Liu CI, et al. Prophylaxis and treatment of recurrent hepatitis B after liver transplantation. Transplantation 2003; 75:S41–S44.

103. Ascher NL, Lake JR, Emond J, et al. Liver transplantation for hepatitis C virus-related cirrhosis. Hepatology 1994; 20:24S–27S.

104. Feray C, Gigou M, Samuel D, et al. The course of hepatitis C virus infection after liver transplantation. Hepatology 1994; 20:1137.

105. Charlton M, Seaberg E, Wiesner R, et al. Predictors of patient and graft survival following liver transplantation for hepatitis C. Hepatology 1998; 28:823–830.

106. Gayowski T, Singh N, Marino IR, et al. Hepatitis C virus genotypes in liver transplant recipients: impact on posttransplant recurrence, infections, response to interferon-alpha therapy and outcome. Transplantation 1997; 64:422–426.

107. Forman LM, Lewis JD, Berlin JA, et al. The association between hepatitis C infection and survival after orthotopic liver transplantation. Gastroenterology 2002; 122:889–896.

108. Feray C, Samuel D, Thiers V, et al. Reinfection of liver graft by hepatitis C virus after liver transplantation. J Clin Invest 1992; 89:1361–1365.

109. Rosen HR, O'Reilly PM, Shackleton CR, et al. Graft loss following liver transplantation in patients with chronic hepatitis C. Transplantation 1996; 62:1773–1776.

110. Rosen HR, Gretch DR, Oehlke M, et al. Timing and severity of initial hepatitis C recurrence as predictors of long-term liver allograft injury. Transplantation 1998; 65:1178–1182.

111. Roayaie S, Schiano TD, Thung SN, et al. Results of retransplantation for recurrent hepatitis C. Hepatology 2003; 38:1428–1436.

112. Berenguer M, Ferrell L, Watson J, et al. HCV-related fibrosis progression following liver transplantation: increase in recent years. J Hepatol; 2000; 32:673–684.

    Evaluation of HCV recurrence and discussion of factors related to disease severity.

113. Machicao VI, Krishna M, Bonatti H, et al. Hepatitis C recurrence is not associated with allograft steatosis within the first year after liver transplantation. Transplantation 2004; 77:84–92.

114. Firpi RJ, Abdelmalek MF, Soldevila-Pico C, et al. One-year protocol liver biopsy can stratify fibrosis progression in liver transplant recipients with recurrent hepatitis C infection. Liver Transpl 2004; 10:1240–1247.

    Article describes a rationale for using protocol liver biopsy to stratify patients for antiviral therapy based on early predictors for disease recurrence.

115. Terrault NA. Prophylactic and preemptive therapies for hepatitis C virus-infected patients undergoing liver transplantation. Liver Transpl 2003; 9(11):S95–S100.

116. Firpi RJ, Abdelmalek M, Soldevila-Pico C, et al. Combination of interferon alfa-2b and ribavirin in liver transplant recipients with histologic recurrent hepatitis C. Liver Transplant 2002; 8(11): 1000–1006.

CHAPTER FORTY-FIVE

45

Primary tumors of the liver

Hashem B. El-Serag

INTRODUCTION

Liver cancer refers to a variety of malignant diseases that are either primary or secondary to the liver. Primary liver cancers include hepatocellular carcinoma (HCC), cholangiocarcinoma (CC), angiosarcoma, and several other rare forms. In addition, the liver is affected by several benign tumors including cavernous hemangioma, fibronodular hyperplasia, and adenoma. The liver is also a frequent site for secondary tumors that metastasize, most frequently from colorectal, breast, and the stomach.

Each year over half a million persons worldwide are affected with primary liver cancer and almost an equal number die of it. HCC accounts for 85–90% of liver cancers. One noteworthy exception is in the Khon Kaen region of Thailand, where due to endemic infestation with liver flukes, the major type of primary liver cancer is intrahepatic CC.[1] Concern about primary liver cancer has been growing, due to the recognition of the magnitude of the problem in many developing countries and a striking increase in the number of cases in the US and other Western countries in recent years. This increase is due largely to an increase in HCC incidence, which has doubled over the last two decades in the US.[2]

PRIMARY LIVER TUMORS

Hepatocellular carcinoma

Epidemiology and risk factors

There are remarkable variations in the incidence of HCC related to age, sex, geography, race, and ethnicity. HCC is rarely seen during the first four decades of life, but becomes more common with increasing age, reaching a peak between the ages of 70 and 75 years. In the United States, Asians are two to three times more likely to have the tumor than African-Americans, who, in turn, are two to four times more likely to be affected than Caucasians. In all ethnic groups, men are two to three times more likely to be affected than women. The sex and ethnicity related differences are partly explained by differences in the prevalence of risk factors such as hepatitis B virus (HBV) and hepatitis C virus (HCV), alcohol, and increased iron stores. The great majority of HCC cases (>80%) occur in either sub-Saharan Africa or in Eastern Asia. In most high-risk areas the dominant risk factor is chronic HBV infection. In Japan, unlike the rest of Asia, the dominant hepatitis virus is HCV. The recent rising incidence rates of HCC reported from

several countries in North America, Europe, and Asia has also been linked to HCV. For example, in the USA, the yearly age-adjusted incidence rate of HCC increased twofold from 1.4 per 100 000 during 1976–1980, to 3.0 per 100 000 during 1996–1998, with at least half of the increase related to HCV.[2]

HCC is unique in that it occurs largely in the context of known risk factors. In most cases, it appears that cirrhosis represents the key mediator. Diseases such as chronic hepatitis C or alcoholism first cause cirrhosis, followed by the development of HCC.

Chronic infection with HCV increases the risk of HCC by 15- to 20-fold. Of HCV-infected patients, approximately 1–3% develops HCC after 2–4 decades of chronic infection. The progression to cirrhosis and HCC among HCV-infected persons is increased with older age, male gender, heavy alcohol intake, HBV coinfection, and possibly obesity and HIV coinfection. Viral factors such as genotype, quasispecies, or viral load do not appear to be important risk factors for HCC. Successful antiviral therapy of patients with HCV-related cirrhosis may reduce the future risk of HCC, especially in those who achieve a sustained virological response.[3] Antiviral therapy may also be effective for secondary prevention in individuals who have undergone resection for HCC.[4]

Chronic HBV carriers (i.e., positive for HBV surface antigen; HBsAg) have a 5- to 15-fold increase in the risk of HCC than the general population. The annual HCC incidence in chronic HBV carriers in Asia ranges between 0.1% and 0.6%. Factors that increase the risk of HCC among HBV carriers include older age, male gender, Asian or African race, cirrhosis, family history of HCC, exposure to aflatoxin B1 (AFB-1), alcohol and tobacco, coinfection with HCV and HDV, and the presence of HBeAg.[3,5] In addition AFB_1, a mycotoxin elaborated by fungi of the *Aspergillus* species, interacts with HBV to increase the risk of HCC. The characteristic genetic change associated with AFB_1 (p53 249[ser] mutation) has been observed in approximately half of the tumors arising in persons living in high AFB-1 areas but in virtually none of the cases seen in Western countries. In HBV carriers, the spontaneous or treatment-induced development of antibodies against HBsAg and HBeAg leads to improvement in the clinical outcome and possible reduction in HCC risk. A significant decline in the incidence of HCC during childhood and adolescence has been reported in high HBV prevalence areas following the introduction of universal childhood hepatitis B vaccination.[6]

Heavy alcohol intake defined as daily ingestion of an amount greater than 50–70 g/day for prolonged time periods is a risk factor for HCC by predisposing to cirrhosis. There is little evidence for a direct carcinogenic effect for alcohol otherwise.

More recently, there is evidence that links HCC with obesity, diabetes, and insulin resistance, factors that are involved in the development of nonalcoholic steatohepatitis (NASH). Case-control studies have indicated that HCC patients with cryptogenic cirrhosis tend to have clinical and demographic features suggestive of non-alcoholic fatty liver disease, namely a predominance of women, diabetes, and obesity.[7] There is a fivefold increase in liver cancer among heavy persons with BMI 35–40 as compared to those with normal BMI.[8] Diabetes has been associated with a two- to three-fold increase in HCC risk, especially with type 2 diabetes, and longer duration of the disease.[9] Diabetes predisposes to fatty liver disease and is also associated with increased levels of insulin and insulin-like growth factors, which are potential cancer promoting factors.

Clinical presentation

HCC may present with right upper quadrant pain, weight loss, and/or worsening liver enzymes in a patient known to have cirrhosis. Rare presenting features include rupture with intra-abdominal bleeding, or extrahepatic manifestations (e.g., hyper-calcemia, hyperglycemia, thyrotoxicosis). Anemia is present in more than half of cases, although rarely erythrocytosis can be seen due to extrarenal synthesis of erythropoietin. In addition to signs of cirrhosis and portal hypertension, a hepatic bruit could be detected in 10–20% of patients with HCC. A quarter of patients presenting with HCC have previously undiagnosed cirrhosis. More patients are being diagnosed with HCC at an asymptomatic stage as a result of widespread use of surveillance imaging studies.

Surveillance for HCC

Rationale

The goal of surveillance of patients with liver cirrhosis is to detect HCC at an early stage when it is more likely to be amenable to therapies that may prolong survival. HCC detected in patients receiving surveillance is likely to be smaller, unifocal and amenable to surgical resection, local ablation or transplantation than tumors not discovered through surveillance. Of those detected by surveillance, 50–75% are unifocal, less than 3 cm in size, and potentially treatable with resection or transplantation. However, the actual resection rate is lower and varies between 35% and 55% with old age, cirrhosis, and comorbidity as the main contraindications. Importantly, it is not clear whether the all-cause or cancer-related mortality are improved by surveil-lance. There is no evidence from prospective randomized trials to indicate the efficacy of HCC surveillance and it is highly unlikely that it will ever be conducted, mainly for practical and ethical reasons. Similarly, the optimal method and frequency of surveil-lance and the cost-effectiveness of surveillance for HCC have yet to be established. However, the majority of hepatologists employ some sort of HCC surveillance, which has become an accepted part of the management of patients with liver disease.[10]

In appropriate candidates (Table 45.1) HCC surveillance may be beneficial. The ideal target population is patients with Child-Pugh's class A cirrhosis and no severe comorbid illness. Patients who are not suitable for potentially curative therapy should not receive HCC surveillance, as they are unlikely to benefit. HCC surveillance is not indicated in chronic liver disease without cirrhosis except in those with HBV. With the exception of areas in the world where HBV is endemic, it is uncommon to find HCC in

Table 45.1 Recommendations for hepatocellular carcinoma (HCC) surveillance

Surveillance for HCC is recommended for the following groups

Cirrhosis of any cause

Adults with chronic hepatitis B, especially if acquired early in life, and/or a family history of HCC

Adults with hereditary hemochromatosis

Previously resected HCC

Metabolic liver diseases known to increase HCC risk (e.g., hereditary tyrosinemia)

Surveillance for HCC is not recommended for the following groups

Healthy individuals with no liver disease (i.e., screening)

Patients with HCV infection and no cirrhosis

Patients who are not candidates for surgical resection, liver transplantation, or ablative therapy

the absence of cirrhosis. Once cirrhosis is established, the annual rate of HCC is between 1% and 6%. In HCV-related cirrhosis, high-baseline AFP and low platelets may reflect increased HCC risk.

Methods of HCC surveillance

The preferred method of HCC surveillance is a combination of serological marker (e.g., AFP) and noninvasive imaging (e.g., ultrasound). Given that the tumor doubling time of HCC is approximately 4–6 months, a commonly recommended surveil-lance frequency is every 6 months. However, a number of studies suggest that a longer surveillance interval (1 year) is as effective as the 6-month interval.

The most commonly used and tested serological marker for HCC surveillance is alpha-fetoprotein (AFP). Approximately 30% of HCC cases do not present with serum AFP elevation, especially in patients with small HCC. On the other hand, modest elevation of AFP levels (10–100 ng/mL) can be seen in patients with chronic viral hepatitis or cirrhosis in the absence of HCC. Therefore, when AFP >20 ng/ml is used alone for HCC surveillance, it has a low sensitivity and specificity of approximately 50–60%, and a very low positive predictive value of 10%. The higher the AFP cut-off level, the higher the specificity and the lower the sensitivity. Thus, the use of AFP alone in HCC surveillance is generally not recom-mended. Measurement of various HCC-specific isoforms of AFP such as Lens culinaris agglutinin A-reactive alpha-fetoprotein improves specificity for HCC but sensivity remains low. However, the development of a routine assay is technically challenging and has prevented widespread clinical application. Another marker, Des-gamma-carboxy prothrombin (DCP), is a form of prothrombin that is deficient in carboxyglutamic acid residues making the molecule inactive as a prothrombin. The combination of AFP and DCP increases the sensitivity for HCC detection slightly over AFP alone.[10,11]

Ultrasound (US) is the most commonly used imaging modality for HCC surveillance. The use of US for HCC surveillance has been examined in healthy HBV carriers and in patients with cirrhosis. The reported sensitivity of US as a surveillance test for HCC ranges between 40% and 70%, the specificity is between 80% and 90%, and the positive predictive value ranges between 15% and 20%. The diagnostic accuracy of US depends partly on the operator's experience and the patient's body habitus. US has poor sensitivity in detecting HCC lesions less than 3 cm, and multifocal or diffuse HCC. Similarly, US does not distinguish large regenerative nodules from HCC. High-grade dysplastic nodules, which develop into HCC in approximately 30% of cases, are usually 1 cm or less in size and are also missed by US. CT scan or MRI is more sensitive in detecting HCC than US.[10,11] The performance and utility of CT or MRI imaging has not been well examined for HCC surveillance; in addition, these tests are more expensive and require the use of a contrast material. These tests are usually reserved for surveillance in preliver transplant settings, and as confirmatory or diagnostic tests in cases of abnormal AFP and/or US.

Surveillance and recall strategy

The European Association for the Study of Liver Disease expert panel proposed a reasonable strategy for surveillance and recall (Fig. 45.1). During surveillance, patients found to have *progressive* elevation of serum AFP levels >20 ng/mL and negative US examination should undergo contrast-enhanced CT scan or MRI to exclude occult lesions.[11]

The detection of a hypo- or hyperechoeic nodule should receive further investigation. In patients with a small mass lesion (<1 cm), serial ultrasound every 3 months is recommended until growth beyond 1 cm is established, since malignancy is only present in these small nodules (<1 cm) in less than 50% of cases, they are difficult to characterize by other imaging studies (CT or MRI), and they are difficult to biopsy.[11]

For mass lesions between 1–2 cm in size, there is a higher chance of HCC. The combined use of fine needle aspiration with biopsy, contrast imaging, and AFP is recommended for diagnosis. For lesions of that size, none of these tests has a high accuracy when used alone. Fine needle aspiration may have a 30–40% false-negative rate for diagnosis, and the diagnostic accuracy of radiologic with or without serological tests is uncertain. Limitations of noninvasive methods include the misclassification of vascular dysplastic nodules as HCC. Furthermore, early HCC that is defined histologically as carcinoma-in-situ may be classified by US as a nodule though it appears hypovascular on CT; hence, it is likely to be missed or misclassified.[11]

For large lesions of 3 cm and more, a biopsy may not be required in the presence of imaging studies with typical HCC findings, especially if multiple imaging studies are used and AFP levels are elevated more than 400 ng/mL. Practitioners should become familiar with local expertise in noninvasive and invasive radiology, as this frequently dictates the choice of testing.

Diagnosis of HCC

HCC diagnosis is usually made by fine needle biopsy of a suspected mass. Surgical biopsy procedures (via laparoscopy) may also be performed. The routine use of biopsy is becoming controversial, particularly in patients who may be potentially cured by surgical resection or liver transplantation. There is a small risk (less than 1%) of spreading HCC along the needle track with percutaneous needle biopsy. In addition, there is 10–20% false-negative rate for biopsy. Biopsy, however, should be attempted for lesions smaller than 2 cm, lesions difficult to distinguish on imaging studies, or in young patients (<40 years) where fibrolamellar carcinoma comprises a large proportion of cases. On the other hand, a biopsy may not be required if the diagnosis of HCC can be made accurately by noninvasive tests. For example, biopsy may not be required in the presence of a mass greater than 3 cm with characteristic features of HCC on imaging studies (e.g., CT scan or MRI) and elevated AFP greater than 400–500 ng/mL. Given the radical nature of some HCC therapies such as liver transplantation, one has to weigh the small risk of tumor seeding with biopsy against transplantation for a false-positive test. For those who satisfy the size, number, and

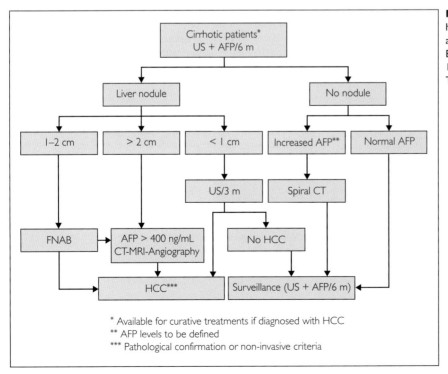

Fig. 45.1 • Surveillance and recall strategy for hepatocellular carcinoma. US, ultrasound; AFP, alpha-fetoprotein; m, months. (Reprinted from El Serag HB et al, Gastroenterology, 2004; 126:460–468. © 2004, with permission from The Amercian Gastroenterological Association.)

* Available for curative treatments if diagnosed with HCC
** AFP levels to be defined
*** Pathological confirmation or non-invasive criteria

liver disease status criteria for resection or transplant, further staging is performed using CT scan of the chest and bone scan.[11,12]

Diagnostic imaging

Noninvasive imaging tools rely on the different vascular supply to distinguish between malignant and benign nodules. HCC derives its blood supply predominantly from the hepatic artery whereas the remainder of the liver receives both arterial and portal blood. In addition, HCC has abundant internal blood vessels. US is usually the first imaging study performed. On US examination, HCC is typically hypoechoic especially if small and a capsule may be noted. Multifocal tumors and daughter nodules are two common features of HCC. Conventional US, while a valuable surveillance test, has limited diagnostic value due to its inability to examine the important feature of abnormal vascularity characteristic of HCC. False-positive results also arise from inability to distinguish HCC from nonmalignant regenerating nodules or premalignant dysplastic nodules. The use of contrast agents containing encapsulated microbubbles increases the sensitivity and specificity of US for both detection and characterization of HCC by being able to demonstrate increased vascularity. The presence of arterial hypervascularization (i.e., contrast enhancement on the arterial phase of an MRI or CT scan) is highly predictive of HCC in the appropriate set-up (e.g., patients with cirrhosis). MRI of HCC is typically hypointense on T-1- and hyperintense on T-2-weighted images. The sensitivity and specificity of contrast-enhanced spiral CT for HCC diagnosis is approximately 70% and 80%, respectively. These figures are slightly higher for MRI. The sensitivity decreases with tumors of less than 2–3 cm, and both CT and MRI fail to detect HCC lesions less than 1 cm in 30–40% of cases. Regenerative and dysplastic nodules usually have normal hepatic arteries and portal veins within the lesion. These lesions are usually homogenous and they are iso or hypointense in T2-weighted MRI, whereas almost all moderately or poorly differentiated HCC demonstrate mild hyperintensity. Radioisotope scans of the liver should not be used due to lack of both sensitivity and specificity. The use of Lipiodol CT scan has been largely abandoned as a result of its low accuracy. Positron emission tomography (PET) is not an effective technique for the detection of HCC. Angiography use is limited at present except as a route for the administration of chemoembolization.[12]

Prognosis of HCC

The prognosis of patients with HCC is generally poor, with a median survival of 7–8 months, a 1-year survival of less than 20%, and a 5-year survival rate of 6%.[13] However, survival of patients with HCC is strongly dependent on the stage of cancer at the time of diagnosis, the underlying severity of liver disease, presence of comorbid conditions, and whether potentially curative therapy is applied. *Carcinoma in situ* is the earliest clinical entity currently recognized; it is a well-differentiated HCC that contains bile ducts and portal veins and by definition has not invaded any structure and is less likely to recur and relapse. For these patients, the 5-year survival rate approaches 90% and 70% following resection and local ablation, respectively. Patients with small HCC (less than 2 cm) have approximately 70% and 50% survival rates at 5 years following resection or percutaneous ablation, respectively.[13,14] The prognosis of patients presenting with advanced HCC is poor, especially in those with cancer-related symptoms, vascular invasion, or extrahepatic spread where survival rates of less than 20% at 3 years have been reported. Lastly, the small number of patients (less than 15% of total) who receive either surgical resection or transplantation in the United states have an overall 5-year survival of up to 40%. United Network for Organ Sharing (UNOS) data indicate that patients treated with liver transplantation have a 57% 5-year survival. Unfortunately, HCC is commonly diagnosed at an advanced stage in patients with decompensated liver disease, making curative therapy very unlikely.[13]

Conventional tumor node metastasis (TNM) is limited by poor accuracy in predicting the prognosis of an individual patient because it excludes variables representing underlying liver function. Therefore, a number of staging systems have been developed to aid in determining individualized prognosis and eligibility for treatment. One recommended staging system is that of Cancer of the Liver Italian Program (CLIP). The CLIP classification shown in Table 45.2 is relatively easy to calculate based on clinical and imaging features and was prospectively validated and shown to predict survival in a wide range of patients with HCC (Table 45.3). It includes four variables: Child-Pugh Class, number and extent of tumor(s), AFP levels, and portal vein thrombosis. CLIP score is also useful in identifying patients who are unlikely to tolerate or benefit from any of the available therapies. Patients with high CLIP scores (virtually all of those with scores 4–6, and most of those with CLIP score of 3) should receive supportive and symptomatic care only.[15] Another commonly cited classification is the Barcelona Clinic Liver Cancer (BCLC), which is useful for giving therapy recommendations, especially for early and intermediate HCC stage (Fig. 45.2).[16]

Treatment of HCC

Unfortunately, less than 15% of patients with HCC receive potentially curative therapy in population-based studies, and even in

Table 45.2 CLIP staging system

Variables	Score		
	0	1	2
Child-Pugh class	A	B	C
Tumor morphology	Single nodule and <50% area*	Multiple nodules and <50% area	Massive or >50% area
AFP (ng/mL)	<400	>400	
Portal vein thrombosis	No	Yes	

The score ranges between 0 and 6.
* Cross-sectional area on imaging.

Table 45.3 HCC prognosis using the CLIP staging system

CLIP score	Median survival (months)	One-year survival	Two-year survival
0	36	84%	65%
1	22	66%	45%
2	9	45%	17%
3	7	36%	12%
4 to 6	3	9%	0%

(Reprinted from Bugianesi E et al, Digestive Liver Disorder, 2004; 36:165–173. © 2004, with permission from Editrice Gastroenterological Italiana S.r.l.)

referral centers less than 30% receive such therapy.[13] Three potentially curative therapies (surgical resection, liver transplantation, nonsurgical local ablation) are recommended for patients with early HCC. Studies on the efficacy of these therapies have demonstrated longer survival rates for patients with tumors less than 3 cm in size as compared to historical survival rates in studies of natural history. However, there is no direct evidence to support this contention. Furthermore, there are no randomized, controlled trials comparing the efficacy of these therapies. Palliative therapy is offered to approximately half of the patients, and of those only a small proportion are able to tolerate and benefit from chemoembolization, the only palliative therapy with somewhat proven benefit. For the rest of patients with advanced liver disease, tumor spread, and poor functional status, only symptomatic and supportive measures should be offered.[14] A recommended approach to treating HCC is outlined in Fig. 45.2; this approach has been formalized by investigators from the Barcelona Clinic Liver Cancer group.[16]

Surgical resection

Resection of HCC should be considered for all patients who have no cirrhosis or Child A cirrhosis, and no extrahepatic spread. Because most HCCs occur in patients with advanced cirrhosis, tumor spread, or both, these patients are at high risk of decompensation if surgical resection is attempted and only a small number of patients can undergo surgical resection. Among patients with Child A cirrhosis, applying more stringent criteria such as normal bilirubin levels and the absence of portal hypertension to determine suitability for surgical resection reduces operative mortality to <5%, but further limits the number of patients who qualify for this therapy. Subjects with no portal hypertension and normal bilirubin have up to 70% survival at 5 years following

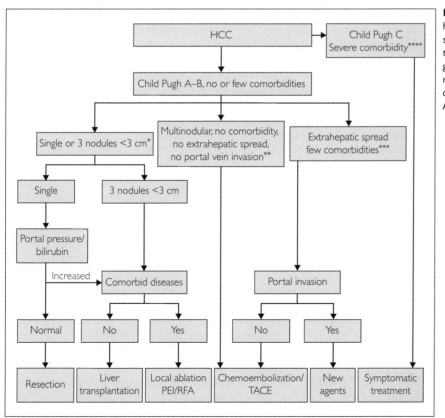

Fig. 45.2 • An algorithm for the treatment of hepatocellular carcinoma. It is based on and is slightly modified from the algorithm proposed by the Barcelona Clinic Liver Cancer (BCLC) group.[2,9] PEI, percutaneous ethanol injection; RFA, radiofrequency ablation; TACE, transarterial chemoembolization. According to BCLC * Stage A, ** Stage B, *** Stage C, and **** Stage D.

resection, which diminishes to 50% in those with portal hypertension and normal bilirubin, and to 25% in patients with portal hypertension and abnormal bilirubin. Significant portal hypertension is indicated clinically by the presence of splenomegaly, low platelet count, or esophageal varices, or by the presence of a hepatic venous pressure greater than 10 mmHg. After surgical resection, there is a high recurrence rate greater than 70% at five years. Larger tumors are associated with increased risk of dissemination and therefore with disease recurrence related to the presence of vascular invasion or additional tumor size. In addition, liver resection does not eliminate the remaining portions of the liver at risk for malignant transformation. The postresection residual liver, often cirrhotic, has the same high potential for HCC. Treatment with interferon after resection in HCV-infected patients is recommended to reduce the risk of recurrence. One regimen that has been shown to be effective is interferon-alpha, 6 MIU intramuscularly daily for 2 weeks, then three times weekly for 14 weeks, and finally twice weekly for 88 weeks.[4] Other agents used to decrease recurrence include retinoids, and lipiodol coupled to 131-Iodine.

Liver transplantation

Orthotopic liver transplantation (OLT) has become an established treatment for HCC, especially when tumor characteristics and hepatic reserve are such that resection cannot be safely performed. Transplantation has the advantage of removing the cancer and the remaining liver tissue that is at risk for the development of new cancer as well as restoring hepatic function. Large tumors, multiple nodules, vascular invasion, and poor differentiation are associated with increased risk of tumor recurrence after transplantation. However, using strict selection criteria (The Milan Criteria) for transplantation, Mazzaferro et al. reported a 75% actuarial survival rate and a low recurrence rate (15%) at 4 years following transplantation in patients with HCC.[17] These selection criteria, which are also adopted by the United Network for Organ Sharing (UNOS), include the presence of solitary tumors less than 5 cm or up to 3 nodules each of less than 3 cm. HCC recurrence is much lower with OLT than that of resection if these criteria are used. These figures are currently diminished independent of tumor recurrence in the HCV infected due to the universal post-transplant recurrence of HCV, with 25% of patients developing cirrhosis within 5 years. Unfortunately, the majority of patients with HCC exceed these criteria and, therefore, are not ideal candidates for transplantation. Transplantation is also limited by the shortage of donor organs. With longer waiting time, contraindications to transplantation develop in up to 50% of patients within 1 year, usually because of progression of HCC. In the United States, there have been recent changes in prioritization for allocation of deceased donor livers that have given a substantial advantage to patients with HCC, and perhaps also resulting in increased frequency of false-positive HCC diagnosis.[18] Chemoembolization, ethanol injection, and radiofrequency ablation are commonly employed while waiting for transplant although the benefit of these procedures is unclear. There are only limited data on survival after living donor liver transplantation but most series show comparable short-term patient survival with that in cadaveric transplants.

Local ablation

In patients who are not eligible for surgical resection or transplantation, ablation of HCC may be accomplished by either chemical (e.g., ethanol) or physical means (e.g., radiofrequency ablation, or microwave coagulation). Ablation is associated with similar recurrence-free survival to that achieved with surgical resection in patients with a single HCC lesion of less than 3 cm. US or CT-guided percutaneous ethanol injection (PEI) used to be the standard ablative technique in patients who have less than 3 lesions that are smaller than 5 cm, with no significant coagulopathy, and no ascites. Tumors smaller than 2 cm in diameter can usually be completely ablated in a single session. Larger tumors require 2 to 3 sessions. Recently, the use of radiofrequency ablation (RFA) has become an established mode of therapy for HCC because of its ability to destroy HCC (up to 5 cm in size) at one session. RFA is performed either via a percutaneous or laparoscopic approach. Despite earlier reports of high rates of RFA needle-track HCC seeding, subsequent studies have failed to corroborate these findings. The most common complications following ablation are local pain or bleeding; however, serious complications are rare and there is virtually no procedure-associated mortality. RFA also carries a small risk of ground pad burns and thermal burns of adjacent viscera, and approximately one-third of patients experience postablation flu-like symptoms 3–5 days after the procedure. Similar to surgical resection, a trial of interferon treatment is recommended following local ablation in HCV-infected patients to decrease of the incidence of recurrent HCC.

Palliative therapy

For patients not suitable for potentially curative therapy, the median survival is 6–7 months. Transarterial chemoembolization (TACE) provides a modest increase in survival in selected patients with unresectable HCC. The beneficial effect is restricted to patients with preserved liver function (Child-Pugh A) without cancer-related symptoms or vascular invasion.[19] Only a small proportion of individuals (10–15%) with HCC are optimal candidates for TACE. In these patients a 2-year survival of 50–60% can be achieved. TACE is performed by injecting chemotherapeutic agents into the hepatic artery, which is then occluded by injection of particulate materials such as Gelfoam, polyvinyl alcohol, blood clots, or microspheres to obstruct flow. Obstruction can also be produced by the placement of metallic coils, but this may reduce the potential for repeated treatment sessions. Extensive tumor necrosis can be achieved in more than 80% of patients. Side effects of chemoembolization include severe pain, liver failure, and formation of liver abscess. TACE is contraindicated when the tumor is diffuse throughout the liver, in the presence of decompensated liver disease, and in the presence of portal vein thrombosis. If the portal blood flow is obstructed by tumoral invasion or reversed by the presence of advanced cirrhosis, the tolerance to arterial obstruction is reduced and the risk of associated mortality is increased. Arterial embolization without chemotherapy has no evidence to support a similar positive impact on survival. The choice of chemotherapeutic agent does not seem to make a large difference in the results, with doxorubicin and cisplatinum being the most commonly used agents.

Systemic agents have been typically studied in the more advanced patients, making outcomes predictably worse. There is no data to support a standard systemic chemotherapy and, in the United States, there is no approved systemic treatment for HCC. No survival benefit has been shown with tamoxifen. Radiofrequency and thermal ablation, transcutaneous alcohol injection, and transarterial internal radiotherapy with Yttrium-90 spheres have been shown to result in significant reduction in size of HCC, but their efficacy in prolonging survival has yet to be demonstrated.[20]

Cholangiocarcinoma

Cholangiocarcinoma (CC) is a malignancy of the bile ducts that is classified depending on its location as either intrahepatic or extrahepatic. Intrahepatic CC can be either peripheral, arising from smaller bile ducts, or central (perihilar). Intrahepatic CC comprises 10–15% of all primary liver tumors in most countries in Europe and North America, and up to 90% of these tumors in Thailand and the Philippines. Recent reports have documented a threefold increase in the incidence and mortality related to ICC in the United States between 1975 and 1999. There are only few risk factors for ICC and they explain a small proportion of all cases; these include primary sclerosing cholangitis, parasitic infestations (*Opisthorcis viverrini*), Thorotrast exposure, choledochal cysts, and possibly chronic liver disease and hepatitis C virus.[21] The management of CC is discussed in detail in Chapter 30.

Other malignant primary liver tumors

Fibrolamellar carcinoma

Fibrolamellar carcinoma (FLC) constitutes approximately 1% of all cases of primary liver cancer and 13% of all cases below the age of 40. There have been conflicting reports on whether this malignancy is a histological variant of HCC or a different biological entity. The epidemiological features in the USA are quite different between FLC and HCC. Patients with fibrolamellar carcinoma are younger (mean age 39 versus 65), more likely female (52% versus 26%), and white Caucasian (85% versus 60%) compared with HCC. The 5-year survival rates are significantly longer in patients with fibrolamellar carcinoma (32%) than those of HCC (7%). Survival following FLC is significantly longer than HCC even after adjusting for age of cancer diagnosis, and receipt of therapy. The presence of intralesional calcification is characteristic of FLC and is a useful distinctive feature from focal nodular hyperplasia.[22] The treatment is similar to that of HCC.

Angiosarcoma

Angiosarcoma or hemangiosarcoma is an aggressive sarcoma of the liver. Although rare, angiosarcoma is the most common malignant mesenchymal tumor of the liver. Some cases have been linked to remote exposure to thorium dioxide, arsenic-containing insecticides, or vinyl chloride monomers. Most patients are first seen with advanced disease that is not amenable to surgery. The results of irradiation and chemotherapy are poor.

Epithelioid hemangioendothelioma

Epithelioid hemangioendothelioma is a low-grade malignancy with a slight female preponderance and possible association with oral contraceptive use. A massive lesion may produce a Budd-Chiari syndrome or veno-occlusive disease. It is commonly misdiagnosed as a non-neoplastic condition such as scar tissue, granulation, cirrhosis, or veno-occlusive disease, especially on small biopsies. The prognosis is variable but generally good in spite of its malignant potential. Treatment is complete surgical resection, but extensive disease involving both lobes of the liver may require total hepatectomy and liver transplantation. The efficacy of chemotherapy and radiotherapy is unclear. Following orthotopic liver transplantation, 33% of hepatic epithelioid hemangioendothelioma recur; the 2-year survival rate is 82%, whereas the 5-year survival is 43%.

HEPATIC METASTASES

Metastases often present with multiple smaller lesions, all approximately the same size, whereas HCC and CC lesions often have a dominant larger mass surrounded by smaller lesions. Metastases are readily imaged by CT, MRI, or US. The diagnosis is typically confirmed by needle biopsy. When a cancer spreads to the liver, it is generally an indication of incurable disease and therapeutic interventions are intended mainly for palliation. The exceptions include some cases of metastatic colorectal carcinoma and in neuroendocrine tumors where the prognosis may not be so poor. Prolonged survival has been reported after surgical resection for metastatic colorectal carcinoma confined to the liver. Five-year survival rates approaching 40% have been reported. Large and repeated resections have been performed with minimal hepatic compromise. Cryoablation is being used primarily for the palliative treatment of colorectal carcinoma metastases. Fluoropyrimidines delivered either systematically or by intrahepatic arterial infusion may produce objective responses in unresectable metastatic colorectal carcinoma.

Neuroendocrine tumors that originate from the gastrointestinal tract frequently metastasize to the liver. These tend to be slowly growing tumors, and their morbidity is attributed mostly to the severe symptoms with which they are associated, including carcinoid and Zollinger-Ellison syndromes. Liver metastases may be surgically resected, and sometimes resection with embolization of the hepatic artery is performed to reduce residual tumor bulk. Traditional chemotherapy is not generally effective because of the slowly growing nature of these malignancies. Interferon-α has been associated with objective tumor responses. Use of the somatostatin analogue octreotide in carcinoid syndrome may result in considerable improvement in symptoms. Patients with metastatic neuroendocrine tumors have been successfully treated with OLT.

BENIGN LIVER TUMORS

Cavernous hemangioma

Cavernous hemangioma is the most common benign tumor of the liver and is found in as many as 10% of livers at autopsy. The great majority of cavernous hemangiomas are small and asymptomatic. The risk of rupture is very small even in patients with giant hemangiomas. Rarely, massive hemangiomas may be a site for intravascular coagulation and result in consumptive coagulopathy (Kasabach-Merritt syndrome).

Hemangiomas are usually discovered incidentally on US examination where the characteristic finding is a solitary round mass with a well-demarcated border, encapsulated appearance, vascular features, and bright echoes within the tumor. However, the sensitivity of US for diagnosis of cavernous hemangioma ranges between 60% and 75%, and specificity ranges between 60% and 80%. The recommended initial diagnostic test is a dynamic CT scan, which has sensitivity between 75% and 85%, and specificity ranging between 75% and 90%. The characteristic feature of cavernous hemangioma on CT scan is a hypodense center with a focal globular enhancement caused by collection of contrast in dilated vascular spaces within the tumor. Technetium-labeled (^{99}Tc) red blood cell single photon emission computed tomographic (SPECT) scanning is often used as a confirmatory test for lesions larger than 3 cm in diameter. MRI has the greatest sensitivity (85–95%) and specificity (85–95%) for diagnosis of hepatic hemangioma but is more expensive than SPECT and should probably be reserved for small and/or deeply positioned lesions. Characteristic findings on MRI include multiple intra-tumoral lobulations and high signal intensity on T2-weighted images. This characteristic 'light-bulb appearance' results from slow-flowing blood through the hemangioma.[23] Needle biopsy should not be performed if a cavernous hemangioma is suspected because of the risk of bleeding.

The great majority of cavernous hemangiomas require no treatment. Routine follow-up is also not necessary for lesions that appear typical with diagnostic imaging. Surgical resection is indicated for lesions causing pain, or for very large tumors (more than 10 cm) to eliminate risk of hemorrhage, thrombosis, and rupture. If surgical resection is not feasible, arteriographic embolization, irradiation, or systemic glucocorticoids have been rarely used.[24]

Focal nodular hyperplasia

Focal nodular hyperplasia is a circumscribed lesion composed of nodules of benign hyperplastic hepatocytes surrounding a central stellate fibrous scar. It is the second most common benign liver tumor. It is seen more often in women than men, although the sex difference is less striking than that of adenoma. A role for oral contraceptive steroids in the development of the lesion has been suggested, but is doubtful. Areas of focal nodular hyperplasia are usually small (less than 5 cm in diameter) and single. Most of these lesions are asymptomatic.

The diagnosis is often difficult. Serum AFP levels are normal. A central scar may be seen in less than half of cases on US or CT. The absence of intralesional calcification (which are present in fibrolamellar carcinoma) and signs of chronic liver disease are helpful features. Dynamic contrast-enhanced Doppler US with intra-arterial infusion of microbubbles shows characteristic findings. Selective hepatic arteriography shows a highly vascular lesion that contains septation in about 50% of cases. However, it is often difficult to differentiate focal nodular hyperplasia from adenoma on the basis of the angiographic findings.[23] MRI has higher sensitivity (70%) and specificity (90%) for focal nodular hyperplasia. Typically, the lesion is iso- or hypointense on T1-weighted images, slightly hyperintense on T2-weighted images, and has a hyperintense central scar on T2-weighted image.

Given that the risk of rupture or development of malignancy is extremely small, no specific treatment is needed for focal nodular hyperplasia although they are often resected as part of diagnostic work-up. Periodic US should be performed if a definite diagnosis of focal nodular hyperplasia has not been established, and a lesion seen to increase in size should be resected. Large symptomatic or complicated lesions should be resected, usually by segmental resection or enucleation. If the lesion is not resected, a trial of discontinuing contraceptive use should be attempted.[24,25]

Hepatic adenoma

Hepatocellular adenomas are rare tumors strongly linked to the use of oral contraceptive steroids. The estimated relative risk for women who use oral contraceptive agents continuously longer than 9 years is 15- to 25-fold higher than controls not using these agents. Sporadic adenomas otherwise are rare, especially in men. Hepatic adenomas are solitary in approximately three-quarters of cases. They are usually asymptomatic but may result in abdominal discomfort or even pain. Worsening pain may indicate impending rupture, an uncommon but dreaded complication. Progression to HCC has been documented in a few cases but is rare.

Hepatic adenomas do not take up contrast used in nuclear scanning due to the absence of Kupffer cells, and the characteristic finding on scintigraphic study is a focal defect in the liver whereas focal nodular hyperplasia is often hyperdense. The sonographic appearance of hepatic adenoma is non-specific unless there is an internal hemorrhage, which produces increased echogenicity acutely. The findings of hepatic adenomas on CT scan and MR imaging are relatively non-specific. The noncontrast-enhanced appearance of hepatic adenoma may be hypodense to the remainder of the liver. With contrast enhancement, the hepatic adenoma often enhances in a centripetal fashion. Hepatic angiography, although seldom used, shows a characteristic 'spoke-wheel appearance' where parallel vessels are seen entering a clearly defined mass from the periphery. One characteristic of hepatic adenoma seen on all imaging studies is the encapsulated lesion with well-defined borders. Serum AFP concentrations are normal. Because adenomas mimic normal liver tissue microscopically, needle biopsy and fine needle aspiration may be of limited value.[24,25]

Oral contraceptives should be discontinued, whether or not the tumor is removed. Discontinuing these medications will result in regression of adenoma in some cases. Hepatic adenoma irrespective of size and symptoms should be removed surgically because of the risk of rupture and cancer. If the adenoma is not resected, then pregnancy should also be avoided.

SUMMARY

Hepatocellular carcinoma (HCC) is the most common primary liver tumor, and it continues to increase in several countries in Europe and North America due to HCV-related chronic liver disease. Surveillance of high-risk patients with AFP and ultrasound may detect HCC in a stage amenable to potentially curative therapy including surgical resection, liver transplantation, and local ablation. Palliative therapy with transarterial chemoembolization may prolong survival in some patients with compensated liver disease and patent portal vein. HCC diagnosis can be made with a combination of several advanced imaging techniques (e.g., triple-phase CT scan, MRI) and serum AFP with or without tissue confirmation. The latter is required for smaller tumors. Several relatively simple models can be used to determine prognosis. Intra-hepatic cholangiocarcinoma constitutes 10–15% of primary liver cancer and has either a peripheral variety that is similar in risk factors and management to HCC, or perihilar (central), for which surgical resection is curative, but is rarely possible. There are several benign liver tumors including hemangioma, fibronodular hyperplasia, adenoma, in descending order of frequency. These have characteristic appearance on imaging studies, and certain unique risk factors. The diagnosis and management of these tumors is discussed in some detail.

REFERENCES

1. McGlynn KA, Tsao L, Hsing AW, et al. International trends and patterns of primary liver cancer. Int J Cancer 2001; 94:290–296.

2. El Serag HB, Davila JA, Petersen NJ, et al. The continuing increase in the incidence of hepatocellular carcinoma in the United States: an update. Ann Intern Med 2003; 139:817–823.

3. El-Serag HB. Epidemiology of hepatocellular carcinoma. Clin Liver Dis. 2001; 5:87–107, vi.

   A contemporary review of the global epidemiology of HCC, with special emphasis on the United States.

4. Shiratori Y, Shiina S, Teratani T, et al. Interferon therapy after tumor ablation improves prognosis in patients with hepatocellular carcinoma associated with hepatitis C virus. Ann Intern Med. 2003; 138:299–306.

5. Lok AS. Prevention of hepatitis B virus-related hepatocellular carcinoma. Gastroenterology 2004; 127(5 Suppl 1):S303–S309.

6. Chang MH, Chen CJ, Lai MS, et al. Universal hepatitis B vaccination in Taiwan and the incidence of hepatocellular carcinoma in children. Taiwan Childhood Hepatoma Study Group. N Engl J Med 1997; 336:1855–1859.

7. Bugianesi E, Zannoni C, Vanni E, et al. Non-alcoholic fatty liver and insulin resistance: a cause-effect relationship? Dig Liver Dis 2004; 36:165–173.

8. Calle EE, Rodriguez C, Walker-Thurmond K, et al. Overweight, obesity, and mortality from cancer in a prospectively studied cohort of US adults. N Engl J Med 2003; 348:1625–1638.

9. El Serag HB, Tran T, Everhart JE. Diabetes increases the risk of chronic liver disease and hepatocellular carcinoma. Gastroenterology 2004; 126:460–468.

10. Collier J, Sherman M. Screening for hepatocellular carcinoma. Hepatology 1998; 27(1):273–278.

    This article provides an evidence-based systematic approach to the pros and cons of HCC surveillance, and is a must read for anyone interested in HCC surveillance.

11. Bruix J, Sherman M, Llovet JM, and EASL Panel of Experts on HCC. Clinical management of hepatocellular carcinoma. Conclusions of the Barcelona-2000 EASL conference. European Association for the Study of the Liver. J Hepatol 2001; 35(3):421–430.

    A very useful article that contains clear tables containing 'cookbook' guidelines, and ample explanation of the rationale behind these guidelines.

12. Befeler AS, Di Bisceglie AM. Hepatocellular carcinoma: diagnosis and treatment. Gastroenterology 2002; 122(6):1609–1619.

    This easy to read article offers a rational expert summary of the current diagnostic and therapeutic options for HCC. This is especially relevant to practitioners in North America.

13. El-Serag HB, Mason AC, Key C. Trends in survival of patients with hepatocellular carcinoma between 1977 and 1996 in the United States. Hepatology 2001; 33(1):62–65.

    This article provides prognosis data from the unique perspective of population-based study as opposed to more optimistic results from referral centers.

14. Llovet JM, Burroughs A, Bruix J. Hepatocellular carcinoma. Lancet 2003; 362(9399):1907–1917.

    An outstanding recent review of various aspects of HCC by some of the world experts on the topic. This is a highly recommended reading.

15. CLIP Investigators. Prospective validation of the CLIP score: a new prognostic system for patients with cirrhosis and hepatocellular carcinoma. The Cancer of the Liver Italian Program (CLIP) Investigators. Hepatology 2000; 31(4):840–845.

    This article details the external validation and comparison of the CLIP score, the most commonly recommended staging system, to the Okuda staging system in patients with cirrhosis and HCC.

16. Bruix J, Llovet JM. Prognostic prediction and treatment strategy in hepatocellular carcinoma. Hepatology 2002; 35(3):519–524.

17. Mazzaferro V, Regalia E, Doci R, et al. Liver transplantation for the treatment of small hepatocellular carcinomas in patients with cirrhosis. N Engl J Med 1996; 334(11):693–699.

    Classical study that gave the genesis to the 'Milan Criteria' for selecting patients with HCC to be treated with liver transplantation.

18. Sharma P, Balan V, Hernandez JL, et al. Liver transplantation for hepatocellular carcinoma: the MELD impact. Liver Transpl 2004; 10(1):36–41.

    This article examines UNOS database for the effects of the allocation system based on the Model for End-stage Liver Disease (MELD) in patients diagnosed with hepatocellular carcinoma.

19. Llovet JM, Bruix J. Systematic review of randomized trials for unresectable hepatocellular carcinoma: Chemoembolization improves survival. Hepatology 2003; 37(2):429–442.

    This is a systematic review and meta-analyses of randomized trials examining TACE. It provides an in-depth look at the methods, conduct, and results of therapy with TACE.

20. Di Maio M, De Maio E, Perrone F, et al. Hepatocellular carcinoma: systemic treatments. J Clin Gastroenterol 2002; 35(5 Suppl 2):S109–S114.

    A thoughtful review of a disparate literature, with careful assessment of the validity of the evidence supporting the use of the major groups of therapy.

21. Shaib Y, El-Serag HB. The epidemiology of cholangiocarcinoma. Semin Liver Dis 2004; 24(2):115–125.

    A useful review of the global epidemiology and risk factors of cholangiocarcinoma, with special emphasis on the United States.

22. McLarney JK, Rucker PT, Bender GN, et al. Fibrolamellar carcinoma of the liver: radiologic-pathologic correlation. Radiographics 1999; 19:453–471.

23. Macdonald GA, Peduto AJ. Magnetic resonance imaging (MRI) and diseases of the liver and biliary tract. Part 1. Basic principles, MRI in the assessment of diffuse and focal hepatic disease. J Gastroenterol Hepatol 2000; 15:980–991.

24. Trotter JF, Everson GT. Benign focal lesions of the liver. Clin Liver Dis 2001; 5(1):17–42, v.

    This article focuses on the origin, diagnosis, and management of focal benign lesions of the liver. The most common lesions include cavernous hemangioma, focal nodular hyperplasia, hepatic adenoma, and nodular regenerative hyperplasia. A number of less frequently occurring lesions are also discussed.

25. Mortele KJ, Ros PR. Benign liver neoplasms. Clin Liver Dis 2002; 6:119–145.

CHAPTER FORTY-SIX

Neonatal jaundice

Mike A. Leonis and William F. Balistreri

INTRODUCTION

Jaundice is a common physical finding encountered during the neonatal period, occurring in about half of infants in the first few days of life. In most instances, neonatal jaundice is a self-limited manifestation of benign physiologic processes. The challenge for the clinician is to recognize the rare instances when jaundice poses a risk to the infant (e.g., acute bilirubin encephalopathy or kernicterus) or represents a sign of serious underlying pathology (e.g., Crigler-Najjar syndrome or cholestasis), so that appropriate therapy can be implemented to avoid long-term deleterious consequences.[1,2]

Bilirubin metabolism and alterations in early life

Bilirubin is formed from the degradation of heme (most of which comes from hemoglobin) in a two-step process (Fig. 46.1). Bilirubin complexes with albumin in the bloodstream and, following delivery to the liver, dissociates in the hepatic sinusoids. Free bilirubin is then taken up by the hepatocytes, where it binds to cytosolic ligandin. In the endoplasmic reticulum, bilirubin is covalently linked with glucuronic acid (and to a lesser extent with glucose and xylose) to form mono- and di-conjugated bilirubin, which is then excreted into the biliary tract. Most excreted conjugated bilirubin is eliminated from the body in feces, although it may be deconjugated by intestinal bacteria, allowing unconjugated bilirubin to be reabsorbed. If any of these pathways are altered due to normal developmental changes or to pathological conditions, hyperbilirubinemia results (Table 46.1).

Infants are particularly prone to hyperbilirubinemia for several reasons. Prior to birth, bilirubin is efficiently cleared by the placenta. After delivery, increased susceptibility of fetal erythrocytes to degradation and immaturity of the bilirubin metabolic pathways in the liver result in neonatal hyperbilirubinemia.[3] Breastfeeding can result in increased serum bilirubin concentrations as well, possibly due to decreased conjugation and increased intestinal absorption of unconjugated bilirubin. Finally, various pathological conditions in infants may increase input into or block flow through the bilirubin metabolic pathway described above.

Initial patient assessment

The neonate with jaundice requires a thorough evaluation, including a detailed examination of the perinatal history and carefully performed physical examination to narrow the differential diagnosis. The temporal onset of jaundice can provide important clues as to whether the infant is truly healthy with physiologic jaundice or whether the jaundice is an early symptom

Table 46.1 Alterations in bilirubin metabolism causing neonatal jaundice

Increased free heme	Hemolysis
	Rapid erythrocyte turnover (common in newborns)
	Extravascular blood (cephalohematoma, intraventricular hemorrhage)
	Polycythemia/plethora
Decreased albumin binding capacity	Hypoalbuminemia
	Displacement by drugs
Decreased bilirubin uptake by hepatocytes	Interference by drugs
	Prematurity
	Cardiovascular lesions causing hepatic hypoperfusion
Decreased ligandin binding capacity	Prematurity
Decreased conjugation of bilirubin	Prematurity
	Gilbert syndrome
	Crigler-Najjar syndrome
	Breastfeeding?
Decreased biliary excretion	Hepatocellular dysfunction (various causes)
	Bacterial sepsis
	Congenital infections
	Prematurity
Increased bacterial deconjugation	Intestinal obstruction
	Delayed passage of meconium
Increased absorption of bilirubin from the intestine	Breastfeeding

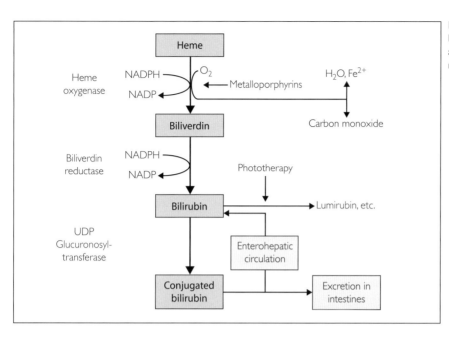

Fig. 46.1 • Metabolism of heme to conjugated bilirubin. The sites of therapeutic interventions and pathways for elimination of bilirubin metabolites are noted.

of a serious pathophysiologic process. The presence of hypopigmented (acholic) stools should raise suspicion for biliary atresia. Historical information such as birth weight, length of gestation, genetic/racial variations, maternal health, perinatal events, and method of early feeding may provide clues. Premature babies are more likely to have physiologic hyperbilirubinemia and are more prone to the development of kernicterus. Newborns of Asian, Greek, and Native American heritage have a higher incidence of hyperbilirubinemia due to the higher prevalence of glucose-6-phospate dehydrogenase deficiency in these populations. Gestational diabetes, maternal drug use, and isoimmunization impact the infant's bilirubin metabolism. Bleeding or bruising during delivery increases degradation of red blood cells, thereby increasing the bilirubin load to be disposed of by an already heavily taxed system.

On physical examination, attention to noteworthy clinical signs is crucial. Sources of increased erythrocyte breakdown (e.g., birth-related hematomas and cephalohematomas) should be identified. Signs of sepsis must be carefully sought with appropriate laboratory investigations. Evidence of hepatomegaly should be sought by measuring the liver span and palpation of the liver edge, and splenomegaly should be assessed by palpation of the spleen. Hydrops caused by Rh isoimmunization is now only rarely encountered in developed countries.

Importance of bilirubin fractionation

When bilirubin metabolism or hepatobiliary excretion is altered, bilirubin accumulates in conjugated (direct-reacting) or unconjugated (indirect-reacting) forms. The differentiation between these forms is an essential first step to diagnose and, if necessary, to treat the cause of hyperbilirubinemia. Serum conjugated bilirubin levels are traditionally considered to be elevated when > 1.5 mg/dL or >20% of the total bilirubin; however, any level should be a cause for suspicion. Because hepatic conjugation of bilirubin is initially low in newborns, it is important to recheck the conjugated bilirubin concentration periodically if jaundice persists beyond 14 days of age.

Additional laboratory investigation of hyperbilirubinemia will be directed by the findings from the history and physical examination. Several laboratory studies are performed routinely in newborns including determination of the newborn's blood type, a Coomb's test for antierythrocyte antibodies, and state-mandated newborn screens. In the United States, screening for hypothyroidism, galactosemia, and hemoglobinopathies are required by most states; a few states also screen for tyrosinemia or cystic fibrosis.[4] It should be emphasized that these tests are population-based screening tests and that the accuracy of results can depend upon clinical factors such as the gestational age and type of feeding. Therefore, clinical suspicion should be high and appropriate studies should be repeated if indicated.

The therapy of hyperbilirubinemia is based on the need to reduce the risk of toxicity of unconjugated bilirubin to the central nervous system, and to identify and treat specific causes of conjugated hyperbilirubinemia which are due to hepatobiliary dysfunction. Severe unconjugated hyperbilirubinemia may be associated with the development of acute bilirubin encephalopathy and/or kernicterus (i.e., the chronic and permanent sequelae of severe bilirubin toxicity). Early recognition and treatment of underlying hepatobiliary disease due to anatomic anomalies or metabolic or toxic insults may delay or prevent hepatic failure, which may obviate the need for liver transplantation. Therefore, prompt recognition, evaluation, and treatment of neonatal jaundice is essential.

UNCONJUGATED HYPERBILIRUBINEMIA

Because neonatal unconjugated hyperbilirubinemia is common and often not indicative of significant pathology, the need for treatment of jaundice depends upon an assessment of the overall risk to the neonate of developing severe hyperbilirubinemia and its potentially long-lasting neurologic sequelae. In practice, therapy is usually begun before extensive laboratory evaluations (other than routine determination of blood type and Coombs' test) are performed. Of the usually benign causes of neonatal unconjugated hyperbilirubinemia, physiologic jaundice and

Table 46.2 Causes of unconjugated hyperbilirubinemia in neonates

Physiologic jaundice

Breast milk jaundice

Crigler-Najjar syndrome, types I and II

Gilbert syndrome

Hemolysis (e.g., glucose-6-phosphate dehydrogenase deficiency)

Drugs

Congenital hypothyroidism/hypopituitarism

Sepsis

Gastrointestinal obstruction

breast milk jaundice refer to normal, nonpathological causes. Metabolic defects, hemolysis, and several other processes may also cause unconjugated hyperbilirubinemia (Table 46.2). Phototherapy is the current initial therapy of choice for unconjugated hyperbilirubinemia in the newborn.[1]

Causes of unconjugated hyperbilirubinemia

Physiologic jaundice and breast milk jaundice

As noted above, immaturity of bilirubin clearance mechanisms in the newborn result in an increase in serum unconjugated bilirubin levels even in normal circumstances. This process is termed *physiologic jaundice*, wherein the serum concentration of unconjugated bilirubin peaks on the third to fourth day of life and then decreases to the normal range by 7 days of age. In premature babies, who have clearance mechanisms which are even more immature, the peak may be higher, later, and more prolonged (several weeks).

In addition to the normal immaturity of the processes involved in bilirubin metabolism and excretion which lead to physiologic jaundice no matter what the infant's diet, feedings with breast milk may give a slightly different pattern. In breast-fed infants, jaundice may begin early as a result of relative starvation before the mother's milk 'comes in,' perhaps resulting in increased enterohepatic circulation of bilirubin.[5] Hyperbilirubinemia peaks in breast-fed infants in the second week and may remain elevated for several weeks. This may be the result of uncharacterized factor(s) present in breast milk or association with common genetic defects in bilirubin UDP-glucuronosyltransferase I (B-UGT) found in Gilbert's syndrome; both scenarios may lead to decreased glucuronidation of bilirubin.[6] Supplementation with formula leads to rapid reduction of the serum bilirubin concentration, and in most cases, breastfeeding should not be discouraged.[1]

Inherited disorders of bilirubin metabolism

Three forms of inherited unconjugated hyperbilirubinemia are recognized in humans: type I and II Crigler-Najjar syndromes, which are both severe and rare, and the milder Gilbert syndrome, which is present in 5–10% of the population. All three syndromes are differentiated from each other at the molecular level by varying degrees of deficiency in B-UGT, the enzyme responsible for formation of conjugated bilirubin in the hepatocyte (see Fig. 46.1).[7,8]

In *type I Crigler-Najjar syndrome*, early and severe jaundice is the result of completely absent B-UGT enzyme activity, with serum unconjugated bilirubin levels reaching as high as 40 mg/dL. Diagnosis is confirmed by the absence of bilirubin diglucuronide in serum or bile, or of B-UGT enzyme in liver biopsy tissue. Phenobarbital is ineffective in inducing bilirubin elimination. Ten to 12 hours of daily phototherapy are often necessary to reduce serum bilirubin concentrations to non-neurotoxic levels, although this becomes less effective as the child ages. Oral calcium phosphate can modestly further decrease bilirubin levels in patients receiving daily phototherapy.[9] Bilirubin levels are poorly controlled by exchange transfusion, but this may be necessary in the neonatal period. Neurologic dysfunction is frequently seen in patients with type I Crigler-Najjar syndrome and is universal without phototherapy; therefore, liver transplantation, which is the only definitive treatment, should be carried out early before neurological sequelae develop.[10] Drugs that displace bilirubin from albumin (e.g., sulfa drugs, salicylates, and penicillin) must be avoided. In the future, this disorder may benefit from advances in gene therapy, hepatocyte transplantation, or the use of heme oxygenase inhibitors; the latter two options are currently being investigated, with encouraging preliminary results.[11,12]

Type II Crigler-Najjar syndrome results from a partial deficiency of B-UGT, and is more variable in its phenotype. In this condition, serum bilirubin levels are less markedly elevated (6–20 mg/dL), and thus the development of neurologic sequelae is less frequent. In type II Crigler-Najjar syndrome, treatment with phenobarbital may induce UGT activity or alternate pathways for bilirubin elimination, thus decreasing serum unconjugated bilirubin concentrations by greater than 25% of the pretreatment level. However, side effects from this medication are common.

In contrast to the Crigler-Najjar syndromes, *Gilbert syndrome* is a mild form of unconjugated hyperbilirubinemia typically presenting after puberty and not requiring treatment. Baseline bilirubin concentrations are <3 mg/dL, and may increase to 6 mg/dL during periods of illness, fasting, or stress. Hepatic UGT enzyme levels are about 20–30% of normal. At the present time, Gilbert syndrome *by itself* is not thought to pose a risk of kernicterus in the newborn period. However, recent studies have revealed that neonates with Gilbert syndrome UGT enzyme mutations, in association with other derangements in bilirubin physiology, are at increased risk of developing significant neonatal jaundice.[6,13]

Molecular analyses have shown that mutations in the UGT1A1 gene, which encodes for B-UGT, leads to diminished B-UGT enzyme activity. Several mutations in the coding region of the UGT1A1 gene cause the more severe Crigler-Najjar syndromes, and heterozygotes for such mutations may manifest a dominant form of Gilbert syndrome. On the other hand, homozygous mutations in the promoter region of the UGT1A1 gene (i.e., the A(TA)$_7$TAA polymorphism, which disrupts the normal A(TA)$_6$TAA sequence) reduces transcription of an otherwise normal UGT protein, and is necessary but not sufficient for the manifestation of Gilbert syndrome.[14] Neonates who are homozygous for the A(TA)$_7$TAA polymorphism have an accelerated increase in neonatal jaundice in the first two days of life and an increased incidence of prolonged hyperbilirubinemia.[15,16] Variability in the presence of polymorphisms in the UGT1A1 gene, as well as additional factors affecting bilirubin production, uptake, or clearance, likely account for the heterogeneous clinical expression of Gilbert syndrome.[14,15,17,18]

Other causes of unconjugated hyperbilirubinemia

Hemolysis, although still common, is no longer a major cause of unconjugated hyperbilirubinemia due to improvements in management of maternal–fetal isoimmune hemolysis.[3] Isoimmune hemolysis most often results from maternal antibodies against fetal erythrocyte antigens, commonly due to ABO or Rh incompatibility. The maternal immunoglobulin G crosses the placenta into the fetal circulation and causes hemolysis, resulting in an increased load of bilirubin to be cleared by the liver. Treatment is by exchange transfusion, which removes the maternal antibodies, heme, and unconjugated bilirubin from the circulation. Hemolysis may also result from glucose-6-phosphate dehydrogenase (G6PD) deficiency and other erythrocyte defects. G6PD deficiency is an X-linked condition most commonly seen in persons of African, Mediterranean, and Asian ancestry.[19] Drugs and infectious agents are the most common triggers of hemolysis in these patients, and these patients are at risk for a sudden rise in their total serum bilirubin (TSB) levels. Interestingly, heterozygous G6PD deficiency synergizes with the presence of the variant UGT1A1 promoter found in Gilbert's syndrome to lead to an increased incidence of neonatal hyperbilirubinemia.[13] Of note, G6PD levels can be elevated in the presence of hemolysis, which can obscure the diagnosis of G6PD deficiency in a hemolyzing infant.[20] Moreover, severe hyperbilirubinemia in patients of African descent should raise the suspicion of G6PD deficiency since this population has lower baseline bilirubin levels compared to the Caucasian population.[1]

Drugs which displace bilirubin from albumin, including sulfa compounds and ceftriaxone, can increase the risk of kernicterus by increasing the free concentration of bilirubin in serum; in addition, ceftriaxone can cause sludging of bile in the gallbladder, decreasing biliary flow. Withdrawal of the offending drug is necessary in each case.

Congenital hypothyroidism may cause jaundice due to unconjugated hyperbilirubinemia, although conjugated hyperbilirubinemia is more commonly observed. Screening of newborns for hypothyroidism is required in the entire United States, but measurement of thyroid hormone levels should be repeated if there is clinical suspicion of an endocrinopathy. Thyroid hormone replacement using thyroxine is the required therapy.

Unconjugated hyperbilirubinemia may also be a sign of sepsis. Prompt evaluation for the presence of sepsis and initiation of antibiotic therapy should be considered.

Gastrointestinal obstruction may cause jaundice in newborns by allowing bacterial deconjugation of conjugated bilirubin, resulting in reabsorption of unconjugated bilirubin. Vomiting, particularly of bilious material, and/or abdominal distention in conjunction with jaundice should prompt consideration of an obstructive process.

Treatment of unconjugated hyperbilirubinemia

The American Academy of Pediatrics recently presented updated clinical practice guidelines for the management of hyperbilirubinemia in full-term newborns,[1] with particular focus on assessing the risk to the newborn of developing complications from severe unconjugated hyperbilirubinemia. Guidelines for the management of unconjugated hyperbilirubinemia in low birthweight (<2500 g) newborns take into account the same general clinical parameters.[21]

Recommendations include encouraging frequent breastfeeding (8–12 times per day) of the infant during the first days of life to decrease dehydration and poor caloric intake, and to systematically assess the infant for the development of jaundice at the time of every vital sign measurement. Every newborn found to be jaundiced in the first 24 hours of life must have their total serum bilirubin (TSB) level determined and re-evaluated frequently. Assessment of risk of developing severe hyperbilirubinemia is guided by the use of percentile-based nomograms based on hour-specific TSB level determinations.[1] The infant and mothers' blood types should be determined in all newborns, as incompatibility with maternal blood type can lead to severe hemolysis. Additional risk factors for the development of severe unconjugated hyperbilirubinemia include the newborn's gestation period, birth weight, age, and additional perinatal factors such as exposure to hypoxia, acidosis, or sepsis.

Phototherapy should be used if the TSB level exceeds the recommended age-specific TSB level, which is stratified by gestational age and the presence of additional risk factors (see Figure 3 in Reference 1). The cause of jaundice in the newborn should be sought if phototherapy is needed or if the degree of rise in TSB levels is not otherwise explained by the history or physical exam (e.g., presence of a large resolving cephalohematoma). Intensive phototherapy can result in a 30–40% decrease in TSB levels by 4 hours, although the degree of change depends on a multitude of factors.[1]

Phototherapy makes use of the fact that bilirubin photoisomerizes when exposed to wavelengths of 420–500 nanometers (blue light), resulting in more polar nontoxic compounds (e.g., lumirubin) which can be excreted by the kidneys and hepatobiliary system without conjugation.[22] A variety of phototherapy systems are commercially available for delivering intense light to as much of the skin surface as possible. In addition, total exposure time, the TSB level at the start of therapy, and the cause of jaundice all influence the response to phototherapy. Phototherapy is not without risk, not to mention inconvenience and expense, and should thus be used judiciously. Depending on the light source used, the newborn's eyes should be protected during phototherapy to prevent possible retinal damage. In addition, overhead phototherapy lamps can cause increased insensible water losses; therefore, the newborn's fluid status must be closely monitored. Phototherapy should be carefully considered for patients with conjugated hyperbilirubinemia, because it can result in 'bronzing' of the skin or blistering; if the latter occurs it is important to consider the possible diagnosis of congenital porphyria.[1]

Certain drugs, such as phenobarbital and rifampin, up-regulate alternative pathways of bilirubin metabolism (i.e., the cytochrome P450 pathway) and may be useful in the treatment of some cases of hyperbilirubinemia.

When unconjugated hyperbilirubinemia is not responsive to intense phototherapy, exchange transfusion, which reduces serum concentrations of bilirubin by dilution, is required. Exchange transfusion is indicated if: (1) at any time the TSB is >25 mg/dL, (2) the TSB level exceeds the recommended age-specific exchange transfusion level (see nomogram [Figure 4 in Reference 1]), (3) the TSB/serum albumin ratio is >6.8–8.0 (depending on gestational age), or (4) the infant is jaundiced and manifests signs of acute bilirubin encephalopathy (e.g., shrill cry, retrocollis and opisthotonos alternating with drowsiness and hypotonia).[1] If criteria for exchange transfusion are reached, it is likely that hemolysis is occurring, although this can be difficult to determine. Measurement of end tidal carbon monoxide levels (ETCO$_c$), although not widely available, allows for the most direct measurement of heme catabolism.[1,13] Because exchange transfusions can cause severe electrolyte and fluid shifts and/or transfusion reactions, they are usually performed in an intensive care setting.

A simpler approach to the treatment of unconjugated hyperbilirubinemia involves the parenteral delivery of metalloporphyrins, which are competitive inhibitors of heme oxygenase, the rate-limiting enzyme in bilirubin production (see Fig. 46.1).[11] By blocking the degradation of heme to bilirubin, intact heme (which is apparently nontoxic) accumulates and is subsequently excreted via the hepatobiliary system. In several studies involving newborns with unconjugated hyperbilirubinemia belonging to three diagnostic groups (i.e., 283 newborns with G6PD deficiency, 517 premature newborns, and 166 full-term infants with breast-feeding jaundice), a single dose of tin mesoporphyrin (Sn-MP) was shown to be safe and efficacious in lowering TSB levels and reducing the need for phototherapy.[23–26] No lasting toxicities have been reported, although skin photosensitivity can occur in those newborns concurrently receiving phototherapy. Thus far, the use of Sn-MP has been approved by the United States FDA only on a compassionate-need basis (e.g., for patients with type I Crigler-Najjar syndrome or newborns with extreme hyperbilirubinemia born to Jehovah's Witness parents who refuse exchange transfusion).[11,27] Further evaluation of this compound is warranted, and if approved, Sn-MP could find immediate use in preventing the need for exchange transfusion in newborns who are not responding to phototherapy.[1,11,23]

Before discharge, every infant should be assessed for the risk of severe hyperbilirubinemia by measurement of a TSB level and/or review of clinical risk factors. Moreover, parents should be educated on how to assess for the development of jaundice and the importance of scheduling a follow-up office visit in the first week of life based on the time of hospital discharge.

Jaundice persisting after the first 2 weeks of life requires re-evaluation, including measurement of the TSB and conjugated bilirubin levels. In the office setting, urine can be tested for bilirubin using a dipstick as a screen; bilirubin must be conjugated for renal excretion. Elevation of serum conjugated bilirubin is suggestive of hepatobiliary pathology and requires prompt evaluation and referral to a specialist.

CONJUGATED HYPERBILIRUBINEMIA (CHOLESTASIS)

A variety of neonatal conditions can result in jaundice due to conjugated hyperbilirubinemia, including obstructive lesions of the extrahepatic biliary tree, endocrine or metabolic defects, infections and familial disorders (Table 46.3). Conjugated hyperbilirubinemia of unknown cause associated with elevation of serum alanine aminotransferase levels is termed idiopathic neonatal hepatitis, which probably represents a heterogeneous group of as yet uncharacterized disorders and often resolves spontaneously.

Causes of neonatal cholestasis

Obstructive lesions of the extrahepatic biliary tree

Biliary atresia is a disorder of infants in which obliteration or discontinuity of the extrahepatic biliary system occurs.[28] Two

forms of biliary atresia are recognized: a *perinatal* (acquired/nonsyndromic) form occurring in about 80% of patients and an *embryonic* (congenital/syndromic) form present in about 10–20% of patients. The perinatal form results from a progressive postnatal obliteration of the extrahepatic biliary system, often including the gallbladder, which results in persistent or worsening jaundice in the first months of life, rather than the normal resolution. The embryonic form manifests with early-onset jaundice and is thought, given the association with other congenital anomalies (e.g., cardiac defects, asplenia or polysplenia, laterality defects, and gastrointestinal malformations), to be due to defective embryogenesis of biliary structures.

Recognition of persistent jaundice due to conjugated hyperbilirubinemia and early evaluation and diagnosis within the first 2 months of life are critical for optimal treatment of infants with biliary atresia. Intrahepatic causes of cholestasis (infectious, metabolic, genetic, and toxic) and choledochal cysts (see below) must be excluded. Depending on the expertise of the treatment center, hepatic ultrasonography, radionuclide scintigraphy, or percutaneous transhepatic cholecystography can aid in diagnosis. A liver biopsy is particularly important, and can show proliferation and expansion of the bile ducts, portal inflammation, bile plugs, and (later) portal or perilobular fibrosis. Diagnosis of biliary atresia is confirmed by intraoperative cholangiogram.

Given the dire natural history of untreated biliary atresia, all cases of biliary atresia require surgical attempts to re-establish bile flow, either by anastomosis of residual, discontinuous but patent, biliary segments (including the gallbladder, if present) or as is the case for most patients, by performing a hepatoportoenterostomy (Kasai procedure). The surgical center's experience in performing the Kasai procedure is an important predictor of success, but perhaps the most important prognostic factor is the age at which the procedure is performed.[28] Bile flow is re-established in about 80% of infants with biliary atresia undergoing a Kasai procedure before 2 months of age, but in less than 20% who have the procedure performed after 3 months of age. Depending upon the degree of bile flow established, progressive cirrhosis and hepatic failure may develop over months to years, which may require liver transplantation, or it may never develop. An important early complication of the Kasai portoenterostomy is the development of ascending cholangitis, which can cause reduced biliary patency and/or sepsis, and should be suspected if the patient presents with fever, lethargy, irritability, acholic stools, jaundice, or abdominal pain. Intravenous antibiotics should be initiated without delay while the patient is evaluated for systemic infection. Prophylactic antibiotics (e.g., trimethoprim-sulfamethoxazole) may be given chronically following the Kasai procedure to reduce the risk of ascending cholangitis. The benefit of using corticosteroids to reduce biliary inflammation either before or after the Kasai procedure, or for ascending cholangitis nonresponsive to antibiotics, has not been definitively established. Recurrent episodes of ascending cholangitis are a predictor of poor outcome of the Kasai procedure, and heighten the need for orthotopic liver transplantation.[28]

Choledochal cysts are congenital dilatations of all or part of the biliary tree. Five types of choledochal cysts are recognized. Type I cysts are the most common and result from diffuse enlargement of the common bile duct. Patients usually present in infancy with jaundice, abdominal pain, and occasionally with a palpable abdominal mass. Diagnosis is usually made by ultrasonography

Table 46.3 Conjugated hyperbilirubinemia in neonates: causes and treatments

Type	Disorder	Specific treatment
Idiopathic	'Neonatal hepatitis'	None (supportive for cholestasis)
Lesions of bile ducts	Biliary atresia	Kasai hepatoportoenterostomy, OLT
	Choledochal cysts	Excision of cyst and gallbladder & hepatoportoenterostomy
	Spontaneous perforation of the bile duct	Surgical repair or enterostomy
	Cholelithiasis	Cholecystectomy if symptomatic
	Hydrops of the gallbladder	Treatment specific to etiology
	Tumors	Excision vs. chemotherapy
Endocrine causes	Congenital hypothyroidism	Thyroxine
	Congenital hypopituitarism	Hormone replacement
Metabolic/genetic causes	Galactosemia	Galactose-free diet
	Hereditary fructose intolerance	Fructose-free diet
	Tyrosinemia	NTBC
	Neonatal iron storage disease	Anti-oxidants (α-tocopherol, N-acetylcysteine, & selenium), Prostaglandin E_1
	Inborn errors of bile acid biosynthesis	Bile acid therapy
	α-1-antitrypsin deficiency	None
	Citrin deficiency	Nutritional management[46]
	Cystic fibrosis	Ursodeoxycholic acid
	Disorders of carbohydrate or lipid storage	Variable
	Progressive familial intrahepatic cholestasis	None
	Alagille syndrome	None
	Trisomy 21 (Down syndrome)	None
	Trisomy 18	None
Infections	Bacterial sepsis	Appropriate parenteral antibiotics
	Hepatitis B	No specific therapy in neonates *Prophylaxis:* hepatitis B immune globulin & vaccine
	Hepatitis C	No specific therapy in neonates
	Syphilis	Penicillin G
	Herpes simplex virus	Acyclovir
	Toxoplasmosis	Pyrimethamine, sulfadiazine, & folinic acid
	Human immunodeficiency virus	Anti-retroviral therapy
	Parvovirus B19	None
	Human herpesvirus-6	None
	Echoviruses	None
	Coxsackieviruses	None
Toxic exposures	Parenteral nutrition	Advance enteral feedings Ursodeoxycholic acid?
	Drugs	Eliminate exposure

although other imaging modalities are effective. Antenatal observation of fetal biliary cystic malformations may become choledochal cysts, but they should raise suspicion of the diagnosis of biliary atresia as well.[29] Surgical excision of the entire cyst, with reconstruction of an extrahepatic biliary conduit, is usually required given the considerably increased risk of developing cholangiocarcinoma from the remnant cystic biliary mucosa.

Several other rare conditions affecting the extrahepatic biliary system may present with neonatal jaundice.[30,31] For example, cholelithiasis has been observed with the use of parenteral nutrition, a history of prior abdominal surgery, sepsis, and hemolytic disease. Treatment of symptomatic cholelithiasis is surgical since the majority of gallstones in infants are insoluble pigment stones unresponsive to medical therapy. Neonatal hydrops of the gallbladder has been associated with parenteral nutrition, sepsis, cystic fibrosis, alpha-1-antitrypsin deficiency, and the fasting state. Spontaneous perforation of the bile duct is a rare problem of infancy and should be considered if acholic stool and abdominal disten-

tion are present, along with other symptoms. Neonatal sclerosing cholangitis has also been reported.[31] Finally, tumors may very rarely cause biliary obstruction and jaundice in the newborn period.

Endocrine and metabolic disorders

Several metabolic disorders present in infancy with conjugated hyperbilirubinemia as a major feature. State-mandated newborn screening programs may assist in the early identification of certain disorders presenting with neonatal cholestasis; however, these screening programs may miss some infants, and additional hormone or metabolite measurements should be performed if clinical suspicion of an endocrinopathy remains. Early diagnosis and treatment, either before or after symptoms develop, is important to prevent or decrease the serious morbidity or mortality of these conditions.

Congenital hypothyroidism or *hypopituitarism* may present with neonatal cholestasis and hepatic dysfunction, with both usually resolving with appropriate hormone replacement therapy.[32]

Galactosemia is a disorder of the metabolism of galactose due to the absence of galactose-1-phosphate uridyltransferase. Thus, following exposure to lactose (which is composed of galactose and glucose) in breast milk or cow's milk-containing formulas, newborns with galactosemia present in the first week of life with the acute onset of lethargy, vomiting and diarrhea, and hypoglycemia. Conjugated hyperbilirubinemia is common. If left untreated, accumulation of hepatotoxic metabolites can lead to hepatic failure and death. Treatment consists of dietary restriction of galactose; although life-saving, such therapy does not eliminate long-term complications of this disorder such as neuropsychological compromise.[33]

Infants with *hereditary fructose intolerance* (due to fructose-1-phosphate aldolase B deficiency) usually have an acute presentation following the introduction of fructose or sucrose to their diet, typically at about 4–6 months of age. This disorder results from the accumulation of metabolites in organs where aldolase B is expressed, which may account for the hepatic dysfunction, diarrhea and vomiting, and proximal renal tubulopathy that is seen. Careful attention to recent dietary changes, extensive biochemical investigations and review of the liver histology (which may show non-specific findings of macrovesicular steatosis) may lead to the diagnosis.[34] The patient is effectively treated by the elimination of all dietary and medicinal sources of fructose or sucrose.

In *hereditary tyrosinemia type I (HT1)*, deficiency of fumarylacetoacetate hydrolase, the final enzyme in the degradation pathway for the amino acid tyrosine, results in accumulation of hepatotoxic metabolites (i.e., succinylacetoacetate [SAA] and succinylacetone [SA]) upstream of the enzyme defect.[35] The acute presentation of HT1 in early infancy leads to acute liver failure; the diagnosis of HT1 can be made by the detection of SA in the urine. A potent inhibitor (i.e., 2-[2-nitro-4-trifluoromethylbenzoyl]-1,3-cyclohexanedione [NTBC]) of 4-hydroxyphenylpyruvate dioxygenase, an early enzyme in the tyrosine degradation pathway, completely blocks accumulation of these hepatotoxic metabolites in patients with HT1. Dietary restriction of phenylalanine and tyrosine is also necessary. Treatment with NTBC prior to the age of 2 years (i.e., for patients with either the acute or chronic presentations of HT1) significantly improves the long-term clinical prognosis of these patients, reducing the subsequent development of hepatocellular carcinoma to about 1% of the affected children, as well as the need for liver transplantation.[36,37]

Neonatal iron storage disease is a familial disorder characterized by massive iron accumulation, possibly due to aberrant placental iron transport. Iron, a strong oxidant, deposits in multiple non-reticuloendothelial tissues, including the liver and pancreas. Acute hepatic failure ensues in the neonatal period due to the toxic iron load. Obtaining an abdominal MRI to detect extrahepatic iron deposition (e.g., in the pancreas) and serum iron studies may aid in the diagnosis of neonatal iron storage disease. Treatment with deferoxamine, an iron chelator, combined with several antioxidant compounds (α-tocopherol, N-acetylcysteine, and selenium) and prostaglandin E_1 (which increases hepatic perfusion) may reduce the extent of hepatic injury and allow recovery, particularly if started within the first week of life.[38] However, liver transplantation remains the mainstay of therapy in most cases.

Interestingly, about 10% of newborns with *neonatal lupus* have hepatobiliary disease, and of these, 20% have fatal clinical courses within the first week of life, with liver pathology consistent with neonatal iron storage disease. The remainder have complete resolution of their hepatobiliary disease.[39]

The *progressive familial intrahepatic cholestasis* (PFIC) *syndromes* encompass a group of disorders shown to be due to *inborn errors of bile acid synthesis* or *bile acid transport*. The major division between these cholestatic patients centers on whether their serum γGT level is low (PFIC1, PFIC2 and those with bile acid synthetic defects) or high (PFIC3). Bile acid synthetic defects often result in the formation of hepatotoxic bile acid intermediates, and can usually be diagnosed by analysis of urine or bile from the cholestatic infant.[40] These rare disorders are often successfully treated by giving bile acids orally, thereby replenishing the bile acid pool, improving bile flow, and down-regulating the aberrant endogenous bile acid synthetic pathways.[41]

Patients with PFIC1 (formerly called Byler's disease) and PFIC2 can present with severe pruritus during infancy and have low-to-normal serum γGT and high serum bile acid levels. The distinction between PFIC1 and PFIC2 is difficult, but may be suggested based on the presence of extrahepatic manifestations (PFIC1) such as diarrhea and characteristic features on liver histology. PFIC1 and PFIC2 are due to defects in the *FIC1* P-type ATPase and the bile salt export pump (BSEP), respectively.[42] Patients with PFIC3 have high serum γGT and bile acid levels, and liver histology showing ductular proliferation; this form tends to present with cholestatic jaundice later in infancy and childhood (and rarely in the first month of life). One-third of PFIC3 patients have defects in the MDR3 phospholipid translocator.[43] Therapy with ursodeoxycholic acid or biliary diversion is variably helpful for PFIC patients; often, liver transplantation is required in the first or second decade of life.

Approximately 10–15% of the infant population with *alpha-1-antitrypsin deficiency* will present in the newborn period with liver disease manifesting as cholestasis. Diagnosis is made by electrophoretic determination of the alpha-1-antitrypsin phenotype. No specific therapy is available, and for most, their liver disease will improve without intervention. However, 5% of alpha-1-antitrypsin deficient patients with liver disease will proceed to liver transplantation by 4 years of age.[44]

Two percent of patients with *cystic fibrosis* may present with neonatal cholestasis as a primary manifestation of disease; however, the natural history of the liver disease in this subset of patients is unknown. Management involves optimizing nutritional status and treatment with ursodeoxycholic acid. The latter may improve cholestasis and slow progression of the hepatic complications of cystic fibrosis.[45]

Over the last decade, 70 East Asian newborns with hyperaminoacidemia (e.g., elevated citrulline, methionine, tyrosine, etc.) and cholestasis have been designated as having *neonatal intrahepatic cholestasis due to citrin deficiency* (NICCD) based on genetic analysis.[46] Elevated serum galactose levels may also be observed. Citrin is an aspartate/glutamate carrier protein which supplies aspartate into the urea cycle.[47] Loss of hepatic citrin protein expression due to numerous frameshift or nonsense mutations in the citrin gene have been identified in patients with adult-onset type 2 citrullinemia (CTLN2).[48] These same CTLN2 mutations have been identified in cholestatic newborns with the biochemical abnormalities noted above, leading to the NICCD designation.[46,49,50] Curiously, most patients with NICCD fully resolve all biochemical abnormalities spontaneously or with minimal dietary restrictions (e.g., the use of lactose-free formulas,

formulas containing medium chain triglycerides (MCT), or supplementation with fat-soluble vitamins). However, several infants have undergone liver transplantation before the age of 1 year.[49,51] Clearly, much remains to be learned about the etiopathogenesis of this patient population. Nevertheless, jaundiced infants with multiple abnormal newborn metabolic screen results (e.g., elevated phenylalanine, methionine, or galactose blood levels) need to be closely observed given their risk of developing end-stage liver disease.[49,50,52]

Infants with carbohydrate or lipid storage or processing disorders (e.g., Niemann-Pick disease type C and congenital disorders of glycosylation [CDG]) may present with cholestasis as well as other systemic signs and symptoms.[53,54] Diagnosis may involve a liver or bone marrow biopsy or cultured fibroblast analysis (for storage disorders), or serum transferrin isoelectrophoresis (for CDG syndromes). For most of these disorders, specific therapy is presently unavailable; however, there are some exceptions (e.g., treatment with mannose for CDG Type 1b).[54]

Other syndromic causes of conjugated hyperbilirubinemia

Alagille syndrome is an autosomal dominant disorder of variable penetrance characterized by the association of several possible clinical features (chronic cholestasis, peculiar facies, congenital heart disease, posterior embryotoxon, and 'butterfly-like' vertebrae) and mutations in the Jagged 1 gene. In a review of 163 children with Alagille syndrome, two-thirds presented with neonatal cholestatic jaundice; of these, most had pruritus and hepatomegaly, and up to a third required liver transplantation.[55] Alleviating symptoms and complications of cholestasis (see below) and monitoring overall liver function are the mainstay of therapy.

Newborns with chromosomal anomalies such as trisomy 21 (Down syndrome) and trisomy 18 may present with cholestatic jaundice which usually resolves without intervention.

Arthrogryposis-renal dysfunction-cholestasis (ARC) syndrome is an autosomal recessive syndrome associated with neonatal cholestasis (with low GGT levels and bile duct hypoplasia) and is usually fatal within the first year of life.[56] Finally, several other syndromes featuring neonatal cholestasis have been described, some in specific ethnic groups.[57]

Infections

Neonatal hyperbilirubinemia may also be caused by bacterial, viral, or parasitic infections, and may be acquired pre-, peri-, or postnatally (see Table 46.3). However, many of these infections are rare compared to other causes of hyperbilirubinemia, and extensive, costly laboratory investigations, or obtaining so-called TORCH (toxoplasmosis, rubella, cytomegalovirus, and herpes simplex) titers, are rarely helpful in the absence of specific historical findings or physical features suggestive of an infectious process occurring in either the mother or newborn.

Bacterial sepsis may present with either an indolent or rapid onset of jaundice, likely due to the release of bacterial toxins which inhibit hepatocyte excretion of conjugated bilirubin. Suspected bacterial infection should be promptly treated with appropriate intravenous antibiotics pending identification of the microbe.

Congenital syphilis manifests a variety of signs and symptoms, including jaundice, which are usually present within the first few weeks of life. Maternal history and laboratory findings, including nontreponemal and treponemal test results on both infant and mother may point to the diagnosis. Intravenous penicillin G is effective therapy for congenital syphilis.[58]

Perinatal transmission of *hepatitis B virus* or *hepatitis C virus* from infected mothers to infants, while quite serious from a long-term perspective because of the high rate of chronic infection which results, rarely if ever manifests as significant neonatal jaundice.

Disseminated *herpes simplex virus* (HSV) infection can involve multiple organs; jaundice, when present, is associated with severe liver dysfunction. Perinatal transmission of HSV infection is highest if active genital lesions are present at the time of delivery; however, three-quarters of HSV-infected newborns are born to mothers without clinical findings or history of HSV infection. Intravenous acyclovir is indicated for all cases of neonatal HSV infection, as the risk of long-term neurologic sequelae and/or death is high.[58]

Congenital *human immunodeficiency virus (HIV) infections* usually present with additional signs and symptoms pointing to this diagnosis. Zidovudine administered to the mother during pregnancy, labor, and delivery, and to the newborn for the first 6 weeks of life, decreases the rate of perinatal transmission of HIV. Breastfeeding by HIV-infected mothers should be avoided. Several antiviral agents are available to treat the HIV-infected newborn.[58] Congenital *cytomegalovirus infection* is fairly common (i.e., about 1% of newborns), and can be a cause of neonatal jaundice, especially in those exposed to maternal primary infection.[58] Several other viral infections may cause neonatal jaundice (see Table 46.3); however, specific treatments for these viral infections do not presently exist.

The parasite *Toxoplasma gondii* is a rare cause of congenital infection. Congenital toxoplasmosis is asymptomatic in 70–90% of newborns; however, jaundice is often a presenting symptom. Prolonged treatment with pyrimethamine, sulfadiazine, and folinic acid is required.[58]

In addition to the congenital, genetic, and infectious processes described above, neonatal cholestasis may develop following exposure to a variety of peri- and postnatal environmental insults. Parenteral nutrition can cause hepatocyte dysfunction and cholestasis, especially in infants who receive limited enteral feedings. Ursodeoxycholic acid may reduce the hepatotoxicity of parenteral nutrition, but data are limited.[41] In this setting, it is important to advance enteral feedings and reduce dependence upon parenteral nutrition to the extent possible. Drugs may also be hepatotoxic and cause jaundice, and thus a careful drug exposure history (including over-the-counter preparations such as acetaminophen) must be obtained. Other perinatal events associated with neonatal cholestasis include asphyxia, prematurity, respiratory distress, and maternal pre-eclampsia.[59] Specific treatments may be available (e.g., N-acetylcysteine for toxicity to acetaminophen); however, often only supportive measures can be taken while the newborn's liver function is closely monitored and consideration is given for the need for liver transplantation.

General considerations in the treatment of neonatal cholestasis

In addition to the specific treatments described above, attention needs to be paid to metabolic, nutritional, and quality-of-life issues that are consequences of cholestasis (Table 46.4). For example, glucose homeostasis may be impaired with hepatic failure, so serum glucose levels should be measured and continuous enteral or parenteral sources of glucose should be provided

Table 46.4 General treatment of cholestasis

Clinical Issue	Treatment Considerations	
Nutrition	Medium-chain triglyceride-containing formula	
	Fat-soluble vitamins (orally):	
	Vitamin A	5000–25 000 IU/day
	Vitamin D (ergocalciferol)	2500 IU/day in infants
	Vitamin E [tocophersolan (TPGS) or α-tocopherol]	25–50 IU/kg/day
	Vitamin K (phytonadione)	2.5 mg every other day
	Nasogastric tube feeds	
Pruritus	Antihistamines (diphenhydramine, hydroxazine)	
	Cytochrome P450 stimulation (phenobarbital, rifampin)	
	Bile salt binding resins (cholestyramine)	
	Bile acid displacement (ursodeoxycholic acid)	
	Opiate antagonists (naltrexone)?	
Ascites/portal hypertension	Diuretics (furosemide, spironolactone)	
	Sodium restriction	

as needed. Cholestasis can lead to fat malabsorption resulting in malnutrition and fat-soluble vitamin deficiencies. Weight gain should be closely monitored and supplemental feedings, including nasogastric tube feedings, should be started if growth is poor. Because absorption of MCT is less dependent upon the presence of intraluminal bile acids, inclusion of or supplementation with MCT in the infant's diet will increase caloric intake and aid in the absorption of fat-soluble vitamins.

Fat-soluble vitamin deficiencies are of concern in patients with chronic cholestasis, and all such patients should be supplemented with oral vitamins A, D, E, and K. Assessment of deficiencies in these vitamins should be made periodically; vitamin K status is the easiest to assess clinically by measuring the prothrombin time. If the prothrombin time is elevated, parenteral vitamin K should be administered. Serum 25(OH) vitamin D levels are the best biologic marker for assessing vitamin D status. Vitamin E status should be evaluated by measuring the ratio between serum vitamin E levels and total lipids, and the retinol to retinol-binding protein molar ratio may be helpful in assessing vitamin A status.[60]

Cholestasis often results in pruritus, which can be the most incapacitating symptom of pediatric chronic liver disease. The exact mechanism of cholestatic-related pruritus is unknown, and therefore targeted therapy has been elusive. Medicinal agents shown to have some effectiveness include antihistamines (diphenhydramine or hydroxazine), stimulators of the cytochrome P450 system (rifampin or phenobarbital), bile salt-binding resins (cholestyramine), and alternative 'displacing' bile acids (ursodeoxycholic acid).[41,61] Opioid antagonists have been shown to control

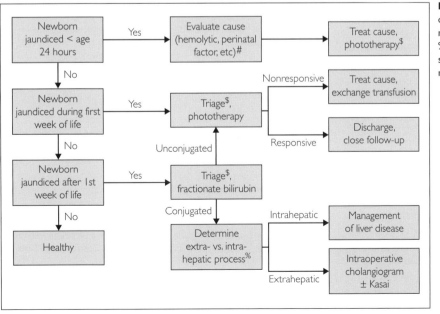

Fig. 46.2 • Algorithm for the management of neonatal jaundice. #, See text. $, See text; management guidelines based on Reference 1. %, Using a combination of findings from radiologic studies and liver biopsy; for more detailed management guidelines, see Reference 2.

cholestasis-induced pruritus in adults, but no studies have been performed in the pediatric age group.[62] Severe pruritus which is refractory to medical therapy may respond to biliary diversion[63,64] or even necessitate hepatic transplantation due to the severely compromised quality of life of the child.

Chronic cholestasis may progress to the development of portal hypertension and ascites. As in other age groups, treatment with diuretics and sodium restriction is needed. Ultimately, however, liver transplantation may be the only effective long-term treatment option.

SUMMARY

Jaundice in the newborn infant requires thoughtful evaluation of the risks this imposes to the newborn's health, followed by targeted treatment based upon the results of this evaluation. Early recognition of whether jaundice is a symptom of significant pathology, with particular attention to differentiating between unconjugated and conjugated hyperbilirubinemia, is the first step towards definitive diagnosis and the initiation of appropriate therapy.[2] An algorithm for the clinical approach to neonatal jaundice is provided in Figure 46.2.

REFERENCES

1. American Academy of Pediatrics Subcommittee on Hyperbilirubinemia. Management of hyperbilirubinemia in the newborn infant 35 or more weeks of gestation. Pediatrics 2004; 114:297–316.

   A comprehensive evidence-based guideline for the clinical assessment and management of unconjugated hyperbilirubinemia in the full-term newborn infant.

2. Moyer V, Freese DK, Whitington PF, et al. Guideline for the evaluation of cholestatic jaundice in infants: recommendations of the North American Society for Pediatric Gastroenterology, Hepatology and Nutrition. J Pediatr Gastroenterol Nutr 2004; 39:115–128.

3. Matsunaga AT, Lubin BH. Hemolytic anemia in the newborn. Clin Perinatol 1995; 22:803–828.

4. [No authors listed]. Newborn screening fact sheets. American Academy of Pediatrics. Committee on Genetics. Pediatrics 1996; 98:473–501.

5. Gartner LM. Neonatal jaundice. Pediatr Rev 1994; 15:422–432.

6. Maruo Y, Nishizawa K, Sato H, et al. Prolonged unconjugated hyperbilirubinemia associated with breast milk and mutations of the bilirubin uridine diphosphate-glucuronosyltransferase gene. Pediatrics 2000; 106:E59.

7. Kaplan M, Hammerman C, Maisels MJ. Bilirubin genetics for the nongeneticist: hereditary defects of neonatal bilirubin conjugation. Pediatrics 2003; 111:886–893.

8. Bosma PJ. Inherited disorders of bilirubin metabolism. J Hepatol 2003; 38:107–117.

9. Van der Veere CN, Jansen PL, Sinaasappel M, et al. Oral calcium phosphate: a new therapy for Crigler-Najjar disease? Gastroenterology 1997; 112:455–462.

10. van der Veere CN, Sinaasappel M, McDonagh AF, et al. Current therapy for Crigler-Najjar syndrome type 1: report of a world registry. Hepatology 1996; 24:311–315.

11. Kappas A. A method for interdicting the development of severe jaundice in newborns by inhibiting the production of bilirubin. Pediatrics 2004; 113:119–123.

    An up-to-date review of research on the use of metalloporphyrins in the treatment of neonatal unconjugated hyperbilirubinemia.

12. Fox IJ, Chowdhury JR, Kaufman SS, et al. Treatment of the Crigler-Najjar syndrome type I with hepatocyte transplantation. N Engl J Med 1998; 338:1422–1426.

13. Kaplan M, Beutler E, Vreman HJ, et al. Neonatal hyperbilirubinemia in glucose-6-phosphate dehydrogenase-deficient heterozygotes. Pediatrics 1999; 104:68–74.

14. Kadakol A, Ghosh SS, Sappal BS, et al. Genetic lesions of bilirubin uridine-diphosphoglucuronate glucuronosyltransferase (UGT1A1) causing Crigler-Najjar and Gilbert syndromes: correlation of genotype to phenotype. Hum Mutat 2000; 16:297–306.

    A thorough review of the correlation of UGT1A1 gene mutations with the varied phenotypes seen in the three clinically-relevant UGT-deficient syndromes.

15. Bancroft JD, Kreamer B, Gourley GR. Gilbert syndrome accelerates development of neonatal jaundice. J Pediatr 1998; 132:656–660.

    The first study to show a correlation between the presence of the Gilbert syndrome genotype and the degree of neonatal hyperbilirubinemia.

16. Monaghan G, McLellan A, McGeehan A, et al. Gilbert's syndrome is a contributory factor in prolonged unconjugated hyperbilirubinemia of the newborn. J Pediatr 1999; 134:441–446.

17. Beutler E, Gelbart T, Demina A. Racial variability in the UDP-glucuronosyltransferase 1 (UGT1A1) promoter: a balanced polymorphism for regulation of bilirubin metabolism? Proc Natl Acad Sci USA 1998; 95:8170–8174.

18. Persico M, Persico E, Bakker CT, et al. Hepatic uptake of organic anions affects the plasma bilirubin level in subjects with Gilbert's syndrome mutations in UGT1A1. Hepatology 2001; 33:627–632.

19. Valaes T. Severe neonatal jaundice associated with glucose-6-phosphate dehydrogenase deficiency: pathogenesis and global epidemiology. Acta Paediatr Suppl 1994; 394:58–76.

20. Kaplan M, Hammerman C. Glucose-6-phosphate dehydrogenase deficiency: a potential source of severe neonatal hyperbilirubinaemia and kernicterus. Semin Neonatol 2002; 7:121–128.

21. Maisels MJ, Watchko JF. Treatment of jaundice in low birthweight infants. Arch Dis Child Fetal Neonatal Ed 2003; 88:F459–F463.

22. Ennever JF, Costarino AT, Polin RA, et al. Rapid clearance of a structural isomer of bilirubin during phototherapy. J Clin Invest 1987; 79:1674–1678.

23. Alexander D. A method for interdicting the development of severe jaundice in newborns by inhibiting the production of bilirubin. Pediatrics 2004; 113:135.

24. Martinez JC, Garcia HO, Otheguy LE, et al. Control of severe hyperbilirubinemia in full-term newborns with the inhibitor of bilirubin production Sn-mesoporphyrin. Pediatrics 1999; 103:1–5.

25. Valaes T, Drummond GS, Kappas A. Control of hyperbilirubinemia in glucose-6-phosphate dehydrogenase-deficient newborns using an inhibitor of bilirubin production, Sn-mesoporphyrin. Pediatrics 1998; 101:E1.

26. Valaes T, Petmezaki S, Henschke C, et al. Control of jaundice in preterm newborns by an inhibitor of bilirubin production: studies with tin-mesoporphyrin. Pediatrics 1994; 93:1–11.

27. Kappas A, Drummond GS, Munson DP, et al. Sn-Mesoporphyrin interdiction of severe hyperbilirubinemia in Jehovah's Witness newborns as an alternative to exchange transfusion. Pediatrics 2001; 108:1374–1377.

28. Sokol RJ, Mack C, Narkewicz MR, et al. Pathogenesis and outcome of biliary atresia: current concepts. J Pediatr Gastroenterol Nutr 2003; 37:4–21.

    A recent comprehensive review of the literature on the pathogenesis, clinical features, and therapeutic outcomes of infants with biliary atresia.

29. Hinds R, Davenport M, Mieli-Vergani G, et al. Antenatal presentation of biliary atresia. J Pediatr 2004; 144:43–46.

30. Heubi JE, Lewis LG, Pohl JF. Diseases of the gallbladder in infancy, childhood, and adolescence. In: Suchy FJ, ed. Liver disease in children. 2nd edn. Philadelphia: Lippincott Williams & Wilkins; 2001:343–362.

31. Balistreri WF, Bove KE, Ryckman FC. Biliary atresia and other disorders of the extrahepatic bile ducts. In: Suchy FJ, ed. Liver disease in children. 2nd edn. Philadelphia: Lippincott Williams & Wilkins; 2001:253–274.

32. Ellaway CJ, Silinik M, Cowell CT, et al. Cholestatic jaundice and congenital hypopituitarism. J Paediatr Child Health 1995; 31:51–53.

33. Schweitzer-Krantz S. Early diagnosis of inherited metabolic disorders towards improving outcome: the controversial issue of galactosaemia. Eur J Pediatr 2003; 162(Suppl 1):S50–S53.

34. Stormon MO, Cutz E, Furuya K, et al. A six-month-old infant with liver steatosis. J Pediatr 2004; 144:258–263.

35. Grompe M. The pathophysiology and treatment of hereditary tyrosinemia type 1. Semin Liver Dis 2001; 21:563–571.

36. Holme E, Lindstedt S. Nontransplant treatment of tyrosinemia. Clin Liver Dis 2000; 4:805–814.

37. Mitchell GA, Grompe M, Lambert M. Hypertyrosinemia. In: Scriver CR, Sly WS, Childs B, et al., eds. The metabolic and molecular bases of inherited disease; 8th edn. New York: McGraw-Hill; 2000: 1777–1805.

38. Flynn DM, Mohan N, McKiernan P, et al. Progress in treatment and outcome for children with neonatal haemochromatosis. Arch Dis Child Fetal Neonatal Ed 2003; 88:F124–F127.

    A small retrospective series suggesting that early treatment of neonatal hemochromatosis with antioxidant cocktail may be beneficial.

39. Lee LA, Sokol RJ, Buyon JP. Hepatobiliary disease in neonatal lupus: prevalence and clinical characteristics in cases enrolled in a national registry. Pediatrics 2002; 109:E11.

40. Setchell KD, O'Connell NC. Disorders of bile acid synthesis and metabolism: A metabolic basis for liver disease. In: Suchy FJ, ed. Liver disease in children; 2nd edn. Philadelphia: Lippincott Williams & Wilkins; 2001:701–733.

41. Balistreri WF. Bile acid therapy in pediatric hepatobiliary disease: the role of ursodeoxycholic acid. J Pediatr Gastroenterol Nutr 1997; 24:573–589.

42. Jacquemin E, Hadchouel M. Genetic basis of progressive familial intrahepatic cholestasis. J Hepatol 1999; 31:377–381.

43. Jacquemin E, De Vree JM. Cresteil D, et al. The wide spectrum of multidrug resistance 3 deficiency: from neonatal cholestasis to cirrhosis of adulthood. Gastroenterology 2001; 120:1448–1458.

    This study expands on this group's earlier observations (in two patients with PFIC3) by determining the MDR3 genotype in 31 patients with PFIC3 and correlating the genotype with clinical features.

44. Francavilla R, Castellaneta SP, Hadzic N, et al. Prognosis of alpha-1-antitrypsin deficiency-related liver disease in the era of paediatric liver transplantation. J Hepatol 2000; 32:986–992.

45. Feranchak AP, Sokol RJ. Cholangiocyte biology and cystic fibrosis liver disease. Semin Liver Dis 2001; 21:471–488.

46. Saheki T, Kobayashi K, Iijima M, et al. Adult-onset type II citrullinemia and idiopathic neonatal hepatitis caused by citrin deficiency: involvement of the aspartate glutamate carrier for urea synthesis and maintenance of the urea cycle. Mol Genet Metab 2004; 81(Suppl 1):S20–S26.

47. Palmieri L, Pardo B, Lasorsa FM, et al. Citrin and aralar1 are Ca(2+)-stimulated aspartate/glutamate transporters in mitochondria. Embo J 2001; 20:5060–5069.

48. Yasuda T, Yamaguchi N, Kobayashi K, et al. Identification of two novel mutations in the SLC25A13 gene and detection of seven mutations in 102 patients with adult-onset type II citrullinemia. Hum Genet 2000; 107:537–545.

49. Tamamori A, Okano Y, Ozaki H, et al. Neonatal intrahepatic cholestasis caused by citrin deficiency: severe hepatic dysfunction in an infant requiring liver transplantation. Eur J Pediatr 2002; 161:609–613.

50. Ohura T, Kobayashi K, Abukawa D, et al. A novel inborn error of metabolism detected by elevated methionine and/or galactose in newborn screening: neonatal intrahepatic cholestasis caused by citrin deficiency. Eur J Pediatr 2003; 162:317–322.

51. Tazawa Y, Kobayashi K, Ohura T, et al. Infantile cholestatic jaundice associated with adult-onset type II citrullinemia. J Pediatr 2001; 138:735–740.

52. Saheki T, Kobayashi K. Mitochondrial aspartate glutamate carrier (citrin) deficiency as the cause of adult-onset type II citrullinemia (CTLN2) and idiopathic neonatal hepatitis (NICCD). J Hum Genet 2002; 47:333–341.

53. McGovern M, Mistry P. The lysosomal storage diseases. In: Suchy FJ, ed. Liver disease in children; 2nd edn. Philadelphia: Lippincott Williams & Wilkins; 2001:687–700.

54. Freeze HH. Congenital disorders of glycosylation and the pediatric liver. Semin Liver Dis 2001; 21:501–515.

55. Lykavieris P, Hadchouel M, Chardot C, et al. Outcome of liver disease in children with Alagille syndrome: a study of 163 patients. Gut 2001; 49:431–435.

56. Eastham KM, McKiernan PJ, Milford DV, et al. ARC syndrome: an expanding range of phenotypes. Arch Dis Child 2001; 85:415–420.

57. Whitington PF, Emerick KM, Suchy FJ. Familial hepatocellular cholestasis. In: Suchy FJ, ed. Liver disease in children; 2nd edn. Philadelphia: Lippincott Williams & Wilkins; 2001:315–325.

58. Pickering LK. Red Book. 2003 Report of the Committee on Infectious Diseases. Vol.: 26 edn. Elk Grove Village: American Academy of Pediatrics; 2003.

59. Jacquemin E, Lykavieris P, Chaoui N, et al. Transient neonatal cholestasis: origin and outcome. J Pediatr 1998; 133:563–567.

60. Cohran VC. Heubi JE. Treatment of pediatric cholestatic liver disease. Curr Treat Options Gastroenterol 2003; 6:403–415.

61. Yerushalmi B, Sokol RJ, Narkewicz MR, et al. Use of rifampin for severe pruritus in children with chronic cholestasis. J Pediatr Gastroenterol Nutr 1999; 29:442–447.

62. Terra SG, Tsunoda SM. Opioid antagonists in the treatment of pruritus from cholestatic liver disease. Ann Pharmacother 1998; 32:1228–1230.

63. Ng VL, Ryckman FC, Porta G, et al. Long-term outcome after partial external biliary diversion for intractable pruritus in patients with intrahepatic cholestasis. J Pediatr Gastroenterol Nutr 2000; 30:152–156.

64. Emerick KM, Whitington PF. Partial external biliary diversion for intractable pruritus and xanthomas in Alagille syndrome. Hepatology 2002; 35:1501–1506.

CHAPTER FORTY-SEVEN

47

The pregnant patient with jaundice

J. Eileen Hay

INTRODUCTION

Most pregnant women are young and healthy. Liver disease is uncommon in this patient population. However, many hemodynamic and metabolic changes occur during a normal pregnancy to support the placenta and fetus; among these physiologic changes are some which mimic features commonly associated with hepatic dysfunction – spider nevi, palmar erythema, increased alkaline phosphatase due to placental production, decreased serum levels of bilirubin and hemoglobin with expanded blood volume.[1–3] Occasionally, pathophysiologic changes occur, including five liver diseases unique to pregnancy and the postpartum period.[4–7] In addition, any liver disease occurring in young females of childbearing age may also occur during pregnancy. Elevation of bilirubin or aminotransferase levels, hepatosplenomegaly, and hepatic tenderness during pregnancy are always abnormal and the causes of these abnormalities fall into three main categories (Table 47.1): (1) liver diseases unique to pregnancy, (2) liver diseases occurring coincidentally in pregnant patients, and (3) pregnancy in patients with chronic liver disease.

Abnormalities in liver tests occur in 5% of pregnancies and jaundice in 0.1% with causes ranging from self-limiting to rapidly fatal.[4,5,7] Most hepatic dysfunction in pregnancy, especially when severe, is due to pregnancy-associated liver diseases.[8] A study of 4377 deliveries found abnormal liver tests in 3% patients. Most cases showed elevated aminotransferase levels, though bilirubin was increased in 17%. Eighty percent of cases were attributed to pregnancy-associated diseases, 12% had pre-existing hepatobiliary disease, and about one-third had sepsis or postpartum problems which may have contributed.[9]

Pregnancy-related liver diseases

The liver diseases unique to pregnancy have characteristic clinical features and timing of onset in relation to pregnancy (see Table 47.1) and they fall into two main categories depending on their association with or without preeclampsia.

The most common of the pregnancy-related liver diseases not associated with preeclampsia are intrahepatic cholestasis of pregnancy (ICP) and hyperemesis gravidarum. ICP presents with severe pruritus, mild jaundice, and biochemical cholestasis limited to the second half of pregnancy.[10–13] Genetic, hormonal, and exogenous factors have been implicated in its etiology.[12,14–17] In the United States, ICP occurs in 0.1% pregnancies, with jaundice in 20% of patients affected by ICP. Hyperemesis gravidarum occurs at a rate between 2 and 10 per 1000 pregnancies and is characterized by

Table 47.1 Causes and timing of liver disease during pregnancy

Disease category	Specific disease	Trimester of pregnancy
Chronic liver disease/portal hypertension	Chronic hepatitis B	1–3
	Hepatitis C	1–3
	Autoimmune disease	1–3
	Wilson's disease	1–3
	Cirrhosis of any cause	1–3
	Extrahepatic portal hypertension	1–3
Liver disease coincidental with pregnancy	Acute viral hepatitis	1–3
	Budd-Chiari	Postpartum
	Gallstones	1–3
	Drug-induced	1–3
Liver disease unique to pregnancy	Cholestasis of pregnancy	2–3
	Hyperemesis gravidarum	1
	Preeclampsia	3, late 2
	HELLP syndrome	3, late 2
	Acute fatty liver of pregnancy	3

intractable nausea and vomiting occurring in the first trimester. High aminotransferase levels occur in 50% of patients and occasionally jaundice, transient hyperthyroidism, and elevated serum fatty acids may occur.[18-20] ICP and hyperemesis are not associated with preeclampsia.

The preeclampsia-associated liver diseases are preeclampsia itself, the HELLP syndrome, and acute fatty liver of pregnancy (AFLP) and there is overlap between these three conditions. These are, like preeclampsia, diseases of the third trimester of pregnancy. Preeclampsia occurs in 5–10% of pregnancies and, although liver involvement is infrequent, it is the most common pregnancy-related cause of hepatic dysfunction – 1.4% of all deliveries in a recent prospective study.[8,21] Severe preeclampsia is complicated in 2–12% cases (0.2–0.6% pregnancies) by hemolysis (H), elevated liver tests (EL), and low platelet count (LP) – the so-called HELLP syndrome.[22-25] Microangiopathic hemolytic anemia causes the classic hepatic lesion of periportal or focal parenchymal necrosis and hemorrhage which may extend into a parenchymal or subcapsular hemorrhage and hepatic rupture. Microvesicular fatty infiltration of the liver in pregnancy (AFLP) causes encephalopathy and hepatic failure, a sudden catastrophic illness occurring almost exclusively in the third trimester.[26-30] In its most severe form, AFLP is reported as uncommon to rare, less than 0.005% pregnancies,[29] although its incidence was considerably higher in a recent prospective study.[9] A large British population study of 48 865 deliveries had 25 cases of HELLP with one maternal death and 3 cases of AFLP.[31] In 46 cases of severe pregnancy-related hepatic dysfunction referred to a tertiary referral center, 70% had AFLP, 15% HELLP syndrome, 2% hepatic rupture associated with preeclampsia, and 13% causes incidental to pregnancy.[32] The etiologies of the pregnancy-associated liver diseases remain obscure but new knowledge is emerging, in particular greater understanding of biliary canalicular transport proteins in ICP[12,13] and of intramitochondrial fatty acid oxidation in AFLP.[17,30,33-37]

Of course, not all liver diseases that present during pregnancy are actually related to the pregnancy. Jaundice in pregnancy may be due to any of the many causes of jaundice in the nonpregnant patient. Viral hepatitis, due to hepatitis A, B, C, D, or E, herpes simplex, cytomegalovirus, or Epstein-Barr virus, is reported to account for 40% of jaundice in pregnant women in the USA.[38-42] The incidence of viral hepatitis is the same in pregnant and nonpregnant populations and during each of the three trimesters of pregnancy (hepatitis A in 1 per 1000, hepatitis B in 2 per 1000). Hepatitis E is an exception. It is an enterically transmitted hepatitis virus that is rare in the USA, but is endemic to large areas of Asia, Africa, and Central America. If infection occurs during the third trimester of pregnancy, a high proportion of women develop fulminant hepatitis and the mortality rate is high, probably influenced by malnutrition.[43,44] In India, 25% of women with fulminant hepatic failure are pregnant and almost all cases are due to acute viral hepatitis, particularly hepatitis B and E.[44-47]

Gallstones are found in 3% pregnant women due to the increased lithogenicity of bile and biliary stasis during pregnancy, but symptomatic in only 0.1–0.3% of pregnancies.[6,48-50] The most frequent clinical presentation is biliary colic and liver tests may be abnormal at the time of presentation. In addition, gallstone pancreatitis (50% of women <30 years old with pancreatitis are pregnant) and, less commonly, acute cholecystitis may occur.[50]

Many women with chronic viral hepatitis, autoimmune hepatitis, or Wilson's disease are of child-bearing age. Although most patients with advanced cirrhosis are amenorrheic and infertile, increased maternal and fetal problems can be expected if pregnancy occurs. However, the majority of women with chronic liver disease are well compensated and capable of pregnancy. Chronic hepatitis B is present in 0.5–1.5% pregnancies and chronic hepatitis C in 2.3%, particularly in some indigent populations. An uncomplicated pregnancy with no disease flare is expected in those with mild disease or disease in remission.[51,52] Discontinuation of D-penicillamine therapy in the pregnant Wilson's patient can result in fulminant disease. The pregnant liver transplant recipient with jaundice represents a unique clinical situation requiring specialized care.

DIAGNOSIS

Diagnostic strategy

Optimal management of the pregnant patient with abnormal liver tests or jaundice requires accurate and usually rapid diagnosis. The following questions are relevant in the approach to such patients (Fig. 47.1):

1) Are there any features of underlying chronic liver disease?
2) Is the presentation compatible with acute viral hepatitis?
3) Are there any features to suggest biliary disease?
4) Is there any history of drugs or toxins?
5) Are there any features of Budd-Chiari syndrome?
6) Is there any evidence or risk factors for sepsis?
7) Does the presentation fit one of the liver diseases unique to pregnancy?

An approach focused on these questions will narrow the investigation. Clinical features and laboratory testing will easily reduce the large number of diagnostic possibilities and allow a diagnosis to be made quickly in most patients. In some, hepatic imaging by ultrasonography or computed tomography, endoscopic retrograde cholangiopancreatography (ERCP) or liver biopsy will be necessary.

Clinical presentation

The clinical presentation and trimester of pregnancy are of vital diagnostic importance (see Table 47.1). Features of chronic liver disease must be sought, risk factors for viral hepatitis elicited, and a history of drugs or potential hepatotoxins (including alcohol) identified. Acute viral hepatitis can occur at any time during pregnancy. Apart from hepatitis E and herpes simplex, the clinical and serologic course of acute hepatitis is identical to the nonpregnant patient. In most cases, the hepatitis does not appear to adversely affect the pregnancy. Though rare, herpes simplex hepatitis must be diagnosed, as specific therapy is life-saving for mother and child. Herpes simplex hepatitis typically occurs as a primary infection in the third trimester and has systemic features with a prodrome and fever, diffuse vesicular rash, vulvar or oropharyngeal vesicular lesions, leukopenia, and coagulopathy. Patients are usually anicteric even with hepatic failure.[53] Although drug therapy is rare in pregnancy, ritodrine, used for the treatment of premature labor, may occasionally cause liver test abnormalities.[54] The clinical features of biliary disease and pancreatitis are the same as in the nonpregnant patient, can occur at any time of gestation, and may recur during the pregnancy. Budd-Chiari syndrome is rare but may occur in pregnancy or, more typically,

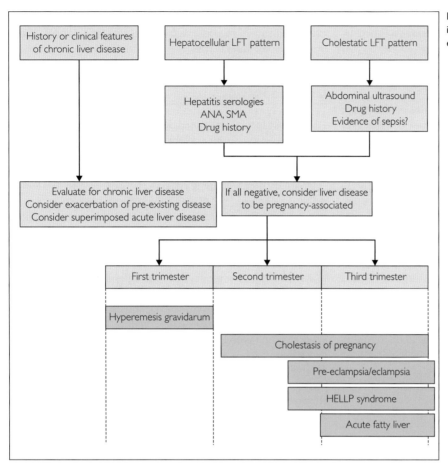

Fig. 47.1 • Approach to abnormal liver tests in the pregnant patient (see text for features of each disease).

in the postpartum period. It has been associated with antiphospholipid antibody syndrome, thrombotic thrombocytopenic purpura, paroxysmal nocturnal hemoglobinuria, myeloproliferative disorders such as essential thrombocytosis, preeclampsia, and septic abortion.[55,56] Cholestatis of sepsis due to pyelonephritis or septic abortion may cause jaundice in early pregnancy and severe Gram-negative sepsis with jaundice may occur in the third trimester.

Hyperemesis gravidarum[19,21,22] is intractable vomiting during pregnancy of such severity as to necessitate intravenous hydration. It occurs in the first trimester, typically between weeks 4 and 10, and may be complicated by jaundice. Risk factors are adolescent pregnancy, multiparity, twins and hydatiform mole. Generally a clinical diagnosis is made but with high aminotransferases, other diseases such as viral hepatitis or drug-induced liver disease must be excluded. In contrast to hyperemesis gravidarum, uncomplicated vomiting in pregnancy does not result in liver dysfunction.

The onset of pruritus around weeks 25–32 in a patient without other signs of liver disease is strongly suggestive of ICP, especially in the multiparous patient with a history of pruritus that resolved after delivery in a previous pregnancy.[11] Occasionally diarrhea or steatorrhea will be present with malabsorption of fat-soluble vitamins. Jaundice occurs in 10–25% patients and usually follows the pruritus by 2–4 weeks. Jaundice without pruritus is rare. The typical clinical picture with consistent liver abnormalities and exclusion of other causes of liver disease usually allows a confident diagnosis to be made. However, ICP is only confirmed by the rapid

postpartum resolution of symptoms and liver test abnormalities.

In the severely ill patient with jaundice in third trimester, preeclampsia, HELLP and AFLP must be considered. Preeclampsia is the triad of hypertension, edema, and proteinuria and may present with right upper abdominal pain, jaundice, and a tender, normal-sized liver.[57] No clinical features distinguish this from the HELLP syndrome (weight gain due to edema (60%), hypertension (80%)) but jaundice is uncommon (5%). Some patients have no obvious preeclampsia. Patients with HELLP also may present with epigastric or right upper quadrant pain (65–90%), nausea, and vomiting (35–50%), a 'flu-like' illness (90%), and/or headache (30%). Most (71%) present between 27 and 36 weeks' gestation, but 11% present earlier and 18% present after this time. Indeed, 30% of cases of HELLP develop in the postpartum period, usually within 48 hours of delivery. Finally, parenchymal hematoma may lead to hepatic rupture and can occur in the late third trimester or postpartum period.

While HELLP is more common in the older multiparous patient, 50% patients with AFLP are nulliparous and there is an increased incidence in twin pregnancies.[27] AFLP occurs almost exclusively in the third trimester from 28 to 40 weeks, but occasionally develops after delivery. About 50% of patients with AFLP have preeclampsia. The presentation varies from asymptomatic to fulminant liver failure with jaundice in most patients. The typical patient has a prodromal illness consisting of 1–2 weeks of anorexia, nausea, vomiting, and right upper quadrant pain. The patient is usually ill and icteric, and examination commonly reveals hypertension, edema, ascites, a small liver (though it may be enlarged initially) and a variable degree of hepatic encephalopathy.[58] Intrauterine death may occur.

Liver tests

Liver tests may help differentiate between a hepatic or cholestatic process, although an elevated alkaline phosphatase is less helpful during pregnancy. High aminotransferase levels are consistent with viral hepatitis (often >1000 IU/mL), flare of autoimmune disease, or AFLP. In AFLP, the AST level can vary from near normal to 1000, but averages about 300 IU/mL. The aminotransferase level is quite variable in patients with hyperemesis gravidarum, intrahepatic cholestasis of pregnancy,[11] acute biliary obstruction, and preeclampsia with or without HELLP syndrome ranging from minimally elevated to 10–20 times the upper limit of normal. Mild elevations of serum bilirubin (<5 mg/dL) are typical of ICP, hyperemesis, preeclampsia, HELLP syndrome, and AFLP and higher levels in the latter conditions may indicate more severe or complicated disease with hemolysis or renal insufficiency. Elevated serum bile acid levels (up to 100 times above normal) are a very sensitive marker of ICP, are always elevated in this disorder, and may correlate with fetal risk.[11,15,59] Diagnostic criteria for viral, autoimmune, and other types of chronic liver disease are the same for pregnant patients as for the nonpregnant.

Hepatitis serology

Hepatitis serology for A, B, and C and serology for Epstein-Barr and cytomegalovirus should be performed in all cases of abnormal liver tests or jaundice during pregnancy. Antibody to hepatitis E virus should be tested if the patient is from or has been a recent traveler to an endemic area.[42] Because the antibody test for hepatitis C may be negative during acute hepatitis, HCV RNA should be tested; HCV RNA has been positive in several pregnant patients who subsequently developed hepatitis C.[60] Serologies, nucleic acid testing of serum and liver, liver biopsy, and cultures may be necessary to diagnose herpes simplex hepatitis.

Imaging of liver and bile ducts

Ultrasonography (US) of the liver and abdomen is safe at any time during pregnancy and can be helpful in the evaluation of biliary tract disease, patency of hepatic and portal veins, AFLP, hematomas, and rupture. In ICP hepatic ultrasonography is usually normal, although gallstones and biliary sludge may be seen.[11] Computed tomography (CT) is more sensitive than US in detecting AFLP, hepatic rupture, and necrosis; however, it should be limited to 1–2 views of the liver to reduce radiation exposure to the fetus. In 34 patients with HELLP, hepatic imaging was abnormal in 16 patients, showing subcapsular hematomas in 13, intraparenchymal hemorrhage in 6, a ruptured capsule in 4, and hepatic infarction in 1.[61] The utility and safety of magnetic resonance imaging (MRI) has yet to be definitely established. Radionucleotide scans during pregnancy are best avoided because of radiation exposure.

To confirm the diagnosis of choledocholithiasis, ERCP can be safely done in the pregnant patient. The fluoroscopy utilized for a typical ERCP usually exposes the patient to radiation well below the fetal safety level but this can be further minimized by shielding of the lower abdomen. Midazolam, meperidine, and glucagon can be given with safety. If indicated, sphincterotomy and stone extraction should be performed at the same time. Hepatic venography is sometimes necessary to confirm Budd-Chiari syndrome in the patient with compatible clinical and US features.

Liver biopsy

Liver biopsy is rarely indicated during pregnancy. In particular, it is not necessary to do a biopsy to differentiate preeclampsia, HELLP, and AFLP, as the therapy is similar, but biopsy may be necessary in some cases to differentiate AFLP from viral hepatitis. A biopsy with special stains for fat (e.g., oil red) is essential for the definitive diagnosis of AFLP. The characteristic histologic appearance is that of microvesicular, and infrequently macrovesicular, fatty infiltration (free fatty acids) predominantly in zone 3. There is lobular disarray with pleomorphism of hepatocytes and mild portal inflammation with cholestasis.[62] The appearance is similar to Reye's syndrome, tetracycline and valproic acid toxicity. This histologic picture, while usually diagnostic, may occasionally be difficult to differentiate from viral hepatitis or preeclampsia. However, the characteristic histologic finding in both the HELLP syndrome and preeclampsia is periportal hemorrhage and fibrin deposition which is absent in AFLP.[23] Periportal hepatocytes are necrotic and thrombi may form in small portal arterioles. In severe disease, areas of infarction may be multiple or diffuse; hemorrhage dissects through the portal connective tissue initially from zone 1, then more diffusely to involve the whole lobule leading to large hematomas, capsular tears, and intraperitoneal bleeding. However, in general, the severity of the histologic findings in HELLP and preeclampsia correlates poorly with the clinical or biochemical picture. Hepatic histology may be necessary for the diagnosis of autoimmune hepatitis and is usually essential for herpes simplex hepatitis with typical intranuclear inclusions. In ICP, the appearance of the liver is nearly normal, even in the presence of high aminotransferase levels, or may show only mild cholestasis and minimal hepatocellular necrosis. The hepatic histologic appearance of hyperemesis gravidarum is usually normal, but rare cholestasis or cell dropout without inflammation may be seen. In ICP or hyperemesis gravidarum, a liver biopsy is done only if necessary to exclude another more serious condition.

Diagnoses of HELLP and AFLP

The rapidity of clinical deterioration usually mandates that the diagnoses of HELLP and AFLP be established quickly in order to minimize maternal and fetal risk and expedite delivery, if indicated. Since both conditions occur during the third trimester in patients with preeclampsia, it is worthwhile reviewing their diagnostic criteria and differentiation.[29,63] Their typical clinical, biochemical, and radiologic features are described above but both require further testing for diagnostic confirmation (Table 47.2). Diagnosis of HELLP syndrome requires the presence of all three criteria: (1) hemolysis with an abnormal blood smear, elevated LDH (>600 IU/L) and increase in indirect bilirubin; (2) AST of >70 IU/L; and (3) platelet count of <100 000 cells/mm³, and, in severe cases, <50 000 cells/mm³.[59] Prothrombin time, APTT, and fibrinogen levels are usually normal with no increase in fibrin-split products, though disseminated intravascular coagulation (DIC) may occasionally be present. Elevation of

Table 47.2 Diagnostic differences between AFLP and HELLP

	AFLP	HELLP
Parity	Nulliparous, twins	Multiparous, older
Jaundice	Common	Uncommon
Mean bilirubin	8 mg/dL	2 mg/dL
Encephalopathy	Present	Absent
Platelets	Low–normal	Low
Protime	Prolonged	Normal
APTT	Prolonged	Normal
Fibrinogen	Low	Normal–increased
Glucose	Low	Normal
Creatinine	High	High
Ammonia	High	Normal
CT scan	Fatty infiltration	Hemorrhage

aminotransferases is highly variable. Hepatic CT scan may show the diagnostic features described above.

In AFLP, typical laboratory abnormalities include a normochromic-normocytic anemia, high WBC count, normal-to-low platelet count, prolonged prothrombin time and APTT, reduced fibrinogen with or without DIC, metabolic acidosis, renal dysfunction (often progressing to oliguric renal failure), hypoglycemia, aminotransferase levels from 100 to 1000 IU/L, mild elevation of bilirubin (<6 mg/dL), high ammonia, and often biochemical pancreatitis.[64] Hepatic CT scan is more sensitive than US to demonstrate fatty infiltration, but a normal scan cannot exclude the diagnosis; the diagnosis is confirmed only by liver biopsy. Nonetheless, in the patient who is severely ill, has coagulopathy, and requires urgent termination of pregnancy, a presumptive diagnosis of AFLP is usually made on the above criteria without the benefit of a liver biopsy. The complications of sepsis, DIC, and major intra-abdominal bleeding are much more common in AFLP than HELLP. Some studies actually suggest a continuum from HELLP to preeclampsia with liver abnormalities to AFLP.[65]

The differential diagnoses of HELLP and AFLP include thrombotic thrombocytopenic purpura[66] and hemolytic-uremic syndrome. In patients who present in the third trimester with acute hepatic failure, the clinical differentiation of AFLP and viral hepatitis, especially hepatitis E in the appropriate geographic setting, can be impossible without positive viral serology or liver biopsy. Hepatitis serology should be performed in all cases but is sometimes not available in time to make clinical decisions.

MANAGEMENT

Hyperemesis gravidarum

Treatment is symptomatic though hospitalization is occasionally necessary for rehydration and nutritional support.[19,20,67] Symptomatic therapy with antihistamines or metoclopramide is often helpful. Oral ginger root or pyridoxine (vitamin B$_6$) may give occasional relief. Short-term high-dose steroids are occasionally used in refractory cases.

Intrahepatic cholestasis of pregnancy

Pruritus improves and liver function normalizes immediately after delivery and, since there is no maternal mortality, management strategies for the mother have focused on symptomatic relief.[12] Pruritus affects maternal well-being to a variable extent from mild distress to suicidal ideation. Steatorrhea may affect maternal nutrition and occasionally cause vitamin K deficiency with resulting coagulopathy that can be problematic for the fetus. In patients on progesterone, withdrawal of that drug may cause remission of the pruritus in some patients prior to delivery.[4,11]

Ursodeoxycholic acid (UDCA) is the agent of choice for treatment of ICP. One gram of UDCA daily in divided doses may give relief of pruritus with parallel improvement in liver tests without adverse maternal or fetal effects.[68] Three small double-blind trials have randomized 29 patients to UDCA (600–1000 mg/d) and compared them to 27 placebo-treated patients.[58,69,70] There was demonstrable clinical and biochemical improvement with UDCA, and fetal outcome was improved with less prematurity.[58,69,70] High-dose UDCA (1.5–2.0 g/d) has recently been shown to relieve pruritus in most cases and reduce abnormal maternal bile acid levels, while remaining safe for the fetus. In addition, babies born to these mothers had almost normal bile acid levels in comparison to babies born to untreated mothers.[71]

Cholestyramine, 8–24 g/d, may sometimes give relief of pruritus after 1–2 weeks but biochemical parameters, maternal malabsorption, and fetal prognosis are not improved. Dexamethasone (12 mg/d for 7 days), by suppressing fetoplacental estrogen production, improves symptoms, liver tests, and fetal lung maturity without apparent adverse effects.[72] Intravenous S-adenosyl-L-methionine (SAMe), an antioxidant, has not proven to be effective as compared to UDCA.[73–75] Similarly, epomediol and silymarin have produced symptomatic relief in a few patients without changes in biochemical markers.[76,77] Benzodiazepines, antihistamines, and phenobarbital are ineffective.

ICP recurs in 45–70% of subsequent pregnancies and occasionally with oral contraceptives. Thus, counseling is indicated. Patients with ICP may develop more gallstones and gallbladder disease. Some rare familial cases of apparent ICP have persisted postpartum, with progression to subsequent fibrosis and cirrhosis.[78,79]

The main risk during the pregnancy with ICP is to the fetus, with a high incidence of premature deliveries, perinatal deaths, and fetal distress.[13] Fetal monitoring for chronic placental insufficiency is essential but will not prevent all fetal deaths.[11,80] Fetal deaths due to acute anoxia[81] can be prevented only by early delivery by 35 weeks or earlier as soon as there is fetal lung maturity. Whether or not UDCA improves fetal outcome remains to be determined.

Preeclampsia

Delivery is the only definitive therapy and should be done urgently whenever complications of preeclampsia are severe.[24] No specific therapy is needed for the hepatic involvement of preeclampsia and its only significance is as an indicator of severe disease with need for immediate delivery to avoid eclampsia, hepatic rupture, or necrosis. The rare patient with hepatic rupture and severe necrosis, complicated by encephalopathy and metabolic acidosis, may need consideration for liver transplantation. Both HELLP and AFLP may complicate preeclampsia.

HELLP syndrome

The management of the patient with HELLP syndrome must be effected without delay[24,25] and first priority is antepartum stabilization of the mother including treatment of hypertension and DIC, and seizure prophylaxis. A hepatic CT scan is helpful to determine whether hepatic infarction, subcapsular hematomas, or hepatic rupture is present. Consideration should be given to transfer to a tertiary referral center.

Delivery is the only definitive therapy. When the patient is near-term and/or there is fetal lung maturity, immediate delivery should be effected. Cesarean section is preferred, though well-established labor should be allowed to proceed in the absence of obstetric complications or DIC. More than 40% of affected women will require cesarean section especially if they are primigravidae, remote from term, or have an unfavorable cervix.[25] Half of patients require blood or blood products to correct hypovolemia, anemia, or coagulopathy, especially those undergoing cesarean section. Careful fluid management is critical since patients have a high risk of renal compromise if they have intravascular volume depletion and pulmonary edema, ascites, and edema with overhydration. Hemodynamic monitoring may be needed in severe cases.[8] Management remote from term is controversial and sometimes in milder cases who are at <34 weeks of gestation a more conservative approach with high-dose glucocorticoids is taken in hopes of prolonging the pregnancy and improving fetal lung maturity.[82] This therapy may also be of benefit to aid maternal stability during the transfer time to a tertiary referral center.

Most patients have rapid and early resolution of HELLP following delivery, with normalization of platelet counts after 5 days. However, some have persisting thrombocytopenia, hemolysis, progressive elevations of bilirubin and creatinine. Persistence of signs for more than 72 hours with either no improvement or development of life-threatening complications is usually taken as an indication for plasmapheresis. Several other modalities have been used in an attempt to treat or reverse the syndrome including plasma volume expansion, antithrombotic agents, steroids, plasmapheresis, plasma exchange with fresh-frozen plasma,[83] and hemodialysis, but no clinical trials have been done. More specific therapy awaits better understanding of the pathophysiologic mechanism.[84] Serious maternal complications are not infrequent and are due to DIC (20%), abruptio placentae (16%) – both of which are associated with fetal mortality – acute renal failure (8%), pulmonary edema (8%), ARDS (1%), severe ascites (8%), or hepatic failure (2%). Due to these complications, present maternal mortality rates range 1–4%, although in the past much higher mortality was seen in severe cases. Most babies do very well though occasionally there may be mild hemolysis.

Most recent experience of hepatic hemorrhage without rupture supports conservative management of hemodynamically stable patients. These patients require close hemodynamic monitoring in an intensive care unit, correction of coagulopathy, and availability of large-volume transfusion of blood and blood products. Even minimal exogenous abdominal trauma, for example from abdominal palpation, convulsions, emesis, or unnecessary transportation, must be avoided. Serial CT scans can be helpful. Most ruptures are preceded by parenchymal hematomas in the right lobe which progresses to a contained subcapsular hematoma. Obviously, suspicion of hepatic rupture mandates immediate surgical or radiologic (embolization) intervention.[85] Liver transplantation has been carried out in the rare patient with severe acute hepatic necrosis and rupture. Maternal mortality from hepatic rupture remains very high at 50% and perinatal mortality rates are 10–60%, mostly from placental rupture, intrauterine asphyxia, or prematurity. Rarely, hepatic rupture is associated with an intra-hepatic tumor (especially an adenoma) rather than with HELLP.

The risk of recurrence of HELLP in subsequent pregnancies is difficult to assess but is estimated at 3–25%.[86] Subsequent deliveries in these patients carry an increased risk of pre-eclampsia, preterm delivery, intrauterine growth retardation, and abruptio placentae.[87]

Acute fatty liver of pregnancy

Early recognition of acute fatty liver of pregnancy (AFLP) with immediate termination of pregnancy and intensive supportive care are essential for both maternal and fetal survival. There are no reports of recovery prior to delivery. Aminotransferases and encephalopathy typically improve within a few day after delivery, but intensive supportive care is needed until recovery occurs. Patients who are critically ill at the time of presentation, who develop complications (encephalopathy, hypoglycemia, coagulopathy, bleeding), or who continue to deteriorate despite emergency delivery, should be transferred to a specialized liver unit.

Delivery is usually accomplished by cesarean section, but the necessity for this has not been tested in randomized trials.[88] Rapid controlled vaginal delivery with fetal monitoring is probably safer if the cervix is favorable and will reduce the incidence of major intra-abdominal bleeding.[54] Following correction of coagulation, epidural anesthesia is probably the best choice for delivery and will allow better ongoing assessment of the patient's level of consciousness. It is probably best to maintain an INR of less than 1.5 and a platelet count of at least 50 000 cells/mm^3 during and after delivery (to prevent postpartum hemorrhage) and administer prophylactic antibiotics. Intra-abdominal bleeding is a poor prognostic sign.[54]

Intensive supportive care requires blood glucose monitoring and 5–20% intravenous glucose as needed for hypoglycemia. Packed cells should be used to correct anemia, platelets for thrombocytopenia, and FFP for coagulopathy or DIC. Bleeding complications especially from the uterus may require large-volume blood transfusion and re-exploration of the abdomen may be needed with occasional ligation of pelvic vessels or hysterectomy. With severe bleeding, FFP is best for the coagulopathy and neither heparin nor antithrombin III is recommended for DIC.[27] H$_2$-blockers should be administered for bleeding prophylaxis since gastrointestinal bleeding is common. Careful fluid management is critical and dialysis should be instituted for renal failure and control of volume, especially when large amounts of volume are required. Lactulose and a high carbohydrate diet have been recommended for management of encephalopathy. Plasmapheresis has been used in some cases though its benefit is unproven. Corticosteroids are ineffective.

Although liver function will start to improve within 3 days of delivery, the disease then enters a cholestatic phase with rising bilirubin and alkaline phosphatase. Depending on the severity and complications, recovery can occur in days or be delayed for months but is eventually complete with no signs of chronic liver disease. With early delivery and advances in supportive management, maternal mortality is now 10–18% and fetal mortality

9–23%.[28,54,63] Infectious and bleeding complications remain the most life-threatening. Liver transplantation has a very limited role here because of the great potential for recovery with delivery which makes the timing of OLT very difficult even in the rare patient who may need it. However, successful liver transplantation has been reported and should be considered in patients whose clinical course continues to deteriorate with advancing fulminant hepatic failure after the first 1–2 days postpartum without signs of hepatic regeneration.[89]

Many patients do not become pregnant again after AFLP, either by choice due to the devastating effect of the illness or by necessity due to hysterectomy to control postpartum bleeding with the AFLP. However, AFLP does not tend to recur in subsequent pregnancies though one such case has been reported. Because LCHAD (long-chain 3-hydroxyacyl-coenzyme dehydrogenase) deficiency in the infant is responsible for many cases of AFLP, later neonatal problems may occur.[35,90] Infants born to mothers with AFLP should be evaluated by a neonatologist and followed closely.

Biliary disease

Biliary colic and cholecystitis are not associated with fetal or maternal mortality. Conservative therapy with bed rest, intravenous fluids, and antibiotics is the preferred initial therapy and is successful in more than 80% of cases, though symptoms are likely to recur.[6] An impacted common bile duct stone or worsening gallstone pancreatitis requires ERCP, sphincterotomy, and stone extraction under antibiotic coverage since maternal health and survival is the best way to ensure good fetal outcome.[91,92] Indications for cholecystectomy during pregnancy are generally considered to be limited to intractable biliary colic, severe acute cholecystitis not responding to conservative measures, and acute gallstone pancreatitis with retained gallstones. These indications occur with a widely variable reported incidence of 0.005–0.1% of pregnancies. Surgery during the first 10 weeks of pregnancy has an abortion risk associated with anesthesia and a potential teratogenic effect of carbon dioxide. In the third trimester, the uterus may impinge into the surgical field and there is an increased risk of premature delivery. Thus, the second trimester is the safest period for surgical intervention with a fetal morbidity of rate of less than 1%. Laparoscopic cholecystectomy with or without ERCP and sphincterotomy can be performed with very little morbidity or mortality between weeks 13 and 32 of pregnancy.[6,92–95] Standard precautions for obstetric anesthesia are required with relative maternal hyperventilation and minimal intra-abdominal CO_2 pressure to minimize changes in maternal $PaCO_2$.

Viral hepatitis

Management of the patient with acute viral hepatitis is supportive with the exception of herpes simplex infection which requires prompt therapy with acyclovir or vidarabine. Early treatment of systemic herpetic infection is life-saving; without treatment 50% of mothers will die. Acute or chronic viral hepatitis are not indications for termination of pregnancy, except in herpes infection which is not responding to antiviral therapy. Congenital malformations in the fetus occur only with early CMV and herpetic infection. Viral hepatitis is not an indication for cesarean section, and breast feeding should not be discouraged.

Perinatal transmission of hepatitis B is highest in those with acute or chronic hepatitis who have high levels of viremia (HBV DNA >10^5 copies/mL), especially with HBeAg positivity in the third trimester (50–80%). The risk of transmission is lower in mothers with low levels of replication, it occurs in 25% of anti-HBe-positive chronic hepatitis patients and only 5% of those with anti-HBe positivity and normal aminotransferase levels (carriers). Infection transmitted to the infant results in chronic infection in 80–90% of babies.[38,39] Transmission of hepatitis B is not transplacental but occurs at the time of delivery and is preventable in about 95% of cases by passive-active immunoprophylaxis of the babies at birth and such treatment is indicated for all infants born to HBsAg-positive mothers (Table 47.3). Breast feeding is not contraindicated even if the mother has active hepatitis B. Vertical transmission of hepatitis A, D, and C is rare, though the latter increases in HIV coinfection.[96,97] Newborns of mothers with hepatitis A in third trimester should be given passive immunoprophylaxis with standard immunoglobulin within 48 hours of birth. Immunoglobulin does not prevent transmission of hepatitis C from infected mothers and is not indicated.

Complications of chronic liver disease

Autoimmune disease is usually relatively quiescent during pregnancy. Disease activity may flare in the late third trimester or early postpartum period and is managed by increasing steroids as necessary. Azathioprine is often used for maintenance of remission in the patient with autoimmune hepatitis and does not need to be stopped during pregnancy. Azathioprine has not been associated with increased fetal risk.

Patients with Wilson's disease must be adequately treated prior to pregnancy and therapy must continue throughout. Discontinuation of chelation therapy risks development of fulminant hepatic failure. D-penicillamine is the best therapy for Wilson's disease and it has been associated with rare congenital defects. Thus, patients should be forewarned of the risks. Trientine is a safe alternative for fetal health, but of less proven efficacy for the mother.[98]

Little is known about the optimal management of the pregnant patient with cirrhosis and portal hypertension since most women with advanced liver disease are infertile.[3,99] The main risk to the mother is massive gastrointestinal bleeding (20–25%). Patients with known esophageal varices should be considered for prophylactic endoscopic therapy, shunt surgery, or even liver transplantation prior to pregnancy. Vaginal deliveries are possible in most

Table 47.3 Prophylaxis regimen for babies of HBsAg-positive mothers

Preparation	Dose	Route of administration
HBIG	0.5 mL	Intramuscularly at birth
HBV vaccine*	0.5 mL(10 μg)	At birth (2 days) 1 month 6 months

* Recombinant vaccine.

patients, but should be done with early forceps or vacuum suction to avoid lengthy labor. In patients known to have large varices or other evidence of portal hypertension, cesarean section is generally recommended since it avoids straining and the resulting increases to portal pressure seen with vaginal delivery. Some studies, however, have suggested that the risk of variceal bleeding is not increased with vaginal delivery. Postpartum hemorrhage occurs in 15–30% of these patients and is reduced by correction of coagulopathy. Other maternal risks are hepatic decompensation, jaundice, thrombocytopenia, and rupture of splenic aneurysms.[10,99] Postpartum bacterial infections are more common in cirrhotics and warrant prophylactic antibiotics. The complications of portal hypertension should be managed as they would be in the non-pregnant patient. However, vasopressin should not be used in the pregnant patient.

The liver transplant recipient

Management of jaundice in the pregnant liver transplant recipient is a unique situation which needs the combined expertise of a high-risk obstetrician and a transplant hepatologist. Pregnancies are more likely to result in early abortions, preterm deliveries, and low birth weight babies when compared to pregnancies in non-transplant patients.[100–105] In some series, preeclampsia and hypertension (less with tacrolimus than cyclosporine) are increased especially in patients with pre-existing renal dysfunction,[31] with occasional reports of ICP (in a multiparous patient whose pre-transplant pregnancies were normal), and HELLP.[106] However, in most cases the outcome of pregnancy is excellent when the pregnancy is planned in the patient with 1–2 years of stable allograft function. Either cyclosporine or tacrolimus-based immunosuppression is acceptable. The main risk to the allograft is probably from acute cellular rejection[105] or recurrent viral hepatitis. Allograft dysfunction may require investigation with ultrasonography and/or a liver biopsy. Immunosuppression requires close monitoring during pregnancy and the dose may need to be increased as plasma volume expands in later pregnancy.[105]

SUMMARY

Pregnant women are typically young and healthy, so liver disease is uncommon. Nonetheless, abnormal liver tests occur in about 5% of pregnancies and require evaluation since the underlying disease may be severe and result in increased risk to the mother and fetus. Several questions usually clarify the diagnosis during the initial evaluation of the patient. These include: (1) Are there any features of underlying chronic liver disease? (2) Is the presentation compatible with acute viral hepatitis? (3) Are there any features to suggest biliary tract disease? (4) Is there any history of the use of potentially hepatotoxic drugs or agents? (5) Are there any features of Budd-Chiari syndrome? (6) Is there evidence or risk factors for sepsis? and, finally, (7) Does the presentation fit one of the liver diseases unique to pregnancy? With the exception of hyperemesis gravidarum liver disease unique to pregnancy, all occur during the third trimester, sometimes during the second trimester, and even occasionally within days after delivery. While a precise diagnosis cannot always be made in severe liver dysfunction in the third trimester, the appropriate management (i.e., delivery) should not be delayed.

REFERENCES

1. Steven MM. Pregnancy and liver disease. Gut 1981; 22:592–614.

2. Bacq Y, Zarka O, Brechot, J-F, et al. Liver function tests in normal pregnancy: a prospective study of 103 pregnant women and 103 matched controls. Hepatology 1996; 23:1030–1034.

   Defines the normal range of liver test during the course of pregnancy.

3. Yip DM, Baker AL. Liver disease in pregnancy. Clin Perinatol 1985; 12:683–694.

4. Knox TA, Olans LB. Liver disease in pregnancy. N Engl J Med 1996; 335:569–576.

5. Wolf JL. Liver disease in pregnancy. Med Clin N Am 1996; 80:1167–1187.

6. Malangoni MA. Gastrointestinal surgery and pregnancy. Gastroenterol Clin N Am 2003; 32:181–200.

7. Sandhu BS, Sanyal AJ. Pregnancy and liver disease. Gastroenterol Clin N Am 2003; 32:407–436.

8. Rahman TM, Wendon J. Severe hepatic dysfunction in pregnancy. Q J Med 2002; 95:343–357.

9. Ch'ng CL, Morgan M, Hainsworth I, et al. Prospective study of liver dysfunction in pregnancy in southwest Wales. Gut 2002; 51:876–880.

10. Bacq Y, Sapey T, Brechot M-C, et al. Intrahepatic cholestasis of pregnancy: a French prospective study. Hepatology 1997; 26:358–364.

    A review of 50 cases of intrahepatic cholestasis of pregnancy characterized by pruritus and jaundice. Exogenous progesterone treatment may be implicated in the pathogenesis. Premature delivery was common.

11. Reyes H, Simon FR. Intrahepatic cholestasis of pregnancy: an estrogen-related disease. Sem Liv Dis 1993; 13:289–301.

12. Mullally BA, Hansen WF. Intrahepatic cholestasis of pregnancy: review of the literature. Obstet Gynecol Surv 2002; 57:47–52.

13. Milkiewicz P, Elias E, Williamson C, et al. Obstetric cholestasis: may have serious consequences for the fetus, and needs to be taken seriously. Br Med J 2002; 324:123–124.

14. Lunzer M, Barnes P, Byth K. Serum bile acid concentrations during pregnancy and their relationship to obstetric cholestasis. Gastroenterology 1986; 91:825–829.

15. Meng L-J, Reyes H, Palma J, et al. Profiles of bile acids and progesterone metabolites in the urine and serum of women with intrahepatic cholestasis of pregnancy. J Hepatol 1997; 7:346–357.

16. Davies MH, Ngong JM, Yucesoy M. The adverse influence of pregnancy upon sulphation: a clue to the pathogenesis of intrahepatic cholestasis of pregnancy? J Hepatol 1994; 21:1127–1134.

17. de Vree JM, Jacquemin E, Sturm E, et al. Mutations in the MDR 3 gene cause progressive familial intrahepatic cholestasis. Proc Natl Acad Sci USA 1998; 95:282–287.

18. Bashiri A, Neumann L, Maymon E, et al. Hyperemesis gravidarum: epidemiologic features, complications and outcome. Eur J Obstet Gynecol and Reprod Biol 1995; 63:135–138.

    A review of 190 cases of hyperemesis gravidarum. Liver disease is uncommon.

19. Kuscu NK, Koyuncu F. Hyperemesis gravidarum: current concepts and management. Postgrad Med J 2002; 78:76–79.

20. Koch KL, Frissora CL. Nausea and vomiting during pregnancy. Gastroenterol Clin N Am 2003; 32:201–234.

21. Alexander J, Cuellar RE, Van Thiel DH. Toxemia of pregnancy and the liver. Sem Liv Dis 1987; 7:55–58.

22. Weinstein L. Syndrome of hemolysis, elevated liver enzymes, and low platelet count: a severe consequence of hypertension in pregnancy. Am J Obstet Gynecol 1982; 142:159–167.

23. Sibai BM, Ramadan MK, Usta I, et al. Maternal morbidity and mortality in 442 pregnancies with hemolysis, elevated liver enzymes and low platelets (HELLP syndrome). Am J Obstet Gynecol 1993; 169:1000–1006.

    A large and detailed review of over 400 cases of HELLP syndrome. Thirty percent of cases occurred post-partum. Maternal mortality was low (1%), but morbidity was great.

24. Barton JR, Sibai BM. HELLP and the liver diseases of preeclampsia. Clin Liver Dis 1999; 3:31–48.

25. Curtin WM, Weinstein L. A review of HELLP syndrome. J Perinatol 1999; 19:138–143.

26. Sheehan HL. The pathology of acute yellow atrophy and delayed chloroform poisoning. J Obstetr Gynecol 1940; 47:49–61.

27. Mabie WC. Acute fatty liver of pregnancy. Gastroent Clin N Am 1992; 21:951–960.

28. Minakami H, Oka N, Sato T, et al. Preeclampsia: a microvesicular fat disease of the liver? Am J Obstetr Gynecol 1988; 159:1043–1047.

29. Riely CA, Latham PS, Romero R, et al. Acute fatty liver of pregnancy. Ann Intern Med 1987; 106:703–706.

30. Reyes H. Acute fatty liver of pregnancy: a cryptic disease threatening mother and child. Clin Liver Dis 1999; 3:69–81.

31. Casele HL, Laifer SA. Association of pregnancy complications and choice of immunosuppressant in liver transplant patients. Transplantation 1998; 65:581–583.

32. Pereira SP, O'Donohue J, Wendon J, et al. Maternal and perinatal outcome in severe pregnancy-related liver disease. Hepatology 1997; 26:1258–1262.

33. Treem WR, Shoup ME, Hale DE, et al. Acute fatty liver of pregnancy, hemolysis, elevated liver enzymes, and low platelets syndrome, and long chain 3-hydroxyacyl-coenzyme A dehydrogenase deficiency. Am J Gastroenterol 1996; 91:2293–2300.

34. Batey RG. Acute fatty liver of pregnancy: is it genetically predetermined? (Editorial) Am J Gastroenterol 1996; 91:2262–2264.

35. Isaacs JD Jr, Sims HF, Powell CK, et al. Maternal acute fatty liver of pregnancy associated with fetal trifunctional protein deficiency: molecular characterization of a novel maternal mutant allele. Ped Res 1996; 40:393–398.

36. Ibdah JA, Bennett MJ, Rinaldo P, et al. A fetal fatty-acid oxidation disorder as a cause of liver disease in pregnant women. N Engl J Med 1999; 340:1723–1731.

37. Yang Z, Yamada J, Zhao Y, et al. Prospective screening for pediatric mitochondrial trifunctional protein defects in pregnancies complicated by liver disease. JAMA 2002; 288:2163–2166.

38. Rustgi VK, Hoofnagle JH. Viral hepatitis during pregnancy. Sem Liv Dis 1987; 7:40–46.

39. Mishra L, Seeff LB. Viral hepatitis, A through E, complicating pregnancy. Gastroenterol Clin N Am 1992; 21:873–887.

40. Snydman DR. Hepatitis in pregnancy. N Engl J Med 1985; 313:1398–1401.

41. Simms J, Duff P. Viral hepatitis in pregnancy. Sem Perinatol 1993; 17:384–393.

42. Hay JE. Viral hepatitis in pregnancy. Viral Hepat Rev 2000; 6:205–215.

43. Mast EE, Krawczynski K. Hepatitis E: an overview. Annu Rev Med 1996; 47:257–266.

44. Acharya SK, Dasarathy S, Kumer TL, et al. Fulminant hepatitis in a tropical population: clinical course, cause, and early predictors of outcome. Hepatology 1996; 23:1448–1455.

45. Lee WM, Sorrell MF. Developing a world view toward acute liver failure. Hepatology 1996; 24:270–271.

46. Hamid SS, Jafri SMW, Khan H, et al. Fulminant hepatic failure in pregnant women: acute fatty liver or acute viral hepatitis? J Hepatol 1996; 25:20–27.

47. Jaiswal SPB, Jain AK, Naik G, et al. Viral hepatitis during pregnancy. Int J Gyn Obstetr 2001; 72:103–108.

48. Landers D, Carmona R, Crombleholme W, et al. Acute cholecystitis in pregnancy. Obstetr Gynecol 1987; 69:131–133.

49. Swisher SG, Schmit PJ, Hunt KK, et al. Biliary disease during pregnancy. Am J Surg 1994; 168:576–581.

50. Valdivieso V, Covarrubias C, Siegel F, et al. Pregnancy and cholelithiasis: pathogenesis and natural course of gallstones diagnosed in early puerperium. Hepatology 1993; 17:1–4.

51. Floreani A, Paternoster D, Zappala F, et al. Hepatitis C virus infection in pregnancy. Br J Obstetr Gynaecol 1996; 103:325–329.

52. Steven MM, Buckley JD, Mackay IR. Pregnancy in chronic active hepatitis. Q J Med 1979; 192:519–531.

53. Fairley I, Wilson J. Herpes hepatitis in pregnancy (case report). J Clin Path 1994; 47:478.

54. De Arcos F, Gratacos E, Palacio M, et al. Toxic hepatitis: a rare complication associated with the use of ritodrine during pregnancy. Acta Obstetr Gynecol Scand 1996; 75:340–342.

55. Hsu HW, Belfort MA, Vernino S, et al. Postpartum thrombotic thrombocytopenic purpura complicated by Budd-Chiari. Obstetr Gynecol 1995; 85:839–843.

56. Segal S, Shenhav S, Segal O, et al. Budd-Chiari syndrome complicating severe preeclampsia in a parturient with primary antiphospholipid syndrome. Eur J Obstetr Gynecol Reprod Biol 1996; 68:227–229.

57. Doshi S, Zucker SD. Liver emergencies during pregnancy. Gastroenterol Clin N Am 2003; 32:1213–1227.

58. Palma J, Reyes H, Ribalta J, et al. Ursodeoxycholic acid in cholestasis of pregnancy: final report of a randomized, double-blind, placebo controlled study (Abstract). Hepatology 1996; 24:373A.

59. Bacq Y, Myara A, Brechot M-C, et al. Serum conjugated bile acid profile during intrahepatic cholestasis of pregnancy. J Hepatol 1995; 22:66-70.

60. Kryczka W, Brojer E, Witczak A, et al. Acute hepatitis C manifesting itself as cholestasis of pregnancy (Abstract). J Hepatol 1997; 26:302.

61. Barton JR, Sibai BM. Hepatic imaging in HELLP syndrome (hemolysis, elevated liver enzymes, and low platelet count). Am J Obstetr Gynecol 1996; 174:1820–1827.

62. Rolfes DB, Ishak KG. Acute fatty liver of pregnancy: a clinicopathologic study of 35 cases. Hepatology 1985; 5:1149–1158.

63. Audibert F, Friedman SA, Frangieh AY, et al. Clinical utility of strict diagnostic criteria for the HELLP (hemolysis, elevated liver enzymes, and low platelets) syndrome. Am J Obstetr Gynecol 1996; 175:460–464.

64. Packros PJ, Peters RL, Reynolds TB. Idiopathic fatty liver of pregnancy: findings in ten cases. Medicine 1984; 63:1–11.

65. Minakami H, Tamada T. Hepatic histopathologic characteristics in HELLP syndrome (hemolysis, elevated liver enzymes, and low platelet count) (Letter). Am J Obstetr Gynecol 1993; 169:1357–1358.

66. Kaiser C, Distler W. Thrombotic thrombocytopenic purpura and HEELP (hemolysis, elevated liver enzymes, and low platelets) syndrome: differential diagnostic problems (Letter). Am J Obstetr Gynecol 1996; 175:506–507.

67. Hamaoui E, Hamaoui M. Nutritional assessment and support during pregnancy. Gastroenterol Clin N Am 2003; 32:59–121.

68. Palma J, Reyes H, Ribalta J, et al. Effects of ursodeoxycholic acid in patients with intrahepatic cholestasis of pregnancy. Hepatology 1992; 15:1043–1047.

69. Diaferia A, Nicastri PL, Tartagni M, et al. Ursodeoxycholic acid therapy in pregnant women with cholestasis. Int J Gynecol Obstetr 1996; 52:133–140.

70. Isla CR, Cappelletti CA, Tielli G, et al. Value of ursodeoxycholic acid in the treatment of intrahepatic cholestasis of pregnancy (Abstract). Gastroenterology 1996; 110:1219A.

71. Mazzella G, Rizza N, Azzaroli F, et al. Ursodeoxycholic acid administration in patients with cholestasis of pregnancy: effects on primary bile acids in babies and mothers. Hepatology 2001;3 3:504–508.

72. Hirvioja M-L, Tuimala R, Vuori J. The treatment of intrahepatic cholestasis of pregnancy by dexamethasone. Br J Obstetr Gynaecol 1992; 99:109–111.

73. Frezza M, Pozzato G, Chiesa L, et al. Reversal of intrahepatic cholestasis of pregnancy in women after high dose S-adenosyl-L-methionine administration. Hepatology 1984; 4:274–278.

74. Ribalta J, Reyes H, Gonzalez MC, et al. S-Adenosyl-L-methoionine in the treatment of patients with intrahepatic cholestasis of pregnancy: a randomized, double-blind, placebo-controlled study with negative results. Hepatology 1991; 13:1084–1089.

75. Floreani A, Paternoster D, Melis A, et al. S-adenosylmethionine versus ursodeoxycholic acid in the treatment of intrahepatic cholestasis of pregnancy: preliminary results of a controlled trial. Eur J Obstetr Gynecol 1996; 67:109–113.

76. Gonzalez MC, Iglesias J, Tiribelli C, et al. Epomediol ameliorates pruritus in patients with intrahepatic cholestasis of pregnancy (Letter). J Hepatol 1992; 16:241–250.

77. Gonzalez M. Reyes H, Ribalta J, et al. Effect of silymarin on pruritus of cholestasis (Abstract). Hepatology 1988; 8:1356.

78. Olsson R, Tysk C, Aldenborg F, et al. Prolonged postpartum course of intrahepatic cholestasis of pregnancy. Gastroenterology 1993; 105:267–271.

79. Leevy CB, Koneru B, Klein KM. Recurrent familial prolonged intrahepatic cholestasis of pregnancy associated with chronic liver disease. Gastroenterology 1997; 113:966–972.

80. Fisk NM, Storey GNB. Fetal outcome in obstetric cholestasis. Br J Obstetr Gynaecol 1988; 95:1137–1143.

81. Alsulyman OM, Ouzounian JG, Ames-Castro M, et al. Intrahepatic cholestasis of pregnancy: perinatal outcome associated with expectant management. Am J Obstetr Gynecol 1996; 175:957–960.

82. Magann EF, Bass D, Chauhan SP, et al. Antepartum corticosteroids: disease stabilization in patients with the syndrome of hemolysis, elevated liver enzymes, and low platelets (HELLP). Am J Obstetr Gynecol 1994; 171:1148–1153.

83. Julius CJ, Dunn ZL, Blazina JF. HELLP syndrome: laboratory parameters and clinical course in four patients treated with plasma exchange. J Clin Apheresis 1994; 9:228–235.

84. Strand S, Strand D, Seifert R, et al. Placenta-derived CD95 ligand causes liver damage in hemolysis, elevated liver enzymes, and liver platelet count syndrome. Gastroenterology 2004; 126:849–858.

85. Terasaki KK, Quinn MF, Lundell CJ, et al. Spontaneous hepatic hemorrhage in preeclampsia: treatment with hepatic arterial embolization. Radiology 1990; 174:1039–141.

86. Sullivan CA, Magann EF, Perry KG Jr, et al. The recurrence risk of the syndrome of hemolysis, elevated liver enzymes, and low platelets (HELLP) in subsequent gestations. Am J Obstetr Gynecol 1994; 171:940–943.

87. Sibai BM, Ramadan MK, Chari RS, et al. Pregnancies complicated by HELLP syndrome (hemolysis, elevated liver enzymes, and low platelets): subsequent pregnancy outcome and long-term prognosis. Am J Obstetr Gynecol 1995; 172:125–129.

Among 152 women with HELLP who subsequently became pregnant, HELLP recurred in only 3%. However, preeclampsia and prematurity were very common.

88. Hou SH, Levin S, Ahda S, et al. Acute fatty liver of pregnancy: survival with early caesarean section. Dig Dis Sci 1984; 29:449–452.

89. Ockner SA, Brunt EM, Cohn SM, et al. Fulminant hepatic failure caused by acute fatty liver of pregnancy treated by orthotopic liver transplantation. Hepatology 1990; 11:59–64.

90. Treem WR, Rinaldo P, Hale DE, et al. Acute fatty liver of pregnancy and long-chain 3-hydroxyacyl-coenzyme A dehydrogenase deficiency. Hepatology 1994; 19:339–345.

The clinical picture and liver histology of women with acute fatty liver of pregnancy is similar to children with metabolic defects in the intramitochondrial beta-oxidation pathway. This study documented a defect in the long-chain 3-hydroxyacyl-coenzyme of fatty oxidation in the infant while the mother was heterozygous.

91. Nesbitt TN, Kay HH, McCoy MC, et al. Endoscopic management of biliary disease during pregnancy. Obstetr Gynecol 1996; 87:806–809.

92. Visser BC, Glasgow RE, Mulinhill KK, et al. Safety and timing of nonobstetric abdominal surgery in pregnancy. Dig Surg 2001; 18:409–417.

93. Martin IG, Dexter SPL, McMahon MJ. Laparoscopic cholecystectomy in pregnancy. A safe option during the second trimester? Surg Endosc 1996; 10:508–510.

94. Steinbrook RA, Brooks DC, Datta S. Laparoscopic cholecystectomy during pregnancy. Surg Endosc 1996; 10:511–515.

95. Sungler P, Heinerman PM, Steiner H, et al. Laparoscopic cholecystectomy and interventional endoscopy for gallstone complications during pregnancy. Surg Endosc 2000; 14:267–271.

A review of surgical and endoscopic management of biliary complications of pregnancy.

96. Varma RR. Course and prognosis of pregnancy in women with liver disease. Sem Liv Dis 1987; 7:59–66.

97. Kurauchi O, Furui T, Itakura A, et al. Studies on transmission of hepatitis C virus from mother to child in the perinatal period. Gynecol Obstetr 1993; 253:121–126.

98. Scheinberg IH, Jaffe ME, Sternlieb I. The use of trientine in preventing the effects of interrupting penicillamine therapy in Wilson's disease. N Engl J Med 1987; 317:209–213.

99. Pajor A, Lehoczky D. Pregnancy in liver cirrhosis. Gynecol Obstetr Invest 1994; 38:45–50.

100. Armenti VT, Herrine SK, Mortiz MJ. Reproductive function after liver transplantation. Liver Transplant 1997; 1:471–485.

101. Armenti VT, Radomski JS, Mortiz MJ. Parenthood after liver transplantation. Liver Transpl Surg 1995; 1:84–88.

102. Radomski JS, Moritz MJ, Munoz SJ, et al. National transplantation pregnancy registry: analysis of pregnancy outcomes in female liver transplant recipients. Liver Transpl Surg 1995; 1:281–284.

103. Laifer SA, Guido RS. Reproductive function and outcome of pregnancy after liver transplantation in women. Mayo Clin Proc 1995; 70:388–394.

104. Cundy TF, O'Grady JG, Williams R. Recovery of menstruation and pregnancy after liver transplantation. Gut 1990; 31:337–338.

105. Jain AB, Reyes J, Marco A, et al. Pregnancy after liver transplantation with tacrolimus immunosuppression: a single center's experience update at 13 years. Transplantation 2003; 65:827–832.

106. Nagy S, Bush MC, Berkowitz R, et al. Pregnancy outcome in liver transplant recipients. Obstetr Gynecol 2003; 102:121–128.

Section

7 Seven

Management of intestinal disorders

Irritable bowel syndrome

Jan Tack

INTRODUCTION

Irritable bowel syndrome (IBS) is a functional gastrointestinal (GI) disorder characterized by episodes of symptoms referring to the large bowel, in the absence of organic disease that readily explains them. IBS is compounded by a cluster of symptoms including abdominal pain or discomfort, bloating, and disordered bowel habits.[1] The pathophysiology of IBS is incompletely understood, but several mechanisms may contribute to IBS symptoms. These include abnormal colonic or small intestinal motility and transit, increased gut sensitivity, low-grade inflammation, psychological and social factors, several intraluminal factors, and abnormalities of certain gastrointestinal hormones. However, each of these abnormalities is at best only present in a subset of IBS patients, and symptom pattern and severity are likely to be determined in a multifactorial way.

SYMPTOMS

Irritable bowel syndrome is characterized by a symptom cluster which includes abdominal pain, often relieved by defecation, distention of the abdomen, a disordered bowel habit, a frequent feeling of incomplete evacuation, mucus in the stool, looser stools with the onset of pain, and more frequent stools with the onset of pain. Relief of symptoms by defecation is a key characteristic feature of IBS. In a subset of patients, aggravation of abdominal symptoms occurs after a meal.[2] In addition, a number of noncolonic features are also highly prevalent in IBS patients. These include upper gastrointestinal symptoms (nausea, vomiting, heartburn, chest pain, etc.), urinary frequency and urgency, incomplete bladder emptying, low back pain, and chronic fatigue.

DEFINITION

No diagnostic markers for IBS exist, so the diagnosis rests on the recognition of characteristic symptom patterns and the exclusion of organic disease. Similarly, there are no biological markers of disease severity, which can only be assessed by reporting of symptom severity. In order to help clinicians recognize and manage IBS, and to allow a more uniform selection of patients entering clinical trials, diagnostic criteria have been proposed. The first symptom criteria were proposed by Manning et al.[3] and these were adapted in the Rome I diagnostic criteria.[4]

The currently accepted symptom criteria were proposed by the Rome II working team (Table 48.1).[1] The definition of IBS according to the 'Rome symptom criteria' has gained international acceptance, at least for application in research, in epidemiological studies, and in clinical trials. A number of observations suggest that the Rome criteria may also have diagnostic usefulness.[5,6] However, at this time it remains to be established whether the criteria alone could be sufficient to make a confident diagnosis of IBS.

EPIDEMIOLOGY

IBS is one of the most frequent conditions that physicians are confronted with. Older population studies often did not use standard diagnostic criteria. Hungin and colleagues applied random-digit-dialing technology to conduct telephone interviews in more than 40 000 subjects 18 years and older in Europe.[7] Using a structured questionnaire to obtain information on IBS,

---

Table 48.1 Rome II criteria for diagnosis of irritable bowel syndrome

At least 12 weeks, which need not be consecutive, in the preceding 12 months of abdominal discomfort or pain that has two of three features:

Relieved with defecation

and/or

Onset associated with a change in frequency of stool

and/or

Onset associated with a change in form (appearance) of stool

Supportive symptoms:

Fewer than three bowel movements per week

More than three bowel movements per day

Hard or lumpy stools

Loose (mushy) stools

Straining during a bowel movement

Urgency

Feeling of incomplete bowel movement

Passing mucus during a bowel movement

Abdominal fullness, bloating or swelling

they demonstrated that the overall prevalence of this disorder varied from 7% (The Netherlands) to 17% (Italy). Mean prevalence rates for undiagnosed IBS ranged from 2.9–6.5% in the combined populations. Females outnumbered males in both diagnosed and undiagnosed populations, averaging 68% and 61%, respectively, in these groups. These findings are consistent with recent epidemiologic studies in the US, Europe, and Australia.[8–10] When standardized criteria were applied to subdivide individuals with symptoms of IBS into diarrhea-predominant, constipation-predominant, or alternating subgroups, 16% were assigned to the constipation-predominant category, 21% to the diarrhea-predominant category, and 63% to the alternating type.[7]

IMPACT OF THE IRRITABLE BOWEL SYNDROME

The morbidity and life expectancy in patients with IBS does not differ from that in the general population,[11] but a considerable impact on daily life is present and quality of life is impaired in IBS patients.[7,12] Patients with IBS experience symptoms that interfere with normal daily activities,[12] for which they repeatedly see physicians, and they have a higher number of days absent from work or school.[13] Direct medical costs in patients with IBS are significantly higher than those in a control population.[14]

PATHOPHYSIOLOGY OF THE IRRITABLE BOWEL SYNDROME

Historically, several hypotheses have been suggested to underlie symptoms in IBS. Until the 1990s, symptoms in functional bowel disorders had mainly been viewed as expressions of altered motor function of the gut. More recently, alterations in visceral sensitivity, infection, and inflammation and abnormalities of the central nervous system have been implicated (Fig. 48.1).

Disorders of colonic and intestinal motility

Alterations in bowel function observed in IBS seem to be related to intestinal and colonic transit times.[15] Older studies have suggested abnormalities of rectosigmoid motility, including more frequent long-duration colonic contractions in IBS[16] and a lower rectal compliance in diarrhea-predominant IBS.[17] However, the

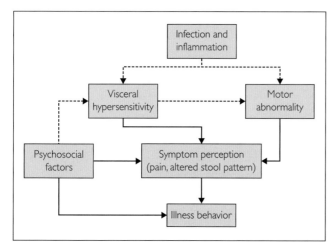

Fig. 48.1 ● Pathophysiological factors in IBS.

relevance of these findings to the IBS symptom complex has not been established. More recently, impaired colonic transit of gas was demonstrated in IBS patients, and this was mainly associated with symptoms of bloating.[18]

Several abnormalities of small bowel motility have also been reported in IBS, but again their relevance is not established. Ileal propulsive waves and clusters of jejunal contractions were reported to be more common in patients with IBS. In response to an intraduodenal infusion of a fatty meal, a correlation was observed between the presence of prolonged propagated contractions and cramping discomfort or pain.[19,20] However, 24-hour manometry studies failed to confirm a consistent correlation.[21]

Visceral hypersensitivity

Over 20 years ago, Ritchie showed that in patients with IBS, the distention volume required to induce pain from the pelvic colon was on average lower than in controls.[22] Visceral thresholds for discomfort and pain in response to isovolumic distention of the colon are lower in IBS patients than in controls. This hypersensitivity to distention is not due to a defective compliance since compliance curves and basal colonic tone were similar in both groups. In the last 15 years, the visceral hypersensitivity hypothesis has been a major area of research with several well-controlled studies showing a reduction in the threshold pressure or volume of colorectal distention required to induce perception or a sensation of discomfort or pain in patients with IBS.[16,17,23] Somatic sensitivity is not enhanced in patients with IBS.[24,25] Additional studies confirmed that rectal hypersensitivity is a feature of IBS and not of other colonic disorders, and that the presence of hypersensitivity has good sensitivity and specificity for the diagnosis of IBS.[26,27]

It is unclear whether the same pathways are involved in the encoding of discomfort and pain (response to noxious stimulation) (specificity theory versus intensity theory). Recent studies evaluating mechanical and electrical stimulation of intestinal afferents in IBS concluded that patients with IBS have selective hypersensitivity of mechanical afferents.[24] Lembo et al. attempted to characterize indirectly the receptors involved in signaling colorectal sensation by using two types of balloon inflation: phasic and ramp.[28] They concluded that phasic distention was the most appropriate stimulus to investigate IBS. Studies using intrarectal lidocaine suggested that mucosal afferents are not the predominant source of the colorectal hypersensitivity in IBS, although they do contribute to the sensory response in controls.[29] This suggests that in IBS, the receptors that become sensitized are high-threshold mechanoreceptors located in the muscle or in the serosa.

Psychosocial factors

Psychosocial factors in IBS relate to a number of topics that have received variable attention in the past. Initial studies were focused at detecting specific personality traits in patients with IBS. Later, the focus was placed on illness behavior and health-seeking behavior. More recently, life events and a history of sexual or physical abuse have received more attention.

IBS is often considered a somatization syndrome, reflecting underlying psychopathology. Patients with IBS have more psychological disturbances than the general population, but less than psychiatric out-patients.[30,31] The prevalence of psychological and psychiatric disturbances is higher in patients with IBS.[32,33] However, the psychological disorders in patients with IBS are non-specific. The observation that only a minority of persons with symptoms suggestive of IBS is seeing a physician led to the hypothesis that psychopathology might not determine the symptoms, but rather who would come to medical attention. Comparative studies demonstrated that those subjects with functional bowel symptoms that see a physician are more focused on their symptoms, which might be indicative of illness behavior.[34–36] Sex differences in seeking medical attention might explain why IBS is more frequent in women, although hormonal factors might also play an important role.[37,38] Finally, a recent epidemiological study suggested that pain is a major factor that drives medical attention seeking.[7]

Patients with IBS experience more stress than asymptomatic controls,[39,40] and patients often experience a temporal relationship between stress and symptoms. Stressful life events do not only precipitate symptoms in IBS, but also in several psychosomatic and somatic disorders. Well-controlled studies are lacking, unfortunately, and in a prospective study a correlation with stress could only be found in 25% of the exacerbations of IBS symptoms.[41] Moreover, about half of a healthy population experiences that stress may alter bowel habits and induce abdominal pain.[34] Hence, the notion that IBS might be stress-induced is far from proven, and may even be hampered by overemphasizing of stressful events when retrospectively seeking a cause or explanation. A possible underlying mechanism is also unclear: whereas IBS is a chronic disorder, and stressful life events often have a chronic impact, only acute stress has been studied experimentally. Moreover, experiments using acute stress have generally failed to elicit typical IBS symptoms.

Recently, several groups have reported a higher prevalence of sexual or physical abuse in patients with functional bowel disorders.[42,43] However, the prevalence is already high in asymptomatic subjects in the general population,[44] thus questioning the specificity of this observation. Sleep disorders are frequently observed in patients with the IBS[45] and, in healthy volunteers, sleep deprivation is able to elicit IBS-like symptoms.[46] Their contribution to IBS pathogenesis remains unelucidated.

Infection and inflammation

In a large retrospective study, Chaudhary and Truelove demonstrated that in about one-third of patients with IBS, symptoms seemed to have started after a gastrointestinal infection.[47] These and other observations are the basis of the hypothesis that inflammation might predispose to the development of IBS.[48] Animal studies were indeed able to demonstrate that a large array of inflammatory mediators, including cytokines and arachidonic acid metabolites, are able to alter neuromuscular function and that inflammation is able to induce persistent neuromuscular dysfunction in the gastrointestinal tract.

Several more recent studies have focused on the potential role of infection and inflammation in IBS. Both in retrospective and in prospective studies, it has now been well established that IBS may follow an acute intestinal infection.[47–51] A group of patients with proven *Salmonella* enteritis were followed prospectively during several months. After two years, 32% of them had symptoms suggestive of IBS.[49] Those patients who developed IBS after a *Salmonella* infection seemed to have more psychological distur-

bances, and they experienced more stressful life events during the months preceding the infection.[50] However, they also had signs of ongoing inflammation.[51]

A marked increase of enteroendocrine cell numbers was reported in the rectum of patients with postinfectious IBS,[52] but their pathophysiological role is incompletely elucidated. Studies investigating postprandial release of 5-HT in IBS were able to demonstrate an increase in only a small subset of the patients.[53,54] In addition to increased enteroendocrine cell numbers, patients with postinfectious IBS also had higher counts of inflammatory cells in the lamina propria.[55] Several recent studies, not all of them focusing on postinfectious IBS, have also reported signs of ongoing low-grade inflammation in IBS.[51,52,55,56] At this very moment, the relevance of these findings needs further confirmation in larger-scale studies in less selected patient groups.

Food allergy and food intolerance

Many patients with IBS report intolerance to different food substances and food often aggravates symptoms.[2] Studies using exclusion diets and gradual reintroduction allowed identification of a group of patients with symptoms that were related to specific food substances.[57] However, as this approach is extremely demanding and often yields conflicting results, exclusion diet testing never gained widespread acceptance.

In a subset of patients with diarrhea-predominant IBS and a history of atopy, IgE-mediated food allergy may contribute to symptom induction.[58] Studies using the mast cell stabilizer cromoglycate showed responsiveness in the same subset of patients.[59–61] IgG antibodies to food commonly occur and are considered physiological. However, a recent study comparing elimination diets based on IgG food antibodies and random control elimination diets demonstrated significantly better symptom relief in the former group.[62] The most common IgG antibodies were directed against yeast, milk, egg, and wheat. Clearly, this area deserves additional studies. For the time being, it seems appropriate to eliminate dietary constituents that are associated with aggravated symptoms on more than one occasion.

CLINICAL APPROACH TO THE IRRITABLE BOWEL SYNDROME

A stepwise algorithm for the management of IBS patients is summarized in Table 48.2. The challenge of diagnosing IBS is the exclusion of organic disease. Certain clinical features can be used to distinguish IBS from organic disease. In patients with a typical history and no alarm symptoms, no added value for additional diagnostic testing has been shown. Although routine blood tests are usually performed their utility has not been proven. In areas with a high prevalence of celiac disease, screening for endomysial antibodies seems logical, although their usefulness in a primary care setting has not been proven. The same is true for examination of stools for parasites and ova. Although many patients report intolerance to diary products, tests for lactase deficiency usually do not contribute to the diagnosis and a trial of lactose elimination is to be recommended. Colorectal cancer is a major differential diagnosis and screening is indicated in those with a family history. Although rectal barostat studies were shown to have good sensitivity and specificity for IBS,[27] routine use in clinical practice cannot be recommended.

Table 48.2 Therapeutic approach to patients with the irritable bowel syndrome

Diagnostic evaluation and physician–patient interaction

Careful history and examination
Determine immediate reason for patient's visit
Cost-effective investigation
Explanation of the disorder
Discuss therapeutic expectations and limitations

Patients with mild symptoms

Education
Reassurance
Life style modifications

Patients with moderate symptoms

Education
Reassurance
Life style modifications
Symptom monitoring and modification
Pharmacotherapy directed at specific symptom(s)

Patients with severe symptoms

Education
Reassurance
Life style modifications
Symptom monitoring and modification
Pharmacotherapy directed at specific symptom(s)
Antidepressants as second-line drugs
Behavioral treatments or psychotherapy
Pain treatment center referral in refractory cases

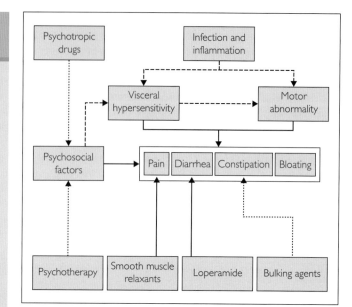

Fig. 48.2 • Classical therapeutic approach to IBS.

STANDARD THERAPEUTIC APPROACH TO THE IRRITABLE BOWEL SYNDROME

Over time, several therapeutic trials in IBS have been reported in the literature. Many of these studies are of poor scientific quality, and systematic reviews until the end of the 1990s concluded that there were no treatment options of proven efficacy.[63,64] In the last few years, studies of better quality have been published. An algorithm of standard therapeutic approach to IBS patients is summarized in Table 2 and is depicted in Figure 48.2.

General measures

Therapy for IBS does not always consist of pharmacological treatment but also includes education and supportive measures. Once the diagnosis of IBS has been made (after the initial examinations and exclusion of organic pathology), the patient should be reassured (with emphasis on the absence of sinister organic pathology) and extensively informed about the nature of his complaints. An empathic approach is recommended. A retrospective analysis from the Mayo Clinic suggests that reassurance and explanation do indeed have a significant clinical impact.[65]

Dietary measures

In diarrhea-predominant IBS, an underlying carbohydrate intolerance (lactose, sucrose, sorbitol, or fructose intolerance) or the existence of a food allergy has to be considered. No studies have demonstrated that carbohydrate intolerance can be the sole cause of typical IBS symptoms, but reducing the intake of carbohydrates can improve symptoms.[66–68] A therapeutic trial with a diet eliminating those carbohydrates can be considered. In constipated patients, a diet rich in fiber may improve symptoms, whereas diarrhea may worsen. Increasing the fiber content of the diet is best done gradually. However, the overall therapeutic impact of a diet rich in fiber is rather disappointing.[69]

Fiber supplements

Fiber supplements are traditionally prescribed to patients with constipation-predominant IBS, and they may improve constipation. The effect of fiber supplements on stool frequency and stool weight are determined more by psychometric variables than by the type or the quantity of the administered fiber.[70] For alleviating abdominal pain, fiber is not superior to placebo, and there is often an adverse influence on symptoms of abdominal pain, bloating, or diarrhea.[71] Alternatively, bulking agents such as psyllium or ispaghula can be prescribed, but their efficacy has not been proven.[72,73]

Antispasmodics and anticholinergics

Antispasmodics cause relaxation of the intestinal smooth muscle cells, mostly by inhibiting the influx of calcium. Placebo-controlled studies show an inconsistent effect.[74] However, meta-analyses of smooth muscle relaxant studies suggest a benefit of these drugs on abdominal pain.[75,76]

Anticholinergics inhibit basal as well as meal-induced gastrointestinal motility by blocking muscarin M2-receptors on the intestinal smooth muscle. In comparison with the impact on motility, the clinical effects of anticholinergics are rather small: in the short term they may improve abdominal pain and rectal urgency, but they often cause systemic anticholinergic side effects; an effect in the long term has not been proven.[77]

Antidiarrheal drugs

Opioids that do not cross the blood–brain barrier (e.g., loperamide) exert their action via mu-receptors on the enteric nervous system, by enhancing nonpropulsive motility and inhibiting propulsive motility. They slow the intestinal transit, inhibit intestinal secretions, inhibit rectal sensitivity, and increase the internal anal sphincter tone. Placebo-controlled trials confirmed the effect of loperamide on diarrhea, rectal urgency, and abdominal pain in IBS.[78,79]

Serotonergic drugs

Serotonin is a key neuromodulator and neurotransmitter in the control of gastrointestine sensorimotor function.[80,81] Seven types of 5-HT receptors have been recognized and they have been termed 5-HT$_{1-7}$. It seems that 5-HT$_{5-7}$ receptors are predominantly distributed in the brain, whereas 5-HT$_{1-4}$ receptors are mainly expressed in the gastrointestine, and involvement of these in many gastrointestinal functions has been shown.[80,81] In particular 5-HT$_3$ and 5-HT$_4$ receptors have been demonstrated to regulate the motor, sensory, and secretor gut response to intraluminal stimuli.[82,83]

Tegaserod, an agonist at the 5-HT$_4$ receptor, was shown to promote small intestinal transit time and to enhance proximal colonic emptying in patients with constipation-predominant IBS.[84] The dose used in this study (4 mg/day) is lower than the dose classically used in the treatment of constipation-predominant IBS (12 mg/day), which established benefit of tegaserod over placebo in constipation-predominant IBS.[85,86] Prucalopride, another 5-HT$_4$-receptor agonist, was also shown to enhance colonic transit time.[87] Several studies have established that tegaserod is able to improve constipation and to provide relief of pain/discomfort and bloating in constipation-predominant IBS.[85,86,88]

Antagonists at the 5-HT$_3$ receptor inhibit colonic transit time.[89] Clinical studies have established that the 5-HT$_3$-receptor antagonist alosetron is able to improve stool pattern and to provide relief of pain/discomfort in diarrhea-predominant IBS.[90] Preliminary data suggest a similar potential for the 5-HT$_3$-receptor antagonist cilansetron.[91] Shortly after its introduction to the American market, alosetron was withdrawn due to suspected side effects of colonic ischemia.[92] The drug has now been reintroduced in a restricted-use program in the US, but is unavailable elsewhere.

Although the use of the 5-HT ligands described above matches their influence on colonic transit, and hence on colonic motor function, recent studies indicate that they might also affect visceral sensitivity (Fig. 48.3). In animal studies, firing of visceral afferents during rectal distention was decreased by pretreatment with tegaserod.[93,94] In humans, using a surrogate marker for pain-related autonomic function, an analgesic effect of tegaserod on rectal sensitivity was suggested, but the classical sensitivity thresholds to balloon distention were not altered.[95] Studies investigating the effect of 5-HT$_3$ antagonists on rectal sensitivity have yielded conflicting results. Granisetron, but not ondansetron or alosetron, decrease the sensitivity to rectal distention in patients with IBS.[96–98] In IBS, pretreatment with alosetron was found to decrease colonic tone and to allow larger intracolonic volumes before thresholds for discomfort were reached.[99] However, as the response to pressure-based stimuli was not significantly altered, it has been argued that these changes reflect relaxation of the

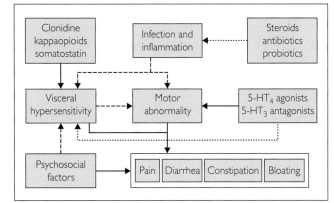

Fig. 48.3 • Mechanistic properties of some newer pharmacological agents in IBS.

colon, without a true antinociceptive action of alosetron.[100] On the other hand, the effects of alosetron on colonic sensitivity are more than a non-specific side effect of antidiarrheal agents, as loperamide was found to have opposite effects on colonic sensitivity to distention.[101]

Tricyclic antidepressants

Tricyclic antidepressants are frequently used to treat patients with IBS, especially those with more severe or more refractory symptoms. Initially, they were used because of the high prevalence of depression in patients with IBS. Several placebo-controlled studies have confirmed the efficacy of low doses of tricyclic antidepressants in IBS.[76,102–105] The largest study that investigated the efficacy of tricyclic antidepressants was less clearly positive,[105] and a significant advantage was only found in those patients that tolerated and continued the medication.

Tricyclic agents have not only antidepressant, but also neuromodulatory and analgesic properties. They are nonselective serotonin reuptake inhibitors and they also have anticholinergic properties. It is still unclear whether they act by influencing the mood, through a central or peripheral neuromodulatory effect or through an analgesic effect. It is also unclear whether their effect in IBS is constituted by their anticholinergic or by their serotonin reuptake inhibitor effects.

Psychotherapy

Because of the rather disappointing effects of standard medical treatment of IBS, and because of the association with psychological disturbances, several forms of psychotherapy have been applied. Rare controlled trials have investigated dynamic psychotherapy, relaxation therapy, cognitive behavioral therapy, and hypnotherapy.

The application of dynamic psychotherapy, in addition to classical medical therapy, significantly increases therapeutic benefit, both for physical and for psychological symptoms.[106,107] A recent study showed equivalence of psychotherapy and tricyclic antidepressants[105] and of psychotherapy and a selective serotonin reuptake inhibitor.[108] Only one controlled trial used relaxation therapy, showing that relaxation therapy was superior to a placebo treatment.[109] Cognitive therapy is superior to an equivalent time of therapeutic contact not involving cognitive therapy, both for physical and for psychological symptoms.[110,111] In a controlled trial, hypnotherapy was better than supportive therapy and placebo medication in a group of refractory IBS patients in improving symptoms of abdominal pain and diarrhea.[112,113] Additional studies showed that hypnotherapy decreases rectal sensitivity to distention.[114]

In spite of these studies, the role of psychotherapy in IBS remains unclear. The studies have used different criteria for patient selection, and different definitions of IBS. Moreover, most studies selected refractory patients, with a higher likelihood of underlying psychological disturbances, for psychotherapy. Because of these methodological problems, the value of psychotherapy has been questioned.[115]

RECENT DEVELOPMENTS IN IBS PHARMACOTHERAPY

Agents that influence colonic motor function

Renzapride, a mixed 5-HT$_3$-receptor antagonist and 5-HT$_4$-receptor agonist, was shown to decrease whole gut transit time in IBS in a dose-dependent manner.[116] Clinical studies in constipation-predominant IBS and in alternating IBS are in progress.

Agents that influence colonic sensitivity

The alpha-2 adrenergic agonist clonidine, which is also used in chronic neuropathic pain, was found to decrease colonic sensitivity to distention.[117] In a double-blind, randomized study in IBS, clonidine 0.1 mg per day was found to provide significant symptom relief over placebo, but at a cost of a high incidence of (cardiovascular) side-effects.[118]

The peripherally acting kappa opioid agonist fedotozine was shown to reduce sensitivity to colonic distention in the absence of an effect on colonic tone, suggesting an antinociceptive activity.[119] Studies in patients with IBS showed a significant improvement of abdominal pain, but further development of the drug was interrupted.[120] Asimadoline, another peripherally acting kappa opioid agonist, decreased pain sensation at lower colonic distending pressures, but not at higher pressures.[121]

Finally, the long-acting somatostatin analogue octreotide was shown to decrease sensitivity to rectal distention, probably by acting at the level of spinal afferents.[122,123] Clinical studies with octreotide or even longer-acting preparations in IBS are lacking.

Agents that act on psychosocial mechanisms

Tricyclic antidepressants are frequently used to treat patients with IBS, especially those with more severe or more refractory symptoms. Initially they were used because of the high prevalence of depression in patients with IBS. Tricyclic agents have not only antidepressant, but also neuromodulatory and analgesic properties. They are nonselective serotonin reuptake inhibitors and they also have anticholinergic properties. Although several placebo-controlled studies have confirmed the efficacy of low doses of tricyclic antidepressants in IBS, it is unclear whether they act by influencing the mood through a central or peripheral neuromodulatory effect, or through an analgesic effect. It is also unclear whether their effect in IBS is constituted by their anticholinergic or by their serotonin reuptake inhibitor effects.

A recent study evaluating the selective serotonin reuptake inhibitor sertralin failed to demonstrate a significantly favorable effect.[124] In a mechanistic study in healthy subjects, the selective serotonin reuptake inhibitor citalopram was found to decrease sensitivity to colonic distention and to inhibit the colonic response to feeding.[125] In a randomized crossover study in IBS patients without depression, citalopram was found to provide significant symptom relief over placebo.[126]

Agents that act on infection and inflammation

The pathophysiological role of the low-grade inflammation requires further studies. In the only, preliminary study, treating patients with post-IBS with prednisolone or placebo for 3 weeks, no benefit of the steroids was found.[127]

The role of intestinal flora in IBS has received attention in some very recent studies (see Fig. 48.3). Pimentel et al. used the lactulose breath test to investigate the presence of bacterial overgrowth in IBS patients. In patients with 'IBS,' specifically referred for this test, they found a prevalence of bacterial overgrowth in 78%, and successful eradication therapy provided symptom relief in a subgroup of these patients, whereas failure of successful eradication did not improve symptoms.[128] However, this was a study in a selected patient group, and the test did not adequately control for rapid small bowel transit. In a follow-up study in 101 patients, bacterial overgrowth was detected in 83%, and in a randomized, controlled study, neomycin treatment was superior to placebo in providing symptom relief.[129] However, the assessment happened at the end of a 7-day treatment and no longer follow-up was reported. Several studies assessed the use of probiotics in IBS. Only a few of these were randomized and controlled.[130–132]

SUMMARY

The pathophysiology of IBS is likely to be heterogeneous. Several classes of agents that are under development for IBS address one or more of these pathophysiological mechanisms (see Fig. 48.2). Agents that act on 5-HT receptors to alter colonic motor function are the most recent additions to clinical practice. Newly developed agents may act on visceral sensitivity, on central nervous system dysfunction, or on intestinal inflammation.

REFERENCES

1. Drossman DA. Rome II: a multinational consensus document on functional gastrointestinal disorders. Gut 1999; 45(Suppl 2):1–5.

2. Ragnarsson G, Bodemar G. Pain is temporally related to eating but not to defecation in the irritable bowel syndrome (IBS). Patients' description of diarrhea, constipation and symptom variation during a prospective 6-week study. Eur J Gastroenterol Hepatol 1998; 10:415–421.

3. Manning AP, Thompson WG. Heaton KZ, et al. Towards a positive diagnosis of the irritable bowel. Br Med J 1978; 2:653–654.

4. Drossman DA, Thompson WG, Talley NJ, et al. Identification of subgroups of functional bowel disorders. Gastroenterol Internat 1990; 3:159–172.

5. Vanner SJ, Depew WT, Paterson WG, et al. Predictive value of the Rome criteria for diagnosing the irritable bowel syndrome. Am J Gastroenterol 1999; 94:2912–2917.

6. Tibble JA, Sighthorsson G, Foster R, et al. Use of surrogate markers of inflammation and Rome criteria to distinguish organic

from nonorganic intestinal disease. Gastroenterology 2002; 123: 450–460.

7. Hungin AP, Whorwell PJ, Tack J, et al. The prevalence, patterns and impact of irritable bowel syndrome: an international survey of 40 000 subjects. Aliment Pharmacol Ther 2003; 17:643–650.

A large epidemiologic study in eight European countries that confirmed the deleterious effects of IBS on lifestyle. IBS was common, though the majority of cases were undiagnosed and the prevalence varied markedly among countries.

8. Saito YA, Schoenfeld P, Locke GR III. The epidemiology of irritable bowel syndrome in North America: a systematic review. Am J Gastroenterol 2002; 97:1910–1915.

9. Badia X, Mearin F, Balboa A, et al. Burden of illness in irritable bowel syndrome comparing Rome I and Rome II criteria. Pharmacoeconomics 2002; 20:749–758.

10. Koloski NA, Talley NJ, Boyce PM. Epidemiology and health care seeking in the functional GI disorders: a population-based study. Am J Gastroenterol 2002; 97: 2290–2299.

11. Owens DM, Nelson DK, Talley NJ. The irritable bowel syndrome: long-term prognosis and the physician-patient interaction. Ann Intern Med 1995; 122:107–112.

12. Hahn BA, Yan S, Strassels S. Impact of irritable bowel syndrome on quality of life and resource use in the United States and United Kingdom. Digestion 1999; 60:77–81.

13. Drossman DA, Zhiming L, Andruzzi E, et al. U.S. householder survey on functional gastrointestinal disorders. Dig Dis Sci 1993; 38:1569–1580.

14. Talley NJ, Gabriel SE, Harmsen WS, et al. Medical costs in community subjects with irritable bowel-type symptoms. Gastroenterology 1995; 109:1736–1741.

A community-based study that demonstrated the costs for medical care incurred by patients with IBS is significantly higher than age- and gender-matched controls.

15. Vassallo M, Camilleri M, Phillips SF, et al. Transit through the proximal colon influences stool weight in irritable bowel syndrome. Gastroenterology 1992; 102:102–108.

16. Whitehead WE, Holtkotter B, Enck P, et al. Tolerance for rectosigmoid distention in irritable bowel syndrome. Gastroenterology 1990; 98:1187–1192.

An important study that demonstrated that IBS patients have visceral but not somatic hypersensitivity.

17. Prior A, Maxton DG, Whorwell PJ. Anorectal manometry in irritable bowel syndrome: differences between diarrhoea and constipation predominant subjects. Gut 1990; 31:458–462.

18. Serra J, Azpiroz F, Malagelada JR. Impaired transit and tolerance of intestinal gas in irritable bowel syndrome. Gut 2001; 48:14–19.

19. Kellow JE, Phillips SF, Miller LJ, et al. Dysmotility of the small intestine in irritable bowel syndrome. Gut 1988; 29:1236–1243.

20. Kellow JE, Gill RC, Wingate DL. Prolonged ambulant recordings of small bowel motility demonstrate abnormalities in the irritable bowel syndrome. Gastroenterology 1990; 98:1208–1218.

21. Schmidt T, Hackelsberger N, Widmer R, et al. Ambulatory 24-hour jejunal motility in diarrhea-predominant irritable bowel syndrome. Scand J Gastroenterol 1996; 31:581–589.

22. Ritchie J. Pain from distension of the pelvic colon by inflating a balloon in the irritable colon syndrome. Gut 1973; 14:125–132.

23. Bradette M, Delvaux M, Staumont G, et al. Evaluation of colonic sensory thresholds in IBS patients using a barostat. Dig Dis Sci 1994; 39:449–457.

24. Accarino AM, Azpiroz F, Malagelada JR. Selective dysfunction of mechanosensitive intestinal afferents in irritable bowel syndrome. Gastroenterology 1995; 108:636–643.

25. Cook IJ, van Eeden A, Collins SM. Patients with irritable bowel syndrome have greater pain tolerance than normal subjects. Gastroenterology 1987; 93:727–733.

26. Mertz H, Naliboff B, Munakata J, et al. Altered rectal perception is a biological marker of patients with irritable bowel syndrome. Gastroenterology 1995; 109:40–52.

27. Bouin M, Plourde V, Boivin M, et al. Rectal distention testing in patients with irritable bowel syndrome: sensitivity, specificity and predictive values of pain sensory thresholds. Gastroenterology 2002; 122:1771–1777.

28. Lembo T, Munakata J, Mertz H, et al. Evidence for the hypersensitivity of lumbar splanchnic afferents in irritable bowel syndrome. Gastroenterology 1994; 107:1686–1696.

29. Plourde V, Lembo T, Shui W, et al. Effects of the somatostatin analogue octreotide on rectal afferent nerves in humans. Am J Physiol 1993; 265:G742–G751.

30. Talley NJ, Phillips SF, Bruce B, et al. Relation among personality and symptoms in nonulcer dyspepsia and the irritable bowel syndrome. Gastroenterology 1990; 99:327–333.

31. Kumar D, Pfeffer J, Wingate DL. Role of psychological factors in the irritable bowel syndrome. Digestion 1990; 45:80–87.

32. Guthrie E, Creed PH, Whorwell PK. Outpatients with irritable bowel syndrome: a comparison of first time and chronic attenders. Gut 1992; 33:361–363.

33. Lydiard RB, Fossey MD, Marsh W, et al. Prevalence of psychiatric disorders in patients with irritable bowel syndrome. Psychosomatics 1993; 34:229–234.

34. Drossman D, McKee DC, Sandler RS, et al. Psychosocial factors in the irritable bowel syndrome. A multivariate study of patients and nonpatients with the irritable bowel syndrome. Gastroenterology 1988; 99:409–415.

35. Whitehead WE, Winget C, Fedoravicius AS, et al. Learned illness behavior in patients with irritable bowel syndrome and peptic ulcer. Dig Dis Sci 1982; 79:283–288.

36. Sandler RS, Drossman DA, Nathan HP, et al. Symptom complaints and health care seeking behavior in subjects with bowel dysfunction. Gastroenterology 1984; 87:314–318.

37. Talley NJ. Diagnosing an irritable bowel: Does sex matter? Gastroenterology 1992; 100:834–837.

38. Whitehead WC, Cheskin LJ, Heller BR, et al. Evidence for exacerbation of irritable bowel syndrome during menses. Gastroenterology 1990; 98:1485–1489.

39. Craig TKJ, Brown GW. Goal frustration and life events in the aetiology of painful gastrointestinal disorder. J Psychomatic Research 1984; 28:411–421.

40. Ford MJ, Miller P, Eastwood J, Eastwood MA. Life events, psychiatric illness and the irritable bowel syndrome. Gut 1987; 28:160–165.

41. Whitehead WC, Crowell MD, Robinson JC. Effects of stressful life events on bowel symptoms: subjects with irritable bowel syndrome compared with subjects without bowel dysfunction. Gut 1992; 33:825–830.

42. Drossman DA, Leserman J, Nachman G, et al. Sexual and physical abuse in women with functional or organic gastrointestinal disorders. Ann Int Med 1990; 113:828–833.

43. Talley NJ, Fett SL, Zinsmeister AR. Self-reported abuse and gastrointestinal disease in outpatients: association with irritable bowel-type symptoms. Am J Gastroenterol 1995; 90:366–371.

44. Talley NJ, Fett SL, Zinsmeister AR, et al. Gastrointestinal tract symptoms and self-reported abuse: a population-based study. Gastroenterology 1994; 107:1040–1049.

45. Kumar D, Thompson PD, Wingate DL. Abnormal REM sleep in the irritable bowel syndrome. Gastroenterology 1992; 103:12–17.

46. Goldsmith G, Levin JS. Effect of sleep quality on symptoms of irritable bowel syndrome. Dig Dis Sci 1993; 38:1809–1814.

47. Chaudhury NA, Truelove SC. The irritable bowel syndrome. Q J Med 1962; 31:307–322.

48. Collins SM. Is the irritable gut an inflamed gut? Scand J Gastroenterol 1992; Suppl. 192:102–105.

49. Bergin AJ, Donnelly TC, McKendrick MW, et al. Changes in anorectal function in persistent bowel disturbance following *Salmonella* gastroenteritis. Eur J Gastroenterol Hepatol 1993; 5:617–620.

50. Gwee KA, Graham JC, McKendrick MW, et al. Psychometric scores and persistence of irritable bowel after infectious diarrhea. Lancet 1996; 347:150–153.

51. Gwee KA, Collins SM, Read NW, et al. Increased rectal mucosal expression of interleukin 1beta in recently acquired post-infectious irritable bowel syndrome. Gut 2003; 52:523–526.

52. Spiller RC, Jenkins D, Thornley JP, et al. Increased rectal mucosal enteroendocrine cells, T lymphocytes, and increased gut permeability following acute *Campylobacter* enteritis and in post-dysenteric irritable bowel syndrome. Gut 2000; 47:804–811.

53. Bearcroft CP, Perrett D, Farthing MJ. Postprandial plasma 5-hydroxytryptamine in diarrhoea predominant irritable bowel syndrome: a pilot study. Gut 1998; 42:4206.

54. Houghton LA, Atkinson W, Whitaker P, et al. Increased platelet depleted plasma 5-hydroxytryptamine (5-HT) concentration following meal ingestion in symptomatic female subjects with diarrhoea predominant irritable bowel syndrome (IBS). Gut 2003; 52:663–670.

55. Chadwick VS, Chen W, Shu D, et al. Activation of the mucosal immune system in irritable bowel syndrome. Gastroenterology 2002; 122:1778–1783.

56. Tornblom H, Lindberg G, Nyberg B, et al. Full-thickness biopsy of the jejunum reveals inflammation and enteric neuropathy in irritable bowel syndrome. Gastroenterology 2002; 123:1972–1979.

57. Jones VA, McLaughlan P, Shorthouse M, et al. Food intolerance: a major factor in the pathogenesis of irritable bowel syndrome. Lancet 1982; 20:1115–1117.

58. Petitpierre M, Gumowski P, Girard JP. Irritable bowel syndrome and hypersensitivity to food. Ann Allergy 1985; 54:538–540.

59. Lunardi C, Bambara LM, Biasi D, et al. Double-blind cross-over trial of oral sodium cromoglycate in patients with irritable bowel syndrome due to food intolerance. Clin Exp Allergy 1991; 21:569–572.

60. Stefanini GF, Prati E, Albini MC, et al. Oral disodium cromoglycate treatment on irritable bowel syndrome: an open study on 101 subjects with diarrheic type. Am J Gastroenterol 1992; 87:55–57.

61. Stefanini GF, Saggioro A, Alvisi V, et al. Oral cromolyn sodium in comparison with elimination diet in the irritable bowel syndrome, diarrheic type. Multicenter study of 428 patients. Scand J Gastroenterol 1995; 30:535–541.

62. Atkinson W, Sheldon T, Shaath N, et al. IgG antibodies to food: a role in irritable bowel syndrome. Gut 2004; 53: 1459–1464.

63. Klein KB. Controlled treatment trials in the irritable bowel syndrome: a critique. Gastroenterology 1988; 59:232–241.

64. Camilleri M. Review article: clinical evidence to support current therapies of irritable bowel syndrome. Aliment Pharmacol Ther 1999; 13(suppl. 2):48–53.

65. Owens DM, Nelson DK, Talley NJ. The irritable bowel syndrome: long-term prognosis and physician-patient interaction. Ann Intern Med 1995; 15:107–112.

66. Symons P, Jones MP, Kellow JE. Symptom provocation in irritable bowel syndrome. Effects of differing doses of fructose-sorbitol. Scand J Gastroenterol 1992; 27:920–924.

67. Fernandez-Banares F, Esteve-Pardo M, de Leon R, et al. Sugar malabsorption in functional bowel disease: clinical implications. Am J Gastroenterol 1993; 88:2044–2050.

68. Ledochowski M, Widner B, Bair H, et al. Fructose- and sorbitol-reduced diet improves mood and gastrointestinal disturbances in fructose malabsorbers. Scand J Gastroenterol 2000; 35:1048–1052.

69. Lambert JP, Brunt PW, Moat NAG, et al. Eur J Clin Nutr 1991; 45:601–609.

70. Tucker DM, Sandstead HH, Logan GM, et al. Dietary fiber and personality factors as determinants of stool output. Gastroenterology 1981; 81:879–883.

71. Cann PA, Read NW, Holdsworth CD. What is the benefit of coarse wheat bran in patients with irritable bowel syndrome? Gut 1984; 25:168–173.

72. Longstreth GF, Fox DD, Youkeles L, et al. Psyllium therapy in the irritable bowel syndrome – a double-blind trial. Ann Int Med 1981; 95:53–56.

73. Prior A, Whorwell PJ. Double-blind study of isphaghula in irritable bowel syndrome. Gut 1987; 28:221–225.

74. Poynard T, Naveau S, Mory B, et al. Meta-analysis of smooth muscle relaxants in the treatment of the irritable bowel syndrome. Alim Pharmacol Ther 1994; 8:499–510.

75. Poynard T, Regimbeau C, Benhamou Y. Meta-analysis of smooth muscle relaxants in the treatment of the irritable bowel syndrome. Alim Pharmacol Ther 2001; 15:355–361.

76. Jailwala J, Imperiale TF, Kroenke K. Pharmacologic treatment of the irritable bowel syndrome: a systematic review of randomized, controlled trials. Ann Intern Med 2000; 133:136–147.

A critical review of the treatments used to treat IBS demonstrating beneficial effects of smooth-muscle relaxants for abdominal pain, loperamide for diarrhea but inconclusive effects of psychotropic agents. The efficacy of bulking agents has not been established.

77. Ivey KJ. Are anticholinergics of use in the irritable bowel syndrome? Gastroenterology 1975; 68:1300–1307.

78. Awouters F, Megens A, Verlinden M, et al. Loperamide – survey of studies on mechanisms of its antidiarrheal activity. Dig Dis Sci 1993; 38:977–985.

79. Lavo B, Stenstam M, Nielsen AL. Loperamide in the treatment of irritable bowel syndrome – a double-blind, placebo-controlled study. Scand J Gastroenterol 1987; 22(Suppl. 130):77–80.

80. Foxx-Orenstein AE, Kuemmerle JF, Grider JF. Distinct 5-HT receptors mediate the peristaltic reflex induced by mucosal stimuli in human and guinea pig intestine. Gastroenterology 1996; 111:1281–1290.

81. Gershon MD. Review article: roles played by 5-hydroxytryptamine in the physiology of the bowel. Aliment Pharmacol Ther 1999; 13(Suppl 2):15–30.

82. Kim DY, Camilleri M. Serotonin: a mediator of the brain-gut connection. Am J Gastroenterol 2000; 95(10):2698–2709.

83. De Ponti F, Tonini M. Irritable bowel syndrome. New agents targeting serotonin receptor subtypes. Drugs 2001; 61(3):317–332.

84. Prather CM, Camilleri M, Zinsmeister AR, et al. Tegaserod accelerates orocecal transit in patients with constipation-predominant irritable bowel syndrome. Gastroenterology 2000; 118:462–468.

85. Muller-Lissner SA, Fumagalli I, Bardhan KD, et al. Tegaserod, a 5-HT$_4$ receptor partial agonist, relieves symptoms in irritable bowel syndrome patients with abdominal pain, bloating and constipation. Aliment Pharmacol Ther 2001; 15:1655–1666.

86. Kellow J, Lee OY, Chang FY, et al. An Asia-Pacific, double-blind, placebo controlled, randomised study to evaluate the efficacy, safety and tolerability of tegaserod in patients with irritable bowel syndrome. Gut 2003, 52:671–676.

A large randomized, controlled study confirming the efficacy of tegaserod in an Asian-Pacific population. The mean proportion of patients with overall satisfactory relief was greater in the tegaserod group than in the placebo group over weeks 1–4 (56% versus 35%) and weeks 1–12 (62% versus 44%).

87. Bouras EP, Camilleri M, Burton DD, et al. Prucalopride accelerates gastrointestinal and colonic transit in patients with constipation without a rectal evacuation disorder. Gastroenterology 2001; 120:354–360.

88. Novick J, Miner P, Krause R, et al. A randomized, double-blind, placebo-controlled trial of tegaserod in female patients suffering from irritable bowel syndrome with constipation. Aliment Pharmacol Ther 2002; 16:1877–1888.

89. Talley NJ, Phillips SF, Haddad A, et al. Effect of selective 5HT$_3$ antagonist (GR38032F) on small intestinal transit and release of gastrointestinal peptides. Dig Dis Sci 1989; 34:1511–1515.

90. Camilleri M, Northcutt AR, Kong S, et al. Efficacy and safety of alosetron in women with irritable bowel syndrome: a randomised, placebo-controlled trial. Lancet 2000; 355:1035–1040.

A large randomized controlled trial examining the efficacy of alosetron for IBS. In this trial 41% of alosetron-treated patients and 29% of placebo-treated patients reported adequate relief for all 3 months of treatment. Alosetron also significantly decreased urgency and stool frequency, and increased stool firmness but was associated with constipation (30% of patients taking alosetron versus 3% in the placebo group).

91. Cara S, Krause G, Biesheuvel E, et al. Cilansetron shows efficacy in male and female non-constipated patients with irritable bowel syndrome in a United States study (Abstract). Gastroenterology 2001; 120:1339.

92. Thompson CA. Alosetron withdrawn from market. Am J Health Syst Pharm 2001; 58:13.

93. Schikowski A, Thewissen M, Mathis C, et al. Serotonin type-4 receptors modulate the sensitivity of intramural mechanoreceptive afferents of the cat rectum. Neurogastroenterol Motil 2002; 14:221–227.

94. Coelho AM, Rovira P, Fioramonti J, et al. Antinociceptive properties of HTF 919 (tegaserod), a 5-HT$_4$ receptor partial agonist, on colorectal distensions in rats (Abstract). Gastroenterology 2000; 118:A835.

95. Coffin B, Farmachidi JP, Ruegg P, et al. Tegaserod, a 5-HT$_4$ receptor partial agonist, decreases sensitivity to rectal distension in healthy subjects. Aliment Pharmacol Ther 2003; 15:577–585.

96. Prior JA, Read NW. Reduction of rectal sensitivity and postprandial motility by granisetron, a 5-HT$_3$ receptor antagonist, in patients with irritable bowel syndrome. Aliment Pharmacol Ther 1993; 7:175–180.

97. Hammer J, Phillips SF, Talley NJ, et al. Effect of a 5-HT$_3$-antagonist (ondansetron) on rectal sensitivity and compliance in health and the irritable bowel syndrome. Aliment Pharmacol Ther. 1993; 7:543–551.

98. Zighelboim J, Talley NJ, Phillips SF, et al. Visceral perception in irritable bowel syndrome. Rectal and gastric responses to distension and serotonin type 3 antagonism. Dig Dis Sci 1995; 40:819–827.

99. Delvaux M, Louvel D, Mamet JP, et al. Effect of alosetron on responses to colonic distension in patients with the irritable bowel syndrome. Aliment Pharmacol Ther 1998; 12:849–855.

100. Camilleri M, Coulie B, Tack JF. Visceral hypersensitivity: facts, speculations and challenges. Gut 2001; 48:125–131.

101. Tack J, Vos R, Gevers AM, et al. Alosetron: more than a constipating drug? A comparison of the effects of alosetron and of loperamide on colonic sensorimotor function in man (Abstract). Gastroenterology 2001; 120:4041.

102. Clouse RE, Lustman PJ, Geisman RA. et al. Antidepressant therapy in 138 patients with the irritable syndrome: a five-year clinical experience. Aliment Pharmacol Therap 1994; 8:409–416.

103. Greenbaum DS, Mayle JE, Vanegeran LE, et al. The effects of desipramine on irritable bowel syndrome compared with atropine and placebo. Dig Dis Sci 1987; 32:257–266.

104. Myren J, Groth H, Larsen SE, et al. The effect of trimipramine in patients with the irritable bowel syndrome – a double-blind study. Scand J Gastroenterol 1982; 17:871–875.

105. Drossman DA, Toner BB, Whitehead WE, et al. Cognitive-behavioral therapy versus education and desipramine versus placebo for moderate to severe functional bowel disorders. Gastroenterology 2003; 125:19–31.

106. Svedlund J, Sjodin I, Ottoson JO, et al. Controlled study of psychotherapy in irritable bowel syndrome. Lancet 1983; 2:589–592.

107. Guthrie E, Creed PH, Dawson D, et al. A controlled trial of psychological treatment for the irritable bowel syndrome. Gastroenterology 1991; 100:450–457.

108. Creed F, Fernandes L, Guthrie E, et al. The cost-effectiveness of psychotherapy and paroxetine for severe irritable bowel syndrome. Gastroenterology 2003; 124:303–317.

For patients with severe IBS, both psychotherapy and paroxetine improve health-related quality of life compared with routine care by a gastroenterologist and general practitioner. Psychotherapy but not paroxetine was associated with significant reduction in healthcare costs compared with usual treatment at 1 year.

109. Blanchard EB, Greene B, Scharff L, et al. Relaxation training as a treatment for irritable bowel syndrome. Biofeedback Self Regulation 1993; 18:125–132.

110. Greene B, Blanchard EB. Cognitive therapy for irritable bowel syndrome. J Consult Clin Psychol 1994; 62:576–582.

111. Payne A, Blanchard EB. A controlled comparison of cognitive therapy and self help groups in the treatment of irritable bowel syndrome. J Consult Clin Psychol 1995; 63:779–786.

112. Whorwell PJ, Prior A, Farragher EB. Controlled trial of hypnotherapy in the treatment of severe refractory irritable bowel syndrome. Lancet 1984; 2:1232–1234.

113. Harvey RF, Hinton RA, Gunary RM, et al. Individual and group hypnotherapy in the treatment of irritable bowel syndrome. Lancet 1989; 1:424–425.

114. Lea R, Houghton LA, Calvert EL, et al. Gut-focused hypnotherapy normalizes disordered rectal sensitivity in patients with irritable bowel syndrome. Aliment Pharmacol Ther 2003; 17:635–642.

115. Talley NJ, Owens BK, Boyce P, et al. Psychological treatments for irritable bowel syndrome – a critique of controlled trials. Am J Gastroenterol 1996; 91:277–286.

116. Meyers NL, Tack J, Middleton S, et al. Efficacy and safety of renzapride in patients with constipation-predominant irritable bowel syndrome (Abstract) UEGW 2002; Geneva.

117. Viramontes BE, Malcolm A, Camilleri M, et al. Effects of an alpha(2)-adrenergic agonist on astrointestinal transit, colonic motility and sensation in humans. Am J Physiol Gastrointest Liver Physiol 2001; 281:G1468–G1476.

118. Camilleri M, Kim DY, McKinzie S, et al. A randomized, controlled exploratory study of clonidine in diarrhea-predominant irritable bowel syndrome. Clin Gastroenterol Hepatol 2003; 1:111–121.

119. Delvaux M, Louvel D, Lagier E, et al. The kappa agonist fedotozine relieves hypersensitivity to colonic distention in patients with irritable bowel syndrome. Gastroenterology 1999; 116:38–45.

120. Dapoigny M, Abitbol JL, Fraitag B. Efficacy of the peripheral kappa agonist fedotozine versus placebo in the treatment of the irritable bowel syndrome: a multicenter dose-response study. Dig Dis Sci 1995; 40:2244–2249.

121. Delgado-Aros S, Chial H, Camilleri M, et al. Effects of a kappa-opioid agonist, asimadoline, on satiation and GI motor and sensory functions in humans. Am J Physiol Gastrointest Liver Physiol 2003; 284:G558–G5566.

122. Chey WD, Beydoun A, Roberts DJ, et al. Octreotide reduces perception of rectal electrical stimulation by spinal afferent pathway inhibition. Am J Physiol 1995; 259:G821–G826.

123. Plourde V, Lembo T, Shui Z, et al. Effects of the somatostatin analogue octreotide on rectal afferent nerves in humans. Am J Physiol 1993; 256:G742–G751.

124. Kuiken SD, Tytgat GNJ, Boeckxstaens GEE. The selective serotonin reuptake inhibitor fluoxetine does not change rectal sensitivity and symptoms in patients with irritable bowel syndrome: A double blind, randomized, placebo-controlled study. Clin Gastroenterol Hepatol 2003; 1:219–228.

125. Tack J, Vos R, Broekaert D, et al. Influence of citalopram, a selective serotonin reuptake inhibitor, on colonic tone and sensitivity in man. 2004; submitted for publication.

126. Broekaert D, Vos R, Gevers AM, et al. A double-blind randomised placebo-controlled crossover trial of citalopram, a selective serotonin reuptake inhibitor, in irritable bowel syndrome (Abstract). Gastroenterology 2000; 120:3250.

127. Dunlop S, Jenkins D, Neal KR, et al. Randomised double-blind placebo-controlled trial of prednisolone in post-infectious irritable bowel syndrome. Aliment Pharmacol Ther 2003; 18:77–84.

128. Pimentel M, Chow EJ, Lin HC. Eradication of small intestinal bacterial overgrowth reduces symptoms of irritable bowel syndrome. Am J Gastroenterol 2000; 95:3503–3506.

   A controversial paper showing an association between bacterial overgrowth and IBS.

129. Pimentel M, Chow EJ, Lin HC. Normalization of lactulose breath testing correlates with symptom improvement in irritable bowel syndrome: a double-blind, randomized, placebo-controlled study. Am J Gastroenterol 2003; 98:412–419.

130. Nobaek S, Johansson ML, Molin G, et al. Alteration of intestinal microflora is associated with reduction in abdominal bloating and pain in patients with irritable bowel syndrome. Am J Gastroenterol 2000; 95:1231–1238.

131. O'Sullivan MA, O'Morain SA. Bacterial supplementation in the irritable bowel syndrome. A randomised double-blind placebo-controlled crossover study. Dig Liver Dis 2000; 32:294–301.

132. Niedzielin K, Kordecki H, Birkenfeld B. A controlled, double-blind, randomized study on the efficacy of *Lactobacillus plantarum* 299V in patients with irritable bowel syndrome. Eur J Gastroenterol Hepatol 2001; 13:1143–1147.

CHAPTER FORTY-NINE

49

Celiac sprue and other malabsorptive disorders

Norton J. Greenberger

INTRODUCTION

Impaired intestinal absorption of nutrients can result from any disease process that affects one or more of the key steps involved in the normal digestion and absorption of nutrients. These diseases include those in which occur defective intraluminal digestion and nutrient processing, impaired uptake in the transport of nutrients across the epithelium of the small intestine, and transport of nutrients from the intestinal mucosa to the systemic circulation. Examples of intraluminal defective processes include bile salt deficiency, pancreatic insufficiency, and bacterial overgrowth syndromes. Celiac sprue exemplifies defective mucosal transport of nutrients because of altered small bowel mucosa. Impaired transport from the mucosa into the systemic circulation can be due to lymphatic obstruction, a disease process within the intestinal mucosa (intestinal lymphangiectasia), or a disease process external to the small bowel per se, such as lymphoma.

The pathophysiologic basis for the symptoms and signs of malabsorptive disorders is depicted in Table 49.1. It should be emphasized that patients with malabsorptive disorders may have gross evidence of malabsorption manifested by typical symptoms and signs, or they may have isolated findings that alone may not suggest the diagnosis of malabsorption. For example, a patient may have edema resulting from hypoalbuminemia but no steatorrhea, diarrhea, weight loss, or weakness. Similarly, a patient with malabsorption might have iron deficiency anemia alone without gross evidence of malabsorption. Accordingly, it is important to consider a malabsorptive disorder when patients have the symptoms or signs detailed in Table 49.1.

Many of the tests useful in the diagnosis of intestinal malabsorption indicate the presence of abnormal digestive or absorptive function and only a few tests may suggest a specific diagnosis.[1] Accordingly, it is necessary to use a combination of tests to establish a diagnosis. Tests commonly used in the differential diagnosis of malabsorptive disorders are described in Table 49.2. To illustrate the use of these tests, the typical findings in a primary malabsorptive disorder (celiac sprue) are compared with those in a classic maldigestive disorder (pancreatic insufficiency).

Table 49.1 Symptoms of malabsorptive disorders

Symptom or sign	Pathophysiology
Diarrhea	Impaired absorption of sodium and water; cathartic effects of unabsorbed fatty acids and bile salts
Weight loss	Impaired absorption of nutrients
Edema	Hypoproteinemia
Anemia	Impaired absorption of iron, folic acid, vitamin B_{12}
Weakness	Anemia, weight loss, electrolyte depletion (hypokalemia)
Amenorrhea	Protein depletion and malnutrition
Hemorrhagic phenomenon	Vitamin K malabsorption
Nocturia	Delayed absorption of water
Glossitis, cheilosis, stomatitis	Vitamin deficiencies
Tetany, paresthesias	Hypocalcemia, hypomagnesemia
Bone pain	Osteoporosis and osteopenia secondary to calcium malabsorption and protein depletion
Peripheral neuropathy	Nutrient deficiency, long-standing vitamin B_{12} deficiency

Table 49.2 Tests useful in the diagnosis of malabsorptive disorders

Typical tests	Malabsorption (celiac sprue)	Maldigestion (pancreatic insufficiency)
Stool studies		
Qualitative analysis	↑ fat	↑ fat, ↑ undigested muscle fibers
Quantitative analysis	>6 g/24 h*	>6 g/24 h*
Specific absorptive tests		
D-Xylose (25 g)	<4.5 g/5 h urine collection	Normal
Schilling test for vitamin B$_{12}$ absorption	Frequently ↓	Frequently ↓ (40–50% abnormal)
Indirect tests		
Serum albumin	Frequently ↓	May be normal
Serum calcium	Frequently ↓	Usually normal
Serum cholesterol	↓	Frequently ↓
Serum iron	Usually ↓	Normal
Serum carotenes	↓	Frequently ↓
Prothrombin time	Frequently prolonged	May be prolonged
Imaging studies		
Small intestine radiographs	Malabsorptive pattern	May be normal; may show pancreatic calcification
CT scan	Unremarkable	May show pancreatic calcification, dilated pancreatic duct, atrophic pancreas
Endoscopic and biopsy studies		
Endoscopy	Abnormal duodenal mucosa	Normal duodenum
Small bowel biopsy	Abnormal	Normal
ERCP/MRCP	Usually not done	Abnormal pancreatic ductal system
Pancreatic function tests		
Secretin test	Abnormal in 10–20%	Abnormal
Bentiromide	Abnormal; xylose test also abnormal	Abnormal but xylose test normal
Miscellaneous		
Urine 5-HIAA	Increased mildly (10–20 mg/24 h)	Normal

CT, computed tomography; ERCP, endoscopic retrograde cholangiopancreatography; MRCP, magnetic resonance cholangiopancreatography; 5-HIAA, 5-hydroxyindoleacetic acid.
* If stool volume exceeds 1200 mL/day, fecal fat excretion can increase to 14 g/day as a direct result of diarrhea.

CELIAC SPRUE

Definition

Celiac sprue is a disorder characterized by malabsorption, abnormal small bowel structure, and intolerance to gluten, a protein found in wheat and wheat products. It has also been referred to as gluten-induced enteropathy. Celiac disease in children and nontropical sprue in adults are probably the same disorder with the same pathogenesis.

Celiac sprue occurs primarily in whites of northern European ancestry. Studies in 2000 American blood donors suggested a prevalence of 1:250 based upon endomysial antibody testing.[2] These findings suggest that the number of undiagnosed celiacs is much higher than the number of patients with classic celiac sprue, and in some studies in children the ratio of undiagnosed to diagnosed celiac disease is 7:1.

One of the largest studies in the United States included 13 354 subjects from 32 states screened for serological evidence of celiac sprue (IgA and IgG antigliadin antibodies, IgA antiendomysial antibody). Three hundred and fifty (2.7%) were positive for antiendomysial antibody.[3] The prevalence of celiac disease was 1:22 for first-degree relatives, 1:39 for second-degree relatives, and 1:68 in symptomatic subjects many of whom presumably carried the diagnosis of irritable bowl syndrome. Mucosal biopsies were abnormal in 116/350 (33%) of subjects. Celiac sprue can be viewed as an 'iceberg' disease, with the majority of cases going clinically undetected with either silent of latent disease.

Pathophysiology

The characteristic lesion in the small intestine of patients with celiac sprue is a blunted and flattened mucosa, expanded lamina propria, and exuberant infiltration of lymphocytes along with abnormalities of the surface epithelium. This lesion, although characteristic, is not specific for the diagnosis of celiac sprue. A 33-amino peptide (alpha gliadin peptide 56-89) has been identified that has several characteristics suggesting that it is the primary initiator of the inflammatory response in celiac sprue. This peptide is particularly resistant to intraluminal gastrointestinal peptidases but can be degraded by enterocytes in controls but only partially in celiac sprue patients. The peptide reacts with tissue transglutaminase and is a potent inducer of gut-derived T-cell lines.[4] The exclusion of wheat gluten, rye, barley, and oat polyamines from the diet results in prompt improvement in absorption along with progression to normalization of the associated small intestinal lesion.[1] The spectrum of manifestations of celiac sprue is broad (Table 49.3), but the severity of disease generally correlates with the length of small intestine that is damaged. When the mucosal lesion is limited to the duodenum and proximal part of the jejunum, overt gastrointestinal symptoms and steatorrhea may be absent and the only manifestation in such patients may be anemia caused by iron deficiency. On the other hand, when most or all of the small intestinal mucosa is involved, symptoms are severe and the malabsorption is generalized.

Diagnosis

Characteristic findings in the diagnosis of celiac sprue are detailed in Table 49.4. The diagnosis is usually based on four features: (1) evidence of malabsorption, (2) an abnormal small bowel biopsy specimen, (3) response to a gluten-free diet (GFD), and (4) abnormal serologic studies and, in particular, a positive test for antiendomysial antibodies. In equivocal cases, a challenge with 30 g of gluten can be carried out, but this provocative test is not usually necessary. In patients with only duodenal involvement, iron deficiency anemia may be the only abnormality found. Indeed, in a series of 39 patients with celiac sprue, anemia was the sole manifestation in 17 patients.[7] Celiac sprue is underdiagnosed and the diagnosis is still delayed even in patients with classic diarrhea.[7,8] Tests useful in the differential diagnosis of celiac sprue are listed in Table 49.2 and are compared with the typical findings in pancreatic exocrine insufficiency.

Table 49.3 The many faces of celiac sprue[5,6]

Classical presentation (diarrhea, weight loss, malabsorption)

Iron deficiency anemia (most common presentation)

Metabolic bone disease (osteopenia, osteoporosis, premature fractures)

Unexplained hypoalbuminemia

Unexplained neuropsychiatric findings (ataxia, depression, epilepsy)

Diabetic diarrhea (5% of diabetics have concurrent celiac sprue)

Irritable bowel syndrome (2.5–5.0% of IBS patients have celiac sprue)

Increased risk of intestinal lymphoma (standardized incidence ratio 1.3)

T-cell enteropathy (harbinger of lymphoma)

Dermatitis herpetiformis

Elevations in serum aminltransfeases

Table 49.4 Diagnosis of celiac sprue

Characteristic findings

Evidence of malabsorption*
    Steatorrhea
    Decreased absorption of D-xylose
    Decreased serum iron, calcium, albumin, cholesterol, carotenes
    Prolonged prothrombin time
Abnormal small bowel biopsy
    Blunted and flattened mucosa, elongated crypts, increased lymphocytic infiltration, abnormal surface epithelium
Response to a gluten-free diet
    Clinical improvement (weight gain, decreased diarrhea)
    Improvement in laboratory studies (see above)
    Improvement in small bowel histology if repeated biopsies are performed (usually not necessary)
Abnormal serologic studies
    Abnormal antiendomysial, tissue transglutaminase, and antigliadin antibodies
Response to gluten challenge
    In equivocal cases challenge with 30 g of gluten can be carried out

Subclinical findings

    Antiendomysial antibody – usually positive in patients with latent celiac sprue; titer correlates with extent and severity of disease
    Dermatitis herpetiformis
    Latent celiac sprue can be unmasked by gastric surgical procedures (subtotal gastrectomy, vagotomy, and pyloroplasty)

* Not all of these abnormalities must be present.

IgA antiendomysial antibodies represent an excellent serologic test for celiac sprue, with a sensitivity of 97% and specificity of 98–99%. Because 2–3% of celiac sprue patients have a selective IgA deficiency, IgA levels should be measured. The enzyme tissue transglutaminase is the antigen for antiendomysial antibody and is reported to have a sensitivity of 95% and specificity of 94% in the diagnosis of celiac sprue. The antiendomysial antibody can also be used as a measure of patient compliance with a gluten free diet (GFD). With strict adherence to a GFD, serum antiendomysial antibodies should not be detected. Conversely, persistent positive antibody tests suggest either willful or inadvertent noncompliance with a GFD.

Epidemiological studies have suggested that irritable bowel syndrome (IBS) affects 2.5–15% of Western populations. Sanders et al. carried out a prospective study in which 300 IBS patients and matched controls were investigated for celiac sprue.[9] Of 66 patients with IBS and positive antibody tests (IgA or IgG antigliadin, IgA antiendomysial) 14 (4.7%) had celiac sprue confirmed by duodenal biopsy. Compared with matched controls, IBS was significantly associated with celiac sprue, with an odds ratio of 7.0. Shabazkhani[10] studied 105 IBS patients and 105 controls. Celiac sprue was diagnosed in 12 IBS patients and in no controls. Of the 12 patients, 3 presented with diarrhea, 4 with constipation, and 5 with alternating constipation and diarrhea. Thus, celiac sprue may be found in 2–5% of patients labeled as IBS, and routine testing for celiac sprue may be indicated in such patients, especially if they have not responded to conventional IBS treatments.

Fine[11] determined the prevalence of occult gastrointestinal bleeding in patients with celiac sprue and found that 15 of 28 patients with sprue had persistently positive tests for occult blood. All these patients underwent an extensive evaluation that included esophagogastroduodenoscopy, colonoscopy, and barium radiography of the small bowel. Importantly, over half of these patients responded to gluten withdrawal with reversal of Hemoccult-positive stool specimens to Hemoccult negativity. The conclusion drawn is that occult gastrointestinal bleeding can be detected in about half of patients with celiac sprue and should be added to the list of factors that can contribute to iron deficiency anemia in such patients.

Treatment

The cornerstone of treatment in celiac sprue is to restrict intake of gluten-containing foods. The major sources of gluten are foods containing wheat, barley, rye, and oats, which are detailed in Table 49.5. Patients with sprue need to be provided detailed information regarding the major sources of gluten. In particular, several foods, including processed foods, salad dressings, and dairy products, as well as snack foods, contain appreciable amounts of gluten. Foods usually substituted for gluten-containing foods are also detailed in Table 49.5.

The vast majority of patients with celiac sprue will respond to a GFD, especially if they adhere rigidly to such a diet. Improvement in surface epithelium has been documented as early as 2 weeks after institution of a GFD. Improvement in tests of intestinal absorptive function can usually be documented within a few months after institution of a GFD. Furthermore, improvement in tests of intestinal absorptive function can usually be correlated with stringent adherence to a GFD. However, improvement in intestinal histology with restoration of normal-appearing villi and crypts may take considerably longer and may not be evident for 6 to 18 months after institution of a GFD. In up to 20% of patients, however, even strict adherence to a GFD may not result in the restoration of normal-appearing small bowel mucosa.

Failure to respond to a GFD should prompt consideration of several factors detailed in Table 49.6. The most likely cause is nonadherence to a strict GFD. Frequently, concurrent conditions may contribute to malabsorption, such as pancreatic insufficiency or bacterial overgrowth syndromes. Failure to respond to a GFD, especially if adherence to a strict diet is not a problem, should always raise the question of an underlying small bowel lymphoma. Cellier et al.[12] studied 21 patients with adult refractory sprue (ARS) and 20 controls to assess the phenotype of intraepithelial lymphocyte and T-cell receptor clonal gene configuration. Sixteen of 19 ARS patients had an aberrant intraepithelial lymphoid (IEL) intestinal population expressing intracytoplasmic CD3 but not surface CD8. Clonal intestinal T-cell receptor gene rearrangements were found in 13/17 (76%) of patients. The patients with an aberrant phenotype all had uncontrolled malabsorption and three subsequently developed overt T-cell lymphoma. The three patients without aberrant clonal IEL made a full recovery with a gluten-free diet plus corticosteroids. The authors suggest that refractory sprue with an aberrant clonal IEL may predispose such patients to develop T-cell lymphoma. Egan and colleagues[13] studied 30 patients with small bowel lymphoma complicating celiac sprue. It is interesting to note that 23 of these patients had celiac sprue and lymphoma diagnosed during the same illness. In this group, 14 of 23 patients were surgical emergencies and were treated with tumor resection and chemotherapy. Nine of the 23 patients were disease-free and alive or died of another cause after 10 to 196 months (mean, 74 months) of follow-up. The authors concluded that celiac-associated lymphoma is a difficult to diagnose, and commonly fatal complication of celiac sprue. An aggressive diagnostic approach is recommended in any patient with celiac sprue who relapses without obvious cause. Small bowel enteroscopy and wireless capsule endoscopy can be used to diagnose T-cell enteropathy, which is frequently the harbinger of an underlying T-cell lymphoma. Long-term survival can be expected in a significant number of these patients and in this series was almost exclusively confined to patients treated with chemotherapy.

Table 49.5 Gluten-containing foods

Major sources of gluten: wheat, barley, rye, malt, oats

Breads, flours, cereals (except those with just rice or corn)

Alcohol-containing beverages (beer, ale, whisky, gin, vodka)

Gravies

Processed meats (sandwich meats, cold cuts, frankfurters, canned meats)

Snack foods (pretzels, trail mix, chips, chip mixes)

Any foods prepared with bread or cracker crumbs

Soup mixes, canned soups (some brands), bouillion cubes

Yogurts (some brands), nondairy creamers, hot chocolate mixes

Foods usually substituted for gluten-containing foods

Other starches (rice cereal and cakes, potato flour, corn products)

Meat, fish, poultry

Milk, cheese, eggs

Yellow and green vegetables

Fruits

Nuts, chocolate

All clear soups, most vegetable soups

Table 49.6 Failure to respond to a gluten-free diet

Diagnosis incorrect

Nonadherence to a strict gluten-free diet

Concurrent conditions contributing to malabsorption

Exocrine pancreatic insufficiency (<10% of celiac sprue patients)

Bacterial overgrowth syndrome

Associated lactose intolerance secondary to lactase deficiency

Underlying small bowel lymphoma

Collagenous sprue

Development of diffuse small bowel ulcerations

Development of lymphocytic/microscopic colitis

In a small subset of patients with sprue a broad band of collagen deposition develops in the subepithelial space, an entity termed *collagenous sprue*.[14] Such patients may not respond to a GFD. Furthermore, they may not respond to corticosteroid therapy. In patients with celiac sprue, corticosteroids often induce normalization of the surface epithelium and improvement in tests of absorptive function. However, in patients with collagenous sprue, such therapy is often ineffective. In a few case reports, patients with collagenous sprue have responded to treatment with immunosuppressive drugs such as 6-mercaptopurine. Diffuse small bowel ulceration, which has been termed *nongranulomatous idiopathic jejunoileitis*,[15,16] has been reported in association with celiac sprue, lymphoma, and hypogammaglobulinemia and is discussed in detail later. It appears to be rare in patients with celiac sprue.

In patients with sprue who have responded to a GFD but in whom diarrhea subsequently develops, lymphocytic/microscopic colitis should be considered.[17] This diagnosis is established by performance of colonoscopy with colonic biopsies; the latter usually reveal evidence of significant lymphocytic infiltration. Patients with lymphocytic/microscopic colitis often respond to treatment with sulfasalazine, 5-aminosalicylic acid analogues, and corticosteroids. A disorder closely related to lymphocytic/microscopic colitis is collagenous colitis. Zins and colleagues[17] surveyed 172 consecutive patients seen at the Mayo Clinic in whom collagenous colitis had been diagnosed. Small bowel biopsies were performed in 45 of the patients, and three were found to have evidence of celiac sprue. Thus, although lymphocytic/microscopic colitis may develop in 10% of patients with celiac sprue, collagenous colitis appeared to have developed in a smaller number.

TROPICAL SPRUE

Definition and epidemiology

Individuals living in tropical regions, including Puerto Rico, India, and parts of Southeast Asia, appear to be at risk for the development of a malabsorption syndrome termed tropical sprue. Earlier reports indicated that the syndrome develops in 10% of US Army recruits stationed in Puerto Rico. Importantly, clinical symptoms may not become apparent in some cases until several months after the individual has returned from an endemic area.

Clinical features and diagnosis

Anorexia, weight loss, impaired tests of intestinal absorptive function, severe fatigue, and pronounced megaloblastic anemia are common findings.[8] Indeed, the megaloblastic anemia can be severe, with hematocrits ranging from 20% to 25%. Small bowel biopsy specimens reveal a characteristic lesion consisting of partial flattening of the intestinal villi, subepithelial lymphocytic infiltration, an expanded lamina propria, and abnormal crypts as in celiac sprue. Also, as in celiac sprue, the lesions seen in proximal small intestinal mucosa are characteristic, although not pathognomonic for tropical sprue. Chronic diarrhea in a tropical environment is most often caused by infectious agents, including *Giardia lamblia*, *Yersinina enterocolitica*, *Cryptosporidia*, *Isospora belli*, *Cyclospora cayetanensis*, and *E. bienusi*, and tropical sprue should not be the final diagnosis until the presence of cysts and trophozoites has been excluded.

Treatment

Patients respond dramatically to treatment with folic acid or antibiotics. Approximately 75% of patients will respond within 2 weeks to folic acid therapy at a dosage of 5 mg orally three times daily for 1 week, followed by a maintenance dosage of 1 mg three times daily. However, approximately one-fourth of patients with tropical sprue will require antibiotic therapy, which usually consists of tetracycline, 500 mg four times daily, or ampicillin, 500 mg four times daily for 2–4 weeks or longer, to ameliorate symptoms.

NONGRANULOMATOUS ULCERATIVE JEJUNOILEITIS

Definition

Nongranulomatous ulcerative jejunoileitis is an unusual disorder that has been reported in association with celiac sprue, hypoalbuminemia, malignant histiocytosis, and hypogammaglobulinemia.[15,16] This disorder is characterized by severe chronic diarrhea and intestinal ulcerations with a propensity to gastrointestinal bleeding and iron deficiency anemia. Additional complications include intestinal obstruction or perforation. The terms nongranulomatous ulcerative jejunoileitis, idiopathic chronic ulcerative enteritis, ulcerative enteritis, and T-cell enteropathy have been used interchangeably and most likely reflect the same entity. Diffuse small intestinal ulceration can complicate the course of previously established celiac sprue (which is usually refractory to gluten withdrawal), or patients can present with multiple small bowel ulcerations and malabsorption without evidence of underlying celiac sprue. It has been demonstrated that in many such patients, the intestinal intraepithelial T cells are monoclonal.[18] Further, accumulating evidence suggests that in refractory celiac sprue and ulcerative enteritis lymphoma can develop when a dominant clone of T lymphocytes undergoes neoplastic transformation.

Clinical features and diagnosis

As noted earlier, patients often have chronic diarrhea, weight loss, and evidence of malabsorption. Hypoproteinemia is a very consistent finding. Acute gastrointestinal bleeding or iron deficiency from chronic bleeding may result from intestinal ulcerations. In a representative series,[15] the duodenum and proximal part of the jejunum were inflamed at endoscopy in six of seven patients, with superficial ulcerations in five patients. On histologic examination, the lamina propria was infiltrated by polymorphonuclear and chronic inflammatory cells, along with varying degrees of villous atrophy. No significant cellular abnormalities were seen in epithelial enterocytes. It is not surprising, therefore, that in earlier studies the disorder was linked to celiac sprue. It is not generally appreciated that lesions may also appear in the colon, and in the study by Ruan and associates,[15] ulcerative lesions similar to those identified in the small bowel mucosa were present in four of five patients. The disorder is termed *nongranulomatous ulcerative enterocolitis* because the typical histologic features of Crohn's disease are not found. In addition, other features of Crohn's disease such as colonic involvement, perirectal disease, fistulas, skin lesions, and arthritis occur rarely or not at all.

Treatment

Gluten-free diets are usually ineffective. Response to corticosteroids (e.g., oral prednisone, 40 mg/day) is highly variable. In earlier reports summarized by Jewell,[16] two-thirds of the patients in whom ulcerative idiopathic enterocolitis developed died within 3 years after the onset of symptoms. However, in the more recent report by Ruan and colleagues,[15] four of nine patients have survived while being maintained on low-dose corticosteroid therapy. These authors conclude that idiopathic nongranulomatous enterocolitis may be manifested as a primary and frequently fatal disease and emphasize that corticosteroid therapy may provide immediate benefit in patients and may be required indefinitely. In patients with established T-cell lymphoma, chemotherapy is frequently prescribed, but generally the results are disappointing.

MALABSORPTION IN DIABETIC PATIENTS

Definition and clinical features

Diarrhea often develops in patients with diabetes, and in addition they exhibit signs and symptoms of malabsorption.[19,20] In this setting it is not sufficient merely to label such patients as having 'diabetic diarrhea.' Rather, it is important to determine the specific cause of the diarrhea in such patients because treatment may be specific. The major causes of diarrhea in malabsorptive diabetic patients are listed in Table 49.7. Concurrent celiac sprue occurs in 4–5% of diabetic patients, in which case a GFD is appropriate and effective. Although abnormalities in tests of pancreatic exocrine function are often seen in diabetic patients, frank pancreatic exocrine insufficiency is unusual. In an adult patient with recent onset of diabetes and stigmata of pancreatic exocrine insufficiency, pancreatic cancer must be excluded. For patients with diabetes and pancreatic exocrine insufficiency secondary to chronic pancreatitis, pancreatic enzyme replacement therapy often improves symptoms. Patients with diabetes are also prone to bacterial overgrowth in the small bowel, which generally responds to antibiotics. Visceral autonomic neuropathy in a diabetic is recognized by the presence of the following constellation of clinical findings: (1) delayed gastric emptying, (2) diarrhea with incontinence of stool,

(3) overflow urinary incontinence, (4) impotence in male subjects, (5) anhidrosis with an inability to perspire over the lower half of the body, and (6) postural hypotension. Autonomic neuropathy develops more frequently in individuals with early-onset type 1 diabetes.

Treatment

The treatment of diarrhea in this disorder requires appropriate diagnostics, as outlined earlier, to define the underlying mechanisms. It is important to optimize control of hyperglycemia and control diarrhea with medications such as clonidine,[21] 0.1–0.3 mg three times daily, or octreotide, 100–300 µg/day. If a patient is found to have steatorrhea, decreasing the fat intake in the diet is also important. It is not generally appreciated that many dietetic foods that are labeled 'sugarless' contain sorbitol, a poorly absorbed polyalcohol sugar. Some dietetic foods contain very large quantities of sorbitol. Accordingly, diabetic patients with diarrhea should be asked specifically about foods and medicines. In this regard, many medicines provided as an elixir contain large amounts of sorbitol. Theophylline and digitalis are two common examples.

CHRONIC PANCREATITIS AND PANCREATIC EXOCRINE INSUFFICIENCY

Clinical features and diagnosis

Diarrhea, maldigestion, and as a consequence, malabsorption often develop in patients with chronic pancreatitis. The important causes of chronic pancreatitis and pancreatic insufficiency are detailed in Table 49.8. The most common cause of chronic pancreatitis and pancreatic exocrine insufficiency is chronic alcoholism. An increasing number of patients formerly categorized as having idiopathic chronic pancreatitis are now being diagnosed with one of several forms of hereditary pancreatitis and cystic fibrosis. Patients with cystic fibrosis are now surviving well into adulthood and include a small subset who do not have pulmonary manifestations but in whom stigmata of malabsorption develop because of pancreatic exocrine insufficiency.[22,23] Thus in any young adult in their 20s with stigmata of pancreatic insufficiency, tests

Table 49.7 Diarrhea and malabsorption in diabetic patients

Cause	Treatment
Concurrent celiac sprue (4–5% of diabetics)	Gluten-free diet (see section on celiac sprue)
Pancreatic exocrine insufficiency	Pancreatic enzyme replacement therapy (see section on pancreatic insufficiency)
Bacterial overgrowth in small bowel	Antibiotics (see section on abnormal bacterial proliferation in small bowel)
Visceral autonomic neuropathy	Optimize control of hyperglycemia
'Sugarless' dietetic foods containing sorbitol	Read labels and avoid sorbitol-containing dietetic foods
Control diarrhea	Clonidine
	Octreotide
	Dietary measures (decrease fat intake)

Table 49.8 Causes of chronic pancreatitis and pancreatic insufficiency

Chronic alcoholism

Idiopathic

Cystic fibrosis

Hereditary pancreatitis

Carcinoma of the pancreas

After gastric surgery
    Subtotal gastric resection with Billroth II anastomosis
    Whipple's procedure

Radiation-associated pancreatic injury

Protein-calorie malnutrition
    Hypoalbuminemia
    Kerala pancreatitis (India)

Shwachman's syndrome

should be carried out to exclude cystic fibrosis. In adults past the age of 50 who have stigmata of pancreatic exocrine insufficiency, it is important to exclude pancreatic carcinoma. The alert or alarm signals include (1) onset of diabetes without an obvious predisposing factor (family history, obesity, or corticosteroid therapy), (2) pseudocyst in the body or the tail of the pancreas

Table 49.9 Pancreatic enzyme replacement therapy

Labeled enzyme content (USP units/capsule)

Product	Lipase	Proteases	Amylase
Creon 5	5000	18 570	16 600
Creon 10	10 000	37 500	33 200
Creon 20	20 000	75 000	66 400
Pancrease MT 4	4000	12 000	12 000
Pancrease MT 10	10 000	30 000	30 000
Pancrease MT 16	16 000	48 000	48 000
Pancrease MT 20	20 000	56 000	44 000
Viokase	8000	30 000	30 000

Dosing schedule before meals

Viokase (conventional)	8 tablets each time
Creon 5 (enteric-coated)	5 capsules each time
Pancrease MT 4 (enteric-coated)	6 capsules each time

Possible side effects

General
Nausea
Bloating
Cramping
Constipation
Diarrhea
High-dose effects
Hyperuricosuria
Hyperuricemia

Data from Physicians' desk reference, 53rd edn. Montvale, NJ: Medical Economics; 1999.

without an obvious insult, or (3) prior episodes of acute pancreatitis after age 60 without any obvious predisposing factor.

Tests useful in the diagnosis of maldigestion secondary to pancreatic insufficiency are summarized in Table 49.2, and differentiation from celiac sprue is discussed in the text.

Treatment

Patients with diarrhea and/or steatorrhea secondary to pancreatic insufficiency usually respond to pancreatic enzyme replacement therapy.[24] Table 49.9 lists the preparations that are available, the content of various enzymes, the recommended dosage, and possible side effects. Patients with pancreatic exocrine insufficiency who are placed on a regimen of pancreatic enzymes should notice a reduction in diarrhea/steatorrhea as well as a gain in weight. If such improvement does not occur, the next step is to decrease the fat content of the diet. If improvement still does not occur, treatment with H_2 blockers or proton pump inhibitors can be initiated in an attempt to decrease premature intragastric inactivation of the pancreatic enzyme preparations. Results have been equivocal, especially inasmuch as many of the newer pancreatic enzyme preparations are microencapsulated and are designed to release their contents when intraluminal pH exceeds 5.5. If the patient fails to respond after all of the aforementioned interventions have been initiated, one should look for concurrent problems that may be confounding the patient's response. Abnormal bacterial proliferation in the proximal part of the small bowel may have developed in patients with prior gastric surgery or gastric hypochlorhydria. In addition, structural diseases of the small bowel such as celiac sprue and Crohn's disease need to be excluded. This recommended approach to treatment of bacterial overgrowth is summarized in Table 49.10.

WHIPPLE'S DISEASE

Definition and clinical features

Whipple's disease is a rare disorder clinically characterized by arthralgia, abdominal pain, diarrhea, and progressive weight loss. Low-grade fever, peripheral lymphadenopathy, and wasting are frequently present. Central nervous system manifestations, including confusion, memory loss, focal cranial nerve signs, and ophthalmoplegia, may be present. Laboratory studies usually reveal the presence of steatorrhea, impaired xylose absorption, abnormal small bowel radiographs, anemia, and hypoalbuminemia. The disease occurs most commonly in males 30–60 years of age. The symptoms usually develop slowly over a period of several months and may initially consist of only vague abdominal complaints. The diagnosis is usually established by demonstrating the presence of mucosal macrophages that give a brilliant magenta appearance with periodic acid-Schiff (PAS) staining. In addition to the PAS-positive macrophages, jejunal biopsy specimens frequently show dilated lymphatics and some degree of blunting of the intestinal mucosa. Current microscopic studies have revealed the presence of rod-shaped structures of bacilliform bodies within and adjacent to the macrophage in the lamina propria, as well as within epithelial cells and polymorphonuclear leukocytes. Although the bacterium has not been cultured, *Tropheryma whippelii* has been identified as a Gram-negative bacillus with distinct morphologic characteristics. Tissue specimens are tested

Table 49.10 Causes of intestinal bacterial overgrowth

Structural abnormalities producing stasis of intestinal contents

Strictures
Regional enteritis
Radiation enteritis
Ischemic enteritis (vasculitis)
Billroth II subtotal gastrectomy
Afferent loop stasis
Dysfunctional Roux-en-Y anastomosis
Multiple small bowel diverticula
Multiple laparotomies resulting in adhesions, partial small bowel obstruction, fistulas

Fistulas

Gastrocolic, gastroileal, jejunoileal, jejunocolic

Motor abnormalities resulting in intestinal hypomotility

Infiltrative disorders
Amyloidosis
Scleroderma
Metabolic disorders
Diabetes mellitus
Hypothyroidism
Truncal vagotomy
Intestinal pseudo-obstruction
Visceral myopathy
Visceral neuropathy
The infiltrative and metabolic disorders noted above
Drugs (chronic narcotic use, tricyclic antidepressants)
Paraneoplastic syndromes

Miscellaneous

Gastric achlorhydria/hypochlorhydria
Pernicious anemia
Total/subtotal gastrectomy
Prolonged use of H_2-receptor antagonists or proton pump inhibitors
Pancreatic insufficiency
Cirrhosis
Hypogammaglobulinemia
Nodular lymphoid hyperplasia
Elderly malnourished patients

by polymerase chain reaction (PCR) for the presence of *T. whippelii* DNA. Such specimens are invariably positive in patients with histologically confirmed disease.

Treatment

Although this disease was invariably fatal in the past, antibiotics have now been shown to produce long remissions. Treatment with tetracycline alone or penicillin alone is not adequate. After initial therapy, relapse rates with these drugs approach approximately 40%. The most frequently used regimen includes tetracycline (500 mg twice daily or three times daily) and trimethoprim-sulfamethoxazole (one double-strength tablet twice daily or three times daily) for at least 1 year.[25] Monotherapy with trimethoprim-sulfamethoxazole is also appropriate. After treatment with anti-

biotics, the bacilliform bodies decrease or disappear, along with a decrease in the number of PAS-positive macrophages. The most reliable indicator of a sustained response to treatment is the failure to demonstrate *T. whippelii* DNA by PCR.[26,27] In patients with an initial clinical response, persistence of *T. whippelii* DNA by PCR is associated with an increased likelihood of relapse. Thus PCR is highly sensitive and specific when used to confirm the diagnosis of Whipple's disease, to identify inconclusive and suspicious cases, and to monitor response to therapy. In patients who have failed to respond to initial therapy or who have relapsed after an initial response, a third-generation cephalosporin such as ceftriaxone should be considered. Recent studies have indicated that central nervous system involvement is more frequent than previously believed. In a representative study, positive results for *T. whippelii* determined by PCR were obtained in 4 of 5 patients with neurologic symptoms but also in 7 of 10 patients without neurologic symptoms examined before therapy and in 3 of 11 patients without neurologic symptoms studied during or after therapy. These studies indicate that testing of cerebrospinal fluid in Whipple's disease yields a high rate of positive results even in patients without neurologic symptoms. Examination of cerebrospinal fluid is, therefore, potentially useful for initial staging and monitoring of the efficacy of therapy.

AMYLOIDOSIS

Definition and clinical features

The small intestine is involved in 75–90% of patients with systemic amyloidosis. Despite intestinal involvement, severe clinical manifestations, including obstruction, ulceration, malabsorption, hemorrhage, protein loss, or diarrhea, occur infrequently. Three pathophysiologic mechanisms are involved: (1) direct infiltration of the small intestinal mucosa, (2) vascular deposits that may produce gastrointestinal ischemia with resultant bleeding and perforation, and (3) amyloid infiltration of the gut autonomic nerve sheaths and muscle layers with resultant altered gut motility and secondary bacterial overgrowth. In a recent study approximately two-thirds of patients with systemic amyloidosis had abnormal absorption of ^{75}Se-labeled homocholic toric acid, which is indicative of bile acid malabsorption.[28] Although small bowel mucosal biopsy specimens may be normal on examination by light and electron microscopy, amyloid can be detected in the submucosal or muscle layers in the vast majority of patients. Small intestinal radiographs may also demonstrate prominent intestinal folds. Abnormal breath hydrogen tests and prolonged oral–cecal transit times have also been demonstrated in patients with systemic amyloidosis.[28]

Treatment

Antibiotic regimens including treatment with trimethoprim-sulfamethoxazole, metronidazole, erythromycin, and clarithromycin have been reported. In addition, treatment with prokinetic drugs such as metoclopramide or erythromycin may improve symptoms. Patients with clinical findings indicative of pseudo-obstruction may not respond to any of the aforementioned treatment modalities.

RADIATION ENTERITIS (see Chapter 54)

SYSTEMIC MASTOCYTOSIS (see Chapter 20)

Definition and clinical features

Systemic mastocytosis is defined by mast cell hyperplasia that in most instances is indolent and non-neoplastic. Type 1, defined as indolent systemic mastocytosis, is most relevant to patients with gastrointestinal manifestations and is characterized by cutaneous manifestations, abdominal pain, ulcer disease, malabsorption, skeletal disease, hepatosplenomegaly, or lymphadenopathy. The diagnosis of mastocytosis is established by demonstrating an increased number of mast cells in gastric, duodenal, small bowel, or colonic mucosal biopsy specimens. An elevated total serum tryptase level (mostly alpha) greater than 20 ng/mL and increased levels of histamine in the urine are additional helpful laboratory tests to consider before bone marrow biopsy. Bone marrow biopsy specimens may reveal dense infiltrates of mast cells. The classic picture of urticaria pigmentosa, bone lesions, hepatosplenomegaly, and lymphadenopathy occurs only infrequently. More often, patients have noted alcohol intolerance which causes flushing, cramping abdominal pain, and episodic diarrhea, and skin examination usually reveals striking dermatographism. The differential diagnosis requires that other disorders that cause flushing, such as carcinoid syndrome, pheochromocytoma, drugs (niacin), and rosacea be excluded.

Systemic mastocytosis can be associated with a secretory diarrhea that is mediated by histamine and mast cell products. Evidence of malabsorption occurs in 30% of patients with systemic mastocytosis and is usually due to intestinal mucosal infiltration by mast cells. Malabsorption is not usually severe and is manifested primarily as minimal to moderate steatorrhea and impaired absorption of D-xylose and vitamin B$_{12}$. Small bowel biopsy specimens typically show moderate blunting of villi and mast cell infiltration.

Treatment

Treatment is directed toward symptoms and usually includes the following: histamine H$_1$ blockers for flushing and pruritus and histamine H$_2$-receptor antagonists to inhibit gastric acid secretion. A mast cell stabilizing agent such as oral cromolyn concentrate is often used for diarrhea and abdominal pain at dosages of 400–800 mg/day.[29] Newer leukotriene inhibitors may prove helpful, but no controlled clinical trials on the use of these agents have been reported. If symptoms persist despite treatment with histamine H$_1$ and H$_2$ blockers and cromolyn, a short course of systemic glucocorticoids may be helpful.

MALABSORPTION CAUSED BY BACTERIAL OVERGROWTH OF THE SMALL BOWEL

Definition and pathophysiology

The proximal portion of the small intestine is usually bacteriologically sterile because of three factors: (1) the acid milieu of the stomach; (2) intestinal peristalsis, which sweeps bacteria to the distal portion of the small bowel; and (3) the secretion of immunoglobulin, which may serve as coproantibodies, into the lumen of the intestine. The major mechanism limiting the growth of bacteria in the small intestine is normal peristalsis. Any disorder leading to impaired intestinal motility may result in abnormal stasis of intestinal contents with ineffective mechanical clearing of bacteria. This process may lead to abnormal bacterial proliferation with resultant changes in bile salt metabolism. An increase in unconjugated bile salts and a decrease in conjugated bile salts contribute to impaired intraluminal micellar lipid formation and fat malabsorption. In addition, intestinal mucosal lesions have been demonstrated in patients with intestinal stasis.[30]

Clinical features and diagnosis

Several malabsorptive disorders have been associated with bacterial overgrowth and are summarized in Table 49.10. Breath tests with ^{14}C-labeled bile acid (^{14}C-xylose) and lactulose are useful screening tests for malabsorption syndrome resulting from abnormal bacterial overgrowth of the small intestine. In the lactulose breath test 20 g of lactulose are given p.o. and serial measurements of breath hydrogen are determined every 15 minutes. If there is abnormal bacterial proliferation in the proximal small bowel, there will be a premature increase in breath hydrogen, i.e., at 30–45 minutes not the usual 60–90 minutes when the lactulose bolus reaches the cecum. The 2-h, 50-g glucose breath test reliably predicts the presence of bacterial overgrowth. A definitive diagnosis is established by demonstrating greater than 10^5 microorganisms per milliliter and polymicrobial organisms on culture of duodenal or jejunal fluid. Other clinical features include (1) modest steatorrhea, usually in the range of 15–30 g of fecal fat per 24 h; (2) macrocytic anemia with megaloblastic bone marrow; (3) impaired absorption of vitamin B$_{12}$ that is not corrected by intrinsic factor; and (4) correction of steatorrhea and impaired B$_{12}$ absorption by appropriate antibiotic therapy.

Treatment

In patients with bacterial overgrowth syndrome secondary to surgically correctable lesions such as strictures and fistulas, surgery is the treatment of choice. In patients with mucosal abnormalities caused by an infiltrative or metabolic disorder or intestinal pseudo-obstruction, several antibiotic regimens may prove helpful, including the following:

1. Metronidazole at a dosage of 10 mg/kg up to 750 mg/day;
2. Trimethoprim-sulfamethoxazole, one double-strength tablet twice daily;
3. Erythromycin, 500 mg daily;
4. Doxycycline, 100 mg twice daily;
5. Quinolones such as ciprofloxacin, 500 mg daily;
6. Clarithromycin, 500 mg daily.

Various authorities recommend treatment for 2–3 weeks of each month, and it is often helpful to rotate antibiotics among the six listed above.

In specific disorders other treatments may prove beneficial. Thus, in patients with scleroderma, octreotide at a dose of 50 μg at h.s. may prove useful. Although patients with hypothyroidism may become euthyroid with thyroid hormone replacement therapy, it may take several months before gut motility is restored to normal. In patients with intestinal pseudo-obstruction caused by chronic narcotic use or tricyclic antidepressants, discontinuation of these medications often suffices to correct their diarrhea and/or steatorrhea. Recent studies have indicated that bacterial overgrowth may be more prevalent than generally appreciated in elderly malnourished patients. In such patients without an obvious cause for their malnutrition, an evaluation for evidence of bacterial overgrowth is prudent.

INTESTINAL LYMPHOMA

Definition and clinical features

Steatorrhea is a manifestation of *primary* intestinal lymphoma. The disease occurs predominately in men, and the mean age of onset of symptoms is the third to fifth decades. The diagnosis should be suspected in patients with malabsorption and the following findings: (1) a malabsorption syndrome in which clinical and biopsy features resemble those of celiac sprue but the response to a GFD is incomplete, (2) the presence of relentless abdominal pain and fever, and (3) signs and symptoms of intestinal obstruction. The usual stigmata of generalized lymphoma, such as hepatomegaly, splenomegaly, palpable abdominal masses, and peripheral lymphadenopathy, are not usually found. The diagnosis can generally be established at laparotomy and can often be made through examination of multiple intestinal mucosal biopsy specimens. Villi may be totally absent, or lesser degrees of blunting and shortening of the villi may be present. In contrast to celiac sprue, however, the lamina propria is usually massively infiltrated with lymphoid cells.

Treatment

The course of primary intestinal lymphoma is highly variable, and with newer regimens patients may live 3–5 years or longer.[31,32] With a definite diagnosis of small intestinal lymphoma, therapy regimens with or without irradiation are the preferred modalities of treatment and may induce remission for many years. In the presence of partial small bowel obstruction, there may well be abnormal bacterial proliferation, and such patients may require antibiotics. Other symptomatic measures such as reduced fat in the diet, low-residue liquid regimens, and avoidance of fructose and high sucrose loads may result in amelioration of symptoms.

HYPOPARATHYROIDISM

Definition and clinical features

Steatorrhea has been documented in several patients with idiopathic hypoparathyroidism. In addition to hypocalcemia, impaired absorption of D-xylose and vitamin B_{12}, decreased serum iron values, and abnormal small intestinal radiographs have been demonstrated in some cases. Reports have summarized data on 68 patients with autoimmune polyendocrinopathy, candidiasis, and ectodermal dystrophy. All the patients had candidiasis at some time, and approximately 80% had hypoparathyroidism. Intestinal malabsorption was present in six patients (9%), and multiple endocrine deficiencies were detected in half of the patients. It was recently demonstrated that malabsorption in a patient with autoimmune polyglandular syndrome type I was caused by a transient and selective loss of small intestinal enteroendocrine cells leading to a deficiency of cholecystokinin.[33] Isolated case studies have reported improvement after treatment with pancreatic enzymes, broad-spectrum antibiotics, and antifungal drugs.

HYPERTHYROIDISM

Definition and clinical features

Diarrhea frequently develops in patients with hyperthyroidism, but few detailed studies have been conducted on intestinal absorptive function in such patients. Mild to moderate steatorrhea and hypoalbuminemia have been reported, but absorption of D-xylose and vitamin B_{12} is frequently normal. Clinical studies suggest that steatorrhea associated with hyperthyroidism is not due to any defect of pancreatic or small intestinal mucosal function. Furthermore, some data support the concept that steatorrhea is due at least in part to hyperphagia, with ingestion of unusually large amounts of fat occurring in association with rapid gastric emptying and intestinal transit.[30] Detailed studies have documented that oral–cecal transit is markedly accelerated in hyperthyroid patients, an abnormality reversed after patients become euthyroid. A report has documented bile acid malabsorption in hyperthyroidism, with improvement in both diarrhea and bile salt absorption occurring after individuals were rendered euthyroid.[34,35]

Treatment

Treatment with β-blockers, reduction of fat intake, and the use of bile acid sequestrants such as cholestyramine may ameliorate the symptoms of diarrhea and steatorrhea. Restoration of the euthyroid state can also be expected to result in sustained improvement in both diarrhea and steatorrhea.

INTESTINAL LYMPHANGIECTASIA

Clinical features and diagnosis

Intestinal lymphangiectasia is characterized by increased enteric loss of protein, hypoproteinemia, edema, lymphocytopenia, malabsorption, and abnormally dilated lymphatic channels in the small intestine. Imaging studies have demonstrated the presence of hypoplastic visceral lymphatic channels, which is believed to result in the obstruction of lymph flow; in turn, obstructed lymph flow causes dilated lymphatic vessels throughout the small bowel wall and mesentery. Hypoproteinemia and steatorrhea are thought to be due to rupture of dilated lymphatic vessels with discharge of lymph into the bowel lumen. The diagnosis of intestinal lymphangiectasia is established on the basis of an abnormal small bowel biopsy specimen showing dilated lacteals in the intestinal mucosa. The primary laboratory finding is hypoproteinemia with decreased levels of albumin, IgM, IgA, IgG, transferrin, and ceruloplasmin. Steatorrhea is usually mild, although fat losses may be as high as 40 g/day. Some patients have hypocalcemia and impaired absorption of vitamin B_{12}. Lymphocytopenia caused by the loss of lymphocytes in lymph is common, with lymphocyte counts ranging from 400 to 1000/mL.

Treatment

In adults, approximately 1500 mL of lymph containing 70 g of fat and 50 g of albumin passes through the thoracic duct each day. Leakage of a small amount of this lymph might be expected to result in considerable loss of protein and fat in the intestinal lumen. High-fat diets given to patients often result in increased steatorrhea and increased enteric protein loss. These features underline the rationale for the institution of a low-fat diet in patients with intestinal lymphangiectasia. A low-fat diet, by decreasing lymph flow, usually results in significant improvement with decreased fecal fat excretion, decreased enteric protein loss, and increased serum calcium and albumin levels. The substitution of medium-chain triglycerides instead of dietary long-chain triglycerides has also been shown to improve enteric protein loss and steatorrhea. It should be noted, however, that significant steatorrhea may persist in patients after institution of a completely fat-free diet, which suggests an increased enteric loss of endogenous fat in such patients. A provocative report[36] described dramatic improvement in serum proteins and the disappearance of duodenal lesions in a 35-year-old woman with lymphangiectasia treated with antiplasmin therapy (*trans*-4-(aminomethyl)cyclohexane carboxylic acid).

SUMMARY

The diagnosis of celiac sprue, the prototype malabsorptive disorder, is summarized in Table 49.4 and treatment in Tables 49.6 and 49.7.

REFERENCES

1. Trier JS. Diagnosis and treatment of celiac sprue. Hosp Pract 1993; 28(4A):41–48.

   An excellent review article with very useful information on treatment.

2. Not T, Horvath K, Hill ID, et al. Celiac disease in the USA: High prevalence of antiendomysium antibodies in healthy blood donors. Scand J Gastroenterol 1998; 33:494.

3. Fasano A, Berti I, Gerarduzzi T, et al. Prevalence of celiac disease in at-risk and not-at-risk groups in the United States. A large multicenter study. Arch Int Med 2003; 163:286.

   A large study including 13 354 subjects from 32 states who were screened for serologic evidence of celiac sprue (IgA and IgG antigliadin antibodies, antiendomysial antibodies). Three hundred and fifty (2.7%) were positive for antiendomysial antibody. The prevalence of celiac disease was 1:22 for first-degree relatives, 1:39 for second degree relatives, and 1:68 in symptomatic subjects many of whom presumably carried the diagnosis of irritable bowel syndrome.

4. Shan L, Molberg O, Parrot I, et al. Structural basis for gluten intolerance in celiac sprue. Science 2002; 123:803.

   A 33 amino acid peptide (alpha gliadin 56-89) has been identified that has several characteristics that it is the primary initiator of the inflammatory response in celiac sprue. This peptide is particularly resistant to intraluminal gastrointestinal peptidases but can be degraded by enterocytes in control subjects but only partially in celiac sprue patients.

5. Hadjivassiliov MM, Grunewald RA, Chattopadhyaym AK, et al. Clinical, radiological, nuerological, and neuropathological characteristics of gluten ataxia. Lancet 1998; 352:1592.

6. Abdo A, Meddings J, Swain J. Liver abnormalities in celiac disease. Clin Gastroenterol Hepatol 2004; 2:167–172.

7. Corazza GR, Frisomi M, Treggiarr EA, et al. Subclinical celiac sprue: increasing occurrence and clues to its diagnosis. J Clin Gastroenterol 1993; 16:16–21.

8. Dickey W, McConnell JB. How many hospital visits does it take before celiac sprue is diagnosed? J Clin Gastroenterol 1996; 23:21–23.

9. Sanders DA, Carter MS, Hurlstone DP, et al. Association of adult celiac disease with irritable bowel syndrome: A case-control study in patients fulfilling Rome II criteria referred to secondary care. Lancet 2001; 358:1504–1508.

   A prospective study in which 300 irritable bowel syndrome patients and matched controls were investigated for celiac sprue. Of 66 patients with IBS and positive antibody tests (IgA or IgG antigliadin, IgA antiendomysial) 14 or 4.7% had celiac sprue confirmed by duodenal biopsy.

10. Shahbazkhani B, Forootan M, Merat S. Coeliac sprue presenting as symptoms of irritable bowel syndrome. Aliment Pharm Ther 2002; 18:231–235.

11. Fine KD. The prevalence of occult gastrointestinal bleeding in celiac sprue. N Engl J Med 1996; 334:1163–1169.

   Fine determined the prevalence of occult gastrointestinal bleeding in patients with celiac sprue and found that 15 of 28 patients had persistently positive tests for occult blood. All of these patients underwent an extensive evaluation that included esophagogastroduodenoscopy, colonoscopy, and barium studies of the small bowel. Importantly, over half of these patients responded to gluten withdrawal with reversal of Hemoccult-positive stool specimens.

12. Cellier C, et al. Refractory sprue, celiac disease and enteropathy associated T-cell lymphoma. Lancet 2000; 356:203–208.

   Sixteen of 19 adult refractory sprue patients had an aberrant intraepithelial lymphoid (IEL) population expressing intracytoplasmic CD3 but not surface CD8. Clonal intestinal T-cell receptor gene rearrangements were found in 13 of 17 patients (76%). The patients with an aberrant phenotype all had uncontrolled malabsorption and 3 subsequently developed overt T-cell lymphoma. The 3 patients without aberrant clonal IEL made a full recovery with a gluten-free diet plus corticosteroids.

13. Egan LJ, Walsh SV, Stevens FM, et al. Celiac associated lymphoma. A single institution experience of 30 cases in the combination chemotherapy era. J Clin Gastroenterol 1995; 21:123–129.

14. Weinstein WM, Saunders DR, Tytgat GN, et al. Collagenous sprue: an unrecognized type of malabsorption. N Engl J Med 1971; 283:1297–1301.

15. Ruan EA, Komorowski RA, Hogan WJ, et al. Nongranulomatous chronic idiopathic enterocolitis: clinicopathologic profile and response to corticosteroids. Gastroenterology 1996; 111:629–637.

16. Jewell DP. Ulcerative enteritis (Editorial). Br Med J 1983; 287:1740.

17. Zins BJ, Truman WJ, Carpenter HA. Collagenous colitis: mucosal biopsies and association with fecal leukocytes. Mayo Clin Proc 70: 1995; 430–433.

18. Ashton-Key M, Diss TC, Paov L, et al. Molecular analysis of T-cell clonality in ulcerative jejunitis and enteropathy associated T-cell lymphoma Am J Pathol 1997; 155:493–498.

19. Valdovinos MA, Camiler M, Zimmerman BR. Chronic diarrhea in diabetes mellitus: mechanisms and an approach to diagnosis and treatment. Mayo Clin Proc 1993; 68:691–702.

20. Fedorak RN, Field M, Chang EB. Treatment of diabetic diarrhea with clonidine. Ann Intern Med 1985; 102:197–199.

21. Mourad FH, Gorard D. Effective treatment of diabetic diarrhea with somatostatin analogue, octreotide. Gut 33: 1992; 1578–1580.

22. Sharer N, Schwarz M, Malone G, et al. Mutations of the cystic fibrosis gene in patients with chronic pancreatitis. N Engl J Med 1998; 339:645–652.

23. Cohn JA, Friedman KJ, Noone PG, et al. Relation between mutations of the cystic fibrosis gene and idiopathic pancreatitis. N Engl J Med 1998; 339:653–658.

24. Greenberger NJ. Enzymatic therapy in patients with chronic pancreatitis. Gastroenterology Clin North Am 1999; 155:493–498.

25. Keinath RD, Merrell DE, Vliestra R, et al. Antibiotic treatment and relapse in Whipple's disease: long-term follow up of 88 patients. Gastroenterology 1985; 88:1867–1873.

26. Ramzan NN, Loftus E Jr, Burgart LJ, et al. Diagnosis and monitoring of Whipple's disease by polymerase chain reaction. Ann Intern Med 1997; 126:520–527;

27. VanHerbay AD, Ken HJ, Schumacher F. Whipple's disease: Staging and monitoring by cytology and polymerase chain reaction analysis of cerebrospinal fluid. Gastroenterology 1997; 113:435–441.

28. Suhr O, Damelsson A, Steen L. Bile acid malabsorption caused by gastrointestinal motility dysfunction. An investigation of gastrointestinal disturbances in familial amyloidosis with polyneuropathy. Scand J Gastroenterol 1992; 27:201–207.

29. Horan RF, Sheffer AC, Austen KF. Cromolyn sodium in the management of systemic mastocytosis. J Allergy Clin Immunol 1990; 85:852–855.

30. McEroy T, Dutton J, James OF. Bacterial contamination of the small intestine is an important cause of malabsorption in the elderly. Br Med J 1983; 287:789–793.

31. Amer MH, El-Akkad S. Gastrointestinal lymphoma in adults: clinical features and management of 300 cases. Gastroenterology 1994; 106:846–858.

32. Domizzo, P, Owen LA, Shepher NA, et al. Primary lymphoma of the small intestine. A clinicopathologic study of 119 cases. Am J Surg Pathol 1993; 17:429–442.

33. Hogenauer C, Meyer RL, Netto GJ, et al. Malabsorption due to cholecystokin deficiency in a patient with autoimmune polyglandular syndrome type I. New Eng J Med 2001; 344:270.

Malabsorption in a patient with autoimmune polyglandular syndrome type I was caused by a selective loss of small intestinal enteroendocrine cells leading to a deficiency cholecystokin.

34. Thomas FB, Caldwell JH, Greenberger NJ. Steatorrhea in thyrotoxicosis: Relation to hypermotility and excessive dietary fat. Ann Intern Med 1973; 74:669–675.

35. Rajn GS, Dawson B, Bardhen KD. Bile acid malabsorption associated with Graves disease. J Clin Gastroenterol 1994; 19:54–56.

36. Mine K, Matsubayashi S, Nakai Y, et al. Intestinal lymphangiectasia markedly improved with antiplasmin therapy. Gastroenterology 1987; 96:1596–1599.

CHAPTER FIFTY

Treatment of acute infectious diarrheas

Ralph A. Giannella

INTRODUCTION

Infections of the intestine are common disorders throughout the world. In developing countries, infectious diarrhea, accompanied by dehydration and malnutrition, is a major cause of morbidity and mortality. It is estimated that, on a worldwide basis, acute infectious diarrheal disease results in approximately five million deaths each year.[1,2] In developed countries with adequate sanitation, acute infectious diarrhea is more often a minor illness. However, even in developed countries acute infectious diarrhea may become a gastrointestinal emergency.[3,4] Infections such as *E. coli* O157:H7, *Vibrio cholerae*, or *Clostridium difficile* may be fatal, especially when accompanied by hypotension, shock, renal failure, intestinal perforation, or hemorrhage. In the United States, the General Accounting Office estimates that approximately 85 million cases of enteric infection, largely food-borne, occur each year and results in thousands of deaths. The cost of these illnesses ranges from US$5 to US$22 billion per year.[5]

An extremely wide spectrum of infectious agents cause enteric infections in man. In the US the commonest causes of acute diarrhea by far are viral agents which are usually undefined. The commonest bacterial enteropathogens are *Campylobacter*, *Shigella*, *Salmonella*, and *E. coli*. Fortunately, most cases are self-limited and do not require investigation or more than supportive treatment.[6]

In this chapter, we will discuss enteric infections in the adult patient. A discussion of enteric infections in the pediatric patient is beyond the scope of this chapter.[7] Two recent reviews are highly recommended.[8,9]

ACQUISITION OF INTESTINAL INFECTIONS

In general, enteric infections are acquired by ingestion of contaminated food or water, or person to person spread via the fecal–oral route. The risk of developing an enteric infection is influenced by the intrinsic virulence of the enteropathogen, the inoculum size, and host susceptibility.[10] Usually, a large inoculum (10^6–10^9 organisms) must be ingested in order to induce clinical disease. However, as few as 10–100 *Shigella*[11] or enterohemorrhagic *E. coli* (EHEC) organisms can cause disease.[12,13] In addition to the organism, one must also take into account host susceptibility, i.e., persons with liver disease have an annual rate of illness from *Vibrio vulnificus* 80 times greater, and a death rate 200 times greater than that of adults without liver disease.[14] Host

factors such as decreased gastric acid secretion, reduced intestinal motility, alteration of normal flora, or an immunosuppressed state may reduce the size of the inoculum required as well as enhance the severity of the illness.[10] Additional conditions predisposing to enteric infections include malignancies, lymphomas, steroid therapy, iron overload, ulcerative colitis, and hemolytic anemias, especially sickle cell anemia.[15,16]

PHYSIOLOGY OF INTESTINAL ABSORPTION AND SECRETION

The gastrointestinal tract is exposed to approximately nine liters of fluid each day, approximately two liters from food and ingested liquid and seven liters from endogenous secretions, including salivary juice, gastric secretion, and bile. Of these nine liters, approximately 0.2 liters is excreted in stool. The bulk of the reabsorbed fluid is reabsorbed in the small intestine.[17] In the small intestine, as in most other tissues, ions flow across membranes by active transport and bulk flow processes and water follows to maintain osmotic equilibrium. With regard to diarrhea, the major relevant ions are sodium and chloride. Two major sodium absorption pathways reside in the enterocytes lining the villus, i.e., the neutral Na^+-Cl^- cotransport pathway (the net result of coupled Na^+-H^+ and Cl-$HCO3^-$ transporters) and Na^+-substrate pathways. The Na^+-substrate pathways are comprised of various cotransporters, i.e., Na^+-glucose and several Na^+-amino acid transporters. In the Na^+-substrate transporters, Na^+ absorption is driven by the accompanying substrate. The coupled Na-Cl transport system is regulated by cyclic nucleotides, i.e., inhibited by cAMP and cGMP. Crypt cells contain Cl^- channels which are also regulated by cyclic nucleotides, i.e., stimulated by cAMP and cGMP. When the channels are opened, Cl^- is secreted into the lumen and water follows.[17]

The villus crypt unit is simultaneously absorbing and secreting. Under normal circumstances, absorption exceeds secretion and the net result is movement of Na^+ and water from the lumen into the vascular compartment. The regulation of absorption and secretion in the intestine is quite complex and dysregulation of either absorption or secretion can result in diarrhea. Diarrhea can result either from the inhibition of absorption and/or the stimulation of secretion.[17] Infection with pathogenic bacteria, viruses, etc. cause diarrhea by various mechanisms.[3,6,10,17] Some of these include the elaboration of enterotoxins, provoking an inflammatory reaction in the intestine, altering the cytoskeleton of the enterocyte, disrupting the intercellular junctions between enterocytes (zona occludens), etc. All of these alter the transport of electrolytes, resulting in the inhibition of absorption and/or the stimulation of secretion. If secretion exceeds absorption in the small intestine and the volume of fluid entering the colon exceeds its reabsorptive capacity, diarrhea results.

In many intestinal infections, the Na$^+$-Cl$^-$ co-transport systems are inhibited or destroyed; the Na$^+$-substrate (glucose and amino acid) pathways, however, are unaffected. This is extremely important and allows the use of the Na$^+$-substrate systems to hydrate the patient by oral means.[3,7,17] This realization has led to the development of oral rehydration solutions (ORS) which have saved the lives of millions of individuals suffering with cholera. The same solutions can be used in many enteric infections and are underutilized.[18] Oral rehydration therapy and solutions are also discussed in Chapter 71.

APPROACH TO THE PATIENT WITH ACUTE DIARRHEA

Two guidelines from the American College of Gastroenterology and the Infectious Disease Society of America are highly recommended to all readers.[19,20] Most episodes of acute diarrhea are self-limited and do not require evaluation. However, the physician consulted by an adult patient with acute diarrhea needs to consider and identify which patients would benefit from specific therapy. Most patients merely need attention to hydration status and rehydration therapy. The decision to evaluate a patient with acute diarrhea should be made on the basis of the patient's general health, the severity and duration of illness, the setting in which the illness was acquired, and the likelihood of finding a pathogen for which a beneficial, specific treatment exists. A succinct but thorough discussion of the approach to the patient with acute diarrhea is recommended to the interested reader.[6]

A useful exercise is to classify patients into two clinical syndromes, i.e., inflammatory and noninflammatory diarrhea (Table 50.1).[6,21] Noninflammatory diarrheas generally do not require extensive evaluation, while patients with inflammatory diarrhea frequently have a specific pathogen and will benefit from antimicrobial therapy.

Noninflammatory diarrhea is characterized by large-volume watery stools and few systemic signs or symptoms. Fever is usually absent or minimal. Microbes causing this syndrome are enterotoxin-producing bacteria, protozoa, or minimally invasive viruses. These enteropathogens generally infect the small intestine, stimulating intestinal secretion which may result in dehydration. The most likely causes of this syndrome include viruses (rotavirus; Norwalk virus), enterotoxigenic *E. coli*, *V. cholerae*, staphylococcal and clostridial food poisoning, *Giardia*, and *Cryptosporidia*.

Inflammatory diarrhea is characterized by multiple, small-volume bowel movements which may contain gross blood. Such patients are usually febrile, have severe abdominal cramping, and may appear toxic and quite ill. Dehydration, however, is less common than with the noninflammatory syndrome. Organisms causing this syndrome usually affect the colon and either invade the mucosa or elaborate cytotoxins which result in an acute inflammatory reaction and the presence of mucus, RBC, and WBC in the stool. The most likely causes of this syndrome include *Salmonella, Shigella, Yersinia, Campylobacter*, enterohemorrhagic *E. coli*, *C. difficile*, and *Entamoeba histolytica*.

Examination of stool for fecal leukocytes or a stool lactoferrin assay is helpful in differentiating these two syndromes.[22,23] A stool positive for fecal leukocytes or lactoferrin indicates an acute inflammatory reaction within the intestine. While infections are the most common cause, ischemia, radiation colitis, or inflammatory bowel disease may also result in positive tests.

Patients who are debilitated, malnourished, immunocompromised, or have severe comorbid illnesses are at increased risk for complications of severe diarrhea. They may require early evaluation and hospitalization. Other patients who require a more aggressive approach include patients with systemic signs and evidence of an inflammatory diarrhea; patients whose illness lasts more than 3–4 days; and patients whose history and physical examination suggest a disease process which will benefit from specific therapy (Table 50.2).[6]

Stool cultures are ordered too frequently. In most laboratories, routine processing detects only three pathogens: *Salmonella, Shigella*, and *Campylobacter*. Because of sporadic shedding and the fact that most episodes of acute diarrhea are caused by viruses, undetectable pathogens, or noninfectious causes, stool cultures are infrequently positive. In fact, the cost per positive result (*Salmonella, Shigella, Campylobacter*) exceeds US$900–1000.[20] Special cultures may be ordered depending upon the epidemiologic setting of the illness.[6] Specific cultures should be ordered if *Vibrio*,

Table 50.1 Inflammatory versus noninflammatory diarrhea

Characteristic	Inflammatory diarrhea	Noninflammatory diarrhea
Fecal leukocytes	Positive	Negative
Clinical presentation	Bloody, small-volume diarrhea; lower left quadrant abdominal cramps; may be febrile and toxic	Large-volume, watery diarrhea; may have nausea, vomiting, cramps, no fever
Causes	*Shigella, Salmonella*, amebic colitis, *Campylobacter*, invasive *Escherichia coli, Yersinia, Clostridium difficile*	Viruses, *Vibrio, Giardia*, Enterotoxigenic *Escherichia coli*, enterotoxin-producing bacteria, staphylococcal and clostridial food poisoning
Site of involvement	Colon	Small intestine
Diagnostic evaluation	Indicated	If severely volume depleted or toxic

Modified from: Park SI, Giannella RA. Approach to the adult patient with acute diarrhea. Gastroenterol Clin North Am 1993; 22:3:483–497.

Table 50.2 Indications for antimicrobial therapy

Shigella infection	Protozoan infection
Vibrio cholerae infection	*Giardia lamblia*
Clostridium difficile infection	*Entamoeba histolytica*
Traveler's diarrhea	Sexually transmitted diseases
Extraintestinal salmonellosis	Gonorrhea
Toxic subjects with salmonellosis	Syphilis
Prolonged *Campylobacter* diarrhea	*Chlamydia* infection
	Herpes simplex

From: Park SI, Giannella RA. Approach to the adult patient with acute diarrhea. Gastroenterol Clin North Am 1993; 22:3:483–497.

Yersinia, or *E. coli* O157:H7 is suspected. If *C. difficile* infection is suspected, a stool cytotoxin assay is the preferred test.[24] When parasitic or protozoal infection is suspected, stool examination for cysts, trophozoites, larvae, or eggs should be performed. Viral infections may be detected by ELISA for rotaviruses and Norwalk viruses but are rarely required in adults. Endoscopy can be used to obtain aspirates and biopsies of the small bowel to detect *Giardia, Cryptosporidia, Microsporidia, Isospora belli,* or *Mycobacterium avium intracellulare.* Flexible sigmoidoscopy can be useful in evaluating patients with proctitis, tenesmus, sexually transmitted diseases, or in identifying *C. difficile* pseudomembranes.[25] In AIDS patients, colonoscopy with biopsy may be required to detect cytomegalovirus ulcers which may be confirmed by the presence of 'inclusion bodies' on biopsy.[25]

With a careful evaluation of the patient and the selective ordering of tests, patients can be managed in a cost-effective manner. This should allow for more effective utilization of the microbiology laboratory and patient resources.

THERAPY OF ACUTE INFECTIOUS DIARRHEA (ALSO SEE CHAPTER 71)

General measures

Treatment should be mainly directed at preventing dehydration and restoring lost volume. Caffeine should be avoided as the inhibition of phosphodiesterase can increase intracellular cAMP, resulting in increased secretion from the gut. Similarly, lactose-containing foods should be avoided since lactase deficiency frequently accompanies intestinal infection.

While rehydration is most commonly done with intravenous fluids, it can also be accomplished with oral fluid-electrolyte therapy. Increased fluid intake may be sufficient in mild diarrhea. When moderate volume depletion occurs, solutions should contain glucose and specific electrolytes to replace diarrheal losses. Appropriately formulated solutions can take advantage of the Na+-substrate coupled absorptive pathways which are preserved in many diarrheal disorders. Home remedies, such as colas, fruit juices, and soft drinks, are suboptimal since they contain inadequate electrolyte concentrations, are frequently hyperosmolar, and thus are poor solutions for either rehydration or

replacement of diarrheal losses. Various oral rehydration solutions are commercially available and these are formulated optimally to take advantage of the Na+-glucose coupled transport mechanism to stimulate Na+ and thus water absorption.[3,6,18,26] Some of these formulations include Infalyte, Rehydrolyte, and Pedialyte, whose compositions are shown in Table 50.3. They are strongly recommended for use in adults as well as children. An effective oral rehydration solution using the World Health Organization recipe can be inexpensively prepared at home.[26]

$\frac{3}{4}$ teaspoon table salt
1 teaspoon baking powder
4 tablespoons sugar
1 cup orange juice
1 liter clean water

Patients with severe dehydration or with hypovolemic shock require intravenous hydration.

Antidiarrheal agents

Many over-the-counter and prescription preparations are available for symptomatic relief of diarrhea and abdominal cramping. Anticholinergics (Bentyl, Donnagel) decrease intestinal motility and may provide relief of abdominal cramps. Diarrhea is not affected. Adsorbents such as kaolin, pectin, and activated charcoal decrease stool liquidity, but not volume. Opiates and their derivatives (codeine, loperamide, dephenoxylate-atropine) slow intestinal motility thereby increasing absorption of salt and water. They are effective and, when properly used, are safe. They are most effective when taken around the clock, i.e., every 6–12 hours.[6,27,28] These drugs should be used with caution in anyone with dysentery, fever, or systemic symptoms, since they can cause significant worsening in patients with *Shigella, Salmonella, Campylobacter,* or *C. difficile.*

A reasonable alternative for mild to moderate acute diarrhea is bismuth subsalicylate.[9,27] Bismuth subsalicylate has antisecretory, antibacterial, and antiinflammatory properties, decreases stool liquidity and frequency, and has few side effects. The bismuth portion of the molecule may block the effect of enterotoxins and has direct bactericidal action while the salicylate portion may promote absorption. The effective dose is 30–60 ml or 2–4 tablets every 30 minutes for eight doses.

Antimicrobial therapy

Antimicrobial therapeutic recommendations (Table 50.4) are based on a review of the literature. However, recommendations are constantly changing. When possible, the choice of antimicrobial agent should be based on a knowledge of the antibiotic sensitivity patterns in one's own community. Two in-depth discussions of enteric infections[29,30] and three recent reviews of acute infectious diarrhea[3,4,9] are highly recommended. In addition, the reader is referred to a very useful pocket guide of antimicrobial therapy which is updated regularly (*Sanford's Guide to Antimicrobial Therapy*).[31]

Most cases of acute infectious diarrhea do not benefit from treatment with antibiotics. Infections in adults that benefit from specific therapy include: some cases of *Salmonella, Shigella,* enteroinvasive *E. coli, C. difficile,* traveler's diarrhea, *Vibrio cholerae, Entamoeba histolytica,* and *Giardia. Yersinia* infections probably do not benefit from treatment unless systemic illness is suspected. Antibiotic therapy is also recommended for prolonged or severe

Table 50.3 Composition of some oral hydration solutions and other clear liquids

	Na	K	Cl	Base mmol/liter	CHO	Osmolarity mosm/l
Rehydration						
WHO solution[a]	90	20	80	10(C)	111	310
Rehydralyte[b]	75	20	65	10(C)	140	305
Maintenance						
Infalyte	50	20	40	10(B)	111	270
Lytren[b]	50	25	45	10(C)	111	290
Pedialyte[b]	45	20	35	10(C)	140	250
Resol[b]	50	20	50	11(C)	111	270
Ricelyte[b]	50	25	45	11(C)	30(D)	200
Clear liquid						
Cola	2	0.1	2	13(B)	730[c]	750
Ginger ale	3	1	2	4(B)	500[c]	540
Apple juice	3	28	30	0	690[c]	730
Chicken broth	250	8	250	0	0	450
Tea	0	0	0	0	0	5

CHO, carbohydrate; B, bicarbonate; C, citrate; D, rice-syrup solids (g/L).
[a] WHO solution can be obtained from Jianas Brothers, 2533 Southwest Blvd. Kansas City, MO 64108-2395.
[b] Ready to use.
[c] Combination of glucose and fructose.
Modified from: Avery ME, Snyder JD. Oral therapy for acute diarrhea: the underused simple solution. N Engl J Med 1990; 323:891–894.

cases of *Salmonella*, *Campylobacter*, *Aeromonas*, or *Plesiomonas* infections (Tables 50.2, 50.4 and 50.5).[4,9]

Empiric therapy may be recommended for persons with traveler's diarrhea and for those patients with a febrile, dysenteric illness, patients with positive fecal leukocytes, immunocompromised patients, and severely ill patients.[3,4,9,19] If *Shigella* or *Campylobacter jejuni* is suspected, a fluoroquinolone is the drug of choice in adults. A more thorough discussion of antibiotic choice is presented in DuPont et al.[19] and Thielman and Guerrant.[9]

SPECIFIC INFECTIONS

Salmonella

In the United States, nontyphoidal salmonellae are the commonest organisms isolated from cases of acute diarrhea.[32] Infection is usually acquired by the ingestion of fecally contaminated food or water. The reservoir of nontyphoidal *Salmonellae* include poultry, cows, pigs, turtles, and other domestic animals and birds.[15,33] Several serotypes of *Salmonella* account for the bulk of infections in the US, i.e., *S. typhimurium* (26% of cases), *S. enteritidis*, *S. heidelberg*, and *S. newport*.

The five clinical syndromes seen with *Salmonella* infection include uncomplicated gastroenteritis, bacteremia, a typhoidal or enteric fever syndrome, localized infection, or an asymptomatic carrier state.[15,33]

Bacteremia occurs in 5–10% of adults, especially with *S. cholerasuis*, and *S. typhi* infection and occurs most often in infants and in the elderly. Localized infections may result in cholecystitis, appendicitis, peritonitis, abscess, pneumonia, osteomyelitis, meningitis, wound infections, or hepatitis.[15,16]

Classic typhoid fever is a more severe illness due to *S. typhi* infection. Gastrointestinal hemorrhage, perforation, sepsis and localized infections may occur and in the preantibiotic era, the mortality rate was 12–16%.[15] Relapse occurs in 8–12% of patients who have not been treated and a chronic carrier state occurs in less than 1% of patients infected with *S. typhi*.

General salmonellosis treatment measures include replacing fluid loss by oral and intravenous routes, and controlling pain, nausea, and vomiting. Typhoid fever and nontyphoidal salmonellosis manifesting an enteric fever syndrome or localized infection should be treated with antibiotics. Antibiotics are not recommended for uncomplicated *Salmonella* gastroenteritis because they do not shorten the illness, significantly prolong the fecal excretion of the organisms, and increase the number of antibiotic-resistant strains.[4,15,34] Antibiotic therapy of nontyphoidal salmonellosis should be reserved for the septicemic, enteric fever, and focal infection syndromes. In addition, patients with lymphoproliferative disorders, malignancies, other immunosuppressive diseases or patients on immunosuppressive medications, pregnant females, patients with prosthetic valves, valvular heart disease, vascular grafts, prosthetic orthopedic devices, hemolytic anemia, infants, and the elderly should be treated with antibiotics.[4,15,35] Adults should be treated with ciprofloxacin 500 mg twice daily for 7 days, TMX 160 mg/SMX 800 mg every 12 hours for 7 days, or ceftriaxone 1 g i.v. twice daily for 7 days, depending on susceptibility testing. Typhoid fever should always be treated with chloramphenicol, amoxicillin, or with ciprofloxacin.

Table 50.4 Antibiotic therapy for bacterial enteropathogens in adults

Organism/syndrome	Recommendation	Alternative drug
Shigella	Ciprofloxacin 500 mg b.i.d. for 3 days	Norfloxacin 400 mg b.i.d. for 3 days TMP-SMX 160 mg/800 mg b.i.d. for 3 days Nalidixic acid 1 g t.i.d.-q.i.d. for 5 days
Salmonella Gastroenteritis – uncomplicated	None	
Gastroenteritis – severe, immunocompromised patients, pregnant women, prostheses, cancer	Ciprofloxacin 500 mg b.i.d. for 7 days	TMP-SMX 160 mg/800 mg b.i.d. for 7 days Ceftriaxone 1 g i.v. b.i.d. for 7 days Tetracycline 500 mg q.i.d. for 7 days
Bacteremia and localized infection	Bacteremia treated for 10–14 days; endocarditis and/or osteomyelitis treated for 4–6 wk or longer	Cefotaxime, especially in meningitis or vascular infection 2 g Q4–6H
	Chloramphenicol 50 mg/kg/d in 4 div. doses (not for use in vascular infections) Ampicillin 1 g q 4–6 h Amoxicillin 1 g q 6–8 h TMP 10 mg/kg/d plus SMX 50 mg/kg/d in 4 divided doses	Ciprofloxacin 750 mg b.i.d. especially long term for prevention of bacteremia relapse in AIDS patients
Enteric-fever	Chloramphenicol 500 mg p.o. or i.v. q 8 h for at least 2 weeks	Amoxicillin 1 g q.i.d. for 2 wk Ciprofloxacin 500 mg b.i.d. for 7–14 days TMP-SMX 160 mg/800 mg 1–2 tabs b.i.d. for 2 wk
Campylobacter jejuni Gastroenteritis – uncomplicated	None	
Gastroenteritis – severe or prolonged	Erythromycin 250 mg b.i.d. for 5 days	Ciprofloxacin 500 mg b.i.d. Norfloxacin 400 mg b.i.d.
Campylobacter fetus	Ampicillin and gentamicin i.v.	Erythromycin 0.25–1.0 g q 6 h
Yersinia enterocolitica	Not usually required Tetracycline 500 mg q.i.d.	Chloramphenicol 50 mg/kg/d in 4 divided doses
	TMP-SMX 160 mg/800 mg b.i.d. Ciprofloxacin 500 mg b.i.d.	Aminoglycosides
Escherichia coli Enteroinvasive	No controlled studies: consider empiric therapy Ciprofloxacin 500 mg b.i.d. Norfloxacin 500 mg b.i.d.	TMP-SMX 160 mg/800 mg b.i.d.
Enterotoxigenic	Ciproflaxacin 500 mg b.i.d. Norfloxacin 500 mg b.i.d. Rifaxamin 500 mg b.i.d. 3 days	TMP-SMX 160 mg/800 mg b.i.d.
Enteropathogenic	No controlled studies: consider empiric therapy Ciproflaxacin 500 mg b.i.d. Norflaxacin 500 mg b.i.d.	TMP-SMX 160 mg/800 mg b.i.d.
Enterohemorrhagic	Unclear if antibiotics are effective. May be harmful.	
Vibrio cholerae	Tetracycline 500 mg p.o.q 6 h for 3 days	Ciprofloxacin 500 mg p.o. b.i.d. for 3 days Doxycycline 300 mg once or 100 mg q.d. for 3 days
Vibrio parahaemolyticus	Supportive therapy only	
V. vulnificus and *V. alginolyticus*	Tetracycline 500 mg q.i.d. 0.5–1.0 g i.v. q 12 h	Chloramphenicol 50 mg/kg/d q.i.d. Penicillin G > 20 000 000 U/d i.v.

Table 50.5 Indications for antibiotic therapy in *Salmonella* gastroenteritis

Lymphoproliferative disorders
  Leukemia
  Lymphoma
Malignancies
Immunosuppression
  AIDS
  Congenital and other acquired immunosuppressive disorders
  Corticosteroid treatment
  Organ transplants
Abnormal cardiovascular system
  Prosthetic heart valves
  Vascular grafts
  Aneurysms
  Valvular heart disease
Prosthetic orthopedic devices
Hemolytic anemia
Extreme ages of life

From: Gorbach SL: Infectious diarrhea. In: MB Taylor, ed Gastrointestinal emergencies. Baltimore: Williams and Wilkins; 1992:440.

Campylobacter

In the United States, *Campylobacter* is the second commonest organism isolated from cases of acute diarrhea.[32] Of the nine species of *Campylobacter*, *C. jejuni* is the commonest isolate in the immunocompetent patient with bacterial diarrhea. *C. fetus* may be isolated in the immunocompromised patient.

Infection is usually acquired by ingestion of contaminated food, most commonly poultry. The usual illness is characterized by abdominal cramps, sometimes extremely severe, fever, and after a lag period, diarrhea. The diarrhea is usually free of visible blood but frank dysentery may result. In most cases the illness is brief, 1–3 days, and the patient recovers without consulting a physician and before a specific diagnosis can be made.[36] However, in many cases, the illness may be more prolonged and last for several weeks. The clinical syndrome of *Campylobacter* infection can closely mimic that of shigellosis, salmonellosis, or infection with enterohemorrhagic *E. coli*, and infection with these organisms cannot be reliably differentiated from one another on clinical grounds.[36]

Specific antimicrobial treatment is unnecessary in many cases which are brief and self-limited. However, when symptoms are prolonged and severe, antimicrobial therapy is beneficial. Erythromycin is the drug of choice in infections with *C. jejuni*, i.e., 250 mg orally four times per day. An alternative effective regimen is the use of a quinolone, e.g., ciprofloxacin 500 mg orally twice daily for 5 days.[3,4,9,36]

Although most cases recover without sequelae, various complications can occur, i.e., Guillain-Barre syndrome, toxic megacolon, pseudomembranous colitis, massive gastrointestinal hemorrhage,

cholecystitis, reactive arthritis, mesenteric adenitis, and appendicitis.[37] Fortunately, these complications are uncommon.

Shigella

Infection occurs by ingestion of contaminated food or water or fecal–oral contamination.

The organism initially invades the colonic mucosa and also produces an enterotoxin-cytotoxin, Shiga toxin.[38] Treatment with antibiotics both shortens the course of disease and the duration of excretion of the organism. Effective regimens include: Ciprofloxacin 500 g every 12 hours for 5 days, or, if susceptible, TMP 160/SMX 800 every 12 hours for 5 days.[3,4,39,40] Resistance to ampicillin is widespread, so treatment should be based on sensitivities.

Complications are unusual, although toxic megacolon, colonic perforation, protein-losing enteropathy, leukemoid reactions, hyponatremia, seizures, the hemolytic uremic syndrome, fulminant dysentery, or Reiter's syndrome may occur.[38,41,42]

E. coli

Five forms of *E. coli* can infect the intestine: enterotoxigenic, enteropathogenic, enteroinvasive, enteroadherent, and enterohemorrhagic *E. coli*.[43] Enterotoxigenic *E. coli* cause infantile diarrhea and traveler's diarrhea in adults. It is an unusual pathogen in the US but extremely common in underdeveloped countries and among travelers. The resulting illness is a watery diarrhea which may cause dehydration. Treatment consists of rehydration and correction of electrolyte abnormalities. Antibiotics, such as ciprofloxacin or trimethoprim-sulfamethoxazole, decrease the duration of diarrhea and fecal excretion of the organism if started early in the illness. Another option is the recently approved (in the US) nonabsorbable antibiotic rifaxamin. Recovery generally occurs within several days.[44]

Enteropathogenic *E. coli* (EPEC) cause diarrhea by an unknown mechanism. They do not produce toxins and are noninvasive. EPEC cause 10% of infantile diarrhea in developing countries. In the US, they are associated with community epidemics and hospital outbreaks. The clinical syndrome consists of fever, malaise, vomiting, and diarrhea, and can last up to 2 weeks. Antibiotic treatment is not required in most cases[45] but may be necessary in severe cases. Ciprofloxacin, TMP/SMX, or nalidixic acid may be effective.

Enteroinvasive *E. coli* are biochemically similar to *Shigella*.[38] Infection results in a similar clinical syndrome of watery diarrhea, followed by tenesmus and dysentery. Diagnosis may be made by tissue culture or DNA probe assays which, unfortunately, are not routinely available. Ciprofloxacin or TMP/SMX may be effective.

Enteroadherent *E. coli* cause an acute diarrheal and a persistent diarrheal illness in infants and children. The importance of these in the US and other developed countries is uncertain.

E. coli O157:H7

Many serotypes of E. *coli* can cause hemorrhagic colitis.[12,13] In the US, approximately 90% of all cases are due to the specific serotype O157:H7. These organisms are collectively called enterohemorrhagic *E. coli* (EHEC). *E. coli* O157:H7 is now widely recognized as a major cause of bloody diarrhea. It is a cause of sporadic and epidemic illnesses throughout the US, usually caused by ingestion of contaminated and undercooked ground beef although a variety of other foods have also been incriminated. The elderly and children seem particularly at risk and exhibit higher mortality rates. The clinical manifestations of EHEC infection include hemorrhagic colitis, nonbloody diarrhea, asymptomatic infection, the hemolytic-uremic syndrome, and thrombotic thrombocytopenic purpura.

After a 3–4 day incubation period, symptoms include severe abdominal cramps and watery diarrhea. Bloody diarrhea follows in many patients in a day or two. Vomiting occurs in one-half and fever is usually absent or low-grade. Recovery occurs in 2–15 days. Sigmoidoscopic and colonoscopic appearance is that of a hemorrhagic colitis, which may be confined to the right colon. Approximately 10% of patients develop severe sequelae such as hemolytic-uremic syndrome (HUS), or thrombotic thrombocytopenic purpura (TTP) which is fatal in 5–10% of patients so afflicted. Treatment is basically supportive. There is no evidence that antibiotic therapy will decrease fecal excretion, duration of illness, or development of complications and there is some evidence that antibiotics might be harmful and enhance the likelihood of developing the hemolytic-uremic syndrome.[46,47]

Clostridium difficile

See Chapter 51.

Vibrios

Of the various Vibrio species, two commonly cause intestinal infection: V. cholerae and V. parahaemolyticus. V. parahaemolyticus is a common cause of food poisoning in the Far East, especially in Japan, and is occasionally seen in coastal areas in the United States. Other species of Vibrio that can cause intestinal infection include V. mimicus, V. fluvialis, V. vulnificus, and several others. Because of their rarity, discussion of these infections is beyond the scope of this chapter.[48,49]

V. cholerae cause a wide spectrum of illness ranging from an asymptomatic infection to a life-threatening, rapidly dehydrating illness which can be fatal in 24–48 hours if not adequately treated. Stool losses of 10–15 liters per day can occur and this syndrome is called cholera gravis. The most important aspect of the treatment of cholera is fluid and electrolyte therapy, prevention of dehydration, and rehydration. This can be done intravenously and/or orally. Oral rehydration solutions were developed as a consequence of understanding the pathophysiology of intestinal fluid loss in cholera and has wide applicability to diarrheal disorders as discussed above. Antibiotic treatment will shorten the duration of illness, the duration of fecal excretion of the organisms, and decrease the magnitude of stool losses. Tetracycline is the currently preferred therapy. In the adult, the recommended regimen is tetracycline 500 mg orally every 6 hours for 3 days. Alternative regimens are ciprofloxacin 500 mg twice daily for 3 days or doxycycline 300 mg once or 100 mg daily for 3 days.[50,51]

V. parahaemolyticus infection, usually acquired by eating contaminated, undercooked or raw seafood, can cause an explosive watery diarrheal syndrome associated with abdominal cramping pain, chills, and fever. A second syndrome is a dysentery-like illness with bloody stools and colitis. The syndrome can be brief and self-limited and usually does not require specific treatment. If the diarrhea is persistent, tetracycline, TMP-SMX, or ciprofloxacin, as above, are recommended.

Yersinia

Of the various species of Yersinia, two cause intestinal infection: Y. enterocolitica and Y. pseudotuberculosis. Infections with Y. enterocolitica are the more common. Y. enterocolitica infections are common in Northern climes, i.e., Finland, Scandinavia, Belgium, Canada, and much less common in the United States. Pork and contaminated dairy products are the most common vehicles of transmission. The manifestations of yersiniosis include acute diarrhea, chronic diarrhea, an appendicitis-like syndrome, septicemia, and localized infections.[52] The chronic diarrhea syndrome can be associated with ileitis and strongly mimic Crohn's disease.[53] Common extraintestinal manifestations include reactive arthritis, erythema nodosum, and autoimmune thyroiditis.[52]

Acute diarrhea and the appendicitis-like syndrome are usually brief and do not warrant antibiotic treatment. Chronic diarrhea, septicemia, and suppurative infections, however, should be treated with antibiotics. The treatment should be based on antibiotic sensitivities, if possible. However, if these are not available or until these are available, therapy with tetracycline, quinolones, or TMP-SMX are recommended. For diarrhea, cirprofloxacin 500 mg orally twice daily for three days, or TMP-SMX orally twice daily for 3 days is recommended. For severe illness, ceftriaxone 2.0 g intravenously per day for 7–10 days is recommended.[52]

Y. pseudotuberculosis infection is less common than those with Y. enterocolitica. The manifestations of infection and possible clinical syndromes are similar to those discussed above. Most uncomplicated infections spontaneously resolve without therapy. If illness is severe, therapy is recommended as above.[52]

Traveler's diarrhea

Traveler's diarrhea is a syndrome and not a specific illness.[54,55] It is a diarrheal syndrome caused by a wide spectrum of infectious agents. A specific infectious agent can be identified in 60–80% of cases. The most common pathogen is enterotoxigenic E. coli (ETEC). Clinical presentations range from a mild to cholera-like diarrhea to a dysenteric syndrome. Other organisms which may cause traveler's diarrhea include Salmonella, Shigella, rotavirus, Giardia lamblia, Entamoeba histolytica, etc. Giardia lamblia infection should be considered in patients with persistent diarrhea. Entamoeba histolytica and shigellosis should be considered in travelers with dysentery.[54,55]

Fortunately, 90% of cases are self-limited and evaluation is unnecessary. However, 1–2% of travelers will have persistent diarrhea lasting longer than 1 month and, in rare cases, diarrhea can last longer than 6 months and become a chronic illness. A specific pathogen should be sought in cases that are prolonged, accompanied by fever, systemic manifestations, the presence of dysentery, occult or gross blood or polymorphonuclear leukocytes on microscopic examination of stool, or cases that occur in the immunocompromised host.[56,57]

The high incidence of bacterial pathogens in traveler's diarrhea makes the use of prophylactic antibiotics very tempting. However, safe eating and drinking habits are the traveler's best method of prophylaxis. Various antibiotic regimens can be used to prevent up to 90% of the episodes of traveler's diarrhea. However, to do so is at the expense of significant possible side effects including skin rashes, photosensitivity, antibiotic-associated colitis, and vaginal candidiasis.[54,55] Furthermore, the broad use of antibiotics risks the development of antimicrobial resistance in the individual patient, bacterial overgrowth, or persistent salmonellosis. Antidiarrheal agents are not useful prophylactically. Prophylaxis should be recommended for certain groups of people, i.e., persons with severe kidney, liver, or heart disease, insulin-dependent diabetes, inflammatory bowel disease, or those with gastrectomy, achlorhydria, or ileostomies, or those taking steroids or suffering with immunosuppressive illnesses.[54,55]

Bismuth subsalicylate significantly decreases the risk of developing traveler's diarrhea.[58] While prophylactic antibiotic therapy has a better success rate, bismuth subsalicylate has a more benign side effect profile. The most effective dosage is 2.1 g per day and should be given four times/day, at meals and at bedtime. Side effects of this drug include transient blackening of the tongue and stool, and constipation. The salicylate portion of the molecule is absorbable and may result in toxicity if taken in excess or in patients already taking salicylates for other reasons. This agent should be avoided in patients with peptic ulcer disease.

The mainstay of treatment for traveler's diarrhea is adequate hydration. Fluids and electrolytes should be repleted. Symptomatic therapy for mild cases should be adequate. Loperamide reduces the frequency and duration of diarrhea as does bismuth subsalicylate. These agents are usually adequate in mild diarrhea. Empiric antimicrobial therapy will shorten the duration and severity of the illness and should be used in cases of moderate severity. Ciprofloxacin 500 mg orally twice daily for 3 days is effective. Trimethoprim-sulfamethoxazole has been recommended in the past; however, resistance of various organisms to this combination is increasing in frequency especially in the developing world.[59,60] Recently, Rifaximin, a nonabsorbable antibiotic, has been shown to be as effective as fluoroquinolones in the treatment of traveler's diarrhea.[61]

Antibiotic therapy for specific enteropathogens is as discussed above.

Protozoan infections

See Chapter 52.

AIDS diarrhea

See Chapter 7.

Sexually transmittted infections

See Chapter 64.

Summary

Specific antibiotic regimens for bacterial enteropathogens in adults are summarized in Table 50.4.

REFERENCES

1. Farthing MJG, Keusch GT. Global impact and patterns of intestinal infection. In: Farthing MJG, Keusch GT, eds. Enteric infection. New York: Raven Press; 1989:3–12.

2. Black RE, Lanata CF. Epidemiology of diarrheal diseases in developing countries. In: Blaser MJ, Smith PD, Ravdin JI, et al., eds. Infections of the gastrointestinal tract. 2nd edn. Philadelphia: Lippincott Williams & Wilkins; 2002:11–29.

3. Robinson PK, Giannella RA, Taylor MB. Infectious diarrheas. In: Taylor MB, ed. Gastrointestinal emergencies. 2nd edn. Baltimore: Williams and Wilkins; 1997:649–675.

4. Wolf D, Giannella R. Antibiotic therapy for bacterial enterocolitis. Amer J Gastroenterol 1993; 88:1667–1683.

5. Irujo C. Food safety initiative underfunded say microbiologists. Washington Fax–life science edition. September 25, 1997.

6. Park S, Giannella R. Approach to the adult patient with acute diarrhea. In: Giannella R, ed. Acute infectious diarrhea. Philadelphia: WB Saunders; 1993:483–497.

   A succinct discussion of an efficient but thorough approach to the patient with acute diarrhea.

7. Laney EW, Cohen MB. Approach to the pediatric patient with diarrhea. In: Giannella R, ed. Acute infectious diarrhea. Philadelphia: WB Saunders; 1993:499–516.

8. Casburn-Jones AC, Farthing MJG. Management of infectious diarrhea. Gut 2003; 296–305.

   A very recent comprehensive and readable review from the United Kingdom.

9. Thielman NM, Guerrant RL. Acute infectious diarrhea. New Engl J Med 2004: 350:38–47.

   A very recent comprehensive and readable review from the United States.

10. Guerrant RL. Principles and syndromes of enteric infection. In: Mandel GO, Bennett JE, Dolin R, eds. Infectious diseases. 4th edn. New York: Churchill Livingstone; 1995:945–962.

11. Levine MM, DuPont HL, Formal SB et al. Pathogenesis of *Shigella dysenteriae 1* (Shiga) dysentery. J Infect Dis 1973; 127:261–270.

12. Cohen M, Giannella R. Hemorrhagic colitis associated with *E. coli* O157:H7. Adv Int Med 1992; 37:173–195.

13. Griffin PM, Mead PS, Sivapalasingam S. *E. coli* O157:H7 and other enterohemorrhagic *E. coli*. In: Blaser MJ, Smith PD, Ravdin JI, et al., eds. Infections of the gastrointestinal tract, 2nd edn. Philadelphia: Lippincott Williams & Wilkins; 2002:627–642.

14. Centers for Disease Control. *Vibrio vulnificus* infections associated with raw oyster consumption, Florida, 1981–1992. MMWR 1993; 42:405–416.

15. Pegues DA, Ohl ME, Miller SI. *Salmonella* including *S. typhi*. In: Blaser MJ, Smith PD, Ravdin JI, et al., eds. Infections of the gastrointestinal tract, 2nd edn. Philadelphia: Lippincott Williams & Wilkins; 2002: 669–695.

16. Black PH, Kunz LJ, Swartz MN. Salmonellosis – A review of some unusual aspects. N Engl J Med 1960; 262: 811–817; 864–870; 921–927.

   A classic and comprehensive review of unusual aspects of salmonellosis.

17. Field M. Intestinal ion transport and the pathophysiology of diarrhea. J Clin Invest 2003; 117:931–943.

   A readable, brief review of the mechanisms of intestinal ion transport and the pathophysiology of diarrhea by an authority.

18. Avery ME, Snyder JD. Oral therapy for acute diarrhea. The underused simple solution. N Eng J Med 1990; 323:891–894.

19. DuPont HL and the Practice Parameters Committee of the American College of Gastroenterology. Guidelines in acute infectious diarrhea in adults. Am J Gastro 1997; 92:1962–1975.

   Guidelines for acute infectious diarrhea from the American College of Gastroenterology. Highly recommended.

20. Guerrant RL, Van Gilder T, Steiner TS, et al. Practice guidelines for the management of infectious diarrhea. Clin Infec Dis 2001; 32:331–350.

Guidelines for acute infectious diarrhea from the Infectious Diseases Society of America. Highly recommended.

21. Giannella RA. Gastrointestinal infections. In: Kelley WN, ed. Textbook of internal medicine. Philadelphia: JB Lippincott Co; 1989:554–562.

22. Calubiran OV, Domenico P, Klein N, et al. The significance of fecal leukocytes in infectious disease. Hospital Physician 1990; 56–62.

23. Huicho L, Campos M, Rivera J, et al. Fecal screening tests in the approach to acute infectious diarrhea. A scientific overview. Pediatr Infect Dis J 1996; 15:486–494.

24. Bartlett JG. Antibiotic-associated diarrhea. New Engl J Med 2002; 346:334–339.

25. Martin SP, Giannella RA. Infectious diseases of the colon. In: Marino AJ, Benjamin SB, eds. Gastrointestinal diseases: an endoscopic approach. Malden MA: Blackwell Science; 1997:593–609.

26. Calligaro I. Treatment of acute diarrhea in children. American Pharmacy 1992; NS32:29–34.

27. Schiller LR. Review article: anti-diarrheal pharmacology and therapeutics. Aliment Pharmacol Ther 1995; 9:87–106.

28. Powell DW, Szauter KE. Nonantibiotic therapy and pharmacotherapy of acute infectious diarrhea. In: Giannella R, ed. Acute infectious diarrhea. Philadelphia: WB Saunders; 1993:22:683–707.

29. Blaser MJ, Smith PD, Ravdin JI, et al. Infections of the gastrointestinal tract, 2nd edn. Philadelphia: Lippincott Williams & Wilkins; 2002.

A comprehensive authoritative textbook devoted to gastrointestinal infections with each chapter written by leaders in the field. Very highly recommended.

30. Surawicz C, Owen RL. Gastrointestinal and hepatic infections. Philadelphia: WB Saunders; 1995.

31. Sanford JP, Gilbert DN, Sande MA. The Sanford guide to antimicrobial therapy. Vienna, VA: Antimicrobial Therapy, Inc; 1996.

32. Preliminary FoodNet Data-Selected Sites, United States, 2002. MMWR 2003; 52:340–343.

33. Baird-Parker AC: Food-borne salmonellosis. Lancet 1990; 336:1231–1235.

34. Sanchez C, Garcia-Restoy E, Garau J, et al. Ciprofloxacin and trimethoprim-sulfamethoxazole versus placebo in acute uncomplicated Salmonella entertitis. A double-blind trial. J Infect Dis 1993; 168:1304–1307.

35. Hamer DH. Bacterial and viral diarrhea. In: Baddour LM, Gorbach SL, eds. Therapy of infectious diseases. Philadelphia: WB Saunders; 2003:399–414.

36. Skirrow MB. Campylobacter. Lancet 1990; 336:921–923.

37. Skirrow MB, Blaser MJ. Campylobacter jejuni. In: Blaser MJ, Smith PD, Ravdin JI, et al., eds. Infections of the gastrointestinal tract. 2nd edn. Philadelphia: Lippincott Williams & Wilkins; 2002:719–739.

38. Keusch GT. Shigella and enteroinvasive E. coli. In: Blaser MJ, Smith PD, Ravdin JI, et al., eds. Infections of the gastrointestinal tract. 2nd edn. Philadelphia: Lippincott Williams & Wilkins; 2002:643–667.

39. Bennish ML, Salam MA, Khan WA, et al. Treatment of Shigellosis. III. Comparison of one or two-dose ciprofloxacin with standard 5 day therapy. A randomized, blinded trial. Ann Intern Med 1992; 117:727–734.

40. Khan WA, Seas C, Dhar U, et al. Treatment of shigellosis. V. Comparison of azithromycin and ciprofloxacin: A double-blind, randomized, controlled trial. Ann Intern Med 1997; 126:697–703.

41. Cohen MB, Giannella RA. Bacterial infections: pathophysiology, clinical features, and treatment. In: Phillips SF, Pemberton JH, Shorter RG, eds. The large intestine: physiology, pathophysiology, and disease. New York: Raven Press; 1991:395–428.

42. Barrett-Conner EB, Conner JB. Extra-intestinal manifestations of shigellosis. Am J Gastroenterol 1970; 53:234–245.

43. Levine MM. E. coli that cause diarrhea. Enterotoxigenic, enteropathogenic, enteroinvasive, enterohemorrhagic, and enteroadherent. J Infect Dis 1987; 155:377–389.

A brief, but still current, discussion of the complex subject of E. coli diarrhea by an authority.

44. Cohen MB, Giannella RA. Enterotoxigenic E. coli. In: Blaser MJ, Smith PD, Ravdin JI, et al., eds. Infections of the gastrointestinal tract. 2nd edn. Philadelphia: Lippincott Williams & Wilkins; 2002:579–594.

45. Donnenberg MS. Enteropathogenic E. coli. In: Blaser MJ, Smith PD, Ravdin JI, et al., eds. Infections of the gastrointestinal tract. 2nd ed. Philadelphia: Lippincott Williams & Wilkins; 2002:595–612.

46. Wong CS, Jelacic S, Habeeb RL, et al The risk of the hemolytic-uremic syndrome after antibiotic treatment of E. coli O157:H7 infections. New Engl J Med 2000; 342:1930–1936.

47. Safdar N, Said A, Gagnon RE, et al. Risk of hemolytic-uremic syndrome after antibiotic treatment of E. coli O157:H7 enteritis: a meta-analysis. JAMA 2002; 288:996–1001.

48. Morris JG, Black RE. Cholera and other Vibrios in the United States. N Eng J Med 1985; 312:343–350.

49. Hardy WG, Klontz KC. The epidemiology of Vibrio infections in Florida, 1981–1993. J Infect Dis 1996; 173:1176–1183.

50. Nalin DR. Cholera and severe toxigenic diarrheas. Gut 1994; 35:145–149.

51. Sanchez JL, Taylor DN. Cholera. Lancet 1997; 349:1825–1830.

52. Cover TL. Yersinia enterocolitica and Y. pseudotuberculosis. In: Blaser MJ, Smith PD, Ravdin JI, et al., eds. Infections of the gastrointestinal tract. 2nd edn. Philadelphia: Lippincott Williams & Wilkins; 2002:699–717.

53. Vantrappen G, Agg HO, Ponette E, et al. Yersinia enteritis and enterocolitis gastroenterological aspects. Gastroenterology 1977; 72:220–227.

54. Farthing MJG, DuPont HJ, Guandalini S, et al. Working team report: Treatment and prevention of traveler's diarrhea. Gastroenterol Internat 1992: 5:162–175.

55. DuPont HJ. Traveler's diarrhea In: Blaser MJ, Smith PD, Ravdin JI, et al., eds. Infections of the gastrointestinal tract. 2nd edn. Philadelphia: Lippincott Williams & Wilkins; 2002:255–265.

A brief but comprehensive discussion of the common problem of traveler's diarrhea by an authority.

56. Giannella RA. Chronic diarrhea in travelers: diagnostic and therapeutic considerations. Rev Infect Dis 1986; 8(suppl 2):223–226.

57. DuPont HL, Capsuto EG. Persistent diarrhea in travelers. Clin Infect Dis 1996; 22:124–128.

58. Steffen R, DuPont HL, Heusser R, et al. Prevention of traveler's diarrhea by the tablet form of bismuth subsalicylate. Antimicrob Agents Chem 1986; 29:625–627.

59. Ericsson CD, Johnson PC, DuPont HL, et al. Ciprofloxacin or trimethoprim-sulfamethoxazole as initial therapy for traveler's diarrhea. A placebo-controlled, randomized trial. Ann Intern Med 1987; 106:216–220.

60. Salam I, Katelaris P, Leigh-Smith S, et al. Randomized trial of single dose ciprofloxacin for traveller's diarrhea. Lancet 1994; 344:1537–1539.

61. DuPont HL, Jiang ZD, Ericsson CD, et al. Rifaximin versus cirprofloxacin for the treatment of traveler's diarrhea: a randomized, double-blind clinical trial. Clin Infect Dis 2001; 33:1807–1815.

CHAPTER FIFTY-ONE

51

Treatment of *Clostridium difficile* diarrhea and colitis

Ciarán P. Kelly and J. Thomas LaMont

INTRODUCTION

Clostridium difficile (*C. difficile*) is a common nosocomial pathogen that infects approximately 15–20% of hospital inpatients in high-risk hospital wards. The most important control measure is to avoid the unnecessary use of antibiotics. *C. difficile* colitis is an infectious disease spread by fecal–oral transmission. Thus, observing standard infection control measures including hand washing, the use of examining gloves and disinfectants, and patient isolation are useful in reducing cross-infection. The majority of patients colonized with *C. difficile* are asymptomatic and do not require any specific therapy. Similarly, patients with mild antibiotic-associated diarrhea may be managed conservatively by stopping the offending antibiotic. Specific treatment is indicated in patients infected by toxigenic *C. difficile* who have severe or persistent diarrhea or evidence of severe colitis. The high efficacy and low cost of metronidazole make it the drug of first choice. Oral vancomycin is also effective but its use may encourage the proliferation of nosocomial, vancomycin-resistant bacteria. Vancomycin is therefore reserved for patients who are intolerant of, or fail to respond to, metronidazole or for patients with severe or refractory *C. difficile* associated diarrhea and colitis. Patients with an ileus may be treated with intravenous metronidazole sometimes supplemented by vancomycin given via nasogastric tube or by enema. Discontinuation of therapy with metronidazole or vancomycin is followed by relapse in approximately 20% of patients, probably related to a defective host immune response as well as continued exposure to antibiotic-resistant spores. A first relapse is treated by a second course of metronidazole or vancomycin. A variety of regimens have been described for the management of multiple relapses including prolonged, tapered and pulsed antibiotic therapy, anion-binding resins, probiotic therapy and passive immunotherapy.

EPIDEMIOLOGY AND PATHOGENESIS

Healthy adults rarely carry *C. difficile* since the normal bacterial population of the colon provides effective colonization resistance.[1,2] Antibiotic therapy changes the colonic microflora allowing *C. difficile* infection to occur (Fig. 51.1).[3] Nearly all antibiotics have been implicated as causing *C. difficile* diarrhea and colitis but prominent offending antibiotics include ampicillin/amoxicillin, second- and third-generation cephalosporins, and clindamycin, given either as single agents or in combination with other antibiotics (Table 51.1).[4,5]

C. difficile is primarily a hospital acquired infection; outpatient cases are increasingly recognized but are nonetheless far less common.[6–8] Hospitalized patients acquire *C. difficile* through fecal–oral spread from other infected patients or from the environment through ingestion of viable bacteria or spores.[6,7,9–11] Surface wipe tests in hospitals indicate that *C. difficile* contaminates bathrooms, soiled linen, bed rails, call buttons, and commodes. The organism resides under finger nails, in skin folds, and on the underside of rings and can be carried unwittingly from patient to patient by healthy hospital personnel.

Pathogenic strains of *C. difficile* release two potent exotoxins: toxin A and toxin B (see Fig. 51.1).[12–15] These toxins cause colonic

Table 51.1 Antimicrobial agents that predispose to *C. difficile* diarrhea and colitis		
Frequently	**Infrequently**	**Rarely or never**
Ampicillin and amoxicillin	Tetracyclines	Parenteral aminoglycosides
Cephalosporins	Sulfonamides	Metronidazole
Clindamycin	Macrolides (including erythromycin)	Bacitracin
	Chloramphenicol	Vancomycin
	Trimethoprim	
	Quinolones	

Reprinted from Kelly CP, LaMont JT. Treatment of *Clostridium difficile* diarrhea and colitis. In: Wolfe MM, ed. Gastrointestinal pharmacotherapy. Philadelphia: WB Saunders; 1993:199–212. With permission from Elsevier Inc © 1993.

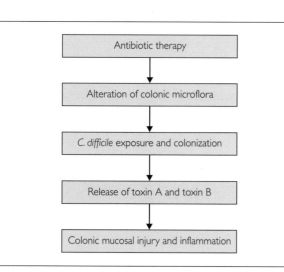

Fig. 51.1 • Pathogenesis of *C. difficile*-associated diarrhea and colitis. (Reproduced from American Journal of Clinical Nutrition 1980; 33:2521–2526. © 1980 with permission from the American Journal of Clinical Nutrition, American Society for Clinical Nutrition.)

mucosal injury and inflammation resulting in diarrhea and colitis.[15,16] Patients colonized by nontoxigenic strains of *C. difficile* do not develop diarrhea or colitis.

Epidemiological studies show that asymptomatic carriage of *C. difficile* is common in adults hospitalized for 3 days or longer.[6,7,17] In high-risk units such as a general medical ward, ICU, or oncology unit over 20% of patients who receive antibiotics are colonized by *C. difficile* during their hospital stay. Many of these are asymptomatic carriers, while approximately 40% develop diarrhea.[6,7,17] Many carriers remain culture positive at the time of discharge to chronic care facilities or to home. Approximately 7% of patients are culture positive on admission to hospital.[6,17] These findings suggest that asymptomatic carriers may be an important reservoir for *C. difficile* and may carry *C. difficile* back and forth between the acute care hospital and chronic care facility.[17–19]

CLINICAL SPECTRUM OF *C. difficile* INFECTION

C. difficile can produce a range of clinical conditions, from asymptomatic carriage to fulminant and fatal pseudomembranous colitis. It is important to recognize the different forms of this infection, because not all patients with positive stool cultures or toxin assays require therapy. Mild diarrhea is common in hospitalized patients treated with antibiotics, and in many patients is not related to *C. difficile*, but to other factors, including osmotic diarrhea from unabsorbed dietary carbohydrate.[20,21]

The infantile carrier state is common in newborns and may persist for up to 1 year.[2,22,23] This presumably reflects inadequate neonatal colonization resistance because of the absence of a mature colonic microflora. Fifty to 75% of healthy infants will have positive stool cultures for *C. difficile*, and, although many of these have toxins A and B in their stools, disease manifestations are rare. In hospitals, asymptomatic adult carriers of *C. difficile* outnumber symptomatic patients.[6,7] Treatment of asymptomatic carriers with metronidazole or vancomycin is not effective.[24] The explanation for the wide differences in host response to this pathogen is not known. Possibilities include variations in the

amount of toxin production by different strains of *C. difficile*, differences in intestinal receptor expression by the host, or differences in the host immune response to *C. difficile* and its toxins.[17,23,24–26]

Diagnosis of *C. difficile* colitis is based upon a history of recent or current antibiotic therapy, development of diarrhea or other evidence of acute colitis, and demonstration of infection by toxigenic *C. difficile*, usually by detection of toxin A or toxin B in a stool sample.[5,27–29]

TREATMENT

Therapeutic agents

The general principles of therapy for *C. difficile*-associated diarrhea are to discontinue, if possible, the inciting antibiotic and, if symptoms and colitis are severe or persist, to administer an antimicrobial agent effective against *C. difficile*.[5,27–29] *C. difficile* is sensitive to a wide range of antibiotics in vitro.[30–37] However, resistance to cefoxitin is common to the point that this antibiotic is used in selective media to culture *C. difficile*.[38] Many clinical isolates are also resistant to clindamycin and this phenomenon has been implicated in some nosocomial outbreaks.[39] A decreased susceptibility to fluoroquinolones amongst *C. difficile* isolates is increasingly recognized with at least partial resistance (related to point mutations in gyrA or gyrB) in 7% of 198 clinical isolates in a series from France.[40] Fortunately, resistance to metronidazole is very rare and to vancomycin essentially nonexistent. In one series all of 186 clinical isolates were sensitive to both metronidazole and vancomycin with MICs in the range of 0.5–4 μg per ml.[38] In a series of 415 Spanish isolates 6% showed intermediate sensitivity to metronidazole (i.e., MIC greater than 16 μg per ml).[41] However, this partial resistance pattern was not clonal and was not sustained in serial culture, suggesting an acquired tolerance rather than genetically determined metronidazole resistance. It is important to note that many agents, including ampicillin and amoxicillin which show in vitro activity against *C. difficile*, are commonly implicated as inducing *C. difficile* colitis in clinical practice (Table 51.2, Fig. 51.2).[31,44] Thus, in vitro sensitivity testing alone is a poor predictor of therapeutic efficacy. The most widely employed animal model has been the Syrian hamster, which invariably develops fatal *C. difficile* cecitis when treated with oral clindamycin. In this model, the efficacy of therapeutic agents is assessed by their ability to protect clindamycin-exposed hamsters.[32,36,43–45] In general, these animal studies have provided a reliable indication of the effectiveness of various therapeutic agents in human disease.

The most widely accepted antimicrobials for the treatment of *C. difficile*-associated diarrhea and colitis are vancomycin and metronidazole (Table 51.3). A number of nonantibiotic agents are under investigation for prevention or treatment of *C. difficile* diarrhea and are discussed below in the section on relapsing disease. One of these agents, tolevamer, is a toxin-binding polymer that has been evaluated in a Phase 2 clinical trial as an alternative to antibiotics for primary therapy of *C. difficile*-associated diarrhea.[45,46] In that study tolevamer 6 g daily was as effective as vancomycin in treating mild to moderately severe *C. difficile*-associated diarrhea. Since tolevamer is a nonantibiotic agent it may prove to be associated with a lower relapse rate than either metronidazole or vancomycin.[46]

Table 51.2 Susceptibility of *C. difficile* isolates to various antimicrobial agents

| | MIC (μg/mL) | |
Agent	Median	Range
Rifampin	0.2	0.2
Metronidazole	0.2	0.2–0.4
Vancomycin	0.2	0.2–0.4
Penicillin G	0.4	0.2–1.6
Ampicillin	0.8	0.2–3.1
Chloramphenicol	0.8	0.2–6.3
Carbenicillin	6.3	0.4–25
Tetracycline	6.3	0.2–50
Cephalothin	6.3	0.2–25
Cotrimoxazole	12.5	0.4≥100
Cephalexin	25	0.8–100
Clindamycin	25	0.2≥100
Gentamicin	25	6.3–100
Cefoxitin	50	0.2–100
Erythromycin	>100	0.2–100

(Modified from Fekety R et al, Review of Infectious Diseases 1981; 3:S273–281. © 1981 with permission from the University of Chicago Press.)

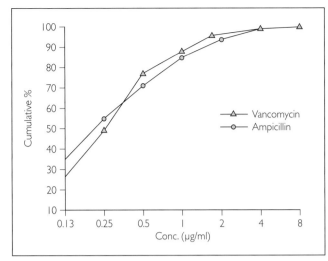

Fig. 51.2 • Susceptibility of 111 strains of *C. difficile* to vancomycin and to ampicillin. (Reproduced from Bartlett JG, Taylor NS, Chang T, et al. Clinical and laboratory observations in *Clostridium difficile* colitis. Am J Clin Nutr 1980; 33:2521–2526.)

Vancomycin

Vancomycin is a tricyclic glycopeptide antibiotic which is purified from cultures of *Nocardia orientalis*. Its bactericidal activity appears to depend upon its ability to bind to the bacterial cell wall, resulting in the inhibition of glycopeptide polymerization at a site different from that affected by the penicillins.[47] Vancomycin is active against Gram-positive organisms, notably staphylococcal and clostridial species. Vancomycin is not active against Gram-negative bacteria, fungi, or yeast, a factor that allows it to be used in conjunction with biotherapies utilizing yeast as described below.

Vancomycin is highly active in vitro against clinical isolates of toxigenic *C. difficile* (see Fig. 51.2) with a MIC100 usually less than 5 μg/mL.[32,35–38] Orally administered vancomycin is not appreciably absorbed through the gastrointestinal tract and is mainly excreted unchanged in the feces. Thus, its pharmacokinetic properties are ideally suited to the treatment of *C. difficile* colitis. Bactericidal concentrations are easily achieved within the colonic lumen, whereas systemic side effects such as ototoxicity and nephrotoxicity are avoided.[37,48–51] Patients receiving oral vancomycin do not require monitoring of serum levels with the possible rare exception of patients with severe extensive colitis and compromised renal function. A number of controlled trials have confirmed the efficacy of oral vancomycin in the treatment of *C. difficile* colitis.[36,48,52,53] Symptomatic improvement is usually evident within 72 hours of initiating therapy, and complete resolution of diarrhea and colitis occurs in the majority of patients (96% overall)[30] by the end of a 10-day treatment period. Despite

Table 51.3 Metronidazole and vancomycin for treatment of *C. difficile* diarrhea

	Metronidazole	Vancomycin
Dose	250–500 mg	125–500 mg
Frequency	t.i.d. or q.i.d.	t.i.d. or q.i.d.
Duration	10–14 days	10–14 days
Route	Oral or intravenous	Oral
Response rate	>96%	>96%
Cost (10 day oral course)	US$20	US$75–$800*
Disadvantages	Systemic side effects Rare partially resistant strains of *C. difficile*	Encourages growth of nosocomial vancomycin-resistant bacteria

* The use of vancomycin prepared for intravenous infusion can greatly reduce the purchase cost of oral vancomycin, especially for the hospital pharmacy.

these impressive results, oral vancomycin therapy for *C. difficile* colitis has three major drawbacks: expense, disease relapse, and risk of encouraging vancomycin resistance amongst nosocomial bacteria.

The current cost for one 125 mg capsule of vancomycin is ≈US$5. Initial regimens used to treat *C. difficile* colitis consisted of a 10-day course of 2 g daily in three or four divided doses, resulting in a current overall treatment cost of US$800. This expense led a number of investigators to use lower-dose regimens, most commonly 125 mg four times daily for 10 days based on the theory that even this lower dose should easily result in bactericidal levels of vancomycin within the colonic lumen (500 µg/mL allowing for a stool volume of 1 liter per day).[36,50,52,53] Fekety et al. prospectively compared the efficacy of vancomycin 500 mg q.i.d. or 125 mg q.i.d. in the treatment of *C. difficile* colitis.[54] They found no significant differences between the two regimens with respect to overall response rate, duration of symptoms (i.e., diarrhea and abdominal pain) after initiation of therapy, persistence of *C. difficile* in the stool, or disease relapse after vancomycin was discontinued (Fig. 51.3).[54] Thus, in mild or moderately severe colitis, 125 mg of vancomycin given orally four times daily for 10 days appears to be adequate. Therapy for 5–7 days is less effective than a 10- to 14-day course. Liquid vancomycin formulated for intravenous use may be considerably less expensive than oral capsules or powder and can be administered orally as a cost-saving measure.

The emergence of nosocomial vancomycin-resistant enterococci (VRE) led to concern regarding transmission of vancomycin resistance to staphylococci and other nosocomial bacterial pathogens.[55] This has led to the recommendation that oral vancomycin therapy be reserved for patients who are intolerant of metronidazole, fail to respond to metronidazole, have severe pseudomembranous colitis, are pregnant, or are under the age of

10 years.[55,56] As a result, despite its efficacy, safety, and nearly ideal pharmacokinetic profile, oral vancomycin has been relegated to become the second-line antimicrobial agent for nosocomial *C. difficile*-associated diarrhea.

Metronidazole

Metronidazole is a synthetic nitroimidazole-derived antibacterial and antiprotozoal agent. Its mechanism of action has not been clearly elucidated, but appears to be related to its ability to disrupt DNA and inhibit nucleic acid synthesis in sensitive organisms.[47] It is active against most obligately anaerobic bacteria, including most strains of pathogenic *C. difficile*.[35,36,57] However, occasional metronidazole-resistant *C. difficile* isolates have been reported, and, enigmatically, metronidazole has been implicated as the offending agent in a small number of cases of *C. difficile* colitis.[41,58–60]

Metronidazole, unlike vancomycin, is well absorbed when administered orally,[57] and systemic side effects may occur. These include nausea and vomiting, a metallic taste, peripheral neuropathy (with prolonged therapy), and a disulfiram-like reaction with alcohol. Fecal concentrations of metronidazole are low or absent in healthy individuals or asymptomatic carriers of *C. difficile*, but higher concentrations are observed in patients with *C. difficile* colitis. Exudation through the inflamed colonic mucosa may be an important mechanism for increasing luminal metronidazole concentrations in active colitis.[61–63] With improvement of diarrhea and colitis, fecal concentrations drop.

Metronidazole was first suggested as a less expensive alternative to vancomycin for the treatment of *C. difficile* colitis in 1978.[64,65] A number of clinical studies have demonstrated that metronidazole therapy results in resolution of diarrhea and colitis in the vast majority of patients treated (98% overall).[30,66–68] Teasley et al. conducted a prospective randomized trial comparing metronidazole (250 mg q.i.d. for 10 days) and vancomycin (500 mg q.i.d. for 10 days) for the treatment of *C. difficile*-associated diarrhea and colitis.[52] Both regimens were equally successful in controlling symptoms and equally likely to be associated with subsequent disease relapse (see Table 51.3). Thus, the combination of high efficacy and low cost (50 cents per 250 mg tablet) has encouraged the recommendation of metronidazole as the drug of first choice in the treatment of *C. difficile* diarrhea and colitis.[5,56] This recommendation gained widespread acceptance following the emergence of VRE.[55,56]

Other antibiotics

Bacitracin, an antibiotic obtained from a strain of *Bacillus subtilis*, is poorly absorbed from the gastrointestinal tract and demonstrates in vitro activity against *C. difficile*. Bacitracin (25 000 units q.i.d. for 7–10 days) has been studied in several clinical trials of *C. difficile* colitis.[30,37,50,69,70] The overall response rate (approximately 80%) is lower, and the relapse rate (>30%) higher, than reported with either metronidazole or vancomycin. Furthermore, bacitracin is considerably more expensive than metronidazole and the oral formulation is not readily available in the United States. For these reasons bacitracin is seldom used to treat *C. difficile* colitis.

Teicoplanin, a glycopeptide antibiotic structurally related to vancomycin, shows equal efficacy to vancomycin in the treatment of *C. difficile* colitis but is also not available in the United States.[34,51,71] Teicoplanin has the advantage of a twice-daily dosage regimen (200 mg b.i.d. for 10 days).[51]

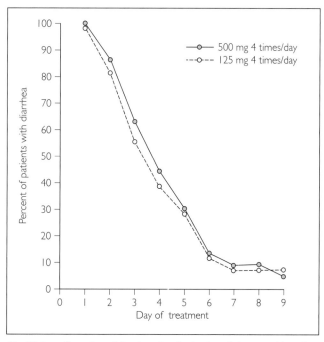

Fig. 51.3 • Cessation of diarrhea after institution of therapy with oral vancomycin 125 mg or 500 mg q.i.d. (Reproduced from Fekety R, Silva J, Kauffman C, et al. Treatment of antibiotic-associated *Clostridium difficile* colitis with oral vancomycin: comparison of two dosage regimens. Am J Med 1989; 86:15–19.)

Initial therapy for *C. difficile* diarrhea and colitis

The first step in the treatment of patients with confirmed or suspected *C. difficile* colitis is to discontinue the antimicrobial agent(s) responsible for initiating the diarrhea (Table 51.4). No further specific therapy will be required in a substantial number of patients, particularly those with mild diarrhea and without symptoms or signs of colitis.[5,56] In patients in whom it is inadvisable to discontinue all antimicrobial therapy because of ongoing infection, the patient's antibiotic regimen should be altered to make use of agents less likely to be associated with *C. difficile* overgrowth and colitis, e.g., parenteral aminoglycosides (see Table 51.2). Agents which reduce colonic motility (e.g., Lomotil or Immodium) should not be used since, in theory, they may delay clearance of toxin from the colon and thereby exacerbate toxin-induced colonic injury. They may also precipitate or exacerbate ileus and toxic dilatation.

Specific therapy to eradicate *C. difficile* should be used in patients with severe presenting symptoms, and in patients whose symptoms persist despite discontinuation of antibiotics. Oral metronidazole (250 mg t.i.d. or q.i.d. for 14 days) is currently the drug of first choice (see Table 51.3).[56] Vancomycin (125 mg q.i.d. for 14 days) is reserved for patients who are intolerant of or fail to respond to metronidazole. Vancomycin may also be used as a first-line agent for patients with severe pseudomembranous colitis, for young children (<10 years), and during pregnancy.[56] Therapy with metronidazole or vancomycin should be continued for at least 10 days. As discussed below, enteric precautions, including hand-washing, should be observed in nosocomial infections to prevent spread of toxigenic *C. difficile* to other susceptible hospital in-patients. It is prudent to warn patients of the substantial risk (≈20%) of symptomatic relapse once therapy is discontinued and to advise them to seek medical attention early should their symptoms recur. It is not necessary to test patients routinely in convalescence for persistence of *C. difficile* or its toxins in the stool. Many patients who respond well to treatment continue to be infected by *C. difficile* and have toxins in their stool but remain asymptomatic. This transition to the asymptomatic carrier state appears to reflect the development of protective immunity to *C. difficile* toxins.[17,25,72] Thus, evaluation for recur-rent infection and further therapy is indicated only if symptoms recur.

Treatment of severe pseudomembranous colitis

Severe pseudomembranous colitis, defined as leading to admission to an intensive care unit, surgery, or death, occurs in approximately 3% of hospital patients with *C. difficile* diarrhea.[73,74] Severe *C. difficile* colitis is frequently associated with abdominal pain, peritoneal signs, massive generalized colonic dilatation, hypo-albuminemia, a markedly elevated (>25 000) or a suppressed (<1500) white blood cell count, and a clinical picture of progressive sepsis.[73-76] Some clinicians prefer to use vancomycin as initial therapy in such severely ill patients.[56] This approach is not based on the results of controlled studies, but on clinical observations that such patients may respond more quickly to vancomycin than to metronidazole, the rationale being that even a marginal difference in the overall efficacy of vancomycin above metronidazole may be critical in these very ill patients.

A common problem in patients with severe colitis is that oral therapy cannot be administered due to recent abdominal surgery, ileus, or colonic dilatation. Under these circumstances metronidazole should be administered intravenously (500 mg, 6 hourly).[77] As discussed earlier, biliary excretion and colonic exudation are sufficient to provide bactericidal concentrations of metronidazole and hydroxymetronidazole in the feces.[61] Intravenous vancomycin is not used because excretion of bactericidal quantities of vancomycin into the gastrointestinal tract has not been demonstrated.[78,89] However, in severely ill patients, intravenous metronidazole may be supplemented by vancomycin administered by nasogastric tube (500 mg 6 hourly) or by enema (500 mg 4 hourly).[56] There are also reports of intracolonic infusion of vancomycin through a soft, flexible, narrow-bore (e.g., 6-French) tube placed over a guidewire at colonoscopy.[80,81] However, in patients with severe colitis, colonoscopy carries a risk of causing colonic perforation.

Patients with severe or prolonged *C. difficile* diarrhea have low serum and fecal antibody levels against *C. difficile* toxins whereas those with mild, brief episodes have higher antitoxin antibody concentrations.[25,26,74,82-87] In one report, intravenous infusion of normal pooled human immunoglobulin increased serum IgG antitoxin levels and this approach may be considered in patients with severe colitis who do not respond to therapy with metronidazole and vancomycin.[88]

For most patients with pseudomembranous colitis, the response to vancomycin or metronidazole is rapid and unequivocal, and clinical improvement should be expected within 72 hours of initiating treatment. Surgical intervention should be considered in severe colitis if no improvement is evident after 4–7 days of appropriate medical therapy or even earlier if the patient's condition continues to deteriorate. CT scan is a useful, noninvasive test to assess the extent and severity of colonic involvement and to look for evidence of colonic perforation, intramural gas, or intra-abdominal abscess formation.

Colectomy for *C. difficile* colitis is rarely required but may be lifesaving in fulminant, refractory, or complicated disease.[73-76,89-91] However, many of these patients already have substantial comorbid disease, making them unfit to undergo surgery or resulting in high perioperative mortality rates. A number of operations have been used including colectomy, subtotal colectomy, sigmoid

---

Table 51.4 Treatment of *C. difficile* diarrhea and colitis

Discontinue inciting antibiotic if possible

Supportive therapy

Confirm diagnosis

Specific therapy if symptoms are severe or persistent:
  Metronidazole orally for 10–14 days (drug of choice)

Vancomycin orally for 10–14 days if:
  Diarrhea does not improve during metronidazole treatment
  Patient cannot tolerate metronidazole
  Patient is pregnant or under the age of 10 years
  Severe diarrhea and colitis

If patient cannot tolerate oral medication:
  Metronidazole 500 mg, 6 hourly, intravenously

Modified from Fekety R. Guidelines for the diagnosis and management of *Clostridium difficile*-associated diarrhea and colitis. American College of Gastroenterology, Practice Parameters Committee. Am J Gastroenterol 1997; 92:739–750.

colectomy, transverse colostomy, cecostomy, and ileostomy. No controlled studies have been or are likely to be performed to determine the optimum surgical approach; however, subtotal colectomy with diverting ileostomy is the usual procedure of choice, as it effectively treats the acute problem and allows subsequent ileorectal anastomosis.[91]

Management of recurrent *C. difficile* diarrhea

One of the most perplexing problems associated with treatment of *C. difficile* diarrhea and colitis is the substantial incidence of recurrence.[5,56,92,93] The variety of innovative therapies described below attests to the fact that no single therapeutic measure is uniformly effective in preventing recurrent diarrhea. Multiple recurrences in the same patient are not uncommon, and more than 10 bouts of recurrence have occurred in some patients. Overall, 15–30% of patients treated with vancomycin or metronidazole relapse after their initial antibiotic therapy is completed.[5,25,56,92,94] The signs and symptoms of recurrence are similar to the initial attack. Patients develop recurrent diarrhea, cramping abdominal pain, or fever, usually 2–10 days after discontinuing therapy. Late recurrences are less common but may occur for up to 2 months after stopping treatment. The diagnosis of recurrent *C. difficile*-associated diarrhea should be confirmed whenever possible by toxin assay or bacterial culture. However, in patients with typical signs and symptoms of recurrence therapy can be reinstituted while awaiting stool assay results. Prompt therapy is especially important in those with a history of severe or protracted *C. difficile* diarrhea and this subpopulation is enriched in those with recurrent infection, presumably because of their now well-documented inadequate immune response to *C. difficile* toxins.[17,25,26,72,82]

The mechanism of symptomatic recurrence appears to involve reinfection either with the same or a different strain of *C. difficile* from that responsible for the initial episode as determined by bacteriologic typing techniques.[95–97] Resistance to metronidazole or vancomycin is seldom an important factor in recurrence.[38] Bartlett et al. were unable to demonstrate in vitro vancomycin resistance in 23 isolates of *C. difficile* from relapsing patients.[98] In some patients, *C. difficile* can be cultured from the stools, even during successful vancomycin therapy, and it is possible that these patients are more likely to relapse than those in whom eradication of the pathogen occurs during therapy.[95] However, *C. difficile* can also be cultured from the stools during and after antibiotic treatment in patients who have responded to therapy and do not relapse. This culture positivity in the face of symptomatic improvement may reflect the persistence of spores that are resistant to antibiotics. In one study, 18 of 22 patients with recurrence were noted to have colonic diverticula.[92] This led to speculation that spores may survive in diverticula where they escape the normal cleansing action of diarrhea and may not be exposed to the high luminal concentration of antibiotics. However, reinfection by bacteria and spores through the fecal–oral route may be a more prevalent mechanism of recurrence.[97]

Conservative therapy

The natural history of antibiotic-associated pseudomembranous colitis is full recovery in many if not most patients following cessation of antibiotics. In a series of 20 patients with clindamycin-associated pseudomembranous colitis, published prior to the discovery of vancomycin as effective therapy, all patients eventually recovered when clindamycin was stopped.[99] An important advantage to this form of management is that recurrence of diarrhea or colitis has not been reported. Anecdotal experience suggests that some patients with mild symptoms of recurrence can be managed conservatively, without specific antibiotic treatment. Obviously, this approach is not appropriate for elderly or infirm patients with moderate or severe symptoms.

Repeat treatment with vancomycin or metronidazole

The most common therapy of recurrence is a second course of the same antibiotic used to treat the initial attack. Some experts recommend a longer course of therapy (e.g., 4–6 weeks) with metronidazole or vancomycin for patients who have relapsed. Most patients respond well to treatment. However, patients with a history of recurrence have a substantial risk of further episodes of *C. difficile* diarrhea after antibiotic therapy is discontinued.[100] In two independent studies, patients with one or more previous recurrence had a subsequent recurrence rate of greater than 50% following standard therapy with metronidazole or vancomycin.[25,101]

Prolonged or tapering and pulsed antibiotic therapy

The use of tapering and pulsed antibiotic regimens is based on the theory that recurrence is caused by persistence of antibiotic-resistant spores that survive antibiotic therapy, and then convert to vegetative toxin-producing forms when antibiotic therapy is discontinued. Administration of vancomycin or metronidazole every other day or every third day allows the spores to vegetate on the off days and then be killed when the antibiotics are taken again. Tedesco et al. treated 22 patients with multiple recurrences of *C. difficile* antibiotic colitis using tapered doses of vancomycin for a 3-week period, followed by every other day therapy for 1 week and every third day for an additional week.[92] All patients responded symptomatically and did not relapse during a mean follow-up period of 6 months. Although this treatment regime is widely used, the rationale is suspect since there is no known mechanism for spores to sense the presence or absence of toxic antimicrobial agents. An alternative explanation is perhaps more plausible: that maintenance therapy over a prolonged period of time reduces the likelihood of reinfection when treatment is eventually terminated. Interestingly, toxin production by *C. difficile* is regulated so as to occur not during the early exponential growth phase of the bacterium but rather in the subsequent stationary phase.[102] Hence, after active *C. difficile* toxin-induced diarrhea and colitis have been controlled by treatment with metronidazole or vancomycin 24–72 hours are needed for the bacteria to reinitiate toxin production, in keeping with the reported clinical efficacy of alternate day therapy.

Binding resins

Because *C. difficile* diarrhea and colitis are caused by luminal toxins, anion-exchange binding resins have been proposed as a possible alternative to antimicrobial therapy. Clinical studies have been performed using two such agents: colestipol and cholestyramine. The response rate to colestipol in patients with *C. difficile* colitis was a disappointing 36% compared to a placebo response rate of 22%.[53] Cholestyramine therapy yielded a somewhat better overall response rate of 68%,[53,103] but this still compares poorly to response rates of over 96% with vancomycin or metronidazole. Therefore, these agents are not used as primary therapy for *C. difficile* colitis.

Cholestipol and cholestyramine have also been used in treating diarrhea recurrence. The usual dosage of cholestipol is 5 g every 12 hours and cholestyramine 4 g three or four times daily for 1–2 weeks. Tedesco treated 11 patients with relapsing *C. difficile* colitis with tapering doses of vancomycin plus cholestipol.[104] Because anion-exchange resins bind vancomycin as well as toxins, they must be taken at least 2 or 3 hours apart from the vancomycin.[105] An advantage of binding-resin therapy is that the bowel flora is not substantially altered, as occurs with vancomycin or metronidazole. This may allow more rapid reconstitution of the normal colonic microflora.

Tolevamer is a soluble anionic polymer designed to bind toxin A and toxin B of *C. difficile*. In preclinical studies tolevamer inhibited the cytotoxicity and enterotoxicity of *C. difficile* toxins and was superior to metronidazole in protecting hamsters from death caused by *C. difficile* cecitis.[45] In a phase II human clinical trial tolevamer showed similar efficacy to vancomycin as primary treatment for mild or moderately severe *C. difficile*-associated diarrhea.[46] Although not yet approved for clinical use, tolevamer holds promise as a safe, effective, nonantibiotic agent for treatment and prevention of *C. difficile* toxin-induced diarrhea and colitis. In theory, the ability of tolevamer to neutralize *C. difficile* toxins without an antimicrobial effect should facilitate reconstitution of the normal colonic bacterial flora, thereby restoring *C. difficile* colonization resistance to reduce or preventing disease recurrence.

Therapy with microorganisms

Reconstitution of the colonic flora in patients with relapsing disease is attractive as a therapeutic option because it addresses the underlying impairment of the colonic microbial barrier and avoids the use of antibiotics, which further delay recolonization by normal colonic flora. Bacteriotherapy has been reported in patients with relapsing *C. difficile* colitis using enemas of fresh feces from a healthy relative or rectal infusions of a mixture of 10 different aerobic and anaerobic bacteria.[106,107] The defined bacterial mixture led to bowel colonization with *Bacteroides* species, as well as prompt loss of *C. difficile* and its toxin from the feces. This observation suggests that *Bacteroides* may be one of the organisms that normally protects against pathogenic colonization with *C. difficile* and that is also capable of eliminating *C. difficile* during recovery. Another reported biotherapy for *C. difficile* diarrhea is the oral administration of a nontoxigenic strain of *C. difficile*. This novel approach was apparently successful in two patients treated for relapsing *C. difficile* diarrhea.[108] Preclinical studies are underway to characterize a nontoxigenic strain of *C. difficile* that may be suited to widespread use in humans as a targeted probiotic against infection with toxigenic *C. difficile*.[109]

Lactobacillus species have been used for many years to treat diarrhea. *Lactobacillus* strain GG has been reported to ameliorate symptoms in patients with relapsing *C. difficile* colitis.[110] However, in a controlled clinical trial *Lactobacillus* GG was not effective in protecting against nosocomial antibiotic-associated diarrhea.[111]

Saccharomyces boulardii is a nonpathogenic yeast used widely in continental Europe and now available in the United States without prescription to prevent antibiotic-associated diarrhea.[112] In a double-blind controlled clinical trial, Surawicz et al. reported that co-administration of oral capsules containing viable *S. boulardii* with antibiotics significantly reduced the incidence of antibiotic-associated diarrhea in hospitalized patients (from 22% on placebo to 9.5% in the *S. boulardii* group, p=0.04).[94] However, only a small minority of patients in this study were positive for stool *C. difficile* toxin. Animal studies suggest that *S. boulardii* may also protect against *C. difficile* toxin-induced colitis.[113–116] A randomized placebo-controlled trial examined the efficacy of *S. boulardii* in combination with either vancomycin or metronidazole in patients with *C. difficile* diarrhea.[101] Patients treated for a first episode of *C. difficile* diarrhea had similar recurrence rates with or without *S. boulardii* treatment group (19% and 24%, respectively, p=0.86). Patients treated with *S. boulardii* who had a history of previous episodes of relapsing *C. difficile* diarrhea had a significantly lower recurrence rate than the placebo group (35% and 65%, respectively, p=0.04). However, in a subsequent study *S. boulardii* (500 mg twice daily for 28 days) only reduced relapse rates (from 50% to 17%, p=0.05) in subjects treated with high-dose vancomycin (2 g per day for 10 days) but not in the groups that received other antibiotic treatment regimens.[117] Taken together, these controlled clinical trials indicate that *S. boulardii* is safe and may be effective in treating some patients with multiple recurrences of *C. difficile*-associated diarrhea but the protective effect is not uniform.

Immunoglobulin therapy

Serum antibodies to *C. difficile* toxin A and B are present in approximately 60% of the United States adult population.[118,119] Passive or active immunization against *C. difficile* toxins protects animals against *C. difficile*-induced colitis.[120–122] Leung et al. reported that six children with relapsing *C. difficile* colitis had low levels of serum IgG antibody directed against toxin A.[85] These children had failed multiple courses of antibiotics. Treatment with intravenous gamma globulin at a dose of 400 mg/kg, which contains high titer IgG antitoxin A, was followed by resolution of their chronic and recurrent *C. difficile* infection and diarrhea. Further study is required before gamma globulin can be recommended as therapy for patients with recurrent *C. difficile* diarrhea; however, similar results have been reported by other investigators and two recent studies have demonstrated a strong association between humoral immune responses to *C. difficile* toxin A and protection against symptomatic and recurrent CDAD.[17,25,123] A *C. difficile* toxoid vaccine has been produced and tested in early clinical trials where it was shown to be immunogenic.[124,125] Furthermore, in a small case series vaccination was also associated with resolution of recurrent CDAD.[126] Thus, passive or active immunization may ultimately prove to be both viable and effective in treating patients with refractory or recurrent disease.[26,127]

An approach to the management of relapsing *C. difficile* diarrhea and colitis

The initial management of recurrence following therapy for *C. difficile* diarrhea and colitis does not differ substantially from treatment of the initial episode (Table 51.5). Other etiologies for the patient's symptoms should be sought and stool samples should be examined to confirm the presence of toxigenic *C. difficile*. Relapsing patients with mild symptoms may be managed conservatively. If symptoms are persistent or severe or if there is evidence of colitis, a 14-day course of metronidazole or vancomycin should be administered. If recurrence again occurs, alternative regimens should be considered. The tapering and

Table 51.5 Approach to management of recurrent *C. difficile* colitis

First relapse

Confirm diagnosis
Symptomatic treatment if symptoms are mild
14-day course of metronidazole or vancomycin

Second relapse

Confirm diagnosis
Prolonged (4–6 week) course of metronidazole or vancomycin
or
Vancomycin taper
    125 mg q6h for 7 days
    125 mg q12h for 7 days
    125 mg qd for 7 days
    125 mg qod for 7 days
    125 mg every 3 days for 7 days

Further relapse

Saccharomyces boulardii in combination with metronidazole
    or vancomycin
or vancomycin in tapering dose as above plus cholestyramine
    4 g b.i.d.*
or vancomycin 125 mg q.i.d. and rifampicin 600 mg b.i.d. for
    7 days
or intravenous immunoglobulin
or therapy with other microorganisms

* Note: this regime is cumbersome since the doses of vancomycin and cholestyramine must be separated in time to prevent adsorption of the vancomycin.
Modified from Linevsky JK, Kelly CP. *Clostridium difficile* colitis. In: LaMont JT, ed. Gastrointestinal infections: diagnosis and management. New York: Marcel Dekker; 1997:293–325.

Table 51.6 Practice guidelines for prevention of *C. difficile* diarrhea

Limit the use of antimicrobial drugs

Wash hands between contact with all patients

Use enteric (stool) isolation precautions for patients with *C. difficile* diarrhea

Wear gloves when contacting patients with *C. difficile* diarrhea or their environment

Disinfect objects contaminated with *C. difficile* with sodium hypochlorite, alkaline glutaraldehyde, or ethylene oxide

Educate the medical, nursing, and other appropriate staff members about the disease and its epidemiology

Fekety R. Guidelines for the diagnosis and management of *Clostridium difficile*-associated diarrhea and colitis. American College of Gastroenterology, Practice Parameters Committee. Am J Gastroenterol 1997; 92:739–750.

pulsed antibiotic regimen described by Tedesco et al. is well tolerated and frequently successful.[92,128] If this fails, a host of alternative approaches have been described and are summarized in Table 51.5.[93] In difficult cases, a variety of different therapies may need to be used before the organism is finally eradicated. In some instances prolonged therapy with oral vancomycin (e.g., 125 mg twice daily) is a pragmatic and effective means to prevent further recurrences. This approach is indicated in frail or elderly individuals where symptomatic recurrence can lead to severe, life-threatening disease or in individuals who have suffered repeated recurrences despite trying multiple antibiotic regimens, probiotics, and other treatments.

PREVENTION OF NOSOCOMIAL OUTBREAKS

The major locus of *C. difficile* infection is the hospital or nursing home.[6,7,10,18,56,129,130] *C. difficile* and its spores can be identified in patient rooms, bathrooms, treatment areas, endoscopy suites, and on soiled linen, stethoscopes, and the hands of hospital personnel.[6,7,10,11] The asymptomatic carriage rate is above 20% in high-risk hospitalized patients, and nosocomial outbreaks and case clustering in wards are common.[6,7,9–11] While it is unlikely that *C. difficile* can ever be eradicated from hospitals, certain environmental control measures may reduce the prevalence and control the spread of this pathogen (Table 51.6).[56]

Hospital inpatients with *C. difficile*-associated diarrhea should be bedded in private rooms whenever possible to reduce patient-to-patient spread. Strict stool precautions and handwashing after patient contact should be observed universally. *C. difficile* can be cultured from the hands of healthcare workers after 60% of contacts with infected patients.[6] A controlled trial of the use of vinyl disposable gloves during patient contact was successful in reducing the incidence of *C. difficile* diarrhea in a hospital setting.[131] Handwashing with soap containing chlorhexidine gluconate also reduced hand carriage of *C. difficile* by healthcare workers. Environmental disinfection with agents effective against *C. difficile*, such as sodium hypochlorite, alkaline glutaraldehyde, or ethylene oxide, should be performed after discharge of infected patients.[56]

Endemic cases and outbreaks of *C. difficile* diarrhea in hospitals result from the close approximation of susceptible individuals, i.e., elderly and infirm patients who frequently receive antibiotics and are exposed to toxigenic *C. difficile* through person-to-person spread or environmental contamination. Antibiotic therapy with metronidazole or vancomycin is effective in treating individual patients but has not been effective as a disease control measure.[24] At present, the incidence of *C. difficile* diarrhea can best be reduced by avoiding the unnecessary use of broad-spectrum antibiotics and by the infection control measures discussed above. In the future, increasing individual and herd immunity to *C. difficile* and its toxins by vaccination or by passive immunotherapy may prove to be an effective means of preventing this troublesome iatrogenic disease.[25,26,74,82,127] Other prophylactic measures such as the use of bacterial and yeast probiotic agents or toxin binders in high-risk hospital patients also warrant further investigation.[45,46,94,109]

REFERENCES

1. Borriello SP. The influence of the normal flora on *Clostridium difficile* colonisation of the gut. Ann Med 1990; 22:61–67.

2. Viscidi R, Willey S, Bartlett JG. Isolation rates and toxigenic potential of *Clostridium difficile* isolates from various patient populations. Gastroenterology 1981; 81:5–9.

3. Linevsky JK, Kelly CP. *Clostridium difficile* colitis. In: LaMont JT, ed. Gastrointestinal infections: diagnosis and management. New York: Marcel Dekker; 1997:293–325.

4. Kelly CP, LaMont JT. Treatment of *Clostridium difficile* diarrhea and colitis. In: Wolfe MM, ed. Gastrointestinal pharmacotherapy. Philadelphia: WB Saunders; 1993:199–212.

5. Kelly CP, Pothoulakis C, LaMont JT. *Clostridium difficile* colitis. N Engl J Med 1994; 330:257–262.

6. McFarland LV, Mulligan ME, Kwok RY, et al. Nosocomial acquisition of *Clostridium difficile* infection. N Engl J Med 1989; 320:204–210.

   Among hospital inpatients receiving antibiotic therapy asymptomatic carriers of *C. difficile* outnumber those with *C. difficile*-associated diarrhea.

7. Johnson S, Clabots CR, Linn FV, et al. Nosocomial *Clostridium difficile* colonisation and disease. Lancet 1990; 336:97–100.

8. Hirschhorn LR, Trnka Y, Onderdonk A, et al. Epidemiology of community-acquired *Clostridium difficile*-associated diarrhea. J Infect Dis 1994; 169:127–133.

9. Nolan NP, Kelly CP, Humphreys JF, et al. An epidemic of pseudomembranous colitis: importance of person to person spread. Gut 1987; 28:1467–1473.

10. Fekety R, Kim KH, Brown D, et al. Epidemiology of antibiotic-associated colitis; isolation of *Clostridium difficile* from the hospital environment. Am J Med 1981; 70:906–908.

11. Kim KH, Fekety R, Batts DH, et al. Isolation of *Clostridium difficile* from the environment and contacts of patients with antibiotic-associated colitis. J Infect Dis 1981; 143:42–50.

12. Larson HE, Price AB, Honour P, et al. *Clostridium difficile* and the aetiology of pseudomembranous colitis. Lancet 1978; 1:1063–1066.

13. Bartlett JG, Chang TW, Gurwith M, et al. Antibiotic-associated pseudomembranous colitis due to toxin-producing clostridia. N Engl J Med 1978; 298:531–534.

   Toxin-producing strains of clostridia, later identified as *Clostridium difficile*, are recognized as being the causative agent in antibiotic-associated diarrhea and colitis.

14. Dove CH, Wang SZ, Price SB, et al. Molecular characterization of the *Clostridium difficile* toxin A gene. Infect Immun 1990; 58:480–488.

15. Barroso LA, Wang SZ, Phelps CJ, et al. Nucleotide sequence of *Clostridium difficile* toxin B gene. Nucleic Acids Res 1990; 18:4004.

16. Pothoulakis C. Pathogenesis of *Clostridium difficile*-associated diarrhoea. Eur J Gastroenterol Hepatol 1996; 8:1041–1047.

17. Kyne L, Warny M, Qamar A, et al. Asymptomatic carriage of *Clostridium difficile* and serum levels of IgG antibody against toxin A. N Engl J Med 2000; 342:390–397.

18. Bender BS, Bennett R, Laughon BE, et al. Is *Clostridium difficile* endemic in chronic-care facilities? Lancet 1986; 2:11–13.

19. Kyne L, Merry C, O'Connell B, et al. Factors associated with prolonged symptoms and severe disease due to *Clostridium difficile*. Age Ageing 1999; 28:107–113.

20. Bartlett JG. Management of *Clostridium difficile* infection and other antibiotic-associated diarrhoeas. Eur J Gastroenterol Hepatol 1996; 8:1054–1061.

21. Rao SS, Edwards CA, Austen CJ, et al. Impaired colonic fermentation of carbohydrate after ampicillin. Gastroenterology 1988; 94:928–932.

22. Hall IC, O'Toole E. Intestinal flora in newborn infants with description of a new pathogenic anaerobe. Am J Dis Child 1935; 49:390–402.

   The first identification of *Clostridium difficile* was as a commensal bacterium in the fecal flora of healthy neonates.

23. Larson HE, Barclay FE, Honour P, et al. Epidemiology of *Clostridium difficile* in infants. J Infect Dis 1982; 146:727–733.

24. Johnson S, Homann SR, Bettin KM, et al. Treatment of asymptomatic *Clostridium difficile* carriers (fecal excretors) with vancomycin or metronidazole. A randomized, placebo-controlled trial. Ann Intern Med 1992; 117:297–302.

25. Kyne L, Warny M, Qamar A, et al. Association between antibody response to toxin A and protection against recurrent *Clostridium difficile* diarrhoea. Lancet 2001; 357:189–193.

   An absent or inadequate host immune response to *C. difficile* toxins is a major risk factor for recurrent *C. difficile*-associated diarrhea.

26. Kyne L, Kelly CP. Prospects for a vaccine for *Clostridium difficile*. BioDrugs 1998; 10:173–181.

27. Eglow R, Pothoulakis C, Itzkowitz S, et al. Diminished *Clostridium difficile* toxin A sensitivity in newborn rabbit ileum is associated with decreased toxin A receptor. J Clin Invest 1992; 90:822–829.

28. Bartlett JG. Clinical practice. Antibiotic-associated diarrhea. N Engl J Med 2002; 346(5):334–339.

29. Thomas C, Stevenson M, Riley TV. Antibiotics and hospital-acquired *Clostridium difficile*-associated diarrhoea: a systematic review. J Antimicrob Chemother 2003; 51(6):1339–1350.

30. Peterson LR, Gerding DN. Antimicrobial agents. In: Rambaud JC, Ducluzeau R, eds. *Clostridium difficile*-associated intestinal diseases. Paris: Springer-Verlag; 1990:115–127.

31. Bartlett JG, Taylor NS, Chang T, et al. Clinical and laboratory observations in *Clostridium difficile* colitis. Am J Clin Nutr 1980; 33:2521–2526.

32. Bartlett JG, Chang TW, Onderdonk AB. Comparison of five regimens for treatment of experimental clindamycin-associated colitis. J Infect Dis 1978; 138:81–86.

33. Clabots CR, Shanholtzer CJ, Peterson LR, et al. In vitro activity of efrotomycin, ciprofloxacin, and six other antimicrobials against *Clostridium difficile*. Diagn Microbiol Infect Dis 1987; 6:49–52.

34. de Lalla F, Privitera G, Rinaldi E, et al. Treatment of *Clostridium difficile*-associated disease with teicoplanin. Antimicrob Agents Chemother 1989; 33:1125–1127.

35. Dzink J, Bartlett JG. In vitro susceptibility of *Clostridium difficile* isolates from patients with antibiotic-associated diarrhea or colitis. Antimicrob Agents Chemother 1980; 17:695–698.

36. Fekety R, Silva J, Toshniwal R, et al. Antibiotic-associated colitis: effects of antibiotics on *Clostridium difficile* and the disease in hamsters. Rev Infect Dis 1979; 1:386–397.

37. Young GP, Ward PB, Bayley N, et al. Antibiotic-associated colitis due to *Clostridium difficile*: double-blind comparison of vancomycin with bacitracin. Gastroenterology 1985; 89:1038–1045.

38. Drummond LJ, McCoubrey J, Smith DG, et al. Changes in sensitivity patterns to selected antibiotics in *Clostridium difficile* in geriatric in-patients over an 18-month period. J Med Microbiol. 2003; 52(Pt 3):259–263.

39. Johnson S, Samore MH, Farrow KA, et al. Epidemics of diarrhea caused by a clindamycin-resistant strain of *Clostridium difficile* in four hospitals. N Engl J Med 1999; 341(22):1645–1651.

40. Dridi L, Tankovic J, Burghoffer B, et al. gyrA and gyrB mutations are implicated in cross-resistance to ciprofloxacin and moxifloxacin in *Clostridium difficile*. Antimicrob Agents Chemother 2002; 46(11):3418–3421.

41. Pelaez T, Alcala L, Alonso R, et al. Reassessment of *Clostridium difficile* susceptibility to metronidazole and vancomycin. Antimicrob Agents Chemother 2002; 46(6):1647–1650.

42. Fekety R, Silva J, Armstrong J, et al. Treatment of antibiotic-associated enterocolitis with vancomycin. Rev Infect Dis 1981; 3(Suppl):S273–S281.

43. Bartlett JG, Onderdonk AB, Cisneros RL, et al. Clindamycin-associated colitis due to a toxin-producing species of *Clostridium* in hamsters. J Infect Dis 1977; 136:701–705.

44. Browne RA, Fekety R Jr, Silva J Jr, et al. The protective effect of vancomycin on clindamycin-induced colitis in hamsters. Johns Hopkins Med J 1977; 141:183–192.

   The in vivo therapeutic efficacy of vancomycin in *C. difficile*-associated diarrhea was first identified in the clindamycin-treated hamster model of antibiotic-associated colitis.

45. Kurtz CB, Cannon EP, Brezzani A, et al. GT160-246, a toxin binding polymer for treatment of *Clostridium difficile* colitis. Antimicrob Agents Chemother 2001; 45(8):2340–2347.

46. Louie T, Peppe J, Watt CK, et al. A phase 2 study of the toxin binding polymer tolevamer in patients with *C. difficile*-associated diarrhea. Gastroenterol 2004;126(S2):A511.

47. [No authors listed]. Metronidazole. In: McEvoy GK ed. American hospital formulary service. Bethesda: American Society of Hospital Pharmacists; 1990.

48. Keighley MR, Burdon DW, Arabi Y, et al. Randomised controlled trial of vancomycin for pseudomembranous colitis and postoperative diarrhoea. Br Med J 1978; 2:1667–1669.

49. Tedesco F, Markham R, Gurwith M, et al. Oral vancomycin for antibiotic-associated pseudomembranous colitis. Lancet 1978; 2:226–228.

50. Dudley MN, McLaughlin JC, Carrington G, et al. Oral bacitracin vs vancomycin therapy for *Clostridium difficile*-induced diarrhea. A randomized double-blind trial. Arch Intern Med 1986; 146:1101–1104.

51. Wenisch C, Parschalk B, Hasenhundl M, et al. Comparison of vancomycin, teicoplanin, metronidazole, and fusidic acid for the treatment of *Clostridium difficile*-associated diarrhea. Clin Infect Dis 1996; 22:813–818.

52. Teasley DG, Gerding DN, Olson MM, et al. Prospective randomised trial of metronidazole versus vancomycin for *Clostridium difficile*-associated diarrhoea and colitis. Lancet 1983; 2:1043–1046.

53. Mogg GA, Arabi Y, Youngs D, et al. Therapeutic trials of antibiotic associated colitis. Scand J Infect Dis Suppl 1980; 41–45.

54. Fekety R, Silva J, Kauffman C, et al. Treatment of antibiotic-associated *Clostridium difficile* colitis with oral vancomycin: comparison of two dosage regimens. Am J Med 1989; 86:15–19.

55. [No authors listed].Recommendations for preventing the spread of vancomycin resistance: recommendations of the Hospital Infection Control Practices Advisory Committee (HICPAC). Am J Infect Control 1995; 23:87–94.

   Metronidazole is the treatment of first choice for *C. difficile*-associated diarrhea with vancomycin as a second-line agent for those who are intolerant of or fail to respond to metronidazole or possibly those with severe disease.

56. Fekety R. Guidelines for the diagnosis and management of *Clostridium difficile*-associated diarrhea and colitis. American College of Gastroenterology, Practice Parameters Committee. Am J Gastroenterol 1997; 92:739–750.

57. Bartlett JG. Metronidazole. Johns Hopkins Med J 1981; 149:89–92.

58. Bingley PJ, Harding GM. *Clostridium difficile* colitis following treatment with metronidazole and vancomycin. Postgrad Med J 1987; 63:993–994.

59. Saginur R, Hawley CR, Bartlett JG. Colitis associated with metronidazole therapy. J Infect Dis 1980; 141:772–774.

60. Thomson G, Clark AH, Hare K, et al. Pseudomembranous colitis after treatment with metronidazole. Br Med J (Clin Res Ed) 1981; 282:864–865.

61. Bolton RP, Culshaw MA. Faecal metronidazole concentrations during oral and intravenous therapy for antibiotic associated colitis due to *Clostridium difficile*. Gut 1986; 27:1169–1172.

62. Krook A. Effect of metronidazole and sulfasalazine on the normal human faecal flora. Scand J Gastroenterol 1981;1 6:587–592.

63. Krook A, Jarnerot G, Danielsson D. Clinical effect of metronidazole and sulfasalazine on Crohn's disease in relation to changes in the fecal flora. Scand J Gastroenterol 1981; 16:569–575.

64. Dinh HT, Kernbaum S, Frottier J. Treatment of antibiotic-induced colitis by metronidazole. Lancet 1978; 1:338–339.

65. Matuchansky C, Aries J, Maire P. Metronidazole for antibiotic-associated pseudomembranous colitis. Lancet 1978; 2:580–581.

66. Cherry RD, Portnoy D, Jabbari M, et al. Metronidazole: an alternate therapy for antibiotic-associated colitis. Gastroenterology 1982; 82:849–851.

67. Johnson TA, Tabbut BR, Page CO. Treatment of antibiotic-associated pseudomembranous colitis with metronidazole. Am J Hosp Pharm 1981; 38:1034–1035.

68. Pashby NL, Bolton RP, Sherriff RJ. Oral metronidazole in *Clostridium difficile* colitis. Br Med J 1979; 1:1605–1606.

69. Chang TW, Gorbach SL, Bartlett JG, et al. Bacitracin treatment of antibiotic-associated colitis and diarrhea caused by *Clostridium difficile* toxin. Gastroenterology 1980; 78:1584–1586.

70. Tedesco FJ. Bacitracin therapy in antibiotic-associated pseudomembranous colitis. Dig Dis Sci 1980; 25:783–784.

71. de Lalla F, Nicolin R, Rinaldi E, et al. Prospective study of oral teicoplanin versus oral vancomycin for therapy of pseudomembranous colitis and *Clostridium difficile*-associated diarrhea. Antimicrob Agents Chemother 1992; 36:2192–2196.

72. Wilcox M, Minton J. Role of antibody response in outcome of antibiotic-associated diarrhoea. Lancet 2001; 357(9251): 158–159.

73. Rubin MS, Bodenstein LE, Kent KC. Severe *Clostridium difficile* colitis. Dis Colon Rectum 1995; 38:350–354.

74. Dallal RM, Harbrecht BG, Boujoukas AJ, et al. Fulminant *Clostridium difficile*: an underappreciated and increasing cause of death and complications. Ann Surg 2002; 235(3):363–372.

75. Morris JB, Zollinger RM Jr, Stellato TA. Role of surgery in antibiotic-induced pseudomembranous enterocolitis. Am J Surg 1990; 160: 535–539.

76. Morris LL, Villalba MR, Glover JL. Management of pseudomembranous colitis. Am J Surg 1994; 60:548–551; discussion 551–552.

77. Friedenberg F, Fernandez A, Kaul V, et al. Intravenous metronidazole for the treatment of *Clostridium difficile* colitis. Dis Colon Rectum 2001; 44(8):1176–1180.

78. Kleinfeld DI, Sharpe RJ, Donta ST. Parenteral therapy for antibiotic-associated pseudomembranous colitis. J Infect Dis 1988; 157:38.

79. Oliva SL, Guglielmo BJ, Jacobs R, et al. Failure of intravenous vancomycin and intravenous metronidazole to prevent or treat antibiotic-associated pseudomembranous colitis. J Infect Dis 1989; 159:1154–1155.

80. Pasic M, Jost R, Carrel T, et al. Intracolonic vancomycin for pseudomembranous colitis. N Engl J Med 1993; 329:583.

81. Apisarnthanarak A, Razavi B, Mundy LM. Adjunctive intracolonic vancomycin for severe *Clostridium difficile* colitis: case series and review of the literature. Clin Infect Dis. 2002; 35(6):690–696. Epub 2002 Aug 26. Review.

82. Kelly CP. Immune response to *Clostridium difficile* infection. Eur J Gastroenterol Hepatol 1996; 8:1048–1053.

83. Aronsson B, Granstrom M, Mollby R, et al. Serum antibody response to *Clostridium difficile* toxins in patients with *Clostridium difficile* diarrhoea. Infection 1985; 13:97–101.

84. Johnson S, Gerding DN, Janoff EN. Systemic and mucosal antibody responses to toxin A in patients infected with *Clostridium difficile*. J Infect Dis 1992; 166:1287–1294.

85. Leung DY, Kelly CP, Boguniewicz M, et al. Treatment with intravenously administered gamma globulin of chronic relapsing colitis induced by *Clostridium difficile* toxin. J Pediatr 1991; 118:633–637.

   Passive immunization may be an effective treatment for recurrent *C. difficile*-associated diarrhea.

86. Mulligan ME, Miller SD, McFarland LV, et al. Elevated levels of serum immunoglobulins in asymptomatic carriers of *Clostridium difficile*. Clin Infect Dis 1993; 16(Suppl 4):S239–S244.

87. Warny M, Vaerman JP, Avesani V, et al. Human antibody response to *Clostridium difficile* toxin A in relation to clinical course of infection. Infect Immun 1994; 62:384–389.

88. Salcedo J, Keates S, Pothoulakis C, et al. Intravenous immunoglobulin therapy for severe *Clostridium difficile* colitis. Gut 1997; 41:366–370.

89. Medich DS, Lee KK, Simmons RL, et al. Laparotomy for fulminant pseudomembranous colitis. Arch Surg 1992; 127:847–852; discussion 852–853.

90. Trudel JL, Deschenes M, Mayrand S, et al. Toxic megacolon complicating pseudomembranous enterocolitis. Dis Colon Rectum 1995; 38:1033–1038.

91. Bradley SJ, Weaver DW, Maxwell NP, et al. Surgical management of pseudomembranous colitis. Am Surg 1988; 54:329–332.

92. Tedesco FJ, Gordon D, Fortson WC. Approach to patients with multiple recurrences of antibiotic-associated pseudomembranous colitis. Am J Gastroenterol 1985; 80:867–868.

   Prolonged, tapered, and pulsed antibiotic therapy may be effective in patients with recurrent *C. difficile*-associated diarrhea and colitis.

93. Kyne L, Kelly CP. Recurrent *Clostridium difficile* diarrhoea. Gut 2001; 49(1):152–153.

94. Surawicz CM, Elmer GW, Speelman P, et al. Prevention of antibiotic-associated diarrhea by *Saccharomyces boulardii*: a prospective study. Gastroenterology 1989; 96:981–988.

95. Walters BA, Roberts R, Stafford R, et al. Relapse of antibiotic associated colitis: endogenous persistence of *Clostridium difficile* during vancomycin therapy. Gut 1983; 24:206–212.

96. Young G, McDonald M. Antibiotic-associated colitis: why do patients relapse? Gastroenterology 1986; 90:1098–1099.

97. Wilcox MH, Fawley WN, Settle CD, et al. Recurrence of symptoms in *Clostridium difficile* infection – relapse or reinfection? J Hosp Infect 1998; 38(2):93–100.

98. Bartlett JG, Tedesco FJ, Shull S, et al. Symptomatic relapse after oral vancomycin therapy of antibiotic-associated pseudomembranous colitis. Gastroenterology 1980; 78:431–434.

99. Tedesco FJ, Barton RW, Alpers DH. Clindamycin-associated colitis. A prospective study. Ann Intern Med 1974; 81:429–433.

100. Kim PH, Iaconis JP, Rolfe RD. Immunization of adult hamsters against *Clostridium difficile*-associated ileocecitis and transfer of protection to infant hamsters. Infect Immun 1987; 55:2984–2992.

101. McFarland LV, Surawicz CM, Greenberg RN, et al. A randomized placebo-controlled trial of *Saccharomyces boulardii* in combination with standard antibiotics for *Clostridium difficile* disease. JAMA 1994; 271:1913–1918.

   In a randomized controlled trial the probiotic yeast *Saccharomyces boulardii*, used in combination with standard antibiotic therapy, reduced relapse risk in patients with recurrent *C. difficile*-associated diarrhea.

102. Dupuy B, Sonenshein AL. Regulated transcription of *Clostridium difficile* toxin genes. Mol Microbiol 1998; 27(1):107–120.

103. Kreutzer EW, Milligan FD. Treatment of antibiotic-associated pseudomembranous colitis with cholestyramine resin. Johns Hopkins Med J 1978; 143:67–72.

104. Tedesco FJ. Treatment of recurrent antibiotic-associated pseudomembranous colitis. Am J Gastroenterol 1982; 77:220–221.

105. Taylor NS, Bartlett JG. Binding of *Clostridium difficile* cytotoxin and vancomycin by anion-exchange resins. J Infect Dis 1980; 141:92–97.

106. Tvede M, Rask-Madsen J. Bacteriotherapy for chronic relapsing *Clostridium difficile* diarrhoea in six patients. Lancet 1989; 1:1156–1160.

107. Persky SE, Brandt LJ. Treatment of recurrent *Clostridium difficile*-associated diarrhea by administration of donated stool directly through a colonoscope. Am J Gastroenterol 2000; 95:3283–3285.

108. Seal D, Borriello SP, Barclay F, et al. Treatment of relapsing *Clostridium difficile* diarrhoea by administration of a non-toxigenic strain. Eur J Clin Microbiol 1987; 6:51–53.

109. Sambol SP, Merrigan MM, Tang JK, et al. Colonization for the prevention of *Clostridium difficile* disease in hamsters. J Infect Dis 2002; 186(12):1781–1789.

110. Gorbach SL, Chang TW, Goldin B. Successful treatment of relapsing *Clostridium difficile* colitis with *Lactobacillus* GG. Lancet 1987; 2:1519.

111. Thomas MR, Litin SC, Osmon DR, et al. Lack of effect of *Lactobacillus* GG on antibiotic-associated diarrhea: a randomized, placebo-controlled trial. Mayo Clin Proc 2001; 76(9):883–889.

112. Elmer GW, Surawicz CM, McFarland LV. Biotherapeutic agents. A neglected modality for the treatment and prevention of selected intestinal and vaginal infections. JAMA 1996; 275:870–876.

113. Elmer GW, McFarland LV. Suppression by *Saccharomyces boulardii* of toxigenic *Clostridium difficile* overgrowth after vancomycin treatment in hamsters. Antimicrob Agents Chemother 1987; 31:129–131.

114. Massot J, Sanchez O, Couchy R, et al. Bacterio-pharmacological activity of *Saccharomyces boulardii* in clindamycin-induced colitis in the hamster. Arzneimittelforschung 1984; 34:794–797.

115. Pothoulakis C, Kelly CP, Joshi MA, et al. *Saccharomyces boulardii* inhibits *Clostridium difficile* toxin A binding and enterotoxicity in rat ileum. Gastroenterology 1993; 104:1108–1115.

116. Toothaker RD, Elmer GW. Prevention of clindamycin-induced mortality in hamsters by *Saccharomyces boulardii*. Antimicrob Agents Chemother 1984; 26:552–556.

117. Surawicz CM, McFarland LV, Greenberg RN, et al. The search for a better treatment for recurrent *Clostridium difficile* disease: use of high-dose vancomycin combined with *Saccharomyces boulardii*. Clin Infect Dis 2000; 31(4):1012–1017. Epub 2000 Oct 25.

118. Kelly CP, Pothoulakis C, Orellana J, et al. Human colonic aspirates containing immunoglobulin A antibody to *Clostridium difficile* toxin A inhibit toxin A-receptor binding. Gastroenterology 1992; 102:35–40.

119. Viscidi R, Laughon BE, Yolken R, et al. Serum antibody response to toxins A and B of *Clostridium difficile*. J Infect Dis 1983; 148:93–100.

120. Corthier G, Muller MC, Wilkins TD, et al. Protection against experimental pseudomembranous colitis in gnotobiotic mice by use of monoclonal antibodies against *Clostridium difficile* toxin A. Infect Immun 1991; 59:1192–1195.

121. Libby JM, Jortner BS, Wilkins TD. Effects of the two toxins of *Clostridium difficile* in antibiotic-associated cecitis in hamsters. Infect Immun 1982; 36:822–829.

122. Lyerly DM, Bostwick EF, Binion SB, et al. Passive immunization of hamsters against disease caused by *Clostridium difficile* by use of bovine immunoglobulin G concentrate. Infect Immun 1991; 59:2215–2218.

123. Wilcox MH. Descriptive study of intravenous immunoglobulin for the treatment of recurrent *Clostridium difficile* diarrhoea. J Antimicrob Chemother 2004; 53(5):882–884.

124. Kotloff KL, Wasserman SS, Losonsky GA, et al. Safety and immunogenicity of increasing doses of a *Clostridium difficile* toxoid vaccine administered to healthy adults. Infect Immun 2001; 69(2):988–995.

Based on the results of this first human clinical trial, vaccination against *C. difficile* toxins may ultimately prove to be effective in protecting at risk individuals from *C. difficile*-associated diarrhea and colitis.

125. Aboudola S, Kotloff KL, Kyne L, et al. *Clostridium difficile* vaccine and serum immunoglobulin G antibody response to toxin A. Infect Immun 2003; 71:1608–1610.

126. Sougioultzis S, Kyne L, Drudy D, et al. *Clostridium difficile* toxoid vaccine in recurrent *C. difficile*-associated diarrhea. Gastroenterol 2004; 126(S2):A512.

127. Giannasca PJ, Warny M. Active and passive immunization against *Clostridium difficile* diarrhea and colitis. Vaccine 2004; 22:848–856.

128. McFarland LV, Elmer GW, Surawicz CM. Breaking the cycle: treatment strategies for 163 cases of recurrent *Clostridium difficile* disease. Am J Gastroenterol 2002; 97(7):1769–1775.

129. McFarland LV. Epidemiology of infectious and iatrogenic nosocomial diarrhea in a cohort of general medicine patients. Am J Infect Control 1995; 23:295–305.

130. McFarland LV, Surawicz CM, Stamm WE. Risk factors for *Clostridium difficile* carriage and *C. difficile*-associated diarrhea in a cohort of hospitalized patients. J Infect Dis 1990; 162:678–684.

131. Johnson S, Gerding DN, Olson MM, et al. Prospective, controlled study of vinyl glove use to interrupt *Clostridium difficile* nosocomial transmission. Am J Med 1990; 88:137–140.

CHAPTER FIFTY-TWO

Treatment of intestinal parasitic diseases

Joachim Richter

INTRODUCTION

History

Parasitism is an essential phenomenon of biological evolution. Palaeoparasitological studies of human fecal samples confirm that man has probably always suffered from *Entamoeba histolytica*, *Giardia intestinalis*, *Ascaris lumbricoides*, and *Capillaria* spp.[1–3] Ancient Egyptian and Chinese mummies were infected by schistosomes.[4]

Acquisition of parasites and parasite–host interactions

Human intestinal parasites comprise two different types of organisms: protozoa and helminths. Most intestinal parasites are acquired by the enteral route (foodborne parasites). Some helminths (schistosomes, hookworms, *Strongyloides* spp.) are acquired percutaneously. The immune response against protozoa differs from the one against helminths: intestinal protozoa induce local IgA antibody production but do not elicit a systemic immune response. When systemic infection occurs, e.g., invasive amebiasis, this is accompanied by neutrophilia. In contrast, helminths induce a particular immune response involving eosinophils because worms are too large for phagocytosis by host cells. This response is predominantly local when the whole cycle of the infective helminth occurs inside the lumen of the gastro-intestinal tract of the human host. In this case, blood eosinophilia is not to be expected, e.g., in pinworm infection. If the life cycle of the helminth includes a systemic larval migration phase, such as in ascariasis or hookworm infection, eosinophilia is seen in peripheral blood.

OBTAINING AND PROCESSING OF BIOLOGICAL SAMPLES FOR DIAGNOSIS

For the diagnosis of an intestinal parasitic infection stool samples and, in most instances, a serum sample are required. Multiple stool samples must be examined, as the stool quantity of a sample examined under the microscope is extremely small and excretion of protozoal cysts or worm ova or larvae may be scanty and irregular.[5–7] Since pinworm ova are deposited in the perianal area but not into feces by the female adult worms, these ova must be searched for on anal cellophane samples. Microscopy of duodenal fluid for *G. intestinalis*, *Fasciola hepatica*, and of duodenal mucosal biopsies for *Giardia* may sometimes contribute to diagnosis although in giardiasis these methods are less sensitive than repeated parasitological stool examinations.[7–9] Microscopic examination of fresh crushed biopsies of rectum and colon is useful in intestinal schistosomiasis, and histopathological methods may also be helpful, e.g., for invasive amebiasis and schistosomiasis.

In order to diagnose an intestinal parasitic infection reliably, several points must be taken into account:
1. Good quality is achieved only if the personnel examining stool samples are properly trained and experienced and sufficient time is available for each examination.[10]
2. Examination of native fresh stools is useful to detect mobile vegetative and erythrophagocytic entamebae, *Giardia* tropho-zoites and *Strongyloides stercoralis* larvae. Examination must be performed within 30 minutes, because morphology of organisms changes and mobility decreases rapidly.
3. A preservative must be added to stools that cannot be examined immediately. Specific enrichment methods are necessary, which concentrate ova and protozoan cysts by centrifugation or other means.[11–14] Detection of some parasites require special methods, e.g., *F. hepatica* (cup sedimentation[15] and *S. stercoralis* [Baermann,[16] Harada Mori,[17] agar plate[18] enrichments]).
4. Staining of stool samples improves the judgment on the morphology of protozoan cysts or helminth ova. Some protozoa require special staining (*Cyclospora cayetanensis*, *Cryptosporidium parvum*).
5. The detection of parasitic copro-antigens is increasingly used for the diagnosis, e.g., of *G. intestinalis*, *C. parvum*, *E. histolytica*, flukes, schistosomes.[19]
6. Identification of specific parasite DNA by PCR techniques (e.g., *G. intestinalis*, *E. histolytica*). These methods are described in detail elsewhere.[16,20,21]

Biological prerequisites

In some instances ova or larvae are not excreted in stools in spite of an active helminthic infection, e.g., in: (1) *infertile or uni-sexual worm infection*; (2) *abortive infection by an animal helminth* unable to develop to the mature stage in humans; (3) infection during the *prepatency period*.
1. *Infertile infections* can only be diagnosed by detection of specific antigens or antibodies in serum or by recovery of adult worms in feces. Inspection of adult worms or of fragments of worms excreted in stools allows specific diagnosis.

2. *Abortive infection by an animal helminth* is suspected when a typical skin eruption occurs immediately or soon after exposure (e.g., 'swimmer's itch' in dermatitis due to worm larvae of avian schistosomes after bathing in contaminated fresh water, cutaneous larva migrans after a stay on a beach with straying dogs or cats). Visceral larva migrans is accompanied by high eosinophilia and confirmed by serological tests.

3. *Prepatency* refers to the time elapsed between infection and the excretion of worm ova or larvae in feces. The prepatency period exceeds the incubation period in those helminthic infections where larvae or immature worms migrate through the host organism before being capable of producing ova. This stage may be accompanied by an acute febrile disease with high eosinophilia, hepatosplenomegaly, migrating pulmonary infiltrates (Loeffler infiltrates) and urticarial skin manifestations. 'Eosinophilic febrile syndrome' is observed frequently in infections due to trematodes (acute schistosomiasis, acute fluke infection) and in several roundworm infections. Prepatency may last up to 8 weeks in schistosomiasis and whipworm infection. During the prepatency period, specific antigens and antibodies must be searched for in serum before ova or larvae appear in stool samples. Sometimes parasitological methods preclude the establishment of a definitive diagnosis or at least do not provide a diagnosis by the time the patient requires treatment.

PROTOZOAL INFECTIONS

Amebiasis

Many different apathogenic ameba colonize man. Two species, *Entamoeba dispar* and *E. moshkovskii*, cannot be differentiated microscopically from potentially pathogenic *Entamoeba histolytica (sensu stricto)*.[7,20] Among the 500 million people in the world estimated to be infected by entamebae of the *E. dispar/ E. histolytica*-complex, 450 million are asymptomatic carriers of *E. dispar*. *E. histolytica s.s.* may show all degrees of virulence from nonpathogenic commensalism to high tissue invasiveness. Around 5 million of the 50 million *E. histolytica s.s.* infections become frankly invasive and are estimated to cause 50 000 to 100 000 deaths per year. The main reservoir of *E. histolytica* is man. Amebae are transmitted via the fecal–oral route either directly by ingestion of contaminated water or food, or via flies and cockroaches carrying the amebae from infected stool to food. Amebiasis occurs worldwide, but is most prevalent in subtropical and tropical developing countries. Incidence is related to poor sanitation and crowding, to using human excrement as fertilizer, and/or to contamination of food by food handlers. Person-to-person transmission occurs among individuals in mental institutions. Other at-risk groups comprise immigrants from highly endemic areas, canal or sewage workers, and prisoners. Among male homosexuals predominantly *E. dispar* is spread by particular sexual practices.

Corticosteroids given for an inflammatory colon disease may convert a commensal into an agent of invasive infection. Young children, pregnant women, and immunocompromised individuals are at risk of severe amebiasis, whereas AIDS does not constitute a predisposing condition for severe disease.

E. dispar and *E. histolytica s.s.* colonize the colon. The detection of entameba cysts most frequently corresponds to *asymptomatic*

intestinal carriage of *E. dispar*. Also *E. histolytica s.s.* carriage usually resolves spontaneously. On the contrary, invasive *E. histolytica* trophozoites penetrate the mucosa, adhere to host cells and ingest these, especially erythrocytes. These trophozoites produce ulcerations of the colon wall and may subsequently reach the liver via the portal circulation. Severity of *amebic colitis* due to invasive trophozoites may range from mild/moderate with increased frequency of stool evacuations and abdominal cramps to overt dysentery with bloodstained mucus. Amebic colitis may be misdiagnosed as ulcerative colitis, especially when there is no history of a recent stay in regions of high endemicity. Ulcers are initially small (3–5 mm) and superficial. As the disease advances, ulcers typically become flask-shaped with undermined borders. The patient becomes prostrate. Although amebic colitis is sometimes accompanied by fever, especially nonfebrile dysentery should raise the suspicion of amebiasis. Sometimes, chronic inflammation leads to colon polyposis. Fulminant ulcerative colitis may develop from confluent ulcers. Deep ulcerations may perforate and lead to peritonitis. In some patients a precarious equilibrium between parasite virulence and the host's immune response results in a localized chronic granulomatous lesion of the colon, called ameboma. Amebomas of the colon may be single or multiple and be misinterpreted as a colonic carcinoma. When presenting as a circular constricting tumor, amebomas lead to intestinal sub-occlusion. Amebomas may bleed either spontaneously or during endoscopy. Biopsy specimens show granulation tissue. Since the number of *E. histolytica* microorganisms is few, amebiasis may be overlooked by a nonexperienced pathologist. If surgery is performed without antiparasitic coverage, life-threatening dissemination may occur.

Extraintestinal amebiasis occurs when trophozoites reach extraintestinal organs after penetration of the colon. Severity of *peritoneal amebiasis* depends on the degree of colon perforation, and clinical signs vary from mild abdominal pain to frank peritonitism, with free intraperitoneal gas. Although *amebic liver abscess* (ALA) (Fig. 52.1) is a relatively rare complication of *E. histolytica* infection, due to the high incidence of *E. histolytica* infection worldwide it is not uncommon. Patients with an ALA may present in every hospital because of its relatively slow evolution during weeks to months. Because of this latency *E. histolytica* is not more detectable in feces in about 50% of ALA cases. Therefore, patients are sometimes suspected to have colonic cancer with a hypoechogenic focus (ALA) taken for a liver metastasis. Patients report abdominal pain irradiating to the right or left shoulder. There is general malaise and in some patients fever. If the abscess is not treated promptly and appropriately it may rupture into the pleural, peritoneal, pericardial space or other contiguous organs. *Pleuropulmonary amebiasis* develops from an ALA in up to 15% of cases. It should be suspected when symptoms of an ALA are followed by severe pain in the lower chest, dyspnea, and nonproductive cough. Bronchohepatic fistulas are characterized by expectoration of dark-brown material. Fortunately, less than 1% of ALAs, especially of the left liver lobe, penetrate into the pericardial cavity: *pericardial amebiasis* leads to cardiac tamponade and shock, requiring immediate pericardial drainage. *Cerebral amebiasis* occurs in less than 0.1% of patients with *E. histolytica s.s*-infection. It should be suspected when patients with amebiasis present because of the abrupt onset of central nervous symptoms. If given in a timely fashion, metronidazole, which penetrates the blood–brain barrier,

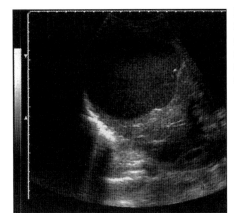

Fig. 52.1 •
Longitudinal ultrasound scan of the right liver lobe, showing a large amebic liver abscess.

improves the prognosis. *Urinary amebiasis* is usually a complication of perforated amebic abscesses or colitis. *Genital amebiasis* may complicate perineal amebiasis or be due to fistula from rectocolitis or an ALA. *Cutaneous amebiasis* may either occur spontaneously in the perineal area or in other sites after surgical intervention. Usually, it presents as an ulceration but in longstanding infection it may mimic verrucous carcinoma.[7]

Diagnosis of amebiasis

Diagnosis of amebiasis relies on the microscopic detection of *Entamoeba histolytica*-like protozoa in stool and subsequent differentiation between *E. histolytica s.s.* and *E. dispar. E. histolytica s.s* infection is proved either by the detection of *E. histolytica* trophozoites phagocyting erythrocytes in fresh native stool samples, by the detection of *E. histolytica* DNA, of specific zymodemes in stool or aspirate cultures (before therapy) or of specific antibodies against *E. histolytica* in serum. Several diagnostic pitfalls have to be considered: (1) microscopy of fresh stool samples has a very low sensitivity; (2) *E. dispar* and *E. histolytica* are not differentiable microscopically unless erythrocytophagic forms are seen; (3) antibodies against *E. histolytica s.s.* develop slowly and may be borderline even in case of overt ALA – an active infection is not differentiable from a past infection because antibodies persist after cure; (4) for exclusion of invasive amebiasis the examination of at least three stool samples enriched by special methods (MIF, SAF, culture) is required. However, negative results do not rule out extraintestinal amebiasis, since amebae have frequently disappeared from the intestine. Amebiasis does not cause eosinophilia. If a liver abscess presents with eosinophilia, a helminthic etiology should be suspected (e.g., visceral larva migrans, acute fascioliasis, or schistosomiasis). Most cases with ALAs present with neutrophilic leukocytosis; only few patients with longstanding infection or additional infection present have leukopenia. Before puncturing a liver abscess, empiric therapy with metronidazole should always be initiated, which also covers anaerobic bacteria. Puncture-aspiration increases the risk of systemic spread and usually does not shorten recovery. Moreover, amebae are rarely found in the (typically chocolate brown) aspirate. Amebae are found in the marginal areas of the abscess, i.e., the last portion of the aspirate. *E. histolytica* antigen detection appears to be more sensitive. Ultrasonography is the method of choice for the diagnosis of ALAs; it should be routinely performed and controlled in patients

with *E. histolytica s.s.*-infections. Ultrasound enables the differentiation from cysts, benign tumors, and malignancies by demonstrating fluctuating echoes inside a hypoechogenic mass with distal enhancement. Frequently, ALA is rather homogenic, well defined, but without a definite outer single or double membrane as seen in cystic echinococcosis. Multiple ALAs may appear as polycyclic or irregularly delimited hypoechogenic foci.[22,23]

No therapy is required to eradicate asymptomatic intestinal carriage (90%) of *E. dispar*. The cost of unnecessary intraluminal intestinal decontamination of the bowel may outweigh that of PCR analysis in specialized centers to rule out *E. histolytica s.s.* infection. In true *E. histolytica s.s.* infection decontamination of the bowel is mandatory. In invasive amebiasis, therapy with a tissue amebicide (metronidazole) must be added to an intraluminal amebicide: oral metronidazole is highly efficacious for treating amebic colitis and ALA, provided sufficient dosage is given (at least 2 g/d for 10 days). Parenteral treatment is required in patients who are not able to absorb metronidazole or who are noncompliant (Table 52.1). ALAs regress slowly, and during the first week of metronidazole therapy may even increase in size. This may be misinterpreted by the clinician as metronidazole resistance. At this stage, decisions should therefore be guided by the clinical status of the patient rather than by the size of an ALA: in most cases the clinical status improves dramatically within 2–3 days of metronidazole therapy. Whereas the specific ELISA antibody test usually becomes negative within 6–12 months posttherapy, this is not the case for IHA, which may persist for more than 10 years.

Giardia intestinalis (syn. Giardia lamblia, Giardia duodenalis)

Giardia intestinalis is a noninvasive intestinal flagellate affecting the small bowel. Giardiasis occurs worldwide but most frequently in areas with poor sanitation. Prevalence in children in the developing world may reach 20–30%. In many poor areas of the world all small children may become infected within their first three years of life. Giardiasis is the most common protozoal infection in industrialized countries with a prevalence 2–5%.[7] In Europe it is particularly common in the St. Petersburg area. In the USA., travelers to national parks and skiers in Colorado are at risk, especially if they drink the apparently clean surface water. Moreover, animals such as dogs, cats, and beavers may also carry *G. intestinalis. Giardia* cysts may resist chlorination of drinking water. *G. intestinalis* is able to multiply inside the host and to cause disease for many years after infection. Hypogammaglobulinemia and IgA-deficiency increase the risk of severe giardiasis. In HIV infection and AIDS carriage rate is increased, but severe cases are rarely seen.

Symptoms of giardiasis resemble the symptoms included in the Rome criteria for irritable bowel syndrome.[24] Uncomplicated giardiasis does not cause any laboratory abnormalities (besides an increased gamma-GT in some cases). Complications include lactase deficiency, malabsorption, and sprue. Giardiasis should be suspected in every prolonged nonfebrile nonbloody diarrhea. Multiple stool examinations, copro-antigen detection, duodenal brushing, or biopsy and fresh examination of duodenal lavage may still miss 2–15% of infections. The yield of copro-antigen tests has usually been compared with microscopy of one stool sample, although examination of a single stool sample is not

Table 52.1 Treatment of intestinal protozoa

Organism	Drug of choice and dose	Alternative
Entamoeba histolytica (sensu stricto)		
Intestinal carriage	Paromomycin 25–35 mg/kg/d in 3 divided doses for 5–10 days	1. Diloxanid furoate 500 mg t.i.d. for 10 days or 2. Iodoquinol 650 mg t.i.d. for 20 days
Invasive *E. histolytica* s.s.	Metronidazole 750 mg, t.i.d. p.o. or in severe cases i.v + paromomycin 25–35 mg/kg/d for 10 days in 3 divided doses for 10 days	Tinidazole 800 mg t.i.d. for 3–5 days + diloxanid furoate 500 mg t.i.d. for 10 days or + iodoquinol 650 mg t.i.d. for 20 days
Colitis, ameboma, extraintestinal amebiasis, liver abscess	Only liver abscesses close to the pericardium: drainage + optionally: chloroquine (salt) 250 mg b.i.d. for 7–20 days	
Balantidium coli	Tetracycline 500 mg q.i.d. for 10 days	Iodoquinol 650 mg t.i.d. for 20 days
Blastocystis hominis	Metronidazol 750 mg t.i.d. for 5–10 days	Iodoquinol 650 mg t.i.d. for 20 days or paromomycin 25–35 mg/kg/d in 3 divided doses for 5–10 days
Cryptospora parvum	Efficacious HAART will result in parasite clearance	Nitazoxanide 500 mg b.i.d. for 3 days
Cyclospora cayetanensis	TMP 160 mg + SMZ 800 mg b.i.d. for 3 days	
Dientamoeba fragilis	Tetracycline 500 mg q.i.d. for 5 days	Iodoquinol 650 mg t.i.d. for 20 days or paromomycin 25–35 mg/kg/d in 3 divided doses for 5–10 days
Giardia intestinalis	Tinidazole 1 g b.i.d. for 2–3 days	Non-responders: 1. Tinidazole 1 g b.i.d. for 6 days 2. Ornidazole 500 mg q.i.d. for 5 days 3. Metronidazole 750 mg t.i.d. for 3–5 days Polyresistant giardiasis: 1. Albendazole 10–15 mg/kg/d for 3 days + Nimorazole 1 g b.i.d. for 5–7 days 2. Nitazoxanide 500 mg b.i.d. for 3 days
Isospora belli	Infection is usually self-limiting; otherwise TMP 160 mg + SMZ 800 mg q.i.d., for 10 days followed by TMP 160 mg + SMZ 800 mg b.i.d. for 20 days	
Microsporidiae	Efficacious HAART will result in parasite clearance	Albendazole 400 mg b.i.d. for 20 days *E. bieneusi*: Fumagillin 20 mg t.i.d., 2 weeks[59]

sufficiently sensitive. The question whether a positive copro-antigen test in a patient negative at stool microscopy should be regarded as a false-positive result due to cross-reaction with other fecal antigens or as a true positive result with falsely negative microscopy is not yet solved, although some studies suggest that the latter assumption is correct.[7,8,25–28] Sensitivity of some copro-antigen tests increases if the test is repeated on another stool specimen and may be influenced by the preservative added to the stool specimen.[28,29] PCR techniques for *Giardia*-specific DNA are being validated. The increased frequency of gastrointestinal symptoms persisting for months after cure of a bacterial gastro-enteritis may be due to occult *Giardia* coinfection.[30] Therefore, in highly suspicious cases, empiric treatment is justified. Tinidazole and ornidazole are more effective than metronidazole. In multiresistance, prolonged tinidazole treatment or combined therapy with a nitro-imidazole+albendazole may be effective (see Table 52.1).[31–33]

Other intestinal protozoa

Balantidium coli, a common ciliated protozoan of pigs, is rarely transmitted to humans, where it can cause chronic recurrent or severe acute diarrhea. *Cyclospora cayetanensis* causes prolonged nonbloody diarrhea and should be suspected when *G. intestinalis* has been ruled out. Facultative pathogens in immunocompe-tent hosts include *Blastocystis hominis*, *Dientamoeba fragilis*, *Cryptosporidium parvum*, microsporidia (*Enterocytozoon bieneusi*, *Encephalitozoon hellem*, *E. intestinalis*, and *E. cuniculi*), *Isospora belli*, *Sarcocystis bovihominis*, and *Sarcocystis suihominis*. In immunocompromised hosts, especially in AIDS patients, these protozoa may cause chronic profuse diarrhea and wasting, sclerosing cholangitis, and acalculous cholecystitis. No treatment is required to eliminate nonpathogenic protozoa, e.g., *Entamoeba coli*, *E. hartmanni*, *Endolimax nana*, and *Iodamoeba bütschlii* from the intestinal tract.

HELMINTHIC INFECTIONS

Intestinal helminthic infections occur worldwide and are related to precarious hygienic conditions. Some of them are restricted to tropical regions because the worms or their intermediate hosts require specific climatic conditions. Suspicion is raised by *exposure*, either by travel to endemic areas or by the ingestion of contaminated food, e.g., marinated or uncooked fish in fish tapeworm infection and anisakiasis. Usually, worms are unable to multiply inside the same host. Therefore, the parasite burden depends on the quantity of worms acquired. Whereas *Ascaris lumbricoides* has a lifespan of less than 2 years, schistosomes may survive for more than 2 decades. Pinworm infection and strongyloidiasis may persist for years because of the possibility of auto-reinfection of the human host who becomes infected by larvae or ova excreted by adult worms harbored in their own intestine.

Symptoms of helminthic infections

Symptoms of intestinal helminthic infections are multifaceted. Most cases with light infections are asymptomatic. *Epigastric pain* occurs in anisakiasis, whereas *diarrhea* and *abdominal cramps* predominate in strongyloidiasis and ascariasis. Excretion of *bloody stools* not accompanied by fever is seen in severe trichuriasis and intestinal schistosomiasis. Intestinal obstruction, abdominal masses, and rectal prolapse may occur in ascariasis and schistosomiasis. Intermittent *biliary obstruction* occurs in fluke infections and ascariasis. Fluke infections occur worldwide but are particularly frequent in Asian countries due to particular alimentary habits. These infections may cause malaise, recurrent cholangitis, biliary calculi, life-threatening bile duct perforation, intra-abdominal hemorrhages and cholangiocarcinoma.[34-36] Indolent gallbladder wall thickening occurs in schistosomiasis. *Hepatosplenomegaly* occurs during larval migration. Periportal and network hepatic fibrosis with portal hypertension occur in hepatosplenic schistosomiasis, which may be complicated by pulmonary hypertension.[37] Macrocytic *anemia* is due to vitamin B$_{12}$ deficiency in fish tapeworm infection, while microcytic anemia is secondary to iron loss in hookworm infection, severe trichuriasis and intestinal schistosomiasis. In developing countries *impaired school performance*, *growth retardation*, and *delayed sexual development* have been related to intestinal worm infections. *Cutaneous manifestations* may resemble allergic rashes, e.g., non-specific urticarial rashes in larval invasion stages. 'Swimmer's itch' is caused by schistosome cercariae. Creeping eruption occurs in cutaneous larva migrans and strongyloidiasis ('larva currens'). Perianal itching is particularly intense in pinworm infection. *Vulvitis* and *adnexitis* may occur in pinworm infection and schistosomiasis. *Scrotal swelling* may be due to intestinal schistosomes.[38] In immunocompromised individuals worm infections may become *generalized*, e.g. *Strongyloides* hyperinfection syndrome. Dry *cough* and migrating pulmonary ('Loeffler') infiltrates are caused by migrating worm larvae, e.g., in ascariasis and strongyloidiasis. Focal symptoms due to *central nervous system* and *ocular involvement* occur in visceral larva migrans, ectopic fluke infections, neuroschistosomiasis, and cysticercosis.[34,37] Neurocysticercosis is life-threatening, and ocular cysticercosis may result in loss of vision. Exposure to other animal tapeworms may result in cystic (*E. granulosus*), polycystic (*E. vogeli*, *E. oligarthrus*) or alveolar echinococcosis (*E. multilocularis*).[39-41]

Therapy of helminthic infections

Modern chemotherapy is usually very effective, and frequently a worm infection is eradicated by a single-dose regimen. In acute infections and some ectopic infections, antiparasitic chemotherapy must be accompanied by corticosteroids to avoid severe systemic adverse events due to the massive antigen presentation resulting from worm death (Table 52.2).

All *roundworms* pathogenic to humans are sensitive to two broad-spectrum drug classes: benzimidazoles and avermectins. Cure of most intestinal nematode infections is achieved by albendazole. Ivermectin is more efficient in strongyloidiasis. Patients with *Strongyloides* hyperinfection syndrome due to HTLV infection or other causes of immunosuppression may require high doses and repeated courses of ivermectin. Care must be taken to avoid auto-reinfection in strongyloidiasis and pinworm infection: pinworm ova may be reingested either with fingers contaminated by scratching the perianal region or after inhalation ('dust-eggs') and subsequent ingestion via the oropharynx. Clothes and blankets must be washed at a temperature of 60°C for 30 minutes at least.

The spectrum of praziquantel includes all *flatworm* infections except *Fasciola* spp. Care must be taken in patients with infection by adult *Taenia solium* to avoid accidental autoinfection resulting in cysticercosis.

Follow-up after therapy

At least three stool samples 2–8 weeks after the end of chemotherapy should be examined. In amebiasis, follow-up examinations must also include abdominal ultrasonography and serology. In pork tapeworm infection, monitoring of eosinophils, serology, and cranial computed tomography are required to rule out concomitant cysticercosis.

PRINCIPAL INDICATIONS, ADVERSE EVENTS, AND CONTRAINDICATIONS OF ANTIPARASITIC DRUGS

Avermectins

Ivermectin, the only avermectin used in humans, is highly efficacious against nematodes, e.g., microfilariae, *S. stercoralis*, *A. lumbricoides*, *Toxocara* spp. and some ectoparasites, especially scabies. Adverse events observed during ivermectin therapy are due to the stimulation of the immune system by dying larvae and not drug toxicity.

Benzimidazoles

Benzimidazoles are usually absorbed best (up to five times better) if taken after a fatty meal. *Albendazole* has a rapid tissue diffusion and a broad spectrum not only against some larval and adult nematodes (hookworms, *A. lumbricoides*, *Loa loa* filariae) but also against the metacestode stage of human cestodes. It is the drug of choice for cysticercosis and echinococcosis. It has some antiprotozoal activity against *G. intestinalis* and the microsporidia *Encephalitozoon* spp. The most important adverse events are reversible hepatitis and bone marrow depression.

Mebendazole is less well absorbed from the intestine than albendazole. It is cheap and particularly useful in intestinal nematode infections, e.g., pinworm, whipworm, and hookworm infections.

Treatment of Intestinal Parasitic Diseases

Table 52.2 Treatment of intestinal helminths

Organism	Drug of choice and dose	Alternative
Angiostrongylus	Prednisone 40–60 mg/kg/d for 3–5 days than tapered + albendazole 7.5 mg/kg b.i.d. for 6 days	Helminths die spontaneously within months, sometimes surgery required
Anisakis spp.	Endoscopic or surgical removal	Albendazole 400 mg b.i.d. for 3 days
Ascaris lumbricoides	Mebendazole 100 mg b.i.d. for 3 days	1. Albendazole 500 mg once 2. Pyrantel 10 mg base/kg once 3. Piperazine 75 mg/kg once for 2–4 days 4. Levamisole 150 mg once
Capillaria philippinensis	Albendazole 200 mg b.i.d. for 10 days	Mebendazole 200 mg b.i.d. for 20 days
Enterobius vermicularis	Mebendazole 100 mg once, repeated after 3 and 6 weeks. In reinfection, treat the whole family or cluster at the same time. Hygienic measures	Pyrvinium 5 mg base/kg once, or pyrantel 10 mg base/kg once as suspension or tablet; repeated after 3 and 6 weeks
Hookworms	Mebendazole 100 mg t.i.d. for 3 days	1. Albendazole 200 mg/d for 3 days 2. Pyrantel embonate 10 mg/kg/d for 3 days
Oesophagostoma bifurcum	Albendazole 5 mg/kg b.i.d. for 5 days	
Strongyloides stercoralis	Ivermectine 0.2 mg/kg/d for 2 days Hyperinfection syndrome: ivermectine 0.2–0.4 mg/kg/d for 2 days, repeated after 2 weeks. Sometimes higher doses and/or combination with albendazole required	1. Albendazole 400 mg b.i.d. for 3 days 2. Mebendazole 200 mg t.i.d. for 3 days
Toxocara catis/canis Cutaneous larva migrans Visceral larva migrans	Topical application of thiabendazole 2% (1 g) + triamcinolone-acetonide 0.1% (0.05 g) + unguentum emulsificans aquosum at 50.0 b.i.d. for 7–10 days Albendazole 7.5 mg/kg/d b.i.d. for 5 days CAVE: do not treat before exclusion of ocular toxocariasis. In case of ocular toxocariasis this must be treated by an experienced ophthalmologist! Corticosteroids may be required to mitigate allergic phenomena during antiparasitic therapy	Albendazole 400 mg/d, for 1–3 days 1. Ivermectin 0.2 mg/kg once or 2. Diethylcarbamazine 0.5 mg/kg/d increasing to 3 mg/kg/d during 7 days
Trichinella spiralis	Prednisone 40–60 mg/kg/d for 3–5 days than tapered + albendazole 7.5 mg/kg b.i.d. for 6 days	Prednisone 40–60 mg/kg/d for 3–5 days then tapered + mebendazole 200–400 mg t.i.d. for 3 days, than 400 mg–500 mg/d for 10 days
Trichostrongylus spp.	Mebendazole 100 mg t.i.d. for 3 days	1. Levamisole 2.5 mg/kg once or 2. Pyrantel embonate 10 mg/kg/d for 3 days
Trichuris trichiura	Mebendazole 100 mg b.i.d. for 3–6 days	1. Albendazole 400 mg/d, for 3 days 2. Oxantel 10 mg/kg once
Flatworms		
Clonorchis sinensis	Praziquantel 25 mg/kg b.i.d. for 1 day	Praziquantel 50 mg/kg once
Diphyllobotrium latum	Praziquantel 10 mg/kg once	Niclosamide 2 g once
Fasciola spp.	Triclabendazole 10 mg/kg once or repeated after 12 h. In acute fascioliasis corticosteroids; in chronic-latent fascioliasis spasmolytics may be required	Bithionol 30–50 mg every other day for 10–15 doses (less effective than triclabendazole)
Fasciolopsis buskii	Praziquantel 15 mg/kg once	
Heterophyes spp.	Praziquantel 20 mg/kg once	
Hymenolepis spp..	Praziquantel 25 mg/kg once	Niclosamide 2 g on day 1, than 1g/d on days 2–7
Opistorchis spp.	Praziquantel 25 mg/kg b.i.d. for 1 day	Praziquantel 50 mg/kg once
Paragonimus spp.	Triclabendazole 10 mg/kg	Praziquantel 25 mg/kg t.i.d. for 3 days
Schistosoma haematobium, Schistosoma intercalatum	Praziquantel 40 mg/kg once	S. haematobium: metrifonate 7.5 mg/kg once repeated after 2 and 4 weeks

Table 52.2 Treatment of intestinal helminths—Cont'd

Organism	Drug of choice and dose	Alternative
Schistosoma mansoni	Praziquantel 40 mg/kg single dose for 1–3 days	Oxamniquine 15–20 mg/kg once or for 2 days
Schistosoma japonicum, Schistosoma mekongi	Praziquantel 30 mg/kg b.i.d. for 1 or 2 days	
Acute schistosomiasis	Severe cases: Prednisone 1 mg/kg/d for 1 week, followed by 0.5 mg/kg/d, and 0.25 mg/kg/d for 1 week. In mild cases, antihistaminics may be sufficient. One day after initiation of prednisone therapy: praziquantel 30 mg/kg b.i.d. for 1 or 2 days, repeated after 6 weeks	Artesunate 50 mg b.i.d., for 5 days (usually not sufficient if therapy is not combined with praziquantel)
Taenia spp.	Praziquantel 10 mg/kg once	Niclosamide 2 g once
Cysticercosis	Albendazole 7.5 mg/kg b.i.d. for 14 days. In cerebral cysticercosis coverage with corticosteroids required, antiepileptic drugs may be necessary. In ocular cysticercosis treatment by an experienced oculist. Antiparasitic treatment may worsen ocular cysticercosis	Praziquantel 50 mg/kg/d in 3 divided doses for 15 days

It has been replaced by albendazole in the treatment of echinococcosis but constitutes an alternative in albendazole hepatitis.

Thiabendazole, due to its side effects, is no longer available for enteral use and has been replaced by albendazole. It is used for topical therapy against cutaneous larva migrans.

Triclabendazole is the drug of choice for trematode infections due to the large liver flukes *Fasciola hepatica*, *F. gigantica*, and the lung flukes *Paragonimus* spp. Its side effects are due to its efficacy rather than to pharmacological toxicity: biliary colics due to the expulsion of liver flukes or parasite fragments through the biliary tract. Triclabendazole is available through the WHO.[35, 42–44]

Nitroimidazoles

Nitroimidazoles are effective against a large spectrum of protozoa, such as *Trichomonas* spp., *E. histolytica*, *G. intestinalis*, *Blastocystis hominis*.

The broad spectrum of *metronidazole* also includes anaerobic bacteria. Adverse events after metronidazole therapy include neurotoxicity and a disulfiram effect. Due to the widespread use and subsequent selection of resistant *G. intestinalis* strains, in giardiasis, metronidazole is less effective than other nitroimidazoles.

Ornidazole is available in Switzerland.

Nimorazole:[45] the author has successfully eradicated multiresistant giardiasis several times by a combined nimorazole-albendazole therapy.

Tinidazole is the drug of choice for treating *G. intestinalis*. It is better tolerated than metronidazole. Tinidazole has recently been approved for use in the United States.

Praziquantel

The wide spectrum of praziquantel includes all adult flatworms except *Fasciola* spp., cysticerci, and echinococcus scolices.[41] Praziquantel at a daily dosage of 60 mg/kg for 3 days will eradicate all infections by adult flatworms except fascioliasis (see Tables 52.1, 52.2). It is very well tolerated, the most frequent adverse events being related to worm death (exacerbation of eosinophilic febrile syndrome, abdominal cramps).

Other antiparasitic drugs

Artesunate

Artesunate, a derivate of *Artemisia annua*, is an excellent antimalarial with activity also on the early larval stages of schistosomes. It may be added to praziquantel for treating acute schistosomiasis and to prevent schistosomal (re-)infection.[46,47]

Bithionol

Bithionol has been the drug of choice for treating fascioliasis until the advent of triclabendazole. Due to its toxicity and necessity of a multidose regimen its indication is restricted to true triclabendazole-resistant fascioliasis or when triclabendazole is not available.[34,35]

Diethylcarbamazine

Diethylcarbamazine (DEC) was the antifilarial drug of choice until the advent of ivermectin. It is an option to treat visceral larva migrans during pregnancy.

Diloxanide furoate

Diloxanide furoate is an intraintestinal amebicide but appears to be less efficacious than paromomycin in eradicating intestinal *E. histolytica* (see below).

Iodoquinol

The most important adverse event of this well-tolerated drug is neurotoxicity. It is contraindicated in thyroid disease.

Levamisole

Levamisole is used in oncology and as an antiparasitic drug. The side effects described in oncology are rare when the low dosages against intestinal helminths such as hookworms are prescribed. It may be given as a suspension in children younger than 2 years.

Niclosamide

Niclosamide is a taenicide which may be given when praziquantel is not available or too expensive. Care has to be taken to exclude concomitant cysticercosis.

Nitazoxanide

Nitazoxanide is registered for cryptosporidiasis in the US. The main adverse events are gastrointestinal. Further studies on its efficacy against *F. hepatica*, *G. intestinalis*, *I. belli*, *T. trichiura*, *H. nana* and *T. saginata* are warranted.[48–50]

Oxamniquine

Oxamniquine has been the mainstay of schistosomiasis control in South America. It is being replaced by praziquantel because of increasing resistance of South American strains of *S. mansoni* and because praziquantel is becoming less expensive than oxamniquine. However, production of oxamniquine should be maintained because of the threat of praziquantel resistance which may arise, due to the increasing use of the latter drug worldwide.[51,52]

Paromomycin

Paromomycin is a topical intraluminal aminoglycoside. Its spectrum includes intraintestinal amebae, anaerobic bacteria, and to a minor extent *G. intestinalis*. The observation that paromomycin is more effective in eradicating intraluminal *E. histolytica s.s.* than diloxanide furoate awaits confirmation in a higher number of patients and other regions than Viet Nam.[53]

Piperazine

Piperazine may be given in intestinal nematode infections such as enterobiasis and ascariasis. It is contraindicated in patients with history of convulsions.

Pyrvinium embonate

Pyrvinium embonate may be given as a suspension and is therefore an alternative for treating enterobiasis in small children from the age of 3 months on.

Pyrantel and oxantel

Pyrantel salts (embonate and pamoate), as well as oxantel, are widely used in veterinary medicine. Although less effective than mebendazole, pyrantel may be used for enterobiasis. Pyrantel is not indicated in children younger than 2 years. Oxantel is not yet approved for human use.

Tetracycline

For gastrointestinal protozoa tetracycline, *not* doxycycline or other derivatives is used, because tetracycline is better concentrated inside the intestinal lumen. Its main collateral effects are photosensitization and mucosal fungal infections. Tetracyclines are contraindicated in children younger than 8 years.

TMP+SMZ

TMP+SMZ is effective in some intestinal protozoal infections, e.g., cyclosporiasis. Contraindications and side effects are not discussed here.

PREGNANCY AND LACTATION

Principally, during *pregnancy* and *lactation*, any kind of drug should be avoided. Since in a number of antiparasitic drugs data on mutagenicity and embryotoxicity are lacking and, on the other hand, many intestinal worm infections are mild and not immediately threatening, therapy may often be postponed until after delivery. On the other hand, in severe invasive amebiasis and acute fascioliasis the risk for mother and fetus by the disease frequently outweighs the theoretical risk of drug therapy during pregnancy. For classification of each drug, see FDA recommendations and references.[54–58]

SUMMARY

An intestinal parasitic disease is to be suspected in every person coming from highly endemic areas or otherwise exposed. Many infections are asymptomatic. Nonfebrile diarrhea may indicate gastrointestinal protozoa, whereas helminthic infections cause multifaceted clinical symptoms. Suspicion is raised by blood eosinophilia but its absence does not rule out a worm infection. Intestinal parasites are identified by repeated stool examinations and/or copro-antigen detection. Proper collection and examination of samples is essential. Parasitological investigations, being noninvasive, should precede invasive endoscopic investigations. Sometimes, differential empiric therapy, taking into account exposure, symptomatology and non-specific laboratory findings, is justified. This applies to high suspicion of giardiasis or helminthic infections during the prepatency stage. Well-tolerated broad-spectrum antiparasitic drugs, such as nitroimidazoles (protozoa), praziquantel (flatworms), ivermectin (roundworms, ectoparasites) and albendazole (roundworms, some flatworms, protozoa), are best suited and applied according to the synopsis of clinical findings obtained. A successful empiric treatment of occult giardiasis may preserve the patient from an odyssey of superfluous endoscopic investigations.

REFERENCES

1. Bouchet F, Petrequin F, Paicheler PC. First paleoparasitologic approach to the Neolithic site in Chalain, Jura, France. Bull Soc Path Exot 1995; 88:265–268.

2. Bouchet F. Recovery of helminth eggs from archeological excavations of the Grand Louvre (Paris). J Parasitol 1995; 81(5):785–787.

3. Gonçalves MLC, Silva VL, Andrade CM, et al. Amoebiasis distribution in the past: first steps using an immunoassay technique. Trans R Soc Trop Med Hyg 2004; 98:88–91.

4. Deelder AM, Miller RL, de Jonge N, et al. Detection of schistosome antigen in mummies. Lancet 1990; I:724–725.

5. Engels D, Sinzinkayo E, Gryseels B. Day-to-day egg count fluctuation in *Schistosoma mansoni* infection and its operational implications. Am J Trop Med Hyg 1996; 54:319–324.

6. Engels D, Sinzinkayo E, Gryseels B. Intraspecimen fecal egg count variation in *Schistosoma mansoni* infection. Am J Trop Med Hyg 1997; 57:571–577.

7. Farthing MJG, Cevallos AM, Kelly P. Intestinal protozoa. In: Cook GC, Zumla A, eds. Manson's tropical diseases. 21st edn. London: Saunders; 2002:1373–1430.

Comprehensive and detailed chapter on infections due to intestinal protozoa in the UK standard textbook of tropical medicine.

8. Goka AK, Rolston DD, Mathan VI, et al. The relative merits of faecal and duodenal juice microscopy in the diagnosis of giardiasis. Trans R Soc Trop Med Hyg 1990; 84(1):66–67.

9. Gupta SK, Croffie JM, Pfefferkorn MD, et al. Diagnostic yield of duodenal aspirate for *G. lamblia* and comparison to duodenal mucosal biopsies. Dig Dis Sci 2003; 48(3):605–607.

10. Brinkmann UK, Powollik W, Werler C, et al. An evaluation of sampling methods within communities and the validity of parasitological examination techniques in the field. Trop Med Parasitol 1988; 39:162–166.

11. Ritchie LS. An ether sedimentation technique for routine stool examinations. Bull US Army Med Dept 1948; 8:326.

12. Teesdale CH, Amin MA. Comparison of the Bell technique and a digestion method for the field diagnosis of schistosomiasis mansoni. J Helminthol 1970; 50:17–20.

13. Katz N, Chaves A, Pellegrino J. A simple device for quantitative thick smear technique in schistosomiasis mansoni. Rev Inst Med Trop S Paulo 1990; 14:97–100.

14. Marti HP, Escher E. SAF – an alternative fixation solution for parasitological specimens. Schweiz Med Wochenschr 1990; 120:1473–1476.

15. Lumbreras H, Cantella R, Bengra R. Acerca de un procedimiento de sedimentación rápida para investigar huevos de *Fasciola hepatica* en las heces, su evaluación y uso en el campo. Rev Med Peruana 1962; 31:167–174.

16. Cheesbrough M. District Laboratory practice in tropical countries. part 1: parasitology, clinical chemistry, management, quality control. Doddington, UK: Tropical Health Technology; 1998.

The standard textbook of laboratory diagnostics in tropical medicine and parasitology for the laboratory technician. Practical performance of methods is described in detail.

17. Harada Y, Mori O. A new method for culturing hook-worm. Trop Dis Bull 1956; 53:343.

18. Koga K, Kasuya S, Khamboonruang C, et al. A modified agar plate method for detection of *Strongyloides stercoralis*. Am J Trop Med Hyg 1991; 45(4):518–521.

19. Espino AM, Finlay CM. Sandwich enzyme linked immunosorbent assay for detection of excretory-secretory antigens in humans with fascioliasis. J Clin Microbiol 1994; 32:190–193.

20. Strickland GT, ed. Hunter's tropical medicine and emerging infectious diseases. 8th edn. London: WB Saunders; 2000.

The US standard textbook of tropical medicine.

21. Moody AH. Clinical laboratory diagnosis. In: Cook GC, Zumla A, eds. Manson's tropical diseases. 21st edn. London: WB Saunders; 2002:1615–1628.

22. Diamond LS, Clark CG. A redescription of *Entamoeba histolytica* Shaudinn, 1903 (amended Walker, 1911) separating it from *Entamoeba dispa* brumpt, 1925. J Euk. Microbiol 1993; 40:340–344.

23. Richter J, Hatz C, Häussinger D. Ultrasound in tropical and parasitic diseases. Lancet 2003; 362:900–902.

24. Mearin F, Roset M, Badia X, et al. Splitting irritable bowel syndrome: from original Rome to Rome II criteria. Am J Gastroenterol 2004; 99 (1):122–130.

25. Addiss DG, Mathews HM, Stewart JM, et al. Evaluation of a commercially available enzyme-linked immunosorbent assay for *Giardia lamblia* antigen in stool. J Clin Microbiol 1991; 29(6):1137–1142.

26. Aldeen WE, Carroll K, Robison A, et al. Comparison of nine commercially available enzyme-linked immunosorbent assays for detection of *Giardia lamblia* in fecal specimens. J Clin Microbiol 1998; 36(5):1338–1340.

27. Aziz H, Beck CE, Lux MF, et al. A comparison study of different methods used in the detection of *Giardia lamblia*. Clin Lab Sci 2001; 14(3):150–154.

28. Hanson KL, Cartwright CP. Use of an enzyme immunoassay does not eliminate the need to analyze multiple stool specimens for sensitive detection of *Giardia lamblia*. J Clin Microbiol 2001; 39(2):474–477.

29. Fedorko DP, Williams EC, Nelson NA, et al. Performance of three enzyme immunoassays and two direct fluorescence assays for detection of *Giardia lamblia* in stool specimens preserved in ECOFIX. J Clin Microbiol 2001; 38(7):2781–2783.

30. Neal KR, Hebden J, Spiller R. Prevalence of gastrointestinal symptoms six months after bacterial gastroenteritis and risk factors for development of the irritable bowel syndrome: postal survey of patients. Br Med J 1997; 314(7083):779–782.

31. Cacopardo B, Patamia I, Bonaccorso V, et al. Efficacia sinergica dell'associazione albendazolo-metronidazolo nella giardiasi refrattaria a monoterapia con metronidazolo. Clinica terapeutica 1995; 146:761–767.

32. Zaat JOM, Mank TG, Assendelft WJJ. A systematic review on the treatment of giardiasis. Trop Med Int Hlth 1997; 2(1):63–82.

Systematic review of all anglophone publications on the treatment of giardiasis until 1997.

33. Nash TE, Ohl CA, Thomas E, et al. Treatment of patients with refractory giardiasis. Clin Infect Dis 2001; 33:22–28.

34. Arjona R, Riancho JA, Aguado JM, et al. Fascioliasis in developed countries: a review of classic and aberrant forms of the disease. Medicine-Baltimore 1995; 74(1):13–23.

35. Richter J, Knipper M, Göbels K, et al. Fascioliasis. Curr Treatment Options Infect Dis 2002a; 4:313–317.

36. Mairiang E, Mairiang P. Clinical manifestations of opistorchiasis and treatment. Acta Trop 2003; 88:221–227.

37. Lambertucci JR. Schistosomiasis mansoni: pathological and clinical aspects. In: Jordan P, Webbe G, Sturrock RF, eds. Human schistosomiasis. Wallingford, Oxon, UK: CAB International; 1993:195–235.

38. Richter J, Stegemann U, Häussinger D. Hydrocele in a young boy with *Schistosoma mansoni* infection. Brit J Urol 2002b; 89:1–2.

39. D'Alessandro A. Polycystic echinococcosis in tropical America: *E. vogeli* and *E. oligarthrus*. Acta Trop 1997; 67:43–65.

40. Gottstein B, Reichen J. Echinococcosis/hydatidosis. In: Cook GC, Zumla A, eds. Manson's tropical diseases. 21st edn. London: WB Saunders; 2002:1561–1582.

41. Kern P. *Echinococcus granulosus* infection: clinical presentation, medical treatment and outcome. Langenbeck's Arch Surg 2003; 388:413–420.

42. Ripert C, Couprie B, Moyou R, et al. Therapeutic effect of triclabendazole in patients with paragonimiasis in Cameroon, a pilot study. Trans R Soc Trop Med Hyg 1992; 86:417.

43. Calvopiña M, Guderian RH, Paredes W, et al. Treatment of human pulmonary paragonimiasis with triclabendazole: clinical tolerance and drug efficacy. Trans R Soc Trop Med Hyg 1998; 92:566–569.

44. Millán JC, Mull R, Freise S, et al., and the Triclabendazole Study Group. Efficacy and tolerability of triclabendazol for the treatment of latent and chronic fascioliasis. Am J Trop Med Hyg 2000; 63:264–269.

45. Levi GC, de Avila CA, Amato Neto V. Efficacy of various drugs for treatment of giardiasis. A comparative study. Am J Trop Med Hyg. 1977; 26(3):564–565.

46. Li S, Swu L, Liu Z, et al. Studies on the prophylactic effect of artesunate on schistosomiasis japonica, Chin Med J 1996; 109:848–853.

47. De Clercq D, Vercruysse J, Verle P, et al. Efficacy of artesunate against *Schistosoma mansoni* infections in Richard Toll, Senegal. Trans R Soc Trop Med Hyg 2000; 94:90–91.

48. Rossignol JF, Abaza H, Friedman H. Successful treatment of human fascioliasis with nitazoxanide. Trans R Soc Trop Med Hyg 1998; 92:103–104.

49. Gilles HM, Hoffman PS. Treatment of intestinal parasitic infections: a review of nitazoxanide. Trends Parasitol 2002; 18(3):95–97.

50. Armadi B, Mwiya M, Musuku J, et al. Effect of nitazoxanide on morbidity and mortality in Zambian children with cryptosporidiosis: a randomised controlled trial. Lancet 2002; 360:1375–1380.

51. Stelma FF, Talla I, Sow S, et al. Efficacy and side effects of praziquantel in an endemic focus of *Schistosoma mansoni*. Am J Trop Med Hyg 1995; 53:167–170.

52. Cioli D. Chemotherapy of schistosomiasis: an update. Parasitol Today 1998; 14:418–422.

53. Blessmann J, Tannich E. Treatment of asymptomatic intestinal *Entamoeba histolytica* infection. N Engl J Med 2003; 347(17):1384.

54. Abdi YA, Gustafsson LL, Ericsson Ö, et al. Handbook for tropical parasitic infections. 2nd edn. London: Taylor & Francis; 1995.

Detailed description of most antiparasitic drugs used until 1995.

55. Gann PH, Neva FA, Gam AA. A randomized trial of single- and two-dose ivermectin versus thiabendazole for treatment of strongyloidiasis. J Infect Dis 1994; 169:1076–1079.

56. Datry A, Hilmasrsdottir I, Mayorga-Sagastume R, et al. Treatment of *Strongyloides stercoralis* infection with ivermectin compared with albendazole; results of an open study of 60 cases. Trans R Soc Trop Med Hyg 1994; 88:344–345.

57. Bradley M, Horton J. Assessing the risk of benzimidazole therapy during pregnancy. Trans R Soc Trop Med Hyg 2001; 95(1):737.

58. Olds GR. Administration of praziquantel to pregnant and lactating women. Acta Trop 2003; 86(2–3):185–195.

Reviews on the use of the most important antihelminthic drugs during pregnancy.

59. Molina JM, Tourneur M, Sarfati C, et al., Agence Nationale de Recherches sur le SIDA 090 Study Group. Fumagillin treatment of intestinal microsporidiosis. N Engl J Med 2002; 20;346(25): 1963–1969.

CHAPTER FIFTY-THREE

53

Treatment of eosinophilic gastroenteritis

James H. Caldwell

INTRODUCTION

Eosinophilic gastroenteritis (EGE) is defined as gastrointestinal tissue eosinophilia associated with digestive tract symptoms in the absence of other disease such as parasitic infection, classic inflammatory bowel disease, gastrointestinal or distant neoplasm, vasculitis, hypereosinophilic syndrome, etc. EGE has been reported in several hundred patients over six decades. About 50% of cases have some allergic association, such as atopic dermatitis, asthma or rhinitis, or allergy to foods or drugs. Earliest reports described an intense gastric eosinophilic inflammatory response to drug or food sensitivity or parasite infection, with radiologic diagnosis and surgical confirmation and treatment the rule. Since then, the clinical features and classification schemes, as well as the treatment options associated with this diagnosis have evolved, as the clinical features, natural history, area of gut involved, and presumed cause have changed. Early in the era of mucosal biopsy a mucosal form was recognized and separated from surgical cases causing obstruction or ascites.[1] Typical examples of this form involved the stomach and small bowel, and 'gastroenteritis' entered the literature as the most common example of the lesion. Emphasis on features of allergic gastroenteropathy in subsequent decades then dominated the literature but because of variable results with dietary approaches in early cases,[2,3] food allergy as an etiology was doubted and corticosteroids remained the mainstay of therapy in most collected series.[4,5] Recent developments that will be addressed in detail in this chapter include: (1) new evidence supporting food hypersensitivity as a cause of typical cases, with unequivocal responses to elimination or elemental diets; (2) growing recognition of eosinophilic esophagitis as a distinct but related entity, with evidence for food allergy versus gastroesophageal reflux disease offering different treatment opportunities; (3) preliminary results of new pharmacologic approaches, especially in eosinophilic esophagitis, with the promise of extension to other forms of eosinophilic gastrointestinal disease; and (4) new developments in understanding the pathogenesis of eosinophilic esophagitis (EE) and other eosinophilic gastrointestinal diseases (EGID) based on insights from new animal models.[6]

Epidemiology

EGE is worldwide in distribution and, with the exception of some unusual forms of intestinal parasitism which should not be mistaken for 'classic' EGE, most descriptions are similar regardless of nation of origin. Most reports suggest a slight to marked preponderance of males, depending on the age range, tissue involved, and incidence of allergy in the population studied. The growing literature on eosinophilic esophagitis has influenced the age range materially since most of these reports come from pediatric centers. Otherwise, the age range includes infancy to the elderly, with the majority of patients identified in childhood, adolescence, or early adulthood. Normal life expectancy is the rule, some cases are self-limited, and death from gastrointestinal crises is rare, especially in typical cases.

PATHOGENESIS AND ETIOLOGY

Food allergy

Early observations suggested a role for IgE-mediated food allergy in patients with EGE[7–9] but failed to account for the difference between this disease and food-mediated anaphylaxis. Studies of eosinophil cytokines suggested their involvement in activation and remission of EGE.[10,11] Rothenberg and coworkers have described animal models of eosinophil accumulation in esophagus and other digestive tissue in response to allergen sensitization that further our understanding of events and factors influencing eosinophil stimulation, tissue accumulation, blood eosinophilia, and the role of eosinophils in organ injury.[12] Mice challenged intranasally with *Aspergillus fumigatus* developed eotaxin and IL-5-dependent airway and esophageal eosinophilia, in contrast to those challenged by oral or intragastric allergen. These results establish a pathophysiological connection between allergic airway disease and eosinophilic esophagitis.[13] Similar studies using oral challenge with enteric-coated beads of ovalbumin result in esophageal, gastric, and small intestinal eosinophilia with pathological and clinical consequences, and demonstrate that oral antigen in the sensitized host is sufficient to produce eosinophilic inflammation of the digestive tract that, like experimental esophagitis, is influenced by eotaxin and IL-5.[14] Further study of human EGID using insights from these models should produce additional understanding of the role of food sensitization in these disorders and lead to advances in therapy.

Other etiologies

Many individual case reports of eosinophilic gastroenteritis meet the criteria described above but have no evidence for hypersensitivity to food allergens. Some are clearly drug reactions and are easily demonstrated.[15] Numerous individual reports from around the world, heavily weighted to patients presenting acutely with ascites, intestinal obstruction, or perforation, probably represent cases of unusual intestinal parasites or sensitization to other unidentified antigens.[16,17] Rare examples of diseases in transition to other illnesses or evolving to hypereosinophilic syndrome, and strictly pediatric conditions such as allergic eosinophilic colitis of infancy will not be discussed further in this chapter.

DIAGNOSIS

Clinical features include upper and lower gastrointestinal manifestations depending on the age of the patient as well as tissue layer and organ involved, and may include growth failure, regurgitation or gastroesophageal reflux, nausea and vomiting, dysphagia, abdominal pain, diarrhea, ascites, and evidence of intestinal obstruction. Peripheral blood eosinophilia is not required for diagnosis but is present to some degree in the majority of cases and is often an important clue to the diagnosis. Patients with mucosal disease often have iron deficiency anemia, hypoalbuminemia, and protein losing enteropathy, and the sedimentation rate may be normal or elevated. Stool examination for exclusion of parasitic disease may show Charcot-Leyden crystals. Radiographic studies may show proximal or midesophageal narrowing, enlarged gastric mucosal folds, thickening of small bowel mucosal folds, and luminal dilatation. Abdominal CT or ultrasound may demonstrate wall thickening, lymphadenopathy, or ascites. Except for EE (see below) endoscopic abnormalities in stomach and duodenum that would trigger biopsies or raise suspicion are not characteristic, but most diagnoses are made by endoscopic biopsies showing predominantly eosinophilic inflammation. Surgical specimens from full-thickness biopsies in cases not diagnosed at endoscopy may be required for histologic diagnosis.[18]

Differential diagnosis

Parasitic infection, drug reactions, systemic connective tissue disease and vasculitis syndromes, mastocytosis, inflammatory bowel disease, celiac disease, acid-peptic disease such as reflux esophagitis and gastric or duodenal ulcer, and hypereosinophilic syndrome should be excluded by appropriate study. These disorders may show mucosal eosinophilic infiltration not distinguishable from EGE on histologic grounds alone as there are no microscopic findings that are pathognomonic for EGE. The diagnosis can only be made by correlation of biopsy findings with the clinical context.[18]

TREATMENT OF EOSINOPHILIC GASTROENTERITIS

First we will consider 'classic' EGE as implied by the terminology in long use, that disorder also referred to as allergic gastroenteropathy which predominantly involves the stomach and small intestine, as this is still the form to which most clinicians refer when the term is used. The discussion of EE and its treatment follows as a separate topic because of the special considerations and issues concerning this form of EGID.

Diet therapy for eosinophilic gastroenteritis

Elimination diet

Complete remission in response to an elimination diet is strong supporting evidence for the role of food allergy in pathogenesis of EGE and this approach represents the most specific therapy.[19] Dietary treatment was generally regarded as ineffective in EGE until individual reports of well-studied individual cases with comprehensive allergic evaluations showed otherwise. A young man with milk allergy and eczema in infancy who developed typical features of proximal mucosal EGE with multiple positive skin tests for food antigens responded completely to a milk-free diet.[3] Another report documented reversal of eosinophilia, decrease in serum IgE, and symptomatic improvement in response to exclusion of beef, lamb, and pork in a 22-year-old man who had previously required intermittent systemic steroids since childhood to obtain remission of relapsing EGE.[9] The complexity of this problem in younger patients is exemplified by the landmark study by Katz and coworkers of a group of young children with iron deficiency, protein-losing enteropathy, and striking gastrointestinal eosinophilia.[20] The younger subgroup had normal IgE levels and responded to milk exclusion, while the older children who had more severe symptoms including growth failure, hyper-IgE, and systemic allergic symptoms failed on exclusion of a single dietary agent and required corticosteroid therapy. Although both groups had histologic criteria for EGE, a difference in response to elimination diet distinguished one group from another and suggested a fundamentally different immunologic response in these two groups. Although the collected experience with elimination diets based on available testing methods is mixed, and often unfavorable, the continued appearance of reports of successful treatment of individual adult cases with elimination diet based on conventional allergy evaluation suggests that this approach has value in selected patients.[21,22]

Elemental diet

Compelling results of elemental diet therapy were documented in an 18-year-old male with lifetime food allergy, corticosteroid dependent EGE, a history of food sensitivity with increased serum IgE and positive radioallergosorbent test for multiple foods, who failed therapy with elimination diet and oral cromolyn. This chronically ill young man became steroid free and growth failure reversed while on an elemental diet. He had been in remission for 22 months at the time of report.[23] Sicherer et al.[24] recently reported 31 children aged 6 months to 17 years, including 17 with cow's milk allergy and 14 with EGE and multiple food allergies (soy, egg, peanut, others). The EGE group, similar to the results of Katz et al.,[20] previously had not responded to milk elimination or to hydrolyzed formula diets. In contrast to the experience with elimination diet, elemental diet therapy in both groups allowed normal growth for up to 40 months. Serial laboratory evaluation showed significant reductions in percentage eosinophilia and increases in iron and hemoglobin in parallel with clinical improvement. Thus, in well-characterized EGE patients in whom there is convincing evidence of allergy to foods, the pathogenetic role of allergy is further established by the response to elimination diet. Reintroduction of specific food groups at intervals with clinical and endoscopic surveillance then allows for maintenance of remission or identification of relapse.[6]

Pharmacotherapy for eosinophilic gastroenteritis

Sodium cromoglicate (cromolyn)

Cromolyn is a histamine-1 receptor antagonist and mast cell-stabilizing drug used by inhalation in asthma and topically in allergic rhinitis and conjunctivitis. An oral form is available and is useful as an adjunct to dietary manipulation in some cases of food allergy[25-27] and in nonallergic conditions mediated by mast cell products.[28] These properties suggested a potential role in management of EGE, and published experience is mixed. Early reports of the use of cromolyn in cases thought to be EGE were negative and reviews concluded that there was no place for its use.[5] Two small series of cromolyn treatment in children and young adults have been published, showing that improvement could be maintained, and in some cases, steroids discontinued, with objective improvement in anemia, hypoalbuminemia, and growth failure.[29,30] In these uncontrolled, unblinded, observational studies, the typical responder was a young person with mucosal gastroenteritis, evidence for IgE mediated food allergy, and incomplete response to dietary elimination. Individual case reports continue to suggest a role for cromolyn in some steroid-dependent or steroid-resistant patients.[31-33] Recent authoritative reviews are divided on the role of this agent, probably reflecting variations in patient material, doses used, compliance issues or adverse experiences with therapy, and the absence of evidence-based data on which to base solid recommendations.[6,34] In addition, purely symptomatic improvement after cromolyn may be due to other than immunologic or biochemical mechanisms.[35]

Ketotifen

Ketotifen, a drug with similar properties to cromolyn sodium that is not available in the USA, has been reported to be beneficial in food allergy[36] and subsequently reported to be useful in patients with eosinophilic gastroenteritis and colitis.[37-39] Preliminary reports of usefulness in inflammatory bowel disease[40,41] suggest other antiinflammatory properties that have not been further described.

Leukotriene inhibitors

Use of these agents as a primary therapy or for steroid sparing seems an attractive possibility because of their usefulness in chronic management of reactive airway disease, and they are mentioned in current reviews of the topic.[6,34,42] Reported experience in EGE is extremely limited and with mixed results. Two patients with positive responses to montelukast have been described, one successful as primary therapy[43] and another for maintenance of steroid-induced remission.[44] A third patient, also steroid dependent with EGE and esophageal stricture, showed reduced peripheral blood eosinophilia but no endoscopic, histologic, or symptomatic improvement after 5 months of this therapy.[45] A single report of success with suplatast tosilate, not available in the USA, has appeared.[46] Since there is wide experience with these agents in airway disease and the safety profile and tolerability are well established, it is likely that additional reports of their use as primary or steroid replacing therapy for EGE will appear.

Corticosteroids

Nearly all reviews of EGE indicate that corticosteroid therapy is first-line treatment, that virtually all patients respond promptly, and that a short course has continued effectiveness in most patients.[1,5,18] A more recent development has been the appreciation and acknowledgment that recurrence is common, requiring repeated courses of steroid treatment or maintenance therapy. Lee et al.[47] reported 2–10-year follow-up of eight patients treated with steroids in doses similar to most of the literature (prednisolone 40 mg/day for initial therapy and 5–10 mg/day for maintenance). Of six patients available for evaluation, four required maintenance steroids. Of the six children reported by Katz et al.[20] who did not respond to milk exclusion, all required alternate day therapy for maintenance of remission during a follow-up of up to 12 years. The experience of 15 patients treated by Chen et al.[22] is representative, with 1 patient having spontaneous remission, another responding to elimination of seafood, and 13 responding to steroids within 2 weeks. Of 11 available for long-term follow-up, 5 relapsed and required re-treatment and 2 required maintenance low-dose prednisolone. These data are consistent with the landmark review of 220 cases published by Naylor.[4] In this report, 90% of patients responded rapidly to 20–40 mg prednisolone daily, 15% relapsed when steroids were tapered to a maintenance dose of 10 mg, and 55% relapsed after cessation of steroid therapy. In the absence of treatment alternatives, continuous, alternate day, or intermittent treatment has been the usual outcome in at least half of the cases of EGE. The risk of adverse effects of corticosteroid therapy is the principal reason for finding safer pharmacologic alternatives when dietary therapy is ineffective or poorly tolerated.[34]

Budesonide

The enteric-coated form of this unique corticosteroid is available for use in patients with ileal and right-sided colonic Crohn's disease. Its use is associated with reduced systemic steroid levels and consequently fewer systemic adverse effects and less adrenal suppression than with systemic steroids.[34] An early report of its application in EGE was in a patient whose disease resembled granulomatous enterocolitis[48] and the nonenteric-coated form originally available has been reported to be effective in maintaining remission in a patient otherwise dependent on prednisone.[49]

EOSINOPHILIC ESOPHAGITIS

Introduction

In an organ that normally does not contain eosinophils, esophageal eosinophilia occurs in a spectrum of diseases from GERD to hypereosinophilic syndrome.[50] Eosinophilic esophagitis (EE) was originally described as a component of EGE[51] and as a cause of dysphagia.[52,53] The radiologic and pathologic features of small series of cases emphasized proximal esophageal narrowing[54] and marked eosinophilic infiltration,[55] and it was speculated that this was an unusual manifestation of gastroesophageal reflux. Later endoscopic and radiologic series included predominantly allergic young male cases with similar features of esophageal eosinophilia regardless of whether there was other organ involvement[56] and in whom there was no evidence for gastroesophageal reflux.[57] Corticosteroid treatment and esophageal dilatation were the principal therapies described in these patients. Eosinophils as a marker of gastroesophageal reflux in esophageal biopsies were first described in children.[58] Consequently, symptoms of regurgitation, vomiting, poor feeding, and growth failure associated with this finding in infants and children with no other cause were also originally considered a manifestation of GERD in this age group.

Diagnosis and treatment

Beginning in 1995 with the landmark study of Kelly et al.[59] which showed improvement in EE attributed to gastroesophageal reflux in infants and children by feeding an elemental formula, the pediatric literature on this lesion has undergone explosive growth. Studies from several centers described a similar syndrome characterized by food hypersensitivity, absence of pH monitoring evidence of gastroesophageal reflux, and failure of medical or surgical antireflux therapy, in whom improvement with elemental or elimination diets or corticosteroids was the rule.[60–62] Radiologic study may show a small-caliber esophagus without a discrete stricture[63] in addition to subtle to marked narrowing, more often proximal than distal, as described above. Occasionally, webs and rings are found that predict some of the sentinel endoscopic findings. These include discrete white plaques,[64] granularity with rings or furrowing,[65] corrugated esophagus or multiple rings,[66] mucosal fragility[67] ('crepe-paper sign'), and a tendency to perforation or long mucosal tears during passage of the scope or as a result of dilatation.[63,67–69] Although a similar endoscopic and histologic appearance in adults has been regarded by some as evidence for gastroesophageal reflux disease, proof of GERD other than compatible histology has not been established. Most such patients are young men with dysphagia and recurrent food impactions without clinical symptoms such as pyrosis or manometric evidence of pathological acid reflux, who are reported to respond to acid suppression and esophageal dilatation.[70] In children, the degree of eosinophilia in number of cells per high-power field (eos/hpf) distinguishes between those who respond to antireflux therapy and those who require elimination diet or corticosteroids, so that the distinction between eosinophilia due to GERD and that of EE was established some years ago.[61,71] Similar criteria (i.e., >24–30 eos/hpf) have been applied by other investigators to the identical condition in adult patients who do not display features of pathological acid reflux and who are managed by dilatation only.[69,72] In addition, there may be some patients with EE in whom coexistent clinical features of GERD play a role so that empirical antireflux therapy combined with other treatments has been advocated.[6]

Dietary treatment of eosinophilic esophagitis

Elimination diets may be designed to restrict certain food groups by trial and error, or may be based on other evidence. Liacouras and coworkers have described the results of a trial in which 26 patients with EE followed restricted diets based on the results of skin prick and patch tests.[73] Milk and egg were the most common foods identified by prick tests and wheat the most common positive food by patch testing. Eighteen had complete and 6 had partial resolution of symptoms by restriction only of foods based on testing, and 2 were lost to follow-up. Esophageal eosinophil counts fell from a mean of 55.5 to 8.4 eos/hpf following dietary therapy. Similar results from the same investigators followed a few days of elemental diet in children and adolescents with EE.[74] In this study EE was rigorously defined during study of 346 patients with symptoms of GERD. Fifty-one had esophageal eosinophilia persisting after 3 months of proton pump inhibitor therapy, repeat EGD and biopsy, and exclusion of those with substantial abnormalities on 24-hour pH study. Symptoms improved significantly after an average of 8 days on the elemental diet, paralleled by esophageal eosinophil counts which fell from a mean of 33.7/hpf to 1.0/hpf after the diet. Although these short-term studies do not clarify the role of diet therapy in the long-term management of these patients, they do establish the role of food sensitivity in pathogenesis and the role of diet in initiating improvement. Furthermore, the allergy test results suggest that some patients may be managed by less than extremely restrictive diets if a single or small group of potentially offending foods is identified.

Pharmacotherapy of eosinophilic esophagitis

Following the demonstration that oral corticosteroids were effective in children with primary EE[61] similar results were achieved with inhaled steroids.[75] These results were extended by Teitelbaum et al., who showed resolution of symptoms with swallowed fluticasone propionate in 11 children who had poor results from antigen-specific diet restriction.[76] Post-treatment biopsies showed significant reduction in esophageal eosinophil counts. Lacking controlled trials, clinicians found that empirical combinations of elimination diets with cromolyn or steroids for resistance, breakthrough, or relapse were successful multimodal therapies for young patients.[65] Not every patient, especially the adolescent or adult, will tolerate long-term extreme dietary restrictions, and the personal experience of the author is that some patients identified in adulthood consider any major change in their self-selected diet to be more trouble than the illness, at least partly because so many adapt to chronic low-grade dysphagia during their early years. For these patients as well as those with initial responses to diet therapy and those who fail diet therapy, pharmacotherapy has appeal as long as it does not confer long-term risks.

Two recent uncontrolled but well-characterized series of consecutive adult patients suggest that effective medical options are available. A 28-month experience at the Mayo Clinic included 21 patients (17 men, 4 women, age range from 28–55 years at diagnosis but onset of symptoms as early as 12 years of age) characterized by chronic dysphagia and food impaction, compatible X-rays, ringed or small-caliber esophagus at endoscopy with >20 eosinophiles/hpf, and resistance to PPI therapy. Six weeks of topical corticosteroid therapy with fluticasone propionate, 220 micrograms/puff b.i.d., swallowed rather than inhaled and followed by a mouthful of water, relieved dysphagia in all patients within 2 weeks, with the duration of response lasting more than 12 months in most.[77] Eight patients with similar features were studied by another unit with long interest in EE.[78] Patients with endoscopic rings or furrows who averaged 56.9 eos/hpf on biopsy were chosen for therapy with montelukast because of prior improvement on steroids or failure of cromolyn or acid suppression therapy. All patients reported some improvement, with five of eight in complete remission on a maintenance dose of 20–40 mg/day, and all choosing to continue medication. Perhaps because there is a change in eosinophil effector activity but no change in numbers of tissue eosinophils with this treatment, relapse after discontinuation of therapy rather than durable response seems to be the rule. The role of this or other leukotriene inhibitors in EE, as in other EGID, as primary or steroid sparing therapy, remains to be established by appropriate controlled studies.

EMERGING THERAPIES FOR EOSINOPHILIC GASTROINTESTINAL DISEASES

Rothenberg has characterized the current clinical and research activity surrounding EE in children as a 'miniepidemic'[6] and the same can be said of adults.[79] A Medline search from 1966 to the present using 'eosinophilic esophagitis' as a search term disclosed a total of 79 references, with 52 of these appearing since 2000. The combination of greatly increased recognition or incidence and the availability of new agents has led to an array of new potential therapies for EE and other EGID. New agents that may be broadly useful in other hypereosinophilic states have the potential for application to EGID.[6] Imatinib mesylate, a tyrosine kinase inhibitor, which has been used in myeloproliferative HES,[80] could have a therapeutic role in gastrointestinal eosinophilic diseases. New approaches to cytokine antagonism include the humanized monoclonal antibody against IL-5, mepolizumab. A pilot study of this agent in four patients with hypereosinophilic syndromes included one patient with eosinophilic esophagitis who experienced striking reduction in tissue eosinophil counts in parallel with clinical and endoscopic improvement following anti-IL-5 infusion.[81]

Other therapeutic considerations

Many individual case reports in recent years confirm that patients meeting diagnostic criteria for EGE occasionally present with various kinds of acute abdominal problems,[16] with abdominal mass,[82] or with ulcer disease or gastric outlet obstruction.[83,84] No new therapeutic or etiologic insights come from these isolated reports. They emphasize the protean nature of disorders lumped under this diagnosis and the fact that some patients are eventually diagnosed only when surgically resected tissue is examined. Empirical antihelminthic therapy before corticosteroids has been advocated in some cases of idiopathic EGE that might be infectious because frequently no parasite can be identified in spite of

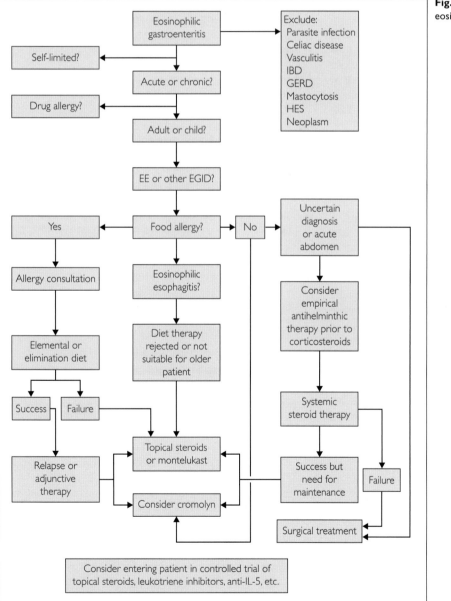

Fig. 53.1 • Algorithm for treatment of eosinophilic gastroenteritis.

multiple stool examinations and other studies.[18] Infections with *Ancylostoma, Enterobius, Eustoma, Toxocara, Strongyloides, Ascaris, Schistosoma,* and *Trichuris* can mimic idiopathic eosinophilic gastroenteritis. For example, a form of eosinophilic ileocolitis common in northeastern Australia was not thought to be infectious until the chance discovery of dog hookworm. A total of 79 affected patients, many of whom underwent exploratory laparotomy and resection for obstruction and uncertain diagnosis, were described, most with positive ELISA assays for *Ancylostoma caninum*.[85] In strongyloidiasis, the parasite most likely to cause chronic illness, empirical steroid therapy can lead to lethal systemic dissemination.[86] Our experience includes two patients in whom diarrhea, abdominal pain, fever, weight loss, and marked eosinophilic leukocytosis developed in middle age. In one patient, a resident of rural Appalachia with symptoms for 3 months and endoscopic evidence of tissue eosinophilia, multiple studies for parasitic infection remained negative. Prior to consideration of steroid therapy she received a 1-week course of mebendazole followed by complete remission. The second patient was seen postmortem after steroid therapy for cutaneous vasculitis was begun at an outside hospital. She was referred for evaluation of idiopathic EGE but died in our emergency department of disseminated sepsis with central nervous system involvement. Her skin lesions had developed after cleaning a basement after a septic tank leak and were not initially recognized as a sign of *Strongyloides* entry. Recent studies showing serologic evidence of *Ascaris*[87] or *Anisakis*[17] infection in cases thought to be 'idiopathic' emphasize the importance of considering occult parasitism in any case without other likely etiologic associations.

SUMMARY

There has been considerable progress since Kelly summed up the dilemma of EGID as 'can a 77-year-old woman with a 12-year history of intermittent cramping epigastric pain, vomiting, a 30 lb weight loss, ankle-swelling edema, diarrhea, a 30% peripheral eosinophil count, and an eosinophilic infiltration of the small intestinal mucosa have the same disease process as a 25-day-old girl with a 1-week history of nonprojectile, nonbilious vomiting, pylorospasm, and eosinophilic infiltration of the lamina propria and submucosa of the gastric antrum?'[88] The development of animal models and other advances in the biology of eosinophilia, plus the increasing prevalence and recognition of eosinophilic esophagitis, have led to new treatment opportunities for the whole family of eosinophilic diseases. A website has been established to act as a registry for patients, a source of information on eosinophilic diseases, and for the dissemination of information about available therapeutic trials.[50] Laching controlled trials to provide evidence-based approaches to treatment, an algorithmic representation of a decision-making approach to the therapy of EGID is shown in Figure 53.1.

REFERENCES

1. Klein NC, Hargrove L, Sleisenger MH, et al. Eosinophilic gastroenteritis. Medicine 1970; 49:299–318.

2. Leinbach GE, Rubin CE. Eosinophilic gastroenteritis: A simple reaction to food allergens? Gastroenterology 1970; 59:874–889.

3. Cello JP. Eosinophilic gastroenteritis – a complex disease entity. Am J Med 1978; 67:1097–1104.

4. Naylor AR. Eosinophilic gastroenteritis. Scott Med J 1990; 35: 163–165.

5. Talley NJ, Shorter RG, Phillips SF, et al. Eosinophilic gastroenteritis: a clinicopathological study of patients with disease of the mucosa, muscle layer, and subserosal tissues. Gut 1990; 31:54–58.

6. Rothenberg ME. Eosinophilic gastrointestinal disorders (EGID). J Allergy Clin Immunol 2004; 113(1):11–28.

   Excellent review with emphasis on pathogenesis of eosinophilia.

7. Greenberger NJ, Tennenbaum JI, Ruppert RD. Protein-losing enteropathy associated with gastrointestinal allergy. Am J Med 1967; 43:777–784.

8. Caldwell JH, Tennenbaum JI, Bronstein HA. Serum IgE in eosinophilic gastroenteritis. Response to intestinal challenge in two cases. N Engl J Med 1975; 292:1388–1390.

9. Verdaguer J, Corominas M, Bas J, et al. IgE antibodies against bovine serum albumin in a case of eosinophilic gastroenteritis. Allergy 1993; 38:542–546.

10. Takahashi T, Nakamura K, Nishikawa S, et al. Interleukin-5 in eosinophilic gastroenteritis. Am J Hematol 1992; 40:295–298.

11. Desremaux P, Bloget F, Seguy D, et al. Interleukin 3, granulocyte-macrophage colony-stimulating factor, and interleukin 5 in eosinophilic gastroenteritis. Gastroenterology 1996; 110:768–774.

12. Hogan SP, Foster PS, Rothenberg ME. Experimental analysis of eosinophil-associated gastrointestinal diseases. Curr Opinion Allergy Clin Immunol 2002; 2:239–248.

13. Mishra A, Hogan SP, Brandt EB, et al. An etiological role for aeroallergens and eosinophils in experimental esophagitis. J Clin Invest 2001; 107(1):83–90.

14. Hogan SP, Mishra A, Brandt EB, et al. A pathological function for eotaxin and eosinophils in eosinophilic gastrointestinal inflammation. Nature Immunol 2001; 2(4):1–8.

15. Lee JY, Medellin MV, Tumpkin C. Allergic reaction to gemfibozil manifesting as eosinophilic gastroenteritis. South Med J 2000; 93:807–808.

16. Tran D, Salloum L, Tshibaka C, et al. Eosinophilic gastroenteritis mimicking acute appendicitis. Am Surg 2000; 66:990–992.

17. del Pozo V, Arrieta I, Tunon T, et al. Immunopathogenesis of human gastrointestinal infection by Anisakis simplex. J Allergy Clin Immunol 1999; 104:637–643.

18. Talley NJ. Eosinophilic gastroenteritis. In: Feldman MF, Friedman LS, Sleisenger MH, eds. Sleisenger & Fordtrans' gastrointestinal and liver disease: pathophysiology/diagnosis/management. 7th edn. Philadelphia: Saunders; 2002:1972–1982.

   Comprehensive treatment in a widely available textbook.

19. Fahrenholz J, Simon R. Food allergy. Curr Treatment Options Gastroenterology 2002; 5:42–59.

20. Katz AJ, Twarog FJ, Zeiger RS, et al. Milk-sensitive and eosinophilic gastroenteropathy: similar clinical features with contrasting mechanisms and clinical course. J Allergy Clin Immunol 1984; 74:72–78.

21. Pfaffenbach B, Adamek RJ, Bethke B, et al. Eosinophilic gastroenteritis in food allergy. Z Gastroenterology 1996; 34(8):490–493.

22. Chen M-J, Chu C-H, Lin S-C, et al. Eosinophilic gastroenteritis: clinical experience with 15 patients. World J Gastroenterology 2003; 9(12):2813–2816.

23. Justinich C, Katz A, Gurbindo C, et al. Elemental diet improves steroid-dependent eosinophilic gastroenteritis and reverses growth failure. J Pediatr Gastroenterol Nutr 1996; 23:81–85.

24. Sicherer SH, Noone SA, Koerner CB, et al. Hypoallergenicity and efficacy of an amino acid-based formula in children with cow's

milk and multiple food hypersensitivities. J Pediatrics 2001; 138:688–693.

25. Gerrard JW. Oral cromoglycate: Its value in the treatment of adverse reactions to foods. Ann Allergy 1979; 2(3):135–138.

26. Edwards AM. Oral sodium cromoglycate: Its use in the management of food allergy. Clin Exp Allergy 1995; 25(Suppl 1):31–33.

27. Zur E, Kaczmarski M. Sodium cromoglycate in the treatment of food hypersensitivity in children under 3 years of age. Pol Merkuriusz Lek 2001; 11:228–232.

28. Soter NA, Austen KF, Wasserman SI. Oral disodium cromoglycate in the treatment of systemic mastocytosis. N Engl J Med 1979; 301:465–469.

29. Caldwell JH. Oral cromolyn therapy for allergic eosinophilic gastroenteritis. Gastroenterology 1984; 86:1038.

30. Whitington PF, Whitington GL. Eosinophilic gastroenteropathy in childhood. J Pediatr Gastroenterol Nutr 1988; 7:379–385.

31. Gioacchino MD, Pizzicannella NF, Falasca F, et al. Sodium cromoglycate in the treatment of eosinophilic gastroenteritis. Allergy 1990; 45:161–166.

32. Van Dellen RG, Lewis JC. Oral administration of cromolyn in a patient with protein-losing enteropathy, food allergy, and eosinophilic gastroenteritis. Mayo Clin Proc 1994; 69:441–444.

33. Perez-Millan A, Martin-Lorente JL, Lopez-Morante A, et al. Subserosal eosinophilic gastroenteritis treated efficaciously with sodium cromoglycate. Dig Dis Sci 1997; 42:342–344.

34. Khan S, Orenstein SR. Eosinophilic gastroenteritis: epidemiology, diagnosis and management. Paediatr Drugs 2002; 4:563–570.

35. Stefanini GF, Saggioro A, Alvisi V, et al. Oral cromolyn sodium in comparison with elimination diet in the irritable bowel syndrome, diarrheic type. Multicenter study of 428 patients. Scand J Gastroenterol 1995; 30(6):535–541.

36. Jay GT, Chow MSS. Focus on ketotifen: a long-acting, H-1 receptor blocker with mast cell stabilizing properties. Hosp Formul 1989; 24:632–645.

37. Melamed I, Feanny SF, Sherman PM, et al. Benefit of ketotifen in patients with eosinophilic gastroenteritis. Am J Med 1991; 90:310–314.

38. Moore D, Lichtman S, Lentz J, et al. Eosinophilic gastroenteritis presenting in an adolescent with isolated colonic involvement. Gut 1986; 27:1219–1222.

39. Katsinelos P, Pilpilidis I, Xiarchos P, et al. Oral administration of ketotifen in a patient with eosinophilic colitis and severe osteoporosis. Am J Gastroenterol 2002; 97(4):1072–1074.

40. Jones NL, Roifman CM, Griffiths AM, et al. Ketotifen therapy for acute ulcerative colitis in children: a pilot study. Dig Dis Sci 1998; 43(3):609–615.

41. Marshall JK, Irvine EJ. Ketotifen treatment of active colitis in patients with 5-aminosalicylate intolerance. Can J Gastroenterol 1998; 12(4):273–275.

42. Daneshjoo R, Talley NJ. Eosinophilic gastroenteritis. Curr Gastroenterol Rep 2002; 4(5):366–372.

43. Neustrom MR, Friesen C. Treatment of eosinophilic gastroenteritis with montelukast. J Allergy Clin Immunol 1999; 104:506.

44. Schwartz DA, Pardi DS, Murray JA. Use of montelukast as steroid-sparing agent for recurrent eosinophilic gastroenteritis. Dig Dis Sci 2001; 46(8):1787–1790.

45. Diakh BE, Ryan CK, Schwartz RH. Montelukast reduces peripheral blood eosinophilia but not tissue eosinophilia or symptoms in a patient with eosinophilic gastroenteritis and esophageal stricture. Ann Allergy Asthma Immunol 2003; 90(1):23–27.

46. Shirai T, Hashimoto D, Suzuki K, et al. Successful treatment of eosinophilic gastroenteritis with suplatast tosilate. J Allergy Clin Immunol 2001; 107(5):924–925.

47. Lee CM, Changchien CS, Chen PC, et al. Eosinophilic gastroenteritis: 10 years experience. Am J Gastroenterol 1993; 88:70–74.

48. Russell MG, Zeijen RN, Brummer RJ, et al. Eosinophilic enterocolitis diagnosed by means of technetium-99m albumin scintigraphy and treated with budesonide (CIR). Gut 1994; 35:1490–1492.

49. Tan AC, Kruimel JW, Naber TH. Eosinophilic gastroenteritis treated with non-enteric coated budesonide tablets. Eur J Gastroenterol Hepatol 2001; 13:425–427.

50. Rothenberg ME, Mishra A, Collins MH, et al. Pathogenesis and clinical features of eosinophilic esophagitis. J Allergy Clin Immunol 2001; 108(6): 891–894.

51. Dobbins JW, Sheahan DG, Behar J. Eosinophilic gastroenteritis with esophageal involvement. Gastroenterology 1977; 72:1312–1316.

52. Landres RT, Kuster GG, Strum WB. Eosinophilic esophagitis in a patient with vigorous achalasia. Gastroenterology 1978; 74:1298–1301.

53. Munch R, Kuhlmann U, Makek M, et al. Eosinophilic esophagitis, a rare manifestation of eosinophilic gastroenteritis. Schweiz Med Wochenschr 1982; 115:731–734.

54. Feczko PJ, Halpert RD, Zonca M. Radiographic abnormalities in eosinophilic esophagitis. Gastrointest Radiol 1985; 10:321–324.

55. Lee RG. Marked eosinophilia in esophageal mucosal biopsies. Am J Surg Pathol 1985; 9:475–479.

56. Vitellas KM, Bennett WF, Bova JG, et al. Idiopathic eosinophilic esophagitis. Radiology 1993; 186:789–793.

57. Attwood SEA, Smyrk TC, Demeester TR, et al. Esophageal eosinophilia with dysphagia. A distinct clinicopathological syndrome. Dig Dis Sci 1993; 38:109–116.

58. Winter HS, Madara JL, Stafford RJ, et al. Intraepithelial eosinophils: A new diagnostic criterion for reflux esophagitis. Gastroenterology 1982; 83:812–818.

59. Kelly KJ, Lazenby AJ, Rowe PC, et al. Eosinophilic esophagitis attributed to gastroesophageal reflux; improvement with an amino acid-based formula. Gastroenterology 1995; 109:1503–1512.

60. Cavataio F, Iacono G, Montalto G, et al. Gastroesophageal reflux associated with cow's milk allergy in infants: which diagnostic examinations are useful? Am J Gastroenterol 1996; 91:1215–1220.

61. Liacouras CA, Wenner WJ, Brown K, et al. Primary eosinophilic esophagitis in children: successful treatment with oral corticosteroids. J Pediatr Gastroenterol Nutr 1998; 26:380–385.

62. Liacouras CA, Markowitz JE. Eosinophilic esophagitis: a subset of eosinophilic gastroenteritis. Curr Gastroenterol Rep 1999; 1:253–258.

63. Vasilopoulos S, Murphy P, Auerbach A, et al. The small-caliber esophagus: an unappreciated cause of dysphagia for solids in patients with eosinophilic esophagitis. Gastrointest Endosc 2002; 55(1):99–106.

64. Straumann A, Spichtin HP, Bernoulli R, et al. Idiopathic eosinophilic esophagitis: a frequently overlooked disease with typical clinical aspects and discrete endoscopic findings. Schweiz Med Wochenschr 1994; 124:1419–1429.

65. Orenstein SR, Shalaby TM, Di Lorenzo C, et al. The spectrum of pediatric eosinophilic esophagitis beyond infancy: a clinical series of 30 children. Am J Gastroenterol 2000; 95:1422–1430.

66. Siafakas CG, Ryan CK, Brown MR, et al. Multiple esophageal rings: an association with eosinophilic esophagitis: case report and review of the literature. Am J Gastroenterol 2000; 95:1572–1575.

67. Straumann A, Rossi L, Simon H-U, et al. Fragility of the esophageal mucosa: a pathognomonic endoscopic sign of primary eosinophilic esophagitis? Gastrointest Endosc 2003; 57(3):407–412.

68. Kaplan M, Mutlu EA, Jakate S, et al. Endoscopy in eosinophilic esophagitis: 'feline' esophagus and perforation risk. Clin Gastroenterol Hepatol 2003; 1(6):433–437.

69. Croese J, Fairley SK, Masson JW, et al. Clinical and endoscopic features of eosinophilic esophagitis in adults. Gastrointest Endosc 2003; 58(4):516–522.

70. Morrow JB, Vargo JJ, Goldblum JR, et al. The ringed esophagus: histological features of GERD. Am J Gastroenterol 2001; 96(4):984–989.

71. Ruchelli E, Wenner W, Voytek T, et al. Severity of esophageal eosinophilia predicts response to conventional gastroesophageal reflux therapy. Pediatr Dev Pathol 1999; 2(1):15–18.

72. Straumann A, Spichtin H-P, Grize L, et al. Natural history of primary eosinophilic esophagitis: a follow-up of 30 adult patients for up to 11.5 years. Gastroenterology 2003;125(6):1660–1669.

Excellent review of long term experience and natural history of adult EE.

73. Spergel JM, Beausoleil JL, Mascarenhas M, et al. The use of skin prick tests and patch tests to identify causative foods in eosinophilic esophagitis. J Allergy Clin Immunol 2002; 109(2):363–368.

74. Markowitz JE, Spergel JM, Ruchelli E, et al. Elemental diet is an effective treatment for eosinophilic esophagitis in children and adolescents. Amer J Gastroenterol 2002; 98(4):777–782.

75. Faubion WA, Perrault J, Burgart LJ, et al. Treatment of eosinophilic esophagitis with inhaled corticosteroids. J Pediatr Gastroenterol Nutr 1998; 27(1):90–93.

76. Teitlebaum JE, Fox VL, Twarog FJ, et al. Eosinophilic esophagitis in children: immunopathological analysis and response to fluticasone propionate. Gastroenterology 2002; 122(5):1216–1225.

Detailed study of results and successes of topical steroid therapy in childhood EE.

77. Arora AS, Perrault J, Smyrk TC. Topical corticosteroid treatment of dysphagia due to eosinophilic esophagitis in adults. Mayo Clin Proc 2003; 78:830–835.

Well-described study of treatment of adult EE.

78. Attwood SEA, Lewis CJ, Bronder CS, et al. Eosinophilic esophagitis: a novel treatment using montelukast. Gut 2003; 52:181–185.

79. Potter JW, Saeian K, Staff D, et al. Eosinophilic esophagitis in adults: an emerging problem with unique esophageal features. Gastrointest Endosc 2004; 59(3):355–361.

80. Gleich GJ, Leiferman KM, Pardanani A, et al. Treatment of hypereosinophilic syndrome with imatinib mesilate. Lancet 2002; 359:1577–1578.

81. Garrett JK, Jameson SC, Thomson B, et al. Anti-interleukin-5 (mepolizumab) therapy for hypereosinophilic syndromes. J Allergy Clin Immunol 2004; 113(1):115–119.

Early description of a promising new therapy for eosinophilic diseases.

82. Shweiki E, West JC, Klena JW, et al. Eosinophilic gastroenteritis presenting as an obstructing cecal mass – a case report and review of the literature. Am J Gastroenterol 1999; 94:3644–3645.

83. Chaudhary R, Shrivastava RK, Mukhopadhyay HG, et al. Eosinophilic gastritis – an unusual cause of gastric outlet obstruction. Indian J Gastroenterol 2001; 20:110.

84. Markowitz JE, Russo P, Liacouras CA. Solitary duodenal ulcer: a new presentation of eosinophilic gastroenteritis. Gastrointest Endosc 2000; 52: 673–676.

85. Walker NI, Croese J, Clouston AD, et al. Eosinophilic enteritis in northeastern Australia. Pathology, association with *Ancylostoma caninum*, and implications. Am J Surg Pathol 1995; 19:328–337.

86. Martinez-Vasquez C, Gonzalez Mediero G, Nunez M, et al. *Strongyloides stercoralis* in the south of Galicia. An Med Interna 2003; 20(9):477–479.

87. Takeyama Y, Kamimura S, Suzumiya J, et al. Eosinophilic colitis with high antibody titre against *Ascaris suum*. J Gastroenterol Hepatol 1997; 12:204–206.

88. Kelly KJ. Eosinophilic gastroenteritis. J Pediatr Gastroenterol Nutr 2000; 30: S28–S35.

CHAPTER FIFTY-FOUR

54

Treatment of radiation-induced enterocolitis: a mechanistic approach

Alan B. R. Thomson, M. T. Clandinin and G. E. Wild

INTRODUCTION

A number of succinct and scholarly reviews have been published on the topic of the effects of radiation damage to the gastrointestinal tract.[1-11] Radiotherapy plays an important role in the curative and palliative treatment of many cancers, notably male and female genitourinary and gynecological malignancies, as well as Hodgkin's disease.[12,13] High-energy photons (>10 MeV) interact with normal tissues through their photoelectric and Compton effects.[14] Photons are electromagnetic waves that are absorbed by tissue, then release their energy to produce fast-moving electrons that subsequently damage normal as well as cancerous tissues. This is largely explained from the partial transfer of the photon energy to electrons, which are ejected from their orbit.[5] Free radicals are formed, such as hydroxyl radicals (OHX),[15] which result in single or double breaks in the DNA,[15] as well as damaging cell membranes[16] through the formation of free radicals from polyunsaturated fatty acids which are present in membrane phospholipids. The amount of energy absorbed after the interaction of the photon with tissue is termed the gray (Gy), defined as the energy absorption of 1 joule per kilogram; 1 Gy is the equivalent of 100 cGy. The total radiation dose is administered in small daily doses, or fractions.

MECHANISMS OF EFFECT OF RADIATION

The main cells damaged in the small intestine and colon are the stem cells in the crypts of Lieberkühn, from which the enterocytes or colonocytes, goblet cells, endocrine cells, Paneth cells or M cells develop. The enterocytes differentiate, migrate to the tip of the villus, then undergo apoptosis and are shed.[17] This process takes place in 5–6 days in the human small intestine. Apoptosis is enhanced by transforming growth factor B1 (TGF-B1), which is produced by radiation.[18] In the colon, TGF-B1 is expressed at the top of the colonic crypts, but the rate of apoptosis is slower in the large as compared with the small intestine. This is explained, at least in part, by the presence of the anti-apoptotic protein bcl-2 in the colon.[19] Furthermore, the rate of apoptosis increases with the dose of radiation, up to 100 cGy, as well as with the fraction size.[20] Radiation increases the expression of the tumor suppressor gene p53, as well as bcl-2 and TGF-B. The levels of the three isoforms of TGF-B are increased in the intestine early after radiation, but the TGF-B1 isoform remains elevated in endothelial and smooth muscle cells as well as in fibroblasts.[21] Following radiation, the percentage of S-phase cells in the crypts as well as the number of crypt cells is reduced, leading to cystic dilation of the crypts and villous atrophy.[22] If there is no further exposure, and if the radiation dose is not too high, crypt cell repair and recovery take place.

The threshold dose above which small bowel radiation complications occur[11,23] appears to be a dose of 4500 cGy. A total dose of 4500–5000 cGy in 180–200 cGy daily fractions can be delivered safely to a standard pelvic field, without causing significant damage to the small intestine.[24] Higher doses of radiation over short intervals administered to a large anatomic volume with a large fraction size contribute to an increased incidence of complications. The direct acute effect of radiation is thought to be cytotoxic, and an acute inflammatory reaction ensues.[25]

Biological actions of radiation

The biological alterations in response to radiation include hyperresponsiveness to secretagogues,[26] as well as increased electrical conductance, which is an indicator of increased epithelial permeability. This increase in permeability after radiation exposure is possibly related to reduced mast cell numbers,[27] or to increased nitric oxide (NO) from enhanced inducible NO synthase.[28] The absorption of nutrients may be impaired.[29-33] In addition, radiation leads to the generation in the small and large intestine of giant migrating contractions, but unaltered migrating motor complexes.[34,35] The cycle length of contractile waves becomes irregular, and aberrant pacemakers in the distal bowel initiate retrograde propagation, thereby resulting in nausea and vomiting.[8,36] The cause of the dysmotility is unknown, but may relate to alterations in various gut peptides such as vasoactive intestinal peptide (VIP), substance P, peptide YY, and motilin.[37] Serotonin may also be involved in the cholinergic hypersensitivity following radiation.[37,38]

CLINICAL PRESENTATIONS

The incidence of acute and chronic radiation enteritis may have increased in recent years because of the enhanced use of radiation as part of a multidisciplinary approach to patients with cancer.[39,40] Within hours to days, but usually by week 3, a substantial proportion of patients (20–70%) develop symptoms of acute radiation sickness, including nausea, vomiting, pain, or diarrhea. The incidence varies depending on characteristics related to the patient, or to the characteristics of the radiotherapy regimen, such as total dose or size of radiation fractions, radiotherapy technique, volume of tissue exposed, or previous concurrent use of chemotherapy.[41] Patient risk factors include previous abdominal surgery, diabetes, hypertension, congestive heart failure, and pelvic inflammatory disease.[41-48] Selective Cox-2 inhibitors enhance the effect of radiation on tumors that express COX-2, but not on Cox-2-lacking tumors.[49] A variety of chemotherapeutic agents enhance radiation effects, so it is not surprising that when chemotherapy is given during or immediately following radiation therapy, the risk of radiation enteritis is increased.[50]

The symptoms may sometimes be severe enough to require the interruption of radiotherapy, but usually these complications can be managed symptomatically (see below), and they resolve within weeks of the completion of therapy.[6,51] The only exception may be in the patient treated concurrently with radiotherapy, under which circumstance fatal sepsis may occur.[52] Retrospective studies suggest that the incidence of chronic radiation enteritis is 1.2–1.5%, and it usually occurs from weeks, months or years after the initiation of radiotherapy.[51,53,54] The development of chronic damage may be more likely to develop in patients who initially suffer from acute radiation damage,[55] suggesting that '...the incidence of adverse chronic effects is proportional to the severity of acute symptoms, implying that the early response to ionizing radiation in some way alters the physiology of the intestine such that it is more susceptible to triggers of inflammation.'[6] These symptoms have an adverse effect on the patient's quality of life, and may be more common than generally reported.[56]

Pathological changes

Pathologically, chronic radiation enteritis is characterized by an obliterative vasculitis, ischemia, fibrosis, telangiectasia and mucosal ulceration.[3,24,55,57] The pathology worsens, and there develops symptoms of hemorrhage, obstruction, perforation, fistulae, abscesses, and malabsorption.[58] In the late phases of radiation damage, arterioles, small arteries, and small veins show hyalinization and obliteration with fibrosis; long segments of intestine may become diffusely narrow, or a short segment may develop signs of concentric constriction.[59]

DIAGNOSIS

The diagnosis of acute radiation enteritis is suspected from the clinical presentation of gastrointestinal symptoms occurring soon after radiation. The possibility of chronic radiation damage must be considered with a high index of suspicion in anyone treated with previous radiotherapy, even when the treatment occurred years previously, because of the latency between radiation exposure and the development of symptoms. Diagnostic investigations are usually not necessary with suspected acute radiation damage. Because of the risk of perforation in the acute setting, colonoscopy must be done cautiously, if at all.[51] In chronic radiation enteritis, in contrast, colonoscopy may be useful to exclude tumor recurrence as a cause of the intestinal symptoms, and may be diagnostically useful with evidence of mucosal ulceration or hyperemia. Mucosal biopsies are useful. An enteroclysis is superior to a small bowel follow-through to demonstrate ulceration and thickening of folds, with a sensitivity and specificity of over 90% for chronic radiation enteritis.[60] A CT scan may be useful to diagnose an abdominal abscess or metastases.[61] If the CT scan is negative but the index of suspicion for an abscess is high, a gallium scan may prove to be useful.[62] In the patient suspected of having a small bowel obstruction, CT enteroclysis is 89% sensitive and 100% specific.[63,64]

RADIOTHERAPY TECHNIQUES TO PREVENT RADIATION DAMAGE

The single most important consideration for the prevention of radiation damage is the use of computerized dosimetry and three-dimensional techniques, with maximum doses administered to the target,[65] and a minimum volume of small bowel exposed to radiation.[66] The total radiation dose[67] and the irradiated volume of the small bowel[68] are major factors responsible for acute and chronic enteritis. Thus, the tolerance of the small bowel and bladder is one of the dose-limiting factors in treating cancer in the pelvis. A 'belly board' may be useful to reduce the volume of the small bowel within a high-dose region.[69] With the belly board, an opening in the top of the table allows the abdomen of the prone patient to fall, helping to displace the small bowel from the pelvis. This reduces the small bowel volume in the treatment portals by about two-thirds.[70] Also helpful is the use of distention of the bladder,[71] or bladder distention plus lower anterior abdominal wall compression with patients in the prone position.[68] A final approach to small bowel displacement is the production of a temporary pneumoperitoneum.[72] The clinical benefit of this approach has not been proven.

Pretreatment small bowel X-ray studies may be useful to modify the radiation regimen and to minimize small bowel complications.[23,73] Actual implementation of this concept was undertaken with a retrospective analysis showing that patients who were simulated with small bowel contrast had significantly fewer radiation-associated adverse effects.[74] This benefit is presumably the result of optimum treatment positioning, minimizing the volume of the small bowel irradiated within the pelvis.

Symptom control

Because acute radiation enteritis is usually of short duration, the patient's symptoms are managed conservatively by the appropriate use of antiemetics, antidiarrheals, and temporary removal of milk from the diet. Severe dehydration may require the use of intravenous replacement therapy, and severe bone marrow depression may require treatment with granulocyte colony stimulating factor (GCSF).[75] With the modern antiemetics, 5-HT$_3$ antagonists (such as ondansetron), the prevention and treatment of nausea is usually possible.[76] An outline of the management of early intestinal symptoms during radiation therapy is given in Table 54.1.

The approach to the patient with early and late radiation enteritis depends upon the nature of the complication (Tables 54.2, 54.3). For example, the malabsorption associated with bacterial overgrowth can be treated with a short course of antibiotics.[77,78] Chronic diarrhea not responding to antidiarrheals such as loperamide may require the use of bile salt binding agents if there is bile salt wastage as a result of ileal damage. In a randomized study, the probiotic *Lactobacillus acidophilus* reduced the incidence of diarrhea.[79] Ondansetron may also be used to reduce the diarrhea.[76] Acetylsalicylate[80] but not olsalazine[81] results in a

Table 54.1 Management of early intestinal symptoms during radiation therapy

Symptoms	Mild	Severe
Nausea, vomiting	**Antiemetics** **Primary** Ondansetron (Zofran); p.o., i.m., i.v. Granisetron (Kytril); p.o., i.v. **Secondary** Metoclopramide (Reglan); p.o., i.v. Trimethobenzamide (Tigan); p.o., i.m. Thiethylperazine (Torecan); i.m. Prochlorperazine (Compazine); p.o., i.m. Scopolamine (Transderm Scop); dermal patch Domperidone (not approved in the USA)	Same drugs plus altered radiation or decreased dose fraction size
Abdominal or rectal cramping and pain	**Antispasmotic, anticholinergics** Dicyclomine (Bentyl); p.o. Hyoscyamine (Levsin, Donnatol); p.o. Scopolamine (Transderm Scop, Donnataal); p.o. Clidinium (Librax); p.o. Glucopyrrolate (Robinul); p.o.	Same drugs plus altered radiation or decreased dose fraction size
	Analgesics and narcotics Acetominophen; p.o. Narcotics (e.g., codeine, meperidine (Demerol); p.o., i.m. Combinations (e.g., Vicodin, Percocet); p.o.	Same drugs plus altered radiation or decreased dose fraction size
Diarrhea	**Antidiarrheal drugs** Loperamide (Immodium); p.o. Diphenoxylate (Lomotil); p.o. Codeine, tincture of opium; p.o. Hydophilic mucilloid preparations; p.o. **Bile acid-sequestering agents** Cholestyramine (e.g., Questran); p.o. Avoid lactose, sorbitol, xylitol, mannitol, and the like in diet	
Tenesum, mucoid or bloody rectal discharge	Antispasmotic, anticholinergic drugs Sedatives Analgesics/narcotics Antidiarrheal drugs Warm sitz bath Low-residue diet	Same drugs plus altered radiation or decreased dose fraction size
Nutritional depletion	Oral elemental diet supplement or total parenteral nutrition	

significant reduction in stool frequency and associated cramping. Occasionally the diarrhea may be unresponsive, and a therapeutic trial with somotostatin or octreotide may prove to be efficacious.[82]

Nutritional support

Poor nutrition may increase the surgical morbidity and mortality.[83,84] For this reason, in patients with radiation enteritis, pre- and postoperative nutritional support is useful.[85] The malnutrition associated with chronic radiation enteritis may be treated with total parenteral nutrition (TPN), and may allow oral feeding to be resumed in about a third of patients. Bounous and coworkers have reported on the protective effect of an elemental diet given before ischemic injury, including a protective effect in patients treated with fluorouracil and during pelvic and abdominal sur-

gery.[86,87] Elemental diets may be protective against radiation injury to the bowel of dogs[88] and humans,[89] as studied in 20 patients fed these diets 3 days before and during radiotherapy given prior to radical cystectomy and ileal conduit for invasive bladder cancer.

When malnutrition is severe and the nutritional well-being of the patient cannot be maintained by oral intake, TPN may be necessary. Intestinal failure may result from extensive radiation injury and small bowel resections, leaving the patient in a situation where they may require home parenteral nutrition (HPN). In a randomized trial of 24 patients with severe radiation injury to the small bowel, nitrogen balance, serum albumin concentration, and small bowel radiographic score over the 8 weeks of the study were much better with TPN than with enteral nutrition with Vivonex-HN; as well, the addition of a daily intravenous dose of methylprednisolone enhanced the beneficial effect of TPN.[90]

Table 54.2 Management of symptomatic intermediate and late radiation enterocolitis

New onset or recurrent	General considerations/treatment
Nausea, vomiting, abdominal cramping pain	Barium radiographs or CT scan to evaluate for stricture, mechanical or functional obstruction, stasis, fistural, ischemia, or recurrent neoplasm Individualize treatment
Watery diarrhea	Hydrophilic mucilloids Antidiarrheal drugs Cholesytramine Avoid disaccharides; use lactase
Weight loss and diarrhea	Evaluate for steatorrhea Stasis with bacterial overgrowth Impaired ileal function Enteroenteric fistula Partial obstruction Recurrent neoplasm Treat underlying cause(s) as found: antibiotics, promotility drugs, medium-chain triglyceride, pancreatic enzymes, surgery, and so on
Symptomatic proctitis: Tenesmus, rectal pain or spasm, mucoid or serosanguinous discharge	Sedatives, analgesics, narcotics Anticholinergics, antispasmotics Warm sitz bath
Rectal incontinence	Antidiarrheal drugs Avoid lactose, sorbitol, and other disaccharides Hydrophilic muilloids Use of perineal pads Balneol lotion for anal irritation Colostomy as last resort
Rectal bleeding	Avoid enemas Iron replacement, transfusion as needed Consider ischemic process

In a retrospective study of 54 patients with radiation enteritis seen at the Mayo Clinic between 1975 and 1999, HPN was started within a median of 20 months (range, 2–432) from the date of radiation therapy.[39] The mean number of intestinal operations for radiation-related complications was 2.2 per patient (range, 0–6), and the causes of intestinal failure resulting from radiation therapy and requiring HPN were intestinal obstruction (27 patients), short bowel syndrome (17), malabsorption (5), fistula (3), and dysmotility (2). The mean duration of use of HPN was 20.4 months (range, 2–108). At last follow-up, 37 patients (68%) were dead, mostly as a result of recurrent cancer; one patient died of catheter sepsis. The overall estimated 5-year probability of survival on HPN, calculated by Kaplan-Meier analysis, was 75%. These rates of survival and complications associated with the use of HPN in patients with radiation enteritis are similar to those in the HPN-treated groups, except for patients with Crohn's disease, who have a better 5-year survival rate.[91]

MEDICATIONS

The mucosal cytoprotective agent, sucralfate, has been shown in a blinded, placebo-controlled study of 70 patients receiving curative-intent radiotherapy for cancer of the prostate or bladder to result in fewer acute or chronic changes of radiation enteritis.[92] Radiation proctitis does not respond well to the use of steroids,[93,94]

sulfasalazine,[95] transexamic acid,[96] or sulcrate enemas.[97] Hemorrhage is not usually severe, will often subside spontaneously, but occasionally may have a poor prognosis.[98] If conservative measures fail to control bleeding, persistent bleeding may require cautery, laser therapy, angiographic embolization, or for proctitis, the topical application of 4% formalin soaked in a gauze.[99–104]

In addition to attempting to prevent radiation enteritis by optimizing the radiotherapy technique, efforts have been made to use radioprotectants.[7] Amifostine (WR 2721) is a promising radiosensitizer. It is a sulfhydryl prodrug formed by membrane-bound alkaline phosphatase oxidation to a symmetrical disulfide or to mixed disulfides to an active metabolite which binds free radicals and stabilizes the DNA.[105–107] There are few adverse effects, and the therapeutic efficacy of the radiation treatment is not affected.[108–111] For example, in a randomized trial in 100 patients with unresectable or recurrent rectal cancer, amifostine given in a dose of 340 mg/m² 15 minutes before each whole-pelvis radiation treatment, the incidence of severe late radiation toxicity was significantly less ($p < 0.03$) in the treated as compared with the control group (0% versus 14%).[107] The WR 2721 appears to be protective out to 24 months, and it needs to be determined if this initial benefit is sustained for longer periods.[107] Amifostine works synergistically with GCSF to enhance hemopoietic reconstitution and to increase survival.[112] Interestingly, amifostine has no benefit for proctitis when delivered per rectum.[113]

Table 54.3 Summary of patient management

Radiation damage to the GI tract is common, occurs both early and late after therapy, and has a significant negative effect on the quality of the patient's life.

The late GI symptoms which develop after radiation treatment need to be investigated by colonoscopy, enteroclysis, CT scan, gallium scan and possibly CT enteroclysis, to exclude tumor recurrence, strictures, ulcers, abscesses and metastases.

Every effort is made to prevent radiation damage, such as by the use of computerized dosimetry and three-dimensional techniques, with maximum doses to the target and a minimum volume of small bowel exposed to radiation.

Treatment of symptoms such as with the use of antidiarrheals including loperamide and ondansetron (a 5-HT$_3$ antagonist), antiemetics, and dietary modifications (e.g., avoidance of milk, cheese, raw vegetables, and *Lactobacillus acidophilus*).

Treatment of specific complications such as diarrhea due to bacterial overgrowth, bile acid wastage, and mucositis with appropriate antibiotics, bile acid sequestering agent, and acetylsalicylate (rarely octreotide may be efficacious).

Nutritional support, including dietary counseling, nutrient supplements, enteral nutrition and occasionally TPN/home parenteral nutrition with or without supplemental methylprednisolone.

Sulcralfate for acute or chronic changes of radiation enteritis.

For persistent bleeding not responding to conservative measures, cautery, laser therapy, angiographic embolization, or 4% formalin topical application.

Consider use of radiosensitized amifostine (WR 2721).

Surgery for obstruction undertaken only when absolutely necessary.

Many patients enjoy benefit from 'complementary' or 'alternate' therapy.

Experimental approaches include hyperbaric oxygen, GLP-2, KGF, TGF-B.

SURGICAL CONSIDERATIONS

A common presentation of chronic radiation enteritis is subacute bowel obstruction arising from the development of a stricture. If this does not settle with temporary bowel rest, nasogastric suction, and intravenous fluid and electrolyte infusions, then surgery may be necessary. Because of the associated morbidity and mortality, surgery is undertaken only when absolutely necessary. This concern is because there is a risk of anastomotic leakage in about one person in two. It may be necessary to consider using intraoperative endoscopic examinations to distinguish between normal and radiation-damaged intestine to identify the appropriate resection margins.[114]

It remains an issue for debate whether intestinal resection or bypass is the optimal surgical approach.[115,116] In a retrospective evaluation of 90 patients from a single center (Freiburg, Germany), the postoperative morbidity was 44%, with a mortality rate of 22%.[117] In a retrospective analysis of the results from 88 patients from another center, postoperative complications occurred in 40%, with fatal outcome in 13%.[118] In a retrospective study from Springfield, Illinois, in 38 patients the morbidity was 45% and the postoperative mortality was 16%.[119] Shiraishi and coworkers[120] report a much higher risk of death for patients treated with intestinal decompression alone, as compared to decompression plus intestinal resection. In a recent retrospective analysis of 83 patients, 76 underwent resection with immediate anastomosis, mostly for obstructive symptoms.[121] In the remaining seven patients, a bypass or viscerolysis was performed. Postoperative mortality was 2.4%, and morbidity was 23%. Within 1 month

12 patients required reoperation, with a morbidity of 41%, whereas morbidity was 54% in the 15 patients who were operated upon later. The most frequent causes of morbidity were anastamotic leakage, wound infection, or intra-abdominal infection. Others have also reported the relentless nature of chronic radiation enteritis, with more than half of the patients who required surgical intervention having further symptoms.[122]

In a small number of patients, stricturoplasty with or without intestinal resection or bypass may serve as a tool to conserve intestinal length, particularly in those patients '...with limited intestinal reserve whose strictures are located within long segments of diseased bowel which, if resected or bypassed, would have significant nutritional or metabolic consequences.'[123] Surgical management of a pelvic fistula may first require a diversion colostomy, followed by a corrective surgical approach (Chapter 24). In rectal cancer patients treated with surgical resection and postoperative radiotherapy, retrospective analysis showed a numerical but not statistical reduction of small bowel obstruction.[124]

If radiation therapy is planned after surgery, the exposure of the small intestine to radiation may be lessened with the displacement of the bowel using various forms of biodegradable mesh.[125–127] In Devereux' series of 60 patients treated with the absorbable sling technique,[127] all patients received postoperative radiotherapy (mean dose, 5500 cGy) in fractions of 180–200 cGy/day;[126] at a mean follow-up of 28 months, no cases of radiation enteritis were seen, but unfortunately there was no control group for comparison. Dasmahapatra and Swaminathan[128] also reported no cases of radiation enteritis a mean of 34 months after placement of a mesh and radiotherapy (mean total dose of 5680 cGy), but again there was no control group. In the series by Rodier and coworkers,[127] radiation enteritis developed in 4 of 60 patients. Thus, the technique appears to be promising, but without a controlled study, the enthusiasm needs to be somewhat cautious. The use of nonirradiated bowel for at least one end of a surgical anastomosis in the patient with radiation enteritis improves the results of resection of the irradiated bowel.[129] The volume of the small bowel exposed to radiation is lessened, and a higher dose of radiation may be delivered.[127,128]

Omentoplasty has been reported[130–133] in which an omental pedicle flap based on the left gastroepiploic vessels is passed along the left paracolic gutter and is sutured into place in the pelvis.[7]

EXPERIMENTAL APPROACHES

In the occasional patient with persistent severe symptoms unresponsive to the usual medical measures, two-thirds of patients may respond to hyperbaric oxygen.[134,135] Rarely, in children with radiation enteritis, small bowel transplantation has been performed, with a 68% 5-year survival rate.[136]

Newer experimental approaches have been examined:[137] keratinocyte growth factor (KGF) reduces intestinal damage caused in mice by chemotherapy or radiotherapy, or a combination of the two,[138–140] is under study as a possible radioprotectant agent for patients with head and neck cancer.[141] Glucagon-like peptide-2 (GLP-2) given to rats or mice before or after chemotherapy reduces intestinal damage.[142,143] Treatment with epidermal growth factor (EGF) before or after radiation limits the severity of mucositis,[144] but the potential benefit of EGF remains controversial, since transogenic mice with overexpression of EGF remain susceptible to intestinal damage.[145] Similarly, it is controversial whether insulin-like growth factor 1 (IGF-1) is beneficial, since IGF-1 reduces intestinal damage when given after methotrexate or radiation therapy but worsens damage when given during chemotherapy.[146–148] Interlukin (IL)-2 may worsen muscositis,[149,150] whereas IL-11 and IL-15 may be protective or therapeutic when given before or after chemotherapy or radiotherapy.[149–153] Transforming growth factor (TGF)-β enhances gut repair and improves several of radiated mice.[153–156] In animal studies, glutamine was shown to be protective to the small bowel,[157–159] but this was not confirmed in a further animal study.[160] In human studies, glutamine supplementation may be of benefit but not to all symptoms, and there is a large variability in the response among individuals.[161–166] The radiation-associated altered apoptosis is associated with the inhibition of epithelial mitosis in the crypts,[167] with protection of the crypt cells with prostaglandins.[151] Vitamin E but not misoprostol is also effective against the morphological changes that develop in the irradiated rat intestine.[168] Fibroblast growth factor given by oral gavage exerted a beneficial effect on only a few parameters in a rat model of enterocolitis.[9] Superoxide dismutase, a free radical scavenger, reduces the morbidity from abdominal radiation,[169] as also do nonsteroidal antiinflammatory drugs,[170] glutathione and antioxidants,[51] a 21-aminosteroid, and a troloxamine.[171] It may be speculated that many (88%) patients receive symptomatic benefit from practitioners of alternative medicine.[56]

A summary of patient management is given in Table 54.3.

REFERENCES

1. Thomson ABR, Churnratanakul S, Wirzba B, et al. Radiation effects on normal intestinal tissue. In: Thomson ABR, Shaffer E, eds. Modern concepts in gastroenterology. Vol. 3. New York: Plenum Medical Book; 1992; Chpt 5:72–77.

2. Churnratanakul S, Wirzba BJ, Lam T, et al. Radiation and the small intestine. Future perspectives for preventive therapy. Surv Dig Dis 1990; 8:45–60.

3. Dubois A, Walker RI. Prospects for management of gastrointestinal injury associated with the acute radiation syndrome. Gastroenterology 1988; 95: 487–493; 500–507.

4. Earnest DL, Triet JS. Radiation enteritis and colitis. In: Sleisenger MH, Fordtran JS, eds. Gastrointestinal disease: pathophysiology, diagnosis and management. 2nd edn. Philadelphia: WB Saunders; 1989:1369–1382.

5. Nguyen NP, Antoine JE. Radiation enteritis. In: Feldman M, Friedman LS, Sleisenger MH, eds. Sleisenger and Fordtran's gastrointestinal and liver disease pathophysiology/diagnosis/management. New York: WB Saunders; 2002: Chapter 102;1994–2004.

6. MacNaughton. Review article: new insights into the pathogenesis of radiation-induced intestinal dysfunction. Aliment Pharmacol Ther 2000; 14:523–528.

A useful and detailed review of pathogenesis.

7. Waddell BE, Radriguez-Bigas MA, Lee RJ, et al. Prevention of chronic radiation enteritis. J Am Coll Surg 1999; 189:611–624.

8. Classen J, Belka C, Paulsen F, et al. Radiation-induced gastrointestinal toxicity. Strahlenther Onkol 1998; 174:(Suppl III):82–84.

9. Szabo S, Sandor Z, Vincze A, et al. Radiation-induced enterocolitis: basic and applied science. Eur J Surg 1998; 582:85–89.

10. Mathes SJ, Alexander J. Radiation injury. Plastic surgical reconstruction: possibilities in surgical oncology I. Surg Oncol Clin N Am 1996; 5(4):809–824.

11. Rodier JF. Radiation enteropathy – incidence, aetiology, risk factors, pathology and symptoms. Tumori 1995; 81 Supple:122–125.

12. Marc E, Sher BA, Baver J. Radiation-induced enteropathy. Am J Gastroenterol 1990; 85:2.

13. Crook J, Esche B, Futter N. Effect of pelvic radiotherapy for prostatic cancer on bowel, bladder, and sexual function: the patient's perspective. Urology 1996; 47(3):387–394.

14. Khan FM. The physics of radiation therapy. In: Interaction of ionizing radiation. Baltimore: Williams & Wilkins; 1994:79.

15. Hall EJ. Radiobiology for the radiologist. In: DNA strand breaks and chromosal aberrations. Philadelphia: JB Lippincott; 1994:15.

16. Haimovitz-Friedman A. Radiation-induced signal transduction and stress response. Radiat Res 1998; 150:S102.

17. Potten CS, Cooth C, Pritchard DM. The intestinal epithelial stem cell: the mucosal governor. Int J Exp Pathol 1997; 78:219.

18. Jones BA, Gores GJ. Physiology and pathophysiology of apoptosis in epithelial cells of the liver, pancreas, and intestine. Am J Physiol 1997; 273:G1174.

19. Metcalfe A, Streuli C. Epithelial apoptosis. Bioessays 1997; 19:711.

20. Wang J, Richter KK, Sung CC, et al. Unregulation and spatial shift in the localization of the mannose 6-phosphate/insulin-like growth factor II receptor during radiation enteropathy development in the rat. Radiother Oncol 1999; 50:205.

21. Wang J, Zheng H, Sung CC, et al. Cellular sources of transforming grow factor-B isoforms in early and chronic radiation enteropathy. Am J Pathol 1998; 5:S69–S75.

22. Becciolini A, Cremonimi D, Fabbrica C, et al. Cell proliferation and differentiation in the small intestine after irradiation with multiple fractions. Acta Radiol Oncol 1986; 25:51–56.

23. Green N, Iba G, Smith WR. Measures to minimize small intestine injury in the irradiated pelvis. Cancer 1975; 35:1633–1640.

24. Kao M-S. Intestinal complications of radiotherapy in gynecologic malignancy – clinical presentation and management. Int J Gynecol Obstetr 1995; 49:S69–S75.

25. Carr KE, Hume SP, Ettarh R, et al. Radiation-induced changes to epithelial and non-epithelial tissue. In: Dubois A, King GL, Livengood D, eds. Radiation and the gastrointestinal tract. Boca Raton: CRC Press; 1994:113.

26. MacNaughton WK, Leach KE, Pred'homme-Lalonde L, et al. Ionizing radiation reduces neurally evoked electrolyte transport in rat ileum through a mast cell-dependent mechanism. Gastroenterology 1994; 106:324–335.

27. Cummins AG, Munro GH, Huntley JF, et al. Separate effects of irradiation and of graft-versus-host reaction on rat mucosal mast cells. Gut 1989; 30:355–360.

28. MacNaughton WK, Aurora AR, Bhamra J, et al. Expression, activity and cellular localization of inducible nitric oxide synthase in rat ileum and colon post-irradiation. Int J Radiat Biol 1998; 74:255–264.

An interesting proposal for one of the mechanisms of radiation-associated damage.

29. Thomson ABR, Cheeseman CI, Walker K. Effect of external abdominal irradiation on the dimensions and characteristics of the barriers to passive transport in the rat intestine. Lipids 1984; 19(6):405–418.

30. Thomson ABR, Cheeseman CI, Walker K. Intestinal uptake of bile acids: effect of external abdominal irradiation. Int J Radiation Oncology Biol Phys 1984; 10:671–683.

31. Thomson ABR, Cheeseman CI, Walker K. Late effects of abdominal radiation of intestinal uptake of nutrients. Radiation Res 1986; 107:344–353.

32. Thomson ABR, Keelan M, Cheeseman CI, et al. Fractionated low doses of abdominal irradiation alters jejunal uptake of nutrients. Int J Radiation Oncology Biol Phys 1986; 12:917–925.

33. Keelan M, Cheeseman C, Walker K, et al. Effect of external abdominal irradiation on intestinal morphology and brush border membrane enzyme and lipid composition. Radiation Res 1986; 105:84–96.

34. Otterson MF, Sarna SK, Lee MB. Fractionated doses of ionizing radiation alter postprandial small intestinal motor activity Dig Dis Sci 1992; 37:709–715.

35. Otterson MF, Sarna SK, Leming SC, et al. Effects of fractionated doses of ionizing radiation on colonic motor activity. Am J Physiol 1992; 263:G518–G526.

36. Summers RW, Flatt AJ, Prihoda MJ, et al. Effect of irradiation on morphology and motility of canine small intestine. Dig Dis Sci 1987; 12:1402–1410.

37. Otterson MF, Koch TR, Zhang Z, et al. Fractionated irradiation alters enteric neuroendocrine products. Dig Dis Sci 1995; 40:1691–1702.

38. Krantis A, Rana K, Harding RK. The effects of gamma-radiation on intestinal motor activity and faecal pellet expulsion in the guinea pig. Dig Dis Sci 1996; 41:2307–2316.

39. Scolapio JS, Ukleja A, Burnes JU, et al. Outcome of patients with radiation enteritis treated with home parenteral nutrition. Am J Gastroenterol 2002; 97(3):662–666.

HPN may be useful nutritional support in selected patients with malnutrition from chronic radiation damage.

40. Galland RB, Spencer J. Natural history and surgical management of radiation enteritis. Br J Surg 1987; 74:742–747.

41. Thomas PRM, Lindblad AS, Stablein DM, et al. Toxicity associated with adjuvant postoperative therapy for adenocarcinoma of the rectum. Cancer 1986; 57:1130–1134.

42. Sher ME, Bauer J. Radiation-induced enteropathy. Am J Gastroenterol 1990; 85:121–128.

43. Coia LR, Myerson RJ, Tepper JE. Late effects of radiation therapy on the gastrointestinal tract. Int J Radiat Oncol Biol Phys 1995; 31:1213–1236.

44. Loludice T, Baxter D, Balint J. Effects of abdominal surgery on the development of radiation enteropathy. Gastroenterology 1977; 72:1093–1097.

45. Maruyama Y, van Nagell JR, Utley J, et al. Radiation and small bowel complications in cervical carcinoma therapy. Radiology 1974; 112:699–703.

46. Potish R. Prediction of radiation-related small-bowel damage. Radiology 1980; 135:219–221.

47. van Nagell JR, Parker JC, Maruyama Y, et al. The effect of pelvic inflammatory disease on enteric complication following radiation therapy for cervical cancer. Am J Obstet Gynecol 1977; 128: 767–771.

48. DeCosse JJ, Rhodes RS, Wentz WB, et al. The natural history and management of radiation induced injury of the gastrointestinal tract. Ann Surg 1969; 170:369.

49. Pyo H, Choy H, Amorino GP, et al. A selective cyclooxygenase-2 inhibitor, NS-398, enhances the effect of radiation in vitro and in vivo preferentially on the cells that express cyclooxygenase-2[1]. Clin Cancer Res 2001; 7:2998–3005.

50. Shehata WM, Meyer RL. The enhancement effect of irradiation by methotrexate: report of three complications. Cancer 1980; 46:1349–1352.

51. Nussbaum ML, Campana TJ, Weese JL. Radiation induced intestinal injury. Clin Plast Surg 1993; 20:573–580.

52. Nguyen NP, Sallah S, Karlsson U, et al. Combined preoperative chemotherapy and radiation for locally advanced rectal carcinoma. Am J Clin Oncol 2000; 23:442.

53. Mann WJ. Surgical management of radiation enteropathy. Surg Clin North Am 1991; 71:977–990.

54. Deveney CW, Lewis FR, Schrock TR. Surgical management of radiation injury of the small and large intestine. Dis Colon Rectum 1976; 19:25–29.

55. Johnson RJ, Carrington BM. Pelvic radiation disease. Clin Radiol 1992; 45:41–42.

56. Gami B, Harrington K, Blake P, et al. How patients manage gastrointestinal symptoms after pelvic radiotherapy. Aliment Pharmacol Ther 2003; 18:987–994.

Chronic gastrointestinal symptoms are common after pelvic radiation and impair patients' quality of life.

57. Hasleton PS, Carr N, Schofield PF. Vascular changes in radiation bowel disease. Histopathology 1985; 9:517.

58. Girvent M, Carlson GL, Anderson I, et al. Intestinal failure after surgery for complicated radiation enteritis. Ann R Coll Surgeons England 2000; 82(3):198–201.

59. Perez CB, Breaux S, Madoc-Jones H. et al., Radiation therapy alone in the treatment of carcinoma of the uterine cervix: Analysis of complications. Cancer 1984; 54:235.

60. Dixon PM, Roulston ME, Nolan DJ. The small bowel enema: a ten year review. Clin Radiol 1993; 47:46.

61. Freed KS, Lo JY, Baker JA, et al. Predictive model for the diagnosis of intra-abdominal abscess. Acad Radiol 1998; 5:473.

62. Lantto E. Investigation of suspected intra-abdominal sepsis: the contribution of nuclear medicine. Scand J Gastroenterol 1994; 203(Suppl):11.

63. Bender GN, Maglinte DDT, Kloppel VR, et al. CT enteroclysis: a superfluous diagnostic procedure or valuable when investigating small-bowel disease? AJR Am J Roentgenol 1999; 172:373.

64. Walsh DW, Bender GN, Timmons JH. Comparison of computed tomography-enteroclysis and traditional computed tomography in the setting of suspected partial small bowel obstruction. Emerg Radiol 1998; 5:29.

65. Kolbl O, Richter S, Flentje M. Influence of treatment technique on dose-volume histogram and normal tissue complication probability for small bowel and bladder. A prospective study using a 3-D planning system and a radiobiological model in patients receiving postoperative pelvic irradiation. Strahlenther Onkol 2000; 176:105–111.

66. Letschert JG, Lebesque JV, de Boer RW, et al. Dose-volume correlation in radiation induced late small bowel complications: a clinical study. Radiother Oncol 1990; 18:307.

67. Potish RA, Jones TK, Levitt SH. Factors predisposing to radiation-related small-bowel damage. Radiology 1979; 132:479–482.

68. Gallagher MJ, Brereton HD, Rostock RA, et al. A prospective study of treatment techniques to minimize the volume of pelvic small bowel with reduction of acute and late effects associated with pelvic irradiation. Int J Radiat Oncol Biol Phys 1986; 12:1565–1573.

69. Rudat V, Flentje M, Engenhart R, et al. The belly-board technique for the sparing of the small intestine. Studies on positioning accuracy taking into consideration conformational irradiation techniques. Strahlenther Onkol 1995; 171:437–443.

70. Shanahan TG, Mehta MP, Bertelrud KL, et al. Minimization of small bowel volume within treatment fields utilizing customized 'belly boards.' Int J Radiat Oncol Biol Phys 1990; 19:469–476.

71. Green N. The avoidance of small intestine injury in gynecologic cancer. Int J Radiat Oncol Biol Phys 1983; 9:1385–1390.

72. Hindley A, Cole H. Use of peritoneal insufflation to displace the small bowel during pelvic and abdominal radiotherapy in carcinoma of the cervix. Br J Radiol 1993; 66:67–73.

73. Gunderson LL, Russell AH, Llewellyn HJ, et al. Treatment planning for colorectal cancer: radiation and surgical techniques and value of small-bowel films. Int J Radiat Oncol Biol Phys 1985; 11:1379–1393.

74. Herbert SH, Solin LJ, Hoffman JP, et al. Volumetric analysis of small bowel displacement from radiation portals with the use of a pelvic tissue expander. Int J Radiat Oncol Biol Phys 1993; 25:885–893.

75. Lyman GH. A novel approach to maintain planned dose chemotherapy on time: a decision-making tool to improve patient care. Eur J Cancer 2000; 36:S15.

76. Henriksson R, Lomberg H, Israelsson G, et al. The effect of ondansetron on radiation-induced emesis and diarrhea. Acta Oncol 1992; 31:767–769.

77. Meyers JS, Ehrenpreis ED, Craig RM. Small intestinal bacterial over-growth syndrome. Curr Treat Options Gastroenterol 2001; 4:7–14.

78. Attar A, Flourie B, Rambaud JC, et al. Antibiotic efficacy in small intestinal bacterial overgrowth-related chronic diarrhea: a crossover, randomized trial. Gastroenterology 1999; 117:794.

79. Salminen E, Elomaa I, Minkkinen J, et al. Preservation of intestinal integrity during radiotherapy using live *Lactobacillus acidophilus* cultures. Clin Radiol 1988; 39:435–437.

80. Mennic AT, Dalley VM, Dinneen LC, et al. Treatment of radiation-induced gastrointestinal distress with acetylsalicylate. Lancet 1975; 2:942–943.

81. Martenson JA, Hyland G, Moertel CG, et al. Olalazine is contraindicated during pelvic radiation therapy: results of a double-blind, randomized clinical study. Int J Radiat Oncol Biol Phys 1996; 35:299–303.

82. Baillie-Johnson HR. Octreotide in the management of treatment-related diarrhoea. Anti-Cancer Drugs 1996; 7(Suppl 1):11–15.

83. Cross MJ, Frazee RC. Surgical treatment of radiation enteritis. Am Surg 1992; 58:132–135.

84. Van Halteren HK, Gortzak E, Taal BG, et al. Surgical intervention for complications caused by late radiation damage of the small bowel: A retrospective analysis. Eur J Surg Oncol 1993; 19:336–341.

85. Joyeux H, Matias J, Gouttebel MC, et al. Therapeutic strategy in 46 cases of radiation injury of the intestine. Chirurgie 1994–95; 120(12):129–133.

86. Bounous G, Gentile JM, Hugon J. Elemental diet in the management of the intestinal lesion produced by 5-fluorouracil in man. Can J Surg 1971; 14:312–324.

87. Bounous G, Lebel E, Shuster J, et al. Dietary protection during radiation therapy. Strahlentherapie 1975; 149:476–483.

88. McArdle AH, Wittnich C, Freeman CR, et al. The use of elemental diet as prophylaxis against radiation injury: histologic and ultrastructural studies. Arch Surg 1985; 120:1026–1032.

89. McArdle AH, Reid EC, Laplante MP, et al. Prophylaxis against radiation injury. The use of elemental diet prior to and during radiotherapy for invasive bladder cancer and in early postoperative feeding following radical cystectomy and ileal conduit. Arch Surg 1986; 121:879–885.

Elemental diets may be useful beyond the nutritional support provided.

90. Loiudice TA, Lang JA. Treatment of radiation enteritis: A comparison study. Am J Gastroenterol 1983; 78(8):481–487.

91. Howard L, Ament M, Fleming CR, et al. Current use and clinical outcome of home parenteral and enteral nutrition therapies in the United States. Gastroenterology 1995; 109:355–365.

92. Henriksson R, Franzen L, Littbrand B. Effects of sucralfate on acute and late bowel discomfort following radiotherapy of pelvic cancer. J Clin Oncol 1992; 10:969–975.

93. Hurtig A. Local hydrocortisone acetate for radiation proctitis. J Postgrad Med 1954; 15:37–39.

94. Blank WA. Irradiation injury to the bowel and rectum. J R Soc Med 1970; 63(Suppl):98–100.

95. Golstein F, Khoury J, Thorton JJ. Treatment of chronic radiation enteritis and colitis with salicylazopyridine and systemic corticosteroids. Am J Gastroenterol 1976; 65:201–208.

96. McElligott E, Quigley C, Hanks GW. Tranexamic acid and rectal bleeding. Lancet 1988; 2:1.

97. Kocker R, Sharma SL, Gupta BB, et al. Rectal sucralfate in radiation proctitis. Lancet 1988; 2:400.

98. Libotte F, Autier P, Delmelle M, et al. Survival of patients with radiation enteritis of the small and the large intestine. Acta Chir Belg. 1995; 95(Suppl 4):190–194.

99. Seow-Choen F, Goh H-S, Eu K-W, et al. A simple and effective treatment for hemorrhagic radiation proctitis using formalin. Dis Colon Rectum 1993; 36:135–138.

100. Yegappan M, Ho YH, Nyam D, et al. The surgical management of colorectal complications from irradiation for carcinoma of the cervix. Ann Acad Med Singapore 1998; 27(5):627–630.

101. Alexander TJ, Dwyer RM. Endoscopic Nd:YAG laser treatment of severe radiation injury of the lower gastrointestinal tract: long-term follow-up. Gastrointest Endosc 1988; 34:407–411.

102. Barbatzas C, Spencer GM, Thorpe SM, et al. Nd:YAG laser treatment for bleeding from radiation proctitis [erratum appears in Endoscopy 1997 Jan;29(1):47 Note: Carbatzas C [corrected to Barbatzas C]]. Endoscopy 1996; 28(6):497–500.

103. O'Conner JJ. Argon laser treatment of radiation proctitis. Arch Surg 1989; 124:749.

104. Buchi KN, Dixon JA. Argon laser treatment of hemorrhagic radiation proctitis. Gastrointest Endosc 1987; 33:27–30.

105. Dorr RT. Radioprotectants: pharmacology and clinical applications of amifostine. Sem Radiat Oncol 1998; 8(Suppl 1):10–13.

106. Mehta MP. Protection of normal tissues from the cytotoxic effects of radiation therapy: focus on amifostine. Semin Radiat Oncol 1998; 8(Suppl1):14–16.

107. Liu T, Liu Y, He S, et al. Use of radiation with or without WR-2721 in advanced rectal cancer. Cancer 1992; 69:2820–2825.

108. Brizel D, Sauer R, Wannenmacher M, et al. Randomized phase III trial of radiation and amifostine in patients with head and neck cancer. Proc Am Soc Clin Oncol 1998; 17:386.

109. Buntzel J, Kuttner K, Russell L, et al. Selective cytoprotection by amifostine in the treatment of head and neck cancer with simultaneous radiochemotherapy (Abstract). Proc Am Soc Clin Oncol 1997; 16:393.

110. Antonadou D, Pepelassi E, Synodinou M, et al. The prophylactic use of amifostine in the prevention of chemoradiation induced mucositis and xerostomia in head and neck cancer (Abstract). Int J Radiat Oncol Biol Phys 1998; 42:224.

111. Montana GS, Anscher MS, Mansbach CM, et al. Topical application of WR-2721 to prevent radiation-induced proctosigmoiditis: a phase I/II trial. Cancer 1992; 69:2826–2830.

112. McDonald S, Meyerowitz C, Rubin P, et al. Preliminary results of a pilot study using WR-2721 before fractionated irradiation of the head and neck to reduce salivary gland dysfunction. Int J Radiat Oncol Biol Phys 1994; 29:747–754.

113. Patchen ML, MacVittie TJ, Souza LM. Postirradiation treatment with granulocyte colony-stimulating factor and preirradiation WR-2721 administration synergize to enhance hemopoietic reconstitution and increase survival. Int J Radiat Oncol Biol Phys 1992; 22:773–779.

114. Kuroki F, Iida M, Matsui T, et al. Intraoperative endoscopy for small intestinal damage in radiation enteritis. Gastroenterol Endosc 1992; 38:196.

115. Hendrix P, Pahow E. Thronic radiation enteritis. Gastroenterologist 1994; 2:70.

116. Nakashima H, Ueo H, Shibuta K, et al. Surgical management of patients with radiation enteritis. Int Surg 1996; 81:415–418.

117. Farthmann EH, Imdahl A, Eggstein S. Radiation enteropathy. Strahlenther Onkol 1994; 170:437–440.

118. Jahnson S, Westerborn O, Gerdin B. Prognosis of surgically treated radiation-induced damage to the intestine. Eur J Surg Oncol 1992; 18(5):487–493.

119. Fenner MN, Sheehan P, Nanavati PJ, et al. Chronic radiation enteritis: a community hospital experience. J Surg Oncol 1989; 41(4):246–249.

120. Shiraishi M, Hiroyasu S, Ishimine T, et al. Radiation enterocolitis: overview of the past 15 years. World J Surgery 1998; 22(5):491–493.

121. Muttillo I, Elias K, Bolognese A, et al. Surgical treatment of severe late radiation injury to the bowel: A retrospective analysis of 83 cases. Hepatogastroenterology 2002; 49:1023–1026.

122. Galland RB, Spencer J. The natural history of clinically established radiation enteritis. Lancet 1985; 1:1257–1258.

123. Dietz DW, Remzi FH, Faxio VW. Strictureplasty for obstructing small-bowel lesions in diffuse radiation enteritis – Successful outcome in five patients. Dis Colon Rectum Dec 2001; 44(12):1772–1777.

124. Mak AC, Rich TA, Schultheiss TE, et al. Late complications of postoperative radiation therapy for cancer of the rectum and rectosigmoid. Int J Radiat Oncol Biol Phys 1994; 28:597–603.

125. Meric F, Hirshl RB, Womer RB, et al. Prevention of radiation enteritis in children, using a pelvic mesh sling. J Pediator Surg 1994; 29:917–921.

126. Devereux DF, Chandler JJ, Eisenstat T, et al. Efficacy of an absorbable mesh in keeping the small bowel out of the human pelvis following surgery. Dis Colon Rectum 1988; 31:17–21.

127. Rodier JF, Janser JC, Rodier J, et al. Prevention of radiation enteritis by an absorbable polyglycolic acid mesh sling. Cancer 1991; 68:2545–2549.

128. Dasmahapatra KS, Swaminathan AP. The use of a biodegradable mesh to prevent radiation associated small bowel injury. Arch Surg 1991; 126:366–369.

129. Galland RB, Spencer J. Surgical management of radiation enteritis. Surgery 1986; 99(2):133–139.

130. Russ JE, Smoron GL, Gagnon JD. Omental transposition flap in colorectal carcinoma: adjunctive use in prevention and treatment of radiation complications. Int J Radiat Oncol Biol Phys 1984; 10:55–62.

131. DeLuca FR, Ragins H. Construction of an omental envelope as a method of excluding the small intestine from the field of postoperative irradiation to the pelvis. Surg Gynecol Obstet 1985; 160:365–366.

132. Lechner P, Cesnik H. Abdominopelvic omentopexy: preparatory procedure for radiotherapy in rectal cancer. Dis Colon Rectum 1992; 35:1157–1160.

133. Choi HJ, Lee HS. Effect of omental pedicle hammock in protection against radiation-induced enteropathy in patients with rectal cancer. Dis Colon Rectum 1995; 38:276–280.

134. Gouello JP, Bouachour G, Person B, et al. Interet de l'oxygenotherapie hyperbare dans la pathologie digestive post radique. La Presse Med 1993; 28:1053.

135. Lak KH, Baker DG, Fellows CF. Hyperbaric oxygen after radiation and its effect on the production of radiation myelitis. Int J Radiat Oncol Biol Phys 1978; 4:457–459.

136. Abu-Elmagd K, Reyes J, Todo S, et al. Clinical intestinal transplantation: new perspectives and immunologic consideration. J Am Coll Surg 1998; 5:512.

137. Duncan M, Grant G. Review article: oral and intestinal mucositis – causes and possible treatments. APT 2003; 18:853–874.

Practical as well as experimental approaches to the care of the patient with mucositis are provided.

138. Farrell CL, Rex KL, Chen JN, et al. The effects of keratinocyte growth factor in preclincial models of mucositis. Cell Prolif 2002; 35(Suppl 1):78–85.

Experimental evidence is growing that a variety of hormones, cytokines, and growth factors may be therapeutically effective, and may eventually find a clinical role.

139. Khan WB, Shui C, Ning S, et al. Enhancement of murine intestinal stem cell survival after irradiation by keratinocyte growth factor. Radiat Res 1997; 148:248–253.

140. Farrell CL, Bready JV, Rex KL, et al. Keratinocyte growth factor protects mice from chemotherapy and radiation-induced gastrointestinal injury and mortality. Cancer Res 1998;58; 933–939.

141. Brizel DM. Future directions in toxicity prevention. Semin Radiat Oncol 1998: 8(Suppl 1):17–20.

142. Boushey RP, Yusta B, Drucker DJ. Glucagon-like peptide (GLP-2) reduces chemotherapy-associated mortality and enhances cell survival in cells expressing a transfected GLP-2 receptor. Cancer Res 2001;61:687–693.

143. Tavakkolizadeh A, Shen R, Abraham P, et al. Glucagon-like peptide 2: a new treatment for chemotherapy-induced enteritis. J Surg Res 2000;91:77–82.

144. McKenna KJ, Ligato S, Kauffman GLJ, et al. Epidermal growth factor enhances intestinal mitotic activity and DNA content after acute abdominal radiation. Surgery 1994;115:626–632.

145. Huang FS, Kemp CJ, Williams JL, et al. Role of epidermal growth factor and its receptor in chemotherapy-induced intestinal injury. Am J Physiol Gastroinest Liver Physiol 2002; 282:G432–G442.

146. Howarth GS, Cool JC, Bourne AJ, et al. Insulin-like growth factor-I (IGF-I) stimulates growth of the damaged intestine in rats, when administered following, but not concurrent with, methotrexate. Growth Factors 1998;15: 279–292.

147. Howarth GS, Fraser R, Frisby CL, et al. Effects of insulin-like growth factor-I administration on radiation enteritis in rats. Scand J Gastroenterol 1997; 32:1118–1124.

148. Howarth GS. Insulin-like growth factor-I and the gastrointestinal system: therapeutic indications and safety implications. J Nutr 2003; 133:2109–2112.

149. Cao S, Troutt AB, Rustum YM. Interleukin 15 protects against toxicity and potentiates antitumour activity of 5-fluorouracil alone and in combination with leucovorin in rats bearing colorectal cancer. Cancer Res 1998; 58:1695–1699.

150. Cao S, Black JD, Troutt AB, et al. Interleukin 15 offers selective protection from irinotecan-induced intestinal toxicity in a preclinical animal model. Cancer Res 1998;58:3270–3274.

151. Cohn SM, Schloemann S, Tessner T, et al. Crypt stem cell survival in the mouse intestinal epithelium is regulated by prostaglandins synthesized through cyclooxygenase-1. J Clin Invest 1997; 99:1367–1379.

152. Orazi A, Du X, Yang Z, et al. Interleukin-11 prevents apoptosis and accelerates recovery of small intestinal mucosa in mice treated with combined chemotherapy and radiation. Lab Invest 1996; 75:33–42.

153. Booth D, Potten CS. Protection against mucosal injury by growth factors and cytokines. N Natl Cancer Inst Monogr 2001;29:16-20.

154. Salminen E, Elomaa I, Minkkinen J, et al. Preservation of intestinal integrity during radiotherapy using live *Lactobacillus acidophilus* cultures. Clin Radiol 1988; 39:435–437.

155. Empey LR, Papp JD, Jewell LD, et al. Mucosal protective effects of vitamin E and misoprostol during acute radiation-induced enteritis in rats. Dig Dis and Sciences 1992; 37(2):205–214.

156. Potten CS, Booth D, Haley JD. Pretreatment with transforming growth factor beta-3 protects small intestinal stem cells against radiation damage in vivo. Br J Cancer 1997;75:1454–1459.

157. Jenson JC, Schaefer R, Nwokedi E, et al. Prevention of chronic radiation enteropathy by dietary glutamine. Ann Surg Oncol 1994; 1:157–163.

158. Fox AD, Kripke SA, De Paula J, et al. Effect of a glutamine-supplemented enteral diet on methotrexate-induced enterocolitis. J Parenter Enteral Nutr 1988; 12:325–331.

159. Klimberg VS, Salloum RM, Kasper M, et al. Oral glutamine accelerates healing of the small intestine and improves outcome after whole abdominal radiation. Arch Surg 1990:125:1040–1045.

160. Gardner ML, Earl SK, Wood D. Elemental diets in the repair of small intestinal damage. Nutrition 1997;13:755–759.

161. Daniele B, Perrone F, Gallo C, et al. Oral glutamine in the prevention of fluorouracil induced intestinal toxicity: a double blind, placebo controlled, randomized trial. Gut 2001;48:28–33.

162. van der Hulst RR, Van Dreel BK, von Meyenfeldt MF, et al. Glutamine and the preservation of gut integrity. Lancet 1993: 341:1363–1365.

163. Tremel H, Kienle B, Weilemann LS, et al. Glutamine dipeptide-supplemented parenteral nutrition maintains intestinal function in the critically ill. Gastroenterology 1994;107:1595–1601.

164. Decker-Baumann C, Buhl K, Frohmuller S, et al. Reduction of chemotherapy-induced side-effects by parenteral glutamine supplementation in patients with metastatic colorectal cancer. Eur J Cancer 1999; 35:202–207.

165. Ziegler TR. Glutamine supplementation in cancer patients receiving bone marrow transplantation and high dose chemotherapy. J Nutr 2001; 131:2578S–2584S.

166. Muscaritoli M, Brieco G, Capria S, et al. Nutritional and metabolic support in patients undergoing bone marrow transplantation. Am J Clin Nutr 2002; 75:183–190.

167. Quastler H. The nature of intestinal radiation death. Radiat Res 1956; 4:303–320.

168. Empey LR, Papp JD, Jewell LD, et al. Mucosal protective effects of vitamin E and misoprostol during acute radiation-induced enteritis in rats. Dig Dis and Sciences 1992; 37(2):205–214.

169. Petkau A. Role of superoxide dismutase in modification of radiation injury. Br J Cancer 1987; 8(Suppl):87.

170. Hanson WR, Houseman KA, Collins PW. Radiation protection in vivo by prostaglandins and related compounds of the arachidonic acid cascade. Pharmacol Ther 1987; 39:347.

171. Delaney JP, Bonsack ME, Felemovicius I. Lumenal route for intestinal radioprotection. Am J Surg 1993; 166:492–501.

CHAPTER FIFTY-FIVE

55

Approach to the patient with short-bowel syndrome

Malcolm K. Robinson, Theresa A. Byrne and Douglas W. Wilmore

INTRODUCTION

The first successful intestinal resection was reported in 1880 and it was only a short time thereafter that the direct relationship between length of bowel resected and long-term survival was understood.[1] In 1935, Haymond analyzed a series of 257 patients who had undergone intestinal resection.[2] He determined that those with resection of one-third or less of small bowel retained near-normal bowel function. However, those who had resection of 50% or more of the small bowel suffered dire consequences and developed 'short-bowel syndrome,' often succumbing to dehydration and malnutrition. Subsequently, several advancements in anesthesia, critical care, and antibiotics made survival of these patients possible. Key to this success was the development of total parenteral nutrition (TPN). Jonathan Rhoads led a team of pioneers in this area from the Department of Surgery at the University of Pennsylvania. This team was the first to make TPN a practical reality in humans and demonstrated that an infant with a short bowel could sustain normal growth and development receiving all nutrients exclusively by vein.[3] Currently, survival for even those with extremely short segments of small intestine is likely with the utilization of TPN.

Although TPN can be life-saving for the patient with short-bowel syndrome (SBS), this treatment is not ideal. There are several TPN-associated complications including liver failure, which is particularly common in children receiving long-term TPN, recurrent central venous catheter sepsis, and venous thromboses. These TPN-related problems are frequently the ultimate cause of death of patients with SBS. Consequently, the goal of treatment of those with this syndrome is to achieve 'nutritional autonomy,' i.e., TPN-independence. This chapter will review the pathophysiology of SBS and outline the medical, nutritional, and surgical approaches to treatment of patients with this condition.

ETIOLOGY

Short-bowel syndrome is defined as that symptom complex which occurs in adults who have less than 200 centimeters of combined jejunum-ileum in continuity following massive small bowel resection.[4] This represents approximately one-third of the normal length of small bowel in adults.[5,6] SBS also occurs in children who have less than 30% of the normal small bowel length for their age.[7] The syndrome is characterized by diarrhea, weight loss, dehydration, malnutrition, and malabsorption of macro- and micronutrients all due to the reduction in effective intestinal absorptive surface area. Note that some patients who have had extensive bowel resections, which leave them with *more* than one-third of their small bowel, may develop symptoms indistinguishable from those who fulfill the technical criteria for SBS. This may occur, for example, in those with Crohn's disease or radiation enteritis in whom the remaining bowel is diseased. These latter patients can be managed in a manner similar to those with the classic definition of SBS.

Extensive small bowel resection in adults may be necessary for treatment of ischemic necrosis, traumatic injury, tumors, inflammatory bowel disease, or iatrogenic injury of the small bowel or mesenteric vasculature.[8,9] In children, necrotizing enterocolitis, intestinal atresia and volvulus, and gastroschisis are the most common causes of SBS.[10]

THE ADAPTIVE RESPONSE

The remaining small bowel adapts following massive intestinal resection in humans by dilating and mildly elongating.[4] This increases absorptive surface area. The microscopic adaptive response probably does not include villous hypertrophy in humans as is observed in animals (e.g., rats). However, there are increased cells per unit length of intestinal villus (i.e., hyperplasia) in SBS patients, which increase nutrient transport and thereby absorptive efficiency.[11] Eventually, there is a compensatory slowing of bowel motility following massive bowel resection, which prolongs transit of food through the intestinal tract and thus increases nutrient contact time with the absorptive surface. Clinically, there is a decrease in diarrhea and a gradual transition from parenteral dependence to enteral autonomy. These changes collectively result in a marked ability of patients to adapt to loss of large segments of bowel.[12]

Under normal circumstances, most nutrients including carbohydrate, protein, and fat are absorbed within the first 150 centimeters of jejunum in the adult. The ileum has certain specialized functions including uptake of vitamin B_{12} and bile salts. Following loss of the jejunum with preservation of the ileum, the ileum adapts and largely assumes those absorptive functions previously carried out by the jejunum. In contrast, massive resection of the ileum is associated with significant malabsorption of vitamin B_{12}, bile salts, and fat even with the jejunum in place. In addition, if the colon remains in continuity with the jejunum following ileal resection, unabsorbed bile salts exacerbate diarrhea due to colonic irritation. Thus, the clinical consequences of resecting jejunum versus ileum are different and, therefore, may require different treatments to allow the patient to become independent of TPN.[12]

The principal, normal functions of the colon are limited to water resorption and elimination of undigested material. However, the colon can take on a critical role in nutrient absorption in the SBS patient. If the colon is in continuity with the small bowel in the SBS patient, undigested soluble fiber and starches pass into the colon where they are fermented by colonic bacteria to form short-chain fatty acids (SCFAs) including butyrate, propionate, and acetate. SCFAs are absorbed by the colon and can provide a significant portion of the daily caloric absorption. In addition, SCFAs promote sodium and water absorption and may improve fluid balance and hydration status.[13]

Thus, the overall adaptive response of the SBS patient is complex and consists of changes in both small and large bowel function, which can potentially overcome the adverse effects of extensive bowel resection. The signals that support adaptation are multiple and are largely triggered by enteral feeding (Fig. 55.1). This adaptive response has been extensively reviewed elsewhere and typically evolves over 1–2 years before the maximal response is achieved.[4,12]

NATURAL HISTORY OF SHORT-BOWEL SYNDROME

Certain features of the natural history of those with SBS are strikingly consistent. Hence, clinicians who regularly care for SBS patients find that there are at least three common factors that play an important role in determining a patient's ability to achieve nutritional autonomy from TPN.[4,8,14]

The first important determinant of whether an SBS patient will achieve TPN independence is the amount of residual jejunum-ileum. Patients with at least 120–150 cm of small bowel may require only short periods (up to 6 months) of enteral or parenteral nutrition support before adequate bowel adaptation occurs, and nutrients can be provided by enteral feedings alone. Patients with more than this length usually have shorter periods of TPN dependence with optimal medical and dietary management, if TPN is required at all.

The second important determinant is the presence or absence of colon in continuity with the jejunum-ileum. As described above, the colon adapts after small bowel resection and can absorb significant amounts of calories as well as additional fluid in the SBS patient. The presence of the ileocecal valve can be an added advantage as this valve slows transit of food through the bowel. Thus, patients with as little as 50 cm of jejunum-ileum in continuity *with* colon have a chance of achieving nutritional autonomy. In contrast, patients *without* colon in continuity require at least 100–120 cm of small bowel to have a reasonable chance of becoming independent from TPN. Patients with lesser amounts of bowel can anticipate life-long requirement for TPN without specialized treatments (described below) or intestinal transplantation.

The third important determinant is whether the remaining bowel is normal or diseased. If mucosal disease if present, as, for example, in patients with active Crohn's disease or radiation enteritis, the adaptive process may be impaired. Consequently, such patients with relatively long segments of residual bowel may be unable to absorb adequate nutrients to sustain themselves by enteral feeding alone.

Planning for the care of the SBS patient should be based on knowledge of these three factors, as the likelihood of success is related to all three. Particularly important is the presence or absence of the colon in continuity with the small bowel. Therapy is often planned based on this feature alone, as is described below. However, the effectiveness of current and potentially new treatments of SBS patients must be evaluated in the context of all three of these factors. SBS patients, although similar in many ways, are not identical and should not be treated as such. Lack of understanding of the interplay of these factors decreases the likelihood of achieving nutritional autonomy and may unnecessarily doom a patient to life-long TPN.

OPERATIVE MANAGEMENT AT INITIAL BOWEL RESECTION

Initial management of the patient with SBS begins at the time when extensive bowel resection is contemplated in the operating room. Decisions made at this time may make the difference between achieving and not achieving TPN independence regardless of what is done postoperatively. It is best to speak of residual bowel length in terms of centimeters rather than percent remaining because the pre-resection length of bowel is often unknown. Thus, at the time of surgery, the surgeon should measure the length of the residual bowel along the antimesenteric border without tension and record the length in centimeters. This information can be used to plan future therapy.

Every effort should be made to preserve as much bowel as possible.[4,14–17] In the patient with bowel ischemia, one should resect the obviously necrotic bowel and leave marginally viable bowel in place. A planned 'second look' within 24 hours is then done to assess the viability of the remaining bowel. Alternatively, one may consider use of fluorescein dye injection or Doppler flow estimation of bowel viability at the initial operation. However,

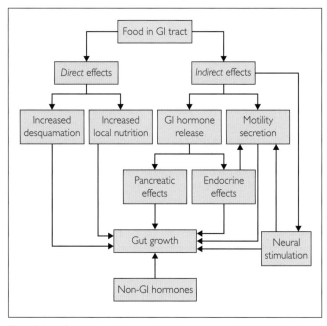

Fig. 55.1 • Regulation of the proliferative response of the intestinal tract. GI, gastrointestinal. (Adapted from Johnson LR. Physiology of the digestive tract. New York: Raven Press; 1987:303.)

these latter two techniques may be less reliable in the hands of those who do not use them regularly. Patients with small bowel strictures (e.g., in patients with Crohn's disease) are better served by stricturoplasty rather than resection where possible. In addition, every effort should be made to preserve the ileocecal valve as this anatomical structure may aid in increasing transit time, thereby enhancing nutrient absorption.

Up to one-third of SBS patients may develop symptomatic cholelithiasis. This may be secondary to TPN or lack of enteral nutrition leading to abnormal bilirubin metabolism and/or bile stasis. Hence, some consider SBS an indication for cholecystectomy although this is not uniformly agreed upon.[4,18] If performed, timing of gallbladder removal requires careful planning. Performing a prophylactic cholecystectomy is ill advised in the unstable patient undergoing emergency bowel resection. In addition, it may be unclear at the initial operation whether long-term TPN will be required. Hence, some advise performing cholecystectomy, if at all, on an elective basis when the patient has been stabilized and long-term prognosis is more predictable.

POSTRESECTION CARE: STANDARD TREATMENT

After the initial bowel resection, SBS patients begin a complex recovery process requiring a variety of therapies to optimize outcome. They progress through a series of phases that can be termed the *perioperative care* phase, the *adaptation and bowel compensation* phase, and the *chronic* phase. For each phase, there is a standard approach to SBS treatment, which includes specific medical, nutritional, and surgical plans. It is imperative to consider each of these treatment modalities carefully when developing an overall plan for SBS therapy. Inattention to any one will undoubtedly result in suboptimal results for the patient. If standard treatment fails or is unlikely to achieve nutritional autonomy, then specialized therapy should be considered.

Acute perioperative care

Perioperative care is the priority in the first 30–90 days after surgery, with the duration of the hospital stay depending on the severity of the illness, associated risk factors, and postoperative complications. Patients should be aggressively rehydrated following extensive bowel resections, as many are hypovolemic. Inadequate resuscitation may cause those patients with marginally perfused bowel to develop necrosis of additional bowel. Most of these patients are also at risk for sepsis and, therefore, require broad-spectrum antibiotics in the perioperative period. Proton pump inhibitors or H_2 antagonists are used to inhibit gastric hypersecretion.[19] Persistently unstable patients should be aggressively evaluated for intra-abdominal abscesses and may requiring CT scanning and possible re-exploration in the operating room to rule out additional intra-abdominal pathology.

TPN should be administered in the immediate postoperative period to help limit the consequences of hypercatabolism in the SBS patient. Most adults will require 1.5 grams of protein and 35 calories per kilogram of body weight per day. As with other critically ill patients, it is important to avoid both under- and overfeeding calories and protein, as inappropriate feeding of either type can be associated with worse outcome. For example, overfeeding calories may predispose one to liver dysfunction.[20] Indirect calorimetry (metabolic cart study) may be required to assess caloric needs, as predictive nutrient-requirement equations (e.g., the Harris-Benedict equation) are often unreliable.

Enteral nutrition is indicated in most, if not all, SBS patients regardless of their short- or long-term requirements for TPN. However, it should be noted that delivery of nutrients to the intestinal lumen increases oxygen consumption by the intestinal mucosa. This can cause bowel necrosis in the patient who has restricted oxygen delivery to the intestine due to mesenteric ischemia.[21] Hence, enteral nutrition should only be started when the SBS patient is hemodynamically stable and the viability of the remaining bowel is assured. This may be several days after the initial operation. In addition, antidiarrheal agents should not be used in the SBS patient until the postoperative ileus resolves and stool output begins.

The adaptation and bowel compensation phase

With recovery from the acute perioperative period, the patient is prepared for discharge to home for convalescence. During the next 2–6 months after the initial operative period, intestinal absorption generally improves as a result of adaptation and bowel compensation. The patient gains strength, and a treatment plan is developed to control SBS-related complications (e.g., dehydration and malnutrition) and support the intestinal adaptive response, which evolves over 6–24 months.

Medical therapy during this phase focuses on minimizing gastric hypersecretion, controlling diarrhea, and repleting electrolyte losses. Massive small bowel resection is associated with hypergastrinemia and increased gastric acid secretion for several months.[22] Hence, H_2 antagonists or proton pump inhibitors should be used in all SBS patients during this time to reduce gastric fluid secretion and the risk of ulcer formation.[19]

Diarrhea is usually a significant problem in SBS patients and necessitates control with antidiarrheal agents such as dyphenoxylate/atropine (Lomotil).[4] If these are ineffective, one can consider use of codeine sulfate or deodorized tincture of opium. However, these latter agents have significant addictive potential and may require increased dosages over time to maintain effectiveness, further increasing this potential for addiction. Octreotide can have a significant impact on stool output in some SBS patients.[23] However, this agent also inhibits the intestinal adaptation process through a number of mechanisms.[24] Hence, octreotide should be reserved for those SBS patients with high output jejunostomies in whom achieving TPN independence is unlikely and there are uncontrollable fluid and electrolyte losses with use of other therapies.[4] Cholestyramine may be used as well in those with less than 100 cm of ileum and colon in continuity with the small bowel. Bile salts that are unabsorbed by the ileum and reach the colon have a cholorrhetic effect, exacerbating fluid losses, which may be improved by a bile salt binder.[4]

In addition to the significant fluid losses observed in SBS patients, there are significant electrolyte losses, particularly potassium and magnesium. These electrolytes need to be repleted aggressively as they may inhibit normal bowel function and precipitate cardiac arrhythmias. It should be noted, however, that enterally administered magnesium and potassium can exacerbate diarrhea and, hence, intravenous administration of electrolytes, with or without TPN, may be necessary if enteral administration is not tolerated.

Nutritional therapy focuses on providing adequate protein and calories to support the adaptive response.[25] Two treatment approaches are possible: the patient is taught to self-administer parenteral nutrition at home or the patient can initiate an enteral feeding program. Frequently, both approaches are appropriate and used during this phase. The old concept of 'bowel rest' in SBS patients should be abandoned in favor of enteral feeding as soon as clinically possible, even if supplemental TPN is required. Enterally administered nutrients are known to enhance the bowel adaptive response in a way that parenterally administered nutrients can not, even if the same number of calories and protein are administered intravenously.[12]

Oral food intake is often associated with nausea and vomiting with subsequent diarrhea. If oral feeding is possible, nausea can be limited by providing frequent small feedings of relatively low-fat foods. Occasionally, antiemetics are required. Diarrhea can be more disabling and is primarily controlled by restricting and controlling type of food intake. The patient begins with a six-feeding diet high in complex carbohydrates (50–60% of total calories) and protein (20% of total calories). Rice, baked potatoes, and pasta balanced with small quantities of chicken, fish, and lean meat serve as the mainstay for this diet. Intake is initially limited to 600 kcal/day. Fluid is limited to 600 mL/day and consists of an electrolyte-containing solution. Commercially available oral solutions include Gatorade® (The Gatorade Co., Chicago, IL), Pedialyte® (Ross Laboratories, Columbus, OH) and Ricelyte® (Mead Johnson, Evansville, IN). Patients with less than 100 cm of jejunum-ileum may benefit from a high-sodium, glucose-containing 'oral rehydration solution.' Of note, glucose promotes sodium and water absorption by solvent drag.[26] As overall tolerance and stool output dictate, the patient is slowly advanced over time (2–6 weeks) to 1000 kcal and 1000 mL per day. This may require adjustment of antidiarrheal medications.

Over a period of several weeks to months, the patient may observe a decrease in stool frequency and a more solid stool consistency as the bowel adaptation process progresses. The quantity of food and liquid should be progressively increased as this occurs with the ultimate goal of providing 120–200% of the usual estimated protein and calorie needs. The additional increase in oral feeding required varies inversely with bowel length and compensates for nutrients lost in the stool.

Surgical therapy during the bowel compensation phase focuses on re-establishing continuity of the remaining intestinal segments.[27] This includes not only reconnecting small bowel segments but also giving consideration to rejoining jejunum-ileum to any remaining colon. As stated previously, significant calorie and fluid absorption can occur in the colon in SBS patients. Colon in continuity with residual small bowel can decrease fluid loses by up to 75% (Fig. 55.2). In addition, the colon can account for up to 50% of daily calorie absorption.[13] The benefits of rejoining small to large bowel are generally realized in patients who have at least one-third of their remaining colon. Colonic calorie and fluid absorption may be limited in those SBS patients with less than one-third of their colons. In addition, problems with copious diarrhea, fecal incontinence and perianal excoriation may outweigh any potential benefits from such a procedure in patients with short colonic segments or extremely short small bowel segments. Hence, under these circumstances an end enterostomy may be preferable. Anastomoses should be done so as to preserve as much bowel as possible and special care should

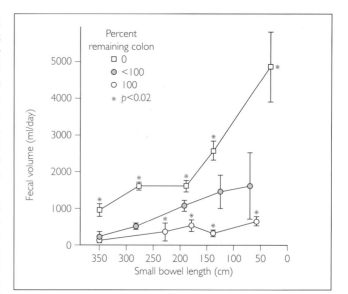

Fig. 55.2 • At any small bowel length, fecal volume increases as the length of colon is reduced. Note the massive fluid losses associated with ostomy patients (0% colon) with less than a 150 cm small bowel. (Adapted from Nordgaard I, Hansen BS, Mortensen PB. Importance of colonic support for energy absorption as small-bowel failure proceeds. Am J Clin Nutr 1996; 64:222–231. © Am J Clin Nutr American Society for Clinical Nutrition.)

be given to preventing iatrogenic enterotomies that could necessitate resection of additional, precious segments of bowel.

It should also be noted that feeding through a jejunostomy tube (j-tube) results in feeding several centimeters distal to the ligament of Treitz, given the location of the tip of the typical j-tube. This distance, which is inconsequential in the usual patient, can make a significant difference in the ability of the SBS patient to achieve nutritional autonomy. Consequently, SBS patients with marginal intestinal adaptation who are receiving j-tube feedings should be converted to gastrostomy tube or oral feedings if there is not disabling gastroparesis or another contraindication to such feedings.

The chronic phase

By 6 months, most patients have reached the chronic phase of their illnesses and the focus is often on *nutritional therapy* at this point. Attempts should be made to sustain patients on an enteral regimen providing 120–200% of estimated needs if tolerated and as described below. However, it may be evident that TPN will be needed for the foreseeable future. If TPN is required, every attempt should be made to encourage enteral intake as well. This optimizes bowel adaptation and helps 'protect' the liver from the consequences of long-term TPN administration.[12,18] Because TPN administration may suppress the appetite, the combined enteral–parenteral feeding regimen may be best accomplished by providing TPN on three or four alternate nights. Dehydration may become a problem in those who are not receiving daily TPN infusions and have high stool output. Under such circumstances, an electrolyte-containing i.v. infusion without nutrients can be provided on the TPN 'off' days. Patients who have increased energy requirements or those in whom weight gain is desired may require TPN on a daily basis. However, this is often only in a small percentage of patients, and may only be required intermittently.

Maintaining adequate nutrition in part entails close monitoring of body weight. Body mass index (BMI, weight [kg]/height [m]²) should be maintained at or above 20 (normal BMI range for adults is 18.5–25) with changes in nutrition prescription as necessary to maintain this goal. A dietary goal is established for each individual patient, and food and fluid intake is closely monitored initially to achieve a successful outcome.

The enteral diet is most satisfactorily composed of 40–60% complex carbohydrate, 20–30% protein, and 20–40% fat.[8,25,28] Simple sugars are excluded, including lactose-containing milk products for most patients. The diet is divided into six small meals of equal size. The patient is taught, through specific meal planning and food preparation guidelines, the specific amount of food to ingest at each meal. In addition, specific fluid volume that will maintain adequate hydration is planned. Isotonic electrolyte-containing fluids are preferred, particularly for the patient with no colon. Both food and fluid records should be maintained and closely monitored until the patient can satisfactorily comply with the diet and fluid prescription. In general, this may take 2–4 weeks of intensive education by trained staff (e.g., a registered dietitian with special interest in the SBS population) for a patient to satisfactorily achieve these goals. Close follow-up is often necessary to assure appropriate and consistent dietary intake.

Enteral feeding regimens must be further refined according to the presence or absence of colon in continuity with jejunum-ileum (Table 55.1).[28] Those SBS patients with colon in continuity should receive a diet high in complex carbohydrates (50–60% of total enteral intake) and protein (20–30%) and low in fat (20%). Such a diet prescription takes advantage of the colon's ability to ferment and absorb the energy-rich byproducts of complex carbohydrates, which have passed undigested through the small intestine. SBS patients with colon in continuity and fat malabsorption are predisposed to increased oxalate absorption and the development of calcium oxalate nephrocalcinosis and nephrolithiasis. Hence, they should also receive an oxalate-restricted diet. Administration of oral calcium can tightly bind oxalate, decrease oxalate absorption, and thereby decrease the risk of oxalate stone formation in the kidneys.

In contrast, those SBS patients *without* colon in continuity should receive a more liberal intake of fat (30–40%) and less carbohydrate (40%) as this prescription may decrease the severity of osmotic diarrhea. These general guidelines are a good starting point for most SBS patients, but a more individualized diet frequently needs to be developed through trial and error and close follow-up with a registered dietitian familiar with dietary management of the SBS patient.

Medical therapy during the chronic phase in SBS patients focuses on identifying micronutrient deficiencies and repleting vitamins, minerals, and electrolytes as necessary while minimizing the risks of solid organ dysfunction and development of bacterial overgrowth.[4] Resection of the distal small bowel where vitamin B_{12} is absorbed necessitates close monitoring of vitamin B_{12} levels in the SBS patient. This vitamin is provided in parenteral forms and may be given in intravenous solutions including TPN, subcutaneously, or intranasally. Fat malabsorption in the SBS patient is associated with malabsorption of the fat-soluble vitamins A, E, and D. Both vitamin A and E can be administered via the enteral route. Vitamin D deficiency is associated with malabsorption of calcium and leads to the osteoporosis and osteomalacia commonly seen in short bowel patients. Patients are encouraged to expose their skin to the sunlight to promote vitamin D biosynthesis. Patients may also need vitamin D supplementation by the parenteral or enteral route with adequate calcium. In addition to calcium, magnesium, another divalent ion, is frequently malabsorbed or lost in the stool. Oral magnesium repletion is possible but may promote diarrhea in large doses. Alternatively, magnesium sulfate can be added to an electrolyte drink and with slow, hourly ingestion, the diarrhea associated with magnesium ingestion may be minimized. Magnesium may also be administered as part of TPN or other intravenous fluids as necessary. Finally, selenium and zinc levels should be monitored in the plasma (or preferentially in the hair, fingernails, or urine) and repleted as these trace elements are often depleted in those with chronic diarrhea.

The great majority of SBS patients have deficiency of linoleic and linolenic acids, the essential fatty acids.[28] Essential fats are generally provided via the enteral route. In those who cannot absorb sufficient fat via the enteral route, 100 grams of fat emulsion are provided intravenously per week. Essential fatty acid levels should be monitored at 6-month intervals on samples of plasma obtained after a 12-hour fast from both enteral and parenteral nutrients. If essential fatty acid deficiency is identified, patients are given additional infusions of a 20% lipid emulsion intravenously each week for 2–5 weeks.

Three major solid organs may become dysfunctional in SBS patients and eventually fail. These are the liver, bones, and kidneys. Hence, it is important to medically manage the SBS patient with

Table 55.1 Diet prescription

Nutrient	Colon	No colon
Carbohydrate	50–60% of total calories (limit simple sugars)	40–50% of total calories restricted simple sugars)
Protein	20–30% of total calories	20–30% of total calories
Fat	20–30% of total calories (primarily as essential fats)	30–40% of total calories (primarily as essential fats)
Fluid	Isotonic or hypo-osmolar fluids	Isotonic, high-sodium oral rehydration solutions
Soluble fiber	5–10 g/day (if stool output>3 L/day)	5–10 g/day (if stool output >3 L/day)
Oxalates	Limited intake	
Meals/snacks	5–6 meals per day	4–6 meals per day

prevention of organ dysfunction in mind. Liver dysfunction was initially described in infants and later reported in adults after extensive bowel resection.[29,30] The pathologic findings of the liver revealed fat infiltration, cholestasis, and fibrosis. These changes have been associated with overinfusion of dextrose, underadministration of lipids, lack of administration of trace substances (e.g., choline and carnitine), and absorption of bacteria or their byproducts from a permeable intestinal tract. Repeated episodes of line sepsis also are associated with liver dysfunction. Although the exact mechanisms of TPN-associated liver dysfunction in the SBS patient remain to be determined, certain medical practices can reduce the risk to the liver. These include good central venous line care to minimize episodes of line sepsis. Enteral feeding, even in the TPN-dependent patient, may 'protect' the liver, as well as cycling TPN and providing TPN on alternate days if possible. One should avoid overfeeding calories, especially dextrose, and provide carnitine – an important element necessary for mitochondrial fat metabolism – as indicated by carnitine levels.

Bone mass is another important index to monitor. It should be assessed at regular intervals (i.e., every 1–2 years) with dual-energy X-ray absorptiometry (DEXA) scanning. Weight-bearing exercise is encouraged to maintain bone mass and vitamin D, calcium, and magnesium are monitored and repleted as described previously to promote bone health as well.

Renal dysfunction in SBS is most likely to occur if there is chronic dehydration or repeated episodes of severe, acute dehydration. Hence, maintaining hydration status is a key element in preserving renal function. Adequate hydration is indicated by a daily urine output of 1500–2000 mL per day in the adult of normal size and with normal renal function. As an alternative to collecting urine over 24 hours to monitor daily urine output, patients can use a urometer to spot-check urine specific gravity. The goal is to maintain specific gravity to less than 1.015. If specific gravity rises above this, patients are instructed to increase oral fluid intake or take additional intravenous fluid.

Bacterial overgrowth and D-lactic acidosis are rare events in patients with colon in continuity with the small bowel remnant.[4] In addition, SBS with dilated loops of small bowel prone to stool stasis can develop significant bacterial overgrowth. Alterations or overgrowth of intraluminal intestinal bacteria may allow more pathogenic bacteria to dominate and contribute to increased diarrhea and alterations in the metabolism and absorption of nutrients. In addition, overgrowth has been found to have a direct effect on normal peristalsis. Such alteration in bacterial flora may be related to change in diet, associated illnesses, or the use of antibiotics for other reasons. Diagnosis of this condition can be difficult but may be facilitated by obtaining a hydrogen breath test or culture of endoscopically obtained aspirates. A 10–14 day course of antibiotics (e.g., metronidazole, ciprofloxacin) is the usual treatment for bacterial overgrowth.

If the patient ingests large quantities of refined sugar, the fermenting organisms may produce increased amounts of D-lactate leading to D-lactic acidosis. This is associated with confusion, fatigue, inability to function, and possibly coma if left untreated. There may be an increased anion gap acidosis with elevated D-lactate. It is critical in making the diagnosis that the physician request a D-lactate level instead of the usual L-lactate which may be tested for. Intravenous fluid, supportive care, and treatment with antibiotics to reduce the bacterial overgrowth usually results in prompt resolution of this condition.

Surgical therapy during the chronic phase focuses on central venous line care. A frequent cause of death in SBS patients is line-associated complications including repeated episodes of line sepsis and venous thrombosis. Hence, line care is critical to the long-term survival of the TPN-dependent SBS patient. The surgeon is often called upon to deal with such issues. While meticulous sterile technique in the operating room decreases the short-term risk of line infection, it is the patient and his/her nurses who are instrumental in reducing long-term infection risk through their meticulous sterile technique while caring for and accessing the central venous catheter.

Patients who have had multiple lines and are running out of venous access sites should be considered for 'antibiotic lock' treatment.[31] This technique involves instillation of a super-concentrated, low volume (e.g., 3 mL) antibiotic solution into the infected catheter lumen or lumens, which stays in the catheter for 12–24 hours. At the end of this time the antibiotic solution is aspirated and the catheter flushed with normal saline. This can be repeated for several days to 2 weeks. An antibiotic to which the infecting organism is sensitive is chosen. The antibiotic lock technique is only effective for internal catheter infections and not 'pocket' or 'tunnel' infections, which are external to the catheter lumen. This procedure has been noted to salvage infected lines in up to 89% of cases, which prevents unnecessary removal of a line with loss of a venous access site in a patient who will need access sites on a long-term, potentially life-long, basis.

Prevention of venous thrombosis associated with venous catheters begins with proper positioning of the catheter by the surgeon. Centers with large-volume central venous line practices have noted that catheters whose tips reside close to atrio-caval junction are less likely to thrombose relative to those that reside more distally (e.g., the subclavian vein). In patients who have limited venous access due to thrombosis of upper body veins, one can consider achieving access via the femoral venous system. In desperate situations, the translumbar approach to the inferior vena cava with assistance of the interventional radiologists has been used with success.[32]

SPECIALIZED CARE

Despite optimal standard treatment, some SBS patients continue to be TPN dependent. These patients should be considered for specialized care. These specialized treatments can be thought of in terms of surgical, medical, and nutritional care, just as is done for standard care of the SBS patient. *Surgical procedures* fall into two categories: those procedures designed to prolong intestinal transit time and those designed to increase functional intestinal absorptive surface area.[27] Procedures designed to prolong transit are generally reserved for patients who have normal bowel caliber, while those designed to improve functional absorptive area are generally designed for those with dilated bowel (Fig. 55.3). These procedures assume that small and large bowel continuity has been restored to the maximal extent possible as described above.

To prolong intestinal transit time, surgeons have created intestinal valves using such techniques as intussuscepting a 2 cm segment of small bowel and securing the intussuscepted segment with sutures to prevent it from slipping back to its normal configuration. Alternatively, reversed 10 cm segments of small or large bowel have been anastomosed in continuity with the small bowel to serve as an antiperistaltic segment. Others have tried a

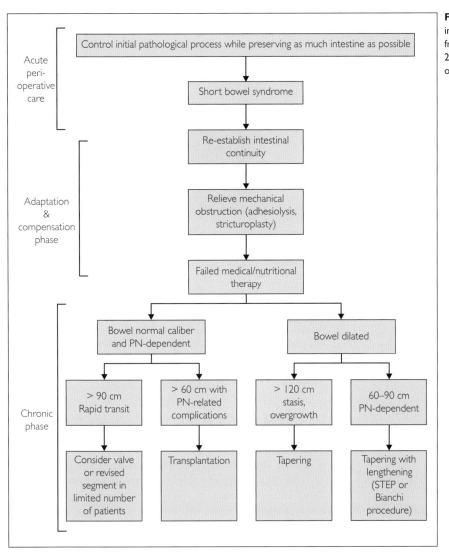

Fig. 55.3 • Algorithm for surgical treatment in SBS. TPN, total parenteral nutrition. (Reprinted from Thompson JS et al, Annals of Surgery, 1995; 222:600–607. © 1995, reprinted with permission of Lippincott, Williams & Wilkins.)

variety of recirculating loops and pouches, as well as retrograde intestinal pacing. Those with experience with these procedures conclude that these procedures are highly inconsistent, fraught with complications, and of limited long-term efficacy. Hence, it is not recommended that such procedures be used on a regular basis.[27]

In contrast, procedures designed to increase functional absorptive capacity of the bowel can be quite successful in the appropriately selected individual *with dilated bowel*. These procedures include relieving mechanical obstruction from intra-abdominal adhesions or strictures with proximal dilatation of the small bowel. To minimize loss of residual bowel, adhesiolysis should be done to minimize iatrogenic enterotomies, and strictures should be preferentially dealt with by stricturoplasty rather than enterectomy.

In those SBS patients with dilated bowel without stricture or other mechanical obstruction, one may perform a tapering enteroplasty with or without lengthening of the bowel. This includes the well-known procedure first described by Bianchi in 1980.[33] The Bianchi procedure consists of dissecting along the mesenteric border of the small intestine to reveal the blood vessels, which independently supply the two halves of the bowel along its longitudinal axis. The bowel is then divided between these vessels along its longitudinal axis so as to create two tubes of equal lengths. These tubes are subsequently anastomosed end to end in an isoperistaltic fashion. The result is an intestinal segment that is twice as long as but half the diameter of the original segment (Fig. 55.4A).

More recently, the serial transverse enteroplasty (STEP) procedure has been used. This involves serial application of a linear stapler from opposite directions, which divides the bowel from the mesenteric and antimesenteric borders. The net result is increase in length and reduction in diameter of the bowel, similar to the Bianchi procedure (Fig. 55.4B). Although the actual surface area of the intestine is not increased with either procedure (at least acutely), the function of the bowel improves and thus absorptive capacity increases significantly. Surgical procedures that improve function of the remnant bowel account for more than half of the specialized surgical treatments for SBS patients and have a reported success rate of 90% in the hands of experienced surgeons.[27]

There is little to offer patients who have failed to achieve nutritional autonomy with standard management and specialized surgical treatments (if indicated) other than intestinal transplantation. However, intestinal transplantation carries high morbidity and mortality despite significant progress in this procedure as discussed below. Consequently, many have attempted to identify

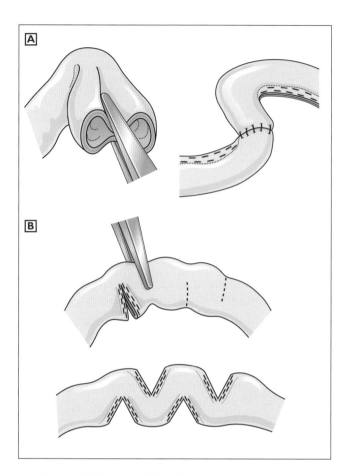

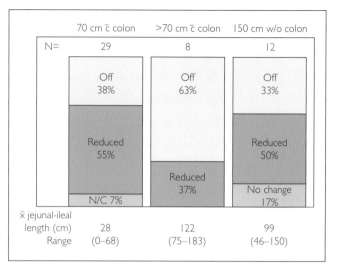

Fig. 55.5 • PN status 1 year following treatment for 49 PN-dependent patients with = 70 cm of small bowel continuity with some colon (n=29), for those >70 cm small bowel in continuity with colon (n=8), and those with =150 cm small bowel and no colon (n=12). 'Off' indicates no PN, 'Reduced' indicates less than what was originally given, and 'No Change-NC' indicates similar volume and calories to that which was originally administered. The mean jejunal-ileal length and the range are also provided). (Reprinted from Byrne TA et al, Transplant Proceedings, 2002; 34:887–890. © 2002 with permission from Elsevier.)

Fig. 55.4 • (A) Bianchi and (B) STEP procedure to taper and lengthen dilated small bowel in SBS patients.

growth factors and nutrients, which may enhance intestinal adaptation through *specialized medical and nutritional regimens* without surgical intervention. The largest clinical experience is with growth hormone and glutamine. Exogenous administration of growth hormone (GH) has been shown in experimental animal models to increase colonic mass, enhance sodium and water absorption in the small and large intestine, increase amino acid transport by enterocytes, and promote mucosal hyperplasia after extensive small bowel resection. Glutamine (GLN), a conditionally essential amino acid in catabolic states, serves as a primary fuel for both enterocytes and colonocytes, accelerates mucosal hyperplasia, and enhances sodium and water absorption following massive enterectomy in animals.

Based on the above experimental evidence, a specialized treatment plan using a combination of GH and GLN with strict adherence to an SBS-appropriate diet was developed.[34] Use of this therapy in a diverse group of nearly 400 SBS patients over the past decade has demonstrated significant efficacy in patients previously thought to have no chance of gaining nutritional autonomy. Subsets of this group have been reported on over the years.[8,14,25] This includes a group of patients with an average of 28 cm of jejunum-ileum anastomosed to colon in whom 38% became TPN independent, and an additional 55% had significant reductions in their TPN utilization (Fig. 55.5). This group of patients is traditionally thought of as the most difficult to treat and least likely to become TPN independent.[4] At least two other groups have found positive effects from using combined GH and

GLN in SBS patients as well.[35,36] This therapy is not without controversy, however. Data from a group of eight patients did not show a benefit from such therapy.[37] Of note, seven of the eight patients in this series had Crohn's disease and six of the eight had no colon. SBS patients with no colon and diseased remnant bowel (whether active or inactive disease) have significant limitations on their ability to adapt, which may explain why no benefit was observed in this small study. In contrast, a more recent prospective, randomized, double-blind, placebo-controlled clinical study in 41 patients further supports use of this therapy in the appropriately selected and motivated patient in whom standard management techniques have failed or are likely to fail.[38] Patients receiving growth hormone and glutamine had a dramatic statistically significant response (Table 55.2). This approach is relatively safe therapy with minimal complications in experienced hands, and long-term efficacy has been achieved. Hence, such therapy should be considered before committing patients to intestinal transplantation or life-long TPN.

INTESTINAL TRANSPLANTATION

Intestinal transplantation is a potential alternative for those SBS patients who have failed all standard and specialized treatments. While life saving for some, it carries a very high morbidity and mortality. Hence, intestinal transplantation should be reserved for those who (1) are not likely to become TPN independent despite maximal standard and specialized treatment, and (2) have potentially life-threatening complications of TPN dependence. One way to predict the likelihood of achieving nutritional autonomy without intestinal transplantation is based on the ratio of jejunal-ileal length to body weight, which was developed based on clinical studies in patients with the shortest segments of bowel. Those with a small bowel/body weight ratio of greater than 0.5 have a 75% chance of TPN independence. Those with a ratio of

Table 55.2 Change in PN dependency with dietary modification, supplemental glutamine (GLN), and recombinant human growth hormone (rhGH)

	Dietary modification with supplemental GLN (n = 9)	Dietary modification with rhGH (n = 16)	Dietary modification with rhGH and supplemental GLN
Decrease in PN volume (liters)	3.8 ± 0.8	5.8 ± 1.0*	7.7 ± 0.8**
Decrease in PN calories (kcal)	2661 ± 439	4323 ± 464*	5745 ± 519**
Decrease in PN frequency (days)	2.0 ± 0.3	3.0 ± 0.5*	4.2 ± 0.4**

Data reported as mean ± SEM.
* p<0.05
** p<0.001 versus dietary modification with supplemental GLN.
From Byrne, TA et al. J Parent Ent Nutr 2003; 27:S17.

0.25 to 0.5 have a 50% chance of achieving autonomy. Those with a smaller ratio are unlikely to ever become free of TPN even with specialized therapy unless offered transplantation. Based on this ratio, a probability of success for standard and progressively aggressive therapies can be predicted (Fig. 55.6).

Currently, it is felt that intestinal transplantation should be reserved for SBS patients with life-threatening problems from liver failure, recurrent venous catheter sepsis or thromboses, and recurrent dehydration secondary to massive fluid loss.[4] A combined intestine/liver transplant may be the only option for survival for patients with end-stage liver disease as a result of TPN dependence due to SBS. Significant advances have been made in improving graft survival in these patients but overall patient survival has largely been unchanged. Graft survival for intestine only and intestine/liver transplant are 60% and 55%, respectively, at 1 year, and 37% and 30% at 5 years. Patient survival for those receiving intestine and intestine/liver transplant are 71% and 62% at 1 year, respectively, and 45% and 37% at 5 years. Eighty percent of surviving patients achieve nutritional autonomy.[39] With less than half of patients having long-term survival after small bowel transplant, improvements in immunosuppressive therapy are clearly necessary to improve long-term outcome.

SUMMARY AND CONCLUSION

It is currently estimated that SBS patients have a 1-year survival that approaches 75% with the algorithm outlined in Figure 55.7. This represents significant progress over the 20% survival rate prior to the TPN era. Critical to potentially achieving nutritional autonomy for the SBS patient are preserving as much bowel as possible during the initial surgical procedure and restoring small bowel and colon continuity (if possible) at the initial or later procedure. Enteral feeding of whole food should be encouraged to enhance intestinal adaptation even if TPN is required. Well-defined problems that develop later, such as intestinal strictures or dilated, poorly functioning bowel, should be corrected surgically. Patients that remain TPN dependent after these measures should be considered for growth factor therapy. Finally, intestinal transplantation should be reserved for those who have life-threatening TPN-related complications in whom maximal, optimized nontransplant therapy has been attempted but failed. Future therapy will focus on new, more potent growth factors, better immunosuppressive therapy for those who do undergo intestinal transplant, and tissue engineering of new intestinal segments.

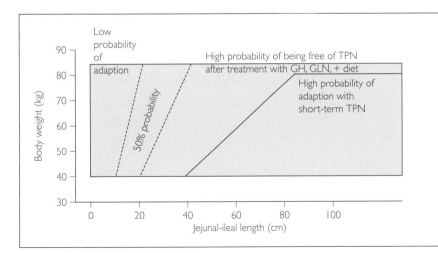

Fig. 55.6 • Chart used to predict the probability of success of weaning from total parenteral nutrition (TPN) a patient with short-bowel syndrome and a portion of the colon in continuity. To determine the predicted outcome for an individual patient, locate the point at which bowel length and body weight cross. The area identified will describe the predicted outcome. GH, growth hormone; GLN, glutamine.

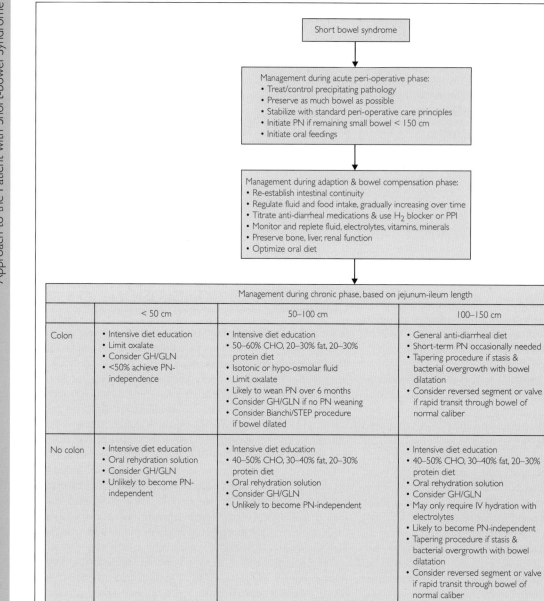

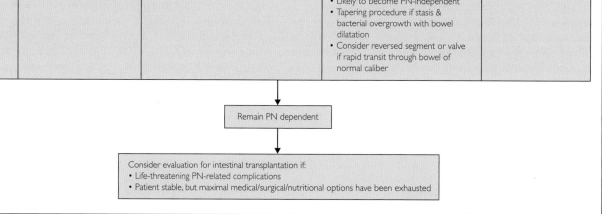

Fig. 55.7 • Algorithm for management of short bowel syndrome. PN, parenteral nutrition; PPI, proton pump inhibitor; GH, growth hormone; GLN, glutamine; CHO, carbohydrate.

REFERENCES

1. Koeberle E. Resection de deux meters d'intestin grel. Bull Acad Med 1881; 8:249–250.

2. Haymond HE. Massive resection of the small intestine. Surg Gynecol Obstet 1935; 51:693–705.

3. Wilmore DW, Dudrick SJ. Growth and development of an infant receiving all nutrients exclusively by vein. JAMA 1968; 203:140–144.

   One of the seminal papers regarding total parenteral nutrition.

4. AGA Technical review on short bowel syndrome and intestinal transplantation. Gastroenterology 2003; 124:1111–1134.

Details theoretical basis for current clinical treatment of patients with short-bowel syndrome.

5. Underhill BML. Intestinal length in man. Br Med J 1955; 4950:1243–1246.

6. Backman L, Hallberg D. Small intestinal length. Acta Chir Scand 1974; 140:57–63.

7. Vanderhoof JA, Langnas AN. Short-bowel syndrome in children and adults. Gastroenterology 1997; 113:1767–1778.

8. Byrne TA, Cox S, Karimbakas M, et al. Bowel rehabilitation: an alternative to long-term parenteral nutrition and intestinal transplantation for some patients with short bowel syndrome. Transplantation Proc 2002; 34:887–890.

9. Thompson JS, Iyer KR, DiBaise JK, et al. Short bowel syndrome and Crohn's disease. J Gastrointest Surg 2003; 7:1069–1072.

10. Andorsky DJ, Lund DP, Lillehei CW, et al. Nutritional and other postoperative management of neonates with short bowel syndrome correlates with clinical outcomes. J Pediatr 2001; 139:27–33.

11. Porus RL. Epithelial hyperplasia following massive bowel resection in man. Gastroenterology 1965; 48:753–757.

12. Robinson MK, Ziegler TR, Wilmore DW. Overview of intestinal adaptation and its stimulation. Eur J Pediatr Surg 1999; 9:200–206.

Details adaptive process following massive small bowel resection in humans.

13. Nordgaard I, Hansen BS, Mortensen PB. Colon as a digestive organ in patients with short bowel. Lancet 1994; 343:373–376.

14. Wilmore DW, Lacey JM, Soultanakis RP, et al. Factors predicting a successful outcome after pharmacologic bowel compensation. Ann Surg 1997; 226:228–292.

15. Robinson MK, Wilmore DW. Short bowel syndrome. In: Holzheimer RG, Mannick JA, eds. Surgical treatment: evidence-based and problem-oriented. Muchen, New York: W. Zuckschwerdt Verlag; 2001:140–145.

16. Thompson JS, Langnas AN, Pinch LW, et al. Surgical approach to short-bowel syndrome: experience in a population of 160 patients. Ann Surg 1995; 222:600–607.

17. Robinson MK. Short bowel syndrome. In: Cameron JL, ed. Current surgical therapy. Philadelphia: Elsevier Mosby; 2004:140–146.

18. Fulford A, Scolapio JS, Aranda-Michel J. Parenteral nutrition-associated hepatotoxicity. Nutr Clin Pract 2004; 19:274–283.

19. Jeppesen PB, Staun M, Tjellesen L, et al. Effect of intravenous ranitidine and omeprazole on intestinal absorption of water, sodium, and macronutrients in patients with intestinal resection. Gut 1998; 43:763–769.

20. Buchman A. Total parenteral nutrition-associated liver disease. J Parent Ent Nutr 2002; 26(5 Suppl):S43–S48.

21. McClave SA, Chang WK. Feeding the hypotensive patient: does enteral feeding precipitate or protect against bowel ischemia? Nutr Clin Pract 2003; 18:279–284.

22. Williams NS, Evans P, King RJ. Gastric acid secretion and gastrin production in the short bowel syndrome. Gut 1985; 26:914–919.

23. Harris AG, O'Dorisio TM, Woltering EA, et al. Consensus statement: octreotide dose titration in secretory diarrhea: diarrhea management consensus development panel. Dig Dis Sci 1995; 40:1464–1473.

24. O'Keefe SJD, Haymond MW, Bennet WM, et al. Long-acting somatostatin analogue therapy and protein metabolism in patients with jejunostomies. Gastroenterology 1994; 107:379–388.

25. Byrne TA, Nompleggi DJ, Wilmore DW. Advances in the management of patients with intestinal failure. Trans Proceed 1996; 28:2683–2690.

26. Fortran JS. Stimulation of active and passive sodium absorption by sugars in the human jejunum. J Clin Invest 1975; 55:728–737.

27. Thompson JS. Surgical rehabilitation of intestine in short bowel syndrome. Surgery 2004; 135:465–470.

Reviews current surgical treatment strategies for patients with short-bowel syndrome.

28. Byrne TA, Veglia L, Camelio M, et al. Beyond the prescription: optimizing the diet of patients with short bowel syndrome. Nutr Clin Pract 2000; 15:306–311.

Details current nutritional management of short-bowel syndrome, including the most complex patients.

29. Dahms BB, Halpin TC. Serial liver biopsies in parenteral nutrition-associated choleostasis of early infancy. Gastroenterology 1981; 81:136–144.

30. Stanko RT, Nathan G, Mendelow H, et al. Development of hepatic choleostasis and fibrosis in patients with massive loss of the intestine supported by prolonged parenteral nutrition. Gastroenterology 1987; 92:197–202.

31. Carratala J. The antibiotic-lock technique for therapy of 'highly needed' infected catheters. Clin Microbiol Infect 2002; 8:282–289.

Reviews technique for preserving infected central venous catheters in patients who have limited vascular access options.

32. Steiger E. Obtaining and maintaining vascular access in the home parenteral nutrition patient. J Parent Ent Nutr 26(5 Suppl): 2002; S17–S20.

33. Bianchi A. Intestinal loop lengthening – a technique for increasing small intestinal length. J Pediatr Surg 1980; 15:145–151.

34. Byrne TA, Persinger RL, Young LS, et al. A new treatment for patients with short-bowel syndrome: growth hormone, glutamine, and a modified diet. Ann Surg 1995; 222:243–255.

Seminal paper regarding treatment of short-bowel syndrome patients with combination of growth hormone, glutamine, and a modified diet.

35. Seguy D, Vahedi K, Kapel N, et al. Low-dose growth hormone in adult home parenteral nutrition-dependent short bowel syndrome patients: a positive study. Gastroenterology 2003; 124:293–302.

36. Ellegard L, Bosaeus I, Nordgren S, et al. Low dose recombinant human growth hormone increases body weight and lean body mass in patients with short bowel syndrome. Ann Surg 1997; 225:88–96.

37. Scolapio JS, Camilleri M, Fleming CR, et al. Effect of growth hormone, glutamine, and diet on adaptation in short-bowel syndrome: a randomized controlled study. Gastroenterology 1997; 113:1074–1081.

38. Byrne TA, Lautz DB, Iyer KR, et al. Recombinant human growth hormone (rhGH) reduces parenteral nutrition (PN) in patients with the short bowel syndrome: a prospective, randomized, double-blind, placebo-controlled study. J Parent Ent Nutr 2003; 27:S17.

Prospective, randomized, placebo-controlled trial demonstrating efficacy of growth hormone with glutamine in the treatment of short bowel syndrome patients.

39. 2000 annual report. The U.S. scientific registry of transplants recipients and the organ procurement and transplantation network. Transplant data 1990–1999. U.S. Department of Health and Human Services Administration, Office of Special Programs, Division of Transplantation, Rockville, MD; United Network of Organ Sharing, Richmond, VA.

CHAPTER FIFTY-SIX

Crohn's disease

Sonia Friedman and Gary R. Lichtenstein

INTRODUCTION

Crohn's disease (CD) is an idiopathic chronic inflammatory disorder of the intestinal tract that can affect any portion(s) of the gastrointestinal tract from the mouth to the anus. Inflammatory bowel disease (IBD) consistent with Crohn's disease was described as long as 300 years ago and single cases were reported during the early part of the nineteenth century. By 1920, American physicians had reported instances of granulomatous lesions of the terminal ileum or ileocecal region in young patients with diarrhea, fevers, and weight loss who were operated on for presumed appendicitis. In 1932, a pivotal paper by Crohn, Ginzburg, and Oppenheim from Mount Sinai Hospital in New York reported 14 cases of 'terminal ileitis,' later referred to as 'regional enteritis.' The concept of a 'Crohn's colitis' was not completely accepted in America until 1959 when it was described as a pathologic entity separate from ulcerative colitis by Lockhart-Mummery and Morson.[1,2]

EPIDEMIOLOGY

The incidence of Crohn's disease is highest in northern countries such as the United Kingdom, Norway, Sweden, and the United States. The incidence rate in the United States is about 7 per 100 000. Countries in southern Europe, South Africa, and Australia have a lower incidence rate with a range of 0.9–3.1 per 100 000. In Asia and South America, Crohn's disease is rare with an incidence rate in a Japanese population of 0.08 per 100 000. In most studies, the incidence of CD reaches its peak in persons between the ages of 15 and 30 years. A second, smaller peak has been observed in persons between the ages of 60 and 80. The incidence and prevalence also varies depending on race and ethnicity. A two- to fourfold increased frequency of CD in Jewish populations has been described in the United States, Europe, and South Africa. The prevalence decreases progressively in non-Jewish Caucasian, African-American, Hispanic, and Asian populations. There is also an increased prevalence in urban rather than rural areas and in high socioeconomic class and white-collar occupations rather than lower socioeconomic class and blue-collar occupations. The male-to-female ratio for CD is 1.1–1.8 to 1.[3]

Smoking is a risk factor for developing Crohn's disease and patients who smoke have a twofold increased risk.[4,5] Oral contraceptives are also linked to CD; the relative risk of CD for oral contraceptive users is about 1.9.[3] Women with Crohn's disease may become more symptomatic around the time of their menstrual cycles[6] but there is no seasonal variation in flares.[7] There is familial aggregation of Crohn's disease and in twin studies, 67% of monozygotic twins are concordant for CD. Eight percent of dizygotic twins are concordant for CD. There is also concordance for anatomic site and clinical type of CD within families. If a patient has either CD or ulcerative colitis (UC), the lifetime risk that a first-degree relative will be affected is slightly less than one in ten. If both parents have either CD or UC, there is a 36% chance that the child will be affected.[8]

PATHOLOGY

Crohn's disease can affect any part of the gastrointestinal tract from the mouth to the anus. Thirty percent to 40% of patients have small bowel disease alone, 40–55% have disease involving both the small and large intestines, and 15–25% have colitis alone. In the 75% of patients with small intestinal disease, the terminal ileum will be involved in 90%. Although rectal sparing is characteristic of Crohn's disease and helps to distinguish it from ulcerative colitis, perianal and perirectal lesions are present in one-third of patients with CD, particularly those with colonic involvement. Crohn's disease may also involve the liver and the pancreas.[9]

Unlike UC, Crohn's disease is a transmural process. Endoscopically, there are aphthous or small superficial ulcerations in mild disease and in more active disease stellate ulcerations and serpiginous ulcerations that fuse longitudinally and transversely to form islands of mucosa that frequently are histologically normal. This 'cobblestoning' is a characteristic finding of CD, both endoscopically and by barium radiography. Pseudopolyps, or long, finger-like inflammatory polyps, can also form in chronic Crohn's disease. Unlike UC where the inflammation is continuous, CD is a segmental disease.[9]

The Vienna Classification of Crohn's disease is an attempt to categorize the three different types of disease behavior (Table 56.1), as well as anatomy and age at diagnosis.

Patients most commonly present with nonstricturing, nonpenetrating disease which often evolves over time to either stricturing (fibrostenotic) or penetrating (fistulizing) disease.[10] Knowing the eventual phenotype at the initiation of therapy might very be helpful in determining the most effective treatment.

The definitive pathologic lesion in Crohn's disease is the noncaseating granuloma. Noncaseating granulomas consist of

Table 56.1 Vienna classification of Crohn's disease

Age at diagnosis	A1	<40 years
	A2	≥40 years
Location	L1	Terminal ileum
	L2	Colon
	L3	Ileocolon
	L4	Upper gastrointestinal
Behavior	B1	Nonstricturing, nonpenetrating
	B2	Stricturing
	B3	Penetrating

aggregations of macrophages and can be seen in all layers of the bowel wall from mucosa to serosa. They can even be seen in lymph nodes, mesentery, peritoneum, liver, and pancreas, probably as an extension of disease from the bowel wall. Although granulomas are a pathognomonic feature of Crohn's disease, only half of cases reveal granulomas on surgical specimens. Other histologic features of CD include submucosal or subserosal lymphoid aggregates, particularly away from areas of ulceration, gross and microscopic skip areas, and transmural inflammation that is accompanied by fissures that penetrate deeply into the bowel wall and sometimes form fistulous tracts.[9]

Population-based cohort studies have shown that 20–40% of patients with Crohn's disease will develop fistulae. Types of fistulae include perianal, enterocutaneous, enteroenteral and fistulas from the bowel to adjacent organs such as the uterus, vagina, and bladder.[11]

DIFFERENTIAL DIAGNOSIS

The differential diagnosis of Crohn's disease is large and includes infectious and noninfectious etiologies (Table 56.2). When initially evaluating a patient who presents with diarrhea and abdominal pain, it is of paramount importance to exclude the presence of an enteric infection. Stool cultures for enteric pathogens and stool evaluation for ova and parasites should be routinely performed. Stool assay for *Clostridium difficile toxin* should be checked if the patient has risk factors such as antibiotic use, immunosuppression, or is a resident in a chronic care facility. Common bacterial infections in addition to *C. difficile* whose symptoms can mimic Crohn's disease include *Campylobacter, Salmonella, Yersinia enterocolitica*, and *Eschericha coli*. Gonorrhea, *Chlamydia*, and syphilis can also cause proctitis. Mycobacterial infections can mimic Crohn's disease of the ileal and cecal area and diagnosis is best made by colonoscopy and biopsy. Cytomegalovirus (CMV) and herpes proctitis can also masquerade as Crohn's disease. Protozoan parasites that can cause diarrhea and abdominal pain include *Isospora belli* and *Entamoeba histolytica*. Colonoscopy and biopsy is the most accurate way to diagnose these clinical entities that can mimic Crohn's disease.

Many noninfectious diseases can mimic Crohn's disease. Diverticulitis usually affects the left colon and can cause fevers, abdominal pain, and fistulas. When the inflammation decreases, colonoscopy can be performed to distinguish between the two diseases. Although patients with diverticular disease can have minimal endoscopic inflammation due to diverticular-associated colitis, significant endoscopic abnormalities are much more likely in Crohn's disease. Ischemic colitis is another disease frequently confused with Crohn's colitis. It should be considered in the elderly or in patients with vascular disease. Patients with ischemic colitis classically present with acute left lower quadrant pain and bloody diarrhea. The ischemic process can be acute or chronic and can leave the colon scarred and strictured. Colonoscopy and biopsy can usually differentiate between the two diseases. Like Crohn's disease, radiation enteritis can also cause diarrhea, malabsorption, stricturing, and intestinal bleeding.

The solitary rectal ulcer syndrome occurs in persons of all ages and may be caused by impaired evacuation and failure of relaxation of the puborectalis muscle. Ulceration may be caused by anal sphincter overactivity, higher intrarectal pressures during defecation, constipation, and digital removal of stool. Patients complain of rectal bleeding, pain, and tenesmus. The ulceration, which can be as large as 5 cm in diameter, is usually seen anteriorly or anteriorlaterally 3–15 cm from the anal verge. Biopsy can usually distinguish this from Crohn's disease of the rectum. Treatment consists of stool softeners and laxatives.

Other types of colidites that can mimic Crohn's disease include NSAID-related colitis, microscopic colitis, diversion colitis, and indeterminate colitis. NSAIDs can cause colon inflammation by themselves or can exacerbate IBD that has already been diagnosed. Microscopic colitis is comprised of two distinct disorders: lymphocytic colitis and collagenous colitis. In either of these two disorders the colon appears normal endoscopically and the diagnosis is made upon pathologic examination. In patients with lymphocytic colitis, histologic examination reveals that intraepithelial lymphocytes are increased. In patients with collagenous colitis, there is a layer of subepithelial collagen deposition in addition to increased intraepithelial lymphocytes. Treatment is similar to that for IBD. Diversion colitis occurs when segments of the large intestine are excluded from the fecal stream. It usually occurs in patients with an ileostomy or colostomy and a Hartmann pouch. This disorder is felt to result from a deficiency of butyrate resulting from the fecal diversion. It is reversible by surgical anastomosis or treatment with topical butyrate. Indeterminate colitis refers to cases of IBD that cannot be categorized as either UC or CD. ANCA/ASCA serologies have been assessed in an effort to distinguish between the two, especially when ileoanal pouch surgery is being considered.

CLINICAL DIAGNOSIS

Ileocolitis

Because the most common site of inflammation is the terminal ileum, the usual presentation of Crohn's disease is a chronic history of recurrent episodes of right lower quadrant pain and diarrhea. Sometimes the initial presentation mimics acute appendicitis with pronounced right lower quadrant pain, a palpable mass, fever, and leukocytosis. Pain is usually crampy and is relieved by defecation. Patients usually have a low-grade fever. High fevers are worrisome for abscess formation. Patients can lose up to 10–20% of their body weight secondary to diarrhea, anorexia, and fear of eating.

On physical exam, an inflammatory mass can be palpated in the right lower quadrant. This mass consists of inflamed bowel and mesentery and enlarged abdominal lymph nodes. On occasion, extension of this mass can cause right ureteral obstruction, hydronephrosis or rarely, an ileopsoas abscess. After a period of

Table 56.2 Diseases mistaken for Crohn's disease

Infectious

Bacterial	Mycobacterial	Parasitic	Viral	Fungal
Salmonella	Tuberculosis	Amebiasis	Cytomegalovirus	Histoplasmosis
Shigella	Mycobacterium avium	Isospora	Herpes simplex	Candida
Toxigenic Escherichia coli		Trichuris trichura	HIV	Aspergillus
Campylobacter		Hookworm		
Yersinia		Strongyloides		
Clostridium difficle				
Gonorrhea				
Chlamydia trachomatis				

Inflammatory	Neoplastic	Drugs and chemicals
Appendicitis	Lymphoma	NSAIDs
Diverticulitis	Lymphosarcoma	Phosphosoda
Diversion colitis	Carcinoma of the ileum	Cathartic colon
Collagenous/lymphocytic colitis	Carcinoid	Gold
Ischemic colitis	Familial polyposis	Oral contraceptives
Radiation colitis/enteritis	Metastatic carcinoma	Cocaine
Solitary rectal ulcer		Chemotherapy
Eosinophilic gastroenteritis		
Neutropenic colitis		
Behçet's syndrome		
Graft-versus-host-disease		

time, the bowel becomes fibrotic and strictured. At first, patients have postprandial abdominal pain and nausea but as the bowel lumen becomes more and more narrow, patients will have the potential for bowel obstruction. Episodes of obstruction are caused by either bowel inflammation and spasm or impaction of food or medication. Usually, episodes resolve by nasogastric decompression and concurrent administration of intravenous fluids. Surgery is required for an obstruction that does not resolve or if the episodes occur too frequently and impair the individual patient's nutrition or quality of life.

Severe inflammation of the ileum and right colon can lead to microperforation with fistulization to the adjacent organs such as the bowel, bladder, or skin. Patients with enterovesical fistulas present with recurrent bladder infections and less commonly pneumaturia or fecaluria. Patients with enterocutaneous fistulas present with purulent drainage through the skin, usually at the site of abdominal surgical scars. An abscess cavity in the mesentery can also form and may need to be drained either surgically or by means of interventional radiology. Fistulas can also form from the ileum to the vagina but are rare in women without a prior hysterectomy.

Colitis and perianal disease

Patients with colitis present with diarrhea, low-grade fevers, weight loss, malaise, and crampy abdominal pain. Rectal bleeding occurs in about half of patients with colonic disease. One to 2% of patients can have massive gastrointestinal bleeding. Diarrhea is often caused by a decrease in rectal compliance due to localized inflammation, and pain is caused by passage of stool through narrowed, spastic, and inflamed bowel. Toxic megacolon is rare in Crohn's colitis but can be seen in severe, short-term disease. Stricturing in the colon can cause bowel obstruction, and patients will need surgery if the obstruction does not resolve. Feculent vomiting is caused by fistulization of the colonic disease to the stomach or duodenum. Only rarely does the fistula initiate in the stomach or duodenum; rather it usually arises from the ileum or colon and extends to the adjacent organs. Rectovaginal fistulas develop in 10% of women with Crohn's colitis.

Perianal disease affects about one-third of patients with Crohn's colitis and consists of anal fissures, fistulas, skin tags, and perirectal abscesses. Patients present with pain, drainage, and sometimes incontinence. Five to 10% of Crohn's patients have only perianal disease without endoscopic evidence of colonic inflammation.

Jejunoileitis

The presence of extensive inflammatory Crohn's disease is associated with malabsorption and steatorrhea due to a loss of digestive and absorptive surface area. Patients with extensive small bowel Crohn's disease can have nutritional deficiencies resulting from many different factors including poor oral intake and enteric losses of protein and other nutrients. Patients can become hypoalbuminemic, hypomagnesemic, hypokalemic, and coagulopathic. Bone fractures can be caused by vitamin D deficiency, hypocalcemia, and prolonged corticosteroid use. The use of specific medications to treat patients with Crohn's disease such as corticosteroids, methotrexate, and cyclosporine are known to decrease bone mineral density. Malabsorption of vitamin B_{12} can cause a megaloblastic anemia and neurologic symptoms.

Active small bowel inflammation also causes diarrhea. Other mechanisms of diarrhea include bacterial overgrowth (which can occur with resection of the ileocecal valve, in obstructive stasis or fistulization), bile acid-induced diarrhea (from a diminished absorptive capacity of a diseased or resected terminal ileum), colonic inflammation with decreased water absorption and increased secretion of electrolytes, and exudation of pus and mucus into a rectum with decreased compliance.

Gastroduodenal disease

Patients with Crohn's disease of the stomach and duodenum classically present with nausea, vomiting, and epigastric pain. Endoscopic biopsies usually reveal an *H. pylori*-negative chronic gastritis. The second portion of the duodenum is more commonly involved than the bulb. Patients can suffer from chronic gastric outlet obstruction.[10]

ENDOSCOPIC, LABORATORY AND RADIOGRAPHIC DIAGNOSIS

Distinguishing endoscopic features of CD are rectal sparing, aphthous ulcerations, cobblestoning, fistulas, ulcers within normal mucosa in early disease, and skip lesions (Fig. 56.1). Inflammatory polyps or pseudopolyps can be seen in areas of previous inflammation that have healed (Fig. 56.2). Colonoscopy and biopsy is useful for initial diagnosis and assessment of disease activity and colon cancer surveillance.[12,13] It is also useful in assessing postoperative recurrence of Crohn's disease.[13] Intubation of the ileocecal valve during colonoscopy allows examination and biopsy of the terminal ileum, and endoscopy is useful to discover possible gastroduodenal involvement in patients with upper tract symptoms. At present, there is a capability of examining the small intestine by means of video capsule endoscopy (wireless capsule endoscopy) in patients suspected of having small bowel Crohn's disease who are symptomatic but have had unremarkable small intestinal radiographic studies.[14] There is no clearly

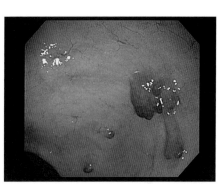

Fig. 56.2 • Endoscopic image of a patient with chronic Crohn's colitis and pseudopolyps.

established role for repeated endoscopy to follow severity of inflammation in CD because endoscopic appearance correlates poorly with clinical remission, either in response to drug therapy, or postoperatively. Laboratory abnormalities commonly encountered are non-specific, including elevated erythrocyte sedimentation rate and C-reactive protein, hypoalbuminemia, anemia, and leukocytosis.

Early radiographic findings in CD of the small bowel include a coarse villous pattern of the mucosa, thickened folds, and aphthous ulcerations. In more advanced disease, strictures, fistulas (Fig. 56.3), inflammatory masses, and abscesses may be detected. The transmural inflammation of CD leads to deep ulceration and fistula formation. The radiographic 'string sign' represents long areas of circumferential inflammation and fibrosis resulting in intestinal strictures (Fig. 56.4). The segmental nature of CD results in wide gaps of normal or dilated bowel between involved segments.

CT findings in CD include mural thickening, mesenteric fat stranding, adenopathy, and perianal disease. CT scanning can also help identify abscesses, fistulas, and sinus tracts. MRI may prove superior for demonstrating pelvic lesions such as ischiorectal abscesses. There may be a role for endoscopic ultrasound in combination with either MRI or surgical evaluation in classifying perianal fistulizing disease.[15]

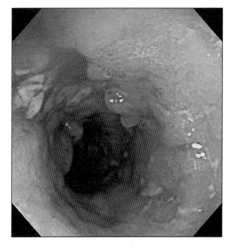

Fig. 56.1 • Endoscopic image of a patient with chronic Crohn's colitis with erythema and ulcerations.

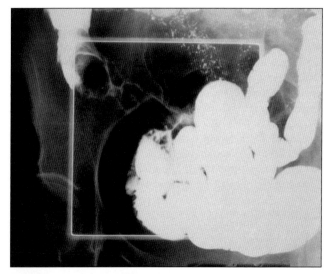

Fig. 56.3 • Small bowel series of a patient with inflammation and fistulization of the terminal ileum.

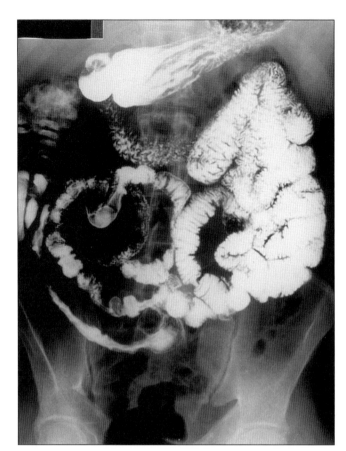

Fig. 56.4 • Small bowel series of a patient with extensive Crohn's disease of the ileum and jejunum. There are small bowel strictures and separation of loops.

SEROLOGIC DIAGNOSIS

There are several serologic markers that may be used to differentiate between CD and UC and that may help to predict the course of disease. Two antibodies that can be detected in the serum of IBD patients are perinuclear antineutrophil cytoplasmic antibody (pANCA) and anti-*Saccharomyces cerevisiae* antibodies (ASCA). A distinct set of antineutrophil cytoplasmic antibodies with perinuclear staining by indirect immunofluorescence are associated more commonly with UC. The antigens to which these antibodies are directed have not been clearly identified but they are clearly distinct from those associated with vasculitis. pANCA positivity is found in about 60–70% of UC patients and 5–10% of CD patients. Five percent to 15% of first-degree UC patients are pANCA positive whereas only 2–3% of the general population is pANCA positive. pANCA positivity is associated with pancolitis, early surgery, pouchitis, or inflammation of the pouch after ileal pouch-anal anastomosis, and primary sclerosing cholangitis. pANCA in CD is associated with colonic disease.[16]

ASCA antibodies recognize mannose sequences in the cell wall mannan of the *Saccharomyces cerevisiae* yeast strain. Sixty percent to 70% of CD patients, 10–15% of UC patients, and 0–5% of non-IBD controls are ASCA positive. About 55% of CD patients are seroreactive to outer-membrane porin C (OmpC), a bacterial antigen. The combined measurement of pANCA and ASCA has been advocated as a valuable diagnostic approach to IBD. In one report, pANCA positivity with ASCA negativity yielded 57%

sensitivity and 97% specificity for UC, whereas pANCA negativity with ASCA positivity yielded 49% sensitivity and 97% specificity for CD. The presence of a positive ASCA antibody has been associated with the presence of small bowel Crohn's disease.[16] These antibody tests may also be additional information that may help decide whether a patient with indeterminate colitis should undergo an ileal pouch-anal anastomosis since there is often a complicated postoperative course in patients with predominant features of Crohn's disease. They can also help when it is important to distinguish Crohn's disease of the ileoanal pouch from refractory pouchitis.

COMPLICATIONS

The most common complications of Crohn's disease are intestinal obstruction, fistula formation, malabsorption, abscess formation, and severe perianal disease. Less common complications include rupture of an intra-abdominal abscess causing peritonitis, and massive hemorrhage. Because Crohn's disease is a transmural process with serosal involvement, this provides a pathway for fistulas to track, with free perforation being a rare complication. Perforation of the gastrointestinal tract can occur as a complication of toxic megacolon or occasionally in the jejunum or ileum. The resulting peritonitis can be fatal.[10]

POSTOPERATIVE RECURRENCE

Of the 70% of Crohn's patients who ultimately need surgery, a majority will experience a recurrence of their disease. Endoscopic recurrence occurs roughly in 70% over 1 year and 85% over 3 years. Recurrence that necessitates another surgery occurs in 25–30% of patients by 5 years and 40–50% after 20 years of postoperative follow-up. Clinical recurrence of symptoms that requires medical and not surgical therapy occurs in 20% at 2 years, 30% by 3 years, and 40–50% by 4 years.[17,18] A perforating indication for initial resection and a longer duration of disease before initial surgery predict an earlier postoperative recurrence.[19,20] Cigarette smoking may also increase the likelihood of postoperative recurrence.[21]

STANDARD MEDICAL THERAPY

There are no trials that compare 'step-up' to 'top-down' therapy in Crohn's disease although knowing the phenotype of the disease should help determine the appropriate therapy. The current practice guidelines recommend using a sequential approach to treatment according to the severity of the clinical presentation and associated complications.[22,23] Medical treatment recommendations are detailed in Table 56.3. Categories of severity include the following:

Mild to moderate disease: Patients who are ambulatory, eating, and drinking without dehydration, toxicity, abdominal tenderness, painful mass, obstruction, or more than 10% of weight loss.

Moderate to severe disease: Patients who have failed to respond to therapies for mild to moderate disease or those with more prominent symptoms of fevers; significant weight loss, abdominal pain, or tenderness; intermittent nausea or vomiting (without obstructive findings); or significant anemia.

Table 56.3 Crohn's disease: medical management

Active disease

Mild to moderate	Moderate to severe	Severe to fulminant
5-ASA (see Table 56.4 for dosing)	5-ASA	i.v. hydrocortisone (300–400 mg/d)
Metronidazole (250–500 mg t.i.d.)	Metronidazole and/or ciprofloxacin	i.v. solumedrol (40–60 mg/d)
Ciprofloxacin (500 mg b.i.d.)	Prednisone (40–60 mg/d)	Infliximab (5–10 mg/kg)
Budesonide (9 mg/d)	Azathioprine/6-MP	TPN
Azathioprine (2–3 mg/kg/d)	Methotrexate (25 mg i.m./week)	
6-MP (1–1.5 mg/kg/d)	Infliximab	
	TPN or elemental diet	

Perianal or fistulizing

Metronidazole and/or ciprofloxacin

Infliximab

Azathioprine or 6-MP

Oral tacrolimus (0.1–0.2 mg/kg/d)

i.v. cyclosporine (4 mg/kg/d)

Maintenance therapy

Inflammatory	Perianal or fistulizing
5-ASA (see Table 56.4 for dosing)	Azathioprine/6-MP
Azathioprine or 6-MP	Infliximab
Methotrexate (15 mg i.m./week)	
Infliximab	

Severe to fulminant disease: Patients with persistent symptoms despite the introduction of corticosteroids as outpatients or those presenting with high fevers, persistent vomiting, evidence of an intestinal obstruction, rebound tenderness, cachexia, or evidence of an abscess.

5-ASA agents

Sulfazalazine and mesalamine are first-line therapies for mild to moderate disease with disease location determining the formulation and delivery system. Most trials demonstrate a 40–60% response rate with these agents. The National Cooperative Crohn's Disease Study (NCCDS)[24] and the European Cooperative Crohn's Disease Study (ECCDS)[25] were the first to show that sulfasalazine is effective in inducing remission in mild to moderate Crohn's ileocolitis and colitis. Although sulfasalazine is more effective at higher doses, at 6 or 8 grams a day up to 30% of patients experience allergic reactions or intolerable side effects such as headache, anorexia, nausea, and vomiting that are attributable to the sulfapyridine moiety. Hypersensitivity reactions, independent of sulfapyridine levels, include rash, fever, hepatitis, agranulocytosis, hypersensitivity pneumonitis, pancreatitis, worsening of colitis, and reversible sperm abnormalities. Sulfasalazine can also impair folate absorption and patients should be supplemented with oral folate.

The development of sulfa-free aminosalicylate preparations has enabled clinicians to provide increasing amounts of the pharmacologically active component of sulfasalazine (i.e., 5-ASA,

mesalamine) to the site of active bowel disease while limiting systemic toxicity. If free mesalamine is administered orally it is absorbed in the jejunum and is not available to be delivered to the inflamed area of the bowel. Consequently, the formulation of various delivery systems to deliver mesalamine to the affected bowel has been undertaken. Pentasa is a mesalamine formulation that uses an ethylcellulose coating to allow water absorption into small beads containing the mesalamine. Water dissolves the 5-ASA, which then diffuses out of the bead into the lumen. In a recent study, disintegration of the capsule occurred in the stomach. The microspheres then dispersed throughout the entire gastrointestinal tract from the small intestine through the distal colon in both the fasted or fed conditions. Approximately 50% of the mesalamine is delivered to the small intestine. Singleton et al. compared the efficacy of Pentasa at 1, 2 or 4 grams a day to placebo in a trial of 310 patients and found that 4 grams a day was statistically superior to placebo.[26] Two further trials comparing Pentasa 2 or 4 g/day versus placebo had a similar benefit with 4 g/day. However, a high placebo response prevented statistical significance. In a meta-analysis by Drs. Hanauer and Stromberg, pooling of results from these three trials was performed, demonstrating that there was a marginally significant benefit of Pentasa 4 g/day over placebo.[27]

Asacol is also an enteric-coated form of mesalamine but has a slightly different release pattern, with 5-ASA liberated at pH >7.0. Approximately 15–30% of the mesalamine in Asacol is delivered to the small bowel. There have been other clinical trials comparing various formulations of mesalamine, including

Asacol, with placebo that suggest a trend towards benefit of the active drug with approximately 45–55% of patients treated with mesalamine placed into clinical remission. Table 56.4 demonstrates the different 5-ASA formulations and appropriate dosages.

The role of 5-ASA in maintaining remission is not as well documented in CD as it has been in UC.[28-35] In a meta-analysis of 15 randomized, controlled trials with 2097 patients, mesalamine significantly reduced the risk of relapse when remission was induced surgically and not medically.[36] Mesalamine was also effective in reducing postoperative endoscopic recurrence of Crohn's disease at 12 months after resection. If remission was induced with corticosteroids, mesalamine was not effective at preventing relapse.[37] Studies are now in progress to see if higher doses of mesalamine (6 g/day) can maintain remission.

Antibiotics

Antibiotics are about as effective as 5-ASA agents in inducing remission in mild to moderate Crohn's disease and, in particular, disease involving the colon.[38] In a 105-patient placebo-controlled trial, metronidazole 10 mg/kg/day or 20 mg/kg/day was associated with significant improvements in disease activity although remission rates were no different than placebo.[39] In the Swedish Cooperative Crohn's Disease Study, metronidazole (400 mg b.i.d.) was slightly more effective than sulfasalazine.[40] Dose-limiting side effects include nausea, headache, anorexia, peripheral neuropathy, and a disulfuram-like reaction. Ciprofloxacin was compared with Pentasa 4 g/day in a single study of 40 patients and equal numbers of patients achieved clinical remission (56% Cipro versus 55% Pentasa).[41] In another study of mild to moderate Crohn's disease, metronidazole and ciprofloxacin were compared with methylprednisolone in a total of 41 patients. Forty-five-and-a-half percent of the antibiotic-treated patients and 63% of the steroid-treated patients went into remission.[42] The difference was not statistically significant. Rifaximin, a nonabsorbable antibiotic currently approved for traveler's diarrhea, may also be beneficial in treating active Crohn's disease.[43]

Evidence for the efficacy of ciprofloxacin and metronidazole in perianal fistulizing disease comes from small case series and widespread clinical response. These agents are first-line therapy for perianal fistulizing disease; however, 50% of fistulas relapse when these agents are stopped.

Corticosteroids

Prednisone and prednisolone are highly effective in moderate to severe Crohn's disease. There is a 60–70% remission compared to a 30% placebo response in active CD. The National and European Cooperative Crohn's disease trials demonstrated the superiority of prednisone and prednisolone compared with placebo.[24,25] The usual starting dose of prednisone is 40 mg/day, but even at low doses these agents can cause severe side effects. Over 50% of Crohn's patients treated acutely with systemic steroids become steroid dependent or steroid resistant, particularly smokers and those with colonic disease. In the Olmstead County population-based study, of 74 patients with CD treated with their first course of corticosteroids, 58% had complete remission, 26% had partial remission, and 16% had no response at 30 days. One-year out-

Table 56.4 Oral 5-ASA preparations

Preparation	Formulation	Delivery	Dosing (per day)
Azo-bond			
Sulfasalazine (500 mg) (Azulfadine)	Sulfapyridine-5-ASA	Colon	3–6 g (acute) 2–4 g (maintenance)
Olsalazine (250 mg) (Dipentum)	5-ASA-5-ASA	Colon	1–3 g
Balsalazide (750 mg) (Colazal)	Aminobenzoyl-alanine-5-ASA	Colon	6.75–9 g
Delayed-release			
Mesalamine (400, 800 mg) (Asacol)	Eudragit S (pH 7)	Distal ileum-colon	2.4–4.8 g (acute) 1.6–4.8 g (maintenance)
Claversal/Mesasal/Salofalk (250, 500 mg)	Eudragit L (pH 6)	Ileum-colon	1.5–3 g (acute) 1.5–3 g (maintenance)
Sustained-release			
Mesalamine (250, 500, 1000 mg) (Pentasa)	Ethylcellulose microgranules	Stomach-colon	2–4 g (acute) 1.5–4 g (maintenance)
Rectal 5-ASA preparations			
Mesalamine suppository (400, 500, 1000 mg) (Canasa)		Rectum	1–1.5 g (acute) 500 mg–1 g (maintenance)
Mesalamine enema (1, 4 g) (Rowasa)	60 mL, 100 mL suspension	Rectum Splenic flexure	1–4 g (acute) 1 g/d to 3 times/week (maintenance)

comes were prolonged response in 32%, corticosteroid dependence in 28%, and operation in 38%.[44] There was no benefit of 5-ASA agents used after a corticosteroid-induced remission[37] and no role for corticosteroids in maintenance of remission.[45] Once clinical remission has been induced, steroids may be tapered according to the time for clinical response. Patients with inflammatory disease who fail oral agents may respond to intravenous corticosteroids in the form of hydrocortisone 300–400 mg/day or methylprednisolone (48–60 mg/day) in either continuous or bolus infusion. There are no data on the superiority of bolus versus continuous infusion.

The side effects from steroids are numerous, including fluid retention, abdominal striae, fat redistribution, hyperglycemia, subcapsular cataracts, myopathy, and emotional disturbances. Bone loss occurs in 31–59% of patients with IBD and steroid therapy compounds this risk, increasing the rate of trabecular bone loss independent of the usual risk factors. The risk of bone loss is increased even with low dose and short duration of therapy. The risk of steroid-induced bone loss is often greatest in the first few weeks of therapy when the highest doses are given and patients should be started on calcium and vitamin D when steroid therapy is initiated.[46] Other factors that contribute to osteoporosis include smoking, sedentary lifestyle, low body mass, family history, and nutritional deficiencies. A 12-month, randomized, double-blind, placebo-controlled trial with a 10 mg daily dose of alendronate significantly increased bone mineral density in patients with CD.[47]

Another often-neglected side effect of steroid therapy is suppression of the hypothalamic-pituitary axis. In a recent paper, 65% of patients had an abnormal cosyntropin test after only 2–3 months of a prednisone taper. Hypothalamic-pituitary-adrenal axis suppression was noted in 30–100% of patients after receiving 2–8 weeks of topical steroid enemas (hydrocortisone, bethamethasone phosphate, or prednisolone). Physicians should be aware of this side effect and consider checking a cosyntropin test before discontinuing steroids.[48] Budesonide is a potent glucocorticoid with first-pass hepatic metabolism that is formulated into microgranules for ileocecal release and possesses a high topical antiinflammatory effect without appreciable systemic activity.[49] It is effective in inducing remission in mild to moderate Crohn's disease of the ileum and right colon.[50–57] In a meta-analysis of 16 studies, budesonide was significantly more effective than placebo or 5-ASA agents for inducing remission for active CD.[58,59] Although it was 13% less effective for induction of remission than conventional corticosteroids (based upon a meta-analysis of prospective randomized, controlled trials published to date), it was less likely to cause corticosteroid-related adverse events. In a dose-ranging, placebo-controlled trial, 9 mg/day was the most effective dose.[52] In a quality of life study, patients taking budesonide had a better quality of life than those taking mesalazine.[60] Although the short-term safety of budesonide is well established, its long-term effect on bone and the hypothalamic-pituitary axis remains to be determined. Patients may be able to switch safely from systemic steroids to budesonide without relapse and therefore reduce steroid side effects.[61] The majority of the literature indicates that lower doses of 3 or 6 mg/day are not of benefit in the maintenance of long-term remission.[62,63] Only a single study showed a benefit of budesonide 6 mg/day over mesalamine 3 g/day in maintaining a remission in steroid-dependent Crohn's disease.[64]

Azathioprine and 6-mercaptopurine

Azathioprine (AZA) and 6-mercaptopurine (6-MP) are purine analogues commonly employed in the management of steroid-dependent Crohn's disease. Azathioprine is rapidly absorbed and converted to 6-MP, which is then metabolized to the active end product, thioinosinic acid, an inhibitor of purine ribonucleotide synthesis and cell proliferation. These agents also alter the immune response via inhibition of natural killer cell activity and suppression of cytotoxic T-cell function. It was thought that these agents took 3–4 months to work but an aggressive dosing regimen may speed up clinical efficacy.[65] Checking thiopurine methyltransferase (TPMT) genotype or phenotype before initiating therapy enables initial dosing at 1.0–1.5 mg/kg/day for 6-MP and 2.0–2.5 mg/kg/day for azathioprine.[66] Adherence can be determined by measuring the levels of 6-thioguanine and 6-methymercaptopurine, end products of 6-MP metabolism. There is currently a large prospective, randomized, controlled trial ongoing evaluating whether conventional medication dosing or use of metabolites is more effective for dosing patients with medication. Azathioprine and 6-MP have enabled two-thirds of CD steroid-dependent patients to be weaned from corticosteroids.[67–69] A meta-analysis of five placebo-controlled trials for a total of 319 patients with quiescent CD found remission rates of 67% among patients treated with azathioprine versus 53% among patients receiving placebo with an overall odds ratio of response of 2.27 (CI, 1.76–2.93).[70] Two trials in this meta-analysis reported that azathioprine has a steroid-sparing effect. Another trial demonstrated that AZA was significantly more effective than placebo in maintaining remission after the cessation of steroids (at 12 weeks) over a period of 15 months.[71]

The optimum duration of therapy is unclear and one retrospective study found a statistically significant increase in relapse rates at 1, 2, 3, and 5 years in patients who discontinued 6-MP while in remission.[72,73] In the only prospective, randomized, placebo-controlled trial that evaluated the ability of patients to remain in remission, at 18 months 21% of placebo-treated patients relapsed versus 8% of azathioprine-treated patients.[74]

The role of these immunomodulators in treating perianal, abdominal wall, and enteroenteric fistulas in CD appears promising. Combining data from three randomized trials for active CD that included 18 patients with fistulas, AZA was associated with a more favorable response rate than placebo. Complete healing or decreased drainage of fistulas was reported in 56% of patients on AZA versus 29% receiving placebo. In addition, in a single trial, 6-MP at a dose of 50 mg/d was more effective than Pentasa or placebo for postoperative prophylaxis of CD.[75]

Although azathioprine and 6-MP are usually well tolerated, pancreatitis occurs in 1–2% of patients, typically presents within the first few weeks of therapy, and is always completely reversible when the drug is stopped. Other side effects include nausea, fever, rash, and hepatitis. Some patients can be switched from 6-MP to AZA and vice versa if the side effect is nausea and vomiting and not fever or pancreatitis. Bone marrow suppression (particularly leukopenia) is dose-related and often delayed, necessitating regular monitoring of the patient's complete blood count. Additionally, 1 in 300 individuals lack thiopurine methyltransferase (TPMT), the enzyme responsible for drug metabolism (i.e., homozygous deficiency) and an additional 11% of the population are heterozygotes with intermediate enzyme activity. Both are at increased risk of toxicity because of increased accumulation of thioguanine metabolites.[65] Because of the small but life-threatening risk of neutropenia in patients who lack TPMT activity, we believe it should be a standard of care to check TPMT phenotype prior to initiating therapy. In a recent analysis of patients who developed leukopenia,[76] it was found that those who are homozygous deficient will have leukopenia within 6 weeks. It should be noted, however, that leukopenia in those individuals who do not lack the enzyme may develop several years later – without any specific identifiable pattern. Thus, complete blood count should be performed at approximately 2, 4, and 8 weeks after initiating therapy, regardless of thiomethylpurine status. Liver enzymes are tested concurrently. The complete blood count should be repeated every 2–3 months thereafter or every 2 weeks after a dose adjustment. 6-MP metabolite levels can be determined after 2–4 weeks of therapy or after a dose change, when a steady state is reached.

Methotrexate

Methotrexate (MTX) inhibits dihydrofolate reductase, resulting in impaired DNA synthesis. Additional antiinflammatory properties may be related to decreased IL-1 production. The efficacy of intramuscular methotrexate as inductive therapy in moderate to severe CD is well established.[77,78] In a 16-week randomized, double-blind, placebo-controlled trial, intramuscular methotrexate 25 mg/week induced remission in 37 of 94 (39.4%) of patients compared with 9 of 47 (19.1%) placebo-treated patients.[79]

Methotrexate has also been effective in maintaining remission for patients who respond in the acute setting. In a randomized, controlled trial using intramuscular methotrexate, 15 mg/week, 65% of patients maintained remission off steroids for 40 weeks.[80] Similar data were seen in two open-label trials. Potential toxicities include leukopenia and hepatic fibrosis, necessitating periodic evaluation of complete blood counts and liver enzymes. The most frequently occurring events are nausea and vomiting, abdominal pain, joint pain, cold symptoms, and fatigue. All patients should be supplemented with folic acid 1 mg/day. Patients receiving more than 1.5 g of methotrexate probably do not need liver biopsies unless they have risk factors for hepatic fibrosis such as diabetes mellitus, alcohol use, and obesity. This, however, has not been studied in a systematic way. Another rare side effect is hypersensitivity pneumonitis. In general, methotrexate is used when 6-MP or azathioprine is ineffective or not well tolerated.

Infliximab

Infliximab, a chimeric monoclonal antibody directed against tumor necrosis factor-α (TNF-α) is approved by the US Food and Drug Administration for use in moderate to severe luminal or fistulizing CD.[81–87] It is effective in patients refractory to 5-ASA agents, antibiotics, 6-MP, and steroids. It is also used as a first-line agent in severe perianal fistulizing disease. For refractory luminal or fistulizing disease, infusions of 5 mg/kg are given at 0, 2, and 6 weeks. In a study of 108 treatment-refractory patients, there was a statistically significant response rate of 65% for active disease compared with 17% for placebo.[85] There are equally good results in patients with perianal fistulizing disease with a response rate of 68% compared with 26% for placebo.[82] Reinfusion, typically every 8 weeks, is necessary to continue therapeutic benefits in many patients.

The development of antibodies to infliximab is associated with an increased risk of infusion reactions and decreased response to treatment.[88] Patients who receive on-demand or episodic infusions are more likely to develop antibodies to infliximab compared to those individuals who are given infliximab on a regular basis (5 mg/kg every 8 weeks) and to lose their response.[89,90] The majority of published studies and the standard of care in clinical practice is to use a three-dose induction regimen followed by maintenance treatment. Immunomodulator use or hydrocortisone pretreatment may also increase therapeutic efficacy.[91,92] No combination of these strategies has been formally tested. Most experts believe that patients should be started on either 6-MP or azathioprine if they are sick enough to warrant treatment with infliximab.[93] It is unclear if and when infliximab can be discontinued. Based upon general treatment principles it seems unlikely that any medication used for maintenance of remission in patients with Crohn's disease (mesalamine, antibiotics, azathioprine, 6-mercaptopurine, methotrexate or infliximab) should be discontinued. This concept will, however, need to be tested to see if continued treatment lessens surgery and stricture formation while maintaining good quality of life for the afflicted patient.

Common (>10%) side effects of infliximab include nausea, headache, upper respiratory infections, fatigue, and fever. More serious side effects include fungal and other invasive opportunistic infections. In a study looking at the safety profile of infliximab in 500 patients from the Mayo Clinic, 43 patients (8.6%) experienced a serious adverse event, of which 30 (6%) were related to infliximab.[94] Serious events attributed to infliximab included acute infusion reactions (3.8%) and serum sickness-like disease (2.8%). Three patients developed drug-induced lupus and one patient developed a new demyelination disorder. Forty-one (8.2%) patients had an infectious event attributed to infliximab and 20 patients had a serious infection (2: fatal sepsis; 8: pneumonia; 6: viral infections; 2: abdominal abscesses; 1: cellulitis; 1: histoplasmosis). Nine patients had a malignant disorder, 3 of which were possibly related to infliximab. A total of 10 deaths were observed. For five of these patients (1%), the events leading to death were possibly related to infliximab. The rate in this retrospective series (of 1% death rate per year) is similar to other large series of patients treated for Crohn's disease prior to the era of infliximab.

There have been 117 reported cases of disseminated tuberculosis related to infliximab. For this reason, patients should be evaluated for TB prior to infliximab therapy. Because the majority of IBD patients are anergic, a thorough evaluation for TB should also include a travel history and a chest X-ray.[95]

Cyclosporine

Cyclosporine A (CSA) alters the immunoinflammatory cascade by acting as a potent inhibitor of T cell-mediated responses. Although CSA acts primarily via inhibition of IL-2 production from T-helper cells, it also decreases recruitment of cytotoxic T cells and blocks other cytokines, including IL-3, IL-4, alpha-interferon, and tumor necrosis factor (TNF). It has a more rapid onset of action than 6-MP and azathioprine. Cyclosporine is used to treat Crohn's disease when infliximab fails or cannot be used.

Intravenous CSA is effective in 80% of patients with refractory fistulas but 6-MP or azathioprine must be used to maintain remission.[96–98] Oral CSA alone is only effective at a higher dose

(7.5 mg/kg/d) in active disease[99] but is not effective in maintaining remission without 6-MP/azathioprine. Neoral® is a microemulsion formulation of cyclosporine that has increased bioavailability due to improved absorption especially in the setting of small bowel disease.

CSA has the potential for significant toxicity, and blood levels as well as renal function should be frequently monitored. Hypertension, gingival hyperplasia, hypertrichosis, paresthesias, tremors, headaches, and electrolyte abnormalities are common side effects. Nephrotoxicity is an important complication of CSA necessitating dose reduction or discontinuation of therapy if there is a significant rise in serum creatinine. Seizures may also complicate therapy, especially if serum cholesterol levels are less than 120 mg/dL. Opportunistic infections, most notably *Pneumocystis carinii* pneumonia, have occurred with combination immunosuppressive treatment, leading to recommendations for prophylaxis in those on CSA in combination with other immunomodulators.

Nutritional therapies

Dietary intraluminal antigens may act as stimuli of the mucosal immune response and patients with active CD respond to bowel rest, along with total enteral or parenteral nutrition (TPN). In fact, bowel rest and TPN are as effective as corticosteroids for inducing remission in patients with active CD although they are not effective as maintenance therapy. Enteral nutrition in the form of elemental or peptide-based preparations is also as effective as corticosteroids or TPN but these diets are not palatable for long periods of time. In addition, enteral diets may provide the small intestine with nutrients vital to cell growth and do not have the complications of TPN.

NOVEL MEDICAL THERAPIES: IMMUNOMODULATORS

Tacrolimus

Tacrolimus has a mechanism of action similar to cyclosporine. Its use, mainly in cardiac and renal transplants, has shown tacrolimus to provide more complete immunosuppression but with limiting side effects. There have been preliminary reports of efficacy in children with refractory IBD and in adult patients with extensive involvement of the small bowel.[100] In a randomized, double-blind, placebo-controlled trial of 48 patients (22 tacrolimus, 26 placebo), 43% of tacrolimus-treated patients had fistula improvement with a dose of 0.2 mg/kg/day. In this study tacrolimus was not more effective than placebo for complete fistula closure.[101] Tacrolimus thus has a potential role as a second-line agent in infliximab-refractory patients who have not had responses to immunomodulatory therapy.

Thalidomide

Thalidomide, a drug originally released as a sedative and antiemetic and discontinued in the 1960s because of its teratogenic effects, has been shown to inhibit TNF production by monocytes and other cells. In several open-label studies, thalidomide was effective in steroid refractory and fistulizing Crohn's disease,[102–104] but randomized, controlled trials still need to be performed. Addi-

tionally, toxicity in these preliminary trials (sedation and peripheral neuropathy) was significant and merits further prospective controlled evaluation.

Mycophenolate mofetil

Mycophenolate mofetil inhibits the de novo pathway of purine synthesis in lymphocytes, disrupting the conversion of inosine monophosphate to guanosine monophosphate (GMP) by reversible inhibition of inosine monophosphate dehydrogenase. The resulting depletion of intracellular GMP suppresses the generation of cytotoxic T cells and formation of antibodies by activated B cells. The compound is well absorbed and highly effective in transplant patients. Patients with CD or UC who received either 500 mg twice a day or 15 mg/kg/d in two divided doses have tolerated the drug well and have experienced benefit with reduction of steroid requirements,[105,106] There have been several cases of drug-induced colitis and a higher incidence of lymphoproliferative disorders reported in a 3-year follow-up study. Mycophenolate mofetil should be considered only as a third-line agent in 6-MP/AZA and MTX-refractory patients.

NOVEL MEDICAL THERAPIES: BIOLOGICS

Adalimumab, CDP870 and CDP571

Adalimumab is a recombinant human monoclonal IgG1 antibody containing only human peptide sequences. Adalimumab binds TNF-α and neutralizes its function by blocking the interaction between TNF and its cell surface receptor. Therefore, it seems to have a similar mechanism of action to infliximab. Adalimumab is currently approved for rheumatoid arthritis. It has shown promise in treating Crohn's disease in one open-label trial.[107] It may be potentially useful in infliximab-allergic patients.[108] CDP571 is a humanized antibody to TNF-α that contains 95% human residues. Initial preliminary evidence suggested that it was potentially beneficial in moderate to severe Crohn's;[109] however, further data suggested that further investigation into the efficacy of this compound was not merited. CDP870 is a PEGylated form of an anti-TNF antibody administered subcutaneously once monthly. Initial data suggested efficacy, especially in patients who have elevated serum C-reactive protein levels.[110] Several fully humanized anti-TNF antibodies in addition to adalimumab are currently being developed.[111]

Natalizumab

Natalizumab is a humanized monoclonal IgG4 antibody to α4 integrin that blocks migration of leukocytes from the circulation into the parenchyma and also blocks activation within inflammatory sites. In a recent large randomized, double-blind, placebo-controlled trial, natalizumab produced a significant improvement in response rates in patients with moderate to severe Crohn's disease.[112,113] This response was sustained for at least 6 months in another large, follow-up six-month trial.[114] The future of natalizumab is unclear, however after recent reports that this therapy can result in JC virus-induced progressive multifocal leukoencephalopathy (PML).[115–117]

TREATMENT OF CROHN'S DISEASE DURING PREGNANCY

In general, patients with quiescent Crohn's disease have fertility rates similar to patients without IBD. The only exception is patients who have had prior surgeries with adhesions and scarring of the fallopian tubes. The chief determinant of disease activity during pregnancy is disease activity at the time of conception. Two-thirds of women with active disease at the time of conception will have continued or worsened symptoms during their pregnancy. If a woman is in remission at the start of her pregnancy, she has a one-third chance of a flare. Most disease exacerbation in the asymptomatic Crohn's patient occurs in the first trimester or after delivery and likely stems from decreased compliance with the maintenance medical regimen, as worries of teratogenicity overshadow symptom control. Patients with quiescent or mild disease can expect normal pregnancies. No study has demonstrated an increased risk of congenital abnormalities, although an increased rate of low birth rate babies has been described in most studies. Although unproven by prospective studies, it is generally considered the standard of care for women with quiescent or mild disease without perianal activity to deliver vaginally and patients with fulminant or active perianal disease to undergo cesarean sections.[8]

Active disease is more dangerous to the fetus than medical therapy for Crohn's disease. Sulfasalazine, mesalamine, and balsalazide are safe for use in pregnancy but folate supplementation must be given with sulfasalazine. No adverse affects have been reported from sulfasalazine in nursing infants. Topical 5-ASA agents are also safe during pregnancy. Corticosteroids are generally safe for use during pregnancy and are indicated for patients with moderate to severe disease activity during pregnancy. The amount of steroids received by the nursing infant is minimal. The safest antibiotics to use for CD in pregnancy are ampicillin, or cephalosporins. Flagyl is probably safe during the second and third trimesters. Ciprofloxacin may impair cartilage development and should be avoided. Because there have been no studies on long-term antibiotics use during pregnancy, antibiotics should only be used for 2–3 weeks at a time.

There have been several studies suggesting minimal or no risk of 6-mercaptopurine and azathioprine during pregnancy but their safety is not firmly established.[118–120] The current recommendation is to continue 6-MP/AZA through a pregnancy if the patient needs it to stay in remission. There are few data on 6-MP/AZA in nursing and they should be avoided in this setting.

There are few data on cyclosporine in pregnancy. In a small number of patients with severe IBD treated with intravenous cyclosporine during pregnancy, 80% of pregnancies were successfully completed without development of renal toxicity, congenital malformations, or developmental defects. In the renal transplant literature, pregnancy patients on oral cyclosporine have babies with a higher incidence of prematurity and low birth weight but also a higher survival rate.[121] Thus cyclosporine should not be used unless the patient would otherwise require surgery. Methotrexate, thalidomide, and mycophenolate mofetil are contraindicated in pregnancy and nursing.

There have been published cases of 131 pregnancies in women with direct exposure to infliximab[122] with outcome data available for 96 of these women. Live births occurred in 67% (64/96),

miscarriages in 15% (14/96), and therapeutic terminations in 19% (18/96).These results are consistent with those observed in a national cohort of healthy women. However, due to the lack of long-term experience with infliximab during pregnancy and nursing, caution should be exercised unless infliximab is truly necessary. Women should stop medication at least 6 months before attempting to conceive.

SURGICAL TREATMENT OF CROHN'S DISEASE

The need for surgery is related to duration of disease and the site of involvement but most patients require at least one operation in their lifetime.[123,124] More than 75% of patients require surgery by 20 years from the onset of symptoms and 90% by 30 years. After the first resection, about 45% will require a second operation, only 25% of whom will require a third operation. Overall, nearly 90% of people undergoing first resections for CD will never require more than one additional operation. The indications for surgery are depicted in Table 56.5.

Small intestinal disease

Surgical options to treat obstructing CD include resection of the diseased segment and strictureplasty. Since Crohn's disease is diffuse, chronic, and recurring with no clear surgical cure, as little intestine as possible is resected. In most cases where a bowel resection is performed, primary anastomosis can be done to restore continuity. In patients who have had multiple small bowel resections and in whom the diseased segment is short, a strictureplasty is the operation of choice. The strictured area of intestine is incised longitudinally, applying traction sutures perpendicular to the bowel, and closing the incision transversely, thus widening the narrowed area. For longer areas of narrowing, the bowel immediately proximal and distal to the stricture can be sutured side to side. Complications of strictureplasty include prolonged ileus, hemorrhage, fistula, abscess, leak, and restricture at the strictureplasty site.[9]

Colorectal disease

Patients with Crohn's colitis come to surgery for intractability, fulminant disease, or severe perianal disease. In the emergency situation, a simple loop ileostomy, or a subtotal colectomy with ileostomy and Hartmann closure of the rectum can be performed. This procedure allows removal of most of the disease-bearing tissue and the establishment of a firm histologic diagnosis and

Table 56.5 Indications for surgery	
CD of small intestine	**CD of colon and rectum**
Stricture and obstruction unresponsive to medical therapy	Intractable disease
	Fulminant disease
	Perianal disease unresponsive to medical therapy
Massive hemorrhage	
Refractory fistula	Refractory fistula
Abscess	Colonic obstruction
Malignancy	Cancer prophylaxis
	Colon dysplasia or cancer

does not preclude sphincter-sparing ileorectal anastomosis. For the elective treatment of colorectal disease, available alternatives include a temporary defunctioning ileostomy, subtotal colectomy, or total proctocolectomy and permanent ileostomy. For patients with segmental involvement, segmental colon resection with primary anastomosis can be performed. Although there is often extensive involvement of the colon and rectum in Crohn's colitis, in 20–25% of patients there is sufficient rectal sparing to consider rectal preservation. In patients with severe perianal disease or rectovaginal fistulas, a proctectomy may be necessary.[9]

DIAGNOSIS AND MANAGEMENT OF EXTRAINTESTINAL MANIFESTATION

Metabolic bone disorders

Low bone mass occurs in 3–30% of IBD patients. The risk is increased by corticosteroids and other medications such as cyclosporine, methotrexate, and TPN. Inflammation mediated by IL-1, IL-6, and TNF and malabsorption also contribute to low bone density. In a large Canadian study, there was an increased incidence of hip, spine, wrist, and rib fractures, 36% in CD and 45% in UC. The absolute risk of an osteoporotic fracture was about 1% per person per year in IBD patients. Fracture rates, particularly in the spine and hip, were the highest among the elderly (age >60).[125] In another case-control study of 156 CD patients and 282 UC patients, the odds ratio of a vertebral fracture was 1.72 and hip fracture 1.59. The disease severity predicted the risk of a fracture even after adjusting for steroid use.[126] In addition, only 13% of IBD patients who had had a fracture were on any kind of antifracture treatment. More than 50% of patients on long-term steroid therapy develop osteoporosis, irrespective of the underlying disease. Up to 20% of bone mass can be lost per year with chronic steroid use. The effect is dosage-dependent and patients on 10 mg/day of prednisone have a significantly lower bone density than those on 0–5 mg/day.[127] In addition to prednisone, one study showed that budesonide may also suppress the pituitary-adrenal axis and thus carries a potential risk of causing osteoporosis.

Osteonecrosis is characterized by death of osteocytes and adipocytes and eventual bone collapse. The pain is aggravated by motion and swelling of the joints. It affects the hips more often than knees and shoulders and in one series, 4.3% of patients developed osteonecrosis within a 6-month period of steroid use.

Diagnosis is made by bone scan or MRI, and treatment consists of pain control, core decompression, and arthroplasty.

The other extraintestinal manifestations are detailed in Table 56.6.

TREATMENT RECOMMENDATIONS

The complete medical treatment recommendations are outlined in Table 56.3. For mild to moderate inflammatory Crohn's disease, 5-ASA agents are the first choice followed by antibiotics and then budesonide. In moderate to severe disease, patients will usually need either prednisone or infliximab to induce a remission. Methotrexate is generally reserved for use in 6-MP/AZA refractory patients. In severe to fulminant disease, most often intravenous steroids, infliximab, or TPN are indicated. Although antibiotics and 6-MP/AZA can be used for perianal fistulas, infliximab is indicated in severe perianal fistulizing disease. Although 5-ASA agents may be marginally effective in maintaining remission, the only two agents consistently proven to maintain remission are 6-MP/AZA and infliximab. For the pregnant Crohn's patient, most medical therapy is safe and patients should continue it throughout pregnancy to maintain remission.

Indications for surgery are detailed in Table 56.5.

SUMMARY

Crohn's disease is an idiopathic granulomatous disease that can affect the entire gastrointestinal tract. The etiology is thought to be an immune-medicated intestinal inflammation with a genetic predisposition. The differential diagnosis is broad but there are certain key features such as noncaseating granulomas, transmural inflammation, cobblestoning, fistulization, and recurrence after surgery that make the diagnosis apparent. There are multiple extraintestinal manifestations, the most important of which are metabolic bone disease, arthritis, skin, eye, and hepatobiliary disorders. Chronic and extensive colitis can lead to colon cancer and patients should undergo colonoscopic surveillance after 8–10 years of disease. While traditional therapy is directed at blocking more general components of the inflammatory cascade, newer therapies are targeted against specific cytokines. The future of Crohn's disease therapy is in pharmacogenomics; the determination by genetic analysis of the correct medication for the correct disease phenotype. The main goal for the future treatment of Crohn's disease

Table 56.6 Extraintestinal manifestations

Category	Clinical course	Treatment
Rheumatologic disorders (5%–20%)[128]		
Peripheral arthritis	Asymmetric/migratory Parallels bowel activity	Reduce bowel inflammation
Sacroiliitis	Symmetric/spine and hip joints Independent of bowel activity	Steroids/injections/methotrexate/anti-TNF
Ankylosing spondylitis	Gradual fusion of spine Independent of bowel activity	Azulfadine/methotrexate/anti-TNF
Dermatologic disorders (10%–20%)[128]		
Erythema nodosum	Hot, red, tender, nodules/extremities Parallels bowel activity	Reduce bowel inflammation

Table 56.6 Extraintestinal manifestations—cont'd

Category	Clinical course	Treatment
Pyoderma gangrenosum	Ulcerating, necrotic lesions Extremities, trunk, face, stoma Independent of bowel activity	Antibiotics/steroids/cyclosporine/infliximab/ dapsone/azathioprine/intralesional steroids/ thalidomide/NOT debridement or colectomy
Pyoderma vegetans	Intertriginous areas Parallels bowel activity	Evanescent; resolves without progression
Pyostomatitis vegetans	Mucous membranes Parallels bowel activity	Evanescent; resolves without progression
Metastatic Crohn's disease	Crohn's disease of the skin Parallels bowel activity	Reduce bowel inflammation
Sweet's syndrome	Neutrophilic dermatosis Parallels bowel activity	Reduce bowel inflammation
Aphthous stomatitis	Oral ulcerations Parallels bowel activity	Reduce bowel inflammation/topical rx
Ocular disorders (1%–11%)[129]		
Uveitis	Ocular pain, photophobia, blurred vision, headache Independent of bowel activity	Topical or systemic steroids
Episcleritis	Mild ocular burning Parallels bowel activity	Topical corticosteriods
Hepatobiliary disorders (10%–35%)[128]		
Fatty liver	Secondary to chronic illness, malnutrition, steroid rx	Improve nutrition/reduce steroids
Cholelithiasis	Patients with ileitis or ileal resection Malabsorption of bile acids, depletion of bile salt pool, secretion of lithogenic bile	Reduce bowel inflammation
Primary sclerosing cholangitis (PSC)	Intrahepatic and extrahepatic Inflammation and fibrosis leading to biliary cirrhosis and hepatic failure; 7%–10% cholangiocarcinoma	ERCP/high dose ursodiol lowers risk of colonic neoplasia
Genitourinary disorders (4%–23%)[128]		
Calculi	Calcium oxalate: following small bowel resection (colon intact) Uric acid: large ileostomy outputs	Hydration/decrease diarrhea Hydration
Ureteral obstruction	Varies from minimal periureteral fibrosis to complete obstructive uropathy	Treatment varies
Other[130]		
Thromboembolic disease (Clinical studies 1.3%–6.4%; postmortem 39%)	Deep vein thrombosis/pulmonary embolus/cerebrovascular accidents/arterial emboli Correlates with classic risk factors for thrombosis	Anticoagulation/thrombolysis
Cardiopulmonary complications	Myocarditis/pleuropericarditis/endocarditis/airway disease/interstitial lung disease/necrobiotic parenchymal nodules/serositis	Treatment varies
Amyloidosis	Reactive to CD; diarrhea/constipation/renal failure	Treatment varies
Pancreatitis	Secondary to duodenal fistulas, ampullary CD, gallstones, PSC, medications (6-MP/AZA/5-ASA), autoimmune, primary CD of the pancreas	Treatment varies

will be to give the correct medication at disease initiation and thereby prevent the sometimes devastating complications. By knowing from the start which subsets of patients will respond to medicines such as 6-MP/AZA, infliximab, or a yet undiscovered novel medication, we may be able to alter the natural history of Crohn's disease itself.

REFERENCES

1. Morson BC, Lockhart-Mummery HE. Crohn's disease of the colon. Gastroenterologia 1959; 92:168–173.

2. Lockhart-Mummery ME, Morson BC. Crohn's disease (regional enteritis) of the large intestine and its distinction from ulcerative colitis. Gut 1960; 1:87–105.

3. Loftus EV. Clinical epidemiology of inflammatory bowel disease: Incidence, prevalence, and environmental influences. Gastroenterology 2004; 126:1504–1517.

4. Sutherland L, Ramcharan S, Bryant H, et al. Effect of cigarette smoking on recurrence of Crohn's disease. Gastroenterology 1990; 98:1123–1128.

5. Cottone M, Rosselli M, Orlando A, et al. Smoking habits and recurrence in Crohn's disease. Gastroenterology 1994; 108:643–648.

6. Kane SV, Sable K, Hanauer SB. The menstrual cycle and its effects on inflammatory bowel disease and irritable bowel syndrome: A prevalence study. Amer J Gastroenterol 1998; 93(10):1867–1872.

7. Lewis JD, Aberra FN, Lichtenstein GR, et al. Seasonal variation in flares of inflammatory bowel disease. Gastroenterology 2004; 126:665–673.

8. Tilson RS, Friedman S. Inflammatory bowel disease during pregnancy. Curr Treat Options Gastroenterol 2003; 6:227–236.

9. Hanauer SB, Sandborn W. The Practice Parameters Committee of the American College of Gastroenterology: Management of Crohn's disease. Am J Gastroenterol 2003; 93(3):625–643.

   Important practice guidelines for treating Crohn's disease.

10. Gasche C, Scholmerich J, Brynskov J, et al. A simple classification of Crohn's disease: report of the Working Party for the World Congresses of Gastroenterology Vienna 1998. Inflamm Bowel Dis 2000; 6(1):8–15.

11. Schwatrz DA, Loftus EV, Tremaine WJ, et al. The natural history of fistulizing Crohn's fisease in Olmsted County, Minnesota. Gastroenterology 2002; 122:875–880.

12. Rutgeerts P. Strategies in the prevention of post-operative recurrence in Crohn's disease. Best Pract Res Clin Gastroenterol 2003; 17(1):63–73.

13. Olaison G, Smedth K, Sjodahl R. Natural course of Crohn's disease after ileocolic resection: Endoscopically visualized ileal ulcers preceding symptoms. Gut 1992; 33:331–335.

14. Mow WS, Lo SK, Targan SR, et al. Initial experience with wireless capsule enteroscopy in the diagnosis and management of inflammatory bowel disease. Clin Gastroenterol Hepatol 2004; 2:31–40.

    Initial experience with capsule endoscopy in Crohn's disease.

15. Schwatrz DA, Wiersema MJ, Dudiak KM, et al. A comparison of endoscopic ultrasound, magnetic resonance imaging, and exam under anesthesia for evaluation of Crohn's perianal fistulas. Gastroenterology 2001; 121:1064–1072.

16. Quinton JF, Sendid B, Reumaux D, et al. Anti-*Saccharamyces cerevisae* mannan antibodies combined with antineutrophil cytoplasmic antibodies in inflammatory bowel disease: Prevalence and diagnostic role. Gut 1998; 42:788.

    Classic paper detailing use of serologic markers in IBD.

17. Sachar DB. The problem of postoperative recurrence of Crohn's disease. Med Clin N Am 1990; 74(1):183–188.

18. Rutgeerts P. Strategies in the postoperative recurrence of Crohn's disease. Best Pract Res Clin Gastroenterol 2003; 17(1):63–73.

19. Greenstein AJ, Lachman F, Sachar DR, et al. Perforating and non-perforating indications for repeated operations in Crohn's disease: Evidence for two clinical forms. Gut 1988; 29:588–592.

20. Rutgeerts P, Geboes K, Vantrappen G, et al. Predictability of the postoperative course of Crohn's disease. Gastroenterology 1990; 9:956–963.

21. Lautenback E, Berlin JA, Lichtenstein GR. Risk factors for early postoperative recurrence of Crohn's disease. Gastroenterology 1998; 115:259–267.

22. Hanauer SB, Present DH. The state of the art in the management of inflammatory bowel disease. Rev Gastroenterol Dis 32003; (2):81–92.

23. Hanauer S. Crohn's disease: Step-up or top-down therapy. Best Pract Res Clin Gastroenterol 2003; 17:131–137.

24. Summers RW, Switz DM, Sessions JT, et al. National cooperative Crohn's disease study: Results of drug treatment. Gastroenterology 1979; 77:847–869.

25. Lochs H, Mayer M, Fleig WE, et al. Prophylaxis of postoperative recurrence of Crohn's disease with mesalamine. The European Cooperative Crohn's Disease Study VI. Gastroenterology 2000; 118:364–373.

26. Singleton JW, Hanauer SB, Gitnick GL, et al. Mesalamine capsules for the treatment of active Crohn's disease: results of a 16-week trial. Gastroenterology 1993; 104:1293–1301.

27. Hanauer SB, Stromber ULF. Oral Pentasa in the treatment of active Crohn's disease: A meta-analysis of double-blind, placebo-controlled trials. Clin Gastroenterol Hepatol 2004; 2:379–388.

28. Camma C, Giunta M, Rosselli. Mesalamine in the maintenance treatment of Crohn's disease: A meta-analysis adjusted for confounding variables. Gastroenterology 1997; 112:1465–1473.

29. Brignola C, Iannone P, Pasquali S, et al. Placebo-controlled trial of oral 5-ASA in relapse prevention of Crohn's disease. Dig Dis Sci 1992; 17(1):29–32.

30. Prantera C, Pallone F, Brunetti G, et al. Oral 5-aminosalicylic acid (Asacol) in the maintenance treatment of Crohn's disease. Gastroenterology 1992; 103:363–368.

31. Thomson ABR, Wright JP, Vatn M, et al. Mesalazine (Mesasal/Claversal) 1.5 g bid. vs. placebo in the maintenance of remission of patients with Crohn's disease. Aliment Pharmacol Ther 1995; 9:673–683.

32. De Franchis R, Omodei P, Ranzi T, et al. A controlled trial of oral 5-aminosalicylic acid for the prevention of early relapse in Crohn's disease. Aliment Pharmacol Ther 1997; 11:845–852.

33. Gendre JP, Mary JY, Florent C, et al. Oral mesalamine (Pentasa) as maintenance treatment in Crohn's disease: A multicenter placebo-controlled study. Gastroenterology 1993; 104:435–439.

34. Sutherland LR, Martin F, Bailey RJ, et al. A randomized, placebo-controlled, double-blind trial of mesalamine in the maintenance of remission of Crohn's disease. Gastroenterology 1997; 112:1069–1077.

35. Mahmud N, Kamm MA, Dupas JL, et al. Olsalazine is not superior to placebo in maintaining remission of inactive Crohn's colitis and ileocolitis: a double blind, parallel, randomized, multicentre study. Gut 2001; 49:552–556.

36. Brignola C, Cottone M, Pera A, et al. Mesalamine in the prevention of endoscopic recurrence after intestinal resection for Crohn's disease. Gastroenterology 1995; 108:345–349.

37. Modigliani R, Colombel JF, Dupas, et al. Mesalamine in Crohn's disease with steroid induced remission: Effect on steroid withdrawal and remission maintenance. Gastroenterology 1996; 110:688–693.

38. Farrell RJ, LaMont JT. Microbial factors in inflammatory bowel disease. Gastoenterol Clin N Am 2002; 31:41–62.

39. Sutherland L, Singleton J, Sessions J, et al. Double-blind, placebo-controlled trial of metronidazole in Crohn's disease. Gut 1991; 32:1071–1075.

40. Ursing B, Alm T, Barany F, et al. A comparative study of metronidazole and sulfasalazine for active Crohn's disease: The cooperative Crohn's disease study in Sweden. Gastroenterology 1982; 83:550–562.

41. Colombel JF, Lemann M, Cassagnou M, et al. A controlled trial comparing ciprofloxacin with mesalazine for the treatment of active Crohn's disease. Am J Gastroenterol 1999; 94(3):674–678.

42. Prantera C, Zannoni F, Lia Scribano M, et al. An antibiotic for the treatment of active Crohn's disease: A randomized, controlled clinical trial of metronidazole plus ciprofloxacin. Am J Gastroenterol 1996; 91(2):328–332.

43. Srinivasan R, Lichtenstein GR. Recent developments in the pharmacological treatment of Crohn's disease. Expert Opin Investig Drugs 2004; 13(4):373–391.

44. Munkholm P, Davidsen M, Langholz E, et al. Frequency of glucocorticoid resistance and dependency in Crohn's disease. Gut 1994; 35:360–362.

45. Faubion WA, Loftus EV, Harmsen WS, et al. The natural history of corticosteroid therapy for inflammatory bowel disease: A population-based study. Gastroenterology 2001; 121:255–260.

46. Plevy SE. Corticosteroid-sparing treatments in patients with Crohn's disease. Am J Gastroenterol 2002; 97(7):1607–1617.

47. Haderslev KV, Tjellesen L, Sorensen HA, et al. Alendronate increases lumbar spine bone mineral density in patients with Crohn's disease. Gastroenterology 2000; 119(3):639–646.

48. Desrame J, Sabate JM, Agher R, et al. Assessment of hypothalamic-pituitary-adrenal axis after corticosteroid therapy in inflammatory bowel disease. Am J Gastroenterol 2002; 97(7):1786–1791.

49. Edsbacker S, Bengtsson B, Larsson P, et al. A pharmacoscintigraphic evaluation of oral budesonide given as controlled-release (Entocort) capsules. Aliment Pharmacol Ther 2003; 17:525–536.

50. Steinhart AH, Feagan BG, Wong CJ, et al. Combined budesonide and antibiotic therapy for active Crohn's disease: A randomized controlled trial. Gastroenterology 2002; 123:33–40.

51. Mantzaris GJ, Petraki K, Sfakianakis M, et al. Budesonide versus mesalamine for maintaining remission in patients refusing other immunomodulators for steroid-dependent Crohn's disease. Clin Gastroenterol Hepatol 2003; 1:122–128.

52. Greenberg GR, Feagan BG, Martin F, et al. Oral budesonide for active Crohn's disease. N Engl J Med 1994; 331(13):836–841.

53. Rutgeerts P, Lofberg R, Malchow H, et al. A comparison of budesonide with prednisolone for active Crohn's disease. N Engl J Med 1994; 331(13):842–845.

Classic paper describing the use of budesonide in Crohn's disease.

54. Tremaine WJ, Hanauer SB, Katz S, et al. Budesonide CIR capsules (once or twice daily divided-dose) in active Crohn's disease: A randomized placebo-controlled study in the United States. Am J Gastroenterol 2002; 97(7):1748–1754.

55. Campieri M, Ferguson A, Doe W, et al. Oral budesonide is as effective as oral prednisone in active Crohn's disease. Gut 1997; 41(2):209–214.

56. Greenberger GR, Feagan BG, Martin F, et al. Oral budesonide as maintenance treatment for Crohn's disease: A placebo-controlled, dose-ranging study. Gastroenterology 1996; 110:45–51.

57. Edsbacker S, Bengtsson B, Larsson P, et al. A pharmacoscintigraphic evaluation of oral budesonide given as controlled-release (Entocort) capsules. Aliment Pharmacol Therapeutics 2001; 17:525–536.

58. Kane SV, Schoenfeld P, Sanborn WJ, et al. Systematic review: the effectiveness of budesonide therapy for Crohn's disease. Aliment Pharmacol Ther 2002; 16:1509–1517.

59. Feagan B, Sandborn W. Initial therapy for mild to moderate Crohn's disease. Mesalamine or budesonide? Rev Gastroenterol Dis 2002; 2(2):9–15.

60. Thomsen O, Cortot A, Jewell D, et al. Budesonide and mesalazine in active Crohn's disease: A comparison of the effects on quality of life. Am J Gastroenterol 2002; 97(3):649–653.

61. Cortot A, Colombel JF, Rutgeerts P, et al. Switch from systematic steroids to budesonide in steroid-dependent patients with inactive Crohn's disease. Gut 2001; 48:186–190.

62. Ferguson A, Campieri M, Doe W, et al. Oral budesonide as maintenance therapy in Crohn's disease: Results of a 12-month study. Aliment Pharmacol Therapeutics 1998; 12:175–183.

63. Green JRB, Lobo AJ, Giaffer M, et al. Maintenance of Crohn's disease over 12 months: Fixed versus flexible dosing regimen using budesonide controlled ileal release capsules. Aliment Pharmacol Ther 2001; 15:1331–1341.

64. Mantzaris GJ, Petraki K, Sfakianakis M, et al. Budesonide versus mesalamine for maintaining remission in patients refusing other immunomodulators for steroid-dependent Crohn's disease. Clinical Gastroenterol Hepatol 12003; :122–128.

65. Seidman EG. Clinical use and practical application of TPMT enzyme and 6-mercaptopurine metabolite monitoring in IBD. Rev Gastroenterol Dis 2003; 3:S30–S38.

Guidelines for using TPMT genetics in IBD patients on 6-MP/azathioprine.

66. Cuffari C. Monitoring azathioprine metabolite levels in IBD: Does it make a difference? Inflamm Bowel Dis Monitor 52003; (2):43–48.

67. D'Haens G, Geboes K, Rutgeerts P. Endoscopic and histologic healing of Crohn's (ileo-) colitis with azathioprine. Gastrointest Endosc 1999; 50(5):667–671.

68. Markowitz J, Grancher K, Kohn N, et al. A multicenter trial of 6-mercaptopurine and prednisone in children with newly diagnosed Crohn's disease. Gastroenterology 2000; 119:895–901.

69. Korelitz BI, Adler DJ, Mendelsohn RA, et al. Long-term experience with 6-mercaptopurine in the treatment of Crohn's disease. Am J Gastroenterol 1993; 88(8):1198–1205.

70. Pearson DC, May GR, Fick GH, et al. Azathioprine and 6-mercaptopurine in Crohn disease: a meta-analysis. Ann Intern Med 1995; 123(2):132–142.

An important meta-analysis of the efficacy of 6-MP/azathioprine in Crohn's disease.

71. Candy S, Wright J, Gerber M, et al. A controlled double blind study of azathioprine in the management of Crohn's disease. Gut 1995; 37:674–678.

72. Kim PS, Zlatanic J, Korelitz BI, et al. Optimum duration of treatment with 6-mercaptopurine for Crohn's disease. Am J Gastroenterol 1999; 94(11):3524–3257.

73. Bouhnik V, Lemann M, et al. Long-term follow-up of patients with Crohn's disease treated with azathioprine or 6-mercaptopurine. Lancet 1996; 347:215–219.

74. Lemann M, Mary JY, Colombel, et al. A randomized, double-blind, controlled withdrawal trial in Crohn's disease patients in long-term remission on azathioprine. Gastroenterology 2005; 128:1812–1818.

75. Hanauer SB, Korelitz BI, Rutgeerts P, et al. Postoperative maintenance of Crohn's disease remission with 6-mercaptopurine, mesalamine, or placebo: a 2-year trial. Gastroenterology 2004; 127:723–729.

76. Colombel JF, Ferrari N, Debuysere H, et al. Genotypic analysis of thiopurine S-methyltransferase in patients with Crohn's disease and severe myelosuppression during azathioprine therapy. Gastroenterology 2000; 118(6):1025–1030.

77. Schroder O, Stein J. Low dose methotrexate in inflammatory bowel disease: Current status and future directions. Am J Gastroenterol 2003; 98(3):530–537.

78. Alfadhli AA, McDonald JW, Feagan BG. Methotrexate for induction of remission in refractory Crohn's disease. Cochrane Database System Review 2003; 1:CD003459.

79. Feagan BG, Rochon J, Fedorak RN, et al. Methotrexate for the treatment of Crohn's disease. N Engl J Med 1995; 332(5):292–297.

One of the initial papers describing the efficacy of methotrexate in treating Crohn's disease.

80. Feagan BG, Fedorak RN, Irvine EJ, et al. A comparison of methotrexate with placebo for the maintenance of remission in Crohn's disease. N Engl J Med 2000; 342(22):1627–1632.

81. Hanauer SB, Feagan BG, Lichtenstein GR, et al. Maintenance infliximab for Crohn's disease: the ACCENT 1 randomized trial. Lancet 2002; 359:1541–1549.

82. Present DH, Rutgeerts P, Targan S, et al. Infliximab, for the treatment of fistulas in patients with Crohn's disease. New Engl J Medicine 1999; 340:1398–1405.

83. Riscart E, Panaccione R, Loftus EV, et al. Infliximab for Crohn's disease in clinical practice at the Mayo Clinic: The first 100 patients. Am J Gastroenterol 2001; 96(3):722–729.

84. D'Haens G, Van Deventer S, Van Hogezand R, et al. Endoscopic and histological healing with infliximab anti-tumor necrosis factor antibodies in Crohn's disease: A European multicenter trial. Gastroenterology 1999; 116:1029–1034.

85. Targan SR, Hanauer SB, Van Deventer SJH, et al. A short-term study of chimeric monoclonal antibody cA2 to tumor necrosis factor α for Crohn's disease. N Engl J Med 1998; 337(15):1029–1035.

One of the initial papers on infliximab and Crohn's disease.

86. Parsi MA, Achkar JP, Richardson S. Predictors of response to infliximab in patients with Crohn's disease. Gastroenterology 2002; 123:707–713.

87. Vermeire S, Luois E, Carbonez A, et al. Demographic and clinical parameters influencing the short-term outcome of anti-tumor necrosis factor (infliximab). Am J Gastroenterol 2002; 97(9):2357–2363.

88. Hanauer SB, Wagner CL, Bala B, et al. Incidence and importance of antibody responses to infliximab after maintenance of episodic treatment in Crohn's disease. Clin Gastroenterol Hepatol 2004; 2:542–553.

89. Sandborn WJ. Preventing antibodies to infliximab in patients with Crohn's disease: Optimize, not immunize. Gastroenterology 2003; 124(4):1140–1145.

90. Baert F, Norman M, Vermeire S, et al. Influence of immunogenicity on the long-term efficacy of infliximab in Crohn's disease. N Engl J Med 2003; 348(7):601–608.

91. Sandborn WJ, Naauer SB. Infliximab in the treatment of Crohn's disease: A users guide for clinicians. Am J Gastroenterol 2002; 97(12):2962–2972.

92. Rutgeerts P, Feagan BG, Lichtenstein GR, et al. Comparison of scheduled and episodic treatment strategies of infliximab in Crohn's disease. Gastroenterology 2004; 126:402–413.

93. Sachar DB. Ten common errors in the management of inflammatory bowel disease. Inflamm Bowel Dis 2003; 9(3):205–209.

Important guide to common errors in treating IBD.

94. Colombel J, Loftus EV, Tremaine WJ. The safety profile of infliximab in patients with Crohn's disease: The Mayo Clinic experience in 500 patients. Gastroenterology 2004; 126:19–31.

Important safety experience with infliximab.

95. Mow WS, Abreau-Martin MT, Papadakis KA, et al. High incidence of anergy in inflammatory bowel disease patients limits the usefulness of PPD screening before infliximab therapy. Clin Gastroenterol Hepatol 2004; 2:309–313.

96. Egan LJ, Sandborn WJ, Tremaine WJ. Clinical outcome following treatment of refractory inflammatory and fistulizing disease with intravenous cyclosporine. Am J Gastroenterol 1998; 93(3):442–448.

97. Present DH, Lichtiger S. Efficacy of cyclosporine in treatment of fistula of Crohn's disease. Dig Dis Sci 1994; 39(2):374–380.

98. Hanauer SB, Smith MB. Rapid closure of Crohn's disease fistulas with continuous intravenous cyclosporine A. Am J Gastroenterol 1993; 88(5):627–630.

99. Brynskov J, Freund L, Rasmussen SN, et al. A placebo-controlled, double-blind, randomized trial of cyclosporine therapy in active chronic Crohn's disease. N Engl J Med 1989; 321(13):845–850.

100. Sandborn WJ. Preliminary report of the use of oral tacrolimus (FK506) in the treatment of complicated proximal small bowel and fistulizing Crohn's disease. Am J Gastroenterol 1997; 92(5):876–879.

101. Sandborn WJ, Present DH, Isaacs KL, et al. Tacrolimus for the treatment of fistulas in patients with Crohn's disease: A randomized, placebo-controlled trial. Gastroenterology 2003; 125:380–388.

102. Ehrenpreis ED, Kane SV, Cohen LB, et al. Thalidomide therapy for patients with refractory Crohn's disease: An open label trial. Gastroenterology 1999; 117(6):1271–1277.

103. Vasiliauskas EA, Kam LY, Abreau-Martin MT, et al. An open-label pilot study of low-dose thalidomide in chronically active, steroid-dependent Crohn's disease. Gastroenterology 1999; 177(6):1278–1287.

104. Sabate JM, Villarejo J, Lemann M, et al. An open-labeled study of thalidomide for maintenance therapy in responders to infliximab in chronically active and fistulizing refractory Crohn's disease. Aliment Pharmacol Therapeutics 2002; 16(6):1117–1124.

105. Neurath M, Wanitschke R, Peters M, et al. Randomized trial of mycophenolate mofetil versus azathioprine for treatment of chronic active Crohn's disease. Gut 1999; 44:625–628.

106. Orth T, Peters M, Schlaak JF, et al. Mycophenolate mofetil versus azathioprine in patients with chronic active ulcerative colitis: A 12 month pilot study. Am J Gastroenterol 2000; 95:1201–1207.

107. Hanauer S, Lukas M, Macintosh D, et al. A randomized double-blind placebo-controlled trial of the human anti TNF-α monoclonal antibody adalimumab for the induction of remission in patients with moderate to severely active Crohn's disease. Gastroenterology 2004; 127(1):332.

108. Youdim A, Vasiliauskas EA, Targan SR. A pilot study of adalimumab in infliximab-allergic patients. Inflamm Bowel Dis 2004; 10:333–338.

109. Sandborn WJ, Feagan BG, Hanauer SB, et al. An engineered human antibody to TNF (CDP571) for active Crohn's disease:

A randomized double-blind placebo-controlled trial. Gastroenterology 2001; 120:1330–1338.

110. Lin WC, Hanauer SB. Emerging biologic therapies in inflammatory bowel disease. Rev Gastroenterol Dis 2004; 4(2):65–85.

111. Korzenik JR. Crohn's disease: Future anti-tumor necrosis factor therapies beyond infliximab. Gastroenterol Clin N Am 2004; 33:285–301.

112. Gordon F, Lai CWY, Hamilton MJ, et al. A randomized placebo-controlled trial of a humanized monoclonal antibody to α4 integrin in active Crohn's disease. Gastroenterology 2001; 121:268–274.

113. Ghosh S, Goldin E, Gordon FH, et al. Natalizumab for active Crohn's disease. N Engl J Med 2003; 348(1):24–32.

114. Sandborn WJ, Colombel J, Enns R, et al. A phase III, double-blind, placebo-controlled study of efficacy, safety, and tolerability of antegren (natalizumab) in maintaining clinical response and remission in Crohn's disease (ENACT-2). Gastroenterology 2004; 127(1):332.

115. Van Assche G, Van Ranst M, Sciot R, et al. Progressive multifocal leukoencephalopathy after natalizumab therapy for Crohn's disease. N Engl J Med 2005; 353.

116. Kleinschmidt-Demasters BK, Tyler KL. Progressive multifocal leukoencephalopathy complicating treatment with natalizumab and interferon beta-1a for multiple sclerosis. N Engl J Med 2005; 353.

117. Langer-Gould A, Atlas SW, Bollen AW, et al. Progressive multifocal leukoencephalopathy in a patient treated with natalizumab. N Engl J Med 2005; 353.

118. Rajapakse R, Korelitz B, et al. Outcome of pregnancies when fathers are treated with 6-mercaptopurine for inflammatory bowel disease. Am J Gastroenterol 2000; 95(3):684–688.

119. Alstead EM, Ritchie JK, Lennard-Jones JE, et al. Safety of azathioprine in pregnancy in inflammatory bowel disease. Gastroenterology 1990; 99:443–446.

120. Francella A, Dyan A, Bodian C, et al. The safety of 6-mercaptopurine for childbearing patients with inflammatory bowel disease: A retrospective cohort study. Gastroenterology 2003; 124:9–17.

121. Armenti V, Ahlswede K, Ahlswede B, et al. National transplantation pregnancy registry outcomes of 154 pregnancies in cyclosporine-treated female kidney transplant recipients. Transplantation 1994; 57:502–505.

122. Katz A, Antoni C, Keenan GF, et al. Outcome of pregnancy in women receiving infliximab for treatment of Crohn's disease or rheumatoid arthritis. Am J Gastroenterol 2004; 99(12):2385–2392.

123. Yazdanpanah Y, Klein O, Gambiez L, et al. Impact of surgery on quality of life in Crohn's disease. Am J Gastroenterol 1997; 92(10):1897–1900.

124. Thirlby R, Fenster F, Lonborg R. Effect of surgery on health-related quality of life in patients with inflammatory bowel disease. Arch Surg 1998; 133:826–832.

125. Bernstein CN, Blanchard JF, Leslie W, et al. The incidence of fracture among patients with inflammatory bowel disease: A population-based cohort study. Ann Intern Med 2000; 133(10):795–799.

126. Van Staa TP, Cooper C, Brusse LS, et al. Inflammatory bowel disease and the risk of fracture. Am J Gastroenterol 2003; 128:1591–1597.

127. Bernstein CN, Lewis WD. Review article: osteoporosis and inflammatory bowel disease. Aliment Parmacol Ther 2004; 19(9):941–952.

128. Isaacs KL. Extraintestinal manifestations. Advanced therapy of inflammatory bowel disease. Hanauer SB, Bayless T, eds. Hamilton: BC Decker; 2001:267–270.

129. Mintz R, Feller ER, Bahr RL, et al. Ocular manifestations of inflammatory bowel disease. Inflamm Bowel Dis 2004; 10(2):135–139.

130. Hoffman RM, Kruis W. Rare extraintestinal manifestations of inflammatory bowel disease. Inflamm Bowel Dis 2004; 10(2):140–147.

CHAPTER FIFTY-SEVEN

Ulcerative colitis

Lawrence J. Saubermann and Francis A. Farraye

INTRODUCTION

Medical therapies for ulcerative colitis (UC) have not changed dramatically in recent years, a striking contrast to the development of new biologic therapies and new strategies for treating Crohn's disease (see Ch. 56). The reasons for this phenomenon are numerous and are due predominately to the current lack of understanding of the pathophysiology of UC. In comparison, Crohn's disease has had an evolutionary increase of new information about the disease process as genetic loci and their role in immunologic dysregulation are being defined.[1,2] Despite this deficit in our understanding of the initiating and perpetuating mediators of UC, there have been significant advances in how gastroenterologists treat patients with this disorder using currently available medications.[3] New and potentially more potent biologic therapies are being investigated for their use in the treatment of UC.[4–6] Along with the appropriate use of available treatments, these new treatments may reduce the significant morbidity and health burden of ulcerative colitis.

DIAGNOSIS OF ULCERATIVE COLITIS

There are no clearly distinguishing features to UC, and it is a diagnosis that must be made clinically after reviewing the patient's history, physical examination, laboratory, radiologic, endoscopic, and pathologic findings. UC is a chronic disease characterized by recurrent episodes of superficial and continuous mucosal colonic inflammation, involving the rectum and extending proximally. As a result, the typical symptoms are the passage of blood and/or mucus per rectum, bloody diarrhea, tenesmus, and in some cases fever. Occasionally, crampy abdominal pain that is relieved with the passage of flatus or bowel movements are also present. Deep visceral pain, nausea, and/or vomiting are more suggestive of Crohn's disease. A number of extraintestinal manifestations involving the skin, eyes, joints, and other organ systems may also be present.[7]

Obtaining a history of environmental and genetic factors can also assist in the diagnosis of UC.[8,9] Travel history and a good medication history are particularly important in evaluating for other causes of acute and chronic diarrhea. Since UC has a familial and an as yet undefined genetic component, a patient's family history can also assist in the differential diagnosis. Another important aspect to the patient's history involves tobacco use.[10] Often, patients relate the onset of their colitis to smoking cessa-tion, and a number of studies have confirmed a correlation between either nonsmoking or cessation of smoking and the onset of UC.[11,12] Prior appendectomy may also confer some protection and lower the risk of developing UC, but does not exclude it as a diagnosis.[13,14] Psychosocial stressors could modulate the disease process and also affect relapse rates.[15] Unlike Crohn's disease, which involves the small intestine, weight loss is not usually as pronounced, and is generally related to a decrease in nutritional intake in an effort to reduce bowel frequency.

On abdominal exam, left lower quadrant tenderness may be present, or if pancolitis is present, the tenderness may extend across the mid-epigastric region to the right side of the abdomen. Frank blood is commonly seen on rectal examination. The presence of anal fistulae or large external 'hemorrhoids' suggests Crohn's disease rather than UC. Peritoneal signs, such as rebound and/or guarding, would imply worsening transmural inflammation in the setting of fulminant ulcerative colitis.

An examination for extraintestinal manifestations may assist in the diagnosis, but are not specific to UC, and may be observed in Crohn's disease or bacterial-associated colitis. These include arthritic, ocular, hepatic, dermatologic, and hematologic disorders.[7]

Laboratory findings commonly include leukocytosis and anemia. The anemia may be normocytic if acute, or microcytic if chronic and related to iron deficiency. Electrolyte disturbances are often present and consistent with chronic diarrhea, such as hypokalemia. Serum protein and albumin levels may be decreased due to the chronic inflammation and protein loss. The presence of increased acute-phase reactants is non-specific and include elevation of the erythrocyte sedimentation rate and C-reactive protein. Serum perinuclear anticytoplasmic antibodies (pANCA) levels tend to be elevated in the setting of UC, as compared to increased anti-*Saccharomyces* antibodies (ASCA) levels in Crohn's disease, but these tests currently lack sufficient sensitivity to be used as the sole basis for diagnosis.[16,17] UC patients who are pANCA positive do appear to have a clinically worse course in terms of their response to treatment and the development of pouchitis following colectomy and ileoanal anastomosis.[18] Elevated liver enzymes in a cholestatic pattern may indicate the presence of primary sclerosing cholangitis, which is present in approximately 3–5% of individuals with UC. Conversely, patients with primary sclerosing cholangitis have a 70–80% chance of having UC.

Initial plain radiographs in the ill patient are useful to exclude free air in the peritoneal cavity, assess for areas of inflammation in the colon, and assist in ruling out intestinal obstruction. On occasion, a loss of haustral folds in the setting of chronic colitis can be seen on abdominal radiographs, though this feature is more easily observed on barium enema. Examination of the sacroiliac joints and intervertebral disc regions can be seen on plain radiographs to enable an assessment for extraintestinal articular manifestations, e.g., sacroiliitis or ankylosing spondylitis. More commonly, computerized tomography (CT) is performed during the initial evaluation in the patient with moderate to severe symptoms. CT will generally demonstrate bowel wall thickening in a distribution consistent with colitis; however, it cannot distinguish colitis that is caused by other etiologies. CT can assist in suggesting Crohn's disease is more likely than UC if pericolonic fat 'stranding', or an abdominal abscess/mass, or small bowel thickening are present.

Endoscopic evaluation is useful to ascertain the location and degree of activity (Fig. 57.1) and to obtain biopsies for histopathologic analysis. Because UC predominantly involves the rectum and extends proximally, a flexible sigmoidoscopy is all that is usually required in the acute setting. A full colonoscopic evaluation can be performed when the disease is less active to assess for pancolitis, as this will impact future surveillance for colorectal cancer, and possibly indicate a more difficult management case.

The histologic analysis of mucosal biopsies demonstrates evidence of chronic inflammation and injury, including branching of the colonic crypts, crypt dropout, and infiltration of the mucosa with plasma cells as well as a large number of lymphocytes (Fig. 57.2). Crypt abscesses are also present, usually in more active disease states, but are not specific. Histology also helps eliminate other possible causes of colitis that must be considered in the differential diagnosis, such as ischemic colitis, infectious colitis, and microscopic colitis.

MEDICATIONS USED TO TREAT ULCERATIVE COLITIS

Sulfasalazine

Sulfasalazine (Azulfidine®) was the first orally administered treatment for UC and has been in clinical use for over 60 years. It is used for the treatment of mild to moderate UC for both the induction and maintenance of remission. However, its therapeutic dosage range is limited due to a significant adverse effect profile at higher doses. Better-tolerated forms of its active

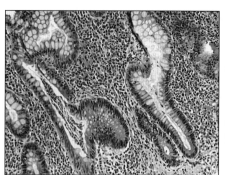

Fig. 57.2 • Ulcerative colitis histology. Mucosal biopsy demonstrating crypt abscess, crypt branching, and infiltration of the lamina propria with lymphocytes and plasma cells.

ingredient 5-aminosalicyclic acid (5-ASA) have been developed and are replacing sulfasalazine as an initial therapy for mild to moderate UC.

Sulfasalazine is a conjugate of 5-ASA linked to a sulfapyridine moiety through an azo-bond that makes the medication poorly absorbed in the upper intestinal tract. In the colon, enteric bacteria cleave the azo-bond, and the 5-ASA portion exerts its local antiinflammatory effects. The precise mechanism of 5-ASA in reducing colonic inflammation is not clear, but appears to involve intracellular inflammatory mediators such as NFκB or PPARγ within the colonic epithelial cells and/or within infiltrating immune cells.

The initial recommended dosage of sulfasalazine in active UC is 3–4 g/day in divided doses, starting at 500 mg twice daily and increasing to the target dose over 1 week. After the induction of remission, the dose is reduced to approximately 2 g/day for maintaining remission. Both enteric coated and nonenteric coated forms are available, and peak serum levels are reached in approximately 12 hours with a half-life of about 7–8 hours.[19] Sulfasalazine is poorly absorbed and possesses limited bioavailability, and what is absorbed is acetylated or hydroxylated in the liver and then conjugated to glucuronic acid for biliary excretion.[19] Acetylation of the medication appears to affect the side effect profile, as it has been shown that those individuals who are slow acetylators generally have more adverse side effects in comparison to rapid acetylators.[20-22] The plasma sulfapyridine concentration is much higher in the slow acetylators and is associated with side effects.[23-25]

Sulfasalazine is approved for use in both adults and children greater than 2 years of age, for both active disease and

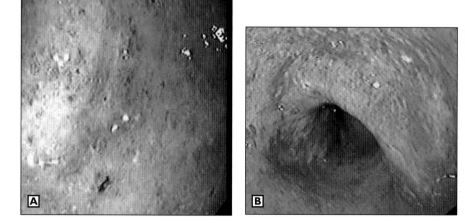

Fig. 57.1 • **(A)** Endoscopic image of mild UC. **(B)** Endoscopic image of moderate to severe UC.

maintenance of remission. Sulfasalazine and the 5-ASA compounds are less effective than corticosteroids for the treatment of active disease. The initial response to sulfasalazine in UC is usually observed within 3–4 weeks of beginning the medication, and will result in clinical improvement or remission in approximately 40–80% of patients with mild to moderate disease.[26] It is contraindicated in those individuals with hypersensitivity to the medication, urinary obstruction (due to poor urinary excretion of acetylated sulfapyridine), and porphyria. Reduced dosages should be given for patients with renal and hepatic impairment. In patients with hypersensitivity reactions to the medication, desensitization strategies have been effective.

The side effect profile for sulfasalazine is significant and almost always related to the sulfapyridine component. These side effects include hematologic changes, such as leukopenia (rarely agranulocytosis), thrombocytopenia, hemolytic or aplastic anemia. Megaloblastic anemia due to folate deficiency is also well described, and all individuals on sulfasalazine should take a folic acid supplement daily. Neurologic effects include headache and less commonly a peripheral neuropathy. Rarely, pancreatitis or hepatotoxicity as a result of a hypersensitivity reaction occurs. Pulmonary infiltrates may develop and are usually associated with a peripheral blood eosinophilia. Male infertility is a common side effect of the medication, and is a result of oligospermia. After stopping the medication, this effect is reversible within 3 months.[27] Dermatologic effects are primarily a pruritic skin rash, with rare cases of erythema multiforme (Stevens-Johnson syndrome). The most concerning reaction with administration of sulfasalazine is a hypersensitivity reaction to the sulfapyridine component. This usually manifests within the first 1–3 weeks of therapy, but may be delayed. Typically, patients present with hepatomegaly, increased liver enzymes, rash, fever, lymphadenopathy, leukocytosis, and eosinophilia, which may progress to liver failure.

As a result of these potential toxic and severe adverse effects of sulfasalazine, monitoring of patients should include baseline and periodic complete blood counts, liver function tests, and electrolytes with renal assessment.

In summary, sulfasalazine remains an important medication for the treatment of mild to moderate ulcerative colitis and is significantly less costly than the other 5-ASA formulations. Simply reducing the dose of the medication can usually treat many of the nonallergic side effects, such as headaches and abdominal discomfort. However, because of its significant adverse side effect profile, this agent is being replaced by newer nonsulfa-based 5-ASA medications (e.g., mesalamine).

Aminosalicylates (5-ASA compounds)

Mesalamine (5-ASA) has become the medication of choice for the treatment of mild to moderate UC.[28] Mesalamine is available in a variety of preparations, including oral, enema, and suppository forms. This class of agents is well-tolerated, allowing dose escalations not possible in most patients receiving sulfasalazine. There are several 5-ASA preparations available that differ in their delivery mechanism. Asacol® (Procter and Gamble) is coated with Eudragit S and is designed to release 5-ASA at a pH of 7.0 in the terminal ileum and cecum. Pentasa® (Shire) is composed of 5-ASA incorporated into a semipermeable membrane that releases 5-ASA throughout the small and large intestine. Colazal® (Salix) is composed of 5-ASA linked to an inert carrier by an azo-bond, while Dipentum® (Celltech) is composed of two 5-ASA molecules linked by an azo-bond. After bacterial cleavage of the azo-bond of Colazal and Dipetum, 5-ASA is released in the colon. Asacol is commonly prescribed at a dose of 2.4 g (two 400 mg tablets three times per day),[29] while Pentasa is given at a dose of 1 g four times a day.[30] The dose for Colazal is 6.75 g (three 750 mg tablets three times a day) while Dipentum is given at 500 mg twice daily. (See Table 57.1 for a description of the various 5-ASA preparations.)

Although generally well tolerated, some side effects have been observed with mesalamine. Mesalamine must be prescribed carefully in the setting of renal impairment as it has been reported to cause interstitial nephritis and/or worsen pre-existing renal insufficiency. It is also contraindicated for those with allergic reactions to salicylates. Rare cases of rash, hepatitis,

Table 57.1. Aminosalicylate preparations

Brand name	Generic name	Tablet form	Usual adult dose	Dosing interval
Aminosalicylates (5-ASA)				
Oral				
Asacol®	Mesalamine	400 mg	2.4–4.8 g q.d.	b.i.d.–q.i.d.
Azulfidine®	Sulfasalazine	500 mg	3.0–6.0 g q.d.	b.i.d.–q.i.d.
Colazal®	Balsalazide disodium	750 mg	6.75 g q.d.	t.i.d.
Dipentum®	Olsalazine sodium	250 mg	2.0 g q.d.	b.i.d.
Pentasa®	Mesalamine	250/500 mg	4.0 g q.d.	q.i.d.
Suppository				
Canasa®	Mesalamine	500/1000 mg	1.0–1.5 g q.d.	q.d.–t.i.d.
Suspension				
Rowasa®	Mesalamine	4 g in 60 mL	4.0 g q.d.	q.d.–b.i.d.

t.i.d., three times a day; b.i.d., two times a day; q.i.d., four times a day; q.d., once a day.

thrombocytopenia, leukopenia, anemia, pericarditis and pleuritis with pericardial and pleural effusions have also been noted. Gastrointestinal complaints occur less often than sulfasalazine, and include nausea, vomiting, dyspepsia, constipation, and rarely, pancreatitis. In contrast to sulfasalazine, however, there does not appear to be any significant effects on sperm counts in men taking mesalamine.

Currently, there are insufficient data to determine whether the new forms of 5-ASA are superior to sulfasalazine in terms of their efficacy,[31–33] and all forms of 5-ASA appear better than placebo in meta-analyses.[26,34–37] In a recent Cochrane review, it was concluded that the newer 5-ASA preparations were superior to placebo in their ability to induce remission and tended toward a therapeutic benefit over sulfasalazine. However, a clinical advantage to using the newer 5-ASA preparations in place of sulfasalazine appeared unlikely given the higher cost of the newer 5-ASA agents.[32] During maintenance therapy, while the newer 5-ASA preparations were superior to placebo, they were statistically inferior to sulfasalazine therapy.[31] Eighty percent of patients who are unable to tolerate sulfasalazine are able to tolerate mesalamine.

Enema administration is very effective in the setting of distal colitis.[38,39] Studies have shown that combination therapy with both oral and rectal administration is better than oral or rectal therapy alone at similar concentrations.[40]

Corticosteroids

In the setting of moderate to severe UC unresponsive to 5-ASAs, corticosteroids can induce remission, but have no role in maintenance therapy.[41] They do not prevent relapses, and a significant percentage of patients are likely to become 'steroid dependent' if they are unresponsive to traditional maintenance regimens. These patients will commonly relapse upon tapering of the steroid preparation. In this setting, the significant side effect profile of chronic steroid use becomes a major issue.

Intravenous corticosteroids are generally administered to the hospitalized patient once other causes for colitis have been excluded. There does not appear to be any significant differences in terms of efficacy among the parenteral preparations used.[42]

Oral corticosteroids are useful in the patient with moderate colitis, and remission rates of approximately 70% are commonly achieved.[43] Oral agents can also be used to transition patients after induction of remission with parenteral corticosteroids for outpatient management. Prednisone and prednisolone are commonly used preparations, with a typical daily dose of 40–60 mg of prednisone or its equivalent. The use of higher doses of corticosteroids does not appear to confer any benefit to patients with mild to moderate disease that are unresponsive to 5-ASA therapy. Topical corticosteroid preparations (enemas and foams) are available for the treatment of distal ulcerative colitis but are less effective than topical 5-ASA formulations.[44]

Steroid-related side effects are significant and can result in serious consequences. They include hypertension, hyperglycemia, osteonecrosis, osteopenia, mood disorders, hypertrichosis, epidermal thinning, and change in adipose distribution. Given the lack of data to suggest that maintenance regimens with corticosteroids are effective in UC, the early addition of an immunomodulator is recommended (discussed below). It is also recommended that calcium supplementation and the use of bisphosphonates be considered due to the risk of osteopenia while taking corticosteroids for prolonged periods of time.[45]

In a population-based study from the Mayo Clinic, of 185 UC patients diagnosed between 1970 and 1993, 34% needed steroids at some time during the course of their illness. Immediate outcomes (30 days) for UC patients treated with steroids were complete remission in 54%, partial remission in 30%, and no response in 16%. At 1 year, 22% of the patients were steroid dependent, 29% underwent colectomy, and the remaining 49% were off steroids.[46]

Therefore, although steroids are very effective in inducing remission in patients with UC, they should be avoided for maintenance therapy.

IMMUNOMODULATORS

Azathioprine and 6-mercaptopurine

Used as immunosuppressive agents in the setting of solid organ transplantation, azathioprine or 6-mercaptopurine (6-MP) are the most commonly used immunomodulators in the treatment of both Crohn's disease and UC. These medications are primarily used in UC patients with moderately to severely active disease for maintenance of remission and also for their steroid-sparing effect. There are limited data regarding the induction of remission in UC with either agent.[47,48] Their exact mechanisms of action are not known, but these agents do affect DNA and RNA synthesis, and a recent report has suggested a possible role in causing T-cell apoptosis.[49]

Although responses can occur as early as 8 weeks, it may take up to several months for patients to respond to azathioprine or 6-MP. Given this latency period, these agents are generally initiated early in the treatment of moderately active UC. A trial in patients with steroid-treated Crohn's disease using an initial intravenous loading dose of azathioprine did not decrease the time to response.[50] More commonly, oral azathioprine is given in the setting of other immunosuppressive agents, such as steroids or cyclosporine, during a moderate or severe episode of colitis, while tapering these other agents.[51]

Azathioprine bioavailability is about 50%, and it is converted rapidly to 6-mercaptopurine (6-MP) in the bloodstream and then into several additional metabolites, of which 6-thioguanine (6-TG) is the therapeutically active metabolite. The metabolism of azathioprine and 6-MP is controlled by thiopurine methyltransferase (TPMT), and those individuals with a genetic decrease in levels of TPMT are prone to toxicity. Approximately 11% of individuals are heterozygous for TPMT mutations, and they have a 50% reduction in their ability to metabolize the medication. About 1 in 300 individuals are homozygous and at risk for severe toxicity. Genetic testing is available for this enzyme and can be performed prior to the initiation of therapy. Regardless of whether TPMT genotype or activity is measured, the patient's complete blood count should be monitored for leukopenia. Monitoring will identify those individuals with genetic deficiencies in TPMT within the first few weeks, at which time the dose can be adjusted accordingly. 6-TG was considered as a potential alternative immunomodulator, but long-term treatment results in nodular hyperplasia and fibrosis in the liver, thereby precluding its use.[52]

Azathioprine is generally initiated at a dose of 0.5–1 mg/kg/day in divided doses, and if tolerated, increased to 2.0–2.5 mg/

kg/day. Initial doses of 6-MP are 50 mg/day, and the standard dose is 1.0–1.5 mg/kg daily. As noted above, an alternative approach is to start at the target dose after assessment of the TPMT genotype or enzyme activity.[53,54] Dosing needs to be adjusted in the setting of renal insufficiency.

The side effects of azathioprine are usually bone marrow suppression. Leukopenia and or thrombocytopenia are dose dependent and reversible. Because this side effect can occur late in the course of treatment, laboratory values need to be followed on a weekly basis initially and then periodically thereafter. Rare red-cell aplasia has also been reported, which may present late in the course of therapy. Gastrointestinal side effects are common in patients taking azathioprine and most commonly include nausea, vomiting, and dyspepsia, all of which may be transient. Some patients who are intolerant to azathioprine due to nausea or headaches can tolerate 6-MP. Pancreatitis is a well-documented adverse effect that occurs in about 3–5% of individuals, and the medication must be discontinued in this setting. Hepatotoxicity is also associated with the use of azathioprine, usually in the form of cholestatic liver disease in the setting of a hypersensitivity reaction. This hypersensitivity reaction is rare and presents as fevers, chills, leukocytosis, renal impairment, and hepatotoxicity, usually within the first few weeks of treatment. Monitoring of liver enzymes is thus recommended during the first few weeks of therapy and then regularly thereafter. Although significant concern had been raised regarding the potential for an increased risk of malignancy with azathioprine use, retrospective reviews have not detected a significant increase in the number of cancers in those taking azathioprine.[55,56]

Azathioprine and 6-MP are both contraindicated in patients on allopurinol. Allopurinol inhibits xanthine oxidase, which metabolizes 6-MP to an inactive metabolite; coadministration can result in severe pancytopenia. In addition, clinicians should be aware of an interaction between 5-ASA preparations and azathioprine or 6-MP. In a study of patients with Crohn's disease receiving azathioprine or 6-MP, the addition of mesalamine or sulfasalazine resulted in an increase in whole blood 6-TG concentrations and a high frequency of mild leukopenia. It is felt that this drug interaction results from the inhibition of TPMT by mesalamine and sulfasalazine.[57]

As noted, azathioprine is primarily used as a maintenance therapy and as a means for reducing steroid dependency. Azathioprine has been demonstrated to be effective at maintenance of disease remission in 80–90% of patients over two years.[58] In addition, it has enabled the discontinuation of corticosteroids in steroid-dependent subjects.[59] In one study, with steroid-dependent active UC, the 1-year relapse rate was 31% on azathioprine as compared to 61% on placebo.[60] In another study in which intravenous cyclosporine was started for severe steroid refractory UC, 10 of 12 subjects responded to azathioprine; only one patient experienced a relapse, while no patient required colectomy by 16 months.[61] Two other studies have confirmed the observation that the addition of azathioprine after induction with intravenous cyclosporine results in a reduction in relapse and the need for colectomy.[62,63] Furthermore, in a double-blind, placebo-controlled study of 44 subjects with active UC, significant reductions in steroid use were again seen in the azathioprine-treated group.[64] The duration of maintenance therapy with azathioprine or 6-MP in patients with UC is unknown.

In summary, azathioprine or 6-MP has become the current medication of choice for long-term maintenance for moderate to severe UC, especially in the steroid-dependent patient. The role of these two agents in the induction of remission is less clear. The use of these drugs requires close monitoring for toxicity, including frequent laboratory measurements, and regular office visits. Table 57.2 summarizes the typical doses of the immunomodulators.

Cyclosporine

In severe cases of ulcerative colitis in the hospitalized patient unresponsive to intravenous corticosteroids, parenteral cyclosporine can be used as a potent and rapidly acting immunosuppressive medication. Cyclosporine has a significant side effect profile and toxicity that limits its long-term use in patients with UC. Consequently, it is reserved for patients with severe colitis

Table 57.2 Corticosteroid and immunomodulator preparations

Brand name	Generic name	Tablet form	Usual adult dose
Corticosteroids			
	Prednisolone		40–60 mg p.o. q.d
	Prednisone		40–60 mg p.o. q.d
	Methylprednisolone		40–60 mg i.v. q.d
	Hydrocortisone		300 mg i.v. q.d
Immunomodulators			
Imuran®	Azathioprine	50 mg	2.0–2.5 mg/kg q.d.
Purinethol®	6-mercaptupurine	50 mg	1.0–1.5 mg/kg q.d.
	Cyclosporine		2.0–4.0 mg/kg i.v. continuous over 24 h
Neoral®	Cyclosporine	25 mg, 100 mg	Twice the i.v. dose given b.i.d.

b.i.d., two times a day; q.d., once a day; i.v., intravenous.

refractory to steroids who would otherwise undergo a colectomy.[65] The starting dose originally described in the randomized controlled trials was 4 mg/kg/day,[65] although recent data have suggested that 2 mg/kg/day has similar efficacy with less toxicity.[66] UC clinical trials have indicated a clear benefit of cyclosporine in severe, steroid-refractory disease. In the original randomized, controlled study of cyclosporine versus placebo in hospitalized UC patients unresponsive to intravenous steroids, the response rate was 82% at a mean of 7 days.[65]

Cyclosporine is bound to lipoproteins in the blood and has a half-life of approximately 8 hours. It is distributed throughout the fatty tissues and is excreted primarily through the biliary system along with its metabolites. Its mechanism of action is unclear, but the drug appears to inhibit second-messenger molecules in T cells, such as cyclophilin and calmodulin, which leads to a down-regulation of inflammatory molecules and leukocyte function.

Patients on intravenous cyclosporine can be changed to an oral preparation; however, due to decreased oral bioavailability, higher doses (typically twice the intravenous dose) are used. High-fat meals may interfere with absorption. Following cyclosporine levels does not appear to be related to efficacy in treatment and are obtained primarily to help avoid toxicity and to evaluate the bioavailability of the medication.

As indicated above, cyclosporine has a number of significant side effects. Nephrotoxicity is commonly observed (up to approximately 25% of individuals) and may occur either early or late. This effect is dose-related and is usually reversible, but irreversible renal toxicity may occur. Oliguria is a common presentation along with a rise in serum creatinine. Patients must be monitored closely for hyperkalemia and hypomagnesemia. Hypertension is another significant and common side effect of cyclosporine use, occurring in up to 50% of individuals, and its use is contraindicated in the setting of uncontrolled hypertension. The onset is typically early and may be associated with the development of headaches. Blood pressure monitoring should be performed at baseline and then every other week initially, followed by monitoring every month thereafter. This effect is also reversible, but can be managed by antihypertensive medications if necessary. Rare cases of hemolytic uremic syndrome, hepatotoxicity in the form of hyperbilirubinemia and seizures have been described. Tremors may be observed while on cyclosporine. Another common side effect is hypercholesterolemia, with hypertriglyceridemia rarely observed.

Other issues that have been noted with cyclosporine use include gingival hyperplasia and an increased risk of opportunistic infection, specifically *Pneumocystis carinii* pneumonia. Prophylaxis against *P. carinii* is recommended in the setting of cyclosporine use when administered with azathioprine/6MP and corticosteroids.

NEW THERAPIES/OTHER MEDICATIONS

A large number of new biologic therapies are being considered for UC. Although none has been approved at this time for UC, active investigation is underway with a number of potential antiinflammatory agents. The antitumor necrosis factor-α (TNF-α) treatments, including mouse-human chimeric (infliximab) and fully humanized antibodies (CDP571), have been used in patients with UC, with mixed results to date. The majority of these studies have been open-label in small numbers of subjects.[67] In one randomized, placebo-controlled study involving infliximab, no benefit was detected at 6 weeks in moderately severe and steroid-resistant

UC.[68] Two recent large multicenter randomized, placebo-controlled studies found that infliximab at doses of 5–10 mg/kg were effective in treating ulcerative colitis refractory to at least one standard therapy including 5-ASA, corticosteroids, or immunosuppressants (Supplement to *Gastroenterology* 2005, 128: A-104, A-105). In the Active Ulcerative Colitis One (ACT 1) trial, clinical response rates at 30 weeks were 52.1% and 50.8% for the 5 mg/kg and 10 mg/kg infliximab groups compared with 29.8% of the placebo. Remission rates were 33.9%, 36.9% and 15.7% respectively. Similar responses were seen in another large multicenter trial (ACT 2).

Another antibody blocking strategy for the treatment of UC involves reducing leukocyte adhesion. The α4 integrin is critical for the recognition and migration of leukocytes through the intestinal endothelium. Two different forms of an antibody that block either the α4 integrin or α4β7 pair of integrins on the surface of leukocytes and prevent their adhesion/migration are being investigated. Initially, 10 subjects were tested with an anti-α4 infusion, and a clinically significant response was noted in 50% of subjects by 2 weeks.[69] However, recent larger studies have been suspended due to the development of progressive multifocal leukoencephalopathy (PML) in several subjects.

Similarly, leukopheresis columns are being tested to remove circulating leukocytes that may be involved in the disease process. Some benefits have been described in reducing steroid dependence over time; however, this approach is still considered experimental.[70,71] Large randomized, controlled trials are ongoing.

Another targeted antibody-based therapy involves antibodies directed against the interleukin-2 receptor alpha-chain (CD25). To date, this approach has been demonstrated to be beneficial in a small clinical trial.[72]

Other biologic treatments include the use of small molecules, such as the ten amino acid antiinflammatory molecule known as RDP58.[73,74] This amino acid molecule inhibits proinflammatory substances like TNF-α and interferon-gamma at a local, intracellular point, rather than in a systemic fashion.[74]

Transdermal nicotine has been considered a possible treatment for UC. The rationale for its use has been the observation that many UC subjects experience their initial episode within weeks to months after the cessation of smoking.[12] In some trials, transdermal nicotine has been shown to be an additional effective therapy to induction regimens.[75–78] However, the side effects are significant, and nicotine must be used cautiously in nonsmoking individuals or in those who may return to smoking and become nicotine dependent.[75] This mode of therapy is not effective for use as a maintenance therapy.[79]

Antibiotics have also been used as additive therapy to induce remission in UC. A double-blind, randomized trial of ciprofloxacin reported a beneficial effect in steroid or aminosalicylate-treated individuals.[80] However, when given alone, it did not appear to be effective.[81] In another trial, metronidazole and tobramycin had no effect on the clinical course of UC.[82]

Intramuscular methotrexate has been demonstrated to be effective in treating Crohn's disease (see Ch. 56). However, in UC when administered orally at doses of 12.5 or 15 mg, no benefit from methotrexate has been demonstrated in the treatment of patients with UC.[83,84]

The unfractionated form of heparin has also been examined in UC and was initially believed to be beneficial; however, further studies have found it to be ineffective as a monotherapeutic agent.[85,86]

A recent study compared the efficacy of the probiotic preparation *Escherichia coli* Nissle 1917 with mesalazine in maintaining remission in patients with UC. The rate of relapse was similar in both groups at 12 months (36.4% in the probiotic group and 33.9% in the mesalazine group).[87]

MEDICAL TREATMENT STRATEGIES

The goals of treating UC are the control of symptoms and the induction and maintenance of clinical remission, while limiting medication-induced side effects. The choice of medical therapy in patients with UC is based on the extent and severity of disease, which can be modified by patient preference and their response to previous therapeutic trials. Traditionally, therapies have been applied using a tiered approach, with increasing efficacy and toxicity at higher levels. Oral and topical therapies are initiated in patients with mild to moderate disease, followed by immunomodulator treatment in patients with moderate to severe disease. As discussed above, there has been a strategic shift in practice in the treatment of UC, primarily to an increase in the use of immunomodulation earlier in the course of the disease to prevent recurrent exacerbations, limit steroid toxicity, and reduce disease morbidity.

Proctitis

Patients with ulcerative proctitis typically present with hematochezia and mucus both with and without bowel movements, tenesmus, and a lack of systemic signs or symptoms. Due to its distal location, topical therapies are very effective,[35] and they cover the affected region well.[88] Patient preference usually determine the form of treatment to be used.

Topical 5-ASA (mesalamine) enemas, suppositories, or foam (not available in United States) are the first-line therapy for induction and maintenance of remission, with reported remission rates of approximately 75%.[89] Doses are generally 500–1000 mg/day for the suppositories and 4 g for the 5-ASA enemas. Nightly enemas or twice daily enemas are often used, but patient preference often dictates the use of 5-ASA suppositories.[90–92] Corticosteroids are available in enema, foam, and suppositories as well.[93,94] Topical corticosteroids can also be used, and while some studies have demonstrated effectiveness equal to topical mesalamine therapies, meta-analyses have indicated a greater derived benefit with mesalamine therapy.[44,93–95] Topical corticosteroids may be useful in those individuals intolerant to mesalamine or in more severe cases of distal colitis.[39,96] Oral 5-ASA medications are generally less efficacious than topical 5-ASA therapies for proctitis.[97] The use of topically administered mesalamine formulations has been demonstrated to be effective for maintenance of remission for proctitis (Fig. 57.3).[98]

Left-sided colitis

Left-sided colitis includes proctosigmoiditis or colitis extending to the splenic flexure. The treatment of left-sided colitis includes both topical and oral forms of 5-ASA, as well as topical corticosteroids.

Induction of remission: Similar to proctitis, the initial induction regimen involves the use of sulfasalazine or 5-ASA-containing compounds.[39,99] Doses range 2–4 g in daily divided doses for 5-ASA and 4 g for sulfasalazine.[100] Topical therapy is commonly used, but oral therapy tends to be preferred by most patients. Enemas effectively treat the more proximal disease-affected areas than suppositories or foam.[35,88] The combination of topical and oral 5-ASA forms is superior to either one alone, possibly a result of either improved compliance, a higher total 5-ASA dose, or a more directed form of localized therapy.[40,101–103]

In patients unable to attain remission with high-dose oral and topical 5-ASA, corticosteroid enemas may be initiated in an attempt to avoid systemic steroids.[96,104–106] However, in the patient with ongoing symptoms in the absence of systemic toxicity, such

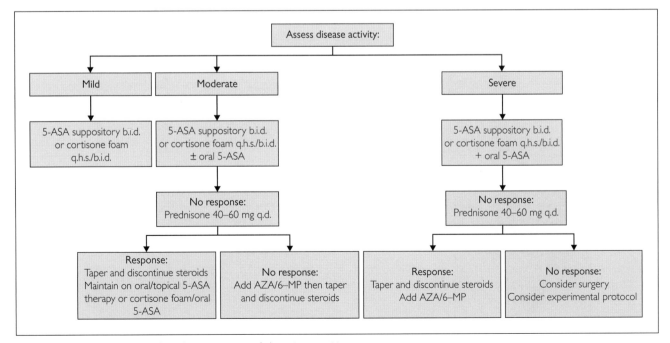

Fig. 57.3 ● A suggested approach to the management of ulcerative proctitis.

as fever, weight loss, or severe abdominal pain, oral corticosteroids should be considered. Typically, they should be prescribed once or twice daily. If symptoms of progression and toxicity are present, hospitalization and the use of intravenous corticosteroids may be necessary (see below in the next section on pancolitis).

Maintenance regimen: After achieving remission, patients are often gradually tapered off their topical 5-ASA formulations in favor of the easier to tolerate oral 5-ASA formulations. In general, the dose of sulfasalazine is often reduced from 4 g to 2 g daily for maintenance to prevent dose-related toxicity. Dose reductions are generally not necessary for the newer mesalamine-based therapies, and the dose of mesalamine typically used to induce remission is now commonly prescribed as the maintenance dose.

In more severe cases of left-sided UC, where the use of oral and topical mesalamine has been maximized, azathioprine or 6-MP can be added in an attempt to induce and maintain a lasting remission. This approach has not been investigated extensively in patients with left-sided colitis; however, its benefit can be inferred from its efficacy in patients with pancolitis. Serial monitoring of complete blood counts and liver enzymes is required at initiation and throughout the course of treatment. Oral folic acid should be administered because of indirect evidence that it may help prevent the development of dysplasia and neoplasia in chronic UC (Fig. 57.4).[107,108]

Pancolitis

Disease extending from the rectum proximal to the splenic flexure is defined as pancolitis or extensive colitis. It is important to assess the disease extent by endoscopy and biopsy in all patients with UC, as individuals who initially present with extensive colitis more commonly require colectomy or develop complications.

Induction regimen: The disease activity determines the form of induction therapy. For mild cases, therapy with sulfasalazine or mesalamine is generally initiated. As in distal colitis, topical therapy is useful as an adjunct to oral therapy. The response rate using this regimen approaches 70–80%, and over 50% of patients will achieve a lasting remission. Sulfasalazine or 5-ASA doses should be maximized to induce remission and to avoid the use of corticosteroids.

In more moderate cases, or when patients are not responding rapidly to maximal 5-ASA treatments, the addition of oral corticosteroids is warranted. Typically, in the outpatient setting, doses are initiated at 40–60 mg/day of prednisone, either in single or twice daily doses.[109] After the patient has achieved remission, steroid doses can be tapered. Although data comparing various steroid tapering strategies are not available, in general, a decrease of 5–10 mg/week is used until a daily dose of 20 mg is achieved, at which time the daily dose is decreased in 5 mg increments per week. Those patients who appear to require corticosteroids early in the course of their disease and relapse as the steroid dose is tapered are candidates for immunomodulator treatment with azathioprine or 6-MP. Owing to their delayed onset of action, these medications should be considered early in the course of the illness.

In severe cases of UC or in those patients not responding to oral corticosteroids, hospitalization may be required. Stool studies should be obtained for enteric pathogens including *C. difficile* and

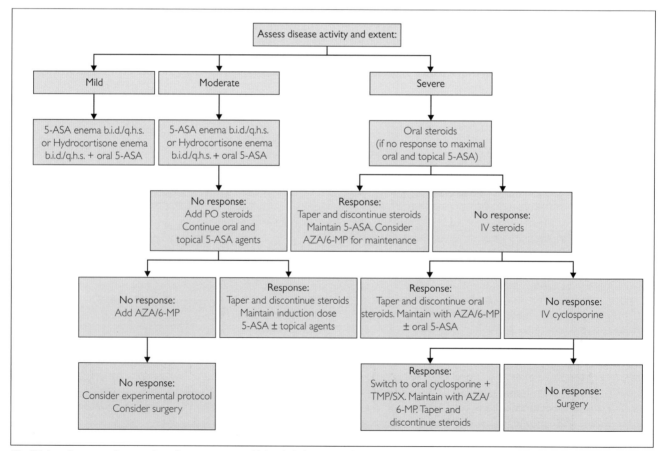

Fig. 57.4 • A suggested approach to the management of left-sided ulcerative colitis.

a limited flexible sigmoidoscopy performed to exclude super-imposed *cytomegalovirus* or other infections. These patients often have weight loss, anemia, fever, abdominal pain, and nocturnal and frequent bowel movements (>10/day). Intravenous steroids should be initiated after an initial evaluation to exclude any contraindication to their use. The starting dose is typically 300 mg/day of hydrocortisone, 32–48 mg of methylprednisolone, or 40–60 mg of prednisone, in divided doses or by continuous infusion. There are no data to suggest that continuous or divided dosing confers any benefit over the other, nor are there data to suggest that higher doses of steroids provide any additional benefit. Steroid enemas or foam may also be added topically to treat tenesmus. In these severe cases, 5-ASA therapy adds little or no benefit and can thus be initially deferred and started once patients begin to show evidence of improvement or at the time of hospital discharge. Surgical consultation should be obtained in all patients admitted with a severe attack of UC.

Hospitalized patients are often fasted in an attempt to reduce the frequency of bowel movements. However, as the small intestinal mucosa is not involved in UC, oral feeding is recommended whenever possible.[110] A low-residue diet may be preferred, but inflammation causes a catabolic state, and caloric supplementation is frequently required. If a patient reports significant nausea, vomiting, or worsening of abdominal pain associated with eating, parenteral nutrition may be considered.

While most patients respond to intravenous corticosteroid administration within the first week, approximately 20–30% of patients are unresponsive. Steroid-refractory individuals are unlikely to improve in response to continued steroid administration.[111] Therefore, after 5–7 days of intensive therapy with intravenous corticosteroids, options include proceeding with colectomy or adding intravenous cyclosporine. Response rates for intravenous cyclosporine of 70–80% have been reported in steroid-refractory patients after 1 week of therapy.[65,112,113] The traditional starting dose is 4 mg/kg/day administered by continuous infusion, although recent data suggest that 2 mg/kg/day may be as effective while reducing side effects.[66] Blood levels are monitored to maintain levels between 200 and 400 ng/ml, despite the fact that these levels do not correlate with a clinical response. Patients must be made aware of risks and benefits prior to initiating therapy, and must be carefully monitored for electrolyte disturbances, cholesterol levels, renal dysfunction, and hypertension. Hypertension can be treated by the concomitant use of calcium channel blockers. Patients are likely to respond during the first 5–7 days, and those who do not respond at 7 days are unlikely to attain remission. Under such circumstances, total proctocolectomy should be recommended. Trials of other immunosuppressive medications, such as methotrexate or mycophenolate mofetil, have either demonstrated no effect or are considered experimental at this time.[83,114]

Maintenance regimen: Individuals with mild pancolitis who respond to aminosalicylates are maintained on the dose used to achieve remission,[29] except in those patients responding to induction doses of sulfasalazine. In such cases, the dose can be tapered from 4 to 2 g/day if the patient experiences side effects.[40,102] For 5-ASA compounds, long-term monitoring is required, including periodic testing of renal function, blood counts, and liver enzymes.

In more moderate pancolitis cases, in which oral corticosteroids are required to achieve remission, it may be more difficult to maintain remission. During the tapering of the steroid dose, it is possible for patients to experience an exacerbation of their disease. Patients should be evaluated for other possible causes of colitis, including infections such as *Clostridium difficile*, enteric pathogens, or cytomegalovirus. Repeat endoscopy can determine if the disease recurrence is localized to the distal colon and rectum, or is more extensive. If localized, topical therapy may be initiated or the dose increased. Efforts should be made to maximize the 5-ASA dose during the steroid taper to reduce disease relapse.

Currently, maintenance with azathioprine or 6-MP is the treatment of choice for corticosteroid-dependent patients.[51,58] The once or twice a day dosing regimen increases compliance. For example, in one study of 35 patients, the combination of azathioprine and sulfasalazine was significantly better than sulfasalazine and placebo in maintaining remission.[115] There are risks associated with the use of these medications, including a slightly increased risk of infection, and individuals must decide with their physician's assistance whether the possible benefits outweigh the risks of therapy. Close monitoring of the blood counts for the development of leukopenia is required, particularly in those with genetic mutations in the TPMT gene, who may achieve toxic blood levels and have bone marrow suppression or severe leukopenia.

Most patients with severe pancolitis who respond to intravenous steroids can be changed to oral preparations and will probably require use of azathioprine or 6-MP to maintain remission. Many of these patients are initiated on the azathioprine or 6-MP during their acute hospitalization. This approach facilitates their transition off oral steroids within 2–3 months as the azathioprine/6-MP is beginning to achieve its efficacy.[51] Those individuals who required intravenous cyclosporine to achieve remission can be changed to oral cyclosporine using twice the intravenous dose.[116] However, due to its significant toxicity, oral cyclosporine should be considered a 'bridge therapy,' and azathioprine or 6-MP should be initiated concurrently with the eventual goal of discontinuing the cyclosporine at a later date.[61,62] Patients on cyclosporine are at risk for *Pneumocystis carinii* pneumonia and, as stated above, should receive prophylaxis with sulfamethoxazole/trimethoprim three times per week. Patients should be re-evaluated during the first week after discharge from the hospital and should then be seen every 2 weeks during the first few months while adjusting medications (Fig. 57.5).

Fulminant colitis

Fulminant or toxic colitis is a medical and surgical emergency. Surgery should not be delayed, and expedited assessments by the emergency room physician, gastroenterologist, and surgeon are required. These patients have severe colitis with significant anemia, fever, abdominal tenderness, and abdominal distention. Very close monitoring is required, and patients may or may not have concomitant colonic dilation.[117]

The presence of colonic dilation on an abdominal radiograph raises the possibility of toxic megacolon, which may also be associated with cytomegalovirus or *C. difficile* infection. The use of antidiarrheal medications, hypokalemia, and other electrolyte disturbances can predispose patients to the development of toxic megacolon. Moreover, the use of corticosteroids may mask symptoms and signs of megacolon, and toxic megacolon should also be considered in those patients whose bowel movements suddenly decrease in the setting of increased abdominal distention.

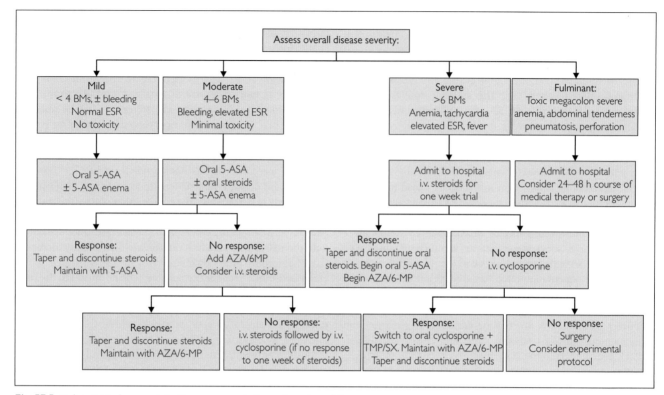

Fig. 57.5 ● A suggested approach to the management of pan ulcerative colitis.

Radiographs may show distention (>6 cm) and/or bowel wall edema ('thumbprinting') in fulminant colitis, and in some cases, pneumatosis may be present. Computerized tomographic scanning is more sensitive than plain X-ray films for identifying free air, pneumatosis, or edema.

The medical aspect to the management of toxic megacolon requires the recognition of the severity of the illness and supportive care. A short trial of intravenous corticosteroids can be administered in some cases, and complete bowel rest with nothing given orally is mandatory. Antibiotics are empirically used as transmural extension is assumed, and the risk of bacterial septicemia and/or bacterial peritonitis is high. Clearly, intensive care monitoring, and administration of crystalloid, colloid, or blood products are given as needed.

Emergency surgery is necessary in those individuals with evidence of perforation, as well as in those who fail to improve rapidly or who deteriorate clinically. Morbidity is greater in those patients who develop colonic perforation; thus, close monitoring with serial radiographs, laboratory testing, and physical examinations should help guide the decision to initiate surgical therapy.

Pregnancy/fertility issues

Infertility in UC is primarily due to male oligospermia that occurs with the use of sulfasalazine. Oligospermia will resolve within 3 months after discontinuing sulfasalazine in favor of a newer 5-ASA agent. Women with UC have normal fertility unless they have undergone proctocolectomy and ileal pouch-anal anastomosis (IPAA).[118]

Pregnancy in the setting of UC has been studied extensively (see Ch. 10), and both the impact of inflammatory bowel disease on pregnancy and the effect of the pregnancy on inflammatory bowel disease have been evaluated. In more active disease states, there is a significant increase in the number of spontaneous abortions, premature and low-birth weight infants. The effect of pregnancy on UC disease activity itself does not appear to be significant, with both exacerbations and remissions noted that might be related to the natural history of the disease. Therefore, the goal of medical therapy is to maintain remission or reduce the level of disease activity, before and during the pregnancy.[119]

The safety of medications used to treat UC during pregnancy has been extensively studied. A recent review of 207 conceptions at an inflammatory bowel disease (IBD) referral center reported no significant effects in patients taking any of the commonly used IBD medications.[120] Most of these drugs are well tolerated during pregnancy, including the 5-ASA compounds and corticosteroids. A prospective evaluation and a case-report study of mesalamine use in UC indicated no significant increase in reported congenital abnormalities.[121,122] Another review of 5-ASA use within a Scandinavian birth registry likewise found no increased risk of congenital malformations.[123] The immunosuppressive medications azathioprine and 6-MP have been categorized as unsafe during pregnancy. However, recent data have found no increased risk to the fetus. Rather, the greater risk appears to be associated with an increase in disease activity during pregnancy.[124,125] Although cyclosporine appears safe to use, it is generally used only during active disease and patients should be changed to another immunomodulator agent once remission has been achieved.

If required to assist in diagnosis and management, sigmoidoscopy can be performed safely in the pregnant patient. Occasionally, surgery is also required to treat fulminant colitis, and should not be avoided if clinically necessary for the safety of the mother. In those patients with an ileal pouch-anal anastomosis, fertility is decreased and the timing of surgery and plans for a family need to be considered.[126]

In conclusion, both planning for and the management of pregnancy in UC should be a coordinated exercise among the patient, the obstetrician, and the gastroenterologist.

SURGERY

The most common indications for colectomy are medically intractable disease, complications of colitis, including dysplasia or cancer, and side effects of medical therapy. In the case of the critically ill toxic colitis patient, urgent surgery is required. Otherwise, a short trial of intravenous corticosteroids is warranted to try to prevent the need for emergency surgery, but lack of improvement during the initial 24–72 hours is generally indicative of a poor prognosis and the need for surgery. Toxic megacolon also requires surgery in most cases and can be viewed as a complication of the extensive disease process.

In the acute setting, proctocolectomy or subtotal colectomy is performed with an end-ileostomy. At a later time, an ileal pouch-anal anastomosis (IPAA) can be performed in appropriate candidates. The IPAA operation is more technically demanding than a total proctocolectomy and ileostomy, and both immediate and long-term complications are associated with this procedure. Nonetheless, this operation achieves the highest patient satisfaction rate, as it allows for construction of an ileal reservoir for stool and defecation through an intact anal sphincter.

A major indication for total proctocolectomy is the association of UC with colonic neoplasia. The prevalence of colonic adenocarcinoma in subjects with UC increases at a rate of about 1% per year after 8–10 years of disease. Thus, 30 years after the onset of UC, the risk of developing cancer is approximately 20%. Risk factors for an increased risk of colonic neoplasia include the extent and duration of disease, concomitant primary sclerosing cholangitis, a family history of colorectal cancer, and as the severity of disease.[127,128] In patients with pancolitis, annual surveillance colonoscopy is recommended after the seventh year of disease, with random biopsies taken at 10 cm intervals, as well as biopsies of any abnormal-appearing mucosa. Indications for proctocolectomy include either flat high-grade or low-grade dysplasia confirmed by an expert pathologist. Recent data support the conservative treatment of polypoid dysplastic lesions that are completely removed and without associated flat dysplasia elsewhere in the colon.[129] Because of the increased risk of colon cancer development in patients with long-standing disease, some individuals may opt for elective surgery given a clear understanding of the risk/benefit ratio. Colectomy represents a 'cure' for UC, and for many individuals a reduction in the use of medication and an improvement in quality of life provide the rationale to consider this option. Nonetheless, because of problems associated with IPAA, every effort must be extended to maximize medical therapy before proceeding with surgery.

Pouchitis

As many as 25% of UC patients will require a colectomy during the course of their illness, and the majority of those having surgery will undergo an IPAA procedure rather than an ileostomy. Inflammation of the pouch (pouchitis) is a well-recognized complication after IPAA.[130] In a large series from the Mayo Clinic, 40% of patients had a single episode of pouchitis, while 15% and 5% experienced intermittent episodes and chronic pouchitis, respectively.[131] Symptoms of pouchitis include increased stool frequency, pelvic and abdominal pain, rectal bleeding, tenesmus, fecal incontinence, and fever. Symptoms alone should not be used to make a diagnosis of pouchitis.[132] The differential diagnosis of pouchitis includes the irritable pouch, 'cuffitis,' Crohn's disease, and anatomical problems with the pouch, including strictures. The evaluation of the symptomatic pouch requires endoscopy, including assessment of the prepouch ileum, and biopsy.[133]

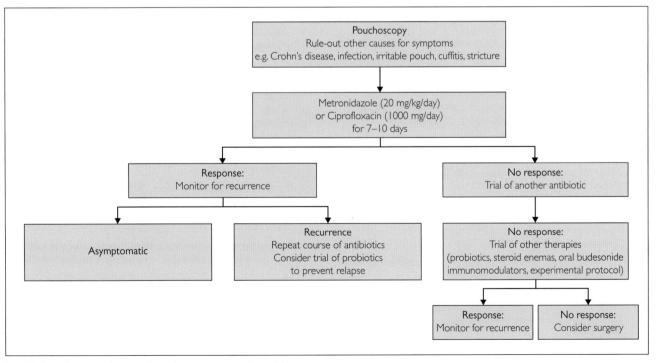

Fig. 57.6 • A suggested approach to the management of pouchitis.

The treatment of pouchitis involves the use of antibiotics. Metronidazole (20 mg/kg/day) and ciprofloxacin (1000 mg/day) are both effective, with the latter showing benefit over the former in one clinical trial.[134] Other treatments have included budesonide enemas[135] and probiotics, either to prevent relapses in patients with chronic pouchitis[136] or to prevent the first episode of pouchitis in patients after IPAA (Fig. 57.6).[137]

SUMMARY

The medical management of ulcerative colitis has not changed significantly in recent years. The biggest advance has been the development of the new generation aminosalicylates that allow for increased dosing with fewer side effects compared with sulfasalazine. There has also been a shift towards the earlier use of immunomodulators as maintenance therapy. Improvements in surgical techniques have led to this option being exercised more frequently in clinically indicated settings. Overall, the management of patients with ulcerative colitis requires an understanding of the disease process as well as a 'team' effort consisting of experienced gastroenterologists, nutritionists, radiologists, surgeons, and pathologists. Treatment algorithms must consider the extent of colonic involvement (Figs 57.3, 57.4, 57.5). It is anticipated that new biologic agents will be added to the treatment armamentarium during the next several years as scientists continue to unravel the pathobiology of this disorder.

REFERENCES

1. Fiocchi C. Inflammatory bowel disease: etiology and pathogenesis. Gastroenterology 1998; 115:182–205.

2. Podolsky DK. Inflammatory bowel disease. N Engl J Med 2002; 347:417–429.

3. Kornbluth A, Sachar DB. Ulcerative colitis practice guidelines in adults (update): American College of Gastroenterology, Practice Parameters Committee. Am J Gastroenterol 2004; 99:1371–1385.

4. Papachristou GI, Plevy S. Novel biologics in inflammatory bowel disease. Gastroenterol Clin North Am 2004; 33:251–269, ix.

5. Lim WC, Hanauer SB. Emerging biologic therapies in inflammatory bowel disease. Rev Gastroenterol Disord 2004; 4:66–85.

6. Hanauer SB. Medical therapy for ulcerative colitis 2004. Gastroenterology 2004; 126:1582–1592.

7. Bernstein CN. Extraintestinal manifestations of inflammatory bowel disease. Curr Gastroenterol Rep 2001; 3:477–483.

8. Danese S, Sans M, Fiocchi C. Inflammatory bowel disease: the role of environmental factors. Autoimmun Rev 2004; 3:394–400.

9. Loftus EV Jr. Clinical epidemiology of inflammatory bowel disease: Incidence, prevalence, and environmental influences. Gastroenterology 2004; 126:1504–1517.

10. Cosnes J. Tobacco and IBD: relevance in the understanding of disease mechanisms and clinical practice. Best Pract Res Clin Gastroenterol 2004; 18:481–496.

11. Logan RF, Edmond M, Somerville KW, et al. Smoking and ulcerative colitis. Br Med J (Clin Res Ed) 1984; 288:751–753.

12. Abraham N, Selby W, Lazarus R, et al. Is smoking an indirect risk factor for the development of ulcerative colitis? An age- and sex-matched case-control study. J Gastroenterol Hepatol 2003; 18:139–146.

13. Florin TH, Pandeya N, Radford-Smith GL. Epidemiology of appendicectomy in primary sclerosing cholangitis and ulcerative colitis: its influence on the clinical behaviour of these diseases. Gut 2004; 53:973–979.

14. Andersson RE, Olaison G, Tysk C, et al. Appendectomy and protection against ulcerative colitis. N Engl J Med 2001; 344:808–814.

15. Hart A, Kamm MA. Review article: mechanisms of initiation and perpetuation of gut inflammation by stress. Aliment Pharmacol Ther 2002; 16:2017–2028.

16. Quinton JF, Sendid B, Reumaux D, et al. Anti-*Saccharomyces cerevisiae mannan* antibodies combined with antineutrophil cytoplasmic autoantibodies in inflammatory bowel disease: prevalence and diagnostic role. Gut 1998; 42:788–791.

17. Sandborn WJ. Serologic markers in inflammatory bowel disease: state of the art. Rev Gastroenterol Disord 2004; 4:167–174.

18. Kuisma J, Jarvinen H, Kahri A, et al. Factors associated with disease activity of pouchitis after surgery for ulcerative colitis. Scand J Gastroenterol 2004; 39:544–548.

19. Klotz U. Clinical pharmacokinetics of sulphasalazine, its metabolites and other prodrugs of 5-aminosalicylic acid. Clin Pharmacokinet 1985; 10:285–302.

20. Das KM, Eastwood MA, McManus JP, et al. Adverse reactions during salicylazosulfapyridine therapy and the relation with drug metabolism and acetylator phenotype. N Engl J Med 1973; 289:491–495.

21. Wadelius M, Stjernberg E, Wiholm BE, et al. Polymorphisms of NAT2 in relation to sulphasalazine-induced agranulocytosis. Pharmacogenetics 2000; 10:35–41.

22. Tanigawara Y, Kita T, Aoyama N, et al. N-acetyltransferase 2 genotype-related sulfapyridine acetylation and its adverse events. Biol Pharm Bull 2002; 25:1058–1062.

23. Sharp ME, Wallace SM, Hindmarsh KW, et al. Acetylator phenotype and serum levels of sulfapyridine in patients with inflammatory bowel disease. Eur J Clin Pharmacol 1981; 21:243–250.

24. Das KM, Eastwood MA. Acetylation polymorphism of sulfapyridine in patients with ulcerative colitis and Crohn's disease. Clin Pharmacol Ther 1975; 18:514–520.

25. Das KM, Dubin R. Clinical pharmacokinetics of sulphasalazine. Clin Pharmacokinet 1976; 1:406–425.

26. Sutherland LR, May GR, Shaffer EA. Sulfasalazine revisited: a meta-analysis of 5-aminosalicylic acid in the treatment of ulcerative colitis. Ann Intern Med 1993; 118:540–549.

27. O'Morain C, Smethurst P, Dore CJ, et al. Reversible male infertility due to sulphasalazine: studies in man and rat. Gut 1984; 25:1078–1084.

28. Sninsky CA, Cort DH, Shanahan F, et al. Oral mesalamine (Asacol) for mildly to moderately active ulcerative colitis. A multicenter study. Ann Intern Med 1991; 115:350–355.

Randomized, blinded, placebo-controlled study showing efficacy of mesalamine in active UC.

29. The Mesalamine Study Group. An oral preparation of mesalamine as long-term maintenance therapy for ulcerative colitis. A randomized, placebo-controlled trial. Ann Intern Med 1996; 124:204–211.

Randomized, blinded, placebo-controlled study showing efficacy of mesalamine in the maintenance of remission in patients with UC.

30. Miner P, Hanauer S, Robinson M, et al. Safety and efficacy of controlled-release mesalamine for maintenance of remission in ulcerative colitis. Pentasa UC Maintenance Study Group. Dig Dis Sci 1995; 40:296–304.

31. Sutherland L, Roth D, Beck P, et al. Oral 5-aminosalicylic acid for maintenance of remission in ulcerative colitis. Cochrane Database Syst Rev 2002; CD000544.

32. Sutherland L, MacDonald JK. Oral 5-aminosalicylic acid for induction of remission in ulcerative colitis. Cochrane Database Syst Rev 2003; CD000543.

33. Ewe K, Eckardt V, Kanzler G. Treatment of ulcerative colitis with olsalazine and sulphasalazine: efficacy and side-effects. Scand J Gastroenterol Suppl 1988; 148:70–75.

34. Zinberg J, Molinas S, Das KM. Double-blind placebo-controlled study of olsalazine in the treatment of ulcerative colitis. Am J Gastroenterol 1990; 85:562–566.

35. Friedman LS, Richter JM, Kirkham SE, et al. 5-Aminosalicylic acid enemas in refractory distal ulcerative colitis: a randomized, controlled trial. Am J Gastroenterol 1986; 81:412–418.

36. Loftus EV Jr, Kane SV, Bjorkman D. Systematic review: short-term adverse effects of 5-aminosalicylic acid agents in the treatment of ulcerative colitis. Aliment Pharmacol Ther 2004; 19:179–189.

37. Kornbluth AA, Salomon P, Sacks HS, et al. Meta-analysis of the effectiveness of current drug therapy of ulcerative colitis. J Clin Gastroenterol 1993; 16:215–218.

38. Biddle WL, Greenberger NJ, Swan JT, et al. 5-Aminosalicylic acid enemas: effective agent in maintaining remission in left-sided ulcerative colitis. Gastroenterology 1988; 94:1075–1079.

39. Cobden I, al-Mardini H, Zaitoun A, et al. Is topical therapy necessary in acute distal colitis? Double-blind comparison of high-dose oral mesalazine versus steroid enemas in the treatment of active distal ulcerative colitis. Aliment Pharmacol Ther 1991; 5:513–522.

40. Safdi M, DeMicco M, Sninsky C, et al. A double-blind comparison of oral versus rectal mesalamine versus combination therapy in the treatment of distal ulcerative colitis. Am J Gastroenterol 1997; 92:1867–1871.

41. Katz JA. Treatment of inflammatory bowel disease with corticosteroids. Gastroenterol Clin North Am 2004; 33: 171–189, vii.

42. Meyers S, Sachar DB, Goldberg JD, et al. Corticotropin versus hydrocortisone in the intravenous treatment of ulcerative colitis. A prospective, randomized, double-blind clinical trial. Gastroenterology 1983; 85:351–357.

43. Kjeldsen J. Treatment of ulcerative colitis with high doses of oral prednisolone. The rate of remission, the need for surgery, and the effect of prolonging the treatment. Scand J Gastroenterol 1993; 28:821–826.

44. Marshall JK, Irvine EJ. Rectal corticosteroids versus alternative treatments in ulcerative colitis: a meta-analysis. Gut 1997; 40:775–781.

45. Bernstein CN, Leslie WD, Leboff MS. AGA technical review on osteoporosis in gastrointestinal diseases. Gastroenterology 2003; 124:795–841.

46. Faubion WA Jr, Loftus EV Jr, Harmsen WS, et al. The natural history of corticosteroid therapy for inflammatory bowel disease: a population-based study. Gastroenterology 2001; 121:255–260.

47. Jewell DP, Truelove SC. Azathioprine in ulcerative colitis: final report on controlled therapeutic trial. Br Med J 1974; 4:627–630.

48. Caprilli R, Carratu R, Babbini M. Double-blind comparison of the effectiveness of azathioprine and sulfasalazine in idiopathic proctocolitis. Preliminary report. Am J Dig Dis 1975; 20:115–120.

49. Tiede I, Fritz G, Strand S, et al. CD28-dependent Rac1 activation is the molecular target of azathioprine in primary human CD4+ T lymphocytes. J Clin Invest 2003; 111:1133–1145.

50. Sandborn WJ, Tremaine WJ, Wolf DC, et al. Lack of effect of intravenous administration on time to respond to azathioprine for steroid-treated Crohn's disease. North American Azathioprine Study Group. Gastroenterology 1999; 117:527–535.

51. Rosenberg JL, Wall AJ, Levin B, et al. A controlled trial of azathioprine in the management of chronic ulcerative colitis. Gastroenterology 1975; 69:96–99.

52. Geller SA, Dubinsky MC, Poordad FF, et al. Early hepatic nodular hyperplasia and submicroscopic fibrosis associated with 6-thioguanine therapy in inflammatory bowel disease. Am J Surg Pathol 2004; 28:1204–1211.

53. Lichtenstein GR. Use of laboratory testing to guide 6-mercaptopurine/azathioprine therapy. Gastroenterology 2004; 127:1558–1564.

54. Cuffari C, Dassopoulos T, Turnbough L, et al. Thiopurine methyltransferase activity influences clinical response to azathioprine in inflammatory bowel disease. Clin Gastroenterol Hepatol 2004; 2:410–417.

55. Warman JI, Korelitz BI, Fleisher MR, et al. Cumulative experience with short- and long-term toxicity to 6-mercaptopurine in the treatment of Crohn's disease and ulcerative colitis. J Clin Gastroenterol 2003; 37:220–225.

56. Fraser AG, Orchard TR, Robinson EM, et al. Long-term risk of malignancy after treatment of inflammatory bowel disease with azathioprine. Aliment Pharmacol Ther 2002; 16:1225–1232.

57. Lowry PW, Franklin CL, Weaver AL, et al. Leucopenia resulting from a drug interaction between azathioprine or 6-mercaptopurine and mesalamine, sulphasalazine, or balsalazide. Gut 2001; 49:656–664.

58. Mantzaris GJ, Sfakianakis M, Archavlis E, et al. A prospective randomized observer-blind 2-year trial of azathioprine monotherapy versus azathioprine and olsalazine for the maintenance of remission of steroid-dependent ulcerative colitis. Am J Gastroenterol 2004; 99:1122–1128.

59. Ardizzone S, Molteni P, Imbesi V, et al. Azathioprine in steroid-resistant and steroid-dependent ulcerative colitis. J Clin Gastroenterol 1997; 25:330–333.

60. Sandborn WJ. Azathioprine: state of the art in inflammatory bowel disease. Scand J Gastroenterol Suppl 1998; 225:92–99.

61. Fernandez-Banares F, Bertran X, Esteve-Comas M, et al. Azathioprine is useful in maintaining long-term remission induced by intravenous cyclosporine in steroid-refractory severe ulcerative colitis. Am J Gastroenterol 1996; 91:2498–2499.

62. Domenech E, Garcia-Planella E, Bernal I, et al. Azathioprine without oral cyclosporine in the long-term maintenance of remission induced by intravenous cyclosporine in severe, steroid-refractory ulcerative colitis. Aliment Pharmacol Ther 2002; 16:2061–2065.

63. Campbell S, Ghosh S. Combination immunomodulatory therapy with cyclosporine and azathioprine in corticosteroid-resistant severe ulcerative colitis: the Edinburgh experience of outcome. Dig Liver Dis 2003; 35:546–551.

64. Kirk AP, Lennard-Jones JE. Controlled trial of azathioprine in chronic ulcerative colitis. Br Med J (Clin Res Ed) 1982; 284:1291–1292.

    Important double-blind, placebo-controlled trial showing benefits of azathioprine in treating UC and reducing steroid use.

65. Lichtiger S, Present DH, Kornbluth A, et al. Cyclosporine in severe ulcerative colitis refractory to steroid therapy. N Engl J Med 1994; 330:1841–1845.

    Landmark study demonstrating benefit of cyclosporine in severe steroid-refractory UC subjects.

66. Van Assche G, D'Haens G, Noman M, et al. Randomized, double-blind comparison of 4 mg/kg versus 2 mg/kg intravenous cyclosporine in severe ulcerative colitis. Gastroenterology 2003; 125:1025–1031.

67. Evans RC, Clarke L, Heath P, et al. Treatment of ulcerative colitis with an engineered human anti-TNF alpha antibody CDP571. Aliment Pharmacol Ther 1997; 11:1031–1035.

68. Probert CS, Hearing SD, Schreiber S, et al. Infliximab in moderately severe glucocorticoid resistant ulcerative colitis: a randomised controlled trial. Gut 2003; 52:998–1002.

69. Gordon FH, Hamilton MI, Donoghue S, et al. A pilot study of treatment of active ulcerative colitis with natalizumab, a humanized monoclonal antibody to alpha-4 integrin. Aliment Pharmacol Ther 2002; 16:699–705.

70. Sawada K, Muto T, Shimoyama T, et al. Multicenter randomized controlled trial for the treatment of ulcerative colitis with a leukocytapheresis column. Curr Pharm Des 2003; 9:307–321.

71. Naganuma M, Funakoshi S, Sakuraba A, et al. Granulocytapheresis is useful as an alternative therapy in patients with steroid-refractory or -dependent ulcerative colitis. Inflamm Bowel Dis 2004; 10:251–257.

72. Creed TJ, Norman MR, Probert CS, et al. Basiliximab (anti-CD25) in combination with steroids may be an effective new treatment for steroid-resistant ulcerative colitis. Aliment Pharmacol Ther 2003; 18:65–75.

73. Murthy S, Flanigan A, Coppola D, et al. RDP58, a locally active TNF inhibitor, is effective in the dextran sulphate mouse model of chronic colitis. Inflamm Res 2002; 51:522–531.

74. Iyer S, Lahana R, Buelow R. Rational design and development of RDP58. Curr Pharm Des 2002; 8:2217–2229.

75. Pullan RD, Rhodes J, Ganesh S, et al. Transdermal nicotine for active ulcerative colitis. N Engl J Med 1994; 330:811–815.

   Randomized, placebo-controlled study that showed a role for transdermal nicotine as an adjunct therapy in inducing remission in patients with UC.

76. Guslandi M, Tittobello A. Outcome of ulcerative colitis after treatment with transdermal nicotine. Eur J Gastroenterol Hepatol 1998; 10:513–515.

77. Thomas GA, Rhodes J, Ragunath K, et al. Transdermal nicotine compared with oral prednisolone therapy for active ulcerative colitis. Eur J Gastroenterol Hepatol 1996; 8:769–776.

78. McGrath J, McDonald J, Macdonald J. Transdermal nicotine for induction of remission in ulcerative colitis. Cochrane Database Syst Rev. 2004; CD004722.

79. Thomas GA. Rhodes J, Mani V, et al. Transdermal nicotine as maintenance therapy for ulcerative colitis. N Engl J Med 1995; 332:988–992.

80. Turunen UM, Farkkila MA, Hakala K, et al. Long-term treatment of ulcerative colitis with ciprofloxacin: a prospective, double-blind, placebo-controlled study. Gastroenterology 1998; 115:1072–1078.

81. Mantzaris GJ, Archavlis E, Christoforidis P, et al. A prospective randomized controlled trial of oral ciprofloxacin in acute ulcerative colitis. Am J Gastroenterol 1997; 92:454–456.

82. Mantzaris GJ, Hatzis A, Kontogiannis P, et al. Intravenous tobramycin and metronidazole as an adjunct to corticosteroids in acute, severe ulcerative colitis. Am J Gastroenterol 1994; 89:43–46.

83. Oren R, Arber N, Odes S, et al. Methotrexate in chronic active ulcerative colitis: a double-blind, randomized, Israeli multicenter trial. Gastroenterology 1996; 110:1416–1421.

   Important study that showed that methotrexate therapy is not effective in the treatment of patients with UC.

84. Mate-Jimenez J, Hermida C, Cantero-Perona J, et al. 6-mercaptopurine or methotrexate added to prednisone induces and maintains remission in steroid-dependent inflammatory bowel disease. Eur J Gastroenterol Hepatol 2000; 12:1227–1233.

85. Ang YS, Mahmud N, White B, et al. Randomized comparison of unfractionated heparin with corticosteroids in severe active inflammatory bowel disease. Aliment Pharmacol Ther 2000; 14:1015–1022.

86. Panes J, Esteve M, Cabre E, et al. Comparison of heparin and steroids in the treatment of moderate and severe ulcerative colitis. Gastroenterology 2000; 119:903–908.

87. Kruis W, Fric P, Pokrotnieks J, et al. Maintaining remission of ulcerative colitis with the probiotic Escherichia coli Nissle 1917 is as effective as with standard mesalazine. Gut 2004; 53:1617–1623.

88. Brown J, Haines S, Wilding IR. Colonic spread of three rectally administered mesalazine (Pentasa) dosage forms in healthy volunteers as assessed by gamma scintigraphy. Aliment Pharmacol Ther 1997; 11:685–691.

89. Gionchetti P, Rizzello F, Venturi A, et al. Comparison of mesalazine suppositories in proctitis and distal proctosigmoiditis. Aliment Pharmacol Ther 1997; 11:1053–1057.

90. Campieri M, Paoluzi P, D'Albasio G, et al. Better quality of therapy with 5-ASA colonic foam in active ulcerative colitis. A multicenter comparative trial with 5-ASA enema. Dig Dis Sci 1993; 38:1843–1850.

91. d'Albasio G, Trallori G, Ghetti A, et al. Intermittent therapy with high-dose 5-aminosalicylic acid enemas for maintaining remission in ulcerative proctosigmoiditis. Dis Colon Rectum 1990; 33:394–397.

92. Campieri M, Corbelli C, Gionchetti P, et al. Spread and distribution of 5-ASA colonic foam and 5-ASA enema in patients with ulcerative colitis. Dig Dis Sci 1992; 37:1890–1897.

93. Farup PG, Hovde O, Halvorsen FA, et al. Mesalazine suppositories versus hydrocortisone foam in patients with distal ulcerative colitis. A comparison of the efficacy and practicality of two topical treatment regimens. Scand J Gastroenterol 1995; 30:164–170.

94. Porro GB, Ardizzone S, Petrillo M, et al. Low Pentasa dosage versus hydrocortisone in the topical treatment of active ulcerative colitis: a randomized, double-blind study. Am J Gastroenterol 1995; 90:736–739.

95. Danielsson A, Lofberg R, Persson T, et al. A steroid enema, budesonide, lacking systemic effects for the treatment of distal ulcerative colitis or proctitis. Scand J Gastroenterol 1992; 27:9–12.

96. Lofberg R, Ostergaard Thomsen O, Langholz E, et al. Budesonide versus prednisolone retention enemas in active distal ulcerative colitis. Aliment Pharmacol Ther 1994; 8:623–629.

97. Gionchetti P, Rizzello F, Venturi A, et al. Comparison of oral with rectal mesalazine in the treatment of ulcerative proctitis. Dis Colon Rectum 1998; 41:93–97.

98. Hanauer S, Good LI, Goodman MW, et al. Long-term use of mesalamine (Rowasa) suppositories in remission maintenance of ulcerative proctitis. Am J Gastroenterol 2000; 95:1749–1754.

99. Pokrotnieks J, Marlicz K, Paradowski L, et al. Efficacy and tolerability of mesalazine foam enema (Salofalk foam) for distal ulcerative colitis: a double-blind, randomized, placebo-controlled study. Aliment Pharmacol Ther 2000; 14:1191–1198.

100. Hanauer SB. Dose-ranging study of mesalamine (Pentasa) enemas in the treatment of acute ulcerative proctosigmoiditis: results of a multicentered placebo-controlled trial. The U.S. Pentasa Enema Study Group. Inflamm Bowel Dis 1998; 4:79–83.

101. Frieri G, Pimpo MT, Palumbo GC, et al. Rectal and colonic mesalazine concentration in ulcerative colitis: oral vs. oral plus topical treatment. Aliment Pharmacol Ther 1999; 13:1413–1417.

102. d'Albasio G, Pacini F, Camarri E, et al. Combined therapy with 5-aminosalicylic acid tablets and enemas for maintaining remission in ulcerative colitis: a randomized double-blind study. Am J Gastroenterol 1997; 92:1143–1147.

   An important study showing the importance of combining oral and topical (enema) therapy in the treatment of patients with UC.

103. Vecchi M, Meucci G, Gionchetti P, et al. Oral versus combination mesalazine therapy in active ulcerative colitis: a double-blind, double-dummy, randomized multicentre study. Aliment Pharmacol Ther 2001; 15:251–256.

104. Bansky G, Buhler H, Stamm B, et al. Treatment of distal ulcerative colitis with beclomethasone enemas: high therapeutic efficacy without endocrine side effects. A prospective, randomized, double-blind trial. Dis Colon Rectum 1987; 30:288–292.

105. Danish 5-ASA Group. Topical 5-aminosalicylic acid versus prednisolone in ulcerative proctosigmoiditis. A randomized, double-blind multicenter trial. Dig Dis Sci 1987; 32:598–602.

106. Mulder CJ, Tytgat GN, Wiltink EH, et al. Comparison of 5-aminosalicylic acid (3 g) and prednisolone phosphate sodium enemas (30 mg) in the treatment of distal ulcerative colitis. A prospective, randomized, double-blind trial. Scand J Gastroenterol 1988; 23:1005–1008.

107. Lashner BA, Heidenreich PA, Su GL, et al. Effect of folate supplementation on the incidence of dysplasia and cancer in chronic ulcerative colitis. A case-control study. Gastroenterology 1989; 97:255–259.

108. Lashner BA, Provencher KS, Seidner DL, et al. The effect of folic acid supplementation on the risk for cancer or dysplasia in ulcerative colitis. Gastroenterology 1997; 112:29–32.

109. Lofberg R, Danielsson A, Suhr O, et al. Oral budesonide versus prednisolone in patients with active extensive and left-sided ulcerative colitis. Gastroenterology 1996; 110:1713–1718.

110. Han PD, Burke A, Baldassano RN, et al. Nutrition and inflammatory bowel disease. Gastroenterol Clin North Am 1999; 28:423–443, ix.

111. Meyers S, Lerer PK, Feuer EJ, et al. Predicting the outcome of corticoid therapy for acute ulcerative colitis. Results of a prospective, randomized, double-blind clinical trial. J Clin Gastroenterol 1987; 9:50–54.

112. D'Haens G, Lemmens L, Geboes K, et al. Intravenous cyclosporine versus intravenous corticosteroids as single therapy for severe attacks of ulcerative colitis. Gastroenterology 2001; 120:1323–1329.

113. Shibolet O, Regushevskaya E, Brezis M, et al. Cyclosporine A for induction of remission in severe ulcerative colitis. Cochrane Database Syst Rev 2005; (1): CD004277.

114. Skelly MM, Logan RF, Jenkins D, et al. Toxicity of mycophenolate mofetil in patients with inflammatory bowel disease. Inflamm Bowel Dis 2002; 8:93–97.

115. Sood A, Kaushal V, Midha V, et al. The beneficial effect of azathioprine on maintenance of remission in severe ulcerative colitis. J Gastroenterol 2002; 37:270–274.

116. Kornbluth A, Present DH, Lichtiger S, et al. Cyclosporine for severe ulcerative colitis: a user's guide. Am J Gastroenterol 1997; 92:1424–1428.

117. Gan SI, Beck PL. A new look at toxic megacolon: an update and review of incidence, etiology, pathogenesis, and management. Am J Gastroenterol 2003; 98:2363–2371.

Excellent recent review of the diagnosis and management of toxic megacolon.

118. Larson DW, Pemberton JH. Current concepts and controversies in surgery for IBD. Gastroenterology 2004; 126:1611–1619.

119. Steinlauf AF, Present DH. Medical management of the pregnant patient with inflammatory bowel disease. Gastroenterol Clin North Am 2004; 33:361–385, xi.

120. Moskovitz DN, Bodian C, Chapman ML, et al. The effect on the fetus of medications used to treat pregnant inflammatory bowel-disease patients. Am J Gastroenterol 2004; 99:656–661.

121. Diav-Citrin O, Park YH, Veerasuntharam G, et al. The safety of mesalamine in human pregnancy: a prospective controlled cohort study. Gastroenterology 1998; 114:23–28.

122. Marteau P, Tennenbaum R, Elefant E, et al. Foetal outcome in women with inflammatory bowel disease treated during pregnancy with oral mesalazine microgranules. Aliment Pharmacol Ther 1998; 12:1101–1108.

123. Norgard B, Fonager K, Pedersen L, et al. Birth outcome in women exposed to 5-aminosalicylic acid during pregnancy: a Danish cohort study. Gut 2003; 52:243–247.

124. Francella A, Dyan A, Bodian C, et al. The safety of 6-mercaptopurine for childbearing patients with inflammatory bowel disease: a retrospective cohort study. Gastroenterology 2003; 124:9–17.

125. Dubinsky MC. Azathioprine, 6-mercaptopurine in inflammatory bowel disease: pharmacology, efficacy, and safety. Clin Gastroenterol Hepatol 2004; 2:731–743.

126. Olsen KO, Juul S, Bulow S, et al. Female fecundity before and after operation for familial adenomatous polyposis. Br J Surg 2003; 90:227–231.

This study demonstrated that ileal pouch-anal anastomosis surgery can have important negative effects on female fecundity.

127. Rutter M, Saunders B, Wilkinson K, et al. Severity of inflammation is a risk factor for colorectal neoplasia in ulcerative colitis. Gastroenterology 2004; 126:451–459.

128. Itzkowitz SH, Harpaz N. Diagnosis and management of dysplasia in patients with inflammatory bowel diseases. Gastroenterology 2004; 126:1634–1648.

129. Odze RD, Farraye FA, Hecht JL, et al. Long-term follow-up after polypectomy treatment for adenoma-like dysplastic lesions in ulcerative colitis. Clin Gastroenterol Hepatol 2004; 2:534–541.

A long-term study that demonstrated that UC patients who develop an adenoma-like DALM may be treated adequately by polypectomy with complete excision and continued endoscopic surveillance.

130. Sandborn WJ, Pardi DS. Clinical management of pouchitis. Gastroenterology 2004; 127:1809–1814.

Excellent recent review on the management of pouchitis.

131. Sandborn WJ. Pouchitis following ileal pouch-anal anastomosis: definition, pathogenesis, and treatment. Gastroenterology 1994; 107:1856–1860.

132. Shen B, Achkar JP, Lashner BA, et al. Endoscopic and histologic evaluation together with symptom assessment are required to diagnose pouchitis. Gastroenterology 2001; 121:261–267.

133. Shen B, Shermock KM, Fazio VW, et al. A cost-effectiveness analysis of diagnostic strategies for symptomatic patients with ileal pouch-anal anastomosis. Am J Gastroenterol 2003; 98:2460–2467.

134. Shen B, Achkar JP, Lashner BA, et al. A randomized clinical trial of ciprofloxacin and metronidazole to treat acute pouchitis. Inflamm Bowel Dis 2001; 7:301–305.

135. Sambuelli A, Boerr L, Negreira S, et al. Budesonide enema in pouchitis – double-blind, double-dummy, controlled trial. Aliment Pharmacol Ther 2002; 16:27–34.

136. Gionchetti P, Rizzello F, Venturi A, et al. Oral bacteriotherapy as maintenance treatment in patients with chronic pouchitis: a double-blind, placebo-controlled trial. Gastroenterology 2000; 119:305–309.

137. Gionchetti P, Rizzello F, Helwig U, et al. Prophylaxis of pouchitis onset with probiotic therapy: a double-blind, placebo-controlled trial. Gastroenterology 2003; 124:1202–1209.

CHAPTER FIFTY-EIGHT

58

Intestinal obstruction

Sareh Parangi and Richard Hodin

MECHANICAL OBSTRUCTION OF THE INTESTINE

Introduction

Definitions: Intestinal obstruction is one of the most common disorders seen by both gastroenterologists and surgeons, and a thorough knowledge of this disorder is important for virtually all physicians. This chapter will review the definition of mechanical obstruction of the intestine, the clinical presentations, the proper evaluation of the patient, and the therapeutic considerations. *Obstruction of the intestine* occurs when there is impairment in the normal flow of luminal contents due to an extrinsic or intrinsic encroachment on the intestinal lumen. A *complete obstruction* is present if there is no passage of intestinal contents beyond the point of obstruction, whereas a *partial obstruction* means some passage of intraluminal contents is occurring distal to the obstruction. An obstruction is described as a *simple obstruction* if only one point of obstruction is seen, whereas in a *closed-loop obstruction* two sites of luminal obstruction exist. *Strangulated obstruction* occurs when the blood flow to the intestine is compromised causing ischemic necrosis of the gut. This is often seen with closed-loop obstructions but can also be present with simple complete obstructions, especially as a late event. *Intestinal pseudo-obstruction* is used to describe a functional obstruction with no mechanical or anatomic cause, such as Ogilvie's syndrome in which colonic pseudo-obstruction is present. *Adynamic ileus* refers to impaired passage of luminal contents due to disordered or absent motility. Both pseudo-obstruction and ileus can mimic a mechanical obstruction. Adynamic ileus usually leads to distended loops of small and large bowel, but vascular compromise of the intestine almost never occurs.

The key to the management of patients with small intestinal obstruction is early diagnosis so that proper therapy can be instituted. Identification of those patients with strangulation is of critical importance since prompt surgical correction is needed in order to minimize morbidity and mortality. Numerous clinical and radiological criteria can be helpful in distinguishing simple from strangulating obstruction, but this differentiation remains a challenge to even the most experienced clinicians (Fig 58.1).

Etiology: Hippocrates describes the entity of small bowel obstruction and early treatment included observation, reduction of hernias when applicable, narcotics for pain, and even the use of mercury or lead ingestion to 'open' areas of occluded small intestine. Praxagoras in 350 BC performed the first operative intervention for a small bowel obstruction by creating an enterocutaneous fistula to relieve the obstruction.[1] In 1912, Hartwell and Hoguet first described the aggressive use of normal saline administration to prolong the life of animals with mechanical obstruction, and to this day fluid resuscitation remains a cornerstone of treatment in every patient with intestinal obstruction.[2] Common causes of intestinal obstruction include adhesive bands, hernias, malignant neoplasms (most commonly colonic or ovarian), inflammatory bowel disease, ischemic strictures, diverticulitis, radiation-related strictures, intussusception, gallstones, bezoars, as well as foreign bodies. Small intestinal obstruction has a variety of etiologies that differ markedly as a function of age (Table 58.1). For example, in the neonate, congenital anomalies such as atresia, malrotation of the midgut with volvulus, duodenal atresia, and imperforate anus are common causes of obstruction, whereas infants are more likely to have strangulated hernias or intussusception. Over 90% of pediatric intussusceptions are idiopathic with no lead-point cause and most present before the first year of age. Males are more likely to be affected. Meconium ileus also accounts for over 30% of all neonatal small bowel obstructions and can be seen in 7–25% of neonates with cystic fibrosis

In contrast, small intestinal obstruction in adults is primarily due to either adhesive bands or groin hernias, whereas large bowel obstruction occurs in the settings of diverticulitis, cancer, or volvulus. Although strangulated hernias were the most common cause of small bowel obstruction in the past, more recent series indicate that adhesive bands are now far more likely to be the etiology. In 1900, Gibson reviewed the reports of 1000 patients with intestinal obstruction and found that 35% were on the basis of strangulated hernias, whereas only about 19% were caused by bands.[3] Similarly, Vick reviewed 6892 patients from Great Britain with acute obstruction between 1925 and 1930 and found that approximately 50% were due to strangulated hernias, whereas adhesions accounted for only 7% of the cases.[4] The increase in elective inguinal hernia repairs coupled with an increase in the number of laparotomies performed in recent decades likely account for a change in etiology of obstruction over time. In 1955, Wangensteen reviewed 1252 cases of obstruction and found only 10% to be due to hernias, compared with 37% due to adhesions.[5] Certain surgical procedures appear more likely to cause a future obstruction due to an adhesive band or matted intestine. Prior colorectal procedures account for one-third of all

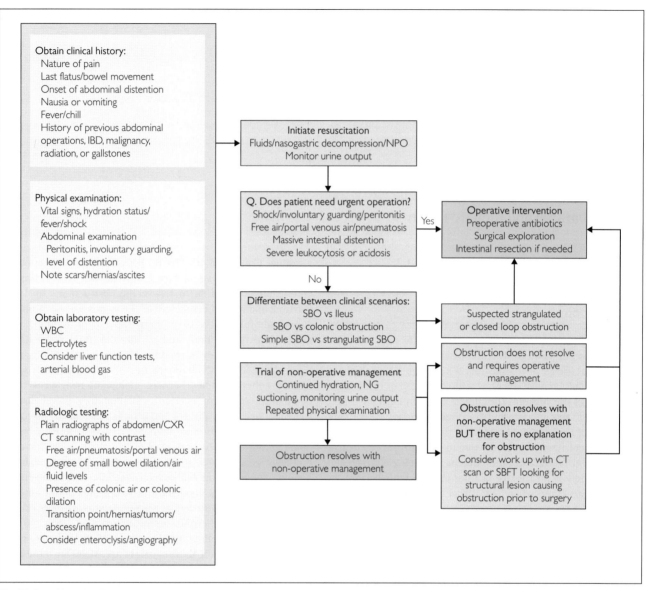

Fig. 58.1 • Algorithm for evaluating the patient with bowel obstruction.

patients who later present with small bowel obstruction.[6] In fact, the risk of an adhesion related small bowel obstruction appears to be around 10% within 1 year of colorectal surgery, and can increase to approximately 30% at 10 years.[7] Other previous operations that are the causative agent of future obstructions are: gynecologic procedures (22%), appendectomy (14%), and hernia repair (10%).[8] Cholecystectomy and foregut surgery appear to be

responsible only for a minority of subsequent small bowel obstructions. Positive trauma laparotomies, especially those from penetrating injuries or those with gross spillage of intestinal contents, also appear to be at high risk for future intestinal obstruction. Of patients diagnosed with an initial presentation of adhesion-related bowel obstruction, 5% present within the first month of the operation, 23% between the first month and the

Table 58.1 Common causes of mechanical bowel obstruction as a function of age			
Neonate	**Infant**	**Young adult**	**Middle age/elderly**
Atresia	Inguinal hernia	Adhesions	Adhesions
Midgut volvulus	Intussusception	Groin hernia	Groin hernia
Meconium ileus	Meckel's diverticulum		Colon cancer
Imperforate anus			Diverticulitis
			Sigmoid volvulus

first year, and approximately 11–12% between the first and fifth year, 11% between the fifth and tenth years, and 12% between the tenth and twentieth year. Fourteen percent of patients present with a bowel obstruction more than 20 years after the initial abdominal operation. The etiology for obstruction also differs geographically, such that large and even small bowel volvulus is relatively common in certain African countries, and less developed countries generally have higher incidences of strangulated hernias.[9]

Pathophysiology of obstruction: In the setting of obstruction, the normal absorptive mechanisms of the small bowel are deranged, such that excess fluid losses occur. Initially, there is vomitus, bowel wall edema, and transudative loss into the peritoneal cavity, but during the late stages of obstruction, venous pressure increases with resultant hemorrhage into the lumen, worsening the problem with hypovolemia. Both small bowel and colonic obstruction result in marked changes in motility, with increased contractions in segments proximal to the obstruction, and decreased motility in segments distal to the obstruction.[10] Swallowed gas and increased intraluminal fluid contents due to both decreased absorptive capacity of the intestine and increased secretion result in increased intraluminal pressure. Increased intraluminal pressure in late complete obstruction or closed-loop obstructions can lead to ischemic necrosis of the mucosa due to its high metabolic needs. Ischemia of the intestine initially leads to a loss in the protective barrier function of the mucosa, but over time there can be necrosis of all layers of the intestinal wall with resultant perforation. In some cases there is a direct compromise to the circulation of the segment of intestine, such as with compression of vessels through a tight hernial ring.

The normal relatively sterile environment of the proximal small intestine is altered under obstructed conditions such that bacterial overgrowth occurs, most notably involving the anaerobes such as *Bacteroides*.[11] The feculant vomiting seen in cases of longstanding distal small bowel obstruction is due to this bacterial overgrowth and is virtually pathognomonic for a high-grade or complete distal mechanical small bowel obstruction. The importance of bacterial overgrowth in the morbidity and mortality of intestinal obstruction has been demonstrated in experimental animals, e.g., germ-free dogs survive intestinal strangulation better than controls.[12] As such, antibiotics may be of benefit in the setting of strangulation, although there is probably no role for antibiotics in patients with simple mechanical bowel obstruction.

Clinical history and presentation

The diagnosis of intestinal obstruction is usually made on clinical grounds with the symptoms of crampy abdominal pain, decreased or absent flatus and stool, nausea and/or vomiting, and signs of abdominal distention on exam. A thorough history should be taken, including the onset and the duration of the current episode of abdominal pain, the last known time flatus and/or stool was passed, when vomiting started, when abdominal distention was noted, the presence of fever or chills, and whether the patient has had similar episodes in the past. The past history should be noted for previous abdominal operations, previous obstructive episodes, inflammatory bowel disease, known gallstone or diverticular disease, known hernias, previous abdominal malignancies, or a history of abdominal irradiation. A history of recent travel or ingestion of a foreign body should be also sought. A prior history of small bowel obstruction is particularly important since

patients with mechanical small bowel obstruction due to adhesions often will experience recurrences of the problem.

The pain described in 85–90% of patients is vague, colicky, and poorly localized; and is due to visceral distention of the intestine as it contracts against a mechanical obstruction. Partial obstructions can lead to intermittent crampy pain, especially soon after meals, but with complete obstruction the crampy pain tends to be more severe. Nausea and vomiting are common features of small bowel obstruction. Reflex vomiting is common and in cases of early or distal obstructions the volume of the vomitus will be quite small, since it takes some time for intestinal contents to back up to the stomach. The vomitus often contains occult blood and appears as 'coffee grounds' in color, probably due to distention of the stomach with resultant mucosal hemorrhage. Evaluation of such patients for gastrointestinal bleeding will not be fruitful and will delay the diagnosis and treatment of the true problem of the mechanical obstruction. The level of the obstruction is often suggested based upon the pattern of the pain, since proximal small bowel obstruction usually causes more frequent cramps, perhaps every 3–5 minutes, whereas more distal small bowel and large bowel obstructions cause less severe cramps with longer durations between episodes. Constant pain, especially if localized, or a history of fever, chills, rigors, or worsening mental status often suggests ischemia and infarction, and patients with these findings in their history should be taken for urgent laparotomy to avoid the mortality that can be as high as 30%.

Physical examination

The patient will often display signs of dehydration with dry mouth and loss of skin turgor. Vomitus can be malodorous and feculent, especially after a few hours of a complete obstruction given overgrowth of both anaerobic and Gram-negative bacteria.[11] The waves of abdominal pain, or colic, can actually be witnessed at the bedside and provide the strongest possible indication of a mechanically obstructed intestine. Occasionally, audible bowels sounds, or borborygmi, are present as a result of strong intestinal muscular contractions. Bowel sounds can be hyperactive during the initial phases of the obstruction, whereas later on the bowel becomes more dilated and bowel sounds can be diminished or even absent. Inspection of the abdomen will usually reveal distention, although the magnitude of distention will be greater with more distal and/or long-standing obstructions. Patients with large bowel obstruction will be especially distended on physical examination due to the large capacity of the colon, whereas proximal jejunal obstruction is generally associated with minimal distention. The presence of surgical scars should be noted, indicating the possibility of intra-abdominal adhesions as the etiology. The abdomen should be carefully and gently palpated from the costal margins to the groins. Any ascites or hepatomegaly should be noted since these can be signs of a malignancy. An abdominal wall hernia might also be evident as the site of the obstruction and common sites of herniation, such as the inguinal and femoral canals, and umbilicus should be palpated carefully since even moderate obesity coupled with distention can make the examination difficult. When hernia contents are soft and easily reducible in the obstructed patient, it is likely that an etiology other than the hernia exists. Any pre-existing hernia will tend to protrude in a patient who develops a bowel obstruction (Fig. 58.2). Tenderness, erythema, or induration in the abdominal wall at the site of a hernia usually indicates ischemia in an incarcerated loop of

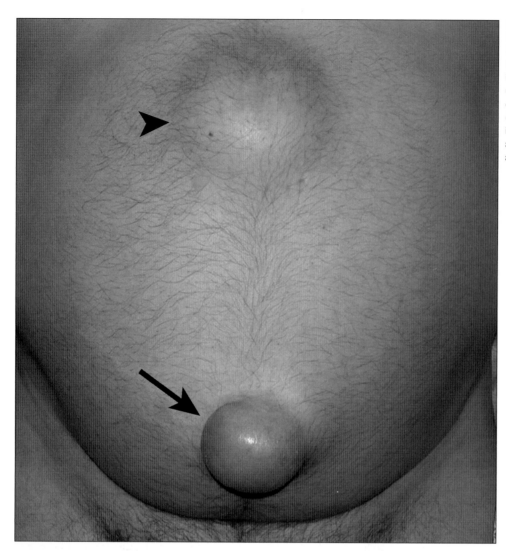

Fig. 58.2 • A distended abdomen is seen in this patient with small bowel obstruction. Patients should be examined carefully to look for incarcerated hernias. An incarcerated umbilical hernia is seen with characteristic changes in skin color (black arrow). A subxiphoid hernia is also more prominent (black arrowhead), given the massive abdominal distention.

bowel but can also denote active inflammatory bowel disease. Although mild, diffuse tenderness is a common feature in patients with distention from a mechanical obstruction, involuntary guarding or other signs of peritoneal irritation are unusual and suggest the possibility of ischemia or infarction of the bowel, perhaps even with perforation. Rectal examination is important in order to detect mass lesions and to check for the presence of stool that is usually absent in cases of mechanical bowel obstruction, especially of long-standing nature. It is important to remember that while the majority of patients are able to provide a thorough history that will aid in establishing a rapid diagnosis, some patients are unable to provide a good history, especially elderly patients who present in a delayed fashion with significant dehydration, tachycardia, oliguria, azotemia, hemoconcentration, increased abdominal compartment pressures, and even shock. The use of repeated physical examinations are essential to detect any changes such as fever, hypotension, or peritoneal signs, findings that should alert the physician to the need for rapid intervention.

Laboratory tests

Laboratory tests are not very helpful in the diagnosis and/or management of patients with bowel obstruction, with most abnormalities being neither sensitive nor specific and often developing late in the course of the obstruction.[13] In partial obstructions or early complete obstructions blood testing is usually normal. Routine blood counts will reveal an elevated hematocrit indicative of intravascular volume depletion. Leukocytosis is sometimes present, but is often the result of hemoconcentration and an acute stress response, rather than actual underlying infection. A markedly elevated white blood cell count (>18 000) should raise the suspicion for strangulation; however, it must be kept in mind that one-third of patients with strangulated small bowel obstructions have white blood cell counts between 10 000 and 14 000. The blood chemistries may reveal elevated blood urea nitrogen and creatinine, indicating hypovolemia with prerenal azotemia. In cases of suspected strangulation and vascular compromise, arterial blood gas measurements are used to evaluate for acidosis. Hyperkalemia can also be a sign of bowel necrosis. Mild elevations in serum levels of pancreatic enzymes such as amylase can be a sign of intestinal perforation or pancreatitis, although these may also be seen with simple obstructions.

Radiologic evaluation

In bowel obstruction radiologic imaging is used for several purposes: to confirm the diagnosis, to help distinguish between simple and strangulating obstructions, to differentiate the various causes of obstruction, to differentiate small and large bowel obstruction, to estimate the degree of obstruction, and to help exclude paralytic ileus. An upright chest radiograph might show free air under the diaphragm, pneumonia, or demonstrate compromised cardiopulmonary status. Plain radiography of the abdomen continues to be used since it is readily available, quick, and is quite sensitive for high-grade or complete obstructions, particularly in cases of a distal obstruction. Supine and upright radiographs should be obtained, but if an upright cannot be obtained then a left lateral decubitus film with the right side up

will allow delineation of both air-fluid levels and free air against the liver. Small bowel loops can be distinguished from colonic loops as the markings of the valvulae conniventes stretch across the entire lumen of the small bowel. Twenty-one percent of patients with suspected small bowel obstruction are in fact obstructed. Overall, the sensitivity and specificity of plain X-rays of the abdomen in obstruction is approximately 65% and 57%, respectively (Fig. 58.3A).[14] Of those patients with non-specific abdominal radiographs, 9% have high-grade obstruction (Fig. 58.4A).[15,16] Small bowel obstruction will lead to dilation of the

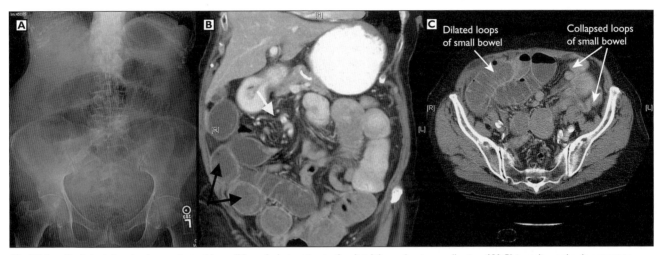

Fig. 58.3 • Radiologic imaging in a patient with small bowel obstruction in the distal ileum due to an adhesion. **(A)** Plain radiographs demonstrate distended loops of small intestine, and no air in the colon. **(B)** Reformatted coronal CT images reveal distended loops of small bowel in the right abdomen (black arrows) with bowel wall edema, and mesenteric swirling and edema (white arrow). **(C)** Standard axial CT images reveal distended loops of small bowel in the right abdomen and collapsed loops of small bowel with no contrast in the left abdomen.

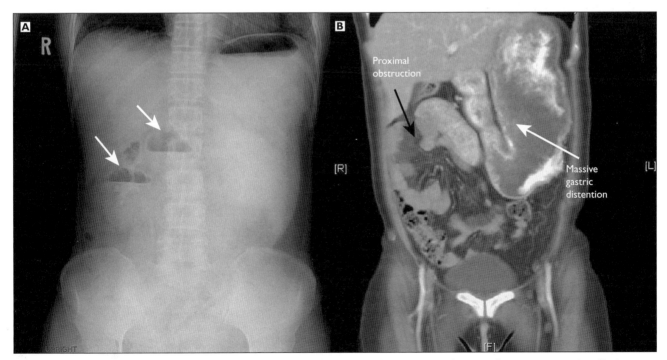

Fig. 58.4 • Radiologic imaging in a patient with proximal small bowel obstruction and massive gastric distention due to a postoperative adhesion. **(A)** Plain radiographs can be deceivingly non-specific in proximal obstruction, revealing only a few air-fluid levels in the right upper quadrant (white arrows). **(B)** Reformatted coronal CT images show a very proximal obstruction (black arrow) with massive gastric distention (white arrow), and edema of the small bowel mesentery.

small bowel with air-fluid levels and a stepladder appearance on an upright film. Although differential air-fluid levels, i.e., air-fluid levels at different heights in the same loop of bowel, have been considered an important finding suggestive of a mechanical obstruction, Harlow et al.[17] found this sign to be very insensitive, since it was present in only 52% of patients with proven mechanical obstruction. In addition, 29% of patients with adynamic ileus had this finding on plain radiographs. In small bowel obstruction of long-standing nature, perhaps greater than 24 hours, all of the air and stool from the colon will have been evacuated and this will be evident on plain abdominal films. However, if the obstruction is in its early phase, or if it is only partial, then some air and stool will be present within the colon, making distinction between an early complete and a partial small bowel obstruction very difficult. In *adynamic ileus* there are dilated loops of small bowel as well as colon, with overall less dilation of the small intestine compared to the colon. *Sentinel loops* of moderately dilated small bowel with impaired motility can be seen adjacent to areas of acute inflammation such as is seen in acute pancreatitis. In cases of acute colonic obstruction (especially with a competent ileocecal valve which does not allow any backward decompression into the distal ileum) the entire colon up to point of obstruction may be massively dilated with haustrae seen as incomplete indentations in the colonic wall. The dilation is often worse in the cecum due to Laplace's law that dictates that the wall tension will be greatest in the area with the largest radius. In advanced cases of strangulation, edematous small bowel can take on a thumbprinted appearance, and air may be seen in the wall of the intestine, portal venous system, or free in the abdominal cavity. Any of these findings on a plain upright X-ray almost always indicates the need for urgent operation.

Abdominal CT scans with intravenous contrast are employed increasingly to evaluate patients with suspected bowel obstruction in whom the plain radiograph alone does not provide a full answer. The CT scan can provide useful information, clearly identifying the dilated proximal and collapsed distal bowel, a feature that is aided by the administration of an oral contrast agent.[18] CT scan of the abdomen usually enables one to confirm the diagnosis of bowel obstruction, often demonstrates its cause, and helps differentiate between small and large bowel obstruction. This modality may be especially helpful in identifying closed-loop obstruction before the onset of strangulation.[19] Bowel obstruction is considered to be present when distended loops of bowel are seen proximal to collapsed loops. When a point of transition from dilated to normal bowel caliber is seen without apparent cause, adhesions are the presumed cause (see Fig. 58.3). Frager et al.[20] compared standard clinical evaluation, including plain radiographs, with CT scans in 90 cases of suspected small bowel obstruction. The correct diagnosis of complete obstruction was made in only 46% of patients by clinical, plain radiographic findings, whereas CT scan was found to be 100% sensitive in these cases (see Fig. 58.4). CT scan was also superior in cases of partial small bowel obstruction. However, false-positive CT scans were obtained in six cases, suggesting that the CT scan criteria for small bowel obstruction may have been too broad. Based upon these and other series in the literature,[15,16] CT scan has replaced the contrast small bowel follow-through in many centers as the primary radiologic tool in cases of suspected mechanical small bowel obstruction. In general, CT scans appear to be better at distinguishing closed-loop obstructions and strangulation and appear to be helpful in demonstrating causative agents such as hernias, tumors, abscesses, and inflammatory diseases (Fig. 58.5). There are similar advantages of CT scan in cases of large bowel obstruction, where tumor masses and pericolic inflammatory changes can be identified. Angiography may be helpful in cases of suspected mesenteric ischemia, especially if the findings on CT angiography are inconclusive or if a therapeutic angiographic intervention is planned.

Enteroclysis is performed by instilling a dilute barium contrast material directly past the pylorus using a small tube and allows for enhanced visualization of the lumen of the obstructed bowel. The frequent intermittent fluoroscopic monitoring during an enteroclysis study along with the volume challenge instilled into the small bowel can be helpful in delineating the cause and location of small bowel obstruction preoperatively, especially in those with low-grade or intermittent obstructions. This modality may also be helpful in ruling out obstruction if the results of other radiologic studies are indeterminate. The drawbacks of enteroclysis include the inability to obtain subsequent CT imaging due to the retained barium, the risk of inspissation and impaction of barium, the operator dependent nature of the procedure, and the inability to examine structures outside the lumen of the bowel. To overcome some of the limitations associated with enteroclysis, CT enteroclysis is now being employed in some centers. This examination involves the infusion of water-soluble contrast material through a nasointestinal tube followed by CT imaging after moderate distention of the small intestine. Interpretation of the CT images allows for a higher reliability given the presence of volume-challenged intestine displayed with cross-sectional imaging. In addition, CT enteroclysis images may be easier to interpret because of the ability to demonstrate bowel loops that may have been superimposed on conventional imaging.[21]

Abdominal ultrasound has been previously touted as a useful test in patients with suspected small bowel obstruction. Ultrasound can detect fluid-filled, dilated small bowel proximal to collapsed bowel and also the presence of peristaltic activity. Ko et al.[22] compared ultrasound with plain radiographs retrospectively in 54 patients with surgically proven obstruction and found that ultrasound was diagnostic in 89% of the cases, compared with 71% by plain X-rays. These authors also found ultrasound to be more accurate than plain films in determining the level and cause of the obstruction. Ogata et al.[23] studied 50 patients with suspected bowel obstruction and found ultrasound to be highly accurate with a sensitivity of 88% and a specificity of 96%. Plain radiographs were very sensitive in this study (96%), but the specificity was only 65%. Ultrasonic evaluation is extremely operator dependent, limiting its value to those who have expertise readily available.

Therapy

All the clinical decision-making skills of the experienced surgeon must come into play in order to make the correct therapeutic decisions when evaluating the patient with bowel obstruction (see Fig. 58.1). Decisions fall into broad categories: (1) determining the extent of fluid resuscitation, initiating nasogastric decompression, and monitoring urinary flow rates; (2) differentiating between the clinical scenarios of adynamic ileus, small bowel, and colonic obstruction based on the clinical and radiologic data; (3) differentiating simple from strangulating obstructions; (4) determining which patients will need an urgent operation after

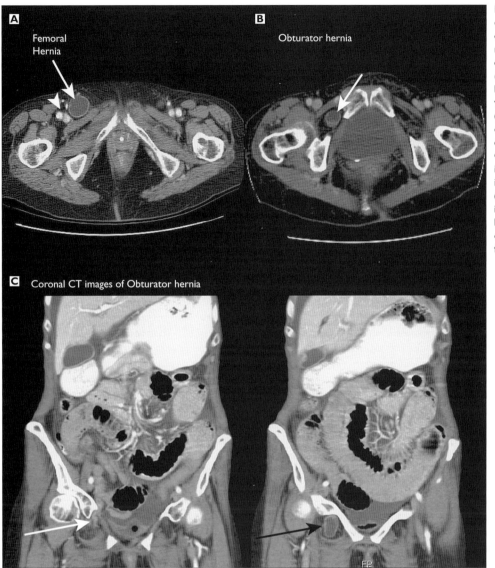

Fig. 58.5 • CT imaging often delineates the cause for mechanical obstructions. **(A)** Axial CT images reveal a femoral hernia with a loop of incarcerated small intestine (white arrow). Note the femoral hernia is medial to the femoral vessels (white arrowhead). **(B)** Obturator hernias are very difficult to distinguish on physical examination; in this standard axial CT image herniated small bowel is seen deep to the femoral vessels in the obturator canal (arrow). **(C)** Reformatted coronal CT images help confirm that small bowel is protruding through the obturator canal into the obturator fossa (arrows).

fluid and electrolyte resuscitation; and (5) determining which patients can be safely managed with nonoperative treatment and repeat examinations.

Fluid resuscitation and intestinal decompression

Fluid resuscitation and correction of acid base and electrolyte imbalances are among the most important interventions done for both patients with obstruction and ileus, and treatment should not be delayed by radiologic imaging. A balanced salt solution or lactated ringers can be used, with potassium supplementation as needed to correct deficits. Adequate fluid replacement will often correct any acid base imbalances and use of intravenous bicarbonate is rarely needed. Continued fluid losses caused by vomiting and nasogastric suctioning should be taken into account. Urinary catheterization will allow close monitoring of urine output as a measure of the adequacy of the fluid replacement. Occasionally, a Swan-Ganz catheter is needed for close monitoring, especially in those with congestive heart failure, marginal pulmonary status, or renal failure.

A nasogastric tube should be used to decompress the stomach in most patients with adynamic ileus and all patients with obstruction, and the patient should not be fed solids or liquids by mouth. This decompression allows for reduced gastric distention, lessens the nausea and vomiting, increases patient comfort, and may reduce the risk of aspiration. The use of long intestinal tubes such as the Cantor or Miller-Abbott tubes is rarely indicated and it is fairly clear from the literature that they add little to the decompression provided by standard nasogastric suctioning.[24,25]

Differentiating adynamic ileus from bowel obstruction

In adynamic ileus, there is usually gas present in both the small bowel and colon, usually with most of the gas seen in the colon. Patients with adynamic ileus usually appear less ill, may be less tender on physical exam, and radiologic studies show gas in the colon as well as the small bowel. The underlying cause of the adynamic ileus is often obvious (recent operation, narcotic use, pain, electrolyte imbalances) but can sometimes be difficult to elucidate. Treatment of the underlying cause for the ileus usually leads to its resolution as both colonic and small bowel motor function returns to normal. Early partial small obstructions can be quite difficult to differentiate from adynamic ileus, and the overall clinical picture and repeated physical examinations and radiologic evaluations are often necessary to differentiate between these two entities. In partial small bowel obstructions operative treatment is rarely indicated prior to a trial of nonoperative management. If the patient continues to pass flatus and no worrisome signs develop on repeat examinations, most patients will respond to nonoperative treatment and exploratory laparotomy can be avoided. It is important to note that when patients with no known etiology for a mechanical obstruction (i.e., they have had no previous abdominal operations and have no hernias) present with partial or complete obstructions, these patients need to be explored if no cause for their obstruction is found, since they could have a small bowel tumor or other intra-abdominal malignancy which can be difficult to diagnose with current technology.

Colonic pseudoobstruction (Ogilvie's syndrome) will result in isolated and often massive colonic dilatation. As in adynamic ileus, the treatment is directed to management of the underlying cause with correction of electrolyte imbalances, mobilization, and withdrawal of drugs such as psychiatric medications and opioids. Both the rapidity of the gaseous distention and the ultimate size of the colon must be taken into consideration in order to avoid a colonic perforation that can be devastating. A cecal diameter of greater than 12 cm, especially if rapidly expanding, should be treated aggressively with colonoscopic deflation and placement of a decompressing catheter or with surgical intervention via an ileostomy or cecostomy.[26] Intravenous administration of the cholinergic agonist neostigmine has been used successfully to aid in colonic decompression in cases of colonic pseudo-obstruction. Cardiac monitoring is necessary when neostigmine is used and in some patients the medication is contraindicated.[27]

Differentiating small from large bowel obstruction

Among the most important distinctions in the patient with a mechanical bowel obstruction is whether the site is within the small or large intestine. This difference is usually evident on plain radiographs, since the characteristic features of dilated colon will not be present in patients with small bowel obstruction. The differentiation between small and large bowel obstruction is critical in regard to both underlying etiologies (see Table 58.1) and clinical management. Regardless of the cause, if non-operative treatment fails, surgical exploration in a patient with mechanical small bowel obstruction will usually allow for adequate and complete treatment, without the need for stoma formation or subsequent surgical intervention. In the case of colonic obstruction, the timing and nature of the surgical intervention can be more complex, and in some cases stoma creation may be needed.

Differentiating simple from strangulating obstruction

The most important issue to be addressed in patients with mechanical small bowel obstruction is whether or not strangulation exists. Series which have compared mortality figures for simple versus strangulating obstruction have clearly demonstrated the importance of early recognition and treatment, since mortality for strangulated cases is generally 2–10 times higher than that for simple obstruction.[9] In those patients with strangulating groin hernias, the signs on physical exam are usually clear and include a firm, tender mass, perhaps with overlying erythema of the skin. In such situations, prompt surgical repair usually with bowel resection is mandatory. However, in those patients with obstruction on the basis of intra-abdominal pathology, the identification of strangulation may be extremely difficult. One of the most common mechanisms for strangulating small bowel obstruction is the *closed loop* which is usually due to adhesions and results in a twisting of a segment of intestine. The *closed loop* is a segment of small bowel occluded at two points along its course by a single constrictive lesion, often occluding both the small bowel and the mesentery. Patients with closed-loop obstruction usually have severe pain early, and the fluid-filled loops of bowel are often not seen on plain abdominal radiographs. It is with this particular group of patients that the experienced clinician is called upon to make a rapid and accurate diagnosis so that surgical intervention might prevent the sequelae of infarction and perforation with resultant peritonitis.

The differentiation between simple and strangulating obstruction has been the subject of numerous studies designed to identify one or more key signs or symptoms that could reliably predict the presence of strangulation. Silen et al.[28] reviewed the case histories of 480 patients with mechanical small bowel obstruction due to causes other than external hernias or mesenteric vascular occlusion. Unfortunately, these authors were not able to easily differentiate simple from strangulating obstruction. For example, although it has been generally taught that those patients with strangulation will have continuous pain, whereas a simple obstruction would cause an intermittent or colicky pain, this was not found to be the case in this series. Similar results were reported by Zollinger and Kinsey[29] who found that constant pain was present in 18% of patients with simple obstruction, and 20% of those with strangulation. So, too, tenderness to palpation is present in most (≈85%) patients with strangulation, but is also present in a majority (≈75%) of patients with simple obstructions.[28] A similar overlap has been documented in regard to other signs such as fever, leukocytosis, and the presence of a mass. Based upon these studies, as well as the anecdotal experience of numerous surgeons, it has generally been accepted that only short periods of observation (<24 hours) are appropriate in patients with mechanical small bowel obstruction, for fear of missing an unsuspected strangulation.

Because clinical criteria are imperfect in regard to differentiating simple from strangulating obstructions, a variety of radiologic tests have been employed. It is clear that plain abdominal radiographs can be extremely helpful in diagnosing a bowel obstruction, but normal X-rays can be seen in up to 20% of those patients with strangulation (see Figs 58.3 and 58.4).[28] The presence of a single loop of dilated small bowel in the setting of acute, severe abdominal pain should raise the suspicion of a strangulated *closed-loop obstruction*. Abdominal CT scan has been reported to be useful in identifying strangulation, usually on the basis of either bowel wall thickening, mesenteric edema, asymmetric enhancement with contrast, pneumatosis, or portal venous gas. Although ascites on the CT scan may be present in patients with closed-loop obstruction without ischemia, or with simple bowel obstruction, it is more commonly seen in patients with strangulation and should be considered a suspicious finding.[19] Figure 58.6 illustrates several of the features of strangulating obstruction detected by CT scan in a patient proven at operation to have a large segment of infarcted small intestine. Frager et al. studied 60 patients with small bowel obstruction on the basis of either adhesions or hernias and found CT scan to be highly sensitive (100%) for the detection of ischemia, but there were 12 false positives (61% specificity).[30] Ogata et al.[31] reported on

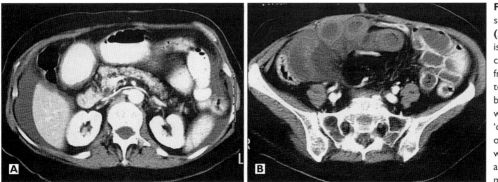

Fig. 58.6 • Features of strangulated small bowel seen on CT scan. **(A)** Dilated proximal small intestine is seen to be filled with the oral contrast agent. A large amount of free ascites fluid is evident adjacent to the liver and spleen. **(B)** Small bowel loops are fluid-filled but without luminal contrast, since the 'closed loop' is completely obstructing. In addition, the bowel wall is quite thickened and there are 'streaky' changes in the adjacent mesentery.

ultrasonography in 231 patients with adhesive small bowel obstruction. An akinetic loop seen on real-time ultrasonography proved to have a high sensitivity (90%) and specificity (93%) for the recognition of strangulation. However, the positive predictive value for strangulation was only 73%. These authors also found that the presence of peritoneal fluid was often an indicator of strangulation, a finding that has also been present in studies using CT scans.[19] It is clear, however, that the diagnosis of a strangulating obstruction remains a difficult one and requires a high degree of suspicion on the part of an experienced clinician.

Nonoperative treatment

The keys to therapy in patients with mechanical bowel obstruction are early diagnosis along with accurate differentiation between simple and strangulating mechanisms. With improved surgical and anesthetic management, the mortality from small bowel obstruction has decreased over the past 50–60 years from approximately 25% to 5%.[9] Initial therapy is geared towards normalization of intravascular fluid and electrolyte abnormalities. The patient should be given nothing by mouth, and nasogastric tube suction can often relieve some of the gastric distention, providing symptomatic improvement. Resolution of the obstruction may occur after adequate hydration and decompression via a nasogastric tube, avoiding the need for surgical intervention. This nonoperative approach is often successful in those patients with partial obstruction from adhesions, those with multiple previous episodes of obstructions, extensive abdominal radiation, widespread carcinomatosis, or obstructions related to impaction of food particles at the sites of luminal narrowing, such as a Crohn's stricture. In addition to standard nasogastric tubes, a variety of long intestinal tubes are available and have been used in an attempt at optimizing luminal decompression. The tubes are generally weighted with a mercury-filled balloon, passed into the stomach, and the patient placed in the right lateral decubitus position in the hopes that peristalsis will carry the tube beyond the pylorus and into the more distal jejunum. Several trials have compared the standard and long tubes and have generally found no significant difference in the percentage of patients ultimately requiring surgical intervention. Fleshner et al. conducted a prospective, randomized trial of short versus long tubes in 55 patients with acute adhesive small bowel obstruction and found no advantage of one tube type over the other.[32] This prospective study confirmed previous retrospective studies in the literature[33,34] which have shown no advantage of long intestinal tubes. Since the long tubes often do not pass into the small intestine and, when they do,

sometimes knot and are difficult to remove, there is probably little indication for their use.

Obstructions due to incarcerated hernias can rarely be relieved by reduction of the hernia contents, a procedure that should be performed cautiously and only by experienced clinicians. Excessive external pressure will lead to significant patient discomfort and, in rare circumstances, an inadvertent reduction 'en masse' may occur, resulting in disappearance of the hernia bulge but persistent bowel obstruction and possible strangulation within the constricting peritoneal sac.

Using a colonoscopically placed rectal tube that allows release of the gaseous distention in the colon proximal to the volvulus can often relieve colonic volvulus, especially of the sigmoid. Recurrence of the volvulus requires surgical intervention. Tumors obstructing the rectum can be treated with lasers or expandable stents under direct colonoscopic or fluoroscopic guidance and can lead to temporary relief of the obstruction to allow for initiation of other necessary treatments, often enabling a one-step surgical intervention at a later date.[35,36]

Operative treatment

Surgical intervention is indicated in those patients with a complete small bowel obstruction who have any signs or symptoms indicative of strangulation or in those patients with simple obstruction that has not resolved within a reasonable period of nonoperative therapy, perhaps 24–48 hours. Most clinicians would agree that constant or severe pain, especially associated with fever or signs of peritoneal irritation, acidosis, or sepsis, should be indications for urgent laparotomy.

The surgical approach to most patients with small bowel obstruction is straightforward and includes the use of perioperative antibiotics and surgical exploration (often laparotomy, sometimes laparoscopy) looking for the cause of the obstruction. A thorough abdominal exploration is performed with adhesiolysis, resection of nonviable intestine, and resection of any lesions that are causing obstruction. The determination of when and how much intestine to remove is usually simple and based upon the purple or black discoloration that occurs in severely ischemic or necrotic intestine. In addition to the normal pink coloration, viable intestine will have mesenteric arterial pulsations and normal motility. In some cases of more limited ischemic damage, the adhesiolysis should be followed by a 10–15 minute period of observation to allow for possible improvement in the gross appearance of the involved segment. Laser Doppler flowmetry has been advocated as an intraoperative method to accurately assess bowel viability.[37] Bulkley et al.[38] studied 71 ischemic bowel segments and found fluorescein ultraviolet fluorescence to be more accurate in determining bowel viability than either standard clinical judgment or Doppler blood flow measurements. In making the judgment as to the extent of resection, it should be kept in mind that a given marginally viable segment of intestine might survive in the short term, only to be followed weeks or months later by stricture formation that requires resection. As such, it is probably best to remove any segment that is not clearly viable by gross examination at the time of adhesiolysis. In most cases, all of the adhesions should be lysed so as to ensure that the obstruction is relieved and perhaps to prevent future recurrences. Under some circumstances, the offending adhesion might be lysed and others left alone, especially if continued adhesiolysis may result in serosal damage or inadvertent enterotomy leading to intestinal leaks or fistulas. When an obstructing lesion is identified, resection with primary anastomosis is performed. If a primary tumor of the small intestine is suspected, the segment of small intestine with its mesenteric lymph nodes should be removed and the entire small intestine should be carefully inspected for second primaries. In the case of a metastatic lesion to the small intestine, either resection or intestinal bypass should be performed, depending on the situation.

Since the advent of minimally invasive surgical techniques in the 1980s, some surgeons have employed a laparoscopic approach to patients with small bowel obstruction.[39,40] In some cases, a single adhesive band can be lysed laparoscopically or a small laparotomy performed overlying the area of obstruction, thereby avoiding a long incision in the abdominal wall. Laparoscopy in the setting of a bowel obstruction can be performed safely, but the 'open' technique for trocar placement is preferred in order to avoid the blind insertion of needles or trocars into the peritoneal cavity when distended loops of bowel are present. Placement of the initial trocar, experience of the surgical team, and sufficient instrumentation are of utmost importance. Ibrahim et al. retrospectively reviewed 33 patients with acute small bowel obstruction managed by laparoscopy.[41] Of those patients with postoperative adhesive obstruction, they were able to successfully lyse the adhesions in 72%. However, these authors reported two iatrogenic intestinal perforations and a variety of other patients who required conversion to laparotomy. Overall, these authors suggested that they were able to spare 67% of their patients a formal laparotomy. More recently Franklin et al.[42] reported on 167 patients with colonic or small bowel obstructions in which 92% were successfully managed using a laparoscopic approach. In this series, there was an operative complication rate of 3.5% including six inadvertent enterotomies, five of which were treated laparoscopically. The overall postoperative complication rate was fairly high (18.6%) and included wound infections, prolonged ileus, recurrent obstruction, sepsis, and death (2.3%). Clearly, patient selection and surgeon experience are the key factors in considering a laparoscopic approach to the patient with mechanical bowel obstruction.

SPECIAL FORMS OF INTESTINAL OBSTRUCTION

Crohn's disease and other strictures

Obstructing strictures are among the most common indications for surgery in patients with Crohn's disease. It is important to recognize that obstruction in Crohn's disease is most often due to impaction of undigested food particles at a site of luminal narrowing. A careful history will often reveal the recent ingestion of poorly digestible foods such as popcorn, peanuts, or very high-fiber-content foods. Such luminal obstructions almost never result in intestinal strangulation and will often resolve with non-operative management. In patients with recurrent episodes of such obstructions or those whose obstructions fail to resolve non-operatively, surgical treatment is indicated. It cannot be assumed a priori that the obstruction is caused by a stricture, however, since many patients with Crohn's disease have undergone multiple previous operations, thus raising the possibility of an adhesive obstruction with its associated increased likelihood of strangulation.

In selected cases of ileal narrowing caused by Crohn's disease, successful balloon dilatation via the colonoscope can be accomplished. This technique is limited, however, due to both anatomic considerations and also the fact that most symptomatic improvements are short lived. The incidence of perforation is appreciable and sometimes difficult to diagnose given the concomitant use of steroids by many of these patients. Couckuyt and colleagues prospectively studied 55 patients with Crohn's disease and ileocolonic strictures who underwent dilation with a hydrostatic balloon. Ninety percent of the procedures were technically successful, although six perforations occurred, two of which required immediate surgical intervention and resection. Many patients required two or more dilatations, and a long-term success rate of 62% was reported during a 33-month follow-up.[43] In some patients with Crohn's disease, a strictureplasty can be performed in lieu of surgical resection in order to widen the narrowed lumen. Large series of strictureplasties have been reported with low rates of recurrent obstructive symptoms and surprisingly few complications. Stebbing et al.[44] reviewed 241 stricutreplasties at 76 operations and reported no operative mortality and septic complications in only 4% of their patients. With a median follow-up of 49 months, they reported recurrence at the site of strictureplasty in only 4 patients. However, 36% of the patients required a second operation, and 13% needed a third operation, usually because of disease in areas remote from the prior strictureplasty. These and other authors have confirmed that strictureplasty is a safe and effective procedure in the setting of small bowel obstruction caused by Crohn's disease.[45–47]

In addition to Crohn's disease, a variety of other processes can lead to stricture formation within the small intestine (Table 58.2). Certain drugs[48,49] are known to cause mucosal ulceration and strictures, most notably enteric-coated potassium chloride preparations[50] and the nonsteroidal antiinflammatory agents.[51] Radiation therapy for intraperitoneal malignancy can lead to stricture formation, especially in those patient who have previously undergone abdominal surgery, which will increase the radiation exposure to segments of intestine that are fixed due to postsurgical adhesions.[52] Because of problems with healing, obstructed segments of irradiated bowel should be either bypassed,[53] or if a resection is performed, at least one end of an anastomosis should include nonirradiated bowel.[54] Mesenteric ischemia can also lead to stricture formation, the distal ileum being at greatest risk since the ileocolic artery is the last branch of the superior mesenteric artery.[55] Various neoplasms can also cause strictures within the small intestine, including carcinoma, carcinoid tumors, lymphoma, etc.[56,57] In most cases of small bowel strictures, the obstructive symptoms are chronic and progressive

Table 58.2 Etiologies of intestinal strictures

Trauma

Ischemia

Tumors

Drugs (potassium, NSAIDs)

Anastomotic

Crohn's disease

Postinflammatory

Infectious (TB)

Radiation

Cystic fibrosis

NSAIDs, nonsteroidal antiinflammatory drugs; TB, tuberculosis.

in nature, and the best surgical approach is resection, whenever technically feasible.

Internal hernias

An internal hernia is a protrusion of any intraperitoneal viscus into a compartment within the abdominal cavity. There is no hernia sac, and most often the herniated viscus is entering a known anatomical space or foramen; some hernias occur in surgically created or congenital defects. Congenital defects causing hernias have been described in the mesenteries of the ileum, transverse colon, sigmoid colon, and that of a Meckel's diverticulum, as well as in the left paracolic gutter, and within the falciform ligament. In one review, 0.2–0.9% of cadavers had incidentally noted internal hernias, most commonly paraduodenal (53%) followed by pericecal (13%) and the foramen of Winslow (8%), supravesical and intersigmoid hernias (6–7% each).[58,59] Transmesenteric hernias occur most commonly in children, along the mesentery of the jejunum. Prenatal ischemic events may be the causative agent as the area of defect is often associated with atretic segments of intestine. In addition to these intraperitoneal defects, a variety of retroperitoneal fossae can also be the site of internal herniation and bowel obstruction. The most common of these is the paraduodenal region, although they also occur in the ileocecal and sigmoid regions, and are thought to arise as abnormalities in the gut rotation which occurs in utero.[59] Intraabdominal hernias are very rare causes of intestinal obstruction.

Internal herniation can be related to surgical defects created by prior operations, e.g., in the paracolic or paraileal spaces adjacent to end stomas, or in a retroanastomotic location. A retroanastomotic hernia occurs through any defect in the mesenteric space left open after completion of an intestinal anastomosis. Hernias can occur after a Bilroth II anastomosis in the space between the gastrojejunostomy and the posterior abdominal wall. Seventy-five percent of iatrogenic hernias manifest in the first postoperative year. The presentation will generally be indistinguishable from other causes of intestinal obstruction, so that an accurate preoperative diagnosis is rarely made. Surgical repair of the defect should be performed along with resection of any nonviable bowel. If discovered incidentally at the time of laparotomy for other reasons, such defects should be repaired to avoid future problems.

Given the increasing number of patients undergoing gastric bypass operations, herniation and volvulus associated with the new anatomy created by Roux-en-Y gastric bypasses deserves special mention. Retrocolic-retrogastric herniation of most of the small intestine has been reported due to internal herniation at the mesenteric defect of the jejunojejunostomy after both laparoscopic and open gastric bypass surgery.[60] This unusual, but not rare complication is potentially life threatening due to possible ischemic necrosis of most of the small bowel as well as perforation of the gastric remnant, which is almost uniformly fatal. Internal hernias appear to be more common after laparoscopic Roux-en-Y gastric bypasses, possibly due to the relative lack of postoperative adhesions. Patients with retrocolic placement of the Roux limb appear to be at highest risk of herniation.[61] Patients often present with intermittent abdominal pain, small bowel obstruction, and normal radiologic studies, including contrast studies and CT scans, but can also present with signs and symptoms of an intraabdominal catastrophe. One retrospective analysis of 2000 consecutive patients who underwent laparoscopic Roux-en-Y gastric bypass found 63 patients with such internal hernias requiring operative intervention, an incidence of 3.1%. The site of internal herniation included: 44 in the mesocolon, 14 in the jejunal mesentery, and 5 in Petersen's space. Twenty percent of these patients had normal small bowel series and/or CT scans.[62] In another study, volvulus and ischemia requiring resection of small intestine was present in over 50% of patients with transmesenteric hernias, and absence of the 'whirl sign' and other radiologic signs of bowel ischemia did not exclude volvulus or ischemia.[63] Diagnosis of internal herniation in this patient population remains extremely challenging given relative lack of experience with this situation, and extreme obesity leading to difficulty with reliability of physical exam findings as well as laboratory findings. A high index of suspicion, diligent patient evaluation with special attention to symptoms, early abdominal CT scanning, communication with the surgical team involved with the patient's gastric bypass (if different from current physician team), and urgent operative intervention are necessary to achieve a successful outcome.

Gallstone ileus

Gallstones account for approximately 1–2% of cases of intestinal obstruction, usually affecting patients older than 60 years.[64] In order to cause obstruction, the gallstone needs to be of large size (>2.5 cm) and therefore can enter the intestinal tract only by a process of ulceration and fistulization. The most common site of entry is a cholecystoduodenal fistula, although stones may also erode into the stomach, jejunum, ileum, colon, or through the distal common bile duct into the duodenum. The gallstone will cause obstruction in the distal ileum or rarely at other areas of intestinal narrowing. The presentation will be that of acute, perhaps recurrent, attacks of small bowel obstruction, and would be suggested by the concurrent radiologic features of intestinal obstruction along with air in the biliary tree. Surgical treatment mandates removal of the stone via enterotomy, or resection in cases where the stone has become severely impacted in the wall of the bowel. Whether or not to perform a cholecystectomy at the time of relief of the obstruction remains controversial,[65] but as long as the gallbladder is emptied of all stones, the chances of recurrent intestinal obstruction are extremely low.[9] Kasahara et al. reviewed 112 cases of gallstone ileus and found a significant mortality (19%) in patients treated with a one-stage procedure (enterotomy plus cholecystectomy), whereas there was no mortality in those treated with enterolithotomy alone, leading these authors to recommend the latter procedure in most patients.[66] In contrast, Clavien et al. reviewed a series of 33 patients and concluded that a one-stage procedure was safe and effective in most patients.[67] Therefore, if the general condition of the patient is good and anatomical factors are favorable, a one-stage procedure can be recommended. In addition to gallstones, other *intraluminal foreign bodies* can rarely cause small bowel obstruction, including various bezoars, worms, and swallowed objects.[68–71]

Intussusception

Intussusception occurs when an entire advancing proximal segment of bowel, usually including part of its mesentery (intussuscipiens) invaginates into a more distal receiving segment of bowel (intussusceptum). Intussusception is the most common cause of childhood obstruction. However, intussusception in young adults and adults is rare, accounting for less than 5% of obstructions. Adult intussusception is usually due to an intrinsic bowel lesion such as a small bowel tumor (primary or metastatic), submucosal lipoma, Meckel's diverticulum, or parasite that usually initiates the process. In addition, intussusception is now being more frequently described at sites of jejuno-jejunal anastomoses such as after a Roux-en-Y gastric bypass.[72] The presenting clinical picture of an adult with intussusception is generally the same as those with other reasons for obstruction; however, episodes of pain and obstruction may be quite intermittent and sometimes more chronic. Radiologic studies aid in the diagnosis, and sometimes a barium enema is helpful, especially in the setting of intussusception where a large bowel tumor is the causative agent. CT findings can be quite classic and include the target sign, a sausage-shaped mass with alternating layers of low and high attenuation which represents the intussuscepted mesentery.[73] In a small number of patients with melanoma, small bowel obstruction with intussusception caused by a metastatic lesion in the small bowel is the first manifestation of disease (Fig. 58.7). Treatment involves surgical exploration and reduction of small bowel intussusceptions with resection of any suspicious lesions or segments of bowel. Large bowel intussusceptions should not be reduced, given a high chance of malignancy, and resection should be performed. Rarely, an enterotomy with resection of a small polyp may be prudent, especially in the setting of Peutz-Jeghers syndrome where multiple polyps may be present throughout the entire small bowel.[9]

Volvulus

Volvulus, or twisting of the intestine, most often occurs in the small bowel, cecum, or sigmoid colon and in the Western hemisphere accounts for approximately 5% of the cases of adult obstruction. A loop of bowel with a disproportionately long mesentery is most at risk for torsion. Often the torsed segment of intestine rapidly becomes a closed-loop obstruction with occlusion of its blood supply. The sigmoid is involved in 7–8% of the cases and the cecum in 10%. Volvulus of the small intestine occurs much more often in newborns and can be associated with congenital anomalies.[74] Volvulus of the stomach can be due to congenital or acquired diaphragmatic defects or large paraesophageal hernias. Most patients present with colicky, intermittent abdominal pain and a grossly distended abdomen, sometimes asymmetric in nature. Radiologic studies are very helpful and often help confirm clinical suspicion. In sigmoid volvulus, a tremendously distended sigmoid loop is seen with a 'bent innertube sign,' and a barium enema will often reveal the sigmoid twist at the base of the mesocolon, above which lies the dilated loop of obstructed sigmoid colon. Treatment of sigmoid volvulus includes attempts at nonoperative reduction with barium enema, or passage of a soft tube past the obstructing point with the aid of sigmoidoscopy. These treatments often result in prompt and dramatic reductions in the size of the distended abdomen. Successful nonoperative reduction allows optimization of cardiopulmonary comorbidity in a high-risk group of patients and converts an emergent to an elective procedure and minimizes operative morbidity as a result.[75] Surgical intervention is recommended if nonoperative reduction methods are unsuccessful, and elective resection of the sigmoid is performed, given the risks of recurrence of the volvulus. Small bowel volvulus remains a difficult and elusive clinical diagnosis even with the aid of CT imaging; immediate operation is mandatory given the risk of ischemia.

Radiologic studies in cecal volvulus will often reveal evidence of small bowel obstruction with great distention of the cecum, which can sometimes be in the left upper quadrant. Distended loops of small bowel can sometimes be seen to the right of the distended cecum. Treatment is usually operative and includes reduction of the twist, and cecopexy or resection of the right colon. Laparoscopy is being considered more often in the setting of uncomplicated cecal volvulus.[76]

Early postoperative obstruction

In the early postoperative period (within 3–4 weeks) following laparotomy for any reason, small bowel obstruction occurs in

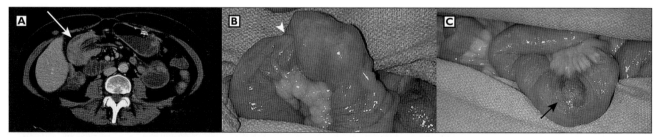

Fig. 58.7 • Metastatic melanoma presenting as intussusception of the small bowel. **(A)** CT imaging in a patient with abdominal pain reveals classic findings of intussusception with a sausage-shaped mass (white arrow) and alternating layers of low and high attenuation representing the intussuscepted mesentery. **(B)** At operation, multiple points of intussusception are found (white arrowhead). **(C)** Each intussusception lead point was a small bowel tumor comprised of metastatic melanoma (black arrow).

approximately 1–5% of patients. The differentiation between obstruction and adynamic ileus can usually be made on clinical grounds, since an ileus rarely persists for more than 5 or 6 days. Clearly, many patients thought to have a 'prolonged ileus' really have some degree of mechanical small intestinal obstruction.[77] The diagnosis of early postoperative obstruction can be made in those patients who initially experience return of bowel function, only subsequently to develop nausea, vomiting, and abdominal distention. Plain radiographs may distinguish adynamic ileus from obstruction, since a predominance of small bowel gaseous distention would not be seen in most cases of ileus. Frager et al. examined 36 patients with CAT scans and reported 100% sensitivity and specificity in distinguishing mechanical small bowel obstruction from paralytic ileus.[78]

It should be noted that the distinction between ileus and mechanical obstruction in the early postoperative period is rarely of clinical consequence, since the treatment will usually be identical, that being nonoperative.[77] This is the case because in early postoperative obstruction the chances of nonoperative resolution appears to be higher and the incidence of strangulation lower than in other clinical settings. Soft, filmy, and broad-based adhesions form early after laparotomy, occasionally leading to some degree of luminal obstruction, a situation that will resolve as the adhesions undergo their natural course of dissolution and reformation. The fact that the adhesions contain little scar tissue probably explains why the incidence of strangulation is so rare in the early postoperative setting. Many clinicians have suggested a relatively long trial of nonoperative therapy, perhaps 3–4 weeks, before considering surgical intervention. Clearly, there are some patients who have more severe forms of obstruction, e.g., twisting of the mesentery or internal herniations, who will require prompt surgical correction, even in the early postoperative period.

In patients with early postoperative obstruction after laparoscopic surgery special consideration must also be given to etiologies other than adhesions or internal hernias as causes of any prolonged ileus or early postoperative small bowel obstruction. Trocar site herniation, trocar insertion injuries to organs, or inadvertent intestinal injury should be strongly considered. In fact, some patients undergoing laparoscopic surgery who go on to have a postoperative complication such as small bowel injury can have very different presenting signs and symptoms, perhaps due to different immune and cytokine responses in those undergoing laparoscopic surgery.[79] Physicians taking care of the patient after laparoscopic surgery must be especially vigilant given the relatively subtle and potentially delayed physical exam findings which may accompany intra-abdominal processes such as internal herniation, or missed small bowel injury. Patients with early postoperative obstruction after laparoscopic surgery should be carefully examined and consideration should be given to an earlier return to the operating room if warranted, which can often be accomplished laparoscopically.

PREVENTION

Attempts to prevent small bowel obstruction have been focused on reducing adhesions, since this is the most common underlying etiology. It is thought that adhesion formation can be reduced by avoiding excessive tissue ischemia, trauma, and manipulation. Since fibrin deposition is one of the initiating events in adhesion formation, various anticoagulants, e.g., heparin and dextran, or thrombolytic agents, e.g., streptokinase and urokinase, have been used, but with minimal success. Several synthetic agents have been developed which may reduce the incidence of adhesions. Becker et al.[80] reported a prospective, randomized study using a bioresorbable membrane (Seprafilm adhesion barrier, modified sodium hyaluronic acid and carboxymethylcellulose; Genzyme) placed anterior to all bowel loops in patients undergoing colectomy/ileoanal pouch procedures with diverting loop ileostomies. At the time of ileostomy closure (8–12 weeks), laparoscopy was used to assess the degree of adhesion formation and showed that 51% of the patients treated with the membrane were free of adhesions, compared to only 5% of control patients. More recently, Beck et al.[81] used Seprafilm in over 1700 patients undergoing abdominal and pelvic surgery in a prospective, randomized, multicenter study with no increase in rates of intra-abdominal abscess, pulmonary embolism or foreign body reaction. However, of note, in those patients in whom an intestinal anastomosis was wrapped with Seprafilm, a higher rate of anastomotic leak, fistula, peritonitis, abscess, and sepsis was seen. Whether or not using such treatments will lower the incidence of chronic adhesions and subsequent small bowel obstruction will need to be determined by further studies. Other chemical and biologic agents (such as Adcon-P) are being rapidly developed and studied for the purpose of reducing postoperative adhesions.[82,83] A decrease in the incidence of adhesive small bowel obstruction is hopefully anticipated as more and more laparoscopic operations replace formal laparotomies, since it is well recognized that laparoscopy leads to minimal adhesion formation. In patients who are to receive postoperative radiotherapy, e.g., following resection of ovarian or rectal cancers, radiation-induced small bowel strictures may be prevented by placement of a pelvic 'sling' at the time of initial laparotomy, thereby restraining the small intestine in the upper abdomen and out of the radiation field.[84]

SUMMARY

Intestinal obstruction is one of the most common disorders seen by both gastroenterologists and surgeons, and a thorough knowledge of this disorder is important for virtually all physicians. The key to the management of patients with small intestinal obstruction is early diagnosis so that proper therapy can be instituted. All the clinical decision-making skills of the experienced surgeon will come into play in order to make the correct therapeutic decisions when evaluating the patient with bowel obstruction. Decisions fall into broad categories: (1) determining the extent of fluid resuscitation, initiating nasogastric decompression, and monitoring urinary flow rates; (2) differentiating between the clinical scenarios of adynamic ileus, small bowel, and colonic obstruction based on the clinical and radiologic data; (3) differentiating simple from strangulating obstructions; (4) determining which patients will need an urgent operation after fluid and electrolyte resuscitation; and (5) determining which patients can be safely managed with nonoperative treatment and repeat examinations. Identification of those patients with strangulation is of critical importance since prompt surgical correction is needed in order to minimize morbidity and mortality. Numerous clinical and radiological criteria can be helpful in distinguishing simple from strangulating obstruction, but this differentiation remains a challenge to even the most experienced clinicians.

REFERENCES

1. Jones RS. Intestinal obstruction. Textbook of surgery. Sabiston DC, ed. Philadelphia: WB Saunders; 1991:835.

2. Hartwell JA, Hoguet JP. Experimental intestinal obstruction in dogs with especial reference to the cause of death and the treatment by large amounts of normal saline solution. JAMA 1912; 59:82.

3. Gibson C. A study of 1000 operations for acute intestinal obstruction. Ann Surg 1900; 32:486.

4. Vick R. Statistics of acute intestinal obstruction. Br Med J 1932; 2:546.

5. Wangenstein O. Intestinal obstructions. Springfield, IL: Charles C. Thomas; 1955.

6. Ellis CN, Boggs HW Jr, Slagle GW, et al. Small bowel obstruction after colon resection for benign and malignant diseases. Dis Colon Rectum 1991; 34:367–371.

7. Beck DE, Opelka FG, Bailey HR, et al. Incidence of small-bowel obstruction and adhesiolysis after open colorectal and general surgery. Dis Colon Rectum 1999; 42:241–248.

8. Asbun HJ, Pempinello C, Halasz NA. Small bowel obstruction and its management. Int Surg 1989; 74:23–27.

9. Ellis H. In: Maingot's abdominal operations. Schwartz SI, Ellis H, (eds). 9th edition. Norwalk, Connecticut: Appleton & Lange; 1989:885–904.

10. Prihoda M, Flatt A, Summers RW. Mechanisms of motility changes during acute intestinal obstruction in the dog. Am J Physiol 1984; 247:G37–G42.

11. Sykes PA, Boulter KH, Schofield PF. The microflora of the obstructed bowel. Br J Surg 1976; 63:721–725.

12. Yale CE, Balish E. Intestinal strangulation in germfree and monocontaminated dogs. Arch Surg 1979; 114:445–448.

13. Sachs SM, Morton JH, Schwartz SI. Acute mesenteric ischemia. Surgery 1982; 92:646–653.

14. Maglinte DD, Gage SN, Harmon BH, et al. Obstruction of the small intestine: accuracy and role of CT in diagnosis. Radiology 1993; 188:61–64.

15. Balthazar EJ, George W. Holmes Lecture. CT of small-bowel obstruction. AJR Am J Roentgenol 1994; 162:255–261.

16. Balthazar EJ. For suspected small-bowel obstruction and an equivocal plain film, should we perform CT or a small-bowel series? AJR Am J Roentgenol 1994; 163:1260–1261.

   This important reference provides a detailed analysis of the usefulness of CT scans as a second-tier study after initial radiologic imaging for bowel obstruction.

17. Harlow CL, Stears RL, Zeligman BE, et al. Diagnosis of bowel obstruction on plain abdominal radiographs: significance of air-fluid levels at different heights in the same loop of bowel. AJR Am J Roentgenol 1993; 161:291–295.

18. Siewert B, Raptopoulos V. CT of the acute abdomen: findings and impact on diagnosis and treatment. AJR Am J Roentgenol 1994; 163:1317–1324.

19. Balthazar EJ, Birnbaum BA, Megibow AJ, et al. Closed-loop and strangulating intestinal obstruction: CT signs. Radiology 1992; 185:769–775.

   This paper provides detailed analysis of radiologic findings associated with closed-loop and strangulated obstructions, a difficult clinical diagnosis.

20. Frager D, Medwid SW, Baer JW, et al. CT of small-bowel obstruction: value in establishing the diagnosis and determining the degree and cause. AJR Am J Roentgenol 1994; 162:37–41.

21. Maglinte DD, Kelvin FM, Rowe MG, et al. Small-bowel obstruction: optimizing radiologic investigation and nonsurgical management. Radiology 2001; 218:39–46.

22. Ko YT, Lim JH, Lee DH, et al. Small bowel obstruction: sonographic evaluation. Radiology 1993; 188:649–653.

23. Ogata M, Mateer JR, Condon RE. Prospective evaluation of abdominal sonography for the diagnosis of bowel obstruction. Ann Surg 1996; 223:237–241.

24. Brolin RE. The role of gastrointestinal tube decompression in the treatment of mechanical intestinal obstruction. Am Surg 1983; 49:131–137.

25. Snyder CL, Ferrell KL, Goodale RL, et al. Nonoperative management of small-bowel obstruction with endoscopic long intestinal tube placement. Am Surg 1990; 56:587–592.

26. Bode WE, Beart RW Jr, Spencer RJ, et al. Colonoscopic decompression for acute pseudoobstruction of the colon (Ogilvie's syndrome). Report of 22 cases and review of the literature. Am J Surg 1984; 147:243–245.

27. Ponec RJ, Saunders MD, Kimmey MB. Neostigmine for the treatment of acute colonic pseudo-obstruction. N Engl J Med 1999, 341.137–141.

   This important paper reports a nonsurgical approach to acute colonic pseudo-obstruction. This is a novel approach and if used properly can result in avoidance of surgery in some patients.

28. Silen W, Hein MF. Strangulation obstruction of the small intestine. Am Surg 1962; 30:1.

29. Zollinger RM, Kinsey D. Diagnosis and management of intestinal obstruction. Am Sur 1964; 30:1.

30. Frager D, Baer JW, Medwid SW, et al. Detection of intestinal ischemia in patients with acute small-bowel obstruction due to adhesions or hernia: efficacy of CT. AJR Am J Roentgenol 1996; 166:67–71.

31. Ogata M, Imai S, Hosotani R, et al. Abdominal ultrasonography for the diagnosis of strangulation in small bowel obstruction. Br J Surg 1994; 81:421–424.

32. Fleshner PR, Siegman MG, Slater GI, et al. A prospective, randomized trial of short versus long tubes in adhesive small-bowel obstruction. Am J Surg 1995; 170:366–370.

33. Brolin RE, Krasna MJ, Mast BA. Use of tubes and radiographs in the management of small bowel obstruction. Ann Surg 1987; 206:126–133.

34. Bizer LS, Liebling RW, Delany HM, et al. Small bowel obstruction: the role of nonoperative treatment in simple intestinal obstruction and predictive criteria for strangulation obstruction. Surgery 1981; 89:407–413.

35. Low DE, Kozarek RA, Ball TJ, et al. Colorectal neodymium-YAG photoablative therapy. Comparing applications and complications on both sides of the peritoneal reflection. Arch Surg 1989; 124:684–688.

36. Ahmad T, Mee AS. Expandable metal stents in malignant colorectal obstruction. Promising, but trials are needed on safety and cost effectiveness. Br Med J 2000; 321:584–585.

37. Johansson K, Ahn H, Lindhagen J. Intraoperative assessment of blood flow and tissue viability in small-bowel ischemia by laser Doppler flowmetry. Acta Chir Scand 1989; 155:341–346.

38. Bulkley GB, Zuidema GD, Hamilton SR, et al. Intraoperative determination of small intestinal viability following ischemic injury: a prospective, controlled trial of two adjuvant methods (Doppler and fluorescein) compared with standard clinical judgment. Ann Surg 1981; 193:628–637.

39. Reissman P, Wexner SD. Laparoscopic surgery for intestinal obstruction. Surg Endosc 1995; 9:865–868.

40. Suter M, Zermatten P, Halkic N, et al. Laparoscopic management of mechanical small bowel obstruction: are there predictors of success or failure? Surg Endosc 2000; 14:478–483.

41. Ibrahim IM, Wolodiger F, Sussman B, et al. Laparoscopic management of acute small-bowel obstruction. Surg Endosc 1996; 10:1012–1014; discussion 1014–1015.

42. Franklin ME Jr, Gonzalez JJ Jr, Miter DB, et al. Laparoscopic diagnosis and treatment of intestinal obstruction. Surg Endosc 2004; 18:26–30.

43. Couckuyt H, Gevers AM, Coremans G, et al. Efficacy and safety of hydrostatic balloon dilatation of ileocolonic Crohn's strictures: a prospective longterm analysis. Gut 1995; 36:577–580.

44. Stebbing JF, Jewell DP, Kettlewell MG, et al. Recurrence and reoperation after strictureplasty for obstructive Crohn's disease: long-term results [corrected]. Br J Surg 1995; 82:1471–1474.

45. Lee EC, Papaioannou N. Minimal surgery for chronic obstruction in patients with extensive or universal Crohn's disease. Ann R Coll Surg Engl 1982; 64:229–233.

46. Tjandra JJ, Fazio VW. Strictureplasty without concomitant resection for small bowel obstruction in Crohn's disease. Br J Surg 1994; 81:561–563.

47. Tjandra JJ, Fazio VW. Strictureplasty for ileocolic anastomotic strictures in Crohn's disease. Dis Colon Rectum 1993; 36:1099–1103; discussion 1103–1104.

48. George CF. Drugs causing intestinal obstruction: a review. J R Soc Med 1980; 73:200–204.

49. Lee FD. Drug-related pathological lesions of the intestinal tract. Histopathology 1994; 25:303–308.

50. Abbruzzese AA, Gooding CA. Reversible small-bowel obstruction: withdrawal of hydrochlorothiazide-potassium chloride therapy. JAMA 1965; 192:781–782.

51. Speed CA, Bramble MG, Corbett WA, et al. Non-steroidal anti-inflammatory induced diaphragm disease of the small intestine: complexities of diagnosis and management. Br J Rheumatol 1994; 33:778–780.

52. Jackson BT. Bowel damage from radiation. Proc R Soc Med 1976; 69:683–686.

53. Mann WJ. Surgical management of radiation enteropathy. Surg Clin North Am 1991; 71:977–990.

54. Galland RB, Spencer J. Natural history and surgical management of radiation enteritis. Br J Surg 1987; 74:742–747.

55. Thaker P, Weingarten L, Friedman IH. Stenosis of the small intestine due to nonocclusive ischemic disease. Arch Surg 1977; 112:1216–1217.

56. Zollinger RM Jr. Primary neoplasms of the small intestine. Am J Surg 1986; 151:654–658.

57. Martin RG. Malignant tumors of the small intestine. Surg Clin North Am 1986; 66:779–785.

58. Janin Y, Stone AM, Wise L. Mesenteric hernia. Surg Gynecol Obstet 1980; 150:747–754.

59. Hansmann GH, Morton SA. Intraabdominal hernias: report of a case and review of the literature. Arch Surg 1939; 39:973.

60. Serra C, Baltasar A, Bou R, et al. Internal hernias and gastric perforation after a laparoscopic gastric bypass. Obes Surg 1999; 9:546–549.

61. Champion JK, William M. Small bowel obstruction and internal hernias after laparoscopic Roux-en-Y gastric bypass. Obes Surg 2003; 13:596–600.

62. Higa KD, Ho T, Boone KB. Internal hernias after laparoscopic Roux-en-Y gastric bypass: incidence, treatment and prevention. Obes Surg 2003; 13:350–354.

    This important paper reviews and provides illustrations of a relatively rare but new kind of internal hernia, becoming increasingly frequent due to the large increase in the number of laparoscopic gastric bypasses.

63. Blachar A, Federle MP, Brancatelli G, et al. Radiologist performance in the diagnosis of internal hernia by using specific CT findings with emphasis on transmesenteric hernia. Radiology 2001; 221:422–428.

64. Stitt RB, Heslin DJ, Currie DJ. Gall-stone ileus. Br J Surg 1967; 54:673–678.

65. Buetow GW, Glaubitz JP, Crampton RS. Recurrent gallstone ileus. Surgery 1963; 54:716–724.

66. Kasahara Y, Umemura H, Shiraha S, eet al. Gallstone ileus. Review of 112 patients in the Japanese literature. Am J Surg 1980; 140:437–440.

67. Clavien PA, Richon J, Burgan S, et al. Gallstone ileus. Br J Surg 1990; 77:737–742.

68. Marc B, Baud FJ, Aelion MJ, et al. The cocaine body-packer syndrome: evaluation of a method of contrast study of the bowel. J Forensic Sci 1990; 35:345–355.

69. Cauchi JA, Shawis RN. Multiple magnet ingestion and gastrointestinal morbidity. Arch Dis Child 2002; 87:539–540.

70. Lees NP, Reid F, Lee SH, et al. Distal small bowel obstruction caused by a migrated self expanding metal oesophageal stent. Eur J Surg Suppl 2003; 588:66–68.

71. Traub SJ, Hoffman RS, Nelson LS. Body packing – the internal concealment of illicit drugs. N Engl J Med 2003; 349:2519–2526.

72. Bocker J, Vasile J, Zager J, et al. Intussusception: an uncommon cause of postoperative small bowel obstruction after gastric bypass. Obes Surg 2004; 14:116–119.

73. Boudiaf M, Soyer P, Terem C, et al. CT evaluation of small bowel obstruction. Radiographics 2001; 21:613–624.

74. Ballantyne GH, Brandner MD, Beart RW Jr, et al. Volvulus of the colon. Incidence and mortality. Ann Surg 1985; 202:83–92.

75. Connolly S, Brannigan AE, Heffeman E, et al. Sigmoid volvulus: a 10-year-audit. Ir J Med Sci 2002; 171:216–217.

76. Madiba TE, Thomson SR. The management of cecal volvulus. Dis Colon Rectum 2002; 45:264–267.

77. Silen W. Cope's early diagnosis of the acute abdomen. New York: Oxford University Press; 1996.

78. Frager DH, Baer JW, Rothpearl A, et al. Distinction between postoperative ileus and mechanical small-bowel obstruction: value of CT compared with clinical and other radiographic findings. AJR Am J Roentgenol 1995; 164:891–894.

79. Bellon JM, Manzano L, Larrad A, et al. Endocrine and immune response to injury after open and laparoscopic cholecystectomy. Int Surg 1998; 83:24–27.

80. Becker JM, Dayton MT, Fazio VW, et al. Prevention of postoperative abdominal adhesions by a sodium hyaluronate-based bioresorbable membrane: a prospective, randomized, double-blind multicenter study. J Am Coll Surg 1996; 183:297–306.

81. Beck DE, Cohen Z, Fleshman JW, et al. A prospective, randomized, multicenter, controlled study of the safety of Seprafilm adhesion barrier in abdominopelvic surgery of the intestine. Dis Colon Rectum 2003; 46:1310–1319.

    This randomized, prospective study analyzes both the benefits and disadvantages of use of Seprafilm as a barrier to adhesion formation.

82. Oncel M, Remzi FH, Senagore AJ, et al. Application of Adcon-P or Seprafilm in consecutive laparotomies using a murine model. Am J Surg 2004; 187:304–308.

83. Oncel M, Remzi FH, Senagore AJ, et al. Liquid antiadhesive product (Adcon-p) prevents post-operative adhesions within the intra-abdominal organs in a rat model. Int J Colorectal Dis 2003; 18:514–517.

84. Rodier JF, Janser JC, Rodier D, et al. Prevention of radiation enteritis by an absorbable polyglycolic acid mesh sling. A 60-case multicentric study. Cancer 1991; 68:2545–2549.

CHAPTER FIFTY-NINE

59

Chronic intestinal pseudo-obstruction

Juan-R. Malagelada

INTRODUCTION

Chronic intestinal pseudo-obstruction (CIP) is a relatively rare condition, conceptually simple to grasp but difficult to manage in practice. The clinical picture of pseudo-obstruction develops when there is protracted failure of intestinal peristalsis to overcome the normal resistance to flow. Consequently, CIP mimics the effects of a chronic, partial obstruction of the bowel, but without mechanical impediment.[1,2]

CIP can result from either reversible or irreversible dysfunction of the gut smooth muscle and/or its neurohormonal regulatory systems.[3] When the dysfunction is caused by diseases restricted to the smooth muscle or enteric nerves, the condition is classified as primary CIP. This classification includes some CIP forms that are genetic hereditary or nonhereditary conditions.[4–6] When the dysfunction is part of a systemic condition, it is classified as secondary. Myopathic pseudo-obstruction refers to CIP caused by enteric smooth muscle degeneration, which may eventually become replaced by collagen, whereas neuropathic pseudo-obstruction refers to CIP caused by neural enteric or extra-enteric disorders.[7,8] Enteric neuropathies in turn may be divided into degenerative (noninflammatory) and inflammatory forms. The latter may be amenable to specific therapy.

CIP was initially a diagnosis restricted to small bowel motor dysfunction. Presently, CIP connotes a broader diagnostic label, encompassing the entire gastrointestinal tract.[9] Furthermore, it is well recognized that even in primary CIP other visceral systems, particularly the vesicourinary, may be affected, probably because their neuromuscular tissue structure and neural control are similar to that of the gastrointestinal tract.

CLINICAL FEATURES

Chronic intestinal pseudo-obstruction is characterized by a stereotyped clinical picture that defines the syndrome. In addition, there may be associated manifestations that depend on the involvement of different regions or organs, the etiology, and related conditions or complications. Knowledge of the various clinical facets of CIP is a prerequisite for effective management.

To facilitate the description of the clinical picture of CIP, it will be arbitrarily divided into three parts:

1. Core clinical manifestations;
2. Clinical peculiarities associated with the involvement of different regions; and
3. Complications.

Core clinical manifestations

Core clinical manifestations correspond to chronic (conventionally defined as longer than 3 months) intestinal obstruction-like symptoms. Chronic intestinal pseudo-obstruction may present abruptly, mimicking the clinical picture of acute mechanical small bowel obstruction, or as repeated subocclusive crisis characterized by colicky-type abdominal pain and abdominal distention. Unfortunately, these symptoms are rather non-specific. Patients may describe other types of pain: pressure-like, painful bloating, and sometimes focal pain. Abdominal distention may refer to the sensation of distention (bloating), to visible distention, or to both. Audible borborygmi may or may not be presented. Unlike complete mechanical obstruction where flatus is virtually absent, patients with CIP may describe either excessive flatulence (albeit usually stating that it brings minor, if any relief to their abdominal symptoms) or no gas expulsion at all. Nausea and vomiting (exceptionally feculent) may be very prominent manifestations in some patients. Disturbances in bowel habit are common but unpredictable. Some patients suffer from diarrhea, others from constipation, and some manifest alternating diarrhea and constipation resembling a severe irritable bowel syndrome. The signs observed on physical examination are also varied and mostly non-specific and include abdominal distention, borborygmi, and high-pitch bowel sounds. In uncomplicated CIP there should be no signs of peritoneal irritation.

Clinical peculiarities associated with specific regional involvement

Chronic intestinal pseudo-obstruction, as a neuromuscular disorder, may involve any segment of gut and even other organs with comparable tissue structure. Alternatively, focal or regional involvement predominates in some patients and determines peculiarities of the clinical presentation.[10] Thus, some patients with esophageal dysmotility may complain mostly of reflux-like or achalasia-like symptoms. In other patients a picture akin to gastroparesis dominates the clinical presentation. These are patients who complain of nausea, vomiting, and other manifestations of delayed gastric emptying. It should be noted, however, that such a gastroparetic picture is as likely to result pathogenetically from altered small bowel motility as from gastric dysmotility, or from a combination of both.[11] Colonic atony and dilatation may be particularly prominent in some patients with CIP, which has led to some confusion with Ogilvie's syndrome.[12] However, the latter denomination should probably be reserved for patients with acute or subacute colonic distention in the context of toxic, neoplastic, or systemic diseases. Patients with megacolon and other forms of colonic neuromuscular contractile failure associated with protracted constipation, as the exclusive or predominant clinical manifestation, should probably also be excluded from CIP classification. However, it is true that some CIP patients present initially as colonic inertia, and only years later (sometimes after colectomy) does it become apparent that the small bowel is also affected. Anorectal dysfunction is a relatively common feature of CIP and, even without distal complaints, manometric studies may disclose abnormalities. Extraintestinal manifestations should be actively investigated in patients with CIP. Urinary tract involvement is particularly common in myopathic CIP and it tends to manifest clinically by recurrent infections and altered micturition.[13] In secondary CIP, drugs, systemic disease, and neurologic disorders may produce accompanying manifestations that should be looked for, since they can help establish the specific etiology of secondary CIP (see below).

Clinical manifestations of complications

In severe CIP, malnutrition and specific deficits may be part of the clinical picture. This situation should be anticipated in patients who tolerate intake poorly, vomit frequently, and suffer from secondary diarrhea and malabsorption. In fact, the latter manifestations are often due to bacterial overgrowth in the small bowel. Specific deficiencies in electrolytes, vitamins, minerals, and metals may produce the corresponding clinical manifestations. However, more commonly, deficits are not clinically obvious and should be actively sought by an appropriate battery of blood and urine tests.[14]

RELEVANT TESTS USED IN THE DIAGNOSIS OF CHRONIC INTESTINAL PSEUDO-OBSTRUCTION

Step 1: Abdominal imaging

A critical step in the diagnosis of CIP is to exclude mechanical obstruction or another specific intestinal lesion responsible for the clinical syndrome, which may be challenging for two main reasons: (1) a 'hidden' lesion causing partial bowel obstruction may be difficult to identify in a distended bowel partially filled with fluid and organic detritus, and (2) conversely, in many patients with CIP presenting with potentially obstructing lesions (commonly, kinks and adhesions from prior abdominal surgeries), it may be difficult to ascertain whether there is partial mechanical obstruction (with secondary proximal neuromuscular dysfunction) or whether the observed postsurgical sequelae in fact represent epiphenomena without pathologic significance.

Abdominal imaging should, therefore, be performed initially in the evaluation of a patient with suspected chronic intestinal pseudo-obstruction. Note, however, that in ill patients certain urgent measures such as decompressing the abdomen and re-establishing fluid and electrolyte balance and nutritional support (see later) may need to be implemented immediately, even prior to diagnostic studies. Note also that imaging procedures are most informative when performed after thorough bowel decompression

obtained either by prolonged fasting and/or via aspiration by nasogastric or nasoenteric tube.

Endoscopy

The main value of endoscopy is the identification of mucosal lesions (e.g., Crohn's ulcers and focal amyloid 'pimples') that might otherwise be missed by radiology. Endoscopy is, therefore, a reasonable *first step* in most patients. The upper intestine should be examined as far distally from the pylorus as possible, and ordinarily should be complemented by colonoscopy and ileoscopy.

Plain abdominal radiology

Plain abdominal radiology may not reliably distinguish between intestinal mechanical obstruction and pseudo-obstruction. However, it is useful to establish the presence of air-filled and dilated loops of bowel and, later, to follow up response to therapy.

Abdominal CT scan

An abdominal CT scan should be obtained early in the diagnostic process. It provides information regarding the magnitude of intestinal dilation, thickness of the intestinal walls and, sometimes crucially, a change in the caliber of the intestinal lumen that may indicate an area of mechanical obstruction. The CT scan may also detect masses or extraintestinal and/or retroperitoneal pathology causing the obstruction.

Gastrointestinal transit with barium contrast

Gastrointestinal transit with barium contrast may help to localize the precise location and magnitude of an occlusive lesion. It may be indicated when the acute crisis has been resolved and signs of peritonitis and ileus are absent. In general, barium contrast should be avoided when there is a possibility of colonic mechanical obstruction or severe inertia, to preclude barium solidification and impaction in the colon.

Enteroclysis

Enteroclysis consists of the administration of barium suspension directly into the small bowel via nasoenteric tube. It is a time-honored procedure that in our hands retains good value in the management of CIP. If enteroclysis shows free flow of barium into the terminal ileum and colon, it is unlikely that a significant mid-small bowel obstructing lesion has been missed.

Step 2: Physiological assessment of intestinal function

Physiological assessment is the logical next step when a mechanical obstructing lesion or other significant intra-abdominal pathology has been reasonably excluded by the imaging procedures in the first step.

Measurement of gut transit

In theory, measurement of small bowel transit speed should be a rewarding diagnostic approach to a condition such as CIP that represents a gut propulsive disturbance. In practice, however, measurements of transit are not that useful and are rarely indicated. Indirect methods such as the lactulose hydrogen breath test, which assesses the time-span from mouth to cecum, may be hampered by technical pitfalls, including spurious early hydrogen peaks caused by small bowel bacterial overgrowth. Direct transit measurements, mostly based on radioscintigraphy, are more accurate since they allow visualization and quantification of whole gut transit of an externally monitored radiolabeled marker(s). However, patients with radiologic evidence of stasis (dilated loops of small bowel, pooling of barium) do not need further documentation of delayed transit. Moreover, in those patients without gross luminal disturbance apparent on contrast studies, changes in transit speed may be difficult to interpret.

On the other hand, in CIP patients in whom colonic stasis predominates, as opposed to small bowel stasis, transit measurements may be of greater practical value by documenting either pancolonic or segmental colonic propulsive defects. Colonic transit can be measured either with radiopaque markers[15,16] or with 'gammagraphic' techniques, a variation of the whole gut transit method encapsulating the gamma-emitting label in an enteric-coated cover to release it in the distal small bowel/cecal area.

Gastrointestinal manometry

Direct measurement of gut contractile activity should, in principle, never be undertaken without: (1) having first decompressed the stomach and small bowel; and (2) without performing the pertinent imaging procedures described above to exclude mechanical obstruction. Failure to take these two preliminary steps may result in erroneous interpretation of the contractile patterns registered manometrically. With this important proviso, it is also true that gastrointestinal manometry may occasionally provide indication of an unsuspected obstruction when it shows postprandial intense minute rhythm activity and/or a characteristic pattern of high amplitude, near simultaneous phasic contractions that may be associated with mechanical impediment (Fig. 59.1). In the absence of mechanical obstruction, gastrointestinal manometry is currently the most sensitive and specific test for the diagnosis of CIP.[17–19] Gastrointestinal manometry is performed by means of an orointestinal tube fitted with perfused pressure ports or electronic sensors that record the phasic pressure waves produced by contractile activity of the stomach, duodenum, and jejunum, both fasting and postprandially. It should be performed after overnight fast. Any medication that may interfere directly or indirectly with intestinal motility (prokinetic agents, calcium channel blockers, opiates, antidepressants, and any other drugs that may interfere with gut neuromuscular activity) should be withdrawn well prior to the test procedure. A test meal is ingested after an initial 3-hour fasting recording interval to evaluate the postprandial motor pattern. The small bowel manometric recording may be used to diagnose pseudo-obstruction when the following alterations are observed:

1. *Myopathic pattern*: The typical recording would show well-coordinated contractile activity, with presence of the interdigestive motor complex in the fasting period and a postprandial pattern following ingestion of a meal, but with phasic pressure waves of decreased amplitude (>20 mmHg) due to weaker contractions by the musculature of the digestive tract (Fig. 59.2).

2. *Neuropathic pattern*: The typical recording would show contractile activity of normal amplitude, but with irregular patterns since, although the muscle remains unaffected, neurohormonal control of activity is disturbed.

Of course, mixed or non-specific manometric patterns do occur. For instance, when a neurogenic or myogenic disorder is severe and has progressed, contractile failure may develop and little pressure activity may be visible in the manometric tracing. Some have claimed that a normal gastrointestinal manometry excludes CIP,[20] but we have seen some symptomatic CIP cases with normal manometry in adults who presented evidence of enteric neuropathy on morphologic study of full-thickness biopsy of the small bowel, who later developed unequivocal manometric abnormalities.

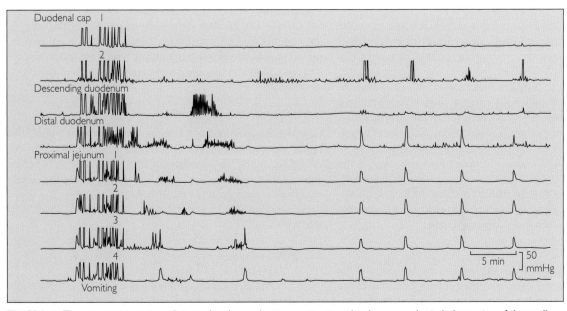

Fig. 59.1 • The manometric pattern that may be observed in some patients with subacute mechanical obstruction of the small bowel. Note the simultaneous, high-amplitude, and repetitive pressure waves detected in the duodenum and jejunum. The patients vomited at the beginning of the recording and a normally progressing interdigestive migrating motor complex-like front developed as a commonly observed postemetic event. Note that absence of this 'mechanical obstruction pattern' does not exclude such a possibility, which should be investigated by the appropriate imaging tests. (Reprinted from Manometric Diagnosis of Gastrointestinal Motility Disorders 1986: p.85. © 1986 with permission from Thieme, New York.)

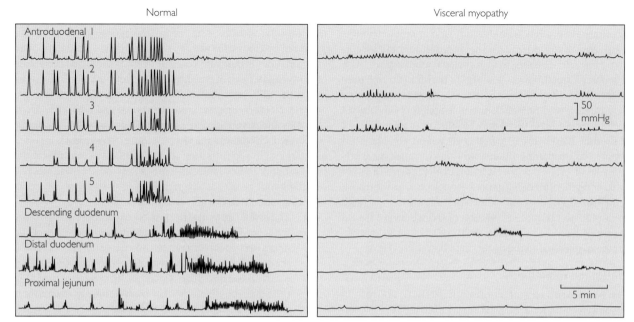

Fig. 59.2 • Typical manometric pattern in a patient with CIP caused by a visceral myopathy (panel on right). Note the normally progressing interdigestive migrating motor complex albeit with a much lower amplitude of phasic pressure waves than in the normal example shown on the left panel. In the advanced stages, very often these vestiges of normal motor activity disappear. (Reprinted from Manometric Diagnosis of Gastrointestinal Motility Disorders 1986: p.85. © 1986 with permission from Thieme, New York.)

Esophageal, colonic and anorectal manometry

Manometry is normally used to characterize the extent of the gut motor disturbance; however, it is rarely used for definitive diagnosis because contractile and/or reflex abnormalities are non-specific. It may be symptom-guided. Esophageal manometry may be useful in cases with dysphagia and/or chest pain, while colonic and/or anorectal manometry may be particularly useful in cases with prominent defecatory disturbance.[21]

Laparoscopy and laparotomy

In patients in whom it is not possible to exclude conclusively the presence of a mechanical subocclusive lesion by conventional testing, it may be necessary to resort to exploratory laparoscopy or laparotomy with direct examination of the abdominal cavity and intestinal loops. Surgical examination should always be conducted by an experienced surgeon and in a specialized center.[22] Furthermore, if no evidence of mechanical obstruction or other significant pathology is apparent at surgery, a full-thickness biopsy of the small intestine should be obtained to examine the myenteric plexus and muscle layers to ascertain the existence of a primary motor disorder. Because many centers lack sufficient experience and/or tools to perform the complex tissue analysis required, referral of the patient to a specialized center for exploratory laparotomy and biopsy is advisable.

Tissue morphology

Full-thickness specimens of the small intestine should be appropriately fixed, processed in sections cut perpendicular to the mucosa, and stained with hematoxylin and eosin, with Mason's trichrome, and processed for various specific techniques, as outlined below. Smooth muscle should be differentiated from fibrosis (and quantified) and smooth muscle cells carefully observed for morphological anomalies. Identification of enteric neuropathies requires a combination of light microscopy,

immunohistochemistry, electromicroscopy, and molecular biology techniques, and it is best performed at specialized centers. It includes assessment of neuronal loss and neuronal degenerative features, assessment of neurochemically distinct subclasses of enteric neurons and assessment of neurotropic factors and related receptors. In inflammatory forms of enteric neuropathies, the immune infiltrate may be characterized by identifying putative messengers involved in lymphocyte recruitment (chemokines) and immune-mediated neuronal damage (cytokines). A normal appearance of smooth muscle and neural tissues does not exclude CIP because some neuromuscular dysfunctions do not evidence into histopathological abnormalities. Furthermore, not all molecular disease mechanisms have been characterized. Positive findings do, however, make such diagnosis of CIP much more tenable.[23,24]

Evaluation of the extension of the disease

Once the diagnosis of small bowel disorder has been established by the above tests, the digestive and extradigestive extent of the condition should be investigated, first, to determine whether other tissues and systems are affected, and second, to help establish the etiology of the gut anormality.

Digestive

This is to be performed, if not obtained yet, during the initial diagnostic evaluation.

1. Esophagus, by esophageal manometry;
2. Stomach, by gastric emptying test; and
3. Colon, via colonic transit time, colonic manometry and/or anorectal manometry.

Extradigestive

1. *Urinary system*: It may be affected in both myopathic and neuropathic pseudo-obstruction. In advanced cases,

appropriate imaging techniques may show a dilated pyelocalyceal system and bladder. In the early stages, the involvement may only be detectable by a urodynamic study.

2. *Cardiovascular system*: It tends to be affected primarily, but not exclusively, in neuropathic pseudo-obstruction. Alterations in cardiac rhythm, orthostatic hypotension, or syncopal symptoms may occur. Abnormalities are investigated via cardiac electrical studies and the tilt table test for autonomic blood pressure regulation.

3. *Autonomous nervous system and central nervous system*: Investigated via CT scan or brain MRI, cutaneous impedance test, variation in heart rate during deep inspiration or Valsalva maneuver.

Diagnosis of complications

Complications in CIP arise from:

1. *Associated extraintestinal neuromuscular dysfunction*: This category chiefly refers to urinary tract abnormalities (ureteral and/or renal collector system dilatation, bladder dysfunction). The urological abnormalities may be clinically silent or manifested by either micturition problems or recurrent urinary tract infections.

2. *Associated autonomic dysfunction*: This complex disorder may produce orthostatic hypotension, accommodative ocular disturbances, or sweating abnormalities (see also secondary CIP).

3. *Complications of bowel dilatation and stasis*: This category includes hydroelectrolytic disturbances, aspiration pneumonia (from vomiting), small bowel bacterial overgrowth, and malnutrition.

Etiologic diagnosis in secondary chronic intestinal pseudo-obstruction

There are many conditions causing or associated with CIP (see elsewhere), and it is therefore important to follow an efficient strategy to reach the correct diagnosis. The diagnostic process may be divided into three steps: priority tests, second-line tests, and 'exceptional' tests.

Priority tests: These include a battery of easily available and relatively inexpensive blood and urine analyses. Check for blood electrolytes (chloride, sodium, potassium, calcium), thyroid hormones (T3, T4, TSH), renal function (blood urea nitrogen, creatinine), metabolism (glucose, glycosylated hemoglobin), collagen-vascular disease (antinuclear antibodies, urinary albumin, urinary sediment), dysproteinemias (protein electrophoresis). One should check initially for occult neoplasia (chiefly small cell carcinoma of the lung) by chest X-ray and antineuroenteric antibodies.

Second line tests: Second-line tests should be performed next, if the initial screening has yielded no apparent cause of CIP. Three types of second-line tests should be considered:

1. Brain imaging to check for intracranial disease (tumor, ischemic lesion, hydrocephalus): CT or MRI.

2. Imaging tests to check for occult malignancy in the thorax (negative chest X-ray) and abdomen, specially retroperitoneal or mesenteric: Usually CT scan of chest and abdomen, abdominal ultrasound, or MRI, depending on the clinical situation.

3. Small bowel/rectal biopsy to check for the possibility of amyloidosis, celiac disease, Whipple's disease, and

lymphoma, and to search for cytomegalovirus or other viral inclusions. These disorders may sometimes produce a clinical picture similar to CIP.

Exceptional tests: Exceptional tests are directed towards identifying conditions that are either rare or infrequently associated with CIP. Such conditions include abdominal vascular disease (arteriography, dynamic CT scan), rare metabolic disorders such as porphyria, heavy metal intoxication, and other even more esoteric conditions. Adds expense; think carefully before ordering.

GOALS OF THERAPY AND WELL-BEING

With the exception of some secondary forms, CIP is a chronic incurable condition. Therefore, the primary goals of therapy should be to alleviate troublesome symptoms, restore well-being, and avoid incapacitation (Table 59.1).[25]

In clinical practice, patients with CIP present with a wide spectrum of clinical severity. Some CIP patients have relatively mild symptoms: abdominal discomfort, distention, and alterations in bowel movement pattern. These mild CIP cases are able to carry on with normal nutrition and activities, and their illness resembles that of nonserious conditions such as irritable bowel syndrome or functional dyspepsia. It is even conceivable that all of these conditions share a common pathophysiology, although this possibility remains to be proven. At the other end of the spectrum are patients with very severe CIP afflicted by protracted vomiting, with a distended abdomen containing dilated loops of bowel and unable to tolerate any oral intake.

Psychological support is a key measure for chronically ill patients with CIP. In particular, patients with moderate and severe forms are often frustrated and depressed over their inability to conduct normal lives. They cannot eat what they want, they experience pain and other uncomfortable symptoms, and their physical and social activities may be significantly curtailed. Knowledge about incurability further discourages patients. Under these somewhat gloomy circumstances, many forms of psychological support are indicated. Physicians responsible for the primary care of the patients should be available and compassionate. Nursing and nutritionist assistance may help build up confidence. Psychotherapist assistance on a regular basis may facilitate coping. There is also an important role for psychopharmacological agents, particularly the newer isomeric serotonin reuptake inhibitor antidepressants with minimal anticholinergic side effects.

In some patients with CIP, the condition may be aggravated (or rarely caused solely by) various drugs that interfere pharmacologically with normal contractile and propulsive gut activity. The most common culprits are opiates, tricyclic antidepressants,

---

Table 59.1 Principles of management of chronic intestinal pseudo-obstruction

Establish a clinical diagnosis

Exclude mechanical obstruction

Differentiate between idiopathic and secondary forms

Perform a physiologic assessment

Outline a therapeutic plan

and anticholinergics. The possibility that drugs are responsible for a flare-up of the CIP syndrome should always be considered and evaluated by drug withdrawal, if feasible. Prevention and treatment of complications is another important facet of pharmacological therapy.

MANAGEMENT OF CHRONIC INTESTINAL PSEUDO-OBSTRUCTION IN THE ACUTE PHASE

Management of CIP may be somewhat arbitrarily, but conveniently, divided between acute exacerbations and maintenance between successive crises. In the acute phase (Table 59.2), standard management guidelines are:

1. Nothing by mouth;
2. Nasogastric or nasoenteric suction to decompress the digestive tract. The latter (via endoscopically guided enteric tube) may be required if there is significant upper intestinal stasis;
3. Parenteral hydration and electrolyte replacement matched to the volume aspirated. In addition, total parenteral nutrition should be considered if oral intolerance persists over 1 week; and
4. Pharmacological treatment of the motor dysfunction.[26,27] In the acute setting, drugs that may be administered parenterally should be used:
   a. *Metoclopramide*: A dopamine D_2-receptor antagonist and $5-HT_4$-receptor agonist with a weaker $5-HT_3$-receptor antagonist action at high doses. It increases the frequency and amplitude of antral contractions, improves antro-pyloric coordination and alleviates nausea and vomiting via central antiemetic action. It has potential side effects at the central nervous system level that restrict its use. It may be administered at doses of 10 mg every 8 hours by slow infusion (since boluses may induce acute anxiety).
   b. *Erythromycin*: Macrolide antibiotics act as motilin agonists. When given intravenously, they are excellent gastric prokinetic agents, inducing a powerful burst of activity that begins in the proximal stomach and extends aborally into the small bowel, resembling phase III of the interdigestive motor complex. Erythromycin is preferentially used as an acute treatment for gastroparesis at 200 mg doses, administered as rapid intravenous infusion every 6–8 hours. When administered orally, its prokinetic effect may be diminished, and some authors caution against its use, as disbacteriosis and resistances may potentially develop. However, other reports suggest that it may be useful.[28] In general, we suggest that it should be replaced by another prokinetic after a maximum treatment period of 10 days.
   c. *Octreotide*: A somatostatin analogue, it acts mainly on the small intestine, inducing activity that resembles phase III of the interdigestive motor complex, hence improving intestinal propulsion and decreasing bacterial overgrowth.[29] The recommended dose is 50 micrograms administered subcutaneously as a single night dose. It may slow down gastric emptying, and therefore, if the patient has gastroparetic symptoms, it should be combined with a prokinetic agent.
   d. *Neostigmine*: Reversible inhibitor of acetylcholinesterase, it may be administered intravenously. Indicated for acute colonic pseudo-obstruction or Ogilvie's syndrome,[30] but it may be tried in small bowel stasis, although its usefulness tends to be limited to point treatment of gas distention. Administered intravenously in a single dose of 0.5–2.5 mg, it may be repeated after several hours if necessary. The alternative (or complement) to neostigmine is colonoscopic decompression, which has a success rate of 75–90% and a relapse rate of 15% in Ogilvie's syndrome.

In severe cases, the above measures may not produce sufficient improvement for patients to maintain their nutritional status without aggravation of their abdominal symptoms. In that case, the application of venting catheters via laparoscopic surgery (gastric and/or jejunal) should be considered to maintain the intestine decompressed and, eventually, to permit nutrient intake and/or to serve as a direct route for enteral nutrition.

MAINTENANCE MANAGEMENT

Diet and lifestyle

During intercrisis periods, the objective is to maintain an adequate nutritional status, while inducing minimal or no abdominal discomfort. The following recommendations should be applied:

1. An oral diet should be administered to the extent tolerated by the patient, with additional formula nutritional supplements to attain the required daily caloric intake.
2. If a significant gastroparesis component exists, adequate nutrition may only be attainable by means of infused enteral nutrition via a gastrostomy or jejunostomy catheter (preferably with its tip located distally to the ligament of Treitz).
3. Home parenteral nutrition (TPN) should be implemented only if the patient does not tolerate oral or enteral feedings. TPN should preferably be administered sporadically, several days a week, to supplement any oral intake that the patient might accept. Shortcomings include growth retardation in children, and complicating hepatobiliary infections and metabolic events.

Table 59.2 Therapeutic plan in chronic intestinal pseudo-obstruction

Treat the cause (rarely possible)

Supporting measures
  Diet modification
  Decompression/drainage
  Correct nutritional, metabolic imbalances
  Avoid narcotic dependence
  Psychological support

Pharmacologic treatment
  Prokinetics
  Antiemetics
  Visceral hypoalgesic agents
  Antibiotics

Surgical approach
  Exceptional
  Focal (resection, plication, bypass)

Repeated vomiting and stasis may damage the esophagogastric mucosa. Therefore, adjuvant treatment with a proton pump inhibitor may be appropriate, even though there is some evidence that these agents mildly slow gastric emptying. Opioid-induced aggravation of CIP may be alleviated by using Alvimopan, a novel peripheral opioid antagonist.[31]

Disease-specific treatment

During maintenance periods, the following drugs should be considered:

1. *Orally-administered prokinetics*: These should be used when a gastroparesis component exists, possibly as an extension of the initial treatment with intravenous erythromycin.
   a. *Metoclopramide* (see above for pharmacological properties): 10 mg orally before meals. Higher doses may be given; however, the risk of dystonic reactions increases.
   b. *Domperidone*: This agent, not available in the US, is a D_2 dopamine receptor antagonist that crosses poorly the blood–brain barrier. Therefore, it acts primarily on gastric peripheral D_2 receptors diminishing proximal gastric relaxation and facilitating gastric emptying. It also acts on the area postrema (partially outside the blood–brain barrier), which confers some antiemetic action. It is given orally at a dose of 10 mg before meals. Side effects are uncommon.
   c. *Cisapride*: This drug is an agonist of gastrointestinal $5-HT_4$ receptors, facilitating the release of acetylcholine and improving gastric and intestinal contractility. It is administered in 5–20 mg doses before meals and at bedtime. A major potential side effect is cardiac arrhythmia manifested as syncope, which precipitated its withdrawal for use in the US. Risk factors include advanced age, prior cardiac pathologies, and coadministration with drugs that use the same metabolic pathway (antiarrhythmics, ketoconazole, erythromycin). Severe dispensing restrictions apply in many countries, including the US.
   d. *Tegaserod*: This agent is a selective partial $5-HT_4$ agonist that promotes propulsive peristaltic activity in the small and large bowel, accelerating bowel transit, which also possesses some antinociceptive properties. It may be useful in patients with predominant constipation, bloating, and abdominal pain. Standard doses are 6 mg orally twice daily or 12 mg as a single morning dose, but higher doses may be tried in a step-up fashion. It does not act at central nervous system levels and significant side effects appear to be rare.
   e. *Sildenafil*: This drug, used for male erectile dysfunction, is an orally active phosphodiesterase type 5 inhibitor that has been shown to promote gastric emptying in diabetic gastroparesis, at 50 mg dose.[32]
2. *Octreotide* (see above for pharmacological properties): It may be administered for an indefinite period at the previously described dosage (50 μg subcutaneously at bedtime); it helps improve motor activity of the small intestine and control bacterial overgrowth. In patients with severe abdominal pain, it may also be administered as a visceral analgesic at doses of 100–200 μg every 8 or 12 hours subcutaneously. However, at such higher doses, it may also aggravate gastroparesis and malabsorption.
3. *Antibiotics*: In patients with bacterial overgrowth (see special section below).
4. *Laxatives*: In cases with associated constipation:
   a. Fiber supplement and bulk-forming agents (unless massive small bowel stasis);
   b. Osmotic laxatives: magnesium salts and polyethylene-glycol-based preparations;
   c. Stool lubricants and softeners;
   d. Conventional contact or irritant laxatives.
      It is probably best to avoid fermentable sugars, such as lactilol and lactulose. When colonic inertia predominates, high doses or the stronger laxatives may be required.
   e. *Misoprostol*, a prostaglandin derivative with antiulcer properties that stimulates propulsive activity in the small bowel and colon, and decreases fluid reabsorption. The usual dose is 400–1200 μg daily and is best administered during the interprandial periods.
   f. *Colchicine*, the well-known antigout agent may be occasionally useful with resistant constipation. Given in setup doses from 1 to 6 mg orally, it may induce diarrhea.

Management of complications

In CIP, bacterial hypercolonization of the mid and upper gut is a major cause of malabsorption and diarrhea. When bacterial overgrowth is considered to be clinically significant, as with associated malabsorption, investigation and subsequent therapy are indicated. The initial test for the evaluation of small bowel bacterial overgrowth in CIP is the hydrogen breath test, preferably with glucose. If the test is abnormal, a 1–2-week course of antibiotic treatment should be prescribed. The following antibiotics may be administered orally: doxycycline, metronidazole, ciprofloxacin, and amoxicillin-clavunalate. After antibiotics, patients may be monitored clinically and by repeat glucose breath test. If treatment is ineffective and bacterial overgrowth is still suspected, a different antibiotic therapy should be tried. If the patient's condition still does not improve, it should probably be concluded that his or her diarrhea is unrelated to the bacterial overgrowth. If the initial glucose breath test is normal, but the clinical presentation is very suggestive of bacterial overgrowth, antibiotic treatment can be given empirically. However, chances for success under such circumstances are less likely. In many patients, antibiotic therapy needs to be re-applied at intervals because of recurrent reinfection of the small bowel, usually 5–10 days monthly with alternating antibiotics.

Mechanical and surgical approaches to palliation

Palliation via special intraluminal catheters and surgical procedures should be contemplated in selected cases. The usefulness of nasogastric or nasojejunal suction in patients with symptomatic luminal pooling in the upper and mid gut has been discussed above. Sometimes, gastric aspiration will suffice, but often it is necessary to intubate the small bowel to achieve successful intestinal decompression. In such cases, endoscopic decompression may allow rapid and effective decompression of a dilated stomach and/or small bowel. However, unless endoscopic decompression is followed by other sustaining therapeutic measures, the benefit may be short lived. Sustaining measures may be pharmacological and/or placement of permanent decompression catheters (see below). In contrast, endoscopic decompression may offer longer-lasting results in acute or subacute dilation of the colon that has not fully responded to neostigmine. Decompression via colonoscopy is most successful and long lasting with aspiration proximal to the hepatic flexure. Whether to leave a decompressing rectal tube in place is debatable, but some data suggest anal retention may be a factor in large bowel gas pooling. Endoscopic colonic decompression, as a relieving maneuver, sometimes may need to be performed repeatedly, occasionally accompanied by percutaneous endoscopic colostomy.[33] Nasogastric or intestinal aspiration may be maintained safely for several days, or even weeks provided nutritional requirements are well covered by parenteral routes. However, some patients with CIP become chronically dependent on gastric and/or intestinal 'venting' to prevent accumulation of air and secretions.[34] This long-term objective is best achieved by surgically placing a gastrostomy or jejunostomy catheter, or sometimes both (a venting gastrostomy and a venting/feeding jejunostomy). The gastrostomy may be performed endoscopically, but jejunostomy usually requires a laparotomy with insertion of silicon or polyurethane tubes into a jejunal loop close to the duodenal-jejunal angle using a subserosal tunnel method. Parenteral nutrition at home should be considered an absolutely last resort because of its inherent morbidity and mortality over extended periods of time. Circumstances that may require diagnostic laparotomy with suspected CIP is discussed above. Therapeutic surgery has a role limited in the palliation of pseudo-obstruction, although in well-selected cases it may be quite helpful.[35] On the other hand, the ill-advised use of surgery may even worsen patients, particularly if repeat 'blank' laparotomies (including lysis of adhesions) are performed. The recommended surgical procedures are diverse but focus specifically on the elimination of stagnant segments via entero-enteric anastomosis, plication, or partial resection. In addition, volvulus may develop in children with pseudo-obstruction and may require surgical correction. In general, the experience with intestinal diversion without resection has been disappointing, at least in pediatric patients. The only exception may be plication and reconstruction of dilated bowel segments in some forms of

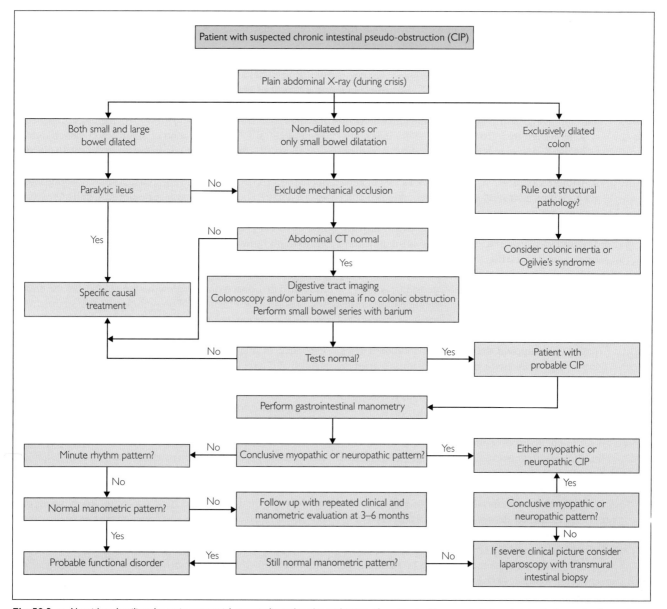

Fig. 59.3 • Algorithm detailing the main sequential steps indicated in the evaluation of a patient with suspected chronic intestinal pseudo-obstruction.

focal myopathic CIP, especially megaduodenum.[36,37] As a rule, such palliative surgical procedures are more appropriate in myogenic than neurogenic CIP. Major obstructive symptoms causing unbearable distress may require segmental resections; these may need to be very extensive and thus require a commitment to enteral or parental feeding. Transplantation may be regarded as the only definitive cure for many forms of CIP. Candidates are patients with end-stage CIP who require total parenteral nutrition to survive. Outcomes of transplantation are still relatively uncertain.[38-40] Surgical palliation is far less effective when it attempts to correct a widespread intestinal motor dysfunction, even if symptoms appear to arise from a circumscribed area. However, severe abdominal bloating or impending obstruction may be considerably alleviated by strategically placed venting stomas. Colectomy is justified in severe colonic dysfunction, although not infrequently the small bowel involvement becomes apparent afterwards. For this reason, we advise to always evaluate gastric and especially small bowel motor function by appropriate manometric and other tests prior to attempting a colonic resection in a patient with colonic inertia who does not manifest clinical evidence of upper and mid gut disfunction.

In particular, it is important to estimate prior to surgery the load of nutrients that the small bowel (or specific areas of the small bowel) is able to accept. This estimation may be accomplished by placing a nasojejunal tube and infusing via a peristaltic pump a semi-elemental formula solution, preferably isosmolar, beginning at low rates (0.25 mL/min) and gradually increasing it to rates of 2 mL/min. In general, an intake of 30 kcal/kg of ideal weight/day is an adequate goal. Since CIP patients tend to be in a stress situation, a 1.5 g/kg/day of proteins should be included. If the patient tolerates such load of enteric feedings without symptoms, the small bowel has sufficient preserved capability to sustain normal nutrition. Nevertheless, there is no guarantee that overt small bowel pseudo-obstruction will not develop over time. Implantation of gastric and intestinal pacemakers aimed at coordinating motility remains, despite considerable technical advances, an investigational approach. Gastric pacing has met, however, with some success in alleviating symptoms in patients with gastroparesis.

SUMMARY

Chronic intestinal pseudo-obstruction (CIP) is a relatively rare condition, conceptually simple to grasp but difficult to manage in practice. CIP is characterized by a stereotypical clinical picture that defines the syndrome. In addition, there may be associated manifestations that depend on the involvement of different regions or organs, the etiology, and related conditions and complications. Knowledge of the various clinical facets of CIP is a prerequisite for effective management. To establish the diagnosis of chronic intestinal pseudo-obstruction, it is essential to exclude conclusively mechanical obstruction along the gastrointestinal tract, chiefly in the small bowel. In patients in whom it is not possible to exclude conclusively the presence of a mechanical subocclusive lesion by conventional test, it may be necessary to resort to exploratory laparoscopy or laparotomy with direct examination of the abdominal cavity and intestinal loops. Management of CIP may be somewhat arbitrarily, but conveniently, divided between acute exacerbations and maintenance between successive crises. Prokinetic drugs and laxatives constitute the mainstay of maintenance therapy. When bacterial overgrowth is considered to be clinically significant, as with associated malabsorption, investigation and subsequent therapy are indicated. Palliation via special intraluminal catheters and surgical procedures should be contemplated in selected cases.

Figure 59.3 provides an overview of the evaluation of patients with chronic intestinal pseudo-obstruction.

REFERENCES

1. Christensen J, Dent J, Malagelada J-R, et al. Pseudo-obstruction. Gastroenterol Internat 1990; 3:107–119.

   A consensus document on what constitutes pseudo-obstruction.

2. Dudley HAF, Sinclair ISR, McLaren IF, et al. Intestinal pseudo-obstruction. J R Coll Surg Edinb 1958; 3:206–217.

3. Di Lorenzo C. Pseudo-obstruction: current approaches. Gastroenterology 1999; 116:980–987.

   Excellent review with emphasis on pediatric CIP.

4. Mueller LA, Camilleri M, Emslie-Smith AM. Mitochondrial neurogastrointestinal encephalomyopathy: manometric and diagnostic features. Gastroenterology 1999; 116:959–963.

   A description of the MNGIE syndrome with documentation of intestinal dysmotility by enteric manometry.

5. Bracci F, Iacobelli BD, Papadatou B, et al. Role of electrogastrography in detecting motility disorders in children affected by chronic intestinal pseudo-obstruction and Crohn's disease. Eur J Pediatr Surg 2003; 13(1):31–34.

6. Pingault V, Girard M, Bondurand N, et al. SOX10 mutations in chronic intestinal pseudo-obstruction suggest a complex physiopathological mechanism. Hum Genet 2002; 111(2):198–206. Epub 2002; Jul 06.

7. Debinski HS, Kamm MA, Talbot IC, et al. DNA viruses in the pathogenesis of sporadic chronic idiopathic intestinal pseudo-obstruction. Gut 1997; 41(1):100–106.

   Evidence linking a viral etiology to cases of sporadic CIP.

8. Jain D, Moussa K, Tandon M, et al. Role of interstitial cells of Cajal in motility disorders of the bowel. Am J Gastroenterol 2003; 98(3):618–624.

9. Lyford G, Foxx-Orenstein A. Chronic intestinal pseudoobstruction. Curr Treat Options Gastroenterol 2004; 7(4):317–325.

   A good updated review on CIP by a group with ample experience.

10. Smith DS, Williams CS, Ferris CD. Diagnosis and treatment of chronic gastroparesis and chronic intestinal pseudo-obstruction. Gastroenterol Clin North Am 2003; 32(2):619–658.

11. Stanghellini V, Camilleri M, Malagelada J-R. Chronic idiopathic intestinal pseudo-obstruction: clinical and intestinal manometric findings. Gut 1987; 28:5–12.

12. Delgado-Aros S, Camilleri M. Pseudo-obstruction in the critically ill. Best Pract Res Clin Gastroenterol 2003; 17(3):427–444.

13. Lapointe SP, Rivet C, Goulet O, et al. Urological manifestations associated with chronic intestinal pseudo-obstructions in children. J Urol 2002; 168(4 Pt 2):1768–1770.

14. Nightingale JM. The medical management of intestinal failure: methods to reduce the severity. Proc Nutr Soc 2003; 62(3):703–710.

15. Sloots CE, Felt-Bersma RJ. Effect of bowel cleansing on colonic transit in constipation due to slow transit or evacuation disorder. Neurogastroenterol Motil 2002; 14:55–61.

16. Fort JM. Azpiroz F, Casellas F, et al. Bowel habit after cholecystectomy: physiological changes and clinical implications. Gastroenterologist 1996; III: 617–622.

17. Malagelada J-R, Camilleri M, Stanghellini V. Manometric diagnosis of gastrointestinal motility disorders. New York: Thieme-Stratton; 1986.

   The original description of human gastrointestinal manometry and its clinical applicability. It contains numerous tracing of actual cases. Useful to learn how to read manometric tracings in the stomach and small bowel.

18. Camilleri M, Parkman H, Quigley EMM, et al. Measurement of gastroduodenal motility in the GI laboratory. Gastroenterology 1998; 115:747–762.

19. Fell JME, Smith VV, Milla PJ. Infantile chronic idiopathic intestinal pseudo-obstruction: the role of small intestinal manometry as a diagnostic tool and prognostic indicator. Gut 1996; 39: 306–311.

   The role of intestinal manometry in the differentiation of myopathic or neuropathic CIP in the first 2 years of life.

20. Cucchiara S, Borrelli O, Salvia G, et al. A normal gastrointestinal motility excludes chronic intestinal pseudoobstruction in children. Dig Dis Sci 2000; 45(2):258–264.

21. Pensabene L, Youssef NN, Griffiths JM, et al. Colonic manometry in children with defecatory disorders: role in diagnosis and management. Am J Gastroenterol 2003; 98(5):1052–1057.

22. Murr MM, Sarr MG, Camilleri M. The surgeon's role in the treatment of chronic intestinal pseudoobstruction. Am J Gastroenterol 1995; 90:2147–2151.

   Important review helping to define the uses of surgery in the management of CIP.

23. Streutker CJ, Huizinga JD, Campbell F, et al. Loss of CD117 (c-kit)- and CD34-positive ICC and associated CD34-positive fibroblasts defines a subpopulation of chronic intestinal pseudo-obstruction. Am J Surg Pathol 2003; 27(2):228–235.

24. Fava M, Borghini S, Cinti R, et al. HOX11L1: a promoter study to evaluate possible expression defects in intestinal motility disorders. Int J Mol Med 2002; 10(1):101–106.

25. Schwankovsky L, Mousa H, Rowhani A, et al. Quality of life outcomes in congenital chronic intestinal pseudo-obstruction. Dig Dis Sci 2002; 47(9):1965–1968.

26. Malagelada JR, Distrutti E. Management of gastrointestinal motility disorders. A practical guide to drug selection and appropriate ancillary measures. Drugs 1996; 52:494–506.

27. Pandolfino JE, Howden CW, Kahrilas PJ. Motility-modifying agents and management of disorders of gastrointestinal motility. Gastroenterology 2000; 118:S32–S47.

28. Emmanuel AV, Shand AG, Kamm MA. Erythromycin for the treatment of chronic intestinal pseudo-obstruction: description of six cases with a positive response. Aliment Pharmacol Ther 2004; 19(6):687–694.

29. Soudah HC, Hasler WL, Owyang C. Effect of octreotide on intestinal motility and bacterial overgrowth in scleroderma. N Engl J Med 1991; 325:1461–1467.

30. Ponce RJ, Saunders MD, Kimmey MB. Neostigmine for the treatment of acute colonic pseudo-obstruction. N Engl J Med 1999; 341:137–141.

31. Schmidt WK. Alvimopan* (ADL 8-2698) is a novel peripheral opioid antagonist. Am J Surg 2001; 182(5A Suppl):27S–38S.

32. Bianco A, Pitocco D, Valenza V, et al. Effect of sildenafil on diabetic gastropathy. Diabetes Care 2002; 25:1888–1889.

33. Thompson AR, Pearson T, Ellul J, et al. Percutaneous endoscopic colostomy in patients with chronic intestinal pseudo-obstruction. Gastrointest Endosc 2004; 59(1):113–115.

34. Pitt HA, Mann LL, Berquist WE, et al. Chronic intestinal pseudo-obstruction. Management with total parenteral nutrition and a venting enterostomy. Arch Surg 1985; 120:614–618.

   It describes the placement and maintenance of intraluminal catheters for intestinal decompression in CIP.

35. Shibata C, Naito H, Funayama Y, et al. Surgical treatment of chronic intestinal pseudo-obstruction: report of three cases. Surg Today 2003; 33(1):58–61.

36. Mansell PI, Tattersall RB, Balsitis M. Megaduodenum due to hollow visceral myopathy successfully managed by duodenoplasty and feeding jejunostomy. Gut 1991; 32:334–337.

37. Loire J, Gouillat C, Partensky C. Megaduodenum in chronic intestinal pseudo-obstruction: management by duodenectomy-duodenoplasty. Gastroenterol Clin Biol 2000; 24(1):21–25.

38. Nishida S, Levi D, Kato T, et al. Ninety-five cases of intestinal transplantation at the University of Miami. J Gastrointest Surg 2002; 6(2):233–239.

   A large series of intestinal transplantation at a specialized US medical center: outcomes, pitfalls, hopes.

39. Iyer K, Kaufman S, Sudan D, et al. Long-term results of intestinal transplantation for pseudo-obstruction in children. J Pediatr Surg 2001; 36(1):174–177.

40. Mousa H, Hyman PE, Cocjin J, et al. Long-term outcome of congenital intestinal pseudoobstruction. Dig Dis Sci 2002; 47(10):2298–2305.

CHAPTER SIXTY

Hirschsprung's disease

Peter J. Milla

INTRODUCTION

History, epidemiology, and presentation

Congenital aganglionosis or Hirschsprung's disease (HSCR) was first described by Harald Hirschsprung in 1887.[1] It occurs in about 1 in 4500 live births, and results in a distal aganglionic segment of bowel of variable length. There is a male predominance of 3.8:1. In about 75% of patients the abnormal segment is restricted to the rectosigmoid colon. In a small minority (about 8%) the condition may be more widespread, involving the whole colon (total colonic aganglionosis) or even the entire gastrointestinal tract.[2–8] In about 7% of those with the short-segment disease there is a familial tendency, increasing to about 21% in patients with total colonic aganglionosis. Most patients present in the first few days of life, 95% failing to pass meconium in the first 24 hours of life. Five percent may present later with constipation and 30% with symptoms of an enterocolitis. Fewer than 1% are not diagnosed until adult life.[8–13]

Presentation varies with the age of the patient and the extent of disease. In the newborn period, bilious emesis, abdominal distention, and failure to pass meconium or abnormal stool frequency are common. Complete intestinal obstruction may occur, and perforation of the cecum or the appendix occurs in 3–5%. If diagnosis is not established in the newborn period, infants may present with constipation. This most often occurs in breast-fed infants.[14] It may be followed by acute obstruction, frequent episodes of fecal impaction, or the development of acute life-threatening enterocolitis. Enterocolitis develops in 15–50% of cases, may be the initial feature of HSCR in up to 12% of patients and is the main cause of death, the mortality reaching 20–50%.[7,15–17]

From infancy until adulthood, mild to severe constipation may be the only symptom of HSCR.[16–20] Because clinical features do not allow complete differentiation between these problems, the diagnosis of HSCR must always be considered in any child, adolescent, adult with severe intractable constipation[11,18,20] or in any child or infant with a history of onset from birth or very shortly thereafter. Where the diagnosis is established in adult life (mean age 26 years, range 11–73), most have had symptoms since childhood and frequently only evacuate their bowel with enemas. Occasionally chronic colitis and pseudopolyps have been reported.[11,12]

Genetics

Hirschsprung's disease can be sporadic or familial, has a complex genetic pattern, and appears to be polygenic or multifactorial.[21–23] A higher incidence of familial involvement has been reported in females and in patients with long segment disease.[8,24,25]

Two major cell signaling systems required for development and maintenance of the enteric nervous system are involved, the RET/GDNF (glial-cell line derived neurotrophic factor[26–31]) and the endothelin systems,[32,33] but mutations in transcription factors known to be important for neuronal development, such as SOX 10,[34] SIPl and, more recently, PMX2B,[35] as-yet undefined genes, may be required for the HSCR phenotype. HSCR may also be associated with Waardenburg syndrome, Smith-Lemli-Opitz syndrome, Down syndrome and multiple endocrine neoplasia syndrome type 2A (MEN 2A).[36] The latter association ties up with the RET abnormalities encountered in Hirschsprung's disease as well as in MEN 2A. The former suggests that there may be a relevant locus on the X chromosome resulting in the Hirschsprung phenotype.

The RET gene, which maps to chromosome IOqll.2[27,29,30] and codes for a cell surface tyrosine kinase receptor, is the major gene involved in human HSCR, and mutations of this gene occur in approximately 50% of familial and sporadic cases of HSCR.[36] As part of the RET-GDNF-GFRal signaling system, RET promotes the survival of neurons, mitosis of progenitor cells, and differentiation of neurons. *Ret-1–* knockout mice have aganglionosis of the small and large intestines and there is an association with renal agenesis. The RET receptor tyrosine kinase consists of an intracellular tyrosine kinase, a transmembrane domain, and an extracellular domain in neurons and neuronal precursor cells. Mutations affecting the intracellular domain affect signaling functions, whereas those affecting the extracellular domain affect ligand binding.[37,38] Multiple mutations resulting in loss of function have been identified that are associated with HSCR, but where they cause a gain of function they are associated with the development of other conditions such as familial medullary thyroid carcinoma (FMTC), multiple endocrine neoplasia (MEN) 2A, and MEN 2E. Around 5% of patients with HSCR will have an associated MEN 2A or FMTC.[38]

Glial-derived neurotrophic factor (GDNF) is a ligand for the RET receptor and requires the co-receptor GFRal for effective signaling.[26,28] It acts on early ENS precursor cells to stimulate differentiation, and in in vitro studies can attract migrating ENS cells.[28] Heterozygosity of *GDNF* may contribute to the severity of the HSCR phenotype, but is not responsible for it. Although not described in humans, the *gdnf*–/– knockout mouse has a similar phenotype to the *ret*–/– mouse. Other members of the GDNF family have now been identified (neurturin, artemin, persephin), but mutations in their genes have not been demonstrated to result in HSCR.

Endothelin signaling system

The endothelin (ET) system in the developing embryo may regulate interactions between gut neural crest and mesenchyme cells. The endothelin family consists of ET-1, ET-2, ET-3, and VIP, but it is ET-3 that is important in ENS development via its interaction with the endothelin receptor-B (ETRB). This has been demonstrated in mouse knockout models. The lethal spotted mouse mutant *(ls/ls)* has distal colonic aganglionosis secondary to a mutation in the *Et-3* gene, and colonic aganglionosis is found to a greater extent in the piebald lethal mouse, which lacks the *ETRB* gene. *ET-3* mutations are associated with approximately 5% of human HSCR cases, with mutations of *ETB* accounting for 5–7% of cases. Mutations of the *ET-3* and *ETRB* genes have been described in the Shah-Waardenburg syndrome, which is characterized by enteric aganglionosis, skin and hair pigmentation defects, and sensorineural hearing loss.[39] As well as ET-3 and ETRB abnormalities, mutations in the endothelin converting enzyme-l can lead to the presentation of aganglionosis, albeit with associated autonomic, craniofacial, and cardiac abnormalities.[39] Mutations of other signaling systems, including the hedgehog signaling system, may have a role in congenital enteric aganglionosis but, given the widespread role of these systems in embryonic development, it is unlikely that enteric aganglionosis would present without many other complex abnormalities.

In familial cases, in all families so far studied *RET* has always been involved, but mutations in at least two other genes are required for expression of the phenotype.[40] Routine screening for *RET* or other mutations is not yet practical and, due to incomplete understanding of the complex genetic nature of the condition, is not yet clinically indicated.

PATHOGENESIS

Developmental basis

The loss of innervation of the distal segment of bowel is due to failure of colonization of the bowel by neural crest cells in early embryonic development from 4 to 10 weeks of gestation.[37] Recent advances in understanding the developmental neurobiology of the enteric nervous system shows that the intrinsic innervation of the gut is developed from neural crest cells from the vagal and sacral neural crest which migrate into and colonize the bowel in a mainly cranio-caudal direction. Within the primitive gut the precursor cells proliferate and differentiate into the multitude of different neurons and glial cells required for the enteric nervous system. This process requires the correct sequence of events coded for by many different genes to occur in both the precursor cells and the environment into which they are moving if a functional nervous system is to develop. Study of animal models and of humans with HSCR has shown that aganglionosis may

result from defects of either the neural crest cells themselves (RET or ETRB) or abnormality of the mesenchymal environment (GDNF or ET-3) into which they are migrating.

Pathophysiology

The aganglionosis in HSCR results in a lack of intrinsic enteric inhibitory nerves, with loss of inhibition of the enteric musculature due to absence of intrinsic nitrergic and peptidergic neurons. This results in a contracted segment of gut with loss of the recto-anal sphincteric reflex. The proximal normal ganglionic bowel is dilated, tapering to the narrowed distal aganglionic bowel.[41]

DIAGNOSIS

The diagnosis needs to be based on the pathologic demonstration of aganglionosis before definitive surgery is undertaken.[5] Because obtaining biopsy specimens involves a degree of risk, and because expert histopathology may not be available, other less invasive techniques such as barium enema and anorectal manometry have been used to select patients who require a biopsy.

Barium enema

The barium enema, although not diagnostic, can be suggestive and supportive.[5] A single-contrast enema is used, and the colon is not prepared. In infants with HSCR, a transition zone from the distal nondilated colon is usually easily detected.[13] However, the absence of a transition zone does not exclude the diagnosis,[10] as it may be absent in 20–30% of patients.[42] In patients with total colonic aganglionosis, the entire colon may appear normal. Barium enema is less helpful in the newborn because a visible transition zone is often not present.

Anorectal manometry

In normal individuals, distention of the rectum causes relaxation of the internal anal sphincter (IAS). This effect is absent in patients with HSCR.[43] After the newborn period, manometry has been shown to accurately diagnose Hirschsprung's disease in 90–100% of patients, with a specificity of 97% and sensitivity of 79%.[44]

In newborns and premature infants the diagnostic accuracy of manometry is lower (from 90% to 70%)[43,44] because it is more difficult to perform, and inaccurate results are more common,[43] with both false-positive and false-negative tests.[44]

Rectal biopsy

Confirming the absence of ganglion cells in the abnormal segment of colon is critical to the diagnosis of HSCR.[45,46] Suction rectal biopsy, which produces a specimen of mucosa and submucosa, is commonly used and allows assessment of the submucous plexus. Accuracy is excellent if the specimen is adequate and if a trained pathologist is available. When ganglion cells are present, the diagnosis of HSCR is excluded even if only one ganglion cell is seen. Inadequate suction rectal biopsies, however, may fail to reveal ganglion cells in up to 39% of patients without HSCR,[45,46] almost always because no submucosa is included in the biopsy. The use of immunohistochemical stains for acetylcholinesterase in combination with hematoxylin and eosin staining can increase the accuracy of diagnosis to a sensitivity of 97–100% with a specificity of 100%. A marked increase in acetylcholinesterase activity is seen in the lamina propria and muscularis mucosae of patients with HSCR.[46,47]

For cases in which suction biopsy has produced equivocal results or is inadequate, it may be necessary to obtain a full-thickness specimen of the rectal wall, which requires a surgical procedure under general anesthesia.[48] Such biopsies allow the evaluation of both the myenteric plexus and submucosal plexus, and some use this procedure to confirm every diagnosis before definitive surgical correction. However, if an experienced pathologist is available and the suction biopsy specimen shows a lack of ganglion cells with abnormal acetylcholinesterase staining, no further diagnostic steps are necessary before definitive surgery is undertaken.

Rectal biopsy is the gold standard and the diagnostic method of choice.

TREATMENT

Initial management

Definitive treatment of HSCR at the present time is surgical.[13–17,49] However, initial medical management to stabilize the patient before surgery is important. Correction of dehydration and electrolyte imbalance, antibiotic therapy for *Clostridia difficile* if enterocolitis is present, and colonic decompression with the use of physiological saline rectal washouts and rectal tubes[50] until the time of surgery may be necessary.

Short segment disease

Definitive surgery

The principle of definitive surgery is to relieve the distal obstruction by resection of the aganglionic segment, followed by a 'pull-through' of ganglionic bowel down to the anus.[5] Traditional surgical treatments consist of either a two- or three-stage operation (an initial colostomy, followed later by a definitive 'pull-through' and/or subsequent closure of the stoma).[51] Usually, the

pull-through is performed at the age of 9–12 months or when the child weighs 8–10 kg.[2]

Three 'pullthrough' operations have stood the test of time: Swenson pull-through (rectosigmoidectomy), Duhamel pull-through (retrorectal transanal pull-through), and Soave pull-through (endorectal pullthrough) (Fig. 60.1).[52] The Swenson pull-through procedure was the first definitive operation to be developed for this disease. It involves resection of the aganglionic segment and anastomosis of the normal ganglionic proximal bowel to a 1–2-cm rectal cuff (see Fig. 60.1).[7,53] It requires a combined abdominoperineal approach, is probably the most difficult technically, and requires extensive pelvic dissection, so injury to the sacral innervation of the bladder and ejaculatory mechanisms may occur. In an effort to avoid the extensive pelvic dissection, other surgical alternatives have been proposed.

In the Duhamel pull-through, the aganglionic rectum is left in place, and normal ganglionic bowel is brought down behind the rectum and through an incision in the posterior rectal wall at the level of the internal anal sphincter.[54]

The pelvic dissection is thus limited to the retrorectal space.[54] The original Duhamel procedure used anastomosis of the ganglionated proximal bowel to the closed native rectum at the anal verge. Dilatation of the rectum by fecal retention in the blind loop resulted in the addition of a proximal suture anastomosis of the anterior native rectum to the pulled through colon,[52] thus creating a rectum of expanded size with an anterior aganglionic wall and a posterior ganglionic wall.

The third alternative is the endorectal pull-through originally described by Soave.[52] In this procedure the mucosal lining of the rectum is removed by submucosal dissection to the anus and the normally innervated colon is passed through the rectal muscular tube for anastomosis within 1 cm of the anal verge (see Fig. 60.1).[52,55] The modified Soave procedure is relatively easy to perform, and the procedure obviates the need for any pelvic dissection.

The incidence of complications is probably determined more by the skill of the individual surgeon and the underlying factors determining the presence of the aganglionosis than the type of operation performed. The outcome of short segment HSCR shows

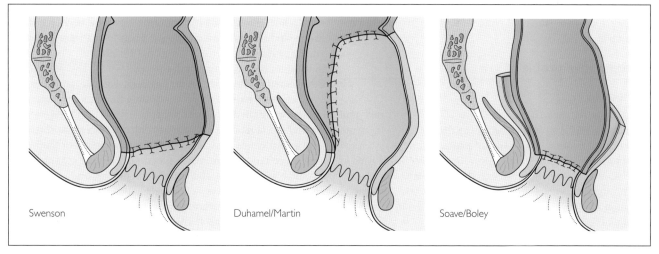

Swenson   Duhamel/Martin   Soave/Boley

Fig. 60.1 • The three major operative procedures for Hirschsprung's disease. The unshaded portion of the rectum is aganglionic, and the shaded pull-through bowel contains ganglion cells. (Modified from Philippart AI. Hirschsprung's disease. In: Aschcraft KW, Holder TM, eds. Pediatric surgery. 2nd edn. Philadelphia: WB Saunders; 1993:358–371.)

disrupted anastomoses (11%) and enterocolitis (16%) to be commoner after Swenson pull-throughs than after Duhamel (2% and 6%, respectively) or Soave (6% and 2%, respectively) operations, but for anal stenosis and incontinence to be much the same (3–5%) whatever operation was done.[2,55]

Long-term outcome

There are few descriptions of the long-term outcome of treatment of HSCR. Undoubtedly, the outcome for total colonic and total intestinal aganglionosis, both morbidity and mortality, is quite different than that for short segment disease and will be considered separately. For short segment HSCR long-term survival is excellent, although sudden death from enterocolitis may occur years after successful surgical reconstruction.[16] Many studies, however, show a higher than anticipated incidence of problems, particularly persistent obstruction, fecal incontinence, or enterocolitis.[5,56–58] Several large studies have shown that between 50% and 75% of patients considered that their pattern of defecation was normal, and about 20% had a degree of fecal incontinence (6% severe) which improved with age. Recurrent enterocolitis occurs in 2–30%, 6% after operation for the first time. Growth overall was comparable to the normal population. Delayed development occurred in 8–10% and behavioral problems in 3%. The functional results were largely determined by the length of the aganglionic segment beyond the rectosigmoid and the degree of neurologic impairment. However, the outcome was less favorable for those who underwent a Swenson pull-through compared to a Soave or Duhamel operation. The increased incidence of abdominal distention, micturition, and sexual dysfunction, together with the anal stenosis and disrupted anastomoses that occur early after operation, has led to the Swenson pull-through being much less popular today.

Surgical advances in the last 10 years have been the demonstration that a primary pull-through operation may be as effective as a staged procedure in the newborn period,[17,51,59,60] and that short-term outcome are the same.[51] Recent reports have also described the surgical treatment of Hirschsprung's disease by laparoscopic surgery,[60,61] either in neonates or in older children. The procedure entails performing the pull-through laparoscopically and the rectal dissection and anastomosis transrectally. The results in small studies are comparable to those of open methods, and the techniques appear to be safe and effective.[60,61] However, long-term studies of either of these techniques are not yet available.

Postoperative problems

Enterocolitis

Enterocolitis remains the major cause of both morbidity and mortality in HSCR with Hirschsprung's disease.[5,9,16,62] It occurs after surgical treatment in 2–33% of patients[14] and is associated with mortality ranging from 0% to 30%.[3,13–15,63] It appears to occur more commonly after Swenson than after Duhamel or Soave pull-through operations. It commonly presents with abdominal distention in 83%, explosive diarrhea in 69%, vomiting in 51%, fever in 34%, lethargy in 27%, rectal bleeding in 5%, and colonic perforation in 2.5%. Chronic diarrhea (longer than 2 weeks) was present in 54% and delayed growth in 44%. The occurrence of explosive diarrhea in any patient with Hirschsprung's disease should suggest the diagnosis, even in the absence of systemic symptoms.[15,16,62] The presence of postoperative enterocolitis needs to be recognized promptly, as a child can initially have mild symptoms followed by a rapidly fulminating course that may lead to death. The diagnosis is aided by abdominal X-ray showing an intestinal cutoff sign and at least two air-fluid levels.[13,63] Endoscopic examination will show colitis and the presence of pseudomembranes if *Clostridia* is present. A barium enema is rarely indicated.[15,62]

The pathogenesis continues to be poorly understood.[64] Fecal stasis and bacterial overgrowth seem important. Associations between enterocolitis and the presence of *Clostridium difficile* have been reported although recent reports indicate that in up to two-thirds of patients, toxin determination for *C. difficile* or stool cultures for other pathogens are negative.[15] Other organisms that have been associated with enterocolitis include rotavirus, retrovirus, *Pseudomonas*, or *Escherichia coli*. If the enterocolitis is secondary to *C. difficile*,[16] the clinical findings may be more fulminant, with rapid progression, shock and prostration, and eventually death.[16]

The treatment of choice includes fluid and electrolyte support, antibiotics, and the use of transrectal decompression either by tube or by sphincter dilatation, or rectal washout.[5,15,16,62] Antibiotics against *C. difficile* and bowel flora should be started empirically as soon as the appropriate cultures are obtained.[16,62] However, it is necessary to remain alert for the occurrence of idiopathic forms of inflammatory bowel disorder in the setting of HSCR.

Fecal incontinence

Fecal incontinence occurs much more commonly than is generally thought. In one long-term study designed specifically to evaluate the extent of incontinence,[57] it was found to be present in 80% of patients. In 53%, fecal incontinence was significant with constant leaking, and in 27% the incontinence was less severe. Contrary to other reports, the incontinence did not diminish with increasing age. The mean age of the patients was 10.1 ± 3.6 years, and the age at definitive surgery, sex of the child, the extent of aganglionosis, the type of surgery, and early or late postoperative complications did not influence the presence or absence of postoperative incontinence. Children with soiling were more likely to have loose stools, a history of anal dilatation, and emotional disturbances.

The pathophysiology of the incontinence is not well understood. Different manometric abnormalities have been described. In one study, 10% of patients were not able to squeeze voluntarily, and impaired rectal sensation was most commonly present after the Duhamel or Swenson pull-through (50%). The presence of the rectoanal inhibitory reflex has been variable and does not correlate with outcome,[49,65,66] indicating that other factors must influence continence in these patients.

Careful evaluation is necessary in order to differentiate between fecal incontinence due to overflow and encopresis or to abnormalities in colonic or anorectal function. Physical examination, colonic transit studies, abdominal radiographs, and colonic and anorectal manometry will allow such differentiation.

Treatment of fecal incontinence is complex. If related to constipation, laxatives and aperients may be helpful. Other treatments have included enemas, bowel management tubes,[67] or more recently, antegrade colonic enemas.[68] On the other hand, if the fecal incontinence is not related to constipation but to anorectal dysfunction, enemas to maintain an empty rectosigmoid together with dietary manipulation and biofeedback therapy are indicated.[56] Where it is associated with excessive propulsive rectosigmoid contractile activity, anticholinergic drugs such as propantheline may help.[69] Where incontinence is very severe and results in serious degradation of quality of life, consideration should be given to reverting to a stoma.

Obstruction

Recurrent obstruction is one of the most common and difficult to manage postoperative symptoms occurring in HSCR.[3] Obstructive symptoms may be related either to an anatomic problem, usually anal stenosis, or to functional disorder.[17,49,56,58] Anal stenosis can usually be managed with dilatation,[8] although a secondary surgical procedure may be necessary, most commonly after a Swenson pull-through. Stenosis in the pulled-through bowel has also been described, both probably secondary to ischemic damage.

Most patients with obstructive symptoms do not have stenosis. In one study in which 107 patients were monitored for at least 4 years, 15% had recurrent episodes of gaseous distention and symptoms suggestive of persisting obstruction in the absence of an anatomically defined lesion. Such symptoms may be as a consequence of a retained aganglionic segment after an inadequate initial operation.[56] The exact incidence of this complication is difficult to establish. The aganglionosis may also be *acquired* or *secondary* after a successful initial operation. Such occurrence is rare but has been well documented.[49,63] This complication has been reported after any of the different corrective procedures, and whilst it may be related to a hypoxic insult[49,63] we now know that aganglionosis may occur following various forms of lymphocytic ganglionitis,[70] which are progressive, and if this is the case, then the original diagnosis of HSCR was incorrect. Further investigation to demonstrate circulating enteric neuronal antibodies of the anti-Hu variety should be undertaken in both children and adults, and treatment of the underlying autoimmune disorder with immunosuppressive drugs commenced. In adults a search for an associated small round cell carcinoma of the lung must also be undertaken.[70] If aganglionosis is suspected, a barium enema may show a transition zone, and four-quadrant rectal suction biopsy at different levels will be necessary to confirm the aganglionosis, or as a consequence of associated neuronal pathology including intestinal neuronal dysplasia.

Some authors have suggested that *intestinal neuronal dysplasia* (IND) type B in children with HSCR may be associated with the presence of obstructive symptoms.[48,49,54] This type of IND is characterized by malformations of the parasympathetic submucous plexus and can be found in a proportion of patients which varies between 1% and 25% in different studies of children with HSCR.[71] Anorectal manometry is not useful in the diagnosis of IND,[72] so diagnosis depends upon a full-thickness rectal biopsy.[48] The value of suction rectal biopsy for the diagnosis of IND is controversial, and recent studies have raised questions about its usefulness and accuracy.[48] The significance of IND as a clinicopathologic entity apart from associated with HSCR is somewhat questionable.[48,72] Whereas some authors suggest that IND may be associated with obstructive symptoms, others believe that its presence may not be significant.[48,71,72] Hanimann and coworkers[71] reported that in 47 cases 11 (23%) had associated IND and that after a mean follow-up of 5 years, no differences in symptoms were seen in patients with IND and those without it. Cord-Udy et al.[48] reported that the histologic criteria of IND were not helpful in predicting clinical outcome and suggested that the finding of IND should not influence clinical management. It is clear, however, that some symptomatic children with HSCR may have motility abnormalities related to neuronal dysplasia in the residual colon. Therefore, in children with HSCR who have undergone definitive surgery and who have obstructive symptoms, it may be necessary to obtain a full-thickness rectal biopsy specimen to exclude the presence of IND. In such children, management should be conservative unless symptoms are severe and clearly associated with the abnormal segment, when surgical resection may be necessary.[73]

Functional obstruction may also be as a consequence of the inflammation associated with enterocolitis. Although the inflammatory process is primarily present in the lamina propria of the mucosa, the neuromusculature as in other inflammatory bowel disorders may become involved.[74] Persistent IAS dysfunction is another possible cause of obstructive symptoms. This dysfunction is sometimes referred as to 'internal sphincter achalasia,'[75] and is related to specific abnormalities in IAS innervation.[41] Because current surgical treatment preserves the IAS, a distinct sphincteric abnormality may explain some of the frequently observed long-term obstructive symptoms.[41,58] It is possible that high IAS tone produces a functional outflow obstruction that with time leads to colonic dilatation and less efficient peristalsis to expel stool.[49,67] Because of sphincteric abnormalities, some authors have suggested that an internal sphincter myotomy or partial myectomy should be performed in patients with postoperative obstructive symptoms that have not responded to medical management.[76–78] Partial myectomy has been shown to significantly decrease IAS pressure.[78] Even though the initial experience suggested a poor response after partial myectomy,[53] recent reports have shown it to be useful in the treatment of these children.[77,78] Sphincter-dividing procedures are not always effective and are sometimes associated with fecal incontinence. With the extensive use of botox in children with skeletal muscle problems and in the treatment of internal sphincteric achalasia,[75] it has been suggested that it could be used to produce a 'medical' myectomy to allow evaluation of a reduction in sphincter pressure without permanent sphincter destruction.[79] Further studies are required to evaluate the role of this potential modality of treatment.

If an anatomic problem such as a stricture or anal stenosis is present, it should be corrected. If aganglionosis is present, the segment should be removed and definitive surgery carried out. If the patient has IND, laxatives, aperients, and prokinetic agents are indicated.[49] If the colonic transit study and anorectal manometry indicate that the obstruction is at the level of the internal sphincter, a partial myectomy or myotomy may be considered.[49] If the symptoms do not improve and there is evidence of colonic distention and malfunction, further surgery needs to be considered. Such surgery may involve performing a new pull-through operation, though redo procedures have a higher incidence of complications. A flowchart of these factors in the pathogenesis of obstruction is shown in Fig. 60.2 in the form of a treatment algorithm.

It may also be necessary at times to create a colostomy or ileostomy if obstructive symptoms or recurrent enterocolitis persists.

In more recent years, antegrade colonic enemas have been developed as a method of treating constipation and fecal incontinence of various causes, including Hirschsprung's disease.[80]

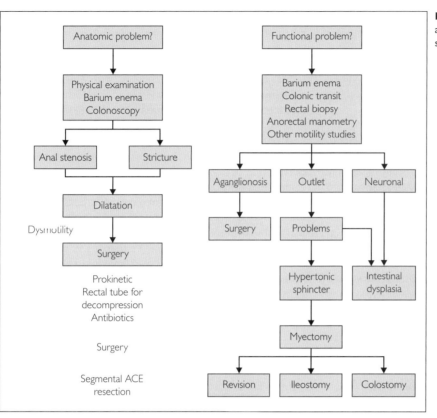

Fig. 60.2 • Algorithm for the evaluation and treatment of patients with obstructive symptoms.

The antegrade colonic enema procedure produces a continent conduit from the skin to the cecum that can be catheterized for self-administration of enemas.[80] This technique can be accomplished either surgically with the use of an appendiceal stump or percutaneously with the insertion of a cecostomy tube under local anesthesia.[80] The procedure tends to be more successful in patients with defects in extrinsic innervation such as spina bifida, but in short-term studies, antegrade colonic enemas have been shown to be effective in children with Hirschsprung's disease in whom a permanent colostomy was being considered for the treatment of refractory constipation or incontinence. There are as yet no long-term follow-up data and the decision as to which course to follow is often determined by patient preference. Success is the product of the patient's motivation to carry out the care required after either of these procedures.

Total colonic and total intestinal Hirschsprung's disease

Definitive surgery

In total colonic and total intestinal HSCR, complications are more frequent and more severe than in patients with shorter segment disease.[49,81–83] The mortality rate is higher and may be as high as 47%.[8,81–83] Improvements in medical management of complications, particularly in parenteral and enteral nutrition, as well as in surgical techniques, have decreased such high mortality rates and allowed the survival of those with total intestinal HSCR. Surgical therapy initially includes an ileostomy, followed at a later stage by an endorectal pull-through along with total colectomy or a long side-to-side anastomosis with the aganglionic distal end of the rectum.[81–83] In total intestinal HSCR a high jejunostomy and gastrostomy are the preferred surgical treatments, followed by long-term home parenteral nutrition and, where and when necessary, intestinal transplantation.

Postoperative problems and long-term outcome

Fecal incontinence occurs in the majority in the early postoperative period, and failure to thrive, malnutrition, and disturbances in electrolyte balance, lipid metabolism, and vitamin B_{12} absorption have all been described.[81] A common problem is that of recurrent obstructive episodes which lead to intestinal dilatation, diarrhea, and postoperative enterocolitis.[81–83] Almost certainly, these episodes are as a result of dysmotility of the apparently normally innervated gut. A number of studies have shown that abnormal motility occurs in the upper gastrointestinal tract well above the aganglionic segment.[84] In such patients, intermittent antibiotics and irrigation via a rectal tube are required chronically for decompression. If it is clear that the patient has a functional obstruction at the level of the sphincter, a partial myectomy may be indicated. This operation should be performed only in patients who have been fully evaluated, inasmuch as fecal incontinence may result after the procedure. In those with severe and recurrent symptoms, it may be necessary to return to a decompression stoma as in patients with intestinal pseudo-obstruction. With aggressive follow-up and nutritional support, as well as treatment of obstructive episodes, most patients who survive will eventually attain normal growth and the ability to feed enterally. Long-term follow-up (12–23 years) has, however, shown that although survivors develop normally and are socially and professionally integrated, fecal incontinence remains a significant problem. All had accelerated passage of stool, but one study has shown that 75% were incontinent at 5 years, 50% at

10 years and 25% at 15 years after definitive surgery in this group of patients with HSCR.[83] Enterocolitis occurred even long after initial repair, so these patients need to be followed closely for many years.

FUTURE DIRECTIONS

The first operative technique for Hirschsprung's disease was described in 1948 by Swenson. While this was widely billed as curative treatment, in reality this, and surgical techniques since that time, have only relieved the obstruction caused by the aganglionic segment of colon. Despite this, progress in surgical techniques and diagnostic methods has allowed the successful survival of the majority of affected children. In spite of this, treatment is inadequate in a significant proportion of children and better treatment modalities are required. Postoperative problems continue to occur, and diagnosis continues to be made late. Effort in the short term needs to be directed to better understanding of the associated enterocolitis, with the lessons learned from other idiopathic inflammatory bowel disorders applied to HSCR. Dysmotility of the ganglionic gut may underlie many postoperative obstructive episodes, yet there are still few systematic studies of these episodes. The principal diagnostic modalities are well understood but are only patchily available in most countries, leading to unnecessary delays in diagnosis and treatment. The availability of long-term home parenteral nutrition has enabled the survival of children with total intestinal aganglionosis. In the short term, the emergence of intestinal transplantation from the realms of experimental treatment will allow these children a better quality of life. Recent research has produced a better understanding of the genetic factors involved and of the developmental neurobiology of the enteric nervous system so that it is now possible to contemplate neuronal replenishment of the aganglionic gut.[85] In the medium to long term, it can be foreseen that autologous neuronal transplantation could replace surgery as the treatment of choice for some forms of HSCR. Undoubtedly, these further refinements will lead to better and more timely treatment of those affected with HSCR.

AUTHOR'S RECOMMENDATIONS

An approach to the child with obstructive symptoms

To establish the cause of the obstruction, simple tests are required. The treatment depends upon accurately delineating the etiology. In general, while evaluation of the patient is in progress, close attention to rectal decompression and treatment of symptoms suggestive of enterocolitis are necessary. Specific therapy should be based on the results of the evaluation, which is presented in the form of an algorithm in Figure 60.2.

REFERENCES

1. Hirschsprung H. Stuhltragheit Neugeborener infolge von Dilatation und Hypertrophie des Colons. Jarb Kinderheilkd 1887; 27:1–9.

   Original clinical description of HSCR still valid today.

2. Kleinhaus S, Boley SJ, Sheran M, et al. Hirschsprung's disease. A survey of the members of the surgical section of the American Academy of Pediatrics. J Pediatr Surg 1979; 14:588–597.

3. Puri P. Hirschsprung's disease: Clinical and experimental observations. World J Surg 1993; 17:374–384.

4. Hoehner JC, Wester T, Pahlman S, et al. Alterations in neurotrophin and neurotrophin receptor localization in Hirschsprung's disease. Pediatr Surg 1996; 31:1524–1529.

5. Reding R, Goyet V, Gosseye S, et al. Hirschsprung's disease: A 20 year experience. Pediatr Surg 1997; 32:1221–1225.

6. Bealer JF, Natuzzi ES, Buscher C, et al. Nitric oxide synthase is deficient in the aganglionic colon of patients with Hirschsprung's disease. Pediatrics 1994; 93:647–651.

7. Swenson O. Early history of the therapy of Hirschsprung's disease: Facts and personal observations over 50 years. J Pediatr Surg 1996; 31:1003–1008.

8. Swenson O, Sherman P, Fisher IN. Diagnosis of congenital megacolon: an analysis of 501 patients. J Pediatr Surg 1973; 8:587–594.

   Largest cohort of patients but diagnostic tools have advanced.

9. Qualman SJ, Pysher T, Schauer G. Hirschsprung disease: Differential diagnosis and sequelae. Perspect Pediatr Pathol 1997; 20:111–126.

10. Hung WT, Chiang TP, Tsai YW, et al. Adult Hirschsprung's disease. Pediatr Surg 1989; 24:363–366.

11. Bassotti G, Mortara G, Lazzaroni M, et al. Adult Hirschsprung's disease mimicking Crohn's disease. Hepatogastroenterology 1995; 42:100–102.

12. Wang TY, Lin TC, Hsu H; Hirschsprung's disease manifested with obstructive colitis in adult: A case report. Chin Med (Taipei) 1996; 58:444–447.

13. Barness PR, Lennard-Jones JE, Hawley PR, et al. Hirschsprung's disease and idiopathic megacolon in adults and adolescents. Gut 1986; 27:534–541.

14. Rudolph C, Benaroch L. Hirschsprung disease. Pediatr Rev 1995; 16:5–11.

15. Elhalaby EA, Coran AG, Blane CE, et al. Enterocolitis associated with Hirschsprung's disease: A clinical-radiological characterization based on 168 patients. Pediatr Surg 1995; 30:76–83.

16. Marry TL, Matlak ME, Hendrickson M, et al. Unexpected death from enterocolitis after surgery for Hirschsprung's disease. Pediatrics 1995; 96:118–121.

   Enterocolitis remains the major cause of mortality.

17. Teitelbaum MD. Hirschsprung's disease in children. Curr Opin Pediatr 1995; 7:316–322.

18. Nurko SS. Constipation. In: Walker-Smith J, Hamilton D, Walker AW, eds. Practical pediatric gastroenterology. Hamilton, Ontario: BC Decker; 1996:95–106.

19. Nurko SS, Garcia-Aranda A, Guerrero VY, et al. Treatment of intractable constipation in children: Experience with cisapride. J Pediatr Gastroenterol Nutr 1996; 22:38–44.

20. Todd I. Adult Hirschsprung's disease. Br J Surg 1977; 64:311–312.

   References 21–44 refer to the genetic revolution in HSCR, mice, men, and experimental studies.

21. Passarge E. The genetics of Hirschsprung's disease. N Engl J Med 1967; 276:138–143.

22. Pingault V, Puliti A, Prehu M, et al. Human homology and candidate genes for the dominant megacolon locus, a mouse model of Hirschsprung disease. Genomics 1997; 39:86–89.

23. Eng C. The RET proto-oncogene in multiple endocrine neoplasia type 2 and Hirschsprung's disease. N Engl J Med 1996; 335:943–951.

24. Many TL, Seo T, Matalak ME, et al. Gastrointestinal function after surgical correction of Hirschsprung's disease: Long-term follow-up in 135 patients. J Pediatr Surg 1995; 30:655–658.

25. Heij HA, de Vries X, Bremer I, et al; Long term anorectal function after Duhamel operation for Hirschsprung disease. Pediatr Surg 1995; 30:430–432.

26. Trupp M, Arinas E, Fainzibla M, et al. Peripheral expression and biological activities of GDNF, a new neurotropic factor for avian and mammalian peripheral neurons. Nature 1996; 381:789–793.

27. Schuchardt A, D'Agati V, Larsson-Blomberg L, et al. Defects in the kidney and enteric nervous system of mice lacking the tyrosine kinase receptor ret. Nature 1994; 367:380–383.

28. Sanchez MP, Selos Santiago I, Frezen J, et al. Renal agenesis and the absence of enteric neurons in mice lacking GDNF. Nature 1996; 382:70–73.

29. Edery P, Lyonnet S, Mulligan LM, et al. Mutation of the ret proto oncogene in Hirschsprung's disease. Nature 1994; 367:378–380.

30. Lyonnet S, Bellono A, Pelet A, et al. A gene for Hirschsprung's disease maps to the proximal long arm of chromosome 10. Nat Genet 1993; 4:346–350.

31. Moore MW, Klein RD, Farinas I, et al. Renal and neuronal abnormalities in mice lacking GDNF. Nature 1996; 382:76–79.

32. Hosoda K, Hammer RE, Richardson JA, et al. Targeted and natural piebald lethal mutations of endothelin B receptor gene produce megacolon associated with spotted coat colour in mice. Cell 1994; 79:1267–1276.

33. Payette RF, Tennyson VM, Pomeranz HD, et al. Accumulation of components of basal laminae: association with the failure of neural crest cells to colonise the presumptive aganglionic bowel of LS/LS mutant mice. Dev Biol 1988; 125:341–360.

34. Kapur RP, Yost C, Palmiter RD. A transgenic model for studying the development of the enteric nervous system in normal and aganglionic mice. Development 1992; 116:167–175.

35. Benailly HK, Lapierre JM, Laudier B, et al. PMX2B, a new candidate gene for Hirschsprung's disease. Clin Genet 2003; 64:204–209.

36. Angrist M, Bolk S, Thiel B. et al. Mutation analysis of the RET receptor tyrosine kinase in Hirschsprung disease. Hum Mol Genet 1995; 4:821–830.

37. Newgreen D, Young HM. Enteric nervous system: development and developmental disturbances – Part 1. Pediatr Dev Pathol 2002; 5:224–247.

38. Mulligan LM, Eng C, Healey CS, et al. Specific mutations of the RET proto-oncogene are related to disease phenotype in MEN 2A and FMTC. Nat Genet 1994; 6:70–74.

39. Edery P, Attie T, Amiel J, et al. Mutation of the endothelin-3 gene in the Waardenburg-Hirschsprung disease (Shah Waardenburg syndrome). Nat Genet 1996; 12:442–444.

40. Bolk S, Pelet A, Hofstra R, et al. A human model for multigenic inheritance: phenotypic expression in Hirschsprung's disease requires both RET gene and a new 9q31 locus. Proc Natl Acad Sci USA 2000; 97:268–273.

Evidence that HSCR is a multigenic disorder.

41. Bealer JF, Natuzzi ES, Flake AW, et al. Effect of nitric oxide on the colonic smooth muscle of patients with Hirschsprung's disease J Pediatr Surg 1994; 29:1025–1029.

42. Taxman TL, Yulish BS, Rothstein FC; How useful is the barium enema in the diagnosis of infantile Hirschsprung's disease? Am J Dis Child 1986; 140:881–884.

43. Lopez-Alonso M, Ribas J, Hernandez J, et al. Efficiency of the anorectal manometry for the diagnosis of Hirschsprung's disease in the newborn period. Eur J Pediatr Surg 1993; 5:160–163

44. Low PS, Quak SH, Prabhakaran K, et al. Accuracy of anorectal manometry in the diagnosis of Hirschsprung's disease. J Pediatr Gastroenterol Nutr 1989; 9:342–346.

45. Hanani M, Udassin R, Ariel I, et al. A simple and rapid method for staining the enteric ganglia: Application for Hirschsprung disease. J Pediatr Surg 1993; 28:939–941.

46. Lake BD, Puri P, Nixon HH, et al. Hirschsprung's disease an appraisal of histochemically demonstrated acetylcholinesterase activity in suction rectal biopsies, an aid to diagnosis. Arch Pathol Lab Med 1978; 102:244–247.

Suction rectal biopsy with acetylcholinesterase staining is the gold standard for the diagnosis of HSCR.

47. Schofield DE, Devine W, Yunis EJ. Acetylcholinesterase-stained suction rectal biopsies in the diagnosis of Hirschsprung's disease. J Pediatr Gastroenterol Nutr 1990; 11:221–228.

48. Cord-Udy CL, Smith VV, Ahmed S, et al. An evaluation of the role of suction rectal biopsy in the diagnosis of intestinal neuronal dysplasia. J Pediatr Gastroenterol Nutr 1997; 24:1–6.

49. Moore SW, Millar AJ, Cywes S. Long term clinical, manometric, and histologic evaluation of obstructive symptoms in the postoperative Hirschsprung's patient. J Pediatr Surg 1994; 29:106–111.

50. Marty TL, Seo T, Sullivan JJ, et al. Rectal irrigations for the prevention of postoperative enterocolitis in Hirschsprung's disease. J Pediatr Surg 1995; 30:652–654.

51. Pierro A, Fasoli L, Kiely EM, et al. Staged pull-through for rectosigmoid Hirschsprung's disease is not safer than primary pull-through. J Pediatr Surg 1997; 32:505–509.

52. Philippart AI. Hirschsprung's disease. In: Ashcraft KW, Holder TM, eds. Pediatric surgery. Philadelphia: WB Saunders; 1993:358–371.

53. Swenson O, Sherman JO, Fisher JH. The treatment and postoperative complications of congenital megacolon: A 25 year follow up. Ann Surg 1975; 182:266–272.

54. Klein MD, Philippart AI. Hirschsprung's disease: Three decades' experience at a single institution. J Pediatr Surg 1993; 10:1291–1294.

55. Tariq GM, Brereton RJ, Wright VM. Complications of endorectal pull-through for Hirschsprung's disease. J Pediatr Surg 1991; 26:1202–1208.

56. Nurko SS. Complications after gastrointestinal surgery: A medical perspective. In: Walker WA, Durie PR, Hamilton JR, et al. eds. Pediatric gastrointestinal disease. Pathophysiology, diagnosis, management. 2nd edn. St Louis: Mosby; 1996:2067–2094.

57. Catto-Smith AG, Coffey CM, Nolan T, et al. Fecal incontinence after the surgical treatment of Hirschsprung's disease. J Pediatr 1995; 127:954–957.

58. Moore SW, Albertyn R, Cywes S. Clinical outcome and long-term quality of life after surgical correction of Hirschsprung's disease. J Pediatr Surg 1996; 31:1496–1502.

59. Cilley RE, Starter MB, Hirschl RB, et al. Definitive treatment of Hirschsprung's disease in the newborn with a one-stage procedure. Surgery 1994; 115:551–556.

60. Georgeson KE, Fuenfer MM, Hardin WH. Primary laparoscopic pull-through for Hirschsprung's disease in infants and children. J Pediatr Surg 1996; 30:1017.

61. Rothenberg S, Chang JH. Laparoscopic pull-through procedures using the harmonic scalpel in infants and children with Hirschsprung's disease. J Pediatr Surg 1997; 32:894–896.

Advances in surgical technique but improvement in outcome controversial.

62. Blane CE, Elhalaby E, Coran AG. Enterocolitis following endorectal pull-through procedure in children with Hirschsprung's disease. Pediatr Radiol 1994; 24:164–166.

63. Moore SW, Neveling U, Kaschula RO. Acquired aganglionosis following surgery for Hirschsprung's disease: A report of five cases during a 33 year experience with pull-through procedures. Histopathology 1993; 22:163–168.

64. Aslam A, Spicer RD, Corfield AP. Children with Hirschsprung's disease have an abnormal colonic mucus defensive barrier independent of the bowel innervation status. J Pediatr Surg 1997; 32:1206–1210.

65. Mishalany HG, Wooley MM. Postoperative functional and manometric evaluation of patients with Hirschsprung's disease. J Pediatr Surg 1987; 22:443–446.

66. Nagasaki A. Anorectal manometry after Ikeda Z-shaped anastomosis in Hirschsprung's disease. Prog Pediatr Surg 1989; 21:59–66.

67. Blair GK, Djonlic K, Fraser GC, et al. The bowel management tube: An effective means for controlling fecal incontinence. Pediatr Surg 1992; 27:1269–1272.

68. Dick AC, McCallion WA, Brown S, et al. Antegrade colonic enemas. Br J Surg 1996; 83:642–643.

69. Di Lorenzo C, Solzi GF, Flores AF, et al. Colonic motility after surgery for Hirschsprung's disease. Am J Gastroenterol 2000; 95:1759–1764.

70. Smith VV, Gregson N, Foggensteiner L, et al. Acquired intestinal aganglionosis and circulating autoantibodies without neoplasia or other neural involvement. Gastroenterology 1997; 112:1366–1371.

71. Hanimann B, Inderbitzin D, Briner J, et al. Clinical relevance of Hirschsprung-associated neuronal intestinal dysplasia. Eur J Pediatr Surg 1992; 2:147–149.

72. Koletzko S, Ballauff A, Hadziselimovic F, et al. Is histological diagnosis of neuronal intestinal dysplasia related to clinical and manometric findings in constipated children? Results of a pilot study. J Pediatr Gastroenterol Nutr 1993; 17:59–65.

   Intestinal neuronal dysplasia in perspective; read in conjunction with reference 48.

73. Ryan DP. Neuronal intestinal dysplasia. Semin Pediatr Surg 1995; 4:18–25.

74. Collins SM. The immunomodulation of enteric neuromuscular function: implications for motility and inflammatory disorders. Gastroenterology 1996; 111:1683–1699.

75. Langer JB, Birnbaum E. Preliminary experience with intrasphincteric botulinum toxin for persistent constipation after pull-through for Hirschsprung's disease. J Pediatr Surg 1997; 32:1059–1062.

76. Kobayashi H, Hirakawa H, Puri P. Abnormal internal anal sphincter innervation in patients with Hirschsprung's disease and allied disorders. J Pediatr Surg 1996; 31:794–799.

77. Blair GK, Murphy JJ, Fraser GC. Internal sphincterotomy in post-pull-through Hirschsprung's disease. J Pediatr Surg 1996; 31:843–845.

78. Bannani SA, Forootan H. Role of anorectal myectomy after failed endorectal pull-through in Hirschsprung's disease. J Pediatr Surg 1994; 29:1307–1309.

79. Nurko S. Botulinum toxin for achalasia: Are we witnessing the birth of a new era? J Pediatr Gastroenterol Nutr 1997; 24:447–449.

80. Shandling B, Chait PG, Richards HF. Percutaneous cecostomy: A new technique in the management of fecal incontinence. J Pediatr Surg 1996; 31:534–537.

81. Hengster P, Pernthaler H, Gassner I, et al. Twenty-three years of follow-up in patients with total colonic aganglionosis. Klin Padiatr 1996; 208:3–7.

82. Endo M, Watanabe K, Fuchimoto Y, et al. Long-term results of surgical treatment in infants with total colonic aganglionosis. J Pediatr Surg 1994; 29:1310–1314.

83. Tsuji H, Spitz L, Kiely EM, et al. Management and long-term follow-up of infants with total colonic aganglionosis. J Pediatr Surg 1999; 34:158–161.

   Outcome of total colonic aganglionosis is worse than short-segment HSCR. Management is a real challenge.

84. Miele E, Tozzi A, Staiano A, et al. Persistence of abnormal gastrointestinal motility after operation for Hirschsprung's disease. Am J Gastroenterol 2000; 95:1226–1230.

85. Bondurand N, Natarajan D, Thapur N, et al. Neuron and glia generating progenitors of the mammalian enteric nervous system isolated from foetal and post-natal gut cultures. Development 2003; 130:6387–6400.

   Perhaps the beginning of the development of alternative forms of treatment.

Diverticular disease of the colon

Bradley R. Davis and Jeffrey B. Matthews

INTRODUCTION

Diverticular disease of the colon was rarely described before the twentieth century, and it was not until 1899 that Graser first correlated the pathological changes with the clinical signs and symptoms.[1,2] Today the diagnosis is extremely common, affecting about 10% of the population over the age of 45 and 65% of those over 80.[3] Its emergence as a significant clinical and pathological disorder (*diverticulitis*) has been attributed to the dramatic reduction in the fiber content of Western diets,[4] and although it remains considerably less common in Asia and Africa, studies of immigrant populations suggest that westernization of diets is associated with an increased frequency of diverticulosis within about 10 years.[5] Some prospective data suggests an inverse relationship, independent of dietary fiber intake, between physical activity and the development of symptomatic diverticular disease in men, although the basis for this is unclear.[6] Although diverticula develop in many people, clinical complications occur in only a small percentage. These complications usually, but not always, develop after age 40, and are usually related to perforation and inflammation or to bleeding. It is estimated that symptomatic diverticulitis will develop in 20% of patients with diverticula,[7] accounting for approximately 455 000 admissions at an annual cost of US$1.9 billion.[8]

Most colonic diverticula are pseudodiverticula and represent mucosal and submucosal herniation through the muscle layers of the colon at areas of intrinsic weakness, where the nutrient arteries enter adjacent to the *teniae*.[1] The diverticula may be single but are usually multiple and can vary in size up to 2 cm. The sigmoid colon is involved in 95% of cases, although 35% of patients also have more proximal disease. Diverticula are distinctly unusual below the pelvic peritoneal reflection. Right-sided diverticulosis is rare in Western countries but is the predominant pattern in Asian populations.[9–11] This condition is distinct from *solitary cecal diverticulum*, although both tend to affect younger patients. True diverticula are quite uncommon in the colon but when present are usually single and right sided. A true diverticulum that appears on the antimesenteric border of the sigmoid colon *(giant sigmoid diverticulum)* may reach enormous size and be visible on plain abdominal films.[12]

The cause of diverticular herniation in the colon is complex and continues to be elucidated. The underlying mechanism is an aberrant balance between intraluminal pressure, elasticity, and tensile strength of the involved colonic segment. Stiffening of the longitudinal muscle layers as a result of excessive deposition of elastin, occurs normally with aging.[13] As the colon attempts to contract against this increased resistance, hypertrophy occurs, with resultant luminal narrowing, a process referred to as *myochosis coli*. Isolated colonic segments are therefore exposed to excessive intraluminal pressure, which is thought to lead to mucosal herniation. Pressures are higher in patients with symptomatic disease than in those with asymptomatic diverticulosis.[14] Measurements of intraluminal pressure also indicate exaggerated responses to food intake and pharmacologic stimulation which may be due in part to segmental abnormalities in cholinergic activity.[15] Indigestible cereal fiber increases the wet weight and diameter of stool and decreases intraluminal pressure, supporting the notion that dietary fiber and diverticular disease are inversely related.[16]

CLINICAL SPECTRUM

Diverticulosis and uncomplicated diverticulitis

The clinical manifestations of diverticular disease are myriad, ranging from asymptomatic diverticulosis to life-threatening free perforation. Some patients with diverticulosis describe recurring episodes of lower abdominal cramping in the absence of clear-cut evidence of inflammation; so-called painful diverticulosis has been ascribed to intermittent functional obstruction associated with the hypersegmentation, although the relationship to the presence of diverticula is unclear. When the lumen of a diverticulum is occluded by a fecalith, inflammatory changes develop, initially in the lymphoid tissue at the apex of a diverticulum but soon spreading to the visceral peritoneum and pericolic fat.[2] The necrotizing inflammatory process occurs without gross perforation and leakage of luminal contents. With further diverticular distention, subsequent vascular ischemia leads to *microperforation*, which usually results in uncomplicated diverticulitis. This is the most common clinical manifestation of diverticular disease, resulting in localized peritonitis and abdominal pain.

Complicated diverticular disease

Complications of diverticulitis have been well described, and a classification scheme has been proposed by Hinchey and colleagues in an effort to stratify diagnosis and treatment (Table 61.1).[17] Most often, a perforation is walled off by surrounding structures and a localized abscess develops. Direct extension and perforation into an adjacent hollow viscous results in fistula formation.

Table 61.1 Staging of perforative complications of diverticular disease

A.	Fistula formation
B.	Inflammation and perforation
Stage I	Sigmoid obstruction, intracolonic or mesenteric abscess
Stage II	Localized pericolic abscess
Stage III	Generalized septic (purulent) peritonitis
Stage IV	Generalized fecal peritonitis

Intestinal obstruction may develop in some instances, either because of compromise of the large bowel lumen by the severe changes within the colonic wall or as a result of kinking of small bowel loops caught up in the inflammatory mass. A free perforation of a diverticulum or peridiverticular abscess may result in generalized peritonitis. Diverticular hemorrhage is discussed later in the chapter.

EVALUATION OF THE PATIENT WITH ACUTE DIVERTICULITIS

Clinical features

Abdominal pain, usually in the left lower quadrant, and fever are the usual initial symptoms of acute diverticulitis (Table 61.2). Nausea and vomiting are uncommon without associated intestinal obstruction. Diarrhea is reported about as frequently as constipation. Urinary function may also be altered if the inflammatory mass abuts the bladder wall. Dysuria, urgency, and urinary frequency may be present, and if fistulization has occurred, the patient may note pneumaturia or foul-smelling urine suggestive of infection with fecal organisms. Examination typically reveals tenderness with some signs of peritoneal inflammation. A tender, fixed mass is often palpable. If the inflammatory mass is confined to the pelvis, the abdominal findings may be minimal. Patients who are more seriously ill will display signs of severe localized or generalized peritonitis associated with symptoms of systemic sepsis. A necrotizing infection may extend extraperitoneally and present by extension into the abdominal wall. Leukocytosis is not invariable. Urinalysis may reveal hematuria, pyuria, or a polymicrobial infection.

Investigation

The diagnosis of acute diverticulitis is often made on clinical grounds with sufficient certainty to direct initial therapy. In practice, however, most patients undergo radiologic or endoscopic investigation (Table 61.3). Useful initial studies include a complete blood count, urinalysis, and abdominal flat and upright X-rays. If the clinical picture is clear, it has been suggested that no other tests are needed to make the diagnosis. However, by relying on clinical parameters alone, the diagnosis may be incorrect in up to one-third of patients.

Sigmoidoscopy may exclude rectal pathology or distal colitis, but within the first few days of assessment most clinicians are reluctant to choose sigmoidoscopy for fear of disrupting a contained perforation. Contrast enema in the acute setting is also controversial. Because of the risk of perforation, minimal pressure should be used and water-soluble contrast should be chosen. The radiologic characteristics of acute diverticulitis on water-soluble contrast enema include: (1) diverticulosis with or without spasm; (2) marked sigmoid irregularity with long luminal strictures or obstruction; and (3) extraluminal extravasation of contrast. These changes are not pathognomonic of diverticular inflammation. The advantages of contrast enema are its low cost and the ability to identify mucosal lesions. Its most important role is in the nonacute setting. Arguably, the most important diagnostic modality in acute diverticulitis is computed tomography (CT).[18,19] It is noninvasive, safe, and can detect complications of diverticular disease. Bowel wall thickening, mesenteric streaking, and pericolic phlegmonous changes in association with diverticulosis indicate the presence of acute diverticulitis (Fig. 61.1). Complicated diverticulitis may be recognized by identifying associated abscesses, fistulas, or intra-abdominal or pelvic free fluid or air. The ability of CT to stratify patients for inpatient versus outpatient management of acute diverticulitis is not established but is of interest.[20–22] Abdominal ultrasound is useful if local expertise in this modality is available.[23] Laparoscopy as a diagnostic modality may be useful, but is rarely necessary.[24]

Differential diagnosis

A number of entities must be considered in the differential diagnosis (Table 61.4). Both diverticular disease and colonic malignancy tend to affect an older population and may coexist in the same individual.[25,26] It may be difficult to distinguish between these possibilities on initial evaluation; however, initial manage-

Table 61.2 Clinical manifestations of acute diverticulitis

Symptoms	Signs	Laboratory findings
Pain, usually LLQ	Fever	Leukocytosis
Fever, chills	Abdominal tenderness	Hematuria
Malaise	Abdominal mass	Pyuria
Anorexia, nausea	Abdominal distention	Polymicrobial UTI
Diarrhea or obstipation	Pelvic or rectal irritation	
Urinary frequency	Local peritoneal irritation	
	Psoas sign	

Table 61.3 Diagnostic investigation in acute diverticulitis

Examination	Major diagnostic findings	Disadvantages
Plain abdominal radiography	Soft tissue density Air-fluid levels	Non-specific
Upright chest radiography	Free intraperitoneal air	False-negative results
Contrast enema	Presence of diverticula Luminal narrowing or spasm Extravasation of contrast Fistulous tract	Perforation Barium peritonitis (water-soluble contrast is preferable)
Colonoscopy/sigmoidoscopy	Presence of diverticula Luminal narrowing or spasm	Risk of perforation
Abdominal and pelvic CT	Presence of diverticula Mural thickening Mesenteric streaking Free intra-abdominal fluid or air Pericolic abscess Air within the urinary bladder	Expense
Abdominal ultrasound	Thickened colonic segment Pericolic abscess Free intra-abdominal fluid	Operator dependent

ment is similar, and one need not go to great lengths to do so. After resolution of the acute situation, a concerted effort must be made to exclude the diagnosis of carcinoma. Crohn's colitis may be manifested as abdominal pain, fever, a tender abdominal mass, and leukocytosis. On occasion it may be surprisingly difficult even on histopathologic examination of a resected specimen to distinguish short segmental Crohn's disease from diverticulitis.[27] Ischemic colitis may closely mimic diverticulitis. Diverticulitis may simulate urinary tract infection as well as pelvic inflammatory disease.[28] Confusion between diverticulitis and appendicitis may occur in a number of circumstances, such as when the sigmoid colon or appendix crosses the midline or when the diverticulitis is right sided.

Recognition of complications

A large peridiverticular abscess is suggested by the presence of a tender mass on palpation of the abdomen, digital examination of the rectum, or pelvic examination in a patient with high, spiking fever. Confirmation is by CT scan (Fig. 61.2A). The most common fistula associated with diverticulitis is colovesical. Typically, such fistulas involve the posterior wall of the bladder. In females, the uterus and broad ligaments protect the bladder, and fistulization

is less common than in males. The diagnosis may be supported by cystoscopy or by barium enema, but CT appears to be the most useful investigation,[29] since air within the bladder is generally considered pathognomonic (Fig. 61.3).[30] Colovaginal fistula, as a complication of diverticulitis, is mostly described in the setting of previous hysterectomy.[31] A colocutaneous fistula may occur after therapeutic drainage or as a result of spontaneous rupture of a paracolic abscess through the abdominal wall. Rarely, a necrotizing infection may extend into the anterior thigh or through the pelvic floor and simulate fistula in ano.[32,33] Coloenteric fistulae are usually asymptomatic but may cause diarrhea as a result of bacterial overgrowth or diversion of small bowel contents into the colon. Intestinal obstruction is most commonly partial and may be due to blockage of either the colon or the small intestine. Obstructive symptoms may dominate the clinical findings. Free perforation of an inflamed diverticulum or peridiverticular abscess results in generalized peritonitis. This catastrophic event is characterized by the sudden onset of severe abdominal pain associated with sepsis. Although free perforation of the colon may be the initial manifestation of diverticular disease, particularly in elderly patients, it may also occur while a patient is under medical

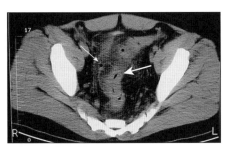

Fig. 61.1 • Acute diverticulitis depicted by contrast computed tomography. Mesenteric thickening and streaking are evident, along with luminal narrowing (large arrow). A small amount of extraluminal gas is also noted (small arrow) and indicates a contained (Hinchey BI) mesenteric abscess.

Table 61.4 Differential diagnosis of acute diverticulitis

Acute appendicitis

Perforated colon carcinoma

Inflammatory bowel disease (Crohn's disease and ulcerative colitis)

Pelvic inflammatory disease

Ischemic colitis

Infectious colitis

Foreign body perforation

Urinary tract infection or nephrolithiasis

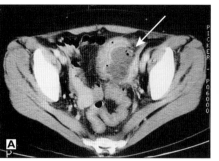

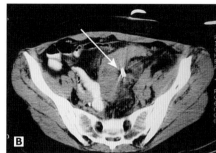

Fig. 61.2 • (A) A contained pelvic abscess (Hinchey B) associated with diverticulitis. Abscess measures 4 cm (arrow). **(B)** A percutaneous catheter has been placed in the abscess (arrow).

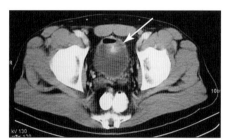

Fig. 61.3 • Colovesical fistula as seen on CT scan of the pelvis. Note the thickening of the bladder wall, the presence of oral contrast, and air within the bladder (arrow).

treatment for acute diverticulitis, in which case rupture of a peridiverticular abscess is the usual etiology.

TREATMENT OF UNCOMPLICATED DIVERTICULOSIS

Dietary modification

In patients with abdominal pain associated with colonic diverticulosis in the absence of signs of acute diverticulitis, enhanced intake of dietary fiber may be of benefit,[34–36] although the efficacy of this practice remains to be convincingly demonstrated.[37] Fiber intake facilitates the passage of softer, bulkier stools, with a resultant decrease in colonic hypersegmentation and intraluminal pressure. Patients should be educated on ways of increasing the bulk in their diet (Table 61.5), and instructed that alleviation of their symptoms may take several months. Unprocessed whole-wheat bran, 10–25 g/day, added to juice, soup, or other liquids is the recommended amount. Often, patients will note bloating and discomfort for several weeks after initiation of this regimen. More palatable approaches include increased intake of high-fiber breakfast cereals or whole-wheat bread. Although fruits and vegetables may also contribute to total dietary fiber intake, substantially

greater amounts are required to achieve the same effect because of their higher content of water. In patients with asymptomatic diverticulosis the addition of dietary fiber, while routinely recommended, has not been shown to reduce the incidence of diverticulitis and the approach to these patients should be individualized.

Bulk additives

As an alternative or in addition to increased dietary fiber intake, a variety of hydrophilic colloid bulk preparations have been introduced into the market, including products based on methylcellulose and ispaghula husk. These substances absorb 25–40 times their weight in water and thereby increase stool volume with the same net effect as dietary fiber. There is no evidence that one preparation is superior to another in terms of reduction in intraluminal pressure or increase in stool volume.[38]

Antispasmodics and analgesics

Agents that affect colonic motility, including musculotropic drugs and anticholinergics, have not been proven to be effective for so-called painful diverticulosis and cannot be recommended. Many opiates raise intraluminal pressure in the sigmoid colon and may predispose to perforation. Although meperidine in usual doses does not appear to share this property, in general the use of such compounds is to be avoided. Like dietary modification, the use of prophylactic antispasmodics has not been demonstrated to reduce the incidence of diverticulitis.

TREATMENT OF UNCOMPLICATED ACUTE DIVERTICULITIS

Medical therapy

In the majority of patients the initial treatment of acute diverticulitis consists of antibiotics and some degree of dietary restriction. Most patients, about 85%, recover completely with medical therapy.[39] Diverticulitis will eventually recur in about one-third, often within the first year after the initial episode; the role of surgery in these patients is discussed later. Unless the symptoms are quite mild, patients should forego oral intake until it becomes certain that urgent surgical or radiologic intervention will not be necessary. Although many advocate complete bowel rest for all patients, such practice is probably unnecessarily restrictive, and clear liquids may be allowed for selected individuals provided that no significant nausea or abdominal distention is present. Nasogastric suction is reserved for patients in whom associated small

Table 61.5 Potential sources of increased dietary bulk

Bulk source	Amount
Unprocessed miller's bran	10–25 g daily with water or juice
High-fiber cereal	One bowl daily
Whole-wheat bread	Five slices daily
Bulk preparations	One tbsp or one tablet once or twice daily
Fruits and vegetables	Several generous portions daily

or large bowel obstruction is suspected. Hospitalized patients are administered intravenous fluids, with careful attention to replace existing intravascular volume deficits and correct electrolyte abnormalities caused by vomiting or diarrhea. Total parenteral nutrition is not needed in most instances, inasmuch as adequate enteral caloric intake is usually achievable within a few days. While there is little evidence to support the role of a specific diet in re-feeding patients recovering from an acute episode, a trial of liquids followed by a more conventional meal with an emphasis on dietary fiber is a reasonable first approach. The role of elemental or semi-elemental diets in patients with diverticulitis has not been examined, but would seem to be a reasonable alternative in patients who are unable to tolerate a more conventional approach.

Broad-spectrum antibiotic therapy directed against both Gram-negative enteric organisms and anaerobic species, especially *Bacteroides fragilis*, is indicated. Intravenous monotherapy is adequate in the majority of cases.[40,41] Antibiotic costs should be considered in the choice of therapy because there is little evidence that newer, more expensive proprietary agents are superior to the more common generic options. Antibiotics should be continued for a minimum of 7 days because early recurrences are usually due to inadequate length of initial therapy.

Narcotic analgesics should be avoided, particularly morphine, which not only increases colonic intraluminal pressure but may also mask signs of spreading peritoneal irritation. If such treatment proves necessary, meperidine should be chosen. Acetaminophen and other antipyretics should also be avoided because recurrent or persistent fever is an important sign of potential complicated diverticulitis. Laxatives and enemas should be avoided. Unless complicated diverticulitis is clinically suspected, radiologic imaging studies are not mandatory, although an initial CT scan may help demarcate those patients who will respond to outpatient treatment.[42] Frequent physical examination of the patient is essential to ensure that an appropriate response to therapy is obtained.

With resolution of the pain and abdominal findings, normal oral intake may resume within 2 to 3 days. There is little evidence to support the use of a low-residue diet in the convalescent period, although this approach is in wide practice. Indeed, it may be perfectly acceptable to begin a high-fiber diet within a few days after resumption of oral intake. It is commonly thought that seeds, nuts, popcorn, and similar items must be scrupulously avoided, but the relationship between recurrent diverticulitis and ingestion of these substances has never been convincingly established.

Outpatient management

Selected patients with uncomplicated diverticulitis may be managed in the outpatient setting, provided that they do not demonstrate potentially worrisome markers for advanced disease such as high fever, shaking chills, signs of local peritonitis, or symptoms of intestinal obstruction.[41] Patients must be able to take fluids and tolerate an oral antibiotic regimen. The approach to antibiotic therapy does not change with outpatient management, with many practitioners opting for monotherapy (ciprofloxacin, amoxicillin/clavulanate), others preferring a combination approach (ciprofloxacin and metronidazole).[40] Detailed instructions for follow-up must be provided, and the physician must be convinced that the patient and family are reliable. Patients are instructed to return if pain or fever fails to resolve quickly or

if fluids are not tolerated. Arrangements for subsequent outpatient investigation to confirm the diagnosis should be made.

TREATMENT OF ACUTE DIVERTICULITIS COMPLICATED BY ABSCESS

Abscess formation as a complication of diverticulitis may occur in as many as 16% of patients.[43] Clinical suspicion may be raised at the initial evaluation or when a patient fails to respond adequately to initial medical management. Hospitalization is mandatory, with complete bowel rest and intravenous fluid administration. Radiologic investigation by CT or ultrasound should be carried out to confirm the presence of a localized abscess. Usually such abscesses are within the leaves of the colonic mesentery, but occasionally a pelvic abscess may form as a result of dependent pooling of a macroscopic perforation.

Percutaneous radiologic catheter drainage

Depending on their location and size, such abscesses may be amenable to percutaneous, radiologically guided catheter drainage. A number of reports attest to the safety and success of this approach,[44–46] although the precise indications remain to be clearly defined. The goal of percutaneous drainage is to gain control of the infection such that later surgery may be performed as a one-stage procedure (see below) without colostomy under more elective circumstances.[41] It is possible that successful percutaneous management of peridiverticular abscess obviates the absolute need for subsequent surgery in certain patients, but this issue is controversial.

It is probably unnecessary to drain small abscesses <2 cm, because they will usually resolve with antibiotics alone or may be resected with the colonic specimen in the few patients who fail to respond to conventional medical management.[47] Larger abscesses may be drained percutaneously if a safe 'window' for catheter access can be identified (see Fig. 61.2B). This approach has proved successful in up to 90% of appropriately selected patients, obviating the need for emergent surgery and its attendant risks.[44] Some patients will never experience future complications associated with their diverticular disease and catheter drainage and antibiotic therapy will prove definitive treatment for them.[48] This is the exception, however, and successful abscess drainage is traditionally followed by elective one-stage resection 6–8 weeks after the resolution of the infectious process. While there are only limited data, this approach is widely accepted with demonstrable benefit to the patient.[49] Catheter dislodgment and the occurrence of a fecal fistula may complicate subsequent management due to inadequate control of infection.[44] In these cases and in patients with complex multilocular abscesses, with an abscess not accessible to percutaneous catheter drainage, or with persistent symptoms after drainage, most clinicians would agree that urgent surgery is necessary.

Operative treatment

In the beginning of the twentieth century, a staged approach to nonelective surgery for acute diverticulitis gained popularity.[50] This involved an initial transverse colostomy, to divert the fecal flow, followed by a delayed segmental resection with anastomosis and finally, after a prolonged period, closure of the colostomy.

This approach has been abandoned due to the unacceptably high morbidity and mortality associated with poor source control and sepsis.[51–53] Today, the majority of surgeons will choose either resection with primary anastomosis, or a Hartmann's procedure. The former is reserved for patients with Hinchey stage I or II perforations (as well as some select stage III) while the latter, which involves resection and creation of an end colostomy, is used for more severe abdominal catastrophes.

In either procedure, the involved colonic segment and associated abscess should be resected. For left-sided disease the entire sigmoid colon is removed to include any proximal thickened and diseased left colon. This can be determined by palpation intra-operatively and it is the presence of muscular hypertrophy (*myochosis coli*) and not diverticula that determine the proximal margin.[41,54] This may be technically challenging, depending on the extent of the left lower quadrant phlegmon. Densely adherent small bowel must occasionally be resected en bloc. It is vitally important to carefully identify both ureters, which may easily become distorted by and caught up within the inflammatory mass. All loculations of fluid should be broken up.

After the involved segment has been resected, the decision to perform an anastomosis largely depends on the inflammatory burden in the pelvis and peritoneal cavity as well as the overall condition of the patient (Fig. 61.4). An anastomosis without proximal diversion should generally be performed only in the setting of an elective or semi-elective operation, in which the bowel is cleansed preoperatively and the patient's sepsis has resolved.[41,55,56] The ability to successfully perform intraoperative colonic lavage, however, as well as advances in postoperative care have led to an increasing body of evidence that a primary anastomosis is acceptable even in the face of select Hinchey stage III perforations. Proponents of this approach cite its safety and cost-effectiveness compared to the traditional two-stage procedures.[57–59] The use of a diverting loop ileostomy to 'protect' a distal anastomosis is usually unnecessary and carries some disadvantages, including the morbidity of the stoma itself, difficulties in stoma management, and the need for a second procedure for stoma closure.

If considerable fecal soilage is present, or the patient is frankly toxic, the operation of choice is a Hartmann procedure. In this case, after excision of the involved colonic segment the proximal portion is brought out through the abdominal wall as an end colostomy and the distal segment is closed as a so-called rectal stump. Alternatively, the distal segment may be exteriorized as a mucous fistula. Both approaches safely remove the source of the acute infection, but it is often not possible to mobilize the distal rectal segment to reach through the abdominal wall. In those cases the rectum should be closed and sutured to the pelvic side-wall to prevent it from shrinking into the pelvis, confounding later attempts to restore intestinal continuity. Mortality rates for the Hartmann procedure performed for complicated diverticulitis in the absence of free perforation are generally reported to be less than 5%.[60,61] The disadvantage of the Hartmann procedure is the second stage, which requires, first, that the rectal stump be identified and properly cleared off (which is occasionally difficult because of postoperative adhesions) and, second, that the proximal part of the bowel be adequately mobilized to reach into the pelvis for a tension-free anastomosis. The latter usually requires

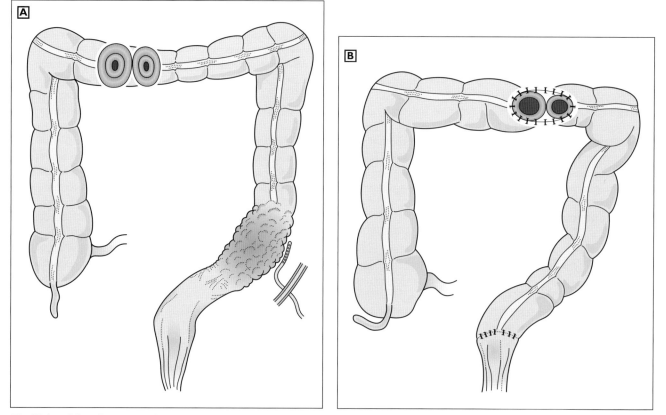

Fig. 61.4 • Selected operations for acute sigmoid diverticulitis. **(A)** Loop transverse colostomy with drainage. **(B)** Resection with primary anastomosis and proximal loop colostomy.

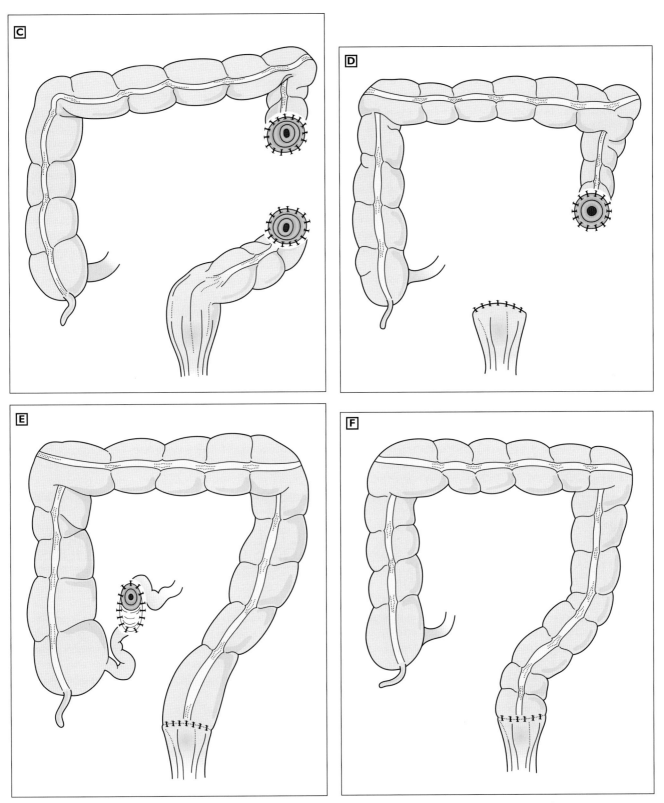

Fig. 61.4 • cont'd **(C)** Resection with end sigmoid colostomy and mucous fistula. **(D)** Hartmann procedure. **(E)** Resection with primary anastomosis and proximal loop ileosotmy. **(F)** Resection with primary anastomosis.

mobilization of the splenic flexure. The second stage of the Hartmann procedure should be deferred at least 3–6 months after the initial resection. In about 30% of patients, reversal of the Hartmann procedure is never undertaken.[62,63]

TREATMENT OF DIVERTICULITIS COMPLICATED BY FISTULA

Perforation of the colon and the subsequent inflammatory reaction can result in the formation of fistulas to adjacent organs in up to 12% of episodes of acute diverticulitis.[63] Such fistula have been described between a myriad of contiguous organs including the ureters, fallopian tubes, and even the pleura,[64–66] but by far the most common involve the bladder and the vagina.[67] After confirmation that the fistula is a result of diverticular disease, the surgical strategy is similar in all cases; resection of the appropriate colonic segment and repair of the involved organ.

Acute diverticulitis associated with a colovesical fistula is generally an indication for surgical management in view of the risks of recurrent urinary tract infection. At surgery, the involved segment is usually densely adherent to the dome of the urinary bladder but may be separated by blunt dissection. Often the fistulous opening in the bladder wall is difficult to identify. It is not necessary to do so, nor is it necessary to oversew the involved segment of bladder unless a large opening is present, as simple Foley catheter drainage for 1 week postoperatively will usually result in spontaneous closure. Occasionally, excision of a small portion of bladder wall will be required. Primary anastomosis without proximal colostomy is appropriate in most cases.[67]

A colovaginal fistula is handled similarly because the fistulous connection is usually to the apex of the vagina in women who have undergone prior hysterectomy. After resection, the residual opening in the upper vaginal wall need not be closed.[68]

A colocutaneous fistula will generally close spontaneously unless distal obstruction or associated infection is present. However, if the underlying septic process cannot be readily controlled, proximal diversion may be appropriate.[69] The most common cause of colocutaneous fistula in the context of acute diverticulitis is prior catheter drainage of a pericolic abscess. If the fistula is well controlled, elective surgery may be undertaken before complete closure. High-output fistulas (>200 mL/day) generally fare poorer than low-output fistulas.[69] A coloenteric fistula should be treated by en bloc resection of the affected segments of small bowel along with the involved colon. Again, primary anastomosis without colostomy is performed.

TREATMENT OF DIVERTICULITIS COMPLICATED BY OBSTRUCTION

Small bowel obstruction associated with acute diverticulitis is managed by intravenous fluids, correction of electrolyte abnormalities, and nasogastric suction. If surgery is undertaken, resection of the adherent small intestinal segment may be required, if it cannot be readily separated from the inflammatory mass.

Large bowel obstruction resulting from sigmoid luminal narrowing presents a more difficult management situation. Even if the obstruction is only partial, preoperative bowel preparation may be impossible. Of greater concern, however, are patients with complete colonic obstruction, in whom the risk of cecal perforation may be substantial. The traditional approach to this situation consists of proximal decompression via cecostomy tube placement or transverse loop colostomy, followed by elective resection of the sigmoid mass. However, current trends favor initial resuscitation followed by expeditious resection of the obstructing mass, either as a Hartmann procedure,[41] as subtotal colectomy, or even with primary anastomosis after on-table colonic luminal lavage.[59,70,71] The specific decision depends on the condition of the patient, the technical ease with which resection can be performed, and the surgeon's preference. The obstruction is not infrequently found to be due to carcinoma rather than diverticulitis.[72]

TREATMENT OF DIVERTICULITIS COMPLICATED BY FREE PERFORATION

Free perforation of a diverticulum or peridiverticular abscess is a surgical emergency. Mortality for this condition approaches 35% in many series, depending on the degree of fecal contamination, the delay before surgery, and the extent of associated comorbid disease. In addition to intravenous fluids and broad-spectrum antibiotics, pressor support may be needed, and invasive cardiovascular monitoring to guide resuscitation may be appropriate. Hartmann resection is the most commonly used procedure and is considered the most conservative approach, with mortality rates ranging from about 10% to 20% depending on the patient mix.[50,73–76] It is reasonable, if anatomic circumstances permit, to bring out the distal end as a mucous fistula to avoid the risk of leakage from the rectal stump in the setting of substantial intraperitoneal soilage. Lavage and drainage of the peritoneal cavity plus transverse loop colostomy, with the diseased segment left in situ, has been advocated for the desperately ill patient,[77] and one small randomized trial comparing this approach with Hartmann resection supports this view.[78] However, many studies suggest either no difference or a higher mortality rate with this approach when compared with resectional procedures.[79–83] Resection is associated with fewer procedures per patient, fewer total hospital days, and fewer infectious complications.[39,82]

Immunocompromised patients with diverticulitis, including transplant patients,[84,85] patients with advanced renal failure,[86] patients receiving corticosteroid therapy,[87] or patients with acquired immunodeficiency syndrome, are particularly prone to free perforation, and mortality is often in excess of 30%.[86,88] Recognition of diverticulitis before perforation in these individuals is often difficult because the usual signs and symptoms are frequently masked.

ELECTIVE TREATMENT OF RECURRENT EPISODES OF ACUTE DIVERTICULITIS

Risk of recurrence

After successful medical management of acute diverticulitis, the risk of further episodes ranges from 7% to 45% depending on the length of follow-up.[89–91] About 50% of recurrences requiring hospital admission will develop in the first year after the initial attack; 90% will develop within 5 years.[92,93] A number of reports suggest that institution of a high-fiber diet may reduce the risk of recurrence, although the data supporting this concept are largely uncontrolled.[94,95] Patients should be encouraged to begin a diet high in bulk and cereal fiber as soon as possible after resumption of normal oral intake. There is no evidence that avoidance of 'blockage foods' such as popcorn, nuts, and so forth will reduce the chance of recurrence, although this advice is often given to patients.

Indications for elective surgery

Indications for surgery in patients with diverticulosis and the operations recommended are shown in Tables 61.6 and 61.7. With each recurrence of acute uncomplicated diverticulitis, patients become less likely to respond to medical therapy, with success decreasing from 70–85% after the first attack to only 6%

Table 61.6 Indications for elective surgery for diverticular disease

After a second well-documented episode of uncomplicated diverticulitis

Failure of resolution of otherwise uncomplicated diverticulitis

After a first episode of acute diverticulitis complicated by abscess

Diverticular disease associated with colovesical fistula

Continued partial obstruction associated with diverticulitis

Inability to exclude carcinoma

after the third. Furthermore, after a second episode of diverticulitis, most patients will have persistent symptoms, and as many as 50% will experience complications. This observation underlies the basis for the recommendation that patients with more than two episodes of uncomplicated acute diverticulitis be considered for elective surgery. Patients with acute complicated diverticulitis should be considered for interval sigmoid resection even if complete resolution of the attack can be accomplished by antibiotics combined, when indicated, with percutaneous catheter drainage; recurrent complications developed in about 85% of such patients in one series as opposed to only 3% of those initially managed by resection.[96] Resection is also indicated for patients with colovesical fistula, and many recommend surgery for those with urinary symptoms even in the absence of a documented fistula. Surgery is also usually considered in the face of continued partial obstruction of the colon, particularly when the possibility of carcinoma cannot be excluded.

Acute diverticulitis in young patients (particularly those less than 40 years) is relatively uncommon and evidence that it is particularly aggressive is largely anecdotal.[97–99] Most of these cases occur in men, with obesity as a common comorbidity.[100,101] While proponents of early elective resection in this population cite the high incidence (up to 66%) of surgical intervention required at the initial episode as an indication of its aggressive behavior, this has not been encountered by all groups. Surgery in these patients is often undertaken for erroneous preoperative diagnoses,[102] and in fact it may be more common for surgery to be required for an elderly rather than a young patient on the first admission.[97,103] Elective surgery for young patients after their first attack of acute diverticulitis, therefore, should only be recommended after careful consideration of the patient and the severity of the initial disease because as yet the natural history has not been clearly elucidated.[102,104]

Results of elective surgery for diverticular disease

Resection is not generally indicated for patients with abdominal pain associated with uncomplicated diverticular disease; the experience of Rennie and associates would suggest that at least 85% will experience persistent symptoms[105] as compared with only 6% after elective resection for patients with objective evidence of diverticulitis.[106] Mortality after elective surgery should be near zero although, for reasons that are not entirely clear, resection for diverticulitis carries a greater morbidity rate than do similar resections for other diagnoses (e.g., cancer).[107] Higher anastomotic leak rates after operations for diverticulitis may be due to the tendency for high intraluminal pressure to develop in patients with diverticular disease, particularly after pharmacologic stimuli such as those associated with reversal of neuromuscular blockade; additionally, leak rates may reflect the presence of infection and technical difficulty in identifying proximal segments that are completely free of diverticula.

Minimally invasive surgery for diverticulitis

Recently, minimally invasive techniques of colonic resection have been used for elective treatment of diverticulitis with low morbidity. The cost of laparoscopic procedures and the operative times are greater than those of conventional surgery, but laparoscopy may lead to a shorter hospital stay with similar morbidity.[108,109] In addition, the use of laparoscopy may ultimately reduce the incidence of postoperative bowel obstruction and hernia formation, due to reduction in adhesion formation and smaller wounds. Further investigation is necessary to define these benefits. As the laparoscopic experience continues to grow, its application in the treatment of diverticular disease will expand to include both complicated and uncomplicated disease.[110–113]

Recurrence after prior resection

Diverticulitis recurs after resection in as many as 4–12% of patients.[114] The incidence of recurrence is thought to be related in part to the adequacy of distal resection; results after limited

Table 61.7 Choice of operation for diverticular disease

Indication	First choice	Alternative
Elective	Resection, primary anastomosis	
Fistula (Hinchey A)	Resection, primary anastomosis, drainage of fistulized organ (i.e., Foley catheter)	Resection, primary anastomosis, repair of fistulized organ
Abscess (Hinchey BI and BII)	Resection, primary anastomosis	Resection, primary anastomosis, proximal diversion
Obstruction	Resection, on-table lavage, primary anastomosis	Hartmann procedure
Perforation (Hinchey BIII)	Hartmann procedure	Resection, primary anastomosis, proximal diversion
Perforation (Hinchey BIV)	Hartmann procedure	Lavage, drainage or suture repair, proximal diversion

sigmoid resection are worse than results after resections that have been extended to the proximal portion of the rectum (at or below the pelvic peritoneal reflection).[54] It is important to remember that patients with recurrences may in fact have had unrecognized Crohn's disease rather than acute diverticulitis at the time of the original operation.[69,115]

TREATMENT OF CECAL OR RIGHT-SIDED DIVERTICULITIS

Cecal diverticula may be congenital or acquired, true diverticula or pseudodiverticula. The incidence of right-sided diverticulitis appears to be higher in Asian populations, where right-sided disease is more common than sigmoid diverticulosis.[9,10,116] Cecal diverticulitis is often mistaken for appendicitis or perforated cecal carcinoma. Acute cecal diverticulitis is usually manifested without a periumbilical pain prodrome, the symptoms are often of several days' rather than hours' duration, and patients tend to be older than patients with appendicitis.[117] Nevertheless, the diagnosis is only occasionally made preoperatively, and at surgery a substantial inflammatory mass is often present. It may be difficult to distinguish between acute cecal diverticulitis and carcinoma at the time of laparotomy, and if so, a right colectomy is indicated. If no evidence of abscess formation is found and cecal carcinoma can be excluded, appendectomy followed by postoperative antibiotics usually suffices.[10,118] Simple diverticulectomy (in cases of a congenital solitary cecal diverticulum) is occasionally possible.[119] An asymptomatic cecal diverticulum found incidentally at surgery may simply be invaginated.

EVALUATION AND TREATMENT OF DIVERTICULAR HEMORRHAGE

Clinical features

While the exact incidence of diverticular hemorrhage is uncertain, it is estimated to account for 40% of lower gastrointestinal bleeding.[120,121] The diagnostic and treatment challenge rests in differentiating diverticular sources of bleeding from other causes such as colitis, vascular ectasias, and neoplasia. While most patients with diverticular bleeding will have a self-limited course, massive hemorrhage does occur in fewer than 5% of patients.[122]

Medical management

A nasogastric tube should be placed to eliminate the chance that the bleeding is due to an upper source, although endoscopy is frequently required to exclude this possibility with certainty. After fluid resuscitation and stabilization, anoscopy and/or rigid sigmoidoscopy should be performed to exclude a hemorrhoidal or low rectal source. Bleeding stops spontaneously in at least 75% of patients,[123] while a number of options for localization and control are available in those patients that continue to bleed. This is covered in detail in Chapter 65, and includes angiography, colonoscopy, and radionuclide scans.[124–126]

Angiography, when positive, can also be used to control diverticular hemorrhage through the selective infusion of vasopressin or through superselective catheter embolization. Vasopressin, an endogenous peptide hormone that causes arterial vasoconstriction in super-physiologic doses, was first described in the treatment of gastrointestinal hemorrhage in 1968.[127] Through selective infusion of vasopressin into the inferior mesenteric artery, diverticular bleeding can be clinically controlled in as many as 90% of patients.[128] While selective infusion limits its systemic effects, the complications associated with vasopressin infusion include colonic ischemia, myocardial ischemia and infarction, bradycardia, and hypertension which can be partly ameliorated by the concomitant use of intravenous nitroglycerin. The rebleeding rate has been reported as high as 43%[128] and overall complication rate as high as 41%.[129] These series are mostly older and do not take into account modern angiographic techniques and the systemic use of nitroglycerin. While vasopressin therapy has remained relatively unchanged, the use of embolization techniques has evolved significantly since its first description for the treatment of lower gastrointestinal hemorrhage in 1974.[130] The unacceptably high occurrence of bowel ischemia and infarction limited its use until the advent of superselective embolization in the early 1990s, a technique that places procoagulant or barrier material selectively into or beyond the marginal artery. This procedure has gained wider acceptance in the past decade and now boasts equivalent or better clinical response rates compared to vasopressin with a significantly lower incidence of complications (15%) and rebleeding (19%). The incidence of colonic ischemia requiring colectomy is negligible (1–5%).[130] The choice between vasopressin or superselective embolization largely depends on local expertise and the patient's overall condition, but it appears that superselective embolization has superseded vasopressin in the medical treatment of lower gastrointestinal hemorrhage.

Surgery for diverticular hemorrhage

Surgery is rarely required in patients whose diverticular hemorrhage ceases spontaneously or through medical intervention, in as much as recurrent episodes are infrequent.[131] Elective surgery may be considered for patients with recurrent hemorrhage, with the threshold for surgery lower in patients whose bleeding site has been localized, allowing for a segmental resection. The outcome for surgery in this setting is excellent.[132] In rare instances, diverticular hemorrhage is so massive that medical stabilization is impossible and emergent surgery must be undertaken to avoid exsanguination. Surgery is also indicated for continued hemorrhage despite medical attempts at control. The loss of four units of blood during the first 24 hours is predictive of at lease a 50% chance of requiring emergency surgery.[133] Preoperative identification of the bleeding site is invaluable so that a limited colectomy may be performed. If such identification proves impossible, intraoperative colonoscopy with the patient in lithotomy position may localize the source,[134] otherwise a subtotal colectomy with an ileorectal anastomosis should be performed. Although the mortality approaches 10% in this setting, the results are more favorable than a blind segmental resection, which is associated with a much higher risk of rebleeding (42% versus 0%) and subsequent complication.[135–137]

SUMMARY

Colonic diverticulosis has become a ubiquitous problem in Western society due in large part to the paucity of dietary fiber ingested in this part of the world. The sigmoid colon is most

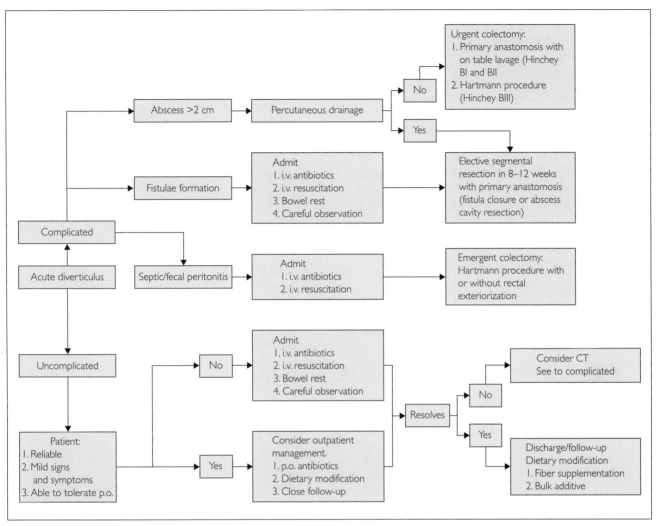

Fig. 61.5 ● Flowchart depicting the management of patients with acute diverticulitis.

frequently affected but any portion of the colon can be involved. As the population ages, an increasing number of patients will be diagnosed with diverticulitis and diverticular bleeding. Acute diverticulitis can often be treated medically with antibiotics and a short period of bowel rest (Fig. 61.5). Repeat episodes are common and current recommendations call for elective colonic resection after two confirmed episodes of uncomplicated diverticulitis. This approach can be individualized on the basis of the severity of the episodes and the general health of the patient. In a subset of patients, complications of their disease will necessitate a more aggressive approach. In patients with free perforation and peritonitis, a Hartmann's procedure is usually required, although stable patients without fecal soilage may be considered for an anastomosis after an on-table colonic lavage. The advances in interventional radiology have allowed many patients with abscess formation to undergo drainage followed by elective one-stage operative resection. Fistulas are managed by resection of the diseased colonic segment and repair of the adjacent organ. Diverticular bleeding is managed by a localizing study followed by selective angiographic ablation of the offending vessel or operative resection.

REFERENCES

1. Fleischner F, Ming S-C, Henken E. Revised concepts on diverticular disease of the colon. I. Diverticulosis: Emphasis on tissue derangement and its relation to the irritable colon syndrome. Radiology 1964; 83:859–871.

   This paper notes the radiographic appearance of sacculations of the colon and symptomatic diverticular disease.

2. Fleischner F, Ming S-C. Revised concepts on diverticular disease of the colon: II. So-called diverticulitis: Diverticular sigmoiditis and perisigmoiditis; diverticular abscess, fistula, and frank peritonitis. Radiology 1965; 84:599–609.

3. Painter NS, Burkitt D. Diverticular disease of the colon, a 20th century problem. Clin Gastroenterol 1975; 4:3–21.

   This paper outlines the research conducted by Burkitt in sub-Saharan Africa and demonstrates the relationship of diverticulosis and the consumption of dietary fiber. He noted a relationship between the consumption of a diet high in fiber content and the paucity of diverticular disease. It should be noted that the people living in this region did not routinely reach the sixth decade of life.

4. Painter N, Burkitt D. Diverticular disease of the colon: A deficiency disease of Western civilization. Br Med J 1971; 1:450–454.

5. Ohi G, Minowa K, Oyama T, et al. Changes in dietary fiber intake among Japanese in the 20th century: A relationship to the prevalence of diverticular disease. Am J Clin Nutr 1983; 38:115–121.

The authors highlight the history of dietary fiber consumption in Japan during the 20th century, noting a 'westernization' trend reflected in a significant decrease in rice consumption. Concomitantly, they report an increase in symptomatic diverticular disease in this same population.

6. Aldoori WH, Giovannucci EL, Rimm EB, et al. Prospective study of physical activity and the risk of symptomatic diverticular disease in men. Gut 1995; 36:276–282.

7. Ozick LA, Salazar CO, Donelson SS. Pathogenesis, diagnosis, and treatment of diverticular disease of the colon. Gastroenterologist 1994; 2(4):299–310.

This review article from the gastroenterology division at Columbia University, College of Physicians and Surgeons, reports on the pathogenesis and treatment of diverticulitis and diverticular bleeding.

8. Everhart JA, et al. The burden of gastrointestinal disease. May 2001. Online. Available: http://www.gastro.org/clinicalRes/burdenreport.html

9. Lo CY, Chu KW. Acute diverticulitis of the right colon. Am J Surg 1996; 171:244–246.

10. Harada RN, Whelan IJ Jr. Surgical management of cecal diverticulitis. Am J Surg 1993; 166:666–671.

11. Wong SK, Ho YH, Leong AP, et al. Clinical behavior of complicated right-sided and left-sided diverticulosis. Dis Colon Rectum 1997; 40:344–348.

12. Roger T, Rommens J, Bailly J, et al. Giant colonic diverticulum: Presentation of one case and review of the literature. Abdom Imaging 1996; 21:530–533.

13. Morson B. The muscle abnormality in diverticular disease of the sigmoid colon. Br J Radiol 1963; 36:385–392.

14. Cortesini C, Pantalone D. Usefulness of colonic motility study in identifying patients at risk for complicated diverticular disease. Dis Colon Rectum 1991; 34:339–342.

15. Golder M, Burleigh DE, Belai A, et al. Smooth muscle cholinergic denervation hypersensitivity in diverticular disease. Lancet 2003; 361:1945–1951.

This article establishes a putative etiology for disturbances in cholinergic smooth muscle activity in the colon as an important effector mechanism in the pathogenesis of diverticulosis.

16. Gear JS, Ware A, Fursdon P, et al. Symptomless diverticular disease and intake of dietary fiber. Lancet 1979; 1:511–514.

17. Hinchey E, Schaal P, Richards G. Treatment of perforated diverticular disease of the colon. Adv Surg 1978; 12:85–109.

In this article Hinchey describes the treatment of perforated diverticulum, discussing the pathogenesis of fecal peritonitis and the tailored approach to the management of these patients based on the amount of peritoneal contamination. His classification schema is still routinely used to describe the extent of peritoneal soilage.

18. Cho KC, Morehouse HT, Alterman DD, et al. Sigmoid diverticulitis: Diagnostic role of CT – comparison with barium enema studies. Radiology 1990; 176:111–115.

The authors prospectively review the results of computed tomography and barium enema examinations of the colon in the diagnosis of diverticulitis. CT was superior not only in the diagnosis of diverticulitis but in confirming alternative pathology when diverticulitis was not found.

19. Birnbaum BA, Balthazar EJ. CT of appendicitis and diverticulitis. Radiol Clin North Am 1994; 32:885–898.

20. Ambrosetti P, Robert J, Witzig JA, et al. Prognostic factors from computed tomography in acute left colonic diverticulitis. Br J Surg 1992; 79:117–119.

21. Ambrosetti P, Grossholz M, Becker C, et al. Computed tomography in acute left colonic diverticulitis. Br J Surg 1997; 84:532–534.

22. Hachigian MP, Honickman S, Eisenstat TE, et al. Computed tomography in the initial management of acute left-sided diverticulitis (published erratum appears in Dis Colon Rectum 1993; 36(2):193). Dis Colon Rectum 1992; 35:1123–1129.

23. Zielke A, Hasse C, Nies C, et al. Prospective evaluation of ultrasonography in acute colonic diverticulitis. Br J Surg 1997; 84:385–388.

24. O'Sullivan GC, Murphy D, O'Brien MG, et al. Laparoscopic management of generalized peritonitis due to perforated colonic diverticula. Am J Surg 1996; 171:432–434.

25. Stefansson T, Ekbom A, Sparen P, et al. Increased risk of left-sided colon cancer in patients with diverticular disease. Gut 1993; 34:499–502.

26. Kajiwara H, Umemura S, Mukai M, et al. Adenocarcinoma arising within a colonic diverticulum (Letter). Pathol Int 1996; 46:538–539.

27. Shepherd NA. Pathological mimics of chronic inflammatory bowel disease. J Clin Pathol 1991; 44:726–733.

28. Naliboff JA, Longmire-Cook SJ. Diverticulitis mimicking a tubo-ovarian abscess. Report of a case in a young woman. J Reprod Med 1996; 41:921–923.

29. Jarrett TW, Vaughan ED Jr. Accuracy of computerized tomography in the diagnosis of colovesical fistula secondary to diverticular disease. J Urol 1995; 153:44–46.

30. Sarr M, Fishman E, Goldman S, et al. Enterovesical fistula. Surg Gynecol Obstet 1987; 164:41–48.

31. Grissom R, Snyder T. Colovaginal fistula secondary to diverticular disease. Dis Colon Rectum 1991; 34:1043–1049.

32. Parks A, Gordon P. Fistula-in-ano: Perineal fistula of intraabdominal or intrapelvic origin simulating fistula-in-ano. Report of seven cases. Dis Colon Rectum 1976; 19:500–506.

33. Rothenbuehler JM, Oertli D, Harder F. Extraperitoneal manifestation of perforated diverticulitis. Dig Dis Sci 1993; 38:1985–1988.

34. Spiller GA, Freeman HJ. Recent advances in dietary fiber and colorectal diseases. Am J Clin Nutr 1981; 34:1145–1152.

35. Brodribb AJ. Treatment of symptomatic diverticular disease with a high-fibre diet. Lancet 1977; 1:664–666.

36. Talbot JM. Role of dietary fiber in diverticular disease and colon cancer. Fed Proc 1981; 40:2337–2342.

37. Ornstein MH, Littlewood ER, Baird IM, et al. Are fibre supplements really necessary in diverticular disease of the colon? A controlled clinical trial. Br Med J 1981; 282:1353–1356.

38. Eastwood MA, Smith AN, Brydon WG, et al. Comparison of bran, ispaghula, and lactulose on colon function in diverticular disease. Gut 1978; 19:1144–1147.

39. Sarin S, Boulos PB. Evaluation of current surgical management of acute inflammatory diverticular disease. Ann R Coll Surg Engl 1991; 73:278–282.

40. Schechter S, Mulvey J, Eisenstat TE. Management of uncomplicated acute diverticulitis: results of a survey. Dis Colon Rectum 1999; 42(4):470–475; discussion 475–476.

41. Wong WD, Wexner SD, Lowry A, et al. Practice parameters for sigmoid diverticulitis. The Standards Task Force American Society of Colon and Rectal Surgeons. Dis Colon Rectum 2000; 43(3):290–297.

The practice parameters published by the American Society of Colon and Rectal Surgeons reviews the pathogenesis and treatment of both complicated and uncomplicated diverticulitis. Updated frequently, they can be found at http://www.fascrs.org

42. Detry R, James J, Kartheuser A, et al. Acute localized diverticulitis: optimum management requires accurate staging. Int J Colorectal Dis 1992; 7:38–42.

43. Bahadursingh AM, Virgo KS, Kaminski DL, et al. Spectrum of disease and outcome of complicated diverticular disease. Am J Surg 2003; 186(6):696–701.

44. Stabile BE, Puccio E, van Sonnenberg E, et al. Preoperative percutaneous drainage of diverticular abscesses. Am J Surg 1990; 159:99–104.

The authors report their experience with 19 patients treated with percutaneous drainage of large paracolic abscesses over a 17-month period. They state that preoperative percutaneous catheter drainage obviates the need for colostomy and multiple-stage surgery in approximately three-fourths of patients with large diverticular abscesses.

45. Montgomery RS, Wilson SE. Intraabdominal abscesses: Image guided diagnosis and therapy. Clin Infect Dis 1996; 23:28–36.

46. Greco R, Kamath C, Nosher J. Percutaneous drainage of peridiverticular abscess followed by primary sigmoidectomy. Dis Colon Rectum 1982; 25:53–55.

47. Ambrosetti P, Robert J, Witzig JA, et al. Incidence, outcome, and proposed management of isolated abscesses complicating acute left-sided colonic diverticulitis. A prospective study of 140 patients. Dis Colon Rectum 1992; 35:1072–1076.

48. Hamy A, Paineau J. Percutaneous drainage of perisigmoid abscesses of diverticular origin. Ann Chir 2001; 126(2):133–137.

49. Piardi T, Ferrari Bravo A, Giampaoli F, et al. Deferred elective colonic resection in complicated acute diverticulitis. Chir Ital 2003; 55(2):153–160.

50. Classen J, Bonardi R, O'Mara C, et al. Surgical treatment of acute diverticulitis by staged procedures. Ann Surg 1976; 184:582–586.

51. Wedell J, Banzhaf G, Chaoui R, et al. Surgical management of complicated colonic diverticulitis. Br J Surg 1997; 84(3):380–383.

52. Rodkey G, Welch C. Changing patterns in the surgical treatment of diverticular disease. Ann Surg 1984; 200:466–478.

53. Hackford A, Schoetz DJ, Coller J, et al. Surgical management of complicated diverticulitis. The Lahey Clinic experience, 1967 to 1982. Dis Colon Rectum 1985; 28:317–321.

This report from the Lahey Clinic reviews the results of 142 patients with complicated diverticulitis treated surgically. Those patients who were able to tolerate a one stage procedure suffered the lowest mortality and morbidity (1% and 13% respectively).

54. Benn PL, Wolff BG, Ilstrup DM. Level of anastomosis and recurrent diverticulitis. Am J Surg 1986; 151:269–271.

This article from the Mayo Clinic highlights the importance of resecting the entire sigmoid colon down to the rectum distally. The proximal margin does not need to be free of all diverticulum, but be of normal caliber and compliance.

55. Moreaux J, Vons C. Elective resection for diverticular disease of the sigmoid colon. Br J Surg 1990; 77:1036–1038.

56. Alanis A, Papanicolaou G, Tadros R, et al. Primary resection and anastomosis for treatment of acute diverticulitis. Dis Colon Rectum 1989; 32:933–939.

57. Regenet N, Pessaux P, Hennekinne S, et al. Primary anastomosis after intraoperative colonic lavage vs. Hartmann's procedure in generalized peritonitis complicating diverticular disease of the colon. Int J Colorectal Dis 2003; 18(6):503–507.

58. Schilling MK, Maurer CA, Kollmar O, et al. Primary vs. secondary anastomosis after sigmoid colon resection for perforated diverticulitis (Hinchey Stage III and IV): a prospective outcome and cost analysis. Dis Colon Rectum 2001; 44(5):699–703.

59. Lee EC, Murray JJ, Coller JA, et al, Intraoperative colonic lavage in non-elective surgery for diverticular disease. Dis Colon Rectum 1997; 40:669–674.

The authors describe the technique used in intraoperative colonic lavage and detail their excellent results in the surgical management of acute diverticulitis.

60. Bell G, Panton O. Hartmann resection for perforated sigmoid diverticulitis. A retrospective study of the Vancouver General Hospital. Dis Colon Rectum 1984; 27:253–256.

61. Eisenstat T, Rubin R, Salvati E. Surgical management of diverticulitis. The role of the Hartmann procedure. Dis Colon Rectum 1983; 26:429–432.

62. Belmonte C, Klas JV, Perez JJ, et al. The Hartmann procedure. First choice or last resort in diverticular disease? Arch Surg 1996; 131:612–617.

63. Wedell J, Banzhaf G, Chaoui R, et al. Surgical management of complicated colonic diverticulitis. Br J Surg 1997; 84:380–383.

64. Cirocco WC, Priolo SR, Golub RW. Spontaneous ureterocolic fistula: a rare complication of colonic diverticular disease. Am Surg 1994; 60(11):832–835.

65. Hain JM, Sherick DG, Cleary RK. Salpingocolonic fistula secondary to diverticulitis. Am Surg 1996; 62(12):984–986.

66. Papagiannopoulos K, Gialvalis D, Dodo I, et al. Empyema resulting from a true colopleural fistula complicating a perforated sigmoid diverticulum. Ann Thorac Surg 2004; 77(1):324–326.

67. Woods R, Lavery I, Fazio V, et al. Internal fistulas in diverticular disease. Dis Colon Rectum 1988; 31:591–596.

68. Bahadursingh AM, Longo WE. Colovaginal fistulas. Etiology and management. J Reprod Med 2003; 48(7):489–495.

69. Fazio V, Church J, Jagelman D, et al. Colocutaneous fistula complicating diverticulitis. Dis Colon Rectum 1987; 30:89–94.

70. Stewart J, Diament R, Brennan T. Management of obstructing lesions of the left colon by resection, on-table lavage, and primary anastomosis. Surgery 1993; 114:502–505.

71. Allen-Mersh TG. Should primary anastomosis and on-table colonic lavage be standard treatment for left colon emergencies? Ann R Coll Surg Eng 1993; 175:195–198.

72. Jackson B. The diagnosis of colonic obstruction. Dis Colon Rectum 1982; 25:603–609.

73. Khan AL, Ah-See AK, Crofts TJ, et al. Surgical management of the septic complications of diverticular disease. Ann R Coll Surg Engl 1995; 77:16–20.

74. Pain J, Cahill J. Surgical options for left-sided large bowel emergencies. Ann R Coll Surg Engl 1991; 73:394–397.

75. Nahrwold D, Demuth W. Diverticulitis with perforation into the peritoneal cavity. Ann Surg 1997; 185:80–83.

76. Berry A, Turner W, Mortensen N, et al. Emergency surgery for complicated diverticular disease: A five-year review. Dis Colon Rectum 1989; 32:849–854.

77. Peoples JB, Vilk DR, Maguire JP, et al. Reassessment of primary resection of the perforated segment for severe colonic diverticulitis. Am J Surg 1990; 159:291–294.

78. Kronborg O. Treatment of perforated sigmoid diverticulitis: A prospective randomized trial. Br J Surg 1993; 80:505–507.

79. Corder AP, Williams JD. Optimal operative treatment in acute septic complications of diverticular disease. Ann R Coll Surg Engl 1990; 72:82–86.

80. Krukowski ZH, Matheson NA. Emergency surgery for diverticular disease complicated by generalized and faecal peritonitis: A review. Br J Surg 1984; 71:921–927.

81. Greif J, Fried G, McSherry C. Surgical treatment of perforated diverticulitis of the sigmoid colon. Dis Colon Rectum 1980; 23:484–487.

82. Finlay I, Carter D. A comparison of emergency resection and staged management in perforated diverticular disease. Dis Colon Rectum 1987; 30:929–933.

83. Nagorney D, Adson M, Pemberton J. Sigmoid diverticulitis with perforation and generalized peritonitis. Dis Colon Rectum 1985; 28:71–75.

84. Carson S, Krom R, Uchida K, et al. Colon perforation after kidney transplantation. Ann Surg 1978; 188:109–113.

85. Lao A, Bach D. Colonic complications in renal transplant patients. Dis Colon Rectum 1988; 31:130–133.

86. Starnes HJ, Lazarus J, Vineyard G. Surgery for diverticulitis in renal failure. Dis Colon Rectum 1985; 28:827–831.

87. Arsura EL. Corticosteroid-association perforation of colonic diverticula. Arch Intern Med 1990; 150:1337–1338.

88. Tyau ES, Prystowsky JB, Joehl RJ, et al. Acute diverticulitis. A complicated problem in the immunocompromised patient. Arch Surg 1991; 126:855–859.

89. Elliott TB, Yego S, Irvin TT. Five-year audit of the acute complications of diverticular disease. Br J Surg 1997; 84:535–539.

90. Munson KD, Hensien MA, Jacob LN, et al. Diverticulitis. A comprehensive follow-up. Dis Colon Rectum 1996; 39:318–322.

91. Sarin S, Boulos PB. Long-term outcome of patients presenting with acute complications of diverticular disease. Ann R Coll Surg Engl 1994; 76:117–120.

92. Parks T. Natural history of diverticular disease of the colon. Clin Gastroenterol 1975; 4:53–69.

93. Colcock B. Diverticular disease. Proven surgical management. Clin Gastroenterol 1975; 4:99–119.

94. Hyland JM, Taylor I. Does a high-fibre diet prevent the complications of diverticular disease? Br J Surg 1980; 67:77–79.

95. Leahy AL, Ellis RM, Quill DS, et al. High-fibre diet in symptomatic diverticular disease of the colon. Ann R Coll Surg Engl 1985; 67:173–174.

96. Farmakis N, Tudor RG, Keighley MR. The 5-year natural history of complicated diverticular disease. Br J Surg 1994; 81:733–735.

97. Ambrosetti P, Robert JH, Witzig JA, et al. Acute left colonic diverticulitis in young patients. J Am Coll Surg 1994; 179:156–160.

98. Anderson DN, Driver CP, Davidson AI, et al. Diverticular disease in patients under 50 years of age. J R Coll Surg Edinb 1997; 42:102–104.

99. Ouriel K, Schwartz SI. Diverticular disease in the young patient. Surg Gynecol Obstet 1983; 156:1–5.

100. Konvolinka CW. Acute diverticulitis under age forty. Am J Surg 1994; 167:562–565.

101. Schauer PR, Ramos R, Ghiatas AA, et al. Virulent diverticular disease in young obese men. Am J Surg 1992; 164:443–448.

102. Spivak H, Weinrauch S, Harvey JC, et al. Acute colonic diverticulitis in the young. Dis Colon Rectum 1997; 40:570–574.

103. Morgan RO, Kaiser M, Koshy J, et al. Incidence and treatment of diverticular disease of the colon among the elderly (Abstract). American Health Services Research Federal Health Services Research Annu Meet Abstr Book 1995; 12:118.

104. Vignati PV, Welch JP, Cohen JL. Long-term management of diverticulitis in young patients. Dis Colon Rectum 1995; 38:627–629.

105. Rennie JA, Charnock MC, Wellwood JM, et al. Results of resection for diverticular disease and its complications. Proc R Sac Med 1975; 68:575.

106. Breen R, Corman M, Robertson W, et al. Are we really operating on diverticulitis? Dis Colon Rectum 1986; 29:174–176.

107. Bokey E, Chapuis P, Pheils M. Elective resection for diverticular disease and carcinoma. Comparison of postoperative morbidity and mortality. Dis Colon Rectum 1981; 24:181–182.

108. Plasencia G, Jacobs M, Verdeja JC, et al. Laparoscopic-assisted sigmoid colectomy and low anterior resection. Dis Colon Rectum 1994; 37:829–833.

109. Bruce CJ, Coller JA, Murray JJ, et al. Laparoscopic resection for diverticular disease. Dis Colon Rectum 1996; 39(Suppl10):1–6.

110. Schlachta CM, Mamazza J, Gregoire R, et al. Could laparoscopic colon and rectal surgery become the standard of care? A review and experience with 750 procedures. Can J Surg 2003; 46(6):432–440.

111. Guller U, Jain N, Hervey S, et al. Laparoscopic vs. open colectomy: outcomes comparison based on large nationwide databases. Arch Surg 2003; 138(11):1179–1186.

112. Senagore AJ, Madbouly KM, Fazio VW, et al. Advantages of laparoscopic colectomy in older patients. Arch Surg 2003; 138(3):252–256.

113. Sher ME, Agachan F, Bortul M, et al. Laparoscopic surgery for diverticulitis. Surg Endosc 1997; 11:264–267.

114. Wolff BG, Ready RL, MacCarty RL, et al. Influence of sigmoid resection on progression of diverticular disease of the colon. Dis Colon Rectum 1984; 27:645–647.

115. Tchirkow G, Lavery I, Fazio V. Crohn's disease in the elderly. Dis Colon Rectum 1983; 26:177–181.

116. Chia J, Wilde C, Ngoi S, et al. Trends of diverticular disease of the large bowel in a newly developed country. Dis Colon Rectum 1991; 34:498–501.

117. Graham S, Ballantyne G. Cecal diverticulitis. A review of the American experience. Dis Colon Rectum 1987; 30:821–826.

118. Ngoi SS, Chia J, Goh MY, et al. Surgical management of right colon diverticulitis. Dis Colon Rectum 1992; 35:799–802.

119. Markham N, Li A. Diverticulitis of the right colon – experience from Hong Kong. Gut 1992; 33:547–549.

120. Puera DA, Lanza FL, Gostout CJ, et al. The American College of Gastroenterology bleeding registry: preliminary findings. Am J Gastroentorol 1997; 92: 924–928.

121. Longstretch GF. Epidemiology and outcome of patients hospitalized with acute lower gastrointestinal hemorrhage: a population-based study. Am J Gastroenterol 1997; 92: 419–424.

122. McGuire JJ Jr, Haynes BW Jr. Massive hemorrhage for diverticulosis of the colon: guidelines for therapy based on bleeding patterns observed in fifty cases. Am Surg 1972; 175:847–855.

123. McGuire HH Jr. Bleeding colonic diverticula. A reappraisal of the natural history and management. Ann Surg 1994; 220:653–656.

124. Browder W, Cerise E, Litwin M. Impact of emergency angiography in massive lower gastrointestinal hemorrhage. Ann Surg 1986; 204:530–536.

125. Sharma R, Gorbien MJ. Angiodysplasia and lower gastrointestinal tract bleeding in elderly patients. Arch Intern Med 1995; 155:807–812.

126. Foutch PG. Diverticular bleeding: Are nonsteroidal anti-inflammatory drugs risk factors for hemorrhage and can colonoscopy predict outcome for patients? Am J Gastroenterol 1995; 90:1779–1784.

127. Nusbaum M, Baum S, Kuroda K, et al. Control of portal hypertension by selective mesenteric arterial drug infusion. Arch Surg 1968; 97:1005–1014.

128. Darcy M. Treatment of lower gastrointestinal bleeding: Vasopressin infusion versus embolization. J Vasc Interv Radiol 2003; 14(5):535–543.

129. DeBarros J, Rosas L, Cohen J, et al. The changing paradigm for the treatment of colonic hemorrhage: superselective angiographic embolization. Dis Colon Rectum 2002; 45(6):802–808.

130. Bookstein JJ, Cholsta EM, Foley D, et al. Transcatheter hemostasis of gastrointestinal bleeding using modified autogenous clot. Radiology 1974; 113:277–285.

131. Parkes BM, Obeid FN, Sorensen VJ, et al. The management of massive lower gastrointestinal bleeding. Am Surg 1993; 59(10):676–678.

132. Ferands PA, Taylor I. Management of acute lower gastrointestinal bleeding in a surgical unit over a four-year period. J Soc Med 1987; 80:79–82.

133. Wright AK, Pellicia O, Higgins EF, et al. Controlled semi-elective, segmental resection for massive colonic hemorrhage. Am J Surg 1980; 139:535–538.

134. Bowden TA Jr, Hooks VH 3rd, Mansberger AR Jr. Intraoperative gastrointestinal endoscopy in the management of occult gastrointestinal bleeding. South Med J 1979; 72(12):1532–1534.

135. Anand AC, Patnaik PK, Bhalla VP, et al. Massive lower intestinal bleeding – a decade of experience. Trop Gastroenterol 2001; 22(3):131-134.

136. Renzulli P, Maurer CA, Netzer P, et al. Subtotal colectomy with primary ileorectostomy is effective for unlocalized, diverticular hemorrhage. Langenbecks Arch Surg 2002; 387(2):67–71.

137. Foutch PG, Zimmerman K. Diverticular bleeding and the pigmented protuberance (sentinel clot): Clinical implications, histopathological correlation, and results of endoscopic intervention. Am J Gastroenterol 1996; 91:2589–2593.

CHAPTER SIXTY-TWO

Vascular insufficiency

Daniel S. Mishkin, Patricia L. Kozuch and Lawrence J. Brandt

INTRODUCTION

Intestinal ischemia refers to the process whereby blood flow to the bowel is decreased with cellular injury consequent to diminished supply of oxygen and nutrients.[1] A vascular emergency of the gastrointestinal tract usually results from a disturbance in the arterial blood supply or venous drainage of the bowel with consequential severe ischemic injury. Severe ischemia manifests as gangrene and perforation or less commonly as stricture formation with intestinal obstruction. Vascular emergencies much more commonly involve the colon than the small intestine, and arterial ischemia is more common than ischemia from venous occlusion.[2]

Vascular insufficiency encompasses a broad spectrum of disease manifestations and severity. The differences may depend on the etiology, speed of onset and duration of the ischemic event, location and length of intestine affected, as well as the specific vasculature involved and its degree of collateral flow. With such a range of possible permutations and combinations it is important to differentiate the etiology if possible and the extent of the injury to better direct therapy. Most cases of colon ischemia resolve spontaneously without sequelae, whereas most small bowel ischemia demands medical/surgical intervention and has serious sequelae or a poor outcome. Therefore, early recognition, diagnosis, and therapy are essential in the management of such patients.

Epidemiology

Acute mesenteric ischemia (AMI) is an uncommon occurrence, accounting for approximately 0.1% of hospital admissions.[1] A rising incidence in the past quarter century has been attributed to a heightened awareness of gastrointestinal ischemic disease as well as to an increase in the number of people at risk for AMI because of population aging and advances in the treatment of cardiovascular diseases, thereby allowing patients to survive what previously were fatal conditions. The overall mortality rate of AMI remains high at 71%; however, survival rates are significantly improved when AMI is diagnosed and treated in an expeditious manner (under 24 hours), especially when mesenteric angiography and splanchnic vasodilators are used early in the management of disease.[3] The most common cause of AMI is superior mesenteric artery emboli (SMAE), accounting for approximately 50% of the cases, with nonocclusive mesenteric ischemia (NOMI) following at 25%. Superior mesenteric artery thrombosis (SMAT, 10%), mesenteric venous thrombosis (MVT, 10%), and focal segmental

ischemia (FSI, 5%) are responsible for the remainder of cases. Colon ischemia (CI) is a frequent disorder of the large bowel in older persons and is the most common form of intestinal ischemic injury. It is estimated to account for 1/100 colonoscopies, 1/700 office visits, and 1/2000 admissions to a tertiary care center. A recent study using medical claims data from a large healthcare organization in the US calculated a crude incidence rate of 7.2 cases per 100 000 person-years of observation in the general population.[4]

Anatomy of the splanchnic circulation

Intestinal ischemia can be classified as acute or chronic and of venous or arterial origin. In acute forms, intestinal viability is threatened, whereas in the chronic forms, blood flow is inadequate to support the functional demands of the intestine. Understanding the anatomy of splanchnic circulations is important to help understand the different types of vascular insults. The celiac axis (CA), superior mesenteric artery (SMA), and inferior mesenteric artery (IMA) supply almost all of the blood flow to the digestive tract. There is marked variability of vascular anatomy among individuals, but typical patterns have emerged from anatomic dissections and abdominal angiography.[5]

The CA arises from the anterior aorta and gives rise to three major branches: (1) the left gastric artery, (2) the common hepatic artery, and its gastroduodenal, right gastroepiploic, and superior pancreaticoduodenal arterial branches, and (3) the splenic artery with its pancreatic and left gastroepiploic arterial branches. The CA and its branches supply the stomach, duodenum, pancreas, and the liver.

The SMA has its origin from the anterior aorta near the neck of the pancreas. It gives rise to four major vessels: (1) the inferior pancreaticoduodenal, (2) middle colic, (3) right colic, and (4) ileocolic arteries, as well as to a series of jejunal and ileal branches, all of which supply their named portions of intestine. These intestinal branches typically form a series of arcades, and from the terminal arcade, numerous straight vessels arise that enter the intestinal wall. These end arteries make the intestine more vulnerable to ischemic insults because of the lack of collateral pathways.

The IMA arises 3–4 cm above the aortic bifurcation close to the inferior border of the duodenum. It branches into the left colic artery and multiple sigmoid branches and terminates as the superior rectal artery. The IMA and its branches supply the large intestine from the distal transverse colon to the proximal rectum. The distal rectum is supplied by branches of the internal iliac (hypogastric) artery.

Abundant collateral circulation to the stomach, duodenum, and rectum accounts for the paucity of ischemic events in these organs. The major anastomosis between the CA and the SMA is formed from the superior pancreaticoduodenal branch of the CA and the inferior pancreaticoduodenal branch of the SMA. These vessels constitute the pancreaticoduodenal arcade and provide blood to the duodenum and the pancreas. The splenic flexure and sigmoid colon have limited anastomoses, and ischemic damage is more common in these locations. There are three potential paths of communication between the SMA and IMA: (1) the marginal artery of Drummond, which is closest to and parallel with the wall of the intestine; (2) the central anastomotic artery, a larger and more centrally placed vessel; and (3) the arc of Riolan, an artery in the base of the mesentery. On angiography, the 'meandering artery' represents a dilated central artery or arc of Riolan and may be diagnostic of an occluded SMA or IMA. It is critical to determine the direction of flow in any meandering artery prior to resection of the IMA, e.g., during aortic aneurysm surgery, lest the IMA be the main vessel supplying blood to the small bowel because of an occluded SMA.

PATHOGENESIS OF INJURY

In addition to the protection offered by collateral blood supply, the bowel has several other mechanisms to prevent ischemic injury. Intestinal blood flow must be reduced by at least 50% from the normal fasting level before oxygen delivery to the intestine becomes compromised.[6] A rich network of intramural submucosal vessels helps protect segments of bowel from ischemia even when SMA blood flow is severely reduced.[7] Further, redistribution of intramural blood supply occurs with ischemia, favoring preservation of the mucosa.[8] It has been demonstrated that the bowel can endure a 75% reduction in its blood supply for up to 12 hours without significant injury.[9] Two mechanisms may account for this observation: first, under normal physiologic conditions, only 20% of the mesenteric capillaries are open and utilizing oxygen at any one time;[10] second, when oxygen delivery is decreased, the bowel adapts by increasing oxygen extraction. When the aforementioned parameters are exceeded, however, these compensatory mechanisms are overwhelmed and no longer protective.

Blood flow to the intestine is regulated by the sympathetic nervous system, humoral factors including angiotensin II and vasopressin, and local factors such as prostaglandins and leukotrienes.[7] The sympathetic nervous system, mainly via α-adrenergic receptors, is of primary importance in maintaining resting splanchnic arteriolar tone. When a major intestinal artery is obstructed, a reduction in pressure in the distal arterial bed below systemic pressure triggers the opening of collaterals. After several hours, however, the distal arteries begin to constrict, resulting in an increased arterial pressure, which consequently decreases collateral flow.

Vasoconstriction initially is reversible, but may become irreversible after a prolonged period, even if the event initiating ischemia has been identified and corrected.[1] So-called nonocclusive mesenteric ischemia (NOMI) from vasoconstriction may be seen clinically as a result of diminished cardiac output or accompany local vascular obstruction such as emboli. Both hypoxia and reperfusion are important etiologic factors in ischemic injury, with the latter playing a greater role when periods of ischemia are short. As the ischemia period lengthens, the hypoxia becomes more detrimental than reperfusion. Reperfusion injury is likely multifactorial, but

oxygen radicals and polymorphonuclear cells are thought to be integral. Such injuries lead to a wide spectrum of microscopic and gross pathologic findings. At one extreme, the milder lesions of nontransmural ischemic injury (mucosal necrosis, submucosal edema, hemorrhage, and ulceration) usually are seen with a more indolent course and ultimately heal. At the other end of this continuum is transmural necrosis (infarction), gangrene, and perforation, findings usually associated with a profound clinical outcome. Lesions of intermediate severity may progress to transmural necrosis or result in fibrosis with stricture formation.[11]

GOALS OF MANAGEMENT

The cardiologists and neurologists have helped further our understanding of the importance of correcting perfusion to critical organs. Limiting hypoxia and, if possible, reperfusion injury are two fundamental aspects also important in patients with vascular insufficiency of the gastrointestinal tract. In this chapter we will address the various forms of intestinal ischemia and their specific management.

ACUTE MESENTERIC ISCHEMIA

Disease spectrum and clinical presentation

Acute mesenteric ischemia (AMI) results from sudden, inadequate blood flow to the gastrointestinal tract. Regardless of the cause of the ischemic insult, the end results are similar – a spectrum of bowel injury that ranges from transient alteration of bowel function to transmural gangrene. Clinical manifestations vary with the extent of ischemic injury and, to a lesser degree, with its cause. It is important to define the cause, as treatment varies accordingly (Table 62.1).

Clinical aspects

Early identification of AMI requires a high index of suspicion, especially in patients older than 50 years who have long-standing congestive heart failure, cardiac arrhythmias, recent myocardial infarction, or hypotension. NOMI increasingly has become recognized after cardiac surgery[12] and in hemodialysis patients.[13] Hypercoagulable states, underlying vasculitides, and intra-abdominal malignancy also have been linked to the development of AMI, particularly acute MVT. Not only are disease entities important as

Table 62.1 Causes and approximate incidences of acute mesenteric ischemia

Cause	Incidence (%)
SMA embolus (SMAE)	50
Nonocclusive mesenteric ischemia (NOMI)	25
SMA thrombosis (SMAT)	10
Mesenteric venous thrombosis (MVT)	10
Focal segmental ischemia	5

(Reprinted from Brandt LJ et al in Feldman M et al ed. Sleisenger and Fordtran's Gastrointestinal and Liver Disease, Philadelphia: W.B. Saunders; 2002, 2321–2340. © 2002, with permission from Elsevier.)

possible precipitants for ischemia, but certain illegal drugs, such as cocaine, and various therapeutic agents, e.g., phenylephrine, amphetamines, triptans, vasopressin, and sodium polystyrene in sorbitol (kayexalate), also have been implicated.[14]

The overwhelming majority of patients with AMI experience abdominal pain during the ischemic episode: an acute onset is usually observed with SMAE as opposed to a more insidious presentation with NOMI. The classic teaching of 'pain out of proportion to findings on physical exam' often is observed in the early stages of AMI, when the abdomen is soft and even nontender. Distention and severe tenderness with rebound and guarding develop as a consequence of bowel infarction. The rapidity with which these findings develop is a function of the severity of the ischemic injury. A small proportion of patients with NOMI do not experience pain, and distention is more common in this group. Patients with SMAE may note forceful bowel evacuation. Occult bleeding is seen in three-fourths of patients with AMI; gross bleeding is rare in patients with AMI and usually indicates right colon involvement. Mental status change in elderly patients is seen in up to 30% of cases.[15] Other late signs and symptoms of intestinal ischemia include nausea, vomiting, hematemesis, fever, obstruction, back pain, and shock.

Diagnostic evaluation

While laboratory tests often are abnormal in patients with AMI, they are neither sufficiently sensitive nor specific to diagnose AMI early enough to improve prognosis. This holds true for serum levels of inorganic phosphate and standard enzyme determinations such as creatinine kinase, lactate dehydrogenase, aspartate transferase and alkaline phosphatase (including the intestinal isoenzyme). More specific enzymes including diamine oxidase, and hexosaminidase also lack sufficient sensitivity and specificity to diagnose AMI.[16] More recently, glutathione S-transferase (a family of cytosolic enzymes widely distributed in the intestine)[17] and intestinal fatty acid binding protein (accounting for 2% of intestinal protein and located at the tips of mucosal villi) have been shown to be promising markers for intestinal ischemia in adults and in neonates with necrotizing enterocolitis.[18,19] Metabolic acidosis is neither sensitive nor specific enough to be used as an aid in diagnosing AMI early, but is common in the presence of intestinal gangrene. Leukocytosis is a common finding in AMI, with an elevated white blood cell count over 15 000/mL seen in more than 75% of patients. Thus, a normal WBC cannot reliably exclude AMI, but neither can an elevated one be used to make the diagnosis, given its lack of specificity.

Radiology

Although poorly sensitive and non-specific, plain films of the abdomen are commonly obtained in evaluating patients with suspected AMI; in most medical centers today, CT scanning has replaced plain film use. There are three relatively specific findings of mesenteric ischemia which are better depicted on CT scans compared with plain films:[20] (1) abnormal gas in the bowel wall or portal system; (2) acute embolic infarction of other intra-abdominal organs; and (3) thrombi in the mesenteric vessels. Early in the course of AMI, abdominal films usually are normal. In late-stage AMI, one may observe an ileus, 'thumbprinting,' formless loops of small bowel, and more rarely portal or mesenteric venous gas.[21] The primary purpose of plain films or CT scans remains to exclude other causes of abdominal pain that might mandate a therapeutic approach

different from that for AMI. Neither a normal abdominal plain film nor a normal CT scan excludes the diagnosis of AMI.

Doppler ultrasound can visualize stenoses or occlusions in the CA or SMA. However, its sensitivity for diagnosing AMI is limited by four significant factors: first, only the proximal portions of the main splanchnic vessels can be studied; second, vessel occlusions or stenoses identified by this technique are not diagnostic of intestinal ischemia, given that complete occlusions in two or even all three vessels can be seen in asymptomatic patients; third, blood flow through the SMA is highly variable, which makes interpretation of this test difficult; and fourth, NOMI, which accounts for approximately 25% of AMI, cannot be diagnosed by Doppler ultrasound.[1]

In patients with AMI, the sensitivity of abdominal CT depends on the underlying cause and severity of ischemia. The spectrum of CT signs for ischemia include bowel lumen dilatation, segmental wall thickening and abnormal bowel wall enhancement, arterial or venous occlusions, and intramural, portal venous, intraperitoneal and retroperitoneal gas.[22] A significant limitation is that the more specific signs of ischemia, such as pneumatosis with portal vein gas, are late manifestations.[23] In one study, the finding of either arterial or venous thrombosis, intramural gas, portal venous gas, focal lack of bowel wall enhancement, or liver or splenic infarcts had a sensitivity and specificity of 64% and 92%, respectively.[24] In another study, the sensitivity of CT for the diagnosis of mesenteric venous thrombosis was approximately 90%.[25]

More recently, CT angiography (CTA) has been shown to be very promising in the diagnosis of AMI. In one study, 62 patients with a clinical suspicion of AMI were evaluated with CTAs for findings suggesting emboli or thrombi in the CA, SMA, or IMA.[26] A finding of any one of pneumatosis intestinalis, venous gas, SMA occlusion, CA and IMA occlusion with distal SMA disease or arterial embolism was 100% specific but only 73% sensitive. The finding of bowel wall thickening in addition to focal lack of bowel wall enhancement, solid organ infarction, or venous thrombosis was 50% sensitive and 94% specific. Independently, the added angiographic findings were believed to alter the course in 19% of patients by making the diagnosis of AMI when CT alone did not. A relatively low mortality rate of 42% in studied patients with documented AMI was observed, paralleling results of older studies that also showed lower mortalities when mesenteric angiography was used diagnostically. While these data are very encouraging, it may fall short of standard angiography in terms of diagnosing NOMI as well as by its inability to allow treatment with intra-arterial vasodilators.

MR angiography (MRA) is another of the newer imaging modalities used to diagnose AMI. MRA provides detailed anatomic information regarding sites of obstruction but at this time, MRA lacks sufficient resolution to diagnose NOMI secondary to low-flow states or to identify distal embolic disease.[27] Delayed phase imaging also permits evaluation of the mesenteric veins. In the future, measuring the absolute value of oxygen saturation between the SMV blood relative to that of the inferior vena cava may be used.[28]

Selective mesenteric angiography has long been the gold standard for diagnosis of AMI, a standard now being challenged by proponents of CTA and MRA. In a review of mesenteric angiography for the diagnosis of AMI, sensitivities in five of six studies have ranged 90–100%; specificity was reported in two of these studies to be 100%.[3] Not only can a diagnosis of AMI and its etiology be established confidently by conventional angiography, but a vascular 'roadmap' in occlusive disease can be obtained that can aid in planning revascularization procedures. Moreover, the angiographic catheter can be used to administer intra-arterial vasodilators such as papaverine. The excellent sensitivity and therapeutic potential of angiography combine to effect a significantly improved mortality rate with reported ranges of 18–53%.[3] Preoperative angiography is, therefore, a valuable tool, although it should never significantly delay what may be life-saving surgery. Disadvantages of traditional angiography are its limited availability and potential renal toxicity as well as its expense and time constraints.

Other diagnostic tests

Laparoscopy may be used as a diagnostic test for mesenteric ischemia with two caveats: first, intraperitoneal pressure exceeding 20 mmHg decreases SMA blood flow;[29] and second, mucosal injury may exist and be unappreciated in the absence of serosal evidence of ischemia.[16] The latter is explained by the mucosal-to-serosal shunting of blood flow that occurs with increased intestinal intraluminal or intraperitoneal pressures.

Upper endoscopy to evaluate for mesenteric ischemia is limited by the reach of the instrument; colonoscopy, however, has become routine in the diagnosis of CI. Although the risk of performing colonoscopy in patients with CI is small, overinflation of the colon, with consequent increase of intraluminal pressure decreases total colon blood flow and renders the colon susceptible to ischemic injury. A decrease in colon blood flow becomes significant with pressure of 30 mmHg or greater and can be decreased significantly by the use of carbon dioxide as the insufflating agent.[30] Intravenous fluorescein has been used both during endoscopy and intraoperatively to define areas of ischemia; the underperfused ischemic areas of bowel demonstrate proportionally less fluorescence than does the bowel with normal blood flow.[16]

Radioisotope studies, laser Doppler flowmetry, reflectance spectrophotometry, and superconducting quantum interference devices (SQUID) are other experimental modalities that have been studied in the diagnosis of intestinal ischemia although not yet been applied clinically.[31]

Therapeutic options

Our approach to the diagnosis and management of AMI is based on several observations. First, if the diagnosis is not made before intestinal infarction, the mortality rate is 70–90%. Second, the diagnosis of both the occlusive and nonocclusive forms of AMI can be made in most patients by angiography. Third, vasoconstriction, which may persist even after the cause of the ischemia is corrected, is the basis of NOMI and a contributing factor in the other forms of AMI. Finally, the vasoconstriction can be relieved by vasodilators infused into the SMA. The cornerstones of our approach, therefore, are the earlier and more liberal use of angiography and the incorporation of intra-arterial papaverine in the treatment of both occlusive AMI and NOMI.

All patients with suspected AMI should undergo volume resuscitation and treatment with broad-spectrum antibiotics as well as correction of any potential contributing causes of AMI such as arrhythmias or congestive heart failure. Bacterial translocation has been shown to occur during AMI owing to loss of mucosal integrity.[32] Experimental studies have shown reduction in the severity and extent of bowel damage with peri-ischemic event fluid resuscitation and antibiotic treatment, covering both Gram-negative and anaerobic organisms.[33]

Occlusive acute mesenteric ischemia: SMAE and SMAT

Superior mesenteric artery emboli (SMAE) generally arise from ventricular or left atrial thrombi, often in the setting of atrial fibrillation. Many patients have a history of peripheral arterial emboli, and synchronous emboli are seen in 20% of patients. Typically, SMAE are found at points of normal anatomic narrowing, frequently just distal to the origin of a major vascular branch. They are classified as 'major' emboli when found proximal to the origin of the ileocolic artery and 'minor' if distal to this point or in one of the distal branches of the SMA. Angiographically, SMAE are characterized by rounded filling defects that result in occlusions to flow; evidence of atherosclerotic disease is seen to a lesser extent with emboli than with thrombosis.

Superior mesenteric artery thrombosis (SMAT) is found most commonly in areas of severe atherosclerotic disease, usually at the origin of the SMA. Twenty percent to 50% of patients with SMAT report postprandial pain compatible with CMI. Coronary artery disease, stroke, and peripheral artery disease are frequent comorbidities. Angiography typically demonstrates an occlusion 1–2 cm distal to the origin of the SMA. Sometimes it can be difficult to differentiate an acute thrombosis from one that is chronic and incidental: the finding of collateral vessels that provide good filling of the SMA argues against an acute thrombosis, and other etiologies for the patient's symptoms should be sought. Alternatively, if collateral vessels cannot be appreciated or adequate collateral filling of the SMA is not seen, then the thrombosis must be considered to be acute and appropriate treatment begun.

Treatment of occlusive AMI is highly dependent upon the presence or absence of peritoneal signs: when such signs are present, a patient must undergo an exploratory laparotomy. Surgical interventions include resection of necrotic bowel with thromboembolectomy, patch angioplasty, endarterectomy and bypass procedures, depending on individual vascular anatomy and cause of the occlusion, e.g., embolus or thrombus.[34] 'Second-look' operations are recommended in an attempt to minimize the amount of bowel that needs to be resected if there is questionable bowel viability during the first surgery. The time in between the index surgery and the second-look procedure is used to maximize bowel survival, e.g., antibiotics, fluid replacement, and correction of adverse comorbidities. Percutaneous transluminal angioplasty also has been successful in one case report of a patient with SMAT and peritoneal signs,[35] but generally is not advocated, given the significant risk of re-thrombosis.

Thrombolytics

In patients without peritonitis, thrombolytics have been used alone successfully to treat SMA emboli and, to a lesser extent, thrombi. The pertinent literature, however, consists of only case reports and small case series; agents that have been used include streptokinase, urokinase, and tissue plasminogen activator (tPA). To date, there have been no randomized controlled trials comparing any of these agents to each other or to other treatments.

Pharmacology of thrombolytics

Plasmin, a key element in the body's endogenous fibrinolytic system, is a protease that dissolves thrombi by breaking down fibrin and other proteins of the clotting cascade including fibrinogen and coagulation factors V and VIII.[36] Plasminogen is converted to plasmin by the cleavage of a single arginyl-valyl bond, also known as the

Arg$_{560}$-Val$_{561}$ 'activator bond.'[37] Endogenous tissue plasminogen activator (tPA) and urokinase serve as plasminogen activators: t-PA converts predominantly fibrin-bound plasminogen to plasmin; urokinase, produced by human kidney cells, helps keep hollow organs such as the ureter, free from thrombi. Fibrinolysis is regulated primarily by inhibitors of both plasmin and plasminogen; however, when thrombolytics are used, these inhibitory controls become overwhelmed, and thus hemorrhage is a feared side effect. Because of its fibrin specificity, tPA is theoretically safer in terms of hemorrhagic risk, but this advantage has not been borne out clinically. Contraindications to thrombolytic therapy relate primarily to increased risk of bleeding, including recent surgery, trauma, severe hypertension, active bleeding or hemorrhagic disorder, previous CVA or active intracranial process, pregnancy or puerperium, aortic dissection, and acute pericarditis.[38]

The largest case series of thrombolytic therapy for AMI evaluated 10 patients who presented with acute abdominal pain of 5–18 hours duration; all had angiographically proven SMAE, two with major and eight with minor emboli.[39] No patients had peritoneal signs and all had normal abdominal plain films. Urokinase (200 000 units) was infused directly into the embolus, followed by infusion of urokinase at 100 000 U/h into the SMA proximal to the embolus until angiographic resolution of the embolus; infusion times ranged between 8 and 32 hours. All patients also were given systemic heparin at 1000 U/h, which was continued for 4 days after urokinase treatment and was followed by warfarin indefinitely, if fibrinolysis was successful. Response to treatment was assessed by repeated clinical assessment and angiography 4–6 h after beginning treatment and thereafter at regular intervals as appropriate, depending on clinical and radiologic results. Resolution of the occlusion was defined by normal angiography or the presence of only tiny nonobstructing emboli with normal blood flow. Follow-up angiography showed successful lysis of emboli in 90% of patients, and resolution of abdominal pain within 1 hour of infusion in 70% of patients. One of these seven patients underwent exploratory laparotomy because of equivocal physical examination findings and was found to have normal bowel. All three patients who continued to have abdominal pain or developed peritoneal signs underwent surgery with bowel resection. One death in this group was believed to be secondary to cardiac insufficiency and was without demonstrable abdominal pathology. The authors of this study believed resolution of abdominal pain within 1 hour to be the most significant factor in predicting the success of fibrinolysis. They cautiously pointed out that, in contrast to classic dogma, duration of symptoms prior to diagnosis and treatment did not predict outcome. No complications occurred from urokinase therapy, and no patient suffered from recurrent embolism or postischemic stenoses in follow-up over an average period of 11 months.

Many questions with regard to fibrinolysis remain to be studied including optimal agent and dose, method of delivery (pulse-spray, intra-embolic, rapidity of infusions), length of treatment, whether treatment should vary depending on emboli location or duration of symptoms, role of adjunctive anticoagulation and its optimal duration, criteria to help define need for surgery and the best means of routine postlytic evaluation.

Vasodilators

In addition to its therapeutic role in NOMI, both canine and human studies have shown vasodilator therapy to be beneficial for AMI secondary to SMAE or SMAT because splanchnic vasoconstriction accompanies acute embolic and thrombotic mesenteric disease. Vasodilators, however, rarely are used alone in these situations unless patients are judged to be poor operative candidates. It has been demonstrated that mesenteric vasoconstriction may develop and persist for hours, causing irreversible 'nonocclusive' ischemia, even after what was believed to be a successful surgery or thrombolytic therapy for SMAE or SMAT.

In a classic study by Boley and colleagues, dogs with iatrogenic SMAE were treated with intra-arterial saline (n=3), intra-arterial papaverine (n=5), intra-arterial streptokinase (n=5) or both papaverine and streptokinase (n=5).[40] Post-treatment angiograms and pathologic examination revealed that although the group treated with streptokinase had the most vigorous response in terms of embolus lysis, the group treated with papaverine had less vasoconstriction, better bowel perfusion, and less bowel necrosis than any of the other three groups. Interestingly, the vasodilator effects of papaverine and the thrombolytic effects of streptokinase were attenuated in the group treated with both agents. Clinically, Boley et al. demonstrated a mortality rate of 54% (compared with 70–80% mortality in traditionally managed patients) when an aggressive approach utilizing early angiography and papaverine was taken in the management of patients with suspected AMI.[41]

Because of these successful experimental and clinical outcomes, papaverine is used frequently both pre- and postoperatively to reduce the splanchnic vasoconstriction that typifies NOMI and accompanies SMAE, SMAT, and even acute MVT. To date, however, no randomized controlled studies have been conducted to confirm the efficacy of this approach. Studies in which embolectomy was performed early in the clinical course without the use of papaverine have had equally successful outcomes; it has been postulated that vasoconstriction had not yet developed in these patients.

Pharmacology of papaverine

Papaverine is a nonselective vasodilator derived from the poppy plant (genus *Papaver*); it inhibits phosphodiesterase, resulting in increased levels of intracellular cyclic AMP, the net effect of which is smooth muscle cell relaxation.[42] In its use as a vasodilator for AMI, papaverine is administered as a bolus dose of 60 mg directly into the SMA, followed by a constant infusion of 30–60 mg/h. Priscoline, an alpha-receptor antagonist, sometimes is administered prior to papaverine to assess mesenteric responsiveness to vasodilation. Few systemic side effects from papaverine occur owing to its high first-pass metabolism (70–90%) and its short half-life of 0.5–2 hours. Some patients with liver disease may exhibit a drop in blood pressure with this dose of papaverine, but the most common cause of hypotension during the papaverine infusion is catheter dislodgment. Patients who have a sudden drop in blood pressure should immediately have the papaverine replaced with a saline or glucose solution and promptly undergo plain film imaging of the abdomen to confirm the catheter's location. Complete AV block is a contraindication to papaverine treatment as large doses may depress AV conduction and result in cardiac arrhythmias.

Proponents of vasodilator therapy recommend that preoperative intra-arterial papaverine be started during the index angiography if possible, and continued for 12–24 hours postoperatively if no second-look surgery is planned, and through the second procedure if one is planned. In either case, angiography should be done before removal of the catheter to confirm that vasospasm does not persist. Complications from repeated angiographic studies include acute tubular necrosis and local hematomas.

Nonocclusive mesenteric ischemia

Nonocclusive mesenteric ischemia (NOMI) results from vasoconstriction that initially serves as a protective mechanism in the setting of a cardiovascular event such as acute myocardial infarction with shock, arrhythmias, congestive heart failure, hypovolemia associated with burns, pancreatitis, hemorrhage, and sepsis; cirrhosis and renal failure/dialysis also are risk factors. Splanchnic vasoconstrictors such as alpha adrenergic agents and digitalis also have been linked to NOMI.[43] The incidence of NOMI has decreased significantly in recent years, likely owing to improved monitoring capabilities of hemodynamic parameters in the intensive care setting as well as the widespread use of vasodilating agents in the management of congestive heart failure and myocardial infarction.[44] Vasoconstriction which initially is reversible may become irreversible if it is not corrected quickly, even after correction of the precipitating cause. Angiographically, four signs help to reliably diagnose NOMI: narrowing at the origins of SMA branches, alternating dilation and narrowing in the intestinal branches (the 'string-of-sausages' sign), spasm of the vascular arcades, and impaired filling of intramural vessels.[45]

An algorithm for management of NOMI proposed by Boley et al. over 25 years ago is still the treatment regimen with the best survival rates. As soon as angiographic diagnosis is established, intra-arterial (SMA) papaverine is initiated with a bolus of 60 mg and then infused at a dose of 30–60 mg/h. If peritoneal signs remain absent or remit within 20–30 minutes after papaverine infusion has begun, then papaverine is continued and repeat angiography is performed in 24 hours to document absence of or improvement in vasospasm. Papaverine infusion may be stopped at this point or continued if vasospasm persists; optimally an angiogram is repeated daily during infusion. If peritoneal signs are newly noted or persist longer than 20–30 minutes after papaverine is started, then exploratory laparotomy is mandated with resection of bowel as needed. Second-look procedures are done if bowel viability is in question. Papaverine is continued intraoperatively and postoperatively for 24 hours or until the time of the second-look operation.[43]

Focal segmental ischemia

Focal segmental ischemia (FSI) is generally not a life-threatening condition as only short segments of bowel are involved and adequate collateral blood flow generally limits transmural necrosis. The etiology of FSI is varied and includes atheromatous emboli, strangulated hernias, immune complex disorders and vasculitis, blunt abdominal trauma, segmental thrombosis, radiation therapy, and oral contraceptives. Limited necrosis may present as acute enteritis, chronic enteritis (often resembling Crohn's disease), or a stricture. The most common presentation is chronic small bowel obstruction with intermittent abdominal pain, distention, and vomiting. Bacterial overgrowth and protein-losing enteropathy also can occur. Definitive treatment of FSI is resection of the involved bowel.[1]

Mesenteric venous thrombosis

Mesenteric venous thrombosis (MVT) may have an acute, subacute, or chronic presentation. Patients with MVT are typically younger than those with other types of mesenteric ischemia. MVT is associated with a myriad of hypercoagulable states, including protein

C, protein S or antithrombin III deficiencies, factor V Leiden mutation, anticardiolipin antibodies, malignancy, estrogens and pregnancy, intra-abdominal inflammation and sepsis, postoperative states, and trauma. MVT secondary to cirrhosis or neoplasm tends to start at the site of obstruction and propagate peripherally, while the centripetal propagation is observed in hypercoagulable states. If collateral blood flow does not permit venous drainage around the obstructed vessel, the bowel will become congested, edematous, cyanotic, and thickened with intramural hemorrhage. Serosanguinous peritoneal fluid heralds early hemorrhagic infarction. Coincidental arterial vasoconstriction may occur and also causes bowel infarction.

Acute MVT presents with abdominal pain in more than 90% of patients and, as with acute arterial ischemia, the pain initially is out of proportion to the physical findings. The mean duration of pain before admission is 5–14 days but may be more than 1 month in as many as 25% of individuals.[46] Other symptoms, including nausea and vomiting, occur in more than 50%. Lower gastrointestinal bleeding, bloody diarrhea, or hematemesis occurs in 15% and indicates bowel infarction. Fecal occult blood is found in more than half the instances during the course of MVT. Initial physical findings vary at different stages and with different degrees of ischemic injury, but guarding and rebound tenderness develop as bowel infarction evolves.

Subacute MVT describes the condition in patients who have abdominal pain for weeks to months but no intestinal infarction. Subacute MVT can be due either to extension of thrombosis at a rate rapid enough to cause pain but slow enough to permit collaterals to develop, thereby preventing infarction, or to acute thrombosis of venous drainage sufficient to permit recovery from ischemic injury. The diagnosis usually is made on imaging studies ordered to diagnose other conditions.

Non-specific abdominal pain usually is the only symptom of subacute MVT, and findings of physical examination and laboratory tests are normal. Some patients who present with subacute MVT ultimately develop intestinal infarction; this blurs the distinction between the acute and subacute forms of MVT. At autopsy, coexistent new and old thromboses have been found in nearly half of patients.

Diagnosis

Standard CT is the current diagnostic test of choice for MVT. Evaluations of the colon are of little value since the colon is rarely involved. Characteristic findings on small bowel series include marked thickening of the bowel wall due to congestion and edema with separation of loops and 'thumbprinting.'

Selective mesenteric arteriography can establish a definitive diagnosis before bowel infarction, can differentiate venous thrombosis from arterial forms of ischemia, and can provide access for vasodilator therapy if indicated. Angiographic findings of MVT include thrombus in the SMV with partial or complete occlusion, failure to visualize the SMV or portal vein, slow or absent filling of the mesenteric veins, arterial spasm, failure of the arterial arcades to empty, reflux of contrast medium into the artery, and prolonged blush in the involved segment.[47]

Ultrasonography, CT, and magnetic resonance imaging (MRI) all have been used to demonstrate thrombi in the SMV and the portal vein.[48–50] CT can diagnose MVT in more than 90% of patients and is the diagnostic study of choice. Specific findings include thickening and enhancement of the bowel wall, enlargement of the SMV, a central lucency in the lumen of the vein (representing a thrombus), a sharply defined vein wall with a rim of increased density, and dilated collateral vessels in a thickened mesentery.

The diagnosis of MVT usually is made at laparotomy, where its hallmarks are serosanguinous peritoneal fluid, dark red to blue-black edematous bowel, thickening of the mesentery, good arterial pulsations in the involved segment, and thrombi in cut mesenteric veins. At this stage, some degree of intestinal infarction invariably has occurred. When persons suspected to have AMI exhibit features suggesting MVT, contrast-enhanced CT is performed before SMA angiography. A history of deep vein thrombosis or a family history of an inherited coagulation defect prompts CT as the first imaging study.

Therapeutic options

Most patients with acute MVT are initially believed to have an arterial form of AMI. Treatment of MVT generally involves surgery, anticoagulation, or both. Surgical intervention includes resection of necrotic bowel, thrombectomy or both; thrombolytics have been used successfully in case reports. In symptomatic individuals, treatment is determined by the presence or absence of peritoneal signs; signs of peritonitis mandate laparotomy and resection of infarcted bowel. If long segments of questionably viable bowel are found and arterial spasm is present, papaverine is infused and if arterial spasm is relieved and the SMV or portal vein is visualized, thrombectomy and a second-look operation may be attempted to determine whether resection should be performed, using similar guidelines as for arterial causes of AMI. Following surgery, heparin should be administered.

A comparison of patients who were treated surgically with those who were treated medically suggested that nonoperative management is a reasonable option provided the diagnosis on CT is certain and there is no transmural necrosis or perforation.[51]

Current recommendations for continued anticoagulation are based on whether an underlying hypercoagulable state is discovered, in which case lifelong coumadin is advocated. If no underlying thrombotic state is found, then anticoagulation is generally recommended for 3–6 months, although this is an arbitrary duration not yet supported by evidence-based data.[1]

The diagnosis and management of intestinal ischemia are summarized in Figure 62.1.

CHRONIC MESENTERIC VENOUS THROMBOSIS

Disease spectrum and clinical presentation

Chronic MVT is seen in patients who are asymptomatic at the time of thrombosis but who may develop gastrointestinal bleeding from varices.[52] Most patients bleed from gastroesophageal varices secondary to thrombosis of the portal or splenic vein, and they have physical findings of portal hypertension. Findings are absent if only the SMV is involved. Laboratory studies may show secondary hypersplenism with pancytopenia or thrombocytopenia.

Diagnostic evaluation

Chronic MVT can be asymptomatic; however, it may manifest as gastrointestinal bleeding, in which case the diagnostic evaluation

is directed towards determining the cause of the bleeding. Endoscopy and appropriate imaging studies should identify the cause and site of bleeding and the extent of thrombosis. While other tests may be used, the most common imaging modality is the CT scan to identify the vascular abnormalities. Papaverine-enhanced selective SMA angiography may further delineate the anatomy, but is more invasive than the other tests currently available.

Therapeutic options

Treatment of chronic MVT is aimed at controlling bleeding, usually from esophageal varices. Sclerotherapy, portosystemic shunts, devascularization procedures, and bowel resection all have a place in treating selected patients. No treatment is indicated for patients with asymptomatic chronic MVT.[1]

COLON ISCHEMIA

Colon ischemia (CI) is a frequent disorder of the large bowel in older persons and is the most common form of intestinal ischemic injury.[53] It comprises a spectrum of clinical manifestations from mild to severe forms (Table 62.2). The initial presentation usually is the same among these types and does not necessarily predict the course of disease, with the exception of ischemia that involves the ascending colon simultaneously with the small intestine. This latter pattern usually is caused by SMAE or NOMI, may have associated shock, and carries a mortality rate of more than 50%.[54,55] In a recent retrospective review of 53 cases of ischemic colitis, it was concluded that CI usually runs a benign course; however, peripheral vascular disease and right colon involvement have been reported to be associated with severe outcomes.[56]

Incidence

The incidence of CI is underestimated, because many patients suffer only mild or transient damage and do not seek medical attention. Also, CI is frequently misdiagnosed and confused with other disorders, notably inflammatory bowel disease. It is estimated to be seen in 1/700 office visits and in the authors' teritiary care hospital accounts for 1/100 colonoscopies and 1/2000 admissions. A recent study using medical claims data from a large healthcare organization in the US calculated a crude incidence rate of 7.2 cases per 100 000 person-years of observation in the general population, in contrast to 42.8 cases per 100 000 person-years for IBS patients. After adjustment for age, sex, and calendar year, the incidence of colon ischemia in people with IBS was 3.4 times higher than in persons without.[4] CI has no sex predilection, and more than 90% of patients with CI of noniatrogenic causes are older than 60 years. CI affecting young persons has been documented in case reports or series of a few patients and has been due to vasculitis, coagulation disorders, illicit use of cocaine, and iatrogenic causes, including a wide variety of medications such as estrogens and progesterones and sodium polystyrene in sorbitol (Kayexalate).[14]

Pathophysiology and etiology

Colon ischemia can result from alterations in the systemic circulation, or anatomic or functional changes in the local mesenteric vasculature (Table 62.3). The colon is relatively vulnerable to hypoperfusion since it has a lower blood flow per gram of tissue than does the rest of the gastrointestinal tract and, in contrast to the small bowel, its physiologic action of defecation is associated with a decrease in blood flow. The colon vasculature also is more sensitive to autonomic stimulation. In addition, the microvasculature plexus of the colon is less developed and is embedded in a relatively thick wall as compared to the small bowel. In most cases, no specific cause for CI is identified, and such episodes are viewed as localized nonocclusive ischemia, perhaps secondary to small vessel disease. Abnormalities on angiography rarely correlate with clinical manifestations of disease, but age-related abnormalities in the splanchnic vessels, including narrowing of small vessels, tortuosity of the long colic arteries, and fibromuscular dysplasia of the superior rectal artery, may be identified.

Once again, vasospasm appears to be another important mechanism of ischemic injury, as the splanchnic vessels respond vigorously to vasoactive substances.[57] Thus, hypotension from dehy-

dration, cardiac failure, sepsis, or hemorrhage may lead to CI, usually within the distribution of the SMA, by compromising flow volume and triggering reflex mesenteric vasoconstriction.

Pathology

The morphologic changes of the colon after an ischemic insult vary with the duration and severity of the injury. The mildest changes include mucosal and submucosal hemorrhage and edema with or without partial mucosal necrosis. Subsequently, these hemorrhages are resorbed or the overlying mucosa is sloughed, thereby evacuating the hemorrhage and creating an ulcer at the site. More severe injury results in more extensive damage, and the submucosa becomes edematous and contains abundant granulation and fibrous tissue. A variable inflammatory component, hemosiderin-laden macrophages, and preferential

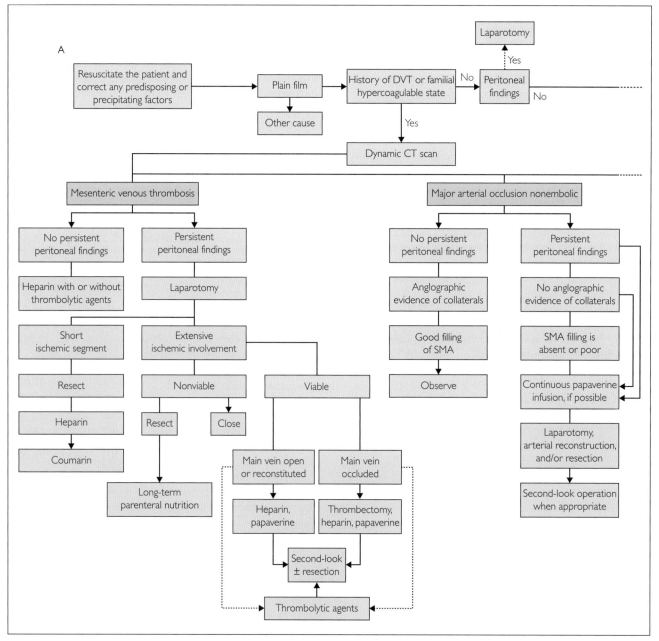

Fig. 62.1 • Algorithm for the diagnosis **(A)** and treatment

injury of the superficial epithelium with relative sparing of the lower crypts is suggestive of ischemic damage.[58] Other findings include pseudomembranes, cryptitis, and crypt abscesses, but these are not prominent, and can overlap with the histopathologic findings associated with IBD.[59] Histologic abnormalities in ischemic colitis are segmental. Occasionally, the inflammatory response and granulation tissue are so abundant as to produce a heaping-up of the mucosa and submucosa that resembles a stricture, constricting or polypoid neoplasm, or a submucosal tumor. With more severe and prolonged ischemia, the muscularis propria is damaged and replaced by fibrous tissue, thus forming a stricture. In the most severe forms of ischemic damage, there is transmural infarction of all layers of the colon, with gangrene and perforation.

Clinical presentation

Colon ischemia usually presents with sudden, crampy, mild, left lower abdominal pain, an urgent desire to defecate, and passage within 24 hours of bright red or maroon blood mixed with the stool. CI can account for approximately 20% of patients who present with lower gastrointestinal bleeding.[60] The pain that accompanies CI usually is not as severe and is felt more in the left lower abdomen when compared with that of AMI. Bleeding usually is not sufficient to require transfusion. Mild to moderate abdominal tenderness usually is present over the involved segment of bowel.

The splenic flexure, descending colon, and sigmoid most commonly are affected (Fig. 62.2). Certain causes tend to affect particular segments of colon: systemic low-flow states, the right colon; local

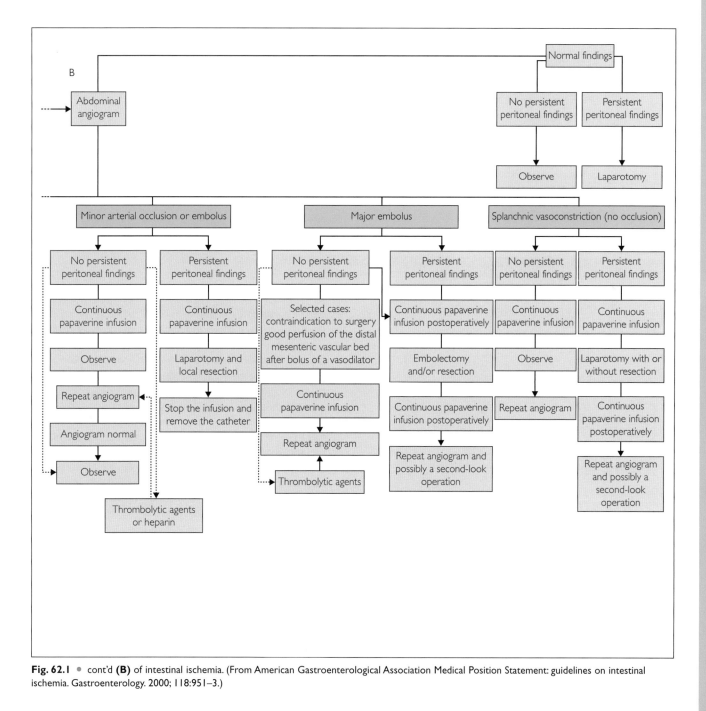

Fig. 62.1 • cont'd **(B)** of intestinal ischemia. (From American Gastroenterological Association Medical Position Statement: guidelines on intestinal ischemia. Gastroenterology. 2000; 118:951–3.)

Table 62.2 Types and approximate incidence of colon ischemia

Type	Incidence (%)
Reversible colopathy	30–40
Transient colitis	15–20
Chronic ulcerating ischemic colitis	20–25
Stricture	10–15
Gangrene	15–20
Fulminant universal colitis	<5

(Reprinted from Brandt LJ et al in Feldman M et al ed. Sleisenger and Fordtran's Gastrointestinal and Liver Disease, Philadelphia: W.B. Saunders; 2002, 2321–2340. © 2002, with permission from Elsevier.)

Table 62.3 Causes of colon ischemia

Inferior mesenteric artery thrombosis

Arterial embolus

Cholesterol emboli

Cardiac failure or arrhythmias

Shock

Pheochromocytoma

Volvulus

Strangulated hernia

Amyloidosis

Pancreatitis

Vasculitis
 Systemic lupus erythematosus
 Polyarteritis nodosa
 Rheumatoid vasculitis
 Buerger's disease
 Takayasu's arteritis
 Kawasaki disease

Hematologic disorders and coagulopathies
 Sickle cell disease
 Polycythemia vera
 Paroxysmal nocturnal hemoglobinuria
 Protein C and S deficiency
 Antithrombin III deficiency
 Activated protein C resistance
 Prothombin 20210A mutation

Infection
 Parasites (*Angiostrongylus costaricensis*)
 Bacteria (*Escherichia coli* O157:H7)
 Viruses (hepatitis B, cytomegalovirus)

Allergy

Trauma, blunt or penetrating

Ruptured ectopic pregnancy

Competitive long-distance running

Iatrogenic causes

Surgical
 Aneurysmectomy
 Aortoiliac reconstruction

Table 62.3 Causes of colon ischemia—cont'd

 Gynecologic operations
 Exchange transfusions
 Colon bypass
 Lumbar aortography
 Colectomy with inferior mesenteric artery ligation
 Colonoscopy and barium enema examination

Medications and drugs
 Digitalis
 Estrogens
 Progestins
 Danazol
 Vasopressin
 Pseudoephedrine
 Phenylephrine
 Sumatriptan
 Methamphetamine
 Ergot
 Gold
 Psychotropic drugs
 Nonsteroidal antiinflammatory drugs
 Oral saline laxatives
 GoLYTELY
 Glycerin enema
 Interferon-α
 Flutamide
 Penicillin
 Immunosuppressive agents
 Alosetron
 Pit viper toxin
 Cocaine

(Reprinted from Brandt LJ et al in Feldman M et al ed. Sleisenger and Fordtran's Gastrointestinal and Liver Disease, Philadelphia: W.B. Saunders; 2002, 2321–2340. © 2002, with permission from Elsevier.)

nonocclusive ischemic injuries, the 'watershed' areas (the splenic flexure and rectosigmoid); and ligation of the IMA, the sigmoid. The length of affected bowel also depends on the cause: atheromatous emboli involve short segments, and nonocclusive injuries involve longer portions of colon.

The most severe extreme is associated with a state of shock in the setting of gangrenous mucosa. These patients present with peritoneal findings when perforation or transmural necrosis has occurred. Fortunately, this is seen in less than 20% of cases.

Fewer than 10% of patients with CI have a distal and potentially obstructing lesion or disorder, including carcinoma of the colon, diverticulitis, volvulus, fecal impaction, postoperative stricture, prior ischemic stenosis, or radiation stricture. Typically, the associated lesion is distal, and there is a segment of normal colon between the distal lesion and the proximal colitis.

Diagnostic evaluation

If CI is suspected and the patient has no signs of peritonitis and an unrevealing abdominal plain film or CT scan, colonoscopy or the combination of sigmoidoscopy and a gentle barium enema should be performed on unprepared bowel within 48 hours of the onset of symptoms.

Findings on plain abdominal films in CI are frequently nonspecific. Distention or pneumatosis typically are seen only with advanced disease. CT findings are predominantly segmental (89%)

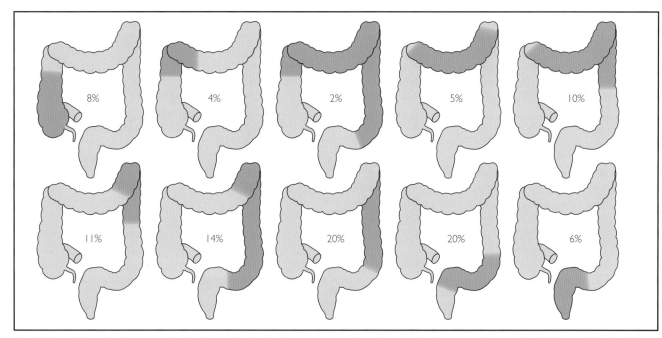

Fig. 62.2 • Schematic of patterns of colon ischemia showing the percentage of involvement of each pattern from a total of 250 cases. (Reprinted from Brandt LJ et al in Feldman M et al ed. Sleisenger and Fordtran's Gastrointestinal and Liver Disease, Philadelphia: W.B. Saunders; 2002, 2321–2340. © 2002, with permission from Elsevier.)

with findings of a wet appearance with heterogeneous areas of edema (61%), a dry appearance with homogeneous thickening (33%), or intramural air.[61] The presence of radiographic findings suggesting ischemia may portend a worse prognosis, signifying a more advanced process.

During colonoscopy and barium enema examination, care should be taken not to overdistend the colon, because high intraluminal pressure diminishes intestinal blood flow and may aggravate ischemic damage, particularly in patients with vasculitis.[62] Colonoscopy is preferable to barium studies because it is more sensitive in diagnosing mucosal abnormalities and biopsy specimens may be obtained.[63] Hemorrhagic nodules seen at colonoscopy represent bleeding into the submucosa and are equivalent to thumbprints seen on barium enema. Segmental distribution of these findings, with or without ulceration, is highly suggestive of CI, but the diagnosis of CI cannot be made conclusively in a single study unless mucosal gangrene is seen. Recently, the correlation has been made between the presence of a single linear ulcer running along the longitudinal axis of the colon, the colon single-stripe sign (CSSS), and ischemic colitis.[64] The presence of the CSSS appears to signify a milder course than a circumferential ulceration. In addition, it appears to have a 75% histopathologic yield in making the diagnosis of ischemic injury. Segmental distribution, abrupt transition between injured and noninjured mucosa, rectal sparing, and rapid resolution are hallmark findings that favor the diagnosis of ischemia.

The initial diagnostic study should be performed within 48 hours, because thumbprinting disappears within days as the submucosal hemorrhages are resorbed or the overlying mucosa sloughs. Studies performed 1 week after the initial study should reflect evolution of the injury – either normalization of the colon or replacement of the thumbprints with a segmental ulcerative colitis-type pattern. Universal colonic involvement, however, favors true ulcerative colitis, whereas fistula formation suggests Crohn's disease. Occasionally,

an abundant inflammatory response can produce heaping-up of mucosa and submucosa that resembles a stricture or neoplasm.

Duplex sonography is an evolving noninvasive technique, which may identify patients with high-grade stenosis of the larger mesenteric arteries. However, significant stenotic vessel changes occur in many asymptomatic patients and do not necessarily indicate mesenteric ischemia. In a retrospective analysis it was noted that the absence of arterial flow in the thickened wall of the ischemic colon may be indicative of more severe colitis.[65]

At the time of symptom onset, colon blood flow typically has returned to normal, so mesenteric angiography usually is not indicated. An exception to this rule is when the clinical presentation does not allow for a clear distinction to be made between CI and AMI. It should be remembered that changes in the right colon implies SMA disease and the possible need for angiography.

Clinical course and management

When CI is diagnosed and physical examination does not suggest gangrene or perforation, the patient is treated expectantly. Parenteral fluids are administered and the bowel is placed at rest. Broad-spectrum antibiotics are given to 'cover' the fecal flora, because in experimental models, antibiotics reduce the extent, depth, and severity of bowel damage. No randomized, controlled, blinded trials have been done to prove the validity of this recommendation. Cardiac failure and arrhythmias are treated, and newly begun medications that may cause mesenteric vasoconstriction (e.g., digitalis and vasopressors) are withdrawn. Decompression of the GI tract can be performed if necessary with a nasogastric or rectal tube. Serial radiographic or endoscopic evaluations of the colon and continued monitoring of the hemoglobin level, white blood cell count, and electrolyte levels are indicated until the patient's condition stabilizes.

Increasing abdominal tenderness, guarding, rebound tenderness, rising temperature, and paralytic ileus indicate colonic infarction and demand immediate laparotomy and colon resection. Mucosal injury may be extensive, despite normal-looking serosa, and the extent of resection should be guided by the distribution of disease as seen on preoperative studies rather than the appearance of the serosal surface of the colon at the time of operation.

Figure 62.3 provides an algorithm for the management of colon ischemia.

Chronic sequelae

In more than half of patients with CI, the disease is reversible. Generally, the symptoms of CI resolve within 48 hours and the colon heals in 1–2 weeks. With severe injury it may take 1–6 months for the colon to heal, but during this time the patient is usually asymptomatic. The remaining patients with CI suffer irreversible damage: gangrene and perforation, segmental ulcerating colitis, stricture, or universal colitis.

Gangrene
Abdominal tenderness with fever and signs of peritonitis suggests infarction and the need for emergent laparotomy.

Segmental ulcerating colitis
Segmental ulcerating colitis may be seen with any of the following clinical patterns: absence of gastroenterologic symptoms but with recurrent fevers and sepsis; continuing or recurrent bloody diarrhea; and persistent or chronic diarrhea with protein-losing colopathy. Patients who are asymptomatic or minimally symptomatic but who also have endoscopic evidence of persistent disease should undergo follow-up colonoscopies to determine whether the colitis is healing, becoming chronic, or whether a stricture is forming. Recurrent fever, leukocytosis, and septicemia suggest unhealed segmental colitis and, if found, mandates elective resection of the ischemic segment of bowel. Patients with persistent diarrhea, bleeding, or protein-losing colopathy of more than 2 weeks'

duration are at high risk of perforation, and early resection is indicated. Patients who present with segmental ulcerating colitis are frequently misdiagnosed as having inflammatory bowel disease. Response to steroid therapy usually is poor and may be associated with an increased incidence of perforation. Some success has been achieved with fatty acid enemas. Short-chain fatty acid enemas were used in a prospective, placebo-controlled trial in patients scheduled for elective aortic graft surgery for arteriosclerosis which resulted in inconclusive data as none of the patients in either group developed ischemic colitis.[66] Patients whose symptoms cannot be controlled medically should have a segmental resection, which usually is curative.

Ischemic stricture
Ischemic strictures that produce no symptoms should be observed. Some disappear over 12–24 months with no therapy. There is limited experience with endoscopic balloon dilation and resection is required for those that cause obstruction.

Universal fulminant colitis
Sudden onset of a 'toxic universal' colitis picture with signs of peritonitis and a rapidly progressive course are typical of universal fulminant colitis, a rare form of CI. Total abdominal colectomy with ileostomy usually is required.

Colon ischemia complicating aortic surgery
Colon ischemia complicates elective aortic surgery in up to 7% and surgery for ruptured abdominal aortic aneurysms in up to 60% of cases.[67] CI is responsible for approximately 10% of deaths after aortic replacement. Factors that contribute to postoperative CI include aneurysmal rupture, hypotension, operative trauma to the colon, hypoxemia, arrhythmias, prolonged cross-clamp time, and improper management of the IMA during aneurysmectomy. Tonometric determination of intramural pH of the sigmoid before

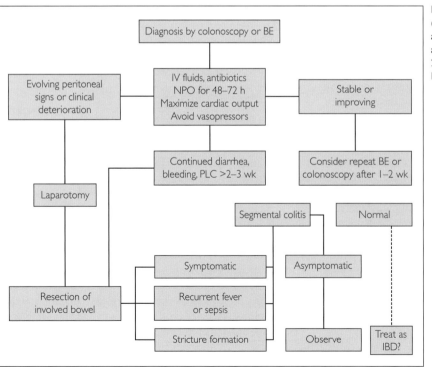

Fig. 62.3 • Management of colon ischemia. (Reprinted from Brandt LJ et al in Feldman M et al ed. Sleisenger and Fordtran's Gastrointestinal and Liver Disease, Philadelphia: W.B. Saunders; 2002, 2321–2340. © 2002, with permission from Elsevier.)

and after cross-clamping the aorta has been used successfully to predict which patients will develop CI after aneurysmectomy.[68] Because postoperative CI is serious and difficult to diagnose early, colonoscopy should be performed within 2 to 3 days after surgery for a ruptured abdominal aortic aneurysm or in patients with a prolonged cross-clamping time, a patent IMA on preoperative aortography, nonpulsatile flow in the hypogastric arteries during surgery, or postoperative diarrhea. If CI is identified, oral feeding and liquids are stopped and antibiotic therapy is begun; clinical deterioration requires reoperation. At surgery, all ischemic colon must be resected.

CHRONIC MESENTERIC ISCHEMIA

Disease spectrum and clinical presentation

Chronic mesenteric ischemia (CMI) is uncommon, accounting for less than 5% of all intestinal ischemic diseases; it almost always is caused by mesenteric atherosclerosis. Abdominal pain is caused by ischemia in the small intestine as blood is 'stolen' from this organ to meet the increased demand for gastric blood flow as food enters the stomach.[69] Patients classically complain of abdominal cramping discomfort that occurs within 30 minutes after eating, gradually increases in severity, and then slowly resolves over 1–3 hours. Although minimal at first, abdominal pain progressively increases and the association of pain with meals leads to fear of eating (sitophobia) with resultant weight loss. Nausea, bloating, episodic diarrhea, and malabsorption or constipation may occur, but it is the weight loss and relation of the abdominal pain to the meals that characterize this syndrome.

Early in the course of disease, if patients do not eat, they remain pain free; pain occurs only after eating or during a meal. Later, pain may become continuous, and this portends intestinal infarction. Physical findings are usually limited, but patients with advanced disease may appear cachectic. Many patients have evidence of cardiac, cerebral, or peripheral vascular disease. The abdomen typically remains soft and nontender even during painful episodes, although significant distention may be appreciated. An abdominal bruit is common but non-specific.

Diagnostic evaluation

The diagnosis of CMI is supported by the demonstration of high-grade stenoses in multiple mesenteric vessels, in patients with unexplained chronic abdominal pain, weight loss, and food aversion.[70] A high clinical index of suspicion is crucial to making the diagnosis, due to the vague nature of the complaints and the lack of a specific diagnostic test. Plain radiographs of the abdomen usually are normal, although vascular calcifications may be present. Endoscopic inspection of the GI tract usually reveals it to be normal, and random biopsies of the upper tract may show only non-specific abnormalities. Barium studies are normal or show non-specific evidence of either malabsorption or a motility disturbance.

A number of tests have been proposed to establish the presence of CMI, including duplex ultrasonography and MR angiography, but none has proven sufficiently sensitive and specific to be diagnostic. Mesenteric duplex ultrasonography has been advocated as a reasonably accurate screening modality for the detection of high-grade CA and SMA stenoses.[71] Elevated 'peak systolic velocity' in the SMA and CA as determined by duplex ultrasonography indicates significant stenosis of >50%;[72,73] this, however, does not establish the diagnosis of CMI.[74,75] Postprandial duplex ultrasonography does not significantly improve upon this yield.[76]

The current gold standard test is dependent on the arteriographic demonstration of an occlusive process of the splanchnic vessels, and, to a great measure, the exclusion of other gastrointestinal disorders. Angiography should show occlusion of two or more splanchnic arteries to allow the diagnosis of CMI; however, such occlusions, even of all three vessels, do not by themselves make the diagnosis of CMI, because they may be present with no corresponding clinical symptoms. In most patients with CMI, at least two of the three splanchnic vessels are either completely obstructed or severely stenosed. In a large review of patients with CMI,[70] 91% had occlusion of at least two vessels and 55% had involvement of all three; 7% and 2% had isolated occlusion of the SMA and CA, respectively.

Magnetic resonance angiography (MRA) appears to provide highly accurate images of the arterial and venous mesenteric vasculature.[77,78] In addition, cine phase-contrast MRA may be able to detect significant abnormalities in mesenteric blood flow.[79,80] Contrast-enhanced MRA has demonstrated excellent sensitivity and specificity for the detection of major splanchnic vessel stenoses and occlusions, although sensitivity is attenuated for smaller peripheral vessels and specificity may be lower for IMA stenosis.[27] Again, the findings of splanchnic artery occlusions alone are insufficient to diagnose CMI; to this end, functional MRA also has been studied. The normal increase in postprandial SMV flow compared to its fasting state has been shown to be less in patients with CMI compared with controls.[79,80] The usefulness of these techniques, especially functional MRA, is currently limited by the need for significant expertise in the use of this highly specialized equipment. At present, MRA should be considered experimental as a diagnostic tool for CMI.

Another modality, balloon tonometry, uses an intraluminal catheter apparatus to indirectly measure the intestinal intramural pH (pH_I) in the jejunum after a test meal. A decrease in pH_I reflects a decrease in oxygen delivery to the gut and results from a shift to anaerobic metabolism with subsequent cellular acidosis; such a decrease in pH_I correlates with abdominal pain and may be a good marker of tissue ischemia. Grum et al. used a canine model to show that pH_I dropped precipitously when blood flow (oxygen delivery) was decreased below 60% of baseline.[81] Tonometry has been applied to predict multiple organ failure and death in the intensive care unit setting,[82] to help diagnose CMI[83,84] and to assess for CI after abdominal aortic surgery.[85]

Therapeutic options

The mainstay of treatment for CMI is surgical bypass, although percutaneous angioplasty and stenting procedures also have been studied. Therapeutic outcomes may be difficult to assess as success has been defined in different ways, including graft patency, relief of symptoms, and long-term survival. As reviewed in one recent article, means of 85% for long-term pain relief, 86% for graft patency, and 7% for mortality rate were found for surgical revascularization.[86] Presently, only retrospective reviews of percutaneous angioplasty and stenting are available and are hampered not only by their inherent suboptimal study design but also by lack of homogeneity in terms of patient population, procedural technique, postprocedural assessment, and length of follow-up. Additionally, it may be difficult to compare surgery with percutaneous procedures as usually more vessels are bypassed in surgery than are treated percutaneously; further, only high-grade stenoses and not partly occluded vessels are treated percutaneously. Although initial success rates for percutaneous angioplasty and stenting are reported to range between 63% and 100%,[87] long-term efficacy is generally less than that for surgery; one recent study reported that patients treated with percutaneous angioplasty and stenting developed recurrent symptoms at a rate of 28% at 1 year and 34% at 3 years.[86] More recently, a study looking at patients treated with only angioplasty plus stenting found success rates equivalent to those of surgery at 15 months (83% symptomatic relief, 94% stent patency, 10% complication rate).[87] However, restenosis and recurrent symptoms occur in one-third to one-half of patients within the first year, making the limited durability of the procedure its greatest limitation. Although experience is limited, a number of reports have described placement of an expandable metal stent to help prevent reocclusion.[88,89] More data are likely needed before definitive conclusions can be reached.

FUTURE DIRECTIONS

The significant morbidity and high mortality of ischemic injury will only be reduced by early diagnosis and treatment. In the future, diagnosis is certain to depend even more on technologically sophisticated imaging studies. At present, therapy consists of intra-arterial vasodilators, thrombolytics, and judicious surgery. The future directions of therapy may include the use of agents to:

1. re-establish blood flow early in the course of disease, e.g., glucagon, angiotensin converting enzyme inhibitor;
2. inhibit platelet aggregation, e.g., iloprost (a synthetic derivative of prostacyclin);
3. vasodilate selectively, e.g., ovine corticotropin releasing factor, sauvagine, and urotensin I;
4. prevent reperfusion injury by inhibiting free radicals, e.g., superoxide dismutase, allopurinol, melatonin, caffeic acid phenethyl ester, ethyl pyruvate;
5. prevent reperfusion injury by inhibiting neutrophil recruitment and adhesion, e.g., antibodies against intercellular adhesion molecule-1, heparin-binding epidermal growth factor, hepatocyte growth factor; and
6. improving mucosal viability, e.g., glycine, glucagonlike peptide-2a, IL-11.

SUMMARY

Intestinal ischemia refers to the process whereby blood flow to the bowel is decreased and cellular injury occurs consequent to diminished supply of oxygen and nutrients. Gastrointestinal ischemia may result from a disturbance in the arterial blood supply or venous drainage of the bowel. Both hypoxia and reperfusion are important etiologic factors in this process. Regardless of its cause, the end results of ischemia are similar – a spectrum of bowel injury that ranges from transient alteration of bowel function to transmural gangrene. The most common cause of AMI is SMAE, followed by NOMI, SMAT, MVT, and FSI. Early on, AMI is characterized by severe abdominal pain, yet a paucity of physical findings.

All patients with suspected AMI should undergo correction of underlying cardiovascular conditions and treatment with broad-spectrum antibiotics. An aggressive approach utilizing early angiography and papaverine in combination with surgery can significantly reduce mortality of AMI. Papaverine is used frequently to reduce the splanchnic vasoconstriction that typifies NOMI and accompanies SMAE, SMAT, and even acute MVT.

CI is a frequent disorder of the large bowel in older persons. Its incidence is underestimated, because most patients suffer only mild, transient damage and do not seek medical attention. Generally, symptoms of CI resolve quickly. Irreversible damage from CI, e.g., gangrene and perforation, segmental ulcerating colitis, or stricture, or universal colitis, is uncommon.

CMI typically is caused by mesenteric atherosclerosis. Patients classically complain of abdominal pain after eating and weight loss. A high clinical index of suspicion is crucial to making the diagnosis, due to the vague nature of the complaints and the lack of a specific diagnostic test. The current gold standard test is dependent on the arteriographic demonstration of an occlusive process of the splanchnic vessels, and the exclusion of other gastrointestinal disorders. Angiography should show occlusion of two or more splanchnic arteries to allow the diagnosis of CMI. The mainstay of treatment for CMI is revascularizing the stenotic vessels either by surgical bypass or percutaneous angioplasty with or without stenting procedures.

REFERENCES

1. Brandt LJ, Boley SJ. Intestinal ischemia. In: Feldman M, Friedman LS, Sleisenger MH, eds. Sleisenger and Fordtran's gastrointestinal and liver disease. Philadelphia: WB Saunders; 2002:2321–2340.

   A complete review of intestinal ischemia with excellent tables.

2. Brandt LJ, Boley SJ. Colonic ischemia. In: Brandt LJ, ed. Clinical practice of gastroenterology. Philadelphia: Current Medicine; 1999:696.

3. Brandt LJ, Boley SJ. AGA technical review on intestinal ischemia. Gastroenterology 2000; 118:954–968.

   This AGA technical review walks a physician through pertinent everyday clinical questions regarding the diagnosis and management of intestinal ischemia. Useful reference to answer specific questions on the subject.

4. Cole JA, Cook SF, Sands BE, et al. Occurrence of colon ischemia in relation to irritable bowel syndrome. Am J Gastroenterol 2004; 99:486–491.

   Recent review indicating a higher than average risk for intestinal ischemia in patients with IBS. An important subject in light of side effect profiles of IBS therapy.

5. Kornblith PL, Boley SJ, Whitehouse BS. Anatomy of the splanchnic circulation. Surg Clin North Am 1992; 72:1–30.

6. Bulkley GB, Kvietys PR, Parks DA, et al. Relationship of blood flow and oxygen consumption to ischemic injury in the canine small intestine. Gastroenterology 1985; 89:852–857.

7. Patel A, Kaleya RN, Sammartano RJ. Pathophysiology of mesenteric ischemia. Surg Clin North Am 1992; 72:31–41.

8. Lundgren O, Svanvik J. Mucosal hemodynamics in the small intestine of the cat during reduced perfusion pressure. Acta Phyiol Scand 1973; 88:551–563.

9. Boley SJ, Brandt LJ, Veith FJ. Ischemic disorders of the intestines. Curr Probl Surg 1978; 15:1–85.

10. Boley SJ, Freiber W, Winslow PR, et al. Circulatory responses to acute reduction of superior mesenteric arterial flow. Physiologist 1969; 12:180.

11. Mitsudo S, Brandt LJ. Pathology of intestinal ischemia. Surg Clin North Am 1992; 72:43–63.

12. Gennaro M, Ascer E, Matano R, et al. Acute mesenteric ischemia after cardiopulmonary bypass. Am J Surg 1993; 166: 231–236.

13. Diamond SM, Emmett M, Henrich WL. Bowel infarction as a cause of death in dialysis patients. JAMA 1986; 256:2545–2547.

14. Cappell MS. Colonic toxicity of administered drugs and chemicals. Am J Gastroenterol 2004; 99:1175–1190.

15. Finucane PM, Arunachalam T, O'Dowd J, et al. Acute mesenteric infarction in elderly patients. J Am Geriatr Soc 1989; 37:355–358.

16. Kurland B, Brandt LJ, Delany HM. Diagnostic tests for intestinal ischemia. Surg Clin North Am 1992; 72:85–105.

17. Khurana S, Corbally MT, Manning F, et al. Glutathione S-transferase: a potential new marker of intestinal ischemia. J Pediatr Surg 2002; 37:1543–1548.

18. Kanda T, Fujii H, Tani T, et al. Intestinal fatty acid-binding protein is a useful diagnostic marker for mesenteric infarction in humans. Gastroenterology 1996; 110:339–343.

19. Guthmann F, Borchers T, Wolfrum C, et al. Plasma concentration of intestinal- and liver-FABP in neonates suffering from necrotizing enterocolitis and in healthy preterm neonates. Mol Cell Biochem 2002; 239:227–234.

20. Yamada K, Saeki M, Yamaguchi T, et al. Acute mesenteric ischemia. CT and plain radiographic analysis of 26 cases. Clin Imaging 1998; 22:34–41.

21. Smerud MJ, Johnson CD, Stephens DH. Diagnosis of bowel infarction: a comparison of plain films and CT scans in 23 cases. AJR Am J Roentgenol 1990; 154:99–103.

22. Lee R, Tung HKS, Tung PHM, et al. CT in acute mesenteric ischaemia. Clin Radiol 2003; 58:279–287.

23. Kernagis LY, Levine MS, Jacobs JE. Pneumatosis intestinalis in patients with ischemia: Correlation of CT findings with viability of the bowel. AJR Am J Roentgenol 2003; 180:733–736.

24. Taourel PG, Deneuville M, Pradel JA, et al. Acute mesenteric ischemia: Diagnosis with contrast-enhanced CT. Radiology 1996; 199:632–636.

25. Rhee RY, Gloviczki P. Mesenteric venous thrombosis. Surg Clin North Am 1997; 77:327–338.

26. Kirkpatrick IDC, Kroeker MA, Greenberg HM. Biphasic CT with mesenteric CT angiography in the evaluation of acute mesenteric ischemia: initial experience. Radiology 2003; 229:91–98.

This study demonstrated the role of CTA in obtaining added important diagnostic information in a relatively noninvasive manner. In this patient population, CTA altered management beyond standard CT in 19% of patients.

27. Laissy JP, Trillaud H, Douek P. MR angiography: noninvasive vascular imaging of the abdomen. Abdom Imaging 2002; 27:488–506.

Thorough review of the role of abdominal MRA with a focus on mesenteric ischemia and the potential for a true functional imaging test. Good discussion of the literature.

28. Li KC, Pelc LR, Dalman RL, et al. In vivo magnetic resonance evaluation of blood oxygen saturation in the superior mesenteric vein as a measure of the degree of acute blood flow reduction in the superior mesenteric artery: findings in a canine model. Acad Radiol 1997; 4:21–25.

29. Kleinhaus S, Sammartano R, Boley SJ. Effects of laparoscopy on mesenteric blood flow. Arch Surg 1978; 113:867–869.

30. Brandt LJ, Boley SJ, Sammartano R. Carbon dioxide and room air insufflation of the colon. Effects on colonic blood flow and intraluminal pressure in the dog. Gastrointest Endosc 1986; 32:324–329.

31. Seidel SA, Bradshaw LA, Ladipo JK, et al. Noninvasive detection of ischemic bowel. J Vasc Surg 1999; 30:309–319.

32. Bennion RS, Wilson SE, Williams RA. Early portal anaerobic bacteremia in mesenteric ischemia. Arch Surg 1984; 199:151–155.

33. Jamieson WG, Pliagus G, Marchuk S, et al. Effect of antibiotic and fluid resuscitation upon survival time in experimental intestinal ischemia. Surg Gynecol Obstet 1988; 167:103–108.

34. Park WM, Gloviczki P, Cherry KJ, et al. Contemporary management of acute mesenteric ischemia: Factors associated with survival. J Vasc Surg 2002; 35:445–452.

35. VanDeinse WH, Zawacki JK, Phillips D. Treatment of acute mesenteric ischemia by percutaneous transluminal angioplasty. Gastroenterology 1986; 91:475–478.

36. Babior BM, Stossel TP. The clotting cascade and its regulation: congenital and acquired clotting factor disorders. In: Babior BM, Stossel TP, eds. Hematology: a pathophysiological approach. New York: Churchill Livingstone; 1994:189–211.

37. Bell WR. Present-day thrombolytic therapy: therapeutic agents – pharmacokinetics and pharmacodynamics. Rev Cardiovasc Med 2002; 3:S34–S44.

38. Hardman JG, Limbrid LE, Molinoff PB, et al. Anticoagulants, thrombolytics, and antiplatelet drugs. In: Hardman JG, Limbrid LE, Molinoff PB, et al., eds. Goodman and Gilman's the pharmacological basis of therapeutics. New York: McGaw-Hill; 1996:1351–1353.

39. Simo G, Echenagusia AJ, Camuex F, et al. Superior mesenteric arterial embolism: local fibrinolytic treatment with urokinase. Radiology 1997; 204:775–779.

40. Boley SJ, Sammartano RJ, Brandt LJ, et al. Intra-arterial vasodilators and thrombolytic agents in experimental superior mesenteric artery embolus. Gastroenterology 1982; 82:1021.

41. Boley SJ, Sprayregan S, Siegelman SS, et al. Initial results from an aggressive roentgenological and surgical approach to acute mesenteric ischemia. Surgery 1977; 82:848–855.

42. Smithline A, Brandt LJ. Drug therapies for mesenteric vascular disease. In: Frishman WH, ed. Cardiovascular pharmacotherapeutics. New York: McGraw-Hill; 1997:1211–1219.

43. Bassiouny HS. Nonocclusive mesenteric ischemia. Surg Clin North Am 1997; 77:319–326.

44. Greenwald DA, Brandt LJ, Reinus JF. Ischemic bowel disease in the elderly. Gastroenterol Clin North Am 2001; 30:445–473.

45. Siegelman SS, Sprayregen S, Boley SJ. Angiographic diagnosis of mesenteric arterial vasoconstriction. Radiology 1974; 122:533–542.

46. Font VE, Hermann RE, Longworth DL. Chronic mesenteric venous thrombosis: Difficult diagnosis and therapy. Cleve Clin J Med 1989; 56:823–828.

47. Clark RA, Gallant TE. Acute mesenteric ischemia: Angiographic spectrum. Am J Radiol 1994; 142:555–562.

48. Matos C, Van Gansbeke D, Zalcman M, et al. Mesenteric vein thrombosis: early CT and ultrasound diagnosis and conservative management. Gastrointest Radiol 1986; 11:322–325.

49. Clavien PA, Huber O, Mirescu D, et al. Contrast enhanced CT scan as a diagnostic procedure in mesenteric ischemia due to mesenteric venous thrombosis. Br J Surg 1989; 76:93–94.

50. Al Karawi MA, Quaiz M, Clark D, et al. Mesenteric vein thrombosis, non-invasive diagnosis and followup (US + MRI) and non-invasive therapy by streptokinase and anticoagulants. Hepatogastroenterology 1990; 37:507–509.

51. Brunaud L, Antunes L, Collinet-Adler S, et al. Acute mesenteric venous thrombosis: case for nonoperative management. J Vasc Surg 2001; 34:673–679.

52. Warshaw AL, Jin GL, Ottinger LW. Recognition and clinical implications of mesenteric and portal vein obstruction in chronic pancreatitis. Arch Surg 1987; 122:410–415.

53. Greenwald DA, Brandt LJ. Colonic ischemia. J Clin Gastroenterol 1998; 27:122–128.

Focused discussion on colon ischemia, its sequelae, and diseases that mimic it.

54. Sakai L, Keltner R, Kaminski D. Spontaneous and shock-associated ischemic colitis. Am J Surg 1980; 140:755–760.

55. Guttormson NL, Bubrick MP. Mortality from ischemic colitis. Dis Colon Rectum 1989; 32:469–472.

56. Medina C, Vilaseca J, Videla S, et al. Outcome of patients with ischemic colitis: review of fifty-three cases. Dis Colon Rectum 2004; 47:180–184.

57. Rosenblum JD, Boyle CM, Schwartz LB. The mesenteric circulation. Anatomy and physiology. Surg Clin North Am 1997; 77:289–306.

58. Sands BE. From symptom to diagnosis: Clinical distinctions among various forms of intestinal inflammation. Gastroenterology 2004; 126:1518–1532.

59. Greenson JK, Odze RD. Inflammatory diseases of the large intestine. In: Odze RD, Goldblum JR, Crawford JM, eds. Surgical pathology of the GI tract, liver, biliary tract, and pancreas. Philadelphia: WB Saunders; 2004:213–246.

60. Newman JR, Cooper MA. Lower gastrointestinal bleeding and ischemic colitis. Can J Gastroenterol 2002; 16:597–600.

61. Balthazar EJ, Yen BC, Gordon RB. Ischemic colitis: CT evaluation of 54 cases. Radiology 1999; 211:381–388.

Extensive experience of CT scan in evaluating patients with proven colon ischemia.

62. Church JM. Ischemic colitis complicating flexible endoscopy in a patient with connective tissue disease. Gastrointest Endosc 1985; 41:181–182.

63. Scowcroft CW, Sanowski RA, Kozarek RA. Colonoscopy in ischemic colitis. Gastrointest Endosc 1981; 27:156–161.

64. Zuckerman GR, Prakash C, Merriman RB, et al. The colon single-stripe sign and its relationship to ischemic colitis. Am J Gastroenterol 2003; 98:2018–2022.

Description of new endoscopic finding (CSSS) and its correlation with ischemic colitis.

65. Danse EM, Van Beers BE, Jamart J, et al. Prognosis of ischemic colitis: Comparison of color Doppler sonography with early clinical and laboratory findings. AJR Am J Roentgenol 2000; 175:1151–1154.

66. Mortensen FV, Jorgensen B, Christiansen HM, et al. Short-chain fatty acid enemas stimulate plasminogen activator inhibitor-1 after abdominal aortic graft surgery: A double-blinded, placebo-controlled study. Throm Res 2000; 98:361–366.

67. Zelenock GB, Strodel WE, Knol JA, et al. A prospective study of clinically and endoscopically documented colonic ischemia in 100 patients undergoing aortic reconstructive surgery with aggressive colonic and direct pelvic revascularization, compared with historic controls. Surgery 1989; 106:771–779.

68. Schiedler MG, Cutler BS, Fiddian-Green RG. Sigmoid intramural pH for prediction of ischemic colitis during aortic surgery: A comparison with risk factors and inferior mesenteric artery stump pressures. Arch Surg 1987; 122:881–886.

69. Poole JW, Sammartano RJ, Boley SJ. Hemodynamic basis of the pain of chronic mesenteric ischemia. Am J Surg 1987; 153:171–176.

70. Moawad J, Gewertz BL. Chronic mesenteric ischemia. Clinical presentation and diagnosis. Surg Clin North Am 1997; 77:357–369.

Review of clinical presentation and diagnostic tests in CMI.

71. Nicoloff AD, Williamson WK, Moneta GL, et al. Duplex ultrasonography in evaluation of splanchnic artery stenosis. Surg Clin North Am 1997; 77:339–355.

72. Harward TR, Smith S, Seeger JM. Detection of celiac axis and superior mesenteric artery occlusive disease with use of abdominal duplex scanning. J Vasc Surg 1993; 17:738–745.

73. Moneta GL, Lee RW, Yeager RA, et al. Mesenteric duplex scanning: A blinded prospective study. J Vasc Surg 1993; 17:79–84.

74. Moneta GL, Yeager RA, Dalman R, et al. Duplex ultrasound criteria for diagnosis of splanchnic artery stenosis or occlusion. J Vasc Surg 1991; 14:511–518.

75. Bowersox JC, Zwolak RM, Walsh DB, et al. Duplex ultrasonography in the diagnosis of celiac and mesenteric artery occlusive disease. J Vasc Surg 1991; 14:780–786.

76. Gentile AT, Moneta GL, Lee RW, et al. Usefulness of fasting and postprandial duplex ultrasound examinations for predicting high-grade superior mesenteric artery stenosis. Am J Surg 1995; 169:476–479.

77. Holland G, Dougherty L, Carpenter J, et al. Breath-hold ultrafast three-dimensional gadolinium-enhanced MR angiography of the aorta and the renal and other visceral abdominal arteries. AJR Am J Roentgenol 1996; 166:971–981.

78. Shirkhoda A, Konez O, Shetty AN, et al. Mesenteric circulation: Three-dimensional MR angiography with a gadolinium-enhanced multiecho gradient-echo technique. Radiology 1997; 202:257–261.

79. Burkart DJ, Johnson CD, Reading CC, et al. MR measurements of mesenteric venous flow: Prospective evaluation in healthy volunteers and patients with suspected chronic mesenteric ischemia. Radiology 1995; 194:801–806.

80. Li KC, Hopkins KL, Dalman RL, et al. Simultaneous measurement of flow in the superior mesenteric vein and artery with cine phase-contrast MR imaging: Value in diagnosis of chronic mesenteric ischemia. Work in progress. Radiology 1995; 194:327–330.

81. Grum C, Fiddian-Green RG, Pittenger GL, et al. Adequacy of tissue oxygenation in intact dog intestine. J Appl Physiol 1984; 56:1065–1069.

82. Taylor DE. Revving the motor of multiple organ dysfunction syndrome: Gut dysfunction in ARDS and multiorgan failure. Respir Care Clin N Am 1998; 4:611–631.

83. Boley SJ, Brandt LJ, Veith FJ, et al. A new provocative test for chronic mesenteric ischemia. Am J Gastroenterol 1991; 86:888–891.

84. Kolkman JJ, Groeneveld AB. Occlusive and non-occlusive gastrointestinal ischaemia: A clinical review with special emphasis on the diagnostic value of tonometry. Scand J Gastroenterol Suppl 1998; 225:3–12.

85. Bjorck M, Hedberg B. Early detection of major complications after abdominal aortic surgery: predictive value of sigmoid colon and gastric intramucosal pH monitoring. Br J Surg 1994; 81:25–30.

86. Kasirajan K, O'Hara PJ, Gray BH, et al. Chronic mesenteric ischemia: Open surgery versus percutaneous angioplasty and stenting. J Vasc Surg 2001; 33:63–71.

Comparison of the difference between percutaneous angioplasty and stenting versus open surgery with regards to early and late complications.

87. Sharafuddin MJ, Olson CH, Sun S, et al. Endovascular treatment of celiac and mesenteric arteries stenosis: Applications and results. J Vasc Surg 2003; 38:692–698.

88. Yamakado K, Takeda K, Nomura Y, et al. Relief of mesenteric ischemia by Z-stent placement into the superior mesenteric artery compressed by the false lumen of an aortic dissection. Cardiovasc Intervent Radiol 1998; 21:66–68.

89. Waybill PN, Enea NA. Use of a Palmaz stent deployed in the superior mesenteric artery for chronic mesenteric ischemia. J Vasc Interv Radiol 1997; 8:1069–1071.

CHAPTER SIXTY-THREE

63

Neoplastic diseases of the small and large bowel

Paul C. Schroy III

INTRODUCTION

Intestinal tumors, particularly those arising in the large bowel, constitute a commonly encountered management challenge to both primary care providers and GI specialists alike. Not surprisingly, appropriate treatment strategies are contingent on a number of factors, including tumor type, site of origin, extent of disease, and natural history. This chapter will focus initially on management issues related to epithelial tumors of the large bowel, i.e., adenomatous polyps and adenocarcinoma, which are by far the most common, clinically significant GI neoplasms. The management of epithelial tumors of the small bowel will be discussed next since treatment options are generally similar to those applied to epithelial tumors of the large bowel. The remainder of the chapter will discuss the management of intestinal lymphomas, carcinoid tumors, and miscellaneous stromal tumors.

COLORECTAL CANCER AND POLYPS

Epidemiology

Adenocarcinoma of the large intestine, commonly referred as colorectal cancer, is by far the most common malignant tumor of the large intestine. Worldwide incidence and mortality rates of colorectal cancer vary considerably.[1] With the notable exception of Japan, industrialized countries are at greatest risk. High rates are found in North America, Australia, New Zealand, and Western Europe, while lower rates are found in Eastern Europe, most South American countries, Asia, and Africa. In the United States, colorectal cancer currently ranks as the fourth most commonly diagnosed malignancy and second leading cause of cancer-related death among males and females. In 2004 alone, there were approximately 146 940 new cases and 56 730 deaths.[2] Incidence rates have declined slightly over the past two decades, but remain in excess of 40 cases per 100 000 population.[2] Declines in incidence have been more dramatic for whites than blacks and for distal cancers compared to proximal cancers.[3] Both cancers of the colon and rectum demonstrate a slight male predominance.[2] An American's lifetime risk of developing colorectal cancer is nearly 6%.[2] Age is an important determinant of risk. Although extremely uncommon in individuals below the age 35 (except with rare predisposing genetic syndromes), the incidence of colorectal cancer increases steadily with age,

beginning around age 40 with an approximate doubling with each successive decade thereafter to around age 80.[1] High-risk groups have been identified and include those with a personal or family history of colorectal cancer or adenomatous polyps, various genetic polyposis and nonpolyposis syndromes, and longstanding inflammatory bowel disease (Table 63.1). Overall 5-year survival rates have improved significantly in recent years, but racial disparities persist. Between 1992 and 1999, overall 5-year survival rates were in excess of 60% for whites but only 53% for blacks.[2] Differences in cancer stage at diagnosis, therapy, or comorbidities rather than tumor biology may account for this discrepancy.[4]

Adenoma–carcinoma sequence

Virtually all colorectal cancers arise from pre-existing adenomas through a process referred to as the 'adenoma–carcinoma sequence.' Only a fraction of adenomas evolve into cancers, however, given the disproportionate prevalence of adenomas relative to lifetime individual risk of colorectal cancer. The conversion rate for adenomas to cancer has been estimated to be on the order of 2.5 polyps per 1000 (0.25%) per year.[5] Cross-sectional studies have identified increased polyp size (>1 cm), villous histology, high-grade dysplasia, and older age (>60 years) as important clinicopathologic determinants of malignant transformation.[6] These determinants alone, however, do not accurately identify all adenomas at risk, since high-grade dysplasia and cancer can be found, albeit rarely, in small tubular adenomas in individuals under the age of 60.[7] Consequently, recent interest has focused on potential molecular determinants of risk, since it is now firmly established that the adenoma–carcinoma sequence is a complex multistage process involving an accumulation of genetic alterations of specific oncogenes, tumor suppressor genes, and/or DNA mismatch repair genes.[8–11]

Another clinically important concept with respect to the adenoma–carcinoma sequence relates to 'polyp dwell time,' i.e., the amount of time it takes for a benign adenoma to transform into an invasive cancer. Although direct observational evidence is lacking, extrapolation of existing data suggest that it takes an average of about 10 years for an adenoma, particularly if <1 cm in diameter, to progress to an invasive cancer.[12,13] An accelerated polyp dwell time, however, may exist in the setting of HNPCC.[14]

Table 63.1 Risk factors for colorectal cancer

Average risk
Age ≥ 50 years, asymptomatic

Increased risk
Familial adenomatous polyposis (FAP)
    Classic FAP
    Gardner's syndrome
    Attenuated FAP
    Turcot's syndrome (medulloblastomas tumors)
MYH-associated adenomatous polyposis
Hereditary nonpolyposis colorectal cancer (HNPCC)
    Site-specific (Lynch syndrome I)
    Cancer family syndrome (Lynch syndrome II)
    Muir-Torre syndrome
    Turcot's syndrome (glioblastoma multiforme tumors)

Family history
Colorectal cancer
Colorectal adenomas < age 60 years

Past history
Colorectal cancer
Colorectal adenomas
Inflammatory bowel disease (IBD)
    Chronic ulcerative colitis
    Crohn's colitis
Hamartomatous polyposis
    Peutz-Jeghers syndrome
    Juvenile polyposis

Primary prevention

Epidemiologic studies have identified a number of modifiable risk factors related to colorectal cancer. Factors associated with an increased risk of the disease include obesity, red meat, alcohol, and tobacco; conversely, factors associated with a decreased risk include physical activity, certain vegetables, and multivitamins with folic acid.[15] These observations suggest that lifestyle modification may be an effective albeit unproven strategy for lowering colorectal cancer risk. Individuals of all ages should be encouraged to exercise at least 30 minutes daily, minimize their consumption of red meat, take a multivitamin containing 0.4 mg of folic acid daily, maintain a healthy weight, consume 5–8 servings of fruits and vegetables daily, limit their alcohol intake to no more than one drink daily, and avoid smoking.

Apart from lifestyle modifications, there is growing interest in chemoprevention as a strategy for reducing colorectal cancer risk. The goal of chemoprevention is to employ safe, well-tolerated, and affordable pharmacological agents and/or natural-occurring compounds to inhibit, reverse, or delay colorectal carcinogenesis. Among the many classes of agents evaluated to date, aspirin (ASA) and the other nonsteroidal antiinflammatory drugs (NSAIDs) have received the most attention (Table 63.2). These agents are believed to exert their activity primarily through inhibition of the enzyme cyclooxygenase, of which there are two isoforms: COX-1 and COX-2. Observational studies and randomized, placebo-controlled trials have demonstrated that both nonselective COX inhibitors (primarily ASA and sulindac) and selective COX-2 inhibitors (celecoxib and rofecoxib) can induce regression but not elimination or prevention of adenomas in familial adenomatous polyposis (FAP) patients.[16–18] Randomized, placebo-controlled trials have also demonstrated that ASA can reduce recurrence of sporadic adenomas following polypectomy but is ineffective in reducing colorectal cancer incidence among healthy individuals, possibly due to an insufficient duration of therapy.[16] In addition to NSAIDs, calcium, selenium, folate, and ursodeoxycholic acid have demonstrated effectiveness in mostly high-risk groups and are currently being evaluated alone or in combination with other agents in prospective randomized trials.[16] Pending completion of these studies, most authorities agree that existing data are insufficient to warrant widespread use of any of these agents solely for the purpose of colorectal chemoprevention, with two notable exceptions: the use of a sulindac or a COX-2 inhibitor as an adjunct to endoscopic surveillance in adult FAP patients[16] and ursodeoxycholic acid in patients with coincident ulcerative colitis and primary sclerosing cholangitis.[19–21]

Table 63.2 Chemopreventive agents and colorectal neoplasia

Strength of evidence	Weakest ⟶ Strongest					
		Observational studies		Randomized human studies		
Agent	Animal studies	Case-control	Cohort studies	Mucosal proliferation	Polyposis patients	Sporadic adenoma
Aspirin/NSAID	↑	↑	↑		↑	↑
COX-2 inhibitors*	↑			↑	↑	•
Vitamins A, C, D	↑	↑	↑	↑	→	→
Calcium	↑	↑	↑	→		↑
Fiber	↑	↑	↑	↑	→	↓
Selenium	↑	↑	→			
Fish oil		↑			↑	
Organosulfer	↑					

* Cyclooxygenase-2
↑ most studies positive; ↓ most studies negative; → studies equivocal; • studies ongoing.

Screening and surveillance (secondary prevention)

There is a strong and persuasive rationale supporting the role of screening as an effective strategy for reducing the mortality and incidence of colorectal cancer.[22] First, as previously discussed, colorectal cancer is a common disease with serious consequences. Second, available screening tests have been shown feasible in general clinical practice, acceptable to patients, and sufficiently accurate in detecting early-stage cancers. Third, sufficient evidence exists to suggest that screening can reduce both the incidence of colorectal cancer through the identification and removal of premalignant adenomas and mortality from colorectal cancer through the detection of early-stage tumors.[23–31] Fourth, decision analyses clearly demonstrate favorable cost-effectiveness ratios for each of the recommended screening modalities,[22,32] comparable to those of other generally accepted screening tests for other diseases. Lastly, estimates of polyp dwell time suggest that there is a sufficiently long 'detectable preclinical phase of disease' to warrant screening.[12,13]

Proponents of colorectal cancer screening widely agree that case finding rather than mass screening is the most appropriate approach for early detection. *Case finding* refers to the performance of screening on individuals at increased risk for the disease of interest. With respect to colorectal cancer, *screening* refers to the identification of asymptomatic individuals who are more likely to have colorectal cancer or adenomas than other asymptomatic individuals from the general population. *Surveillance*, on the other hand, refers to the periodic monitoring of patients at increased risk of colorectal cancer due to pre-existing colorectal disease, e.g., patients with a history of colorectal cancer, adenomas, or inflammatory bowel disease. Patients in whom age (>50 years) is the only risk factor are considered to be of 'average risk,' whereas those with other risk factors, such as a positive family history or inflammatory bowel disease, are considered to be at 'increased risk' (see Table 63.1). Ascertainment of risk is fundamental to appropriate clinical decision-making and provides a framework by which to discuss current recommendations for colorectal cancer screening and surveillance.

Screening guidelines for average-risk individuals

Fecal occult blood testing, sigmoidoscopy, double-contrast barium enema, and colonoscopy have been advocated by most authoritative groups as appropriate screening tests for 'average-risk' individuals, beginning at age 50.[33–36] The different tests vary with respect to effectiveness, strength of supporting evidence, risk of complications, complexity and cost (Table 63.3). The digital rectal examination has not been shown to be an effective screening test for colorectal cancer and hence is not included in these guidelines. Moreover, the common practice of using the digital rectal examination as a means of obtaining a stool sample for fecal occult blood testing should be discouraged, because of concerns about test performance. Several studies have suggested that performing fecal occult blood testing at the time of a digital rectal examination does not increase false-positivity rates and therefore may be useful in noncompliant patients.[37–39] Each of these studies concluded that a diagnostic colonoscopy should be performed for all positive tests, regardless of the method of stool collection. Because of concerns about sensitivity, however, conventional home-based testing on spontaneously passed stools is recommended for those testing negative by digital rectal examination.

Annual Fecal Occult Blood Testing (FOBT): It has long been recognized that occult bleeding is an early sign of colorectal cancer. The most commonly performed tests to detect occult bleeding exploit the fact that hemoglobin possesses peroxidase activity, which can be easily detected at the bedside by the addition of a hydrogen peroxide reagent to a guaiac-impregnated slide (e.g., Hemoccult II, Hemoccult II Sensa). These guaiac-based tests are not specific for blood; peroxidase- and pseudoperoxidase-containing foods such as red meat and certain vegetables will also produce a positive test. Three separate randomized controlled trials have demonstrated that FOBT followed by diagnostic colonoscopy significantly reduces colorectal cancer mortality by 15–18% if performed biannually and 33% if performed annually.[23–25,27] FOBT also reduces the incidence of colorectal cancer.[28] The major limitations of FOBT relate to test sensitivity and specificity. Although randomized controlled trials reported programmatic sensitivities of 72–78% for nonhydrated slides and 88–92% after hydration,[23,25] point sensitivity for nonhydrated slides may be <25% for both cancer and advanced adenomas.[40,41] False-negative tests are largely attributable to the fact that not all neoplasms bleed and those that do may bleed only intermittently.

Recommendations for performing home-based FOBT have been proposed. Preparation of two slides from each of three successive stools, prompt analysis after collection, and repeated testing on an annual basis maximizes test sensitivity without compromising specificity. Strict adherence to certain dietary restrictions, especially red meat, is also recommended when using the more sensitive guaiac-based tests (e.g., Hemoccult II and Hemoccult Sensa) to minimize false-positive results,[42,43] which translate into unnecessary diagnostic studies and their attendant risks and costs. Nonsteroidal antiinflammatory drugs, other than low-dose (<325 mg daily) aspirin, and Vitamin C should also be avoided, if

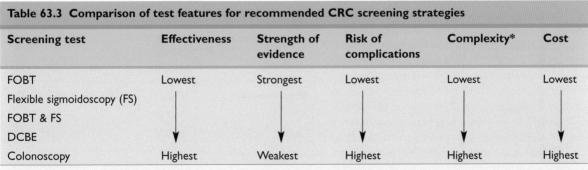

Table 63.3 Comparison of test features for recommended CRC screening strategies

Screening test	Effectiveness	Strength of evidence	Risk of complications	Complexity*	Cost
FOBT	Lowest	Strongest	Lowest	Lowest	Lowest
Flexible sigmoidoscopy (FS)					
FOBT & FS					
DCBE	↓	↓	↓	↓	↓
Colonoscopy	Highest	Weakest	Highest	Highest	Highest

* Complexity involves patient satisfaction, preparation, and convenience, as well as facilities and equipment needed.

possible, since they may produce false-positive and false-negative results, respectively. Iron supplements should not affect test sensitivity or specificity but can darken the stool and thereby interfere with interpretation of the blue color change of a positive test. Rehydration of slides is not recommended even though it enhances sensitivity because of reduced specificity. Diagnostic evaluation with colonoscopy is indicated if any one of the six slides is positive.[44,45]

Immunochemical tests for fecal hemoglobin (e.g., HemeSelect, InSure, FlexsureOBT and Immudia Hem Sp) offer an alternative strategy for detecting occult bleeding. Unlike guaiac-based tests, immunochemical tests use monoclonal and/or polyclonal antibodies to detect the intact globin protein portion in human hemoglobin and therefore obviate the need for strict dietary restrictions. Moreover, since globin is degraded as it traverses the UGI tract, immunochemical tests are specific for occult bleeding from the colon and rectum.[46] Studies to date suggest that these tests perform well compared to guaiac-based tests, but data from large scale screening trials of average-risk patients are limited.[42,47–50] Two-tier combination tests, which employ the guaiac-based approach as an initial screen and the immunochemical test for confirmation, have been advocated as a potential means of dealing with the problems of sensitivity and specificity but have yet to gain widespread endorsement.[47,48]

Sigmoidoscopy every 5 years: Another commonly employed screening test for 'average-risk' individuals is sigmoidoscopy. The rationale for sigmoidoscopy is that it permits direct visualization of the distal large bowel and biopsy of any abnormal lesions. Several types of sigmoidoscopes are available, including the 25 cm rigid scope, the 35 or 60 cm flexible fiberoptic scope, and the 60 cm flexible videoscope. Flexible instruments afford a significantly higher diagnostic yield than the rigid scopes and have demonstrated much better patient tolerance and acceptance.[51] Three case-control studies have provided the strongest evidence to date that sigmoidoscopy is an effective screening test.[26,29,30] These studies suggest that periodic sigmoidoscopy, as infrequently as every 5–10 years, can reduce mortality from colorectal cancers arising in the distal large bowel by 59–80%. Sigmoidoscopy may also reduce the incidence of colorectal cancer through the identification and removal of adenomas.[30] The major disadvantage of sigmoidoscopy is that only the distal half the large bowel can be visualized and hence only about half of all colorectal cancers and adenomas can be detected by this technique alone; however, if colonoscopy is performed for any adenoma or cancer detected at sigmoidoscopy, detection rates for advanced neoplasia are in the range of 70–80%.[41,52]

Colonoscopy every 10 years: Colonoscopy is the only screening strategy that allows direct visualization of the entire large bowel, biopsy of suspicious lesions not amenable to endoscopic removal, and polypectomy. In experienced hands, cecal intubation is achieved in up to 98.6% of screening colonoscopies.[53] Overall sensitivity for polyps and cancer is ~90%, ranging from 75% to 85% for polyps <1 cm in diameter to 95% for larger polyps and cancers; specificity approaches 100% for all lesions.[22] Failure to reach the cecum and suboptimal bowel preparation account for the majority of missed lesions. While there is no direct evidence that colonoscopy is an effective screening test, superior detection rates compared to FOBT and sigmoidoscopy,[41,52,54] and extrapolation of data from the FOBT trials,[23–25,27] screening sigmoidoscopy studies,[26,29,30] and National Polyp Study[12] provide compelling,

albeit indirect, evidence that screening colonoscopy can reduce both the incidence and mortality of colorectal cancer. The major disadvantages of colonoscopy relate to higher procedural costs and risk of complications (Table 63.4) than other screening modalities.

Double-Contrast Barium Enema (DCBE) every 5 years: DCBE offers a less expensive, less invasive, and safer alternative to colonoscopy for evaluating the entire colon. Enthusiasm for DCBE as a screening test has diminished because of concerns about performance. The most recent studies suggest a sensitivity of 85% for cancers, 52% for polyps 6–10 mm in size and 48% for polyps >1 cm in size.[55,56] Although historical data suggest that specificity for cancers is high (>99%), false-positive rates for polyps are in the range 5–10% for large polyps and 50% for small polyps.[22] In addition to concerns about performance, there is no direct evidence that DCBE is an effective screening test for colorectal cancer. Indirect evidence is derived from a single case-control study suggesting that screening barium enema was associated with a 33% reduction in colorectal cancer mortality.[57] The need for follow-up colonoscopy to evaluate abnormal findings is another important limitation.

Novel Strategies: Two new screening strategies have emerged in recent years. *Virtual colonoscopy* is a novel imaging technique in which helical computed tomography (CT) is used to generate two- and three-dimensional displays of the colon and rectum. The procedure is performed after standard preparation and air insufflation, which may be uncomfortable, but requires no sedation, analgesia, or recovery time. Although few data are available regarding the performance characteristics of virtual colonoscopy for detecting colorectal cancers, sensitivities for detecting polyps ≥1 cm have ranged 75–91% for mostly high-risk cohorts[58–60] and 55–94% for average-risk patients.[61,62] *Stool-based DNA testing* is another emerging screening strategy in which spontaneously passed stools are assayed for molecular alterations commonly associated with colorectal neoplasia. Published studies to date suggest that stool-based DNA testing has a sensitivity in the range of 62–91% for detecting colorectal cancers and 50–82% for advanced adenomas; specificity has been in the range of 93–100%.[63–66] Although existing data would suggest that both strategies are less cost-effective than colonoscopy,[67,68] they offer less invasive alternatives that may entice otherwise nonadherent patients to undergo screening.

In summary, a compelling body of evidence has accumulated to suggest that while screening is a cost-effective strategy for reducing both colorectal cancer mortality and incidence in average-risk patients, existing data are insufficient for identifying a single best strategy.[32] Consequently, the American Cancer

Table 63.4 Major complication rates of screening tests

Screening test	Complication rate (perforation and hemorrhage)	Death
Barium enema	1/10 000	<1/50 000
Sigmoidoscopy	1–2/10 000	<1/10 000
Colonoscopy	1–3/1000	1–3/10 000

Note: Major complications with colonoscopy are more frequent if polypectomy is performed. (Reprinted from Winawer SJ et al, Gastroenterology, 1997; 112:594–642. © 1997, with permission from The American Gastroenterological Association.)

Society,[34] US Multisociety Task Force,[36] and many professional societies now endorse several colorectal cancer screening options including: annual FOBT, flexible sigmoidoscopy every 5 years, DCBE every 5 years, or colonoscopy every 10 years (Table 63.5). The combined strategy of annual FOBT plus sigmoidoscopy every 5 years is also recommended, based primarily on evidence from a nonrandomized controlled trial demonstrating that the two modalities together were more effective than either alone.[31] The US Preventive Services Task Force makes similar recommendations, but because of insufficient evidence, fails to define optimal screening intervals for the various strategies other than annual FOBT.[35] Neither virtual colonoscopy nor fecal DNA testing are recommended due to insufficient effectiveness and cost data. Selection of a recommended strategy needs to be individualized on the basis of potential risks and benefits, compliance issues, availability, and local expertise. Decisions about when to stop screening also needs to be individualized, but, in general, screening should be discontinued in patients with significant comorbidity and/or when the lead time between screening and its benefits (~10 years) is longer than the patient's life expectancy.

Screening and surveillance guidelines for individuals at increased risk

Up to 25% of all cases of colorectal cancer occur in individuals with predisposing factors other than age (see Table 63.1). Since each of these factors is associated with an increased risk of colorectal cancer, more aggressive screening and surveillance strategies may be warranted (see Table 63.5). The guidelines proposed herein are based primarily on the US Multisociety Task Force recommendations,[36] which vary in selected instances from those proposed by other authoritative groups, such as the American Cancer Society[34] and the American College of Gastroenterology.[33]

Family History: Family history of colorectal cancer is a well-established risk factor for colorectal cancer and may account for 15–20% cases. More recent studies suggest that the same is true for individuals with a family history of adenomas,[69,70] especially if the affected relatives' polyps exhibited advanced histology.[71] The actual degree of risk is determined by the closeness of the relationship, the age of onset, and the number of affected relatives.[72] Individuals at the highest risk have two or more first-degree relatives (parent, sibling, or offspring) with colorectal cancer at any age of onset, or one first-degree relative with colorectal cancer diagnosed before the age of 55, or an adenoma diagnosed before the age of 60. Individuals at intermediate risk have only a single first-degree relative affected at age >60 or a second-degree relative with colorectal cancer.[72,73] Cancers arising in the setting of a family history tend to develop at an earlier age,[74] but are otherwise similar to sporadic tumors with respect to natural history. Data regarding the anatomic distribution of familial cancers are conflicting; whereas some studies suggest a predilection for the proximal colon, most suggest a distribution similar to that of sporadic cancers.[72]

Based on these observations, both the US Multisociety Task Force and American Cancer Society recommend that individuals with two or more first-degree relatives with colorectal cancer at

Table 63.5 Colorectal cancer screening and surveillance recommendations

Indication	Recommendations
Average risk	Any one of the following beginning at age 50: Annual fecal occult blood testing (FOBT) Flexible sigmoidoscopy every 5 yrs Annual FOBT plus flexible sigmoidoscopy every 5 yrs Double-contrast barium enema every 5 yrs Colonoscopy every 10 yrs
Two FDRs with CRC, or a single FDR with CRC or adenomatous polyps diagnosed at age <60	Colonoscopy every 5 years beginning at age 40, or 10 years younger than earliest diagnosis, whichever comes first
Single FDR with CRC or adenomatous polyps diagnosed at age ≥60, or 2 second-degree relatives with CRC	Same options as for average risk beginning at age 40
HNPCC	Genetic counseling and testing* Colonoscopy every 1–2 years beginning at age 20 and then yearly after age 40†
FAP and variants‡	Genetic counseling and testing* Flexible sigmoidoscopy yearly beginning at puberty if "classic" form† Colonoscopy yearly beginning 10 years before the youngest affected relative if "attenuated" form†
Personal history of CRC	Colonoscopy within 6 months of curative resection if incomplete examination performed preoperatively; repeat at 3 years and then every 5 years if normal
Personal history of colorectal adenoma(s)	Colonoscopy every 3 to 5 years after removal of index polyps
Inflammatory bowel disease	Colonoscopy every 1–2 years beginning after 8 years of pancolitis or after 15 years if only left-sided disease.

FDR, first-degree relative, FAP, familial adenomatous polyposis; HNPCC, hereditary nonpolyposis colorectal cancer
* Recommended for affected individuals meeting clinical criteria and the first-degree relatives of individuals testing positive.
† Recommended for affected individuals meeting clinical criteria, regardless of genetic testing, and all first-degree relatives who test positive, refuse testing or in whom genetic testing is indeterminate (i.e., affected relative tests negative).
‡ Variants include Gardner's syndrome, attenuated FAP, and some families with Turcot's syndrome.

any age, or a single first-degree relative with colorectal cancer or adenomas diagnosed at age <60 should undergo colonoscopy every 5 years beginning at age 40, or 10 years younger than the earliest diagnosis in the family, whichever comes first (see Table 63.5).[34,36] The Multisociety Task Force also recommends that individuals with a single first-degree relative diagnosed with colorectal cancer or adenomatous polyps at age >60, or two second-degree relatives (e.g., grandparents, aunts/uncles, cousins) with colorectal cancer should undergo any of the screening tests recommended for average-risk individuals beginning at age 40.[36] The American College of Gastroenterology guidelines also recommend colonoscopy beginning at age 40, or 10 years before the youngest affected relative, for individuals with a family history of colorectal cancer affecting one or more first-degree-relatives regardless of age of diagnosis but extend the interval from every 5 years to every 10 years if the affected relative was >60 years of age. Recommendations for individuals with a family history of adenomas are similar to those at average risk, i.e., colonoscopy beginning at age 50.[33]

Familial Adenomatous Polyposis (FAP): FAP is a rare genetic condition that accounts for less than 1% of colorectal cancer cases.[75] The disease is caused by mutations of the adenomatous polyposis (*APC*) gene on chromosome 5 and characterized by the appearance of hundreds of colorectal adenomas during the second or third decade of life and a risk of colorectal cancer that approaches 100% by the fifth decade if left untreated. In addition to colorectal polyposis, FAP patients are at risk of a variety of benign extracolonic manifestations, including extracolonic polyps (fundic gland gastric polyps and adenomas of the small bowel), desmoid tumors, cutaneous lesions (lipomas, fibromas, and epidermal cysts), osteomas, odontomas, congenital hypertrophy of the retinal pigment epithelium, adrenal adenomas, and nasopharyngeal angiofibroma. FAP patients are also at risk of extracolonic malignancies, most notably periampullary cancer of the duodenum. The term Gardner's syndrome has been applied to FAP patients with extracolonic manifestations. Two other conditions have been linked to mutations of the *APC* gene and are believed to be FAP variants: an attenuated form in which affected individuals typically present later in life with far fewer (<100), predominantly right-sided adenomas;[76] and Turcot's syndrome, which is another rare genetic condition characterized by colorectal adenomatous polyposis and brain tumors (medulloblastomas).[77] Recently, a novel autosomal recessive polyposis syndrome indistinguishable from classic or attenuated FAP has been described in which mutations of the base excision repair gene, mutY homologue (*MYH*), is causal.[78]

The diagnosis of FAP is made clinically by the identification of colorectal adenomatous polyposis. Genetic testing for mutations of the *APC* gene will confirm the diagnosis in 80–90% of affected individuals. Individuals with both classic FAP (>100 adenomas) and the attenuated form (20–100 adenomas) are candidates for genetic testing. Individuals testing negative for *APC* mutations should be tested for *MYH* mutations.

Members of affected kindreds have a high probability of inheriting these diseases because of their autosomal dominant mode of transmission and hence warrant aggressive screening at an early age (see Table 63.5). At-risk family members should be offered genetic counseling and, if agreeable, undergo genetic testing around the time of puberty (ages 10–12). Whenever possible, affected relatives should be tested first to validate the presence of

an *APC* mutation, since up to 20% of FAP kindreds will have false-negative tests by the commercially available in vitro synthesized protein assay.[79] Kindreds testing negative by this assay should consider alternative genetic testing methods, e.g., direct sequencing, to define their mutational status and identify gene carriers. At-risk individuals testing positive should undergo yearly sigmoidoscopy until around age 40 rather than colonoscopy since the distribution of adenomas is uniform through the large bowel. The only exception would be in kindreds with the variant forms of FAP in which case annual colonoscopy is recommended since there is a predilection for proximal colonic involvement. Yearly sigmoidoscopy is also indicated for at-risk individuals who refuse or for whom genetic testing is unavailable. Individuals testing negative warrant no special follow-up, unless the kindred's mutational status was never defined or found to be falsely negative, in which case screening sigmoidoscopy is also indicated.[36,80]

The goal of sigmoidoscopy is to document the appearance of adenomas so that the timing of prophylactic colectomy can be determined. The preferred surgical options include colectomy with ileorectal anastomosis (IRA) or total colectomy with mucosal proctectomy and ileal pouch–anal anastomosis (IPAA). Total proctocolectomy with IPAA is a 2-stage procedure that is technically more challenging but eliminates the subsequent risk of cancer in the retained rectal segment; alternatively, colectomy with IPAA is technically easier with fewer complications but carries a risk of rectal cancer that steadily increases over time. Although procedures that eliminate the rectum and thus the risk of subsequent rectal cancer have been advocated by many,[81] colectomy with IPA may be an appropriate procedure for (1) young patients with few rectal adenomas and family history of a mild phenotype and (2) patients with attenuated FAP.[82] Patients opting for rectal-sparing procedures require close surveillance with flexible sigmoidoscopy and removal or fulguration of all polyps every 3–6 months. Patients undergoing total colectomy with IPAA also require periodic endoscopic surveillance because of the risk of adenoma formation at the anastomosis or in the pouch.[83] Maintenance therapy with NSAIDs such as sulindac, celecoxib or rofecoxib has been shown to cause regression of rectal stump polyps but has not been shown to reduce the subsequent risk of cancer.[84–86] Because FAP patients are also at increased risk of duodenal cancers, especially in the periampullary region, surveillance of the upper GI tract with both front and side-viewing endoscopes is also warranted every 1–3 years once the diagnosis of colorectal polyposis is established.

Hereditary Nonpolyposis Colorectal Cancer (HNPCC): HNPCC is a distinct autosomal dominant genetic disorder that accounts for 3–6% of colorectal cancer cases. The syndrome is characterized by early-onset colorectal cancer (average age, 44 years) in the absence of polyposis, predominance (60–80%) of tumors proximal to the splenic flexure, and an excess of both synchronous and metachronous colorectal cancers. The estimated lifetime risk of colorectal cancer is in the range of 80%, with approximately 50% of cases occurring before age 50. In addition to colorectal cancer, affected individuals are predisposed to a variety of extracolonic cancers arising in the endometrium, ovaries, stomach (especially in Asian countries such as Japan and Korea), small intestine, pancreas, biliary tract and upper uroepithelial tract (ureters and renal pelvis), brain (Turcot's syndrome), and skin (Muir-Torre syndrome). Historically, the term 'site-specific' HNPCC (Lynch syndrome I) was used to describe kindreds with disease confined

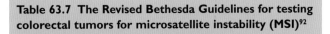

to the colon and rectum and 'cancer family syndrome' (Lynch syndrome II) for those with both CRC and extracolonic malignancies. Despite the absence of polyposis, HNPCC-associated colorectal cancers are believed to arise from pre-existing adenomas. Affected individuals have a propensity to develop a finite number of predominantly right-sided, 'flat' adenomas at a young age. The adenomas are often villous with components of high-grade dysplasia and exhibit an accelerated rate of malignant transformation, which may be as short as 2–3 years, compared to 8–10 years for sporadic adenomas. Notwithstanding the aggressive nature of HNPCC-associated adenomas, HNPCC-associated cancers have a better prognosis stage for stage than those arising in the general population. HNPCC is caused by germline mutations in one of several DNA mismatch repair (MMR) genes. To date, seven distinct MMR genes have been identified, including *hMLH1*, *hMSH2*, *hMSH3*, *hMSH6*, *PMS1*, *PMS2*, and *EXO1*. Mutations of *hMLH1* and *hMSH2* account for nearly 90% of MMR mutations; the remaining 10% involve mostly *hMSH6*.[87–89]

Clinical criteria for identifying patients at risk of HNPCC have been proposed. The original criteria, now known as Amsterdam I criteria (Table 63.6), were predicated on an accurate family history of colorectal cancer that includes number of affected relatives, degree of closeness, and age of diagnoses.[90] The Amsterdam I criteria were later revised to include extracolonic cancers (Amsterdam II criteria [see Table 63.6]).[91] Less stringent revised Bethesda criteria have also been proposed in an effort to increase identification of high-risk individuals (Table 63.7).[92]

The identification of susceptibility loci has promoted genetic testing as the screening strategy of choice for HNPCC. Revised guidelines for the use of genetic testing were proposed in 2004 (see Table 63.6).[92] These new guidelines recommend analysis of tumors from affected high-risk individuals for microsatellite instability (MSI), the phenotypic hallmark of defective DNA mismatch repair, or expression of *hMLH1* and *hMSH2* staining by immunohistochemistry (IHC), as the preferred initial diagnostic strategy. Individuals whose tumors exhibit MSI at two or more markers of a standardized 5-marker panel (MSI-high tumors) or lost of expression of *hMLH1* and *hMSH2* staining by IHC should

undergo direct germline testing for *hMLH1* and *hMSH2* mutations. Direct germline testing without MSI or IHC analysis remains an option for high-risk individuals if tissue testing is not feasible (e.g., affected proband's tumor is unavailable) or if there is a strong clinical suspicion and MSI/IHC testing is negative. If a deleterious mutation is identified, at-risk family members should be referred for genetic counseling and testing if agreeable. If no mutation is identified in a proband with an MSI-high tumor and/or a strong clinical history, the genetic test is deemed non-informative and both the proband and all at-risk relatives should be counseled as if HNPCC was confirmed and high-risk surveillance should be undertaken. Although not specifically stated in the recommendations, germline analysis for *hMSH6* mutations should be considered for kindreds with clustering late-onset MSI-low or microsatellite-stable colorectal cancers and gynecologic malignancies.

Surveillance colonoscopy is recommended every 1–2 years starting around the age of 20, or 10 years before the youngest affected relative, and yearly after age 40 for individuals testing positive by one of the genetic screening assays (see Table 63.5).[34,36,80] A similar strategy should be considered for at-risk individuals who refuse genetic testing or in whom testing is inappropriate, i.e., those from affected kindreds with false-negative results. The rationale for frequent colonoscopy rather than sigmoidoscopy is the predilection for proximal involvement and the accelerated rate of malignant transformation. When combined with endoscopic polypectomy, surveillance colonoscopy has been shown to reduce both the incidence and mortality of colorectal cancer in families with HNPCC.[93] Because of the excessive occurrence of both incident and metachronous cancers, prophylactic subtotal colectomy has been proposed as an alternative to surveillance colonoscopy for mutation-positive individuals. Since there are no evidence-based data to support one approach over the others, aggressive surveillance is generally preferred, except in selected

Table 63.7 The Revised Bethesda Guidelines for testing colorectal tumors for microsatellite instability (MSI)[92]

Tumors from individuals should be tested for MSI or loss of MLH1/MSH2 by immunohistochemistry in the following situations:
Colorectal diagnosed in a patient <50 years of age
Presence of synchronous, metachronous colorectal, or other HNPCC-associated tumors*, regardless of age
Colorectal cancer with histologic features indicative of HNPCC † diagnosed in a patient <60 years of age
Colorectal cancer diagnosed in one or more first-degree relatives with an HNPCC-related tumor, one of which was diagnosed at age <50.
Colorectal cancer diagnosed in two or more first- or second-degree relatives with HNPCC-related tumors, regardless of age

* HNPCC-associated tumors include colorectal, endometrial, stomach, ovarian, pancreas, ureter and renal pelvis, biliary tract, brain (usually glioblastoma), and small bowel cancers, as well as sebaceous gland adenomas and keratoacanthomas (Muir-Torre syndrome).
† Presence of tumor-infiltrating lymphocytes, Crohn's-like lymphocytic reaction, mucinous/signet-ring differentiation, or medullary growth pattern.
(Adapted from Umar A, Boland CR, Terdiman JP, et al. Revised Bethesda Guidelines for hereditary nonpolyposis colorectal cancer (Lynch syndrome) and microsatellite instability. J Natl Cancer Inst 2004; 96:261–268.)

Table 63.6 Clinical criteria for hereditary nonpolyposis colorectal cancer (HNPCC)

Amsterdam I criteria

≥3 relatives with colorectal cancer plus all of the following:
One affected relative is a first-degree relative of the other two
Colorectal cancer involving at least two generations
One or more cancers diagnosed before age 50
Familial adenomatous polyposis excluded
Tumors should be verified by pathological examination

Amsterdam II criteria

≥3 relatives with an HNPCC-associated cancer (colorectal, endometrium, small bowel, ureter, or renal pelvis), one of whom is a first-degree relative of the other two, plus all of the following:
Two or more successive generations affected
One or more cancers diagnosed before age 50
Familial adenomatous polyposis excluded
Tumors should be verified by pathological examination

situations where surveillance is not technically feasible or mutation carriers refuse colonoscopic surveillance but agree to sigmoidoscopic surveillance of the rectal remnant.[94]

Subtotal colectomy is the surgical procedure of choice for lesions not amenable to endoscopic removal or frank cancers. Because of the high rate of metachronous cancers in HNPCC patients, which have been estimated to be as high as 40% at 10 years and 72% at 40 years depending on the length of colon remaining after surgery,[95] surveillance sigmoidoscopy is recommended every 1 or 2 years following subtotal colectomy or partial colectomy, respectively. Evidence supporting this recommendation is derived from studies demonstrating an accelerated rate of malignant transformation in HNPCC and two post-resection surveillance studies demonstrating a high rate of metachronous cancers within 2–5 years of follow-up.[96,97] Surveillance for gynecologic malignancies, particularly endometrial cancer and ovarian cancer, with yearly pelvic examinations, transvaginal ultrasonography, endometrial sampling, and CA-125 levels beginning at age ~25 is also recommended, but of unproven effectiveness.[88] Prophylactic hysterectomy with bilateral salpingo-oophorectomy should be considered at the time of colectomy for women who no longer wish to bear children. With the exception of endometrial cancer, surveillance guidelines for extracolonic malignancies have not been established and hence recommendations need to be individualized on the basis of a particular kindred's cancer profile and the reliability of existing modalities for early detection of the various types of malignancies.

Prior Colorectal Cancer: Patients undergoing resection with curative intent of a colorectal cancer are at risk not only of tumor recurrence at the surgical anastomosis, but also a 5–10% cumulative risk of metachronous cancers after 15 years of follow-up.[98] Approximately 30% of such patients will also develop metachronous adenomas.[99] Since metachronous cancers undoubtedly arise from pre-existing adenomas, periodic surveillance to identify and remove metachronous adenomas should be effective in reducing the incidence of subsequent cancers. Complete evaluation of the colon, preferably by colonoscopy, within 1 year of resection is recommended by the American Cancer Society but not by the US Multisociety Task Force, except in cases where a complete preoperative colonoscopy was never performed (see Table 63.5).[34,36] The rationale for the 1-year follow-up examination recommended by the American Cancer Society, regardless of whether a complete preoperative colonoscopy is performed, relates in part to early detection of anastomotic recurrences, which occur in approximately 3% of cases.[99] Conversely, the US Multisociety Task Force recommendations presumably reflect the fact that most anastomotic recurrences are accompanied by recurrent intra-abdominal disease, thus decreasing the likelihood of long-term benefit from presymptomatic detection.[100] Both groups recommend a surveillance examination after 3 years and, if normal, every 5 years thereafter.[34,36]

Prior Adenomas: Individuals with a history of colorectal adenomas are also at risk of both metachronous adenomas and cancer. Depending on the surveillance interval employed, anywhere from 12% to 60% of patients will have additional adenomas at follow-up colonoscopy.[99] Polyp characteristics at baseline, including size ≥1 cm, tubulovillous or villous histology, and multiplicity, identify those at greatest risk.[101] The National Polyp Study provided the first strong evidence that colonoscopic polypectomy and postpolypectomy surveillance is effective in reducing the subsequent

incidence of colorectal cancer.[12] This study has also demonstrated that postpolypectomy surveillance colonoscopy every 3 years was as effective as yearly examinations in detecting adenomas with advanced pathology, i.e., size ≥1 cm in diameter, villous histology, and/or high-grade dysplasia, or multiple adenomas (≥3).[102] A subsequent study found that patients with only 1 or 2 small (<1 cm) tubular adenomas were at low risk for advanced adenomas at the 3-year follow-up examination.[103] Based on these observations, an interval of at least 3 years is recommended before the initial follow-up examination after colonoscopic removal for patients with advanced adenomas or multiple adenomas; the first follow-up examination can be deferred for 5 years for patients with only 1 or 2 small tubular adenomas (Fig. 63.1).[36] A shorter interval, however, may be warranted in patients with multiple adenomas, malignant polyps or large sessile lesions to ensure total eradication, as well as in those with HNPCC because of the shorter polyp dwell time. Patients found to have advanced adenomas or multiple small adenomas at follow-up continue to warrant surveillance colonoscopy every 3 years, whereas all others can defer subsequent examinations for at least 5 years.[36] Surveillance is currently not indicated for patients with hyperplastic polyps; however, surveillance is recommended for individuals with polyps containing histologic features of both hyperplastic and adenomatous polyps, so-called 'serrated adenomas.'[104]

Inflammatory Bowel Disease: Although estimates of risk vary widely, ulcerative colitis and Crohn's colitis are both associated with an increased risk of colorectal cancer. Duration and extent of disease are the most important determinants of risk in both diseases.[105–107] Severity of inflammation and family history may

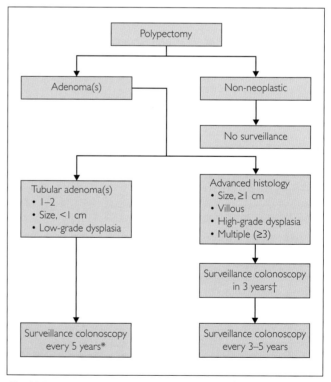

Fig. 63.1 • Algorithm for colonoscopic surveillance of patients with colorectal polyps. *No surveillance is also an option for patients with only 1–2 small (<1 cm), tubular adenomas with low-grade dysplasia. † A shorter interval (3–12 months) may be warranted in patients with malignant polyps, large sessile adenomas or multiple adenomas.

also be important risk factors.[108,109] Patients with coincident primary sclerosing cholangitis are at higher risk than those with ulcerative colitis alone.[110] Despite debates over cost-effectiveness, endoscopic surveillance has been advocated as an alternative to prophylactic proctocolectomy as a means of reducing this risk. The goal of surveillance in this setting is to detect dysplasia and early cancers rather than adenomatous polyps. Colonoscopy with biopsy every 1–2 years is recommended beginning after 8 years of disease in patients with pancolitis or after 15 years of disease in patients with only left-sided involvement (see Table 63.5).[36] Four 'large' biopsies should be obtained from normal-appearing mucosa at 10 cm intervals throughout the large bowel and all suspicious mass lesions to achieve a diagnostic accuracy of >90%.[111,112] Histologic review should be performed by a pathologist experienced in colitis-associated dysplasia, and confirmed by a second pathologist if dysplasia is found, because of the difficulties in distinguishing low-grade dysplasia from reactive inflammatory or reparative changes. For this reason, surveillance has limited utility in the setting of active inflammation and should be deferred. Results should be classified as negative for dysplasia, indefinite for dysplasia, or positive for low-grade or high-grade dysplasia, according to established criteria.[113] Management strategies for each are listed in Figure 63.2. The presence of high-grade dysplasia is a definite indication for proctocolectomy since 30–40% of resected specimens harbor a cancer either adjacent to or distant from the site of biopsy.[114] Although controversial, proctocolectomy should also be considered for those with low-grade dysplasia, especially if a gross lesion is present, based on data suggesting that coincident cancer may be present in up to 40% of resected

specimens and that the 5-year predictive value for high-grade dysplasia or cancer may be in the range of 50%.[115–117] Patients with low-grade dysplasia who refuse surgery as well as those with indefinite dysplasia should undergo a follow-up examination in 6 months and then yearly thereafter if repeat biopsies remain negative for dysplasia. Proctocolectomy should also be considered for patients with longstanding colitis who refuse surveillance or in whom the presence of multiple pseudopolyps hinders surveillance efforts or interpretation of findings.

Adenomas can arise in patients with inflammatory bowel disease and need to be distinguished from 'dysplasia-associated lesions or masses' (DALMs), which carry a high risk of cancer and constitute a strong indication for colectomy.[118,119] The currently recommended approach is to perform a polypectomy plus biopsies of the surrounding mucosa, in addition to surveillance biopsies from the remaining colon. If there is no evidence of dysplasia or cancer in the surrounding mucosa or elsewhere, polypectomy alone is sufficient and routine surveillance should be continued; if dysplasia or cancer is seen, colectomy should be performed.[120]

Miscellaneous Conditions: The Peutz-Jeghers syndrome (PJS) and juvenile polyposis syndrome (JPS), both rare familial hamartomatous polyposis syndromes, are associated with an increased risk of colorectal cancer. Because of this increased risk, which may be as high as 20% for PJS and 68% for JPS, aggressive surveillance is warranted. Colonoscopy is the surveillance procedure of choice and is recommended every 3 years beginning at age 18 for PJS and every 1–2 years beginning at age 15–18 for JPS. Prophylactic colectomy is also an option, especially for JPS patients with a large polyp burden.[121]

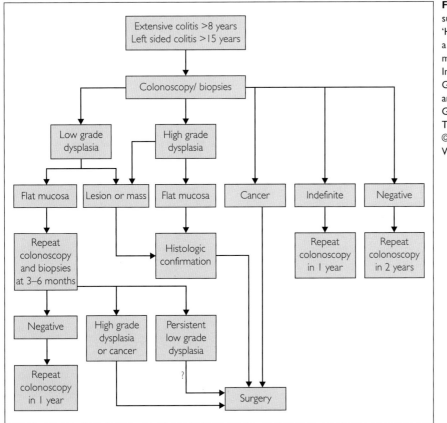

Fig. 63.2 • Algorithm for colonoscopic surveillance of patients with ulcerative colitis. 'Histologic confirmation' refers to agreement by a second experienced pathologist that the biopsy meets the criteria for dysplasia as defined by the Inflammatory Bowel Disease Morphology Study Group.[111] (Reprinted from Ahnen DJ, Dysplasia and chronic ulcerative colitis, in Rustgi A (ed), Gastrointestinal Cancers: Biology Diagnosis and Therapy, Philadelphia, JB Lippincott, 1995, 399. © 1995, reprinted with permission of Lippincott Williams & Wilkins.)

Diagnosis

Symptomatic Patients: Colonoscopy is the diagnostic procedure of choice for patients with symptoms that suggest the presence of colorectal cancer or polyps. GI bleeding is the most common of these symptoms and has a high predictive value for colorectal cancer, especially for patients over the age of 40. The overall yield of colonoscopy for cancer in such patients is about 11% for those with nonemergent rectal bleeding, 8% for those with acute lower GI hemorrhage, 10% for those with melena and a negative upper endoscopy, and 8% for those with iron deficiency anemia, compared to about 0.7% for average-risk patients undergoing screening colonoscopy.[99] The yield for nonemergent rectal bleeding is noteworthy since it pertains to both patients with 'suspicious' bleeding (dark red blood, blood mixed with or streaked on stool, and/or blood associated with a change in bowel habits or mucus discharge) and those with 'outlet'-type bleeding (bright red blood seen during defecation or after defecation on the toilet paper, or in the toilet water).[122] Persistent nonbleeding symptoms of short duration, such as abdominal pain and altered bowel habits, also have a relatively high predictive value for colorectal cancer, but the overall yield of colonoscopy (~3%) is significantly less than for bleeding or iron deficiency anemia.[99] Since adenomas are prevalent in the general population and rarely cause symptoms, it is not surprising that the yield of colonoscopy is fairly similar for both symptomatic and asymptomatic patients.[53] Flexible sigmoidoscopy, CT colography ('virtual colonoscopy') and/or DCBE are alternative diagnostic strategies that afford a lower diagnostic yield, but should be considered in symptomatic patients who are unsuitable candidates for colonoscopy because of unstable comorbid illness or in whom colonoscopy is unsuccessful. FOBT has no role in the evaluation of symptomatic patients.[123]

Positive FOBT: To maximize test sensitivity, a positive guaiac-based FOBT is defined as the presence of peroxidase activity (blue discoloration) in one or more slide windows. Retesting is not recommended even for individuals who failed to comply with dietary or medication (e.g., aspirin or NSAIDs) restrictions. Prompt diagnostic evaluation is warranted for anyone testing positive because of the high probability of finding an early-stage cancer or large adenoma, which is estimated to be in the range of 20–40%.[45] Colonoscopy is the diagnostic procedure of choice by virtue of its superior sensitivity and specificity compared to other modalities, provision for endoscopic biopsy or polypectomy, and proven effectiveness in reducing colorectal cancer mortality when used in this setting. DCBE, preferably combined with flexible sigmoidoscopy, is recommended for patients who refuse colonoscopy or in whom colonoscopy is unsuccessful because of poor preparation, patient intolerance, or technical difficulties that preclude visualization of the entire colon.

'Positive' Screening Sigmoidoscopy: The finding of any cancer or polyp ≥1 cm in diameter constitutes a positive screening sigmoidoscopy and warrants follow-up colonoscopy to remove polyps and search for synchronous neoplastic lesions in the more proximal colon (Fig. 63.3).[36] Since polyps of this size are almost always adenomatous, it is preferable to defer pathologic assessment until the time of polypectomy to avoid sampling errors and reduce costs. Polypectomy is best performed at the time of colonoscopy because of the risk, albeit remote, of electrocautery-induced explosions in an inadequately cleansed bowel.[124] Cancers

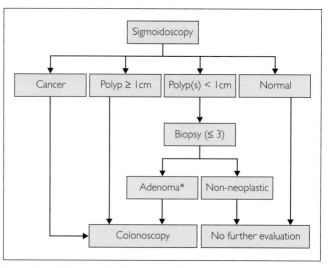

Fig. 63.3 • Algorithm for diagnostic evaluation of a 'positive' screening sigmoidoscopy. *No further evaluation is also an option for patients with 1–2 small (<1 cm), tubular adenomas with low-grade dysplasia.

should be biopsied either at the time of sigmoidoscopy or at colonoscopy.

Whether adenomas <1 cm in diameter, especially if tubular and without high-grade dysplasia, also constitute a positive finding requiring subsequent colonoscopy is controversial. The controversy stems from studies suggesting that small tubular adenomas are uncommonly associated with more advanced neoplastic lesions proximally[125,126] and portend a risk of colorectal cancer no greater than that of the general population.[127] These observations are offset by conflicting data on the true prevalence of advanced proximal lesions in this setting (range, <1–16%),[125] the tendency to underestimate polyp size endoscopically,[128] and insufficient data on potential confounders such as patient age at diagnosis or family history. Moreover, many would argue that a future risk no greater than that of the general population is a less than optimal outcome since the rationale for colorectal cancer screening is to reduce the overall risk of colorectal cancer and its attendant morbidity and mortality, as previously discussed. Pending resolution of this controversy, it is recommended polyps <1 cm of size should be biopsied at the time of sigmoidoscopy and evaluated histopathologically (see Fig. 63.3).[36,129] If numerous small polyps are seen, biopsies should be obtained from a representative sample (3–5 polyps). New technologies such as magnifying colonoscopy with dye staining (chromoendoscopy)[130] and laser-induced fluorescence spectroscopy[131] show promise in discriminating between neoplastic and non-neoplastic polyps and may ultimately obviate the need for histopathologic assessment, but are currently of unproven clinical value. Small adenomas with advanced pathology (i.e., villous change or high-grade dysplasia) are a clear-cut indication for follow-up colonoscopy since the risk of significant proximal neoplasms is comparable to that of larger adenomas.[125,126] Decisions regarding colonoscopy for small tubular adenomas without high-grade dysplasia need to be individualized on the basis of age, family history, comorbidity, availability, and psychological needs. Distal hyperplastic polyps have no malignant potential[132] nor prognostic significance,[125,133,134] and hence require no further work-up.

Management of colorectal polyps

Colonoscopic polypectomy has been shown to reduce the incidence of colorectal cancer and is therefore indicated for patients with adenomas. Endoscopic techniques are preferred since they are safe, effective, and far less costly than surgery. Choice of techniques depends on polyp size and configuration, endoscopist experience and expertise, and equipment availability.

Patient Preparation: Prior to performing colonoscopic polypectomy, the bowel needs to be cleansed using laxatives such as sodium phosphate (e.g., Fleet phosphosoda®) with or without enemas, or large volumes (4 liters) of balanced electrolyte solutions containing polyethylene glycol (e.g., Golytely®, Nulytely®, Colyte®). The balanced electrolyte solutions are recommended for elderly patients and those with specific disorders such as renal insufficiency and congestive heart failure.[135] Clear liquids, or other residue-free diets, for 24–48 hours prior to cleansing and discontinuation of iron-containing medications one week in advance will improve the quality of the preparation. In the absence of a pre-existing bleeding disorder, aspirin and most NSAIDs in standard doses do not increase the risk of significant bleeding after colonoscopy with biopsy or polypectomy and therefore do not need to be discontinued. Management of patients on warfarin needs to be individualized depending on the indication for anticoagulation, risk of thromboembolic disease, and recommendations of the referring provider. Available evidence suggests that temporary interruption of therapy for 3–5 days prior to the procedure followed by prompt reinstitution after polypectomy is appropriate for most patients, including most patients with mechanical valves and nonvalvular atrial fibrillation.[136] Prophylactic antibiotics to prevent infectious endocarditis are no longer recommended for routine colonoscopy or colonoscopy with polypectomy, even among high-risk patients (i.e., those with prosthetic valves, a prior history of infectious endocarditis, or surgically constructed systemic-pulmonary shunts or conduits).[137]

Diminutive Polyps: The majority of diminutive polyps, arbitrarily defined as polyps <1 cm in diameter, are adenomatous and therefore should be fulgurated or removed if seen at colonoscopy.[138] Historically, the 'hot biopsy' technique using either monopolar or bipolar electrocautery has been the preferred treatment modality for polyps <6 mm in size since it permits simultaneous biopsy and fulguration. Bipolar electrocautery has the theoretical advantage of causing less thermal injury to the bowel wall than monopolar electrocautery but comparative trials of safety and efficacy are lacking. Eradication rates are significantly higher (83% versus 42%) if a 1–2 mm rim of visible necrosis (whitening) is achieved during cautery.[139] Complications of hot biopsy include immediate or delayed hemorrhage (0.41%), perforation (0.05%) and 'postcoagulation' syndrome due to transmural thermal injury.[140] Post-polypectomy bleeding may occur acutely or 7–10 days later after sloughing of the cautery-induced eschar. Caution is warranted when performing hot biopsies in the right colon because of its thinner wall and greater risk of perforation.[140] Caution is also warranted in patients on low-dose aspirin because of the risk of major hemorrhage.[141] Snare excision with ('hot') or without ('cold') electrocautery is a safe and effective alternative to the hot biopsy technique in patients without coagulopathy.[142,143] Neodymium:YAG laser ablation has been advocated in the treatment of selected cases with multiple diminutive polyps, such as elderly patients or FAP patients with recurrent rectal stump polyps

after colectomy with ileorectal anastomosis.[144] Apart from the small risk of perforation, the major disadvantage of laser ablation is that no specimen is available for histopathologic evaluation.

Pedunculated Polyps: Snare excision with electrocautery is the preferred method for removing larger polyps on a stalk or pedicle. Ideally, pedunculated polyps should be transected using a continuous 'coagulation' current approximately one-third of the way down the stalk away from the polyp head to ensure complete eradication, maximize histopathologic interpretation, and minimize complications.[142] Submucosal injection of the base of the stalk with 2–3 ml of sterile saline permits more complete excision of the stalk if desired.[145] Very large pedunculated polyps may require 'piecemeal' snare excision. Once transected, the polyp should be retrieved and sent for histopathologic evaluation. The major complication of snare polypectomy is bleeding, which occurs in 0.3%–6.1% of cases.[146] If bleeding occurs, standard endoscopic therapies (e.g., injection therapy, thermocoagulation, or electrocoagulation) are often successful; alternatively, band ligation,[147] EndoLoop application,[148] and use of endoscopic clipping devices[149] can also be employed.

Sessile Polyps: Snare excision with electrocautery is also the procedure of choice for sessile polyps, i.e., polyps without an identifiable stalk or pedicle. Sessile polyps can assume a wide array of configurations including the typical diminutive type, narrow-based 'marble' type, larger broad-based 'mountain' type, 'clam shell' type which wraps around a fold, and very flat 'carpet' type, as well as a mixed or 'extended' type. Despite the lack of a stalk or pedicle, most sessile polyps have a base smaller than the widest diameter of the lesion and are therefore amenable to transection with a single application of the snare.[142] The maximum size base that may be ensnared in a single application is around 2.0–2.5 cm provided that tightening of the wire loop results in bunching of the base to 1.0–1.5 cm; otherwise the polyp should be removed in a piecemeal fashion.[142] Endoscopic mucosal resection, using either the 'strip biopsy' ('lift-and-cut') or 'suck-and-cut' technique, facilitate the safe removal of very flat and/or large sessile lesions; both employ a submucosal injection of 2–3 ml of saline to separate mucosal and submucosal lesions from the muscularis propria.[145,150] Residual polyp tissue can be safely fulgurated by noncontact delivery of inert argon gas using the so-called Argon Plasma Coagulator.[151,152] As with any polypectomy, the major complications associated with endoscopic removal of sessile polyps include bleeding (0.3–6.1%) and perforation (0.1–0.3%). The actual incidence of perforation varies depending partly on polyp location (right-sided > left-sided) and possibly size, configuration, and location. Transmural thermal injury without free perforation, sometimes referred to as a 'post-coagulation' or 'serosal burn' syndrome, is another complication that occurs less frequently than bleeding and is characterized by signs and symptoms of localized peritonitis but without evidence of free air on plain abdominal X-ray.[153] Bleeding complications can often be managed endoscopically, whereas free perforations with pneumoperitoneum generally require surgical repair. The postcoagulation syndrome often responds to conservative treatment including nothing by mouth and intravenous antibiotics for 24–72 h. Aggressive follow-up with repeat colonoscopy 3–6 months after successful excision is indicated, particularly for polyps with advanced pathology, to ensure total eradication.[129]

Malignant Polyps: Polyps containing invasive cancer, defined as the presence of malignant cells extending through the muscularis mucosae, are referred to as malignant polyps. Existing literature regarding the appropriateness of endoscopic therapy for these lesions relies mostly on considerations of risk of residual cancer and/or death versus the risk of surgery. Pathologic criteria have been identified that permit stratification into 'favorable' and 'poor' prognostic categories (see Table 63.7). The risk of residual cancer or nodal metastases for endoscopically resected polyps with favorable criteria ranges from ~0.3% for malignant pedunculated polyps to 1.5% for malignant sessile polyps, versus 8.5% and 14.4% for malignant pedunculated and sessile polyps, respectively, with poor prognostic factors.[154,155] When compared to the overall 2% risk of death from elective colonic resection,[129] these data suggest that endoscopic therapy alone is sufficient for both pedunculated and sessile malignant polyps with favorable histology. Nevertheless, a follow-up colonoscopy should be performed in 3 months to check for residual disease at the site of polypectomy, particularly if sessile. Subsequent surveillance examinations can generally be deferred for 3 years as recommended for those with benign adenomas. Because the incidence of recurrent cancer is small, no other follow-up laboratory (e.g., serum carcinoembryonic antigen [CEA] determinations) or imaging studies are indicated. Recommendations for those with malignant polyps with poor prognostic features need to be individualized on the basis of age, comorbidity, and polyp site.

Surgical Management: Surgical resection is indicated for patients with benign or malignant polyps that are not amenable to complete endoscopic resection. Endoscopic injection of 0.5–1.0 ml of a 1:10 or 1:100 dilution of sterile India ink:saline proximal and distal to the lesion or in all four quadrants of the surrounding lumen facilitates intraoperative localization.[156] In general, formal segmental colectomy including lymph node resection should be performed for all lesions arising above the peritoneal reflection. A less aggressive approach may be appropriate for high-risk patients due to advanced age or comorbidity, or for benign lesions arising below the peritoneal reflection that would otherwise require an abdominoperineal resection.

Surgical treatment of localized colorectal cancer

Surgical resection is the only potentially curative treatment for colorectal cancer. Although colon and rectal tumors are histologically indistinguishable, differences in regional anatomy, venous and lymphatic drainage, accessibility, and response to treatment provide a rationale for discussing surgical management of each separately.

Preoperative Evaluation and Staging: Once the diagnosis is established, all patients should undergo an assessment of surgical risk and extent of disease work-up in order to optimize treatment planning and determine prognosis. Visualization of the entire colon, preferably with colonoscopy, should be performed in all patients because of the 2–7% risk of a second primary cancer and 30–50% risk of synchronous adenomas.[99] A careful physical examination should be performed looking for evidence of locally advanced (i.e., palpable abdominal mass) or metastatic (e.g., Virchow's node, nodular hepatomegaly, or ascites) disease. The digital rectal examination is particularly important for patients with rectal cancers to confirm location, assess configuration (exophytic versus primary ulcerated) and mobility, and detect palpable perirectal nodes if present. A routine chest radiograph should be obtained since colorectal cancers often metastasize to the lungs. Preoperative laboratory tests should include a complete blood count, serum liver function tests, and serum CEA measurement. CEA has no value as a screening or diagnostic test but serves as a useful marker of residual or recurrent disease postoperatively if elevated preoperatively.

The utility of preoperative computed tomography (CT) of the abdomen for staging cancers arising proximal to the peritoneal reflection is controversial. Conceptually, more precise preoperative staging could facilitate surgical planning with respect to the need for simultaneous hepatic resection and/or placement of a hepatic artery chemotherapy infusion catheter in patients presenting with liver metastases at the time of initial diagnosis. In practice, however, CT findings rarely influence surgical decision-making.[157] Regardless, contrast-enhanced dynamic CT offers a reasonably accurate method for detecting liver metastases, with a sensitivity of ~75% and specificity of ~90%.[157–159] Intraoperative ultrasonography offers a reliable alternative to CT for detecting liver metastases, but requires dedicated equipment and operator expertise.[160] Lastly, magnetic resonance imaging (MRI) may be as accurate as CT for detecting liver metastases but is less accurate for detecting extrahepatic disease and therefore is not recommended routinely.[161]

Preoperative imaging studies are essential in the evaluation of patients with rectal cancers, since stage of disease strongly influences the choice of surgical procedure and the role of adjuvant radiation and/or chemotherapy. Depth of invasion, lymph node status, and presence of metastatic disease are important factors in this decision-making process. With respect to staging using the TMN classification system (Table 63.8), endoscopic ultrasound (EUS) is superior to other imaging modalities for assessing depth of invasion (T stage) and lymph node status (N stage). EUS has an overall accuracy in the range of 80–95% for T-staging and 70–80% for N-staging, using surgical pathology as the gold standard.[162,163] MRI is comparable to CT for assessing T or N stage.[163] Abdominal CT is still the modality of choice for assessing extent of disease outside the pelvis (M stage).

Surgical Treatment of Colon Cancer: Curative resection of colon cancers requires wide excision of the primary tumor and en bloc removal of draining lymph nodes, lymphatics, and contiguous structures (Fig. 63.4).[164] The actual extent of resection varies according to anatomic location and vascular supply (Fig. 63.5). Adequate resections should include a tumor-free margin of at least 5 cm from both the proximal and distal edges of the tumor. More extensive resections may be warranted in patients with

---

Table 63.8 Favorable criteria for colonoscopic polypectomy alone in the treatment of malignant colorectal polyps[129]

Complete excision and submitted in toto for pathologic review
'Clean' (≥1 mm) margin of excision
Well or moderately differentiated
No lymphatic involvement
No vascular involvement
Negative follow-up colonoscopy 3 months postpolypectomy

(Adapted from Bond JH, for the Practice Parameters Committee of the American College of Gastroenterology: Polyp guideline: diagnosis, treatment, and surveillance for patients with nonfamilial colorectal polyps. Am J Gastroenterol 2000; 95:3053–3063.)

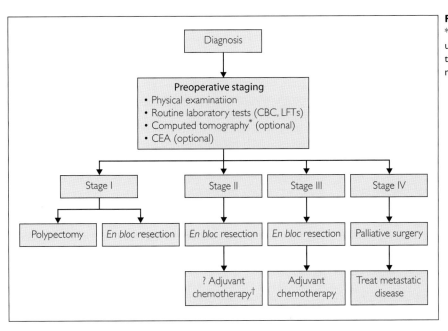

Fig. 63.4 ● Management of colon cancer. *Magnetic resonance imaging and intraoperative ultrasound are alternatives to computed tomography. †Efficacy of adjuvant chemotherapy not established for stage II disease.

synchronous cancers or adenomas not amenable to endoscopic removal, patients with obstructing cancers of the sigmoid and rectosigmoid, and selected patients with a significant cumulative risk of metachronous cancers such as those with FAP, HNPCC, or ulcerative colitis. At least 12 nodes should be examined histologically to accurately determine nodal status.[165] Patients

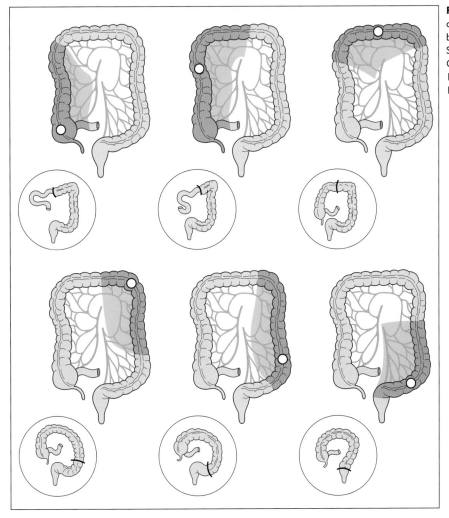

Fig. 63.5 ● Surgical resection of colorectal cancer based on location of the primary tumor, blood supply, and lymphatic drainage. (From Schrock T. Large intestine. In: Way LW, ed. Current surgical diagnosis and treatment. 10th edn. New York: Lange Medical Publishers; 1994.)

presenting with complete obstruction may require a temporary diverting loop colostomy prior to resection, whereas those with partial obstruction can often be managed with standard elective resection and primary anastomosis. The surgical management of patients presenting with perforation varies depending on whether they present with acute peritonitis, which constitutes a surgical emergency requiring prompt resuscitation and resection, or fixation to adjacent structures, in which case elective en bloc resection is preferred. Prophylactic oophorectomy is no longer recommended.[135] Laparoscopic resection in experienced hands affords comparable disease-free and overall survival to open colectomy at the cost of longer operative time but decreased hospital stay and direct costs.[166–168]

Surgical Treatment of Rectal Cancer: Multiple approaches to the surgical management of rectal cancers have been advocated depending on tumor type, stage of disease, and patient comorbidity (Fig. 63.6). Most rectal adenomas and as many as 5% of distal cancers may be treated by local excision alone.[169] A transanal approach is preferred for small (<4 cm), mobile tumors confined to the mucosa (T1) or submucosa (T2) located within 6–8 cm of the anal verge and limited to one quadrant of the rectal circumference. More proximal lesions in the rectum may require transsphincteric,[170] transsacral, or parasacral[171] approaches. EUS is particularly valuable in identifying lesions amenable to local excision. Ideally, the excision should extend to the level of the perirectal fat and provide a >5 mm margin of grossly normal tissue to facilitate pathologic assessment of depth of invasion, margin status, and possible nodal involvement. T1 and T2 cancers with 'favorable' histology, i.e., well or moderately differentiated without venous or lymphatic invasion, have 5-year actuarial recurrence-free survival rates in the range of 90% after local excision, which is comparable to that achieved with abdomino-perineal resection.[172] Conversely, T1 or T2 lesions with adverse pathologic features (positive margins, poorly differentiated or signet-cell histology, lymphatic or vascular invasion, or perineural invasion) and all T3 lesions are associated with a high incidence of local failure and should be treated aggressively with total

mesorectal excision and low anterior resection or abdomino-perineal resection. Alternatively, high-risk lesions in patients for whom radical surgery is not indicated because of unacceptable comorbidity should be treated with local excision followed by adjuvant chemoradiation. Endoscopic approaches including laser therapy,[173] electrocautery fulguration,[174] or, most recently, endoscopic photodynamic therapy,[175] as well as endocavitary irradiation (brachytherapy)[176] have been advocated as options to surgical excision in such patients, but at the cost of higher recurrence rates and, in some cases, higher complication rates. Another disadvantage of ablative therapy is that there is no tissue specimen for pathologic review.

Unfortunately, most rectal cancers are not amenable to local excision or ablation due to adverse pathology or advanced disease and must be treated with radical resection (see Fig. 63.6). Recent advances in surgical technique have resulted in both improved local control, thus reducing the severe morbidity associated with recurrent pelvic disease, and improved survival. 'Total mesorectal excision,' a technique that involves meticulous, sharp dissection of the rectal mesocolon to provide adequate radial margins of the perirectal soft tissues, combined with low anterior resection or abdominoperineal resection has been shown to markedly reduce local recurrence rates to less than 10%.[177] The introduction of circular stapling devices, along with the understanding that distal spread along the bowel wall is rare, has facilitated the implementation of rectal-sparing procedures that obviate the need for permanent colostomy without compromising outcome in patients with low-lying lesions. Low anterior resection with primary colorectal anastomosis can generally be performed successfully for tumors located 5 cm or more from the anal verge. Abdominoperineal resection with a permanent colostomy remains the surgical treatment of choice for distal lesions that cannot be treated by low anterior resection. Coloanal anastomosis is an attractive alternative for sphincter preservation but should be reserved for patients with early-stage lesions with good sphincter tone as assessed by preoperative manometric testing. Increased stool frequency, nocturnal movements, urgency, and episodic

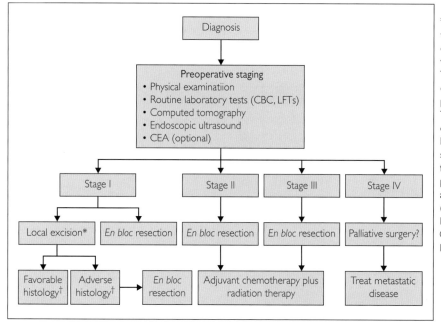

Fig. 63.6 • Management of rectal cancer. *Cancers suitable for local excision include those that are less than 3–4 cm in size, occupy less than one quadrant, located within 6–8 cm of the anal verge, and mobile.† 'Favorable histology' refers to T1 or T2 cancers that are well or moderately differentiated without vascular, lymphatic, or perineural invasion; 'adverse histology' refers to T1 or T2 lesions that are poorly differentiated or signet-cell type and/or exhibit vascular or lymphatic invasion, perineural invasion, or positive surgical margins. Laser ablation, electrocautery fulguration, endocavitary irradiation, or photodynamic therapy are options to abdominoperineal resection for palliation. (Reprinted from Umar et al, Journal of the National Cancer Institute, 2004; 96: 261–268. © 2004, with permission from Oxford University Press.)

'clustering' are common after low anterior resection with colorectal or coloanal anastomosis, but generally improve over time. Dietary manipulations, bulking agents, antidiarrheal medications, and/or the creation of a colonic pouch reservoir at the time of restorative reconstruction may reduce the problems.

Outcomes: Prognosis is closely dependent upon pathologic stage of disease at the time of initial laparotomy, as defined by depth of invasion, lymph node status, and presence or absence of metastatic disease (see Table 63.8).[178–180] Following a potentially curative resection, 5-year survival rates range from 80% for stage I disease, to 60% for stage II, to 40% for stage III disease.[181–184] Other potentially useful prognostic factors include presence of blood or lymphatic vessel invasion; residual tumor following surgery with curative intent (especially if related to positive surgical margins), preoperative CEA, histologic grade, and radial margin status (for resection specimens with nonperitonealized surfaces).[165]

Postoperative Surveillance: Patients undergoing curative surgical resection are at risk of both recurrent and metachronous disease and therefore require close postoperative follow-up. As previously discussed, colonoscopy should be performed within 1 year (preferably 3–6 months) of resection if not completed prior to surgery because of technical difficulties or obstruction. For patients in whom preoperative colonoscopy was successful, surveillance at 1 year is optional, but should be considered for those with suboptimal (<5 cm) surgical margins because of the increased risk of anastomotic recurrence.[34,36]

The utility of other surveillance strategies remains controversial. Serial measurements of CEA every 3–6 months for up to 5 years may be useful in monitoring patients with elevated values preoperatively, but only if the patient and surgeon are willing to proceed with 'second-look' surgery if a greater than twofold elevation is detected postoperatively. CEA-directed 'second-look' surgery is of questionable survival benefit for most eligible patients, but may be of value in patients with resectable liver metastases.[185] Periodic physician visits every 3–6 months for the first 3 years and annually thereafter is warranted to identify suspicious signs and symptoms but has no significant impact on outcome. Serial imaging with chest radiography, CT, or MRI is also of unproven benefit as a routine surveillance strategy, but is clearly indicated in the evaluation of symptomatic patients or patients with abnormal physical findings or laboratory tests (e.g., abnormal liver functions test or elevated CEA).[186,187] Serial imaging, however, may be of value for patients at high risk of local or systemic relapse, since early detection prior to the onset of symptoms portends a favorable prognosis for patients with recurrent disease potentially amenable to surgical intervention.[188]

Adjuvant therapy

Rationale: Nearly 40% of patients undergoing curative surgery will relapse and ultimately die of their disease if treated with surgery alone.[189] Consequently, additional therapeutic modalities delivered soon after curative resection has been advocated as a rational means of improving patient outcome. Clinical data suggesting that adjuvant therapy is effective in delaying tumor recurrence and improving overall survival in certain high-risk patients supports this rationale.

Colon Cancer: Combination chemotherapy with 5-fluorouracil (5-FU), a fluoropyrimidine that binds to thymidylate synthetase and inhibits DNA synthesis, and levamisole, an antihelminthic with putative immunostimulatory activity, was the first regimen to demonstrate a significant survival benefit for stage III (Dukes' C) patients in the adjuvant setting.[190] A 1990 National Cancer Institute (NCI)-sponsored consensus conference felt that the evidence was sufficiently compelling to recommend 5-FU plus levamisole as the standard of care for patients with resected stage III colon cancer.[191] Subsequent data from other cooperative trials have demonstrated that combination therapy with 5-FU plus leucovorin (folinic acid), the regimen of choice for patients with advanced colorectal cancer, was also effective in prolonging disease-free and overall survival in stage III patients.[192–195] Leucovorin has no intrinsic antitumor activity but enhances 5-FU activity by potentiating binding to thymidylate synthetase. Despite a lack of compelling evidence of superior efficacy, 5-FU/LV has emerged as the most widely used regimen. Pooled data suggest that 5-FU/LV increases 5-year disease-free survival from 42% to 58% and overall 5-year survival from 51% to 64%.[196] Response rates appear to be higher among tumors lacking microsatellite instability (MSI), i.e., 'microsatellite stable tumors' and MSI-low tumors than MSI-high tumors, thus suggesting that MSI status may be an important predictor of response.[197] Major toxicities include leukopenia, neutropenia, stomatitis, and diarrhea. The addition of oxaliplatin, a third-generation platinum derivation, to 5-FU/LV may be more effective than 5-FU/LV alone but its impact on overall survival remains undefined;[198] even if validated, concerns about potential neurotoxicity may limit its use among most stage III patients. Adjuvant therapy is not routinely recommended for stage II (Dukes' B2) disease but should be considered in patients with inadequately sampled nodes, T4 lesions, perforation, or poorly differentiated histology.[199]

Rectal Cancer: Unlike colon cancers arising proximal to the peritoneal reflection, effective adjuvant therapy for rectal cancers must take into account both the high risk of local recurrence as well as systemic relapse. The actual incidence of local recurrence is dependent on pathologic stage, ranging from ~8% for stage I (Dukes' A, B1) cancers to ~25% for stage II (Dukes' B2) cancers to over 50% for stage III (Dukes' C) cancers.[181] Total mesorectum excision has reduced the rate of local recurrence to <10% for both stage II and III disease in experienced hands,[177] but has yet to gain full acceptance by the surgical community at-large. Because of the high local recurrence rate in stage II and III disease, a number of studies, many of which predate the introduction of TME, were undertaken to explore the role of adjuvant radiation therapy delivered either preoperatively or postoperatively. These studies demonstrated that adjuvant radiation therapy as a single modality was effective in reducing local recurrence rates but had little impact on systemic recurrence or survival. Subsequent studies were therefore undertaken to assess the efficacy of combined modality treatment with combination chemotherapy and radiation therapy. Besides addressing the issue of systemic relapse, this approach had the potential of further improving local control through the use of chemotherapeutic agents with radiosensitizing properties (e.g., 5-FU). Data from two such trials demonstrated that combined modality therapy with postoperative 5-FU/semustine chemotherapy and pelvic irradiation was in fact effective in improving both local control and overall survival compared to surgery alone.[200,201] These data prompted the previously noted 1990 NCI-sponsored consensus conference to recommend that standard postoperative care for patients with stage II (Dukes' B2) and stage III (Dukes' C) rectal cancers should include six cycles of fluorouracil-based combination chemotherapy plus concurrent conventional (1.8–2.0 Gy per fraction up to a total dose of 45–50.4 Gy) radiation therapy (see Fig. 63.6).[195] Because of the potential leukemogenicity of semustine, 5-FU by prolonged infusion alone or the 5-FU/LV combination rather than 5-FU plus semustine has become the chemotherapeutic regimen of choice in this setting. Improvements in technique, such as delivery to multiple fields, computerized treatment planning, and customized blocking have lessened the risk of radiation-induced small bowel and bladder toxicity.

When administered in the preoperative (neoadjuvant) setting, chemoradiation increases the potential for sphincter-sparing surgery and is frequently recommended for patients with distal mobile rectal tumors not amenable to local excision.[184,202] Preoperative radiation therapy has also been shown to reduce local recurrence rate to less that 5% when combined with total mesocolon excision.[203]

Treatment of advanced colorectal cancer

Surgery: Up to 25% of patients with colorectal cancer have metastatic disease at initial presentation and an additional 40–50% of patients treated with potentially curative resections relapse locally or at distant sites.[2,189] Although most patients with metastatic disease have multifocal involvement, ~10% of patients with isolated metastatic disease or local relapse may be candidates for salvage surgery (Fig. 63.7). Hepatic resection of liver metastases is associated with a median survival of 20–40 months and a 5-year survival rate of 24–38%.[204–208] Operative mortality is low (<5%) in experienced hands. Optimal candidates have a prolonged disease-free interval after resection of their primary cancer, fewer than four metastases, limited liver involvement, no symptoms, and good hepatic function. The presence of extrahepatic disease, whether resected or not, is a poor prognostic factor and serves as a relative contraindication to hepatic resection. Preoperative diagnostic laparoscopy[209] or positron emission tomography (PET scanning)[210] can aid in patient selection. Repeat hepatic resection for isolated liver recurrences may be of

benefit in selected cases.[211,212] Cryosurgery[213] and radiofrequency ablation[214] have also been used to treat both resectable and unresectable liver metastases. Unlike hepatic resection, these approaches preserve normal hepatic parenchyma and therefore may have a role in the treatment of patients with underlying cirrhosis, multifocal metastases, or isolated liver recurrence after hepatic resection.

Surgery may also have a role in the management of selected patients with isolated lung metastases and recurrent pelvic disease. Wedge resection or segmentectomy of lung metastases in patients with no other identifiable sites of relapse reportedly yield 5-year survival rates of 14–45%.[215–217] Surgery has also been shown to achieve both local control and improve survival of patients with pelvic recurrences. Successful outcome often requires en bloc resection of surrounding tissues, including bladder, uterus, ureter, and/or sacrum. Eligible patients most likely to benefit have no symptoms, small tumors, clear surgical margins, and low CEA levels.[218] Intraoperative radiation therapy combined with systemic chemotherapy may enhance local control and survival in patients with positive margins or small areas of gross residual disease.[219]

Lastly, surgery with a palliative intent should be performed in patients with advanced incurable disease to prevent obstruction or bleeding. Endoscopic approaches and/or radiotherapy strategies may be options in high-risk patients or those with rectal lesions who may otherwise require an abdominoperineal resection, as discussed below.

Chemotherapy: Despite its limited efficacy, chemotherapy remains the mainstay of treatment for advanced colorectal cancer (see Fig. 63.7). 5-FU is the most active single agent with response rates in the range of 20% whether administered orally, intravenous bolus, or continuous intravenous infusion. Responses tend to be of short duration, often measured in months, and long-term benefit is rare. Toxicities vary according to dose and mode of administration, but include myelosuppression, vomiting, diarrhea, and stomatitis. Irinotecan, a topoisomerase 1 inhibitor, and oxaliplatin, are also active agents, but tend to more toxic than 5-FU and hence reserved for 5-FU treatment failures.[220,221]

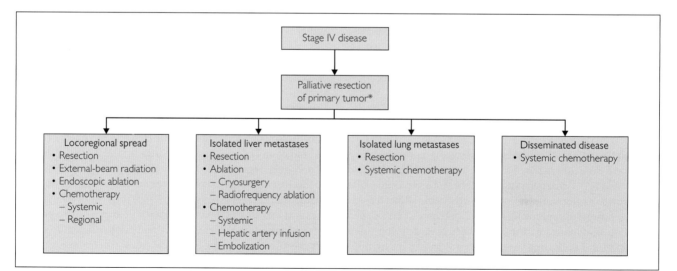

Fig. 63.7 • Treatment options for advanced colorectal cancer. *Laser ablation, electrocautery fulguration, endocavitary irradiation, or photodynamic therapy are options to abdominoperineal resection for palliation.

Combination chemotherapy has replaced single-agent therapy as the standard of care for patients with advanced, unresectable colorectal cancer. During the 1990s, 5-FU/LV emerged as the preferred regimen based on data from a number of randomized trials demonstrating superior response rates to 5-FU alone.[222] Addition of irinotecan to 5-FU/LV ('IFL' regimen) was later shown to be even more effective than 5-FU/LV in terms of response rates (39–49% vs. 21%), time-to-progression (6.7–7.0 v.s. <4.4 months), and overall survival (14.8–17.4 vs. < 14.4 months). Addition of oxaliplatin to 5-FU/LV ('FOLFOX' regimen) also demonstrated superior response rates and time-to-progression but comparable overall survival. Consequently, both have replaced 5-FU/LV as first-line therapy for patients with metastatic colorectal cancer. Both regimens are more toxic than 5-FU/LV. The major dose-limiting toxicities are diarrhea and neutropenia for IFL and sensory neuropathy for FOLFOX.[223] For patients who are not considered appropriate candidates for either FOLFOX or IFL, either intravenous 5-FU/LV or oral *capecitabine*, an oral fluoropyrimidine, is an acceptable alternative for first-line treatment.[224,225] Patients who fail to respond or relapse after first-line chemotherapy may be candidates for salvage therapy with cetuximab, a monoclonal antibody directed against the epidermal growth factor receptor (EGFR), alone or in combination with irinotecan for EGFR-expressing metastatic disease refractory to irinotecan, or bevacizumab, a monoclonal antibody directed against vascular endothelial growth factor, in combination with IFL.[226,227]

Selective infusion of chemotherapeutic agents directly into the hepatic artery via implantable pumps has been shown to be an effective strategy in the treatment of patients with metastatic disease confined to the liver (see Fig. 63.7). Randomized trials to date have consistently demonstrated superior objective response rates with hepatic artery infusion of floxuridine (FUDR) compared with systemic 5-FU, FUDR, or 5-FU/LV therapy (42–62% versus 9–21%), but have yet to conclusively demonstrate a survival advantage. Hepatic artery infusion with FUDR combined with systemic 5-FU/LV has also been shown to decrease local recurrence and improve 2-year survival following resection of hepatic metastases. The two major limitations of this approach are hepatobiliary toxicities, including chemical hepatitis and sclerosing cholangitis, and systemic relapse. The hepatobiliary complications are often reversible after temporary discontinuation of therapy but permanent damage to the biliary tree has been reported. Addition of dexamethasone has been shown to reduce the incidence of hepatobiliary complications without compromising efficacy. Gastroduodenal ulceration is another potential toxicity that usually results from inadvertent perfusion and drug delivery to stomach and duodenum. In an attempt to reduce systemic relapse, several studies have been initiated to examine the efficacy of combination therapy with intra-arterial FUDR plus systemic chemotherapy with irinotecan- or oxaliplatin-based regimens.[228]

Radiation Therapy: Radiation therapy has an important role in the management of patients with inoperable or recurrent rectal cancers (see Fig. 63.7). In patients with inoperable tumors, doses of 45–60 Gy delivered in 180-rad fractions combined with concomitant chemotherapy may be effective in 'down-staging' the lesion, thereby permitting resection with curative intent. Radiation therapy also affords satisfactory palliation of pain or bleeding in patients with inoperable disease.[229,230] Intracavitary radiation therapy (brachytherapy) is another option in such patients.[176]

Endoscopy: Endoscopic approaches may also have a palliative role in the management of patients with advanced colorectal cancers, particularly those with significant comorbidity and/or those with rectal lesions that may otherwise require an abdominoperineal resection (see Fig. 63.7).

Neodymum:YAG laser ablation,[173] electrocautery fulguration[174] and photodynamic therapy[175] have been used successfully to recanalize obstructing lesions and control bleeding in patients in whom surgery is not an option. Endoscopic placement of self-expandable metal stents have also been shown to be of value in the management of malignant strictures.[231]

SMALL BOWEL ADENOMAS AND ADENOCARCINOMAS

Epidemiology

Adenocarcinoma is the most common malignancy of the small bowel with an annual incidence of 3.9 cases per million persons per year.[232] Despite its rarity, incidence rates appear to be rising, especially among black males.[233] The disease is more common among blacks than whites and exhibits a slight male predominance. Peak incidence is in the sixth and seventh decades. As in the colon, small bowel adenocarcinomas are believed to arise from pre-existing adenomas, which may occur sporadically or in the setting of a genetic syndrome such as FAP/GS, HNPCC, or Peutz-Jeghers syndrome. The true prevalence of small bowel adenomas is not well defined due to the fact that most are asymptomatic and not evident clinically. Apart from small bowel adenomas, Crohn's disease and celiac sprue are two other well-recognized predisposing conditions associated with an increased risk of small bowel cancer.[234]

Treatment

Adenomas: Adenomas of the small bowel should be treated because of their premalignant status. Appropriate therapy is dependant on a number of factors, including location, size, shape (sessile or pedunculated), and histologic type (tubular or villous). Isolated duodenal adenomas, with the exception of ampullary lesions, are usually amenable to endoscopic removal or ablation.[235] The management of ampullary adenomas is more controversial. The controversy stems mostly from concerns over the risk of occult carcinoma (35–60%) and risk, albeit low, of malignant transformation. Pancreaticoduodenectomy (Whipple procedure) is the most definite therapy but at the expense of higher morbidity (25–65%) and mortality (0–10%). Local surgical excision (surgical ampullectomy) is a less risky procedure (morbidity, 0–25%; mortality, <1%) but because of higher recurrence rates (5–30%), requires postoperative endoscopic surveillance. Snare ampullectomy is a newer endoscopic technique for which fewer data are available. Endoscopic removal is safer than pancreaticoduodenectomy and less invasive than surgical excision but often requires adjunctive ablative modalities (e.g., fulguration) and multiple procedures (mean, 2.0 procedures) to ensure complete excision; moreover, recurrence rates approach 30%, thus mandating continued endoscopic surveillance. Ultimately, choice is driven by availability of local expertise, patient willingness to undergo long-term surveillance, medical comorbidities, and overall life expectancy.[236]

Adenomas arising in the setting of FAP pose a special management problem because of their multicentricity. Even though the cumulative risk of developing adenomas in the duodenum approaches 100%, the overall probability of progression is relatively low with a risk of periampullary carcinoma in the range of 4%. Consequently, endoscopic surveillance with biopsy generally every 1–5 years, depending on polyp size, number and histology, is recommended rather than excision. Polyps ≥1 cm in size with induration, ulceration, or rapid growth are likely to harbor high-grade dysplasia and should be removed either endoscopically or surgically. Prophylactic duodenal resection is recommended for patients with multiple polyps and the finding on villous change of high-grade dysplasia. The procedure of choice in such patients is a pancreas- and pylorus-sparing duodenectomy, which carries a very low mortality (2.3%) in experienced hands.[75] Chemoprevention therapy with celecoxib (800 mg daily) may also be beneficial in patients with mild or moderate polyposis.[237]

Adenocarcinomas: Surgical resection is the only potentially curative treatment for adenocarcinomas of the small bowel. Since nearly all small bowel adenocarcinomas arise in the duodenum, pancreaticoduodenectomy may be necessary, particularly for tumors involving the first or second portions.[238,239] Wide segmental resection has been shown to be equally effective if technically feasible and is the procedure of choice for adenocarcinomas involving the third or fourth portions of the duodenum, jejunum, or ileum.[240–242] Tumors arising in the terminal ileum may also require a right colectomy. Palliative resection or bypass should be considered if curative resection is not feasible. Biliary bypass and gastrojejunostomy afford reasonable long-term palliation with low operative morbidity and mortality in patients with unresectable periampullary lesions.[243]

Survival rates for small bowel adenocarcinomas are comparable to those of colorectal cancer.[240,242] Depth of mural penetration, nodal involvement, presence or absence of distant metastases, and perineural invasion are important prognostic determinants.[241] Because most small bowel tumors typically present at an advanced stage, overall-5-year survival rates are in the range of 31–54% for adenocarcinomas of the duodenum and 15–30% for adenocarcinomas of the jejunum and ileum.[240,242,244] A role for adjuvant therapy has yet to be defined, and neither chemotherapy nor radiation therapy are effective in improving survival in patient the treatment of advanced disease.

INTESTINAL LYMPHOMAS

Classification and epidemiology

The GI tract is the predominant site of extranodal non-Hodgkin's lymphomas (NHLs). *Primary* intestinal NHLs, operationally defined as lymphomas in which the main bulk of disease is confined to the small or large bowel necessitating treatment directed at that site, are relatively rare, accounting for 12% of small bowel malignancies[245] and less than 0.5% of colonic malignancies.[246] *Secondary* GI involvement, however, is relatively common and may be seen in 10% of patients with limited stage,[247] high-grade NHLs at the time of diagnosis and up to 60% of those dying from NHL.[248]

Primary GI lymphomas are a heterogeneous group of unique B- and T-cell lymphoid malignancies with distinctive epidemiologic and clinicopathologic features.[249] The majority arise from B

cells residing in the marginal zone of mucosa-associated lymphoid tissue and hence referred to as 'extranodal marginal zone B-cell lymphoma of the MALT type' in the REAL classification system, or simply '*MALT lymphomas*.' Predisposing factors include various autoimmune and immunodeficiency syndromes, inflammatory bowel disease and possibly nodular lymphoid hyperplasia.[250] *Immunoproliferative small intestinal disease* ('IPSID') is a specialized type of MALT lymphoma that occurs almost exclusively in the Middle East and is characterized by alpha heavy chain paraproteinemia, malabsorption, and an association with *Campylobacter jejuni* infection.[251,252] *Mantle cell lymphomas* are a less common but aggressive type of primary B-cell GI lymphoma that is distinguished by the presence of multiple nodules or polypoid tumors scattered throughout the colon and small intestine ('lymphomatous polyposis').[253] *Burkitt's* and *Burkitt-like lymphomas* are other rare forms of B-cell lymphoma that frequently occur in the association with chronic Epstein-Barr infection,[254] the human immunodeficiency virus (HIV)[255] syndrome, or post-transplantation immunosuppressive therapy.[256] The majority of T-cell primary GI lymphomas arise in the small bowel and occur in the setting of longstanding celiac sprue, hence the term '*enteropathy-associated T-cell lymphoma (EATL).*'[257] The remaining primary T-cell lymphomas are collectively referred to as '*T-cell lymphomas unassociated with enteropathy.*'

Treatment

Treatment strategies for intestinal lymphomas are contingent upon several factors including type, stage at diagnosis (Table 63.9), extent of intestinal involvement, and presentation. Exploratory laparotomy is often required to establish the diagnosis, particularly in the case of small bowel lymphomas, or manage acute complications such as perforation or obstruction. Once the diagnosis is confirmed, intraoperative sampling of periaortic lymph nodes and liver and splenectomy has been advocated by some for staging purposes. Intraoperative enteroscopy may also be of value in assessing extent of involvement. As a general rule, most patients have advanced disease at diagnosis and thus require multimodality therapy including some combination of surgery, radiation therapy, and/or chemotherapy. Unfortunately, because of their rarity, treatment recommendations are defined largely by case series rather than clinical trials.

B-cell Western-Type- MALT Lymphomas: Western-type intestinal MALT lymphomas are unique in that they behave as focal tumors

Table 63.9 Staging of primary intestinal non-Hodgkin's lymphomas

Stage IE	Involvement of a localized segment of bowel without nodal involvement
Stage IIE	Involvement of a localized segment of bowel with involvement of regional nodes
Stage IIIE	Involvement of bowel and lymph nodes on both sides of the diaphragm; spleen may be involved (stage IIIES)
Stage IV	Diffuse involvement of more than one extralymphatic organs or tissues, with or without nodal involvement

amenable to radical resection when detected early. Consequently, en bloc resection of involved bowel and contiguous nodes with curative intent is treatment of choice for patients with stage IE or IIE disease. Even after curative resection, however, 5-year survival rates are only in the range of 45% for stage IE disease and 17% for stage IIE disease.[258] Moreover, relapses occurring 5–10 years after resection are not uncommon. Patients most likely to relapse include those with nodal involvement, extension beyond the bowel wall, and high-grade histology. In an effort to improve survival rates, both radiation therapy and chemotherapy are often used postoperatively despite limited efficacy data. Radiation therapy appears to reduce local recurrence rates when used in the adjuvant setting, but has little impact on survival because of high recurrence rates outside the radiation portals.[259] Radiation therapy also carries a significant risk of acute and chronic morbidity resulting from radiation enteritis and vasculitis. Alternatively, combination chemotherapy has been shown to improve both disease-free and overall survival compared with surgery alone.[260,261] Since dose-intensive seven-drug regimens appear to be only marginally more effective but far more toxic than 'first-generation' therapy with cyclophosphamide-hydroxy-daunorubicin-vincristine-prednisone (CHOP), adjuvant chemotherapy with CHOP should be considered as standard treatment for patients with stage IE or IIE disease following curative resection outside the realm of a clinical trial.

Combination chemotherapy is the treatment of choice for patients with advanced (stage IIIE and IV) disease. As in the adjuvant setting, CHOP is the preferred regimen outside the realm of a clinical trial. Response rates are comparable to those observed for extraintestinal NHLs, but overall prognosis is poor, with 5-year and 10-year survival rates of approximately 50% and 20%, respectively.[262] Radiation therapy provides effective palliation for extensive, unresectable disease, but is unlikely to impact on overall survival. The role of palliative surgical resection in patients with extensive or advanced disease prior to chemotherapy to prevent subsequent bleeding or perforation remains controversial.[260,263,264]

B-cell IPSID-type MALT Lymphomas: Unfortunately, few data are available concerning the optimal treatment of IPSID-type MALT lymphomas. Surgery is rarely indicated due to the diffuse extent of intestinal involvement. If diagnosed early at a pre-lymphomatous stage, regression has been observed in a 33–71% of patients following a 6-month course of antibiotic therapy with tetracycline alone or the combination of metronidazole plus ampicillin.[251] Most patients, however, ultimately relapse and present with an aggressive high-grade histology. Radiation therapy and/or chemotherapy combined with nutritional support are the mainstays of treatment for patients with established disease. Although early reports suggested that overall prognosis for such patients was poor, more recent studies suggest that 5-year survival rates as high as 70% may be achieved with combination chemotherapy (cyclophosphamide, vincristine, procarbazine, and prednisolone [COPP] regimen) plus tetracycline to control diarrhea and malabsorption.[265]

Mantle Cell Lymphomas: Systemic chemotherapy is the treatment of choice for mantle cell lymphomas because of their propensity to present with stage IV disease involving multiple sites throughout the GI tract, peripheral lymph nodes, spleen, liver, and bone marrow. Anthracycline-based multidrug regimens, such as doxorubicin-teniposide-cyclophosphamide-prednisolone

(AVmCP), have yielded the best results with response rates of 80% and predicted 5-year survival rates of 59%. Intensification with total body irradiation and autologous stem cell transplantation has been advocated for younger patients responding to first-line chemotherapy, but again the experience to date has been limited.[266] Surgery has a relatively limited role in the management of this disease, but may be of value in patients presenting with bowel-obstructing lesions. Anecdotal success, however, has been reported in rare patients with localized disease treated with surgery and abdominal irradiation.[253]

Burkitt's and Burkitt-like Lymphomas: These tumors present typically as bulky mass lesions with or without ulceration. In children, the disease has a predilection for the ileocecal region. The prognosis has improved considerably in recent years and may approach 80% with the use of aggressive, multidrug chemotherapy regimens and CNS prophylaxis.[267] Resection is often required to alleviate symptoms or avoid perforation during chemotherapy. Selected patients with poor-risk disease may benefit from autologous bone marrow transplantation.[268]

In adults, Burkitt-like lymphomas can arise at any site in the GI system, but are most common in the ileocecal region and rectum in adults. Treatment options and outcomes are comparable to those for children.[269,270] Although the prognosis for HIV-associated Burkitt-like lymphomas was historically poor and related more to the underlying HIV syndrome than the lymphoma itself, improved outcomes have been observed with intensive chemotherapy since the introduction of highly active retroviral therapy.[271]

Enteropathy-associated T-cell Intestinal Lymphoma (EATL): Compared to B-cell lymphomas, particularly of the MALT type, EATL is almost always of high-grade histology. Surgery and chemotherapy are the mainstays of treatment but 5-year survival rates are only in the range of 10–20%.[272,273] Because poor nutritional and performance status adversely affect outcome, appropriate therapy should include aggressive management of the malabsorptive state and maintenance on a gluten-free diet.

INTESTINAL CARCINOIDS

Epidemiology

Carcinoid tumors of the small and large intestine are rare. The most common sites of involvement include the appendix, rectum, and small intestine. Carcinoids of both the appendix and rectum are often incidental findings at the time of appendectomy or endoscopy, respectively, and hence their epidemiology is poorly defined; conversely, small bowel carcinoids have a more aggressive natural history and a better-defined epidemiology. The annual incidence of small bowel carcinoids is approximately 2.8 cases per million persons per year.[234] Like small bowel adenocarcinoma, incidence rates appear to be rising, especially among black males.[233] Median age at diagnosis is around 60 years and there is a slight male predominance. Small bowel carcinoids are often multicentric, but show a predilection for the distal ileum. Most patients have regional nodal metastases at the time of diagnosis.

Treatment

Table 63.10 provides a summary of treatment of intestinal carcinoid tumors.

Table 63.10 Treatment of intestinal carcinoid tumors

Localized disease
Surgery

Symptomatic metastatic disease
Hepatic resection
Hepatic artery occlusion
Ligation
Embolization
Liver transplantation
Chemotherapy ± hepatic artery occlusion
Single-agent (5-FU, doxorubicin, dacarbizine, cisplatin)
Combination (e.g., 5-FU plus streptozotocin)

Palliation of carcinoid syndrome
Octreotide (150–500 μg t.i.d.)
Cyproheptadine (4–8 mg t.i.d.)

Local Disease: Surgery is the treatment of choice for localized intestinal carcinoids, regardless of site of origin. Local excision is adequate for tumors <2 cm arising in the appendix or rectum provided that there is no evidence of muscular invasion or metastatic disease; more radical resection is indicated for larger (≥2 cm) for invasive tumors. Curative radical resection is also indicated for any small bowel carcinoid, regardless of size, and most colonic carcinoids, because of the increased risk of metastatic disease.[274]

Advanced and Metastatic Disease: Approximately 70% of patients with carcinoid tumors of the small bowel or colon present with advanced-stage disease.[275] Surgical palliation is often effective in relieving symptoms, such as intermittent abdominal pain, diarrhea, and/or weight loss, related to partial small bowel obstruction or mesenteric ischemia. Resection of hepatic metastases may also provide symptomatic relief in selected patients with the malignant carcinoid syndrome and may prolong survival.[276] Liver transplantation is also an option, with reported 5-year survival rates as high as 69% in highly selected patients.[277]

Hepatic artery occlusion by surgical ligation or percutaneous embolization is alternative treatment strategy for symptomatic patients with carcinoid tumors metastatic to the liver who are not candidates for hepatic resection. Objective regression with partial to complete relief of symptoms has been observed in 60% of patients treated with hepatic occlusion alone and 80% if combined with systemic chemotherapy.[278] Duration of response, however, is relatively short (range, 4–18 months). The major risks, apart from transient abdominal pain, nausea, vomiting, and fever, include hepatorenal syndrome, carcinoid syndrome, and death (0–2%).[274,279]

Chemotherapy is rarely of benefit in the treatment of advanced or metastatic carcinoid tumors. Most studies find that fewer than 25% of patients treated with single agents (5-FU, doxorubicin, dacarbizine, and cisplatin) or combined regimens (e.g., 5-FU/streptozotocin), will achieve an objective response; moreover, response rates tend to be of short duration (4–7 months) and toxicity is high.[280] Consequently, chemotherapy should be reserved for patients with significant symptoms or disability from their disease or who exhibit poor prognostic signs, such as impaired liver function or clinically evident carcinoid heart disease. Sequential hepatic artery occlusion and chemotherapy has been advocated as a more effective therapy than either modality alone.[278]

Carcinoid Syndrome: The malignant carcinoid syndrome is characterized by clinical manifestations of flushing, diarrhea, asthma, and right heart failure in the setting of bulky metastatic liver disease and an elevated urinary 5-HIAA level. Octreotide (Sandostatin) at doses of 150–500 μg administered subcutaneously three times a day has emerged as the treatment of choice for this syndrome. In one series, octreotide caused a significant reduction of flushing and diarrhea in 87% of treated patients.[281] Tumor regression has also been observed in a small percentage of patients. Unfortunately, however, the median duration of response was just over 1 year. The major side effects of treatment include steatorrhea, especially at high doses, and cholelithiasis in up to 50% of patients after long-term treatment. The ^{111}In-DPTA octreotide scan (Octreoscan) is useful not only in staging disease but can also identify those patients most likely to respond to treatment with octreotide.[282] Indications for treatment include disability or severe impairment of life directly attributable to a hormonal syndrome. Cyproheptadine (Periactin), an agent with both antihistamine and antiserotonergic activity, may provide symptomatic relief of diarrhea in patients with mild disease at doses of 4–12 mg three times daily but rarely improves flushing.[283] Tricuspid valve replacement is associated with high perioperative morbidity and mortality but may be of value in patients with refractory right heart failure.[284]

Prognosis: Tumor site, size, stage, and histology are important prognostic determinants. Overall 5-year survival rates are highest for tumors arising in the appendix (86%) and rectum (72%) and poorest for those in the colon (42%) and small intestine (55%). The poorer survival rates for colonic and small bowel tumors is largely due to the fact that most present with advanced-stage disease.[275]

INTESTINAL STROMAL TUMORS

Historically, most mesenchymal tumors of the GI tract were classified as leiomyomas or leiomyosarcomas because they arose from the muscular layer and exhibited a spindle-shaped morphology. In recent years, up to 94% of these tumors have been reclassified as 'gastrointestinal stromal tumors (GISTs).' GISTs are characterized by the presence of spindle-shaped or round, epithelioid cells expressing CD117 (KIT), a cell membrane receptor with tyrosine kinase activity encoded for by the c-kit protooncogene. GISTs are believed to arise from interstitial cells of Cabral. The terms leiomyoma or leiomyosarcoma are reserved for tumors comprised of spindle-shaped cells lacking KIT expression. GISTs account for <1% of GI malignancies. Approximately 25% arise in the small bowel and 11% in the colon. Histology alone is unreliable for classifying tumors as benign or malignant. A high mitotic index (>5 mitosis per 50 high-power fields (HPF)) and tumor size (>5 cm) are reliable determinants of malignant potential. The presence of necrosis and detectable c-kit mutations are other important predictors of malignant potential.[285,286]

The management of intestinal stromal tumors depends upon the confidence in the diagnosis, tumor location, tumor size, and clinical presentation. Surgical resection without lymphadenectomy is the mainstay of therapy for localized disease. Patients with advanced unresectable, metastatic, or recurrent KIT-positive tumors should be treated with imatinib mesylate (400 mg daily), a selective inhibitor of receptor tyrosine kinase. Response rates, as defined by tumor regression or stable disease, are in the range of 80%.[287,288] PET scanning is the preferred imaging modality for staging and assessing response to therapy. Surgery should be considered for responders with recurrent or previously unresectable disease to delay or minimize the chance of developing imatinib resistance; dose escalation is indicated for nonresponders. Since imatinib has no antitumor activity against KIT-negative tumors,[289] combination chemotherapy with doxorubicin-based regimens[290] or *gemcitabine* plus *docetaxel*[291] should be considered in patients with advanced unresectable or metastatic leiomyosarcomas. Resection of isolated liver or pulmonary metastases may have a role in the treatment of selected patients, but long-term survival is uncommon. Overall 5-year survival rates for GISTs range from 20% to 70% following curative surgical resection, depending on tumor size and completeness of resection. The prognosis for patients with metastatic disease remains poor pending data on the effectiveness of imatinib and newer chemotherapeutic regimens.[285,286]

Kaposi's sarcoma (KS) is a unique mesenchymal malignancy of the GI tract that occurs almost exclusively in HIV-infected homosexual males. Intestinal involvement is often indolent, but may, on rare occasion, cause symptoms such as pain or hemorrhage, or life-threatening complications such as intestinal obstruction, intussusception, or perforation. Systemic therapy with liposomal doxorubicin, liposomal daunorubicin, paclitaxel, and interferon-alpha are currently approved for the treatment for patients with visceral disease, but have yet to demonstrate a survival benefit.[292] Survival rates are higher among patients receiving both highly active retroviral therapy and chemotherapy than chemotherapy alone.[293] Surgery and radiation therapy have had anecdotal success in the treatment of selected patients with localized, symptomatic disease, and/or life-threatening complications. Endoscopic sclerotherapy has also demonstrated anecdotal success in patients with severe GI hemorrhage.[294] Although prognosis for HIV-related KS was historically poor, overall 3-year survival rates have improved to >80% since the introduction of highly active retroviral therapy.[295]

SUMMARY

The appropriate management of neoplastic diseases of the small and large bowel is contingent on a number of factors, including tumor type, site of origin, extent of disease, and natural history. Screening and surveillance have been shown to be effective strategies for reducing both colorectal cancer incidence and mortality but are of unproven benefit for other intestinal neoplasms. Consequently, early detection prior to the development of advanced life-threatening disease is the key to a favorable outcome for patients with small neoplasms of all types and colorectal carcinoid tumors, lymphomas, and stromal tumors. Benign lesions not amenable to endoscopic removal or ablation should be treated surgically. Regardless of type or location, surgical resection is also the treatment of choice for virtually all localized malignant tumors. Chemotherapy is the mainstay of treatment for more advanced disease, but long-term survival is rare. Radiation therapy may be of value in selected patients with rectal cancers, especially in the adjuvant setting, and localized intestinal lymphomas. Palliative measures to control pain, bleeding, obstruction, and malnutrition should be considered in patients presenting with advanced, incurable disease to maximize quality of life and reduce hospital stay.

REFERENCES

1. Schottenfeld D, Winawer SJ. Cancers of the large intestine. In: Schottenfeld D, Fraumeni JF, eds. Cancer epidemiology and prevention. 2nd edn. New York: Oxford University Press; 1996:813–840.

2. Jemal A, Tiwari RC, Murray T, et al. Cancer statistics, 2004. CA Cancer J Clin 2004; 54(1):8–29.

3. Ries LA, Wingo PA, Miller DS, et al. The annual report to the nation on the status of cancer, 1973–1997, with a special section on colorectal cancer. Cancer 2000; 88(10):2398–2424.

4. Bach PB, Schrag D, Brawley OW, et al. Survival of blacks and whites after a cancer diagnosis. JAMA 2002; 287:2106–2113.

5. Eide TJ. Risk of colorectal cancer in adenoma-bearing individuals within a defined population. Int J Cancer 1986; 38:173–176.

6. O'Brien MJ, Winawer SJ, Zauber AG, et al. The National Polyp Study. Patient and polyp characteristics associated with high-grade dysplasia in colorectal adenomas. Gastroenterology 1990; 98:371–379.

7. Williams GT, Arthur JF, Bussey HJ, et al. Metaplastic polyps and polyposis of the colorectum. Histopathology 1980; 4:155–170.

8. Vogelstein B, Fearon ER, Hamilton SR, et al. Genetic alterations during colorectal-tumor development. N Engl J Med 1988; 319:525–532.

9. Fearon ER, Vogelstein B. A genetic model for colorectal tumorigenesis. Cell 1990; 61:759–767.

10. Ilyas M, Straub J, Tomlinson IP, et al. Genetic pathways in colorectal and other cancers. Eur J Cancer 1999; 35:335–351.

11. Jass JR, Whitehall VL, Young J, et al. Emerging concepts in colorectal neoplasia. Gastroenterology 2002; 123:862–876.

    An excellent review of emerging data supporting the existence of a 'serrated' pathway for the evolution of colorectal neoplasia that is driven by inhibition of apoptosis and the subsequent inactivation of DNA repair genes by methylation of the MLH1 DNA repair gene.

12. Winawer SJ, Zauber AG, Ho MN, et al. Prevention of colorectal cancer by colonoscopic polypectomy. The National Polyp Study Workgroup. N Engl J Med 1993; 329:1977–1981.

    A landmark study demonstrating that colonoscopic removal of adenomatous polyps was an effective strategy for reducing the incidence of colorectal cancer, thereby providing indirect evidence for the use of colonoscopy as a screening test.

13. Hofstad B, Vatn M. Growth rate of colon polyps and cancer. Gastrointest Endosc Clin N Am 1997; 7:345–363.

14. Jass JR, Stewart SM. Evolution of hereditary non-polyposis colorectal cancer. Gut 1992; 33:783–786.

15. Tomeo CA, Colditz GA, Willett WC, et al. Harvard Report on Cancer Prevention. Volume 3: prevention of colon cancer in the United States. Cancer Causes Control 1999; 10:167–180.

16. Hawk ET, Umar A, Viner JL. Colorectal cancer chemoprevention – an overview of the science. Gastroenterology 2004; 126:1423–1447.

17. Asano T, McLeod R. Nonsteroidal anti-inflammatory drugs (NSAID) and aspirin for preventing colorectal adenomas and carcinomas. Cochrane Database Syst Rev 2004; 2:CD004079.

18. Higuchi T, Iwama T, Yoshinaga K, et al. A randomized, double-blind, placebo-controlled trial of the effects of rofecoxib, a selective

cyclooxygenase-2 inhibitor, on rectal polyps in familial adenomatous polyposis patients. Clin Cancer Res 2003; 9:4756–4760.

19. Tung BY, Emond MJ, Haggitt RC, et al. Ursodiol use is associated with lower prevalence of colonic neoplasia in patients with ulcerative colitis and primary sclerosing cholangitis. Ann Intern Med 2001; 134:89–95.

20. Hawk ET, Viner JL. Chemoprevention in ulcerative colitis: narrowing the gap between clinical practice and research. Ann Intern Med 2001; 134:158–160.

21. Pardi DS, Loftus EV Jr, Kremers WK, et al. Ursodeoxycholic acid as a chemopreventive agent in patients with ulcerative colitis and primary sclerosing cholangitis. Gastroenterology 2003; 124:889–893.

22. Winawer SJ, Fletcher RH, Miller L, et al. Colorectal cancer screening: clinical guidelines and rationale. Gastroenterology 1997; 112:594–642.

23. Mandel JS, Bond JH, Church TR, et al. Reducing mortality from colorectal cancer by screening for fecal occult blood. Minnesota Colon Cancer Control Study. N Engl J Med 1993; 328:1365.

A landmark study demonstrating that fecal occult blood testing is an effective strategy for reducing colorectal cancer mortality.

24. Hardcastle JD, Chamberlain JO, Robinson MH, et al. Randomised controlled trial of faecal-occult-blood screening for colorectal cancer. Lancet 1996; 348:1472–1477.

25. Kronborg O, Fenger C, Olsen J, et al. Randomised study of screening for colorectal cancer with faecal-occult-blood test. Lancet 1996; 348:1467–1471.

26. Selby JV. Screening sigmoidoscopy for colorectal cancer. Lancet 1993; 341:728–729.

27. Mandel JS, Church TR, Ederer F, et al. Colorectal cancer mortality: effectiveness of biennial screening for fecal occult blood. J Natl Cancer Inst 1999; 91:434–437.

28. Mandel JS, Church TR, Bond JH, et al. The effect of fecal occult-blood screening on the incidence of colorectal cancer. N Engl J Med 2000; 343:1603–1607.

29. Newcomb PA, Norfleet RG, Storer BE, et al. Screening sigmoidoscopy and colorectal cancer mortality. J Natl Cancer Inst 1992; 84:1572–1575.

30. Muller AD, Sonnenberg A. Prevention of colorectal cancer by flexible endoscopy and polypectomy. A case-control study of 32,702 veterans. Ann Intern Med 1995; 123:904–910.

31. Winawer SJ, Flehinger BJ, Schottenfeld D, et al. Screening for colorectal cancer with fecal occult blood testing and sigmoidoscopy. J Natl Cancer Inst 1993; 85:1311–1318.

32. Pignone M, Saha S, Hoerger T, et al. Cost-effectiveness analyses of colorectal cancer screening: a systematic review for the U.S. Preventive Services Task Force. Ann Intern Med 2002; 137:96–104.

A widely referenced economic analysis that finds that while all currently recommended colorectal cancer screening strategies are more cost-effective than no screening, a single optimal strategy cannot be determined from the available data.

33. Rex DK, Johnson DA, Lieberman DA, et al. Colorectal cancer prevention 2000: screening recommendations of the American College of Gastroenterology. American College of Gastroenterology. Am J Gastroenterol 2000; 95:868–877.

34. Smith RA, von Eschenbach AC, Wender R, et al. American Cancer Society guidelines for the early detection of cancer: update of early detection guidelines for prostate, colorectal, and endometrial cancers. Also: update 2001 – testing for early lung cancer detection. CA Cancer J Clin 2001; 51:38–75.

35. Pignone M, Rich M, Teutsch SM, et al. Screening for colorectal cancer in adults at average risk: a summary of the evidence for the U.S. Preventive Services Task Force. Ann Intern Med 2002; 137:132–141.

36. Winawer S, Fletcher R, Rex D, et al. Colorectal cancer screening and surveillance: clinical guidelines and rationale – Update based on new evidence. Gastroenterology 2003; 124:544–560.

Updated, evidence-based screening and surveillance recommendations for individuals at average and increased risk of colorectal cancer.

37. Eisner MS, Lewis JH. Diagnostic yield of a positive fecal occult blood test found on digital rectal examination. Does the finger count? Arch Intern Med 1991; 151:2180–2184.

38. Bini EJ, Rajapaksa RC, Weinshel EH. The findings and impact of nonrehydrated guaiac examination of the rectum (FINGER) study: a comparison of 2 methods of screening for colorectal cancer in asymptomatic average-risk patients. Arch Intern Med 1999; 159:2022–2026.

39. Burke CA, Tadikonda L, Machicao V. Fecal occult blood testing for colorectal cancer screening: use the finger. Am J Gastroenterol 2001; 96:3175–3177.

40. Ahlquist DA, Wieand HS, Moertel CG, et al. Accuracy of fecal occult blood screening for colorectal neoplasia. A prospective study using Hemoccult and HemoQuant tests. JAMA 1993; 269:1262–1267.

41. Lieberman DA, Weiss DG. One-time screening for colorectal cancer with combined fecal occult-blood testing and examination of the distal colon. N Engl J Med 2001; 345:555–560.

An important study suggesting that the yield for detecting advanced colorectal neoplasia by screening sigmoidoscopy alone is comparable to that of flexible sigmoidoscopy plus fecal occult blood testing.

42. Rozen P, Knaani J, Samuel Z. Performance characteristics and comparison of two immunochemical and two guaiac fecal occult blood screening tests for colorectal neoplasia. Dig Dis Sci 1997; 42:2064–2071.

43. Sinatra MA, St John DJ, Young GP. Interference of plant peroxidases with guaiac-based fecal occult blood tests is avoidable. Clin Chem 1999; 45:123–126.

44. [No authors listed]. American College of Physicians. Suggested technique for fecal occult blood testing and interpretation in colorectal cancer screening. Ann Intern Med 1997; 126:808–810.

45. Ransohoff DF, Lang CA. Screening for colorectal cancer with the fecal occult blood test: a background paper. American College of Physicians. Ann Intern Med 1997; 126:811–822.

46. Rockey DC, Auslander A, Greenberg PD. Detection of upper gastrointestinal blood with fecal occult blood tests. Am J Gastroenterol 1999; 94:344–350.

47. Allison JE, Tekawa IS, Ransom LJ, et al. A comparison of fecal occult-blood tests for colorectal-cancer screening. N Engl J Med 1996; 334:155–159.

48. Young GP, St John DJ, Winawer SJ, et al. Choice of fecal occult blood tests for colorectal cancer screening: recommendations based on performance characteristics in population studies: a WHO (World Health Organization) and OMED (World Organization for Digestive Endoscopy) report. Am J Gastroenterol 2002; 97:2499–2507.

49. Greenberg PD, Bertario L, Gnauck R, et al. A prospective multicenter evaluation of new fecal occult blood tests in patients undergoing colonoscopy. Am J Gastroenterol 2000; 95:1331–1338.

50. Ko CW, Dominitz JA, Nguyen TD. Fecal occult blood testing in a general medical clinic: comparison between guaiac-based and immunochemical-based tests. Am J Med 2003; 115:111–114.

51. Winawer SJ, Miller C, Lightdale C, et al. Patient response to sigmoidoscopy. A randomized, controlled trial of rigid and flexible sigmoidoscopy. Cancer 1987; 60:1905–1908.

References

52. Imperiale TF, Wagner DR, Lin CY, et al. Risk of advanced proximal neoplasms in asymptomatic adults according to the distal colorectal findings. N Engl J Med 2000; 343:169–174.

53. Rex DK, Lehman GA, Hawes RH, et al. Screening colonoscopy in asymptomatic average-risk persons with negative fecal occult blood tests. Gastroenterology 1991; 100:64–67.

54. Lieberman DA, Weiss DG, Bond JH, et al. Use of colonoscopy to screen asymptomatic adults for colorectal cancer. Veterans Affairs Cooperative Study Group 380. N Engl J Med 2000; 343:162–168.

A widely publicized study demonstrating both the feasibility of screening colonoscopy and its superiority over flexible sigmoidoscopy for detecting significant colorectal neoplasia.

55. Rex D. Barium enema and colon cancer screening: finally a study. Am J Gastroenterol 1997; 92:1570–1572.

56. Winawer SJ, Stewart ET, Zauber AG, et al. A comparison of colonoscopy and double-contrast barium enema for surveillance after polypectomy. National Polyp Study Work Group. N Engl J Med 2000; 342:1766–1772.

57. Scheitel SM, Ahlquist DA, Wollan PC, et al. Colorectal cancer screening: a community case-control study of proctosigmoidoscopy, barium enema radiography, and fecal occult blood test efficacy. Mayo Clin Proc 1999; 74:1207–1213.

58. Fenlon HM, Nunes DP, Clarke PD, et al. Colorectal neoplasm detection using virtual colonoscopy: a feasibility study. Gut 1998; 43:806–811.

59. Fletcher JG, Johnson CD, Welch TJ, et al. Optimization of CT colonography technique: prospective trial in 180 patients. Radiology 2000; 16:704–711.

60. Yee J, Akerkar GA, Hung RK, et al. Colorectal neoplasia: performance characteristics of CT colonography for detection in 300 patients. Radiology 2001; 219:685–692.

61. Pickhardt PJ, Choi JR, Hwang I, et al. Computed tomographic virtual colonoscopy to screen for colorectal neoplasia in asymptomatic adults. N Engl J Med 2003; 349:2191–2200.

62. Cotton PB, Durkalski VL, Pineau BC, et al. Computed tomographic colonography (virtual colonoscopy): a multicenter comparison with standard colonoscopy for detection of colorectal neoplasia. JAMA 2004; 291:1713–1719.

63. Ahlquist DA. Molecular stool screening for colorectal cancer. Using DNA markers may be beneficial, but large scale evaluation is needed. Br Med J 2000; 321:254–255.

64. Dong SM, Traverso G, Johnson C, et al. Detecting colorectal cancer in stool with the use of multiple genetic targets. J Natl Cancer Inst 2001; 93:858–865.

65. Traverso G, Shuber A, Levin B, et al. Detection of APC mutations in fecal DNA from patients with colorectal tumors. N Engl J Med 2002; 346:311–320.

66. Tagore KS LM, Yucaitis JA, Gage R, et al. Sensitivity and specificity of a stool DNA multitarget assay panel for the detection of advanced colorectal neoplasia. Clin Colorectal Cancer 2003; 3:47–53.

67. Song K, Fendrick AM, Ladabaum U. Fecal DNA testing compared with conventional colorectal cancer screening methods: a decision analysis. Gastroenterology 2004; 126:1270–1279.

68. Ladabaum U, Song K, Fendrick AM. Colorectal neoplasia screening with virtual colonoscopy: When, at what cost, and with what national impact? Clin Gastroenterol Hepatol 2004; 2:554–563.

69. Winawer SJ, Zauber AG, Gerdes H, et al. Risk of colorectal cancer in the families of patients with adenomatous polyps. National Polyp Study Workgroup. N Engl J Med 1996; 334:82–87.

70. Ahsan H, Neuget AI, Garbowski GC, et al. Family history of colorectal adenomatous polyps and increased risk for colorectal cancer. Ann Intern Med 1998; 128:900–905.

71. Lynch KL, Ahnen DJ, Byers T, et al. First-degree relatives of patients with advanced colorectal adenomas have an increased prevalence of colorectal cancer. Clin Gastroenterol Hepatol 2003; 1:96–102.

72. Johns LE, Houlston RS. A systematic review and meta-analysis of familial colorectal cancer risk. Am J Gastroenterol 2001; 96:2992–3003.

73. Slattery ML, Kerber RA. Family history of cancer and colon cancer risk: the Utah Population Database. J Natl Cancer Inst 1994; 86:1618–1626.

74. Fuchs CS, Giovannucci EL, Colditz GA, et al. A prospective study of family history and the risk of colorectal cancer. N Engl J Med 1994; 331:1669–1674.

75. Cruz-Correa M, Giardiello FM. Familial adenomatous polyposis. Gastrointest Endosc 2003; 58:885–894.

76. Soravia C, Berk T, Madlensky L, et al. Genotype-phenotype correlations in attenuated adenomatous polyposis coli. Am J Hum Genet 1998; 62:1290–1301.

77. Hamilton SR, Liu B, Parsons RE, et al. The molecular basis of Turcot's syndrome. N Engl J Med 1995; 332:839–847.

78. Lipton L, Tomlinson I. The multiple colorectal adenoma phenotype and MYH, a base excision repair gene. Clin Gastroenterol Hepatol 2004; 2:633–638.

A summary of the genetic and clinical features of the colorectal adenomas and cancers that occur in the recently described MYH-associated polyposis syndrome.

79. Powell SM, Petersen GM, Krush AJ, et al. Molecular diagnosis of familial adenomatous polyposis. N Engl J Med 1993; 329:1982–1987.

80. Giardiello FM, Brensinger JD, Petersen GM. AGA technical review on hereditary colorectal cancer and genetic testing. Gastroenterology 2001; 121:198–213.

81. Nugent KP, Northover J. Total colectomy and ileorectal anastomosis. In: Phillips RKS, Spigelman AD, Thompson JPS, eds. Familial polyposis and other polyposis syndromes. London: Edward Arnold; 1994:79–91.

82. Bulow C, Vasen H, Jarvinen H, et al. Ileorectal anastomosis is appropriate for a subset of patients with familial adenomatous polyposis. Gastroenterology 2000; 119:1454–1460.

83. van Duijvendijk P, Vasen HF, Bertario L, et al. Cumulative risk of developing polyps or malignancy at the ileal pouch-anal anastomosis in patients with familial adenomatous polyposis. J Gastrointest Surg 1999; 3:325–330.

84. Giardiello FM, Hamilton SR, Krush AJ, et al. Treatment of colonic and rectal adenomas with sulindac in familial adenomatous polyposis. N Engl J Med 1993; 328:1313–1316.

85. Cruz-Correa M, Hylind LM, Romans KE, et al. Long-term treatment with sulindac in familial adenomatous polyposis: a prospective cohort study. Gastroenterology 2002; 122:641–645.

86. Steinbach G, Lynch PM, Phillips RK, et al. The effect of celecoxib, a cyclooxygenase-2 inhibitor, in familial adenomatous polyposis. N Engl J Med 2000; 342:1946–1952.

87. Chung DC, Rustgi AK. The hereditary nonpolyposis colorectal cancer syndrome: genetics and clinical implications. Ann Intern Med 2003; 138:560–570.

88. Lynch HT, de la Chapelle A. Hereditary colorectal cancer. N Engl J Med 2003; 348:919–932.

89. Rustgi AK. Hereditary gastrointestinal polyposis and nonpolyposis syndromes. N Engl J Med 1994; 331:1694–1702.

90. Vasen HF, Mecklin JP, Khan PM, et al. The International Collaborative Group on Hereditary Non-Polyposis Colorectal Cancer (ICG-HNPCC). Dis Colon Rectum 1991; 34:424–425.

91. Vasen HF, Watson P, Mecklin JP, et al. New clinical criteria for hereditary nonpolyposis colorectal cancer (HNPCC, Lynch syndrome) proposed by the International Collaborative Group on HNPCC. Gastroenterology 1999; 116:1453–1456.

92. Umar A, Boland CR, Terdiman JP, et al. Revised Bethesda Guidelines for hereditary nonpolyposis colorectal cancer (Lynch syndrome) and microsatellite instability. J Natl Cancer Inst 2004; 96:261–268.

   A comprehensive review of MSI testing for HNPCC and revised guidelines for genetic testing.

93. Jarvinen HJ, Aarnio M, Mustonen H, et al. Controlled 15-year trial on screening for colorectal cancer in families with hereditary nonpolyposis colorectal cancer. Gastroenterology 2000; 118:829–834.

94. Lynch HT. Is there a role for prophylactic subtotal colectomy among hereditary nonpolyposis colorectal cancer germline mutation carriers? Dis Colon Rectum 1996; 39:109–110.

95. Scaife CL, Rodriguez-Bigas MA. Lynch syndrome: implications for the surgeon. Clin Colorectal Cancer 2003; 3:92–98.

96. Lanspa SJ, Jenkins JX, Cavalieri RJ, et al. Surveillance in Lynch syndrome: how aggressive? Am J Gastroenterol 1994; 89: 1978–1980.

97. de Vos tot Nederveen Cappel WH, Nagengast FM, Griffioen G, et al. Surveillance for hereditary nonpolyposis colorectal cancer: a long-term study on 114 families. Dis Colon Rectum 2002; 45:1588–1594.

98. Cali RL, Pitsch RM, Thorson AG, et al. Cumulative incidence of metachronous colorectal cancer. Dis Colon Rectum 1993; 36:388–393.

99. Rex DK. Colonoscopy: a review of its yield for cancers and adenomas by indication. Am J Gastroenterol 1995; 90:353–365.

100. Malcolm AW, Perencevich NP, Olson RM, et al. Analysis of recurrence patterns following curative resection for carcinoma of the colon and rectum. Surg Gynecol Obstet 1981; 152:131–136.

101. Kronborg O, Fenger C. Prognostic evaluation of planned follow-up in patients with colorectal adenomas. An interim report. Int J Colorectal Dis 1987; 2:203–207.

102. Winawer SJ, Zauber AG, O'Brien MJ, et al. Randomized comparison of surveillance intervals after colonoscopic removal of newly diagnosed adenomatous polyps. The National Polyp Study Workgroup. N Engl J Med 1993; 328:901–906.

   A seminal study demonstrating that postpolypectomy surveillance every 3 years is as effective as surveillance after 1 and 3 years for detecting colorectal neoplasia.

103. Noshirwani KC, van Stolk RU, Rybicki LA, et al. Adenoma size and number are predictive of adenoma recurrence: implications for surveillance colonoscopy. Gastrointest Endosc 2000; 51:433–437.

104. Longacre TA, Fenoglio-Preiser CM. Mixed hyperplastic adenomatous polyps/serrated adenomas. A distinct form of colorectal neoplasia. Am J Surg Pathol 1990; 14:524–537.

105. Bernstein CN, Blanchard JF, Kliewer E, et al. Cancer risk in patients with inflammatory bowel disease: a population-based study. Cancer 2001; 91:854–862.

106. Ekbom A, Helmick C, Zack M, et al. Increased risk of large-bowel cancer in Crohn's disease with colonic involvement. Lancet 1990; 336:357–359.

107. Eaden JA, Abrams KR, Mayberry JF. The risk of colorectal cancer in ulcerative colitis: a meta-analysis. Gut 2001; 48:526–535.

108. Rutter M, Saunders B, Wilkinson K, et al. Severity of inflammation is a risk factor for colorectal neoplasia in ulcerative colitis. Gastroenterology 2004; 126:451–459.

109. Askling J, Dickman PW, Karlen P, et al. Family history as a risk factor for colorectal cancer in inflammatory bowel disease. Gastroenterology 2001; 120:1356–1362.

110. Soetikno RM, Lin OS, Heidenreich PA, et al. Increased risk of colorectal neoplasia in patients with primary sclerosing cholangitis and ulcerative colitis: a meta-analysis. Gastrointest Endosc 2002; 56:48–54.

111. Rubin CE, Haggitt RC, Burmer GC, et al. DNA aneuploidy in colonic biopsies predicts future development of dysplasia in ulcerative colitis. Gastroenterology 1992; 103:1611–1620.

112. Levine DS, Reid BJ. Endoscopic biopsy technique for acquiring larger mucosal samples. Gastrointest Endosc 1991; 37:332–337.

113. Riddell RH, Goldman H, Ransohoff DF, et al. Dysplasia in inflammatory bowel disease: standardized classification with provisional clinical applications. Hum Pathol 1983; 14:931–968.

114. Bernstein CN, Shanahan F, Weinstein WM. Are we telling patients the truth about surveillance colonoscopy in ulcerative colitis? Lancet 1994; 343:71–74.

115. Connell WR, Lennard-Jones JE, Williams CB, et al. Factors affecting the outcome of endoscopic surveillance for cancer in ulcerative colitis. Gastroenterology 1994; 107:934–944.

116. Lindberg B, Persson B, Veress B, et al. Twenty years' colonoscopic surveillance of patients with ulcerative colitis. Detection of dysplastic and malignant transformation. Scand J Gastroenterol 1996; 31:1195–1204.

117. Ullman T, Croog V, Harpaz N, et al. Progression of flat low-grade dysplasia to advanced neoplasia in patients with ulcerative colitis. Gastroenterology 2003; 125:1311–1319.

118. Blackstone MO, Riddell RH, Rogers BH, et al. Dysplasia-associated lesion or mass (DALM) detected by colonoscopy in long-standing ulcerative colitis: an indication for colectomy. Gastroenterology 1981; 80:366–374.

119. Odze RD, Farraye FA, Hecht JL, et al. Long-term follow-up after polypectomy treatment for adenoma-like dysplastic lesions in ulcerative colitis. Clin Gastroenterol Hepatol 2004; 2:534–541.

120. Friedman S, Odze RD, Farraye FA. Management of neoplastic polyps in inflammatory bowel disease. Inflamm Bowel Dis 2003; 9:260–266.

121. Dunlop MG. Guidance on gastrointestinal surveillance for hereditary non-polyposis colorectal cancer, familial adenomatous polyposis, juvenile polyposis, and Peutz-Jeghers syndrome. Gut 2002; 51(Suppl 5):V21–V27.

122. Church JM. Analysis of the colonoscopic findings in patients with rectal bleeding according to the pattern of their presenting symptoms. Dis Colon Rectum 1991; 34:391–395.

123. Niv Y, Sperber AD. Sensitivity, specificity, and predictive value of fecal occult blood testing (Hemoccult II) for colorectal neoplasia in symptomatic patients: a prospective study with total colonoscopy. Am J Gastroenterol 1995; 90:1974–1977.

124. Monahan DW, Peluso FE, Goldner F. Combustible colonic gas levels during flexible sigmoidoscopy and colonoscopy. Gastrointest Endosc 1992; 38:40–73.

125. Farraye FA, Wallace M. Clinical significance of small polyps found during screening with flexible sigmoidoscopy. Gastrointest Endosc Clin N Am 2002; 12:41–51.

126. Pinsky PF, Schoen RE, Weissfeld JL, et al. Predictors of advanced proximal neoplasia in persons with abnormal screening flexible sigmoidoscopy. Clin Gastroenterol Hepatol 2003; 1:103–110.

127. Atkin WS, Morson BC, Cuzick J. Long-term risk of colorectal cancer after excision of rectosigmoid adenomas. N Engl J Med 1992; 326:658–662.

128. Fennerty MB, Davidson J, Emerson SS, et al. Are endoscopic measurements of colonic polyps reliable? Am J Gastroenterol 1993; 88:496–500.

129. Bond JH. Polyp guideline: diagnosis, treatment, and surveillance for patients with colorectal polyps. Practice Parameters Committee of the American College of Gastroenterology. Am J Gastroenterol 2000; 95:3053–3063.

130. Kudo S, Tamura S, Nakajima T, et al. Diagnosis of colorectal tumorous lesions by magnifying endoscopy. Gastrointest Endosc 1996; 44:8–14.

131. Cothren RM, Sivak MV Jr, Van Dam J, et al. Detection of dysplasia at colonoscopy using laser-induced fluorescence: a blinded study. Gastrointest Endosc 1996; 44:168–176.

132. Fenoglio CM, Pascal RR. Colorectal adenomas and cancer: pathologic relationships. Cancer 1982; 50(11 Suppl): 2601–2608.

133. Provenzale D, Garrett JW, Condon SE, et al. Risk for colon adenomas in patients with rectosigmoid hyperplastic polyps. Ann Intern Med 1990; 113:760–763.

134. Rex DK, Smith JJ, Ulbright TM, et al. Distal colonic hyperplastic polyps do not predict proximal adenomas in asymptomatic average-risk subjects. Gastroenterology 1992; 102:317–319.

135. Nelson DB, Barkun AN, Block KP, et al. Technology status evaluation report. Colonoscopy preparations. May 2001. Gastrointest Endosc 2001; 54:829–832.

136. Eisen GM, Baron TH, Dominitz JA, et al. Guideline on the management of anticoagulation and antiplatelet therapy for endoscopic procedures. Gastrointest Endosc 2002; 55:775–779.

137. Hirota WK, Petersen K, Baron TH, et al. Guidelines for antibiotic prophylaxis for GI endoscopy. Gastrointest Endosc 2003; 58: 475–482.

138. Waye JD, Lewis BS, Frankel A, et al. Small colon polyps. Am J Gastroenterol 1988; 83:120–122.

139. Vanagunas A, Jacob P, Vakil N. Adequacy of 'hot biopsy' for the treatment of diminutive polyps: a prospective randomized trial. Am J Gastroenterol 1989; 84(4):383–385.

140. Wadas DD, Sanowski RA. Complications of the hot biopsy forceps technique. Gastrointest Endosc 1988; 34:32–37.

141. Dyer WS, Quigley EM, Noel SM, et al. Major colonic hemorrhage following electrocoagulating (hot) biopsy of diminutive colonic polyps: relationship to colonic location and low-dose aspirin therapy. Gastrointest Endosc 1991; 37:361–364.

142. Waye JD. Techniques of polypectomy: hot biopsy forceps and snare polypectomy. Am J Gastroenterol 1987; 82:615–618.

143. Tappero G, Gaia E, De Giuli P, et al. Cold snare excision of small colorectal polyps. Gastrointest Endosc 1992; 38:310–313.

144. Mathus-Vliegen EM, Tytgat GN. Nd:YAG laser photocoagulation in colorectal adenoma. Evaluation of its safety, usefulness, and efficacy. Gastroenterology 1986; 90:1865–1873.

145. Karita M, Tada M, Okita K, et al. Endoscopic therapy for early colon cancer: the strip biopsy resection technique. Gastrointest Endosc 1991; 37:128–132.

146. Dominitz JA, Eisen GM, Baron TH, et al. Complications of colonoscopy. Gastrointest Endosc 2003; 57:441–445.

147. Slivka A, Parsons WG, Carr-Locke DL. Endoscopic band ligation for treatment of post-polypectomy hemorrhage. Gastrointest Endosc 1994; 40(2 Pt 1):230–232.

148. Rey JF, Marek TA. Endo-loop in the prevention of the post-polypectomy bleeding: preliminary results. Gastrointest Endosc 1997; 46:387–389.

149. Parra-Blanco A, Kaminaga N, Kojima T, et al. Hemoclipping for postpolypectomy and postbiopsy colonic bleeding. Gastrointest Endosc 2000; 51:37–41.

150. Conio M, Repici A, Demarquay JF, et al. EMR of large sessile colorectal polyps. Gastrointest Endosc 2004; 60:234–241.

151. Zlatanic J, Waye JD, Kim PS, et al. Large sessile colonic adenomas: use of argon plasma coagulator to supplement piecemeal snare polypectomy. Gastrointest Endosc 1999; 49:731–735.

152. Regula J, Wronska E, Polkowski M, et al. Argon plasma coagulation after piecemeal polypectomy of sessile colorectal adenomas: long-term follow-up study. Endoscopy 2003; 35:212–218.

153. Bedogni G, Bertoni G, Ricci E, et al. Colonoscopic excision of large and giant colorectal polyps. Technical implications and results over eight years. Dis Colon Rectum 1986; 29:831–835.

154. Cranley JP, Petras RE, Carey WD, et al. When is endoscopic polypectomy adequate therapy for colonic polyps containing invasive carcinoma? Gastroenterology 1986; 91:419–427.

155. Coverlizza S, Risio M, Ferrari A, et al. Colorectal adenomas containing invasive carcinoma. Pathologic assessment of lymph node metastatic potential. Cancer 1989; 64:1937–1947.

156. Ginsberg GG, Barkun AN, Bosco JJ, et al. Endoscopic tattooing: February 2002. Gastrointest Endosc 2002; 55:811–814.

157. McAndrew MR, Saba AK. Efficacy of routine preoperative computed tomography scans in colon cancer. Am Surg 1999; 65:205–208.

158. Freeny PC, Marks WM, Ryan JA, et al. Colorectal carcinoma evaluation with CT: preoperative staging and detection of postoperative recurrence. Radiology 1986; 158:347–353.

159. Balthazar EJ, Megibow AJ, Hulnick D, et al. Carcinoma of the colon: detection and preoperative staging by CT. AJR Am J Roentgenol 1988; 150:301–306.

160. Parker GA, Lawrence W Jr, Horsley JS 3rd, et al. Intraoperative ultrasound of the liver affects operative decision making. Ann Surg 1989; 209:569–576; discussion 576–577.

161. Rummeny EJ, Wernecke K, Saini S, et al. Comparison between high-field-strength MR imaging and CT for screening of hepatic metastases: a receiver operating characteristic analysis. Radiology 1992; 182:879–886.

162. Tio T. Gastrointestinal TNM cancer staging by endosonography. New York: Igaku-Shoin; 1995.

163. Kwok H, Bissett IP, Hill GL. Preoperative staging of rectal cancer. Int J Colorectal Dis 2000; 15:9–20.

164. Nelson H, Petrelli N, Carlin A, et al. Guidelines 2000 for colon and rectal cancer surgery. J Natl Cancer Inst 2001; 93:583–596.

165. Compton C, Fenoglio-Preiser CM, Pettigrew N, et al. American Joint Committee on Cancer Prognostic Factors Consensus Conference: Colorectal Working Group. Cancer 2000; 88:1739–1757.

166. Lacy AM, Garcia-Valdecasas JC, Delgado S, et al. Laparoscopy-assisted colectomy versus open colectomy for treatment of non-metastatic colon cancer: a randomised trial. Lancet 2002; 359:2224–2229.

167. Leung KL, Kwok SP, Lam SC, et al. Laparoscopic resection of rectosigmoid carcinoma: prospective randomised trial. Lancet 2004; 363:1187–1192.

168. The Clinical Outcomes of Surgical Therapy Study Group. A comparison of laparoscopically assisted and open colectomy for colon cancer. N Engl J Med 2004; 350:2050–2059.

Data from a multicenter, randomized trial suggesting that laparoscopically assisted colectomy is an acceptable alternative to open colectomy for colorectal cancer.

169. Killingback M. Local excision of carcinoma of the rectum: indications. World J Surg 1992; 16:437–446.

170. Mason AY. Transsphincteric approach to rectal lesions. Surg Annu 1977; 9:171–194.

171. Westbrook KC, Lang NP, Broadwater JR, et al. Posterior surgical approaches to the rectum. Ann Surg 1982; 195:677–685.

172. Willett CG, Compton CC, Shellito PC, et al. Selection factors for local excision or abdominoperineal resection of early stage rectal cancer. Cancer 1994; 73:2716–2720.

173. Unger SW, Stern JD, Arroyo PJ, et al. Endoscopic Nd-YAG laser treatment of colorectal neoplasms. A four-year longitudinal study. Am Surg 1990; 56:153–157.

174. Hoekstra HJ, Verschueren RC, Oldhoff J, et al. Palliative and curative electrocoagulation for rectal cancer. Experience and results. Cancer 1985; 55:210–213.

175. Patrice T, Foultier MT, Yactayo S, et al. Endoscopic photodynamic therapy with hematoporphyrin derivative for primary treatment of gastrointestinal neoplasms in inoperable patients. Dig Dis Sci 1990; 35:545–552.

176. Sischy B. The use of endocavitary irradiation for selected carcinomas of the rectum: ten years experience. Radiother Oncol 1985; 4:97–101.

177. MacFarlane JK, Ryall RD, Heald RJ. Mesorectal excision for rectal cancer. Lancet 1993; 341:457–460.

178. Dukes C. The classification of cancer of the rectum. J Pathol; 35:323–332.

179. Astler U, Culler F. The prognostic significance of direct extension of carcinoma of the colon and rectum. Ann Surg 1954: 846–851.

180. American Joint Committee on Cancer. Manual for staging of cancer. 4th ed. Philadelphia: JB Lippincott; 1992.

181. Rich T, Gunderson LL, Lew R, et al. Patterns of recurrence of rectal cancer after potentially curative surgery. Cancer 1983; 52:1317–1329.

182. Cohen AM, Tremiterra S, Candela F, et al. Prognosis of node-positive colon cancer. Cancer 1991; 67:1859–1861.

183. Willett CG, Tepper JE, Cohen AM, et al. Failure patterns following curative resection of colonic carcinoma. Ann Surg 1984; 200: 685–690.

184. Minsky BD, Mies C, Rich TA, et al. Potentially curative surgery of colon cancer: patterns of failure and survival. J Clin Oncol 1988; 6:106–118.

185. Sardi A, Nieroda CA, Siddiqi MA, et al. Carcinoembryonic antigen directed multiple surgical procedures for recurrent colon cancer confined to the liver. Am Surg 1990; 56:255–259.

186. Berman JM, Cheung RJ, Weinberg DS. Surveillance after colorectal cancer resection. Lancet 2000; 355:395–399.

187. Pfister DG, Benson AB 3rd, Somerfield MR. Clinical practice. Surveillance strategies after curative treatment of colorectal cancer. N Engl J Med 2004; 350:2375–2382.

188. Chau I, Allen MJ, Cunningham D, et al. The value of routine serum carcino-embryonic antigen measurement and computed tomography in the surveillance of patients after adjuvant chemotherapy for colorectal cancer. J Clin Oncol 2004; 22:1420–1429.

189. Kievit J. Follow-up of patients with colorectal cancer: numbers needed to test and treat. Eur J Cancer 2002; 38:986–999.

190. Laurie JA, Moertel CG, Fleming TR, et al. Surgical adjuvant therapy of large-bowel carcinoma: an evaluation of levamisole and the combination of levamisole and fluorouracil. The North Central Cancer Treatment Group and the Mayo Clinic. J Clin Oncol 1989; 7:1447–1456.

191. NIH Consensus Conference. Adjuvant therapy for patients with colon and rectal cancer. JAMA 1990; 264:1444–1450.

192. Wolmark N, Rockette H, Fisher B, et al. The benefit of leucovorin-modulated fluorouracil as postoperative adjuvant therapy for primary colon cancer: results from National Surgical Adjuvant Breast and Bowel Project protocol C-03. J Clin Oncol 1993; 11:1879–1887.

193. Francini G, Petrioli R, Lorenzini L, et al. Folinic acid and 5-fluorouracil as adjuvant chemotherapy in colon cancer. Gastroenterology 1994; 106:899–906.

194. O'Connell MJ, Mailliard JA, Kahn MJ, et al. Controlled trial of fluorouracil and low-dose leucovorin given for 6 months as postoperative adjuvant therapy for colon cancer. J Clin Oncol 1997;15:246–250.

195. International Multicentre Pooled Analysis of Colon Cancer Trials (IMPACT) investigators. Efficacy of adjuvant fluorouracil and folinic acid in colon cancer. Lancet 1995; 345:939–944.

196. Gill S, Loprinzi CL, Sargent DJ, et al. Pooled analysis of fluorouracil-based adjuvant therapy for stage II and III colon cancer: who benefits and by how much? J Clin Oncol 2004; 22:1797–1806.

197. Ribic CM, Sargent DJ, Moore MJ, et al. Tumor microsatellite-instability status as a predictor of benefit from fluorouracil-based adjuvant chemotherapy for colon cancer. N Engl J Med 2003; 349:247–257.

198. Andre T, Boni C, Mounedji-Boudiaf L, et al. Oxaliplatin, fluorouracil, and leucovorin as adjuvant treatment for colon cancer. N Engl J Med 2004; 350:2343–2351.

199. Benson AB 3rd, Schrag D, Somerfield MR, et al. American Society of Clinical Oncology recommendations on adjuvant chemotherapy for stage II colon cancer. J Clin Oncol 2004; 22:3408–3419.

200. Gastrointestinal Study Group. Prolongation of the disease-free interval in surgically treated rectal carcinoma. N Engl J Med 1985; 312:1465–1472.

201. Fisher B, Wolmark N, Rockette H, et al. Postoperative adjuvant chemotherapy or radiation therapy for rectal cancer: results from NSABP protocol R-01. J Natl Cancer Inst 1988; 80:21–29.

202. Rouanet P, Fabre JM, Dubois JB, et al. Conservative surgery for low rectal carcinoma after high-dose radiation. Functional and oncologic results. Ann Surg 1995; 221:67–73.

203. Kapiteijn E, Marijnen CA, Nagtegaal ID, et al. Preoperative radiotherapy combined with total mesorectal excision for resectable rectal cancer. N Engl J Med 2001; 345:638–646.

204. Scheele J, Stang R, Altendorf-Hofmann A, et al. Resection of colorectal liver metastases. World J Surg 1995; 19:59–71.

205. Nordlinger B, Guiguet M, Vaillant JC, et al. Surgical resection of colorectal carcinoma metastases to the liver. A prognostic scoring system to improve case selection, based on 1568 patients. Association Francaise de Chirurgie. Cancer 1996; 77:1254–1262.

206. Jamison RL, Donohue JH, Nagorney DM, et al. Hepatic resection for metastatic colorectal cancer results in cure for some patients. Arch Surg 1997; 132:505–510; discussion 511.

207. Fong Y, Fortner J, Sun RL, et al. Clinical score for predicting recurrence after hepatic resection for metastatic colorectal cancer: analysis of 1001 consecutive cases. Ann Surg 1999; 230:309–318; discussion 318–321.

208. Iwatsuki S, Dvorchik I, Madariaga JR, et al. Hepatic resection for metastatic colorectal adenocarcinoma: a proposal of a prognostic scoring system. J Am Coll Surg 1999; 189:291–299.

209. Jarnagin WR, Conlon K, Bodniewicz J, et al. A clinical scoring system predicts the yield of diagnostic laparoscopy in patients with potentially resectable hepatic colorectal metastases. Cancer 2001; 91:1121–1128.

210. Strasberg SM, Dehdashti F, Siegel BA, et al. Survival of patients evaluated by FDG-PET before hepatic resection for metastatic colorectal carcinoma: a prospective database study. Ann Surg 2001; 233:293–299.

211. Adam R, Bismuth H, Castaing D, et al. Repeat hepatectomy for colorectal liver metastases. Ann Surg 1997; 225:51–60; discussion 60–62.

212. Yamamoto J, Kosuge T, Shimada K, et al. Repeat liver resection for recurrent colorectal liver metastases. Am J Surg 1999; 178:275–281.

213. Sotsky TK, Ravikumar TS. Cryotherapy in the treatment of liver metastases from colorectal cancer. Semin Oncol 2002; 29:183–191.

214. Solbiati L, Livraghi T, Goldberg SN, et al. Percutaneous radio-frequency ablation of hepatic metastases from colorectal cancer: long-term results in 117 patients. Radiology 2001; 221:159–166.

215. McAfee MK, Allen MS, Trastek VF, et al. Colorectal lung metastases: results of surgical excision. Ann Thorac Surg 1992; 53:780–785; discussion 785–786.

216. McCormack PM, Burt ME, Bains MS, et al. Lung resection for colorectal metastases. 10-year results. Arch Surg 1992; 127:1403–1406.

217. Inoue M, Ohta M, Iuchi K, et al. Benefits of surgery for patients with pulmonary metastases from colorectal carcinoma. Ann Thorac Surg 2004; 78:238–244.

218. Hoffman JP, Riley L, Carp NZ, et al. Isolated locally recurrent rectal cancer: a review of incidence, presentation, and management. Semin Oncol 1993; 20:506–519.

219. Gunderson LL, O'Connell MJ, Dozois RR. The role of intra-operative irradiation in locally advanced primary and recurrent rectal adenocarcinoma. World J Surg 1992; 16:495–501.

220. Rougier P, Van Cutsem E, Bajetta E, et al. Randomised trial of irinotecan versus fluorouracil by continuous infusion after fluorouracil failure in patients with metastatic colorectal cancer. Lancet 1998; 352:1407–1412.

221. Armand JP, Boige V, Raymond E, et al. Oxaliplatin in colorectal cancer: an overview. Semin Oncol 2000; 27(5 Suppl 10):96–104.

222. Meta-analysis Group in Cancer. Efficacy of intravenous continuous infusion of fluorouracil compared with bolus administration in advanced colorectal cancer. Meta-analysis Group In Cancer. J Clin Oncol 1998; 16:301–308.

223. Coutinho AK, Rocha Lima CM. Metastatic colorectal cancer: systemic treatment in the new millennium. Cancer Control 2003; 10:224–238.

224. Van Cutsem E, Twelves C, Cassidy J, et al. Oral capecitabine compared with intravenous fluorouracil plus leucovorin in patients with metastatic colorectal cancer: results of a large phase III study. J Clin Oncol 2001; 19:4097–4106.

225. Hoff PM, Ansari R, Batist G, et al. Comparison of oral capecitabine versus intravenous fluorouracil plus leucovorin as first-line treatment in 605 patients with metastatic colorectal cancer: results of a randomized phase III study. J Clin Oncol 2001; 19:2282–2292.

226. Cunningham D, Humblet Y, Siena S, et al. Cetuximab monotherapy and cetuximab plus irinotecan in irinotecan-refractory metastatic colorectal cancer. N Engl J Med 2004; 351:337–345.

227. Hurwitz H, Fehrenbacher L, Novotny W, et al. Bevacizumab plus irinotecan, fluorouracil, and leucovorin for metastatic colorectal cancer. N Engl J Med 2004; 350:2335–2342.

228. Cohen AD, Kemeny NE. An update on hepatic arterial infusion chemotherapy for colorectal cancer. Oncologist 2003; 8:553–566.

229. Dobrowsky W, Schmid AP. Radiotherapy of presacral recurrence following radical surgery for rectal carcinoma. Dis Colon Rectum 1985; 28:917–919.

230. Pacini P, Cionini L, Pirtoli L, et al. Symptomatic recurrences of carcinoma of the rectum and sigmoid. The influence of radiotherapy on the quality of life. Dis Colon Rectum 1986; 29:865–868.

231. Baron TH, Kozarek RA. Endoscopic stenting of colonic tumours. Best Pract Res Clin Gastroenterol 2004; 18:209–229.

232. Weiss NS, Yang CP. Incidence of histologic types of cancer of the small intestine. J Natl Cancer Inst 1987; 78:653–656.

233. Severson RK, Schenk M, Gurney JG, et al. Increasing incidence of adenocarcinomas and carcinoid tumors of the small intestine in adults. Cancer Epidemiol Biomarkers Prev 1996; 5:81–84.

234. Schottenfeld D, Winawer SJ. Cancers of the small intestine. In: Schottenfeld D, Fraumeni JF, eds. Cancer epidemiology and prevention. New York: Oxford University Press; 1996:806–812.

235. Perez A, Saltzman JR, Carr-Locke DL, et al. Benign nonampullary duodenal neoplasms. J Gastrointest Surg 2003; 7:536–541.

236. Martin JA, Haber GB. Ampullary adenoma: clinical manifestations, diagnosis, and treatment. Gastrointest Endosc Clin N Am 2003; 13:649–669.

237. Phillips RK, Wallace MH, Lynch PM, et al. A randomised, double blind, placebo controlled study of celecoxib, a selective cyclooxygenase 2 inhibitor, on duodenal polyposis in familial adenomatous polyposis. Gut 2002; 50:857–860.

238. Lai EC, Doty JE, Irving C, et al. Primary adenocarcinoma of the duodenum: analysis of survival. World J Surg 1988; 12:695–699.

239. Chareton B, Coiffic J, Landen S, et al. Diagnosis and therapy for ampullary tumors: 63 cases. World J Surg 1996; 20:707–712.

240. Barnes G Jr, Romero L, Hess KR, et al. Primary adenocarcinoma of the duodenum: management and survival in 67 patients. Ann Surg Oncol 1994; 1:73–78.

241. Lowell JA, Rossi RL, Munson JL, et al. Primary adenocarcinoma of third and fourth portions of duodenum. Favorable prognosis after resection. Arch Surg 1992; 127:557–560.

242. Ouriel K, Adams JT. Adenocarcinoma of the small intestine. Am J Surg 1984; 147:66–71.

243. Lillemoe KD, Sauter PK, Pitt HA, et al. Current status of surgical palliation of periampullary carcinoma. Surg Gynecol Obstet 1993; 176:1–10.

244. Rose DM, Hochwald SN, Klimstra DS, et al. Primary duodenal adenocarcinoma: a ten-year experience with 79 patients. J Am Coll Surg 1996; 183:89–96.

245. North JH, Pack MS. Malignant tumors of the small intestine: a review of 144 cases. Am Surg 2000; 66:46–51.

246. Fan CW, Changchien CR, Wang JY, et al. Primary colorectal lymphoma. Dis Colon Rectum 2000; 43:1277–1282.

247. Paryani SB, Hoppe RT, Cox RS, et al. Analysis of non-Hodgkin's lymphomas with nodular and favorable histologies, stages I and II. Cancer 1983; 52:2300–2307.

248. Ehrlich AN, Stalder G, Geller W, et al. Gastrointestinal manifestations of malignant lymphoma. Gastroenterology 1968; 54:1115–1121.

249. Isaacson PG. Gastrointestinal lymphoma. Hum Pathol 1994; 25:1020–1029.

250. Haber DA, Mayer RJ. Primary gastrointestinal lymphoma. Semin Oncol 1988; 15:154–169.

251. Fine KD, Stone MJ. Alpha-heavy chain disease, Mediterranean lymphoma, and immunoproliferative small intestinal disease: a review of clinicopathological features, pathogenesis, and differential diagnosis. Am J Gastroenterol 1999; 94:1139–1152.

252. Lecuit M, Abachin E, Martin A, et al. Immunoproliferative small intestinal disease associated with *Campylobacter jejuni*. N Engl J Med 2004; 350:239–248.

253. Ruskone-Fourmestraux A, Delmer A, Lavergne A, et al. Multiple lymphomatous polyposis of the gastrointestinal tract: prospective clinicopathologic study of 31 cases. Groupe D'etude des Lymphomes Digestifs. Gastroenterology 1997; 112:7–16.

254. Magrath I. The pathogenesis of Burkitt's lymphoma. Adv Cancer Res 1990; 55:133–270.

255. Cote TR, Biggar RJ, Rosenberg PS, et al. Non-Hodgkin's lymphoma among people with AIDS: incidence, presentation and public health burden. AIDS/Cancer Study Group. Int J Cancer 1997; 73:645–650.

256. Swinnen LJ. Treatment of organ transplant-related lymphoma. Hematol Oncol Clin North Am 1997; 11:963–973.

257. Loughran TP Jr, Kadin ME, Deeg HJ. T-cell intestinal lymphoma associated with celiac sprue. Ann Intern Med 1986; 104:44–47.

258. Radaszkiewicz T, Dragosics B, Bauer P. Gastrointestinal malignant lymphomas of the mucosa-associated lymphoid tissue: factors relevant to prognosis. Gastroenterology 1992; 102:1628–1638.

259. Contreary K, Nance FC, Becker WF. Primary lymphoma of the gastrointestinal tract. Ann Surg 1980; 191:593–598.

260. Salles G, Herbrecht R, Tilly H, et al. Aggressive primary gastrointestinal lymphomas: review of 91 patients treated with the LNH-84 regimen. A study of the Groupe d'Etude des Lymphomes Agressifs. Am J Med 1991; 90:77–84.

261. Daum S, Ullrich R, Heise W, et al. Intestinal non-Hodgkin's lymphoma: a multicenter prospective clinical study from the German Study Group on Intestinal non-Hodgkin's Lymphoma. J Clin Oncol 2003; 21:2740–2746.

262. Fisher RI, Dahlberg S, Nathwani BN, et al. A clinical analysis of two indolent lymphoma entities: mantle cell lymphoma and marginal zone lymphoma (including the mucosa-associated lymphoid tissue and monocytoid B-cell subcategories): a Southwest Oncology Group study. Blood 1995; 85:1075–1082.

263. List AF, Greer JP, Cousar JC, et al. Non-Hodgkin's lymphoma of the gastrointestinal tract: an analysis of clinical and pathologic features affecting outcome. J Clin Oncol 1988; 6:1125–1133.

264. Rackner VL, Thirlby RC, Ryan JA Jr. Role of surgery in multimodality therapy for gastrointestinal lymphoma. Am J Surg 1991; 161: 570–575.

265. Akbulut H, Soykan I, Yakaryilmaz F, et al. Five-year results of the treatment of 23 patients with immunoproliferative small intestinal disease: a Turkish experience. Cancer 1997; 80:8–14.

266. Khouri IF, Romaguera J, Kantarjian H, et al. Hyper-CVAD and high-dose methotrexate/cytarabine followed by stem-cell transplantation: an active regimen for aggressive mantle-cell lymphoma. J Clin Oncol 1998; 16:3803–3809.

267. Patte C, Philip T, Rodary C, et al. High survival rate in advanced-stage B-cell lymphomas and leukemias without CNS involvement with a short intensive polychemotherapy: results from the French Pediatric Oncology Society of a randomized trial of 216 children. J Clin Oncol 1991; 9:123–132.

268. Ladenstein R, Pearce R, Hartmann O, et al. High-dose chemotherapy with autologous bone marrow rescue in children with poor-risk Burkitt's lymphoma: a report from the European Lymphoma Bone Marrow Transplantation Registry. Blood 1997; 90:2921–2930.

269. Soussain C, Patte C, Ostronoff M, et al. Small noncleaved cell lymphoma and leukemia in adults. A retrospective study of 65 adults treated with the LMB pediatric protocols. Blood 1995; 85:664–674.

270. Bishop PC, Rao VK, Wilson WH. Burkitt's lymphoma: molecular pathogenesis and treatment. Cancer Invest 2000; 18:574–583.

271. Wang ES, Straus DJ, Teruya-Feldstein J, et al. Intensive chemotherapy with cyclophosphamide, doxorubicin, high-dose methotrexate/ifosfamide, etoposide, and high-dose cytarabine (CODOX-M/IVAC) for human immunodeficiency virus-associated Burkitt lymphoma. Cancer 2003; 98:1196–1205.

272. Egan LJ, Walsh SV, Stevens FM, et al. Celiac-associated lymphoma. A single institution experience of 30 cases in the combination chemotherapy era. J Clin Gastroenterol 1995; 21:123–129.

273. Gale J, Simmonds PD, Mead GM, et al. Enteropathy-type intestinal T-cell lymphoma: clinical features and treatment of 31 patients in a single center. J Clin Oncol 2000; 18:795–803.

274. Kulke MH, Mayer RJ. Carcinoid tumors. N Engl J Med 1999; 340:858–868.

275. Modlin IM, Sandor A. An analysis of 8305 cases of carcinoid tumors. Cancer 1997; 79:813–829.

276. Que FG, Nagorney DM, Batts KP, et al. Hepatic resection for metastatic neuroendocrine carcinomas. Am J Surg 1995; 169:36–42; discussion 42–43.

277. Le Treut YP, Delpero JR, Dousset B, et al. Results of liver transplantation in the treatment of metastatic neuroendocrine tumors. A 31-case French multicentric report. Ann Surg 1997; 225:355–364.

278. Moertel CG, Johnson CM, McKusick MA, et al. The management of patients with advanced carcinoid tumors and islet cell carcinomas. Ann Intern Med 1994; 120:302–309.

279. Caplin ME, Buscombe JR, Hilson AJ, et al. Carcinoid tumour. Lancet 1998; 352:799–805.

280. Moertel CG, Hanley JA. Combination chemotherapy trials in metastatic carcinoid tumor and the malignant carcinoid syndrome. Cancer Clin Trials 1979; 2:327–334.

281. Kvols LK, Moertel CG, O'Connell MJ, et al. Treatment of the malignant carcinoid syndrome. Evaluation of a long-acting somatostatin analogue. N Engl J Med 1986; 315:663–666.

282. Lamberts SW, Bakker WH, Reubi JC, et al. Somatostatin-receptor imaging in the localization of endocrine tumors. N Engl J Med 1990; 323:1246–1249.

283. Moertel CG, Kvols LK, Rubin J. A study of cyproheptadine in the treatment of metastatic carcinoid tumor and the malignant carcinoid syndrome. Cancer 1991; 67:33–36.

284. Connolly HM, Nishimura RA, Smith HC, et al. Outcome of cardiac surgery for carcinoid heart disease. J Am Coll Cardiol 1995; 25:410–416.

285. Pidhorecky I, Cheney RT, Kraybill WG, et al. Gastrointestinal stromal tumors: current diagnosis, biologic behavior, and management. Ann Surg Oncol 2000; 7:705–712.

286. Davila RE, Faigel DO. GI stromal tumors. Gastrointest Endosc 2003; 58:80–88.

287. van Oosterom AT, Judson I, Verweij J, et al. Safety and efficacy of imatinib (STI571) in metastatic gastrointestinal stromal tumours: a phase I study. Lancet 2001; 358:1421–1423.

288. Demetri GD, von Mehren M, Blanke CD, et al. Efficacy and safety of imatinib mesylate in advanced gastrointestinal stromal tumors. N Engl J Med 2002; 347:472–480.

A seminal study demonstrating that inhibition of the KIT signal-transduction pathway is a promising treatment for advanced gastrointestinal stromal tumors.

289. Verweij J, van Oosterom A, Blay JY, et al. Imatinib mesylate (STI-571 Glivec, Gleevec) is an active agent for gastrointestinal stromal tumours, but does not yield responses in other soft-tissue

sarcomas that are unselected for a molecular target. Results from an EORTC Soft Tissue and Bone Sarcoma Group phase II study. Eur J Cancer 2003; 39:2006–2011.

290. Edmonson JH, Marks RS, Buckner JC, eet al. Contrast of response to dacarbazine, mitomycin, doxorubicin, and cisplatin (DMAP) plus GM-CSF between patients with advanced malignant gastrointestinal stromal tumors and patients with other advanced leiomyosarcomas. Cancer Invest 2002; 20:605–612.

291. Hensley ML, Maki R, Venkatraman E, et al. Gemcitabine and docetaxel in patients with unresectable leiomyosarcoma: results of a phase II trial. J Clin Oncol 2002; 20:2824–2831.

292. Dezube BJ, Pantanowitz L, Aboulafia DM. Management of AIDS-related Kaposi sarcoma: advances in target discovery and treatment. AIDS Read 2004; 14:236–238, 243–244, 251–253.

293. Holkova B, Takeshita K, Cheng DM, et al. Effect of highly active antiretroviral therapy on survival in patients with AIDS-associated pulmonary Kaposi's sarcoma treated with chemotherapy. J Clin Oncol 2001; 19:3848–3851.

294. Lew EA, Dieterich DT. Severe hemorrhage caused by gastrointestinal Kaposi's syndrome in patients with the acquired immunodeficiency syndrome: treatment with endoscopic injection sclerotherapy. Am J Gastroenterol 1992; 87:1471–1474.

295. Nasti G, Talamini R, Antinori A, et al. AIDS-related Kaposi's sarcoma: evaluation of potential new prognostic factors and assessment of the AIDS Clinical Trial Group Staging System in the HAART Era – the Italian Cooperative Group on AIDS and Tumors and the Italian Cohort of Patients Naive From Antiretrovirals. J Clin Oncol 2003; 21:2876–2882.

CHAPTER SIXTY-FOUR

Treatment of sexually transmitted anorectal diseases

Ron Fried and Christina M. Surawicz

INTRODUCTION

Sexually transmitted diseases (STDs) include protozoal, helminthic, bacterial, and viral infections. Sexual behavior is a major factor in the transmission of infectious disease, and anal-receptive sexual practices, as well as manual and oral contact with the partner's anus, may cause direct person-to-person transmission of infectious agents. Safer sex practices in male homosexuals have altered the epidemiologic patterns of STDs. In a recent review of cases of clinical proctitis from the municipal STD clinic in San Francisco, gonorrhea and chlamydia were the most common STDs, followed by herpes and syphilis.[1] Promiscuity and failure to use condoms remain important risk factors in both homosexuals and heterosexuals. Clinical syndromes can be divided into enteritis, proctocolitis, and proctitis. The enteritic syndrome consists of watery or bloody diarrhea, often accompanied by weight loss and abdominal pain. Many of the pathogens involved, such as *Giardia lamblia*, do not cause proctitis or proctocolitis and are therefore not discussed further. Proctitis, or inflammation of the rectum, and proctocolitis, or inflammation of the colon and rectum, are the subjects of this chapter.

CLINICAL SPECTRUM

Proctitis

Acute proctitis is most commonly associated with recent anal-receptive intercourse with an infected partner. It produces symptoms of anal mucopurulent discharge or bleeding, pain, tenesmus, diarrhea, and occasionally constipation. It is associated with sigmoidoscopic findings of erythema and friable mucosa in the rectum, that is, below 15 cm. The pathogens most frequently involved are *Neisseria gonorrhoeae*, *Chlamydia trachomatis* (non-lymphogranuloma venereum [LGV] types), herpes simplex virus (HSV) type II, and *Treponema pallidum*. Multiple pathogens may be found in the same individual. Routine evaluation should include a test for syphilis such as a VDRL antigen test, smears and culture for *N. gonorrhoeae*, and a rectal swab for *C. trachomatis*. If diarrhea is present, proctitis may also be part of the spectrum of enteritis or proctocolitis. In this case, stool cultures for bacterial pathogens such as *Shigella* and *Campylobacter* and stool for ova and parasite examination are indicated, and flexible sigmoidoscopy must be considered.

Proctocolitis

Proctocolitis is present when sigmoid inflammation extends above 15 cm. It is usually caused by ingested pathogens, most frequently *Shigella*, *Campylobacter*, and *Entamoeba histolytica*. Other pathogens include *C. trachomatis* (LGV types), *Escherichia coli*, *Salmonella*, and *Yersinia*. Common symptoms are those of proctitis just noted, but watery or bloody diarrhea, crampy pain, and bloating can also be present. In individuals treated with antibiotics within the last 2 months, antibiotic-associated colitis secondary to *Clostridium difficile*, with or without pseudomembranes, must also be considered.

Perianal disease, warts, and malignancies

Perianal symptoms can include a spectrum from itching to inflammation. Symptoms of perianal disease include pruritus, pain, and tenesmus. Perianal itching may be caused by *Enterobius vermicularis* (pinworm or threadworm) infestation.

Condylomata acuminata, caused by the human papillomavirus (HPV), consist of anal and genital warts. HPV is the most common STD. Characteristic lesions are pink to white papules occurring in clusters and occasionally in large masses. They are found in the perianal region but commonly extend into the anal canal (Fig. 64.1). Over 60 types of HPV are known, some of which have oncogenic potential, especially types 16 and 18. Dysplastic lesions may be precursors of squamous cell anal cancer in men and cervical carcinoma in women. The frequency of squamous cell carcinoma of the anus is increased in homosexual men (Fig. 64.2).

DIAGNOSIS

History

Proctitis symptoms include anal discharge or bleeding and anorectal pain or tenesmus. Diarrhea may be related to the proctitis but more often indicates an enteric syndrome or proctocolitis. A careful but explicit history concerning sexual preferences and practices is essential, and physicians should not be reluctant to ask such questions. Specifically, anal-receptive intercourse and oral or manual contacts with the partner's anus are common ways for person-to-person transmission of pathogens to occur. The term 'gay bowel syndrome' is misleading because women can also acquire similar infections after heterosexual anal intercourse.

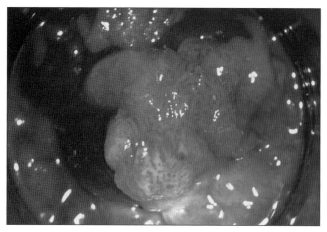

Fig. 64.1 • Colposcopically magnified anoscopic view of internal anal warts showing the characteristic multilobular appearance of these lesions in the internal anal canal. (Courtesy of James Sayer, R.N.)

Physical examination and endoscopy

Anoscopy identifies changes in the distal rectal mucosa and anal canal. Noninfectious diseases such as an anal fissure or hemorrhoids can be detected. Anoscopy allows one to obtain adequate specimens for identification of many sexually transmissible intestinal infections. Flexible sigmoidoscopy is helpful in determining the extent of mucosal changes in the left colon and to obtain mucosal biopsy tissue.

Rectal swab

Rectal swabs are a simple means of detecting anorectal infection with *N. gonorrhoeae* or *C. trachomatis*. A sterile cotton swab is passed through the anal canal and rotated a few times for 10 seconds. Swabs showing visible pus are more likely to yield cultures positive for *N. gonorrhoeae* than are swabs coated with feces. It is not clear whether the diagnostic yield is improved if swabs are taken through the rectoscope. Swabs should be placed directly into appropriate transport media. A positive Gram stain for *N. gonorrhoeae* on a microscopic slide is diagnostic, but direct staining with Gram stain misses approximately 50% of gonococcal infections.

Histology

Biopsy of specific lesions is usually indicated to determine whether they are inflammatory, infectious, or malignant. Biopsy specimens from the rectal mucosa in cases of proctitis often reveal nonspecific inflammatory changes. Some causative pathogens may be detected on hematoxylin and eosin (H&E) stains or with additional techniques such as immunofluorescence for HSV and immunohistology or in situ hybridization for cytomegalovirus (CMV) and HSV. Polymerase chain reaction (PCR) is becoming increasingly useful for detecting some pathogens, but is expensive and not widely available.

Serology

Serologic confirmation of the diagnosis may be helpful in diagnosing infections caused by *C. trachomatis*, *T. pallidum*, and HSV and in some cases of amebiasis. Diagnosis of acute infection by

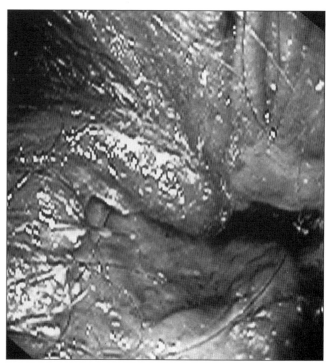

Fig. 64.2 • Ulceration at the anal canal in a homosexual man who was human immunodeficiency virus negative. Biopsy revealed squamous carcinoma of the anus.

serologic testing is specific if an increase in titer over time is observed.

SPECIFIC DISEASES

Bacterial

Gonorrheal proctitis

In acute gonorrheal proctitis, common symptoms are a creamy rectal discharge, rectal bleeding, hematochezia, and anal dyspareunia. Symptoms, however, are most often atypical, and an asymptomatic carrier status is common. In one study, 53% of patients with positive cultures for *N. gonorrhoeae* were asymptomatic.[2] Sigmoidoscopy may be unrevealing, or there may be evidence of mild proctitis with erythema and friability, especially around the anorectal junction. Perirectal abscess or fistulas, rectal stricture, and septicemia are rare complications of anorectal gonorrhea. Swabs should be placed directly on Thayer-Martin media or into special transport media and a second swab smeared onto a microscope slide and stained with Gram stain. Swabs obtained through an anoscope under direct visualization may have a higher diagnostic yield than blind swabs. The diagnosis is based on positive cultures from rectal swabs or Gram stains showing gram-negative intracellular diplococci.

Treatment of anorectal gonorrhea is cefixime, 400 mg orally once, or ceftriaxone, 125 mg intramuscularly once. Ciprofloxacin, in a single oral dose of 500 mg, or ofloxacin 400 mg orally once, or levofloxacin 250 mg orally, may be equally effective in uncomplicated gonorrhea,[3] but the emergence of resistant strains has been a cause for concern. The Centers for Disease Control (CDC) recommends that fluoroquinolones, no longer be used as first-line therapy for gonorrhea in men who have sex with men (MSM).[4] These drugs should be combined with doxycycline, 100 mg orally twice daily for 7 days, or azithromycin, 1 g orally once, because concurrent *Chlamydia* infection is common.[5] Follow-up culture after 7–10 days is highly recommended to verify cure. Persistence of symptoms after the eradication of gonococci may be related to concomitant infection with *C. trachomatis*.

Chlamydial proctitis

C. trachomatis, the agent of LGV, accounts for up to 20% of cases of proctitis in homosexual men.[6] LGV strains L1, L2, and L3 are responsible for most cases of proctitis. Typical symptoms consist of bloody or mucopurulent rectal discharge, diarrhea, and less commonly, rectal pain, tenesmus, and obstipation. Diarrhea and fistula formation may occur and mimic Crohn's disease. Chronic infection may lead to perirectal abscesses, fistulas, and rectal strictures. Tender, enlarged inguinal lymph nodes can be observed. An asymptomatic carrier state is found in 2–5% of cases. The diagnosis is based on culture of the organisms from rectal swabs and a monoclonal antibody test for chlamydial antigen in infected cells. Swabs are placed directly into a transport medium containing 0.2 mol/L sucrose-phosphate and then plated onto McCoy cells. Rectal biopsies show a distinctive granulomatous inflammation with giant cells and crypt abscesses. The organisms can sometimes be demonstrated in rectal biopsy specimens by Giemsa stain. Serologic examination by complement fixation titer or microimmunofluorescent tests is diagnostic if a fourfold rise in titer is observed.

The treatment of choice is doxycycline, 100 mg orally twice daily for 14 days, with erythromycin, 500 mg orally three times daily for 14 days or azithromycin, 1 g orally once, as an alternative. Tetracycline, 500 mg four times daily for 21 days is recommended if an LGV strain is present.

Anorectal syphilis

Cases of anorectal syphilis in homosexual men decreased during the 1980s because of the propagation of safer sex practices. The disease is now just as common in heterosexual male or female patients. After sexual contact with an infected partner, a chancre forms in the perianal area, the anal canal, or the rectal mucosa. Chancres begin as a papule and later erode into an ulcer. The incubation period is usually 3 weeks but ranges 10–90 days. *T. pallidum* penetrates a break in the skin or the intact mucosa. Perianal chancres are often painless, but lesions in the anal canal cause pain, possibly because of secondary infection. Primary syphilitic lesions in the anal canal can be mistaken for anal fissures or fistulas. Enlarged, tender inguinal lymph nodes are often found. The chancre itself is indurated. Syphilitic proctitis produces a purulent discharge. Endoscopically, anal or rectal ulcerations are observed, and diffuse involvement of the rectosigmoid has been reported. The diagnosis is made by detection of the organism by darkfield microscopy from material taken from a lesion. Serologic diagnosis depends on detecting antibodies to nontreponemal and treponemal antigens, including the VDRL and rapid plasmin reagent tests. These tests become positive a few weeks after the infection. Positive tests should be confirmed with a fluorescent treponemal antibody absorption test.

Treatment is with penicillin G, 2.4 million U intramuscularly once. In syphilis of more than one year's duration, penicillin G 2.4 milllion U is recommended weekly for three doses. In patients allergic to penicillin, doxycycline, 100 mg orally twice daily for 14 days, is recommended. Alternatively, ceftriaxone 1g i.m./i.v. can be given for 8–10 days. See Table 64.1 for other treatment regimens. Re-examination after 3 and 6 months is necessary to confirm treatment success.

Spirochetosis

Nontreponemal spirochetes can be found in the colon, appendix, and rectum. The prevalence of *colorectal spirochetosis* in the human colon varies from 1.9% to 6.9% in unselected populations to 30–36% in homosexual men.[7]

Spirochetes can be detected by careful microscopic examination of the luminal surface of colonic biopsy specimens stained with standard H&E. H&E stains reveal a thickened (3 μm) blue band that coats the surface of the epithelial and goblet cells and extends a short distance into the crypts. Silver stains make the diagnosis of spirochetosis easier (Fig. 64.3). Because spirochetes generally do not cause inflammatory changes in the mucosa, their presence may be underestimated if no biopsies are taken. At least two different types of spirochete are known. The larger *Spirocheta eurygyrata* is 4–10 μm in length and 0.2–0.5 μm in diameter and has irregular coils. The smaller organism is up to 6 μm in length and 0.2 μm in diameter, with regular coils. It has been termed *Brachyspira aalborgii* and *Treponema* D 60.

It remains unclear whether these organisms are pathogens or, more likely, represent commensal flora. Although most larger surveys suggest no pathogenic role for these organisms, various case reports indicate that they may occasionally cause symptoms. However, even if invasiveness of the organism is demonstrated histologically, symptoms may improve without specific therapy.[8] In a Danish study, spirochetes were found in 15 of 300 consecutive colon biopsies (5%). The persistence of symptoms after elimination of spirochetes by neomycin and bacitracin argued against a pathogenic role of the organism in this study.[9] Spirochetosis has been found in 9.6–12.6% of appendectomy specimens from patients suspected of having appendicitis but in whom the appendix was normal, compared to lower rates in patients with pathologically proven appendicitis, thus suggesting a possible role for the organism in appendicitis-like syndromes.[10,11]

If no other reason for an individual's symptoms is found, treatment with metronidazole may be considered.[12]

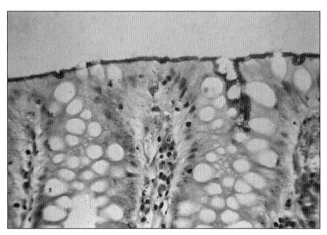

Fig. 64.3 • Silver stain of colorectal mucosa showing spirochetosis on the superficial mucosa seen as a dark layer of organisms coating the surface of the epithelium and extending a short distance into the upper crypt lumen.

Table 64.1 Treatment of proctitis and sexually transmissible diseases of the colon

Organisms	Standard treatment	Alternative treatment	Special points
BACTERIAL			
N. gonorrhoeae	Cefixime 400 p.o. once or ceftriaxone 125 mg i.m. once plus doxycycline 100 mg p.o., b.i.d. for 7 d or azithromycin 1 g p.o. once	Ciprofloxacin 500 mg p.o. once or ofloxacin 400 mg p.o. once or levofloxacin 250 mg p.o. once plus doxycycline 100 mg p.o., bid for 7 d or azithromycin 1 g p.o. once	Concurrent infection with C. trachomatis is common Strains resistant to quinolones have been observed in Asiatic countries
C. trachomatis	Doxycycline 100 mg p.o. b.i.d. for 14 d	Erythromycin 500 mg p.o. t.i.d. for 14 d or azithromycin 1 g p.o. once	Erythromycin preferred during pregnancy
C. trachomatis (LGV strains)	Doxycycline 100 mg p.o. b.i.d. for 21 d	Tetracycline 500 mg q.i.d. for 21 d	
T. pallidum	Penicillin G 2.4 million units i.m. once or doxycycline 100 mg p.o. b.i.d. for 14 d In syphilis of more than one year's duration: Penicillin G 2.4 million units i.m. weekly for 3 doses or doxycycline 100 mg p.o. b.i.d. for 28 d	Tetracycline 500 mg p.o. q.i.d. for 14 d or ceftriaxone 1 g i.m. i.v. q.d. for 8–10 d	Treatment suggestions for primary and secondary syphilis only Reexamination after 3 and 6 months to confirm treatment success
Spirochetosis	Metronidazole 500 mg t.i.d. for 10 d		Rarely indicated, because symptoms improve without therapy in most cases
VIRAL			
Herpes simplex virus	Symptomatic treatment locally	Acyclovir 400 mg p.o. five times daily for 10 d for more severe disease	Topical application of acyclovir six times a day for 7 d may accelerate healing of lesions
Cytomegalovirus	Ganciclovir, 5 mg/kg q 12 h i.v. as induction therapy for 14–21 d, followed by maintenance treatment with ganciclovir 5 mg/kg q 24 h i.v.	Foscarnet 90 mg/kg q 12 h i.v. as induction therapy for 14–21 days, followed by maintenance treatment with foscarnet 90 mg/kg q 24 h i.v.	In immunocompromised patients
PARASITES			
Entamoeba histolytica	Metronidazole 750 mg p.o. t.i.d. for 10 d plus diloxanide furoate 500 mg p.o. t.i.d. for 10 d	Metronidazole 750 mg p.o. t.i.d. for 10 d plus paramomycin (25–30 mg/kg/day) p.o. in three divided doses (or 500 mg p.o. t.i.d.) for 7 d or iodoquinol 650 mg p.o. t.i.d. for 20 d	Asymptomatic carriers are treated with a luminal amebicide only (iodoquinol or paromomycin or diloxanide furoate) to prevent transmission
Enterobius vermicularis	Mebendazole 100 mg p.o. once, repeat after 2 weeks	Pyrantel 11 mg/kg p.o. once, (up to 1 g) repeat after 2 and 4 weeks	Household members and sexual contacts should also be treated

Viral

Herpes simplex proctitis

Herpes simplex virus (HSV) proctitis is associated with anal pain and tenesmus, discharge, and constipation. Infection is due to HSV type 2 (90%) more than HSV type 1 (10%). Urinary retention and lower abdominal or buttock pain are commonly observed. Sexual transmission is by direct skin-to-skin contact. Because of pain, anal examination may be possible only after local anesthesia.

In the anal canal the characteristic lesions are small focal ulcerations that are sometimes confluent. Rectosigmoidoscopy may reveal ulcers and vesicles. Biopsy samples show acute and chronic inflammatory changes with focal microabscesses and superficial ulcerations. In material taken from the ulcer base, multinucleated giant cells can be demonstrated by Giemsa stain. The diagnosis of HSV proctitis is confirmed by isolation of HSV from rectal swabs or biopsy specimens. PCR is being used and is more sensitive than culture. Seroconversion is diagnostic if a fourfold titer rise is observed.

Treatment of mild HSV proctitis is symptomatic, with sitz baths, analgesics, and the application of ointments or suppositories containing a local anesthetic. Local steroids should be avoided. Oral acyclovir remains the mainstay treatment; the dose is 400 mg five times daily for 10 days, recommended for moderate disease. Intravenous therapy may be needed for very severe disease. For genital herpes, acyclovir, famciclovir and valaciclovir all have similar efficacy and side effect profiles.[13] Topical application of acyclovir six times per day for 7 days may also accelerate healing of lesions. Suppressive treatment of genital herpes can reduce transmission to sexual partners.[14] Vaccines for genital herpes are being developed.

Human papilloma infection

Condylomata acuminata, anal and genital warts, have been known since ancient times. They are formed by many small raised points, in contrast to the flat condylomata lata of secondary syphilis. Warts are caused by HPV, the most common sexually transmitted viral infection in the United States.[15] HPV usually infects the basal cells of squamous epithelium but may also infect transitional and cuboidal epithelium. Infectious viral particles are produced only by completely differentiated cells of the upper epithelium because cellular differentiation is necessary for the HPV growth cycle.[16] Infection with HPV can result in clinical or latent infection and in some cases may lead to the subsequent development of cancer.[17]

Receptive anal intercourse is common in patients with anal warts, and conceivably coital trauma allows latent virus in the anorectal region to enter the anal epidermis. Anal dysplasia has been demonstrated in 12% of homosexual men with internal warts.[18]

Symptoms of condylomata acuminata include pruritus, bleeding, anal wetness, and pain, although warts are frequently asymptomatic. Large warts may interfere with defecation. On clinical examination, raised papillary lesions are seen on the vulva and the perianal region. In over 50% of men, condylomata acuminata extend into the anal canal.[19]

A variety of nucleic acid hybridization techniques are used for the detection and typing of HPV infection. Exfoliated epithelial cell samples or tissue biopsies, either fresh or fixed, can be analyzed. The diagnosis of condyloma acuminatum, however, is a clinical one. Visual inspection and anoscopy or colposcopy reveal the extent of the lesions, which may determine the best therapeutic approach. Colposcopy also visualizes flat subclinical lesions on the cervix and the internal anal canal. The detection of HPV DNA and HPV antibodies in the sera of patients has been described,[20] but the clinical significance of a positive result in the absence of a lesion and the relevance of persistent HPV detection are not clear.

Of the more than 60 types of HPV, some 30 are found in anogenital diseases. Several types of HPV have oncogenic potential (types 16, 18, 45, and 56) and are the causal agent of most genital tract squamous cell cancers in women.[21] HPV infection, mainly with types 16 and 18, is also related to anal squamous cell cancer in men.[22] The development of malignancy may depend on several cofactors such as other STDs and smoking.[23,24] Immunosuppression confers an increased risk of HPV-related neoplasia. Anal dysplasia has been reported to be significantly more common in human immunodeficiency virus (HIV)-positive than HIV-negative homosexual men.[18] There is increasing interest in developing methods to screen HIV-infected persons for prevention or early detection of anal squamous cell cancer.[25]

Treatment of external condylomata acuminata is often performed topically. Single small perianal lesions may be treated with podophyllin in a 25% compound of tincture of benzoin. Treatment may require several sessions at weekly intervals. In more extensive disease, surgical excision or ablation with the CO_2 laser, electrocautery, or cryosurgery is the treatment of choice. In any of these approaches, recurrence is frequent. Intralesional interferon-α may be a useful adjunct to surgical methods to decrease recurrence.[26] In a placebo-controlled study, injection of interferon-α, 500 000 IU, into four quadrants of the anal canal reduced the recurrence rate from 39% to 12% during a mean follow-up period of 3.8 months. Vaccines are being developed, and show great promise.

Because of the high rate of recurrence, frequent follow-up visits are recommended. Recurrence may result from latent infection, for which there is no therapy. It is not known whether the treatment of partners or the use of condoms prevents reinfection.

Cytomegalovirus proctocolitis

Serologic evidence of previous contact with CMV is found in more than 90% of homosexual patients.[27] In immunocompetent individuals, the infection rarely becomes symptomatic. Acute ulcerative proctocolitis has been reported.[28]

Treatment is necessary if gastrointestinal manifestations occur because of immunosuppression (see below).

Parasites (protozoal and helminthic)

Amebiasis

Symptoms of amebiasis are often non-specific and can include bloating, abdominal cramping, and diarrhea. E. histolytica can be found in 20% of homosexual men.[29] Many of these patients are asymptomatic. Unusual features in asymptomatic homosexual men include the absence of serum antibodies and the presence of cysts rather than trophozoites in the stool. Long-term follow-up has suggested that symptomatic episodes in these patients are rare and therefore therapy for asymptomatic patients is not required.[30] The diagnosis is based on the presence of amebic trophozoites in the stool. If three separate stool samples are taken, the sensitivity is 90%. Serologic tests (enzyme-linked immunosorbent assay or indirect hemagglutination) may be helpful in diagnosing invasive disease,[31] but the test can remain positive for as long as 10 years after an episode. Sigmoidoscopy may show non-specific inflammatory changes with erythema, edema, and friability. Shallow ulcers covered with a yellowish exudate can be found. Histologically, inflammatory changes are non-specific. Amebae can be found at the mucosal surface or in the adjacent exudate associated with an ulcer.

The treatment of choice for invasive amebiasis is metronidazole, 750 mg orally three times daily for 7–10 days, plus diloxanide furoate (Furamide), 500 mg orally three times daily for 10 days. Instead of diloxanide furoate, which is no longer available in the United States, paromomycin, 25–30 mg/kg/day in three divided doses for 7 days (or 500 mg p.o. t.i.d.), or iodoquinol, 650 mg orally three times daily for 20 days, can be given.[32] Asymptomatic carriers should be treated with a luminal amebicide (iodoquinol, paromomycin, or diloxanide furoate) to prevent transmission.

Enterobius vermicularis

E. vermicularis, called pinworm in the United States and threadworm in Great Britain, resides in the colon. Eggs are deposited by the female worm in the perianal area. Most patients remain asymptomatic, but severe pruritus may develop. Stool surveys of homosexual men have shown a low prevalence of *E. vermicularis*, but the true prevalence may be much higher because the eggs are usually present only in the perianal area. Although pinworms generally cause only perianal symptoms, eosinophilic colitis has been described.[33] The diagnosis is made by microscopic exami-

nation of cellophane tape that has been pressed against the unwashed skin of the perianal area.

Treatment is a single dose of mebendazole (Vermox), 100 mg orally. Household members and sexual contacts should also be treated to prevent reinfection, and treatment should be repeated after 2 weeks. In case of recurrent pinworm infestation, a 3-month course of mebendazole, 100 mg once per month, should be considered.

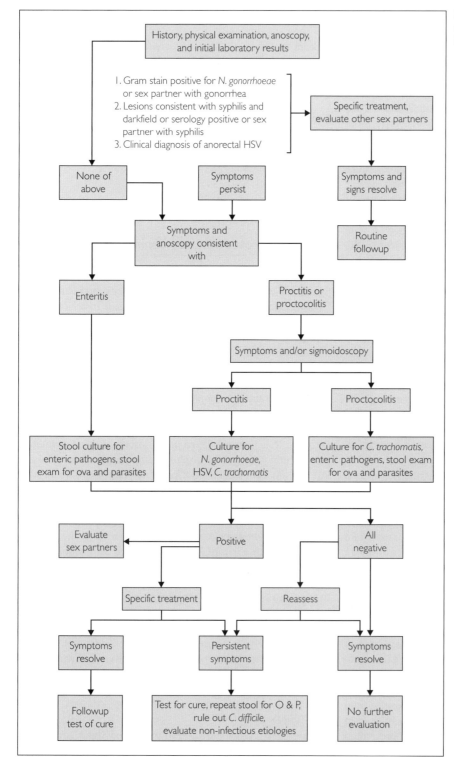

Fig. 64.4 ● Algorithm for evaluation of enteric symptoms after anal-receptive intercourse. HSV, herpes simplex virus; O & P, ova and parasites.

Anorectal lesions and proctocolitis in HIV-infected patients

HIV-infected patients with CD4-positive T-lymphocyte counts above 100 are subject to the same infections as HIV-negative patients. In patients with CD4 counts of less than 100, the most common viral cause of colitis is CMV, which can cause painful colitis or proctitis. Symptoms include crampy abdominal pain, diarrhea, bleeding, fever, and often tenesmus. Focal or diffuse colitis can be present, and ulcers can occur. Because antibodies to CMV are commonly found in patients with high-risk sexual practices, serology is not helpful and the diagnosis of colitis must be based on positive biopsies from the rectosigmoid or colonic mucosa.

Treatment with ganciclovir, 5 mg/kg intravenously every 12 h, is recommended. In a placebo-controlled, double-blind study in 62 patients, symptoms resolved during the first week of therapy. Ganciclovir-treated patients were also able to maintain body weight, in contrast to controls.[34] Induction therapy is given for 14–21 days, followed by maintenance treatment with ganciclovir, 5 mg/kg every 24 h. If CMV infection is resistant to ganciclovir, foscarnet, 90 mg/kg i.v. every 12 h, is given as induction therapy for 14–21 days, followed by maintenance treatment at a dose of 90 mg/kg every 24 h.[35]

In patients with acquired immunodeficiency syndrome, viral infections (HSV and condylomata acuminata) tend to follow a more aggressive course. Treatment, however, is the same as in HIV-negative patients. However, longer courses of therapy may be necessary.

Noninfectious proctitis

Trauma to the anorectum may occur after the insertion of foreign objects, as well as the hand or forearm, as part of sexual practices. Symptoms are similar to those with infectious causes of proctitis, and differentiation from infectious proctitis may be difficult. The presence of polymorphonuclear leukocytes in Gram-stained smears from rectal swabs usually does not occur in traumatic proctitis and indicates an infectious cause. Secondary infection of traumatic proctitis with colonic pathogens may occur. Treatment of traumatic proctitis is symptomatic, with sitz baths, ointments or suppositories containing a local anesthetic, and softening of the stool with bulk agents or stool softeners. Allergic proctitis may be caused by lubricants, including KY Jelly.[36] Soaps, oil, or medicinal cream may be directly irritating to the rectal mucosa. Suppositories containing 5-acetylsalicylic acid or steroids may accelerate the healing and resolution of symptoms.

GENERAL TREATMENT SUGGESTIONS

Patients should be educated on potential risks of sexual practices and counseled on ways to adopt safer sexual behavior. First-line treatment is symptomatic or empirical according to the clinical syndrome. When laboratory diagnostic capabilities are available, treatment decisions should be based on the specific diagnosis. Partners of patients with STDs should be evaluated for any diseases diagnosed in the index patient.

Acute proctitis of recent onset among persons who have recently practiced receptive anal intercourse is usually sexually acquired. The most common causes of proctitis in MSM are gonorrhea and chlamydia, followed by herpes and syphilis.[1] Thus, empirical

therapy is indicated, and should treat *N. gonorrhoeae* and *Chlamydia trachomatis* infections.[37] One regimen is ceftriaxone 125 mg i.m. (or another agent effective against rectal and genital gonorrhea) plus doxycycline 100 mg orally twice a day for 7 days.

Patients with suspected or documented herpes proctitis should be managed in the same manner as those with genital herpes (see treatment of HSV proctitis). If painful perianal ulcers are present or mucosal ulcers are seen on anoscopy, empiric therapy should include a regimen for treating genital herpes. Considering the frequency of HSV and the increased risk of HIV associated with HSV, empiric therapy for HSV should be considered.[38,39] Antiviral therapy has been nicely summarized in a recent review.[40] Finally, control of these infections requires changes in behavior and increased education.[41]

SUMMARY AND CONCLUSIONS

In patients with gastrointestinal symptoms and a history of anal-receptive intercourse, three infectious syndromes can be distinguished: enteritis, proctocolitis, and proctitis. Each of these syndromes may be caused by a certain range of pathogens. In immunocompromised patients, additional diseases must be considered. Figure 64.4 shows a useful algorithm for evaluation of these syndromes.

Clinical examination, a rectal swab with incubation in specific transport media, and Gram staining of mucus or pus from a rectal swab in combination with rectosigmoidoscopy are helpful in differentiating specific diseases. In the case of anorectal disease, stool cultures and serologic examination are of minor importance. Good treatments are available for most sexually transmitted anorectal diseases. An important role for the treating physician, however, is to educate patients about the possible risks of certain sexual practices and their prevention.

ACKNOWLEDGMENT

The authors would like to acknowledge the expert input of Jennifer Chang, Pharm D, Seattle, WA.

REFERENCES

1. Klausner JD, Kohn R, Kent C. Etiology of clinical proctitis among men who have sex with men. Clin Infect Dis 2004; 38(2):300–302.

2. Rompalo AM, Price CB, Roberts PL, et al. Potential value of rectal-screening cultures for *Chlamydia trachomatis* in homosexual men. J Infect Dis 1986; 153:888–892.

3. Echols RM, Heyd A, O'Keeffe BJ, et al. Single-dose ciprofloxacin for the treatment of uncomplicated gonorrhea: A worldwide summary. Sex Transm Dis 1994; 21:345–352.

4. Centers for Disease Control and Prevention. Increases in fluoroquinolone-resistant *Neisseria gonorrhoeae* among men who have sex with men – United States, 2003, and revised recommendations for gonorrhea treatment, 2004. MMWR Morb Mortal Wkly Rep 2004; 53(16):335–338.

5. Sexually transmitted diseases treatment guidelines. MMWR Morb Mortal Wkly Rep 2002; 51(RR-6):1–78.

   Emphasis on epidemiological aspects of STDs and education and counseling of patients and their partners.

6. Quinn TC, Corey L, Chaffee RH, et al. The etiology of anorectal infections in homosexual men. Am J Med 1981; 71:395–406.

This is the classic article describing the spectrum of anorectal infections and the three distinct clinical syndromes and correlation with microbial etiology.

7. Surawicz CM, Roberts PL, Rompalo A, et al. Intestinal spirochetosis in homosexual men. Am J Med 1987; 82:587–592.

8. Padmanabhan V, Dahlstrom J, Maxwell L, et al. Invasive intestinal spirochetosis: A report of three cases. Pathology 1996; 28:283–286.

9. Nielsen RH, Orholm M, Petersen JO, et al. Colorectal spirochetosis: Clinical significance of the infestation. Gastroenterology 1983; 85:62–67.

10. Lee FD, Kraszewski A, Godon J, et al. Intestinal spirochetosis. Gut 1971; 12:126–133.

11. Henrik-Nielsen R, Lundbeck FA, Teglbjaerg PS, et al. Intestinal spirochetosis of the vermiform appendix. Gastroenterology 1985; 88:971–977.

12. Cotton DWK, Kirkham N, Hicks DA. Rectal spirochaetosis. Br J Vener Dis 1984; 60:106–109.

13. Apoola A, Radcliffe K. Antiviral treatment of genital herpes. Int J STD AIDS 2004; 15:429–433.

14. Sacks SL. Famciclovir suppression of symptomatic and symptomatic recurrent anogenital herpes simplex virus shedding in women; a randomized, double-blind, double-dummy, placebo-controlled, parallel-group, single-center trial. J Infect Dis 2004; 189:1341–1347.

15. Stone KM. Epidemiologic aspects of genital HPV infection. Clin Obstet Gynecol 1989; 32:112–116.

16. Broker TR. Structure and genetic expression of papillomaviruses. Obstet Gynecol Clin North Am 1987; 14:329–348.

17. Syrjanen KJ. Epidemiology of human papillomavirus infections and their association with genital squamous cell cancer. APMIS 1989; 97:957–970.

18. Kiviat NB, Critchlow CW, Holmes KK, et al: Association of anal dysplasia and human papillomavirus with immunosuppression and HIV infection among homosexual men. AIDS 1993; 7:43–49.

19. Carr G, William DC. Anal warts in a population of gay men in New York City. Sex Transm Dis 1977; 4:56–57.

20. Gissmann L. Immunologic responses to human papillomavirus infection. Obstet Gynecol Clin North Am 1996; 23:625–639.

21. Munoz N, Bosch FX. HPV and cervical cancer: Review of case-control and cohort studies. In: Munoz N, Bosch FX, Shah KV, et al., eds. The epidemiology of human papillomavirus and cervical cancer. Vol 119. Lyon, France: IARC; 1992: 251–261.

22. Vincent-Salomon A, de la Rochefordiere A, Salmon R, et al. Frequent association of human papillomavirus 16 and 18 DNA with anal squamous cell and basaloid carcinoma. Mod Pathol 1996; 9:614–620.

23. Daling JR, Madeleine MM, Johnson LG, et al. Human papillomavirus, smoking, and sexual practices in the etiology of anal cancer. Cancer 2004; 101:270–280.

Epidemiological studies of anal cancer (population-based, cased-controlled) provide further evidence for the likely etiology of HPV and associated risk factors of cigarette smoking, anal intercourse, and numbers of lifetime sexual partners.

24. Daling JR, Sherman KJ, Hislop TG, et al. Cigarette smoking and the risk of anogenital cancer. Am J Epidemiol 1992; 135:180–189.

25. Berry JM, Palefsky JM, Welton ML. Anal cancer and its precursors in HIV-positive patients: perspective and management. Surg Oncol Clin N Am 2004; 13:355–373.

26. Fleshner PR, Freilich MI. Adjuvant interferon for anal condyloma. Dis Colon Rectum 1994; 37:1255–1259.

27. Drew WL, Mintz L, Miner RC, et al. Prevalence of cytomegalovirus infection in homosexual men. J Infect Dis 1981; 143:188–192.

28. Diepersloot RJA, Kroes ACM, Visser W, et al. Acute ulcerative proctocolitis associated with primary cytomegalovirus infection. Arch Intern Med 1990; 150:1749–1751.

29. Allason-Jones E, Mindel A, Sargeaunt P, et al. *Entamoeba histolytica* as a commensal intestinal parasite in homosexual men. N Engl J Med 1986; 315:353–356.

30. Allason-Jones E, Mindel A, Sargeaunt P, et al. Outcome of untreated infection with *Entamoeba histolytica* in homosexual men with and without HIV antibody. Br Med J 1988; 297:654–657.

31. Flores BM, Reed SL, Ravdin JI, et al. Serologic reactivity to purified recombinant and native 29-kilodalton peripheral membrane protein of pathogenic *Entamoeba histolytica*. J Clin Microbiol 1993; 31:1403–1407.

32. Drugs for parasitic infections. The Medical Letters Drugs and Therapeutics. New Rochelle: The Medical Letter, Inc; 2002.

33. Liu LX, Chi J, Upton MP, et al. Eosinophilic colitis associated with larvae of the pinworm *Enterobius vermicularis*. Lancet 1995; 346:410–412.

34. Dieterich DT, Kotler DP, Busch DF, et al. Ganciclovir treatment of cytomegalovirus colitis in AIDS: A randomized, double-blind, placebo-controlled multicenter study. J Infect Dis 1993; 167:278–282.

35. Romanowski B, Aoki FY, Martel AY, et al. Efficacy and safety of famciclovir for treating mucocutaneous herpes simplex infection in HIV-infected individuals. AIDS 2000; 14(9):1211–1217.

36. Fisher AA, Brancaccio RR. Allergic contact sensitivity to propylene glycol in a lubricant jelly. Arch Dermatol 1979; 115:1451.

37. Rompalo AM. Diagnosis and treatment of sexually acquired proctitis and proctocolitis: an update. Clin Infect Dis 1999; 28(Suppl 1):S84–S90.

Recommends empirical therapy for acute proctitis in MSM, covering *N. gonorrhoeae* and *C. trachomatis* infections.

38. Celum CL. The interaction between herpes simplex virus and human immunodeficiency virus. Herpes 2004; 11(Suppl 1):36A–45A.

Reviews interactions of HSV and HIV; with the former increasing the risk of acquiring HIV, coinfected individuals are at increased risk of HSV reactivation.

39. Renzi C, Douglas JM Jr, Foster M, et al. Herpes simplex virus type 2 infection as a risk factor for human immunodeficiency virus acquisition in men who have sex with men. J Infect Dis 2003; 187:19–25.

40. DeClercq E. Antiviral drugs in current clinical use. J Clin Virol 2004; 30:115–133.

Excellent review of chemotherapy for viral infections; important given large number of new antiviral therapies.

41. Donovan B. Sexually transmissible infections other than HIV. Lancet 2004; 363:545–556.

65

Lower gastrointestinal bleeding

Adam Slivka and Robert E. Schoen

INTRODUCTION

Lower gastrointestinal (LGI) bleeding can be defined as bleeding with an origin distal to the ligament of Treitz. It accounts for approximately 0.5% of all short-term hospital admissions in the United States.[1] Improvements in diagnostic testing, including advancements in endoscopic techniques, radionuclide scanning, and angiography, have increased the success rate for identifying a source for LGI bleeding over the past 20 years from 70% to approximately 90%.[2–4]

LGI bleeding, unlike upper gastrointestinal (GI) bleeding, requires more diagnostic tests and a much greater expenditure of time and resources to localize the source. The average length of stay for LGI bleeding in one Canadian series was 7.5 days.[5] Small bowel bleeding, in particular, is associated with an even greater amount of resource utilization, in comparison to upper or colonic bleeding.[6] The difficulty in localization of LGI bleeding is due to the presence of fecal material in the colon, the large surface area of the colon, and the inaccessibility of the small intestine to direct endoscopic examination. The recent development and dissemination of wireless capsule endoscopy (CE) has allowed for a more detailed examination of the entire small bowel in a noninvasive fashion and has identified sources of LGI bleeding previously considered of obscure origin. The clinical features of LGI bleeding are dependent on the rate and quantity of blood loss and span the spectrum from Hemoccult-positive stools in an asymptomatic individual to an exsanguinating hemorrhage manifested as profound shock. The choice of diagnostic evaluation is based on the condition of the patient, local availability and expertise, and the appropriateness of the diagnostic modality to the specific situation. This chapter focuses on the therapeutic approach to LGI bleeding. We review the clinical entities associated with LGI bleeding; outline an approach to patients with LGI bleeding, including the patient history, physical examination, and initial management; and focus on diagnostic evaluation and therapeutic options, including consideration of newer modalities for the treatment of LGI hemorrhage.

ETIOLOGY AND TREATMENT

Diverticulosis

Diverticular bleeding is one of the most common causes of LGI bleeding (Table 65.1), although data obtained before the availability of angiography and colonoscopy, which relied on barium studies,

may have overestimated its true incidence.[1] The incidence of diverticulosis increases with age and affects 50% of individuals older than 60 years who are consuming a Western diet.[7–9] Only 3–5% of patients with diverticular disease will bleed significantly.[4,10,11]

Diverticula develop from herniation of the colonic mucosa through defects in the muscularis propria, usually at the site of perforating vessels entering the bowel wall from the mesentery. As diverticula expand, the arterioles (vasa recta) that penetrate the colonic mucosa become increasingly exposed and are prone to rupture.[12]

Bleeding is likely to be independent of an inflammatory process in as much as significant hemorrhage occurs only rarely in the settling of diverticulitis.[13] The frequency with which diverticulosis is encountered decreases as one moves from the distal to the proximal end of the colon; involvement of the sigmoid colon is seen in the approximately 90% of individuals with diverticulosis, whereas the right colon is affected in only 15%.[14] A striking geographic distribution in the prevalence of diverticulosis is also evident, with Western countries being affected at a much higher rate than Asia and Africa, where the prevalence is less than 1% of the total population.[15,16] The putative factors that contribute to this marked variation are presumably related to the amount of fiber in the diet which, by affecting intraluminal pressure, may reduce the proclivity for diverticula formation.[17–19]

Diverticular bleeding can be massive. One study reported a mean transfusion requirement of 6–7 U of blood for diverticular hemorrhage.[20] Although the majority of diverticula are localized to the sigmoid colon, diverticular bleeding emanates from the right colon in approximately 70% of cases.[21] Typically, patients have a sudden onset of painless rectal bleeding, with bright red blood or maroon stool. Although the vast majority of this bleeding is self-limited, one large study has suggested that younger patients have a lower propensity for spontaneous resolution than do patients older than 40 years.[22] Recurrent hemorrhage occurs in approximately 40% of patients during the first year of follow-up.[23,24]

Nuclear scintigraphy and arteriography are positive in fewer than 50% of cases[20,25–31] in as much as diverticular bleeding has often ceased by the time that the patient is referred for radiologic studies. If active arterial bleeding is demonstrated during angiography, therapy can be applied successfully in over 90% of cases with either infusion of vasopressin (0.2–0.4 U/min) or embolization with absorbable gelatin sponge (Gelfoam) or coils.[20,32–36] During angiography, the superior mesenteric artery should be the first vessel selectively injected because the most common site of bleeding

Table 65.1 Common causes of lower gastrointestinal bleeding

Diverticulosis

Vascular anomalies
  Angiodysplasia
  Hemorrhoids
  Dieulafoy's lesions
  Radiation enterocolitis
  Portal enterocolopathy
  Varices
  Arterioenteric fistulas

Inflammatory and immune
  Ulcerative colitis
  Crohn's disease
  Vasculitis
  Diversion colitis
  Infectious diarrhea
  Graft-versus-host disease
  Mechanical and traumatic
  Postpolypectomy/postbiopsy
  Solitary rectal ulcer
  NSAID-induced enterocolopathy

Neoplasia
  Polyps
  Primary malignancy
  Metastatic cancer

Ischemia
  Arterial thrombus
  Arterial embolus
  Venous thrombus

Meckel's diverticulum

Endometriosis

NSAID, nonsteroidal antiinflammatory drug.

is in the right colon. If superior mesenteric artery injection fails to demonstrate a bleeding site, efforts should be made to inject the inferior mesenteric artery to determine whether the left colon is the source.

Colonoscopy is an important component in the evaluation of possible diverticular bleeding. Emergency purge colonoscopy may be used as the initial study in patients with suspected acute diverticular hemorrhage.[37] It may be performed in the acute setting concurrently with initial resuscitation and stabilization. Theoretically, one can visualize both active bleeding from diverticula and stigmata of recent hemorrhage during colonoscopy.[38] A shallow ulceration adjacent to a diverticulum with an adherent clot or visible vessel is indicative of recent hemorrhage. Savides and colleagues[39] reported successful colonoscopic hemostasis of diverticular hemorrhage in three patients by coaptive coagulation of identified visible vessels with a multipolar probe. A retrospective study of 13 patients who underwent successful colonoscopic hemostatic management of acute diverticular bleeding with adrenaline injection and/or multipolar electrocoagulation found that 5/13 (38%) re-bled within 30 days, 4 of whom required surgery, and an additional 3 patients (23%) had late re-bleeding.[40] At present, published experience with these modalities is limited, and no prospective data comparing colonoscopic therapy with conservative management or surgery are available. Colonoscopic therapy for diverticular bleeding may be

attempted by experienced endoscopists when encountered in the acute setting. The authors suspect that interventions with hemoclips may be the safest modality for therapeutic intervention, but because of the difficulties in identifying the precise source of diverticular bleeding, it is our opinion that endoscopic therapy is unlikely to become a successful mode of therapy for the majority of cases of diverticular hemorrhage. For patients with continued hemorrhage that cannot be controlled with other modalities or in patients with recurrent bleeding, surgical management is definitive. Accurate preoperative localization reduces operative morbidity and mortality.[41–43]

Small bowel diverticulosis

Bleeding from small bowel diverticula is uncommon, with scattered case reports and small series found in the literature.[44–47] The mechanism of formation of these diverticula, which are most commonly seen in the jejunum, is unknown, but presumably due to increased intraluminal pressure, perhaps related to an underlying myopathy or neuropathy.[48–50] Like colonic diverticular bleeding, hemorrhage may be seen when ulceration at the neck of a diverticulum erodes into penetrating arterioles.[51] Bleeding is painless and may be manifested as massive hematochezia or intermittent melena; hematemesis is less common.[52–54] Localization of a small bowel source may be made at enteroscopy, angiography, or nuclear scanning, and the presence of small bowel diverticulosis detected during routine barium studies, along with documented small intestinal bleeding, should raise suspicion for this diagnosis.[47] With accurate localization, surgical resection with primary anastomosis is curative.[44,53,54] In the rare instance when active small diverticular bleeding is encountered during enteroscopy, coaptive coagulation or injection therapy may be used.

Vascular anomalies

Angiodysplasia

Vascular lesions of the colon are the most common source for lower intestinal bleeding.[1] Vascular lesions and diverticulosis combined account for two-thirds of hemodynamically significant LGI bleeding.[4] They are also commonly identified small bowel lesions in patients with obscure GI bleeding undergoing wireless capsule endoscopy.[55] As noted in a comprehensive review,[1] the terminology for vascular lesions is not standardized. This section will consider angiodysplasia as ectatic changes in normal submucosal veins and mucosal capillaries. The lesions are thought to progress from venous ectasia located in the submucosal area to mucosal involvement of dilated veins, which is followed by progressive dilation of mucosal capillaries and, finally, in end-stage lesions, by dilation of arterioles, thus forming small arteriovenous fistulas.

Identification of vascular lesions can be made either angiographically or endoscopically. However, in the vast majority of patients who have colonic angiodysplasia identified as their source of GI bleeding by colonoscopy, antecedent angiography had failed to detect lesions consistent with that diagnosis.[56,57]

The endoscopic appearance of angiodysplasia has been described as flat or slightly raised red lesions that range in size from 2 to 10 mm in diameter. A spider-like appearance or fern-like margins have been described (Fig. 65.1), and a tortuous feeding arteriole or prominent straight vein may be seen.[1,57,58] With regard to their endoscopic appearance, as was highlighted in an editorial,[59] the

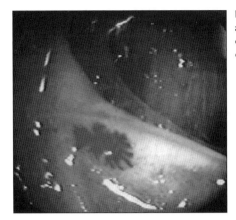

Fig. 65.1 • A jejunal angiodysplasia encountered during enteroscopy.

lack of objectivity in the past literature raises serious concerns regarding what constitutes an angiodysplastic lesion. Photography at colonoscopy has not been used to objectively categorize the appearance of angiodysplastic lesions in a blinded fashion. Therefore, it can be assumed that lesions created from scope tip trauma, suction trauma, nasogastric tube trauma, and submucosal hemorrhage may have been mistakenly identified as angiodysplasia in many previously reported series.

The vast majority of angiodysplastic lesions are found in the right colon of elderly individuals. Multiple lesions are often found.[1,60] The predominance of angiodysplasia in the right colon is hypothesized to be the result of increased wall tension in this part of the colon.[61]

The clinical manifestation of bleeding from colonic angiodysplasia includes hemodynamically significant hematochezia (approximately 15%), melena (up to 26%), Hemoccult-positive stool (up to 47%), and iron deficiency anemia (up to 51%).[1,4,57,62] The probability of recurrent hemorrhage is unpredictable, although median values from pooled series indicate that approximately 50% of patients will re-bleed. The diagnosis is frequently delayed, and active bleeding at angiography is seen in fewer than 20% of patients.[4,62–64] Colonoscopy remains the best single test for the diagnosis and treatment of colonic angiodysplasia.

When evaluating a patient for angiodysplasia during colonoscopy, care must be taken to avoid mucosal trauma. Some investigators believe that the use of meperidine is contraindicated during colonoscopy in search of angiodysplasia because meperidine may cause a transient decrease in colonic blood flow and thus result in blanching of angiodysplastic lesions.[64,65] It has been suggested that the administration of naloxone may improve the detection of angiodysplasia during colonoscopy; however, this practice has

not gained wide acceptance.[66] The overall sensitivity of colonoscopy in detecting angiodysplasia is variable, but generally approaches 80%.[38,57,59]

Thermal ablation is the most widely accepted technique for treatment of bleeding angiodysplasia.[67–76] The success of colonoscopic therapy has ranged between 50% and 90%, although re-bleeding remains a significant problem and may be encountered in up to 50% of patients. Early reports described the use of hot biopsy forceps for thermal ablation of angiodysplasia.[67–69,71,75] However, this technique should be discouraged because monopolar therapy is associated with increased depth of tissue injury, which is not needed for these superficial lesions and may increase the risk of perforation, particularly in the right colon. These initial series were followed by reports of the use of both argon and Nd:YAG lasers. More recent reports demonstrate the effectiveness of thermal devices such as multipolar electrocoagulation and the argon plasma coagulator (Table 65.2).[58,70,72,77] We recommend these modalities as the most cost-effective and convenient forms of therapy for the management of colonic angiodysplasia. Unlike therapy for upper GI bleeding from ulcers, where the principle of coaptive coagulation of submucosal arterioles is critical, lower energy for short duration with minimal pressure is all that is required to ablate these superficial lesions. Care must be taken to avoid deeper tissue injury, particularly in the right colon, where perforation may be seen in 2.4% of patients.[60] If these lesions are found at angiography and active bleeding is present, therapy can be administered in the form of vasopressin infusion or transcatheter embolization.

Several case reports and small series describe the use of conjugated estrogens or other synthetic preparations to treat individuals with bleeding presumed to be due to angiodysplasia.[78–81] Two prospective controlled studies[82,83] offer conflicting results, the larger of which[83] failed to demonstrate reduced bleeding with hormonal therapy. Finally, for isolated lesions that defy attempts at endoscopic hemostasis or that re-bleed on multiple occasions, bowel resection may prove definitive.

Hemorrhoids

Hemorrhoids occur in over 50% of individuals in the United States, and bleeding internal hemorrhoids are the most common cause of LGI hemorrhage in adults.[84,85] A number of explanations for the pathogenesis of hemorrhoids have been proposed.[86–89] Hemorrhoidal bleeding may be significant, but in the absence of a bleeding diathesis, it rarely causes hemodynamically compromising hemorrhage. Iron deficiency anemia associated with hemorrhoidal bleeding has been reported.[86] The presence of hemorrhoids in a patient with hematochezia should not dissuade

Table 65.2 Endoscopic thermal therapy for angiodysplasia and radiation proctitis

Instrument	Energy	Duration	Apposition
BICAP probe	10–15 W	1 s pulses	Light
Heater probe	5–15 J	2-s pulses	Light
Nd:YAG laser	40–60 W	0.2–1 s	Noncontact (1–4 mm)
Argon plasma coagulator			
Right colon	35–40 W Flow, 0.4–1.4 L/min	1 s	Noncontact (1–4 mm)
Rectum	60–80 W Flow, 1.4–2 L/min	1 s	Noncontact (1–4 mm)

one from further evaluation (such as flexible sigmoidoscopy or colonoscopy) to exclude additional colonic pathology because of the high prevalence of colonic polyps. Rigid proctoscopy is superior to flexible sigmoidoscopy in diagnosing bleeding internal hemorrhoids.[90]

A variety of modalities have been used to treat recurrent hemorrhoidal bleeding.[85,91–100] Conservative therapy consists of topical antiinflammatory agents and increased fiber in the diet. Stool softeners may be palliative for patients with obstipation. Rubber band ligation can be performed on internal hemorrhoids and may be applied during flexible endoscopy. However, caution must be taken to avoid banding external hemorrhoids because of the risk of forming anal strictures. Successful treatment with injection sclerotherapy, cryosurgery, electrocoagulation laser ablation, and photocoagulation has been described.[91–100] Thermal modalities may be delivered directly at anoscopy or during flexible endoscopy. Finally, excisional therapy may be required.

Dieulafoy's lesions

Dieulafoy's lesions are a recognized source of upper GI bleeding[101–104] and are discussed in Chapter 21. These lesions are characterized by congenitally and/or acquired abnormally enlarged or caliber-persistent arterioles running within the submucosa. They have also been described as a source of bleeding in the small bowel and colon.[105–112] Therapy for these lesions should start with submucosal[113] circumferential adrenaline injection (1:10 000) in a quantity of 2–20 mL. Coaptive coagulation should be applied. Alternatively, mechanical devices such as the band ligator or hemoclips can be used. We caution against the use of sclerosant agents, including absolute alcohol, in the colon and small bowel because the depth of injury is more difficult to control.[114] Surgical backup is advisable when attempting to treat these lesions.

Radiation colopathy

Incidental exposure of the bowel to therapeutic radiation, used to treat solid tumors or during preparation for bone marrow transplantation, may result in chronic bowel injury that is frequently manifested as LGI bleeding. Two potential mechanisms explain the etiology of the bleeding: (1) direct injury to the endothelium causing thrombosis of end arterioles and resulting ischemic damage;[115] and (2) the development of mucosal telangiectasias, probably a consequence of chronic ischemia, which occurs in up to 55% of patients.[116] Symptoms, typically bleeding, may occur between 6 and 18 months after exposure and are rarely seen in patients who receive a total radiation dose of less than 4000 rad.[116–119] A common scenario is rectal bleeding and tenesmus in an elderly man after radiation therapy for prostate cancer.

Although medical therapy with systemic or local steroids, sucralfate enemas, and oral sulfasalazine has been reported to be useful in the treatment of radiation enterocolonopathy,[120,121] their efficacy remains speculative. Endoscopic treatment consists of ablation of vascular lesions with the Nd:YAG or argon plasma coagulator or other thermal devices.[73,122–124] Multiple lesions covering large surface areas are commonly detected, and several treatment sessions are sometimes required. It is the authors' opinion that radiation colitis should be treated endoscopically and that no reliable data suggest a benefit to adjuvant medical therapy, even immediately after thermal ablation. The authors prefer using a multipolar probe (Table 65.3) and applying gentle tangential pressure with the tip of the probe in a 'painting' maneuver (Fig. 65.2) or using the argon plasma coagulator. Finally, surgical treatment may be considered but is associated with significant morbidity and a high incidence of anastomotic complications.[124,125]

Portal hypertensive colopathy

Mucosal lesions have been reported in the upper GI tract of patients with portal hypertension, including esophageal, gastric, and duodenal varices; portal hypertensive gastropathy; and gastric antral vascular ectasia (watermelon stomach). Similar lesions have also been reported to occur in the proximal portion of the small bowel and the colon of patients with portal hypertension, and have been postulated to contribute to LGI bleeding.[126–131] Kozarek and associates described colonoscopic findings in 20 patients with portal hypertension and LGI bleeding.[127] Seventy percent of these patients had multiple vascular ecstatic lesions, whereas 20% had a more diffuse process consisting of mucosal granularity, erythema, and friability. Biopsies of these lesions showed mucosal edema and dilated capillaries with minimal chronic inflammation, thus supporting the presumed diagnosis of portal hypertensive colopathy. Two patients with hemorrhagic ecstatic lesions were successfully treated with

---

Table 65.3 Clinical findings versus age for common causes of lower gastrointestinal bleeding

Clinical finding	Cause of bleeding			
	Child	Young adult	Middle-age	Elderly
Abdominal pain	IBD Intussusception	IBD	IBD	Ischemia
Painless	Meckel's diverticulum Juvenile polyp	Meckel's diverticulum Polyp	Diverticulosis Polyp Malignancy	Angiodysplasia Diverticulosis Polyp Malignancy
Diarrhea	IBD Infection	IBD Infection	IBD Infection	Ischemia Infection
Constipation/dyschezia	Fissure	Hemorrhoids Fissure Rectal ulcer	Hemorrhoids Fissure	Malignancy Hemorrhoids Fissure

IBD, inflammatory bowel disease.

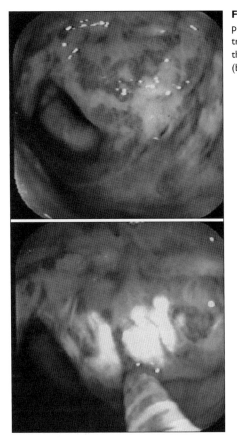

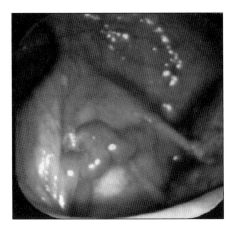

Fig. 65.2 • Radiation proctitis (above) treated with a bipolar thermal probe (below).

Fig. 65.3 • Colonic varix in a patient with cirrhosis and portal hypertension.

heater probe therapy. However, as with portal hypertensive gastropathy, it is likely that effective therapy will consist of modalities directed at lowering portal pressure or alleviating the underlying liver disease. Thus for acute bleeding, pharmacologic management with somatostatin or vasopressin should be initiated, and surgical shunts, transjugular intrahepatic portocaval shunts, or orthotopic liver transplantation should be considered for refractory cases. Colonoscopic therapy should be attempted in rare cases in which point hemorrhage is visualized. Although not formally evaluated, therapy with nonselective β-blockers aimed at decreasing the resting pulse by 25% appears reasonable.

Colonic and small bowel varices

Another source of LGI bleeding in portal hypertensive patients is colonic (Fig. 65.3) or small intestinal varices. Varices are less common in the small intestine and rare in the colon, but are occasionally seen in the rectum. An autopsy study suggested an incidence of 0.07% for colonic varices in patients with portal hypertension.[132] A number of case reports have described LGI bleeding from colonic varices, with the most common site being the rectosigmoid region.[133–137] In patients who have undergone colostomy or enterostomy, peristomal varices may develop and can bleed significantly. The vast majority of patients with small bowel or colonic varices have portal hypertension related to chronic liver disease.[133–137] However, a variety of other etiologies have been reported, including portal vein obstruction, congestive heart failure, mesenteric vein thrombosis, postoperative adhesions, splenic vein thrombosis, and familial colonic varices in the absence of portal hypertension.[137–144] During colonoscopy, these lesions are identified as enlarged submucosal vascular structures and may demonstrate the typical stigmata of recent or impending hemorrhage (hemocystic spots, red wales, or adherent clots).[133] Colonoscopic sclerotherapy for actively bleeding varices has been advocated, as have band ligation, shunt surgery, and surgical devascularization.[133,145–147] The authors have had experience with banding varices, even in the right colon, with good success. The optimal treatment modality is unknown, but as with portal hypertensive colonopathy, pharmacologic, radiologic, and surgical modalities for lowering portal pressure are the mainstays of therapy.

Arterioenteric fistulas

Arterioenteric fistulas are a rare cause of catastrophic intestinal bleeding.[148–152] Most common in the aorta, these lesions may be subdivided into primary and secondary fistulas. The former are less common and involve the primary erosion of an abdominal aortic aneurysm into the intestinal lumen. Seventy-five percent of cases occur in the third and fourth portion of the duodenum; however, erosion into more distal parts of the small bowel and colon has been reported.[149,151] Secondary fistulas occur after aortic reconstructive surgery, possibly as a result of inflammatory reactions from a suture line or from erosion of the graft itself through the intestinal lumen, most commonly occurring in the proximal portion of the graft.[148] An infected prosthesis may predispose to this condition and is associated with an increase in mortality.[152] Clinically, it has been suggested that patients may have a 'herald bleed' that precedes an exsanguinating hemorrhage by hours to days. It is, however, impossible to verify this pattern because of the low incidence of preoperative diagnosis (one-third of cases) and the rare occurrence of this condition in general. If suspected, computed tomography with contrast aortography should be performed. Once the diagnosis is made, plans for prompt operative repair should be initiated because endotherapy has no role in the treatment of arterioenteric fistulas.[148,153,154] Even with prompt surgery, the overall mortality associated with bleeding from aortoenteric fistulas exceeds 50%.

Other vascular lesions

A variety of vascular lesions may be found in isolation or in association with systemic diseases, including angioma, hamartoma, hemangioma, hemangioendothelioma, hemangiosarcoma, blue rubber bleb nevi, dystrophic angiectasia, and hemorrhagic telangiectasia (Rendu-Osler-Weber syndrome). A more detailed description of these unusual conditions can be found in comprehensive reviews.[155]

Inflammatory and immune causes

Inflammatory bowel disease

GI blood loss is a common feature of inflammatory bowel disease; however, massive GI hemorrhage requiring transfusion and manifested as shock is relatively uncommon.[156–158] Interestingly, the incidence of such bleeding is similar for Crohn's disease and ulcerative colitis and has been reported in up to 6% of cases.[159–167] Although bleeding may subside with the rapid institution of aggressive medical therapy, profuse bleeding has been used as an indication for surgery, more frequently in ulcerative colitis than Crohn's disease, where total colectomy is curative. Massive bleeding in patients with Crohn's disease is more likely to be found in the colon, and one study supports early colectomy for massive LGI bleeding in Crohn's disease because of a significant incidence of re-bleeding and poor outcome in those treated nonoperatively.[156] In that study, because of significant inflammation throughout the colon, localization studies were of limited value, and the precise point of bleeding was not found in the majority of patients. Furthermore, the delay in instituting definitive therapy increased blood transfusion requirements and resulted in greater patient morbidity. For these reasons, in patients with defined inflammatory bowel disease who have hemodynamically significant bleeding, an emergent attempt at localization of the site of bleeding is essential and early surgical consultation mandatory.[168]

Vasculitis

A variety of systemic vasculitides can precipitate GI hemorrhage.[169–186] Vascular inflammation leads to mucosal ischemia and ulceration and results in pain and/or bleeding. Obviously, the presence of significant small intestinal ischemia with resultant infarction must be treated as a surgical emergency. The presence of GI involvement in systemic vasculitis in the absence of life-threatening hemorrhage or small bowel ischemia warrants consideration of systemic therapy with immunosuppressive agents.

Diversion colitis

When colonic mucosa is surgically isolated from the normal fecal effluent, it may become inflamed and ulcerated, cause abdominal pain, mucoid discharge, and rectal bleeding, and is termed diversion colitis.[187–189] This sequence of events occurs most commonly in the rectosigmoid colon after a diverting colostomy. Histologically and endoscopically, the findings may be indistinguishable from those of inflammatory bowel disease. The presumed pathogenic mechanism is short-chain fatty acid deficiency and is supported by the resolution of symptoms and gross injury after the administration of 60 mL enemas twice daily for 1 month made up of short-chain fatty acids consisting of sodium acetate (60 mmol/L), sodium propionate (30 mmol/L), and sodium N-butyrate (40 mmol/L), pH adjusted to 7.0[190,191] Restoration of normal fecal flow results in complete resolution of this condition.[192]

Infectious diarrhea

Any enteroinvasive infection is capable of disrupting mucosal integrity to the point of causing LGI hemorrhage. Although the bleeding is rarely hemodynamically significant, in patients with an underlying coagulopathy or an immunocompromised state, bleeding may be massive and is usually seen arising from focal ulceration.[193]

Graft-versus-host disease

In both its acute and, less commonly, chronic form, graft-versus-host-disease may cause hemodynamically significant GI hemorrhage.[194–196] Bleeding is exacerbated by the coagulopathy that is often present in the patient population susceptible to this entity. In one case report, segmental erosive ulcerative lesions in the jejunum, terminal ileum, and cecum were responsible for massive hemorrhage.[195] Management consist of immunosuppressive therapy and blood product support in as much as these patients are rarely candidates for surgery.

Mechanical and traumatic causes

Postpolypectomy and postbiopsy bleeding

LGI bleeding may be seen as a complication of colonoscopy after biopsy or polypectomy (Fig. 65.4).[197–202] Bleeding after biopsy or polypectomy may occur immediately or be delayed by over 2 weeks after the procedure. Immediate bleeding is easier to manage than delayed bleeding for the following reasons: (1) immediate recognition of bleeding, (2) immediate localization of bleeding, (3) immediate application of hemostatic therapy, (4) a prepared colon, and (5) more ready access to other modalities, including angiography and surgery. If hemorrhage occurs after removal of a pedunculated polyp, the easiest and fastest hemostatic maneuver is to gently grasp the stalk with the snare and provide continuous pressure for several minutes. The snare is then carefully released to see whether bleeding recurs. If it does, repeat pressure is applied for 10 min while preparation for additional measures ensues.[203] We prefer to inject the stalk at its base with 2–20 mL of either normal saline or 1:10 000 adrenaline. The injection should be submucosal and a 'ballooning up' of the mucosa should be easily visible. Thermal coaptive coagulation with a BICAP or heat probe may then be applied to the cut surface. Alternatively, band ligation or hemoclips may be used. For bleeding sessile polypectomy sites, injection followed by thermal therapy or use of hemoclips is appropriate. Prophylactic placement of endoloops may be applied to the stalk of large pedunculated polyps prior to snare excision.

The majority of postpolypectomy delayed bleeding resolves spontaneously without requiring blood transfusions or further intervention. For patients who continue to bleed and require intervention, colonoscopy can be used to locate and treat the site of hemorrhage. A small subset of patients will require surgery. In the opinion of the authors, colonoscopy should be the first diagnostic/therapeutic modality used in the localization and

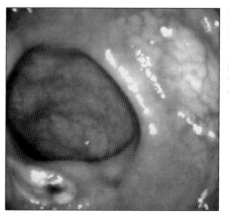

Fig. 65.4 • A flat red spot within a cautery ulcer 1 week after snare polypectomy complicated by delayed bleeding.

management of delayed postpolypectomy hemorrhage. The authors prefer to prepare patients with a polyethylene glycol electrolyte lavage solution. It has been suggested, however, that the procedure may be performed effectively even without prior oral purge[204] because the site of bleeding is predictable and the luminal blood may act as a cathartic to cleanse the bowel distal to the bleeding site. A variety of treatments may be applied to a bleeding polypectomy site, including adrenaline injection (2–20 mL) and the application of thermal methods, for example, a BICAP probe at 15–20 W. Newer devices that may be useful in preventing and treating postpolypectomy hemorrhage include the Endoloop, a detachable plastic loop left at the base of a polyp, and endoscopically delivered hemostatic clips.[77] One report described the adaptation of band ligation to arrest delayed bleeding polypectomy stalks that had failed traditional management.[205]

With regard to the prevention of postpolypectomy bleeding, one study examining the type of current used during polypectomy suggested that pure coagulative current was associated with an increased risk of delayed bleeding when compared with the use of blended current.[198] The cold snare technique is an alternative to snare cautery for the removal of small polyps (=5 mm).[206] Because of the absence of cautery, there is no possibility of progressive injury associated with the heating process, and delayed hemorrhage should not occur. However, the incidence of significant early bleeding after cold snare polypectomy has not been reliably documented but it is presumed to be infrequent. Patients are often instructed to stop aspirin prior to colonoscopy to decrease the incidence of postpolypectomy bleeding. However, a large case-controlled study found no significant increase in postpolypectomy bleeding attributed to aspirin.[207] In contrast, warfarin and plavix are contraindications to polypectomy.

NSAID-associated lower intestinal bleeding

The use of nonsteroidal antiinflammatory drugs (NSAIDs) may be associated with LGI bleeding[208] (see Ch. 19) by two distinct mechanisms: (1) an increased propensity for hemorrhage arising from existing lesions because of platelet inhibitory activity, and (2) a direct toxic mucosal effect giving rise to bleeding. Evidence exists to support both mechanisms as a cause of bleeding distal to the ligament of Treitz in patients with a history of NSAID intake.[209–215] Although better established as a cause of upper GI hemorrhage, epidemiologic studies have documented that patients evaluated for LGI bleeding from all causes are more likely to have a history of NSAID use when compared with control patients, with an odds ratio of approximately 2.0.[209] These studies did not take into account the source of the hemorrhage. A post hoc analysis of a randomized controlled trial of Naprosyn, a nonselective NSAID, and Rofecoxib, a COX-2 selective agent, in 8076 patients with rheumatoid arthritis found that serious lower GI events occurred at a rate of 0.9%/yr accounting for 40% of all serious GI events in patients taking a nonselective NSAID. The incidence of serious lower GI events was 54% lower with the use of the COX-2 selective agent.[210] In addition to bleeding, patients who use NSAIDs appear to be at a greater risk for idiopathic small intestinal and colonic perforations.[215] Although discrete NSAID-induced ulcers are found in these patients, a more diffuse lesion, similar to NSAID gastritis, may also be seen distal to the ligament of Treitz.[211–213] Diaphragmatic webs secondary to NSAID intake have also been described, and endoscopically, NSAID-induced injury can resemble inflammatory bowel disease. Finally, reports of exacer-

bation of pre-existing inflammatory bowel disease, with an increased propensity for hemorrhage, have also been noted.[216] Any patient with LGI bleeding should be questioned regarding the history of NSAID intake, including careful queries about over-the-counter preparations. Neither misoprostol nor omeprazole has proved effective in treating or preventing NSAID-associated LGI bleeding. The cornerstone of therapy remains discontinuation of use of the offending agent.

Neoplasia

Colonic or small bowel adenomas or adenocarcinomas rarely cause significant acute LGI bleeding.[41] Left-sided lesions, particularly in the rectum, are more likely to produce hematochezia, but it is rarely hemodynamically significant. A recent morphologic study determined that bleeding correlated with the surface area of colonic polyps and that the mechanism of bleeding was due to microerosion of neoplastic tissue through a thin surface epithelium.[217] If this erosion occurs in a small arteriole, bleeding may be significant. The diagnosis may be made at colonoscopy or angiography and treatment usually consists of surgical resection, or angiographic embolization in nonoperative candidates. Finally, for large villous lesions that produce significant GI bleeding, endoscopic therapy consisting of snare cautery excision or thermal ablation may result in diminished blood loss.[218]

Other nonepithelial neoplastic diseases may be characterized by significant bleeding, notably leiomyomas and leiomyosarcomas of the small bowel.[219–224] These lesions frequently grow to a large size before obstructive-type symptoms appear, and it is not uncommon for a significant portion of the tumor to extend into the extramural portion of the intestine, producing a so-called 'dumbell' tumor. Bleeding occurs when the tumor outgrows its blood supply, with resultant central necrosis and ulceration, which may involve a small feeding arteriole. The optimal therapy is surgical excision. Endoscopic ablative therapies and even diagnostic biopsies are ill advised because massive bleeding may ensue and endoscopic sampling is rarely adequate for diagnosis.

Unlike primary GI malignancy, metastatic tumors may be accompanied by significant bleeding.[225–229] Virtually all cancers have been reported to metastasize to the GI tract, with lung and breast cancer occurring most commonly because of their high prevalence. As a percentage, melanoma has the highest proclivity for GI metastases, with up to 50% of patients demonstrating GI metastatic disease at autopsy and the small intestine being the most common site.[227] In addition, melanoma metastatic to the intestine is reported to have a significant propensity to bleed. Renal cell carcinoma is another malignancy with a tendency to metastasize to the GI tract (Fig. 65.5), and metastatic disease has been reported in the stomach, duodenum, small intestine, and colon.[226,228–230] Therapy for massive bleeding from GI metastatic disease consists of angiographic embolization or surgical resection. Endoscopic ablation using multipolar electrocoagulation, the argon plasma coagulator, or photodynamic therapy may be effective in providing palliation.

Mesenteric ischemia

Gastrointestinal hemorrhage may be one of the initial manifestations of mesenteric ischemia.[137] In cases with acute occlusive mesenteric ischemia, pain precedes hemorrhage in the majority of patients.[231,232] Therefore, if the diagnosis is delayed until the onset of bloody diarrhea, which is indicative of small bowel necrosis, mortality increases significantly and surgical intervention is

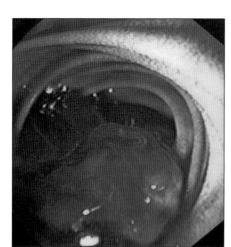

Fig. 65.5 • A large, bleeding renal cell carcinoma metastasis in the jejunum encountered during enteroscopy in the evaluation of recurrent lower gastrointestinal bleeding.

mandatory. In contrast, bloody diarrhea is a common sequela of mesenteric venous thrombosis and ischemic colitis.[233–237] Compared to small bowel ischemia, patients with colonic ischemia are older, more likely to present with overt bleeding, and are somewhat less likely to report abdominal pain.[238] Although endoscopy is important in establishing the diagnosis of ischemic colitis, endoscopic therapy for bleeding is rarely required.

Meckel's diverticulum

The most common complication of Meckel's diverticulum is hemorrhage, which usually occurs during childhood but has also been reported in adults.[137] Ectopic gastric mucosa within a diverticula produces acid that causes ulceration and hemorrhage in the adjacent ileal mucosa.[137,239,240] Traditionally, these are located within 100 cm of the ileocecal valve. The diagnosis is based on a high index of suspicion in the appropriate clinical setting and may be confirmed during angiography or suggested by a technetium pertechnetate scan that demonstrates heterotopic gastric mucosa, most commonly in the right lower quadrant.[241,242] Surgical resection is the definitive therapy.

Endometriosis

Endometriosis is a relatively common disease and affects up to 10% of menstruating women.[137,243–245] Endometrial implants on the serosa of the colon have been associated with lower quadrant abdominal pain and diarrhea. More significant involvement may cause extrinsic compression resulting in obstructive symptoms.[244,246] Colonic bleeding may arise when serosal implants expand through the entire thickness of the bowel to the mucosa and typically occur in the rectosigmoid region.[247–249] The most common manifestation is cyclic hematochezia.[250] Mucosal abnormalities may be seen during endoscopic evaluation, but pathognomonic endoscopic findings have not been described.[137,244] The findings are confirmed by biopsy, and although hormonal suppression may be attempted,[251,252] surgical resection of the involved area is the treatment of choice.

DIAGNOSTIC EVALUATION

Patient assessment

As in the management of acute upper GI hemorrhage, the most important step in the initial management of patients with LGI bleeding is assessment of the degree of volume loss and initiation of fluid resuscitation. Thus, determination of vital signs with assessment for orthostatic changes and physical stigmata of hypovolemia (pallor, loss of skin turgor, and drying of the mucous membranes) should be undertaken immediately on arrival at the emergency department. If signs of hemodynamic compromise are evident, two large-bore intravenous catheters should be inserted, preferably in large antecubital veins. Through these catheters, initial blood work, including type and cross-match, coagulation profile, hemogram, platelet count, and routine chemistry studies, can be obtained before the initiation of fluid resuscitation.

After this initial assessment, a more directed history and physical examination may help in differentiating potential causes of the bleeding to guide the subsequent diagnostic evaluation.

Characteristics of bleeding

Patients with LGI bleeding may describe stool characteristics that help determine the site of bleeding. It must be emphasized, however, that the character of the stool reflects not only the origin and volume of blood loss but bowel transit time as well.[253,254] Hematochezia is defined as the passage of bright red blood per rectum and generally suggests an LGI source. Nevertheless, between 5% and 20% of patients with upper GI bleeding may have hematochezia attributable to both the large quantity of blood and the rapid transit through the small intestine and colon.[37,41,255] These patients will usually have signs and symptoms of severe hemodynamic compromise. Melena is defined as 'tarry' stool that results from the bacterial degradation of intestinal hemoglobin and is described as the hallmark of upper GI bleeding. However, melena can be seen in small intestinal bleeding, as well as right-sided colonic bleeding, provided that colonic transit is slow. Patients with a history of melena should be questioned for iron and bismuth ingestion because these metals will also turn the stool black. However these substances will *not* result in a Hemoccult-positive stool. A maroon stool with clots usually suggests a colonic source but may be seen with massive small intestinal or upper GI bleeding. Blood dripping into the toilet after a bowel movement suggests an anal or perianal source, whereas blood-streaked stool usually indicates a source in the left colon. The validity of the subjective reporting of the color of stool by patients and physicians was evaluated with the use of an objective color card.[256] Considerable divergence was noted, although the objective instrument was more helpful in differentiating upper GI from colorectal bleeding than were traditional methods. Part of the difficulty is the proliferation of terms used to describe blood, for example, 'port-wine stool,' 'dark red,' or 'red-maroon.' To improve reporting consistency, it is the practice of the authors to instruct physicians in training and others to confine their description to black, maroon, or red.

PATIENT HISTORY

The cause of LGI hemorrhage varies with age (see Table 65.1). In very young patients, the history may uncover features consistent with inflammatory bowel disease, hereditary telangiectasia, Meckel's diverticulum, and juvenile polyps. In middle-aged patients, bleeding may emanate from hemorrhoids, polyps, inflammatory bowel disease, diverticula, and less often, malignancy. In the elderly, angiodysplasia, malignancy, ischemia, diverticulosis, and polyps are most common. The presence or absence of abdominal pain is a key feature of the history that can help differentiate the etiology of bleeding. Diffuse abdominal pain can be seen in ischemic bowel and inflammatory bowel disease (most often Crohn's disease). Dyschezia suggests a perirectal source and is more common with fissures than with hemorrhoids. Painless bleeding is common with diverticula, angiodysplasia, malignancy, polyps, and Meckel's diverticulum. A history of bloody diarrhea may suggest ulcerative colitis or infectious colitis, whereas a history of recent constipation may suggest hemorrhoidal bleeding, fissures, or a left-sided colonic malignancy. Other features of the history that should be elicited during the initial evaluation include the use of aspirin or NSAIDs; previous colonoscopy, sigmoidoscopy, or barium enema; the presence of symptoms suggesting extraintestinal manifestations of inflammatory bowel disease; a history of abdominal or vascular surgery or radiation therapy; and a family history of GI bleeding or GI malignancy.

PHYSICAL EXAMINATION

Findings on the initial physical examination will also be helpful. The skin should be examined for telangiectasias and extraintestinal manifestations of inflammatory bowel disease, including pyoderma gangrenosum and erythema nodosum, as well as cutaneous lesions indicative of vasculitis, such as palpable purpura and cutaneous infarcts, that might point to systemic disease. Looking for peripheral stigmata of portal hypertension is critical because finding positive signs broadens the differential diagnosis to include intestinal and colonic varices and portal hypertensive enterocolonopathy. Examination of the cardiovascular system should focus on the presence of peripheral pulses, as well as hemodynamic signs reflecting volume status. Examination of the abdomen should note the presence of any scars from previous surgery. Auscultation for abdominal bruits may indicate the presence of an aneurysm, arterioenteric fistula, or a vascular tumor. The characteristics of bowel sounds may also occasionally be helpful in that patients with small bowel bleeding will frequently have hyperactive bowel sounds (borborygmus) because of the rapid transit of a large volume of blood through the intestinal tract. The absence of bowel sounds in association with severe pain suggests an ischemic process. The abdomen should be palpated for hepatosplenomegaly, for the presence of focal or diffuse peritonitis, and for the presence of masses that might indicate malignancy or aneurysm. Finally, a digital rectal examination should be performed to assess the texture and color of the stool. Anascopy to detect the presence of rectal lesions may also be helpful.

INITIAL MANAGEMENT

As in upper GI bleeding, patients with significant LGI hemorrhage frequently require 'team' management, with multidisciplinary input from the consultation services of gastroenterologists, surgeons, and interventional radiologists. No standard algorithm exists for the management of patients with severe LGI bleeding. Rather, the management of such patients is frequently dependent on the availability and expertise at the individual institution. Gastroenterologists can offer rapid-purge colonoscopy, which has the potential to be both diagnostic and therapeutic. Nuclear medicine may be consulted for radionuclide scanning, and interventional radiologists should be notified if angiography might be considered. Finally, surgical consultation should be requested for all cases of severe LGI hemorrhage so that surgical options can be discussed at an early phase and patient care coordinated appropriately.

After fluid resuscitation and a history and physical examination, passage of a nasogastric tube to localize the site of bleeding should be considered. Gastric contents should be aspirated and examined for evidence of red blood, coffee-ground material, or bile. The absence of significant blood or coffee-ground material in the presence of bile significantly diminishes but does not exclude the possibility of hemorrhage proximal to the ligament of Treitz. Even if signs of upper GI bleeding are not seen, the possibility of a duodenal source must still be considered because up to 16% of patients with clear (although not bilious) gastric lavage fluid may have a duodenal site of bleeding subsequently identified.[257–259] Occult blood testing of a nasogastric aspirate is never indicated because simple passage of the tube frequently causes minor mucosal trauma to the nasal passages, posterior oropharynx, esophagus, and gastric lining and results in a positive test. An elevated blood urea nitrogen/serum creatinine ratio of 25:1 or greater is strongly suggestive of an upper source for bleeding,[260] although a recent study questions the discriminative ability of this ratio to differentiate upper from lower GI bleeding in patients with hematochezia.[261] If a bilious aspirate is obtained during nasogastric lavage, one may proceed cautiously under the premise that the source of bleeding is distal to the ligament of Treitz, provided the patient has no history of melena and an elevated blood urea nitrogen/serum creatinine ratio is not noted on initial laboratory testing. However, if an upper GI source of hemorrhage is suspected, urgent upper endoscopy should be performed.[262] If emergency purge colonoscopy is to be considered, the nasogastric tube should be left in place to facilitate the administration of a colonic lavage solution. If the history and physical examination suggest that the site of hemorrhage may be emanating from the anal canal or rectum, rigid anoscopy or flexible sigmoidoscopy can be performed to exclude lesions in this area. In this setting, however, reflux of blood from the rectum into the sigmoid colon, particularly in the setting of profuse bleeding, may make accurate interpretation of an unprepared proctosigmoidoscopy difficult, and in most instances one could proceed to colonoscopy.

The diagnostic strategy to use when evaluating patients with LGI hemorrhage varies with the patient's age, the rate of bleeding, and the available expertise. The natural history of LGI bleeding is similar to that of upper GI hemorrhage in that bleeding will cease spontaneously in up to 80% of cases.[25,41] Re-bleeding occurs in approximately 25% of cases but depends on the etiology of the bleed.[25] Mortality from LGI bleeding is proportional to the transfusion requirement and is dependent on accurate localization of the bleeding before definitive therapy.[41–43] Therefore, in patients with ongoing bleeding and hemodynamic instability, the localizing modality chosen should be available immediately and should be highly accurate to decrease the transfusion requirement and to provide information for subsequent definitive treatment, which includes surgery in up to two-thirds of cases.[20,26,55,153] The advantages and disadvantages of the various diagnostic modalities available for patients with LGI hemorrhage are reviewed in the following sections.

Barium studies

Barium studies have no role in the evaluation of acute LGI bleeding. A barium study cannot demonstrate active bleeding, is often technically inadequate in critically ill patients, and can obscure the results of subsequent angiography or colonoscopy. Barium studies should be used only in a nonemergency setting after other attempts have failed to localize a potential bleeding source.

Radionuclide scanning

Radionuclide scanning has been used in the diagnostic evaluation of patients with GI bleeding for over 30 years with conflicting results.[148] The concept is to inject a radioactive substance into the blood that can be detected as it enters the GI tract in a patient with active GI bleeding. Two agents have been extensively studied: technetium-99m sulfur colloid is an agent that is rapidly cleared from plasma by the reticuloendothelial system and accumulates in the liver and spleen, and technetium-99m-labeled red blood cells remain in the circulation for up to 48 h, thus allowing repeated visualization, which may be helpful in patients with intermittent bleeding. One advantage of the sulfur colloid technique is that it demonstrates a better signal-to-noise ratio for early studies (low background activity) and can thus demonstrate bleeding rates as low as 0.05–0.1 mL/min. The disadvantage of this modality is that rapid uptake in the liver and spleen makes localization difficult, particularly with bleeding sites in the upper part of the abdomen and transverse colon. For these reasons, since the mid-1980s, technetium-labeled red blood cell scans have become the procedure of choice at most institutions. Initial studies using this technique reported a sensitivity of approximately 90% for the detection of active GI bleeding.[263-267] Tagged red blood cell scans can detect from 0.1 to 0.5 mL/min of bleeding. However, subsequent studies have yielded conflicting results. For patients with positive radionuclide studies who undergo more definitive localization (arteriography, endoscopy, or surgery), the nuclear study is found to be inaccurate in 25–60% of cases.[27-30] Incorrect localization by radionuclide study has the additional disadvantage of misdirecting subsequent therapy and thus resulting in undesirable surgical outcomes in up to 42% of patients.[28]

In one study evaluating 153 patients with GI bleeding, 59% had positive technetium red blood cell scintigraphy.[31] These patients went on to have definitive diagnostic procedures, and nuclear scintigraphy had correctly identified the site of bleeding in 75%. In subsequent subgroup analysis, if the scan was positive within 2 h, the accuracy in localization of bleeding improved to 86%, and when upper GI bleeding was excluded, the radionuclide study was positive in 100% of patients (n=19). A more recent review of 16 studies found an average positive rate of 45%, and an accuracy in defining the location of bleeding in 78%.[268] Radionuclide scanning is often used as a gatekeeper to assess the utility of more invasive testing such as angiography. However, widely variable reports on the diagnostic accuracy of this procedure raise concern about the frequently used policy of routine nuclear scintigraphy before arteriography, particularly in patients who are massively bleeding and in whom rapid diagnosis and therapy are needed.

The authors advise particular caution in attaching significance to delayed scans. Such scans may demonstrate an enhanced signal in the right colon or more distally; such signal enhancement may occur as a result of prior bleeding rather than localize the source of the hemorrhage to this region. As with other diagnostic modalities, the availability and expertise of those performing and interpreting the scintigraphic scans are crucial, and such factors must be included in determining the algorithm that is used in the management of patients with LGI bleeding.

Angiography

Selective mesenteric angiography has remained a cornerstone in the localization and treatment of LGI hemorrhage for over 20 years.[148] Experimental studies have documented that angiography can detect bleeding at a rate as low as 0.5 mL/min, but more typically, its sensitivity is 1.0–2.0 mL/min.[269] Retrospective analyses have demonstrated variable diagnostic accuracy, with the site of active bleeding identified in up to 72% of cases.[3,20,26] Active arterial bleeding is required for positive angiographic localization. Most LGI bleeding is intermittent, and this property contributes to the lack of uniform success. Attempts have been made to improve the diagnostic accuracy of a negative study by pharmacologic manipulation of the patient's natural hemostatic mechanisms, systemic heparinization, intra-arterial vasodilators, or the use of thrombolytic agents during angiography.[207,271] At present, studies using such agents are small, and more experience is required to determine whether the presumed increase in bleeding complications that will ensue justifies their widespread use.

In addition to providing anatomic localization to direct subsequent therapy, angiography offers the benefit of local therapy, provided that selective arterial catheterization can be achieved. Hemostatic modalities include the infusion of vasopressin or selective embolization of an identified bleeding site with gelatin sponges, vascular coils, or polyvinyl alcohol particles. Vasopressin is a potent constrictor of arteriolar smooth muscle and, when infused at a rate of 0.2–0.4 U/min, has been shown to be effective in controlling acute arterial bleeding within 30 min of initiation.[269,272-276] This therapy has been demonstrated to be effective in up to 91% of patients with bleeding from diverticular disease or angiodysplasia.[20,32,33] Complications of this therapy include electrolyte disturbances from antidiuretic hormone activity (hyponatremia and water retention), cardiovascular complications including bradycardia and epicardial arterial spasm, systemic hypertension and resulting peripheral ischemia, and local complications including bowel ischemia and local catheter-related complications.[34] Finally, recurrent bleeding after discontinuation of vasopressin infusion may be seen in a minority of patients.

Embolization, initially developed in the 1970s and used in cases of failed therapy with vasopressin, has become increasingly popular in recent years because of the lack of requirement for an indwelling catheter and no systemic toxicity.[34-36] Unfortunately, results of pooled series using embolization therapy for colonic bleeding have demonstrated an infarction rate of 15%.[277-280] It is hypothesized that this increased rate, when compared with upper GI and small bowel embolization, is due to decreased collateral flow in the intramural arterial blood supply of the colon.[281] The increased rate of infarction has led to the practice of superselective catheterization before embolization, with a lower infarction rate in more recent series. Microcoils for embolization are commonly being used as they allow reliable arterial blockade, but distal flow is maintained.[282]

Emergency purge colonoscopy

The role of colonoscopy in the evaluation of acute GI bleeding has traditionally been reserved for patients in whom clinical evidence suggests that bleeding has stopped. In the 1970s and 1980s, reports on the use of colonoscopy in the setting of active LGI bleeding began to appear.[283–286] These early studies describe the use of colonoscopy without prior bowel cleansing. More recently, colonoscopy has been used after an oral purge, which may be initiated shortly after the patient's evaluation in the emergency department and completed within 3–6 h.[287,288] The most commonly described technique involves instilling the purge solution, most commonly polyethylene glycol, through a naso-gastric tube at a rate of 1 L every 30–45 min until the rectal effluent is clear or pink. Jensen and Machicado[38] advocate the adjuvant use of metoclopramide, 10 mg intravenously every 3 h, to facilitate gastric emptying. They describe adequate preparation with the instillation of 4–8 L over a period of 3–5 h. During this period, patients can be resuscitated in the intensive care unit with fluids and blood products as necessary. The advantages of emergency purge colonoscopy include: (1) performance of the procedure at the bedside in an intensive care unit where patients receive close monitoring and continued hemodynamic support, (2) a high rate of diagnostic accuracy when compared with radiologic imaging techniques, and (3) the ability to perform therapeutic intervention. In a series of 100 patients who were admitted to an intensive care unit with severe hematochezia, Jensen and colleagues[38] reported a diagnostic yield of 74% for colonoscopy. Eleven percent had an upper GI source documented at endoscopy, whereas 9% had indirect evidence for small bowel bleeding. No site was identified in 6% of their patients. Although diverticulosis was seen in over 70% of this patient population (mean age, 77 years), right colonic angiodysplasia was the most common source of hemorrhage and accounted for 41% of bleeding colonic lesions. More recent series of major LGI bleeding[289] support diverticulosis as the most likely etiology (≈30%), and angiodysplasia responsible for only 10% of bleeding episodes, with other common causes attributable to inflammatory and ischemic colitis (15%), cancer or polyp (13%), and anorectal causes (11%). Ten percent of LGI bleeding is due to an upper source.

Colonoscopy has several obvious advantages over emergent angiography. In particular, it is safer and permits a diagnosis. Like angiography, the opportunity for therapeutic intervention exists. No formal trial comparing urgent colonoscopy with angiography has been performed. In a study of urgent colonoscopy with endoscopic intervention for diverticular bleeding, therapy with adrenaline and coagulation (10–15 watt, 1 second bursts) were found to decrease the need for surgical intervention compared to historical controls.[289] In that study, 10/48 (21%) had definite signs of diverticular hemorrhage, and all 10 were successfully managed with endoscopic treatment.[289] However, the cumulative published experience with endoscopic control of diverticular bleeding is paltry[290] and in one study of 13 patients, nearly 40% re-bled within 30 days.[41] In a more recent series from the Mayo Clinic evaluating 78 patients with LGI bleeding due to diverticulosis, only 12 patients (15%) had active bleeding or stigmata of bleeding such as a visible vessel, and endoscopic therapy was attempted in only 7/12 patients, or 9% overall. Furthermore, the timing of colonoscopy, termed urgent if attempted within 12 hours of admission, did not correlate within increased yield of detecting active bleeding.[291] Thus, although potentially useful, endoscopic control of diverticular bleeding is likely to impact on only a small percentage of patients.

Given the safety, diagnostic capability, and potential therapeutic efficacy, urgent purge colonoscopy is probably the best first step in assessment of LGI bleeding (see Fig. 65.6 below).

Capsule and double balloon endoscopy

The development of capsule endoscopy (CE) has been a major breakthrough in the visualization of the small intestine and should be added to the litany of diagnostic tools used in the evaluation of LGI bleeding in hemodynamically stable patients, when endoscopy and colonoscopy fail to identify a source. The small bowel poses a unique challenge to the endoscopist because of its length and looped configuration. Conventional methods to screen the small bowel include small bowel follow-though, enteroclysis, push enteroscopy, sonde endoscopy, and intraoperative enteroscopy. All of these modalities are fraught with limitations.[292–300] Double balloon enteroscopy, which promises to permit endoscopic visualization of the largest length of small bowel yet, is another new diagnostic tool. In the largest series using the instrument, manufactured by Fujinon, about one-half to two-thirds of the small bowel was visualized using either an anterograde or a retrograde approach.[301] Using both approaches allowed visualization of the entire small bowel in 24/28 subjects. The diagnostic yields were high; 76% of 66 patients with obscure GI bleeding had a source identified. Endoscopic hemostasis, biopsy, and stents can be employed, and initial complication rate of 1.1% in 178 patients was reported.[301] Further experience, with a wider array of practitioners, is expected in the coming years.

Most of the published studies of capsule endoscopy have focused on the diagnostic yield in patients with occult GI bleeding, which has ranged from 45% to 70%.[297,302–306] CE has been shown to have a superior diagnostic yield compared to small bowel follow-through[303] and push enteroscopy.[297,302–304] However, the diagnostic yield, though important, can be misleading given the difficulty in interpreting potentially non-specific findings. It is often difficult to differentiate a true positive from a false positive, and a true negative from a false negative.[207] This is especially important with regard to angiodysplasias, which are the most commonly reported diagnostic finding. A recent study focused on clinical outcomes of patients undergoing capsule endoscopy found that although the diagnostic yield was 42%, a positive outcome at 6.7 months mean follow-up was seen in only 7 of 43 (16%) of patients.[307] The timing and utility of capsule endoscopy in inpatients with acute LGI bleeding has not been systematically evaluated and awaits further study.

Enteroscopy

Recent advances in instrumentation have allowed for the endoscopic evaluation of part or all of the small intestine. Most commonly used in the evaluation of chronic obscure GI bleeding but occasionally used during active GI bleeding when upper endoscopy and colonoscopy have failed to yield a diagnosis, enteroscopy can be performed via one of two methodologic approaches: 'push' or 'pull.' Pull enteroscopy, more correctly referred to as sonde enteroscopy, uses a 5 mm fiberoptic scope that is 275–300 cm long.[292,308–312] It is passed intranasally, and an upper endoscope is used to position this instrument in the proximal portion of the small intestine. A balloon is inflated, and with the assistance of prokinetic agents and time, peristalsis carries this scope down variable lengths of the small intestine. In one study of 545 cases, the colon was reached in 10% of cases, the distal ileum in 40%, the proximal ileum in 20% the distal jejunum in 20%, and the proximal jejunum in 5% of cases over a mean of 7 h.[308] Once maximal insertion has been obtained, the balloon is deflated, the scope is withdrawn slowly, and the small bowel is visualized for bleeding. The yield of positive results with this technique ranges from 30% to 60%.[292,308-312] If one evaluates these data with scrutiny, a new diagnosis was established in only one-quarter of these cases. The most common finding is angiodysplasia, which was seen in approximately 75% of cases, with tumors accounting for

15%, and a variety of other etiologies making up the final 10%. A major disadvantage of sonde enteroscopy is the inability to obtain a biopsy or apply endoscopic therapy.

Push enteroscopy was initially performed with a pediatric colonoscope.[313-315] Reportedly, the scope could be passed up to 60 cm beyond the ligament of Treitz. Recently, enteroscopes measuring 200–240 cm have been designed to be used with or without an overtube.[316-318] The overtube is used to straighten the scope and prevent looping in the greater curvature of the stomach to improve the depth of insertion. One study comparing push enteroscopy with and without an overtube documented an increase in depth

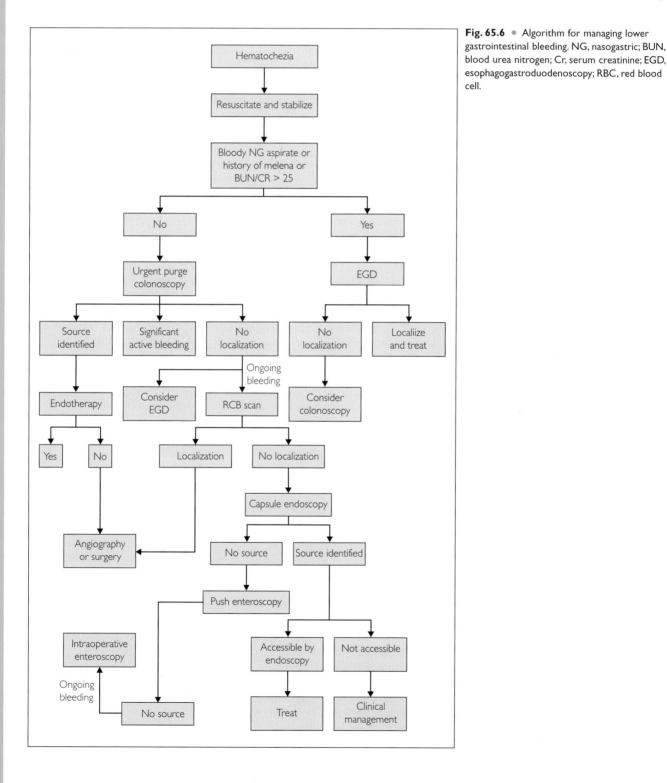

Fig. 65.6 ● Algorithm for managing lower gastrointestinal bleeding. NG, nasogastric; BUN, blood urea nitrogen; Cr, serum creatinine; EGD, esophagogastroduodenoscopy; RBC, red blood cell.

of insertion beyond the ligament Treitz from 11 to 108 cm with the use of an overtube.[319] The diagnostic yield of push enteroscopy has varied between 30% and 60%, with angiodysplasia accounting for the vast majority of bleeding lesions.[320–323] Biopsy forceps and bipolar probes have been designed to be used with these enteroscopes. Complications of enteroscopy include mucosal trauma attributed to the overtube, including pharyngeal and esophageal perforation. In addition, pancreatitis resulting from trauma to the papilla has been reported.

Intraoperative endoscopy

For patients in whom active GI bleeding is documented but a source cannot be identified, intraoperative enteroscopy may localize bleeding sites and aid in directing surgical therapy. During this procedure, an endoscope may be passed by mouth or via an enterotomy. The bowel is manually pleated over the scope by the surgeon while the endoscopist examines the mucosa during the pleating maneuver. In a study of 44 patients at the Mayo Clinic, intraoperative endoscopy identified lesions in 70% of subjects, lesions that had not been localized preoperatively.[324] The mean time in surgery was 3.5 h, and five patients died of complications directly related to the surgery. Other complications were seen in nine patients and included a prolonged ileus, wound infection, and adhesions. In addition, 52% of the patients had recurrent hemorrhage, and the overall success rate in achieving hemostasis in this difficult group of patients was 41%. In another study,[325] good concordance was noted between findings on small bowel enteroscopy and intraoperative endoscopy. However, during the latter procedure, a high incidence of complications was noted, particularly mucosal ulceration and perforation and one terminal episode of small bowel ischemia. Profound ileus was noted in all patients (average of 4.6 days), and the re-bleeding rate was 45%. Thus, although intraoperative enteroscopy can be used when other localizing modalities have failed to demonstrate a source of bleeding, an extraordinarily high complication rate with prolonged postoperative ileus should be expected.

TREATMENT ALGORITHM FOR ACUTE LOWER INTESTINAL BLEEDING

Finally, based on the data presented in this chapter, we offer an algorithm (Fig. 65.6) for a rational treatment approach to patients with severe LGI bleeding. It must be emphasized that the algorithm chosen for a particular center will be dependent on the available local expertise. Further prospective studies are required to determine the most cost-effective strategies for managing LGI hemorrhage.

REFERENCES

1. Reinus JF, Brandt LJ. Vascular ectasias and diverticulosis. Gastroenterol Clin North Am 1994; 23:1–20.

2. Hunt PH. Rectal bleeding. Clin Gastroenterol 1989; 7:719–740.

3. Caos A, Benner KG, Manier J, et al. Colonoscopy after Golytely preparation in acute rectal bleeding. J Clin Gastroenterol 1986; 8:46–49.

4. Boley SJ, DiBiase A, Brandt LJ, et al. Lower intestinal bleeding in the elderly. Am J Surg 1979; 137:57–64.

5. Comay D, Marshall JK. Resource utilization for acute lower gastrointestinal hemorrhage. Ontario GI bleed study. Can J Gastroenterol 2002; 16(10):677–682.

Medical-economic study quantifying high resource utilization for patients admitted with acute lower gastrointestinal bleeding.

6. Prakash C, Zuckerman GR. Acute small bowel bleeding: a distinct entity with significantly different economic implications compared with GI bleeding from other locations. Gastrointest Endosc 2003; 58(3):409–412.

7. Painter NS, Burkitt DP. Diverticular disease of the colon. A deficiency disease of Western civilization. Br Med J 1971; 2:450–454.

8. Parks TG. Natural history of diverticular disease of the colon. A review of 521 cases. Br Med J 1969; 4:639–642.

9. Thompson WG, Patel DG, Tao N, et al. Does uncomplicated diverticular disease produce symptoms? Dig Dis Sci 27: 1982; 605–608.

10. Bowder W, Cerise EJ, Litwin MS. Impact of emergency angiography in massive lower gastrointestinal bleeding. Ann Surg 1986; 204:530–536.

11. Quinn WC. Gross hemorrhage from presumed diverticulosis of the colon. Ann Surg 1961; 153:851–853.

12. Meyers MA, Volberg G, Katzen B, et al. The angioarchitecture of colonic diverticula. Radiology 1973; 108:249–261.

13. Goodwin FH, Collins EN. Diverticulosis of the colon. Radiology Cleve Clin Q 1948; 15:194–205.

14. Horner JL. A study of diverticulitis of colon in office practice. Gastroenterology 1952; 21:223–228.

15. Keelye KJ. Alimentary disease in the Batu. Med Proc 1958; 4:281–285.

16. Narasaka T, Watanabe H, Yamagata S, et al. Statistical analysis of diverticulosis of the colon. Tohoku J Exp Med 1975; 114:271–275.

17. Burkitt DP. A deficiency of dietary fiber may be one cause of certain colonic and venous disorders. Am J Dig Dis 1976; 21:104–108.

18. Eastwood MA, Smith AN, Brydon WG, et al. Colonic function in patients with diverticular disease. Lancet 1978; 1:181–182.

19. Wynne-Jones G. Flatus retention is the major factor in diverticular disease. Lancet 1975; 2:211–212.

20. Bowder W, Cerise EJ, Litwin MS. Impact of emergency angiography in massive lower gastrointestinal bleeding. Ann Surg 1986; 205:530–536.

21. Lichtiger S, Kornbluth A, Saloman P, et al. Lower gastrointestinal bleeding. In: Taylor MB, ed. Gastrointestinal emergencies. Baltimore: Williams & Wilkins; 1992:258–373.

22. Ouriel K, Knightly JJ. Diverticular disease in the young patients. Surg Gynecol Obstet 1963; 156:1–5.

23. Ulin AW. Massive hemorrhage from diverticulitis of the colon. Ann Intern Med 1959; 50:1395–1406.

24. Quinn WC. Gross hemorrhage from presumed diverticular disease of the colon: Results of treatment of 103 patients. Ann Surg 1961; 153:851–860.

25. Nath PL, Sequeira JC, Weltzman AF, et al. Lower gastrointestinal bleeding: Diagnostic approach and management conclusions. Am J Surg 1981; 141:478–481.

26. Uden P, Jiborn H, Johnson K. Influence of selective mesenteric arteriography on the outcome of emergency surgery for massive lower gastrointestinal hemorrhage: A 15 year experience. Dis Colon Rectum 1986; 29:561–566.

27. Bentley DE, Richardson JD. The role of tagged red blood cell imaging in the localization of gastrointestinal bleeding. Arch Surg 1991; 126:821–824.

28. Hunter JM, Pezim ME. Limited value of technetium 99m-labeled red cell scintigraphy in localization of lower gastrointestinal bleeding. Am J Surg 1990; 159:504–506.

29. Ryan P, Styles CB, Chimel R. Identification of the site of severe colon bleeding by technetium-labeled red-cell scan. Dis Colon Rectum 1992; 35:219–222.

30. Voeller GR, Bunch G, Britt LG. Use of technetium-labeled red blood cell scintigraphy in the detection and management of gastrointestinal hemorrhage. Surgery 1991; 110:799–804.

31. Dusold R, Burke K, Carpentier W, et al. The accuracy of technetium ^{99m}labeled red cell scintigraphy in localizing gastrointestinal bleeding. Am J Gastroenterol 1994; 89:345–348.

32. Athanasoulis CA, Baum S, Rösch J, et al. Mesenteric arterial infusions of vasopressin for hemorrhage from colonic diverticulosis. Am J Surg 1975; 129:212–216.

33. Baum S, Athanasoulis CA, Walman AC. Angiography in the diagnosis and therapy of hemorrhage from the large bowel. Radiology 1975; 15:421–433.

34. Gomes AS, Lois JF, McCoy RD. Angiographic treatment of gastrointestinal hemorrhage: Comparison of vasopressin infusion and embolization. Am J Gastroenterol 1986; 146:1031–1037.

35. Rösch J, Dotter CT, Brown MJ. Selective arterial embolization: A new method for control of acute gastrointestinal bleeding. Radiology 1972; 102:303–306.

36. Clark RA, Colley DP, Eggers FM. Acute arterial gastrointestinal hemorrhage: Efficacy of transcatheter control. Am J Gastroenterol 1981; 136:1185–1189.

37. Jensen DW, Machicado GA. Diagnosis and treatment of severe hematochezia: The role of urgent colonoscopy after purge. Gastroenterology 1988; 95:1564–1574.

38. Jensen DM, Machicado GA. Diagnosis and treatment of severe hematochezia. Gastroenterology 1988; 95:46–49.

39. Savides T, Jensen DM, Machido G, et al. Colonoscopic hemostasis for recurrent diverticular hemorrhage associated with a visible vessel: A report of three cases. Am J Gastroenterol 1994; 40:70–73.

40. Bloomfeld RS, Rockey DC, Shetzline MA. Endoscopic therapy of acute diverticular hemorrhage. Am J Gastroenterol 2001; 96(8):2367–2372.

41. DeMarkels MP, Murphy JR. Acute lower gastrointestinal bleeding. Med Clin North Am 1993; 77:1055–1100.

42. Elta GH. Approach to the patient with gross gastrointestinal bleeding. In: Yamada T, Alpers DH, Owyang C, et al., eds. Textbook of gastroenterology, vol 1. Philadelphia: JB Lippincott; 1991:591.

43. Potter GD, Sellin JH. Lower gastrointestinal bleeding. Gastrointest Endosc Clin North Am 1988; 17:341–356.

44. Civetta JM, Daggett WM. Gastrointestinal bleeding from jejunal diverticula. Ann Surg 1967; 166:976–979.

45. Coran AG, Brooks JR. Gastrointestinal bleeding from jejunal diverticulosis. JAMA 1965; 191:139–140.

46. Kozoll D, McHahon JA, Kiely JP. Massive gastrointestinal hemorrhage due to jejunal diverticula. JAMA 1951; 142:1258–1260.

47. Wilcox RD, Shatney CH. Massive rectal bleeding from jejunal diverticula. Surg Gynecol Obstet 1987; 165:425–428.

48. Rankin FW, Martin WJ Jr. Diverticula of the small bowel. Ann Surg 1934; 100:123–135.

49. Benson RE, Dixon DF, Waugh JM. Nonmeckelian diverticula of the jejunum and ileum. Ann Surg 1943; 118:377–393.

50. Krishnamurthy S, Kelly M, Rohrmann C, et al. Jejunal diverticulosis: A heterogeneous disorder caused by a variety of abnormalities of smooth muscle or myenteric plexus. Gastroenterology 1983; 85:538–547.

51. Silen W, Brown WH, Orloff MJ, et al. Complications of jejunal diverticulosis. Arch Surg 1960; 80:597–601.

52. Altemeier WA, Bryant LR, Wulsin JH. The surgical significance of jejunal diverticulosis. Arch Surg 1963; 86:732–744.

53. Echkhouser FE, Zelenock GB, Freier DT. Acute complications of jejunoileal pseudodiverticulosis: Surgical implications and management. Am J Surg 1979; 138:320–323.

54. Thomas CS Jr, Tinsley EA, Brockman SK. Jejunal diverticula as a source of massive upper gastrointestinal bleeding. Arch Surg 1967; 95:89–92.

55. Pennazio M, Santucci R, Rondonotti E, et al. Outcome of patients with obscure gastrointestinal bleeding after capsule endoscopy: Report of 100 consecutive cases. Gastroenterology 2004; 126:643–653.

Performance outcomes of capsule endoscopy in patients with obscure bleeding showing highest yields in patients with ongoing overt bleeding, intermediate yields with iron deficiency anemia and guaiac positive stools, and lower yields in previous overt bleeding.

56. Buchman TG, Bulkely GB. Current management of patients with lower gastrointestinal bleeding. Surg Clin North Am 1987; 61:651–664.

57. Richter JM, Hedbert SE, Athanasoulis CA, et al. Angiodysplasia: Clinical presentation and colonoscopic diagnosis. Dig Dis Sci 1984; 29:481–485.

58. Trudel JL, Fazio VW, Sivak MV. Colonoscopic diagnosis and treatment of arteriovenous malformations in chronic lower gastrointestinal bleedings: Clinical accuracy and efficacy. Dis Colon Rectum 1988; 31:107–110.

59. Gostout LJ. Angiodysplasia and aortic valve disease: Let's close the book on this association (Editorial). Gastrointest Endosc 1995; 42:491–493.

60. Foutch PG. Angiodysplasia of the gastrointestinal tract. Am J Gastroenterol 1993; 80:807–818.

61. Boley SJ, Brandt LJ. Vascular ectasias of the colon – 1986. Dig Dis Sci 1986; 31(Suppl 9):26–42.

62. Britt L, Warren L, Moore O. Selective management of lower gastrointestinal bleeding. Am Surg 1983; 49:121–125.

63. Tedesco FJ, Griffin JW Jr, Khan AQ. Vascular ectasia of the colon: Clinical, colonoscopic and radiographic features. J Clin Gastroenterol 1980; 2:233–238.

64. Potter GD, Sellin JH. Lower gastrointestinal bleeding. Gastroenterol Clin North Am 1988; 17:341–355.

65. Machicado GA, Jensen DM. Upper gastrointestinal angiomata: Diagnosis and treatment. Gastrointest Endosc Clin North Am 1991; 1:24–62.

66. Deal SE, Zfass AM, Duckworth PF, et al. Arteriovenous malformations (AVMS): Are they concealed by meperidine (Abstract)? Am J Gastroenterol 1991; 86:1351.

67. Rogers BHG. Endoscopic diagnosis and therapy of mucosal vascular abnormalities of the gastrointestinal tract occurring in elderly patients and associated with cardiac, vascular, and pulmonary disease. Gastrointest Endosc 1980; 26:134–138.

68. Howard OM, Buchanan JD, Hunt RH. Angiodysplasia of the colon: Experience of 16 cases. Lancet 1982; 2:16–19.

69. Richter JM, Christensen MR, Colditz GA, et al. Angiodysplasia: Natural history of efficacy of therapeutic interventions. Dig Dis Sci 1989; 34:1542–1546.

70. Jensen DM, Machicado GA. Bleeding colonic angioma: Endoscopic coagulation and follow-up (Abstract). Gastroenterology 1985; 88:1433.

71. Roberts PL, Schoetz DJ, Coller JA. Vascular ectasia: Diagnosis and treatment by colonoscopy. Am Surg 1988; 54:56–57.

72. Rutgeerts R, Van Gompel F, Gebos K, et al. Long-term results of treatment of fascicular malformations of the gastrointestinal tract by neodymium-YAG laser photocoagulation. Gut 1985; 26:586–593.

73. Cello JP, Grendell JH. Endoscopic laser treatment for gastrointestinal vascular ectasias. Ann Intern Med 1986; 104:352–354.

74. Mathus-Vlicgcn EMH. Laser treatment of intestinal vascular abnormalities. Int J Colorectal Dis 1989; 4:20–25.

75. Wadas DD, Sanowski RA. Complications of the hot biopsy forceps technique. Gastrointest Endosc 1988; 34:32–37.

76. Naveau S, Aubert A, Poynard T, et al. Long-term results of treatment of vascular malformations of the gastrointestinal tract by neodymium:YAG laser photocoagulation. Dig Dis Sci 1990; 35:821–826.

77. Waye JD. New methods of polypectomy. Gastrointest Endosc Clin North Am 1997; 7:413–422.

78. McGee RR. Estrogen-progesterone therapy for gastrointestinal bleeding in hereditary hemorrhagic telangiectasias. South Med J 1979; 315:731–735.

79. Broner MH, Pate MB, Cunningham JT, et al. Estrogen-progesterone therapy for bleeding gastrointestinal telangiectasis in chronic renal failure: An uncontrolled trial. Ann Intern Med 1986; 105:371–374.

80. Granieri R, Mazzulla JP, Yarborough GW. Estrogen-progesterone therapy for recurrent gastrointestinal bleeding secondary to gastrointestinal angiodysplasia. Am J Gastroenterol 1988; 83:556–558.

81. Van Cutsem E, Rutgeerts P, Gebos K, et al. Estrogen-progesterone treatment of Osler-Weber-Rendu disease. J Clin Gastroenterol 1988; 10:676–679.

82. Van Cutsem E, Rutgeerts P, Vantrappen G. Treatment of bleeding gastrointestinal vascular malformations with oestrogen-progesterone. Lancet 1990; 335:953–955.

83. Lewis B, Salomon P, Rivera-MacMurray S, et al. Does hormonal therapy have any benefit for bleeding angiodysplasia? J Clin Gastroenterol 1992; 15:99–103.

84. Hass PA, Has GP, Schnultz S, et al. The prevalence of hemorrhoids. Dis Colon Rectum 1983; 26:435–439.

85. Smith LE. Hemorrhoids: A review of current techniques and management. Gastroenterol Clin North Am 1987; 16:79–91.

86. Kluiber RM, Wolff BG. Evaluation of anemia caused by hemorrhoidal bleeding. Dis Colon Rectum 1994; 37:1006–1007.

87. Thomson WH. The nature of haemorrhoids. Br J Surg 1975; 62:542–552.

88. Hass PA, Fox TA, Hass GP. The pathogenesis of hemorrhoids. Dis Colon Rectum 1984; 27:442–450.

89. Bernstein WC. What are hemorrhoids and what is their relationship to the portal venous system. Dis Colon Rectum 1983; 26:829–834.

90. Korkis AM, McDougal CJ. Rectal bleeding in patients less than 50 years of age. Dig Dis Sci 40:1520–1523. 1995;

91. Faulconer HJ. Hemorrhoids: Alternative treatments. J Ky Med Assoc 1988; 86:617–620.

92. Ferguson EF. Alternative in the treatment of hemorrhoidal disease. South Med J 1988; 81:606–610.

93. Peral RK, Abcarian H. Nonoperative therapy of hemorrhoids. Infect Surg 1989; 8:411–417.

94. Zinberg SS, Stern DH, Furman DS, et al. A personal experience in comparing three nonoperative techniques for treating internal hemorrhoids. Am J Gastroenterol 1989; 84:488–492.

95. Yu JC, Eddy HG Jr. Laser: A new modality for hemorrhoids. Am J Gastroenterol Colon Rectum Surg 1985; 1:9–10.

96. Schrock TR, Guthrie JF, Shub HA, et al. Lasers in colon and rectal surgery. Perspect Colon Rectum Surg 1989; 2:55–69.

97. Sim AJW, Muries JA, Mackenzie I. Comparison of rubber band ligation and sclerosant injection for first and second degree hemorrhoids: A prospective clinical trial. Acta Chir Scand 1981; 147:717–720.

98. Kilbourne JN. Internal hemorrhoids: Comparative value of treatment by operative and by injection methods. Ann Surg 1934; 99:600–608.

99. Ponsky JL, Mellinger JD, Simon IB. Endoscopic retrograde hemorrhoidal sclerotherapy using 23.4% saline: A preliminary report. Gastrointest Endosc 1991; 37:155–158.

100. Senapati A, Nicholls RJ. A randomized trial to compare the results of injection sclerotherapy with a bulk laxative in the treatment of bleeding hemorrhoids. Int J Colorectal Dis 1988; 3:124–126.

101. Juler GL, Labitzke HG, Lamb R, et al. The pathogenesis of Dieulafoy's gastric erosion. Am J Gastroenterol 1984; 79:195–199.

102. Stark ME, Gostout CJ, Balm RK. Clinical features and endoscopic management of Dieulafoy's disease. Gastrointest Endosc 1992; 38:545–550.

103. Polit SA. The Dieulafoy gastric erosion: an infrequently recognized cause of upper gastrointestinal hemorrhage in the elderly. J Am Geriatr Soc 1990; 38:53–55.

104. Golden SP, Deluca VA, Marignani P. Endoscopic treatment of Dieulafoy's lesion of the duodenum. Am J Gastroenterol 1990; 85:452–454.

105. Abdulian JD, Santor MJ, Chen YK, et al. Dieulafoy-like lesion of the rectum presenting with exsanguinating hemorrhage: Successful endoscopic sclerotherapy. Am J Gastroenterol 1993; 88:1939–1941.

106. Barbier P, Luder P, Triller J, et al. Colonic hemorrhage from a solitary minute ulcer. Gastroenterology 1985; 88:1065–1068.

107. Ma CK, Padda H, Pace EH, et al. Submucosal arterial malformation of the colon with massive hemorrhage: Report of a case. Dis Colon Rectum 1989; 32:149–152.

108. Richards WO, Grove-Mahoney D, Williams LF. Hemorrhage from a Dieulafoy-type ulcer of the colon: A new cause of lower gastrointestinal bleeding. Am Surg 1988; 54:121–124.

109. Matuchansky C, Babin P, Abadie JC, et al. Jejunal bleeding from a solitary large submucosal artery: Report of two cases. Gastroenterology 1978; 75:110–113.

110. Chen KTK. Intestinal bleeding from a caliber-persistent submucosal artery in the ileum. J Clin Gastroenterol 1985; 7:289–291.

111. Vetto JT, Richman PS, Kariger K, et al. Cirsoid aneurysms of the jejunum: An unrecognized cause of massive gastrointestinal bleeding (Review). Arch Surg 1989; 124:1460–1462.

112. Juler GL, Labizke HG, Lamb R, et al. The pathogenesis of Dieulafoy's gastric erosion. Am J Gastroenterol 1984; 79:195–200.

113. Pishori T, Khurshaidi N, Khan SM, et al. Massive lower gastrointestinal bleeding due to Dieulafoy lesion of the colon. Indian J Gastroenterol 2003; 22(2):66–67.

114. Chung IK, Kim EJ, Lee MS, et al. Bleeding Dieulofoy's lesions and the choice of endoscopic method: comparing the hemostatic efficacy of mechanical and injection methods. Gastrointest Endosc 2000; 52:721–724.

115. Carr ND, Pullen BR, Hasleton PS, et al. Microvasculary studies in human radiation bowel disease. Gut 1984; 25:448–454.

116. Den Hartog Jager FCA, Van Haastert M, Batterman JJ, et al. The endoscopic spectrum of late radiation damage of the rectosigmoid colon. Endoscopy 1985; 17:214–216.

117. Kinsella TJ, Bloomer WD. Tolerance of the intestine to radiation therapy. Surg Gynecol Obstet 1980; 115:273–284.

118. Decosse JJ, Rhodes RS, Wentz WB, et al. The natural history and management of radiation-induced injury of the gastrointestinal tract. Ann Surg 1969; 170:369–384.

119. Reichelderfer M, Morrissey JF. Colonoscopy in radiation colitis. Gastrointest Endosc 1980; 26:41–43.

120. Goldstein F, Khoury J, Thornton JJ. Treatment of chronic radiation enteritis and colitis with salicylazosulfapyridine and systemic corticosteroids. Am J Gastroenterol 1976; 65:201–208.

121. Ladas SD, Raptis SA. Sucralfate enemas in the treatment of chronic postradiation proctitis. Am J Gastroenterol 1989; 84:1587–1589.

122. Alexander TJ, Dwyer RM. Endoscopic Nd:YAG laser treatment of severe radiation injury of the lower gastrointestinal tract: Long-term follow-up. Gastrointest Endosc 1988; 34:407–411.

123. Buchi KN, Dixon JA. Argon laser treatment of hemorrhagic radiation proctitis. Gastrointest Endosc 1987; 33:27–30.

124. O'Connor JJ. Argon laser treatment of radiation proctitis. Arch Surg 1989; 124:749.

125. Gelfand MD, Tepper M, Katz LA, et al. Acute irradiation proctitis in man: Development of eosinophilic crypt abscesses. Gastroenterology 1968; 54:401–411.

126. Rabinovitz M, Schade RR, Dindzans VJ, et al. Colonic disease in cirrhosis: An endoscopic evaluation in 412 patients. Gastroenterology 1990; 99:195–199.

127. Kozarek RA, Botoman VA, Bredfeldt JE, et al. Portal colopathy: Prospective study of colonoscopy in patients with portal hypertension. Gastroenterology 1991; 101:1192–1197.

128. Viggiano TR, Gostout CJ. Portal hypertensive intestinal vasculopathy: A review of the clinical, endoscopic and histopathologic features. Am J Gastroenterol 1992; 87:944–946.

129. Ganger DR, Preston A, Sankary H. Colonic lesions in portal hypertension (Letter). Gastrointest Endosc 1993; 39:212–213.

130. Thiruvengadam R, Gostout CJ. Congestive gastroenteropathy: An extension of nonvariceal upper gastrointestinal bleeding in portal hypertension. Gastrointest Endosc 1989; 35:504–507.

131. Tseng-Nip T, Wai-Wah NG, Shou-Dong L. Colonic mucosal changes in patients with liver cirrhosis. Gastrointest Endosc 1995; 42:408–412.

132. Feldman M Jr, Smith VM, Warner CG. Varices of the colon. JAMA 1962; 179:729–730.

133. Gudjonsson H, Zeiler D, Gamelli RL, et al. Colonic varices: Report of an unusual case diagnosed by radionuclide scanning, with review of the literature. Gastroenterology 1986; 91:1543–1547.

134. Levy JS, Hardin JH, Shipp H, et al. Varices of the cecum as an unusual cause of gastrointestinal bleeding. Gastroenterology 1957; 33:637–640.

135. Vescia FG, Babb RR. Colonic varices: A rare but important cause of gastrointestinal hemorrhage. J Clin Gastroenterol 1985; 7:63–65.

136. Boley SJ. Early diagnosis of acute mesenteric ischemia. Hosp Pract 1981; 16:63–71.

137. Miller LS, Barbarevech C, Friedman LS. Less frequent causes of lower gastrointestinal bleeding. Gastroenterol Clin North Am 1994; 23:21–52.

138. Klein SD, Hellinger JC, Siverstein ML, et al. Isolated cecal varices as the source of massive lower GI bleeding patient with cirrhosis. Am J Gastroenterol 2003; 98(1):220–221.

139. Moncure AC, Waltman AC, Vandersalm TJ, et al. Gastrointestinal hemorrhage from adhesion-related mesenteric varices. Ann Surg 1976; 183:24–29.

140. Burbige EJ, Tarder G, Carson S, et al. Colonic varices, a complication of pancreatitis and splenic vein thrombosis. Am J Dig Dis 1978; 23:752–755.

141. Iredale JP, Ridings P, McGinn FP, et al. Familial and idiopathic colonic varices: An unusual cause of lower gastrointestinal hemorrhage. Gut 33: 1992; 1285–1288.

142. Atin V, Sabas A, Cotano JR, et al. Familial varices of the colon and small bowel. Int J Colorectal Dis 1993; 8:4–8.

143. Philippakis M, Karkanias G, Sakorafas GH, et al. Massive gastrointestinal bleeding secondary to intestinal varices. Eur J Surg 1992; 158:379–381.

144. Morini S, Carus F, De Angelis P. Familiar varices of the small and large bowel. Endoscopy 1993; 25:188–190.

145. Weiserbs DB, Zfass AM, Messmer J. Control of massive hemorrhage from rectal varices with sclerotherapy. Gastrointest Endosc 1986; 32:419–421.

146. Orosco H, Takahashuit, Mescado MA, et al. Colorectal variceal bleeding in patients with extrahepatic portal vein thrombosis and idiopathic portal hypertension. J Clin Gastroenterol 1992; 139–143.

147. Wang M, Desigan G, Dunn D. Endoscopic sclerotherapy for bleeding rectal varices. A case report. Am J Gastroenterol 1985; 80:779–780.

148. Shapiro MJ. The role of the radiologist in the management of gastrointestinal bleeding. Gastroenterol Clin North Am 1994; 23:123–181.

149. Nagy WS, Marshal JB. Aortoenteric fistulas. Recognizing a potentially catastrophic cause of gastrointestinal bleeding. Postgrad Med 1993; 93(8):211–212, 219–222.

150. Kalman DR, Barnard GF, Massimi GJ, et al. Primary aortoduodenal fistula after radiotherapy. Am J Gastroenterol 1995; 90:1148–1150.

151. Perez-Cuadrado E, Silva Gonzelez C, Vazquez Dourado R, et al. Lower digestive hemorrhage by aortoenteric fistula: Ileoscopic diagnosis. Endoscopy 1994; 26:515–516.

152. Peck JJ, Eidemiller LR. Aortoenteric fistulas. Arch Surg 1992; 127:1191–1193.

153. Schrock TR. Colonoscopic diagnosis and treatment of lower gastrointestinal bleeding. Surg Clin North Am 1989; 69:1309–1325.

154. Mark AS, Moss AA, McCarthy S, et al. CT of aortoenteric fistulas. Invest Radiol 1985; 20:272–275.

155. Boley SF, Brandt LJ, Mitsudo SM. Vascular lesions of the colon. In: Stollerman GH, ed. Advances in internal medicine. Chicago: Year Book; 1984.

156. Robert JR, Sachar DB, Greenstein J. Severe gastrointestinal hemorrhage in Crohn's disease. Ann Surg 1991; 213:207–211.

157. Fallis LS. Massive intestinal hemorrhage in regional enteritis. Report of a case. Am J Surg 1941; 53:512–513.

158. Rubin M, Lynwood Herrington J, Schneider R. Regional enteritis with major gastrointestinal hemorrhage as the initial manifestation. Arch Intern Med 1980; 140:217–219.

159. Block GE, Moosa AR, Simonowitz D, et al. Emergency colectomy for inflammatory bowel disease. Surgery 1977; 82:531–536.

160. Edwards FC, Truelove SC. The course and prognosis of ulcerative colitis. Gut 1964; 5:1–26.

161. Farmer RG. Clinical features and natural history of inflammatory bowel disease. Med Clin North Am 1980; 64:1103–1115.

162. Smith JN, Winship DH. Complications and extraintestinal problems in inflammatory bowel disease. Med Clin North Am 1980; 64:1161–1171.

163. Robert JH, Sachar DB, Greenstein AJ. Management of severe hemorrhage in ulcerative colitis. Am J Surg 1990; 159:550–555.

164. Farmer RG, Hawk WA, Turnbul RB. Indication for surgery in Crohn's disease. Analysis of 500 cases. Gastroenterology 1976; 71:245–250.

165. Sparbert M, Kirsner JB. Recurrent hemorrhage in regional enteritis. Report of 3 cases. Am J Dig Dis 1966; 2:652–657.

166. Greenstein AJ, Kark AE, Creiling DA. Crohn's disease of the colon. II. Controversial aspects of hemorrhage, anemia and rectal involvement in granulomatous disease involving the colon. Am J Gastrocntcrol 1975; 63:40–48.

167. Homan WP, Tang CK, Thorbjarnarson B. Acute massive hemorrhage from intestinal Crohn's disease. Arch Surg 1976; 111:901–917.

168. Kozaenik JR. Massive lower gastrointestinal hemorrhage in Crohn's disease. Curr Treat Options Gastroenterol 2000; 3(3):211–216.

169. Fauci AS, Haynes BF, Katz P. The spectrum of vasculitis: Clinical, pathologic, immunologic, and therapeutic considerations. Ann Intern Med 1978; 89:660–676.

170. Harvey MH, Neoptolemos JP, Fossard DP. Abdominal polyarteritis nodosa – a possible surgical pitfall? Br J Clin Pract 1984; 38:282–283.

171. Guillevin L, Le TH, Godeau P, et al. Clinical findings and prognosis of polyarteritis nodosa and Churg-Strauss angiitis: A study in 165 patients. Br J Rheumatol 1988; 27:258–264.

172. Cabal E, Holtz S. Polyarteritis as a cause of intestinal hemorrhage. Gastroenterology 1971; 61:99–105.

173. Cremm JJ, Gumpel JM, Peachey RDG. Schönlein-Henoch purpura in adults. Q J Med 1970; 39:461–483.

174. Cappell MS, Gupta AM. Colonic lesions associated with Henoch-Schönlein purpura. Am J Gastronterol 1990; 85:1186–1088.

175. Goldman LP, Lindenberg RL. Henoch-Schönlein purpura: Gastrointestinal manifestations with endoscopic correlation. Am J Gastroentrol 1981; 75:357–360.

176. Pinkney JH, Clarke G, Fairclough PD. Gastrointestinal involvement in Wegener's granulomatosis. Gastrointest Endosc 1991; 76:534–537.

177. Camilleri M, Pusey CD, Chadwick VS, et al. Gastrointestinal manifestations of systemic vasculitis. Q J Med 1983; 206:141–149.

178. Soko RJ, Farrell MK, McAdams AJ. An unusual presentation of Wegener's granulomatosis mimicking inflammatory bowel disease. Gastroenterology 1984; 87:426–432.

179. Laing TJ. Gastrointestinal vasculitis and pneumatosis intestinalis due to systemic lupus erythematosus: Successful treatment with pulse intravenous cyclophosphamide. Am J Med 1988; 85:555–558.

180. Gore RM, Marn CS, Ujiki GT, et al. Ischemic colitis associated with systemic lupus erythematosus. Dis Colon Rectum 1983; 26:449–451.

181. Kurlander DJ, Kirsner JB. The association of chornic 'nonspecific' inflammatory bowel disease with lupus erythematosus. Ann Intern Med 1964; 60:799–803.

182. Scott DG, Bacon PA, Tribe CR. Systemic rheumatoid vasculitis. A clinical and laboratory study of 50 cases. Medicine (Baltimore) 1981; 60:288–297.

183. Burt RW, Berensen MM, Samuelson CO, et al. Rheumatoid vasculitis of the colon presenting as pancolitis. Dig Dis Sci 1983; 28:183–188.

184. Case records of the Massachusetts General Hospital (case 40-1984). N Engl J Med 1984; 311:904–911.

185. Reza MJ, Roth BE, Pops MA, et al. Intestinal vasculitis in essential mixed cryoglobulinemia. Ann Intern Med 1974; 81:632–634.

186. Neil GA, Weinstock JV. Gastrointestinal manifestations of systemic diseases. In: Yamada T, Alpers DH, Owyang C, et al., eds. Textbook of gastroenterology, vol 2. Philadelphia: JB Lippincott; 1991:2135–2157.

187. Bosshardt RT, Abel ME. Proctitis following fecal diversion. Dis Colon Rectum 1984; 27:605–607.

188. Ma CK, Gottlieb C, Haas PA. Diversion colitis: A clinicopathologic study of 21 cases. Hum Pathol 1990; 21:429–436.

189. Murray FE, O'Brien MJ, Birkett DH, et al. Diversion colitis – pathologic findings in a resected sigmoid colon and rectum. Gastroenterology 1987; 93:1404–1408.

190. Agarwal VP, Schimmel EM. Diversion colitis: A nutritional deficiency syndrome? Nutr Rev 1989; 47:257–261.

191. Harig JM, Soergel KH, Komorowski RA, et al. Treatment of diversion colitis with short-chain fatty acid irrigation. N Engl J Med 1989; 320:23–28.

192. Glotzer DJ, Glick ME, Goldman H. Proctitis and colitis following diversion of the fecal stream. Gastroenterology 1981; 80:438–441.

193. Jensen DM, Machicado GA. Colonoscopy for diagnosis and treatment of severe lower gastrointestinal bleeding. Routine outcomes and cost analysis. Gastrointest Endosc Clin North Am 1997; 7:477–498.

194. Saito H, Oshimi K, Nagasako K, et al. Endoscopic appearance of the colon and small intestine of a patient with hemorrhagic enteric graft-vs.-host disease. Dis Colon Rectum 1990; 33:695–697.

195. Murayama T, Nakagawa T, Matsushita K, et al. Hemorrhage colitis with unusual colonoscopy features, complicated with chronic graft-versus-host disease after allogenic bone marrow transplantation. Bone Marrow Transplant 1995; 15:1451–1453.

196. Shabahang M, Pasquale MD, Bitterman P, et al. Massive hematochezia secondary to graft-versus-host disease and cytomegalovirus. Am J Gastroenterol 1984; 89:632–633.

197. Macrae FA, Tan KG, Williams CG. Towards safer colonoscopy: A report of 5000 diagnostic or therapeutic colonoscopies. Gut 1983; 24:376–383.

198. Van Gossum A, Cozzoli A, Adler M, et al. Colonoscopic snare polypectomy: Analysis of 1485 resections comparing two types. Gastrointest Endosc 1992; 38:472–475.

199. Waye JD. Gastrointestinal polypectomy. In: Geenen JE, Fleisher DE, Waye JD, eds. Techniques in therapeutic endoscopy. 2nd edn. Philadelphia: JB Lippincott; 1992.

200. Gilbert DA, Hallstrom AP, Shaney SL, et al. The national ASGE colonoscopy survey – complications of colonoscopy. Gastrointest Endosc 1984; 30A:156.

201. Rosen L, Bub D, Reed J. Hemorrhage following colonoscopic polypectomy. Dis Colon Rectum 1993; 36:1126–1131.

202. Nivatvongs S. Complications in colonoscopic polypectomy: Lessons to learn from an experience with 1576 polyps. Am Surg 1988; 54:61–63.

203. Matsushita M, Kajiro K, Takawuwa H, et al. Infective use of a detachable snare for colonoscopic polypectomy of large polyps. Gastrointest Endosc 1998; 47:496–499.

204. Rex DK, Lewis BS, Waye JD. Colonoscopy and endoscopic therapy for delayed post-polypectomy hemorrhage. Gastrointest Endosc 1992; 38:127–129.

205. Slivka A, Parsons WG, Carr-Locke DC. Endoscopic band ligation for treatment of post-polypectomy hemorrhage. Gastrointest Endosc 1994; 40:230–232.

206. Tappero G, Gaiai E, Deiuli P, et al. Cold snare excision of small colorectal polyps. Gastrointest Endosc 1992; 38:310–313.

207. Yousfi M, Gostout CJ, Baron TH, et al. Postpolypectomy lower gastrointestinal bleeding: potential role of aspirin. Am J Gastroenterol 2004; 99(9):1785–1789.

   Large case-control study of postpolypectomy bleeding showing no increased risks with prior aspirin use.

208. Laine L, Connors LG, Reicin A, et al. Serious lower gastrointestinal clinical events with nonselective NSAID or coxib use. Gastroenterology 2003; 124(2):288–292.

209. Hold S, Rigoglioso V, Sidhu M, et al. Nonsteroidal anti-inflammatory drugs and lower gastrointestinal bleeding. Dig Dis Sci 1993; 38:1619–1621.

210. Lana A, Sekar MC, Hirschowitz BI. Objective evidence of aspirin use in both ulcer and nonulcer upper and lower gastrointestinal bleeding. Gastroenterology 1992; 103:862–869.

211. Hall RI, Petty AH, Cobden I, et al. Enteritis and colitis associated with mefanimic acid. Br Med J 1983; 287:1182.

212. Ravi S, Keat AC, Keat EC. Colitis caused by non-steroidal anti-inflammatory drugs. Postgrad Med J 1986; 62:773–776.

213. Uribe A, Johnasson C, Slezak P, et al. Ulcerations of the colon associated with naproxen and acetylsalicylic acid treatment. Gastrointest Endosc 1986; 32:242–244.

214. Varma J. Do nonsteroidal anti-inflammatory drugs cause lower gastrointestinal bleeding? A brief review. J Am Board Fam Pract 1989; 2:119–122.

215. Langman MJS, Morgan L, Worral A. Use of anti-inflammatory drugs by patients admitted with small or large bowel perforations and hemorrhage. Br Med J 1985; 290:347–349.

216. Kaufmann HJ, Taubin HL. Nonsteroidal anti-inflammatory drugs activate quiescent inflammatory bowel disease. Ann Intern Med 1987; 107:513–516.

217. Uno Y, Munakata A. Endoscopic and histologic correlates of colorectal polyp bleeding. Gastrointest Endosc 1995; 41:460–467.

218. Maciel J, Barbosa J, Junior A. Endoscopic Nd:YAG laser surgery in the treatment of villous adenomas of the rectum. Hepatogastroenterology 1994; 41:58–60.

219. Hansen CP, Colstrup H, Mogensen AM. Recurrent gastrointestinal bleeding due to leiomyosarcomas of the small intestine. Eur J Surg 1991; 157:227–229.

220. Akwaria OE, Dozois RR, Weiland LH, et al. Leiomyosarcoma of the small and large bowel. Cancer 1978; 42:1375–1384.

221. Chitasso PJP, Fazio VW. Prognostic factors of 28 leiomyosarcomas of the small intestine. Surg Gynecol Obstet 1982; 155:197–202.

222. Christou NV, Stein LA, Meakins JC. Recurrent gastrointestinal bleeding due to smooth muscle tumors of the small intestine. Can J Surg 1979; 22:95–98.

223. Martin RG. Malignant tumors of the small intestine. Surg Clin North Am 1986; 66:779–785.

224. Wilson JM, Melvin DB, Gray GF, et al. Primary malignancies of the small bowel: A report of 96 cases and a review of the literature. Ann Surg 1974; 180:175–179.

225. Fecxzko PJ, Collins DD, Mezwa DG. Metastatic disease involving the gastrointestinal tract. Radiol Clin North Am 1993; 31:1359–1373.

226. Heymann AD, Vieto JO. Recurrent renal carcinoma causing intestinal hemorrhage. Am J Gastroenterol 1978; 69:582–585.

227. Ihde JK, Coit DG. Melanoma metastatic to stomach, small bowel, or colon. Am J Surg 1991; 162:208–211.

228. Lynch-Nyhan A, Fishman EK, Kadir S. Diagnosis and management of massive gastrointestinal bleeding owing to duodenal metastasis from renal cell carcinoma. J Urol 1987; 138:611–613.

229. Short TP, Thomas E, Joshi PN, et al. Occult gastrointestinal bleeding in renal cell carcinoma: Value of endoscopic evaluation. Am J Gastroenterol 1993; 88:300–302.

230. Zerbib F, Becouarn Y, Stockle E, et al. Colonic metastasis of a renal carcinoma. A case report. Tumori 1992; 789:219–220.

231. Bergan JJ, Dry L, Conn J, et al. Intestinal ischemic syndromes. Ann Surg 1969; 169:120–126.

232. Peters JH, Reilly PM, Merine DS, et al. Vascular insufficiency. In: Yamada T, Alpers DH, Owyang C, et al., eds. Textbook of gastroenterology, vol 2. Philadelphia: JB Lippincott; 1991:2188–2217.

233. Berg B, Groth C, Magnusson G, et al. Gastrointestinal complications in 248 kidney transplant recipients. Scand J Urol Nephrol Suppl 1975; 29:19–20.

234. Donaldson JK, Stout BF. Mesenteric thrombosis. Am J Surg 29:208-217, 1935.

235. Ottinger LW, Austen WG. A study of 136 patients with mesenteric infarction. Surg Gynecol Obstet 1967; 124:251–261.

236. Abel ME, Russell TR. Ischemic colitis: Comparison of surgical and nonoperative management. Dis Colon Rectum 1983; 26:113–115.

237. Williams LF, Wittenbert J. Ischemic colitis: A useful clinical diagnosis, but is it ischemic? Ann Surg 1975; 182:439–446.

238. Ullery BS, Boyko AT, Banet GA, et al. Colonic ischemia: an under-recognized cause of lower gastrointestinal bleeding. Emerg Med 2004; 27(1)1:1–5.

239. Eisenberg D, Sherwood CE. Bleeding Meckel's diverticulum diagnosed by arteriography and radioisotope imaging. Am J Dig Dis 1975; 20:573–576.

240. Ghahremani GG. Radiology of Meckle's diverticulum. Crit Rev Diagn Imaging 1986; 26:1–43.

241. Duszynski DO, Jewett TC, Allen JE. Tc-99m pertechnetate scanning of the abdomen with particular reference to small bowel pathology. Am J Radiol 1971; 113:258–262.

242. Thompson JN, Hemingway AP, McPherson GAD, et al. Obscure gastrointestinal hemorrhage of small-bowel origin. Br Med J 1984; 288:1663–1665.

243. Forsgren H, Lindhagen J, Melander S, et al. Colorectal endometriosis. Acta Chir Scand 1983; 149:431–435.

244. Bozdech JM. Endoscopic diagnosis of colonic endometriosis. Gastrointest Endosc 1992; 38:568–570.

245. Sampler ER, Slagle GG, Hand AM. Colonic endometriosis: Its clinical spectrum. South Med J 1984; 77:192–194.

246. Collin GR, Russel JC. Endometriosis of the colon: Its diagnosis and management. Am Surg 1990; 45:274–279.

247. Prystowsky JB, Stryker SJ, Ujicki GT, et al. Gastrointestinal endometriosis. Incidence and indications for resection. Arch Surg 1988; 123:855-858.

248. Meyers WC, Kelvin FM, Jones RS. Diagnosis and surgical treatment of colonic endometriosis. Arch Surg 1979; 114:1169–1175.

249. Levitt MD, Hodby KJ, Van Merwyk AJ, et al. Cyclical rectal bleeding in colorectal endometriosis. Aust NZ J Surg 1989; 59:941–943.

250. Weed JC, Ray JE. Endometriosis of the bowel. Obstet Gynecol 1987; 69:727–730.

251. Markham SM, Carpenter SE, Rock JA. Extrapelvic endometriosis. Obstet Gynecol Clin North Am 1989; 16:193–219.

252. Markham SM, Welling DR, Larsen KS, et al. Endometriosis of the rectum treated with a long-term GnRH agonist and surgery. NY State J Med 1991; 91:69–71.

253. Daniel WA, Eagan S. The quantity of blood required to produce a tarry stool. JAMA 1939; 113:2232.

254. Schiff L, Stevens RJ, Shapro N, et al. Observations on the oral administration of citrated blood in man II. The effect on the stools. Am J Med Sci 1942; 203:409–412.

255. Wara P, Stodkilde H. Bleeding pattern before admission as a guideline for emergency endoscopy. Scand J Gastroenterol 1985; 20:72–78.

256. Zuckerman GR, Trellis DR, Shennan TM, et al. An objective measure of stool color for differentiating upper from lower gastrointestinal bleeding. Dig Dis Sci 1995; 40:1614–1621.

257. Silverstein FE, Gilbert DA, Tedesco FJ, et al. The national ASGE survey on upper gastrointestinal bleeding. Part I: Study design and baseline data. Gastrointest Endosc 1981; 27:73–79.

258. Silverstein FE, Gilbert DA, Tedesco JF, et al. The national ASGE survey on upper gastrointestinal bleeding. Part II: Clinical prognostic factors. Gastrointest Endosc 1981; 27:80–93.

259. Gilbert DA, Silverstein FE, Tedesco JF, et al. The national ASGE survey on upper gastrointestinal bleeding. Part III: Endoscopy in upper gastrointestinal bleeding. Gastrointest Endosc 1981; 27:94–101.

260. Snook JA, Holdstock GE, Bamforth J. Value of a simple biochemical ratio in distinguishing upper and lower sites of gastrointestinal hemorrhage. Lancet 1986; 1:1064–1065.

261. Chalasani N, Clark S, Wilcox CM. Blood urea nitrogen to creatinine concentration in gastrointestinal bleeding: A reappraisal. Am J Gastroenterol 1997; 92:1796–1799.

262. Zuccaro G. Management of the adult patient with acute lower gastrointestinal bleeding. Am J Gastroenterol 1998; 93:1202–1208.

263. Alavi A, Dann RW, Baum S, et al. Scintigraphic detection of acute gastrointestinal bleeding. Radiology 1977; 124:753–756.

264. Alavi A, Ring EJ. Localization of gastrointestinal bleeding: Superiority of ^{99m}Tc sulfur colloid compared with angiography. Am J Gastroenterol 1981; 137:741–748.

265. Bunker SR, Lull RJ, Tanasescu DE, et al. Scintigraphy of gastrointestinal hemorrhage: Superiority of ^{99m}Tc red blood cell over ^{99m}Tc sulfur colloid. Am J Gastroenterol 1984; 143:543–548.

266. McKusick KA, Froelich J, Callahan, RJ, et al. ^{99m}Tc red blood cells for detection of gastrointestinal bleeding: Experience with 80 patients. Am J Gastroenterol 1981; 137:1113–1118.

267. Winzelberg GG, McKusick KA, Froelich JW, et al. Detection of gastrointestinal bleeding with ^{99m}Tc-labeled red blood cells. Semin Nucl Med 1981; 12:139–146.

268. Zuckerman GR, Prakash C. Acute lower intestinal bleeding. Part I: clinical presentation and diagnosis. Gastrointest Endosc 1998; 48:606–617.

A review article including assessment of the efficacy of RBC scanning for localization of LGI bleeding.

269. Nusbaum M, Younis MT, Baum S, et al. Control of portal hypertension. Selective mesenteric arterial infusion of vasopressin. Arch Surg 1974; 108:342–347.

270. Koval G, Benner KG, Rosch J, et al. Aggressive angiographic diagnosis in acute lower gastrointestinal hemorrhage. Dig Dis Sci 1987; 32:248–253.

271. Rösch J, Keller GS, Wawrukiewicz AS, et al. Pharmacoangiography in the diagnosis of recurrent massive lower gastrointestinal bleeding. Radiology 1982; 145:615–619.

272. Athanasoulis CA, Walman AC, Simmons JT, et al. Effects of intravenous vasopressin on canine mesenteric arterial blood flow, bowel oxygen consumption, and cardiac output. Am J Gastroenterol 1978; 130:1033–1039.

273. Baum S, Rösch J, Dotter CT, et al. Selective mesenteric arterial infusions in the management of massive diverticular hemorrhage. N Engl J Med 1973; 288:1269–1272.

274. Galloway SJ, Casarella WJ, Shimkin PM. Vascular malformations of the right colon as a cause of bleeding in patients with aortic stenosis. Radiology 1974; 113:11–15.

275. Baum S, Nusbaum M. The control of gastrointestinal hemorrhage by selective mesenteric arterial infusion of vasopressin. Radiology 1971; 98:497–505.

276. Rösch J, Dotter CT, Rose RW. Selective arterial infusion of vasoconstrictors in acute gastrointestinal bleeding. Radiology 1971; 99:27–36.

277. Lawler G, Bircher M, Spencer J, et al. Embolisation in colonic bleeding. Br J Radiol 1985; 58:83–84.

278. Rosenkrantz H, Bookstein JJ, Rosen RJ, et al. Postembolic colonic infarction. Radiology 1982; 142:47–51.

279. Uflacker R. Transcatheter embolization for treatment of acute lower gastrointestinal bleeding. Acta Radiol 1987; 28:425–430.

280. Walker WJ, Goldin AR, Shaff MI, et al. Per catheter control of hemorrhage from the superior and inferior mesenteric arteries. Clin Radiol 1980; 31:71–80.

281. Ross JA. Vascular patterns of small and large intestine compared. Br J Surg 1952; 39:330–339.

282. DeBarros J, Rosas L, Cohen J, et al. The changing paradigm for the treatment of colonic hemorrhage: superselective angiographic embolization. Dis Colon Rectum 2002; 45:802–808.

283. Dehyle P, Blum AL, Nuesch JH, et al. Emergent colonoscopy in the management of the acute perianal hemorrhage. Endoscopy 1974; 6:229–232.

284. Rossini FP, Ferrari A. Emergent colonoscopy: In: Hunt RH, Waye JD, eds. Colonoscopy: techniques, clinical practice and color atlas. London: Chapman & Hall; 1981:289–299.

285. Treat MR, Forde KA. Colonoscopy, technetium scanning, and angiography in acute rectal bleeding – an algorithm for their combined use. Surg Gastroenterol 2:135–138. 1983;

286. Vellacott KD. Early endoscopy for acute lower gastrointestinal hemorrhage. Ann R Coll Surg Engl 68:243–244. 1986;

287. Caos A, Benner KJ, Manier J, et al. Colonoscopy after Golytely preparation in acute rectal bleeding. J Clin Gastroenterol 1988; 95:1569–1574.

288. Gostout CJ, Wang KK, Ahlquist DA, et al. Acute gastrointestinal bleeding – experience of a specialized management team. J Clin Gastroenterol 1992; 14:260–267.

   A recent review article on endoscopic management of diverticular bleeding.

289. Jensen DM, Machicado GA, Jutabha R, et al. Urgent colonoscopy for the diagnosis and treatment of severe diverticular hemorrhage. N Engl J Med 2000; 342(2):78–82.

   A prospective study evaluating the role of emergent colonoscopy for LGI bleeding.

290. Elta GH. Urgent colonoscopy for acute lower-GI bleeding. Gastrointest Endosc 2004; 59(3):402–408.

291. Smoot RL, Gostout CJ, Rajan E, et al. Is early colonoscopy after admission for acute diverticular bleeding needed? Am J Gastroenterol 2003; 98(9):1996–1999.

292. Waye JD. Endoscopy of the small bowel: Push, sonde and intraoperative. Endoscopy 1994; 26:60–63.

293. Foutch PG. Angiodysplasia of the gastrointestinal tract. Am J Gastroenterol 1993; 88:807–818.

294. Nolan DJ, Traill ZC. The current role of the barium examination of the small intestine. Clin Radiol 1997; 52:809–820.

295. Maglinte DD, Kelvin FM, O'Connor K, et al. Current status of small bowel radiography. Abdom Imaging 1996; 21:247–257.

296. Batram CI. Small bowel enteroclysis: cons. Adbom Imaging 1996; 21:245–246.

297. Appleyard M, Fireman Z, Glukhovsky A, et al. A randomized trial comparing wireless capsule endoscopy with push enteroscopy for the detection of small bowel lesions. Gastroenterology 2000; 119:1421–1438.

298. Swain P. The role of enteroscopy in clinical practice. Gastrointest Endosc Clin N Am 1999; 9:135–144.

299. Seensalu R. The sonde exam. Gastrointest Endosc Clin N Am 1999; 9:37–59.

300. Zaman A, Sheppard B, Katon RM. Total peroral intraoperative enteroscopy for obscure GI bleeding using a dedicated push enteroscope: diagnostic yield and patients outcome. Gastrointest Endosc 1999; 40:506–510.

301. Yamamoto H, Kita H, Sunada K, et al. Clinical outcomes of double-balloon endoscopy for the diagnosis and treatment of small-intestinal diseases. Clin Gastroenterol Hepatol 2004; 2:1010–1016.

   Provides the latest information on double balloon enteroscopy.

302. Lewis BS, Swain P. Capsule endoscopy in the evaluation of patients with suspected small intestinal bleeding: results of a pilot study. Gastrointest Endosc 2002; 56:349–353.

303. Costamagna G, Shah SK, Riccioni ME, et al. A prospective trial comparing small bowel radiographs and video capsule endoscopy for suspected small bowel disease. Gastroenterology 2002; 123:999–1005.

304. Adler DG, Knipschield M, Gopstout C. A prospective comparison of capsule endoscopy and push enteroscopy in patients with GI bleeding of obscure origin. Gastrointest Endosc 2004; 59:492–498.

305. Eu C, Remke S, May A, et al. The first prospective controlled trial comparing wireless capsule endoscopy and push enteroscopy in chronic gastrointestinal bleeding. Endoscopy 2002; 34:685–689.

306. Scapa E, Jacob H, Lewkowicz S, et al. Initial experience of wireless capsule endoscopy for evaluating occult gastrointestinal bleeding and suspected small bowel pathology. Am J Gastroenterol 2002; 97:2776–2779.

307. Rastogi A, Schoen RE, Slivka A. Diagnostic yield and clinical outcomes of capsule endoscopy. Gastrointest Endosc 2004; 60(6):959–964.

   One of the first articles to quantify the benefit of capsule endoscopy on patient outcome.

308. Faigel DO, Fennerty MB. 'Cutting the cord' for capsule endoscopy. Gastroenterology 2002; 123:1385–1388.

309. Berner JS, Mauer K, Lewis BS. Push and sonde enteroscopy for the diagnosis of obscure gastrointestinal bleeding. Am J Gastroenterol 1994; 89:2139–2142.

310. Hoffman JS, Cave DR, Birkett D. Intra-operative enteroscopy with a sonde intestinal fiberscope. Gastrointest Endosc 1994; 40:229–230.

311. Lewis BS, Wenger JS, Waye JD. Small bowel enteroscopy and intraoperative enteroscopy for obscure gastrointestinal bleeding. Am J Gastroenterol 1991; 86:171–174.

312. Lewis BS, Waye JD. Chronic gastrointestinal bleeding of obscure origin: Role of small bowel enteroscopy. Gastroenterology 1988; 94:1117–1120.

313. Gostout CJ, Schroeder KW, Burton DD. Small bowel enteroscopy: An early experience in gastrointestinal bleeding of unknown origin. Gastrointest Endosc 1991; 37:5–8.

314. Foutch PG, Sawyer R, Sanowski RA. Push enteroscopy for diagnosis of patients with gastrointestinal bleeding of obscure origin. Gastrointest Endosc 1990; 36:337–341.

315. Barkin J, Schonfeld W, Thomsen S, et al. Enteroscopy and small bowel biopsy: An improved technique for the diagnosis of small bowel disease. Gastrointest Endosc 1985; 31:215–217.

316. Parker HW, Agayoff JD. Enteroscopy and small bowel biopsy using a peroral colonoscopy (Letter). Gastrointest Endosc 1983; 29:139–140.

317. Dabezies MA, Fisher RS, Krevsky B. Video small bowel enteroscopy: Early experience with a prototype instrument. Gastrointest Endosc 1991; 37:60–62.

318. Dykman DD, Killian SE. Initial experience with the Pentax VSB-P2900 enteroscopy. Am J Gastroenterol 1993; 88:570–573.

319. Chong J, Tagle M, Barkin JS, et al. Small bowel push-type fiberoptic enteroscopy for patients with occult gastrointestinal bleeding or suspected small bowel pathology. Am J Gastroenterol 1994; 80:2143–2146.

320. Barkin JS, Resner DK. First generation video enteroscope: Fourth generation push-type small bowel enteroscopy utilizing an overtube. Gastrointest Endosc 1994; 40:743–747.

321. Barkin JS, Reiner DK, Lewis BS, et al. Diagnostic and therapeutic jejunostomy with the SIF-10L enteroscope: Long is really better (Abstract). Gastrointest Endosc 1990; 36:214.

322. Barkin JS, Lewis BS, Reiner DK, et al. Diagnostic and therapeutic jejunostomy with the SIF-10L enteroscope: Long is really better. Gastrointest Endosc 1992; 38:55–58.

323. Zuccaro G, Barthel JS, Slivka MV. Use of a 165 cm push enteroscope in the evaluation of GI bleeding of unknown etiology (Abstract). Gastrointest Endosc 1991; 37:274.

324. Ress AM, Benacci JC, Sarr MG. Efficacy of intraoperative enteroscopy in diagnosis and prevention of recurrent occult gastrointestinal bleeding. Am J Surg 1992; 163:94–99.

   A synopsis of intraoperative enteroscopy which gives pause to widespread use of the technique.

325. Lewis BS, Wenger JS, Waye JD. Small bowel enteroscopy and intraoperative enteroscopy for obscure gastrointestinal bleeding. Am J Gastroenterol 1991; 86:171–174.

CHAPTER SIXTY-SIX

66

Hemorrhoids and other anorectal disorders

Eric J. Dozois and John H. Pemberton

INTRODUCTION

This chapter deals with the management of hemorrhoids and other anorectal disorders. Physicians from various specialties will encounter and treat patients with anorectal disease. The majority of patients will present with symptoms such as bleeding, pain, discharge, and pruritus. A carefully taken medical history will often lead to the diagnosis that then can be confirmed by physical examination. Patients are often reluctant to seek medical care because of fear or embarrassment associated with this part of the anatomy. Benign and malignant anorectal disorders have similar presenting features and patients with malignant disease may delay consultation because their symptoms are commonly attributed to hemorrhoids or other benign conditions. Complicating this is the fact that commercial preparations are readily available, making self-treatment easy.

The reported prevalence rates of anal diseases vary widely depending on the method of evaluation and definition. A survey of benign anal disease symptoms, in a randomly selected American population, showed that a history of hemorrhoids and recurrent anal symptomatology were highly prevalent, and yet 80% of subjects with anal symptoms had not consulted a physician.[1] Due to its high prevalence, the economic impact of anorectal disorders are substantial.

HEMORRHOIDS: BACKGROUND

The word 'hemorrhoid' is derived from the Greek *haimorrhoos*, meaning flowing of blood (*haima* equals blood, *rhoos* equals flowing). The word 'pile' comes from the Latin 'pila' meaning ball or pill. The cause of hemorrhoidal disease is unknown. The prevalence of hemorrhoidal disease varies from 4% of the general population to 36.4% in general practice.[2] The annual rate of office visits for hemorrhoidal disease is 12 for every 1000 patients in the United States, its prevalence is similar between the sexes, and increases with age until the seventh decade.[3,4] Numerous theories concerning the pathogenesis of hemorrhoids have been proposed, but the exact mechanism remains elusive.[5] Constipation and straining were once accepted as the major cause of hemorrhoidal disease, but this is considered to be a gross oversimplification.[6] Straining excessively to pass a bowel movement is a common practice described by patients with hemorrhoidal disease.

In the upper anal canal there are vascular cushions continuous with the rectal columns above. Classically, three vascular cushions are described, two on the right and one on the left, but their arrangement varies greatly. The function of anal cushions is not clearly understood, but there is good evidence to suggest that they provide the final watertight seal to the anal canal.

Clinically, classification of hemorrhoids is described as four distinct 'degrees' depending on the extent of prolapse (Fig. 66.1). First-degree hemorrhoids are anal cushions that do not descend below the dentate line on straining, but may develop symptoms of bleeding. Second-degree hemorrhoids are when anal cushions protrude below the dentate line on straining, but retract automatically when the straining ceases. Third-degree hemorrhoids are when the anal cushions descend below the anal verge on straining or defecation and remain prolapsed until they are digitally replaced. Fourth-degree hemorrhoids is a term used by some to describe anal cushions permanently outside the anal verge.

Hemorrhoidal disease can give rise to varying degrees of bleeding, anal swelling, pain, discomfort, discharge, and pruritus. Bleeding is the most common presenting complaint. Hemorrhoids in themselves rarely cause anal pain unless there is thrombosis. Diagnosis of internal hemorrhoids is usually based on symptoms, which include painless bleeding or prolapse. Bleeding is described as bright red spotting on toilet paper or dripping in the toilet bowl and normally occurs at the end of defecation and is separate from the stool.

Evaluation of patients suspected of having hemorrhoids includes digital rectal examination and palpation of the entire circumference of the anal canal to rule out point tenderness and anorectal masses. Anoscopy, which can be safely done in the office, is an accurate method for examining the anal canal and distal rectum. One of the most advantageous ways to diagnose and grade hemorrhoids is to have the patient sit on a toilet seat and strain and observe the amount and distribution of prolapse.

HEMORRHOIDS: PRINCIPLES OF TREATMENT

Nonsurgical therapy

Dietary manipulation, with the aim to achieve a bulky stool that is easy to pass, is a simple and reasonable first-line approach in the patient with grades I or II hemorrhoids. Bulk-forming agents such as Citrucel® or Metamucil® are often prescribed, but compliance can be poor. Senapati and Nichols[7] reported a prospective randomized trial of 43 patients with bleeding hemorrhoids who

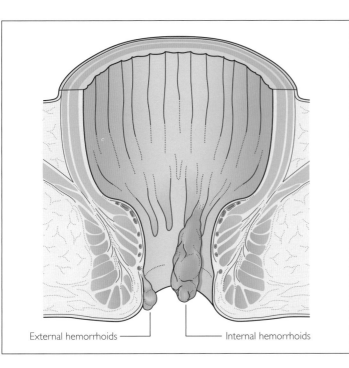

Fig. 66.1 • Prolapsed internal hemorrhoid. (By permission of Mayo Foundation.)

External hemorrhoids — — Internal hemorrhoids

were allocated to receive either a bulk laxative together with injection sclerotherapy or a bulk laxative alone. No significant difference in bleeding at 6 months was detected, which tends to render the more invasive procedures meaningless. Use of warm sitz baths, topical anesthetics, and steroid suppositories can be added for temporary symptomatic relief.

Office procedures

When measures described above fail, office-based treatment can be effective to provide symptomatic relief. Office procedures such as sclerotherapy, rubber band ligation, cryosurgery, infrared coagulation, bipolar diathermy, and anal dilatation have been described to treat grades I–III disease. Mucosal fixation to the underlying muscle, creating submucosal fibrosis or full-thickness ulceration, is the main goal of a majority of these treatments. Injection sclerotherapy is done by the injection of phenyl solution. Five percent phenyl in almond or arachis oil is drawn up from individual 10 ml vials to allow for about 3 cc of injection into the base of each vascular cushion. Five percent quinine and urea hydrochloride is the most commonly used solution in the United States, whereas 5% phenyl in oil is the most common injection used in the United Kingdom. This treatment can be painful and thus complications result from an inappropriate injection site or submucosal extravasation. Overall, the results have been disappointing in large published series.[8]

Rubber band ligation may be the most common office-based procedure done in the United States for grades I–III hemorrhoids. In the authors' experience, we have found hemorrhoidal banding to be effective and straightforward for patients suffering from grade I, II and selected grade III hemorrhoids. A small rubber band, or O-ring, is applied tightly around the neck of a tongue of mucosa, which is pulled into the barrel of an applicator (Fig. 66.2). Ischemic sloughing then follows 5–7 days after application. The hemorrhoid apex should be grasped at least 6 mm above the dentate line so as not to cause significant discomfort to the patient. If one places a rubber band too close to the dentate line,

considerable pain and discomfort will result. Complications of hemorrhoidal banding have been described, with pain being the most common complication. Some patients experience vasovagal fainting and urinary retention. There have been fatal cases of *Clostridium* infection after banding of hemorrhoids, first described by O'Hara.[9] Overall, the results of rubber band ligation therapy for patients with first- and second-degree hemorrhoids have been good. Rothberg et al. reported symptomatic control of internal hemorrhoids in 80% of cases treated with a five- to fifteen-year follow-up in 595 patients after rubber band ligation.[10] Ligation can be done safely in up to two hemorrhoidal groups per session. If more than two groups need to be treated, waiting 2–3 weeks between sessions will often avoid significant discomfort to the patient.

Surgical therapy

For grade IV and large grade III hemorrhoids, and those others that do not improve with conservative measures, surgical therapy may be the only option for cure. The surgeon's choice of technique is primarily based on personal experience and technical training. The options for surgical therapy include anal stretch procedures, closed hemorrhoidectomy, open hemorrhoidectomy, laser hemorrhoidectomy, Whitehead hemorrhoidectomy, and stapled hemorrhoidectomy.

Open hemorrhoidectomy, which involves surgical excision only of the prolapsed hemorrhoidal group, is the operation most widely used in the United Kingdom and is based on a technique originally described by Milligan (Fig. 66.3A).[11] Another common technique is *closed hemorrhoidectomy*, which also involves excision of the hemorrhoidal tissue, but is followed by closure of the wounds with suture material. This technique is popular in the United States and was first described by Ferguson (Fig. 66.3B).[12] The aim of the open and closed hemorrhoidectomy is to remove as much of the hemorrhoid as possible without sacrificing anoderm or internal sphincter muscle. Closure of the wound is

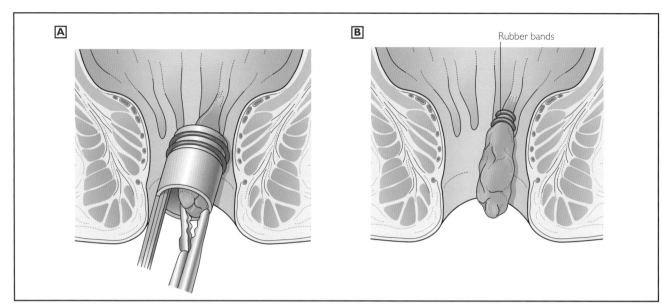

Fig. 66.2 • **(A)** Hemorrhoid banding instrument applied to prolapsed hemorrhoid. **(B)** Postbanding result with rubber bands at base of hemorrhoid. (By permission of Mayo Foundation.)

considered to be an important part of the Ferguson technique to minimize postoperative serous discharge. A randomized trial[13] comparing open and closed hemorrhoidectomy involving 67 patients showed that there was no difference in pain scores, analgesic requirement, and length of hospitalization. Complete wound healing took longer after closed hemorrhoidectomy compared with open hemorrhoidectomy, and complication rates were similar in both groups.

Unfortunately, surgical intervention can be accompanied by a high incidence of complications including urinary retention, hemorrhage, constipation, fecal impaction and severe, debilitating pain. Therefore, attention has been focused on a less painful method of surgical treatment of hemorrhoids. Modification of conventional techniques include the addition of lateral internal sphincterotomy, anal dilation, and anal sphincter relaxants. However, these techniques have not significantly reduced postoperative pain.[14] Regardless of the surgical technique, prophylactic metronidazole has been shown to suppress postoperative pain, increases patient satisfaction, and allows them to return to work earlier.[15]

Most recently, circular stapled rectal hemorrhoidectomy, sometimes known as circular stapled rectal mucosectomy, has emerged as a potentially less painful alternative. This minimally invasive surgical approach recently introduced in the United States, called *Procedure for Prolapse and Hemorrhoids* (PPH), may help patients recover from surgery faster and with less pain when compared to the conventional surgical approaches described above. Stapled hemorrhoidectomy, as initially advocated by Longo

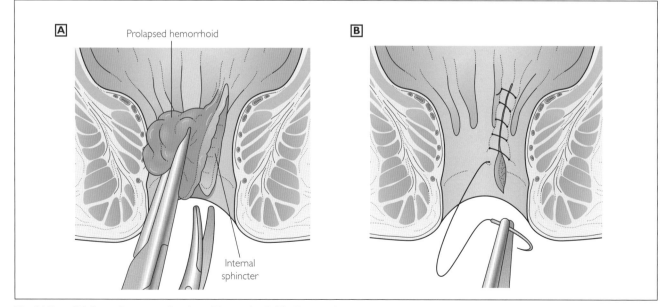

Fig. 66.3 • **(A)** Surgical excision of prolapsed hemorrhoid. **(B)** Closure of postexcision wound. (By permission of Mayo Foundation.)

and colleagues, has been hailed as a significant breakthrough in the way surgical excision of hemorrhoids is performed; both dramatically decreasing the level of postoperative pain and shortening healing time after operation.[16] The operation reduces the size of the internal hemorrhoids by interrupting their blood supply, therefore reducing the size of the vascular cushions and reducing the available rectal mucosa for potential prolapse. Whereas conventional surgical hemorrhoidectomy involves excision of hemorrhoidal tissue, anoderm, and perianal skin, stapled hemorrhoidectomy simply excises an anulus of rectal mucosa above the pathologic rectal mucosa, hemorrhoids. Circumferential grade III or IV hemorrhoids are necessary for application of this technique.

Several randomized, controlled trials have been performed comparing stapled hemorrhoidectomy to conventional excisional hemorrhoidectomy. Most of the trials have shown a decrease in postoperative pain, length of hospital stay, and rapid return to regular activities when compared to conventional hemorrhoidectomy.[17,18] However, stapling increases operative costs, advanced surgical skills are necessary, and there is a learning curve. Moreover, complications of stapled hemorrhoidectomy have been described and include rectovaginal fistula, near-fatal sepsis, anal stricturing, and bleeding.[19,20]

Technique

Currently, surgeons must be trained and certified in the use of the device through programs sponsored by the manufacturer. The procedure starts with dilation of the anal canal and then a purse-string suture is placed 4 cm above the dentate line. Subsequently, the circular stapler is introduced transanally. The anvil of the device is positioned proximal to the purse-string suture, and the suture is tied down to the anvil. Retraction of the suture pulls the attached rectal mucosa into the stapler (Fig. 66.4). Closure of the anvil and firing of the stapler simultaneously excises the ring of mucosa proximal to the hemorrhoids, thus interrupting the blood supply but maintaining continuity of rectal mucosa.[21]

Thrombosed external hemorrhoids

Acute thrombosis is a complication of external hemorrhoids (see Fig. 66.1) and it occurs in the inferior anal plexus under the squamous mucosa. The cause is unknown, but it is postulated that when distended veins lose their connective support, they are prone to thrombosis.[22] Stasis in the veins, with clot formation and acute swelling, may be intensely painful during the first 48 hours. This pain and swelling may be continuous and incapacitating for several days, then gradually subside over the next 3–4 weeks. Treatment is usually nonsurgical and consists of bed rest, dietary changes, local hygiene, sitz baths, stool softeners, and analgesics. If acute thrombosis fails to respond to conservative measures, a surgical approach should be considered. Decapitation of the hemorrhoidal group, with complete removal of the offending clot, is essential to prevent early recurrence.[23] Internal anal sphincter hypertonicity seems to play a role in the pain caused by external hemorrhoids, and topical nitrates and nifedipine have been used to relax the internal sphincter in this setting with good symptomatic relief.[24,25]

ANAL FISSURE

Anal fissure is one of the most common causes of severe anal pain. The patient's symptoms can be highly distressing, often out of proportion to the findings on physical examination. An anal fissure is a linear, longitudinal tear or ulcer situated in the anal canal and extending from below the dentate line to the margin of the anus. The etiology of primary anal fissure is largely speculative, but it is generally agreed that the initiating factor is passage of a large stool that tears the anoderm, resulting in a linear tear that manifests as a fissure. Alternatively, an anal fissure can be instigated by passage of an explosive diarrheal stool. In both instances, trauma to the anal canal seems to be the causative factor. Although the initiating factor in fissure development may be traumatic, its perpetuation is due to an abnormality of internal sphincter tone, leading to chronicity. Investigators have

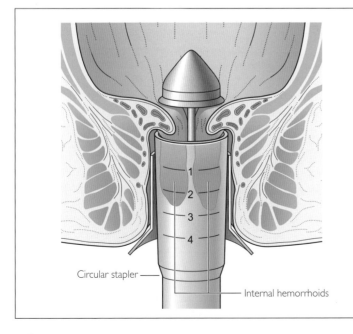

Circular stapler

Internal hemorrhoids

Fig. 66.4 • Stapling device for hemorrhoidectomy. (By permission of Mayo Foundation.)

demonstrated high resting pressures and overshoot contractions of the internal sphincter muscle in patients with fissures.[26–28]

Fissures can be classified as either acute or chronic and may be primary, idiopathic, or secondary. Secondary anal fissures, often having atypical locations in the anorectum, may be associated with Crohn's disease, ulcerative colitis, sexually transmitted diseases, AIDS, tuberculosis, or leukemia. Atypically located ulcers tend to be in the lateral quadrant and may be found to be proximal to the dentate line. In the acute phase a primary anal fissure is a mere cut or crack in the anal epithelium, causing severe anal pain and spasm. Chronic fissures are distinguished from their acute precursor by several features including a sentinel pile, an indurated anal ulcer that often exposes fibers of the internal sphincter muscle, and a hypertrophied anal papilla. The vast majority of fissures encountered in clinical practice are of primary idiopathic origin. The lesion is usually encountered in younger and middle-aged adults, but may occur at the extremes of age. Anal fissure is the most common cause of rectal bleeding in infants. Men and women are affected equally, but women are more likely to develop an anterior fissure. Anterior fissures account for 10% of all fissures in women versus only 1% of fissures in men.[29]

Diagnosis of an acute fissure is often made by history alone, with the patient describing severe anal pain during defecation. Patients may describe the pain as sharp or searing. Anorectal examination, by gently spreading the buttocks and inspecting the anal verge, often confirms the diagnosis. A linear tear or ulcer in the anterior or posterior midline is seen in the epithelium distal to the dentate line. Patients are often too tender for digital rectal examination or anoscopy. Once the fissure is identified, any attempts at instrumentation of the anus or anorectum should be deferred until treatment can be initiated.

Nonsurgical therapy

Conservative, nonsurgical measures, including topical steroids, local anesthetics, and bulk laxatives, successfully heal *acute* fissures in about 90% of instances.[30] Although used alongside specific medical and surgical therapy to minimize relapse, these measures alone heal less than 40% of *chronic* anal fissures. One study showed a poor response to conservative therapy in fissures demonstrating features of chronicity, such as sentinel tag or hypertrophied anal papilla.[31] Treatment of anal fissures begins with avoidance of constipation and breaking the repetitive cycle of hard stool, pain, and spasm. Bulk-forming agents should be initiated and the dosage adjusted to maintain formed but soft stool that is atraumatic to the anoderm during passage. Warm sitz baths are also beneficial in relieving spasm of the fissure. Local application of anesthetic ointments may provide temporary symptomatic relief. It has been shown, though, that symptomatic relief is better among patients treated with sitz baths and bran than in patients treated with lidocaine or hydrocortisone ointment.[32]

Pharmacologic treatment of anal fissure disease has dramatically changed treatment algorithms. There have been two forces behind this: (1) concern over rates of incontinence after surgery, and (2) a deeper understanding of the pharmacology and physiology of the anal sphincter has allowed a reasonable approach to manipulation of sphincter tone.[33] Topical nitroglycerin has recently been used in the treatment of anal fissures with the knowledge that nitric oxide mediates internal anal sphincter relaxation. Loder et al.[34] studied the effects of glycerol trinitrate on anal pressure in patients presenting for physiologic assessment of anal disorders. The authors demonstrated that the application of 0.2% glycerol trinitrate ointment to the anus resulted in a significant decrease in maximum resting anal pressure from pretreatment baseline values, which was not observed in the control patients given a placebo. The role of nitroglycerine paste in chronic anal fissure remains uncertain. Although it showed early promise, initial enthusiasm has been tempered somewhat by concern over medium-term relapse, headache, and tachyphylaxis.[35] As a topical preparation there are inevitable difficulties with regulating dose, and noncompliance may be common. The impressive results of early trials have been countered by reports suggesting that healing rates and patient satisfaction are low.[36]

There are alternatives to nitroglycerin, including both oral and topical calcium channel blockers. Topical 0.1% diltiazem, given twice per day, has shown promise as an effective therapy with minimal side effects. In a randomized trial of 50 patients, 2% diltiazem demonstrated more profound reduction in mean resting pressures (23% versus 15%) and better healing (65% versus 38%) with fewer side effects (0% versus 33%) than with oral diltiazem.[37] Topical diltiazem appears to produce similar fissure healing with fewer side effects than nitroglycerin. It also appears to heal 48–75% of fissures that have failed to heal with nitroglycerin therapy.[38]

Most recently, botulinum toxin has been utilized as a treatment for chronic anal fissure. Botulinum toxin A is an exotoxin produced by the bacterium *Clostridium botulinum* and is a potent neurotoxin that causes botulism in humans. Jost et al.[39] first reported its use in 1993 and others since have shown its effectiveness in the treatment of chronic anal fissure.[40] The results of a recent randomized, double-blind, placebo-controlled trial comparing botulinum toxin and nitroglycerin paste suggested that botulinum toxin should be considered as a first-line therapy for the treatment of chronic anal fissure.[41] Complications of botulinum toxin have been described and includes transient incontinence to flatus and perianal hematoma. Technique for application of botulinum toxin varies but typically involves 1–3 injections into the internal sphincter muscle in different quadrants with up to 20 units of botulinum.

Surgical therapy

Despite the improved efficacy of medical therapy for anal fissure disease, surgery remains an option for patients who fail. Because chronic anal fissures are associated with high resting anal pressures from underlying hypertonia of the internal anal sphincter, a lateral internal sphincterotomy performed surgically reduces the anal resting pressure leading to healing of the fissure. In experienced hands, the procedure is simple and can be done in the outpatient setting with reproducible results. Studies have shown healing rates of more than 95% in patients with chronic anal fissures.[42] Complications of this procedure, including infection and bleeding, are uncommon and self-limiting. However, varying degrees of fecal incontinence has been reported since the initial description of the procedure. Nyam and Pemberton looked at the long-term results of lateral internal sphincterotomy for chronic anal fissure with particular reference to the instance of fecal incontinence.[43] In their results they showed that fissures were healed at a minimum of 3 weeks after surgery in 96% of patients. Recurrence rate for fissures was 8%, with two-thirds of those recurrent fissures healing with conservative management. Ninety-eight percent of patients were satisfied with the outcome of surgery, but some degree of fecal incontinence occurred in 45% of patients at some time during the postoperative period. Incontinence to flatus, mild soiling, and gross incontinence occurred in 31%, 39%, and 23% of patients, respectively. However, by the time of the survey (a mean of >five years after sphincterotomy) 6% report incontinence to flatus, 8% had minor fecal soiling, and 1% experienced loss of solid stool. Importantly, only 3% of patients stated that incontinence had ever affected their quality of life.

ANORECTAL ABSCESS AND FISTULA-IN-ANO

In 90% of patients, the etiology of anorectal abscess and fistula-in-ano is due to non-specific infection of anal glands. At the level of the dentate line, the ducts of the anal glands empty into the anal crypts. According to the cryptoglandular theory, abscesses result from obstruction of the anal glands and ducts.[44] Other etiologies are responsible for the remaining 10% of anorectal suppuration and are listed in Table 66.1. Of these, Crohn's disease is the most common etiology the surgeon is likely to encounter.

Anorectal abscess

Anorectal abscesses can be classified by their position in potential anorectal spaces (Fig. 66.5). In order of frequency of occurrence, these spaces are perianal, ischiorectal, intersphincteric, and

Table 66.1 Etiology of anorectal abscess and fistula-in-ano

Cryptoglandular

Immunocompromised state

Infection
  Hidradenitis (dermatitides)
  Tuberculosis
  Actinomycosis
  Human immunodeficiency virus

Malignancy
  Leukemia
  Lymphoma
  Carcinoma

Crohn's disease

Anal fissure

Foreign body intrusion

Trauma

Radiation

(By permission of Mayo Foundation.)

supralevator. Perianal and ischioanal abscesses almost always present with perianal pain, swelling, induration, and erythema. Fever is occasionally reported. On physical examination the diagnosis is usually quite apparent. There will be noticeable tender swelling that may be accompanied by erythema, induration, and fluctuance. Supralevator, intersphincteric, and postanal abscesses can prove to be more difficult to diagnosis on physical exam alone because they are not externally visible. Presenting complaints of

Fig. 66.5 • Location of anorectal abscesses. (By permission of Mayo Foundation.)

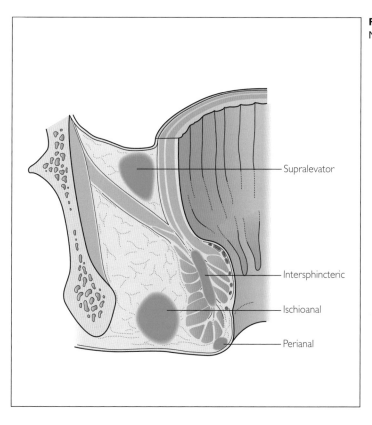

Supralevator

Intersphincteric

Ischioanal

Perianal

severe rectal pain accompanied by urinary symptoms and fever may be suggestive of the diagnosis. Digital examination, if possible, may reveal induration. Patients may be in too much pain to withstand an adequate examination, and thus an examination under anesthesia will be required to make the diagnosis. Diagnostic radiographic investigations can aid the clinician in delineating the extent and location of abscesses. For patients with complex abscesses or fistula-in-ano, CT or MRI scan of the pelvis may be helpful to delineate the extent of the infection and fistula tracts.

Surgical therapy

The treatment of anorectal abscesses is always surgical drainage. With adequate drainage, antibiotics are not necessary. Administration of antibiotics in the hope of curing an abscess is almost always futile and only serves to delay appropriate surgical therapy. Antibiotics do have an adjunctive role, however, in patients with significant cellulitis, immunosuppression, prosthetic valve, rheumatoid heart disease, and diabetes. Drainage of perianal and ischiorectal abscess can usually be accomplished in the office or emergency room under local anesthesia. There is the occasional patient with extreme pain and anxiety in whom general or regional anesthesia may be required. Once the patient is positioned appropriately, the area of abscess is prepared, and local anesthetic is infiltrated into the skin area around rather than directly over the most fluctuant portion of the abscess because the acid environment may preclude adequate anesthesia. A cruciate incision is made and the edges are excised, allowing the purulent material to be expressed. All loculations should be broken up digitally or with an appropriate instrument, and then the cavity packed with gauze. It is important to make the site of the incision as close as possible to the anus, minimizing the complexity of a possible future fistula. It should be stressed that this procedure can be extremely uncomfortable to the patient and large complex abscesses may be better drained under regional or general anesthesia for patient comfort. An alternative method of treatment that has been described for select abscesses is catheter drainage.[45] Once the stab incision is made to drain the purulent material, a soft mushroom catheter is inserted into the abscess cavity to ensure its complete drainage (Fig. 66.6). The patient is instructed on the method of irrigation through the catheter and the patient is seen 7–10 days postoperatively. If the drainage has ceased, the catheter is removed.

A controversial issue exists as to whether primary fistulotomy should be performed simultaneously with drainage. Reluctance to do so is based on the premise that a search for an internal opening in the presence of acute inflammation may lead to creation of false passages resulting in neglect of the main source of infection.[46] Between one-third and two-thirds of patients presenting with anorectal abscesses for the first time will not develop a fistula, thus rendering primary fistulotomy an unnecessary procedure that could result in needless disturbance of continence.[46] A prospective, randomized study that compared drainage alone with drainage and fistulotomy for perianal abscess revealed that incision and drainage alone demonstrated no significant recurrence when compared with concomitant fistulotomy, although there was a tendency toward recurrence in the former.[44] If the internal opening of a low transsphincteric fistula is readily apparent at the time of abscess drainage, primary fistulotomy is feasible. Exceptions to performing fistulotomy should be considered in patients with Crohn's disease, HIV infection, elderly patients, high transsphincteric fistulas, and anterior fistulas in women. The decision to perform a primary fistulotomy should be individualized and should only be attempted by a surgeon with sound knowledge of anorectal anatomy. Postoperatively, the patient should start twice-daily sitz baths. Usually there is no need to repack the wound. Follow-up is done in 10–14 days in the office.

In some patients, anorectal abscess will progress to a life-threatening necrotizing infection that manifests as extensive

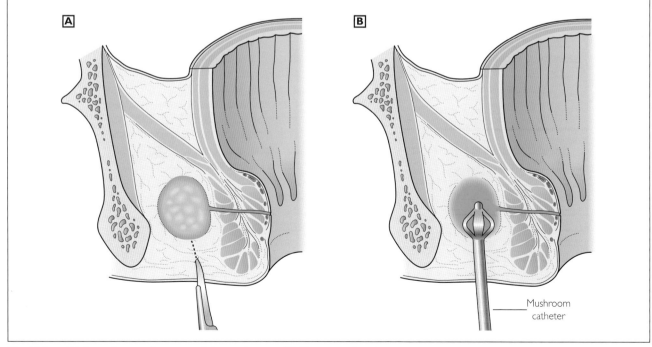

Fig. 66.6 • **(A)** Surgical approach to perianal abscess drainage. **(B)** Placement of mushroom catheter. (By permission of Mayo Foundation.)

perineal and scrotal cellulitis along with subcutaneous emphysema. This condition is a surgical emergency. Patients need to be resuscitated with fluids and given broad-spectrum antibiotics to treat both aerobic and anaerobic bacteria, and wide surgical debridement of the infected tissue should be undertaken as soon as possible, usually accompanied by fecal diversion.

Anorectal infections can also occur in patients with hematologic disease such as leukemia. The risk of infection developing in this population is related to the varying duration of neutropenia that often is associated with chemotherapy.[47] The most common symptom in these patients is fever. Pain and urinary retention can also occur and should raise the suspicion for occult anorectal infection. Because of the neutropenia, the area of infection may be poorly demarcated with erythema and fluctuance appearing late in the infection. Therefore, any patient with perianal pain must be assumed to have an infection. Antibiotics primarily directed at Gram-negative aerobic bacteria should be prescribed immediately, although the type of bacteria cultured from these infections is dependent of the flora of a given institution. It is somewhat controversial whether a wide incision with surgical drainage is helpful or whether the best approach is aspiration of the abscess. In a study by Glenn et al., aspiration and antibiotics was found to be effective, with surgical drainage recommended only if there was obvious fluctuance.[48]

Fistula-in-ano

A fistula is defined as an abnormal communication between two epithelial-lined surfaces. Fistulas are classified by their relationship to the anal sphincter mechanism (Fig. 66.7A). The most widely used classification, as outlined by Parks[49] describes fistulas and the abscess from which they can arise: intersphincteric (perianal), transsphincteric (ischioanal), extrasphincteric, and suprasphincteric (supralevator).

A patient with fistula-in-ano will generally give a history of an abscess that has drained spontaneously or been surgically decompressed. Patient may complain of chronic drainage or bleeding due to the presence of granulation tissue or will describe a pattern of intermittent, crescending pain, which is only relieved when the fistula starts to drain. If the fistula is secondary to proctocolitis, Crohn's disease, actinomycoses, or anorectal carcinoma, additional bowel symptoms will be present. Systemic diseases such as acquired immune deficiency syndrome, and lymphoma should be considered and excluded by appropriate investigations if clinically warranted.[50]

Diagnostic investigations for patients presenting with fistula-in-ano should include careful anoscopic examination; sigmoidoscopy should be done to exclude possible internal openings and exclude underlying pathology such as proctitis or Crohn's disease. Endorectal ultrasound, with or without hydrogen peroxide injection, and MRI can be useful for evaluation. Examination under anesthesia is often required to define presence of the extent of fistula in terms of internal and external openings and multiple tracts. Fistulogram is usually reserved for complex or recurrent fistulas.

Surgical therapy

The treatment of fistulas begins with drainage of any infection. After the abscess cavity is healed and the fistula remains, an attempt is made preoperatively to define the internal and external openings. Multiple techniques have been described for treatment. The two main techniques described are: (1) fistulotomy, in which

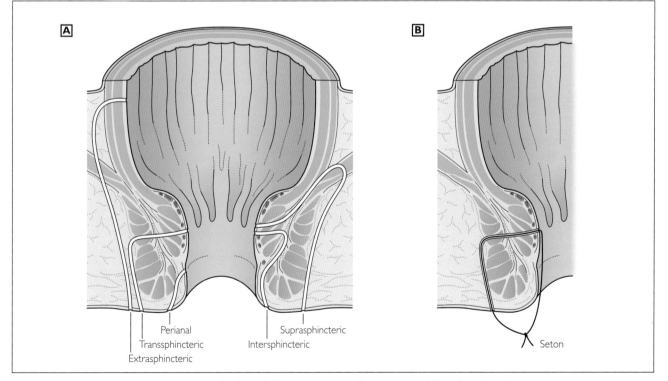

Fig. 66.7 ● **(A)** Parks classification of anorectal fistulas. **(B)** Placement of seton. (By permission of Mayo Foundation.)

the whole tract is cut open and allowed to heal by secondary intention, or (2) fistulectomy which includes complete excision of the tract. Other techniques described to close fistula include fibrin glue injection, cutting Setons, or mucosal advancement flaps.

Perianal fistulas occur in up to 50% of patients with Crohn's disease. For patients with anal fistula and Crohn's disease, a treatment plan must be agreed upon by the surgeon and the gastroenterologist because the origin of many of these fistulas is ulceration of the distal portion of the anorectum and not necessarily a cryptoglandular infection. Patients should undergo appropriate medical therapy directed at treating the underlying Crohn's disease after sepsis has been addressed. Superficial, low transsphincteric and low intersphincteric fistulas are usually treated by fistulotomy and antibiotics. High transsphincteric, suprasphincteric, and extrasphincteric fistulas are usually treated with noncutting Setons (see Fig. 66.7B), antibiotics, and azathioprine or 6-mecaptopurine and, in many cases, infliximab.[51]

PRURITUS ANI

Pruritus ani is a common proctologic problem characterized by intense itching localized in the anus and perianal skin. Pruritus ani may result from an underlying disorder of the epithelium, anorectal pathology, or may be idiopathic. The incidence of a benign or malignant anorectal condition associated with pruritus ani has varied among previous studies. Smith et al. found benign anorectal pathology in 25% of patients in their series.[52] Daniels et al, not only found benign pathology in 50% of patients but also found coexisting anorectal neoplasia in 16%.[53] Fecal contamination of the perineum, irritant chemicals in feces, allergies to locally applied agents, components of diet, and even psychosomatic factors have been suggested as possible etiologies, but are not conclusively proved to be of relevance.[54] Suggested exacerbating factors include diet, coffee, tea, dairy products, chocolate, tomatoes, poor personal hygiene or soiling, and stress.[52] Contact sensitivity may be an important factor in pruritus ani. Daffen et al. have shown that the majority of patients with longstanding pruritus ani have an underlying dermatosis. Patch testing may be an important part of the investigation of these patients as there is a high incidence of sensitization to previously used topical preparations, as was shown in this series.[55] A multidisciplinary approach with the assistance of a dermatologist may improve outcome in this difficult to treat group of patients.

In patients with pruritus ani, physical exam will reveal chronic skin changes secondary to inflammation with thickening of anal folds and mild erythema are common. When the condition is severe, small excoriations of the skin are observed.

The main approach to therapy for pruritus ani is diet and hygiene modification. Limiting the intake of coffee, carbonated and alcoholic beverages, and spicy foods, especially tomatoes, is suggested. The addition of extra dietary fiber helps completeness of defecation and therefore allows for better anal and perianal cleanliness. Advice regarding hygiene and drying methods are usually given, but lead to poor results.[56] Recently, capsaicin, which is a natural alkaloid derivative from plants, has been described as an effective and safe treatment. A study by Lysy et al.[57] looked at the effects of capsaicin on patients suffering from pruritus ani. Thirty-one of 44 patients treated experienced relief during capsaicin treatment. Their conclusions were that capsaicin is a new, safe, and highly effective treatment for severe, intractable idiopathic pruritus ani.

If conservative measures fail to cure the problem, a biopsy should be considered to exclude the presence of serious anorectal pathology such as Bowen's or Paget's disease. Biopsies can be done in the office with a 3 or 6 mm punch biopsy. For patients with severe idiopathic pruritus, not responding to conservative medical therapy, intradermal methylene blue injection has been shown to provide some relief. Patients are given general anesthesia, placed in lithotomy position, and perianal skin is prepared. Ten millileters methylene blue mixed with 7.5 mL marcaine is injected using a 22-gauge spinal needle. The methylene blue is infiltrated intradermally along skin furrows, incorporating any areas of excoriated tissue. Intradermal methylene blue injection has been shown by electron microscopy to destroy dermal nerve endings.[58] When used previously for pruritus ani, it provided relief of symptoms, but was associated with skin necrosis in 25% of patients. Newer techniques have been described using smaller total volume and local anesthetic; in a small series, this was not associated with skin necrosis.[59]

PILONIDAL SINUS DISEASE

Pilonidal sinus disease is a common condition with an incidence of approximately 26 per 100 000 and is seen mainly in young adult males.[60,61] There are many theories about the cause of this disease, but generally no consensus has been reached.[62,63]

Clinically, the lesion is asymptomatic until it becomes infected. The diagnosis is made on the basis of one or more small openings in the midline over the sacrococcygeal region approximately 3.5–5 cm superior to the anal orifice. Hair may be found protruding from the sinus opening. A subacutely or chronically infected cyst may be associated with tenderness and discharge of purulent fluid.

Surgical therapy

There still exists a great deal of diversity of opinion on how treatment may best be accomplished. Many surgical techniques are used to treat pilonidal sinus, such as marsupialization, excision and primary closure, Z-plasty, simple VY advancement flap, and the Limberg flap closure. Presently, recurrence is the major problem for all of the procedures. The ideal surgical treatment of pilonidal sinus should result in a patient's comfort and provide a high chance of cure with a low recurrence rate. The most popular approach seems to be radical block excision of the cyst by the open method in which the wound heals by secondary intention. Marsupialization is another popular technique and in this procedure the skin is incised, the tissue of granulation is scraped, and the edges of the skin wound and cyst are approximated, first described by Buie.[64]

Another theoretical option is to flatten or to lateralize the natal cleft to avoid median recurrences. In this context, surgical techniques with asymmetric or oblique incisions such as a Karydakis flap and other asymmetric procedures have been described. Other full skin flap techniques such as the VY-plasty or the Z-plasty techniques also cover the wound defect by moving full-thickness skin and subcutaneous tissue into the midline defect. The idea of the flap technique is to flatten the natal cleft, which should decrease the recurrence rate.

The authors' approach for primary pilonidal cysts that are infected is to do a simple unroofing or laying open technique using an incision off the midline of the sacrococcygeal area followed by coring out of the sinus tract and debriding the granulation and debris in the sinus. For multiply recurrent or difficult to heal pilonidal cysts the authors have used the Z-plasty with good success.

RECTAL PROLAPSE AND SOLITARY RECTAL ULCER SYNDROME

Rectal prolapse is a problem that has plagued both physicians and patients for many centuries. Rectal prolapse can present at any age range, starting with newborns. Elderly women are afflicted most commonly. The etiology of rectal prolapse has never been fully explained and it occurs six times more frequently in women than in men.[65] Anatomic factors associated with rectal prolapse include abnormally deep cul-de-sac, loss of sacral attachments, redundancy of rectosigmoid, and weak anal sphincter muscles. Quite commonly, rectal prolapse is not an isolated finding and patients may present with associated constipation or incontinence. A thorough history, physical examination, and endoscopic or radiographic assessment of the anorectum are required prior to undertaking any treatment. Careful patient evaluation will not only confirm rectal prolapse and exclude underlying lesions, but also determine the presence of fecal incontinence, constipation, comorbid illnesses, and whether additional testing is needed. Most patients will require colonoscopy or barium enema to rule out concurrent colonic disease. Fecal incontinence can be further evaluated with transanal ultrasound, anorectal manometry, and pudendal nerve terminal motor latency as indicated. Patient with symptoms of rectal outlet obstruction may benefit from evaluation with dynamic proctography.

Surgical therapy

The treatment of rectal prolapse is surgical and aims to restore both normal anatomy and bowel function. Over the years, many procedures have been described to treat rectal prolapse and currently the optimal surgical approach remains elusive. The ideal surgical procedure repairs the prolapse, corrects any functional problems, is minimally invasive, cost-effective, and has a low morbidity.

In general, two surgical approaches are offered to patients, transperineal or transabdominal. For transperineal procedures, the two most common are perineal proctosigmoidectomy (Altemeier procedure) with or without levatorplasty, and the Delorme procedure. The operative technique for both these procedures has been described in the literature.[66] Varying results have been reported, with the most concerning complication of each being recurrence rate. Recurrence rates range anywhere from 30% to 50%.[67]

The other approach to rectal prolapse is transabdominal, and procedures such as rectopexy with or without sigmoid resection have been described. Fixation, or rectopexy, of the rectum is achieved with some form of mesh or sutures. More recently, minimally invasive transabdominal approaches have included laparoscopic surgical techniques including suture rectopexy, stapled rectopexy, posterior mesh rectopexy with artificial material, and resection of sigmoid colon with colorectal anastomosis with or without rectopexy.[68] Significant differences in favor of laparoscopy are noted with regard to narcotic requirements and pain

and mobility scores. Moreover, recurrence rates appear to be equal between both groups.

Direct comparison of the results of perineal versus abdominal approach for rectal prolapse has been done. A comprehensive review of all papers on rectal prolapse in a Medline search by Eu and Seow Choen was published in 1997.[67] After reviewing the literature, they concluded that the recovery of continence after prolapse surgery is related to the approach and that abdominal approaches seem to yield better results than perineal procedures. Perineal procedures usually provide a 45–60% chance of improvement in continence, while abdominal procedures generally result in a 60–90% chance. Recurrence rates for perineal procedures were; Delorme, 5–21%, and perineal proctosigmoidectomy, 0–50%. For the abdominal approach, the ranges were Ripstein, 0–13%; suture rectopexy, 0–4%; anterior resection, 4–9%; and resection rectopexy, 2–8%.

No procedure perfectly addresses rectal prolapse. However, the abdominal approach appears to provide a higher success rate, along with greater chance of functional improvement. In patients with mild to moderate constipation and/or redundant sigmoid colon, precise resection with preservation of the compliant rectum can be achieved. Likewise, in patients with slow transit constipation, diagnosed by scintigraphic techniques or sitz marker studies, and having no pelvic floor defect, a colectomy with ileorectal anastomosis and rectopexy can be done. Incontinence improves in a certain percentage of patients. Whether suture or mesh rectopexy is performed depends on the preference and comfort of the surgeon. With the improvement of medical postoperative care and the addition of laparoscopic prolapse surgery, a majority of patients can safely undergo preferred abdominal approach for their rectal prolapse.

Solitary rectal ulcer syndrome

The term solitary rectal ulcer syndrome (SRUS) is used to describe a spectrum of clinical pathological abnormalities which can affect both adults and children. Though the etiology remains obscure, it appears to be closely related to patients with rectal prolapse. The typical features of SRUS include passage of blood and mucus from the rectum associated with straining and a feeling of incomplete emptying. Evidence of rectal prolapse, either internal or external, is often seen. Sigmoidoscopic appearance varies from erythema to ulceration or polypoid lesion. They commonly are solitary but may be multiple and are found in the anterior rectal wall. Histologic evidence of fibrous obliteration of the lamina propria with distortion of the muscularis mucosa and extension of smooth muscle fibers into lamina propria is seen. Patients will complain of pain, rectal bleeding, and mucous discharge. A biopsy should always be taken to rule out underlying malignancy.

Treatment for SRUS is conservative (nonsurgical) or surgical. Conservative treatment involves application of local agents to the area of ulceration. Topical steroids and sulfasalazine enemas are generally not effective.[69] Patients have also been treated with sucralfate enemas with some success.[70] Other treatments such as human fibrin sealant, dietary manipulation, and biofeedback have been described. Biofeedback in these patients is to correct pelvic floor defecatory behavior, regulate toileting habits, encourage them to stop laxatives, suppositories and enemas, and attempt to address any psychologic factors that may be relevant. Surgical approach included prolapse procedures such as rectopexy, Delorme procedure, and resection.[71] Behavior techniques directed towards defecatory habits help in a substantial portion of patients and should now form the first line of treatment. However, long-term results of such treatment are still not known. Most commonly performed operation, rectopexy, helps about 50% of patients, but it increases symptoms in some. Surgery has only a very minor role and should be reserved for those with intractable symptoms that fail a concerted effort with behavioral therapy and have evidence of prolapse. Progress is likely to come from a greater understanding of the role played by psychological and neuro-muscular factors in the pathogenesis of solitary rectal ulcer syndrome.

CONDYLOMA AND OTHER LESIONS OF THE ANAL CANAL AND ANAL MARGIN

Human papillomavirus (HPV) is responsible for a common perianal disorder known as anal condylomata or venereal warts. Warts in the anal canal or perianal skin can be asymptomatic or present with mild bleeding and itching. History concerning sexual practices and human immunodeficiency virus status should be obtained. In general, a small number of perianal condylomata can be treated in the office with cryotherapy, injection of inter-feron, or application of dicloric ascitic or podophyllin. However, if the patient has diffuse perianal condyloma or has intra-anal disease, carbon dioxide laser ablation or surgical excision with or without electrocoagulation at the base is recommended. Care needs to be taken to avoid extensive resection and cauterization as it may lead to anal canal stenosis. Staged application of the technique is done to safely clear patients who present with large numbers of warts. The anal condyloma and skin should be reviewed pathologically to rule out the presence of squamous cell carcinoma. Certain serotypes of HPV are associated with squamous cell carcinoma, and these patients need to be followed carefully.

Other lesions of the anal canal and anal margin include epider-moid carcinoma, melanoma, adenocarcinoma, sarcoma, basal cell carcinoma, verrucous carcinoma, and Kaposi's sarcoma. Poten-tial malignant lesions of the anal margin include Bowen's disease, Paget's disease, Bowenoid papillosus, and leukoplakia. Malignant anal lesions compromise only 1–5% of large bowel cancers, and benign anal neoplasms are even rarer.

Patients with anal margin lesions will usually describe symp-toms such as mass, bleeding, pain, discharge, and itching. Despite what should be an obvious lesion, patients are often diagnosed late or misdiagnosed as having anal fissures, hemorrhoids, eczema, or abscess.[72] Any suspicious lesion in the anal canal or anal margin should be biopsied to confirm diagnosis, especially if local treatments have been unsuccessful to treat what has been thought to be a benign condition such as anal fissure or pruritus ani.

Potentially malignant lesions such as Paget's disease and Bowen's disease are generally treated with wide local excision after mapping a lesion to differentiate the extent. Wide local excision should achieve clear margins and incomplete excision results in a high recurrence rate. More-radical surgery such as abdominoperineal resection is usually only necessary if the lesion is locally invasive to the sphincter muscles or anal canal.

Malignant lesions such as squamous cell carcinoma and basal cell carcinoma can also be treated with wide local excision with a goal to achieve clear margins if the lesion is not too extensive and too invasive into the anal canal. Epidermoid or squamous cell carcinoma is the most common anal neoplasm. Additional names for this lesion include transitional cell, cloacogenic carcinoma, and mucoepidermoid carcinoma. Likely the most significant risk factors for anal cancer is infection with human papillomavirus (HPV, type 16, 18, and 53).[73] The majority of anal cancer patients have traditionally been females in their seventh decade of life. The exact location, size, and fixity of any anal lesion in the presence of inguinal adenopathy must be documented prior to its treatment. Anoscopy or rigid proctoscopy provides direct visualization and ability to biopsy the lesion and is an inexpensive method to examine and biopsy the anal canal. Initial clinical staging of these lesions can be accomplished with intraluminal ultrasonography, com-puterized tomography scanning, and magnetic resonance imaging. Treatment of anal cancer has largely been surgery, radiation, and chemotherapy, and a combination of these modalities. Surgical options included abdominoperineal resection and transanal excision. Currently, abdominoperineal resection is indicated only after failure of chemoradiotherapy or in patients who cannot receive radiotherapy, as in patients who have had previous pelvic radiation for prostate or cervical cancer. Local transanal excision should be reserved for lesions that are well differentiated, less than 2 cm in diameter, and located in the distal anal canal. Anal carcinomas are radiosensitive and an overwhelming majority of patients now are treated with multimodality therapy including 5 fluorouracil, mitomycin C, and radiotherapy. Chemotherapy is given at the same time as radiotherapy according to standard-ized protocols. Melanoma, adenocarcinoma, and sarcoma treat-ment must be individualized depending on the location and extent of disease.

Leukoplakia is a whitish thickening of the mucous membranes that may represent a precancerous dermatosis. Itching, bleed-ing, and discharge are common complaints. Microscopically, the lesion appears as hyperkeratosis and squamous metaplasia.[74] Patients should be treated symptomatically, and regular follow-up is indicated due to its questionable malignant potential. Any suspicious lesion should be biopsied to exclude malignancy.

ANORECTAL PROBLEMS IN PATIENTS WITH HUMAN IMMUNODEFICIENCY VIRUS

Human immunodeficiency virus (HIV) infection leads to a series of problems in the anorectal area, some related specifically to HIV and others that are unrelated and common problems seen in patients without HIV. Perianal problems associated with HIV include herpetic ulcerations, cytomegalovirus, and condyloma. The approach to HIV patients with anorectal pathology should start with a thorough history, including previous history of benign anorectal conditions or infectious problems of the anal area. Sexual history and degree of immunosuppression must be care-fully assessed. Patients oftentimes will have a significant amount of pain in the anorectum and examination under anesthesia to further clarify and biopsy suspicious lesions may be necessary. In patients with anal condyloma there should be a high index of suspicion for underlying squamous cell carcinoma. Fissures in HIV-positive patients can be typical or atypical in nature. Typical fissures are located in the posterior midline and are found below the dentate line. Atypical fissures can be located anywhere in the anal canal, usually proximal to the dentate line and associated with deep, pocketing ulceration. All fissures and anal ulcers should be biopsied to rule out malignancy. Herpetic and CMV ulcerations can be multiple and extensive. Diagnosis should be confirmed with appropriate tests.

There has been some controversy about surgical treatment in patients who are HIV positive. There has been some controversy in the treatment of benign, anorectal problems in HIV-positive patients. In general, patients that are not significantly immuno-suppressed and receiving antiviral therapy can tolerate hemor-rhoidectomy and even lateral internal sphincterotomy for anal fissure with good results and no significantly increased morbidity compared to HIV-negative patients.[75] Certainly, one would prefer to treat these patients with conservative measures, but if surgery was indicated for intractable symptoms, properly selected patients can receive operations with good outcomes.

SUMMARY

Hemorrhoids and other anorectal disorders are common condi-tions that afflict many patients each year. Approach to treatment should start with a systematic work-up and end with an accurate diagnosis. A multitude of diagnostic approaches are available to the clinician and examination under anesthesia by a surgeon should always be considered for difficult to assess patients before treatment is applied. Though most lesions are benign, the possi-bility of malignancy in this area should always be considered, evaluated, and excluded. Treatment algorithms range from conservative measures to aggressive approaches that involve surgical intervention. Therapy should be directed in the appro-priate manner depending on the patient's overall condition, as in the Crohn's or HIV patient. The ultimate goal in treating these patients should be to minimize morbidity and decrease recurrent disease.

REFERENCES

1. Nelson RL, Abcarian H, Davis FG, et al. Prevalence of benign anorectal disease in a randomly selected population. Dis Colon Rectum 1995; 38:341–344.

2. Hulme-Moir M, Bartolo DC. Hemorrhoids. Gastroenterol Clin North Am 2001; 183–197.

3. Johanson JF, Sonnenberg A. The prevalence of hemorrhoids and constipation: An epidemiologic study. Gastroenterology 1990; 98:380–386.

4. Johanson JF, Sonnenberg A. Temporal changes in the occurrence of hemorrhoids in the United States and England. Dis Colon Rectum 1991; 34:585–591.

5. Loder PB, Kamm MA, Nicholls RJ, et al. Haemorrhoids: pathophysiology and aetiology. Br J Surg 1994; 81:946–954.

6. Brisinda G. How to treat haemorrhoids: Prevention is best: Haemorrhoidectomy needs skilled operators. Br Med J 2000; 321:582–583.

7. Senapati A, Nichols RJ. Randomized trial to compare the results of injection sclerotherapy with a bulk agent alone in the treatment of bleeding haemorrhoids. Int J Colorect Dis 1988; 3:124–126.

8. Khoury GA, Lake SP, Louis MCA, et al. A randomized trial to compare single with multiple phenol injection treatment for haemorrhoids. Br J Surg 1985; 72:741–742.

9. O'Hara VS. Fatal clostridial infection following hemorrhoidal banding. Dis Colon Rectum 1980; 23:570–571.

10. Rothberg R, Rubin RJ, Eisenstat TE, et al. Rubber band ligation hemorrhoidectomy, Long-term results. Am Surg 1983; 49:167–168.

11. Milligan ETC, Morgan C, Naughton Jones LF, et al. Surgical anatomy of the anal canal and the operative treatment of hemorrhoids. Lancet 1937; 2:1119.

12. Ferguson JA, Mazier WP, Ganchrow MI, et al. The closed technique of hemorrhoidectomy. Surgery 1971; 70:480–484.

13. Ho YH, Seow-Choen F, Tan M, et al. Randomized controlled trial of open and closed hemorrhoidectomy. Br J Surg 1997; 84:1729–1730.

   This article by Hull and colleagues compares the healing after open versus closed hemorrhoidectomy. It is a prospective, randomized comparison of both the open and closed hemorrhoidectomy technique. They randomized 33 patients in the open group, 33 to the closed group. Conclusions were that complete wound healing took longer after closed hemorrhoidectomy by approximately three weeks. Their conclusion was that open hemorrhoidectomy leads to faster and more reliable wound healing, although this did not result in less pain or fewer complications.

14. Seouw-Choen F. Stapled haemorrhoidectomy: pain or gain. Br J Surg 2001; 88:1–3.

   This article by Seow-Choen nicely covers literature on stapled hemorrhoidectomy and discusses the issues related to pain and complications following this technique. It also covers applicability and costs.

15. Carapeti EA, Kamm MA, McDonald PJ, et al. Double-blind, randomized controlled trial of effects of metronidazole on pain after day-case hemorrhoidectomy. Lancet 1998; 351:169–172.

16. Longo A. Treatment of hemorrhoids disease by reduction of mucosal and hemorrhoidal prolapse with a circular suturing device: A new procedure. Proceedings of the Sixth World Congress of Endoscopic Surgery, Rome, Italy, 3–6, June 1998; 778–784.

17. Rowsel M, Bellow M, Hemingway DM. Circumferential mucosectomy (stapled haemorrhoidectomy) versus conventional hemorrhoidectomy: Randomized controlled trial. Lancet 2000; 355:779–781.

18. Mehigan BJ, Monson JR, Hartley JE. Stapling procedure for haemorrhoids versus Milligan Morgan haemorrhoidectomy: randomized controlled trial. Lancet 2000; 355:782–785.

19. Molloy RG, Kingsmore D. Life threatening pelvic sepsis after stapled haemorrhoidectomy (Letter). Lancet 2000; 355:810.

20. Pescatori M. Stapled rectal prolapsectomy (Letter). Dis Colon Rectum 2000; 43:876–878.

21. Beattie G, Loudon M. Circumferential stapled anoplasty in the management of hemorrhoids and mucosal prolapse. Colorect Dis 2001; 2:170–175.

22. Haas PA, Fox TA Jr, Haas GP. The pathogenesis of hemorrhoids. Dis Colon Rectum 1984; 27:442–450.

23. Oh C. Acute thrombosed external hemorrhoids. Mount Sinai J Med 1989; 56:30–32.

24. Perrotti P, Antropoli C, Melino D, et al. Conservative treatment of acute thrombosed external hemorrhoids with topical nifedipine. Dis Colon Rectum 2001; 44:405–409.

25. Gorfine SR. Treatment of benign anal disease with topical nitroglycerin. Dis Colon Rectum 1995; 38;453–456.

26. Chowcat NL, Araujo JG, Boulos PB. Internal sphincterotomy for anal fissure: long-term effects on anal pressure. Br J Surg 1986; 73:915–916.

27. Gibbons CP, Read MW. Anal hypertonia in fissures: cause or effect? Br J Surg 1986; 73:443–445.

28. Nothmann BJ, Schuster MM. Internal anal sphincter derangement with anal fissures. Gastroenterology 1974; 67:216–220.

29. Goligher JC. Anal fissure. In: Surgery of the anus, rectum and colon. 4th edn. London: Tyndall; 1984.

30. Keighley MR, Williams NS. Fissures in ano. In: Surgery of the anus, rectum and colon. 2nd edn. Keighley MR, Williams NS, eds. Vol. 1. Philadelphia: WB Saunders; 1999:428–455.

31. Lock MR, Thomson JP. Fissure-in-ano: the initial management and prognosis. Br J Surg 1977; 64:355–358.

32. Jensen SL. Treatment of first episode of acute anal fissure: prospective randomized trial of lignocaine ointment versus hydrocortisone ointment or warm sitz baths plus bran. Br Med J 1986; 292:1167–1169.

33. O'Kelly T, Brading A, Mortensen N. Nerve mediated relaxation of the human internal anal sphincter: the role of nitric oxide. Gut 1993; 34:689–693.

34. Loder PB, Kamm MA, Nicholls RJ, et al. Reversible chemical sphincterotomy by local application of glyceryl trinitrate. Br J Surg 1994; 81:1386–1389.

35. Carapeti EA, Kamm MA, McDonald PJ, et al. Randomized controlled trial shows that glyceryl trinitrate heals anal fissures, higher doses are not more effective, and there is a higher recurrence rate. Gut 1999; 44:727–730.

36. Hyman NH, Cataldo PA. Nitroglycerin ointment for anal fissures: effective treatment or just a headache? Dis Colon Rectum 1999; 42:383–385.

37. Jonas M, Neil KR, Abercrombie JF, et al. A randomized trial of oral versus topical diltiazem for chronic anal fissure. Dis Colon Rectum 2001; 44:1074–1078.

38. Griffin N, Acheson AG, Jonas M, et al. The role of topical diltiazem in the treatment of chronic anal fissures that have failed glycerol trinitrate therapy. Colorect Dis 2002; 4:430–435.

39. Jost WH, Schimrigk K. Botulinum toxin in therapy of anal fissure (Letter). Lancet 1995; 345:188–189.

40. Maria G, Cassettea E, Gui D, et al. A comparison of botulinum toxin and saline for the treatment of chronic anal fissure. N Eng J Med 1998; 338:217–220.

41. Brisinda G, Maria G, Bentivoglio AR, et al. A comparison of injections of botulinum toxin and topical nitroglycerin ointment for the treatment of chronic anal fissure. N Eng J Med 1999; 341:65–69.

   Brisinda and colleagues compared two non-surgical treatments for anal fissure disease, of Botulin-toxin injection and of 0.2% nitroglycerin ointment. Their conclusions were that both topical nitroglycerin and Botulin-toxin were an effective alternative to surgery for patient with chronic anal fissure. Botulin-toxin was more effective than nitroglycerin.

42. Lewis TH, Corman ML, Prager ED, et al. Long-term results of open and closed sphincterotomy for anal fissures. Dis Colon Rectum 1988; 31:368–371.

43. Nyam DCNK, Pemberton JH. Long-term results of lateral internal sphincterotomy for chronic anal fissure with particular reference to incidence of fecal incontinence. Dis Colon Rectum 1999; 42(10):1306–1310.

   This paper by Dr. Nyam and Dr. Pemberton looks at the long-term results of over 500 patients who underwent lateral internal sphincterotomy for chronic anal fissure. Particular reference was made to the incidence of fecal incontinence. Their conclusions were that the operation heals and relieves symptoms of chronic anal fissure in nearly all patients, but that incontinence does occur frequently. Most episodes of incontinence they reported were minor and transient, but the fact remains that a small subgroup will have persistence of fecal incontinence over time.

44. Tang CL, Chew SP, Seow-Cheon F. Prospective randomized trial of drainage alone vs drainage and fistulotomy for acute perianal abscess with proven internal opening. Dis Colon Rectum 1996; 39:1415–1417.

45. Beck DE, Fazio VW, Lavery IC, et al. Catheter drainage of ischiorectal abscesses. South Med J 1988; 81:444–446.

46. Vasilevsky CA, Gordon PH. The incidence of recurrence of abscesses or fistula-in-ano following anorectal suppuration. Dis Colon Rectum 1984; 2:126–130.

47. Barnes SG, Sattler FR, Ballard JO. Perirectal infections in acute leukemia: Improved survival after incision and debridement. Ann Inter Med 1984; 100:515–518.

48. Glenn J, Cotton D, Wesley CR, et al. Anorectal infections in patients with malignant diseases. Rev Infect Dis 1988; 10:42–52.

49. Park AG. Pathogenesis and treatment of fistula-in-ano. Br Med J 1961; 1:463–469.

50. Wexner SD, Rosensface L, Robert PL, et al. Practice parameters for treatment of fistula-in-ano: Supporting documentation. Dis Colon Rectum 1996; 39:1363–1372.

51. Schwartz DA, Pemberton JH, Sandborn WJ. Diagnosis and treatment of perianal fistulas in Crohn disease. Ann Intern Med 2001; 135:906–918.

52. Smith LE, Henrichs D, McCullah RD. Prospective studies on the etiology and treatment of pruritus ani. Dis Colon Rectum 1982; 25:358–363.

53. Daniel GL, Longo WE, Vernava AM . Pruritus ani. Causes and concerns. Dis Colon Rectum 1994; 37:670–674.

54. Jones DJ. ABC of colorectal diseases, pruritus ani. Br Med J 1992; 305:575–577.

55. Dasan S, Neill SM, Donaldson DR, et al. Treatment of persistent pruritus ani in a combined colorectal and dermatological clinic. Br J Surg 1999; 86:1337–1340.

56. Mazier WP. Hemorrhoids, fissures and pruritus ani. Surg Clin North Am 1994; 74:1277–1292.

57. Lysy J, Sistiery-Ittah M, Israelit Y, et al. Topical capsaicin – a novel and effective treatment for idiopathic intractable pruritus ani: a randomized, placebo controlled crossover study. Gut 2003; 52:1323–1326.

   In this study by Lyse et al, they were able to show that 31 out of 41 patients treated with Capsaicin for pruritus ani experienced relief during treatment. They also showed that patients maintained on Capsaicin were able to remain symptom free for a period of several months. The conclusion of this article is that Capsaicin is a new, safe and effective treatment for intractable idiopathic pruritus ani. Mechanism of action appears to be desensitization of neurons in the perianal region.

58. Eusebio EB, Graham J, Mody N. Treatment of intractable pruritus ani. Dis Colon Rectum 1990; 33:770–772.

59. Farouk R, Lee PWR, Shortnote. Intradermal methylene blue injection for the treatment of intractable idiopathic pruritus ani. Br J Surg 1997; 84:670.

60. Akinci OF, Bozer M, Uzunkoy A, et al. Incidence and aetiological factors in pilonidal sinus among Turkish soldiers. Eur J Surg 1999; 165:339–342.

61. Da Silva JH. Pilonidal cyst: cause and treatment. Dis Colon Rectum 2000; 43:1146–1156.

62. Bascom J. Pilonidal disease: long term results of follicle removal. Dis Colon Rectum 1983; 26:800–807.

63. Douglas HC, Gunther SE. Taxonomic position of *Corynebacterium acnes*. J Bacteriol 1946; 52:15–23.

64. Buie LA. Practical proctology, Philadelphia: WB Saunders; 1937.

65. Gordon PH, Rectal procidentia. In: Gordon PH, Nivatvongs S, eds. Principles and practice of surgery for colon, rectum, and anus. St. Louis, MO: Quality Medical Publishing, Inc.; 1992:449–481.

66. Gregorcyk S, Huber P. The surgical treatment of fecal incontinence in rectal prolapse. In: Stanton F, Zimmer P, eds. Female pelvic reconstructive surgery. Dallas TX, London, UK: Springer Publishers; 2002:245–248.

67. Eu KW, Seow Choen F. Functional problems in adult rectal prolapse and controversies in surgical treatment. Br J Surg 1997; 84:904–911.

This article on functional problems associated with rectal prolapse nicely outlines the fact that rectal prolapse is a multi-factorial problem and that surgeons considering surgical management need to consider the pathophysiology of the pelvic floor and anorectal anatomy. Their conclusion was that surgical management has certainly evolved through the minimally-invasive approaches but successful management depends on adequate attention to associated functional problems.

68. Senagore AJ. Management of rectal prolapse: the role of laparoscopic approaches. Sem Laparosc Surg 2003; 10:197–202.

This article by Dr. Senegore nicely reviews the different treatment options for surgical repair of rectal prolapse. The paper specifically compares laparoscopic and open approaches for rectal prolapse and per this review demonstrates that any open transabdominal surgical approach for rectal prolapse can be accomplished laparoscopically and that patients often benefit from the advantage of a minimally invasive approach.

69. Martin CJ, Parks TG, Biggart JD. Solitary rectal ulcer syndrome in Northern Ireland 1971–1980. Br J Surg 1981; 68:744–747.

70. Kochhar R, Mehta SK, Agarwal R, et al. Sucralfate enema in ulcerative rectosigmoid lesions. Dis Colon Rectum 1990; 33:49–51.

71. Sitzler PJ, Kamm MA, Nicholls RJ. Surgery for solitary rectal ulcer syndrome. Int J Colorect Dis 1996; 11:136.

This paper by Dr. Sitzler et al nicely outlines the surgical approach to patients with solitary rectal ulcer syndrome. The study retrospectively reviewed 81 patients who underwent surgery for solitary rectal ulcer syndrome in a ten-year period. At a median follow up of 38 months they had four failures in this group of patients. Their conclusion was that anti-prolapse operations resulted in satisfactory long-term outcome in about 60% of patients having surgery for solitary rectal ulcer syndrome. They also noted that the results of anterior resection for this disorder were disappointing.

72. Jensen SL, Hagen K, Shokouh-Amiri MH, et al. Does an erroneous diagnosis of squamous cell carcinoma of the anal canal and anal margin at first physician visit influence prognosis? Dis Colon Rectum 1987; 30:345–351.

73. Saclarides TJ, Klem D. Genetic alterations and virology of anal cancer. Sem Colon Rectal Surg 1995; 6:131–134.

74. Corman ML. Premalignant and malignant dermatoses. Colon and rectal surgery. Philadelphia, PA: Lippincott; 1989:421–422.

75. Safavi A, Gottesman L, Dailey TH. Anorectal surgery in the HIV+ patient: update. Dis Colon Rectum 1991; 34:299–304.

Section
Eight

Therapy of Symptoms/
Symptom-oriented management/
Symptom-based treatments

CHAPTER SIXTY-SEVEN

67

Acute abdominal pain

Janice G. Rothschild

INTRODUCTION

The ability to evaluate and assess acute abdominal pain is fundamental to the practice of the general surgeon and other practitioners whose care includes the treatment of the abdomen. This has been true since Zachary Cope described the 'necessity of making a … diagnosis, usually predominantly by means of history and physical examination.'[1] The American College of Surgeons has reaffirmed that 'knowledge of these classic presentations is basic to successful diagnosis.'[2] Patients with acute abdominal pain, defined as pain of less than 48 hours duration, account for 10% of emergency room visits or 8 million patients per year in the United States. Abdominal pain is the most common surgical emergency, and it necessitates the largest use of ancillary services and countless work days lost as well as hospital days spent at costs upward of US$600 a day. Two to three percent of all office visits to the general internist are for the evaluation of abdominal pain,[2–4] but only 13% of patients with acute abdominal pain ultimately are found to have a diagnosis requiring emergency surgical intervention. Up to 41% of patients leave the emergency department with a diagnosis of abdominal pain of unknown etiology or non-specific abdominal pain (NSAP),[5] almost uniformly of no future significance.[6,7] The importance of identifying the minority of patients who actually have an acute problem requiring intervention is clear and it is the subject of this chapter.

It has been 'confidently asserted that a large number of acute abdominal conditions can be diagnosed by considering the patient's history.'[1] For the most part, the history is one of abdominal pain and, therefore, the evaluator requires an understanding of the components and pathophysiology of abdominal pain. Seventy-five percent of patients requiring surgical intervention carry one of the four most common surgical diagnoses. Understanding the source of these patients' pain simplifies decision-making and leads to the diagnosis in the majority of cases.[8]

PATHOPHYSIOLOGY AND CHARACTERISTICS OF ABDOMINAL PAIN

Intraperitoneal pain can be of three types:
  Colicky pain;
  Inflammatory pain;
  Ischemic pain.

Colicky pain

The intestine is innervated by the autonomic nervous system and that innervation involves a plexus of sensory neuroreceptors located between the muscular layers. Myelinated A-delta and unmyelinated C-fibers respond to mechanical stimuli, primarily stretch. Other noxious stimuli such as burning, crushing, or cutting are not perceived. Afferent fibers converge into one of three ganglia: celiac, superior mesenteric, and inferior mesenteric.[9] The innervation of the biliary and urinary viscera is similar to that of the gastrointestinal tract.

The clinical manifestations of obstruction are highly reproducible – i.e., the patient will complain of crampy, intermittent 'pressure pain' or colic. In cases of intestinal obstruction, the colicky pain is transmitted by one of the three ganglia and the pain will be perceived as periumbilical or poorly localized, since all of the afferent fibers converge into those three ganglia. In the case of ureteral or gallbladder obstruction, the colicky pain will be more focally perceived within the nerve distribution of these organs, i.e., flank to groin or right-upper quadrant, respectively. The intermittent frequency of the bouts of pain will be determined by the frequency of the organ's peristalsis. The patient presenting with crampy, gas-like, poorly localized pain can reliably be recognized to be suffering from intestinal obstruction.

Inflammatory pain

In contrast to colicky pain, inflammatory pain is neurologically mediated in a different way and it presents clinically in a different way as well. Inflammatory pain can result from a primary inflammatory disorder or from transmural progression of an initially obstructive disorder. Myelinated A-delta fibers, found in serosal structures in the peritoneum, mediate inflammatory pain. There is a one-to-one correlation between the somatic fibers involved and the location of the stimulus. The pain caused by an inflammatory stimulus is perceived as sharp, localized, and steady. The focus of inflammation is easily identified and the pain is exacerbated by anything that moves the offending organ, i.e., the peritoneum. The patient who complains of severe, steady, usually worsening pain, localized to a certain quadrant can be reliably diagnosed as having an inflammatory condition that involves an organ in that quadrant.

Ischemic pain

A complex interaction of regulatory and protective factors, mediated through sensory neuroreceptors, assures an adequate blood flow to the intestine. Blood flow to the intestine is maintained in spite of variations in cardiac output, blood pressure, and volume. This is accomplished through the complementary mechanisms of (1) a densely overlapping mesenteric and mucosal vascular network, (2) a perfusion rate that is the highest in the body, on a tissue weight basis, and (3) an extensively distributed autonomic nervous system that regulates intestinal blood flow.

Furthermore, on a local level, blood flow is maintained through other compensatory mechanisms. These include the interaction of autoregulation, escape, oxygen countercurrent, and redistribution mechanisms.[9]

Massive hemorrhage, a persistent drop in systemic blood pressure, or local atherosclerosis can overcome even these redundant protective mechanisms and lead to a decrease in blood flow to the mucosa. Ischemia can be caused by an embolus in a large vessel, thrombosis at the site of severe atherosclerosis, a decrease in blood flow related to systemic disease, or venous thrombosis related to trauma or hypercoagulability. In each of these situations, the result is anoxic injury to the intestine which causes a steadily worsening pain. Not until the ischemic injury becomes transmural, with secondary peritoneal irritation, will there be the physical finding of tenderness.

HISTORY AND PHYSICAL EXAMINATION

Diagnosis based on history and physical examination

Given the finite number of causes for abdominal pain in the majority of patients, the subtleties of history and physical examination are of paramount importance in determining the etiology of that pain. A review of a data base of over 10 000 patients presenting with abdominal pain showed that structured data sheets help prevent omission of important historical information.[2,3] It remains important, however, that the examiner allow the patient to provide the information without suggestion and leading questions. Structured data sheets (Fig. 67.1) have been shown to improve data collection and improve diagnosis.

Several characteristics of the pain can aid in defining its etiology. It is important to define the duration and mode of onset of the patient's pain. The onset of pain can vary considerably. It may be rapidly progressive over hours, gradually progressive, long-standing or acute, or an acute exacerbation of an indolent long-standing pain. It is also important to characterize the pain. The patient may describe the pain as crampy, continuous, sharp or pressure-like. The location of the pain should also be defined, i.e., focal versus poorly localized; radiating versus referred; or variable in its location and migrating from one site to another. These characteristics of pain are all indicative of potential etiologies. The evaluator should determine if the pain is related to diet, activity, menstrual cycle, or other initiating or exacerbating factors. These may include movement, coughing, or lying flat.

By convention, the history has usually included questions regarding the presence or absence of nausea, vomiting, fever, and diarrhea. Unfortunately, these complaints are less specific and, therefore, less significant. They are so universal in their presentation, with nearly any gastrointestinal or intra-abdominal disease entity, that they lose their value in defining the source of the pain.

The severity of the pain can be a difficult factor to interpret. Unless an objective assessment of the degree of distress can be determined, it is difficult to differentiate the severity of the pain from the severity of the patient's reaction to that pain.

The features of the physical examination can result in a pattern of findings that either supports or refutes the tentative diagnosis that has developed from the history. Physical examination begins with a general assessment of the patient. This assessment should include evaluation of the presence or absence of obvious toxicity or apparent distress, the notation of whether the patient is writhing in pain, lying motionless in a fetal position, or lying flat on the bed. Each of these findings may indicate the presence of different pathologies.

Inspection of the abdomen can be instrumental in eliminating or suggesting certain diagnoses. A patient with a right-lower quadrant scar is unlikely to have appendicitis, since the scar may indicate that a prior appendectomy has been done. Similarly, a right subcostal scar may indicate a prior cholecystectomy. A midline scar should lead the examiner to a discussion of prior surgeries that can exclude certain diseases or make others more likely, i.e., small bowel obstruction secondary to adhesions or recurrence of a malignancy.

Visible hernias can provide the examiner with a diagnosis and elucidate a treatment plan. Stigmata of liver disease, evidence of retroperitoneal bleeding, visible peristalsis or pulsations can each suggest underlying pathological diagnoses.

The utility of auscultation of the abdomen, like the non-specific historical factors of nausea and vomiting, is often overstated. While rushes or high-pitched bowel sounds in a clinical setting consistent with small bowel obstruction can be supportive of that diagnosis, the absence of bowel sounds, difficult to confirm unless the examiner is patient, is much less helpful.

Bimanual examination is an integral part of any female patient's evaluation. Cervical motion tenderness or a palpable, tender adnexal mass should lead to consideration of gynecologic diagnoses that do not require surgery. Evidence of pelvic fluid should raise concerns of an ectopic pregnancy.

Another examination considered integral to the evaluation of abdominal pain is the digital rectal examination (DRE). It has always been deemed crucial in the evaluation of the acute abdomen. Recent evidence, however, revealed that of 100 patients with acute abdominal pain and no evident anorectal pathology, DRE did not alter the clinical diagnosis or initial management in any of the patients.[10] Perhaps routine DRE should be questioned or abandoned as a standard requirement in the evaluation of the patient with abdominal pain.

The examiner may elicit evidence of peritonitis by any maneuver that generates peritoneal motion, i.e., coughing, laughing, or moving the bed. Only inflammation of the peritoneum generates pain or tenderness. Therefore, a maneuver that elicits tenderness confirms the presence of peritoneal inflammation, i.e., peritonitis. The finding of guarding, or muscular spasm, on palpation of the abdomen confirms the presence of peritonitis.

Rigidity, diffuse rectus spasm, is diagnostic of diffuse peritonitis. Guarding confined to a specific quadrant or generalized rigidity may direct one to surgical exploration unless one of the few non-operative causes for peritonitis is identified.

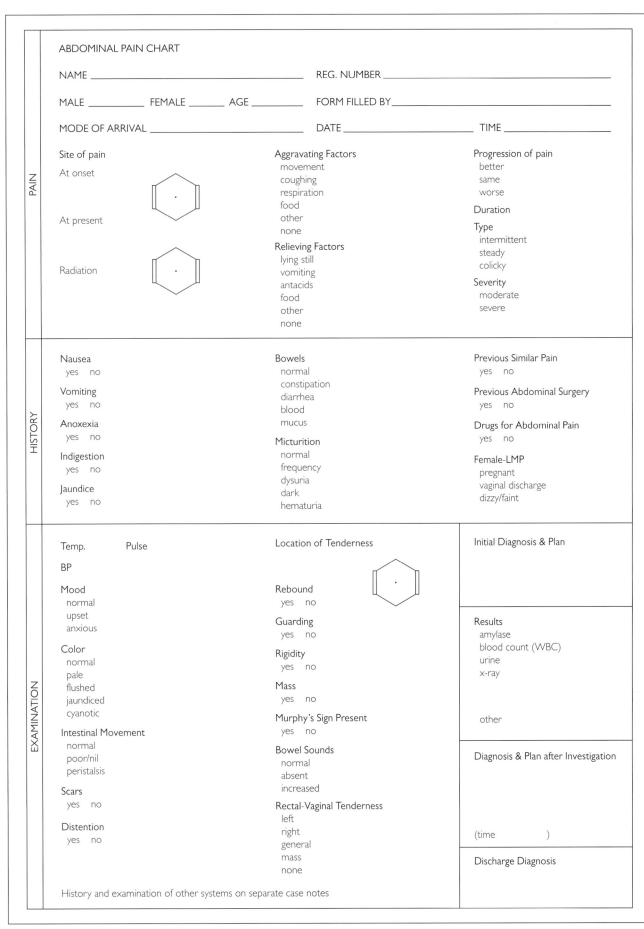

ABDOMINAL PAIN CHART

NAME _____ REG. NUMBER _____

MALE _____ FEMALE _____ AGE _____ FORM FILLED BY _____

MODE OF ARRIVAL _____ DATE _____ TIME _____

PAIN

Site of pain

At onset

At present

Radiation

Aggravating Factors
movement
coughing
respiration
food
other
none

Relieving Factors
lying still
vomiting
antacids
food
other
none

Progression of pain
better
same
worse

Duration

Type
intermittent
steady
colicky

Severity
moderate
severe

HISTORY

Nausea
yes   no

Vomiting
yes   no

Anoxexia
yes   no

Indigestion
yes   no

Jaundice
yes   no

Bowels
normal
constipation
diarrhea
blood
mucus

Micturition
normal
frequency
dysuria
dark
hematuria

Previous Similar Pain
yes   no

Previous Abdominal Surgery
yes   no

Drugs for Abdominal Pain
yes   no

Female-LMP
pregnant
vaginal discharge
dizzy/faint

EXAMINATION

Temp.   Pulse

BP

Mood
normal
upset
anxious

Color
normal
pale
flushed
jaundiced
cyanotic

Intestinal Movement
normal
poor/nil
peristalsis

Scars
yes   no

Distention
yes   no

Location of Tenderness

Rebound
yes   no

Guarding
yes   no

Rigidity
yes   no

Mass
yes   no

Murphy's Sign Present
yes   no

Bowel Sounds
normal
absent
increased

Rectal-Vaginal Tenderness
left
right
general
mass
none

Initial Diagnosis & Plan

Results
amylase
blood count (WBC)
urine
x-ray

other

Diagnosis & Plan after Investigation

(time   )

Discharge Diagnosis

History and examination of other systems on separate case notes

Fig. 67.1 ● Abdominal pain chart.

Are further tests necessary?

A patient with abdominal pain or peritoneal findings on physical examination who presents with or develops hemodynamic instability should be brought immediately to the operating room following resuscitation. No further testing is necessary. Similarly, in a hemodynamically stable patient, a complete history and physical examination may yield enough information to warrant surgical exploration without further testing (Fig. 67.2).

Most disease states which cause peritonitis require surgical treatment and further testing is not needed. However, there are a limited number of disease states which generate peritonitis that should not be treated surgically and it is the evaluator's responsibility to exclude those few diagnoses. Among these are pancreatitis, which is easily identified by hyperamylasemia in the majority of instances, and pyelonephritis, generally diagnosed by urinalysis. While not a cause of peritonitis, but included in the differential of upper abdominal pain, an inferior myocardial infarction can be ruled out by electrocardiogram.

DIAGNOSTIC TESTING

Although a 'large number of ... conditions can be diagnosed ... by the history,'[1] some diagnoses require confirmation to allow planning for surgery. Additionally one-third of patients do not present in a classic manner and will require further testing to establish the diagnosis. Uncertainty may persist even after a thorough evaluation and further testing will be needed. We will discuss the utility of testing in these situations.

Computer aided diagnosis

Multiple trials have shown that computer aided diagnosis is a helpful adjunct to clinical diagnosis.[3,11] The results of several

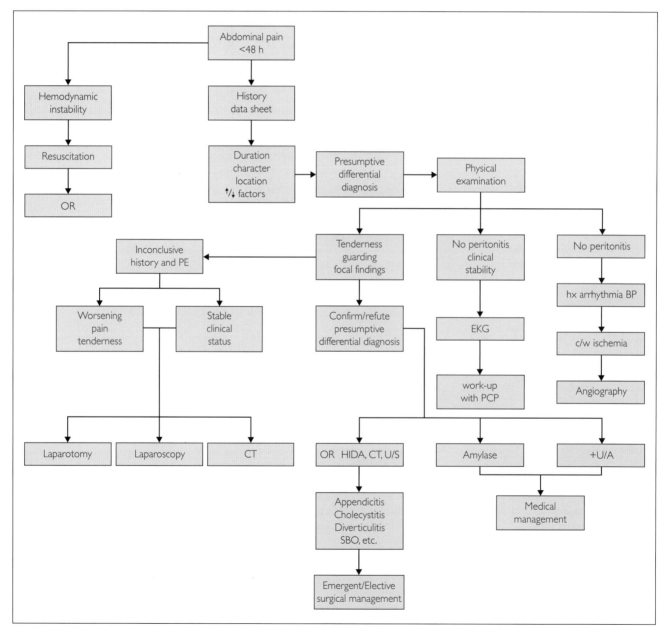

Fig. 67.2 ● Algorithm for treatment of abdominal pain.

trials published in the United Kingdom have shown that a strict intake sheet, input from a computer program, and feedback based on that program, increases diagnostic accuracy from 45% to 63%. This increased diagnostic accuracy is maintained regardless of whether the assessment was done by a resident or an experienced surgeon. In the results of one trial, the negative laparotomy rate decreased by half, perforation rate of appendicitis fell from 23% to 11% and mortality fell 22% when computer aided diagnosis was used. The economic impact of avoided laparotomy and prevented or decreased hospital stay was commensurate. That study did not determine whether the improvement was due to the standardized history and physical examination, already noted to improve diagnostic accuracy, due to the standardized feedback, or due to or the computer program itself.

Hepato-iminodiacetic acid scan

Although localization of tenderness is discriminatory in up to 85% of patients with cholecystitis,[8] it is necessary to confirm a diagnosis of acute cholecystitis prior to initiating plans for surgery. Singer showed that no single clinical or laboratory finding and no combination of clinical and laboratory findings identified all patients with ultimately proven cholecystitis.[12] A history of fever or leukocytosis was absent 90% and 40% of the time, respectively. A Murphy's sign was absent in 10% and not documented in the majority. Murphy's sign, however, was the single most predictive factor for acute cholecystitis. Gruber showed that the majority of patients lacked fever, leukocytosis, or both.[13] It is, therefore, necessary to confirm the diagnosis of cholecystitis with a radiologic test.[14]

Hepatobiliary scintigraphy was shown in 1975 to be an accurate test for patency of the cystic duct.[15,16] In a meta-analysis evaluating the sensitivity and specificity of various tests for biliary tract disease, hepato-iminodiacetic acid (HIDA) scanning showed the best sensitivity and specificity, up to 97%, for acute cholecystitis.[17] Real-time sonography can show both primary and secondary signs of cholecystitis. These include gallbladder wall thickening, gallstones, and pericholecystic fluid. The most significant secondary sign is a sonographic Murphy's sign. However, sonography is sensitive for acute disease in only 80% of patients and, therefore, it is inferior to HIDA scanning for acute cholecystitis.[18] When the issue is whether or not the patient has acute cholecystitis, and surgical planning will rely on the diagnosis, HIDA scan is the test of choice.

Computed tomography

Few tests generate as much controversy among surgeons and emergency room physicians as the computed tomography (CT) scan. Most diagnoses and dispositions can be determined on the basis of a careful history and physical examination. The purpose of any further testing is, therefore, to confirm a likely diagnosis. Where does CT scan fit into this algorithm?

In a review of resource usage, when asked the subjective question of which test provided the most useful information, emergency department physicians cited CT scan 31% of the time. CT scanning was shown to lead to a change in diagnoses or disposition 37–41% of the time.[19] Interestingly, this correlates with the percentage of patients presenting with atypical symptoms not readily diagnosed by classic history and physical examination alone.[8]

CT scanning can be used to confirm the diagnosis of small bowel obstruction or urolithiasis and, for this purpose, it has greater sensitivity and specificity than flat plate X-ray of the abdomen.[20] When considering the utility of CT scanning in the absence of a specific indication – i.e., as a routine test at the outset of evaluation – CT was found to increase the physicians' level of diagnostic certainty, reduce hospital admissions by 24%, lead to more timely surgery in 11%, and to rule out significant disorders in 26%.[21] Ng showed that ordering abdominal/pelvic CT scan, in the absence of a specific indication, reduced hospital stay by 1.1 day, a nonsignificant difference. While CT significantly reduced the incidence of missed diagnosis,[22] Ng concluded that 'computed tomography should be used with caution in acute abdominal pain and that it is probably best reserved for patients with pain of unknown cause. Computed tomography is not infallible and clinical evaluation and review remain critical'.

Taken together, these studies suggest that CT scan may be confirmatory for a suspected diagnosis of small bowel obstruction, urolithiasis, and appendicitis. It may save time in developing a treatment plan. When a diagnostic dilemma persists, CT scan may save time and lead to earlier clarification of a diagnosis and initiation of treatment.

Ultrasound

Many of the most common acute abdominal conditions are better delineated by CT scan than by ultrasound.[23] Where does ultrasound fit in the evaluation of acute abdominal pain?

One of the most common indications for ultrasound is the need to define the presence or absence of cholelithiasis. In a meta-analysis by Shea,[17] ultrasound was found to be superior to other tests for the diagnosis of cholelithiasis. In the absence of inflammation, a patient presenting with right-upper quadrant pain and fatty food intolerance is usually given the presumptive diagnosis of biliary colic. When the question to be answered is whether gallstones are present, the examination of choice is ultrasound. The finding of cholelithiasis in this setting may be sufficient to plan for elective surgery in the future.

There are several other advantages of ultrasound relative to CT in the acute setting. Ultrasound does not involve radiation and in younger children and suspected pregnancies it may be the examination of choice. The dynamic qualities of ultrasound may provide advantage in the visualization of peristalsis. Ultrasound provides immediate feedback between the examiner and the patient. This feedback can allow the clinician to adjust and alter the examination as findings become evident.[24] The mobility and flexibility of ultrasound also adds to its utility. It is becoming a frequently available examination within the emergency department.

Although patients with abdominal aortic aneurysm (AAA) frequently present with back rather than abdominal pain, ultrasound can be helpful in the diagnosis of AAA. In the setting of a stable patient with a suspected AAA, ultrasound can confirm the presence of an aneurysm or identify a patient with a leaking aneurysm.

Angiography

After excluding the three most common causes of acute abdominal pain, i.e., appendicitis, cholecystitis, and small bowel obstruction, there remain a minority of patients in whom a diagnosis remains unclear. Among this group are patients with ischemic bowel.

When an elderly patient with a history of hemodynamic instability or arrhythmia presents with abdominal pain and minimal objective findings, ischemic bowel should be considered. In the absence of peritonitis, an angiogram is the diagnostic procedure of choice in this setting. It can confirm the diagnosis and it may identify the cause of the ischemia. If embolic disease is identified, surgical exploration is required. If a diagnosis of venous thrombosis is made, medical treatment should be initiated. When a diagnosis of nonocclusive mesenteric ischemia is identified, pharmacological treatment may be initiated.

Laparoscopy

When these diagnostic maneuvers do not clarify the diagnosis, the patient may be admitted for clinical observation. In 40–50% of patients, a diagnosis of non-specific abdominal pain is ultimately made. If the clinical status of a patient deteriorates during the period of observation, further evaluation or intervention is required. If the pain or tenderness worsens, further evaluation is also indicated. One option for further evaluation is laparoscopy.

Defining the role and utility of laparoscopy in the management of acute abdominal pain is a process that is still in evolution. Some studies have shown that a definitive diagnosis can be made laparoscopically in 70–98% of patients in whom a radiologic diagnosis cannot be made,[25,26] and that a definitive therapeutic procedure can be performed in 44% of these patients by laparoscopy. In 38%, a definitive diagnosis not requiring further surgery can be made by laparoscopy but, in the remainder of patients, laparotomy was required to assess or treat the patient.

Tests of little value

The flat plate and upright radiograph of the abdomen are among the tests proven to be of no utility in the diagnosis of patients with abdominal pain. Of 1780 examinations, only 10% showed a radiographic abnormality, and 30% of these abnormalities consisted of only a generalized or localized ileus. Clinical factors likely to correlate with an abnormal flat plate radiograph are distention, a history of abdominal surgery, and increased high-pitched bowel sounds.[27] Variables with a statistically significant likelihood for predicting a normal radiograph include mild abdominal pain, a history of ulcer disease, and a pain duration of greater than one week.[27] Of 237 patients in Anyanwu's study, 10% of examinations were diagnostic for the underlying abnormality and 90% were nondiagnostic.[28] In a prospective analysis of 100 consecutive abdominal radiographs, 98% of the radiographs were negative or had findings unrelated to the current clinical problem. Ninety-three percent of the small number of positive radiographs were related to the acute problem in patients with renal colic, ingestion of a foreign body, and a previously noted surgical condition such as incarcerated hernia, metastatic carcinoma, or fecal impaction.[29] In comparing the flat plate X-ray with the CT scan for patients with undefined abdominal pain, the CT scan was found to provide increased sensitivity and specificity for the confirmation of small bowel obstruction and urolithiasis.[20] In a study evaluating flat plate radiography with CT scan in the diagnosis of appendicitis, CT was found to improve specificity and sensitivity at one-fifth the cost per correct diagnoses.[30] Thus, for the most part, plain abdominal radiographs appear to have little value in the diagnosis or treatment of patients with abdominal pain. They may provide confirmatory evidence of bowel obstruction but even the diagnosis of urolithiasis, which can, in fact, be made on flat plate radiography, is more frequently made by CT scan.

Similarly, an upright chest X-ray has very limited value in the evaluation of the patient with abdominal pain. When the findings are that of a rigid abdomen, or diffuse peritonitis, exploration is warranted regardless of the X-ray findings if the diagnosis of pancreatitis has been excluded. In a patient with a history of ulcer disease, an upright chest X-ray is likely to confirm a diagnosis of a perforated ulcer by revealing pneumoperitoneum and this positive finding would support a plan for surgical exploration. On the other hand, a negative X-ray would be unlikely to change the disposition of a patient. Chest X-ray may have a role in the evaluation of the patient with abdominal pain to exclude a supradiaphragmatic source, such as pneumonia, but it otherwise provides little decision-making value in the evaluation of the patient with abdominal pain.

Another highly insensitive, although universally used test, is the white blood cell count. In the presence of peritonitis, neither elevated nor normal values should alter the treatment plan. In an audit of over 10 000 cases the white blood cell count was found to be 'useless … between the extremes, that is a cut-off of 10 000 is of no value.'[4] 'Both [fever and leukocytosis] added little more than supportive evidence … of an acute surgical abdomen.'[5]

EVALUATION OF THE IMMUNOCOMPROMISED PATIENT

Comment should be made about a group of patients for whom the preceding discussion may not pertain: immunocompromised patients. Immunocompromised patients include the elderly, malnourished, patients with malignancies, transplant patients, patients on immunosuppressive treatment, and AIDS patients. They can be difficult to evaluate from two perspectives. First, they can present with the usual surgical diseases, but later in the evolution of the disease process because of an impaired immune and inflammatory response.[31,32] Second, they can present with a host of diseases that are unique to the immunocompromised state.

Among the more commonly seen patients in this group are the elderly. In the elderly population, history and physical examination and routine laboratory evaluations are not as reliable as they are in younger patients. Often, because of a deficit in short-term memory, the elderly patient is unable to give a clear history. Furthermore, a lack of alteration of vital signs, even in the presence of severe pathology, is not unusual in this population.[33,34] The lack of utility of measuring the white blood cell count, previously noted in the average-age patient, is even more true in this population. In an analysis of 10 000 patients, only 39% of patients greater than 65 who ultimately required surgery had a white blood cell count of greater than 10 000.[5] Bender evaluated the presentation of the acute abdomen in elderly patients.[33] Forty-four percent of patients were admitted with an incorrect diagnosis, compared to 18% in the surgical population as a whole. These patients were frequently admitted with a diagnosis of dehydration, gastroenteritis, or abdominal pain of unknown etiology and this resulted in a delay in diagnosis. Ultimately, 51% of the patients greater than 65 years old required immediate operation.[5] Morbidity in this group was notably high, 33%, with a mortality rate of 18%. This elevated morbidity and mortality rate was generally attributable to delay in diagnosis resulting in sepsis and multiorgan system failure.

It is possible that CT may improve these statistics. In a study of 100 patients greater than 65 years old, CT scan altered the suspected diagnosis in 45%, the decision for surgery in 12%, and the decision for admission in 26%.[35] There are no data from this group, however, to document whether these changes improved outcome.

Immunocompromised patients also present with a host of disease states that are not typically seen in the general population. In a patient presenting with a known immunodeficient state, CMV disease, lymphoma, Kaposi's sarcoma, candidal diseases, neutropenic colitis, and other opportunistic infections should be considered and addressed aggressively and early. Also to be considered are disease states that may mimic intra-abdominal sepsis including uremic pericarditis, lower lobe pneumonia, CMV infection, and neutropenic colitis that do not require surgery.[31,32] Therefore, 'an aggressive diagnostic approach should be taken because of the mild and atypical presentation in these patients.' An increased index of suspicion and the willingness to intervene early may be appropriate in the care of these patients because they may deteriorate rapidly and may be 'moribund within hours.'[32]

SUMMARY

In summary, while acute abdominal pain is among the most frequent complaints of patients presenting to the emergency room, only a small minority of patients require acute surgical intervention. We have discussed the means of identifying these patients.

Primary among these is the detailed history and physical examination. With an understanding of the origins and pathophysiology of abdominal pain, and an understanding of the significance of associated physical findings, most surgical patients can be identified by means of the history and physical examination alone.

The role of further testing is also discussed. If uncertainty remains following the development of a tentative differential diagnosis, the appropriate diagnostic test can be chosen. The relative benefits and weaknesses of these diagnostic tests, and their role in the evaluation and management of the patient with abdominal pain, is also discussed.

REFERENCES

1. Silen W. Cope's early diagnosis of the acute abdomen, 18th edn. New York: Oxford University Press; 1991.

   Classic description of symptoms and signs of the acute abdomen.

2. Delcore R, Cheung LY. Acute abdominal pain. In: ACS Surgery: principles and practice 2004:253–268.

   In depth, comprehensive discussion of all etiologies, manifestations and management of acute abdominal pain.

3. deDombal FT. The OMGE acute abdominal pain survey. progress report, 1986. Scand J Gastroenterol 1988; 144(suppl):35–42.

   This and the other entries in the series discusses presentation and analysis of over 10 000 patients with abdominal pain in multicenter, multinational registry.

4. Graff LG, Robinson D. Abdominal pain and emergency department evaluation. Em Med CI No Amer 2001; 19(1):123–136.

   Discussion of the emergency physicians' approach to the acute abdomen.

5. Brewer RJ, Golden GT, Hitch DC. Abdominal pain, an analysis of 1000 consecutive cases in a university hospital emergency room. Am J Surg 1976; 131:219–223.

6. Gray DWR, Collin J. Non-specific abdominal pain as a cause of acute admission to hospital. Br J Surg 1987; 74:239–242.

7. Jess P, Bjerregaard B, Brynitz S, et al. Prognosis of acute nonspecific abdominal pain. a prospective study. Am J Surg 1982; 144:338–340.

8. Staniland JR, Ditchburn J, deDombal FT. Clinical presentation of acute abdominal pain: study of 600 patients. Br Med J 1972; 3:393–398.

9. Johnson LR. Gastrointestinal physiology. St. Louis: CV Mosby Co; 1977:28–34; 139–151.

10. Manimaran N, Galland RB. Significance of routine digital rectal examination in adults presenting with abdominal pain. Ann R Coll Surg Engl 2004; 86:292–295.

11. Adams ID, Chan M, Clifford PC, et al. Computer aided diagnosis of acute abdominal pain: a multicentre study. Br Med J 1986; 293:800–804.

    This and associated sources support the use of standardized intake sheets and computer aided diagnosis.

12. Singer AJ, McCracken G, Henry MC, et al. Correlation among clinical, laboratory, and hepatobiliary scanning findings in patients with suspected acute cholecystitis. Ann Em Med 1996; 28(3):267–272.

13. Gruber PJ, Gottesfeld S, Silverman RA. The presence of fever and leukocytosis in acute cholecystitis (Abstract). Acad Emerg Med 1994; 1:A25.

14. Trowbridge RL, Rutkowski NK, Shojania KG. Does this patient have acute cholecystitis? JAMA 2003; 289(1):80–86.

15. Eikman EA, Cameron JL, Colman M, et al. A test for patency of the cystic duct in acute cholecystits. Ann Int Med 1975; 82:318–332.

16. Bednarz GM, Kalff V, Kelly MJ. Hepatobiliary scintigraphy. increasing the accuracy of the preoperative diagnosis of acute cholecystitis. Med J Aust 1986; 145:316–318.

17. Shea JA, Berlin JA, Escarce JJ, et al. Revised estimates of diagnostic test sensitivity and specificity in suspected biliary tract disease. Arch Int Med 1994; 154:2573–2581.

    Comprehensive meta-analysis of the utility, sensitivity, and specificity of frequently ordered biliary tract evaluations.

18. Ralls PW, Colletti PM, Lapin SA, et al. Real-time sonography in suspected acute cholecystitis. prospective evaluation of primary and secondary signs. Rad 1985; 155:767–771.

19. Nagurney JT, Brown DF, Chang Y, et al. Use of diagnostic testing in the emergency department for patients presenting with non-traumatic abdominal pain. J Emerg Med 2003; 25(4):363–371.

20. Ahn SH, Mayo-Smith WW, Murphy BL, et al. Acute nontraumatic abdominal pain in adult patients: abdominal radiography compared with CT evaluation. Rad 2002; 225:159–164.

21. Rosen MP, Sands DZ, Longmaid HE, et al. Impact of abdominal CT on the management of patients presenting to the emergency department with acute abdominal pain. AJR Am J Roetgenol 2000; 174:1391–1396.

22. Ng CS, Watson CJ, Palme CR, et al. Evaluation of early abdominopelvic computed tomography in patients with acute abdominal pain of unknown cause: prospective randomized study. Br Med J 2002; 325:1387–1389.

    Randomized prospective evaluation of the role and effect of CT scanning on the evaluation of the patient with abdominal pain.

23. Puylaert JB, van der Zant FM, Rijke AM. Sonography and the acute abdomen: practical considerations. AJR Am J Roetgenol 1997; 168:179–186.

24. Puylaert JB. Ultrasonography of the acute abdomen: gastrointestinal conditions. Radiol Clin N Am 2003; 41:1227–1242.

25. Cuesta MA, Eiksbouts QA, Gordijin PJ, et al. Diagnostic laparoscopy in patients with acute abdomen of uncertain etiology. Surg Endosc 1998; 12:915–917.

    Discussion of the expansion of the role of diagnostic laparoscopy in the management of the patient with abdominal pain in whom a treatment decision is not readily made.

26. Salky BA, Edye MB. The role of laparoscopy in the diagnosis and treatment of abdominal pain syndromes. Surg Endosc 1998; 12:911–914.

27. Eisenberg RL, Heineken P, Hedgcock MW et al. Evaluation of plain abdominal radiographs in the diagnosis of abdominal pain. Ann Surg 1983; 197(4):464–469.

28. Anyanwu AC, Moalypour SM. Are abdominal radiographs still overutilized in the assessment of acute abdominal pain? a district general hospital audit. J R Coll Surg Edin 1998; 43:267–270.

29. McCook TA, Ravin CE, Rice RP. Abdominal radiography in the emergency department: a prospective analysis. Ann Em Med 1982; 11(1):23–24.

30. Rao PM, Rhea JT, Rao JA et al. Plain radiography in clinically suspected appendicitis: diagnostic yield, resource use, and comparison with CT. Am J Emerg Med 1999; 17(4):325–328.

31. Scott-Conner CE, Fabrega AJ. Gastrointestinal problems in the immunocompromised host. a review for surgeons. Surg Endosc 1996; 10:959–964.

32. Nylander WA. The acute abdomen in the immunocompromised host. Surg Clin N Amer 1988; 68(2):457–470.

33. Bender JS. Approach to the acute abdomen. Med Clin N Amer 1989; 73(6):1413–1422.

34. Parker JS, Vukor LF, Wollan PC. Abdominal pain in the elderly: use of temperature and laboratory testing to screen for surgical disease. Fam Med 1996; 28(3):193–297.

35. Esses D, Birnbaum A, Bijur P. Ability of CT to alter decision making in elderly patients with acute abdominal pain. Am J Emerg Med 2004; 22(4).

CHAPTER SIXTY-EIGHT

68

Noncardiac chest pain

Ronnie Fass and Ram Dickman

INTRODUCTION

Background

Noncardiac chest pain (NCCP) is defined as recurring angina-like retrosternal chest pain of noncardiac origin. While different underlying mechanisms have been identified for this condition, gastroesophageal reflux disease (GERD) is by far the most common cause. Clinical history does not reliably distinguish between cardiac and esophageal cause of chest pain.[1] Furthermore, because of the nature of the symptoms in patients with NCCP that are described as squeezing or burning substernal chest pain, which may radiate to the back, neck, arms, and jaws, most of patients are evaluated initially by a cardiologist.[2] A history of retrosternal chest discomfort, pressure or heaviness that lasts several minutes, pain that is induced by exertion, emotion, exposure to cold, or a large meal, and pain that is relieved by rest or nitroglycerin usually signifies typical cardiac angina. Any two of these clinical characteristics are suggestive of atypical cardiac angina, and only one or none of these characteristics is indicative of NCCP. Although chest pain may signify a cardiac event, only 15–34% of ambulatory patients who present with chest pain are ultimately diagnosed with coronary artery disease.[3]

The impact of NCCP on reported quality of life is likely to match other functional gastrointestinal disorders, such as irritable bowel syndrome (IBS). Although the overall prognosis of patients with NCCP is favorable, the natural history is characterized in most patients by the persistence of symptoms, repeated admissions, chronic use of medications, repeated cardiac catheterizations, and impaired quality of life.[4]

Epidemiology

Only a few studies have estimated the prevalence of NCCP in the general population. The mean annual prevalence of NCCP in six population-based studies was approximately 25%. These studies differ in many aspects, including definition of NCCP, geography, sample size, and ethnicity.[5] However, some of the important findings of these different population-based studies include a high prevalence rate of NCCP in the general population, decreased prevalence of NCCP with increasing age, and similar prevalence rates among males and females. To further illustrate how common NCCP is, it is estimated that approximately 65 million individuals in the US population are afflicted with NCCP (mean prevalence of 24%), making NCCP the most common atypical extraesophageal manifestation of GERD, and consequently a significant economic burden on the healthcare system.[6] While NCCP is very common in the general population, the percentage of subjects seeking medical attention and the motivating factors that drive patients to become avid and, at times, relentless healthcare users are unclear.

PATHOGENESIS

Main mechanisms related to noncardiac chest pain

The different mechanisms underlying NCCP are not fully understood and can often overlap. The most common esophageal source for NCCP is GERD. Other important etiological factors include esophageal dysmotility, visceral hyperalgesia, psychological comorbidity, autonomic dysfunction, and possibly abnormal central processing of intraesophageal stimuli (Table 68.1).

Gastroesophageal reflux disease-related noncardiac chest pain

Gastroesophageal reflux disease (GERD), the most common cause of NCCP, may be present in up to 60% of patients.[2] Typical reflux

---

Table 68.1 The different proposed underlying mechanisms of noncardiac chest pain

Gastroesophageal reflux

Esophageal dysmotility

Abnormal mechano-physical properties
   Hyperactive
   ↓ compliance

Sustained longitudinal muscle contractions

Visceral hypersensitivity

Altered central processing of visceral stimuli

Altered autonomic activity

Psychological abnormalities
   Panic attack
   Anxiety
   Depression

symptoms (heartburn or acid regurgitation) have been shown to be significantly and independently associated with the presence of NCCP. In a study by Locke et al., NCCP was reported more often in those experiencing frequent heartburn symptoms at least once a week (37%) as compared with those with infrequent heartburn (30.7%) and persons reporting no heartburn (7.9%).[7] Eslick et al.[5] performed a population-based study to determine the prevalence of NCCP and discovered that among subjects with NCCP, 53% experienced heartburn and 58%, acid regurgitation. The prevalence of erosive esophagitis in patients with GERD-related NCCP has been reported to be as low as 10% and as high as 70%.[8-12]

Studies have shown that the percentage of NCCP patients with abnormal pH test is approximately 50%. Fass et al.[13] reported that 41.1% of patients with NCCP had abnormal pH values in a study involving 37 patients. Beedassy et al.[14] evaluated 104 patients with NCCP and reported that 48% had an abnormal ambulatory 24-hour esophageal pH monitoring. Of the 104 patients, 52 reported chest pain during their pH study, but only 23 (44%) had an abnormal pH test. Thus, no relationship between overall abnormal pH values and chest pain was demonstrated.

Beedassy et al.[14] also showed that patients with a positive symptom index (percentage of symptoms that correlates with acid reflux events) were significantly more likely to have an abnormal pH study. Of the 52 patients with chest pain, 10 had a positive symptom index (SI), and 42 had a negative symptom index. Of those with a positive symptom index, 80% had an abnormal pH study compared with 36% of those with a negative symptom index.

In many North American studies, patients with GERD-related NCCP have typical reflux symptoms in addition to their chest pain.[15] In contrast, Chinese patients with GERD-related NCCP rarely present with classic reflux symptoms. A study by Wong et al.[16] evaluated patients with NCCP. Only 1 of the 19 patients with abnormal 24-hour esophageal pH monitoring had typical symptoms of GERD (heartburn or regurgitation). Another possible explanation for lack of GERD symptoms report in this study is the absence of the word 'heartburn' in the Chinese language.

Esophageal dysmotility-related noncardiac chest pain

The distribution of esophageal motility disorders in patients presenting with non-GERD-related NCCP has been scarcely studied. In a commonly cited study, 255 (28%) of 910 NCCP patients evaluated by esophageal manometry were found to have an esophageal motility disorder.[17] By far the most common motor disorder was nutcracker esophagus, followed by non-specific esophageal motility disorders, diffuse esophageal spasm, hypertensive LES, and achalasia. Although this experience reflects one tertiary referral center with a major interest in esophageal motor disorders, the finding of high prevalence of nutcracker esophagus in NCCP patients is common and highly intriguing. Manometrically defined as high amplitude contractions in the distal esophagus (>180 mmHg), nutcracker esophagus remains an area of intense controversy. Investigators have long argued about the clinical relevance of such a manometric phenomenon.[18] However, Achem et al. reported that most patients with chest pain associated with nutcracker esophagus responded symptomatically to antireflux treatment.[19] Normalization of the nutcracker motility phenomenon was documented only in the minority of the patients, suggesting

that GERD was the likely cause of their symptoms rather than the high amplitude contractions in the distal esophagus. Using the Clinical Outcomes Research Initiative (CORI) database, Dekel et al. evaluated 160 NCCP subjects from academic, private, and VA medical centers that underwent evaluation by esophageal manometry.[20] Similar to the study by Katz et al., 70% of the patients had normal esophageal manometry. However, of those with abnormal esophageal motility, 61% were found to have a hypotensive LES and 10% a hypertensive LES, non-specific esophageal motility disorder, and nutcracker esophagus. It is likely that more patients with GERD ended up in the study by Dekel et al. due to the higher prevalence rate of hypotensive LES. Figure 68.1 summarizes the two currently available studies describing the distribution of esophageal motility abnormalities among patients with NCCP.[20]

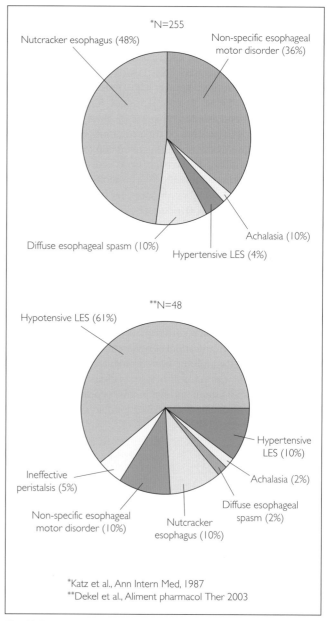

Fig. 68.1 • Distribution of esophageal dysmotility disorders in patients with NCCP and abnormal esophageal manometry.

Esophageal hypersensitivity (visceral hyperalgesia)

The mechanisms of pain in patients with non-GERD-related NCCP are not fully understood. Numerous studies that focused primarily on this group of patients have consistently documented an alteration in pain perception regardless of the presence or absence of esophageal dysmotility. Peripheral and central sensitization of esophageal sensory afferents and spinal cord neurons has been suggested to result in heightened responses to innocuous and noxious intraesophageal stimuli.[21,22] It has been postulated that inflammation or other injuries to the esophageal mucosa set off a cascade of events that leads to upregulation of receptors, which, in turn, induces the development of visceral hypersensitivity through peripheral and central sensitization.[22] The presence of esophageal hypersensitivity can be demonstrated long after the original stimulus has disappeared and the mucosa has healed. It is still unclear what factors determine the long-term persistence of esophageal hypersensitivity.

Rao et al.[23] performed graded balloon distentions of the esophagus using impedance in 16 consecutive patients with NCCP (normal esophageal evaluations) and 13 healthy control subjects. Patients who experienced chest pain during the balloon distention were subsequently restudied after receiving intravenous atropine. Balloon distentions reproduced chest pain at lower sensory thresholds than controls in most NCCP subjects. Similar findings were documented after atropine administration despite a relaxed and more deformable esophageal wall. The investigators concluded that hyperalgesia, rather than motor dysfunction, is the predominant mechanism accounting for functional chest pain of presumed esophageal origin.

Autonomic dysfunction

Several studies have documented altered autonomic function in patients with NCCP. In one study, Tougas et al.[24] assessed autonomic activity using power spectral analysis of heart rate variability before and during esophageal acidification of patients with NCCP and matched healthy control subjects. Of the patients with NCCP, 68% were considered acid sensitive (developed angina-like symptoms during esophageal acidification). The acid-sensitive patients had a higher baseline heart rate and lower baseline vagal activity than acid-insensitive patients. During acid infusion, vagal cardiac outflow increased in acid-sensitive, but not in acid-insensitive, patients. The role that altered autonomic function plays in the pathogenesis of NCCP remains speculative. As stated by Tougas,[25] in most cases in which both central and autonomic factors are involved, it is the former that most likely leads to the occurrence of the latter.

Psychological comorbidity

As with other functional bowel disorders, psychological comorbidity is common in patients with NCCP. In some patients, chest pain is a component of a host of symptoms that characterize panic attacks.[26] In a large study of 441 consecutive ambulatory patients presenting with chest pain to the emergency department of a heart center, 25% were diagnosed as suffering from a panic attack.[27] It has been estimated that 17–43% of patients with NCCP suffer from a psychological abnormality, primarily anxiety, panic disorder, and hypochondriasis.[28] Song et al.[29] evaluated the psychological profiles of 113 patients with chest pain and a variety of esophageal motility abnormalities, 23 symptomatic control subjects (similar symptoms but without esophageal motility abnormalities), and 27 asymptomatic control subjects. All participants were assessed by the Beck Depression Inventory, Spielberger State-Trait Anxiety Inventory, and the psychosomatic symptom checklist. Patients with esophageal symptoms and either hypertensive lower esophageal sphincter, nutcracker esophagus, or hypotensive contractions exhibited increased somatization, anxiety, and depression. Among esophageal symptoms, chest pain was closely correlated with psychometric abnormalities.

Higher ratings on anxiety and depression scales influence pain reporting and may contribute to the psychosocial morbidity suffered by these patients. For example, Lantinga et al. found that patients with NCCP had higher levels of neuroticism and psychiatric morbidity before and after cardiac catheterization than those with coronary artery disease.[30] This finding appears to have prognostic significance because these patients display less improvement in pain, more frequent pain episodes, greater social maladjustment, and more anxiety disorders than do individuals with relatively low initial levels of psychosocial disturbance.

DIAGNOSIS

Diagnostic tools in noncardiac chest pain

Presently, a large variety of tests can be used to evaluate patients with NCCP (Table 68.2). The tests are designed to evaluate patients for gastroesophageal reflux, esophageal dysmotility, and the presence of visceral hypersensitivity. Most of the tests are invasive, costly, and inconvenient to patients and commonly not readily available for many physicians. These drawbacks are compounded by a lack of consistent data about the value of these tests in NCCP. Furthermore, in patients with suspected GERD-related NCCP, the recent introduction of the proton pump inhibitor (PPI) test (discussed below) has gained general popularity as a sensitive, noninvasive, readily available, and cost-effective test. Consequently, the employment of these invasive tests for diagnosing GERD-related NCCP has markedly declined.

Table 68.2 Diagnostic tests for noncardiac chest pain

Gastroesophageal reflux

Acid perfusion test (Bernstein test)
Ambulatory 24-hour esophageal pH monitoring
Barium swallow
Proton pump inhibitor (PPI) test
Upper endoscopy

Esophageal dysmotility

Bethanechol test
Esophageal manometry
Edrophonium (Tensilon) test
Ergonovine test
High-frequency intraluminal ultrasonography
Pentagastrin test

Visceral hypersensitivity

Balloon distention test
Electrical stimulation
Impedance planimetry
Brain imaging

Upper endoscopy

Upper endoscopy, while an accurate test for diagnosing esophagitis and its sequelae, has not been shown to be useful in the initial evaluation of NCCP because only 10–25% of patients are found to have evidence of mucosal injury.[31] Interestingly, despite the limited clinical value, endoscopy is commonly used as the first-line test by community-based gastroenterologists.[10] In patients with NCCP with concomitant alarm symptoms such as anorexia, weight loss, dysphagia, odynophagia, hematemesis, and others, urgent upper endoscopy is indicated.

Ambulatory 24-hour esophageal pH monitoring

Ambulatory 24-hour esophageal pH monitoring with symptom correlation is commonly used to evaluate patients with NCCP.[32] Approximately 50–60% of NCCP patients have increased esophageal acid exposure and a positive symptom index or a positive symptom index alone. Hewson et al.[32] examined 100 consecutive patients with NCCP and detected abnormal esophageal acid exposure in 48 patients (48%). Of the 83 patients with spontaneous chest pain during the pH testing, 37 patients (46%) had abnormal reflux parameters, and 50 patients (60%) had a positive symptom index. The authors concluded that 24-hour esophageal pH monitoring with symptom index is the single best test for evaluating patients with NCCP. In contrast, Dekel et al.[33] demonstrated that positive symptom index is a relatively uncommon phenomenon in NCCP patients because many patients do not experience chest pain during the pH study.

Ambulatory 24-hour esophageal pH monitoring is invasive, costly, inconvenient, and uncomfortable for many patients and is unavailable to many physicians. Reported sensitivity and specificity in GERD patients has ranged from 60–96% and 85–100%, respectively.[34] However, no studies have assessed the sensitivity of the test in NCCP.

Recently, a new ambulatory 24-hour esophageal pH monitoring wireless system (Bravo pH system®, Medtronic, Shoreview, Minnesota) has been introduced to the market. This system is a new USDA class I approved, 'catheterless' pH monitoring system. It involves the attachment of a radiotelemetry pH capsule to the mucosal wall of the esophagus (per oral or transnasally) that simultaneously measures pH and transmits data to a pager-sized receiver, thereby circumventing the need for a nasally placed catheter. The Bravo wireless ambulatory pH recording system has been shown to be well tolerated and reliable and provides reproducible results over a period of 48 hours,[35] and may prove to be helpful in further clarifying the role of GERD in NCCP. A recent study demonstrated that the 48-hour recording provided by the wireless pH capsule improves the assessment of the relationship between symptoms and acid reflux events.[36]

Presently, the precise role of pH testing in patients with NCCP is unclear. Many physicians will perform the test if patients with NCCP continue to be symptomatic despite 2–3 months of PPI therapy. The pH test is done while on therapy to ensure proper acid suppression. However, a recent study by Vaezi et al.[37] demonstrated that more than 90% of the patients with extraesophageal manifestations on double-dose PPI treatment have a completely normal pH test, questioning the value of the test in this situation.

Esophageal manometry

Various esophageal motility abnormalities may present with chest pain only, or more commonly with other esophageal-related symptoms. They include diffuse esophageal spasm, nutcracker esophagus, achalasia, long-duration contractions, multipeaked waves, and hypertensive LES.[38] However, esophageal manometry appears to have a relatively poor sensitivity in evaluating patients with NCCP, with most patients demonstrating normal esophageal motor function. Furthermore, patients rarely experience chest pain during esophageal manometry even if esophageal dysmotility is documented,[39] raising the question about any relationship between documented esophageal dysmotility and chest pain. Unlike GERD, effective drugs are not available that can easily correct motility abnormalities and consequently can be used to demonstrate causal relationship. Some authorities suggest the use of motility abnormalities as a marker for an underlying esophageal motor disorder that may be responsible for patients' symptoms.[39] Although ambulatory 24-hour esophageal manometry has been suggested as a means to improve test sensitivity in NCCP, when examined systematically, a significant number of patients (27–43%) reported no symptoms at all during the 24-hour recording. Moreover, in only 13–24% of the patients were the investigators able to relate the pain episodes to a recorded esophageal dysmotility.[40,41] These results question the routine use of ambulatory 24-hour esophageal manometry in clinical practice for the evaluation of patients with NCCP. Presently, patients who do not respond to antireflux treatment (non-GERD-related NCCP) are likely to undergo esophageal manometry. However, with the exception of achalasia, NCCP patients with other esophageal motility abnormalities respond to pain modulators better than to any of the smooth muscle relaxants.

The proton pump inhibitor test

The limitations of the currently available diagnostic modalities for GERD make a therapeutic trial with a proton pump inhibitor (PPI) an attractive option. The test uses a short course of high-dose PPI as an aid in diagnosing GERD. Overall, the PPI therapeutic trial is a simple, readily available, and clinically practical diagnostic tool.[42] However, no standardized use of the PPI therapeutic trial is documented in the literature. Furthermore, the clinical need for the PPI therapeutic trial increases as the true prevalence of GERD decreases in patients presenting with symptoms suggesting various esophageal (erosive esophagitis, nonerosive reflux disease, and noncardiac chest pain) and extraesophageal (pharyngeal, laryngeal, and pulmonary) manifestations of GERD.[42] The main requirement of the therapeutic trial is to achieve significant symptomatic improvement within a relatively short period of drug administration. To date, only PPIs have been used in studies assessing therapeutic trials, because of their profound acid inhibition and relatively consistent effect on typical and atypical GERD-related symptoms.[10,43–48]

The sensitivity of a therapeutic trial is determined by several factors, including symptoms assessed, duration of drug administration, dose of medication, and symptom score parameters (Table 68.3). Therapeutic trials have been tested in patients with typical symptoms of GERD, those with nonerosive reflux disease,

Table 68.3 Factors that determine the sensitivity of a proton pump inhibitor therapeutic trial

Type of reflux medication used

Dosage

Treatment duration

Definition of a positive test (symptom score cut-off, change in symptom grading, receiver operating characteristics curve analysis)

GERD-related symptom evaluated

Adapted from Fass R, European Journal of Gastroenterology and Hepatology, 2001; 13:S49–50. © 2001, reprinted with permission of Lippincott Williams & Wilkins.

individuals with GERD and noncardiac chest pain, and patients with suspected extraesophageal manifestations.[10,43–51] However, the assessment of sensitivity and specificity of a therapeutic trial in patients with different GERD-related symptoms is generally hampered by the lack of a 'gold standard' to use as a comparator. High doses of PPI have typically been tested regardless of the patient subgroup being evaluated. Schindlbeck et al..[44] demonstrated that omeprazole (40 mg), given for a period of 7 days to patients with GERD, had a sensitivity of only 27.2%, whereas 80 mg daily increased the sensitivity to 83%. The symptoms assessed have also influenced the dose of medication used in a therapeutic trial. In patients with NCCP or extraesophageal manifestations of GERD, larger doses (3–4 times the standard dose) were required to achieve high response rates.[10,46–51]

The duration of a therapeutic trial among studies has ranged from 1 day to 4 weeks. Shorter durations have been used in patients with typical and atypical symptoms of GERD (7–14 days), and longer durations (up to 4 weeks) in those with extraesophageal manifestations. The optimal duration of testing has yet to be determined. However, in at least one study (20 mg of omeprazole twice daily) in patients with typical symptoms of GERD, the maximum number of responders to PPI appeared to be evident by day 5, with few, if any, additional responders afterwards.[45] Whether larger doses of a PPI may achieve even earlier maximal symptom improvement is unknown.

Another important factor determining the sensitivity of a therapeutic trial is the definition of a positive test. In most studies, a symptom score cutoff was used; if the symptom assessment scores for heartburn, chest pain, or other symptoms improved by more than 50–75% (depending on the study), the test was considered positive. As with any diagnostic test, the optimal cutoff is critical in defining test accuracy,[42] and the parameters used among studies that evaluated therapeutic trials for GERD were chosen arbitrarily. Rarely, studies calculated the Receiver Operator Curve (ROC) by varying the percent reduction in the symptom tested to ascertain the optimal value for detecting patients with GERD.[10,42,48] This cutoff point provides the greatest sensitivity, specificity, positive predictive value, and accuracy of the therapeutic trial.

As with any other test, the sensitivity of a therapeutic trial depends on the prevalence of the disease in the patient population being evaluated. Obviously, the therapeutic trial has minimal utility in patients with erosive esophagitis, in whom acid reflux is almost always the underlying cause. However, as the likelihood

of a particular syndrome being attributable to reflux decreases, the potential value of a therapeutic trial increases. The sensitivity of the PPI test for GERD-related NCCP ranged from 69–95% and the specificity from 67–86% (Table 68.4)[10,46,47,52–55] The doses of PPIs used ranged from 60–80 mg daily for omeprazole; 30–90 mg for lansoprazole; and 40 mg for rabeprazole. The trial duration ranged from 1 to 28 days.

When using the PPI test, there was a significant correlation between the extent of esophageal acid exposure in the distal esophagus as determined by ambulatory 24-hour esophageal pH monitoring and the change in symptom intensity score after treatment, suggesting that the higher the esophageal acid exposure, the greater the response to the PPI test in patients with GERD-related NCCP.[56] Moreover, an economic analysis showed that the PPI test for GERD-related NCCP is a cost-saving approach primarily due to a significant reduction in the usage of various costly and invasive diagnostic tests.[10]

Acid perfusion test (Bernstein test)

The acid perfusion test was introduced as an objective method to identify esophageal chemosensitivity to acid.[57] A nasogastric tube is passed into the stomach, and after gastric contents are aspirated, the tube is withdrawn to a distance 30 cm from the nares to the tip.[58] This maneuver assumes that the solution is delivered at a level near the junction of the upper and middle thirds of the esophagus. The tube is connected to an intravenous bottle, and 0.9% NaCl (control) is perfused for 10–15 minutes at a rate of 6–7.5 mL per minute. This perfusion is followed by administration of 0.1 N HCl acid, at a similar rate, for 30 minutes or until discomfort is induced.[58] If symptoms appear, the test is discontinued and 0.9% NaCl is once again given. The acid perfusion test was originally devised to distinguish between chest pain of cardiac and esophageal origin. However, since the initial description, many modifications have been instituted.

Many attempts were made to change the test from a qualitative to a quantitative tool. Fass et al.[13] placed a manometry catheter 10 cm above the upper border of the LES to ensure sufficient exposure of the esophageal mucosa to acid. Saline was infused initially for 2 minutes and then without the patient's knowledge, 0.1 N HCl acid was infused for 10 minutes at a rate of 10 mL per minute. Patients were instructed to report whenever their typical symptoms were reproduced. Esophageal chemosensitivity was assessed by both the duration for induction of typical symptom perception (in seconds) and the total sensory intensity rating reported by the subject at the end of acid perfusion by using a verbal descriptor scale. The scale consisted of a 20-cm vertical bar flanked by descriptors of increasing intensity (no sensation, faint, very weak, weak, very mild, mild, moderate, barely strong, slightly intense, strong, intense, very intense, and extremely intense). Placement of words along the side of the scale was determined from their relative log intensity rating in a normative study. The validity of these scales for assessing the perceived intensity of visceral sensations has been confirmed.

An acid perfusion test intensity score (cm × sec) was then calculated as follows:

$$(I \times T) / 100$$

where I is the total intensity rating at the end of the acid perfusion and T is the duration of typical symptom perception during the

Table 68.4 Proton pump inhibitor therapeutic trials in NCCP

First author	Dosing schedule	Patients (n)	Symptom improvement (%)	Sensitivity (%)	Specificity (%)
Young	Omeprazole 80 mg/day × 1 day	30	75	90	80
Squillace	Omeprazole 80 mg/day × 1 day	17	50	69	75
Xia	Lansoprazole 30 mg/day × 4 weeks	68	50	92	67
Pandak	Omeprazole 40 mg twice daily × 2 weeks	37	50	90	67
Fass	Omeprazole (40 mg in the morning and 20 mg in the evening) for 7 days	37	50	78	86
Fass	Lansoprazole (60 mg in the morning and 30 mg in the evening) for 7 days	40	50	78	82
Fass	Rabeprazole (20 mg in the morning and 20 mg in evening) for 7 days	20	50	83	75

test. For convenience, the score was divided by 100. The test is highly specific, but the sensitivity ranges from 6% to 60%. A negative test has no clinical relevance and does not exclude esophageal origin.

Presently, the acid perfusion test is rarely performed in clinical practice because of its limited diagnostic value in uncomplicated GERD, NCCP, and other esophageal disorders. Because of the low sensitivity and the emergence of noninvasive and highly sensitive modalities, such as the PPI test and empirical therapy with PPI, many authorities consider the acid perfusion test to be obsolete.

Edrophonium test

Edrophonium (Tensilon®) is a cholinesterase inhibitor that increases cholinergic activity at muscarinic receptors.[59] A short-acting drug, edrophonium pharmacologic action is manifested 30–60 seconds after injection and lasts an average of 10 minutes. The aim of the edrophonium test is to induce greater esophageal body amplitude contractions in the hope of provoking the patient's typical chest pain.[60] The test is performed by injecting either 80 mg/kg or 10 mg edrophonium intravenously, which is immediately followed by 5–10 swallows of 5–10 mL of water over a period of 5–10 minutes. Commonly, subjects experience pain within 5 minutes after administration of the edrophonium test, which usually resolves quickly because of its rapid metabolism.

Side effects are due chiefly to excessive cholinergic stimulation and may include increased salivation, nausea, vomiting, and abdominal cramps. Overall, side effects are minimal and the antidote atropine is rarely needed. The drug seems to have no effect on coronary artery diameter.[61] The sensitivity of the edrophonium test has varied from 9% to 55%,[62,63] and the precise sensitivity is unknown because of the lack of a 'gold standard.' The mechanism by which edrophonium induces chest pain in NCCP patients is unclear, but may be related to hypersensitivity to augmented esophageal motor activity.

Overall, it seems that if the edrophonium test is positive, the esophagus is the likely origin of chest pain. However, owing to a lack of differences in esophageal contractile activity after the edrophonium test between NCCP patients and normal healthy subjects, several authorities have suggested that the test be performed with concomitant esophageal manometric studies.

Other provocative tests

The bethanechol test is presently rarely performed in clinical practice because of its questionable diagnostic value and frequent side effects. Bethanechol chloride, a cholinergic agonist, is a synthetic ester that is structurally and pharmacologically related to acetylcholine. Doses of 40–50 mg/kg have been administered subcutaneously, inducing chest pain in 12–33% of NCCP patients.[64] Doubling the dose to two injections of 50 mg/kg (15-minute intervals) increases sensitivity to 77% but at the cost of severe side effects. Side effects reported after the bethanechol test included symptomatic bradycardia requiring atropine treatment, hypotension, headache, increased salivation, sweating, and nervousness, among others. A history of other medical problems, such as asthma, epilepsy, cardiac or vascular disorders, hypotension, and Parkinson's disease, should be elicited and, if present, the test should be avoided.

The intravenous ergonovine stimulation test has been demonstrated to induce augmentation of esophageal contractions and chest pain in many NCCP patients.[65] Ergonovine is a sympathomimetic agent that had been used by cardiologists to diagnose coronary arterial spasm. The drug has been shown to induce chest pain in patients with NCCP and demonstrated similar sensitivity to edrophonium. Presently, however, ergonovine is rarely used for esophageal testing due to potential serious side effects, including severe cardiac events, including death.

Balloon distention

Balloon distention has been used primarily for research purposes to determine perception thresholds for pain. This modality has been used extensively in studies of various functional bowel disorders, most notably irritable bowel syndrome, functional dyspepsia, and NCCP.[66–68] More than 40 years ago, intraesophageal balloon distention in humans was reported to produce pain referred to the chest.[67] Early data indicated that, in patients with documented ischemic heart disease, balloon distention of the esophagus produced pain indistinguishable from anginal pain, but without ECG changes.[69] These effects may be explained by the convergence of sensory pathways at the level of spinal cord or in the midbrain. Despite this similarity in pain, it appears that esophageal balloon distention itself has no effect on coronary function or blood flow.[70]

Balloon distention was reintroduced during the mid-1980s in a seminal study that evaluated perception thresholds for pain in patients with NCCP.[66] The latex balloon was attached to a manometric catheter and filled with air. The balloon was positioned 10 cm above the LES and distended in a stepwise fashion using a hand-held syringe. A further development in the balloon distention technique was the introduction of a pump that was powered by compressed air.[71] The pump ensured inflation at a predetermined rate, which was difficult to achieve with a hand-held syringe. However, neither system was able to provide concomitant pressure measurements that would be helpful to determine whether the balloon remained within the esophageal lumen during each inflation. This determination was particularly critical in protocols that inflated balloons within the distal portion of the esophagus. Concomitant pressure measurements would be helpful to detect the migration of the balloon into the gastric fundus by demonstrating a sudden decrease in intraluminal pressure despite continued increases in balloon volume.

The introduction of the electronic barostat, a computer-driven volume-displacement device, has helped to ensure proper location of the balloon, regardless of the inflation method used.[72] The basic principal of the barostat is to maintain a constant pressure within the balloon/bag in the lumen despite muscular contractions and relaxations.[72,73] To maintain a constant pressure, the barostat aspirates air with contractions and injects air with relaxations. Presently, many prefer the use of a polyethylene bag over a latex balloon. Bags are infinitely compliant and show no increase in intra-bag pressure until about 90% of the maximum bag volume has been achieved.[72,74] In contrast, latex balloon resist inflation and as a result show a rapid increase in intra-balloon pressure with small volumes of distention.[13,72,75] When the pressure increases above the elastance threshold, the balloon becomes plastic and accommodates large volumes of air with very little change in pressure.[72,74] For tubular organs in the gastrointestinal tract, such as the esophagus, experts recommend the use of a cylindrical bag (rather than spherical) with a fixed length.[13,72]

Various distention protocols have been used in different studies. Like any other technique that assesses esophageal sensation, balloon distention has yet to be standardized. Slow-ramp distention is an ascending method that involves slow (rate varies from one study to another) increases in volume or pressure of the balloon, usually until the desired perceptual response has been reported by the subject.[13,76,77] In contrast, phasic distentions are rapid inflations of the balloon that can be delivered in random sequence or double-random staircase.[13] The latter includes two series of distention stimuli (staircases), and the computer alternates between the two staircases on a random basis.[13,72,77] With the tracking method, the barostat is programmed to deliver a series of intermittent phasic stimuli separated by interpulse rest period within an interactive stimulus tracking procedure.[13,78,79] If the subject indicates a sensation below the tracked intensity, the following stimulus will increase in pressure. If the subject reports

the desired sensation, the following pressure step is randomized to stay the same or decrease. The random element is placed to mask the relationship between ratings and subsequent stimulus change, and thus decreases potential scaling bias.[71]

Commonly, qualitative and quantitative perceptual responses are evaluated during balloon distention studies. Qualitative perceptual responses include symptom reports in response to balloon distention, such as chest pain.[13,80] Quantitative perceptual responses are commonly obtained during slow-ramp distention and include the minimal distention volume or pressure at which the individual first reports moderate sensation (innocuous sensation), discomfort, and pain (aversive sensation).[13] Discomfort threshold is commonly defined as the first unpleasant esophageal sensation, and pain threshold is defined as the first sensation of pain.[13]

Balloon studies are primarily designed to assess the presence of visceral hyperalgesia in various esophageal disorders. Early studies demonstrated that pain develops with balloon distention more frequently in NCCP patients than in normal control subjects and that their pain occurs at smaller volumes.[66,71,81] Balloon distention has been used commonly to assess the effect of various drugs on esophageal sensory perception. Imipramine, octreotide, and nifedipine have all been shown to increase the perception threshold for pain in normal controls or patients with NCCP.[82–86]

Impedance

Originally, impedance planimetry was developed to measure the cross-sectional area of the ureter.[87,88] Over the years, the technique was further perfected and was recently used to describe the biomechanical characteristics of the human esophagus.[89–91] The sensing system includes a thin latex balloon, which was used by some investigators to assess esophageal sensory thresholds. Balloon pressure was increased stepwise by 5 cm H_2O increments from 0 to determine sensory thresholds for pain in several studies.[23,90,92] After each inflation, the balloon was completely deflated for a period of 3 minutes. Balloon distentions were maintained for 3–5 minutes each. In this protocol, at each level of distention, the cross-sectional area was measured and sensory response determined using a verbal descriptor. Grade 1 was considered to be a sensation of fullness, grade 2 was considered moderate discomfort, and grade 3 was considered severe pain. In validating this technique, the authors found that the threshold pressure required to induce a sensation of fullness varied between 20 and 50 cm of H_2O.[90]

Multichannel intraluminal impedance

The recent introduction of improved impedance probes with integrated pH sensors has allowed further assessment of esophageal function, as well as refluxate composition and its relationship to symptoms.[93,94] Because the electrical conductivity of the esophageal muscular wall, air, and any given bolus is different, the presence of different substances in the esophageal luman provides a different impedance pattern.[94] With a highly conductive bolus (e.g., saliva), the impedance decreases; with a poorly conductive material (e.g., air) the impedance increases.[95,96]

The combination of impedance catheter and a pH probe provides a unique opportunity to study physiologic events within the esophagus and their relationship to symptoms. In addition, the recording assembly can disclose the characteristics of the gastric refluxate (acid, nonacid, gas, and mixed gas and liquid). The value of such a technique has been demonstrated by recent studies that documented that nonacid reflux is not uncommon in GERD patients and may lead to classic heartburn symptoms.[93,94] The value of the multichannel intraluminal impedance in evaluating patients with NCCP remains to be elucidated.

Brain imaging

In addition to cortical evoked potentials, other techniques have been increasingly used to evaluate brain–gut relationship in patients with esophageal disorders, including those with NCCP. These techniques include positron emission tomography (PET) and functional magnetic resonance imaging (fMRI). The gastrointestinal tract is intricately connected to the central nervous system by pathways that are continuously sampling and modulating gut function.[97]

PET scanning is an established method to study the functional neuroanatomy of the human brain.[98,99] Radiolabeled compounds allow the study of biochemical and physiologic processes involved in cerebral metabolism.[97] Tomographic images represent spatial distribution of radioisotopes in the brain. Regional cerebral blood flow is studied with labeled water ($H_2^{15}O$) and glucose metabolism with ^{18}Fl-labeled fluorodeoxyglucose. Unlike PET, fMRI does not require radioisotopes and hence is considered a safer imaging technique. fMRI detects increases in oxygen concentration in areas of heightened neuronal activity.[99–101] This imaging technique is best suited for locating the site but not the sequence or duration of neuronal activity. Overall, fMRI provides both anatomic and functional information.

To date, only a few studies have attempted to assess the cortical process of esophageal sensation in humans. Aziz et al. examined the human brain loci involved in the process of esophageal sensation using PET and distal esophageal balloon distention in eight healthy volunteers.[102] Nonpainful stimuli elicited bilateral activation along the central sulcus, insular cortex, and the frontal and parietal operculum. Painful stimuli resulted in intense activation of the same areas and additional activation of the right anterior insular cortex and anterior cingulated gyrus. The former is important in affective processing, while the latter in pain processing and generating an affective and cognitive response to pain.[103–105]

Further studies are needed to assess cerebral activation in patients with different esophageal disorders. In addition, it would be of great interest to determine whether there are differences in central processing of an intraesophageal stimulus in patients with NCCP. It is also important to begin to examine the role of psychophysiologic states such as stress, anxiety, and depression and their effects on central nuclei involved with perception of esophageal stimuli.

Psychological evaluation

Some patients with NCCP require psychological evaluation by an expert psychologist or psychiatrist because of the high prevalence rate of psychological abnormalities in this group of patients. Deciding who should be referred is determined on an individual basis, but the likely candidates are those who appeared to be refractory to therapeutic interventions or those that display clear features of a psychological disorder. Physicians can use a struc-

tured psychiatric interview to determine whether any psychological comorbidity is present.[106] Various diagnostic psychological tools, such as the Symptom Checklist-90R (SCL-90R) and the Beck Depression Inventory questionnaires, can be used at the clinical level. However, such tools are unlikely to find a place in a busy GI practice. Regardless, when evaluating a patient with NCCP, the presence of a coexisting psychological comorbidity should always be entertained.

TREATMENT

Overview

The treatment of NCCP should address the likely mechanism underlying the patient's symptoms (Table 68.5). Antireflux treatment has been repeatedly shown to be effective in relieving symptoms of patients with GERD-related NCCP. For patients with non-GERD-related NCCP, pain modulators are the mainstay of therapy.

Treatment of gastroesophageal reflux disease-related noncardiac chest pain

Treatment of GERD-related NCCP (see also Ch. 13) should involve lifestyle modifications and pharmacologic intervention. Elevating the head of the bed at night, reducing fat intake, stopping smoking, and avoiding foods that exacerbate gastroesophageal reflux have been shown to decrease reflux-related symptoms.[107] There are few trials, however, that have assessed the usefulness of acute or maintenance therapy with antireflux medications in patients with GERD-related NCCP.

Small, uncontrolled studies have compared histamine H_2 antagonists (H_2RAs) to placebo or omeprazole. The efficacy of H_2RAs has ranged from 54% to 83%.[31] However, when compared with PPIs, they have demonstrated a limited response. In a small,

---

Table 68.5 Medical therapeutic modalities for noncardiac chest pain

Gastroesophageal reflux
Proton pump inhibitors

Omeprazole (Prilosec)	20 mg p.o. b.i.d.
Rabeprazole (Aciphex)	20 mg p.o. b.i.d.
Pantoprazole (Protonix)	40 mg p.o. b.i.d.
Lansoprazole (Prevacid)	30 mg p.o. b.i.d
Esomeprazole (Nexium)	40 mg p.o. b.i.d.

Esophageal dysmotility

Diltiazem (Cardizem)	60 mg–90 mg p.o. q.i.d
Nifedipine (Adalate/Procardia)	10 mg–30 mg p.o. t.i.d.
Isosorbide dinitrate (Isordil)	10 mg–20 mg po b.i.d.–t.i.d.

Visceral hypersensitivity

Tricyclics (commonly used)	
Nortriptyline (Aventyl/Pamelor)	50 mg p.o. q.h.s.
Amitriptyline (Elavil/Endep)	
Doxepin (Sinequan)	
Trazodone (Desyrel)	100 mg–150 mg p.o. q.d.
Sertraline (Zoloft)	50 mg–200 mg p.o. q.d.

uncontrolled study by Stahl et al.,[108] 13 patients with NCCP and GERD were treated with high-dose ranitidine (150 mg four times daily). Seven patients had failed lower doses of ranitidine previously. All patients improved with high doses of ranitidine, although two patients had to have their dose increased to 300 mg orally four times daily. DeMeester et al.[109] followed 23 patients with abnormal esophageal acid exposure and NCCP for 2–3 years. Twelve patients were treated medically with antacids and cimetidine, and 11 patients were treated with a surgical anti-reflux procedure. Of the medically treated patients, five (42%) were chest pain free at follow-up. These results are not surprising because H_2RAs have limited antisecretory properties (see Ch. 1). A further shortcoming is that tolerance to these drugs generally develops within 2 weeks of repeated administration.[110] PPI therapy, in contrast, produces a more profound and longer duration of acid suppression, and tolerance has not been observed.

When omeprazole 20 mg twice daily was administered over a period of 8 weeks to NCCP patients in a double-blind, placebo-controlled trial, the patients who received omeprazole had a significant reduction in the number of days with chest pain and chest pain severity score when compared with patients who received placebo. Although data regarding the efficacy of PPIs in NCCP are available only with omeprazole, it is highly likely that all other PPIs will demonstrate similar efficacy.[111] Patients with GERD-related NCCP should be treated with at least double the standard PPI dose until symptoms remit, followed by dose tapering to determine the lowest dose that can control patient's symptoms. As with other extraesophageal manifestations of GERD, NCCP patients may require more than 2 months of therapy for optimal symptom control. Long-term PPI treatment has been shown to be highly effective.[112] Borzecki et al.[113] developed a decision tree to compare empirical treatment for NCCP patients with H_2RAs or standard dose PPI for 8 weeks with initial investigations (upper endoscopy or upper gastrointestinal series). Empiric treatment was more cost-effective, with a cost of US$849 per patient versus US$2187 per patient with the initial investigation strategy.

Laparoscopic fundoplication relieves heartburn and acid regurgitation in most patients with GERD, but its effect on chest pain is less clear. DeMeester et al.[109] found a temporal correlation in 12 of 23 patients who had acid reflux as a cause of NCCP. Pain resolved in the 12 patients treated surgically (8 patients) or by acid reducing agents (4 patients). Patti et al.[114] reviewed patients who underwent laparoscopic fundoplication for GERD who complained of chest pain in addition to heartburn and acid regurgitation. Overall, chest pain improved in 85% of the patients after laparoscopic fundoplication. Improvement increased to 96% in patients whose chest pain correlated with GERD most of the time. Farrell et al.[115] evaluated the effectiveness of antireflux surgery for patients with atypical manifestations of GERD. Chest pain improved in 90% of patients after laparoscopic fundoplication, with symptom resolution in 50% of the patients. Although surgical studies demonstrated a high success rate of antireflux surgery in GERD-related NCCP patients, the patients included were carefully selected.

Several endoscopic techniques designed to bolster the antireflux barrier at the gastroesophageal junction are currently under investigation (see Ch. 13).[116] There are three basic types of endoscopic treatments: suturing, radiofrequency, and injection.[117] The published data report only short-term outcomes of a limited number of patients with usually mild disease. No studies to date have specifically evaluated patients with GERD-related NCCP. Consequently, these endoscopic methods are considered experimental and should not be routinely performed even in patients with confirmed GERD-related NCCP. The effect of endoscopic therapies in GERD-related NCCP patients should definitely be studied, primarily because several recent anecdotal reports suggested a good response to endoscopic therapy.

Treatment of esophageal dysmotility-related noncardiac chest pain

Directing treatment to esophageal dysmotility in patients with NCCP remains a controversial area. In recent years, it has been recognized that the role of esophageal manometry in patients with non-GERD-related NCCP is limited primarily to diagnosing achalasia. It appears that NCCP patients with other spastic motility disorders respond better to pain modulators than to medications that alter esophageal motility. Furthermore, response to pain modulators in NCCP patients is essentially unrelated to the presence or absence of esophageal dysmotility.

Generally, treating esophageal motility abnormalities in patients with NCCP is a less rewarding practice primarily because of the paucity of clinically effective motility-related drugs that are currently available. In patients with nutcracker esophagus, antireflux treatment should be tried first before smooth muscle relaxants are considered.[118] Symptom resolution in these patients is unrelated to improvement in esophageal motility.

Smooth muscle relaxants have a very limited role if any in patients with NCCP and documented esophageal motor disorder. Data supporting the usage of nitrates are scarce and not uncommonly based on anecdotal experience. Sublingual nitroglycerin and long-acting nitrate preparations appear to have no effect on esophageal amplitude contractions of healthy subjects.[119] However, 0.4 mg sublingual nitroglycerin was reported to have a transient effect on esophageal dysmotility with relief of chest pain in a case report.[120] Reports about the value of long-acting nitrates in patients with NCCP and esophageal dysmotility are conflicting. In a study published in 1977, the authors reported complete symptom resolution of chest pain during a period of up to four years.[121] However, others could not confirm a long-term effect.[122] Calcium channel blockers, although commonly used in clinical practice, appear to also have a very limited effect on esophageal dysmotility in patients with NCCP. Their use appears to be complicated by side effects, such as hypotension, constipation, pedal edema, and others. Diltiazem in doses of 60–90 mg four times daily has been shown to improve chest pain score significantly better than placebo in small trials of patients with NCCP and documented nutcracker esophagus on esophageal manometry.[123,124] Nifedipine in doses of 10–30 mg three times daily demonstrated a limited symptomatic response in these patients.[125] Symptom improvement lasted only 2 weeks and was noted after a lag time of 3 weeks. By the end of the sixth week, the drug appeared to completely lose its efficacy. Limited effects of calcium channel blockers were also documented in the other spastic motility disorders that were described in association with NCCP.

Data regarding the use of other therapeutic modalities in NCCP patients with esophageal dysmotility are even scarcer. The antispasmodic cimetropium bromide has been shown to be efficacious in eight NCCP patients with nutcracker esophagus.[126] Hydralazine, an antihypertensive drug that directly dilates peripheral vessels, has been shown in five patients to improve chest pain and dysphagia, as well as to decrease the amplitude and duration of esophageal contractions.[122]

Botulinum toxin injection into the LES was used in several uncontrolled trials for patients with NCCP and spastic motility disorders.[127] It appears that botulinum toxin injection leads to a significant symptomatic improvement in patients with spastic esophageal motility disorders whose major complaint is chest pain. However, the mean duration of symptom response in one study was only 7 months. The authors used 100 units of botulinum toxin injected in five circumferential injections of 20 units each at the gastroesophageal junction.

Pneumatic dilation and long esophageal myotomy with or without fundoplication are reserved for severely symptomatic patients with well-documented spastic motility disorder, severe dysphagia, and weight loss.

Treatment of visceral hypersensitivity

During the last decade, pain modulators (visceral analgesics) have become the mainstay of therapy in non-GERD-related NCCP. Tricyclic antidepressants, trazodone, selective serotonin reuptake inhibitors (SSRIs) and theophylline have all been shown to improve symptoms in NCCP patients.

Several tricyclics have been assessed in NCCP patients. The mechanism by which tricyclics reduce visceral pain is poorly understood. Some studies suggested a central mediating effect,[128] while others claimed a potential peripheral effect. The tricyclic antidepressants (TCAs) demonstrate a varied receptor affinity (acetylcholine, histamine-1, and α-adrenergic).[129] Nortriptyline and desipramine are secondary amines (metabolites of tertiary amines) that have less affinity for receptors that result in bothersome side effect.[129] The tertiary amines include amitriptyline, imipramine, and doxepin. Imipramine has been shown to increase esophageal perception thresholds for pain in normal subjects without affecting esophageal tone, suggesting a visceral analgesic effect.[83] Similar effects have been noted in NCCP patients, independent of cardiac, esophageal, or psychiatric testing at baseline.[82] TCAs provide long-term effect in NCCP patients, although the drop-out rate due to side effects may reach 30%.[130]

Treatment with TCAs should be administered at bedtime, staring with a low dose (10–25 mg) and then increased by 10–25 mg increments per week to a maximal non-mood altering dose of 50–75 mg per day.[129] Because of the varied effect of TCAs on the different respective receptors, failure of one TCA to improve symptoms is not indicative of future failure of other TCAs.

The use of SSRIs in NCCP has been very limited. As with TCAs, a neuromodulatory effect has been proposed to mediate their effect on visceral pain. Varia et al.[131] performed a randomized trail that assessed the efficacy, tolerability, and safety of the SSRI sertraline in patients with NCCP in a double-blind, placebo-controlled trial that included 30 subjects. Patients were randomly selected to receive sertraline or placebo in doses starting at 50 mg and adjusted to a maximum dose of 200 mg. By using intention-to-treat analysis, investigators have demonstrated that patients receiving sertraline reported a significant reduction in their pain scores compared with those who received placebo, regardless of concomitant improvement in psychological scores.[132] This study further confirms the potential role of SSRIs in treating patients with NCCP. As with TCAs, the effects of SSRIs on visceral pain perception appears to be independent of their effect on mood.

Low-dose trazodone (100–150 mg/day), an antidepressant and anxiolytic, has been shown to improve symptoms in NCCP patients with esophageal contraction abnormalities, without affecting esophageal amplitude contractions.[133] Information about other compounds with visceral analgesic effect has been limited to isolated reports in the literature. Infusion of theophylline in an open-labeled trial alleviated chest pain in patients with functional chest pain of presumed esophageal origin.[134] It is assumed that theophylline improves esophageal pain by blocking adenosine receptors. Octreotide, a somatostatin analogue, given subcutaneously (100 μg) has been shown to increase esophageal perception thresholds to balloon distension in normal subjects,[135] an effect unrelated to changes in esophageal compliance.

Treatment of psychological comorbidity

Reassurance has been emphasized as an important mode of therapeutic intervention in patients with NCCP. However, symptoms are seldom relieved by reassurance only, resulting in the need for an additional therapeutic modality.[136] Several anxiolytics have been evaluated in NCCP patients, mostly members of the benzodiazepine family. Alprazolam and clonazepam have been demonstrated to reduce panic attack frequency, as well as chest pain episodes and anxiety scores.[137,138] However, benzodiazepines should be cautiously used in NCCP patients, primarily due to their addictive effect. Buspirone is an anxiolytic without dependency potential, but reported experience in NCCP patients is still unavailable.[129]

Young patients and males with NCCP appear to be open to medical psychological treatment.[139] However, management of psychological comorbidity in these patients should be reserved to experts in the field. Optimal management includes prescribing medications for panic attack, depression, and anxiety.

Several studies have suggested that behavioral therapy can be effective in patients with NCCP. Hegel and colleagues published a report in which three patients with chest pain and anxiety disorders were treated with relaxation training and controlled diaphragmatic breathing exercises, which were instituted during increasingly complex activities.[140] Two of the patients had substantial reductions in the frequency and intensity of their chest pain that was maintained for 12 months after treatment. Klimes et al. performed the only controlled study of behavioral treatment of patients with chest pain.[141] This treatment of 31 patients consisted of education, controlled breathing, training in relaxation and diversion of attention from pain, and the practice of newly learned skills in their home environment. When compared with the waiting list controls, the treatment program produced significant improvement in chest pain episodes, functional disability, and psychological distress that was maintained for 46 months after treatment.

Future treatment in noncardiac chest pain

Research into the underlying mechanisms that result in the development of NCCP ultimately may lead to novel therapeutic modalities in the future. Future research will continue to focus on mechanisms for pain in NCCP patients, primarily the role of the central and peripheral sensitization in enhancing perception of intraesophageal stimuli. Alosetron, a 5-hydroxytryptamine (5HT) type 3 antagonist, which was previously available for the treatment of female patients with diarrhea-predominant irritable bowel syndrome, raised the hope for a therapeutic potential in patients with NCCP.[142] This class of drugs appears to have a pain-modulatory effect, probably by altering the initiation, transmission, or processing of extrinsic sensory information from the gastro-intestinal tract. The role of the new partial 5HT type 4 agonist, tegaserod, in modulating pain that originates from the gastro-intestinal tract is less clear.

Phosphorylation of N-methyl-D-asparate (NMDA) receptors expressed by dorsal horn neurons leads to central sensitization via increase in their excitability and receptive field size.[143] Potentially, this central sensitization may be prevented or even reversed by antagonism of NMDA receptors within the spinal cord. However, it is important to note that central nervous system mechanisms that mediate visceral hyperalgesia are sensitive to both NMDA-receptor blockers and non-NMDA-receptor antagonists.[144]

Other neuromodulators such as fedotozine and asimadoline, kappa opioid receptor agonists (produce a peripheral antinociceptive effect in patients with IBS), neurokinin receptor antagonists, NK$_1$ and NK$_2$ (reduce gut motility and pain) and cholecystokinin-A receptor antagonist, loxiglumide (visceral analgesic effect in patients with IBS), may all have a future role in non-GERD-related NCCP.

Lastly, reversible acid pump inhibitors are likely to be introduced into the market by the end of 2010. This class of drugs possesses a more rapid onset of action, independent of meal stimulation, than presently available PPIs, a more predictable dose-response effect, and similar antisecretory properties. They will require extensive evaluation, but it is hoped that these agents may play an important role in GERD-related NCCP as a diagnostic tool ('APA test') or as an improved short- and long-term treatment for GERD-related NCCP.

AUTHORS' RECOMMENDATIONS

Patients with NCCP should be evaluated by a gastroenterologist only after a comprehensive evaluation has excluded a cardiac cause. Patients referred for NCCP are initially evaluated for alarm symptoms (dysphagia, odynophagia, weight loss, anorexia, etc.). If present, patients should undergo an upper endoscopy to exclude a mechanical cause for their symptoms. If patients lack

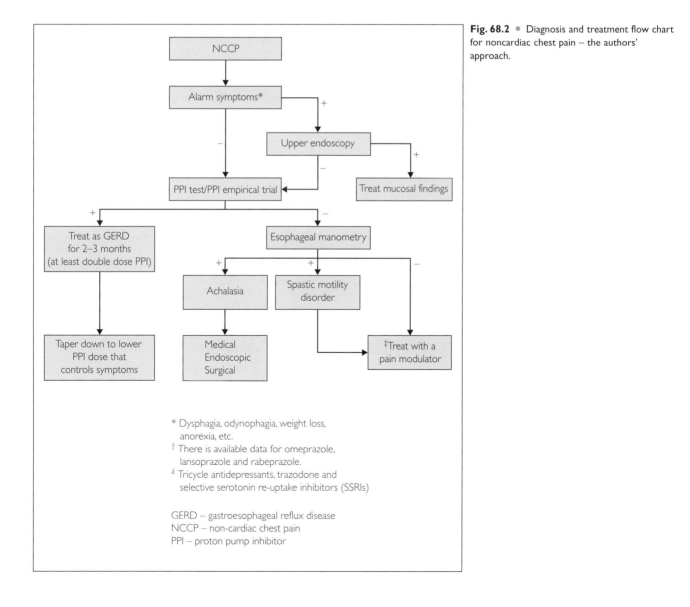

Fig. 68.2 • Diagnosis and treatment flow chart for noncardiac chest pain – the authors' approach.

alarm symptoms, they should be subjected to the PPI test, with duration of the test determined by the frequency of symptoms. If weekly symptoms are present, the PPI test should be administered over a period of 7 days (double dose in the morning before breakfast and single dose before dinner). If symptoms improve during the PPI test, patients are treated for an additional 2–3 months with a PPI twice daily. Subsequently, the PPI dose should be tapered down to the lowest dose that controls their symptoms. If patients demonstrate a lack of any response to the PPI test, esophageal manometry should be ordered to specifically exclude achalasia. In those without achalasia, whether or not other spastic motility disorders are present, pain modulators should be prescribed. The authors prefer nortriptyline due to fewer side effects and improved tolerability by patients. The medication is given at bedtime at a starting dose of 10 mg and subsequently increased by 10 mg increments per week to a therapeutic goal of 50 mg daily. If patients develop side effects during therapy with nortriptyline, another TCA should be prescribed. Patients who demonstrated an underlying psychological comorbidity should be referred to a psychologist or psychiatrist with knowledge in the field for further evaluation. Figure 68.2 depicts the authors' diagnostic and therapeutic approach to NCCP.

SUMMARY

NCCP is the most common atypical/extraesophageal manifestation of GERD. Diagnosis in the last decade has shifted to noninvasive modalities – the PPI test or the PPI empirical trial. The role of pH testing has been questioned and the role of esophageal manometry has been limited to diagnosing achalasia.

The availability of highly potent antireflux medications has improved our ability to treat patients with GERD-related NCCP. In those patients with non-GERD-related NCCP, whether or not esophageal dysmotility is present, pain modulation remains the cornerstone of therapy.

REFERENCES

1. Nevens F, Janssens J, Piessens J, et al. Prospective study on prevalence of esophageal chest pain in patients referred on an elective basis to a cardiac unit for suspected myocardial ischemia. Dig Dis Sci 1991; 36(2):229–235.

2. Richter JE. Chest pain and gastroesophageal reflux disease. J Clin Gastroenterol 2000; 30(3 Suppl):S39–S41.

3. Katerndahl DA, Trammell C. Prevalence and recognition of panic states in STARNET patients presenting with chest pain. J Fam Pract 1997; 45(1):54–63.

4. Eslick GD, Talley NJ. The natural history of non-cardiac chest pain (NCCP): A four-year prospective cohort study (Abstract). Gastroenterology 2004; 126(4 Suppl 2):A-310, #M1321.

5. Eslick GD. Noncardiac chest pain: epidemiology, natural history, health care seeking, and quality of life. Gastroenterol Clin North Am 2004; 33(1):1–23.

6. Eslick GD, Coushed DS, Talley NJ. Review article: the burden of illness of non-cardiac chest pain. Aliment Pharmacol Ther 2002; 16(7):1217–1223.

7. Locke G III, Talley NJ, Fett S, et al. Prevalence and clinical spectrum of gastroesophageal reflux: a population-based study in Olmsted County, Minnesota. Gastroenterology 1997; 112:1448–1456.

8. Fass R, Winters GF. Evaluation of the patient with noncardiac chest pain: is gastroesophageal reflux disease or an esophageal

motility disorder the cause? Medscape Gastroenterol 2001; 3(6):1–10.

9. Cherian P, Smith LF, Bardhan KD, et al. Esophageal tests in the evaluation of non-cardiac chest pain. Dis Esophagus 1995; 8:129–133.

10. Fass R, Fennerty MB, Ofman JJ, et al. The clinical and economic value of a short course of omeprazole in patients with noncardiac chest pain. Gastroenterology 1998; 115(1):42–49.

Seminal article that demonstrated for the first time the usefulness of the PPI test in diagnosing GERD-related NCCP.

11. Hsia PC, Maher KA, Lewis JH, et al. Utility of upper endoscopy in the evaluation of noncardiac chest pain. Gastrointest Endosc 1991; 37:22–26.

12. Frobert O, Funch-Jensen P, Jacobsen NO, et al. Upper endoscopy in patients with angina and normal coronary angiograms. Endoscopy 1995; 27:365–370.

13. Fass R, Naliboff B, Higa L, et al. Differential effect of long-term esophageal acid exposure on mechano sensitivity and chemosensitivity in humans. Gastroenterology 1998; 115(6):1363–1373.

14. Beedassy A, Katz PO, Gruber A, et al. Prior sensitization of esophageal mucosa by acid reflux predisposes to reflux-induced chest pain. J Clin Gastroenterol 2000; 31:121–124.

15. Richter JE. Extraesophageal presentations of gastroesophageal reflux disease: an overview. Am J Gastroenterol 2000; 95 (Suppl):S1–S3.

16. Wong W, Lai KC, Lau C, et al. Upper gastrointestinal evaluation of Chinese patients with non-cardiac chest pain. Aliment Pharmacol Ther 2002; 16:465–471.

17. Katz PO, Dalton CB, Richter JE. Esophageal testing in patients with noncardiac chest pain or dysphagia: results of three years' experience with 1161 patients. Ann Intern Med 1987; 106:593–597.

Commonly cited article about the distribution of esophageal motility abnormalities in patients with NCCP.

18. Kahrilas PJ. Nutcracker esophagus: Editorial: An idea whose time has gone? Am J Gastroenterol 1993; 88:167–169.

19. Achem SR, Kolts BE, Wears R, eet al. Chest pain associated with nutcracker esophagus: a preliminary study of the role of gastroesophageal reflux. Am J Gastroenterol 1993; 88(2):187–192.

20. Dekel R, Pearson T, Wendel C, et al. Assessment of oesophageal motor function in patients with dysphagia or chest pain – the Clinical Outcomes Research Initiative experience. Aliment Pharmacol Ther 2003; 18(11–12):1083–1089.

21. Hollerbach S, Bulat R, May A, et al. Abnormal cerebral processing oesophageal stimuli in patients with noncardiac chest pain (NCCP). Neurogastroenterol Motil 2000; 12:555–565.

An interesting study that compared cortical-evoked potential responses and heart rate variability in both healthy subjects and patients with NCCP in response to electrical esophageal stimulation.

22. Aziz Q. Acid sensors in the gut: a taste of things to come. Eur J Gastroenterol Hepatol 2001; 13:885–888.

23. Rao SS, Hayek B, Summers RW. Functional chest pain of esophageal origin: hyperalgesia or motor dysfunction. Am J Gastroenterol 2001; 96(9):2584–2589.

24. Tougas G, Spaziani R, Hollerbach S, et al. Cardiac autonomic function and oesophageal acid sensitivity in patients with non-cardiac chest pain. Gut 2001; 49(5):706–712.

25. Tougas G. The autonomic nervous system in functional bowel disorders. Gut 2000; 46:861–869.

26. Potokar JP, Nutt DJ. Chest pain: panic attack or heart attack? Int J Clin Pract 2000; 54(2):110–114.

27. Fleet RP, Dupuis G, Marchand A, et al. Panic disorder in emergency department chest pain patients: prevalence, comorbidity, suicidal ideation and physicians' recognition. Am J Med 1996; 101:371–380.

28. Van Peski-Oosterbaan AS, Spinhoven P, Van der Does AJW, et al. Cognitive change following cognitive behavioural therapy for non-cardiac chest pain. Psychother Psychosom 1999; 68:214–220.

29. Song CW, Lee SJ, Jeen YT, et al. Inconsistent association of esophageal symptoms, psychometric abnormalities and dysmotility. Am J Gastroenterol 2001; 96:2312–2316.

30. Lantinga LJ, Sprafkin RP, McCroskery JH, et al. One-year psychosocial follow-up of patients with chest pain and angiography normal coronary arteries. Am J Cardiol 1988; 62(4):209–213.

31. Fang J, Bjorkman D. A critical approach to noncardiac chest pain: pathophysiology, diagnosis and treatment. Am J Gastroenterol 2001; 96:958–968.

32. Hewson EG, Sinclair JW, Dalton CB, et al. Twenty-four-hour esophageal pH monitoring: the most useful test for evaluating noncardiac chest pain. Am J Med 1991; 90:576–583.

33. Dekel R, Martinez-Hawthorne SD, Guillen R, Fass R. Evaluation of symptom index in identifying gastroesophageal reflux disease-related noncardiac chest pain. J Clin Gastroenterol 2004;3 8:24–29.

34. Eslick GD, Fass R. Noncardiac chest pain: evaluation and treatment. Gastroenterol Clin North Am 2003; 32:531–552.

35. Pandolfino JE, Richter JE, Ours T, et al. Ambulatory esophageal pH monitoring using a wireless system. Am J Gastroenterol 2003; 98:740–749.

36. Prakash C, Clouse RE. Extended pH monitoring with the Bravo capsule increases diagnostic yield in chest pain patients (Abstract). Gastroenterology 2004; 126(4 Suppl 2):A-321, #M1376.

37. Vaezi M, Richter J, Stasney CR, et al. A randomized, double-blind, placebo-controlled study of acid suppression for the treatment of suspected laryngopharyngeal reflux (Abstract). Gastroenterology 2004; 126(4 Suppl 2):A-22, #160.

38. Kahrilas PJ, Clouse RE, Hogan WJ. An American Gastroenterological Association medical position statement on the clinical use of esophageal manometry. Gastroenterology 1994; 107:1865–1884.

39. DiMarino AJJ, Allen ML, Lynn RB, et al. Clinical value of esophageal motility testing. Dig Dis Sci 1998; 16:198–204.

40. Breumelhof R, Nadorp JHSM, Akkemans LMA, et al. Analysis of 24-hour esophageal pressure and pH data in unselected patients with noncardiac chest pain. Gastroenterology 1990; 99:1257–1264.

41. Lam HGT, Dekker W, Kan G, et al. Acute noncardiac chest pain in a coronary care unit: evaluation by 24-hour pressure and pH recording of the esophagus. Gastroenterology 1992; 102:453–460.

42. Fass R. Empirical trials in treatment of gastroesophageal reflux disease. Dig Dis Sci 2000; 18:20–26.

Comprehensive review of the clinical and economic value of the PPI test in general and specifically in NCCP.

43. Schenk BE, Kuipers EJ, Klinkenberg-Knol EC, et al. Omeprazole as a diagnostic tool in gastroesophageal reflux disease. Am J Gastroenterol 1997; 92:1997–2000.

44. Schindlbeck NC, Klauser AG, Voderholzer WA, et al. Empiric therapy for gastroesophageal reflux disease. Arch Intern Med 1995; 155:1808–1812.

45. Johnsson F, Weywadt L, Solhaug JH, et al. One-week omeprazole treatment in the diagnosis of gastro-oesophageal reflux disease. Scand J Gastroenterol 1998; 33:15–20.

46. Young MF, Sanowski RA, Talbert GA, et al. Omeprazole administration as a test for gastroesophageal reflux (Abstract). Gastroenterology 1992; 102:192.

47. Squillace SJ, Young MF, Sanowski RA. Single dose omeprazole as a test for noncardiac chest pain (Abstract). Gastroenterology 1993; 107:A197.

48. Fass R, Ofman JJ, Gralnek IM, et al. Clinical and economic assessment of the omeprazole test in patients with symptoms suggestive of gastroesophageal reflux disease. Arch Intern Med 1999; 159:2161–2168.

49. Metz DC, Childs ML, Ruiz C, et al. Pilot study of the oral omeprazole test for reflux laryngitis. Otolaryngol Head Neck Surg 1997; 116:41–46.

50. Ours TM, Kavuru MS, Schilz RJ, et al. Prospective, double-blind study comparing omeprazole 40 mg bid vs. placebo in patients with chronic cough and GE reflux. Am J Gastroenterol 1998; 93:1621.

51. Jaspersen D, Diehl KL, Geyer P, et al. Omeprazole test for gastro-oesophageal reflux-related chronic persistent cough (Abstract). Gastroenterology 1999; 116:A168.

52. Pandak WM, Arezo S, Everett S, et al. Short course of omeprazole: A better first diagnostic approach to noncardiac chest pain than endoscopy, manometry, or 24-hour esophageal pH monitoring. J Clin Gastroenterol 2002; 35:307–314.

53. Xia HH, Lai KC, Lam SK, et al. Symptomatic response to lansoprazole predicts abnormal acid reflux in endoscopy-negative patients with non-cardiac chest pain. Aliment Pharmacol Ther 2003; 17:369–377.

54. Fass R, Pulliam G, Hayden CW. Patients with non-cardiac chest pain (NCCP) receiving an empirical trial of high dose lansoprazole, demonstrate early symptom response – a double blind, placebo-controlled trial (Abstract). Gastroenterology 2001; 122:A580, #W1175.

55. Fass R, Fullerton H, Hayden CW, et al. Patients with noncardiac chest pain (NCCP) receiving an empirical trial of high dose rabeprazole, demonstrate early symptom response – a double blind, placebo-controlled trial (Abstract). Gastroenterology 2002; 122:A580, #W1175.

56. Fass R, Fennerty MB, Johnson C, et al. Correlation of ambulatory 24-hour esophageal pH monitoring results with symptom improvement in patients with noncardiac chest pain due to gastroesophageal reflux disease. J Clin Gastroenterol 1999; 28(1):36–39.

57. Bernstein LM, Baker LA. A clinical test for esophagitis. Gastroenterology 1958; 34(5):760–781.

58. Richter JE, Hewson EG, Sinclair JW, et al. Acid perfusion test and 24-hour esophageal pH monitoring with symptom index. Comparison of tests for esophageal acid sensitivity. Dig Dis Sci 1991; 36(5):565–571.

59. London RL, Ouyang A, Snape WJJ, et al. Provocation of esophageal pain by ergonovine or edrophonium. Gastroenterology 1981; 81:10–14.

60. Nostrant TT. Provocation testing in noncardiac chest pain. Chest pain of undetermined origin. Am J Gastroenterol 1991; 5A:S56–S64.

61. Richter JE, Hackshaw BT, Wu WC, et al. Edrophonium: a useful provocative test for oesophageal chest pain. Ann Intern Med 1985; 103:14–21.

62. De Caestecker JS, Pryde A, Heading RC. Comparison of intravenous edrophonium and oesophageal acid perfusion during oesophageal

manometry in patients with non-cardiac chest pain. Gut 1988; 29:1029–1034.

63. Ghillebert G, Janssens J, Vantrappen G, et al. Ambulatory 24 hour intraesophageal pH and pressure recordings v provocation tests in the diagnosis of chest pain of oesophageal origin. Gut 1990; 31(7):738–744.

64. Benjamin SB, Richter JE, Cordova CM, et al. Prospective manometric evaluation with pharmacologic provocation of patients with suspected esophageal motility dysfunction. Gastroenterology 1983; 84:893–901.

65. Richter JE, Bradley LA, Castell DO. Esophageal chest pain: current controversies in pathogenesis, diagnosis, and therapy. Ann Intern Med 1989; 110:66–78.

66. Richter JE, Barish CF, Castell DO. Abnormal sensory perception in patients with esophageal chest pain. Gastroenterology 1986; 91:845–852.

A pivotal study that demonstrated lower perception thresholds for pain using graded balloon distension protocol in patients with non-GERD-related NCCP as compared to healthy controls.

67. Ritchie J. Pain from distension of the pelvic colon by inflating a balloon in the irritable colon syndrome. Gut 1973; 14:125–132.

68. Mertz H, Walsh JH, Sytnik B, et al. The effect of octreotide on human gastric compliance and sensory perception. Neurogastroenterol Motil 1995; 7:175–185.

69. Lipkin M, Sleisenger MH. Studies of visceral pain: measurements of stimulus intensity and duration associated with the onset of pain in esophagus, ileum and colon. J Clin Invest 1958; 37:28–34.

70. Yakshe PN, et al. Does provocative esophageal testing influence coronary blood flow or coronary flow reserve? Preliminary results of concurrent esophageal and cardiac testing (Abstract). Gastroenterology 1993; 104:A227.

71. Barish CF, Castell DO, Richter JE. Graded esophageal balloon distension. A new provocative test for noncardiac chest pain. Dig Dis Sci 1986; 31:1292–1298.

72. Whitehead WE, Delvaux M. Standardization of barostat procedures for testing smooth muscle tone and sensory thresholds in the gastrointestinal tract. The Working Team of Glaxo-Wellcome Research, UK. Dig Dis Sci 1997; 42(2):223–241.

73. Azpiroz F, Malagelada JR. Physiological variations in canine gastric tone measured by an electronic barostat. Am J Physiol 1985; 248:G229-G237.

74. Toma TD, Zighelboim J, Phillips ST, et al. Methods for studying intestinal sensitivity and compliance: in vitro studies of balloons and a barostat. Neurogastroenterol Motil 1996; 8:19–28.

75. Khan MI, Feinle C, Read NW. Investigating gastric and sensory response to distention: comparative studies using flaccid bags and latex balloons. 2nd United European Gastroenterology Meeting. 1992; 13:175.

76. Hu WHC, Martin CJ, Talley NJ. Intraesophageal acid perfusion sensitizes the esophagus to mechanical distension: a barostat study. Am J Gastroenterol 2000; 95:2189–2194.

77. Sun W, Read NW, Prior A, et al. Sensory and motor responses to rectal distention vary according to rate and pattern of balloon inflation. Gastroenterology 1990; 99:1008–1015.

78. Munakata J, Naliboff B, Harraf F, et al. Repetitive sigmoid stimulation induces rectal hyperalgesia in patients with irritable bowel syndrome. Gastroenterology 1997; 112:55–63.

79. Whitehead WE, Crowell MD, Shone D, et al. Sensitivity to rectal distension: validation of a measurement system (Abstract). Gastroenterology 1993; 104:A600.

80. Pehlivanov N, Liu J, Mittal RK. Sustained esophageal contraction: a motor correlate of heartburn symptom. Am J Physiol Gastrointest Liver Physiol 2001; 281(3):G743–G751.

81. Clouse RE, McCord GS, Lustman PJ, et al. Clinical correlates of abnormal sensitivity to intraesophageal balloon distension. Dig Dis Sci 1991; 36:1040–1045.

82. Cannon RO III, Quyyumi AA, Mincemoyer R, et al. Imipramine in patients with chest pain despite normal coronary angiograms. N Engl J Med 1994; 330(20):1411–1417.

83. Peghini PL, Katz PO, Castell DO. Imipramine decreases oesophageal pain perception in human male volunteers. Gut 1998; 42:807–813.

84. Castell DO, Wood JD, Frieling T, et al. Cerebral electrical potentials evoked by balloon distension of the human esophagus. Gastroenterology 1990; 98:662–666.

85. DeVault KR. Nifedipine does not alter barostat determined esophageal smooth muscle tone (Abstract). Gastroenterology 1995; 108:A591.

86. Smout AJ, DeVore MS, Dalton CB, et al. Effects of nifedipine on esophageal tone and perception of esophageal distension. Dig Dis Sci 1992; 37:598–602.

87. Harris JH, Therkelsen EE, Zinner NR. Electrical measurement of urethral flow. In: Boyarsky S, Tanagho EA, Gottschalf CW, et al., eds. Urodynamics. London: Academic Press; 1971:465–472.

88. Rask-Andersen H, Djurhuus JC. Development of a probe for endoureteral investigation of peristalsis by flow velocity and cross-section area measurement. Acta Chir Scand Suppl 1976; 472:59–65.

89. Silny J, Knigge KP, Fass J, et al. Verification of the intraluminal multiple electrical impedance measurement for the recordings of gastrointestinal motility. J Gastrointest Motil 1993; 5:107–122.

90. Rao SSC, Hayek B, Summers RW. Impedance planimetry: an integrated approach for assessing sensory, active, and passive biomechanical properties of the human esophagus. Am J Gastroenterol 1995; 90:431–438.

91. Orvar KB, Gregersen H, Christensen J. Biomechanical characteristics of the human esophagus. Dig Dis Sci 1993; 38:197–205.

92. Randich A. Visceral nerve stimulation and pain modulation. In: Joshn LR, ed. Physiology of the gastrointestinal tract. 3rd edn. Amsterdam: Elsevier; 1993:126–139.

93. Sifrim D, Holloway R, Silny J, et al. Acid, nonacid, and gas reflux in patients with gastroesophageal reflux disease during ambulatory 24-hour pH-impedance recordings. Gastroenterology 2001; 120:1588–1598.

94. Vela MF, Camacho-Lobato L, Srinivasan R, et al. Simultaneous intraesophageal impedance and pH measurement of acid and nonacid gastroesophageal reflux: effect of omeprazole. Gastroenterology 2001; 120:1599–1606.

95. Silny J. Intraluminal multiple electric impedance procedure for measurement of gastrointestinal motility. J Gastrointest Motil 1991; 3:151–162.

96. Fass J, Silny J, Braun J, et al. Measuring esophageal motility with a new intraluminal impedance device. First clinical results in reflux patients. Scand J Gastroenterol 1994; 29:693–702.

97. Aziz Q, Thompson DG. Brain-gut axis in heath and disease. Gastroenterology 1998; 114:559–578.

98. Hartshorne MF. Positron emission tomography. In: Orrison WW, Lewine JD, Sanders JA, et al., eds. Functional brain imaging. St. Louis, MO: Mosby-Year Book; 1995:187–212.

99. Aine CJ. A conceptual overview and critique of functional nueroimaging techniques in humans: I. MRI/FMRI and PET. Crit Rev Neurobiol 1995; 9:229–309.

100. Smout AJ, DeVore MS, Castell DO. Cerebral potentials evoked by esophageal distension in human. Am J Physiol 1990; 259:G955–G959.

101. Sanders JA, Orrison WW. Functional magnetic resonance imaging. In: Orrison WW, Lewine JD, Sanders JA, et al., eds. Functional brain imaging. St. Louis, MO: Mosby-Year Book; 1995:239–326.

102. Aziz Q, Andersson JL, Valind S, et al. Identification of human brain loci processing esophageal sensation using positron emission tomography. Gastroenterology 1997; 113:50–59.

103. Minshohima S, Maorrow TJ, Koeppe RA. Involvement of insular cortex in central autonomic regulation during painful thermal stimulation. J Cereb Blood Flow Metab 1995; 15:1355–1358.

104. Talbot JD, Marrett S, Evans AC, et al. Multiple representations of pain in human cerebral cortex. Science 1991; 251:1355–1358.

105. Vogt BA, Sikes RW, Vogt LJ. Anterior cingulate cortex and the medial pain system. In: Vogt BA, Gabriel M, eds. Neurobiology of cingulate cortex and limbic thalamus. Boston: Birkhauser; 1994:313–344.

106. Clouse RE. Psychiatric disorders in patients with esophageal disease. Med Clin North Am 1991; 75:1081–1096.

107. Storr M, Meining A, Allescher HD. Pathophysiology and pharmacological treatment of gastroesophageal reflux: effect of omeprazole. Dig Dis Sci 2000; 18:93–102.

108. Stahl WG, Beton RR, Johnson CS, et al. Diagnosis and treatment of patients with gastroesophageal reflux and noncardiac chest pain. South Med J 1994; 87:739–742.

109. DeMeester TR, O'Sullivan GC, Bermudez G, et al. Esophageal function in patients with angina-type chest pain and normal coronary angiograms. Ann Surg 1982; 196:488–498.

110. Jones R, Bytzer P. Acid suppression in the management of gastro-oesophageal reflux disease: an appraisal of treatment options in primary care. Aliment Pharmacol Ther 2001; 15:765–772.

111. Fass R. Chest pain of esophageal origin. Curr Opin Gastroenterol 2002; 18:464–470.

112. Fass R, Malagon I, Schmulson M. Chest pain of esophageal origin. Curr Opin Gastroenterol 2001; 17:376–380.

113. Borzecki AM, Pedrosa MC, Prashker MJ. Should noncardiac chest pain be treated empirically? A cost-effectiveness analysis. Arch Intern Med 2000; 160:844–852.

114. Patti MG, Molena D, Fisichella PM, et al. Gastroesophageal reflux disease (GERD) and chest pain: results of laparoscopic antireflux surgery. Surg Endosc 2002; 16:563–566.

115. Farrell TM, Richardson WS, Trus TL, et al. Response of atypical symptom as of gastro-oesophageal reflux to antireflux surgery. Br J Surg 2001; 88:1649–1652.

116. Moss SF, Armstrong D, Arnold R, et al. GERD 2003: a consensus on the way ahead. Digestion 2002; 67:111–117.

117. Waring JP. Surgical and endoscopic treatment of gastroesophageal reflux disease. Gastroenterol Clin North Am 2002; 31(Suppl): S89–S109.

118. Fass R. Noncardiac chest pain. In: Fass R, ed. GERD/dyspepsia fast facts. Philadelphia, PA: Hanley & Belfus; 2004:183–196.

119. Kikendall JW, Mellow MH. Effect of sublingual nitroglycerin and long-acting nitrate preparations on esophageal motility. Gastroenterology 1980; 79:703–706.

120. Orlando RC, Bozymski EM. Clinical and manometric effects of nitroglycerin in diffuse esophageal spasm. N Engl J Med 1973; 289(1):23–25.

121. Swamy N. Esophageal spasm: clinical and manometric response to nitroglycerine and long acting nitrates. Gastroenterology 1977; 72(1):23–27.

122. Mellow MH. Effect of isosorbide and hydralazine in painful primary esophageal motility disorders. Gastroenterology 1982; 83:364–370.

123. Cattau EL Jr, Castell DO, Johnson DA, et al. Diltiazem therapy for symptoms associated with nutcracker esophagus. Am J Gastroenterol. 1991; 86:272–276.

124. Richter JE, Spurling TJ, Cordova CM, et al. Effects of oral calcium blocker, diltiazem, on esophageal contractions. Studies in volunteers and patients with nutcracker esophages. Dig Dis Sci. 1984; 29:649–656.

125. Richter JE, Dalton CB, Bradley LA, et al. Oral nifedipine in the treatment of noncardiac chest pain in patients with the nutcracker esophagus. Gastroenterology. 1987; 93:21–28.

126. Bassotti G, Gaburri M, Imbimbo BP, et al. Manometric evaluation of cimetropium bromide activity in patients with the nutcracker oesophagus. Scand J Gastroenterol 1988; 23(9):1079–1084.

127. Miller LS, Pullela SV, Parkman HP, et al. Treatment of chest pain in patients with noncardiac, nonreflux, nonachalasia spastic esophageal motor disorders using botulinum toxin injection into the gastroesophageal junction. Am J Gastroenterol. 2002; 97:1640–1646.

128. Mertz H, Fass R, Kodner A, et al. Effect of amitryptyline on symptoms, sleep and visceral perception in patients with functional dyspepsia. Am J Gastroenterol 1998; 93:160–165.

129. Clouse RE. Psychotropic medications for the treatment of functional gastrointestinal disorders. Clin Perspect Gastroenterol 1999; 2:348–356.

130. Prakash C, Clouse RE. Long-term outcome from tricyclic antidepressant treatment of functional chest pain. Dig Dis Sci 1999; 44(12):2373–2379.

131. Varia I, Logue E, O'connor C, et al. Randomized trial of sertraline in patients with unexplained chest pain of noncardiac origin. Am Heart J 2000; 140(3):367–372.

First study to evaluate in a randomized fashion, the efficacy of the SSRI sertraline on symptoms of patients with NCCP.

132. Krishnan KR. Selected summary: Chest pain and serotonin: a possible link. Gastroenterology 2001; 121:495–496.

133. Clouse RE, Lustman PJ, Eckert TC, et al. Low-dose trazodone for symptomatic patients with esophageal contraction abnormalities. A double-blind, placebo-controlled trial. Gastroenterology 1987; 92(4):1027–1036.

An important study that reported about the efficacy of a visceral analgesic, the antidepressant trazodone, on symptoms of NCCP patients with esophageal contraction abnormalities.

134. Rao SS, Mudipalli RS, Mujica V, et al. An open-label trial of theophylline for functional chest pain. Dig Dis Sci 2002; 47(12):2763–2768.

135. Johnston BT, Shils J, Leite LP, et al. Effects of octreotide on esophageal visceral perception and cerebral evoked potentials induced by balloon distension. Am J Gastroenterol 1999; 94(1):65–70.

136. Clouse RE, Carney RM. The psychological profile of non-cardiac chest pain patients. Eur J Gastroenterol Hepatol 1995; 7(12): 1160–1165.

137. Beitman BD, Basha IM, Trombka LH, et al. Pharmacotherapeutic treatment of panic disorder in patients presenting with chest pain. J Fam Pract 1989; 28(2):177–180.

138. Wulsin LR, Maddock R, Beitman B, et al. Clonazepam treatment of panic disorder in patients with recurrent chest pain and normal coronary arteries. Int J Psychiatry Med 1999; 29(1):97–105.

139. Van Peski-Oosterbaan AS, Spinhoven P, Willem Van Der Does AJ, et al. Noncardiac chest pain: interest in a medical psychological treatment. J Psychosom Res 1998; 45(5):471–476.

140. Hegel MT, Abel GG, Etscheidt M, et al. Behavioral treatment of angina-like chest pain in patients with hyperventilation syndrome. J Behav Ther Exp Psychiatry 1990; 20(1):31–39.

141. Klimes I, Mayou RA, Pearce MJ, et al. Psychological treatment for atypical non-cardiac chest pain: a controlled evaluation. Psychol Med 1990; 20(3):605–611.

142. Burbige EJ. Use of a 5-HT$_3$ antagonist in a patient with noncardiac chest pain (Abstract). Gastroenterology 2001; 96(9):S183, #579.

143. Sarkar S, Aziz Q, Woolf CJ, et al. Contribution of central sensitisation to the development of non-cardiac chest pain. Lancet 2000; 356:1154–1159.

144. Cervero F. Visceral hyperalgesia revised (Commentary). Lancet 2000; 356:1127–1128.

CHAPTER SIXTY-NINE

69

Dyspepsia

Ray E. Clouse

INTRODUCTION

Dyspepsia is common, the symptoms occurring in up to 40% of the population and the diagnosis representing nearly 5% of patients seen by the primary care physician.[1–5] In the United States, the point prevalence approximates 25% once patients with typical reflux symptoms are excluded.[6] The best approach to the patient with uninvestigated dyspepsia remains a topic of debate, a debate initially fueled by the uncertain appropriateness of empirical treatment without endoscopic evaluation in conjunction with a strong desire for cost containment.[7] However, outcomes from therapeutic trials with antisecretory drugs now are well established. Likewise, optimal management of *Helicobacter pylori* (*H. pylori*) infection within the context of dyspepsia is better understood, as the benefits of detection and treatment have been evaluated thoroughly. The large body of literature on dyspepsia has led to useful, practical algorithms for managing patients with this common problem.

What is dyspepsia?

No simple or uniform definition exists, and, if used in practice, the term should be clarified at least partially in the patient's record.[8,9] The central feature is a pain or discomfort in the upper abdomen.[9] Although virtually any abdominal pain or abnormal abdominal sensation has been included in some definitions,[10] dyspepsia currently implies a complex of discomforts typical of those originating in the stomach or gastroduodenal region, such as epigastric pain, nausea, upper abdominal fullness or bloating, and early satiety. Heartburn and other symptoms of gastroesophageal reflux disease can be a component of the presentation, but, in order to exclude gastroesophageal reflux as the principal pathological abnormality, these features should be eclipsed by other symptoms. Specific precipitating (e.g., food ingestion) or ameliorating factors (e.g., antacid ingestion) are not diagnostic requirements, are variably present, and have little predictive value for the underlying cause.[11–13] The definition of dyspepsia includes patients with intermittent or constant symptoms and does not specify duration of complaints. Patients with brief, self-limited dyspepsia do not require investigation and will not be discussed further. The majority of patients with chronic symptoms (more than 3 months) will have no explanation detected for the dyspepsia complex and will meet conventional criteria for functional dyspepsia.[9]

The differential diagnosis of dyspepsia

The broad symptom definition results in a large differential diagnosis (Table 69.1). Despite the breadth of possibilities, three diagnoses represent more than 80% of patients who ultimately undergo evaluation: functional dyspepsia, peptic ulcer disease, and gastroesophageal reflux disease.[14] Of these, functional dyspepsia is the most common, a diagnosis made in more than half of patients, especially in younger subjects. Peptic ulcer disease, the hallmark structural disorder responsible for dyspepsia, is found in no more than 15–20% of dyspepsia patients and is declining in prevalence.[14,15] Even when reflux symptoms are not dominant components of the presentation, gastroesophageal reflux disease is the ultimate explanation for dyspepsia in at least 10% of patients, a finding relating to the poor accuracy of typical symptoms toward predicting reflux disease.[12,16,17] Reflux disease is not excluded by a normal endoscopy, particularly when reflux-like symptoms dominate the presentation.[16,18]

Some upper abdominal symptoms that accompany intermittent colic can resolve with cholecystectomy, but chronic dyspepsia should not be attributed routinely to cholelithiasis.[19,20] Dyspepsia in a patient with cholelithiasis is not a harbinger of subsequent cholecystitis or other gallstone complications and has an undependable response to surgery.[19] When the history includes more than five discrete episodes of abdominal pain or when the symptom history exceeds 3 months (characteristic features of dyspepsia patients), the likelihood of complete symptomatic response to cholecystectomy is sharply reduced.[21,22] Although dyspepsia symptoms often improve transiently with cholecystectomy,[23] relapse occurs in nearly half of patients within 2 years.[22] Data are insufficient to recommend cholecystokinin-cholescintigraphy with calculation of gallbladder ejection fraction for further clarification of optimal operative candidates.[24] Current consensus suggests not seeking gallstones or gallbladder dysfunction and not performing cholecystectomy for symptom management in the typical patient with dyspepsia who has no other clinical features of biliary colic or biliary tract disease.

H. pylori infection (see Ch. 18) unaccompanied by peptic ulcer disease now is considered a potential explanation for dyspepsia despite the body of epidemiological and treatment outcome data that refute a significant association between symptoms and simple infection.[25] For example, up to half of patients with unexplained dyspepsia in the United States and other Western countries harbor *H. pylori* infection, yet cross-sectional studies demonstrate

Table 69.1 The differential diagnosis of dyspepsia

Gastrointestinal tract disorders

Peptic ulcer disease

Gastroesophageal reflux disease

Gastric and esophageal neoplasms

Gastroparesis (diabetic, postvagotomy, from connective tissue disease or other causes of pseudo-obstruction)

Infiltrative gastric disorders (Ménétrier's syndrome, Crohn's disease, eosinophilic gastroenteritis, sarcoidosis, amyloidosis)

Malabsorptive disorders (celiac disease, lactose intolerance)

Chronic erosive (varioliform) gastritis

Gastric infections (cytomegalovirus, tuberculosis, syphilis, fungi)

Parasitic infections (*Giardia lamblia*, *Strongyloides stercoralis*)

Chronic gastric volvulus

Chronic intestinal ischemia

Irritable bowel syndrome

Non-specific food intolerance

Helicobacter pylori infection

Medications

Ethanol

Aspirin and other nonsteroidal antiinflammatory drugs

Antibiotics (macrolides, metronidazole)

Theophylline

Digitalis

Corticosteroids

Iron, potassium supplements

Niacin, gemfibrozil

Narcotics

Colchicine

Quinidine

Estrogens

Levodopa

Alendronate

Orlistat

Acarbose

Nitrates

Loop diuretics

ACE inhibitors

Herbal preparations

Pancreaticobiliary disorders

Chronic pancreatitis

Pancreatic neoplasms

Biliary colic

Other abdominal processes

Intra-abdominal malignancy

Abdominal wall pain

Pregnancy

Systemic disorders

Diabetes mellitus

Thyroid disease

Hyperparathyroidism

Adrenal insufficiency

Connective tissue diseases

Renal insufficiency

Cardiac ischemia

Modified from: McQuaid K. Dyspepsia. In: Feldman M, Friedman LS, Sleisenger MH, eds. Gastrointestinal disease. Pathophysiology, diagnosis, management. 7th edn. Philadelphia: WB Saunders; 2002:102–118.

no consistent increase in the rate of infection in dyspepsia patients when compared with appropriate controls.[25–27] The severity of gastritis associated with infection correlates poorly with the level of symptoms, and the symptom profile does not differ between infected and noninfected patients.[28,29] Furthermore, outcome following antibiotic treatment reveals the unpredictable relationship of bacterial eradication with symptom response.[30–34] Two comprehensive meta-analyses reached conflicting conclusions regarding the utility of *H. pylori* eradication in improving otherwise unexplained dyspepsia,[35,36] but inclusion of all evaluable studies suggests a small but significant treatment advantage.[37] The number-needed-to-treat has been calculated at 15, supporting a limited but potentially true role of infection in dyspepsia production.[35] Nevertheless, uniform recommendations for diagnosing *H. pylori* and treating the infection in patients with no other symptom explanation are not yet available.[37,38]

AN OVERVIEW OF FUNCTIONAL DYSPEPSIA

The clinician confronted with a dyspeptic patient should be thoroughly familiar with the current understanding of functional dyspepsia if a rational management approach to this problem is expected.[9,39] Such familiarity is needed for several reasons. First, the diagnosis is the most common among dyspeptic patients who undergo medical evaluation. Second, the economic burden of investigating dyspepsia is strongly affected by the costs involved in evaluating functional dyspepsia, as the outcome of investigation will be negative. Third, the perceived treatment response to empirical therapy in uninvestigated dyspepsia is highly influenced by the unpredictable natural history and spontaneous symptom resolution seen in the large subset of patients with functional dyspepsia. Additionally and of substantial importance, functional dyspepsia may be best managed within the construct of a comprehensive biopsychosocial model, as is true for other functional gastrointestinal disorders.[9,40] The proposed pathogenetic mechanisms and clinical manifestations of this disorder have been described in detail.[9,39]

Functional dyspepsia typically is diagnosed when persistent or recurrent upper abdominal pain or discomfort is present for at least 3 months and no biochemical or structural abnormality is available to explain the symptoms.[9] Symptoms commonly are aggravated by food ingestion.[41,42] The diagnosis rests on a normal endoscopy and lack of evidence that the symptoms are exclusively related to bowel habit or otherwise suggest irritable bowel syndrome.[9] Because of the cumulative evidence that *H. pylori* infection and its associated gastritis can produce dyspepsia, persistent symptoms, despite infection treatment, is required to establish the functional diagnosis. Subtypes of functional dyspepsia have been described depending on associated symptoms.[9] In ulcer-like dyspepsia, pain is the dominant feature, whereas in dysmotility-like dyspepsia, pain is present but overshadowed by other discomforts, such as early satiety, upper abdominal fullness or bloating, belching, or nausea. Although the ulcer-like group may be more responsive to antisecretory therapy,[43] subtyping otherwise is of questionable importance with the presentation shifting from one subtype to the other over time.[39,44] As many as one-third of patients with functional dyspepsia also have symptoms of irritable bowel syndrome, and, in long-term follow-up, dominant symptoms commonly migrate from one presumed organ region to another.[45-47] Symptoms spontaneously resolve in at least 30% of patients, and treatment response rates to placebo range up to 70%.[48-51]

As found in irritable bowel syndrome (see Ch. 48) and functional chest pain (see Ch. 68), a variety of physiological and psychosocial associations are present that may participate in producing symptoms and healthcare-seeking behavior (Table 69.2).[9,39,52] No singular abnormality is representative of all functional dyspepsia patients, suggesting that, if the associations are relevant at all, the pathogenesis of this disorder is multifactorial. The abnormalities listed in the table do not segregate by dyspepsia subtype, but several mechanisms have been linked to specific symptom clusters (see Table 69.2).[39] Exaggerated sensitivity to gastric distention is one of the most commonly observed physiological abnormalities in functional dyspepsia, a finding that reflects up-regulation of multimodal afferent pathways for both pain and the variety of discomforts associated with the dyspepsia complex.[52-55] Gastric distention sensitivity is not necessarily directly related to symptoms; however, patients with functional dyspepsia show the same degree of sensitivity at a variety of tested sites (esophagus, intestine, rectum) as patients with irritable bowel syndrome.[56,57] None of the physiological abnormalities is a proven treatment target for the majority of patients with functional dyspepsia,[39,58] reflecting both the limited understanding of pathogenesis and heterogeneity of the condition. Management approaches remain at an empirical level in most cases.

When studied with psychometric measures, functional dyspepsia patients are more distressed in general than normal subjects, a finding that is explained only partially by the presence of medical illness.[59-66] The patients are bothered by anxiety and family distress as much as by dyspepsia and have poorer social and work functioning than patients with disease-defined ('organic' or 'structural') gastrointestinal illness.[59,65,67] As with physiological abnormalities, however, none of the findings is sufficiently discriminatory to narrow the differential diagnosis in a dyspeptic patient. Studies employing psychiatric diagnosis have demonstrated high rates of affective and anxiety disorders, findings that may be more relevant to referral centers than primary care practices.[68,69] The observations are similar to those made in irritable bowel syndrome and are not unexpected considering apparent interconversion of functional dyspepsia and irritable bowel syndrome over time.[46]

In irritable bowel syndrome, the increase in anxiety and affective disorders may relate to a background tendency for somatization, a relationship only recently explored in functional dyspepsia.[62,63,70-74] Somatization rather than physiological testing predicted dyspepsia in a community sample, and typical features of somatization predicted many of the dyspepsia symptoms in a factor analysis of patients.[72,73] Somatization disorder, as well affective and anxiety disorders, may contribute to the symptomatic state through cognitive mechanisms (e.g., increased worry about symptoms, fear of stomach cancer, unrestricted endorsement of symptoms) or possibly by accentuating abnormal physiology (e.g., enhanced perception of physiologic events, autonomic dysfunction, alteration of gastric emptying).[75-77] Such interactions resemble those proposed for other functional disorders and

Table 69.2 Physiological and psychosocial factors associated with functional dyspepsia

Factor category and type	Associated symptoms*
Motor dysfunction	
Postprandial antral hypomotility	Fullness, nausea, vomiting
Delayed gastric emptying and antral distention (in 30–40% of patients)	Fullness, nausea, vomiting
Abnormal fundic accommodation and intragastric food distribution (in ≈40% of patients)	Early satiety, weight loss
Small bowel dysmotility	
Abnormal gastric myoelectric activity (up to 60% of patients)	
Visceral sensory dysfunction	
Hypersensitivity to gastric distention (in 50–60% of patients)	Pain, belching, weight loss
Extragastric visceral hypersensitivity	
Abnormal intestinogastric reflexes (with defective gastric relaxation, increased gastric distention sensitivity, and symptoms with duodenal distention, lipid infusion, and acidification)	Nausea
Psychosocial factors and CNS dysregulation	
Exaggerated or negative life stress perception and poor coping skills	
Abnormal psychological scale scores (primarily on anxiety, depression, and somatization measures)	Many dyspepsia symptoms
Psychiatric disorder (anxiety and affective disorders, somatization disorder)	
History of physical and/or sexual abuse	
Efferent vagal dysfunction	

* Symptom associations are not consistently observed in all studies.

potentially are amenable to therapeutic manipulation for improving global outcome.

INITIAL APPROACH TO DYSPEPSIA

A search for the 'best' initial approach to dyspepsia is driven by a desire for both optimal patient outcome as well as cost-effective patient care. Fortunately, most dyspepsia episodes are mild and self-limited, and only a minority of sufferers seek medical attention.[6,78] Within the patient group, the high proportion of subjects with functional dyspepsia significantly influences the decision-making process. Empirical treatments for organic causes of dyspepsia could be unnecessarily tried or prolonged in functional dyspepsia patients if accurate diagnosis were not pursued; expensive diagnostic tests could be considered wasted on these same patients for whom the investigative work-up typically is unrevealing. A logical balance between therapeutic trials and investigation is the correct approach, but what guidelines help the clinician reach this balance?

A careful history and physical examination looking for indicators of serious organic dyspepsia is the essential first step. Such 'alarm features' include new onset of dyspepsia in an older individual and a variety of potentially ominous symptoms or signs (Table 69.3), any of which should mandate investigation over therapeutic trials.[15] Patients with personal histories of gastric surgery, malignancy, or peptic ulcer disease, or with family histories of gastric cancer merit investigation, as do those with chronic symptoms or symptoms that have rapidly recurred following an empirical treatment trial.[79] The initial history and physical examination also should focus on features that might suggest one of the unusual causes of dyspepsia. If the history strongly suggests a drug or particular food intolerance, then an elimination trial is appropriate as an early diagnostic and potentially therapeutic maneuver. In the average case, however, the differential diagnosis remains limited to functional dyspepsia and common organic causes of dyspepsia. Following are several issues relevant to the clinician in evaluating and managing dyspepsia, suggested cost containment strategies, and current consensus opinion on the appropriate initial approach to dyspepsia.

Table 69.3 Alarm features in the patient with dyspepsia

Age >55 years (new onset)

Anorexia or early satiety

Persistent vomiting

Progressive dysphagia or odynophagia

Rectal bleeding or melena

Anemia or occult gastrointestinal bleeding

Weight lost of >10% body weight

Jaundice

Abdominal mass or lymphadenopathy

Previous gastric surgery or malignancy

Previous history of peptic ulcer disease

Family history of upper gastrointestinal malignancy

Modified from: Talley NJ. Dyspepsia. Gastroenterology 2003; 125:1219–1226, and Talley NJ, Vakil N. Guidelines for the management of dyspepsia and functional dyspepsia. Am J Gastroenterol 2005; in press.

To diagnose or treat: important issues for the clinician

How useful is the symptom history?

Unfortunately, the medical history is inadequate for predicting endoscopic findings.[13,80–86] Symptoms can only partially discriminate functional dyspepsia from peptic ulcer disease.[87–90] Likewise, at least 5–10% of dyspepsia patients will have reflux esophagitis at endoscopy, even when typical reflux symptoms are not dominant complaints.[14] When heartburn is a dominant finding, the likelihood of detecting reflux disease is little better than the toss of a coin.[15,91] Even determining the subtype of dyspepsia in unselected patients has limited value in predicting final endoscopic diagnoses, with the diagnosis rates of structural diseases varying little across presentations.[9,13,90] In the absence of alarm features, malignancy is very unlikely.[41,85,90] Alarm features were missing from the presentation in only 3% of patients <55 years of age with gastric or distal esophageal malignancies in one large survey.[41] Although sensitive to malignancy, the positive predictive value of alarm features is low,[54,55,92] which reflects the fact that malignancies are uncommon in dyspepsia patients, representing no more than 1–3% of subjects when all ages are considered.[14]

Certain unrecognized clues to organic disease may exist in the history, as the rate of organic causes of dyspepsia increases in the group selected for endoscopy by gastroenterologists compared with the group sent for open access endoscopy by primary care physicians. The difference, however, may reflect a selection bias related to referral. Because functional dyspepsia patients presenting for evaluation often have characteristic features of anxiety, depression, somatization disorder, and other functional bowel disorders, one might suspect some predictive value of nondyspeptic symptoms in identifying the functional dyspepsia subgroup.[63,66,73,93] This assertion remains incompletely tested, however, and relying on such symptoms in decision-making probably is as unsafe as relying on characteristics of the dyspepsia itself. Although the symptom history is inaccurate, an important predictor of organic disease is age.[94,95] Nearly all gastric and esophageal malignancies are found in patients over 45 years of age, and rates of peptic ulcer as well as esophagitis are greater in an older age group, at least in some series.[94,96,97] Because malignancy is rare in the United States in young patients, recent recommendations have suggested increasing the age threshold for endoscopy to 55 years for previously uninvestigated or new-onset dyspepsia in the absence of other alarm features.[37,98,99] The threshold needs adjustment when regional or population differences in malignancy prevalence are present.

Should the investigative work-up be extensive or limited?

If a specific explanation for dyspepsia is desired, then endoscopy is the uncontested procedure of choice. Endoscopy is more accurate than barium radiography in detecting structural lesions, and biopsy capability extends the utility of endoscopy in the small percentage of patients with suspected gastric malignancy or other unusual causes for dyspepsia.[80,100] In the presence of typical symptoms and absence of colic episodes, a pain distribution suggesting a pancreatic origin, or other indicators of pancreatic or biliary tract disease, imaging of the pancreas or biliary tract is not advised routinely. Likewise, because of the unlikely association of cholelithiasis with dyspepsia, as mentioned previously, and low utility of the test in diagnosing other causes of dyspepsia, routine ultrasound examination of the gallbladder is not recommended.[101,102]

In the context of typical symptoms, the investigation safely can be limited to endoscopy. Naturally, investigation must be tailored to clinical suspicion for organic disease, especially in elderly patients with recent dyspepsia onset or any other alarm features. Somato-parietal pain characteristics (sharp, lancinating pain; pain with superficial or radicular features) should trigger further investigation for abdominal wall, skeletal, or neuropathic processes.[103] Ambulatory pH monitoring could complement endoscopy in excluding gastroesophageal reflux disease and would detect the minority of patients with presumed functional dyspepsia who actually have reflux disease;[104,105] therapeutic trials with antisecretory therapy usually are, however, sufficient. During the long-term follow-up of patients given the diagnosis of functional dyspepsia, a diagnosis usually made with endoscopy alone, new diagnoses of serious consequence surface infrequently. There is little overt physical danger of extending the evaluation to include imaging studies of the upper abdomen, the morbidity being more financial than physical. However, repeated or extensive testing of patients with functional dyspepsia may provide the wrong message, leading patients to believe that even more thorough evaluation could uncover the actual cause. A more satisfactory resolution of symptoms in functional gastrointestinal disorders, in general, occurs when such a goal is not implied.

It also appears that determining the physiological abnormalities in patients with functional dyspepsia has little value, either for diagnosis or management.[39,49,50,106] Visceral sensory abnormalities, if detected, are not sufficiently specific for functional dyspepsia to reassure the patient beyond what can be accomplished from the symptom history and endoscopic findings alone. Gastric emptying studies are of little value in the average case.[37,39] Treatment trials using prokinetic agents have not demonstrated consistently a differential response in relation to baseline gastric emptying.[39] Likewise, the outcome of prokinetic treatment in patients with delayed emptying is not predicated on normalization of this finding.[15] Consequently, little evidence exists that ordering a gastric emptying study would alter management;[107] the study may be of benefit for patients with refractory dysmotility-like symptoms.[108,109] If delayed emptying is detected, causes of autonomic neuropathy or visceral muscle dysfunction should be considered and further evaluated if suspected. Demonstration of impaired gastric accommodation could trigger therapeutic trials of fundus-relaxing agents, but presently this approach is empirical.[37]

A limited psychiatric evaluation is justified, as it is in any patient presenting with a chronic pain condition. The interview should look for cardinal symptoms of anxiety states, major depression, and somatization disorder. These diagnoses are sufficiently prevalent in patients with functional dyspepsia that their management may ultimately be required for satisfactory symptom reduction and long-term global improvement.[63,68,69] High levels of somatization can be suspected when a patient endorses many symptoms on a review-of-systems checklist or from a complicated medical history beginning at an early age that includes multiple unexplained somatic symptoms or syndromes.[93,110] Extensive psychiatric evaluation, including referral for formal psychometric testing or psychiatric consultation, is not routinely advised, as the contribution of psychiatric factors to dyspepsia presentations remains unclear in many cases. As for physiological abnormalities in functional dyspepsia, the extent of psychiatric evaluation

and the contribution of psychiatric treatment to overall management may be greatest in the subset of patients who are refractory to other management approaches.[40]

What is the role of H. pylori infection and its treatment?

H. pylori infection has two potentially relevant roles in dyspepsia: its pathogenetic importance in peptic ulcer disease and its limited, direct association with symptoms. In the absence of nonsteroidal antiinflammatory drugs (NSAIDs), several studies have reported that more than 90% of duodenal and gastric ulcers are associated with *H. pylori* infection.[111] Because of the beneficial effects of *H. pylori* eradication on the course of peptic ulcer disease, appropriate antibiotic therapy is unquestionably recommended in the infected dyspepsia patient with a documented history of ulcers or active ulceration at the time of evaluation (see Ch. 18).[112] The presence of both active ulcer disease and infection can be determined at endoscopy, but infection also can be established using less expensive, noninvasive office methods. In the United States and other Western countries wherein the prevalence of *H. pylori* infection approaches 30–50% in patients presenting with dyspepsia,[26] the accuracy of serological testing from locally validated assays approximate 90%.[113–115] Sensitivity and specificity of the urea breath test exceed 95%, but because of its greater expense this test is less commonly performed. A stool-based antigen test also has high accuracy and may be the most practical office-based test.[116,117]

Most ulcers occur in infected patients, and treating the infection without further investigation can sharply reduce endoscopic workload.[118,119] Treating the infection without endoscopic evaluation also provides sufficient reassurance in young patients without other alarm features,[120] and evidence continues to mount that 'test and treat' strategies for *H. pylori* are at least as effective as endoscopic evaluation or usual care in terms of outcomes for most young patient populations with dyspepsia.[121–126] Whereas empirical antisecretory therapy is an acceptable initial approach for uninfected patients without alarm features, recent data also favor detecting and treating *H. pylori* infection over this management option.[127] Prescribing antibiotics without testing for infection is not advised.

Potential disadvantages of 'test and treat' strategies are evident in some patient groups and impact the success of this approach. Ulcers are found in <1–2% of patients with negative serology in the absence of NSAID use,[118,128] but most gastric malignancies also are encountered in patients with *H. pylori* infection, and establishing their diagnosis would be delayed without initial investigation. A negative result from serological or stool-antigen testing is not completely reassuring: nearly 1 in 4 malignancies presenting with dyspepsia have been found in the uninfected group, and other organic causes for dyspepsia, particularly esophagitis, are not predicted by serological testing.[129]

Treatment for *H. pylori* without further investigation also will result in antibiotic treatment of the 50–70% of patients without any structural lesion other than the gastritis related to infection. A sustained symptomatic response for dyspepsia unassociated with peptic ulcer disease occurs in a very small minority, confusion regarding the correct diagnosis persists, and endoscopy ultimately may become necessary in a substantial proportion of patients. Concerns of antibiotic resistance with widespread use have not dissipated.[130] On the other hand, decreased healthcare resource utilization, social morbidity, and symptoms are observed in long-term follow-up of some treated patients.[131] Likewise, the appearance of new symptoms over 1 year is more common in asymptomatic infected patients than in those with negative serology.[132] Chronic antisecretory therapy, the alternative for many untreated patients, may lead to infection progression into more proximal gastric regions with the potential for more serious sequelae.[133,134] To determine whether knowing the presence of infection actually is useful in planning the approach to a dyspeptic patient, many factors (e.g., accuracy of the test for infection, likelihood of structural diagnoses, outcome of their management, cost of endoscopy) simultaneously must be taken into consideration. Because of the difficulty in estimating all potential outcomes, statistical models using decision analysis methods have been particularly useful for such applications (see below).[135]

What are the risks of empirical antisecretory therapy in patients without alarm features?

A 4–8 week treatment course with a proton pump inhibitor is effective for many patients with dyspepsia and an acceptable initial management approach for patients without alarm features, many of whom will never need investigation.[136] Proton pump inhibitors have supplanted H_2-receptor antagonists in this cost-containing approach,[79] and prokinetic agents with established efficacy in this role presently are unavailable in the United States. Risks of empirical antisecretory treatment primarily are restricted to undertreatment and leaving undiagnosed a serious medical condition, such as malignancy. The diagnosis of ulcer disease could be established with endoscopy at relapse, and, in fact, most of the diagnoses responsible for dyspepsia persist or relapse after discontinuation of therapy. At least 80% of patients with significant reflux esophagitis will relapse within 6–12 months of medication discontinuation, and relapse rarely has morbid consequences.[137] Relapse with functional dyspepsia also can be expected in at least two-thirds of patients in relatively short follow-up.[48,138,139] The high relapse rates of the common causes for dyspepsia result in most patients undergoing endoscopy within 1 year, thereby reducing the likelihood of undermanaging common conditions responsible for this presentation.[140]

Of greater concern is the risk of overlooking malignancy. Considering the use of empirical trials, it appears that the outcome of gastric malignancy differs minimally across regions where the use of endoscopy varies widely.[141] However, two reports have suggested that the detection of early gastric cancers is improved by an approach to dyspepsia that includes primary endoscopy without the delays imposed by therapeutic trials.[142,143] These conclusions were restricted to subjects >40 years of age. Consequently, early diagnosis may have merit independent of cost analysis that should influence the approach to dyspepsia patients, particularly those of older age or with other alarm features.

Cost containment strategies

Because of the number and complexity of potential outcomes from fully investigating dyspepsia versus treating the patient with investigation limited to noninvasive *H. pylori* testing, statistical models using decision analysis have been used to help arrive at the most appropriate approach.[135] The value of the findings depends on the accuracy and completeness of the assumptions used in the model as well as the applicability of the decision tree to a clinical setting. The contribution of individual parameters to

the outcome difference between strategies is determined, and the assumptions can be adjusted post hoc to measure the magnitude of change required to modify the conclusions. Because assumptions can be wrong, overlooked, or inappropriately valued, criticism of the clinical usefulness of decision analysis is expected and important.[14] However, these models can guide the design of clinical trials to test strategies and help modify assumptions, demonstrate whether a clinical factor (e.g., the cost of endoscopy) could realistically be adjusted sufficiently to affect the conclusion, and certainly help with consensus building.

Principal findings from eight earlier decision analyses in dyspepsia are summarized in Figure 69.1.[144–151] Preferred strategies may vary depending on whether a cost comparison or some other outcome is given the greatest consideration, and, of course, the conclusions are dependent on the actions taken after the initial decision. The figure reveals the trends, but results across trials rarely are directly comparable. Studies differ in tested hypotheses, assumptions used in the calculations, nature and extent of the projected outcomes, and costs applied. Nevertheless, most differences in outcome can be reconciled.[14] Empirical symptomatic management and immediate investigation appear nearly equally costly. Testing for *H. pylori* before further evaluation probably is useful if infected patients are then treated, but the minimal advantage to the large number of infected patients with dyspepsia and no evidence of peptic ulcer disease limits this benefit. Antibiotic treatment of infected patients, delaying endoscopy until the symptomatic response is determined, appears superior to immediate endoscopy. The conclusions are influenced by the cost of endoscopy, the rate of relapse from treatment in the functional dyspepsia group, and the threshold for accepting an outcome advantage.

Two recent decision analyses demonstrate the stronghold that empirical antisecretory therapy with proton pump inhibitors is beginning to have over *H. pylori* testing, at least in some clinical settings.[152,153] Antisecretory therapy followed by endoscopic evaluation for treatment failures was the least costly strategy in an analysis limited to young subjects in a primary care setting.[152] More subjects were symptom-free at 1 year, however, if empirical antisecretory therapy was combined with the *H. pylori* 'test and treat' approach before investigation. The cost advantages of empirical antisecretory therapy are predicated on the background rate of *H. pylori* infection and resultant peptic ulcer disease in the studied population: as the rate of infection drops below 20%, empirical antisecretory therapy dominates over the 'test and treat' approach in uninvestigated subjects.[153] Prompt endoscopy becomes the most effective initial management step in all models only when it can be offered and at an unreachably low cost.[154]

Clinical trials have addressed the benefits of early investigation and add some support to the findings from decision analysis. In one report, costs were insignificantly different for symptomatic H_2-receptor antagonists with ad lib endoscopy versus immediate investigation.[155] A separate but similar study favored prokinetic drugs and selective use of endoscopy over mandatory investigation.[147] In contrast, others have shown that a reduction in health concerns, unnecessary medication treatment, and other measures of healthcare resource utilization can occur after endoscopic diagnosis;[140,156–159] measures of general satisfaction with care and social functioning, such as time lost from work, may be improved when investigation is not delayed.[140,160] Normal findings at endoscopy with physician reassurance can sharply reduce

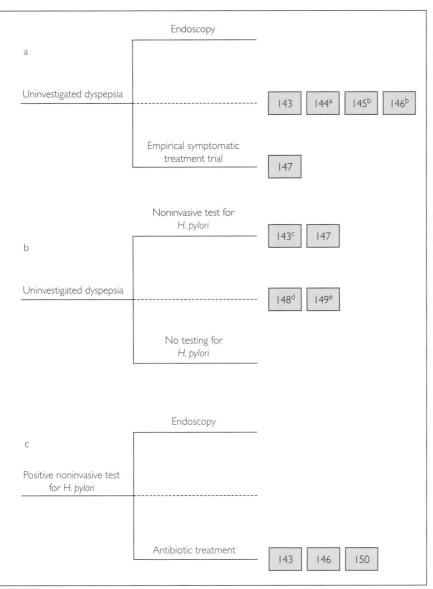

Fig. 69.1 • General conclusions from decision analysis in patients with functional dyspepsia. Strategies are compared in patients presenting with uninvestigated dyspepsia (**a, b**) and in patients who test positively for the presence of *Helicobacter pylori* infection (**c**). References in boxes indicate studies that favored the adjacent strategy. In some reports, the difference between strategies was considered insignificant (—).
[a] Cost favors empirical therapy at the expense of increased mortality (upper gastrointestinal radiography used for screening followed by endoscopy when required). [b] Endoscopy favored when rates of organic diagnoses are higher; empirical treatment favored when likelihood of organic disease is low. [c] Strategy advantage if positive test followed by antibiotic treatment. [d] Positive serology followed by endoscopy and antibiotic treatment if ulcer detected versus symptomatic treatment; would take >8 years to appreciate an advantage of testing. [e] Similar outcome across strategies, but if 5–10% of functional dyspepsia patients responded to treatment, testing would be worthwhile.

health preoccupation and further consultation with the effects lasting for at least 6 months.[140,161,162] Most satisfaction, however, comes from symptom improvement, independent of investigation, diagnosis, or specific treatment.[163] Collectively, these studies reveal the cost similarities between early investigation and symptomatic therapy, at least in younger subjects. In dyspepsia patients presenting over age 50 years to primary care physicians, prompt endoscopy had symptomatic benefits with reduced use of proton pump inhibitors and presumably cost advantages.[164] Data from clinical trials are not yet sufficient to fully support or refute the suggested value of detecting and treating *H. pylori* infection or empirical antisecretory therapy in the initial management of dyspepsia from a cost containment standpoint.

Current consensus opinion

Testing of management strategies, in both clinical and theoretical applications, has changed the recommended approach to dyspepsia.[15,37,165,166] In a medical position statement of the American Gastroenterological Association, the marginal benefits of delayed investigation, the value of *H. pylori* treatment on improving the course of peptic ulcer disease, and the unlikelihood of serious organic disease in a young patient group figured heavily in the final consensus opinion.[166] A recent opinion offered by the American College of Gastroenterology builds on this consensus by incorporating newer information to re-position antisecretory therapy in populations with low prevalence rates of *H. pylori* infection and adjust the recommended age threshold for prompt endoscopy.[37] The modified management algorithm closely parallels much of current practice and differs in some important ways from previous recommendations (Fig. 69.2). First, early endoscopic evaluation is suggested in patients presenting with dyspepsia who are >55 years in age. Second, treatment of detected *H. pylori* infection should be considered in dyspeptic patients of all ages, even if peptic ulcer disease is not documented.

These recommendations are appealing and seem practical. The patient is screened for alarm features (see Table 69.3) and characteristics that would alter the differential diagnosis. Younger patients with non-specific dyspepsia symptoms are tested for *H. pylori* infection using a well-validated local method,

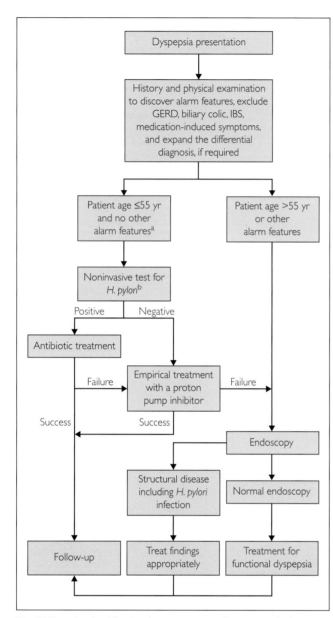

Fig. 69.2 • An algorithm for the management of patients with dyspepsia undergoing initial evaluation. Alarm features are listed in Table 69.3. Success or failure refers to symptom response. [a] Age threshold for prompt endoscopy rather than therapeutic trials needs downward adjustment in regions or populations with higher malignancy risk at lower age. [b] Empirical therapeutic trial with a proton pump inhibitor can precede testing for *Helicobacter pylori* if the prevalence of infection is predicted as <20%. Modified from American Gastroenterological Association: American Gastroenterological Association medical position statement: evaluation of dyspepsia. Gastroenterology 1998; 114:579, and from Talley NJ, Vakil N. Guidelines for the management of dyspepsia and functional dyspepsia. Am J Gastroenterol 2005; in press.

treated with antibiotics if positive, and reevaluated in 1–2 months. Patients without infection or who do not respond to *H. pylori* eradication are offered an empirical trial of symptomatic management with a proton pump inhibitor and also are reevaluated after 2 months of treatment. Those who fail to improve or rapidly relapse after treatment is discontinued are investigated with endoscopy. The approach assumes a modest background prevalence of infection and that gastric cancer is uncommon. In regions or

populations wherein the rate of *H. pylori* infection is low (<20%), the empirical antisecretory trial can be considered before testing for infection.[37] Subjects over the age of 55 years are investigated with endoscopy at presentation; discovered disorders are treated appropriately, and the presence of *H. pylori* infection can be determined at the time of endoscopy. Patients with no diagnosis at endoscopy can be managed using the treatment options for functional dyspepsia. In all cases, cautious observation is required, as dyspepsia can be an important indicator of serious disease. The availability and likelihood of follow-up should be taken into consideration if empirical treatment is chosen over initial investigation.

MANAGEMENT OF FUNCTIONAL DYSPEPSIA

Management of functional dyspepsia can be frustrating, reflecting the poor understanding of mechanisms involved in symptom production, likely heterogeneity of causes, and consequent lack of highly effective medical treatments.[39,58] Worldwide, the most commonly prescribed medications reduce gastric acid or alter gastric motor function, potentially affecting physiological factors that are relevant only to a subgroup of patients with functional dyspepsia. Overall, the results from such treatments have been unimpressive, and no medication is of undisputed efficacy.[39,50] To effectively manage more patients, the disorder probably best is considered within a biopsychosocial context – comprehensively considering all potential contributors to symptoms (see Table 69.2). Correction of biological (physiological) abnormalities may work for some patients, whereas manipulation of psychosocial factors may be more beneficial for others. Common regional treatment

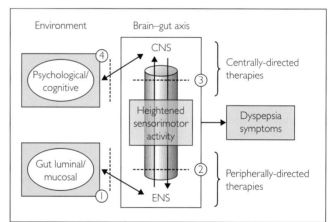

Fig. 69.3 • Treatment targets for managing functional dyspepsia. Up-regulated sensorimotor activity is susceptible to initiating, provoking, or perpetuating stimuli at both central (psychological/cognitive) and peripheral (gut luminal/mucosal) levels. The dashed lines (**1–4**) represent common treatment targets that may have varying utility from patient to patient. For example, some patients may respond to meal adjustments (**1**), medications affecting gastric motility or peripheral gastroduodenal sensitivity (**2**), modification of central signal processing and autonomic response (**3**), or reduction of anxiety/depression effects on symptom reporting (**4**). CNS, central nervous system; ENS, enteric nervous system; GI, gastrointestinal. Adapted from Clouse RE. Central nervous system approaches for treating functional gastrointestinal disorders: how, when, and why? J Pediatr Gastroenterol Nutr 2004; 39(3):S763–S765.

targets are similar for functional dyspepsia as for other pain- and discomfort-based functional gastrointestinal disorders (Fig. 69.3).

The morbidity from functional dyspepsia results from symptoms and their effects on measures of daily functioning. Success of treatment, in lieu of a cure for this disorder, can therefore be measured not solely through effects on symptoms but also in improvement in quality of life.[9,67,167] The clinician should avoid harm that can be induced by chronic medication use (including financial strain, medication side effects, drug dependence) while providing appropriate reassurance of the typically remitting or nonprogressive course of the disorder.[9,44,168] Basic management guidelines are listed in Table 69.4, and the expectations from specific treatments are described in the following sections.

Treatments used in peptic ulcer disease

Treatments for peptic ulcer disease have been studied extensively for functional dyspepsia (see Chs 1 and 20). A significant benefit of H_2-receptor antagonists only has been found in about one-half of the treatment trials, and some of this effect has been attributed to improvement by patients with gastroesophageal reflux disease who were included in the study populations.[49,50,169,170] Similar conclusions have been drawn for proton pump inhibitors, wherein the benefits primarily are restricted to patients with reflux symptoms as part of the dyspepsia presentation.[43,171,172] The mechanism by which acid suppression would reduce nonreflux symptoms is not conspicuous, as hypersensitivity to intraluminal acid does not appear mechanistically important in most patients.[173,174] Likewise, acid suppression has not produced symptomatic relief in patients with duodenal acid sensitivity.[175] Short-term treatment cycles or PRN use of over-the-counter antisecretory medications can be used as 'crutch' therapy without scientific basis, especially

Table 69.4 General management principles for functional dyspepsia

Try to establish a confident clinical diagnosis but avoid overtesting

Determine the reason for this presentation and address specific concerns and fears (e.g., recent diet or medication change, new cancer fears)

Use reassurance appropriately and explain potential physiological mechanisms for the symptoms

Explore and manage psychological contributors to symptoms and global impairment

Recommend avoidance of potential exacerbating factors, such as nonsteroidal antiinflammatory drugs, alcohol, coffee, caffeine and other identified dietary precipitants (e.g., capsaicin-containing foods, high-fat meals)

Inquire of the patient's interest in medication treatment, but set realistic treatment goals looking for increased coping and adaptation to chronic symptoms

Schedule planned follow-up to determine the course of the illness and response to intervention

Modified from: Talley NJ, Collin-Jones D, Koch KL, Koch M, Nyrén O, Stanghellini V. Functional dyspepsia: a classification with guidelines for diagnosis and management. Gastroenterol Int 1991; 4:145, and McQuaid K. Dyspepsia. In: Feldman M, Friedman LS, Sleisenger MH, eds. Gastrointestinal disease. Pathophysiology, diagnosis, management. 7th edn. Philadelphia: WB Saunders; 2002:102–118.

for the subset with some reflux-like symptoms, but prolonged treatment courses are expensive and ill advised.

Typical regimens used for the eradication of *H. pylori* infection have the limited benefits demonstrated only by meta-analysis.[35] However, patients who know they are infected probably will request treatment, and the physician may feel that infection treatment will alleviate some of the anxiety associated with the illness. Despite inconclusive evidence that it would help, the consensus has shifted toward treating the infection in patients with no other recognized cause for dyspepsia after explaining limitations of the approach.[14,37,165] Bismuth compounds alone also have been studied in patients with functional dyspepsia and may be superior to placebo in reducing short-term symptoms.[49,50] These drugs could be tried in short courses for symptom relief. Neither antacids nor sucralfate are of proven benefit.[161]

Prokinetic agents

Prokinetic agents have appeal because of their potential to affect a physiologic abnormality observed in some functional dyspepsia patients (see Ch. 2). Cisapride has been the most studied prokinetic agent, has reduced symptoms more effectively than placebo in most instances, and may be superior to H_2-receptor antagonists.[49,176–179] Benefits are seen in 60–90% of cisapride-treated patients. Although the outcome has been fairly consistent, many of the reported trials are suspected to have included reflux patients in the study populations. Cisapride enhances gastric emptying through peripheral acetylcholine release, but it has been difficult to demonstrate that symptom improvement correlates with drug-induced changes in gastric emptying.[58,180,181] Cisapride also enhances gastric accommodation to a meal,[183] a potential alternative mechanism of action in functional dyspepsia. The availability of cisapride is restricted because of the risk of cardiac arrhythmias. In areas where the medication can be prescribed, short courses can be offered to suitably screened patients who fail antisecretory treatment.

The dopamine antagonists metoclopramide and domperidone possess antiemetic properties as well as peripheral effects to enhance gastric emptying. These drugs interfere with dopamine transmission in the chemoreceptor trigger zone of the area postrema, a hypothalamic region external to the blood–brain barrier that projects to the brainstem vomiting center.[182] Domperidone does not cross the blood–brain barrier and appears superior to placebo in patients with a variety of disorders associated with nausea and vomiting, including functional dyspepsia.[58,179,184,185] The drug is most effective in reducing dysmotility-like symptoms, but less experience in functional dyspepsia is available than for cisapride, and the outcomes have not been subject to as much scrutiny. Metoclopramide also significantly improves similar symptoms but is no more effective than domperidone; long-term treatment can be accompanied by significant extrapyramidal side effects, as this drug does cross the blood–brain barrier.[49,50] As for cisapride, the benefits of domperidone are not readily explained by improvement in gastric emptying, and other antiemetic effects may be more responsible.[186] Erythromycin and tegaserod, other prokinetic agents, have not been tested adequately in functional dyspepsia. Tegaserod both accelerates gastric emptying and improves gastric accommodation to a meal and may prove useful in symptom management.[187]

Antidepressants

Antidepressants have the same potential uses in functional dyspepsia as they do in irritable bowel syndrome and functional chest pain (see Chs 48 and 68).[188] The drugs could work directly on dyspepsia symptoms or indirectly by altering disturbed cognitive mechanisms in psychiatric disorder that influence the clinical presentation (see Fig. 69.3). As an example of direct effects, antidepressants improve functional chest pain and painful diabetic neuropathy independent of effects on emotional functioning.[189,190] These medications may decrease visceral hypersensitivity by reducing central amplification of peripheral signals, although the precise mechanism of action remains uncertain.[191–193] As an example of indirect action, antidepressants in a patient with active major depression could diminish an abnormal focus on dyspepsia symptoms while improving global well-being and other aspects of daily functioning affected by depression.

Despite the common impression that they may be effective, evidence substantiating the use of antidepressants in functional dyspepsia is limited. Open-label treatment with low daily dosages of tricyclic antidepressants (e.g., 25–50 mg/d of amitriptyline or nortriptyline) produced symptomatic improvement in 84% and complete symptomatic remission in 51% of patients with unexplained nausea and vomiting, most of whom had other characteristics typical of functional dyspepsia.[194] Responses were determined from a retrospective chart review and may have been biased by the investigators. Preliminary data from another open-label study suggest that amitriptyline was more effective than antisecretory drugs or *H. pylori* eradication in suppressing symptoms of functional dyspepsia.[195] Likewise, amitriptyline at 50 mg/day was effective in one small placebo-controlled trial.[196] Side effects from tricyclic antidepressants, even at low dosage, are sufficiently common that up to half of patients will need a drug change or drug discontinuation. Whether selective serotonin reuptake inhibitors (SSRIs) or other newer antidepressants would have the same benefits as tricyclic agents remains unknown, as SSRIs can induce some dyspepsia symptoms yet also enhance meal-induced gastric accommodation.[197] One placebo-controlled trial of a combined serotonin- and adrenaline-acting nontricyclic antidepressant agent improved abdominal symptoms in patients with a variety of functional gastrointestinal disorders including dyspepsia.[198] As a minimum, antidepressants other than the tricyclic agents can be useful to manage depression or anxiety and provide indirect benefits on global measures.

Although long medication courses are discouraged in managing functional dyspepsia, tricyclic antidepressants in low daily dosage may be an exception for patients with particularly severe, refractory, or otherwise morbid syndromes.[188] It is equally important in this same patient group to remain vigilant for significant active psychiatric disorder that might be interfering with symptom and global improvement. A low-dose antidepressant regimen would undertreat major depression and potentially delay the required intervention. Studies in other models wherein psychiatric disorders commonly coexist with a medical illness show that a singular focus on the medical problems is insufficient to treat major depression when present.[199] An algorithm for initiating antidepressants in patients with dyspepsia should take into consideration the severity of symptoms (to justify potential side effects), degree of somatization expressed by the patient, and the presence or absence of anxiety or depressive disorders (Fig. 69.4).[200]

Intolerable side effects in patients with high levels of somatization require initiation with very low tricyclic antidepressant dosages (e.g., <10 mg/day) and slow dosage escalation, shifting to nonpharmacological therapies sooner rather than later. All subjects should have tricyclic antidepressant dosages advanced into the psychiatric dosing range or as tolerated by side effects before considering treatment a failure if response is incomplete at lower dosages.[200,201]

Psychological and behavioral treatments

The simplest psychological treatment is reassurance, possibly the most widely employed and effective treatment for functional dyspepsia. Reassurance is most helpful when provided systematically using a six-step approach.[202,203] A detailed description of the symptom is first elicited. Reassurance should be withheld at this step because it can inhibit the patient from expounding on the history or can reflect the physician's own anxiety, rending it ineffective or counterproductive. The second step requires a conscious attempt to allow the patient to describe his or her feelings associated with the symptom – the affective meaning of the symptom. Next, the patient is examined, an interaction that increases the effectiveness of subsequent reassurance. Following this, a diagnosis is made. Because some degree of testing may be required to establish the diagnosis, the early steps involved in reassurance cannot always be completed in one office visit. The final steps involve explaining the presumed mechanisms involved in producing the symptom, and then providing reassurance. Effective reassurance after negative endoscopy in dyspepsia patients significantly reduces the use of symptomatic medication treatment over time.[140]

If somatization disorder is suspected by a dramatic history of medically unexplained symptoms in multiple organ systems, management of the patient with functional dyspepsia should be tailored toward management of somatization disorder.[72,204,205] A compassionate physician–patient relationship will discourage 'doctor shopping' and can protect the patient from iatrogenic morbidity arising out of excessive investigation and treatment. The patient should be seen on a regular basis with thorough but conservative evaluation of complaints. Decisions to investigate or treat symptoms should be based on objective findings as much as is feasible. Acknowledging the patient's suffering and reassuring that serious or disabling illness is unlikely are more productive strategies than suggesting the complaints are 'all in your head.' Additionally, stressing long-term follow-up rather than diagnostic studies will allay patient fears while avoiding costly and potentially morbid tests. This approach can dramatically reduce healthcare resource use by somatization disorder patients without sacrificing health or satisfaction with healthcare.[206]

Referral for psychological or behavioral treatments probably is best suited for (1) patients with a suspected or recognized psychiatric disorder in whom specific psychiatric treatment is one goal; (2) patients who remain refractory to other treatments and who are sufficiently impaired to merit referral; and (3) patients who prefer these treatment approaches to conventional pharmacotherapy. The last in particular is justified considering the modest efficacy of medications. A remote history of physical or sexual abuse, if discovered in the interview process, does not necessarily influence the decision for referral, as the relationship of such findings to symptom production is unknown, and

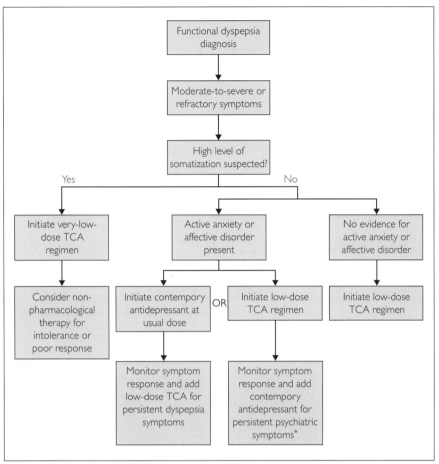

Fig. 69.4 • An algorithm for appropriate initiation of antidepressants in patients with functional dyspepsia. High levels of somatization can be detected by patient endorsement of many symptoms on a review-of-systems checklist or from features of somatization disorder in the medical history. Contemporary antidepressants include the selective serotonin reuptake inhibitors (SSRIs). * Monitoring for toxicity with tricyclic antidepressant (TCA) levels is required if the TCA is used in conjunction with medications that interfere with normal cytochrome p450 activity, such as SSRIs. Modified from Clouse RE. Antidepressants for irritable bowel syndrome. Gut 2003; 52:598–599.

therapeutic outcome data are unavailable. Both cognitive behavioral and psychodynamic-interpersonal psychotherapy appear effective in reducing dyspepsia symptoms.[207–209] Hypnotherapy also had a sustained benefit in a controlled investigation.[210] Stress reduction techniques and deep muscle relaxation training may be tried, as these techniques have proved beneficial for patients with other refractory functional gastrointestinal disorders.

Other treatments

Anticholinergics and other antispasmodics commonly are used in clinical practice for dyspepsia symptoms, but they have been tested in few clinical trials.[49,50] Limited results suggest no measurable benefit over placebo. The reader should be reminded, however, that these same medications are used commonly and with clinical conviction in other functional disorders, yet evidence of efficacy is not demonstrated easily. Anticholinergics influence gastric accommodation, and other fundus-relaxing agents are being studied for their potential benefits in dyspepsia or to provide clues leading toward new drug development. Sildenafil relaxes the proximal stomach, and clinical trials with this or other phosphodiesterase inhibitors are being considered.[211] Serotonin appears important in reflex control of gastric accommodation, and the value of selective 5-HT receptor agonists is being explored.[197] Buspirone, a nonselective 5-HT$_1$-receptor agonist marketed for its antianxiety properties, enhanced accommodation and reduced dyspepsia symptoms in one controlled study, but sites of action could have been multiple.[212] As mentioned previously, the enhanced accom-

modation response to a meal observed with tegaserod may represent a biologically plausible explanation for exploring this prokinetic agent in dyspepsia.[187]

Heightened visceral sensitivity is demonstrated in half of patients with functional dyspepsia, similar to findings in other functional gastrointestinal illnesses.[213] Fedotozine, a kappa opioid agonist that works on peripheral nociceptors, decreases gastric distention sensitivity and was superior to placebo in reducing symptoms of functional dyspepsia in a large, European multicenter trial.[214,215] This drug is not yet available in the United States, but may prove to have some role in symptom management. Ondansetron also may influence visceral perception, and limited data indicate potential effects of this drug on some dyspepsia symptoms.[216] Alosetron, another 5-HT$_3$-receptor antagonist, also had effects on dyspepsia symptoms but was not fully studied before it was removed from general use.[217] Cholecystokinin-receptor antagonists reduce sensitivity to duodenal lipid infusion and are being investigated for use in dyspepsia.[218,219] Several herbal preparations, one combining peppermint oil and caraway, appeared superior to placebo in reducing dyspepsia symptoms, but studies replicating the initial findings are lacking.[220,221] Pancreatic enzyme replacement has been tried on empirical grounds, but the approach appears ineffective.[222]

SUMMARY

Dyspepsia is a common complaint resulting in high healthcare resource utilization. A large body of clinical research has led to rational treatment algorithms with cost containment in mind.

Decisions for early endoscopy versus empirical antisecretory treatment trials or applying a 'test and treat' strategy for *H. pylori* infection rest on patient age and presence of other alarm features at presentation. Subjects 55 years of age or less can be managed initially without endoscopic evaluation; older subjects should be evaluated promptly and treated depending on endoscopic findings. Once identified, *H. pylori* infection should be treated before embarking on other therapeutic approaches. The bulk of patients presenting with chronic dyspepsia will have no specific explanation detected and will be diagnosed with functional dyspepsia. Treatment targets for this heterogeneous condition are multiple, as is typical of the functional gastrointestinal disorders, and empirical treatment trials often are required. Both pharmacological and nonpharmacological management approaches have shown some benefit.

REFERENCES

1. Knill-Jones RP. Geographical differences in the prevalence of dyspepsia. Scand J Gastoenterol 1991; 26(Suppl 182):17.

2. Locke GR 3rd. The epidemiology of functional gastrointestinal disorders in North America. Gastroenterol Clin N Am 1996; 25(1):1.

3. Grainger SL, Klass HJ, Rake MO, et al. Prevalence of dyspepsia: the epidemiology of overlapping symptoms. Postgrad Med J 1994; 70(821):154.

4. Penston JG, Pounder RE. A survey of dyspepsia in Great Britain. Aliment Pharmacol Ther 1996; 10(1):83.

5. El-Serag HB, Talley NJ. The prevalence and clinical course of functional dyspepsia. Aliment Pharmacol Ther 2004; 19:643.

6. Talley NJ, Zinsmeister AR, Schleck CD, et al. Dyspepsia and dyspepsia subgroups: a population-based study. Gastroenterology 1992; 102:1259.

7. Sonnenberg A. Economic analysis of dyspepsia. Eur J Gastroenterol Hepatol 1997; 9(4):323.

8. Heading RC, Wager E, Tooley PJ. Reliability of symptom assessment in dyspepsia. Eur J Gastroenterol Hepatol 1997; 9(8):779.

9. Talley NJ, Stanghellini V, Heading RC, et al. Functional gastroduodenal disorders. In: Drossman DA, Corazziari E, Talley NJ, et al., eds. Rome II: The functional gastrointestinal disorders. diagnosis, pathophysiology and treatment: a multinational consensus. Mclean, VA: Degnon Associates; 2000.

This chapter from the most recent version of the Rome criteria for functional gastrointestinal disorders provides a comprehensive overview of the epidemiology, pathophysiology and management of functional dyspepsia.

10. Crean GP, et al. Ulcer-like dyspepsia. Scand J Gastroenterol 1982; 17(Suppl 79):9.

11. Talley NJ, McNeil D, Piper DW. Discriminant value of dyspeptic symptoms: a study of the clinical presentation of 221 patients with dyspepsia of unknown cause, peptic ulceration, and cholelithiasis. Gut 1987; 28:40.

12. Adang RP, Ambergen AW, Talmon JL, et al. The discriminative value of patient characteristics and dyspeptic symptoms for upper gastrointestinal endoscopic findings: a study on the clinical presentation of 1,147 patients. Digestion 1996; 57:118.

13. Talley NJ, Weaver AL, Tesmer DL, et al. Lack of discriminant value of dyspepsia subgroups in patients referred for upper endoscopy. Gastroenterology 1993; 105(5):1378.

14. Talley NJ, Silverstein MD, Agreus L, et al. AGA technical review: evaluation of dyspepsia. Gastroenterology 1998; 114:582.

A complete discussion of the factors involved in reaching the appropriate approach to managing dyspepsia is provided in this technical review commissioned by the American Gastroenterological Association.

15. Talley NJ. Dyspepsia. Gastroenterology 2003; 125:1219.

The contemporary approach to dyspepsia and its management are described in this case-based discussion; the author offers editorial comment along with an evidence-based literature review.

16. Klauser AG, Schindlbeck NE, Muller-Lissner SA. Symptoms in gastro-oesophageal reflux disease. Lancet 1990; 335:205.

17. Berstad A, Hatlebakk JG. The predictive value of symptoms in gastro-oesophageal reflux disease. Scand J Gastroenterol 1995; 211;1.

18. Pfeiffer A, Aronbayev J, Schmidt T, et al. Gastric emptying, esophageal 24-hour pH and gastric potential difference in non-ulcer dyspepsia. Gastroenterol Clin Biol 1992; 16:395.

19. Kraagg N, Thijs C, Knipschild P. Dyspepsia – how noisy are gallstones? A meta-analysis of epidemiologic studies of biliary pain, dyspeptic symptoms, and food intolerance. Scand J Gastroenterol 1995; 30(5):411.

20. Talley NJ. Gallstones and upper abdominal discomfort. Innocent bystander or a cause of dyspepsia? J Clin Gastroenterol 1995; 20(3):182.

21. French EB, Robb WAT. Biliary cholic. Br Med J 1963; 5350:135–138.

22. Ros E, Zambon D. Postcholecystectomy symptoms: a prospective study of gallstone patients before and two years after surgery. Gut 1987; 28:1500.

23. Weinert CR, Arnett D, Jacobs D Jr, et al. Relationship between persistence of abdominal symptoms and successful outcome after cholecystectomy. Arch Intern Med 2000; 160:989.

24. DiBaise JK, Oleynikov D. Does gallbladder ejection fraction predict outcome after cholecystectomy for suspected chronic acalculous gallbladder dysfunction? A systematic review. Am J Gastroenterol 2003; 98:2605.

25. Talley NJ, Hunt RH. What role does *Helicobacter pylori* play in nonulcer dyspepsia? Arguments for and against *H. pylori* being associated with dyspeptic symptoms. Gastroenterology 1997; 113(Suppl):S67.

26. McQuaid K. Dyspepsia: In: Sleisenger MH, Fordtran JS, eds. Gastrointestinal disease. Pathophysiology, diagnosis, management. 6th edn. Philadelphia: WB Saunders; 1997:105.

27. Veldhuyzen van Zanten S, Malatjalian D, Tanton R, et at. *Helicobacter pylori* infection as a cause of gastritis, duodenal ulcer, gastric cancer and nonulcer dyspepsia: a systematic overview. Can Med Assoc J 1994; 150:177.

28. Lai ST, Fung KP, Ng FH, et al. A quantitative analysis of symptoms of non-ulcer dyspepsia as related to age, pathology, and *Helicobacter* infection. Scand J Gastroenterol 1996; 31(11):1078.

29. De Groot GH, de Both PS. Cisapride in functional dyspepsia in general practice. A placebo-controlled, randomized, double-blind study. Alimen Pharmacol Ther 1997; 11(1):193.

30. Elta GH, Scheiman JM, Barnett JL. Long-term follow-up of *Helicobacter pylori* treatment in non-ulcer dyspepsia patients. Am J Gastroenterol 1995; 90(7):1089.

31. Veldhuyzen van Zanten SJ. The role of *Helicobacter pylori* infection in non-ulcer dyspepsia. Alimen Pharmacol Ther 1997; 11:63.

32. Gilvarry J, Buckley MJ, Beattie S, et al. Eradication of *Helicobacter pylori* affects symptoms in non-ulcer dyspepsia. Scand J Gastroenterol 1997; 32(6):535.

33. Talley NJ. A critique of therapeutic trials in *Helicobacter pylori*-positive functional dyspepsia. Gastroenterology 1994; 106(5):1174.

34. Laheij RI, Jansen JB, van de Lisdonk EH, et al. Review article: symptom improvement through eradication of *Helicobacter pylori* in patients with non-ulcer dyspepsia. Aliment Pharmacol Ther 1996; 10(6):843.

35. Moayyedi P, Soo S, Deeks J, et al. Eradication of *Helicobacter pylori* for non-ulcer dyspepsia (Cochrane Review). Cochrane Database Syst Rev 2003; 1:CD002096.

A small but significant value of *H. pylori* eradication in patients with no other explanation for dyspepsia is determined by this systematic review of controlled trials.

36. Laine L, Schoenfeld P, Fennerty MB. Therapy for *Helicobacter pylori* in patients with nonulcer dyspepsia. A meta-analysis of randomized controlled trials. Ann Intern Med 2001; 13:361.

37. Talley NJ, Vakil N. Guidelines for the management of dyspepsia and functional dyspepsia. Am J Gastroenterol 2005; in press.

This comprehensive review commissioned by the Practice Parameters Committee of the American College of Gastroenterology provides the most recent consensus information on the best management of dyspepsia and suggests nuances in the algorithm compared with previous recommendations.

38. McQuaid K. Dyspepsia. In: Feldman M, Friedman LS, Sleisenger MH, eds. Gastrointestinal disease. Pathophysiology, diagnosis, management. 7th edn. Philadelphia: WB Saunders; 2002:102–118.

39. Tack J, Bisschops R, Sarnelli G. Pathophysiology and treatment of functional dyspepsia. Gastroenterology 2004; 127:1239.

A complete contemporary analysis of the pathophysiological associations with functional dyspepsia, their relationships to symptoms, and the outcome of treatment trials is included in this review.

40. Drossman DA. Diagnosing and treating patients with refractory functional gastrointestinal disorders. Ann Intern Med 1995; 123:688.

41. Bisschops R, Geypens B, Ghoos I, et al. Timing of symptoms in relation to the meal in pain-predominant versus discomfort-predominant dyspepsia. Gastroenterology 2000; 118:2544.

42. Arts J, Caenepeel P, Demedts I, et al. Influence of erythromycin on gastric emptying and meal-related symptoms in functional dyspepsia with delayed gastric emptying. Gut 2004; in press.

43. Talley NJ, Meineche-Schmidt V, Pare P, et al. Efficacy of omeprazole in functional dyspepsia: double-blind, randomized, placebo-controlled trials (the Bond and Opera studies). Aliment Pharmacol Ther 1998; 12:1055.

44. Malagelada JR. Functional dyspepsia. Insights on mechanisms and management strategies. Gastroenterol Clin North Am 1996; 25(1):103.

45. Talley NJ. Spectrum of chronic dyspepsia in the presence of the irritable bowel syndrome. Scand J Gastroenterol 1991; 182:7.

46. Agreus L, Svardsudd K, Nyren O, et al. Irritable bowel syndrome and dyspepsia in the general population: overlap and lack of stability over time. Gastroenterology 1995; 109(3):671.

47. Heikkinen M, Pikkarainen P, Takala J, et al. Etiology of dyspepsia: four hundred unselected consecutive patients in general practice. Scand J Gastroenterol 1995; 30(6):519.

48. Talley NJ, Weaver AL, Zinsmeister AR, et al. Onset and disappearance of gastrointestinal symptoms and functional gastrointestinal disorders. Am J Epidemiol 1992; 136(2):165.

49. Talley NJ. Drug treatment of functional dyspepsia. Scand J Gastroenterol 1991; 26(Suppl 182):47.

50. Holtmann G, Talley NJ. Functional dyspepsia. Current treatment recommendations. Drugs 1993; 45(6):918.

51. Kay L. Prevalence, incidence and prognosis of gastrointestinal symptoms in a random sample of an elderly population. Age Ageing 1994; 23(2):146.

52. Whitehead WE. Psychosocial aspects of functional gastrointestinal disorders. Gastroenterol Clin North Am 1996; 25(1):21.

This comprehensive overview of psychological and psychiatric findings in patients with functional gastrointestinal disorders is applicable to understanding these features and their relationships to symptoms in functional dyspepsia patients.

53. Lémann M, Dederding JP, Flourié B, et al. Abnormal perception of visceral pain in response to gastric distension in chronic idiopathic dyspepsia. The irritable stomach syndrome. Dig Dis Sci 1991; 36(9):1249.

54. Mearin F, Cucala M, Azpiroz F, et al. The origin of symptoms on the brain-gut axis in functional dyspepsia. Gastroenterology 1991; 101(4):999.

55. Vandenberghe J, Vos R, Janssens J, et al. Visceral hyperalgesia in functional dyspepsia (FD): pain-specific or multimodal afferent pathways? Gastroenterology 2002; 122(Suppl 1):A34.

56. Holtmann G, Goebell H, Talley NJ. Functional dyspepsia and irritable bowel syndrome: is there a common pathophysiological basis? Am J Gastroenterol 1997; 92(6):954.

57. Trimble KC, Farouk R, Pryde A, et al. Heightened visceral sensation in functional gastrointestinal disease is not site-specific. Evidence for a generalized disorder of gut sensitivity. Dig Dis Sci 1995; 40(8):1607.

58. Talley NJ. Functional dyspepsia – should treatment be targeted on disturbed physiology? Aliment Pharmacol Ther 1995; 9(2):107.

59. Haug TT, Wilhelmsen I, Berstad A, et al. Life events and stress in patients with functional dyspepsia compared with patients with duodenal ulcer and healthy controls. Scand J Gastroenterol 1995; 30(6):524.

60. Langeluddecke P, Goulston K, Tennant C. Psychological factors in dyspepsia of unknown cause: a comparison with peptic ulcer disease. J Psychosom Res 1990; 34:215.

61. Jain AK, Gupta JP, Gupta S, et al. Neuroticism and stressful life events in patient with non-ulcer dyspepsia. J Assoc of Phys Ind 1995; 43(2):90.

62. Wilhelmsen I, Haug TT, Ursin H, et al. Discriminant analysis of factors distinguishing patients with functional dyspepsia from patients with duodenal ulcer. Significance of somatization. Dig Dis Sci 1995; 40(5):1105.

63. Talley NJ, Phillips SF, Bruce B, et al. Relation among personality and symptoms in nonulcer dyspepsia and the irritable bowel syndrome. Gastroenterology 190; 99:327.

64. Talley NJ, Fung LH, Gilligan IJ, et al. Association of anxiety, neuroticism and depression with dyspepsia of unknown cause. A case-controlled study. Gastroenterology 1986; 90:886.

65. Haug TT, Wilhelmsen I, Ursin H, et al. What are the real problems for patients with functional dyspepsia? Scand J Gastroenterol 1995; 30(2):97.

66. Haug TT, Svebak S, Wilhelmsen I, et al. Psychological factors and somatic symptoms in functional dyspepsia. A comparison with duodenal ulcer and healthy controls. J Psychosom Res 1994; 38(4):281.

67. Talley NJ, Weaver AL, Zinsmeister AR. Impact of functional dyspepsia on quality of life. Dig Dis Sci 1995; 40(3):584.

68. Kane FJ Jr. Strohlein J, Harper RG. Nonulcer dyspepsia associated with psychiatric disorder. South Med J 1993; 86:641.

69. Magni G, DiMario F, Bernasconi G, et al. DSM-III diagnosis associated with dyspepsia of unknown cause. Am J Psychiatry 1987; 114:1222.

70. Jonsson BH, Theorell T, Gotthard R. Symptoms and personality in patients with chronic functional dyspepsia. J Psychosom Res 1995; 39(1):93.

71. Andersson SI, Hovelius B, Molstad S, et al. Dyspepsia in general practice: psychological findings in relation to Helicobacter pylori serum antibodies. J Psychosom Res 1994; 38(3):241.

72. Fischler B, Vandenberghe J, Persoons P, et al. Evidence-based subtypes in functional dyspepsia with confirmatory factor analysis: psychosocial and physiopathological correlates. Gastroenterology 2001; 120:268.

73. Castillo EJ, Camilleri M, Locke GR, et al. A community-based, controlled study of the epidemiology and pathophysiology of dyspepsia. Clin Gastroenterol Hepatol 2004; 2:985.

74. Jones MP, Maganti K. Symptoms, gastric function, and psychosocial factors in functional dyspepsia. J Clin Gastroenterol 2004; 38:866.

75. Bennett EJ, Kellow JE, Cowan H, et al. Suppression of anger and gastric emptying in patients with functional dyspepsia. Scand J Gastroenterol 1992; 27:869.

76. Haug TT, Svebak S, Hausken T, et al. Low vagal activity as mediating mechanism for the relationship between personality factors and gastric symptoms in functional dyspepsia. Psychosom Med 1994; 56:181.

77. Clouse RE, Carney RM. The psychologic profile of non-cardiac chest pain patients. Eur J Gastroenterol Hepatol 1995; 7:1160.

78. Drossman DA, Li Z, Andruzzi E, et al. U.S. householder survey of functional gastrointestinal disorders. Prevalence, sociodemography, and health impact. Dig Dis Sci 1993; 38(9):1569.

79. Health and Public Policy Committee, American College of Physicians. Endoscopy in the evaluation of dyspepsia. Ann Intern Med 1985; 102:266.

80. Dooley CP, Larson AW, Stace NH, et al. Double-contrast barium meal and upper gastrointestinal endoscopy: a comparative study. Ann Intern Med 1984; 101:538.

81. Stevenson GW, Norman G, Frost R, Somers S. Barium meal or endoscopy? A prospective randomized study of patient preference and physician decision making. Clin Radiol 1991; 44:317.

82. Bytzer P. Diagnosing dyspepsia: any controversies left? Gastroenterology 1996; 110(1):302.

83. Bytzer P, Schaffalitzky de Muckadell OB. Prediction of major pathologic conditions in dyspeptic patients referred for endoscopy. A prospective validation study of a scoring system. Scand J Gastroenterol 1992; 27(11):987.

84. Bytzer P, Moller-Hansen J, Schaffalitzky de Muckadell OB, et al. Predicting endoscopic diagnosis in the dyspeptic patient. The value of predictive score models. Scand J Gastroenterol 1997; 32(2):118.

85. Bytzer P, Hansen JM, Havelund T, et al. Predicting endoscopic diagnosis in the dyspeptic patient: the value of clinical judgment. Eur J Gastroenterol Hepatol 1996; 8(4):359.

86. Adang RP, Ambergen AW, Talmon JL, et al. The discriminative value of patient characteristics and dyspeptic symptoms for upper gastrointestinal endoscopic findings: a study on the clinical presentation of 1,147 patients. Digestion 1996; 57(2):118.

87. Kang JY, Ho KY, Yeoh KG, et al. Chronic upper abdominal pain due to duodenal ulcer and other structural and functional causes: its localization and nocturnal occurrence. J Gastroenterol Hepatol 1996; 11(6):515.

88. Muris JW, Starmans R, Pop P, et al. Discriminant value of symptoms in patients with dyspepsia. J Fam Pract 1994; 38(2):139.

89. Johnsen R, Bernersen B, Straume B, et al. Prevalences of endoscopic and histological findings in subjects with and without dyspepsia. Br Med J 1991; 302(6779):749.

90. Stanghellini V, Tosetti C, Paternico A, et al. Predominant symptoms identify different subgroups in functional dyspepsia. Am J Gastroenterol 1999; 94:2080.

91. Moayyedi P, Axon AT. The usefulness of the likelihood ratio in the diagnosis of dyspepsia and gastroesophageal reflux disease. Am J Gastroenterol 1999; 94:3122.

92. Mertz H, Fullerton S, Naliboff B, et al. Symptoms and visceral perception in severe functional and organic dyspepsia. Gut 1998; 42:814.

93. Brown WH, Chey WD, Elta GH. Number of responses on a review of systems questionnaire predicts the diagnosis of functional gastrointestinal disorders. J Clin Gastroenterol 2003; 36:222.

94. Williams B, Luckas M, Ellingham JH, et al. Do young patients with dyspepsia need investigation? Lancet 1988; 2:1349.

95. Adang RP, Vismans JF, Talmon JL. Appropriateness of indications for diagnostic upper gastrointestinal endoscopy: association with relevant endoscopic disease. Gastrointest Endosc 1995; 42(5):390.

96. Bytzer P, Talley NJ. Dyspepsia. Ann Intern Med 2001; 134:815.

97. Voutilainen M, Mantynen T, Kunnamo I, et al. Impact of clinical symptoms and referral volume on endoscopy for detecting peptic ulcer and gastric neoplasms. Scand J Gastroenterol 2003; 38:109.

98. Gillen D, McColl KE. Does concern about missing malignancy justify endoscopy in uncomplicated dyspepsia in patients aged less than 55? Am J Gastroenterol 1999; 94:2329.

99. Canga C, Vakil N. Upper GI malignancy, uncomplicated dyspepsia and the age threshold for early endoscopy. Am J Gastroenterol 2002; 97:600.

100. Shaw PC, van Romunde KL, Griffioen G, et al. Peptic ulcer and gastric carcinoma: diagnosis with biphasic radiography compared with fiberoptic endoscopy. Radiology 1987; 163:39.

101. Klauser AG, Voderholzer WA, Knesewitsch PA, et al. What is behind dyspepsia? Dig Dis Sci 1993; 38:147.

102. Heikkinen MT, Pikkarainen PH, Takala JK, et al. Diagnostic methods in dyspepsia: the usefulness of upper abdominal ultrasound and gastroscopy. Scand J Prim Health Care 1997; 15(2):82.

103. Costanza CD, Longstreth GF, Lin AL. Chronic abdominal wall pain: clinical features, healthcare costs, and long-term outcome. Clin Gastroenterol Hepatol 2004; 2:395.

104. Wayman J, Griffin SM, Campbell FC. Is functional dyspepsia largely explained by gastro-oesophageal reflux disease? Baillières Clin Gastroenterol 1998; 12:463.

105. Farup PG, Hovde O, Torp R, et al. Patients with functional dyspepsia responding to omeprazole have a characteristic gastro-oesophageal reflux pattern. Scand J Gastroenterol 1999; 34:575.

106. Talley NJ, Shuter B, McCrudden G, et al. Lack of association between gastric emptying of solids and symptoms in nonulcer dyspepsia. J Clin Gastroenterol 1989; 11:625.

107. Veldhuyzen van Zanten SJ, Jones MJ, Verlinden M, et al. Efficacy of cisapride and domperidone in functional (nonulcer) dyspepsia: a meta-analysis. Am J Gastroenterol 2001; 96:689.

108. Malagelada J-R. Gastrointestinal motor disturbances in functional dyspepsia. Scand J Gastroenterol 1991; 26(Suppl 182):29.

109. Malagelada J-R. When and how to investigate the dyspeptic patient. Scand J Gastroenterol 1991; 26(Suppl 182):70.

110. American Psychiatric Association. Diagnostic and Statistical Manual of Mental Disorders – DSM-IV. Washington DC: American Psychiatric Association; 1994.

111. Peck RM Jr, Blaser MJ. Pathophysiology of Helicobacter pylori-induced gastritis and peptic ulcer disease. Am J Med 1997; 102:200.

112. Soll AH. Consensus conference. Medical treatment of peptic ulcer disease. Practice guidelines. Practice Parameters Committee of the American College of Gastroenterology. JAMA 1996; 275(8):622.

113. Cutler AF. Diagnostic tests for *Helicobacter pylori* infection. Gastroenterologist 1997; 5(3):202.

114. Thijs JC, van Zwet AA, Thijs WJ, et al. Diagnostic tests for *Helicobacter pylori*: a prospective evaluation of their accuracy, without selecting a single test as the gold standard. Am J Gastroenterol 1996; 91:2125.

115. Loy CT, Irwig LM, Katelaris PH, et al. Do commercial serological kits for *Helicobacter pylori* infection differ in accuracy? A meta-analysis. Am J Gastroenterol 1996; 91:1138.

116. Vaira D, Vakil N, Managatti M, et al. The stool antigen test for the detection of *Helicobacter pylori* after eradication therapy. Ann Intern Med 2002; 136:280.

117. Vaira D, Vakil N. Blood, urine, stool, breath, money and *Helicobacter pylori*. Gut 2001; 48:287.

118. Sobala GM, Crabreee JE, Pentith JA, et al. Screening dyspepsia by serology to *Helicobacter pylori*. Lancet 1991; 338:94.

119. Mendall MA, Jazrawi RP, Marrero JM. Serology for *Helicobacter pylori* compared with symptom questionnaires in screening before direct access endoscopy. Gut 1995; 36(3):330.

120. Patel P, Khulusi S, Mendall MA, et al. Prospective screening of dyspeptic patients by *Helicobacter pylori* serology. Lancet 1995; 346:1315.

121. Chiba N, Veldhuyzen van Zanten SJ, Sinclair P, et al. Treating *Helicobacter pylori* infection in primary care patients with uninvestigated dyspepsia: the Canadian adult dyspepsia empiric treatment-*Helicobacter pylori* positive (CADET-Hp) randomized controlled trial. Br Med J 2002; 324:1012.

122. Allison JE, Hurley LB, Hiatt RA, et al. A randomized controlled trial of test-and-treat strategy for *Helicobacter pylori*: clinical outcomes and health care costs in a managed care population receiving long-term acid suppression therapy for physician-diagnosed peptic ulcer disease. Arch Intern Med 2003; 163:1165.

123. Lassen AT, Pedersen FM, Bytzer P, et al. *Helicobacter pylori* test-and-eradication versus prompt endoscopy for management of dyspepsia patients: a randomized trial. Lancet 2000;.356:455.

124. Heaney A, Collins JS, Watson RG, et al. A prospective randomized trial of a 'test and treat' policy versus endoscopy based management in young *Helicobacter pylori* positive patients with ulcer-like dyspepsia referred to a hospital clinic. Gut 1999; 45:186.

125. McColl KE, Murray LS, Gillen D, et al. Randomised trial of endoscopy with testing for *Helicobacter pylori* compared with non-invasive *H. pylori* testing alone in the management of dyspepsia. Br Med J 2002; 324:999.

126. Jones RJ, Tait C, Sladen G, Weston-Baker J. A trial of a test-and-treat strategy for *Helicobacter pylori* positive dyspepsia patients in general practice. Int J Clin Pract 1999; 53:413.

127. Manes G, Menchise A, De Nucci C, et al. Empirical prescribing for dyspepsia: randomized controlled trial of test and treat versus omeprazole treatment. Br Med J 2003; 326:1118.

128. Fraser AG, Ali MR, McCullough S, et al. Diagnostic tests for *Helicobacter pylori* – can they help select patients for endoscopy? NZ Med J 1996; 109(1018):95.

129. Hansson LE, Engstrand L, Nyren O, et al. Prevalence of *Helicobacter pylori* infection in subtypes of gastric cancer. Gastroenterology 1995; 109:885.

130. Malfertheiner P, Megraud F, O'Morain C, et al, and the European *Helicobacter pylori* Study Group (EHPSG). Current concepts in the management of *Helicobacter pylori* infection: the Maastricht 2000 Consensus Report. Aliment Pharmacol Ther 2002; 16:167.

131. Lazzaroni M, Bargiggia S, Sangaletti O, et al. Eradication of *Helicobacter pylori* and long-term outcome of functional dyspepsia. A clinical endoscopic study. Dig Dis Sci 1996; 41(8):1589.

132. Rosenstock S, Kay L, Rosenstock C, et al. Relation between *Helicobacter pylori* infection and gastrointestinal symptoms and syndromes. Gut 1997; 41(2):169.

133. Kuipers EJ, Uyterlinde AM, Pena AS, et al. Increase of *Helicobacter pylori*-associated corpus gastritis during acid suppressive therapy: implications for long-term safety. Am J Gastroenterol 1995; 90:1401.

134. Graham DY, Operkun AR, Yamaoka Y, et al. Early events in proton pump inhibitor-associated exacerbation of corpus gastritis. Aliment Pharmacol Ther 2003; 17:193.

135. Pauker SG, Kassirer JP. Decision analysis. N Engl J Med 1987; 316:250.

136. Moayyedi P, Soo S, Deeks J, et al. Pharmacological interventions for non-ulcer dyspepsia (Cochrane Review). Cochrane Database Syst Rev 2003; 1:CD001960.

The cumulative outcomes of a variety of drug treatments for functional dyspepsia are described in this systematic database review.

137. Hetzel DJ, Dent J, Reed WD, et al. Healing and relapse of severe peptic esophagitis after treatment with omeprazole. Gastroenterology 1988; 95:903.

138. Jones R, Lydeard S. Dyspepsia in the community: a follow-up study. Br J Clin Pract 1992; 46(2):95.

139. Talley NJ, McNeil D, Hayden A, et al. Prognosis of chronic unexplained dyspepsia: a prospective study of potential predictor variables in patients with endoscopically diagnosed non-ulcer dyspepsia. Gastroenterology 1987; 92:1060.

140. Bytzer P, Hansen JM, Schaffalitzky de Muchadell OB. Empirical H$_2$-blocker therapy or prompt endoscopy in management of dyspepsia? Lancet 1994; 343(8901):811.

141. Holdstock G, Bruce S. Endoscopy and gastric cancer. Gut 1981; 22:673.

142. Hallissey MT, Allum WH, Jewkes AJ, et al. Early detection of gastric cancer. Br Med J 1990; 301:513.

143. Sue-Ling HM, Johnston D, Martin IG, et al. Gastric cancer: a curable disease in Britain. Br Med J 1993; 307:591.

144. Silverstein MD, Petterson T, Talley NJ. Initial endoscopy or empirical therapy with or without testing for *Helicobacter pylori* for dyspepsia: a decision analysis. Gastroenterology 1996; 110(1):72.

145. Read L, Pass TM, Komaroff AL. Diagnosis and treatment of dyspepsia: a cost-effectiveness analysis. Med Decis Making 1982; 2:415.

146. Sonnenberg A, Townsend WF, Müller AD. Evaluation of dyspepsia and functional gastrointestinal disorders: a cost-benefit analysis of different approaches. Eur J Gastroenterol Hepatol 1995; 7(7):655.

147. Ebell MH, Warbasse L, Brenner C. Evaluation of the dyspeptic patient: a cost-utility study. J Fam Pract 1997; 44(6):545.

148. Fendrick AM, Chernew ME, Hirth RA, et al. Alternative management strategies for patients with suspected peptic ulcer disease. Ann Intern Med 1995; 123:260.

149. Briggs AH, Sculpher MJ, Logan RP. Cost effectiveness of screening for and eradication of *Helicobacter pylori* in management of dyspeptic patients under 45 years of age. Br Med J 1996; 312(7042):1321.

150. Sonnenberg A. Cost-benefit analysis of testing for *Helicobacter pylori* in dyspeptic subjects. Am J Gastroenterol 1996; 91(9):1773.

151. Ofman JJ, Etchason J, Fullerton S, et al. Management strategies for *Helicobacter pylori*-seropositive patients with dyspepsia: clinical and economic consequences. Ann Intern Med 1997; 126(4):280.

152. Spiegel BM, Vakil N, Ofman JJ. Dyspepsia management in primary care: a decision analysis of competing strategies. Gastroenterology 2002; 122:1270.

153. Ladabaum U, Chey WD, Scheiman JM, et al. Reappraisal of non-invasive management strategies for uninvestigated dyspepsia: a cost-minimalization analysis. Aliment Pharmacol Ther 2002; 16:1491.

154. Talley NJ. Review article: dyspepsia: how to manage and how to treat? Aliment Pharmacol Ther 2002; 16(Suppl 4):95.

155. Goulston KJ, Dent OF, Mant A, et al. Use of H_2-receptor antagonists in patients with dyspepsia and heartburn: a cost comparison. Med J Aust 1991; 155(1):20.

156. Hungin AP, Thomas PR, Bramble MG, et al. What happens to patients following open access gastroscopy? An outcome study from general practice. Br J Gen Pract 1994; 44(388):519.

157. Bodger K, Daly MJ, Heatley RV. Prescribing patterns for dyspepsia in primary care: a prospective study of selected general practitioners. Aliment Pharmacol Ther 1996; 10(6):889.

158. Quadri A, Vakil N. Health-related anxiety and the effect of open-access endoscopy in US patients with dyspepsia. Aliment Pharmacol Ther 2003; 17:835.

159. Rabeneck L, Wristers K, Souchek J, et al. Impact of upper endoscopy on satisfaction in patients with previously uninvestigated dyspepsia. Gastrointest Endosc 2003; 57:295.

160. Goodson JD, Lehman JW, Richter JM, et al. Is upper gastrointestinal radiography necessary in the initial management of uncomplicated dyspepsia? A randomized controlled trial comparing empiric antacid therapy plus patient reassurance with traditional care. J Gen Intern Med 1989; 4:367.

161. Lewin van den Brock NT, Numans ME, Buskens E, et al. A randomized controlled trial of four management strategies for dyspepsia: relationships between symptom subgroups and strategy outcome. Br J Gen Pract 2001; 51:619.

162. Howell S, Talley NJ. Does fear of serious disease predict consulting behaviour amongst patients with dyspepsia in general practice? Eur J Gastroenterol Hepatol 1999; 11:881.

163. Kurata JH, Nogawa AN, Chen YK, et al. Dyspepsia in primary care: perceived causes, reasons for improvement, and satisfaction with care. J Fam Pract 1997; 44(3):281.

164. Delaney BC, Wilson S, Roalfe A, et al. Cost effectiveness of initial endoscopy for dyspepsia in patients over age 50 years: a randomized controlled trial in primary care. Lancet 2000; 356:1965.

165. Anonymous. Current European concepts in the management of *Helicobacter pylori* infection. The Maastricht Consensus Report. European *Helicobacter Pylori* Study Group. Gut 1997; 41(1):8.

166. American Gastroenterological Association. American Gastroenterological Association medical position statement: evaluation of dyspepsia. Gastroenterology 1998; 114:579.

The initial algorithm for management of dyspepsia that has been in widespread use is described in this position statement of the American Gastroenterological Association.

167. Talley NJ. Quality of life in functional dyspepsia. Scand J Gastroenterol 1996; 221:21.

168. Lindell GH, Celebioglu F, Graffner HO. Non-ulcer dyspepsia in the long-term perspective. Eur J Gastroenterol Hepatol 1995; 7(9):829.

169. Dobrilla G, Comberlato M, Steele A, et al. Drug treatment of functional dyspepsia. A meta-analysis of randomized controlled trials. J Clin Gastroenterol 1989; 11:169.

170. Redstone HA, Barrowman N, Veldhuyzen van Zanten SJ. H_2-receptor antagonists in the treatment of functional (nonulcer) dyspepsia: a meta-analysis of randomized controlled clinical trials. Aliment Pharmacol Ther 2001; 15:1291.

171. Carlsson R, Bolling E, Jerndal P, et al. Factors predicting response to omeprazole treatment in patients with functional dyspepsia. Gastroenterology 1996; 110:A76.

172. Meineche-Schmidt V, Krag E, Christensen E. Identification of omeprazole response in dyspepsia. Data analysis of a Danish multicenter trial in general practice. Gastroenterology 1995; 108:A165.

173. George AA, Tsuchiyose M, Dooley CP. Sensitivity of the gastric mucosa to acid and duodenal contents in patients with nonulcer dyspepsia. Gastroenterology 1991: 101(1):3.

174. Bates S, Sjoden P-O, Fellenius J, et al. Blocked and non-blocked acid secretion and reported pain in ulcer, nonulcer dyspepsia, and normal subjects. Gastroenterology 1989; 97:376.

175. Schwarz MP, Samsom M, van Berge Henegouwen GP, et al. Effect of inhibition of gastric acid secretion on antropyloroduodenal motor activity and duodenal acid hypersensitivity in functional dyspepsia. Aliment Pharmacol Ther 2001; 15:1921.

176. Barone JA, Jensen LM, Colazzi JL, et al. Cisapride: A gastrointestinal prokinetic drug. Ann Pharmacother 1994; 28(4):488.

177. Carvalhinhos A, Fidalgo P, Freire A. Cisapride compared with ranitidine in the treatment of functional dyspepsia. Eur J Gastroenterol Hepatol 1995; 7(5):411.

178. Wiseman LR, Faulds D. Cisapride. An updated review of its pharmacology and therapeutic efficacy as a prokinetic agent in gastrointestinal motility disorders. Drugs 1994; 47:116.

179. Finney JS, Kinnersley N, Hughes M, et al. Meta-analysis of antisecretory and gastrokinetic compounds in functional dyspepsia. J Clin Gastroenterol 1998; 26:312.

180. Corinaldesi R, Stanghellini V, Raiti C, et al. Effect of chronic administration of cisapride on gastric emptying of a solid meal and on dyspeptic symptoms in patients with idiopathic gastroparesis. Gut 1987; 28:300.

181. Jian R, Ducrot F, Ruskone A, et al. Symptomatic, radionuclide and therapeutic assessment of chronic idiopathic dyspepsia: a double-blind placebo-controlled evaluation of cisapride. Dig Dis Sci 1989; 34:657.

182. Tack J, Broeckaert D, Coulie B, et al. The influence of cisapride on gastric tone and the perception of gastric distention. Aliment Pharmacol Ther 1998; 12:761.

183. Mitchelson F. Pharmacological agents affecting emesis: a review (part I). Drugs 1992; 43(3):295.

184. Brogden RN, Carmine AA, Heel RC, et al. Domperidone. A review of its pharmacological activity, pharmacokinetics and therapeutic efficacy in the symptomatic treatment of chronic dyspepsia and as an antiemetic. Drugs 1982; 24:360.

185. Veldhuyzen van Zanten SJ, Jones MJ, Verlinden M, et al. Efficacy of cisapride and domperidone in functional dyspepsia: a meta-analysis. Am J Gastroenterol 2001; 96:689.

186. Davis RH, Clench MH, Mathias JR. Effects of domperidone in patients with chronic unexplained upper gastrointestinal symptoms: a double-blind, placebo-controlled study. Dig Dis Sci 1988; 33:1505.

187. Tack J, Vos R, Janssens J, et al. Influence of tegaserod on proximal gastric tone and on the perception of gastric distention. Aliment Pharmacol Ther 2003; 18:1.

188. Clouse RE. Antidepressants for functional gastrointestinal syndromes. Dig Dis Sci 1994; 39:2352.

189. Clouse RE, Lustman PJ, Eckert TC, et al. Low-dose trazodone for symptomatic patients with esophageal contraction abnormalities. Gastroenterology 1987; 92:1027.

190. Max MB, Culnane M, Schaefer SC, et al. Amitriptyline relieves diabetic neuropathy pain in patients with normal or depressed mood. Neurology 1987; 37:589.

191. Peghnini P, Katz P, Castell D. Imipramine increases pain and sensation thresholds to esophageal balloon distension in humans. Gastroenterology 1997; 112:A255.

192. Gorelick A, Koshy S, Hooper F, et al. Differential inhibitory effects of tricyclic antidepressant agents on pain evoked by nociceptive somatic and viceral stimuli (Abstract). Dig Dis Sci 1996; 41:1888.

193. Mertz H, Pickens D, Morgan V. Amitriptyline reduces activation of the anterior cingulated cortex in irritable bowel syndrome patients during rectal pain. Gastroenterology 2003;.124(Suppl 1):A47.

194. Prakash C, Lustman PJ, Freedland KE, et al. Tricyclic antidepressants for functional nausea and vomiting: clinical outcome in 37 patients. Dig Dis Sci 1998; 43(9):1951–1956.

195. Randall CW, Kwong M. Differences in therapeutic response among patients with ulcer and nonulcer dyspepsia. Gastroenterology 1997; 112:A265.

196. Mertz H, Fass R, Kodner A, et al. Effect of amitriptyline on symptoms, sleep, and visceral perception in patients with functional dyspepsia. Am J Gastroenterol 1998; 93:160.

197. Tack J, Broeckaert D, Coulie B, et al. Influence of the selective serotonin re-uptake inhibitor, paroxetine, on gastric sensorimotor function in man. Aliment Pharmacol Ther 2003; 17:603.

198. Tanum L, Malt UF. A new pharmacologic treatment of functional gastrointestinal disorder. A double-blind placebo-controlled study with mianserin. Scand J Gastroenterol 1996; 31(4).

199. Lustman PJ, Griffith RS, Clouse RE, et al. Efficacy of cognitive therapy for depression in NIDDM: Results of a controlled clinical trial. Diabetes 1997; 46:13A.

200. Clouse RE. Antidepressants for irritable bowel syndrome. Gut 2003; 52:598.

201. Clouse RE, Lustman PJ. Antidepressants for irritable bowel syndrome. In: Camilleri M, Spiller RC, eds. Irritable bowel syndrome: diagnosis and treatment. London: WB Saunders; 2002:161.

202. Clouse RE, Randall CW. Irritable bowel syndrome. Does making a confident diagnosis reassure an unhappy patient? In: Barkin JS, Rogers AI, eds. Difficult decisions in digestive diseases. 2nd edn. St. Louis: Mosby; 1994:399.

203. Sapira JD. Reassurance therapy. What to say to symptomatic patients with benign diseases. Ann Intern Med 1972; 77:603.

204. Monson RA, Smith GR. Somatization disorder in primary care. N Engl J Med 1983; 308:1464.

205. Murphy GE. The clinical management of hysteria. JAMA 1982; 247:2559.

206. Smith GR, Monson RA, Ray DC. Psychiatric consultation in somatization disorders: a randomized controlled study. N Engl J Med 1986; 314:1407.

207. Haug TT, Wilhelmsen I, Svebak S, et al. Psychotherapy in functional dyspepsia. J Psychosom Res 1994; 38(7):735.

208. Soo S, Moayyedi P, Deeks J, et al. Psychological interventions for non-ulcer dyspepsia. Cochrane Database Syst Rev 2001; 4:CD002301.

209. Hamilton J, Guthrie E, Creed F, et al. A randomized controlled trial of psychotherapy in patients with chronic functional dyspepsia. Gastroenterology 2000; 119:661.

210. Calvert EL, Houghton LA, Cooper P, et al. Long-term improvement in functional dyspepsia using hypnotherapy. Gastroenterology 2002; 123:1778.

211. Sarnelli G, Sifrim D, Janssens J, et al. Influence of sildenafil on gastric sensorimotor function in man. Am J Physiol 2004; 287(5):G988–992.

212. Tack J, Piessevaux H, Coulie B, et al. A placebo-controlled trial of buspirone, a fundus-relaxing drug, in functional dyspepsia: effect on symptoms and gastric sensory and motor function. Gastroenterology 1999; 116:A325.

213. Mayer EA, Gebhart GF. Basic and clinical aspects of visceral hyperalgesia. Gastroenterology 1994; 107(1):271.

214. Cofin B, Bouhassira D, Chollet R, et al. Effect of the kappa agonist fedotozine on perception of gastric distention in healthy humans. Aliment Pharmacol Ther 1996; 10(6):919.

215. Fraitag B, Homerin M, Hecketsweiler P. Double-blind dose-response multicenter comparison of fedotozine and placebo in treatment of nonulcer dyspepsia. Dig Dis Sci 1994; 39(5):1072.

216. Maxton DG, Morris J, Whorwell PJ. Selective 5-hydroxytryptamine antagonism: a role in irritable bowel syndrome and functional dyspepsia? Aliment Pharmacol Ther 1996; 10(4):595.

217. Talley NJ, Veldhuyzen van Zanten SJ, Saez LR, et al. A dose-ranging, placebo-controlled, randomized trial of alosetron in patients with functional dyspepsia. Aliment Pharmacol Ther 2001; 15:525.

218. Feinle C, D'Amato M, Read NW. Cholecystokinin-A receptors modulate gastric sensory and motor responses to gastric distension and duodenal lipid. Gastroenterology 1996; 110:1379.

219. Feinle C, Meier O, Otto B, et al. Role of duodenal lipid and cholecystokinin A receptors in the pathophysiology of functional dyspepsia. Gut 2001; 48:347.

220. May B, Kuntz HD, Kieser M, et al. Efficacy of a fixed peppermint oil/caraway oil combination in non-ulcer dyspepsia. Arzneimittel-Forschung 1996; 46(12):1149.

221. Tatsuta M, Iishi H. Effect of treatment with liu-jun-zi-tang (TJ-43) on gastric emptying and gastrointestinal symptoms in dyspeptic patients. Aliment Pharmacol Ther 1993; 7(4):459.

222. Gullo L, Priori P, Pezzilli R. Is chronic pancreatitis a cause of dyspepsia? Ital Gastroenterol 1995; 27(9):494.

CHAPTER SEVENTY

Nausea and vomiting

Kenneth L. Koch

INTRODUCTION

Nausea is one of the most debilitating symptoms experienced by human beings. By many patients' accounts, nausea is worse than pain. Nausea is a queasy, sick-to-the stomach sensation that may progress from mild to moderate to severe with the accompanying urge to vomit. Vague epigastric distress or discomfort is also frequently present during nausea. Autonomic nervous symptoms include cold sweats and pallor.[1] Nausea is a major symptom within the common syndrome known as functional dyspepsia.[1–3]

While the 'urge to vomit' is one description of nausea, the symptom of nausea is actually much more complex. Three dimensions of nausea have been described: (1) gastrointestinal distress such as epigastric discomfort or queasiness; (2) somatic symptoms such as sweating and lightheadedness; and (3) emotional distress such as hopelessness and worry.[4]

Vomiting is the forceful expulsion of gastric content through the mouth. The vomiting reflex begins with retrograde peristaltic contractions of the duodenum which move through the stomach in an orad direction through the relaxed lower esophageal sphincter.[5] During contraction of abdominal muscles and suspension of respiration, the gastric contents are forcibly ejected from the esophagus and the mouth. Vomiting relieves nausea, albeit temporarily, in many cases depending on the precipitating cause(s) of the nausea.

MECHANISMS OF NAUSEA

Inflammation of the mucosa

Inflammation of the esophagus, stomach, or duodenum due to peptic ulcer diseases such as gastroesophageal reflux, gastric or duodenal ulceration or gastritis, is associated with nausea.[6,7] Vagal afferent fibers in the mucosa carry signals to the central nervous system via the nucleus tract solitarius and connect to higher-level neurons. Chronic nausea due to atypical gastroesophageal reflux disease was markedly diminished in patients who were treated with proton pump inhibitor therapy or underwent fundoplication.[6] Patients with burning epigastric pain and nausea due to duodenal ulcer disease had gastric dysrhythmias, myoelectrical abnormalities that occur in patients (and healthy subjects) who have nausea. The gastric dysrhythmias and nausea disappeared as the peptic ulcer was healed

with acid suppression therapy.[7] There are many other examples throughout the gastrointestinal tract where mucosal inflammation is associated with nausea (for example, appendicitis, ulcerative colitis, diverticulitis).

Gastric dysrhythmias and gastroparesis

The gastrointestinal neuromuscular wall is comprised of smooth muscle cells, the interstitial cells of Cajal (ICC), and the nerves of the enteric nervous system.[8,9] Drugs, inflammation, or immune processes may damage these three major components of the gastrointestinal wall responsible for contraction and relaxation. Damage to or loss of one or more of these components (such as the ICC) may lead to neuromuscular dysfunction with loss of contractility or loss of relaxation with or without electrical dysrhythmias.[9] Neuromuscular damage of the stomach and duodenum may result in symptoms of nausea and vomiting.[10] These symptoms also occur in patients with small intestinal dysmotility secondary to myopathies and neuropathies of the small bowel.[11] Irritable bowel syndrome, a neuromuscular disorder affecting colon function, results in constipation, and in some of these patients there is also an element of dyspepsia and nausea.[12]

Nausea is experienced in conditions where disturbances of gastric electrical activity occur. The normal gastric myoelectrical rhythm of 3 cpm is established by the ICCs in the stomach.[13,14] Gastric dysrhythmias are termed bradygastrias (0–2.5 cpm), tachygastrias (3.75–10 cpm), and mixed gastric dysrhythmias (non-specific or mixtures of tachygastria and bradygastria).[15,16] Gastric dysrhythmias precede the onset of nausea induced during motion sickness[17] and thus are not electrical abnormalities caused by nausea. Gastric dysrhythmias and nausea symptoms are elicited in healthy individuals during motion sickness,[17] infusion of morphine,[18] glucagon,[19] and hyperglycemia.[20] Gastric dysrhythmias recorded in women with first trimester nausea and vomiting of pregnancy correlated with the presence of nausea; and the dysrhythmias were not present after delivery.[21] Gastric dysrhythmias and nausea symptoms in patients with diabetic gastroparesis resolved with domperidone therapy, whereas the rate of gastric emptying did not improve.[22] Gastric dysrhythmias recorded in patients with dyspepsia or idiopathic gastroparesis also improved after a variety of prokinetic therapies.[23,24]

Gastroparesis is present in some patients with gastric dysrhythmias.[25,26] Delay in emptying of a meal and nausea symptoms may be due to multiple neuromuscular dysfunctions of the stomach.

Neuromuscular dysfunctions of the stomach are summarized in Figure 70.1. Patients with gastroparesis have less nausea but more fullness and vomiting.[27]

Mechanical obstruction

Mechanical obstruction of the gastrointestinal tract in any region may cause nausea and vomiting. Gastric outlet obstruction is the most obvious mechanical obstruction but may be overlooked in some patients.[28] The key point is that patients with a mechanical obstruction have a pain component associated with the nausea and vomiting. Mechanical obstruction should be considered when abdominal pain *precedes* the nausea and vomiting. Abdominal pain *after* nausea and vomiting is frequently due to tenderness in the abdominal musculature due to the vomiting and/or retching.

Chronic mesenteric ischemia

Chronic mesenteric ischemia is another mechanism of nausea and vomiting. In a subset of patients with chronic mesenteric ischemia, gastric dysrhythmias and gastroparesis are present.[29] This entity is important to consider because the gastroparesis is reversible with revascularization procedures. There are many causes of nausea as listed below, but the precise mechanisms of nausea and vomiting remain difficult to determine.

MECHANISMS OF VOMITING

If nausea from any cause reaches a particular threshold, then the vomiting reflex is elicited. During the development of severe nausea of motion sickness, the sympathetic nervous system is activated and plasma adrenaline (epinephrine) increases significantly compared with baseline.[30] Vagal tone is withdrawn as shown by loss of respiratory sinus arrhythmia and increase in skin conductance.[31] The vomiting reflex requires an intact vagus nerve and is considered a parasympathetic reflex as cholinergic

output is required for the retrograde peristaltic contractions that drive intragastric contents from the stomach into the esophagus.

Mechanisms of vomiting have been described in detail in the dog.[32] In response to infusion of apomorphine, contractions begin in the distal duodenum and move orad into the stomach.[33] The retrograde contraction continues into the antrum and corpus and moves towards the fundus. The lower esophageal sphincter relaxes and respiration is suppressed. When the abdominal muscles contract in conjunction with the reverse peristaltic wave in the antrum and corpus, the gastric contents are forcefully emptied into the esophagus and propelled through the relaxed upper esophageal sphincter and through the mouth. The vomiting reflex is blocked by vagotomy and atropine, reflecting the parasympathetic nervous system mechanism of vomiting.[33]

Mechanisms of vomiting in most gastrointestinal disorders have not been studied in detail. Vomiting due to cancer chemotherapy agents is decreased (but not eliminated) by pretreatment with 5-HT$_3$ antagonists such as ondansetron[34] and indicates that 5-HT$_3$ pathways are relevant to the vomiting reflex. Nausea and upper GI symptoms from gastrointestinal disorders, however, are much less controlled by these agents.[35]

Nongastrointestinal stimuli may elicit vomiting. Central nervous system diseases and disorders such as brain tumors, meningitis, migraine headache, and seizure disorders[36,37] may present with vomiting. These central nervous system abnormalities elicit nausea through central nervous system pathways; however, studies of gastrointestinal dysfunction in association with central nervous system disorders are rarely performed.

Finally, *vomiting* must be differentiated from *regurgitation* which is the gentle return of gastric contents into the mouth. Regurgitation is commonly seen in gastroesophageal reflux and may also indicate esophageal obstruction or esophageal motility abnormalities such as achalasia.[1] *Rumination* is the effortless return of solid gastric content into the mouth.[38] There is no associated abdominal pain or discomfort, heartburn, or nausea. The eliminated food is not bitter and is generally reswallowed. *Retching*, on

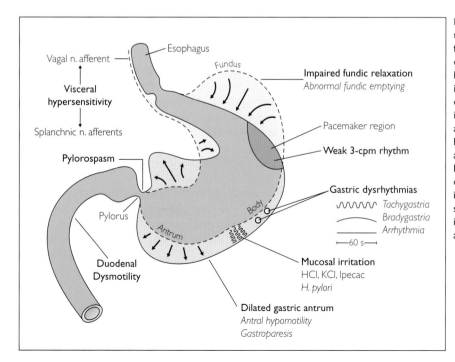

Fig. 70.1 • Neuromuscular abnormalities of the stomach associated with nausea and functional dyspepsia symptoms (epigastric discomfort, early satiety, and vomiting). Neuromuscular abnormalities of the fundus include impaired relaxation and abnormal fundic emptying. Abnormalities of the body and antrum include gastric dysrhythmias, antral dilatation, antral hypomotility and gastroparesis. Pylorospasm and small bowel dysmotility may also play a role in these symptoms. Mucosal irritation from acid and a variety of drugs or *Helicobacter pylori* may also play a role in some patients with nausea and dyspepsia symptoms. Visceral hypersensitivity and nausea in other patients may be mediated by vagal afferent and/or splanchnic afferent nerves.[40]

the other hand, is a vomiting episode during which no gastric content is expelled.

DIAGNOSIS OF NAUSEA AND VOMITING

Clinical features and differential diagnosis

The patient who presents to the gastroenterologist with acute or chronic nausea and vomiting is often a diagnostic and therapeutic challenge. Table 70.1 lists a differential diagnosis of nausea and vomiting with thirteen major categories to consider. The diseases and disorders in Table 70.1 may present either in an acute or chronic fashion.

Table 70.1 Differential diagnosis of nausea and vomiting

Mechanical obstruction
  Stomach, duodenum, small bowel, colon
  Hepatobiliary and pancreatic duct diseases
Peptic disease
  Esophagus – GERD
  Stomach – gastritis, ulcer, *Helicobacter pylori*
  Duodenum – duodenitis, ulcer
Peritoneal irritation (peritonitis, cancer, irradiation)
Carcinoma
  Gastric, ovarian
  Hypernephroma
  Paraneoplastic syndrome
Metabolic–hormonal
  Diabetes mellitus
  Uremia, hypercalcemia
  Addison's disease
  Hyperthyroidism, hypothyroidism
  Pregnancy
Drugs
  Levodopa, digitalis, phenytoin, cardiac antiarrhythmic agents, NSAIDS, antibiotics, chemotherapy agents, morphine, nicotine, progesterone/estrogen
Ischemic gastroparesis (chronic mesenteric ischemia)
Gastric neuromuscular disorders
  Idiopathic gastroparesis
  Gastric dysrhythmias
  Bradygastrias
  Tachygastrias
  Mixed dysrhythmias
Postoperative*
  Vagotomy
  Partial/total gastrectomy
  Fundoplication, fundic resection
Intestinal pseudo-obstruction (visceral neuropathy/myopathy)

Table 70.1 Differential diagnosis of nausea and vomiting—Cont'd

Scleroderma, amyloidosis
Idiopathic
CNS disease
  Migraine, cerebral vascular insufficiency
  Tumors, vestibular nerve–brainstem lesions
  Infections
  Parkinson's disease
Psychological/psychiatric disorders
  Anorexia nervosa, bulimia nervosa
  Rumination, psychogenic nausea (vomiting)
Idiopathic nausea and vomiting (adults; cyclical vomiting syndrome in children)

GERD, gastroesophageal reflux disease; NSAIDS, nonsteroidal anti-inflammatory drugs; CNS, central nervous system.
*With gastroparesis or dumping syndrome.

Several key clinical points should be highlighted.

First, it is important to determine whether the patient has a recurring and specific *pain* in association with the nausea and vomiting. If pain precedes the nausea and vomiting episode, particular care should be taken to exclude structural abnormalities of the gastrointestinal tract (e.g., mechanical obstructions or inflammation or ulceration) that may cause the pain.

Second, if nausea occurs with weight loss, then an underlying malignancy, chronic mesenteric ischemia, gastroparesis, or other neuromuscular disorder of the gastrointestinal tract should be considered.

Third, in patients with no structural or laboratory abnormalities, nausea and early satiety may be due to gastric dysrhythmia with decreased gastric compliance/relaxation. These are key symptoms of functional dyspepsia.[39,40] Gastric emptying is normal in 50–75% of these patients.[26,41] Prolonged fullness after a meal and/or the vomiting of undigested or 'chewed' food 30 minutes to hours after ingestion suggests gastroparesis. Hematemesis, on the other hand, indicates mucosal lesions, while bile-stained vomitus suggests small bowel obstruction. Feculent vomitus suggests the presence of colo-intestinal fistula.

Fourth, heartburn and constipation are associated with nausea. In some patients gastroesophageal reflux disease presents atypically with prominent nausea and little or no heartburn.[6] On the other hand, patients with constipation and abdominal discomfort due to the irritable bowel syndrome may also have gastric dysrhythmias and 20–30% of these patients have delayed gastric emptying.[42] Thus, patients with the irritable bowel syndrome may also have dyspepsia and objective findings of gastric dysrhythmias and gastroparesis.

Physical examination

The general appearance of the patient with nausea and vomiting may be normal or may indicate chronic illness, weight loss, or dehydration. Vital signs should be recorded and orthostatic hypotension excluded. Skin turgor should be assessed. Nystagmus, postural instability, optic disc edema, or stiff neck suggest central nervous system causes of symptoms.

The abdominal examination should be directed toward areas of specific tenderness or pain, masses, or organomegaly. A succussion splash indicates retained gastric content and is detected with gentle to-and-fro pressure applied to the epigastric area. Healed abdominal incisions from laparoscopic or open surgeries should be carefully examined. Painful, tender areas of the scar may be associated with the symptom of nausea. A positive Carnett's sign further suggests an abdominal wall syndrome.[41] Auscultation of the abdomen should be done routinely to detect abdominal bruits suggestive of mesenteric artery stenosis. Rectal and pelvic examinations should be performed.

Basic diagnostic tests

Basic tests include complete blood count, electrolyte, and liver function tests. An upright and supine film of the abdomen may be helpful in patients who have abdominal distention and nausea. Abnormal patterns of gas in the stomach, small bowel, or colon may help to uncover a specific cause of the nausea and vomiting such as obstruction or obstipation. In patients who have postprandial symptoms, an ultrasound of the gallbladder, pancreas, and liver may reveal abnormalities that explain the symptoms.

If blood tests and ultrasound are normal, then an upper endoscopy or upper GI barium series is often ordered by the referring physician. An algorithm for evaluation of these patients by the gastroenterologist is shown in Figure 70.2. Upper endoscopy will exclude significant mucosal abnormalities of the esophagus, stomach, and duodenum. An aggressive work-up is endorsed when the patient has pain, weight loss, hemoccult positive stool, or anemia. Small bowel series, enteroclysis, or colonoscopy may also be needed during the work-up of pain and anemia in the patient with nausea. Computed tomographic scan of the abdomen will detect abdominal masses or extraluminal lesions. Computed tomography of the head may be needed if central nervous signs are detected. In many patients referred to the gastroenterologist with chronic nausea symptoms, all of these tests are normal. If patients with unexplained nausea and bloating have normal basic diagnostic tests, then gastric neuromuscular disorders should be considered as described below.

Tests of gastric neuromuscular function: electrogastrogram and gastric emptying

If mucosal, structural, and biochemical tests are normal, it is important to evaluate gastric neuromuscular function in patients with chronic nausea and vomiting (see Fig. 70.2). Two non-invasive tests of gastric contractile and myoelectrical activity are

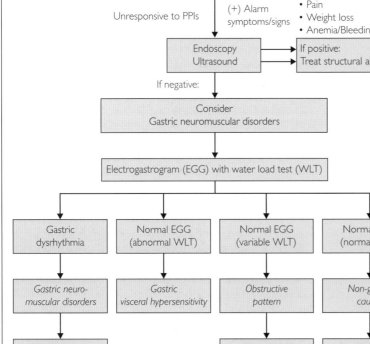

Fig. 70.2 • Diagnostic evaluation and treatment approach based on gastric neuromuscular function for patients with nausea and vomiting. If physical examination, biochemical tests, and standard diagnostic tests (including endoscopy and ultrasound) are normal, then gastric neuromuscular disorders should be considered in patients with nausea and vomiting. Results of electrogastrogram (EGG) with water load test (WLT) identify patients with gastric dysrhythmias and those with normal electrical rhythms. The water load test is also used to determine normal or abnormal gastric capacity and relaxation. See text for details. IBS, irritable bowel syndrome; CNS, central nervous system; GERD, gastroesophageal reflux disease.

performed – the solid-phase gastric emptying study and the electrogastrogram (EGG). By diagnosing specific and objective neuromuscular disorders, the gastroenterologist can provide rational treatment strategies for the patients with unexplained nausea and vomiting as discussed below.

Electrogastrography is the noninvasive method for recording EGGs.[15] The EGG signal reflects gastric myoelectrical (pacemaker) activity and is obtained by placing electrocardiographic-like electrodes on the abdominal surface in the epigastrium. In adults and children with gastric neuromuscular abnormalities of the stomach, gastric dysrhythmias such as bradygastrias, tachygastrias, or mixed dysrhythmias may be recorded, rather than the normal 3 cpm myoelectrical pattern.

Solid-phase gastric emptying studies are performed in nuclear medicine departments. Scrambled eggs labeled with technetium 99 are a common test meal in the United States. When the emptying of the meal is delayed compared to control values, a diagnosis of gastroparesis is established.[43] However, the cause of the gastroparesis is not defined by this test. Mechanical obstruction of the stomach must be excluded, for example, because this is a reversible cause of gastroparesis. Table 70.2 lists causes of gastroparesis which should be considered when the objective diagnosis is made. One-third to one-half of patients with dysmotility-like functional dyspepsia or nausea symptoms have delayed gastric emptying.[26,44] On the other hand, approximately 50% of these patients have normal gastric emptying.

EGG and gastric emptying tests are utilized to diagnose and organize treatment of unexplained nausea and vomiting. The EGG signal reflects the normal 3 cpm pacemaker activity of the stomach or gastric dysrhythmias: bradygastrias (0–2.5 cpm), tachygastrias (3.75–10 cpm) and mixed dysrhythmias which are a combination of bradygastria and tachygastria.[15] The water load test is a provocative, noncaloric test of gastric capacity performed during the EGG recording. During the water load test, the patient ingests water until full over a 5-minute period. This test is reproducible within healthy control subjects and patients with dyspepsia symptoms.[16] On average, healthy subjects ingest almost 600 ml of water, whereas dyspepsia patients ingest approximately 350 ml of water.[16] The EGG test identifies patients with gastric dysrhythmias or normal gastric myoelectrical activity. In addition, normal or abnormal results of the water load test reflect overall gastric capacity or relaxation.[26,45]

Results obtained from the EGG with water load test are shown in Figure 70.2. Patients diagnosed with gastric dysrhythmias have gastric neuromuscular disorders. Patients with tachygastria averaged approximately 30% emptying of a standard technetium-labeled egg meal at 2 hours, whereas patients with bradygastria emptied 60% of the meal in 2 hours.[46] Thus, tachygastria is the more detrimental rhythm to gastric emptying than bradygastria.[46,47] Mixed dysrhythmias are reported in high incidence in patients with gastroesophageal reflux disease and dyspepsia symptoms.[48]

On the other hand, approximately 45–60% of patients with nausea or dyspepsia of unknown cause have *normal* EGG recordings.[26,44] In symptomatic patients who have normal 3 cpm EGG activity and a normal water load test, nongastric causes of symptoms should be considered. Nongastric causes of these symptoms include atypical GERD, gallbladder dyskinesia, occult pancreatic disorders, or the irritable bowel syndrome and CNS disorders.[1]

In some patients the EGG is normal, but <300 ml of water is ingested during the water load test.[26,45] These patients have gastric visceral hypersensitivity to a very small volume of ingested water and decreased stretch or relaxation of the gastric neuromuscular wall in response to the water load. Poor gastric capacity for nutrient test meals has also been reported.[49–51] Stretch of the fundus *and* antrum may elicit symptoms. Distention of the antrum evokes nausea.[52]

A unique, 'normal' 3 cpm EGG pattern is present in patients with mechanical obstruction of the stomach and gastroparesis. The normal 3 cpm signal is extraordinarily regular and high amplitude. The discordant findings of strong 3 cpm EGG signal *and* gastroparesis raises the possibility of mechanical obstruction.[28] Normal 3 cpm EGG activity and gastroparesis is also possible with 'electromechanical dissociation.'

Table 70.3 shows four pathophysiological categories of gastric myoelectrical and emptying abnormalities based on the EGG and gastric emptying tests. Gastric dysrhythmia and gastroparesis represent Category 1, patients with severe gastric and electro-contractile abnormalities. If gastroparesis is confirmed by a solid-phase gastric emptying test, then the *cause* of the gastroparesis should be investigated (see Table 70.2). Gastric dysrhythmia, but *normal* gastric emptying represents Category 2. Category 2 patients have a gastric electrical disorder, but overall gastric emptying remains normal. Category 3 patients have normal 3 cpm EGG activity *and* normal gastric emptying. The normal 3 cpm EGG pattern is associated with normal gastric emptying.[26,47] In Category 4 patients, normal 3 cpm EGG activity *and* gastroparesis are present.

Table 70.2 Causes of gastroparesis

1. **Mechanical obstruction**
   Pylorus, duodenum, small intestine, colon

2. **Postgastric surgery**
   Vagotomy/antrectomy, Roux-en-Y, fundoplication

3. **Metabolic/endocrine disorders**
   Diabetic mellitus, hypothyroidism, hyperthyroidism, adrenal insufficiency

4. **Medications**
   Anticholinergics, narcotics, L-dopa, progesterone, calcium channel blockers

5. **Chronic mesenteric ischemia**

6. **Psychogenic disorders**
   Anorexia nervosa, bulimia

7. **Smooth muscle disorders**
   Hollow viscus myopathy, scleroderma muscular dystrophy

8. **Neuropathic disorders**
   Hollow viscus neuropathy, Parkinson's, paraneoplastic syndrome, Shy-Drager

9. **Postviral gastroparesis**
   Idiopathic gastroparesis with or without gastric dysrhythmias

Table 70.3 Treatment of nausea and vomiting based on gastric electrical and emptying test results

Category 1	Category 2	Category 3	Category 4
Test results Gastric dysrhythmia and gastroparesis	**Test results** Gastric dysrhythmia and normal emptying	**Test results** Normal gastric rhythm and emptying	**Test results** Normal gastric rhythm and gastroparesis
Diagnosis Severe gastric myoelectro-contractile disorder	**Diagnosis** Gastric myoelectrical disorder	**Diagnosis** Visceral hypersensitivity nongastric causes	**Diagnosis** Mechanical obstruction[†] Electro-contractile dissociation
Treatment Nausea/Vomiting Diet Prokinetic agents G-tube/J-tube Hyperalimentation Acustimulation Gastric pacemaker	**Treatment** Nausea/Vomiting Diet Prokinetic agents ?Anti-arrhythmic agents	**Treatment** Nausea/Vomiting Diet ?Neurosensory agents Tricyclic agents Drugs for fundic/antrum relaxation Further workup for nongastric causes	**Treatment** Surgery[†] Nausea/vomiting **Diet** Prokinetic agents

G-tube, gastrostomy tube; J-tube, jejunostomy tube.
[†] Mechanical obstruction in Diagnosis section relates to Surgey in Treatment section.

MEDICAL THERAPIES FOR NAUSEA AND VOMITING

In this section, the treatment of nausea and vomiting will focus on the patients seen by gastroenterologists. Disorders listed in Table 70.1 that have specific treatments have been excluded. Common disorders causing nausea and vomiting such as esophagitis or gastric ulceration and obstructions have been diagnosed and treated or eliminated by standard diagnostic tests for these disorders. Table 70.3 indicates drug, diet, and nondrug treatment approaches based on the four gastric pathophysiological categories described above. Table 70.4 lists specific pharmacologic and non-pharmacologic agents and endoscopic treatments for nausea and vomiting. The drugs are arbitrarily separated into neuromuscular agents, which are known to increase gastric contractility, and neurosensory agents whose mechanism of action is generally related to neural receptors.

Benzamides

Metoclopramide

Metoclopramide (Reglan) has been prescribed by gastroenterologists for over 25 years. Metoclopramide is a potent antiemetic and antinausea drug with multiple mechanisms of action that include dopamine (D_2) receptor antagonist activity, serotonin 5-hydroxytryptamine type 3 (5-HT_3) antagonist activity, 5-HT_4 agonist activity and some anticholinesterase activity.[53] Metoclopramide is used for nausea and vomiting associated with functional dyspepsia, diabetic and idiopathic gastroparesis, although it has not been studied in double-blind, placebo-controlled trials.

The dosage of metoclopramide is 10–20 mg by mouth 30 minutes before meals and before bedtime. The drug can be given by mouth, intravenously, or intramuscularly. Because it can be given intravenously, it is frequently used for hospitalized patients with nausea and vomiting. Central nervous system side effects of metoclopramide are significant, particularly fatigue, depression,

Parkinson's-type side effects, and tardive dyskinesia with chronic use. These side effects may be seen in 20–30% of patients.

Cisapride

Cisapride (Propulsid) is a substituted benzamide approved and then withdrawn from the market by the FDA because of serious but rare cardiac dysrhythmias, including torsade des pointes and ventricular fibrillation. Cisapride is available through compassionate clearance applications with Jansen Pharmaceutical. Cisapride is a 5-HT_4 receptor agonist that releases acetylcholine from cholinergic motor neurons and increases the rate of gastric emptying.[54] The drug also relaxes the fundus of the stomach. Cisapride does not cross the blood–brain barrier and does not produce the depression or neurological side effects of metoclopramide.

Cisapride improved symptoms in diabetic gastroparesis in some, but not all patients. Cisapride eradicated gastric dysrhythmias and improved symptoms in patients with functional dyspepsia. Dosage of cisapride is 10–20 mg by mouth 30 minutes before each meal and before bedtime. Side effects include crampy abdominal pain and diarrhea. Thus, the drug may be prescribed at a lower dose, such as 5 mg 3–4 times per day when initiating treatment. Cisapride at a dose of 5–10 mg 3 times a day significantly reduced dyspepsia symptoms including nausea, compared with placebo.[55]

Domperidone

Domperidone (Motilium) is a substituted benzamide and peripheral dopamine (D_2) antagonist.[56] Domperidone does not cross the blood–brain barrier and does not evoke central nervous system side effects like metoclopramide. Domperidone binds D_2 receptors in the circumventricular organs of the fourth ventricle and area postrema and in the stomach.[56]

Treatment with domperidone decreased nausea and vomiting related to diabetic gastroparesis. In a study by Koch et al., domperidone corrected gastric dysrhythmias and reduced nausea while the rate of gastric emptying did not improve.[22] This study

Table 70.4 Drug and nondrug therapies used to treat symptoms of nausea and vomiting

Drug	Mechanisms of action	Dosage	Side effects/adverse effects
NEUROMUSCULAR AGENTS			
Substituted benzamides Metoclopramide	Dopamine (D_2) receptor antagonist, 5-HT_3-receptor antagonist, 5-HT_4 agonist	5–20 mg before meals and at bedtime	Extrapyramidal symptoms, dystonic reactions, anxiety, drowsiness, hyperprolactinemia
Cisapride*	5-HT_4-receptor agonist	5–20 mg before meals	Cardiac dysrhythmias, diarrhea, abdominal discomfort
Domperidone†	D_2-receptor antagonist (peripheral)	10–20 mg before meals and at bedtime	Hyperprolactinemia
Macrolides Erythromycin	Motilin agonist	75–250 mg q.i.d.	Nausea, diarrhea, abdominal cramps, rash
Serotonin agonists Tegaserod	Partial 5-HT_4 agonist	2–6 mg t.i.d.	Diarrhea, abdominal pain
NEUROSENSORY AGENTS			
Serotonin antagonists Ondansetron	5-HT_3 antagonist	4.0–8.0 mg b.i.d., p.o., i.v.	Headache, increased LFTs
Granisetron	5-HT_3 antagonist	2 mg q.d.	Headache, increased LFTs
Phenothiazines Prochlorperazine	CNS sites	5–10 mg t.i.d., p.o.	Hypotension
Antihistamines Aromethazine	CNS, H_1 antagonist	25 mg b.i.d., p.o.	Drowsiness
Dimenhydrinate	H_1 antagonist	50 mg q.i.d., p.o.	Drowsiness
Cyclizine	H_1 antagonist	50 mg q.i.d., p.o.	Drowsiness
Butyrophenones Droperidol	Central dopamine antagonist	2.5–5.0 mg i.v., q 2 h	Sedation, hypotension
Antidepressants Amitriptyline	CNS sites	50 mg q.h.s.	Constipation
Benzodiazepines Borazepam	CNS sites	0.5–1.0 mg q.i.d., p.o.	Drowsiness, lightheadedness
NONDRUG THERAPIES			
Acupuncture	Spinal/vagal	Variable	Local tenderness
Acupressure	Afferents		
Acustimulation	Endorphins		
Gastric electrical stimulation	?Vagal Afferents?	12 cpm, 330 microsec 5 mA	Pocket infection
Gastric pacing	Control dysrhythmias Improve gastric emptying	3 cpm, 300 millisec 4 mA	Pocket infection
ENDOSCOPIC THERAPIES			
Botox injection of pylorus	Relax pyloric muscle	20 U per quadrant	None
Balloon dilation of pylorus	Stretch pyloric muscle	N/A	Perforation, bleeding
Radiofrequency ablation	Improve yield pressure, improve gastric myoelectrical activity	N/A	Transient dysphagia

* Compassionate clearance use only.
† Not approved in the United States.

indicated that eradication of gastric dysrhythmias was more relevant to symptom reduction than increasing the rate of gastric emptying. In patients with diabetic gastropathy, domperidone significantly improved symptoms compared with placebo. The drug also provided sustained relief of nausea in patients with nausea and vomiting with or without gastroparesis for an average of 18 months.[57]

Domperidone dosage is 10–20 mg by mouth 4 times per day. Side effects are related to increase in prolactin release from the posterior pituitary. Breast tenderness and galactorrhea are seen in approximately 5% of patients. Domperidone is not approved in the United States, although it is an over-the-counter drug in many countries.

Macrolides

Erythromycin

Erythromycin is a macrolide antibiotic that increases the rate of gastric emptying in patients with diabetic and idiopathic gastroparesis.[58] Erythromycin stimulates strong antral contractions in healthy individuals and these contractions are associated with nausea and abdominal cramps. These same side effects are often a limiting factor in treating patients with nausea and vomiting.[59]

The erythromycin molecule is similar to the gut hormone motilin, which is located on nerve and smooth muscle in the gastric antrum. Motilin-like molecules such as erythromycin increase gastric emptying by stimulating the motilin receptor and increasing gastric contractility.[58] Macrolide compounds also stimulate contractions in the small bowel and may produce abdominal cramps and diarrhea. In one report only 30% of patients who were given erythromycin for nausea, vomiting, and gastroparesis were able to tolerate the drug because of side effects.[59] Erythromycin is prescribed in doses ranging from 75–250 mg by mouth 4 times a day. Intravenous infusions may be used in hospitalized patients with gastric stasis.

Serotonin agonists

Tegaserod

Tegaserod is an amino guanidine-indole which resembles serotonin and is a partial 5-HT$_4$ agonist.[60] Tegaserod improves constipation-predominant irritable bowel syndrome in women.[61] Tegaserod also increases the rate of gastric emptying and may have beneficial effects in the treatment of dyspepsia-like symptoms with or without gastroparesis.[62] The FDA has not approved the use of tegaserod for gastroparesis or dyspepsia symptoms.

Tegaserod is prescribed 6 mg b.i.d. for constipation-predominant irritable bowel syndrome. Doses from 2 mg t.i.d. to 6 mg q.i.d. have been prescribed in studies of dyspepsia and gastroparesis. The drug has no reported effect on cardiac electrical rhythms and no central nervous system side effects. Common side effects are abdominal cramps and diarrhea which are temporary and routinely resolve after several days of therapy.

5-HT$_3$ serotonin antagonists

In patients with normal endoscopy, normal gastric emptying, and normal gastric electrical activity, the cause of the symptoms may relate to visceral hypersensitivity, central nervous system mechanisms, or as yet unidentified pathophysiologies. A variety of non-specific antinausea therapies are available. The 5-HT$_3$ antagonist drugs are effective in controlling vomiting related to cancer chemotherapy drugs[34] and postoperative nausea and vomiting.[63] In nausea and vomiting related to the gastrointestinal tract, these same drugs are generally ineffective. There are no studies indicating that they are of benefit for patients with gastroparesis or dyspepsia.

Ondansetron

Ondansetron was the first drug to significantly decrease the nausea and vomiting induced by cancer chemotherapy agents. Ondansetron is a specific 5-HT$_3$ antagonist. 5-HT$_3$ receptors are present in the area postrema of the brain, as well as vagal afferent nerve fibers from the stomach and duodenum, but the precise mechanism of action of this drug is not known.[34]

Ondansetron tablets may be prescribed at doses of 4–8 mg, although doses as high as 32 mg a day may be used. The drug is available for intravenous infusion and severely nauseated patients with GI disorders may be given a short empirical trial of intravenous ondansetron. No studies are available to confirm effectiveness in this clinical setting.

Granisetron

Granisetron is a 5-HT$_3$ receptor antagonist also approved for the treatment of nausea and vomiting due to cancer chemotherapy drugs. There are no studies of granisetron in gastrointestinal disorders of nausea and vomiting.

Phenothiazines

Prochlorperazine

Prochlorperazine (Compazine) is the drug commonly chosen for empiric treatment of mild to moderate nausea of unknown cause. The drug has non-specific actions in the central nervous system. It is prescribed at a dose of 5–10 mg orally 3–4 times a day for short periods of time. Prochlorperazine may be given in intramuscular injections or suppository form. The side effects of prochlorperazine are many and range from hypotension to spastic torticollis and dystonia to tardive dyskinesia.

Antihistamines

Promethazine

Promethazine (Phenergan) is used to treat mild to moderate nausea. This is an antihistamine (H$_1$ antagonist) drug which frequently induces drowsiness and limits daily activities. Some patients with gastric dysrhythmias or unexplained nausea respond to promethazine when other drugs fail to help them. Promethazine may also be given in a subcutaneous or intravenous form. When necessary, intramuscular injections are also possible. Doses range from 12.5 to 25 mg every 4–6 hours.

Dimenhydrinate and cyclizine

Histamine$_1$ antagonists are a class of drugs used to treat motion sickness. These drugs have not been studied in patients who have nausea and vomiting due to gastrointestinal neuromuscular disorders. Dimenhydrinate and cyclizine decrease gastric dysrhythmias and motion sickness symptoms, indicating that the drug also may act on the peripheral end-organ target – the stomach.[64] Side effects are drowsiness.

Butyrophenones

Droperidol

Droperidol (Inapsine) is a D$_2$ antagonist and potent antiemetic administered subcutaneously, intramuscularly, or intravenously. Droperidol is useful for the hospitalized patient with severe nausea and vomiting where control of these symptoms and some level of sedation is needed (personal observations). No controlled studies have been published on the efficacy of droperidol in treating nausea and vomiting from gastric neuromuscular disorders.

Antidepressant drugs

Amitriptyline

Amitriptyline (Elavil) reduced unexplained nausea and vomiting in a series of patients who received 50 mg q.h.s. Side effects include constipation.[65]

DIET THERAPY FOR NAUSEA AND VOMITING

Dietary recommendations for patients with disturbed gastric neuromuscular function are as important as selecting a rational drug for treatment of nausea and vomiting. From a neuromuscular standpoint, the impaired stomach is unable to receive, mix, or empty ingested food in a regular, efficient, and comfortable manner. Indeed, most patients with gastric neuromuscular abnormalities have increased nausea, gastric fullness, distention, and bloating after ingestion of food. Therefore, it is important that the gastroenterologist provide some counseling in terms of diet for these patients.

Intravenous hydration is needed for the patients who become hypovolemic. The Nausea and Vomiting Diet is a common-sense approach that patients easily grasp. The diet assists them in directing daily dietary choices based on their symptoms. The diet lists foods which are easily mixed and emptied from the stomach.

Intravenous hydration

Patients with recalcitrant nausea and vomiting may become dehydrated. In severe cases, the patients present to the emergency department and require intravenous fluids and possibly hospitalization to replace fluid losses and remedy electrolyte deficiencies. When intravenous hydration is completed and nausea is decreased to some extent, the Nausea and Vomiting Diet is begun.

Nausea and Vomiting (gastroparesis) Diet

The Steps 1–3 of the Nausea and Vomiting Diet are outlined in Table 70.5.[1] The diet is reviewed with the patient to educate them in regards to selection of foods which will require the least gastric neuromuscular work. By reducing the amount of gastric work of mixing and emptying foodstuffs for patients with known neuromuscular impairment of the stomach, symptoms such as nausea and vomiting are decreased. The food selection will depend on how the patient is feeling on a particular day or series of days.

Step 1 is begun when the severe nausea and vomiting has resolved to some extent. Hydration is completed and various drug treatments are usually employed during this time. The patient is instructed to sip liquids that contain salt and water such as Gatorade or bouillon. Patients with severe nausea and vomiting may only be able to ingest 1–2 ounces of these liquids at a time

Table 70.5 Nausea and Vomiting Diet

Diet	Goal	Avoid
Step 1: Sports drinks and bouillon For severe nausea and vomiting: • Small volumes of salty liquids, with some caloric content to avoid dehydration • Multiple vitamin	1000–1500 cc/day in multiple servings (e.g., 120 cc servings over 12–14 h) Patient can sip 30 cc at a time to reach approximately 120 cc/h	Citrus drinks of all kinds; highly sweetened drinks
Step 2: Soups If sports drink or bouillon tolerated: • Soup with noodles or rice and crackers • Peanut butter, cheese, and crackers in small amounts • Caramels or other chewy confection • Ingest above foods in at least 6 small-volume meals/day • Multiple vitamin	Approximately 1500 calories/day to avoid dehydration and maintain weight (often more realistic than weight gain)	Creamy, milk-based liquids
Step 3: Starches, chicken, fish If Step 2 is tolerated: • Noodles, pastas, potatoes (mashed or baked), rice, baked chicken breast, fish (all easily mixed and emptied by the stomach) • Ingest solids in at least 6 small-volume meals/day • Multiple vitamin	Common foods that patient finds interesting and satisfying and that evoke minimal nausea/vomiting symptoms	Fatty foods that delay gastric emptying; red meats and fresh vegetables that require considerable trituration; pulpy fibrous foods that promote formation of bezoars

with a goal of 1.0–1.5 liters each day to prevent dehydration. A chewable multivitamin should be taken daily. If these liquids are successfully kept down over the course of 24 hours, then the patient may advance to Step 2. (Note that Step 1 is *not* a clear liquid diet which in most hospitals includes orange juice, grapefruit juice, and other citric acid-containing liquids.)

Step 2 of the gastroparesis diet emphasizes soups, such as broth with noodles or rice. Creamy milk-based soups are often difficult to mix and empty for the stomach impaired by gastric neuromuscular dysfunction. Soups and crackers should be consumed 4–6 times per day in small amounts. Yogurt may be tried in small amounts. A multivitamin is also taken daily. (Note that Step 2 is *not* a full liquid diet which in most hospitals includes milkshakes, puddings, and other milk-based foods which are not tolerated by many patients with gastric neuromuscular disorders.)

Protein drinks have a beneficial effect in patients with nausea and vomiting of pregnancy and nausea associated with motion sickness. High-protein compared with high-fat or high-carbohydrate drinks reduced nausea of pregnancy significantly and reduced gastric dysrhythmias.[66] Similar results were found when high-protein drinks were ingested prior to exposure to an optokinetic rotating drum.[67] Thus, protein drinks may be used in the Step 2 diet. If Step 2 is well tolerated, then the patient may advance to Step 3.

Step 3 of the Nausea and Vomiting Diet emphasizes the ingestion of starches and white meats such as chicken and fish. Potatoes, pasta, rice, and breads may be ingested in six small meals per day. Chicken breast or turkey breast or fish are added in small amounts. Starches are emptied from the stomach more rapidly than proteins, which are emptied more rapidly than fats. Thus, the emphasis of Step 3 is on starches and white meats. A multivitamin is also taken each day. Fried, fatty foods should be avoided, because they delay gastric emptying, and fresh fruits and vegetables contain fiber that are the most difficult foodstuffs to empty from the stomach.[43] These fibers become phytobezoars in patients with the most severe gastroparesis. (Note that Step 3 is *not* a regular diet which in most hospitals includes red meats and fresh vegetables which are difficult to empty for patients with gastric neuromuscular disorders.)

Once the patient understands the rationale for Steps 1, 2, and 3 of the diet, food selections can be adjusted by the patient depending on their symptoms during a particular day. The goal is to ingest enough liquids to avoid dehydration and enough calories to maintain weight or perhaps gain some weight, while minimizing postprandial nausea and other dyspepsia symptoms.

Gastrostomy and jejunostomy

Additional steps must be taken for patients with severe and recalcitrant nausea and vomiting with greater than 10% weight loss or weight loss below ideal weight, despite drug therapies and diet counseling. The physician may consider the placement of a gastrostomy tube for venting and a jejunostomy tube for small bowel enteral nutrition.

The patient can vent the stomach through an endoscopically placed gastrostomy tube and thereby avoid vomiting episodes and the abdominal discomfort and fatigue associated with recurrent vomiting. Medications and electrolyte solutions may be given through the gastrostomy tube. The venting gastrostomy improves the quality of life for these patients. Skin infection at the site of the gastrostomy tube often occurs.

A duodenal extension tube for jejunal feeding may be placed through the gastrostomy tube, but these tubes are frequently returned to the stomach with any episode of vomiting. Thus, duodenal extensions are usually very short-lived. A separate jejunostomy tube, placed by the surgeons or inserted percutaneously by the gastroenterologist, are more secure sites for enteral feeding. Successful enteral feeding gives patients respite from the frequent nausea and postprandial distress induced by the ingestion of food by mouth.

Central hyperalimentation

Central hyperalimentation should be reserved for the rare patient who is unable to tolerate jejunal feedings and in whom weight loss continues to be a significant problem. Patients with gastrointestinal neuromuscular dysfunction are susceptible to central line infections. Therefore, this approach to nutrition should be considered a last resort.

NON-DRUG THERAPY FOR NAUSEA AND VOMITING

Nondrug therapy refers to acupuncture, acustimulation, gastric electrical stimulation, and a variety of therapies delivered with endoscopic methods. At the present time there is a paucity of effective drugs for the treatment of nausea and vomiting and therefore other means, such as devices, are needed to reduce the noxious symptoms.

Acupuncture, acupressure, and acustimulation

Acupuncture involves insertion and rotation of acupuncture needles in specific sites to reduce nausea and vomiting. In acupressure the stimulation is provided with finger pressure or other devices applied to the acupuncture point. Acupuncture and acupressure decrease nausea and vomiting related to cancer chemotherapy and postoperative nausea and vomiting when stimulation of P6 is used.[68,69] Nausea and gastric dysrhythmia were decreased during acupuncture therapy at P6 in patients with chronic nausea and vomiting.[70]

Acustimulation refers to electrical stimulation of P6 or other acupuncture points with electrical current passed through the electrodes. Acustimulation at P6 decreases symptoms of motion sickness and gastric dysrhythmias induced by a rotating drum.[71] Acustimulation with a portable wrist band device also decreased nausea of pregnancy.[72] The mechanism of action of acupuncture, acupressure, and acustimulation is unknown but somatovisceral reflexes are likely involved. Combinations of acustimulation with drug therapy have not been studied.

Gastric electrical stimulation

Gastric electrical stimulation refers to low-amplitude, 12 cpm stimulation of brief duration applied by electrodes sutured onto the gastric antrum and connected to an implantable stimulation device. In patients with refractory nausea and vomiting, significant improvement in the rate of nausea and vomiting was reported.[73] These studies confirmed preliminary studies that showed this faster frequency of stimulation decreased nausea.[74] The mechanism of beneficial effect is unknown. On the other hand, pacing the stomach at the normal slow wave rhythm did not improve gastric emptying. Hocking et al. showed no improvement in gastric emptying during gastric pacing of patients who had various surgical resections.[75] An array of electrodes placed around the stomach induced sequential gastric contractions and improved the rate of gastric emptying in dogs.[76] Further studies are required to define the optimal stimulation parameters and the patients best suited to this approach to treatment.

Endoscopic therapy for nausea and vomiting due to gastric neuromuscular disorders

Botox injection of the pylorus has been reported to improve nausea and vomiting from idiopathic and diabetic gastroparesis.[77] Balloon dilation of the pylorus is used to treat stenoses due to chronic ulcer disease and postsurgical anastomoses that have become strictured. Radiofrequency ablation used to treat patients with GERD and dyspepsia resulted in improvement in gastric myoelectrical activity and emptying.

FUTURE DIRECTIONS

Effective treatment of nausea and vomiting is presently very poor for many patients. Thus, there are great opportunities for development of drugs, diet, and nondrug therapies for the treatment of nausea and vomiting. The improvement in therapies must be based on improved knowledge of the pathophysiology of nausea. Drugs that eradicate gastric dysrhythmia are needed, but it is unclear if these drugs should be directed towards peripheral targets – interstitial cells of Cajal, enteric neurons, or smooth muscle cells. Other drugs are needed to affect vagal afferent or efferent pathways, autonomic nervous system control centers in the hypothalamus, and more cortical level areas of the central nervous system.

For the gastroenterologist, a pragmatic approach ideally involves the use of drugs to eradicate objective abnormalities such as gastric dysrhythmias, gastric relaxation or fundic relaxation abnormalities, or gastroparesis, and to record the accompanying reduction in symptoms. Drugs that improve gastric rhythmicity and gastric emptying will be discovered and many of these drugs will relate to the serotonin family of receptors. Selected novel macrolides will improve antral contractions and the rate of gastric emptying. Dopamine-2 antagonists such as domperidone are very helpful in the treatment of nausea and hopefully new D_2 agents will be discovered.

Studies are needed to evaluate specific nutrients that provide calories *and* promote improved neuromuscular function (nutriceuticals). The high-protein meals described above had beneficial effects on nausea and specific proteins may have positive effects. Herbs such as ginger may also help some patients with nausea and more studies are needed.

Treatment of nausea and vomiting with electrical stimulation provided by pacemaker-type devices is an exciting area of therapy. More research is needed to obtain optimal stimulation parameters and patient selection, but this area will advance and help with the most difficult patients. Endoscopic therapies will also evolve as pacemakers will be implanted via endoscopy. Radiofrequency ablation technologies may be used to treat gastric dysrhythmias much like it is used for control of cardiac dysrhythmias. The role of the pylorus in nausea and vomiting will become clearer and the use of dilation or Botox-type therapies will become more rational.

AUTHOR'S RECOMMENDATIONS AND SUMMARY

In patients with unexplained nausea and vomiting, the first step is to consider the broad differential diagnosis of the causes of nausea and vomiting. After structural and metabolic abnormalities are eliminated, the digestive system should be evaluated with the focus eventually on stomach neuromuscular dysfunction. When mucosal abnormalities are eliminated, then gastric neuromuscular disorders should be considered. Results of electrogastrography and gastric emptying tests establish objective pathophysiological diagnoses and rational treatment can be designed.

My first therapeutic steps for patients with nausea and vomiting and gastric dysrhythmia or gastroparesis include selecting a standard drug such as metoclopramide at low doses (5–10 mg t.i.d.) for 3–4 weeks. If there is no response, then I will increase the dosage (20 mg t.i.d.) and assess symptoms in another 4 weeks. If there is no improvement, I will change to tegaserod as discussed above and go through the same process, beginning with a low dose (2 mg b.i.d.) and advancing to a high dose (6 mg t.i.d.) over 4–8 weeks. If there is no improvement, my next drug selection would be domperidone and then erythromycin. If these drugs do not help, I will move to the antihistamine drugs and try them in a sequential fashion. I instruct the patients in the gastroparesis diet at the first visit and follow up with more details about the diet at later visits.

In patients who have very poor water load tests, indicating poor gastric relaxation or capacity, I will also prescribe calcium channel blockers or nitrates 30 minutes before the meals in an effort to relax the gastric smooth muscle and improve postprandial symptoms such as bloating and distention. If the EGG and gastric emptying tests are normal, then I consider nongastric causes of the symptoms and consider other diagnostic tests. In these patients, I also will prescribe amitriptyline.

If symptoms continue and weight loss develops with frequent vomiting, I may then offer a gastrostomy tube for venting purposes. A jejunal feeding tube may be necessary if weight loss is significant. Advanced therapies such as gastric electrical stimulation are discussed.

If the patient requires hospitalization, then rigorous hydration is provided. Intravenous metoclopramide is started. I will consider intravenous droperidol if hydration and metoclopramide are not helpful in reducing symptoms. Compazine suppository and phenergan by suppository or intravenous route may also be necessary to quell nausea and vomiting early in the hospital course. When vomiting has decreased, usually in 1–2 days, I will begin Step 1 of the nausea and vomiting gastroparesis diet. This diet is often very helpful even in the absence of documented gastroparesis.

The approach to the diagnosis and treatment of patients with chronic and unexplained nausea and vomiting remains very problematic. If nausea could be totally controlled in the future, then vomiting would cease to be a symptom to consider. For now, there is much to be learned to advance our understanding of the diagnosis and therapy of these patients.

ACKNOWLEDGMENTS

The author wishes to acknowledge the excellent secretarial assistance of Renea Donley in the preparation of this manuscript.

REFERENCES

1. Koch KL. Approach to the patient with nausea and vomiting. In: Yamada T, ed. Textbook of gastroenterology. 2nd edn. Philadelphia, PA: JB Lippincott; 1995:731–749.

2. Fischler B, Tack J, DeGucht V, et al. Heterogeneity of symptom pattern, psychosocial factors, and pathophysiological mechanisms in severe functional dyspepsia. Gastroenterology 2003; 124:903–910.

   Factor analysis was utilized to determine relationships of physiological and psychological mechanisms in patients with functional dyspepsia. Four major factors described this population. Factor 1 was characterized by nausea, vomiting, early satiety, and weight loss. This study emphasized that nausea and vomiting are distinct symptoms from other upper GI symptoms (i.e., bloating, abdominal pain, belching) in patients with functional dyspepsia.

3. Talley NJ, Stanghellini V, Heading RC, et al. Functional gastroduodenal disorders. In: Drossman DA, ed. Rome II: functional gastrointestinal disorders: diagnosis, pathophysiology, and treatment – a multinational consensus. McLean, VA: Deganon Associates; 2000:299–350.

4. Muth ER, Stern RM, Thayer JF, et al. Assessment of the multiple dimensions of nausea. The Nausea Profile (NP). J Psychosom Res 1996; 40:511–520.

5. Lang IM, Sarna SK, Condon RE. Gastrointestinal motor correlates of vomiting in the dog: Quantification and characterization as an independent phenomenon. Gastroenterology 1986; 90:40.

6. Brzana RJ, Koch KL. Gastroesophageal reflux disease presenting with intractable nausea. Ann Intern Med 1997; 126:704–707.

   Heartburn secondary to gastroesophageal reflux is common; but in some patients nausea is the predominant symptom of GERD. In this study esophageal pH results showed that nausea correlated with acid reflux events. Nausea was successfully treated with proton pump inhibitors and, in one case, fundoplication.

7. Geldorf H, Van Der Schee EJ, Smout AJPM, et al. Myoelectrical activity of the stomach in gastric ulcer patients: An electrogastrographic study. J Gastrointest Motil 1989; 1:122.

8. Kim TW, Beckett EAH, Hanna R, et al. Regulation of pacemaker frequency in the murine gastric antrum. J Physiol (London) 2002; 538:145–157.

9. Huisinga JD. Physiology and pathophysiology of the interstitial cell of Cajal: From bench to bedside II. Gastric motility: lessons from mutant mice on slow waves and innervation. Am J Physiol 2001; 281:G1129–G1134.

10. He CL, Soffer EE, Ferris CD, et al. Loss of interstitial cells of Cajal and inhibitory innervation in insulin-dependent diabetes. Gastroenterology 2001; 121:427–434.

    This clinical and pathological report documented loss of interstitial cells of Cajal, the pacemaker cells of the stomach, in diabetic gastroparesis. Loss of the ICC in diabetes may account for gastric dysrhythmias and gastroparesis in these patients and indicates new pathophysiological mechanism(s) for this disorder.

11. De Giorgio R, Guerrini S, Barbara G, et al. Inflammatory neuropathies of the enteric nervous system. Gastroenterology 2004; 126:1872–1883.

12. Thompson WG, Longstreth G, Drossman DA, et al. Functional bowel disorders and functional abdominal pain. In: Drossman DA, ed. Rome II: functional gastrointestinal disorders. 2nd edn. McLean, VA: Deganon Associates; 2000:351–397.

13. Hinder RA, Kelley KA. Human gastric pacesetter potential: Sight of origin, spread, and response to gastric transection and of proximal vagotomy. Am J Surg 1997; 133:29–33.

14. Chen JDZ, Schirmer BD, McCallum RW. Serosal and cutaneous recordings of gastric myoelectrical activity in patients with gastroparesis. Am J Physiol 1994; 266:G90–G98.

15. Koch KL, Stern RM. Handbook of electrogastrography. New York: Oxford Press; 2003.

16. Koch KL. The stomach: electrogastrography. In: Schuster M, Crowell M, Koch KL, eds. Atlas of gastrointestinal motility. Ontario, Canada: BC Decker; 2002:185–201.

17. Stern RM, Koch KL, Stewart WR, et al. Spectral analysis of tachygastria recorded during motion sickness. Gastroenterology 1987; 92:92–97.

18. Koch KL, Xu L, Bingaman S, et al. Effects of ondansetron on morphine-induced nausea, vasopressin and gastric myoelectrical activity in healthy humans. Gastroenterology 1993; 104:A535.

19. Abell TM, Malagelada J-R. Glucagon-evoked gastric dysrhythmias in humans shown by an improved electrogastrographic technique. Gastroenterology 1985; 88:1932–1940.

20. Hasler WL, Soudah HC, Dulai G, et al. Mediation of hyperglycemia-evoked gastric slow-wave dysrhythmias by endogenous prostaglandins. Gastroenterology 1995; 108:727–736.

21. Koch KL, Stern RM, Vasey M, et al. Gastric dysrhythmias and nausea of pregnancy. Dig Dis Sci 1990; 35:961–968.

22. Koch KL, Stern RM, Stewart WR, et al. Gastric emptying and gastric myoelectrical activity in patients with symptomatic diabetic gastroparesis: Effect of long-term domperidone treatment. Am J Gastroenterol 1989; 84:1069–1075.

23. Bersherdas K, Leahy A, Mason I, et al. The effect of cisapride on dyspepsia symptoms and the electrogastrogram in patients with non-ulcer dyspepsia. Aliment Pharmacol Ther 1998; 12:755–759.

24. Cucchiara S, Minella R, Riezzo G, et al. Reversal of gastric electrical dysrhythmias by cisapride in children with functional dyspepsia: report of three cases. Dig Dis Sci 1992; 37:1136–1140.

25. Rothstein RD, Alavai A, Reynolds JC. Electrogastrography in patients with gastroparesis and effect of long-term cisapride. Dig Dis Sci 1993; 38:1518–1524.

26. Koch KL, Hong S-P, Xu L. Reproducibility of gastric myoelectrical activity and the water load test in patients with dysmotility-like dyspepsia symptoms and in control subjects. J Clin Gastroenterol 2000; 31(2):125–129.

27. Stanghellini V, Tosetti C, Paternico A, et al. Risk indicators of delayed gastric emptying of solids in patients with functional dyspepsia. Gastroenterology 1996; 110:1036–1042.

28. Brzana RJ, Bingaman S, Koch KL. Gastric myoelectrical activity in patients with gastric outlet obstruction and idiopathic gastroparesis. Am J Gastroenterol 1998; 93:1083–1089.

29. Liberski SM, Koch KL, Atnip RG, et al. Ischemic gastroparesis: Resolution of nausea, vomiting and gastroparesis after mesenteric artery revascularization. Gastroenterology 1990; 99:252–257.

30. Koch KL, Stern RM, Vasey MW, et al. Neuroendocrine and gastric myoelectrical responses to illusory self-motion in man. Am J Physiol 1990; 258:E304–E310.

31. Uitjtdehaage SHJ, Stern RM, Koch KL. Effects of eating on vection-induced motion sickness, cardiac vagal tone and gastric myoelectrical activity. Psychophysiology 1992; 29:193–201.

32. Lang IM, Sarna SK, Condon RE. Gastrointestinal motor correlates of vomiting in the dog: Quantification and characterization as an independent phenomenon. Gastroenterology 1986; 90:40–47.

33. Lang IM, Sarna SK, Dodds WJ. The pharyngeal, esophageal, and proximal gastric responses associated with vomiting. Am J Physiol 1993; 265:G963–G972.

34. Cubeddu LX, Hoffmann IS, Fuenmayor NT, et al. Efficacy of ondansetron (GR 38032F) and the role of serotonin in cisplatin-induced nausea and vomiting. N Engl J Med 1990; 322:810.

35. Neilsen OH, Hvid-Jacobsen K, Lund P, et al. Gastric emptying and subjective symptoms of nausea: Lack of efforts of a 5-hydroxytryptamine, antagonist ondansetron on gastric emptying in patients with gastric stasis syndrome. Digestion 1990; 46:89.

36. Koch KL. Gastroparesis. In: Quigley EMM, Pfeiffer RF, eds. Neuro-gastroenterology. Philadelphia: Elsevier; 2004:163–180.

37. Camilleri M. Disorders of gastrointestinal motility and neurological diseases. Mayo Clin Proc 1990; 65:825–846.

38. O'Brien MD, Bruce BK, Camilleri M. The rumination syndrome: Clinical features other than manometric diagnosis. Gastroenterology 1995; 108:1024–1029.

39. Koch KL, Stern RM. Functional disorders of the stomach. Sem Gastrointest Dis 1996; 4:185–195.

40. Talley NJ, Stanghellini V, Heading RC, et al. Functional gastroduodenal disorders. Gut 1999; 45(II):1137–1142.

41. Carnett JB. Intercostal neuralgia as a cause of abdominal pain and tenderness. Surg Gynecol Obstet 1926; 12:625–635.

42. Van Der Voort IR, Osmanoglou E, Seybold M, et al. Electrogastrography as a diagnostic tool for delayed gastric emptying in functional dyspepsia and irritable bowel syndrome. Neurogastroenterol Motil 2003; 15:467–473.

43. Lin HC, Hasler WL. Disorders of gastric emptying. In: Yamada Y, ed. Textbook of gastroenterology. Philadelphia, PA: JB Lippincott; 1995:1318–1346.

44. Parkman H, Miller M, Trate D, et al. Electrogastrography and gastric emptying scintigraphy are complementary for assessment of dyspepsia. J Clin Gastroenterol 1997; 24:214–219.

45. Chial HJ, Camilleri C, Delgado-Aros S, et al. A nutrient drink test to assess maximum tolerated volume and postprandial symptoms. Effects of gender, body mass index, and age in health. Neurogastroenterol Motil 2002; 14:249-253.

46. Koch KL, Xu L, Hong S-P. Spectrum of gastric dysrhythmias and gastric emptying in 54 patients with chronic unexplained nausea and vomiting. Gastroenterology 2000; 118(4):A849.

47. Abell TL, Camilleri M, Hench VS, et al. Gastric electromechanical function and gastric emptying in diabetic gastroparesis. Eur J Gastroenterol Hepatology 1991; 3:163–167.

48. Noar MK, Koch KL. Effect of radiofrequency ablation on gastric dysrhythmias and gastric emptying in patients with gastroesophageal reflux disease (GERD) and functional dyspepsia. Gastroenterology 2003; 124:A98.

49. Geldof H, Van Der Schee EJ, Van Blankenstein M, et al. Electrogastrographic study of gastric myoelectrical activity in patients with nausea and vomiting. Gut 1986; 27:2799–2808.

50. Boeckxstaens GE, Hirsch DP, Van Locase DEN, et al. Impaired drinking capacity in patients with functional dyspepsia: Relationship with proximal stomach function. Gastroenterology 2001; 121:1054–1063.

51. Tack J, Piessevaux H, Caenepeel P, et al. Role of impaired gastric accommodation to a meal in functional dyspepsia. Gastroenterology 1998; 115:1346–1352.

52. Ladabaum U, Koshy SS, Woods ML, et al. Differential symptomatic and electrogastrographic effects of distal and proximal human gastric distention. Am J Physiol 1999; 275:G418–G424.

Balloon distention of the antrum in healthy volunteers elicited nausea and gastric dysrhythmias, particularly bradygastrias. This study indicated that stretch or distention of the antrum was a mechanism of nausea and gastric dysrhythmias, a mechanism that may also be relevant in nausea of gastroparesis or functional dyspepsia.

53. Albibi R, McCallum RW. Metoclopramide: pharmacology and clinical application. Ann Intern Med 1983; 98:86–95.

54. Wiseman LR, Faulds D. Cisapride: An updated review of its pharmacology therapeutics efficacy as a prokinetic agent in gastrointestinal motility disorders. Drugs 1994; 47:116–152.

55. Veldhuyzen van Zanten SJO, Jones MJ, Verlinden M, et al. Efficacy of cisapride and domperidone in functional (nonulcer) dyspepsia: a meta-analysis. Am J Gastroenterol 2001; 96:689–696.

56. Brogden RN, Carmine AA, Heel RC, et al. Domperidone: A review of its pharmacological activity, pharmacokinetics and therapeutic efficacy in the symptomatic treatment of chronic dyspepsia and as an antiemetic. Drugs 1982; 24:360–400.

57. Patterson DJ, Abell T, Rothstein R, et al. A double-blind multi-center comparison of domperidone and metoclopramide in the treatment of diabetic patients with symptoms of gastroparesis. Am J Gastroenterol 1999; 93:1230–1234.

58. Janssens J, Peeters TL, Vantrappen G, et al. Improvement of gastric emptying in diabetic gastroparesis by erythromycin. Preliminary studies. New Engl J Med 1990; 322:1028–1031.

59. Richards RD, Davenport K, McCallum RW. The treatment of idiopathic and diabetic gastroparesis with acute intravenous and chronic oral erythromycin. Am J Gastroenterol 1993; 88:203.

60. Camilleri M. Tegaserod. Aliment Pharmacol Ther 2001; 15:277–289.

61. Muller-Lissner SA, Fumagalli I, Bardhan KD, et al. Tegaserod, a 5-HT4 receptor partial agonist, relieves symptoms in irritable bowel syndrome patients with abdominal pain, bloating and constipation. Aliment Pharmacol Ther 2001; 15:1655–1656.

62. Tougas G, Chen Y, Luo D, et al. Tegaserod improves gastric emptying in patients with gastroparesis and dyspeptic symptoms. Gastroenterology 2003; 124:A54.

63. McKenzie R, Kovac A, O'Connor T, et al. Comparison of ondansetron versus placebo to prevent post-operative nausea and vomiting in women undergoing ambulatory gynecologic surgery. Anesthesiology 1993; 78:21.

64. Muth ER, Jokerst M, Stern RM, et al. Effects of dimenhydrinate on gastric tachyarrhythmia and symptoms of vection-induced motion sickness. Aviat Space Environ Med 1995; 66:1041–1045.

65. Prakash C, Lustman PJ, Freedland KE, et al. Tricyclic antidepressants for functional nausea and vomiting: clinical outcome in 37 patients. Dig Dis Sci 1998; 43:1951–1956.

66. Jednak MA, Shadigian EM, Kim MS, et al. Protein meals reduce nausea and gastric slow wave dysrhythmic activity in first trimester pregnancy. Am J Physiol 1999; 277:G855–G861.

High-protein meals were given to women with nausea of pregnancy. In contrast to high-carbohydrate and high-fat meals, the high-protein meals decreased nausea and reduced gastric dysrhythmias significantly. Protein meals represent new potential therapies for nausea.

67. Levine ME, Muth ER, Williamson MJ, et al. Protein-predominant meals inhibit development of gastric tachyarrhythmia, nausea in the symptoms of motion sickness. J Aliment Pharmacol Ther 2004; 19:583–590.

68. Dundee GW, Yang J, McMillan C. Non-invasive stimulation of the P6 (Neiguan) antiemetic acupuncture point in cancer chemotherapy. J R Soc Med 1991; 84:210–212.

69. Dundee JW, Ghaly RG, Bill KM, et al. Effect of stimulation of the P6 antiemetic point on post-operative nausea and vomiting. Br J Anaesth 1989; 63:612–618.

70. Koch KL, Bingaman S, Xu L, et al. Acute effects of acustimulation at Neiguan point on nausea and gastric myoelectrical activity in patients with chronic nausea. Gastroenterology 1997; 112:A763.

71. Hu S, Stern RM, Koch KL. Electrical acustimulation relieves vection-induced motion sickness. Gastroenterology 1992; 102:1854–1858.

72. Evans AT, Samuels SN, Marshall C, et al. Suppression of pregnancy-induced nausea and vomiting with sensory afferent stimulation. J Reproduct Med 1993; 38:603–606.

73. McCallum RW, Chen JD, Lin Z, et al. Gastric pacing improves emptying and symptoms in patients with gastroparesis. Gastroenterology 1998; 114:456–461.

74. Abell T, Hocking M, McCallum R, et al. Gastric electrical stimulation for medically refractory gastroparesis. Gastroenterology 2003; 125:421–428.

Gastric electrical stimulation was applied to the stomach via electrodes sutured to the subserosal area of the antrum in 33 patients with chronic gastroparesis. At 6 and 12 months after implantation, vomiting frequency was reduced significantly and overall symptom severity was decreased and quality of life scores were increased.

75. Hocking MP, Vogel SB, Sninsky CA. Human gastric myoelectrical activity and gastric emptying following gastric surgery and with pacing. Gastroenterology 1992; 103:1821–1826.

76. Mintchev MP, Sanmiguel CP, Amars M, et al. Microprocessor-controlled movement of solid gastric content using sequential neuro-electrical stimulation. Gastroenterology 2000; 118:258–263.

77. Miller LS, Szych GA, Kantor SB, et al. Treatment of idiopathic gastroparesis with injection of Botulinum toxin into the pyloric sphincter muscle. Am J Gastroenterol 2002; 97:1653–1660.

CHAPTER SEVENTY-ONE

71

Constipation and diarrhea

Charlene M. Prather

BACKGROUND

Perceptions regarding what constitutes normal or abnormal bowel habits vary greatly. Although most consider a daily bowel habit to be the norm, less than 40% of individuals in population-based studies fit this definition.[1] One-third of women defecate less than once daily, and 7% of men and 4% of women move their bowels more than once daily.[1] Patient reports of constipation and diarrhea are equally problematic. Many patients with symptoms compatible with diarrhea report a normal bowel habit.[2] In addition, there exists a higher prevalence of constipation when using self-reports compared to the more rigorous definitions used by the Rome II criteria (see below and Ch. 48).[3,4] The application of potential treatment regimens begins with a careful understanding of the perceived problem in bowel habit, rather than solely accepting the presence of diarrhea or constipation by self-report alone.

When measured using radiopaque markers, normal intestinal transit ranges from more than 12 hours to less than 120 hours, with little difference between males and females.[5] Normal stool frequency varies from 2 per day to 3 per week,[6,7] and varies by sex and race/ethnicity.[8,9] Women report fewer stools per week than men, and whites report more frequent stools than non-whites. Stool frequency provides only one measure of the bowel habit, with stool consistency and ease of passage also playing a role. Excessive looseness or hardness to the stool may be reported as diarrhea or constipation, respectively, regardless of the stool frequency. Similarly, fecal incontinence may be described as diarrhea in the setting of normal stool frequency. In addition, patients are more likely to describe straining or the passage of hard stools as constipation than considering infrequent defecation to represent constipation.[9] In contrast, the most common physician definition of constipation uses stool frequency with less than three bowel movements per week indicating constipation.

Given the variety of symptoms that may be reported as constipation, a standard definition has been developed by a group of international experts incorporating both frequency and the variety of symptoms reported by patients. These are known as the Rome II criteria:

Two or more of the following for at least 3 months:[4]
straining more than 25% of the time;
hard stools more than 25% of the time;
incomplete evacuation more than 25% of the time;
two or fewer bowel actions in 1 week.

This definition provides criteria for functional constipation, that is, constipation without other cause.

Constipation may result from a variety of underlying causes including inadequate dietary fiber, structural abnormalities, medical conditions, and medications (Tables 71.1 and 71.2). Additional categories of constipation include constipation as part of irritable bowel syndrome, slow transit constipation, and dyssynergic defecation. Constipation may be acute or chronic. Acute constipation includes a bowel habit alteration related to situational changes such as reduced dietary fiber, travel, bed rest, or new medications.[10-12] By definition, chronic constipation has been defined as symptoms present for 3 months or longer.[4] Individuals with a variety of medical conditions including diabetes mellitus, hyperparathyroidism, Parkinson's disease, and multiple sclerosis frequently experience constipation.[13-16] Structural abnormalities such as colonic strictures or neoplasia may also present with constipation. Although structural abnormalities are uncommon in the typical patient with chronic constipation, in the setting of new-onset or progressive constipation in a person at risk for colon neoplasia, appropriate screening is imperative.

Diarrhea typically refers to abnormal looseness of the stool and may include increased stool frequency. Acute diarrhea often results from infectious etiologies, while chronic diarrhea refers to symptoms that have been present for more than 4 weeks.[17] Chronic diarrhea may be categorized as secretory or osmotic

Table 71.1 Medications commonly implicated as contributing to constipation

Iron supplements

Calcium supplements

Calcium channel blockers

Clonidine

Progesterone

Opiates

Nonsteroidal antiinflammatory drugs

Bupropion

Nefazodone

Oxybutynin

Ondansetron

Table 71.2 Medical conditions frequently associated with constipation

Endocrine or metabolic
Diabetes mellitus
Hypothryoidism
Hypercalcemia
Uremia

Neurologic
Cerebrovascular disease
Parkinson's disease
Multiple sclerosis
Spinal cord injury
Autonomic dysfunction

Mechanical
Colon cancer
Colon stricture
Anal stenosis
Intussusception

Depression

Pregnancy

Scleroderma

based on the stool osmotic gap, inflammatory or infectious diarrhea, and fatty diarrhea.[18] The differential diagnosis for chronic diarrhea is large; however, a careful history and a few diagnostic tests help to categorize the type of diarrhea, narrowing the diagnostic possibilities. The following Rome II criteria are used to make the diagnosis of 'functional diarrhea' in patients for whom an investigation into the underlying cause of the diarrhea reveals no obvious cause:

At least 12 weeks, common which need not be consecutive, in the preceding 12 months of:[4]

Loose (mushy) or water stools;
Present >¾ of the time; *and*
No abdominal pain.

Constipation and diarrhea are common digestive complaints. The prevalence of constipation is estimated at 15% of the population,[19] while chronic diarrhea reported by 3–5% of the population.[18] Constipation and/or diarrhea are seen in irritable bowel syndrome in association with abdominal pain (see Ch. 48). Irritable bowel syndrome affects 14–20% of the population.[20,21] The presence of abdominal pain or discomfort associated with an altered bowel habit helps to differentiate irritable bowel syndrome from other causes of chronic diarrhea or chronic constipation. The presence of altered bowel function results in significant impairment to an individual's quality of life.[22,23]

Disorders of bowel function are first approached with a history and physical examination aimed at determining the underlying causes or category. Patients lacking worrisome features such as fever, weight loss, gastrointestinal bleeding, or an abnormal physical examination are candidates for initial empirical therapy. Persistent symptoms despite symptomatic therapy necessitate further evaluation to identify the underlying cause in order to more appropriately target treatment.

TREATMENT OF CONSTIPATION

Constipation is most often treated with an empirical trial of increased dietary fiber, the addition of a bulking agent, or osmotic laxative. Patients who fail to respond may be considered for further diagnostic evaluation. Before embarking on further diagnostic testing or treatment, fecal impaction should be excluded, particularly in patients of limited mobility and/or decreased cognition. The need for a colonic structural examination is based predominantly on the need for a colorectal cancer screening or the presence of worrisome features such as rectal bleeding. Laboratory tests commonly requested but for which there is little evidence to support their routine use include a complete blood count, thyroid function, calcium, and serum albumin. Other testing is based on the underlying clinical suspicion of a metabolic abnormality. Determination of the underlying category of constipation requires physiologic testing. Fortunately, few patients with chronic constipation require these tests, with physiologic testing reserved for patients who fail to respond to initial treatments. Colonic transit is most commonly assessed using radiopaque markers. Using the single capsule method, the retention of >20% of the markers at 120 hours indicate slowed colonic transit.[24] The presence of dyssynergic defecation (sometimes called 'pelvic floor dysfunction' or 'obstructed defecation') may be suspected in a patient with failure to expel a 50 mL water-filled balloon placed in the rectum. This balloon expulsion testing is used as a screening test for a defecatory disorder.[25] Confirmation of dyssynergic defecation may be determined by anorectal manometry, EMG (showing paradoxical contraction of the anal sphincter during strain), or defecography. Despite physiologic testing, most patients are found to have normal colonic transit, with approximately 40% of patients found to have slow transit or defecatory disorders.[26]

Principles of treatment

Despite folklore to the contrary, there exists little evidence to support increased fluid intake or exercise in the treatment of constipation.[27,28] The first step in treating patients with constipation focuses on increasing dietary fiber intake to the American Dietetic Association recommended 20–35 g of fiber per day.[29] The average American consumes far less than this amount. The slow addition of dietary fiber (increasing by approximately 5 g/day each week) may minimize the production of abdominal bloating and gas commonly reported by patients. Patients unable to increase their dietary fiber may use commercially available fiber supplements or bulking agents. Patients failing to respond to, or intolerant of, fiber supplementation may be treated with an osmotic laxative or prokinetic agent (e.g., 5-HT$_4$ agonist). Stimulant laxatives are reserved for patients with medication-induced (e.g., opioid) or very refractory constipation (Table 71.3). The treatment of constipation associated with irritable bowel syndrome is discussed in Chapter 48.

Fiber and bulking agents

Increased fiber intake results in improved colonic transit and stool output.[30] Fiber is an indigestible carbohydrate that retains water

Table 71.3 Agents commonly used in the treatment of constipation

Bulk laxatives	
Dietary fiber	20–35 grams per day
Psyllium	3–12 grams per day
Hydrolyzed guar gum	3–6 grams per day
Methylcellulose	3–12 grams per day
Osmotic laxatives	
Magnesium oxide	15–30 ml once or twice daily
Magnesium citrate	150–300 ml as needed
Lactulose	15–60 mL once or twice daily
Sorbitol 70%	15–60 mL once or twice daily
Polyethylene glycol	17–34 grams once or twice daily
Stimulant laxatives	
Bisacodyl	5–15 mg per day by mouth; 10 mg suppository
Senna	187 mg per day
Cascara sagrada	325 mg per day
Lubricating agent	
Mineral oil	5–20 mL per day
Prokinetic agent	
Tegaserod	6 mg twice daily
Miscellaneous	
Misoprostol	200 μg two to four times daily
Colchicine	0.6 mg three times per day

in the intestine and provides substrate for bacterial digestion.[31] Both mechanisms serve to increase stool bulk. Although wheat fiber is most commonly recommended, multiple sources of dietary fiber, including fruits, vegetables, legumes and other grains provide beneficial effects. Although called 'fiber supplements,' commercially available products work as bulking agents and include psyllium husk, carboxymethylcellulose, and calcium polycarbophil. Psyllium is the most commonly available and most studied bulking agent. Psyllium is natural plant product derived from the ground seeds of the herb *Plantago psyllium*. It forms a gel when mixed with water. Psyllium at a dose of 10 g/day increases stool weight, improves stool frequency, and the ease of defecation.[32] Psyllium is available in capsules, wafers, and powder formulations. The amount of fiber in these preparations varies greatly from 0.53 g/capsule, 6 g/2 wafer serving, and 3–6 g/powder serving. A variety of commercial preparations are available including generic store brands, Fiberall®, Hydrocil Instant®, Metamucil®, Perdiem®, and Konsyl®. Psyllium is considered to be a generally safe product although rare allergic reactions have occurred.[33] Other bulking agents include the hydrolyzed guar gum and synthetic polymers methylcellulose, carboxymethylcellulose, and calcium polycarbophil. Hydrolyzed guar gum (Benefiber®) is a soluble fiber in a powder formulation with 3 g fiber per serving. Few studies are available examining its efficacy although it does appear to improve stool form and constipation.[34,35] The synthetic polymers methylcellulose, carboxymethylcellulose, and calcium polycarbophil

work as bulking agents, increasing water in the stool and are resistant to bacterial degradation. Methylcellulose (Citrucel®) increases stool frequency and water content at a dose of 4 g/day.[36] Calcium polycarbophil has a hydrophilic capacity of 60–100 times its weight and has been theorized to improve both constipation and diarrhea, although few well-controlled human studies exist.[37] The synthetic bulking agents result in less gas production due to the lack of intestinal bacterial degradation, which may benefit some patients intolerant of the other products.[38]

Stool softeners

Stool softeners (e.g., docusate) are reported to work by improving stool consistency and easing defecation. Although commonly used in practice, there is little evidence to support their use.[39] When compared to psyllium, psyllium was found to be more effective.[40] Mineral oil has also been used, particularly in the pediatric population.[41] There is little evidence for efficacy of mineral oil in the adult population and mineral oil may result in anal leakage of oil, fat-soluble vitamin malabsorption, and lipoid pneumonia.[42,43] Thus, in adults, mineral oil and stool softeners are not recommended in the usual treatment of constipation.

Osmotic laxatives

Osmotic laxatives are poorly absorbed or nonabsorbed ions or substances that hold onto water in the intestines to maintain an isosmolar state with the plasma. Osmotic laxatives include magnesium- and phosphate-containing salts, sugar alcohols (e.g., sorbitol), lactulose, and polyethylene glycol. *Magnesium-containing salts* are poorly absorbed ions that have long been used in the treatment of constipation. Surprisingly little peer review data exists supporting the efficacy of magnesium containing salts for the treatment of constipation. However, the ingestion of magnesium in normal subjects produces a progressive increase in stool weight with 7.3 g increase in fecal weight for every millimole increase in stool magnesium.[44] Clinical experience and patient reports indicate that magnesium-containing laxatives do work for many patients, at least in the short term. Caution is necessary due to the potential for magnesium toxicity when recommending magnesium-containing laxatives to the elderly, even in the setting of apparent normal renal function, and magnesium ingestion should be avoided in patients with significant renal disease.[45,46] With proper monitoring, magnesium-containing laxatives can be used safely. The usual dose of milk of magnesia is 30–60 mL (2.4–4.8 g) once or twice daily. When used chronically, especially at higher doses, serum magnesium levels should be measured periodically. Magnesium-containing laxatives are also available as a sparkling liquid (magnesium citrate, 17.5 g/10 ounce bottle) and in pill formulations (100–500 mg tablets or capsules). All produce diarrhea in a dose-dependent manner.

Sodium sulfate and phosphate salts are used as osmotic laxatives. They are better absorbed systemically than the magnesium-containing laxatives and require caution, particularly for individuals with renal disease, liver disease, or heart failure. Sodium phosphate has long been used as a cathartic for colon examinations (i.e., barium enema and colonoscopy). The use of sodium-containing osmotic laxatives has not been well studied for the treatment of chronic constipation.

Polyethylene glycol (PEG) with or without electrolytes has been used both as a colonic purgative for diagnostic colon exams and as a laxative in chronic constipation. PEG increases stool frequency and the water content of stool.[47,48] PEG is well tolerated with evidence of intermediate to long-term efficacy (3–6 months).[49,50] PEG has been well studied in children with chronic constipation, showing efficacy and safety.[51] Open-label studies of PEG in opiate-induced constipation and pregnancy-induced constipation also suggest evidence of improved stool frequency.[52,53] In general, PEG appears to be as or more efficacious than lactulose, another osmotic laxative, and has been shown to be better tolerated.[54,55] PEG does not undergo bacterial fermentation, resulting in less gas formation.[56] Polyethylene glycol is available with or without electrolytes. The usual dose is 17 g of PEG in 8 ounces liquid daily to twice daily. When PEG is given with electrolytes (e.g., GoLYTELY®, NuLytely®) the usual dose is 8–16 ounces per day. GoLYTELY contains sodium sulfate, which also exerts an osmotic effect. The sodium sulfate can be absorbed when GoLYTELY is administered in small quantities that may reduce its effectiveness as a laxative.

Lactulose is a poorly absorbed synthetic disaccharide used in the treatment of portal systemic encephalopathy and constipation. The small intestine lacks a dissacharidase to hydrolyze lactulose, greatly limiting its absorption. It remains in the gastrointestinal tract where it is fermented by the colonic bacterial flora. Lactulose improves stool frequency and is more efficacious than bulking agents.[57–59] The usual dose of lactulose is 15–30 mL/day (10–20 g). Some patients object to the sweetness of the liquid formulation. An alternative crystalline powder lactulose formulation (Kristalose® 10 and 20 g/packet) has minimal perceptible taste. Lactulose is equally efficacious with sorbitol.[60] *Sorbitol* is a sugar alcohol with laxative properties. Sorbitol is used at a concentration of 70%, 15–30 mL once or twice daily. Sorbitol is generally less expensive than lactulose.[60] The use of both sorbitol and lactulose may be limited by patient complaints of excessive gaseousness, thought to results from bacterial fermentation.

Stimulant laxatives

The chronic use of stimulant laxatives has long been frowned upon by the medical community due to concerns over toxicity to the colon (cathartic colon) and potential for dependence. A toxic effect of stimulant laxatives on colonic muscle or nerve has been placed in doubt and has little relevance with currently available laxative preparations.[61] Stimulant laxatives include anthraquinones, diphenylmethane derivatives, and ricinoleic acid. Stimulant laxatives are generally reserved for refractory cases of constipation and when first-line therapies (e.g., fiber and osmotic agents) have failed. Stimulant laxatives work through irritant or stimulatory effects on gastrointestinal epithelium, muscle, and/or nerve.

Anthraquinone laxatives derive from plants and constitute the 'natural' ingredient in many herbal laxative preparations. Anthraquinone laxatives include senna pods, cascara sagrada, aloes, and rhubarb root. These laxatives have no effect in the small bowel and require bacterial metabolism in the colon for activity. The active compounds produced by the colonic bacteria have secretory and motor effects.[62] Few anthraquinone laxatives have been evaluated in randomized clinical trials. A combination product containing aloe, celandin, and psyllium was found effective over a 2-week period compared to placebo.[63] Senna is commonly used in clinical practice and provides improved stool frequency and increased stool weight in combination with psyllium compared to psyllium alone.[64] *Cassia alata* (wild senna) has been shown to increase stool passage at 24 hours compared to placebo, although side effects were noted in 16–25% of subjects.[65] Senna is available commercially and by prescription as granules, syrup, or tables. The usual dose is 30 mg once or twice daily. Nausea, bloating, and abdominal cramps are common side effects. When used long term, the colon becomes discolored from deposition of a lipofuscin pigment in the lamina propria, a condition termed 'melanosis coli.'[66] In addition to its association with anthraquinone laxatives, this colonic discoloration may also be seen with another stimulant laxative, bisacodyl. This colonic discoloration is now considered a harmless condition that disappears with cessation of these stimulant laxatives. Many of the over-the-counter herbal laxative preparations contain additional inactive ingredients and substances of unknown or potentially harmful effect. Pure senna preparations have been used successfully in elderly persons and in the postpartum period without significant safety concerns.[67,68]

Diphenylmethane derivates include bisacodyl, sodium picosulfate, and phenolphthalein. Phenolphthalein is no longer available due to findings of carcinogenicity in animals and concern regarding possible carcinogenicity in humans. Like the anthraquinones, bisacodyl and sodium picosulfate also require conversion to active compounds in the intestine.[62] Bisacodyl is converted by intestinal enzymes and has effects in the small intestine and colon. Sodium picosulfate is converted by bacteria in the colon to its active compound. Bisacodyl administered intraluminally in the colon induces near immediate high amplitude propagated contractions.[69] It increases colonic water and electrolyte secretion.[70] Bisacodyl is available as an oral tablet (10–15 mg per day) or suppository (10 mg p.r.). Sodium picosulfate is not readily available in the United States but may be found in Mexico, South America, Europe, and Asia (Lubrilax®, Sur-lax®, and Laxoberon®). The oral preparations of bisacodyl typically exert their effect in 6–8 hours. The suppositories act more rapidly with effects in 15–30 minutes. The predictability (at least in the short term) of the suppository effect has led to the use of bisacodyl in patients with constipation due to neurologic conditions, such as spinal cord injury.

Ricinoleic acid induces net water secretion into the colon.[71] Animal studies using direct instillation of ricinoleic acid into the small intestine resulted in a temporary increase in small bowel motor activity.[72] Ricinoleic acid is derived from castor oil after undergoing hydrolysis by lipase in the small intestine.[73] Common side effects include abdominal pain and cramping, limiting its routine use.

Prokinetic agents

Tegaserod, a 5-HT$_4$ partial agonist, is the only prokinetic approved for the treatment of constipation. Tegaserod accelerates transit in the small intestine and colon.[74] In a 12-week trial, tegaserod improved symptoms of constipation and was found to be safe and well tolerated.[75] Tegaserod is dosed 6 mg b.i.d. and is given 20–30 minutes before a meal. Occasionally, individuals treated with tegaserod have developed a marked increase in stool frequency (diarrhea). The medication should be discontinued until the diarrhea resolves and if the constipation persists, restarted at a lower dose. Tegaserod is also available in 2 mg tablets. No other prokinetics are approved for use in chronic constipation. Cisapride is now of historical interest in the United States due to the potential for the development of cardiac dysrhythmias. Cisapride also acts at the 5-HT$_4$ receptor site to stimulate the release of acetylcholine. When it was available, it induced a modest effect in improving constipation symptoms.[76,77] Other prokinetic agents include cholinergic agonists, such as bethanechol or pyridostigmine. These non-specific cholinergic agonists produce significant side effects including excessive salivation, abdominal cramping, vomiting, and bladder irritability. They are rarely used in the treatment of constipation. Neostigmine has a role in the treatment of hospitalized patients with acute colonic pseudo-obstruction, but is not used to treat constipation.[78]

Miscellaneous agents

Misoprostol

Patients with refractory chronic constipation may be treatment with the prostaglandin analogue, misoprostol. A frequent side effect of prostaglandin stimulation is diarrhea.[79] Patients with refractory constipation treated with various doses of misoprostol had an increased number of days with bowel movements.[80] The starting dose is 200 µg two to four times daily. This drug is used to induce early medical abortions and is contraindicated in women who are pregnant or planning to become pregnant.

Colchicine

A common side effect of colchicine when used to treat gout is the development of diarrhea. A double-blind trial of 0.6 mg colchicine t.i.d. showed increased stool frequency and accelerated colonic transit.[81] Although uncommon, chronic colchicine use is associated with bone marrow toxicity and agranulocytosis. Colchicine is only recommended in severe constipation for which other options have failed.

Opioid antagonists

Opioid antagonists have been studied as a treatment for constipation for the past two decades with contradictory reports.[82,83] Naloxone may play a role in opioid-induced constipation, although some patients may experience a diminished analgesic effect even with oral naloxone.[84] The opiate antagonists naltrexone, methyltrexone and, more recently, alvimopan continue to be studied as potential agents for the treatment of opiate-induced constipation.[85–88]

Glycerin suppositories

Glycerin suppositories have long been available for use as a laxative. They work through a local irritant and osmotic effect, stimulating defecation. Controlled studies are not available to assess their effectiveness.

Enemas

Enemas, and the more recently renewed practice of 'colonics,' have no support in the medical literature for the treatment of chronic constipation. Tap water or lubricant (e.g., mineral oil) enemas have been used in the initial treatment of fecal impaction. Many case reports outline the hazards of enema therapy, particularly with osmotic/saline products.[89–91] Enema use in children with encopresis is considered counterproductive by some experts.[92] Enema use should be reserved for treatment of more severe, acute constipation and as a preparation for therapeutic examinations. Warm tap enemas are considered safest. The risk of electrolyte disturbances with phosphate and other electrolyte-containing enemas requires caution and careful observation for signs of complications. The use of water-soluble contrast enemas have been used for diagnostic (to exclude colonic perforation) and therapeutic purposes in fecal impaction.[93] The water-soluble contrast material is hyperosmotic, providing a laxative effect.

Antegrade enemas

Several uncontrolled studies report successful use of cecostomy for antegrade enemas in the treatment of refractory constipation in children and adults.[94–96] An indwelling tube is placed into the colon surgically or endoscopically. The tube is flushed with water or PEG at scheduled intervals. The procedure has been reported as particularly effective in individuals with neurogenic bowel and overflow incontinence, such as from myelomeningolocele, but has also been used in neurologically intact individuals.[97]

Special categories of constipation

Slow transit constipation

Patients with slow transit constipation who have failed aggressive medical management may benefit from subtotal colectomy with ileorectal anastomosis.[26] This surgery removes the entire colon, with only a segment of rectum remaining for the anastomosis with the ileum. Lesser degrees of colonic resection are less routinely successful.[98] Less than 10% of patients with slow transit constipation require surgical intervention.[99] Although long-term satisfaction in patients undergoing surgery for slow transit constipation is high, side effects are common, including diarrhea, occasional bowel incontinence. and bowel obstruction.[99–101] A key to success includes excluding patients with coexistent dys-synergic defecation. Results with this surgery are not as good with patients who have coexistent upper gastrointestinal tract motility disorders or significant psychologic disturbance.[102] This surgery, more recently, has been successfully performed using the laparoscopic approach.[103]

Dyssynergic defecation

Biofeedback techniques using auditory and visual feedback, train the patient to use the muscles involved in defecation in a coordinated fashion. This training is typically performed by a trained nurse, physical therapist, or occupational therapist. An intra-rectal probe with a pressure sensor or EMG strip is attached by means of a cord to a computer. Contraction and relaxation of the anal sphincter muscle can be visualized on the computer screen. The therapist provides education and advice to the patient, assisting in the proper relaxation of the external anal sphincter muscle and puborectalis and coordination with straining. The overall success of therapy is nearly 70%.[104] Botulinum type A toxin has been used in uncontrolled trials to treat patients with a poorly relaxing puborectalis with a modest degree of success.[105] The primary treatment of dyssynergic defecation remains biofeedback.

Pregnancy

Constipation affects many pregnant women due to the effects of iron-containing vitamins, hormonal changes (e.g., progesterone), and the enlarging uterus. First-line therapies include increasing dietary fiber and bulking agents. Fiber supplements are effective and have few adverse effects.[106,107] PEG has also been used in pregnancy and may be considered in patients failing to respond to fiber.[53] PEG absorption is negligible, making it an ideal agent for use in pregnancy.[108] Nonetheless, insufficient data exist to determine what effect PEG may have on the developing fetus, and it carries a pregnancy category C classification. The stimulant laxative senna when used short-term appears safe for use in pregnancy.[109] There are no data to support the role of increased fluid intake or exercise in improving constipation in pregnancy.

Combination and 'rescue' therapy

Few therapeutic trials report using combination therapy other than the use of bulking agents with stimulant laxatives. Combination therapy is commonly used in clinical practice for patients refractory to standard doses of single agents. Frequently used combinations include combining an osmotic agent such as PEG with a prokinetic such as tegaserod. Stimulant laxatives are often used as 'rescue' therapy 2–3 times per week in patients going longer than 2–3 days without defecation. Some patients with constipation complain of feeling excessively full and uncomfortable if they do not have a daily bowel movement. The presence of excessive stool may be assessed by a plain abdominal radiograph. In the absence of excessive stool loading in the colon, the reported uncomfortable sensation may relate to overlap with irritable bowel syndrome symptoms. Rather than escalating laxative use, therapies directed at the irritable bowel syndrome, including neuromodulation, may be more appropriate.

TREATMENT OF DIARRHEA

In the absence of fever, bloody stool, or severe abdominal pain, diarrhea may initially be treated empirically with symptomatic therapies while the underlying cause is investigated. As the diagnostic process uncovers the specific cause of the diarrhea, therapy is appropriately targeted to the underlying condition. Diarrheal disorders remain an important cause of morbidity and mortality in the United States and worldwide, particularly in children.[110,111] The first step when treating diarrhea focuses on restoring hydration and electrolyte balance. Most patients with diarrhea are able to tolerate oral intake, with intravenous fluids required in only the most severe cases. Antidiarrheal agents include opiates to inhibit intestinal transit, agents to improve the stool form, and more potent antisecretory agents such as octreotide for the more severe, chronic cases of diarrhea. The treatment of diarrhea associated with irritable bowel syndrome is discussed in Chapter 48.

Rehydration techniques

Oral rehydration solutions take advantage of the cotransport of glucose and sodium across the intestinal epithelium.[112] A reduction in diarrheal deaths is associated with use of oral rehydration solutions.[113] The original composition of the World Health Organization (WHO) oral rehydration solution was near isosmotic (311 mOsm) and relatively high in sodium (90 mM).[114] Although life saving and effective due to improved hydration, diarrhea was not reduced and some patients developed hypernatremia. The optimal composition of oral rehydration solutions continues to be debated.[115] More recently, the WHO has recommended reduced osmolarity oral rehydration solutions as the preferred treatment for diarrhea.[116] The lower sodium and reduced osmolarity formulation advantages include reduced stool output and less need for intravenous fluids.[117,118] In addition to sodium and glucose, oral rehydration solutions contain chloride, potassium, and citrate. Oral rehydration solutions possess several advantages over sports drinks, fruit juice, or soda. Most sports drinks contain minimal or no sodium and most are also hyperosmolar. The lack of sodium reduces their ability to hydrate and the hyperosmolarity serves to increase diarrhea. In addition, many juices contain significant amounts of sorbitol and all contain fructose. These agents exert an osmotic effect, which counterproductively may increase the amount of stool output.[119] Oral rehydration solutions are used most commonly for acute diarrhea. They may also be helpful for patients with moderate or severe chronic diarrhea, reducing the risk of dehydration and need for intravenous fluids.

The first-line treatment for mild to moderate dehydration from diarrhea is administration of an oral rehydration solution (Table 71.4). The amount of fluid required depends on the degree of baseline dehydration and ongoing losses. Sports drinks, juice, and soda are not adequate for rehydration due to the low sodium content and high osmolarity. Individuals unable to tolerate oral intake require intravenous fluids and electrolytes. Patients who are not dehydrated do not require special oral rehydration solutions.

Over-the-counter products

A variety of over-the-counter products exist for treating diarrhea; however, the two most widely available active ingredients are bismuth subsalicylate or loperamide. Activated attapulgite 600 mg was previously shown to improve stool consistency and reduce stool frequency in a randomized, controlled trial.[120] However, the commercially available product, Kaopectate®, and generic equivalents that originally contained attapulgite, have

Table 71.4 Composition of commonly available solutions used for rehydration

Rehydrating solutions	Na mEq/L	K mEq/L	Glucose g/L	mOsm/L
Pedialyte	45	20	25	270
WHO (low osmolarity formulation)	75	20	75	245
Ceralyte	70	20	40	220
Gatorade*	20	3	50	330
Orange juice*	<1	54	118	>600

* Not recommended for use in rehydration due to low sodium content and high osmolarity.

changed their formulation due to the presence of lead in the attapulgite.[121] Kaopectate now contains bismuth subsalicylate, the active ingredient that is also in Pepto-Bismol®. Bismuth subsalicylate has modest activity in reducing the severity and duration of acute diarrhea.[122,123] Bismuth has antimicrobial properties and has been used predominantly for mild travelers' diarrhea and infectious diarrhea in children.

Loperamide, also an over-the-counter product, is an opioid agonist devoid of central opiate effects. The antidiarrheal effects of loperamide include an antisecretory effect, improved fluid absorption, and reduced colonic transit.[124,125] Loperamide is more effective that bismuth subsalicylate in acute diarrhea.[126] Due to the lack of central effects, loperamide is well tolerated with few side effects.[127] In addition to efficacy in the symptomatic treatment of acute diarrhea, loperamide also has efficacy in chronic diarrhea.[128,129] Loperamide is helpful for controlling mild to moderate chemotherapy-induced diarrhea and appears to have some effect in improving anal sphincter tone, reducing episodes of fecal incontinence.[130,131] A combination produce of loperamide and simethicone was found more effective in relieving 'gas' symptoms in patients with acute diarrhea.[132] Overall, loperamide is a safe, effective antidiarrheal for treating symptoms of acute and chronic diarrhea. Loperamide (and other antimotility agents) should not be used in the setting toxin-mediated diarrhea or dysentery and is not recommended for young children. The directions on the package suggest taking 4 mg at the onset of diarrhea, with 2 mg after each loose stool, and a maximum of 8 mg per day. In chronic diarrhea, a prophylactic dose of 2–4 mg twice daily or taking this medication prior to meals may be more effective, taking advantage of its ability to reduce oral–cecal transit.[133] The maximum dose is 16 mg/day, although doses up to 32 mg/day have been used for more severe chronic diarrhea.[134]

Opioid agonists

Opioid agonists other than loperamide used in the treatment of diarrhea include a diphenoxylate/atropine combination, codeine, morphine, and tincture of opium. Unlike loperamide, these are controlled substances, requiring a prescription. Opium and its derivatives interact with mu receptors in the gut, inhibiting intestinal secretion and transit, and increasing absorption.[135] Opiates are extremely effective in controlling diarrhea, although physician concerns regarding abuse potential and central side effects have limited their more widespread use. Codeine delays orocecal and ascending colon transit.[136] Codeine is effective in controlling diarrhea, although side effects are more common than with loperamide.[137–139] Tincture of opium has long been used for the treatment of diarrhea. It is somewhat more difficult to obtain, as many pharmacies no longer routinely carry this medication. The opiate agonist diphenoxylate is combined with the anticholinergic agent, atropine. This combination product is as or slightly less effective than loperamide, but causes greater side effects.[139–141] The opiate agonists are effective in reducing stool frequency and improving stool form. Loperamide is preferred due to the lack of central side effects. For diarrhea refractory to loperamide, deodorized tincture of opium or codeine may be more effective. Once an effective dose of an opiate agonist has been reached, further dose escalation is unusual. Except for loperamide, the potential for opiate abuse must be recognized, but fortunately is rare when treating chronic diarrheal conditions.

Alpha-2 adrenergic agonist

Use of the alpha-2 adrenergic agonist clonidine to control diabetic diarrhea has been described for over two decades.[142] Clonidine slows gut transit, increasing intestinal absorption.[143,144] It appears to be most useful for the treatment of unexplained, diabetic diarrhea, with lesser effects when studied in infectious diarrhea.[145] Due to frequent side effects, including the potential for bradycardia and reduced blood pressure, careful monitoring is required. Relatively large doses may be needed for control of diarrhea. Starting doses begin at 0.1 mg daily to twice daily and may be increased progressively up to 0.3 mg three times per day. Should the medicine need to be withdrawn, it must be tapered to avoid rebound hypertension. Other alpha-2 adrenergic agonists are not readily available in the United States. Although clonidine may be useful in the treatment of diabetic diarrhea, it is unclear whether it is effective in other diarrheal disorders.

Octreotide

Octreotide, a somatostatin analogue, is a potent inhibitory of gastrointestinal hormones. Octreotide blocks the secretion of electrolytes, increases electrolyte absorption, and prolongs intestinal transit.[146,147] Octreotide has been used in a variety of severe, refractory diarrheal disorders including AIDS enteropathy, diabetic diarrhea, chemotherapy-induced diarrhea, graft-versus-host disease and postintestinal resection diarrhea. The majority of randomized, controlled trials evaluating efficacy occurred in chemotherapy-related diarrhea and AIDS enteropathy. A variety of dosing schedules have been used. Octreotide must be injected subcutaneously or given intravenously. Once an established dose of octreotide has been determined, the patient may be changed to the long-acting, microencapsulated form of octreotide (Sandostatin LAR®) that is administered intramuscularly every 4 weeks. Due to the effects of octreotide in inhibiting pancreatic secretion, at higher doses pancreatic insufficiency may develop, requiring pancreatic enzyme supplementation. The starting dose of octreotide is 50 μg subcutaneously three times per day, increasing the dose by 50–100 μg three times daily until a beneficial effect is seen. The maximum recommended dose is 500 μg three times per day. Octreotide LAR is administered intramuscularly every 4 weeks. When octreotide LAR is first started, the subcutaneous thrice-daily injections are continued for the first 2 weeks. When either formulation of octreotide is initiated, patients are monitored for evidence of hyper- or hypoglycemia and pancreatic insufficiency. Long-term use of octreotide is associated with the development of gallstones, although acute cholecystitis has infrequently been reported. Due to the expense and mode of administration, octreotide is reserved for use in the more severe and refractory cases of diarrhea.

See Table 71.5 for a list of agents commonly used in the treatment of diarrhea.

Probiotics

Probiotics are microbial agents beneficial to the health of a host (see Ch. 3).[148] A variety of studies have shown the efficacy of probiotics in children and adults with acute, infectious diarrhea.[149] A variety of probiotics, including various combinations of 'beneficial' bacteria and yeast, are available. Microbial agents

Table 71.5 Agents commonly used in the treatment of diarrhea

	Dose
Oral rehydration solutions	
WHO	1–6 L per day
Pedialyte	1–6 L per day
Ceralyte	1–6 L per day
Over-the-counter	
Bismuth subsalicylate	2 tablets or 30 mL four times a day
Loperamide	2–4 mg four times a day
Opiates	
Diphenoxylate/atropine	2.5 mg (diphenoxylate); one to two tablets up to four times per day
Codeine sulfate	30–90 mg up to four times per day
Tincture of opium	5–20 gtts up to three times per day
Morphine sulfate	5–15 mg up to three times per day
Alpha-2 adrenergic agonist	
Clonidine	0.1–0.3 mg two to three times per day
Bile acid binder	
Cholestyramine	4 g two to four times per day
Somatostatin analogue	
Octreotide	50 μg SQ three times daily, titrating to 500 μg three times daily
Octreotide LAR	10–30 mg i.m. every 4 weeks

SQ, subcutaneous; i.m., intramuscular

that appear to have beneficial effects in the treatment of infectious diarrhea or antibiotic-associated diarrhea, based on two meta-analyses, include the bacteria *Lactobacillus casei GG*, live *Enterococcus LAB strain SF68*, *Lactobacillus acidophilus*, and the yeast *Saccharomyces boulardii*.[149,150] The efficacy of probiotics in infectious diarrhea and antibiotic-associated diarrhea was consistent across the various studies. However, the optimal dose, type of preparation, or strain of probiotic remains unclear. Different probiotics may be appropriate depending on the underlying cause of diarrhea and host factors. Probiotics are considered food supplements and are not tightly regulated by the government. Although generally considered safe, rare cases of bacteremia or fungemia have been reported. Further studies are needed to determine the most effective probiotics for different types of diarrhea and what doses are most effective.

Other agents

Due to their constipating effects, calcium channel blockers have been proposed for the treatment of chronic diarrheal disorders, although they have not been carefully studied for efficacy in the clinical setting. Cholestyramine is a bile acid binder which has been used for the treatment of bile acid diarrhea, postcholecystectomy diarrhea, and diarrhea occurring after ileal resection.[151,152]

Bile acids not absorbed in the ileum act as a cathartic on the colon, an effect that can be reduced with cholestyramine. Other medications should not be given with cholestyramine due to its ability to also bind other drugs. Zinc supplementation has been shown to reduce the frequency and severity of diarrhea in children.[153] It is unclear if zinc supplementation is beneficial in the treatment of diarrhea in individuals who are not zinc deficient. Dietary recommendations have included avoidance of alcohol, milk, caffeine, and high-osmolarity liquids (e.g., juices, regular soda, sports drinks) and poorly absorbed sugars (e.g., sorbitol, fructose). The ingestion of these substances may produce diarrhea in susceptible individuals, and elimination may be helpful in controlling chronic diarrhea. The impact of specific dietary measures (other than oral rehydration solutions) in treating acute diarrhea is unclear. Zaldaride maleate, a calmodulin inhibitor with antisecretory properties, improves travelers' diarrhea.[154,155] It is not yet available in the United States. Another agent, racecadotril, an inhibitor of enkephalinase, has been proposed as a treatment for acute diarrhea with efficacy similar to loperamide.[156–158]

SUMMARY

The usual treatment of constipation begins by eliminating exacerbating factors, such as constipating medications and initiation of an empiric trial of increased dietary fiber and/or a bulking agent. Patients who fail to respond to or are intolerant of these measures may next be treated with an osmotic laxative or prokinetic. The most commonly used osmotic laxatives include polyethylene glycol, magnesium salts, lactulose, and sorbitol. Polyethylene glycol appears to be the best tolerated and safest of this group. Lactulose and sorbitol are equally effective, although sorbitol is less expensive on a dose per dose basis. Magnesium salts (e.g., milk of magnesia) when used chronically require monitoring to prevent or detect magnesium toxicity. The only currently available prokinetic for the treatment of chronic constipation is tegaserod. Patients refractory to these measures should be considered for further evaluation, including physiologic testing. The use of stool softeners or enemas in the treatment of chronic constipation is discouraged due to a lack of efficacy (stool softeners) and risk for dependence or toxicity (enemas).

Patients with refractory constipation may be treated with combination therapy (e.g., osmotic laxative plus prokinetic) and/or the addition of a stimulant laxative. Tolerance does develop with stimulant laxatives such that higher doses are required to obtain the same effect. Prior concerns regarding stimulant laxatives damaging the colon appear to have been overstated. Stimulant laxatives cause more side effects, including abdominal pain. Stimulant laxatives most commonly used include senna and bisacodyl. Few patients have problems when these are used two to three times per week. Misoprostol and colchicine are reserved for the most refractory cases of constipation. Patients with slow-transit constipation who fail to respond to these measures may benefit from surgery with ileorectostomy. In the setting of dyssynergic defecation, biofeedback retraining of the pelvic floor muscles improves symptoms in 70% of patients. When pain is a predominant complaint in addition to the complaints of constipation, consider the diagnosis of irritable bowel syndrome and direct therapy towards this condition (e.g., neuromodulation).

Most patients with acute diarrhea respond to treatment with rehydration and observation. Antibiotics may occasionally be used if indicated by the clinical situation. Patients with chronic diarrhea should be evaluated to determine the underlying category and/or medical problem. Therapy is first directed at correcting fluid and electrolyte abnormalities. Oral rehydration solutions are ideal for this, providing adequate sodium in a formulation that enhances water absorption. Patients unable to tolerate oral intake require intravenous fluid replacement. With persistent symptoms and in the absence of dysentery, the opiate agonist loperamide should next be tried. The efficacy of loperamide may be improved by administering it before events that precipitate increased stool output (e.g., meals). Bismuth subsalicylate is modestly effective and has been most studied in the treatment of travelers' diarrhea.

Patients with more severe or refractory diarrhea should undergo further clinical assessment to determine an underlying cause. Once an underlying condition is identified, directed therapy is initiated (e.g., pancreatic enzymes in pancreatic insufficiency). When stronger antidiarrheal agents are required, the next step is use of other opiate antagonists. Diphenoxylate is equally effective with loperamide. Codeine, deodorized tincture of opium, and morphine are effective in many cases of refractory diarrhea. The use of these agents is limited due to concerns regarding opiate dependency and side effects (especially sedation). Severe secretory diarrhea may be treated with octreotide or long-acting octreotide. The conditions most commonly requiring octreotide are endocrine secreting tumors (e.g., carcinoid), chemotherapy-induced diarrhea, and AIDS enteropathy. The long-acting octreotide represents a significant advance in the treatment of these patients with an intramuscular injection required only every 4 weeks. A variety of other agents have been tried with varying degrees of success. Cholestyramine, a bile acid binder, may be useful in bile acid diarrhea, postcholecystectomy diarrhea, and in the setting of prior ileal resection. Clonidine may be effective for diabetic diarrhea. Probiotics appear promising in the treatment of some cases of infectious antibiotic-associated diarrhea. Few dietary measures consistently improve diarrhea. Susceptible individuals may benefit from reduced intake of caffeine (especially coffee), milk products, juices, poorly absorbed sugars (e.g., sorbitol, mannitol), or hyperosmotic liquids.

REFERENCES

1. Heaton KW, Radvan J, Cripps H, et al. Defecation frequency and timing, and stool form in the general population: a prospective study. Gut 1992; 33:818–824.

2. Talley NJ, Weaver AL, Zinsmeister AR, et al. Self-reported diarrhea: what does it mean? Am J Gastroenterol 1994; 89:1160–1164.

3. Pare P, Ferrazzi S, Thompson WG, et al. An epidemiological survey of constipation in Canada: definitions, rates, demographics, and predictors of health care seeking. Am J Gastroenterol 2001; 96:3130–3137.

4. Drossman DA, Corazziari E, Talley NJ, et al. Rome II: The functional gastrointestinal disorders. Degnon Associates, 2000.

5. Evans RC, Kamm MA, Hinton JM, et al. The normal range and a simple diagram for recording whole gut transit time. Int J Colorect Dis 1992; 7:15–17.

6. Martelli H, Devroede G, Arhan P, et al. Some parameters of large bowel motility in normal man. Gastroenterology 1978; 75:612–618.

7. Connell AM, Hilton C, Irvine G, et al. Variation of bowel habit in two population samples. Br Med J 1965; 2:1095–1099.

8. Zuckerman MJ, Guerra LG, Drossman DA, et al. Comparison of bowel patterns in Hispanics and non-Hispanic whites. Dig Dis Sci 1995; 40:1763–1769.

9. Sandler RS, Drossman DA. Bowel habits in young adults not seeking health care. Dig Dis Sci 1987; 32:841–845.

10. Dukas L, Willett WC, Giovannucci EL. Association between physical activity, fiber intake, and other lifestyle variables and constipation in a study of women. Am J Gastroenterol 2003; 98:1790–1796.

11. Mearin F, Zarate N, Sardi JA, et al. Traveler's constipation. Am J Gastroenterol 2003; 98:507–509.

12. Kinnunen O. Study of constipation in a geriatric hospital, day hospital, old people's home and at home. Aging Clin Experiment Res 1991; 3:161–170.

13. Maleki D, Camilleri M, Burton DD, et al. Pilot study of pathophysiology of constipation among community diabetics. Dig Dis Sci 1998; 43:2373–2378.

14. Ashraf W, Pfeiffer RF, Park F, et al. Constipation in Parkinson's disease: objective assessment and response to psyllium. Movement Dis 1997; 12:946–951.

15. Hinds JP, Eidelman BH, Wald A. Prevalence of bowel dysfunction in multiple sclerosis. A population survey. Gastroenterology 1990; 98:1538–1542.

16. Gardner EC Jr, Hersh T. Primary hyperparathyroidism and the gastrointestinal tract. South Med J 1981; 74:197–199.

17. Schiller LR. Chronic diarrhea. Gastroenterology 2004; 127:287–293.

18. Fine KD, Schiller LR. AGA technical review on the evaluation and management of chronic diarrhea. Gastroenterology 1999; 116:1464–1486.

   Classic review covering the diagnostic evaluation of chronic diarrhea and providing general recommendations for treatment.

19. Stewart WF, Liberman JN, Sandler RS, et al. Epidemiology of constipation (EPOC) study in the United States: relation of clinical subtypes to sociodemographic features. Am J Gastroenterol 1999; 94:3530–3540.

20. Drossman DA, Li Z, Andruzzi E, et al. U.S. householder survey of functional gastrointestinal disorders. Prevalence, sociodemography, and health impact. Dig Dis Sci 1993; 38:1569–1580.

21. Talley NJ, Zinsmeister AR, Van Dyke C et al. Epidemiology of colonic symptoms and the irritable bowel syndrome. Gastroenterology 1991; 101:927–934.

22. Simren M, Brazier J, Coremans G, et al. Quality of life and illness costs in irritable bowel syndrome. Digestion 2004; 69:254–261.

23. Halder SL, Locke GR 3rd, Talley NJ, et al. Impact of functional gastrointestinal disorders on health-related quality of life: a population-based case-control study. Aliment Pharmacol Ther 2004; 19:233–242.

24. Hinton JM, Lennard-Jones JE, Young AC. A new method for studying gut transit times using radioopaque markers. Gut 1969; 10:842–847.

25. Beck DE. Simplified balloon expulsion test. Dis Colon Rectum 1992; 35:597–598.

26. Nyam DC, Pemberton JH, Ilstrup DM, et al. Long-term results of surgery for chronic constipation. Dis Colon Rectum 1997; 40:273–279.

27. Meshkinpour H, Selod S, Movahedi H, et al. Effects of regular exercise in management of chronic idiopathic constipation. Dig Dis Sci 1998; 43: 2379–2383.

   A well-done physiologic study showing the lack of effect of an exercise program in a group of patients with chronic constipation.

Although commonly recommended as a treatment for constipation, there are no clinical trials showing exercise to improve symptoms of constipation.

28. Chung BD, Parekh U, Sellin JH. Effect of increased fluid intake on stool output in normal healthy volunteers. J Clin Gastroenterol 1999; 28:29–32.

29. Marlett JA, McBurney MI, Slavin JL, American Dietetic Association. Position of the American Dietetic Association: health implications of dietary fiber. J Am Dietetic Assoc 2002; 102:993–1000.

30. Badiali D, Corazziari E, Habib FI, et al. Effect of wheat bran in treatment of chronic nonorganic constipation. A double-blind controlled trial. Dig Dis Sci 1995; 40:349–356.

31. Bijlani RL. Dietary fibre: consensus and controversy. Progress Food Nutr Sci 1985; 9:343–393.

32. Ashraf W, Park F, Lof J, et al. Effects of psyllium therapy on stool characteristics, colon transit and anorectal function in chronic idiopathic constipation. Aliment Pharmacol Ther 1995; 9:639–647.

Carefully performed physiologic studies in a group of patients with chronic constipation showing that psyllium fiber improves stool frequency, consistency, and weight. Study subjects received 10 g of fiber per day in divided doses.

33. Khalili B, Bardana EJ Jr, Yunginger JW. Psyllium-associated anaphylaxis and death: a case report and review of the literature. Ann Allergy Asthma Immunol 2003; 91:579–584.

34. Patrick PG, Gohman SM, Marx SC, et al. Effect of supplements of partially hydrolyzed guar gum on the occurrence of constipation and use of laxative agents. J Am Dietetic Assoc 1998; 98:912–914.

35. Takahashi H, Wako N, Okubo T, et al. Influence of partially hydrolyzed guar gum on constipation in women. J Nutr Sci Vitaminol 1994; 40:251–259.

36. Hamilton JW, Wagner J, Burdick BB, et al. Clinical evaluation of methylcellulose as a bulk laxative. Dig Dis Sci 1988; 33:993–998.

37. Danhof IE. Pharmacology, toxicology, clinical efficacy, and adverse effects of calcium polycarbophil, an enteral hydrosorptive agent. Pharmacotherapy 1982; 2:18–28.

38. Bianchi M, Capurso L. Effects of guar gum, ispaghula and microcrystalline cellulose on abdominal symptoms, gastric emptying, orocaecal transit time and gas production in healthy volunteers. Dig Liver Dis 2002; 34(Suppl 2):S129–S133.

39. Goodman J, Pang J, Bessman AN. Dioctyl sodium sulfosuccinate – an ineffective prophylactic laxative. J Chronic Dis 1976; 29:59–63.

40. McRorie JW, Daggy BP, Morel JG, et al. Psyllium is superior to docusate sodium for treatment of chronic constipation. Aliment Pharmacol Ther 1998; 12:491–497.

41. Sondheimer JM, Gervaise EP. Lubricant versus laxative in the treatment of chronic functional constipation of children: a comparative study. J Pediat Gastroenterol Nutr 1982; 1:223–226.

42. Clark JH, Russell GJ, Fitzgerald JF, et al. Serum beta-carotene, retinol, and alpha-tocopherol levels during mineral oil therapy for constipation. Am J Dis Child 1987; 141:1210–1212.

43. Ciravegna B, Sacco O, Moroni C, et al. Mineral oil lipoid pneumonia in a child with anoxic encephalopathy: treatment by whole lung lavage. Pediatr Pulmonol 1997; 23:233–237.

44. Fine KD, Santa Ana CA, Fordtran JS. Diagnosis of magnesium-induced diarrhea. N Engl Med J 1991; 324:1012–1017.

45. Dharmarajan TS, Patel B, Varshneya N. Cathartic-induced life threatening hypermagnesemia in a 90-year-old woman with apparent normal renal function. J Am Geriatr Soc 1999; 47:1039-10–40.

46. Schelling JR. Fatal hypermagnesemia. Clin Nephrol 2000; 53:61–65.

47. Andorsky RI, Goldner F. Colonic lavage solution (polyethylene glycol electrolyte lavage solution) as a treatment for chronic constipation: a double-blind, placebo-controlled study. Am J Gastroenterol 1990; 85:261–265.

48. DiPalma JA, DeRidder PH, Orlando RC, et al. A randomized, placebo-controlled, multicenter study of the safety and efficacy of a new polyethylene glycol laxative. Am J Gastroenterol 2000; 95:446–450.

49. Corazziari E, Badiali D, Bazzocchi G, et al. Long term efficacy, safety, and tolerability of low daily doses of isosmotic polyethylene glycol electrolyte balanced solution (PMF-100) in the treatment of functional chronic constipation. Gut 2000; 46:522–526.

50. Badiali D, Corazziari E. Use of low dose polyethylene glycol solutions in the treatment of functional constipation. Ital J Gastroenterol Hepatol 1999; 31(Suppl 3):S245–S248.

51. Loening-Baucke V. Polyethylene glycol without electrolytes for children with constipation and encopresis. J Pediatr Gastroenterol Nutr 2002; 34:372–377.

52. Freedman MD, Schwartz HJ, Roby R, et al. Tolerance and efficacy of polyethylene glycol 3350/electrolyte solution versus lactulose in relieving opiate induced constipation: a double-blinded placebo-controlled trial. J Clin Pharmacol 1997; 37:904–907.

53. Neri I, Blasi I, Castro P, et al. Polyethylene glycol electrolyte solution (Isocolan) for constipation during pregnancy: an observational open-label study. J Midwifery Women's Health 2004; 49:355–358.

54. Gremse DA, Hixon J, Crutchfield A. Comparison of polyethylene glycol 3350 and lactulose for treatment of chronic constipation in children. Clin Pediatr 2002; 41:225–229.

55. Attar A, Lemann M, Ferguson A, et al. Comparison of a low dose polyethylene glycol electrolyte solution with lactulose for treatment of chronic constipation. Gut 1999; 44:226–230.

Randomized, comparative trial of PEG versus lactulose showing greater improvement with PEG and fewer adverse symptoms, including less flatus.

56. Bouhnik Y, Neut C, Raskine L, et al. Prospective, randomized, parallel-group trial to evaluate the effects of lactulose and polyethylene glycol-4000 on colonic flora in chronic idiopathic constipation. Aliment Pharmacol Ther 2004; 19:889–899.

57. Bass P, Dennis S. The laxative effects of lactulose in normal and constipated subjects. J Clin Gastroenterol 1981; 1:23–28.

58. Rouse M, Chapman N, Mahapatra M, et al. An open, randomised, parallel group study of lactulose versus ispaghula in the treatment of chronic constipation in adults. Br J Clin Pract 1991; 45:28–30.

59. Kot TV, Pettit-Young NA. Lactulose in the management of constipation: a current review. Ann Pharmacother 1992; 26:1277–1282.

60. Lederle FA, Busch DL, Mattox KM, et al. Cost-effective treatment of constipation in the elderly: a randomized double-blind comparison of sorbitol and lactulose. Am J Med 1990; 89:597–601.

61. Muller-Lissner SA. Adverse effects of laxatives: fact and fiction. Pharmacology 1993; 1:138–145.

62. Lennard-Jones JE. Constipation. In: Feldman M, Friedman LS, Sleisenger MH, eds. Gastrointestinal and liver disease. 7th edn. St. Louis: Saunders; 2002:181–210.

63. Odes HS, Madar Z. A double-blind trial of a celandin, aloevera and psyllium laxative preparation in adult patients with constipation. Digestion 1991; 49:65–71.

64. Marlett JA, Li BU, Patrow CJ, et al. Comparative laxation of psyllium with and without senna in an ambulatory constipated population. Am J Gastroenterol 1987; 82:333–337.

65. Thamlikitkul V, Bunyapraphatsara N, Dechatiwongse T, et al. Randomized controlled trial of *Cassia alata* Linn. for constipation. J Med Assoc Thailand 1990; 73:217–222.

66. Mennecier D, Vergeau B. Melanosis coli? N Engl J Med 2004; 350:8.

67. Maddi VI. Regulation of bowel function by a laxative/stool softener preparation in aged nursing home patients. J Am Geriatr Soc 1979; 27:464–468.

68. Shelton MG. Standardized senna in the management of constipation in the puerperium: A clinical trial. S Af Med J 1980; 57:78–80.

69. Herve S, Savoye G, Behbahani A, et al. Results of 24-h manometric recording of colonic motor activity with endoluminal instillation of bisacodyl in patients with severe chronic slow transit constipation. Neurogastroenterol Motility 2004; 16:397–402.

70. Ewe K. Effect of bisacodyl on intestinal electrolyte and water net transport and transit. Perfusion studies in men. Digestion 1987; 37:247–253.

71. Ramakrishna BS, Mathan M, Mathan VI. Alteration of colonic absorption by long-chain unsaturated fatty acids. Influence of hydroxylation and degree of unsaturation. Scand J Gastroenterol 1994; 29:54–58.

72. Stewart JJ, Bass P. Effects of ricinoleic and oleic acids on the digestive contractile activity of the canine small and large bowel. Gastroenterology 1976; 70:371–376.

73. Schiller LR. Review article: the therapy of constipation. Aliment Pharmacol Ther 2001; 15:749–763.

Comprehensive review covering most available agents used in the treatment of constipation and the rationale for their use.

74. Prather CM, Camilleri M, Zinsmeister AR, et al. Tegaserod accelerates orocecal transit in patients with constipation-predominant irritable bowel syndrome. Gastroenterology 2000; 118:463–468.

75. Johanson JF, Wald A, Tougas G, et al. Effect of tegaserod in chronic constipation: a randomized, double-blind, controlled trial. Clin J Gastroenterol Hepatol 2004; 2:796–805.

76. Nurko S, Garcia-Aranda JA, Worona LB, et al. Cisapride for the treatment of constipation in children: A double-blind study. J Pediatr 2000; 136:35–40.

77. Schutze K, Brandstatter G, Dragosics B, et al. Double-blind study of the effect of cisapride on constipation and abdominal discomfort as components of the irritable bowel syndrome. Aliment Pharmacol Ther 1997; 11:387–394.

78. Ponec RJ, Saunders MD, Kimmey MB. Neostigmine for the treatment of acute colonic pseudo-obstruction. N Engl J Med 1999; 341:137–141.

79. Chassany O, Michaux A, Bergmann JF. Drug-induced diarrhoea. Drug Safety 2000; 22:53–72.

80. Roarty TP, Weber F, Soykan I, et al. Misoprostol in the treatment of chronic refractory constipation: results of a long-term open label trial. Aliment Pharmacol Ther 1997; 11:1059–1066.

81. Verne GN, Davis RH, Robinson ME, et al. Treatment of chronic constipation with colchicine: randomized, double-blind, placebo-controlled, crossover trial. Am J Gastroenterol 2003; 98:1112–1116.

82. Fotherby KJ, Hunter JO. Idiopathic slow-transit constipation: whole gut transit times, measured by a new simplified method, are not shortened by opioid antagonists. Aliment Pharmacol Ther 1987; 1:331–338.

83. Sykes NP. An investigation of the ability of oral naloxone to correct opioid-related constipation in patients with advanced cancer. Palliative Med 1996; 10:135–144.

84. Liu M, Wittbrodt E. Low-dose oral naloxone reverses opioid-induced constipation and analgesia. J Pain Sympt Management 2002; 23:48–53.

85. Yuan CS, Foss JF, O'Connor M, et al. Methylnaltrexone for reversal of constipation due to chronic methadone use: a randomized controlled trial. JAMA 2000; 283:367–372.

86. Yuan CS. Clinical status of methylnaltrexone, a new agent to prevent and manage opioid-induced side effects. J Supp Oncol 2004; 2:111–117.

87. Holzer P. Opioids and opioid receptors in the enteric nervous system: from a problem in opioid analgesia to a possible new prokinetic therapy in humans. Neurosci Letts 2004; 361:192–195.

88. Greenwood-Van Meerveld B, Gardner CJ, Little PJ, et al. Preclinical studies of opioids and opioid antagonists on gastrointestinal function. Neurogastroenterol Motility 2004; 16(Suppl 2):46–53.

89. Harrington L, Schuh S. Complications of Fleet enema administration and suggested guidelines for use in the pediatric emergency department. Pediatr Emerg Care 1997; 13:225–226.

90. Gattuso JM, Kamm MA. Adverse effects of drugs used in the management of constipation and diarrhoea. Drug Safety 1994; 10:47–65.

91. Sweeney JL, Hewett P, Riddell P, et al. Rectal gangrene: a complication of phosphate enema. Med J Aust 1986; 144:374–375.

92. Gleghorn EE, Heyman MB, Rudolph CD. No-enema therapy for idiopathic constipation and encopresis. Clin Pediatr 1991; 30:669–672.

93. Culp WC. Relief of severe fecal impactions with water-soluble contrast enemas. Radiology 1975; 115:9–12.

94. Wills JC, Trowbridge B, Disario JA, et al. Percutaneous endoscopic cecostomy for management of refractory constipation in an adult patient. Gastrointest Endosc 2003; 57:423–426.

95. Youssef NN, Barksdale Jr E, Griffiths JM, et al. Management of intractable constipation with antegrade enemas in neurologically intact children. J Pediatr Gastroenterol Nutr 2002; 34:402–405.

96. Rongen MJ, van der Hoop AG, Baeten CG. Cecal access for antegrade colon enemas in medically refractory slow-transit constipation: a prospective study. Dis Colon Rectum 2001; 44:1644–1649.

Case series of 12 subjects with severe refractory constipation treated with antegrade enemas through a tube placed laparoscopically into the cecum or terminal ileum. Eight of the 12 patients received long-lasting benefits, with four requiring further surgery for colectomy or ileostomy.

97. Van Savage JG, Yohannes P. Laparoscopic antegrade continence enema in situ appendix procedure for refractory constipation and overflow fecal incontinence in children with spina bifida. J Urol 2000; 164:1084–1087.

98. Pfeifer J, Agachan F, Wexner SD. Surgery for constipation: a review. Dis Colon Rectum 1996; 39:444–460.

99. Rex DK, Lappas JC, Goulet RC, et al. Selection of constipated patients as subtotal colectomy candidates. J Clin Gastroenterol 1992; 15:212–217.

100. Knowles CH, Scott M, Lunniss PJ. Outcome of colectomy for slow transit constipation. Ann Surg 1999; 230:627–638.

101. Pemberton JH, Drelichman ER. Quality of life after subtotal colectomy for constipation: selection of the right patient, operation, and tools to measure outcome. Dis Colon Rectum 2003; 46:1720–1721.

102. Redmond JM, Smith GW, Barofsky I, et al. Physiological tests to predict long-term outcome of total abdominal colectomy for intractable constipation. Am J Gastroenterol 1995; 90:748–753.

103. Young-Fadok TM. Raising the bar. Laparoscopic resection of colorectal cancer. Surg Endosc 2001; 15:911–912.

104. Enck P. Biofeedback training in disordered defecation. A critical review. Dig Dis Sci 1953; 38:1953–1960.

105. Ron Y, Avni Y, Lukovetski A, et al. Botulinum toxin type-A in therapy of patients with anismus. Dis Colon Rectum 2001; 44:1821–1826.

106. Anderson AS, Whichelow MJ. Constipation during pregnancy: dietary fibre intake and the effect of fibre supplementation. Human Nutr Applied Nutr 1985; 39:202–207.

107. Jewell DJ, Young G. Interventions for treating constipation in pregnancy. Cochrane Database of Systematic Reviews 2001; 2.

108. Tytgat GN, Heading RC, Muller-Lissner S, et al. Contemporary understanding and management of reflux and constipation in the general population and pregnancy: a consensus meeting. Aliment Pharmacol Ther 2003; 18:291–301.

109. Greenhalf JO, Leonard HS. Laxatives in the treatment of constipation in pregnant and breast-feeding mothers. Practitioner 1973; 210:259–263.

110. Haskins R, Kotch J. Day care and illness: evidence, cost, and public policy. Pediatrics 1986; 77:951–982.

111. Kosek M, Bern C, Guerrant RL. The global burden of diarrhoeal disease, as estimated from studies published between 1992 and 2000. Bull World Health Org 2003; 81:197–204.

112. Duggan C. Oral rehydration solution. Doctors must increase use and acceptance of oral rehydration solution. Br Med J 2001; 323:3.

113. Victora CG, Bryce J, Fontaine O, et al. Reducing deaths from diarrhoea through oral rehydration therapy. Bull World Health Org 2000; 78:1246–1255.

 Publication from the World Health Organization outlining the evidence supporting the use of oral rehydration solutions in reducing morbidity and mortality from acute, infectious diarrhea.

114. Rao MC. Oral rehydration therapy: new explanations for an old remedy. Ann Rev Physiol 2004; 66:385–417.

 Comprehensive review outlining the physiologic rationale for using oral rehydration solutions in diarrhea treatment. Basic mechanisms, including illustrations of the cellular processes targeted by the oral rehydration solutions.

115. Nalin DR, Hirschhorn N, Greenough W 3rd, et al. Clinical concerns about reduced-osmolarity oral rehydration solution. JAMA 2004; 291:2632–2635.

116. World Health Organization. Reduced osmolarity oral rehydration salts (ORS) formulation. New York, NY: UNICEF House; July 18, 2001.

117. el-Mougi M, Hendawi A, Koura H, et al. Efficacy of standard glucose-based and reduced-osmolarity maltodextrin-based oral rehydration solutions: effect of sugar malabsorption. Bull World Health Org 1996; 74:471–477.

118. Duggan C, Fontaine O, Pierce NF, et al. Scientific rationale for a change in the composition of oral rehydration solution. JAMA 2004; 291:2628–2631.

119. Lifshitz F, Ament ME, Kleinman RE, et al. Role of juice carbohydrate malabsorption in chronic nonspecific diarrhea in children. J Pediatr 1992; 120:825–829.

120. Zaid MR, Hasan M, Khan AA. Attapulgite in the treatment of acute diarrhoea: a double-blind placebo-controlled study. J Diarrhoeal Dis Res 1995; 13:44–46.

121. Attorney General Lockyer announces approval of settlement in major lead contamination case: Proposition 65 lawsuit results in reformulation of Kaopectate: http://caag.state.ca.us/newsalerts/2003/03-080.htm, 2003.

122. Gorbach SL. Bismuth therapy in gastrointestinal diseases. Gastroenterology 1990; 99:863–875.

123. Chowdhury HR, Yunus M, Zaman K, et al. The efficacy of bismuth subsalicylate in the treatment of acute diarrhoea and the prevention of persistent diarrhoea. Acta Paediatrica 2001; 90:605–610.

124. Awouters F, Megens A, Verlinden M, et al. Loperamide. Survey of studies on mechanism of its antidiarrheal activity. Dig Dis Sci 1993; 38:977–995.

125. Schiller LR, Santa Ana CA, Morawski SG, et al. Mechanism of the antidiarrheal effect of loperamide. Gastroenterology 1984; 86:1475–1480.

126. DuPont HL, Flores Sanchez J, Ericsson CD, et al. Comparative efficacy of loperamide hydrochloride and bismuth subsalicylate in the management of acute diarrhea. Am J Med 1990; 88:15S–19S.

127. Ericsson CD, Johnson PC. Safety and efficacy of loperamide. Am J Med 1990; 88:5S–9S.

128. Barbezat GO, Clain JE, Halter F. A double-blind trial of loperamide in the treatment of chronic diarrhoea. S Af Med J 1979; 55:502–503.

129. Bergman L, Djarv L. A comparative study of loperamide and diphenoxylate in the treatment of chronic diarrhoea caused by intestinal resection. Ann Clin Res 1981; 13:402–405.

130. Gebbia V, Carreca I, Testa A, et al. Subcutaneous octreotide versus oral loperamide in the treatment of diarrhea following chemotherapy. Anti Cancer Drugs 1993; 4:443–445.

131. Sun WM, Read NW, Verlinden M. Effects of loperamide oxide on gastrointestinal transit time and anorectal function in patients with chronic diarrhoea and faecal incontinence. Scand J Gastroenterol 1997; 32:34–38.

132. Kaplan MA, Prior MJ, Ash RR, et al. Loperamide-simethicone vs loperamide alone, simethicone alone, and placebo in the treatment of acute diarrhea with gas-related abdominal discomfort. A randomized controlled trial. Arch Family Med 1999; 8:243–248.

133. Keeling WF, Harris A, Martin BJ. Loperamide abolishes exercise-induced orocecal liquid transit acceleration. Dig Dis Sci 1993; 38:1783–1787.

134. Camilleri M, Prather CM, Evans MA, et al. Balance studies and polymeric glucose solution to optimize therapy after massive intestinal resection. Mayo Clin Proc 1992; 67:755–760.

135. De Luca A, Coupar IM. Insights into opioid action in the intestinal tract. Pharmacol Therapeut 1996;169:103-15.

136. Barrow L, Steed KP, Spiller RC, et al. Quantitative, noninvasive assessment of antidiarrheal actions of codeine using an experimental model of diarrhea in man. Dig Dis Sci 1993; 38:996–1003.

137. King RF, Norton T, Hill GL. A double-blind crossover study of the effect of loperamide hydrochloride and codeine phosphate on ileostomy output. Aust NZ J Surg 1982; 52:121–124.

138. O'Brien JD, Thompson DG, McIntyre A, et al. Effect of codeine and loperamide on upper intestinal transit and absorption in normal subjects and patients with postvagotomy diarrhoea. Gut 1988; 29:312–318.

139. Palmer KR, Corbett CL, Holdsworth CD. Double-blind cross-over study comparing loperamide, codeine and diphenoxylate in the treatment of chronic diarrhea. Gastroenterology 1980; 79:1272–1275.

140. Harford WV, Krejs GJ, Santa Ana CA, et al. Acute effect of diphenoxylate with atropine (lomotil) in patients with chronic diarrhea and fecal incontinence. Gastroenterology 1980; 78:440–443.

141. Jaffe G. A comparison of lomotil and imodium in acute non-specific diarrhoea. J Int Med Res 1977; 5:195–198.

142. Fedorak RN, Field M, Chang EB. Treatment of diabetic diarrhea with clonidine. Ann Intern Med 1985; 102:197–199.

143. Rubinoff MJ, Piccione PR, Holt PR. Clonidine prolongs human small intestine transit time: use of the lactulose-breath hydrogen test. Am J Gastroenterol 1989; 84:372–374.

144. Schiller LR, Santa Ana CA, Morawski SG, et al. Studies of the antidiarrheal action of clonidine. Effects on motility and intestinal absorption. Gastroenterology 1985; 89:982–988.

145. Rabbani GH, Butler T, Patte D, et al. Clinical trial of clonidine hydrochloride as an antisecretory agent in cholera. Gastroenterology 1989; 97:321–325.

146. Hogenauer C, Aichbichler B, Santa Ana C, et al. Effect of octreotide on fluid absorption and secretion by the normal human jejunum and ileum in vivo. Aliment Pharmacol Ther 2002; 16:769–777.

Human balance studies assessing the effect of octreotide on electrolyte secretion and absorption. The greatest effect was seen in the inhibition of basal and sham feeding-related chloride and water secretion.

147. Szilagyi A, Shrier I. Systematic review: the use of somatostatin or octreotide in refractory diarrhoea. Aliment Pharmacol Ther 2001; 15:1889–1897.

148. Marteau PR, de Vrese M, Cellier CJ, et al. Protection from gastrointestinal diseases with the use of probiotics. Am J Clin Nutr 2001; 73(Suppl 2):430S–436S.

149. Allen SJ, Okoko B, Martinez E, et al. Probiotics for treating infectious diarrhoea. Cochrane Database of Systematic Reviews 2004; 2.

Systematic review of studies using probiotics in the treatment of infectious diarrhea. This review assesses the quality of the individual studies. Those studies of sufficient quality were included in a meta-analysis. The meta-analysis showed evidence of efficacy for several probiotics. Questions still remain about which probiotic strains are best, what dose to use, and in what clinical setting. *Lactobacillus* appears to be effective in preventing childhood antibiotic associated diarrhea. *Saccharomyces boulardii* has efficacy in the treatment of *Clostridium difficile* diarrhea.

150. Cremonini F, Di Caro S, Nista EC, et al. Meta-analysis: the effect of probiotic administration on antibiotic-associated diarrhoea. Aliment Pharmacol Ther 2002; 16:1461–1467.

151. Arlow FL, Dekovich AA, Priest RJ, et al. Bile acid-mediated postcholecystectomy diarrhea. Arch Intern Med 1987; 147:1327–1329.

152. Eusufzai S. Bile acid malabsorption in patients with chronic diarrhoea. Scand J Gastroenterol 1993; 28:865–868.

153. Baqui AH, Black RE, El Arifeen S, et al. Effect of zinc supplementation started during diarrhoea on morbidity and mortality in Bangladeshi children: community randomised trial. Br Med J 2002; 325:9.

154. Silberschmidt G, Schick MT, Steffen R, et al. Treatment of travellers' diarrhoea: zaldaride compared with loperamide and placebo. Eur J Gastroenterol Hepatol 1995; 7:871–875.

155. Okhuysen PC, DuPont HL, Ericsson CD, et al. Zaldaride maleate (a new calmodulin antagonist) versus loperamide in the treatment of traveler's diarrhea: randomized, placebo-controlled trial. Clin Infect Dis 1995; 21:341–344.

156. Huighebaert S, Awouters F, Tytgat GN. Racecadotril versus loperamide: antidiarrheal research revisited. Dig Dis Sci 2003; 48:239–250.

157. Prado D, Global Adult Racecadotril Study G. A multinational comparison of racecadotril and loperamide in the treatment of acute watery diarrhoea in adults. Scand J Gastroenterol 2002; 37:656–661.

158. Matheson AJ, Noble S. Racecadotril. Drugs 2000; 59:829–835.

Treatment of fecal incontinence

Adil E. Bharucha

INTRODUCTION AND EPIDEMIOLOGY

Fecal incontinence (FI) is the recurrent uncontrolled passage of fecal material, of one month or greater duration, in an individual with a developmental age of at least 4 years. The prevalence of FI in the community ranges from 2–15%, is similar in men and women, and increases with aging.[1] FI can substantially impair quality of life and contribute to institutionalization. The prevalence of FI in nursing home residents is 25–47%. It is important to ask patients at risk for incontinence (e.g., patients with diarrhea) about the symptom because they may not volunteer the information spontaneously.

MECHANISMS OF NORMAL AND DISORDERED CONTINENCE

Several factors acting in concert maintain fecal continence (Table 72.1). Anatomical factors include the anal sphincters and levator ani (i.e., the pelvic floor), rectal curvatures, and transverse rectal folds (Fig. 72.1). In addition to the anorectal mechanisms listed in Table 72.1, disturbances of stool consistency, mental faculties, and mobility often contribute to FI, particularly in patients who have impaired anorectal continence mechanisms.

Anal pressures are generally reduced in incontinent patients. However, anal pressures may be normal, underscoring the importance of normal stool consistency, rectal compliance, and sensation for maintaining continence. When rectal sensation is impaired, stool can enter the anal canal, and leak before the external sphincter contracts.[2,3] Other patients may have exaggerated rectal sensation, perhaps a marker of coexistent irritable bowel syndrome.[3] Exaggerated rectal sensation can be associated with reduced rectal compliance, repetitive rectal contractions during rectal distention, external sphincter weakness, and exaggerated anal sphincter relaxation during rectal distention. The pathophysiology of fecal incontinence in various disorders is reviewed in detail elsewhere.[1]

ETIOLOGY

Disorders associated with pelvic floor weakness and/or diarrhea may cause FI (Table 72.2). Prior to endoanal ultrasound, unexplained sphincter weakness in women was considered 'idiopathic,' or attributed to a pudendal neuropathy. Endoanal ultrasound revealed clinically occult internal and external anal sphincter injury in FI, and after vaginal delivery in women. Since 'idiopathic' FI generally presents several decades after vaginal delivery, it is conceivable that in addition to anal sphincter trauma caused by vaginal delivery, other factors as yet poorly defined, but including aging, menopause, chronic straining, and disordered bowel habits, likely predispose to FI.

In men, FI is often attributable to local causes, e.g., anal fistulae, poorly healed surgical scars, or proctitis after radiotherapy for prostate cancer. Another cause of idiopathic fecal soiling in men is a long, high-pressure anal sphincter that entraps small pieces of stool during defecation and subsequently expels them, causing perianal soiling and discomfort.[4]

CLINICAL EVALUATION

A carefully elicited history is invaluable for identifying the etiology and pathophysiology of FI, to establish rapport with the patient, and to guide diagnostic testing and treatment. The terms staining, seepage (i.e., leakage of small amounts of stool), and soiling (i.e., of clothes or bedding) are used to reflect the nature and severity of FI. The terms 'urge' and 'passive' FI refer to exaggerated or no awareness of the desire to defecate before the incontinent episode, respectively. Urge and passive FI are associated with more severe weakness of the external and internal anal sphincter, respectively. Recent data suggest that urge FI is also associated with reduced rectal capacity and increased rectal sensation.[5] Bowel habits, stool form, and consistency should preferably be characterized by pictorial stool scales.[6] A multisystem examination should be guided by the history and knowledge of underlying diseases. The digital rectal examination is useful to assess for anal sphincter defects, anal resting pressure, and voluntary contraction of the sphincter and puborectalis when subjects squeeze. Puborectalis contraction manifest as upward and anterior movement of the muscle (i.e., a 'lift'). Examination in the seated position on a commode may be more accurate than the left lateral decubitus position for characterizing rectal prolapse, pouch of Douglas hernia, or excessive perineal descent.

DIAGNOSTIC TESTING

Diagnostic testing is guided by the patient's age, probable etiologies, symptom severity, impact on quality of life, and response to conservative medical management. The strengths and limitations of these tests have been detailed elsewhere.[1,7] Endoscopy to identify mucosal pathology is probably necessary

Table 72.1 Anorectal factors maintaining continence

Factor (method of assessment)*	Physiological functions	Pathophysiology
Internal anal sphincter (anal manometry)	Smooth muscle responsible for maintaining ≈70% resting anal tone. Resting tone is maintained by myogenic factors and tonic sympathetic excitation.	Resting and squeeze pressures are ↓ in most women with FI. Conversely, ↑ sphincter pressures have been implicated to hinder evacuation, predisposing to FI in some men with FI.
External anal sphincter (anal manometry, anal EMG [for neural integrity])	Tonically active striated muscle which predominantly contains Type I (slow-twitch) fibers in humans. Maintains ≈30% of resting anal tone and relaxes during defecation. Voluntary or reflex contraction (i.e., 'squeeze' response) closes the anal canal, preserving continence.	Internal and external sphincter weakness is often caused by sphincter trauma. Obstetric or iatrogenic injury are common causes of sphincter trauma. Diseases affecting upper or lower motor neuron pathways can also weaken the external sphincter.
Puborectalis (defecography, dynamic pelvic MRI)	Maintains a relatively acute anorectal angle at rest. Contracts further to preserve continence during 'squeeze.'	Not widely recognized prior to advent of MRI, which reveals puborectalis atrophy and/or impaired function in a subset of incontinent patients.
Rectal compliance (Barostat testing)	By relaxing (i.e., accommodating), the rectum can hold more stool until defecation is convenient.	Rectal compliance is ↓ in ulcerative and ischemic proctitis. Rectal capacity is ↓ in 'idiopathic' FI.
Rectal sensation (latex balloon, barostat testing)	Rectal distention evokes the desire to defecate and is also critical for initiating the squeeze response when continence is threatened.	↓ rectal sensation occurs in FI, may impair evacuation and continence, and can be ameliorated by biofeedback therapy. ↑ rectal sensation may contribute to the symptom of urgency in FI.
Anal sensation (electrosensitivity, temperature change)	The exquisitely sensitive anal mucosa will periodically 'sample' and ascertain whether rectal contents are gas, liquid, or stool when the anal sphincters relax.	The extent to which a normal or disordered anal sampling reflex contributes to fecal continence or FI are unclear.

* Italicized tests are used in research studies, but not widely available, nor used in clinical practice.
↓ = reduced; ↑ = increased.

for incontinent patients with significant, particularly recent-onset diarrhea or constipation. The extent of examination (i.e., sigmoidoscopy or colonoscopy) and consideration of mucosal biopsies are guided by the patient's age, comorbidities, and differential diagnosis. The indications for, and extent of, diagnostic testing in incontinent patients are evolving. For ambulatory, otherwise healthy patients, anorectal manometry and an endoanal ultrasound are useful to document severity of weakness, and identify abnormal sphincter morphology, respectively, particularly when consideration is being given to surgical repair of anal sphincter defects. Though evacuation proctography is not widely utilized, it can characterize puborectalis contraction, confirm a coexistent evacuation disorder, and/or document severity of clinically suspected excessive perineal descent or a rectocele. Endoanal MRI is more accurate than endoanal ultrasound for characterizing external sphincter atrophy.[5] Dynamic MRI can concurrently image the bladder, genital organs, and anorectum in real time without radiation exposure. However, pelvic MRI is relatively expensive and not widely available. Anal sphincter EMG should be considered for incontinent patients with an underlying disease associated with a neuropathy, e.g., diabetes mellitus, clinical suspicion of a proximal neurogenic process, or sphincter weakness unexplained by morphology as visualized by ultra-sound. Delayed pudendal nerve terminal motor latencies (PNTML) are widely used as a surrogate marker for pudendal neuropathy. Initial studies suggested that patients with a pudendal neuropathy would not fare as well after surgical repair of sphincter defects compared to patients without a neuropathy. However, the accuracy of delayed PNTML as a marker for pudendal neuropathy has been questioned on several grounds.[7] The test only measures conduction velocity in the fastest conducting nerve fibers, and there are inadequate normative data. Test reproducibility is unknown, and sensitivity and specificity are poor. In contrast to initial studies, recent studies suggest the test does not predict improvement, or lack thereof, after surgical repair of anal sphincter defects.

MANAGEMENT

The management must be tailored to clinical manifestations, and includes treatment of underlying diseases, and other approaches detailed in Table 72.3.

Modification of bowel habits by simple measures is often extremely effective for managing FI. By taking loperamide or diphenoxylate before social occasions, or meals outside the home, incontinent patients may avoid having an accident outside the

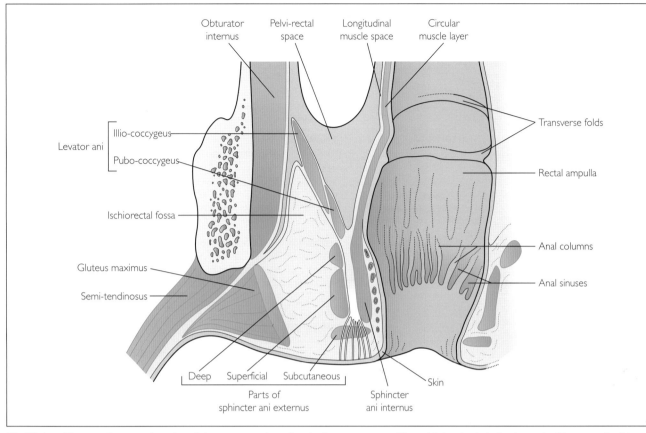

Fig. 72.1 • Diagram of a coronal section of the rectum, anal canal and adjacent structures. The pelvic barrier includes the anal sphincters and pelvic floor muscles. (Reproduced with permission from Bharucha AE. Fecal incontinence. Gastroenterology 2003; 124:1672–1685.)

home, and gain confidence in their ability to participate in social activities.[8] Diarrhea after a cholecystectomy, or attributable to microscopic colitis may respond to cholestyramine (4 g twice daily). Cholestyramine interferes with the absorption of several medications and fat-soluble vitamins. Supplementation with fat-soluble vitamins may be required with long-term use of cholestyramine. The serotonin 5-HT$_3$ antagonist alosetron (Lotronex™, GlaxoSmithKline, Research Triangle Park, NC), available under a restricted-use program, is an alternative option when functional diarrhea is not controlled by other agents. Patients with constipation, fecal impaction and overflow FI may benefit from a

regularized evacuation program, incorporating timed evacuation by digital stimulation and/or bisacodyl/glycerol suppositories, fiber supplementation, and selective use of oral laxatives as detailed in reviews.[9]

Biofeedback therapy is based on the principle of operant conditioning. Using a rectal balloon-anal manometry device, patients are taught to contract the external anal sphincter when they perceive balloon distention; perception may be reinforced by visual tracings of balloon volume and anal pressure, and the procedure is repeated with progressively smaller volumes. In uncontrolled studies, continence improved in ≈70% of patients with FI.[10] A

Table 72.2 Etiology of fecal incontinence
Anal sphincter weakness
Injury – obstetric trauma, related to surgical procedures, e.g., hemorrhoidectomy, internal sphincterotomy, fistulotomy, anorectal infection
Nontraumatic – scleroderma, internal sphincter thinning of unknown etiology
Neuropathy – stretch injury, obstetric trauma, diabetes mellitus
Anatomical disturbances of the pelvic floor – fistula, rectal prolapse, descending perineum syndrome
Inflammatory conditions – Crohn's disease, ulcerative colitis, radiation proctitis
Central nervous system disease – Dementia, stroke, brain tumors, spinal cord lesions (generally at or below T12), multiple system atrophy (Shy Drager's syndrome), multiple sclerosis
Diarrhea – irritable bowel syndrome, post-cholecystectomy diarrhea

Reproduced with permission from Fecal Incontinence, Gastroenterology 2003.

Table 72.3 Management of fecal incontinence

Intervention	Side effects	Comments	Mechanism of action
Incontinence pads*	Skin irritation	Disposable products provide better skin protection than nondisposable products. Underpad products were slightly cheaper than bodyworn products.	Provide skin protection and prevent soiling of linen; polymers conduct moisture away from the skin.
Antidiarrheal agents* Loperamide (Imodium) up to 16 mg/day in divided doses Diphenoxylate – 5 mg q.i.d.	Constipation	Titrate dose; administer before meals and social events.	↑ fecal consistency, ↓ urgency; ↑ anal sphincter tone.
Enemas**	Inconvenient; side effects of specific preparations		Rectal evacuation decreases likelihood of FI.
Biofeedback therapy using anal canal pressure or surface EMG sensors** [26] Rectal balloon for modulating sensation		Prerequisites for success include motivation, intact cognition, absence of depression, and some rectal sensation.	Improved rectal sensation and coordinated external sphincter contraction; ± ↑ anal sphincter tone.
Sphincteroplasty for sphincter defects** [16]	Wound infection; Recurrent FI (delayed)	Restricted to isolated sphincter defects without denervation.	Restore sphincter integrity.
Sacral nerve stimulation**	Infection	Preliminary uncontrolled trials promising.	Unclear; ↑ anal sphincter tone; may modulate rectal sensation.
Artificial sphincter gracilis transposition**	Device erosion, failure and infection	Either artificial device or gracilis transposition with/without electrical stimulation.	Restore anal barrier.

* Grade A; ** Grade B; *** Grade C therapeutic recommendations. Grades A or B are supported by at least one randomized, controlled trial, or one high-quality study of nonrandomized cohorts. Grade C recommendations are expert opinions generally derived from basic research, applied physiological evidence, or first principles, but not necessarily based on controlled or randomized trials.

↑ = increased; ↓ = reduced; ± = possible.

(Adapted from chapter on GI dysmotility and sphincter dysfunction In: John H Noseworthy, ed. Neurological therapeutics: principles and practice. London: Martin Dunitz Ltd; 2003.)

recent study randomized 171 incontinent patients to four groups: (1) standard medical/nursing care (i.e., advice only); (2) advice plus verbal instruction on sphincter exercises; (3) hospital-based computer-assisted sphincter pressure biofeedback; or (4) hospital biofeedback plus use of a home EMG biofeedback device.[11] Overall, 75% reported improved symptoms and 5% were cured; improvement was sustained at 1 year after therapy; symptoms, resting, and squeeze pressures improved to a similar degree in all four groups. These results underscore the importance patients attach to understanding the condition, practical advice regarding coping strategies (e.g., diet and skin care), and nurse–patient interaction.

Biofeedback therapy has relatively modest effects on anal resting and squeeze pressures.[10] The improvement in anal pressures is not correlated to symptom improvement. Perhaps these modest effects are attributable to inadequate biofeedback therapy, lack of reinforcement, and assessment of objective parameters at an early stage after biofeedback therapy. In contrast, sensory assessments, i.e., preserved baseline sensation, and improved sensory discrimination after biofeedback therapy, are more likely to be associated with improved continence after biofeedback therapy.

Incontinence Products: This category includes perineal protective devices and anal plugs. Perineal protective devices include disposable and reusable bodyworns, and disposable and reusable underpads (also called bedpads). A Cochrane review identified six suitable controlled trials from 132 citations on this topic.[12] The authors concluded that disposable bodyworns perform better than nondisposable bodyworns in preventing skin condition problems, and that either bodyworns or underpads containing superabsorbent materials perform better than bodyworns or underpads containing fluff pulp cores. These studies predominantly focused on urinary, rather than fecal incontinence. Many patients with mild fecal incontinence line their underwear with toilet paper, progressing to a panty liner, pad, or diaper for symptoms of incremental severity. Anal plugs are used for fecal incontinence in the UK, but are not available in the US. Anal plugs for fecal incontinence have been evaluated in two published studies.[13,14] These plugs are made of polyurethane sponge wrapped in a water-soluble coat and sized to approximate a conventional suppository. After the water-soluble coat dissolves in the anal canal, the plug expands to full size. In 1 study, 64% of 14 patients were continent for feces when they used the plug.[13] Patient compliance was suboptimal; the plug occasionally slipped out in 43%, and 71% experienced discomfort to a varying degree. Plugs need to be removed before bowel movements, and are probably not suitable for patients with frequent bowel movements. Anorectal physiology studies did not predict benefit, nor inconvenience of using a plug. Perhaps patients with reduced recto-anal sensation are less likely to be encumbered by the plug-induced desire to defecate.

Pharmacological approaches: Phenylephrine, an α_1-adrenergic agonist applied to the anal canal increased anal resting pressure by 33% in healthy subjects and incontinent patients. In a randomized, double-blind, placebo-controlled crossover study of 36 patients with FI, phenylephrine did not significantly improve incontinence scores or resting anal pressure compared to placebo.[15]

Surgical approaches: Continence improved in up to 85% of patients with sphincter defects after an overlapping anterior sphincteroplasty. For reasons that are unclear, continence deteriorates thereafter; <50% of patients are continent at 5 years after the operation.[16] Dynamic gracioplasty and artificial anal sphincter procedures are restricted to a handful of centers worldwide and often complicated by infections and device problems which may require reoperation, including removal of the device.[17,18] A colostomy is the last resort for patients with severe FI.

Minimally -invasive approaches: Sacral nerve stimulation is an FDA-approved device implanted in >3000 patients with urinary incontinence in the US. Observations from European studies suggest that sacral nerve stimulation augmented squeeze pressure more than resting pressure may also modulate rectal sensation and significantly improved continence.[19] Sacral stimulation is conducted as a staged procedure; patients whose symptoms respond to temporary stimulation over ≈2 weeks proceed to permanent subcutaneous implantation of the device. The procedure for device placement is technically straightforward, and device-related complications are less frequent or significant relative to more invasive artificial sphincter devices discussed above.

Table 72.4 Summary of fecal incontinence

Distressing symptom attributable to one or more disordered continence mechanisms.

A majority of patients have internal and/or external sphincter weakness. Rectal sensory disturbances (i.e., increased or reduced) and altered bowel habits (i.e., constipation and/or diarrhea) are also important.

Common causes include anal sphincter injury resulting from obstetric or iatrogenic trauma and/or pudendal neuropathy caused by obstetric injury or chronic straining.

Patients are often embarrassed to discuss the symptom with a physician.

Careful characterization of symptoms is useful for gauging severity, understanding pathophysiology, and guiding management.

Diagnostic testing is guided by clinical features. Anal manometry and ultrasound evaluate sphincter function and structure, respectively. Endoscopy necessary if mucosal disease process a consideration.

Simple measures (i.e., empathy, patient education, management of altered bowel habits, and biofeedback therapy [for sphincter tone and/or rectal sensation]) are often helpful.

Long-term success rates after surgical repair of anal sphincter defects is poor. More invasive approaches (e.g., gracioplasty) involve considerable morbidity.

Colostomy may be the only option for patients with symptoms refractory to other measures.

INCONTINENCE AFTER CHILDBIRTH

Approximately 20–30% of women will have urinary incontinence and ≈10% of women will have fecal incontinence 3 months after vaginal delivery.[1] Over 80% of women with a third-degree obstetric tear have bowel symptoms.[20] There are few controlled studies of therapeutic options for postpartum fecal incontinence. In a trial primarily designed to assess urinary incontinence, a smaller percentage of women who were taught to do pelvic floor exercises (8–10 sessions/day) at home had any fecal incontinence (4%) compared to controls at 12 months (10.5%).[21] However, the proportion of women with severe fecal incontinence at 12 months was not significantly different in the active treatment and control groups. Another study demonstrated that augmented biofeedback (i.e., audiovisual feedback and electrical stimulation) was superior to sensory retraining for fecal incontinence.[22] Whether pelvic floor exercise can prevent postnatal fecal incontinence is unknown. After birth, obstetricians will generally repair third-degree obstetric tears recognized in the postnatal period by end-to-end repair. Early studies suggest that an overlapping repair, favored by colorectal surgeons, is also feasible in the immediate postdelivery period and may produce better results.[23] There is no consensus on how to manage subsequent deliveries in women who have sustained anal sphincter injuries previously.[24] One option is a caesarean section, perhaps after repairing the sphincter. The alternative option is to allow another vaginal delivery, based on the premise that the sphincter has already been damaged. However, fecal incontinence may deteriorate after a second vaginal delivery in women with pre-existing incontinence.[25]

SUMMARY

The treatment of fecal incontinence is summarized in Table 72.4.

REFERENCES

1. Bharucha A. Fecal incontinence. Gastroenterology 2003; 124:1672–1685.

   A comprehensive review on fecal incontinence.

2. Buser WD, Miner PB Jr. Delayed rectal sensation with fecal incontinence. Successful treatment using anorectal manometry. Gastroenterology 1986; 91:1186–1191.

   The beneficial effects of biofeedback therapy in fecal incontinence are attributable to modulation of rectal sensation.

3. Sun WM, Donnelly TC, Read NW. Utility of a combined test of anorectal manometry, electromyography, and sensation in determining the mechanism of 'idiopathic' faecal incontinence. Gut 1992; 33:807–813.

   Patients with fecal incontinence have one or more of a variety of anorectal sensori-motor disturbances.

4. Parellada CM, Miller AS, Williamson ME, et al. Paradoxical high anal resting pressures in men with idiopathic fecal seepage. Dis Colon Rectum 1998; 41:593–597.

5. Bharucha AE, Fletcher JG, Harper CM, et al. Relationship between symptoms and disordered continence mechanisms in women with idiopathic fecal incontinence. Gut. 2005; 54:546–555.

   This comprehensive evaluation of anorectal and pelvic floor functions in fecal incontinence demonstrates that the symptom of urgency is associated with reduced rectal capacity and increased rectal sensitivity.

6. Lewis SJ, Heaton KW. Stool form scale as a useful guide to intestinal transit time. Scand J Gastroenterol 1997; 32:920–924.

7. American Gastroenterological Association. American Gastroenterological Association Medical Position Statement on Anorectal Testing Techniques. Gastroenterology 1999; 116: 732–760.

   A thorough review of the indications, strengths, and limitations of anorectal testing.

8. Read M, Read NW, Barber DC, et al. Effects of loperamide on anal sphincter function in patients complaining of chronic diarrhea with fecal incontinence and urgency. Dig Dis Sci 1982; 27:807–814.

9. Locke GR, 3rd, Pemberton JH, Phillips SF. American Gastroenterological Association Medical Position Statement: guidelines on constipation. Gastroenterology 2000; 119:1761–1766.

10. Bharucha AE. Outcome measures for fecal incontinence: anorectal structure and function. Gastroenterology 2004; 126:S90–S98.

11. Norton C, Chelvanayagam S, Wilson-Barnett J, et al. Randomized controlled trial of biofeedback for fecal incontinence. Gastroenterology 2003; 125:1320–1329.

   The largest, controlled study of biofeedback therapy for fecal incontinence. Underscores the importance of patient education for improving symptoms.

12. Shirran E, Brazzelli M. Absorbent products for the containment of urinary and/or faecal incontinence in adults. Cochrane Database of Systematic Reviews 2000; CD001406.

13. Christiansen J, Roed-Petersen K. Clinical assessment of the anal continence plug. Dis Colon Rectum 1993; 36:740–742.

14. Mortensen N, Humphreys MS. The anal continence plug: a disposable device for patients with anorectal incontinence. Lancet 1991; 338:295–297.

15. Carapeti EA, Kamm MA, Phillips RK. Randomized controlled trial of topical phenylephrine in the treatment of faecal incontinence. Br J Surg 2000; 87:38–42.

16. Bachoo P, Brazzelli M, Grant A. Surgery for faecal incontinence in adults. Cochrane Database of Systematic Reviews. 2000; CD001757.

17. Chapman AE, Geerdes B, Hewett P, et al. Systematic review of dynamic graciloplasty in the treatment of faecal incontinence. Br J Surg 2002; 89:138–153.

18. Wong W, Congliosi S, Spencer M, et al. The safety and efficacy of the artificial bowel sphincter for fecal incontinence: results from a multicenter cohort study. Dis Colon Rectum 2002; 45:1139–1153.

19. Rosen HR, Urbarz C, Holzer B, et al. Sacral nerve stimulation as a treatment for fecal incontinence. Gastroenterology 2001; 121:536–541.

   Sacral nerve stimulation is a promising option for fecal incontinence; US multicenter trials are in progress.

20. Sultan AH, Kamm MA, Hudson CN, et al. Third degree obstetric anal sphincter tears: risk factors and outcome of primary repair. Br Med J 1994; 308:887–891.

21. Meyer S, Hohlfeld P, Achtari C, et al. Pelvic floor education after vaginal delivery. Obstetr Gynecol 2001; 97:673–677.

22. Fynes MM, Marshall K, Cassidy M, et al. A prospective, randomized study comparing the effect of augmented biofeedback with sensory biofeedback alone on fecal incontinence after obstetric trauma. Dis Colon Rectum 1999; 42:753–758; discussion 758–761.

23. Sultan AH, Monga AK, Kumar D, et al. Primary repair of obstetric anal sphincter rupture using the overlap technique [see comment]. Br J Obstetr Gynaecol 1999; 106:318–323.

24. Sultan AH, Kamm MA. Faecal incontinence after childbirth. Br J Obstetr Gynaecol 1997; 104:979–982.

25. Fynes M, Donnelly V, Behan M, et al. Effect of second vaginal delivery on anorectal physiology and faecal continence: a prospective study [see comments]. Lancet 1999; 354:983–986.

26. Norton C, Hosker G, Brazzelli M. Biofeedback and/or sphincter exercises for the treatment of faecal incontinence in adults. Cochrane Database of Systematic Reviews. 2000; CD002111.

Index

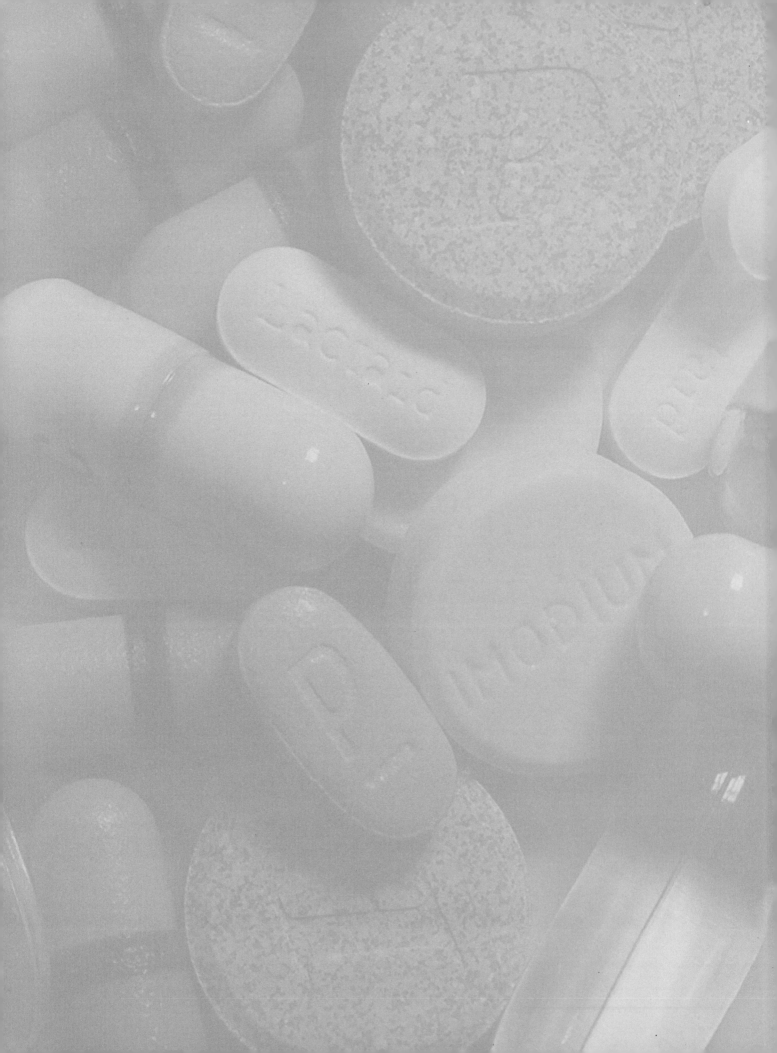